PRACTICAL STRATEGIES
IN PEDIATRIC DIAGNOSIS
AND THERAPY

PRACTICAL STRATEGIES

IN PEDIATRIC DIAGNOSIS

AND THERAPY

EDITED BY:

Robert M. Kliegman, MD
Professor and Chairman
Department of Pediatrics
Medical College of Wisconsin
Children's Hospital of Wisconsin
Milwaukee, Wisconsin

ASSOCIATE EDITORS:

Michael L. Nieder, MD
Assistant Professor of Pediatrics
Case Western Reserve University
  School of Medicine
Rainbow Babies and Childrens Hospital
Cleveland, Ohio

Dennis M. Super, MD
Assistant Professor of Pediatrics
Case Western Reserve University
  School of Medicine
MetroHealth Medical Center
Cleveland, Ohio

W.B. SAUNDERS COMPANY
A Division of Harcourt Brace & Company
Philadelphia London Toronto Montreal Sydney Tokyo

W.B. SAUNDERS COMPANY
A Division of Harcourt Brace & Company

The Curtis Center
Independence Square West
Philadelphia, Pennsylvania 19106

Library of Congress Cataloging-in-Publication Data

Practical strategies in pediatric diagnosis and therapy / edited by Robert M. Kliegman; associate editors, Michael L. Nieder, Dennis M. Super.—1st ed.

p.   cm.

ISBN 0–7216–5161–5

1. Pediatrics—Decision-making.   2. Pediatrics.   I. Kliegman, Robert.
II. Nieder, Michael L.   III. Super, Dennis M.   [DNLM: 1. Pediatrics.
2. Decision Making.   WS 200 P895 1996]

RJ47.P724 1996   618.92—dc20

DNLM/DLC   95–10279

Practical Strategies in Pediatric Diagnosis and Therapy   ISBN 0–7216–5161–5

Printed in the United States of America.

Last digit is the print number: 9   8   7   6   5   4   3   2   1

This book is dedicated to those master clinician-educators
who have inspired us with their clinical wisdom, enthusiasm, empathy, and insight.
At no time in the history of pediatrics
have these adaptable master clinician-educators been needed more than now,
to inspire young students and residents
and to provide encouragement and clinical guidance
to the practicing pediatrician.

CONTRIBUTORS

Trina M. Anglin, M.D., Ph.D.
Associate Professor of Pediatrics, University of Colorado School of Medicine. Associate Chief, Section of Adolescent Medicine, Department of Pediatrics, The Children's Hospital, Denver, Colorado.
Sexually Transmitted Diseases

Lotta Anveden-Hertzberg, M.D.
Fellow in Pediatric Surgery, Department of Pediatric Surgery, St. Görans Hospital, Karolinska Institute, Stockholm, Sweden.
Abdominal Masses

James E. Arnold, M.D.
Associate Professor of Otolaryngology–Head and Neck Surgery and Pediatrics, Case Western Reserve University School of Medicine. Chief, Pediatric Otolaryngology, Rainbow Babies and Childrens Hospital, University Hospitals of Cleveland, Cleveland, Ohio.
Airway Obstruction in Children

Stephen C. Aronoff, M.D.
Professor, Department of Pediatrics, West Virginia University School of Medicine. Chief, Pediatric Infectious Diseases, West Virginia University Children's Hospital, Morgantown, West Virginia.
Fever of Unknown Origin

Jane P. Balint, M.D.
Assistant Professor of Pediatrics, Medical College of Wisconsin. Pediatric Gastroenterologist, Children's Hospital of Wisconsin, Milwaukee, Wisconsin.
Jaundice

William F. Balistreri, M.D.
Dorothy M. M. Kersten Professor of Pediatrics, University of Cincinnati School of Medicine. Director, Division of Pediatric Gastroenterology and Nutrition, Children's Hospital Medical Center, Cincinnati, Ohio.
Jaundice

Gloria Ana Berenson, M.D.
Assistant Professor, Case Western Reserve University School of Medicine. Physician, Rainbow Babies and Childrens Hospital, University Hospitals of Cleveland, Cleveland, Ohio.
Constipation

Brian W. Berman, M.D.
Associate Professor, Department of Pediatrics, Case Western Reserve University School of Medicine. Chief, Division of General Academic Pediatrics, Rainbow Babies and Childrens Hospital, University Hospitals of Cleveland, Cleveland, Ohio.
Lymphadenopathy; Pallor and Anemia

James B. Besunder, D.O.
Assistant Professor of Pediatrics, Case Western Reserve University School of Medicine. Chief, Division of Pediatric Critical Care and Pharmacology, MetroHealth Medical Center, Cleveland, Ohio.
Delirium and Coma

R. Alexander Blackwood, M.D., Ph.D.
Assistant Professor, Department of Pediatrics, University of Michigan Medical School. Attending Physician, Section on Pediatric Infectious Diseases, University of Michigan Medical Center, C.S. Mott Children's Hospital, Ann Arbor, Michigan.
Recurrent Infection

Andrew Bleasel, M.B.B.S.
Staff Neurologist, Westmead Hospital and Royal Alexandra Hospital for Children, Sydney, Australia.
Paroxysmal Disorders

Jeffrey R. Botkin, M.D.
Associate Professor, Department of Pediatrics and Adjunct Associate Professor, Department of Internal Medicine, University of Utah School of Medicine. Medical Director, Medical/Surgical Unit, Primary Children's Medical Center, Salt Lake City, Utah.
Applying Ethical Principles to Clinical Decision Making

Laurence A. Boxer, M.D.
Professor, Department of Pediatrics, University of Michigan Medical School. Director, Pediatric Hematology/Oncology, University of Michigan Medical Center, C.S. Mott Children's Hospital, Ann Arbor, Michigan.
Recurrent Infection

J. Timothy Boyle, M.D.
Associate Professor of Pediatrics, Case Western Reserve University School of Medicine. Chief, Division of Pediatric Gastroenterology and Nutrition, Rainbow Babies and Childrens Hospital, University Hospitals of Cleveland, Cleveland, Ohio.
Hepatomegaly

Paula Brinkley, M.D., M.P.H., M.A.
Field Coordinator, Health Frontiers (Labs), Vientiane, Laos.
Understanding the Importance of Cultural Beliefs and Behaviors in Clinical Practice

Ben H. Brouhard, M.D.
Professor of Pediatrics, Ohio State University College of Medicine, Columbus, Ohio. Director, Pediatric Nephrology and Research Programs, Department of Pediatrics, Cleveland Clinic Foundation, Cleveland, Ohio.
Hematuria

Bruce H. Cohen, M.D.
Associate Professor, Ohio State University College of Medicine, Columbus, Ohio. Director, Neuro-Oncology Program, Cleveland Clinic Foundation, Cleveland, Ohio.
Headaches in Childhood

Warren Cohen, M.D.
Associate Professor of Pediatrics and Neurology, Case Western Reserve University School of Medicine. Chief, Division of Rehabilitative Pediatrics and Developmental Disabilities, Rainbow Babies and Childrens Hospital, University Hospitals of Cleveland. Medical Director, Health Hill Hospital for Children, Cleveland, Ohio.
Hypotonia and Weakness

W. Thomas Corder, M.D.
Associate Professor, Department of Pediatrics, West Virginia University School of Medicine. Attending Physician, Section of Ambulatory/Adolescent Pediatrics, West Virginia University Children's Hospital, Morgantown, West Virginia.
Fever of Unknown Origin

Robert J. Cunningham III, M.D.
Pediatric Nephrologist, Cleveland Clinic Children's Hospital, Cleveland, Ohio.
Proteinuria

Leona Cuttler, M.D.
Associate Professor, Departments of Pediatrics and Pharmacology, Case Western Reserve University School of Medicine. Attending Physician, Rainbow Babies and Childrens Hospital, University Hospital of Cleveland, Cleveland, Ohio.
Short Stature

Steven J. Czinn, M.D.
Associate Professor of Pediatrics, Division of Pediatric Gastroenterology and Nutrition, Case Western Reserve University School of Medicine. Attending Physician, Rainbow Babies and Childrens Hospital, University Hospitals of Cleveland, Cleveland, Ohio.
Gastrointestinal Bleeding

Stephen M. Downs, M.D., M.S.
Assistant Professor of Pediatrics and Biomedical Engineering, University of North Carolina at Chapel Hill School of Medicine, Chapel Hill, North Carolina.
Diagnostic Strategies and Clinical Decision Making

Jack S. Elder, M.D.
Professor of Urology and Pediatrics, Case Western Reserve University School of Medicine. Director of Pediatric Urology, Rainbow Babies and Childrens Hospital, University Hospitals of Cleveland, Cleveland, Ohio.
Acute and Chronic Scrotal Swelling; Ambiguous Genitalia

Thomas Ferkol, M.D.
Assistant Professor, Department of Pediatrics, Case Western Reserve University School of Medicine. Attending Physician, Rainbow Babies and Childrens Hospital, University Hospitals of Cleveland, Cleveland, Ohio.
Respiratory Distress

Robert L. Findling, M.D.
Assistant Professor of Psychiatry, Pediatrics, and Adolescent Health, Case Western Reserve University School of Medicine. Attending Physician, and Medical Director, Child and Adolescent Psychopharmacology Clinic, University Hospitals of Cleveland, Cleveland, Ohio.
Unusual Behaviors

Jonathan Flick, M.D.
Associate Professor of Pediatrics, Temple University School of Medicine. Chief, Section of Gastroenterology and Nutrition, St. Christopher's Hospital for Children, Philadelphia, Pennsylvania.
Diarrhea

Michael W. L. Gauderer, M.D.
Clinical Professor of Surgery, University of South Carolina School of Medicine, Columbia, South Carolina; and Medical University of South Carolina, Charleston, South Carolina. Professor of Bioengineering, Clemson University, Clemson, South Carolina. Chief, Department of Pediatric Surgery, Children's Hospital, Greenville Hospital System, Greenville, South Carolina.
Abdominal Masses

Kenneth Graff, M.D.*
Assistant Professor of Pediatrics, University of Colorado School of Medicine. Attending Physician, The Children's Hospital, Department of Emergency Medicine, Denver, Colorado.
Fever Without Focus

Marjorie Greenfield, M.D.
Associate Professor of Reproductive Biology and Pediatrics, Case Western Reserve University School of Medicine. Physician, Department of Obstetrics and Gynecology, University MacDonald Women's Hospital, Cleveland, Ohio.
Menstrual Problems and Vaginal Bleeding

Peter L. Havens, M.S., M.D.
Associate Professor, Pediatrics, Medical College of Wisconsin. Director, Pediatric HIV Care Program, Children's Hospital of Wisconsin, Milwaukee, Wisconsin.
Applying the Medical Literature to Clinical Decision Making

Daniel M. Hoffman, M.D.
Chief Resident in Urology, Case Western Reserve University School of Medicine, Cleveland, Ohio.
Ambiguous Genitalia

Ellen Hrabovsky, M.D.
Professor of Surgery and Pediatrics, West Virginia University School of Medicine, Morgantown, West Virginia.
Acute and Chronic Abdominal Pain

Carl E. Hunt, M.D.
Professor and Chairman, Department of Pediatrics, Medical College of Ohio, Toledo, Ohio.
Apnea and Sudden Infant Death Syndrome

Vera F. Hupertz, M.D.
Assistant Professor of Pediatrics, Division of Pediatric Gastroenterology and Nutrition, Case Western Reserve University School of Medicine. Attending Physician, Rainbow Babies and Childrens Hospital, University Hospitals of Cleveland, Cleveland, Ohio.
Gastrointestinal Bleeding

___

*Deceased.

Robert N. Husson, M.D.
Assistant Professor of Pediatrics, Harvard Medical School. Associate in Medicine, Children's Hospital, Boston, Massachusetts.
Fever and AIDS

David Jaffe, M.D.
Associate Professor of Pediatrics, Washington University School of Medicine. Medical Director, Emergency Services, St. Louis Children's Hospital, St. Louis, Missouri.
Fever Without Focus

Candice E. Johnson, M.D., Ph.D.
Associate Professor of Pediatrics, Case Western Reserve University School of Medicine. Attending Physician, MetroHealth Medical Center, Cleveland, Ohio.
Dysuria

Satish C. Kalhan, M.B.B.S., F.R.C.P., D.C.H.
Professor of Pediatrics Case Western Reserve University School of Medicine. Attending Physician, Division of Neonatology, Rainbow Babies and Childrens Hospital, University Hospitals of Cleveland, Cleveland, Ohio.
Hypoglycemia

Carolyn M. Kercsmar, M.D.
Associate Professor, Department of Pediatrics, Case Western Reserve University School of Medicine. Director, Children's Asthma Center, Rainbow Babies and Childrens Hospital, University Hospitals of Cleveland, Cleveland, Ohio.
Respiratory Distress

Douglas S. Kerr, M.D., Ph.D.
Professor, Pediatrics, Biochemistry, and Nutrition, Case Western Reserve University School of Medicine. Associate Pediatrician, Rainbow Babies and Childrens Hospital, University Hospitals of Cleveland, Cleveland, Ohio.
Failure to Thrive and Malnutrition

Jill E. Korbin, Ph.D.
Professor, Department of Anthropology, Case Western Reserve University, Cleveland, Ohio.
Understanding the Importance of Cultural Beliefs and Behaviors in Clinical Practice

Robert M. Lembo, M.D.
Associate Professor, Clinical Pediatrics, New York University School of Medicine. Associate Attending Physician in Pediatrics, Bellevue Hospital Center, New York, New York.
Fever and Rash

David A. Lewis, M.D.
Assistant Professor of Pediatrics, Division of Pediatric Cardiology, and Director, Graduate Medical Education, Medical College of Wisconsin, Milwaukee, Wisconsin.
Syncope and Dizziness

Jerome Liebman, M.D., D.M.D., M.S.
Professor of Pediatrics (Pediatric Cardiology), Case Western Reserve University School of Medicine. Pediatrician, Rainbow Babies and Childrens Hospital, University Hospitals of Cleveland, Cleveland, Ohio.
Heart Murmur

Gregory S. Liptak, M.D., M.P.H.
Associate Professor, University of Rochester School of Medicine and Dentistry. Medical Director, Andrew J. Kirch Center, Rochester, New York.
Mental Retardation and Developmental Disability

Colin D. Marchant, M.D.
Associate Professor, Department of Pediatrics, Tufts University School of Medicine. Attending Pediatrician, Division of Pediatric Infectious Diseases, Floating Hospital for Infants and Children at New England Medical Center, Boston, Massachusetts.
Earache

Peter Margolis, M.D., Ph.D.
Assistant Professor of Pediatrics and Epidemiology, University of North Carolina, Chapel Hill, North Carolina.
Diagnostic Strategies and Clinical Decision Making

Jay H. Mayefsky, M.D., M.P.H.
Associate Professor of Pediatrics, Finch University of Health Sciences/The Chicago Medical School. Senior Attending Physician, Cook County Hospital, Department of Pediatrics, Chicago, Illinois.
Meningismus and Meningitis

Robin E. M. Miller, M.D.
Fellow, Department of Pediatric Hematology/Oncology, Rainbow Babies and Childrens Hospital, University Hospitals of Cleveland, Cleveland, Ohio.
Neck Masses in Childhood

Brigitta U. Mueller, M.D.
Assistant Professor of Pediatrics, Uniformed Services University of the Health Sciences. Visiting Scientist, Pediatric Branch, Division of Clinical Sciences, National Cancer Institute, Bethesda, Maryland.
Fever and Neutropenia

Arthur J. Newman, M.S., M.D.
Professor of Pediatrics, Case Western Reserve University School of Medicine. Chief, Pediatric Rheumatology, Rainbow Babies and Childrens Hospital, University Hospitals of Cleveland, Cleveland, Ohio.
Arthritis

Michael L. Nieder, M.D.
Assistant Professor and Vice Chairman, Department of Pediatrics, Case Western Reserve University School of Medicine. Director, Residency Training Program in Pediatrics, Rainbow Babies and Childrens Hospital, University Hospitals of Cleveland, Cleveland, Ohio.
Neck Masses in Childhood

Amy Jo Nopper, M.D.
Resident in Dermatology, Medical College of Wisconsin, Milwaukee, Wisconsin.
Rashes and Skin Lesions

David M. Orenstein, M.D.
Professor of Pediatrics, Professor of Health, Physical, and Recreational Education (Exercise Physiology), University of Pittsburgh School of Medicine. Director, Pediatric Pulmonary/Cystic Fibrosis Center, Children's Hospital of Pittsburgh, Pittsburgh, Pennsylvania.
Cough

Susan R. Orenstein, M.D.
Associate Professor of Pediatrics, University of Pittsburgh School
of Medicine. Attending Physician, Pediatric Gastroenterology,
Children's Hospital of Pittsburgh, Pittsburgh, Pennsylvania.
Vomiting and Regurgitation

Ruth P. Owens, M.D.
Associate Professor of Pediatrics, Division of Pediatric Endocrinology, Case Western Reserve University School of Medicine. Attending Physician, Division of Pediatric Endocrinology, Rainbow
Babies and Childrens Hospital, University Hospitals of Cleveland, Cleveland, Ohio.
Disorders of Puberty

Emory M. Petrack, M.D., M.P.H.
Chief, Pediatric Emergency Medicine, Department of Pediatrics,
Case Western Reserve University School of Medicine. Director,
Pediatric Emergency Department, Rainbow Babies and Childrens
Hospital, University Hospitals of Cleveland, Cleveland, Ohio.
The Irritable Infant

Philip A. Pizzo, M.D.
Professor of Pediatrics, Uniformed Services University of the
Health Sciences. Chief, Pediatrics; Head, Infectious Disease Sec-
tion; and Acting Director, Division of Clinical Sciences, National
Cancer Institute, Bethesda, Maryland.
Fever and Neutropenia

John F. Pope, M.D.
Assistant Professor of Pediatrics, Case Western Reserve University
School of Medicine. Associate Director, Pediatric Intensive Care
Unit, MetroHealth Medical Center, Cleveland, Ohio.
Delirium and Coma

Linda G. Rabinowitz, M.D.
Associate Professor of Pediatrics, Medical College of Wisconsin,
Milwaukee, Wisconsin.
Rashes and Skin Lesions

Lisa Reebals, M.S.N., M.A. (R.N.)
Certified Pediatric Nurse Practitioner, Ambulatory Pediatric and
Adolescent Clinic, MetroHealth Medical Center, Cleveland,
Ohio.
*Understanding the Importance of Cultural Beliefs and Behaviors
in Clinical Practice*

Robert M. Reece, M.D.
Clinical Professor of Pediatrics, Tufts University School of Medicine. Director, Child Protection Program, and Director, Institute
for Professional Education, Massachusetts Society for the Prevention of Cruelty to Children. Attending Physician, The Floating Hospital for Children, and New England Medical Center,
Boston, Massachusetts.
Child Abuse

Thomas F. Riley, M.D.
Assistant Clinical Professor of Pediatrics, State University of New
York at Buffalo (SUNY) School of Medicine. Attending Physi-
cian, Division of Neonatology, Children's Hospital of Buffalo,
Buffalo, New York.
Hypoglycemia

Michael J. Rivkin, M.D.
Assistant Professor of Neurology, Harvard Medical School. Assis-
tant in Neurology, Children's Hospital, Boston, Massachusetts.
Stroke in Childhood

Dennis P. Ruggerie, D.O.
Director, Pediatric Critical Care Services, Deaconess Medical Cen-
ter. Pediatric Cardiologist, Department of Pediatrics, Great Falls
Clinic, Great Falls, Montana.
Heart Failure

John R. Schreiber, M.D.
Associate Professor, Department of Pediatrics, Case Western Reserve University School of Medicine. Chief, Division of Infectious Diseases, Rainbow Babies and Childrens Hospital, University Hospitals of Cleveland, Cleveland, Ohio.
Lymphadenopathy

Peter V. Scoles, M.D.
Professor, Department of Orthopaedics, Case Western Reserve Uni-
versity School of Medicine. Attending Physician, Department
of Orthopedics, University Hospitals of Cleveland, Cleveland,
Ohio.
Back Pain in Children and Adolescents

J. Paul Scott, M.D.
Professor of Pediatrics, Medical College of Wisconsin. Attending
Physician, Children's Hospital of Wisconsin, Milwaukee, Wis-
consin.
Bleeding and Thrombosis

Stanford T. Shulman, M.D.
Professor of Pediatrics and Associate Dean for Academic Affairs,
Northwestern University Medical School. Chief, Division of In-
fectious Diseases, Children's Memorial Hospital, Chicago, Illi-
nois.
Sore Throat

Susan B. Shurin, M.D.
Professor of Pediatrics, Case Western Reserve University School
of Medicine. Chief, Pediatric Hematology–Oncology, Rainbow
Babies and Childrens Hospital, University Ireland Cancer Center,
University Hospitals of Cleveland, Cleveland, Ohio.
Splenomegaly

Garry Sigman, M.D.
Clinical Assistant Professor, Pritzker School of Medicine, University of Chicago, Chicago, Illinois. Director, Adolescent Medicine, Lutheran General Children's Hospital, Park Ridge, Illinois.
Chest Pain

Nimi Singh, M.D., M.P.H.
Fellow, Adolescent Medicine, University of Washington School of
Medicine, and Children's Hospital and Medical Center, Seattle,
Washington.
*Understanding the Importance of Cultural Beliefs and Behaviors
in Clinical Practice*

Frank Smith, M.D.
Associate Professor of Pediatrics, State University of New York at
Syracuse (SUNY) Health Science Center, College of Medicine,
Syracuse, New York.
Cyanosis

Dennis M. Super, M.D., M.P.H.
Associate Professor of Pediatrics, Case Western Reserve University
School of Medicine. Attending Physician, MetroHealth Medical
Center, Cleveland, Ohio.
*Decision Making and Choosing the Optimal Therapy; Eye Disor-
ders*

Robert R. Tanz, M.D.
Associate Professor of Pediatrics, Northwestern University Medical School. Director of Continuity Clinic, Division of General Academic Pediatrics, Children's Memorial Hospital, Chicago, Illinois.
Sore Throat

George H. Thompson, M.D.
Professor, Orthopaedic Surgery and Pediatrics, Case Western Reserve University School of Medicine. Director, Pediatric Orthopaedic Surgery, Rainbow Babies and Childrens Hospital, University Hospitals of Cleveland, Cleveland, Ohio.
Gait Disturbances

Philip Toltzis, M.D.
Assistant Professor of Pediatrics, Case Western Reserve University School of Medicine. Attending Physician, Rainbow Babies and Childrens Hospital, University Hospitals of Cleveland, Cleveland, Ohio.
Fever and AIDS

George F. Van Hare, M.D.
Associate Professor of Pediatrics and Medicine, Case Western Reserve University School of Medicine. Director, Pediatric Arrhythmia Service, Rainbow Babies and Childrens Hospital, University Hospitals of Cleveland, Cleveland, Ohio.
Palpitations and Arrhythmias

Mark A. Wainstein, M.D.
Chief Resident in Urology, Case Western Reserve University School of Medicine, Cleveland, Ohio.
Acute and Chronic Scrotal Swelling

Theodore Reeves Warm, M.D.
Associate Professor of Child Psychiatry, Case Western Reserve University School of Medicine. Teaching Consultant in Pediatrics, Rainbow Babies and Childrens Hospital, University Hospitals of Cleveland, Cleveland, Ohio.
Unusual Behaviors

Martha Wright, M.D.
Assistant Professor of Pediatrics, Case Western Reserve University School of Medicine. Associate Director, Pediatric Emergency Medicine, Rainbow Babies and Childrens Hospital, University Hospitals of Cleveland, Cleveland, Ohio.
Bites

Elaine Wyllie, M.D.
Head, Pediatric Epilepsy Program, The Cleveland Clinic Foundation, Cleveland, Ohio.
Paroxysmal Disorders

Robert Wyllie, M.D.
Head, Section of Pediatric Gastroenterology, The Cleveland Clinic Foundation, Cleveland, Ohio.
Constipation

PREFACE

Most academic medical centers and pediatric residency training programs have multiple educational conferences, such as professor rounds, patient management conference, clinicopathologic conference, and senior resident-intake rounds. In these high-quality learning activities, one or more experienced master clinician-educators provides a verbal approach to a particular patient-based issue related to diagnostic or therapeutic challenges. The advice given is often derived from the knowledge accumulated over many years of clinical experience and years of careful analysis of the medical literature. The ultimate synthesis of the facts about the patient's situation with the clinician's practical experience and knowledge of the literature often results in the obvious diagnosis or most appropriate treatment strategy. These master clinician-educators provide a certain wisdom that gives clarity to confusing clinical cases and helps to reconcile discrepancies between practice and theory.

In addition, the master clinician-educators tend to focus on the importance of taking a detailed history and performing a complete physical examination. The chief complaint directs the questioning during the history, while the physical examination focuses on clues obtained by the history. Laboratory studies are then employed to support the diagnosis, not make a diagnosis.

It is a goal of this book to put into a written text the verbal teaching rounds–based approaches toward clinical problem solving of the many expert clinician-educators who present at teaching conferences. The combination of clinical experience and evidenced-based strategies will provide guidance in developing a differential diagnosis and then a specific diagnosis in addition to the appropriate therapy of common pediatric problems. Because of the nature of clinical practice, this book is arranged in chapters that cover specific chief complaints. Patients do not usually come to the physician with a chief complaint of cystic fibrosis; rather, they may present with a cough, respiratory distress, or chronic diarrhea.

This text is intended to help the reader begin with a specific chief complaint that may encompass many disease entities. In a user-friendly, well-tabulated, and illustrated approach, the text will help the reader differentiate between the many disease states causing a common chief complaint. The inclusion of many original tables and figures should help the reader to identify distinguishing features of diseases and to work through a diagnostic and/or therapeutic approach to the problem using various decision trees. Modified, adapted, and borrowed artwork and tables from other outstanding sources have been added as well. The combination of all of these illustrations and tables will help provide a quick visual guide to the differential diagnosis or treatment of the various diseases under discussion.

We also believe that this textbook will help the pediatric provider successfully survive in our emerging managed care environment. The need for evidence-based medicine and comfort with our ability to identify important diagnostic clues from the patient's history and physical examinations are more important then ever. These tools will always be valuable and will contribute to the clinician's ability to work with the development of care pathways and utilization review.

We greatly appreciate the hard work of our contributing authors. Writing a chapter in this type of format is quite different from the format in a disease-based book. In addition, we greatly appreciate the efforts of Judy Fletcher and Dolores Meloni of W. B. Saunders, whose patience and expertise contributed to the publication of this book. The authors also wish to make a special acknowledgment to Dr. Brendan M. Reilly for his courtesy and assistance. Finally, we acknowledge the support and at times sacrifice of our families and friends—Sharon, Jonathan, Rachel, Alison, and Matthew Kliegman; Mary and Leonard Nieder; and Encie, Emily, Elisa, Ellen, and Eric Super—whose understanding helped make the time and effort put into this book meaningful.

ROBERT M. KLIEGMAN
MICHAEL L. NIEDER
DENNIS M. SUPER

CONTENTS

*Deceased.

SECTION ONE

PRINCIPLES

1 Diagnostic Strategies and Clinical Decision Making

Peter Margolis   Stephen M. Downs

There are three important aspects of diagnosis and clinical decision making:

1. Medical decisions involve uncertainty.
2. Estimating the probability of an outcome numerically can help in making better decisions.
3. Absolute certainty is not needed to make an appropriate decision.

MEDICAL DECISIONS INVOLVE UNCERTAINTY

A 16-month-old girl presents with a fever of 39.3°C of one day's duration. She has had upper respiratory symptoms for the previous two days and last night awoke several times crying. Her past medical history is unremarkable. She is fully immunized. On examination, she is fussy but consolable. She seems only mildly interested in her surroundings but watches you as you move around the examination room. Her physical findings are completely normal.

A likely guess is that the patient has a viral infection. Although you may not think she has meningitis, there is a concern about the possiblity of "occult bacteremia." A urinary tract infection is another possibility. You can consider the following strategies: (1) treat presumptively after obtaining blood and urine cultures, (2) watch and wait, or (3) obtain a complete blood count and urinalysis and use the results of these tests to choose between treatment and watchful waiting.

In thinking about the decision, realize that antibiotics are indicated if the probability that the child has a bacterial infection is reasonably high. At the same time, try to avoid exposing her to the discomfort of blood drawing and bladder catheterization and to the risk of an allergic reaction to antibiotics. The parents should not have to purchase antibiotics if the patient does not need such treatment. The question to be decided is: How high would the chance of occult bacteremia have to be to make it worthwhile imposing the pain, risk, and cost of blood drawing and antibiotics?

One approach to the decision (strategy No. 3) would be to obtain more laboratory tests. For example, if the child had a normal white blood cell count, you may be more certain that she did not have a bacterial infection; however, you cannot be absolutely certain. Even with additional tests, such as an erythrocyte sedimentation rate or a C-reactive protein, you could not be absolutely certain about the absence of infection. Although additional data may help to reduce the uncertainty, the clinician would have to decide whether the risk of infection was low enough to observe the patient without treating.

Alternatively, if it were known that none of the available tests was adequate to rule out occult infection to one's satisfaction, the clinician might decide to treat presumptively while awaiting culture results (strategy No. 2). This approach would avoid the cost of additional testing but would still unnecessarily expose a certain percentage of children to the risk of an allergic reaction to antibiotics and impose on their parents the cost of antibiotics.

This case illustrates the uncertainty involved in medical decisions. Unfortunately, the clinician can never be absolutely certain about the diagnosis when choosing a management strategy, no matter how many tests are performed. The case also suggests how having information about tests, probabilities of outcomes, and risks may lead the clinician to select one strategy over another. For example, a clinician would certainly want to treat a child pending culture results if the risk of occult bacteremia were 50%. By contrast, if the risk were less than 1 in 1000, a physician would not treat but instead would observe the child. This implies that somewhere between these extremes there is a risk of occult bacteremia at which the decision would change from watchful waiting to treating. This point, at which one management strategy appears better than another, is called a *decision threshold*. Thresholds exist between treating presumptively and testing, and between testing and watchful waiting (see below).

ESTIMATING AND USING PROBABILITIES

Clinicians usually describe uncertainty about the probability of outcomes with words like "not very likely" or "occasionally." Unfortunately, such terminology may complicate communication because different clinicians use the same words to describe different probabilities.

A more useful approach to expressing uncertainty about a patient's true state is to use probabilities. Most people are familiar with probabilities because of their use in day-to-day activities. For example, there is a 50% chance that a coin flip will come up heads. There is a 1 in 6 (17%) chance that a role of the dice will come up with the number 3. Probabilities are numbers between 0 and 1 that reflect our belief that an event will occur or that something is true. They are typically expressed as percentages, or proportions.

Probabilities can also be used to express uncertainty about medical outcomes. For example, the chance that a child under 2 years of age with no obvious focus of infection has bacteremia is between 2% and 5%. This probability is also known as a *prevalence*. In other words, no more than 5% of children who have these findings on presentation to the physician will have occult bacteremia. In the context of diagnostic testing, the prevalence of disease is also called a *pre-test probability*, or *prior probability*.

Once the results of a diagnostic test are known, more information is available so it is possible to better evaluate the probability that a patient has a disease. For example, if the white blood cell count is greater than 15,000, the chance that the child described in the above case has occult bacteremia is higher, about 15%. However, if the white blood cell count is less than 15,000, the chances of occult bacteremia are lower, about 2%. This probability—the probability of disease after the results of a test are known—is the *post-test probability*, or *predictive value*.

Interpreting probabilities as the proportion of diseased individuals in a population has little meaning for any individual patient because a given patient either does or does not have a disease. Thus, probabilities may also be thought of as a measure of how much certainty a clinician has in a diagnosis. Using probabilities to express certainty allows clinicians to combine their own clinical judgment with empirical data. Compared with more global expressions of probability, such as "likely" or "possibly," numeric probabilities permit a more accurate assessment of the information that is available when diagnostic tests are used.

Approaches to Estimating Post-test Probabilities

If information is available about the pre-test probability and about the accuracy of a diagnostic test, it is possible to estimate a patient's post-test probability of disease. The post-test probability allows clinicians to know how confident they can be about the diagnosis after the test results are known.

2 × 2 TABLES AND BRANCHING TREES

To estimate the post-test probability, the pre-test probability and test accuracy data need to be combined. Figure 1–1 shows several approaches to performing this calculation to answer the question "What is the probability of streptococcal pharyngitis in a child who has a positive throat culture?" In the illustration, any given child has a 15% probability of having group A streptococci. In other words, in a population of 1000 children with sore throats and a prevalence of streptococcal pharyngitis of 15%, 150 children would have group A streptococci and 850 would not.

Calculating the proportion of children with positive streptococcal throat cultures who have group A streptococci requires assigning actual numbers of patients to the branches of the tree or the 2 × 2 table. This is accomplished by multiplying the number of children with and without disease by the sensitivity and specificity. In the example, when the test characteristics (sensitivity and specificity) are applied to the pre-test probability, the likelihood that group A streptococci are present in children with a positive culture increases from 15% to 61%. Thus, the probability that a child with a positive culture actually has streptococcal infection is 61%. (This post-test probability is also known as the *positive predictive value* of the throat culture.)

Conversely, if the test is negative, the probability that a child with a negative throat culture has group A streptococci is 2%. Thus, there is a 98% chance that a child with negative test results *does not* have streptococcal pharyngitis. (This post-test probability is known as the *negative predictive value* of the throat culture).

This example illustrates again how knowledge of the post-test probability gives us more information about the actual likelihood of disease than a qualitative assessment of probabilities. In addition,

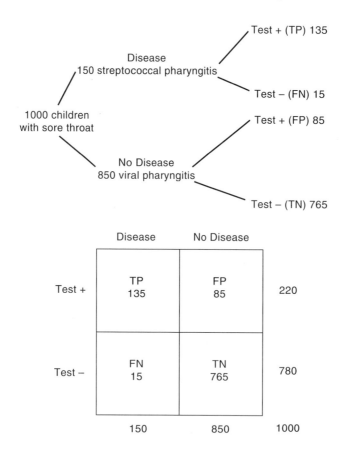

Post-test probability if test is + (positive predictive value) = TP/TP + FP = 135/220 = 61%

Post-test probability if test is − (negative predictive value) = TN/TN + FN = 15/780 = 98%

Figure 1–1. Two methods for calculating post-test probabilities of streptococcal pharyngitis among children presenting with sore throat. Calculations assume the following test characteristics of throat culture: sensitivity = 90%, specificity = 90%. Calculation of number of true-positive (TP) test results: number of diseased children (150) × sensitivity (90%) = number of true positives (135). Calculation of number of true-negative (TN) test results: number of non-diseased children (805) × specificity (90%) = number of true negatives (765). FP = false-positive result; FN = false-negative result.

the post-test probabilities are neither 100% nor 0%. Therefore, even after the test results are known, the diagnosis remains uncertain.

LIKELIHOOD RATIOS

Another approach to assessing how information from a diagnostic test provides evidence about the likelihood of disease is to calculate the post-test probability using *odds* rather than probabilities. This approach uses a ratio of test sensitivity and specificity and thus does not require completion of a 2×2 table or branching tree; as a result, it is faster and easier to use.

An odds is a ratio of two proportions; it is the likelihood that an event will occur compared with the likelihood that it will not. Most people are familiar with the use of odds in gambling. For example, the likelihood that a horse will win a race, compared with the likelihood that it will lose, is the odds of winning. An odds is just another way of expressing probability. For example, a 4:1 odds is the same as an 80% probability. The child with a 15% chance of having group A streptococci has a 15:85 odds of having streptococcal pharyngitis.

A likelihood ratio (LR) can be calculated as the proportion of diseased patients with a particular test result divided by the proportion of nondiseased patients with the same test result (Fig. 1–2). For tests with dichotomous results (positive or negative), there are two likelihood ratios. A ''positive'' likelihood ratio is the proportion of diseased patients with a positive test (sensitivity), divided by the proportion of non-diseased patients with a positive test (1 − specificity). Conversely, a negative likelihood ratio is the proportion of diseased patients who test negative (1 − sensitivity), divided by the proportion of non-diseased patients who test negative (specificity). The numerator always contains an expression related to diseased patients (sensitivity); the denominator always refers to non-diseased patients (specificity).

To calculate a post-test probability, the pre-test odds of disease are multiplied by the likelihood ratio. However, the pre-test probability must first be converted to an odds. After the post-test odds are calculated, the number is converted back to a post-test probability. To use a likelihood ratio to compute the post-test probability from the streptococcal pharyngitis example:

1. Convert the pre-test probability to pre-test odds:

$$\text{pre-test odds} = \text{pre-test probability}/1 - \text{pre-test probability } (P/1 - P)$$
$$= .15/1 - .15 = .15/.85 = .18$$

2. Compute the likelihood ratio (LR):

$$LR = \text{sensitivity}/1 - \text{specificity}$$
$$= .90/1 - .90 = .90/.10 = 9$$

3. Compute the post-test odds:

$$\text{post-test odds} = LR \times \text{pre-test odds}$$
$$= 9 \times .18 = 1.6$$

4. Convert the post-test odds to post-test probability:

$$\text{post-test probability} = \text{post-test odds}/1 + \text{post-test odds } (x/1 + x)$$
$$= 1.6/1 + 1.6$$
$$= 1.6/2.6 = 62\%$$

Although this formula appears complicated, by rounding numbers it is possible to do the calculation mentally. Alternatively, one can use a nomogram to accomplish the calculation (Fig. 1–3).

Likelihood ratios can be used for tests that have multiple cutoff points, as illustrated in Table 1–1. These ratios make it easy to account for the fact that patients with more abnormal findings are more likely to be diseased than patients who have fewer abnormal findings. For example, children with white blood cell (WBC) counts over 25,000 are more likely to be bacteremic than children with WBC counts of 15,000. Finally, likelihood ratios may be easier to use in sequential testing because several likelihood ratios can be multiplied directly; this assumes that the diagnostic tests under consideration are independent of one another (see later, Combining Tests).

Influence of Pre-test Probability and Test Characteristics on Post-test Probability

PRE-TEST PROBABILITY

Clinicians are accustomed to finding positive test results in patients who present with classic symptoms of a disease. For example, we would not be surprised if an 18-year-old sexually active female presenting with dysuria, frequency, and urgency had positive urine culture results. This observation occurs because of the relationship between pre-test probability and post-test probability. The higher the pre-test probability, the higher the post-test probability; thus, interpretation of a test result depends on what is already known.

To illustrate this relationship numerically, consider again the

---

$$\text{positive likelihood ratio} = \frac{\text{probability of positive test in diseased patients}}{\text{probability of positive test in non-diseased patients}}$$

$$= \frac{\text{sensitivity}}{1 - \text{specificity}}$$

$$\text{negative likelihood ratio} = \frac{\text{probability of negative test in diseased patients}}{\text{probability of negative test in non-diseased patients}}$$

$$= \frac{1 - \text{sensitivity}}{\text{specificity}}$$

Calculation of post-test probability using likelihood ratios:

$$\text{pre-test probability} \times LR = \text{post-test probability}$$

Figure 1–2. Likelihood ratios.

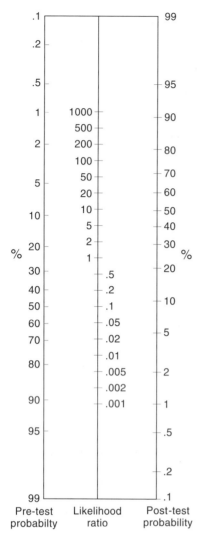

Figure 1–3. Nomogram for calculating the post-test probability of disease. The middle scale is the likelihood ratio (sensitivity ÷ 1 − specificity). To use the nomogram, place a ruler on the right-hand scale at the point that corresponds to the prior probability of disease. Adjust the angle until the ruler lies on the middle scale at the point corresponding to the likelihood ratio. Read the post-test probability from the left-hand scale of the table. (Adapted with permission from New England Journal of Medicine, Fagan TJ. Nomogram for Bayes' formula. 1975;293:257.)

Table 1–1. Likelihood Ratio (LR) for a Test with Multiple Cut-off Points: The White Blood Cell Count As an Indicator of Bacteremia

WBC Count	Sensitivity	Specificity	−LR	+LR
≥ 5,000	1.00	.07	0	1.1
≥10,000	.92	.43	.19	1.6
≥15,000	.65	.77	.45	2.8
≥20,000	.38	.92	.67	4.8
≥25,000	.23	.97	.79	7.7

hematocrit values have only about a 7% chance of having anemia. However, a child with a normal hematocrit value has a 0.7% probability of having anemia:

$$.03/.97 \times .1/.44 = .007/1.007 = .007$$

Thus, when the pre-test probability is low, a positive test result does little to rule in disease. However, a negative test result does help to rule out disease. The relationship between pre-test probability and disease is illustrated in Figure 1–4.

SENSITIVITY AND SPECIFICITY

The other determinant of post-test probability is the quality of the test being used. The more accurate the test, the greater the accuracy with which clinicians can predict whether or not a patient is diseased.

Information about the quality of diagnostic tests is summarized by two measures: sensitivity and specificity (Fig. 1–5). *Sensitivity* measures how often patients with a disease have positive test findings. It is the number of diseased patients with positive results divided by the total number of diseased patients. Tests that have high sensitivity will have few false-negative results. Therefore, when a highly sensitive test is used, patients who test negative have a very low chance of having disease. Sensitive tests are said to be useful in ruling out disease. One way of remembering when sensitive tests are useful is by the mnemonic *snout* (*s*ensitive tests rule *out* disease).

Sensitive tests are most useful when the consequences of missing a diagnosis can be devastating. Thus, lumbar punctures are useful in ruling out meningitis. When there are no cells and no organisms in the cerebrospinal fluid (CSF), the probability of bacterial meningitis is extremely low. Nuchal rigidity, by contrast, is not a sensitive test for meningitis. Young patients with meningitis may not exhibit a stiff neck. Thus, a supple neck in a young child may not rule out meningitis.

Specificity measures how often patients without disease can have negative test results. It is the number of non-diseased patients with negative results divided by the total number of non-diseased patients. Tests with high specificity produce few false-positive results. When a highly specific test is used, patients who test positive are very likely to be diseased. Thus, a positive result on a specific test is said to rule in disease. The mnemonic for this is *spin* (*sp*ecific tests rule *in*). Specific tests are commonly used when it is important to know definitely that a patient has a disease; an example might be before beginning an aggressive or risky therapy, as in obtaining a biopsy specimen of a tumor to confirm malignancy before subjecting a patient to chemotherapy.

Unfortunately, few sensitive tests are highly specific and few specific tests are highly sensitive. Even when cells are present in the CSF, the patient may not have bacterial meningitis because viral meningitis also causes CSF pleocytosis. Such patients have

hypothetical group of children presenting with sore throat. If the prevalence or pre-test probability of streptococcal pharyngitis were 50%, the probability that a child with a positive culture actually had group A streptococcal pharyngitis would be 90%; using likelihood ratios

$$.50/1 − .5 \times 9 = 9; 9/1 + 9 = 90\%$$

In other words, when the clinical suspicion of disease is high, a positive test confirms a diagnosis. In this setting, a child with a negative culture would still have a 10% probability of streptococcal infection. Thus, when the pre-test probability is high, a negative result may not necessarily rule out disease.

In contrast, when the prevalence of disease is low, a positive test result does not greatly increase the probability of disease. This situation is common when one is screening for disease. For example, the prevalence of iron deficiency anemia in children is approximately 3%. Because the sensitivity of a capillary hematocrit is about 90% and the specificity about 44%, children with abnormal

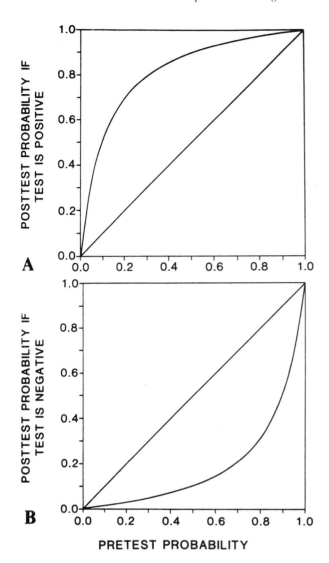

Figure 1–4. *A, B,* Relationship between pre-test probability and post-test probability of disease. The sensitivity and specificity of the test were assumed to be 90% for the examples, with the post-test probability of disease corresponding to a positive test result and the post-test probability of disease corresponding to a positive test result. (From Sox H. *Common Diagnostic Tests.* Philadelphia: American College of Physicians, 1990:20.)

false-positive test results. Thus, there is often a trade-off between sensitivity and specificity.

Estimating the Pre-test Probability of Disease

Making the best use of diagnostic tests requires a knowledge of a test's accuracy as well as the pre-test probability of disease. A patient's pre-test probability is related to demographic characteristics, such as age, sex, and patterns of signs and symptoms. Pre-test probabilities can be estimated on the basis of data in the medical literature as well as personal experience.

Estimates of pre-test probabilities based on personal experience are most likely to be accurate for conditions that are commonly encountered. One way to learn to estimate probabilities is to think about a hypothetical group of 100 patients with a particular group

of presenting findings. If it were possible to create 100 such patients, how many would be diseased? This approach uses probabilities as characteristics of groups of patients that may be used to estimate one's belief that an individual patient either does or does not have a disease. Again, probabilities are one way of expressing the degree of certainty a clinician has about the diagnosis.

Unfortunately, approaches to estimating probabilities based on personal experience are subject to errors in judgment. This is because physicians may not accurately remember or apply the information they need to make probabilistic assessments. This is particularly true for outcomes that are very rare.

Information from the published literature can also be used to assess the probability that a patient has a disease. For example, adult patients who present with fever, pharyngeal exudates, tender anterior cervical nodes, and no cough have about a 40% chance of having a positive group A streptococcal throat culture. In contrast, adults with none of these findings have about a 5% chance.

Published studies are most likely to be useful if the patients studied are similar to the patients one sees in practice. For example, the prevalence of disease among patients referred to tertiary care centers is likely to differ from the prevalence among patients seen in private practice. Thus, clinicians in community practice may not want to generalize to their practice information from studies of patients in tertiary care settings. Such generalization may lead to overestimates of the prevalence of disease (see Chapter 2).

Information in studies is also most likely to be accurate if all patients who presented were included. If certain types of patients were excluded or not enrolled, the reported probability of disease will differ from that which would be present if all patients had been included.

Assessing the Accuracy of Diagnostic Tests

Determining a patient's post-test probability of disease also requires having information about the accuracy of the diagnostic test being used. Published studies of diagnostic tests are the most reliable guide to the selection of which tests to use. When these studies are improperly designed or conducted, however, their results may lead to inaccurate conclusions about a test's accuracy and utility. Readers of the medical literature should be aware of a number of pitfalls, and they should be able to recognize these problems and understand how they may influence reported results.

For reasons described above, studies of diagnostic tests should describe the criteria for selecting patients as well as the clinical setting in which the study was conducted (e.g., private practice, tertiary care center). A description of the proportion of eligible patients enrolled will help the reader decide whether the study sample was representative of the population to which the results should be applied (see Chapter 2). In addition, the eligibility criteria for studies of diagnostic tests should produce a sample of patients with a wide spectrum of disease severity. This is necessary because diagnostic tests may detect a marker of disease common to many illnesses rather than something specific to the disease in question. For example, a study of the erythrocyte sedimentation rate (ESR) that included only children with juvenile rheumatoid arthritis in the

$$\text{sensitivity} = \frac{\text{number of diseased patients with positive test}}{\text{total number of diseased patients}} = \frac{TP}{TP + FN}$$

$$\text{specificity} = \frac{\text{number of healthy patients with negative test}}{\text{total number of healthy patients}} = \frac{TN}{TN + FP}$$

Figure 1–5. Definitions of sensitivity and specificity. TP = true positive; TN = true negative; FN, false negative; FP, false positive.

sample would conclude that the ESR is sensitive and specific for the diagnosis of juvenile rheumatoid arthritis. However, if the sample included a broad range of patients with fever of unknown origin, the ESR would appear much less specific for this diagnosis. In short, the population in which the test is studied should resemble the patient to whom the test is to be applied.

The diagnostic test itself needs to be performed accurately and interpreted by someone blinded to the diagnosis. The frequency of uninterpretable results should also be reported. Often patients with uninterpretable results are those in whom the diagnosis is uncertain, yet these may be the types of patients in whom the test is most likely to be used. Excluding these subjects generally makes the test seem better than it really is.

Assessing the accuracy of a test involves comparing it with a more definitive standard of diagnosis, or "gold standard." The observed accuracy will be incorrect if the gold standard is less than perfect. In principle, assessing a test's accuracy seems simple. In practice, it may be difficult to make this comparison in all cases. Identifying a meaningful gold standard may be difficult because it is not always possible to apply the gold standard to all patients. For example, in studying a test for appendicitis, it would be impossible to operate on patients with negative test results. Although close follow-up of patients with negative tests may be possible in many studies, one should be wary of gold standards that do not produce definitive conclusions.

The gold standard should also be applied equally to all members of the study population. Clinicians as well as investigators have a strong and natural tendency to study patients with positive test results more vigorously than patients who have negative test results. This means that patients with positive results will have the gold standard applied more often than patients who test negative. Such an unequal application of the gold standard is called *work-up* or *verification bias*. It produces a falsely elevated sensitivity. The effect on specificity depends on what happens to patients with negative test results. If the gold standard is not applied and patients are assumed to be disease-free, some patients with false-negative results will be classified as "true negatives." This will produce a falsely elevated specificity. If patients who test negative are excluded from the analysis, the specificity will appear lower than it really is.

Finally, the gold standard needs to be interpreted without knowledge of the test results. Failure to blind those interpreting the gold standard may lead to overestimates of the test accuracy. A summary of criteria for evaluating studies of diagnostic tests is presented in Table 1–2.

Table 1–2. Criteria for Evaluating Studies of Diagnostic Tests

Selecting the Patient Sample
Were the inclusion and exclusion criteria described?
Was the spectrum of disease representative of the patient population of interest?
Was the setting described?

Diagnostic Test
Were the performance and interpretation of the test blinded?
Were uninterpretable results reported and their impact on the results considered?

Gold Standard
Was the interpretation of the gold standard independent of the diagnostic test?
Was the interpretation of the gold standard blinded?
Were all patients in the study population equally likely to receive the gold standard of treatment and be included in the study?
Was the same gold standard applied to all patients?

Table 1–3. Test Characteristics of Leukocyte Esterase, Nitrite, and White Blood Cell Count in Diagnosing Urinary Tract Infection in Children

	Sensitivity (%)	Specificity (%)
Leukocyte esterase (small)	75	90
Nitrite	90	45
Leukocyte esterase *or* nitrite positive*	97.5	41
Leukocyte esterase *and* nitrite positive†	67.5	93.5

Assuming independence of tests:
*Combined sensitivity = 100% − {(1 − sensitivity^{LE}) × (1 − sensitivity^{nitrite})} = 100% − (25% × 10%) = 97.5%. Combined specificity = specificity^{LE} × specificity^{nitrite} = 90% × 45% = 41%.
†Combined sensitivity = sensitivity^{LE} × sensitivity^{nitrite} = 75% × 90% = 67%. Combined specificity = 100% − {(1 − specificity^{LE}) × (1 − specificity^{nitrite})} = 100% − (10% × 65%) = 93.5%.

Combining Tests

Because few tests are highly sensitive and specific, clinicians often combine the results of several tests to evaluate a possible diagnosis. For example, in evaluating the possibility of a urinary tract infection by urinalysis, clinicians sometimes use a combination of the urinary leukocyte esterase and nitrite tests.

Table 1–3 shows the characteristics of these tests when they are used alone as well as a hypothetical example of how the sensitivity and specificity of the tests change when the criterion for a positive test is an abnormality of *any* of them and when the criterion is an abnormality of *all* of them. When the criterion for a positive test is an abnormality of any of the tests, the combined sensitivity is higher than for any test individually; however, the overall specificity is lower. Thus, combining tests in this way *(parallel testing)* is useful for ruling out disease. When the criterion for a positive test is an abnormality on both of the individual tests, the overall specificity increases but the overall sensitivity decreases. Combining tests in this fashion *(serial testing)* is therefore useful for confirming the presence of disease. When some test results are positive and some are negative, there is an intermediate probability of disease and the interpretation depends on the consequences of calling the results positive or negative (see later, Defining Decision Thresholds for Taking Action).

Table 1–3 also presents a calculation of the overall test characteristics if the tests are independent of one another. Tests that are independent of one another provide more information when they are combined than tests that contain some of the same information. For example, computed tomography (CT) scans and magnetic resonance imaging (MRI) provide much of the same information about structural lesions of the brain. Therefore, the result of an MRI may not add much additional information to the CT scan because CT and MRI are not independent tests. Combining tests is most useful when two tests are independent.

The calculation of post-test probability when multiple tests are used is simplified by the use of likelihood ratios. To obtain the post-test probability for positive tests, the likelihood ratios for each test are multiplied. The post-test probability will be correct only if the tests are independent.

Clinical Prediction Rules

Information from multiple tests can be combined to estimate the post-test probability. However, combining tests in this way assumes that each test contributes independent bits of information to the estimate. This assumption is at best an approximation and is often a bad one. Another approach to using multiple pieces of information that does not make such an assumption is called clinical prediction rules, or diagnostic decision rules. Clinical prediction rules summarize the value of groups of clinical findings, not just one.

Clinicians have always used combinations of findings in diagnosing illness and assessing prognosis. Clinical aphorisms, such as the association of Cushing triad (hypertension, bradycardia, and tachypnea) with increased intracranial pressure and the association of colicky abdominal pain and ''currant jelly'' stools with intussusception, are examples of how expert clinicians have recognized the combinations or patterns of findings that help to predict the presence of disease or its prognosis.

Clinical prediction rules differ from such clinical aphorisms because they depend on empirical assessments of the value of each piece of information from studies of large numbers of patients. Thus, they measure more accurately the relative importance of each piece of information in a constellation of clinical findings. The advantage of this type of information is that it may help clinicians understand how much emphasis to place on each piece of clinical information. The disadvantage is that such scores can be difficult to remember.

One example of a clinical prediction rule is the PRISM score. This test was developed to help clinicians predict the prognosis of children admitted to the intensive care unit. The score uses a group of 14 measures of physiologic stability (e.g., arterial blood gas results, blood pressure, and electrolyte disturbances) and weights each according to its importance in predicting mortality. In this case, the test predicts the likelihood of an outcome of disease—*prognosis*—rather than the identification of a disease—*diagnosis*.

Clinical prediction rules are developed using statistical techniques to determine which of the many findings that may be associated with an outcome are most important. Such techniques include *logistic regression modeling, recursive partitioning*, and *bootstrap modeling*. Because the development of such rules relies on modeling, they may be subject to chance variations that occur in the samples of patients selected in which they were developed. Clinical prediction rules can be regarded as more reliable when their findings have been replicated in new samples of patients. In addition, they tend to be more accurate when developed to predict biologic outcomes for which a fairly clear-cut gold standard exists (meningitis, death), rather than an outcome such as the need for hospitalization, which may be influenced by social factors, such as bed availability, patient preferences, and physician judgment. An advantage of this type of score is that it may help clinicians understand how much emphasis to place on each piece of clinical information. A disadvantage is that such scores may be difficult to remember and thus difficult to use in clinical practice.

ABSOLUTE CERTAINTY IS NOT NEEDED

Choosing among alternative management strategies, such as diagnostic testing and watchful waiting, would be easy if a patient's diagnosis were always obvious and the response to therapy completely predictable. Nonetheless, diagnosis and prognosis are fraught with uncertainty. Even after diligent (and sometimes expensive) data collection and thoughtful interpretation of all available clinical data, knowledge of the patient's diagnosis and prognosis remains imperfect. Yet clinicians make decisions in the face of this uncertainty. At some point, clinicians take action: operate, prescribe therapy, or commit the patient to a tincture of time.

Because all medical decisions must be made in the face of uncertainty, the challenge is to know when one is *certain enough* to take action. When is the probability of disease high enough to

justify treatment or low enough to safely ignore it? These judgments are typically made intuitively, but some techniques render decision making explicit. This explicit approach involves enumerating the alternative strategies and their possible consequences. By laying out the relationships between interventions and outcomes, the key issues and trade-offs in complex decisions can be seen with greater clarity.

Decision Trees Describe Problems and Expected Outcomes

Let's use a familiar example; a 10-year-old boy with fever, vomiting, and acute lower abdominal pain. On examination, he has poorly localized abdominal tenderness with some rebound tenderness. The obvious concern is that the patient may have appendicitis.

Deciding on a management plan for this patient involves enumerating alternative plans and their possible consequences. The exact consequence that will result from each alternative plan is, of course, uncertain at the time the decision must be made. By representing this uncertainty with probabilities, the clinician can explore in a more precise way the possible consequences of our actions.

Let's consider two alternative actions: (1) proceed directly to the operating room and remove the boy's appendix, or (2) observe the patient overnight and operate if he is not improved after the next 12 hours, sooner if his condition deteriorates. If surgery is performed, there is a small but real possibility (~1 in 10,000) that the boy will die of anesthetic or surgical complications. If he survives surgery, however, he will return to good health, without the appendix, regardless of whether or not the appendix was inflamed.

The outcome of the second alternative depends on whether the boy has appendicitis or a benign, self-limited, nonspecific cause of abdominal pain, such as a viral syndrome. If the patient has appendicitis, there is about a 35% chance that his appendix will rupture during the observation period. In that event, he must have the ruptured viscus removed in the operating room. This surgery poses a higher risk of death (~1 in 1000) from the appendicitis, peritonitis, and surgical or anesthetic complications.

If the patient is lucky, though, the appendix will not rupture. In this case, the boy will undergo surgery at no greater risk than if the physician had chosen to operate earlier. Finally, this patient may not have appendicitis at all. In this case, let's assume that his status improves during observation and that he returns to good health, avoiding surgery altogether.

Thus, there are two alternatives (operate or observe) and three outcomes (recovery without surgery, recovery after surgery, and surgical death). This oversimplifies the situation; nonetheless, it is becoming difficult to identify and utilize all the factors needed to make a rational decision. To make the task easier, it is possible to use a tool known as a *decision tree*. Figure 1–6 shows such a tree in the case of appendicitis. Every important event is represented as a branch on this tree. There are two types of branch points, or nodes. The first is a *decision node*, represented by a square. Branches from a decision node represent the alternatives among which the decision maker may choose. In the appendicitis tree, the alternatives are to operate (upper branch) or to observe (lower branch).

If the operate option is taken, the patient will either die or survive surgery. These two possibilities are depicted as branches from a round *chance node*, so called because the branch that is taken is not in the control of the decision maker but is uncertain until after the decision is made.

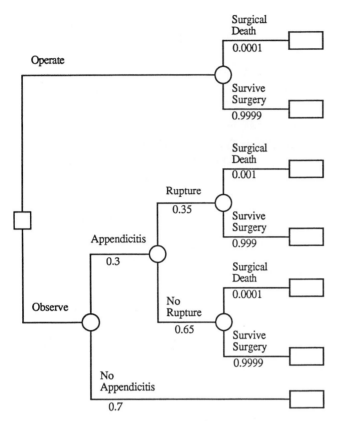

Figure 1–6. The appendicitis decision tree. Branches off the square decision node represent the alternatives from which the clinician can choose. Branches from the round chance nodes are events that may or may not happen. A probability is associated with each branch. The rectangular terminal nodes represent the possible outcomes that the patient faces.

The tree also depicts what may happen if the clinician chooses to observe the patient. If the observe option is taken, the tree represents, with branches at a chance node, the possibility that patient does or does not have appendicitis. If the patient has appendicitis, the appendix may rupture, as indicated by the next chance node. After both the rupture and no rupture branches, the possibility of surgical death or survival is shown. Finally, the lowest branch depicts the possibility that the patient does not have appendicitis and is allowed to recover without surgery. Each of the branches from a chance node is associated with a probability—the probability that the event indicated by the branch will happen. Because the branches at a node represent all the possible outcomes at that point, their probabilities add up to 1.

Each of the final branches ends in a rectangle known as a *terminal node*. Terminal nodes represent the possible outcomes faced by the patient. By representing the decision problem with a decision tree, one can describe the alternatives and outcomes and the probabilistic relationship between them. Organizing the decision in this way clarifies the trade-offs inherent in each strategy: an increased risk of unnecessary surgery for a decreased risk of a ruptured appendix.

This explicit representation can suggest a course of action. This is done by assigning a *value* to each possible outcome, which reflects the desirability of the outcome. Using the value of the outcome and the probability of the outcome, one can compare alternative strategies by determining the *expected value* of each course of action. The expected value is the average value of the possible outcomes weighted by their probabilities. In this case, we can assign a value of 1 to each outcome in which the child survives and a value of zero to a surgical death. Calculation of the expected

value is performed by *averaging out and folding back* the decision tree. This process begins at each terminal node. It is accomplished by multiplying the value of the terminal node by the probability of the outcome at that node. Each of the products is summed over all the branches at the chance node. This sum then becomes the value of that chance node (see circles in Fig. 1–7). The process is repeated until the decision node is reached.

For example, in the "Operate" branch in Figure 1–7, averaging out and folding back would be carried out as follows: the value of "Surgical Death" is 0. Zero times the probability of "Surgical Death" (0.0001) is 0. The value of "Survive Surgery" is 1. One times the probability of "Survive Surgery" (0.9999) is 0.9999. The sum of these expected values, 0.9999, becomes the (expected) value of the "Operate" option. This is shown in the circle pointing to the chance node. Similarly, in the "Rupture" branch following "Observation," the value of "Surgical Death" is 0. Zero times the probability of "Surgical Death" (0.001) is 0. The value of "Survive Surgery" is 1. One times the probability of "Survive Surgery" (0.999) is 0.999. The sum of these expected values, 0.999, becomes the (expected) value of the "Rupture" branch. The value of the "No Rupture" branch, calculated in the same fashion, is 0.9999. The value of "Rupture" (0.999) times the probability of "Rupture" (0.35) is 0.3497. The value of "No Rupture" (0.9999) times the probability of "No Rupture" (0.65) is 0.6499. The sum of these, 0.9996, becomes the (expected) value of the "Appendicitis" branch, and so on.

This process is continued until the expected values of the alternatives at the decision node can be compared. In this example, the option of operating immediately offers a greater probability of survival (0.99990 versus 0.99989). Happily, the child is likely to

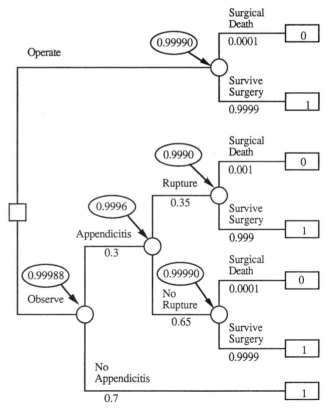

Figure 1–7. Using the decision tree to calculate probability of survival for different alternatives. In the *Observe* branch, the expected value *Rupture* is calculated as follows: value of surgical death × probability of surgical death + value of surviving surgery × probability of surviving surgery; (0 × 0.001) + (1 × 0.999) = .999.

survive either way. Nonetheless, choosing to observe this patient entails a 2 in 100,000 higher risk of death.

This example illustrates a simple but powerful basis for rational medical decision making. The best decision is the one in which the patient has the best average outcome, where the "average" is weighted by the probability. Because it is impossible to predict with 100% certainty how any individual patient will do, describing alternative management strategies and finding the one with the highest expected outcome often makes the best decision clear.

Using New Diagnostic Information

Physicians often have more data on hand than their subjective probability assessments. Diagnostic test results are a good example. Information from diagnostic tests can be represented explicitly in the decision-making process. To include the results of a diagnostic test in a decision tree requires the combination of test sensitivity and specificity with the pre-test probability of disease to calculate the so-called post-test probability.

In the appendicitis example, a physician may want to use the WBC count to help decide whether the patient with fever and abdominal pain has appendicitis. A WBC count of less than 15,000/mm³ has 70% sensitivity and 80% specificity in identifying appendicitis in this clinical situation. Thus, a new alternative—using the WBC count to decide between operating and observing—can be added to the decision tree (Fig. 1–8). If the WBC count is above 15,000/mm³, proceed to surgery. If it is below this cutoff, observe the patient.

To evaluate this alternative in the decision model, we must first determine the likelihood that the patient will have an elevated WBC count. The probability of a positive result can be determined by adding the cells in the first row of a 2 × 2 table (see Fig. 1–1) or by observing that this probability is the sum of the proportion of true positives (sensitivity × prevalence) plus the proportion of false positives [(1 − specificity) × (1 − prevalence)], or 35%. If the pre-test probability is 30%, the sensitivity is 70% and the specificity is 80%, this calculation is

$$[(0.70 \times 0.30) + (1 - 0.8) \times (1 - 0.7) = 0.21 + 0.14 = 0.35]$$

Thus, if we use the WBC to decide on surgery, there is a 35% chance that the count will be above 15,000 (the probability attached to the "Test Positive" branch in Figure 1–8) and the patient will go to surgery.

After determining the probability of an elevated WBC count, we next calculate the post-test probability of appendicitis. If the WBC count is below 15,000, the probability of appendicitis is 14%. This can be calculated using the formula for a negative likelihood ratio:

$$\frac{probability}{1 - probability} \times \frac{1 - sensitivity}{specificity} =$$

$$\frac{0.3}{1 - 0.3} \times \frac{0.3}{0.8} = 0.43 \times 0.375 = 0.16$$

$$and \ldots 0.16 = \frac{14\%}{1 + 0.16}$$

This value is attached to the "Appendicitis" branch that follows the "Test Negative" branch. With these new numbers, we can evaluate the expanded tree as we did before to determine the risk of death associated with the new strategy, testing (see Fig. 1–8). We find that using the test offers the highest probability of survival (0.99993). Testing reduces the risk of death by 3 in 100,000 over operating presumptively.

Defining Decision Thresholds for Taking Action

By considering the alternatives, the outcomes, and the probabilities that link them, we can make a rational management decision in the face of substantial uncertainty. However, our results so far apply specifically to this child, in whom we have estimated a 30% probability of appendicitis. A physician may face similar dilemmas frequently in a typical practice. How can we apply this hard work when a similar case arises again?

To generalize the results of this analysis to other patients, note that the basic decision problem is the same for all cases. It is the estimate of the probability of appendicitis that varies from patient to patient, depending on clinical presentation, examination, and laboratory results. For example, if we are faced with a playful 5-year-old girl who has vague abdominal pain, vomiting and diarrhea, and a low-grade fever, we might estimate her probability of appendicitis to be only 5%. If this is substituted for the 30% probability in the tree in Figure 1–8, the result of evaluating the tree changes. "Observation" becomes the alternative with the highest expected survival.

This implies that at some probability between 5% and 30%, both alternatives ("Observation" and "Test") offer the same survival. This probability is known as the *threshold probability*. Above the threshold, testing is best. Below the threshold, observation offers a higher expected survival. By solving the tree using different values for the probability of appendicitis, a process known as *sensitivity analysis*, we can determine the threshold probability. In this case, it is 8%.

The physician can use this 8% value in evaluating other patients who present with abdominal pain. If the physician believes that the probability of appendicitis is below 8%, observation may be best. If the clinical presentation suggests a probability above 8%, testing will offer the higher probability of survival.

There is an analogous threshold probability above which operating presumptively is best and below which diagnostic testing is best. As an example, if the 10-year-old's abdominal pain is localized to the right lower quadrant and obvious rebound tenderness develops, we would feel more confident of the diagnosis of appendicitis. If there is a 50% probability of appendicitis, the probability of survival is below the likelihood of surviving when we act presumptively without knowing the WBC count.

This implies that obtaining additional information by diagnostic testing may not always be the best alternative. It may seem counterintuitive that obtaining additional information (in the form of the WBC count) could be dangerous to the patient, but in some cases it is. By assessing how the results of the model change at differing prevalence values of appendicitis (a sensitivity analysis), we find that if a patient's probability of appendicitis is below 8%, observing offers a higher chance of survival than relying on the WBC count. If the probability of appendicitis is above 48%, choosing to operate presumptively offers the highest chance of survival.

The reason for this result is that tests are not perfect. When a test is performed, there is a chance that a patient with the disease will be labeled as not having the disease (a false negative result) or that a healthy patient will be labeled as having the disease (a false positive result).

The risk of incorrect classification of patients increases in three settings:

1. When the sensitivity or specificity of a test is poor.
2. When the likelihood of disease is very low.
3. When the likelihood of disease is very high.

As the pre-test probability of disease increases, the negative predictive value of a test becomes lower. Thus, more and more negative test results of patients are false negatives. Likewise, when the pre-test probability is low the positive predictive value is low

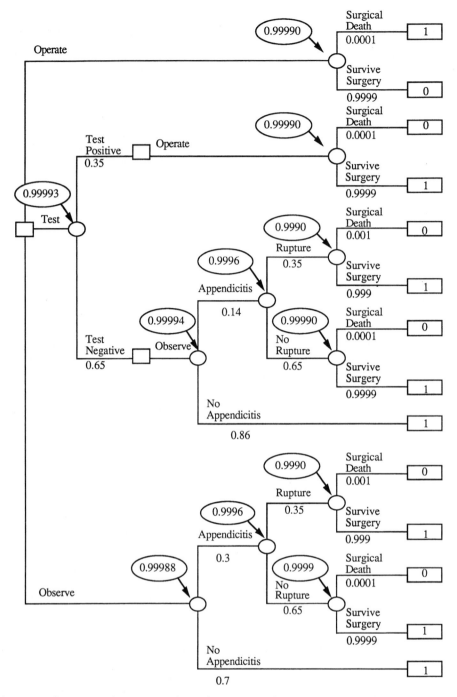

Figure 1–8. The use of diagnostic information, such as a test result, can be incorporated into a decision tree. Manipulations of prior probability, sensitivity, and specificity are used to determine the effect of the test on the probabilities in the tree (see text). The tree is solved exactly as shown in Figure 1–7.

and more and more positive test results of patients are false positives. In fact, when the disease prevalence is very low, as in a population-based screening program, most positive test results may be false positives.

If the chance of this kind of mislabeling of patients is high and the consequences of being mislabeled are significant (in the case of unnecessary surgery or a ruptured appendix), relying on the test is ill advised. In our example, this situation occurs when the probability of appendicitis is below the testing threshold (8%) or above the surgery threshold (48%). These thresholds have been depicted in what is termed a *threshold bar* (Fig. 1–9).

When the probability of disease falls into the "Observe" range, the risk is so low that a test will be misleading; observing the patient is the lowest risk option. When the probability is in the "Operate" region, the chance of a false negative makes the test too risky and presumptive appendectomy is better. When the risk is in the intermediate "Test" region, testing is best.

Several factors may affect the relative size of the regions in the threshold bar (Fig. 1–10). For example, a test with near perfect (100%) sensitivity and specificity would result in a very wide "Test" region. A test with poor (near 50%) sensitivity and specificity would result in a narrower testing region. A relatively benign

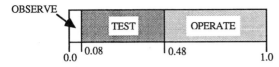

Figure 1-9. The threshold bar illustrates the decision thresholds at which the best alternative changes. When the probability of disease falls into the "Observe" region, observation is the best alternative. For probabilities in the "Test" region, it is best to use a diagnostic test to choose a course of action. In the "Operate" region, the risk of disease is high enough that it is best to operate presumptively (see text).

condition for which treatment was dangerous or of low efficacy would result in a wide "Observe" region. If the therapy were quite harmless and cheap and if the disease were dangerous, the "Operate" region would dominate.

Many features of a clinical decision affect the decision thresholds. But once the thresholds are established, the clinician who is able to express uncertainty in probabilities can apply the thresholds to individual cases in the clinical practice. For example, the child with classic symptoms of appendicitis is likely to have a prior probability of disease above 50% (within the "Operate" region). Therefore, operating, rather than testing or observing, offers this patient the highest likelihood of survival. In contrast, the child with a probability of disease below 8% is so unlikely to have appendicitis that observing is better than relying on the WBC count. In intermediate cases, when the clinician's estimate of the likelihood of disease is between 8% and 48%, a WBC count offers the highest likelihood of survival.

Trade-offs and Utilities

It may oversimplify the problem of ruling out appendicitis to say that the best strategy is always the one in which the patient has the highest probability of surviving ("expected survival"). Other factors may also be important. For example, surgery is associated with discomfort and a period of hospitalization. Both of these outcomes are worse when the appendix ruptures. Another of the clinician's goals may be to keep costs as low as possible. Thus, accommodating these additional outcomes requires a finer gradation of outcomes and the values, or preferences, we place on them.

To compare additional outcomes, we require a trade-off of risks and benefits. For the appendicitis decision tree (see Fig. 1–6), surgery offers a higher survival than patient observation but also requires (100% probability) surgery. In contrast, observation offers a slightly lower probability of survival but also involves a much lower (30%) chance that the patient will require surgery (Table 1–4). Balancing a number of conflicting objectives represents a fundamental challenge for the decision maker: How much additional risk of death is to be tolerated to avoid surgery?

Although this question is difficult to answer, it is inescapable because a trade-off is made whenever a physician makes a decision. For example, if the physician chooses to observe a patient that the clinician believes has a 30% probability of appendicitis, the patient's likelihood of surgery is reduced to less than 1 in 3 (see Table 1–4). However, the patient also faces an additional 2 in 100,000 risk of death.

How physicians and patients regard the various outcomes influences which strategy they choose. Usually, however, when management decisions are made, the trade-offs between outcomes are implicit. Expressing the trade-offs explicitly may help to clarify the best decision. For example, surgery is certainly worse than recovery without surgery. To avoid unnecessary surgery in this case, however, the patient has a slightly increased risk of death. Some physicians would take a 1 in 5000 risk of a patient's dying

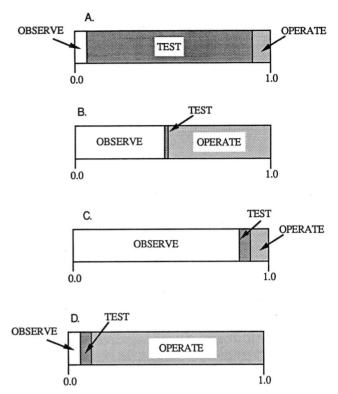

Figure 1-10. Examples of how the threshold bar changes in different settings. *A,* A test with near perfect (100%) sensitivity and specificity. *B,* A test with poor (near 50%) sensitivity and specificity. *C,* A relatively benign condition for which treatment is dangerous or of little efficacy. *D,* The therapy is quite harmless and cheap, and the disease dangerous.

(approximately the risk that the same 10-year-old will die in an automobile accident) in order to avoid an unnecessary surgery. If this is the case, patient observation is preferred to surgery.

In Table 1–4, the "Surgery" option eliminates 2 deaths per 100,000 population over "Observe," at the "cost" of 70,000 additional surgeries. Thus, choosing surgery involves an additional 70,000 surgeries for every 2 deaths prevented. For the patient who chooses surgery rather than take a 2 in 70,000 chance of death, presumptive surgery is the better alternative. However, the clinician may tolerate a 1 in 5000 risk to avoid surgery. Because a risk of death that is less than 1 in 5000 is preferable to surgery and since observing involves a risk of 2 in 70,000 (or 1 in 35,000) to avoid surgery, the observation strategy is better than presumptive surgery for this person.

However, the testing alternative offers the best alternative in this situation. In Table 1–4, testing reduces both the number of surgeries and the number of deaths compared with surgery. Thus, testing is said to be a *dominant* alternative to surgery. In contrast to the "Observe" strategy, however, testing poses a trade-off: testing avoids 5 deaths at a "cost" of 14,000 surgeries compared with observing. This ratio is equivalent to avoiding nearly 2 deaths per

Table 1-4. Numbers of Surgeries and Deaths Expected per 100,000 Patients Managed with the Surgery, Test, and Observe Alternatives

Strategy	Surgeries	Deaths
Surgery	100,000	10
Test	44,000	7
Observe	30,000	12

5000 surgeries, and the clinician's threshold was 1 death per 5000 surgeries. Therefore, testing is still best.

The process of incorporating trade-offs between risks and benefits in evaluating a decision can be simplified by assigning a value directly to the surgery outcome. Because recovery without surgery is better than surgery and recovery following surgery is better than death, we need a value that is intermediate between no surgery and death. The value should also capture the decision maker's willingness to take a 1 in 5000 (but no greater) risk of the patient's dying in order to avoid surgery.

Because the clinician would rather accept a 1 in 5000 risk of a patient's death to avoid surgery, surgery may be said to reduce the value of an outcome by 1 in 5000 on a scale when recovery without surgery is 1 and death is 0. Thus, we can assign values as follows:

- 1, recovery without surgery
- 0, surgical death 1 in 5000, or 0.9998, surgery

Values assigned in this way are called *utilities*. Utilities can be assessed for any outcome in a decision tree. As a rule, the utility of the best (most preferred) outcome is 1 and the least preferred outcome is 0. The utility of intermediate outcomes is assessed by determining how much of a chance a person would take of experiencing the worst outcome to avoid the intermediate outcome.

When utilities are used as the values in the terminal nodes, the tree can be analyzed exactly as before, by multiplying probabilities by utilities. The strategy that has the highest expected utility is the best alternative for the individual whose preferences are captured in the utilities. In the example, where recovery without surgery is 1, recovery after surgery is 0.9998, and surgical death is 0, testing has the highest expected utility. Thus, for the clinician who tolerates a 1 in 5000 risk of death to avoid surgery, testing is still the best alternative.

A simplified version of assessing trade-offs can be applied quickly in the clinical setting. The management of febrile infants is one clinical dilemma in which such an assessment may be helpful. Data suggest that a 6-month-old child with a temperature above 39°C and no apparent focus of infection has a 3% likelihood of occult bacteremia (see Chapter 59). Of children with occult bacteremia, 70% of cases resolve spontaneously. Of the remaining 30%, about 20% will have meningitis. Thus, 2 in every 1000 infants with high fever (3% × 30% × 20%) will have meningitis. Assuming that treating an infant with fever and no source with antibiotics at presentation reduces the risk of meningitis by half, we can express the dilemma as an *explicit* trade-off. To prevent one case of meningitis, we would have to treat 1000 febrile infants. To make a management decision for a febrile 6-month-old child, the physician must choose between giving antibiotics, which are likely to be unnecessary, or accepting an additional 1 in 1000 risk of development of meningitis. If the physician (and parent) tolerates a 1 in 1000 risk of meningitis to avoid antibiotic treatment, observing the child is best. Otherwise, presumptive treatment is the better choice.

Cost-Effectiveness and Decision Analysis in the Literature

Decision analyses can be useful in defining decision thresholds to be used in clinical encounters; however, several caveats apply:

1. Does the scenario evaluated in the model closely resemble your own?

2. Does the model leave out what is considered to be important outcomes? A missing outcome is important if including it would be likely to change the results of the analysis. Missing outcomes are especially dubious if they are missing from one alternative and not another.

3. Are the probability estimates well supported and reasonable, given the clinical setting that *you* face?

4. Were utilities modeled in a way that reflects the clinician's (or patient's) preferences for the outcomes? In particular, does it consider the patient's willingness to avoid undesirable outcomes by taking risks of less desirable outcomes?

5. Finally, does the study include sensitivity analyses to examine how the results change when probability and utility values are varied?

REFERENCES

Bates AS, Margolis PA, Evans AT. Verification bias in studies evaluating diagnostic tests. J Pediatr 1993;122:585.

Berwick DM, Fineberg HV, Weinstein MC. When doctors meet numbers. Am J Med 1981;71:991.

Black ER, Panzer RJ, Mayewski RJ, et al. Characteristics of diagnostic tests and principles for their use in quantitative decision making. *In* Panzer RJ, Black ER, Griner PF (eds). Diagnostic Strategies for Common Medical Problems. Philadelphia: American College of Physicians, 1991:1–16.

Bryant GD, Normal GR. Expressions of probability: Words and numbers. N Engl J Med 1980;302:411.

Downs SM, McNutt RA, Margolis PA. Management of infants at risk for occult bacteremia: A decision analysis. J Pediatr 1991;118:11–20.

Fagan T. Nomogram for Bayes' theorem. N Engl J Med 1975;293:257.

Jaffe DM, Fleisher GR. Temperature and white blood cell count as indicators of bacteremia. Pediatrics 1991;87:670.

Jaffe DM, Tanz RR, Davis AT, et al. Antibiotic administration to treat possible occult bacteremia: A prospective clinical trial. N Engl J Med 1987;317:1175.

Kassirer JP. Our stubborn quest for uncertainty. N Engl J Med 1989;320:1489.

Komaroff AL, Pass TM, Aronson MD, et al. The prediction of streptococcal pharyngitis in adults. J Gen Intern Med 1986;1:1.

Pauker SG, Kassirer JP. The threshold approach to medical decision making. N Engl J Med 1980;302:1109.

Polk HC, Stone HH, Gardner B. Basic Surgery, 2nd ed. East Norwalk, Conn: Appleton-Century-Crofts, 1983.

Pollack MM, Ruttman UE, Getson PR. Pediatric risk of mortality (PRISM) score. Crit Care Med 1988;16:1110.

Ransohoff DF, Feinstein AR. Problems of spectrum and bias in evaluating the efficacy of diagnostic tests. N Engl J Med 1978;299:926.

Robbins SL, Cottran RS. The Pathologic Basis of Disease. Philadelphia: WB Saunders, 1979.

Rudolph AM. Pediatrics, 18th ed. East Norwalk, Conn: Appleton-Lange, 1987.

Sackett DL. A primer on the precision and accuracy of the clinical examination. JAMA 1992;267:2638.

Sox HX, Blatt MA, Higgins MC, et al. Medical Decision Making. Stoneham, Mass: Butterworths, 1988.

Yip R, Binkin NJ, Fleshood L, et al. Declining prevalence of anemia among low-income children in the United States. JAMA 1987;258:1619.

Young PC, Hamill B, Wasserman RC, et al. Evaluation of the capillary microhematocrit as a screening test for anemia in pediatric office practice. Pediatrics 1986;78:206.

Wasson JH, Sox HC, Neff RK, et al. Clinical prediction rules: Applications and methodologic standards. N Engl J Med 1985;313:793.

Weinstein MC, Fineberg HV. Clinical Decision Analysis. Philadelphia: WB Saunders, 1980.

2 Applying the Medical Literature to Clinical Decision Making*

Peter L. Havens

Clinical epidemiology, a discipline that offers a system of thought, can be used to solve problems that arise in clinical medicine. The major focus of the application of epidemiologic thought in study design or study criticism is the avoidance of systematic error *(bias)* and identification of confounding effects between variables. Statistics offers methods of computation and numbers manipulation that can assess the effects of random error and control for confounding variables in the analysis of study results.

The study of epidemiology and statistics helps us to learn enough about the design, implementation, and analysis of clinical studies so that sources of error can be identified. Knowing where to look for errors and what kind of errors are possible makes it more likely that those errors will be found when one is reading pertinent literature. Finding errors in study design, implementation, or analysis is crucial to avoid mistakes in inferences made as the results of published clinical studies are applied to problems in patient management.

Table 2–1 outlines a series of questions that may be helpful to ask when one is reading a clinical study. There are five major issues that these questions address:

1. What population was studied?
2. What measurements were made?
3. What was the design of the study that related the measurements to the population?
4. What non-random errors were made in selection of study subjects *(selection bias)*, what measurements were performed on those subjects *(observation/measurement bias),* and what hidden errors might there have been *(confounding)*?
5. What statistical techniques were used in the analysis of the study to report the main results, and what techniques were used to assess the effects of both random and systematic error on those results?

STUDY POPULATIONS

The actual patients in a study may differ dramatically from what was initially conceptualized as the intended population. The differences between the conceptual study population and actual study sample may be important as one tries to interpret the study's results. One approach to understanding problems associated with study populations is shown in Figure 2–1.

When an investigator starts to design a study, the investigator may plan to study everyone with a given disease. This group of "everyone with disease" is the "target population." For example, one might want to study the effects of an antibiotic in children with otitis media. "All children with otitis media" is the conceptual definition of the target population. The investigator begins by exactly specifying the members of this group, both clinically and demographically.

However, not all children with otitis media are available to any single investigator. Therefore, an investigator studies subjects who are available in both time and place. The population that is accessible may differ dramatically from the conceptualized target population. A study performed with subjects with otitis media at a university hospital emergency room may differ from one performed at a suburban private practice. Understanding the difference between the conceptualized target population and the accessible population is important in interpreting study results.

Even the accessible population may be too large to study completely. Therefore, investigators often study a sample of the accessible population. The most ideal method of sampling the accessible population is called *random sampling*, since all statistical tests of significance assume that the method of sampling was random. However, a common method of sampling for clinical trials is *consecutive sampling*; all subjects coming to the investigator's clinic during a certain period of time are entered into the study. Other methods of sampling from a population are outlined in Table 2–2.

After the accessible population is sampled, one has the intended sample of study subjects. For example, these might all be patients

Table 2–1. Questions to Ask of a Report of a Clinical Study: Outline for a Study Critique

Collection of Data
1. Why was the study done (and who paid for it)? What were the prior hypotheses?
2. What type of study was done?
3. How was the size of the study population determined?
4. How was the ratio of cases to controls determined?
5. Could there have been bias in the selection of study subjects? How might selection bias affect the data?
6. Could there have been bias in the collection of information and performance of measurements? How might observation or measurement bias affect the data?
7. What provisions were made to minimize confounding?

Analysis of Data
1. What methods were used to measure the association between exposure and disease?
2. What methods were used to measure the stability of the association between exposure and disease?
3. What methods were used to control for confounding?

Interpretation of Data
1. What were the major results of the study?
2. How might bias have affected these results?
3. How might random misclassification have affected these results?
4. To whom may the results of this study be generalized?
5. Is the interpretation of the data conservative?

Modified with permission from Monson RR. Occupational Epidemiology, 2nd ed. Boca Raton, Fla, CRC Press, 1990. With permission.

*This chapter is adapted from Chapter 2, Dr. Peter Havens, *Nelson Textbook of Pediatrics*, 15th ed, W. B. Saunders, 1995.

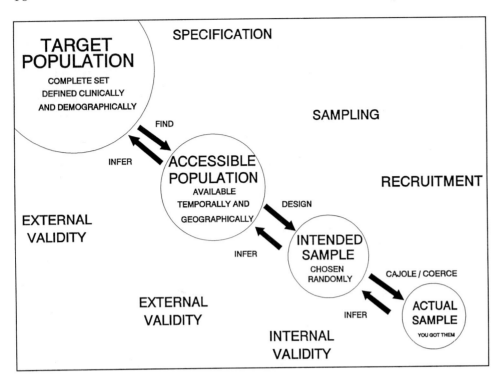

Figure 2–1. Subjects actually enrolled in a study may differ in important ways from the population the investigators initially intended to study. Nonrandom errors in subject selection are called *selection bias* and can result in studies that lead to improper inference when study results are applied to populations other than the study population.

with otitis media coming to the emergency department over a 1-year period. This study sample may not be particularly representative of the initially conceptualized target population. The *generalizability (external validity)* of a study is a measure of how representative the intended sample is of the target population. The results of a study of otitis media in patients who come to a subspecialty otorhinolaryngology clinic for evaluation may not be very generalizable to care of patients with otitis media seen in a primary care office practice. The subspecialty clinic patient sample may have many different problems from those seen in patients in an office practice. Such a study would be said to have "low" generalizability or "poor external validity."

Once an investigator has defined the population sample intended for study, the job of recruitment remains: enrolling those subjects

Table 2–2. Methods of Sampling from a Target Population*

Class	Type	Definition	Problems and Benefits
Probability		Uses a random process to guarantee each unit of population has a specified chance of selection.	The only valid method if you are expecting to do significance tests.
	Simple random	Enumerate every member of the population, then select a sample at random.	Requires enumeration of the entire population. Minimizes potential for sampling bias.
	Stratified random	Identify groups of interest, then randomize within those groups.	A good, nonbiased way to increase precision in subgroup analyses.
	Systematic	Select sample by a "periodic" approach (e.g., every other . . . odd birthdays . . .)	No advantages over random number table. Not really random, open to alteration and bias.
	Cluster	Take a random sample of a natural (temporal or geographic) grouping of members of the population.	Biased if the "natural grouping" is not representative of whole population.
Non-probability		Uses something other than a random process to generate a sample from a population.	All are open to bias and diminish applicability of statistical tests of significance.
	Consecutive	Take all members of the accessible population over the time of the study.	Easy, but may not be a representative sample if the time of the study is short.
	Convenience	Use members of the accessible population who are the easiest to reach.	Strong potential for bias. Volunteers are healthier than others.
	Judgmental	Include those you want, and exclude the ones you don't want.	Very little relation to a random probability sample, don't you think? The potential for systematic error is enormous.

*All statistical significance tests depend on choosing a probability sample from a population of interest.

into a study. The difference between the intended sample and the actual sample can be significant. What leads people to refuse participation in a study may not be random; rather, there may be certain recurring problems that lead to the study of a biased sampling of intended study subjects.

Internal validity is a measure of how representative the actual sample is compared with the intended sample. If sampling at this level is unbiased, the study is said to have "good internal reliability." However, if all patients with severe otitis media refuse to enter a study while patients with mild otitis media agree to be in a study, the subjects actually in the study would be different from those initially intended for inclusion. This would result in a systematic error in choosing study subjects (selection bias) even if the intended sample had been an unbiased representative sample of the population of interest.

Figure 2–2 suggests how far wrong one can go in sampling from a target population. If the actual sample is in the middle of the target population (as shown on the left in Figure 2–2), the study is said to have good internal validity and high generalizability. The diagram on the right in Figure 2–2, however, represents a study in which the actual subjects studied differed greatly from the target population. Such a study has poor internal validity, and the results would be poorly generalizable to a different population of patients.

MEASUREMENTS

Variables

After a sample population is identified for study, the investigator decides on the variables to be measured. The conceptual definition of the variables of interest may be different from the operational definition of the actual measurements. The relationship between these two definitions also affects the internal validity of the study. In the theoretical study of otitis media, ear pain in a child with a bulging, opaque, immobile eardrum will constitute the conceptual definition of otitis media. The operational definition may include

agreement on diagnostic criteria between two certified otoscopists, or it may involve tympanometry, as a way to objectively standardize the definition of otitis media (see Chapter 9). Understanding the differences between the conceptual definition and operational definition used in a study can help as one tries to generalize the results of a study to clinical practice. Operational definitions of disease used for clinical trials may be much narrower than definitions used for diagnosis in clinical practice, limiting the external validity of some trials.

Truly continuous variables have an infinite number of potential values (age, weight, blood pressure). Certain types of continuous variables (*ordered discrete variables*) differ from truly continuous variables. Even though they represent ordered categories with quantifiable intervals between the categories, there is not an infinite number of potential values between each ordered discrete variable. An example is the number of feedings per day.

Categorical variables sort study subjects into different unordered groups. Examples of categorical variables are gender, race, and vital status (dead or alive). *Ordinal variables* are a special type of categorical variable that sort study subjects into categories that have some relative ranking. An example is an asthma score that might identify patients with mild, moderate, or severe asthma.

Categorical variables are often used to measure and report the presence of disease in populations. In fact, this is one of the major goals of epidemiology, which has been described by MacMahon as "the study of the distribution and determinants of disease frequency in man." Measures of disease frequency are reported as *rates*.

The information content of the statement "ten people died of this illness" is greatly enhanced by adding the number of people at risk for the illness and over what period of time the risk was present. The *incidence rate* has as its numerator the number of newly affected individuals and as its denominator the person-time of observation (number of people at risk for the disease for a certain duration of time). The *cumulative incidence rate* has the number of newly affected persons in the numerator and the number at risk in the denominator. Time is not explicitly stated in the cumulative incidence rate, but it is often an annual rate.

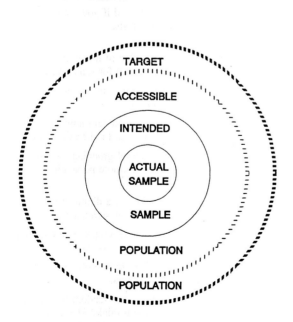
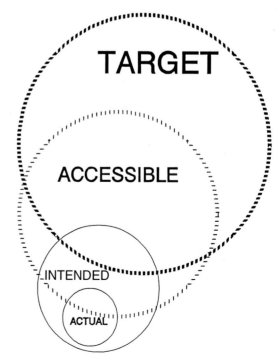

Figure 2–2. The study depicted on the right has poor internal validity and poor generalizability (external validity) because of the large differences between subjects in the actual sample from those in the population initially intended for study.

PRECISION

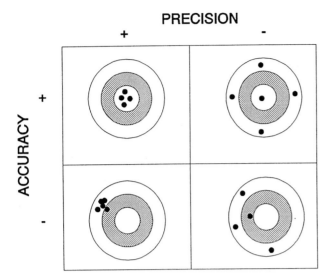

PRECISION AND ACCURACY OF MEASUREMENT VARIABLES

	Precision (Random Error)	Accuracy (Systematic Error, Bias)
Definition	The degree to which a variable has nearly the same value when measured several times.	The degree to which a variable actually represents what it is supposed to represent.
Assessment	Use statistical analysis to compare variation between repeated measurements. Look for standard deviation or 95% confidence interval.	Use epidemiologic thought. Compare measurements with a reference standard.
Importance	Allows detection of differences between groups at "statistically significant" levels.	Allows detection of "clinically significant" differences between groups and identification of studies in which bias leads to the wrong answer.

Figure 2–3. The difference between precision and accuracy of measurements is shown.

Incidence rates reflect new cases. *Prevalence rates* have the total number of cases in the numerator (independent of time of disease onset) and total number at risk in the denominator. In diseases for which the exact onset may be difficult to determine (e.g., cancers), it may be difficult to distinguish between incident and prevalent cases.

The *mortality rate* is a special kind of cumulative incidence rate, with deaths in the numerator and population in the denominator. The *case-fatality rate*, another special type of cumulative incidence rate, has deaths in the numerator and number of people with a specific disease in the denominator.

In the same way that selection bias can lead to errors in choosing study subjects, non-random or systematic errors can be a problem in measurements performed on study subjects. Systematic (non-random) errors in measurement are referred to as measurement bias or observer bias.

The degree to which a measurement actually represents what it was intended to represent is called *accuracy*, or *validity*. Non-random error that may lead to the wrong answer is called *measurement bias*. Errors that lead to finding an association when none actually exists are called *alpha errors*. Special types of measurement bias are *observer bias*, a consistent distortion in the perception or reporting of the measurement by an observer; and *subject bias*,

a consistent distortion of the measurement by the study subject. Comparing results of one study with a "gold standard" measurement is necessary to assess the accuracy of a study.

The *precision (reliability)* of a variable is an indicator of the extent to which a measurement gives the same results when it is performed several times. Problems with precision result in random errors. This type of error may lead to finding "no association" even when an association may exist. This is called *beta error*.

A pictorial interpretation of the relationship between precision and accuracy and the importance of those two concepts in design and interpretation of clinical studies is shown in Figure 2–3. Note that it is possible to have a precise answer that is the wrong answer. It has been thought that it is better to find "no difference" (even if one exists) than to precisely describe an inaccurate answer. Although precision is helpful, accuracy is the most important consideration.

Statistical Inference for Non-statisticians

If epidemiology is useful for controlling or identifying non-random error, statistics are important for controlling the effects of random error in a study. Each time a clinician evaluates a patient, it is somewhat akin to performing a clinical trial with a sample size of one. Clinicians often are in the position of comparing what happens with a patient to what has been reported in the literature. Inferences about a patient are based on comparing measured patient variables to reported reference values. The validity of the inference from reported value to single patient data depends in part on how well the reference study was designed and implemented and on how closely the patient in question matches the subjects in the comparison study. To decide whether a single patient is significantly different from those reported in the literature also requires an understanding of statistical inference.

Suppose an 8-year-old female patient presents with recurrent urinary tract infections (UTIs). A clinician measures the blood pressure and wants to know whether that measurement is higher than usual for other girls with her condition. There is no study that has evaluated all other such girls. There may be a study in which an investigator measures the blood pressure in a sample of 10 subjects from the universe of girls with recurrent UTIs (Fig. 2–4). The individual blood pressure values are summed and divided by the number of subjects in the study, and the mean blood pressure in those 10 girls is reported. The mean value from the subjects in the study sample estimates the mean blood pressure in the target

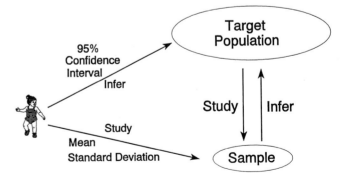

$$\text{95\% Confidence Interval} = \text{Mean} \pm 1.96 \,(\text{Standard Deviation})/\sqrt{N}$$

Figure 2–4. From the results of a study we know the mean and standard deviation of a measurement in the study sample. From this we make inferences about the mean in the target population. It is the 95% confidence interval that allows this inference to be made.

population; this is called the *point estimate* of the main result of the study. The *standard deviation* of the sample mean is also calculated as a way to describe the variability (random error) associated with the measurement.

To know how the single patient value compares with those of the 10 patients in the study, the clinician compares the patient value with the mean blood pressure value in the study sample. If the patient's value is higher than the mean, a comparison is made between the patient value and the range of values encompassed by the standard deviation that was reported in the study. If the single patient's value falls within the range of values reported in the study, that is reassuring.

Finding a patient's blood pressure within the range of values encompassed by the standard deviation of the blood pressure of the 10 study subjects may be reassuring as far as it goes, but it does not tell how the patient's value compares with values in all subjects in the universe of girls with recurrent UTIs. A study with 10 subjects is a small study. The sample studied might not be representative of all girls with recurrent UTIs. What is really of interest is the whole range of values in the population of all girls with recurrent UTIs and how the single patient's value compares with that.

Because an individual investigator cannot study all the subjects in a population of interest, multiple small studies are often performed. Clinicians cannot read all those studies, but they need to know how the mean value reported in one study compares with the

mean values in the other reported studies. The 95% confidence interval allows an answer to the question, "if the same study were to be repeated over and over again, what is the range of answers that would be found 95 times out of 100?" The 95% confidence interval is a function of the standard deviation (SD) and the number of patients in a study and is calculated as

$$\text{mean} \pm \frac{1.96 \, (\text{SD})}{\sqrt{N}}$$

where N is the number of subjects in the study.

Studies with many subjects (large N) have narrower 95% confidence intervals than do smaller studies. As the standard deviation increases (random variation in measurements increases), so does the length of the 95% confidence interval. If an investigator uses a precise measurement that reproducibly gives the same result with very little error and if there is little variability in the population sample being studied, a precise measure of the main effect, with a narrow 95% confidence interval, can be obtained using very few subjects. If the method of measurement is not very precise or if there is wide variability in the sample being studied, the 95% confidence limit will be very wide.

The example above uses a continuous variable. The summary statistic used to report the point estimate of the main effect in a study with a single continuous variable is the *mean* or *median*. The estimate of the uncertainty associated with that point estimate is the standard deviation, or 95% confidence interval (Table 2–3).

Table 2–3. **Reporting Results of Measurements**

Variable Type	Number of Groups	Estimate of Main Effect	Measurement of Variability of the Main Effect Estimate	Comment
Continuous	Single group	Mean	Standard deviation, 95% confidence interval	Mean = sum of all values/number of values. Sensitive to the effects of a few high or low values (outliers). Check for a graph of the data to identify such outliers.
		Median	Range, interquartile range	Median = value in the middle of a range of values (half above and half below the median). For data that are not uniformly distributed, the median is a more accurate representation of central tendency than the mean.
	Two groups	Mean difference	95% confidence interval	Mean difference = group 1 mean − group 2 mean.
Categorical	Single group	Rate (risk)	95% confidence interval	Rate = number affected/number at risk. If the 95% confidence interval includes 0, the risk is not significantly different from 0.
	Two groups	Risk difference	95% confidence interval	Risk difference = rate 1 − rate 2. If the 95% confidence interval includes 0, the risk is not statistically significantly different between the two groups being compared.
		Relative risk (rate ratio)	95% confidence interval	Relative risk = rate 1/rate 2. If the 95% confidence interval includes 1, the risk is not statistically different between the two groups being compared.
		Odds ratio	95% confidence interval	Odds ratio is calculated from data collected in a case-control study. Closely approximates the relative risk for rare outcomes. If the 95% confidence interval includes 1, the risk is not statistically significantly different between the two groups being compared.

Studies with a categorical variable as their main measurement report a rate of illness as the point estimate of the main result. Estimates of rates have the potential for error and need to be reported with a 95% confidence interval. The 95% confidence interval has the same meaning with a categorical variable as it does with a continuous variable: If the study were repeated many times, the risk estimate generated by each of those studies would fall within the range of values encompassed by the 95% confidence interval 95 times out of 100.

Studies are often performed to measure differences between subjects in two groups. Such studies have main effects that report the size of the difference between the groups. This is called the *effect size.* Examples of various summary statistics are given in Table 2–3.

The 95% confidence interval suggests the range that would include the point estimate of the main effect found in a study if the study were performed over and over again. Many studies compare findings in two groups when the question of interest is stated as: ''Is the value in group 1 so much different than the value in group 2 that the populations from which they were sampled are really different?''

The probability that the samples in the two groups came from the same target population is called the *P* value (for probability). When the *P* value is less than .05, it is inferred that the probability that the study group values were sampled from the same population is less than 5%. There is a statistically significant difference between the values in the two groups because they were different enough that they probably represent samples of different target populations.

Statistical significance depends on the same parameters as the 95% confidence interval: the standard deviation and the sample size. Studies with smaller standard deviations or more subjects in each group are more likely to be able to show differences than studies with larger standard deviations or fewer subjects. A study with a precise measurement and many subjects may find a ''statistically'' significant difference between two groups, but the size of the difference itself may be very small. Such a small difference may not be ''clinically'' significant.

CAUSATION, CONFOUNDING, AND CLINICAL TRIAL DESIGN

Causation

Clinical investigators perform studies to understand what causes the presence of disease and what may cause the patient to get better. The relationship between cause and effect is sometimes unclear. Finding an association between variable A and outcome B does not establish that variable A causes outcome B. The association may not be real. Such a spurious association may be caused by the presence of bias in sampling or measurement. Likewise, false associations can be caused by random error. Some studies reveal associations that really do exist. The challenge is understanding the precise relationship between variable A and outcome B. Often the question is, ''Does A cause B?''

Confounding

Criteria exist that can be applied to an association to assess the possibility that variable A causes outcome B (Table 2–4). If some or all of these criteria are met, it is likely that the identified association represents a causative link. Even if the criteria outlined in Table 2–4 are met, one major barrier to establishing a cause and effect relationship still exists. This is the possibility of a *confounding variable* that might explain the apparent relationship.

Table 2–4. Criteria for Assessing Causation

Criterion	Comment
Strength	Exposures that are very strongly associated with an outcome are more likely to be causal than are exposures that are weak.
Consistency	Associations that are consistently found in many different settings, and by many different investigators, are more likely to be causal.
Specificity	If a variable is associated with only one outcome and the outcome is only associated with a single possible cause, the relationship is more likely causal.
Temporality	Causes must precede effects. This is the only one of these criteria that is absolutely necessary to suggest causation.
Biologic gradient	If an increasing amount of exposure is associated with an increased rate or severity of disease, a dose-response relationship exists and causality is more likely.
Plausibility	It is always encouraging if your hypotheses sound reasonable. However, some epidemiologic findings are truly new, in which case biologic knowledge may need to expand to be able to explain the relationship.
Coherence	A causal association is strengthened if data from epidemiology fit in with data from other areas (e.g., pathology).
Experiment	If a possible cause is removed from a population and disease frequency declines, the likelihood of a causal link is strengthened.
Analogy	If a similar association has been shown to be causal, the association under investigation may be more likely to be causal.

From Hill A-B. The environment and disease: Association of causation. Proc Royal Soc Med 1965:58:295–300.

A confounding variable is one that is associated with the *predictor variable,* associated with the *outcome variable* independent of its association with the predictor variable, and is not an intermediate in the causal pathway from exposure to disease. In the presence of confounding variable C, variable A appears to be associated with outcome B. In fact, the illusion of an association occurs only because the confounding variable C is associated independently with both A and B.

It is often difficult to identify confounding variables in a study. One needs to critically examine every reported association and carefully consider the possibility that an association between two variables may be caused by their mutual relationship with a third, possibly unidentified, variable. Certain clinical studies are more likely to have problems with confounders than others.

Trial Design

There are multiple potential study designs. Three major study design types include:

- Cohort studies
- Case-control studies
- Cross-sectional (prevalence) studies

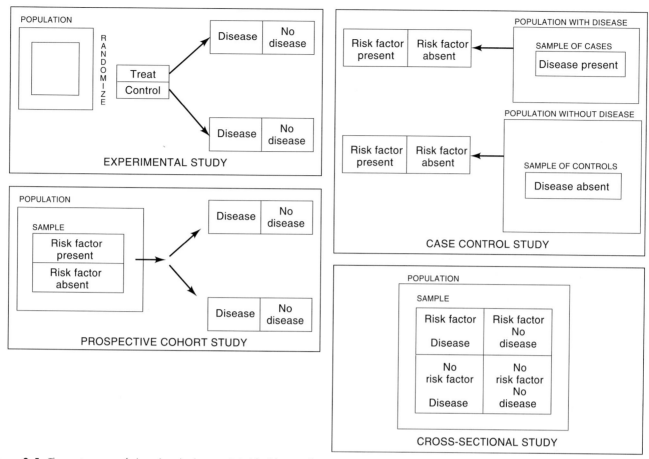

Figure 2–5. The major types of clinical study designs. (Modified from Hulley SB, Cummings SR. Designing Clinical Research: An Epidemiologic Approach. Baltimore: Williams & Wilkins, 1988.)

Study design type affects the ability to infer causality from any association that might be found. Study design also can affect the likelihood that apparent associations suffer from bias or confounding.

COHORT STUDIES

An *experimental study* (Fig. 2–5; Table 2–5) is a special type of cohort study in which an investigator first chooses a sample popula-

tion to study and then assigns subjects to exposed or unexposed categories. A randomized clinical trial identifies a group of willing participants and randomly assigns them to treatment A or treatment B. Such experiments give information about cause and effect that may be impossible to ascertain from other study designs. This design minimizes the potential for confounding because exposure category assignment is carried out by the investigator in a random fashion and not left to the will of study subjects. Selection bias is low, and measurement bias can be reduced by blinding investigators and study subjects to the group assignments. Such experiments

Table 2–5. Advantages and Disadvantages of the Major Types of Observational Studies

	Prospective Cohort	Retrospective Cohort	Cross-Sectional	Case-Control	Nested Case-Control
Sequence of events clear	Yes	(Yes)	No	No	Yes?
Sampling (selection) bias	No	No	No	Yes	No
Bias in risk factor measurement (recall bias)	No	Maybe	Yes	Yes	No
Survivor bias	No	No	Yes	Yes	Yes
Loss to follow-up	Yes	Yes	No	No	Yes
Hypothesis generation	No	No	Yes	Yes	No
Examine multiple associations	Yes	Yes	Yes	Yes	No
Examine >1 outcome	Yes	Yes	Yes	No	No
Study rare diseases	No	No	No	Yes	Yes
Cost in time	Large	Less	Cheap	Cheap	Cheap
Cost in money	Large	Less	Cheap	Cheap	Cheap
Statistic generated	Incidence rate	Incidence rate	Prevalence rate	Odds ratio	Odds ratio

are expensive to perform, and if there is a long delay between exposure and disease, subjects may be lost to follow-up.

Experimental studies may be poorly generalizable because subjects who are willing to participate in a randomized trial may differ from the general population. Therapies used in a clinical trial might be applied with more rigor than in usual clinical practice. The ethics of withholding therapy from one group in an experiment sometimes pose a difficult problem.

In a *prospective* cohort study (see Fig. 2–5 and Table 2–5), subjects in the study sample are divided according to the presence or absence of an exposure or risk factor. Subjects in an observational cohort study have already chosen their exposure category prior to the study. Subjects in the two groups are followed forward in time, and the presence or absence of the outcome of interest is assessed. At the end of a prospective cohort study, one can estimate the cumulative incidence rate of disease in the population of interest and measure the frequency of disease in exposed and unexposed subjects. Comparison of disease rates in exposed and unexposed subjects can be made using the relative risk or risk difference (see Table 2–3).

Prospective cohort studies can show a clear temporal relationship between exposure and outcome. Selection bias and measurement bias in assessing exposure group are minimal. If the investigator who makes the outcome determination is blinded to the exposure group of the subjects, the possibility of measurement bias in assessing outcome is likewise minimal.

Prospective cohort studies have high costs in both time and money. Because the investigator does not control membership in the exposed or unexposed category, confounding is possible. Loss to follow-up may be significant in a cohort study of a disease that progresses slowly from exposure to outcome determination. Loss to follow-up can lead to bias.

Cohort studies can be performed retrospectively as well. Subjects are identified by the presence or absence of exposure that occurred in the past, but both exposure and disease have occurred prior to the study being performed. Retrospective cohort studies are less expensive in time and money than prospective cohort studies, but there are problems of recall bias and confounding.

CASE-CONTROL STUDIES

In a case-control study, subjects are separated into two groups according to the presence or absence of disease. Subjects in each group are evaluated for risk factors for those diseases and the association between risk factor, and disease is measured using the odds ratio. Case-control studies are useful for studying rare diseases and are inexpensive. The possibility of selection bias and bias in risk factor measurement *(recall bias)* is large, at times limiting their usefulness. When carefully designed and performed, these studies are useful for generating hypotheses and examining the possibility of multiple-risk factor associations with the disease. For rare diseases, the odds ratio that is generated by a case-control study is a good estimate of the relative risk that might be generated by a cohort study.

Sampling bias is one of the major threats to validity of a case-control study. Subjects are easy to identify because they have the specific disease. An appropriate control subject is often difficult to identify. Subjects in the control group must have the same potential for development of the disease as the case subjects. Making this determination is sometimes very difficult. If an investigator has already completed a cohort study, it is possible to conduct a case-control study within the same sample. Since these subjects were all chosen as members of a single population group, the chance for sampling bias is diminished. Such a study is called a *nested* case-

	Disease Present	Disease Absent	
Test Positive	a	b	a + b
Test Negative	c	d	c + d
	a + c	b + d	

A = true positives; b = false positives; c = false negatives; d = true negatives.

Sensitivity = a/a + c; specificity = d/b + d; positive predictive value = a/a + b; negative predictive value = d/c + d.

Figure 2–6. Results of a cross-sectional study to evaluate a diagnostic test.

control study; it combines the advantages of a cohort study and a case-control study.

CROSS-SECTIONAL STUDIES

A cross-sectional study, sometimes called a *prevalence study*, samples from a population of interest and simultaneously measures

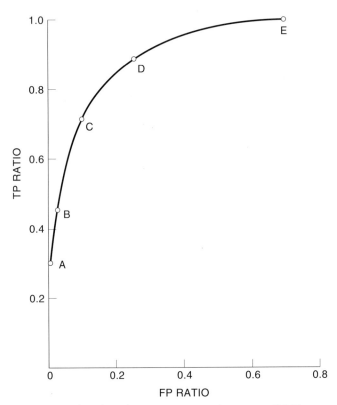

Figure 2–7. A hypothetical receiver operating characteristic (ROC) curve. The vertical scale is the sensitivity (true-positive ratio), and the horizontal scale is (1 − specificity), the false-positive ratio. At one extreme point, A, the test has poor sensitivity but good specificity. At the other extreme, E, the test has high sensitivity but poor specificity. (From McNeil BJ, Keeler E, Adelstein SJ. Primer on certain elements of medical decision making. Reproduced with permission from New England Journal of Medicine, 1975;293:211.)

the presence of risk factors and outcomes. A cross-sectional study can calculate prevalence rates and compare the prevalence of disease in exposed and unexposed subjects. Because time does not pass between assessment of exposure and disease, the temporal relationship between exposure and disease is unclear. Assessing the causal nature of associations found in a prevalence study is often difficult. Cross-sectional studies are inexpensive. They are useful for generating hypotheses and examining multiple associations between potential risk factors and a disease of interest.

Cross-sectional studies are susceptible to a specific type of bias called *incidence-prevalence bias.* A cross-sectional survey is more likely to identify prevalent disease than incident disease, especially if people with the disease live a long time. This is important to remember in interpreting the results of cross-sectional studies.

DIAGNOSTIC TESTS

The study performed to identify the usefulness of a diagnostic test is a special form of cross-sectional study. Such studies measure the ability of a test to identify patients with a specific disease. The generalized form of the results of such a study are shown in Figure 2–6 (see p. 22).

The *sensitivity* of a test is the measurement that answers the question "Of all people with disease, how many will have a positive test?" The *specificity* of a test answers the question "Of all people without disease, how many will have a negative test?" The *positive predictive* value answers the question "Of all people with a positive test, how many will have the disease?" The *negative predictive* value answers the question "Of all people with a negative test, how many will not have the disease?"

Developers of diagnostic tests are often focused on maximizing either sensitivity or specificity (see Chapter 1). The decision to call a diagnostic test positive is somewhat arbitrary, especially for continuously varying laboratory values. Deciding on the cutoff value that defines a positive test is a trade-off between increasing sensitivity at the expense of specificity, or vice versa. For example, if an elevated serum alanine aminotransferase (ALT) concentration is used to define liver toxicity from a given therapeutic agent, the question becomes, "How high an ALT really defines 'toxic'?" Choosing a very high cutoff value may increase the specificity of the test at the expense of decreasing sensitivity. This relationship is shown graphically in Figure 2–7, which shows the plots of sensitivity by specificity for a theoretical diagnostic test. In Figure 2–7, as a cutoff value is chosen to increase sensitivity, the specificity diminishes. The curve in the figure is called a *receiver operating characteristic* (ROC) *curve.* The area under the ROC curve is an excellent indicator of the total usefulness of the specific diagnostic test. Diagnostic tests with a sensitivity of 1 and a specificity of 1 have an area under the ROC curve of 1.

An important aspect of the choice of the cutoff value that defines a positive test is related to the situations to which the test results will be applied. Screening tests for identifying human immunodeficiency virus (HIV) infection are designed to be very sensitive in order to screen out HIV-infected persons from the blood donor pool. A sensitive cutoff is thus chosen to ensure that all potentially positive samples are identified. Although choosing a low cutoff for the determination of a positive screening test increases the sensitivity, it results in decreased specificity and leads to identifying some persons as positive even though they are not truly HIV-infected. That is why all HIV screening tests need to be followed by a very specific test (the Western blot) to distinguish true-positive from false-positive screening results (see Chapter 55).

Users of diagnostic tests often need to know the test's positive and negative predictive values as much as the sensitivity and specificity. Clinicians may find a positive test result and ask how likely it is that this patient with a positive test result actually has the disease. Unfortunately, the positive predictive value alone cannot answer that question. For a diagnostic test of given sensitivity and specificity, the positive predictive value of the test can be calculated only for the population in which the data were generated. The positive predictive value may be different in another popula-

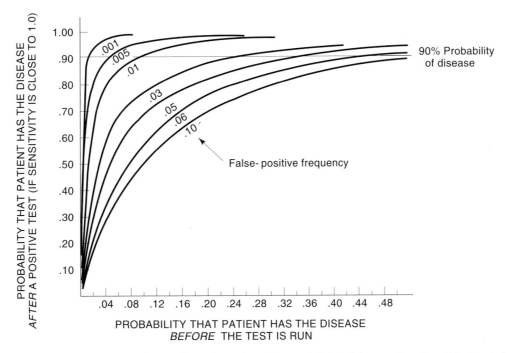

Figure 2–8. The relationship between positive predictive value and prevalence (prior probability) of disease. (From Katz MA. A probability graph describing the predictive value of a highly sensitive diagnostic test. Reproduced with permission from New England Journal of Medicine, 1974;291:1115.)

tion because the prevalence of disease in a population sample influences the positive predictive value of a diagnostic test.

The relationship between prevalence and positive predictive value is described by Bayes' theorem (Fig. 2–8). The test's positive predictive value is lower in a population with a low disease prevalence than it is in a population in which the disease is very common. The population prevalence of disease is called the *prior probability of disease,* a number used to estimate how likely it is that a patient has a disease before the test is performed.

Studies evaluating diagnostic tests are at risk for the same errors as in other cross-sectional studies. Selection bias is a common problem; initial studies of a test are performed in populations of patients with high prevalence of disease, resulting in overestimation of the usefulness of the test when it is applied to patients in a population with a lower prevalence of disease. Errors can also be made in the determination of subjects with disease. The best studies are those in which a true gold standard measurement exists for comparison with the new test.

REFERENCES

Hulley SB, Cummings SR. Designing Clinical Research: An Epidemiologic Approach. Baltimore: Williams & Wilkins, 1988.

Hill AB. The environment and disease: Association or causation? Proc Soc Med 1965;58:295.

Katz MA. A probability graph describing the predictive value of a highly sensitive diagnostic test. N Engl J Med 1974;291:1115.

MacMahon B, Pugh TF. Epidemiology: Principles and Methods. Boston. Little, Brown & Co, 1970.

McNeil BJ, Keeler E, Adelstein SJ. Primer on certain elements of medical decision making. N Engl J Med 1975;293:211.

Miettinen O. Confounding and effect modification. Am J Epidemiol 1974;100:350.

Sackett DL, Haynes RB, Buyatt GH, et al. Clinical Epidemiology: A Basic Science for Clinical Medicine, 2nd ed. Boston: Little, Brown & Co, 1991.

Streiner DL, Norman GR, Blum HM. PDQ Epidemiology. Toronto: BC Decker, 1989.

3 Decision Making and Choosing the Optimal Therapy

Dennis M. Super

TOOLS IN DECISION MAKING

Clinicians are faced with the need to make multiple management decisions for their patients. These decisions revolve around either altering the natural history of or preventing that disease. The tools for making these decisions consist of:

- Evaluation of the medical evidence from the literature
- The process of decision analysis
- Ethical ramifications in decision analysis
- Incorporation of patient and parental beliefs into the decision-making process

For any intervention to be successful, all four tools must be incorporated into the decision-making process. The integration of these tools in altering the natural history of a disease process is central to the decision-making process.

OPTIONS IN DECISION MAKING

The following case is a common occurrence in a pediatric office.

T.G.S., a 24-month-old child, presents for a health maintenance examination. The history and physical findings are normal; however, the parents are concerned regarding the recent television documentary on the effects of low-level lead poisoning on intelligence. The family lives in a home that is more than 60 years old.

In addition, the family has no health insurance and they are of limited financial means. In their community, there is no government agency that monitors lead exposure. The current practice of screening for lead poisoning consists of adding a free erythrocyte protoporphyrin level to the hematocrit obtained at 12 months of age in families who live in homes built before 1980. This laboratory test is inexpensive and easy to perform. The child's free erythrocyte protoporphyrin obtained at 12 months of age was in the normal range.

Several questions are raised by this case:

- Do low plasma levels of lead cause neurotoxicity?
- How should one screen for lead poisoning?
- How should the neurologic deficiencies secondary to low to moderate lead levels be treated?

In addressing the above issues, the clinician has three options: (1) using one's past experience; (2) deferring the decision to an expert; or (3) evaluating the evidence in the literature. Each has its own advantages and disadvantages.

Option 1: The Use of One's Past Experience

The use of past experience is the easiest option to implement. Hence, it is the one that is most often used in the clinical practice of medicine.

By using the free erythrocyte protoporphyrin, the physician in the example has not had a single case of symptomatic lead poisoning in the practice during the past 10 years. In addition, the patients in the clinician's practice who were detected by this process and who had lead levels in the 25 to 45 μg/dl range did not appear to have an increased prevalence of either behavioral or learning problems. On the basis of this prior experience, this physician would reassure the family that there have been no cases of developmental delay or hyperactivity noted in the children in the physician's practice who had a normal free erythrocyte protoporphyrin. Hence, the child will be fine.

With this option, the clinician continues to practice the same way until a series of treatment failures or knowledge of a new therapy forces one to reappraise the management for this condition. Choosing the appropriate therapy with this option may be accomplished by either the intuitive or the analytical method.

THE ANALYTICAL METHOD

With the analytical method, the clinician develops a decision tree built on the probability of the success of a treatment (see Chapter 1). The probability estimates for success may come either from the physician's own experience or from the literature. This process was illustrated in Chapter 1 on when to perform surgery in a patient with abdominal pain. The process is most useful when the outcomes are limited, the problem is straightforward, and the probability estimates are well known. This is the method used in computer-assisted programs in decision analysis. Results from such models are very reproducible when using a verified decision tree. However, if the wrong decision tree is chosen for a patient, the potential for a serious error is great. For example, in a patient presenting with abdominal pain, if the history of cough and fever, coupled with left lower lobe rales and decreased breath sounds, is missed, the appendicitis instead of the pneumonia decision tree may be chosen. If the wrong decision tree is chosen, the patient is at risk for undergoing an unnecessary surgical procedure.

THE INTUITIVE METHOD

In the intuitive process, the clinician makes a clinical judgment. This ''educated guess'' is based on all the nuances of a specific case, coupled with the information from one's past experience and the medical literature. The intuitive method is used in complex situations with multiple outcomes and with therapies that have an uncertain probability of success. Because of the complexity and uncertainty of a condition, an analytical decision tree would be difficult to construct. Unfortunately, because this situation is a common occurrence in medicine, the intuitive model is the one most commonly used in the practice of medicine. Its success is in part based on experience and continuous self-education.

One benefit of the intuitive method is that it is quick. Also, the potential for a major error in choosing the best therapy is less compared with the analytical method. For example, there may be a subtle characteristic to the abdominal pain that would direct the experienced clinician away from surgery that would not be captured by the decision tree approach. The disadvantage of the intuitive method is that it is more prone to cognitive bias than the analytical method.

COGNITIVE BIAS

Cognitive bias deals with the process of how one obtains information, coupled with the ways in which experience alters an opin-

ion of a therapy. As with any bias, these problems cause a systematic deviation from the truth and hence interfere with choosing the correct and best therapy.

The problems in obtaining information deal with:

- Confirmatory bias
- Ignoring negative information
- Framing

In *confirmatory bias*, if a study confirms one's opinion of the superiority of one therapy over another, the clinician is more likely to believe the results of that study. For example, in one survey on how pediatricians judge the scientific merit of a study, 89% reported that they compare the findings with their own experience. Only 27% evaluate the methods section of the article.

Another problem with evaluating the medical literature is *ignoring negative information*. A clinician is more likely to read a study showing positive results than one which shows no difference.

The third source of bias is how the outcome is *framed*. In framing, the same therapy can be presented as either a ''five-year survival rate of 75%'' or a ''five-year death rate of 25%.'' Even though the chance of success is the same, clinicians and parents are more likely to choose this therapy if it is presented in the more favorable manner using survival rates rather than death rates.

Once a therapy is selected, one's impression of that therapy is shaped by one's clinical experience. *Heuristics* (''rules of thumb'') is one such force that can alter our perception of a therapy. The biases associated with heuristics are:

- Availability
- Anchoring
- Representativeness

Availability heuristic refers to the ease of recalling a past event. The most recent case or the most sensational outcome affects one's impression of how successful past interventions have been. With *anchoring heuristic*, once an impression is formed regarding the utility of a treatment regimen, the future outcomes of reapplying that intervention only slightly change the impression of that intervention. For example, the probability of a person's experiencing an allergic reaction to penicillamine (used in oral chelation of lead) is 10%. By the rules of probability, there is a 1% chance ($0.1 \times 0.1 = 0.01$) that the first two patients to receive this treatment in one's practice may experience that complication. Because of this initial experience, the clinician might be unwilling to treat a third patient with this medication. However, if a second clinician treats 20 patients, there is a 12% chance [$(1.0 - 0.1)$ to the 20th power $= 0.12$] that none of these patients will have a complication. If the 21st patient has an allergic reaction to penicillamine, the second clinician would still believe that this therapy is relatively safe and continue to use this intervention. Even though the chance of a complication has been similar in both groups (10%), the timing of when that complication occurred affects the clinician's impression about that medication and alters subsequent treatment strategies.

Representativeness heuristic is the association of the outcome with the intervention. In this bias, the intervention did not cause the outcome but was just temporally related to the outcome. For example, in the above case, we assume that the allergic reaction or the reduction in serum lead was caused by penicillamine. These outcomes could be caused by other factors besides penicillamine. The allergic reaction may be secondary to a different allergen, or the reduction of the lead level may be secondary to another intervention (lead abatement in the home) or to the expected variation (patient versus laboratory) in analysis of the lead levels.

Other types of cognitive bias from clinical experience that may alter an impression of a therapy are:

- Ego bias
- Value-induced bias
- Hindsight bias

With *ego bias*, if a wrong opinion regarding a treatment option is formed, the clinician may become defensive regarding that opinion and become even more hesitant about changing management. This can become a major source of bias, especially with experts who have vested their careers in a certain treatment.

In *value-induced bias*, the concern regarding a certain complication or treatment failure overshadows the actual risk-benefit ratio. With any condition, the probability estimates for complications and treatment successes are fixed. In developing the risk-benefit ratio, relative values are then assigned to these probabilities. The relative values for certain outcomes are inflated, hence producing a biased risk-benefit ratio.

In *hindsight bias*, the clinician reviews the outcome with respect to the treatment chosen. Knowledge regarding this outcome then adversely influences the opinion regarding the therapy. For example, if an adverse reaction occurs, the clinician may conclude that it was obvious that the wrong treatment was chosen, forgetting the uncertainty and the complexity of the original decision-making process. This oversimplification of the decision-making process is a cause of malpractice suits.

Option 2: Deferring the Decision to an Expert

When the clinician has little experience with or when an individual's current practice is challenged by treatment failures or new innovations in medicine, the clinician may turn to experts for advice. This expert advice may come from a colleague in one's own practice, an academician, or practice policies. When this option is used to address the issue of neurotoxicity from low-level lead exposure, the following scenario unfolds.

With Option 2, the family is told that the physician will discuss the issues of low-level lead exposure and intelligence with the regional experts on lead poisoning and that the physician will telephone them in the morning with the consensus. After a discussion of this case with two experts, both recommend using lead levels and not the free erythrocyte protoporphyrin (FEP) to screen for lead toxicity. The first expert recommends chelation for lead levels above 25 μg/dl. The second expert recommends monthly monitoring of plasma lead levels when they are above 25 μg/dl, coupled with chelation when the level exceeds 45 μg/dl. Being confused by these two divergent recommendations, the physician turns to the 1991 statement by the Centers for Disease Control (CDC), *Preventing Lead Poisoning in Young Children*. This report states that the minimal medical management for children with lead levels between 25 and 44 μg/dl includes decreasing exposure to lead, frequent monitoring of plasma lead, correcting iron deficiency, and maintaining appropriate calcium intake. Because of the lack of evidence, decisions regarding chelation are left to the discretion of the clinician.

THE USE OF EXPERTS

With Option 2, the decision is relegated to a third party. These experts have formulated their decisions according to their interpretation of the medical literature, coupled with their experience in managing patients. Unfortunately, this decision-making process is subject to the problems of cognitive bias. Because of these issues, experts may frequently disagree. For example, when 30 directors of tertiary care lead clinics were surveyed on how they would initially manage a child with a lead level of 25 μg/dl, 52% would not recommend chelation whereas 20% would. The remaining would perform a calcium disodium ethylenediaminetetraacetic acid (EDTA) provocation test and base their decision on the results from that study.

In addition, the types of patients seen in a tertiary care center may not represent the same patients seen in a general pediatric practice. The patients in subspecialty clinics are often difficult and complex cases that the primary care provider may have been unsuccessful in treating. Hence, these patients have a greater probability of having experienced complications after the standard therapy or from the original disease process. For example, prior to 1978, most research studies on the prevalence of subsequent epilepsy in children with febrile seizures were based on the experiences of subspecialty clinics in tertiary care centers. The prevalence of epilepsy was as high as 77%; this suggested that children with febrile seizures were at great risk for development of epilepsy. It was not until community-based studies that reflected the types of patients seen in a general practice were performed that the prevalence of epilepsy following simple febrile seizures actually ranged from 2% to 3% (see Chapter 2). This is similar to the prevalence in children without febrile seizures.

PRACTICE POLICIES

An alternative to deferring the management to a local expert is the use of practice policies, such as the 1991 statement from the CDC on preventing lead poisoning. These policies may be developed by professional societies, federal agencies, health maintenance organizations, or even one's own group practice. Based on the flexibility in choosing treatment modalities, the types of practice policies include:

- Standards
- Guidelines
- Options

Policy standards are rigid protocols that the clinician must follow in all cases. In order for standards to be written, there must be unequivocal evidence in the medical literature to substantiate the superiority of one treatment over another. In addition, there must be virtual agreement (i.e., >95%) among patients that the benefits afforded by this intervention exceed those offered by other modalities. Standards offer the clinician no flexibility in management. Deviation from policy standards places the clinician at risk for litigation in the event that an undesirable outcome should occur. Because of the legal ramifications of policy standards, if any of the above criteria are not met, the proposed standard should be downgraded to a guideline.

Policy guidelines are more flexible than standards. The medical literature would support these recommendations; however, the evidence would not be conclusive for all situations or types of patients. When offered the therapy proposed by the guidelines, most patients (60% to 95%) would agree that the proposed therapy is both beneficial and the best one for them. The purpose of guidelines is to furnish the health care provider with a framework for approaching most patients with this problem. However, guidelines also allow one the freedom to customize a treatment plan to the specific situation.

Policy options are the most flexible of the practice policies. With policy options, either the medical literature does not support one therapy over another or the therapy has not yet been evaluated in a systematic fashion. Approximately half of the patients (40% to 60%) would accept the therapy. The main function of options is to inform the clinician about the spectrum of treatments that are available when there is no consensus regarding management.

The clinical ramifications of practice policies are quite significant. The goal of these policies is to enhance patient care. The achievement of this goal depends on the quantity and the quality of the evidence, coupled with the interpretation of the data. If a clinician should choose a substandard therapy, only a few patients in that individual's practice would have the adverse outcome. However, if this same mistake occurred in the formulation of a practice policy, the frequency of these adverse outcomes would be multiplied by the number of clinicians following these policies. Before any organization or clinician accepts a practice policy, the policy must be well designed. A well-designed policy contains the following components:

- Comprehensive discussion of the problem
- Appropriate methods used in evaluation of the treatment modalities
- A discussion of the potential problems of using the policy

The first part of the policy must contain a comprehensive literature search describing the disease process, all the treatment modalities, and all clinically relevant outcomes. The outcomes should include measures of morbidity that are important to the patient in addition to the societal and economic costs.

In the second part of the policy, all evidence regarding the treatments is presented, relative values coupled with the justifications for these values are stated, and the statistical methods used to compare the outcomes are reported. Not only should the policy include all the evidence, but the deficiencies of the data should also be stressed. The patient characteristics must be reported to reduce the problem of extrapolating the results beyond that which is permitted by the data. When relative values are determined for the outcomes, the values should be determined not by how easy they are to measure but by the importance of the outcome to the patient. For example, it is easy to measure 5-year survival rates in patients undergoing cancer chemotherapy. To a patient, however, the important outcome may be quality years of life, which is more difficult to measure. When one is assessing the methods of a policy, the statistical techniques for comparing the various outcomes (a meta-analysis, cost-effectiveness study), coupled with the strategies for dealing with the deficiencies (missing data, indirect outcomes) of the evidence, must be stated.

The third part of the policy deals with problems and inadequacies, including:

- Fitting the policies to specific cases
- Disagreements with policies on the same topic from different organizations
- Comparison of the policy with other disease states
- The influence of future studies on the policy

Because the evidence in guidelines and options is not conclusive, the management of individual cases may differ and different policies on the same condition may be developed. In these policy statements, the policy should offer the clinician suggestions on how to manage various situations that may not be well substantiated in the literature. For example, in the 1991 CDC recommendations on lead chelation, guidelines for chelation are presented for lead levels greater than or equal to 45 μg/dl; however, because the data are less conclusive in supporting chelation for lead levels between 25 and 44 μg/dl, only options are presented.

If a policy disagrees with another organization's policy, that policy should state what the disagreements are and why the clinician should follow their policy.

Because the dollars allocated for health care are finite, a policy should compare its cost-benefit ratio with that for other disease processes. This information would assist the clinician in deciding whether the increased costs (chelation therapy with lead levels between 25 and 44 μg/dl) justify the transfer of funds from other programs (counseling programs to prevent teenage pregnancy).

Finally, a policy should state the authors' credentials as well as the process for revising the policy. A policy should be revised at set intervals. In addition, the experts drafting these policies may know of research studies in progress that may affect the recommen-

dations; hence, they may state that the revision date is based on the estimated completion of those studies.

Option 3: Evaluating the Evidence in the Literature

With this option, the clinician formulates an opinion of the evidence supporting a treatment decision. The strength of this option is that the clinician reviews the actual evidence and formulates an opinion on the data without relying on someone else's interpretation. The clinician then knows exactly how strong the evidence is to support a decision. Often the evidence to support a decision is inconclusive or does not exist for a particular situation. One problem is that patients believe that medicine is infallible and therefore expect success with each intervention. If failure should occur, the parents may perceive that the failure was secondary to negligence and not to the treatment itself. Therefore, when facts regarding the limitations of interventions are shared with the patient and parents, they may be more active in the decision-making process and more understanding of treatment failures.

The systematic evaluation of the medical literature is rarely used in the clinical practice of medicine. When pediatricians have been surveyed regarding the process they use in incorporating a recent clinical advancement into their practice of medicine, only 17% reported that they conducted a literature search for additional information. The common strategies for seeking additional information are to informally discuss the advancement with colleagues (71%) or with someone who has experience with the new therapy (51%). Some reasons why so few pediatricians conducted literature searches include insufficient time, coupled with the lack of formal training in evaluating the evidence in the literature.

THE LITERATURE SEARCH

In the past, searching the literature for relevant articles consisted of going to the medical library and scanning the *Index Medicus* under key words for pertinent articles. For example, the key words for finding articles on lead toxicity are "Lead Poisoning." With the advent of personal computers, this search can be performed with software packages *(Medline, Grateful Med)*. With software the clinician may access the National Library of Medicine (Medlars) and search for pertinent articles. Besides finding references for relevant articles, users can also obtain abstracts summarizing the methods and pertinent findings. After scanning the titles and the abstracts of the articles, the clinician can decide which articles should be reviewed in their entirety.

An alternative to performing one's own search is to utilize the services of the medical librarian. The clinician describes the clinical problem, and the librarian conducts the search. From this list of references and their corresponding abstracts, the clinician can select the articles for the librarian to obtain.

Since the two experts consulted in Option 2 have disagreed and since the 1991 CDC guidelines are equivocal, a clinician may decide to do a computer literature search to determine whether any new or additional evidence has been published since 1991. The results of this search are presented in Figure 3–1. A review of this printout shows that 27 of the 44 research articles are in journals that the clinician receives by subscription. On reading the abstracts of these research articles, the clinician may be concerned because of the sparsity of studies using the more powerful analytical tools, such as meta-analyses and randomized clinical trials. Most of these studies used weaker designs, such as cross-sectional and observational studies. Despite this limitation, the clinician proceeds to examine the evidence.

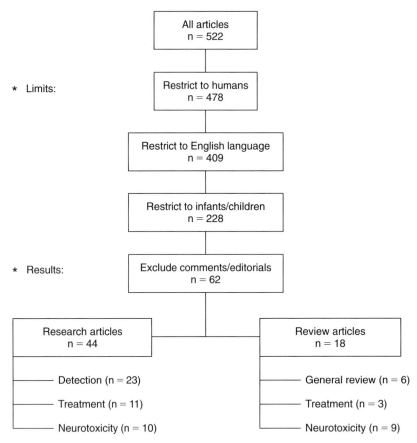

* Search parameters: Lead Poisoning/bi, co, di, dt, ep, et, me, pc, th

Definitions of abbreviations:

bi: biosynthesis
co: complications
di: diagnosis
dt: drug therapy
ep: epidemiology

et: etiology
me: metabolism
pc: prevention/control
th: therapy

* Data base searched: 1990 to 1994

Figure 3–1. Medline search for lead poisoning.

CRITIQUING THE EVIDENCE

Once the information is obtained, the next step in evaluating the literature is knowing how to critique the articles. Most pediatricians base their impression of the scientific soundness of an article by comparing the results with their own clinical experience. Other strategies in evaluating the literature with the corresponding frequency of usage are (1) reliance on the peer review process, (2) informal discussions with colleagues, and (3) reliance on the author's reputation. Because of most clinicians' lack of formal training in evaluating the medical literature, few clinicians can critique an article properly and thus this important option is underutilized in the decision-making process. Before one can apply the evidence from the literature, one must understand the natural history of an illness.

THE NATURAL HISTORY OF A DISEASE

To reduce the morbidity of a disease, one needs to understand its evolution. This understanding is based on the concepts of risk factors, prognostic factors, and causation. In studying the disease's natural history, one allows the disease process to progress without interventions. However, the goal of medicine is to alter this process by deciding when to intervene and by choosing the optimal therapy.

Overview

With any disease process, the patient is well at first. At this point, the patient becomes exposed to risk factors that cause the disease. These risk factors in a susceptible patient cause the biologic development of the disease. In this phase, the disease is present but the patient is asymptomatic. In addition, the disease cannot be detected by any diagnostic test. As the disease progresses, the severity increases to the point that it can be detected by a diagnostic test. Because the patient is asymptomatic, however, only an active screening process can detect the disease. As the disease progresses further, the patient becomes symptomatic and seeks medical care. Once the disease develops, prognostic factors predict the morbidity and mortality of the disease process. The same factor can be both a risk and a prognostic factor.

This model is applied to the neurotoxicity secondary to lead exposure (Fig. 3–2). In the first step, the patient is healthy but exposed to a series of risk factors associated with disease development. The risk factors shown are some of the factors that may influence the development of disease. If a person is exposed to these risk factors, the disease develops (Step 2) at a cellular level that is undetectable by diagnostic tests. For example, there may be a threshold lead level that triggers an alteration in cellular proliferation and function. This threshold can vary among patients and depends on the interaction of the other risk factors along with the duration and timing of the exposure (i.e., prenatal or postnatal). Once the disease has developed, many of these same risks can influence the prognosis.

As the disease evolves, the neurologic examination reveals subtle changes that may be detected only with sophisticated intelligence tests (Step 3). Because of the difficulty in performing and inter-

preting such tests, a surrogate screening test has been chosen that is associated with these neurologic findings. This test is the plasma lead level, which is also a risk and prognostic factor. If the body lead burden rises, the patient will have abdominal pain, irritability, and lethargy (Step 4). The final outcome is determined by the influence of the prognostic factors on the therapeutic interventions.

Barriers to Understanding Disease Development

Some of the barriers to understanding the evolution of a disease process are:

- Identifying the risk and prognostic factors

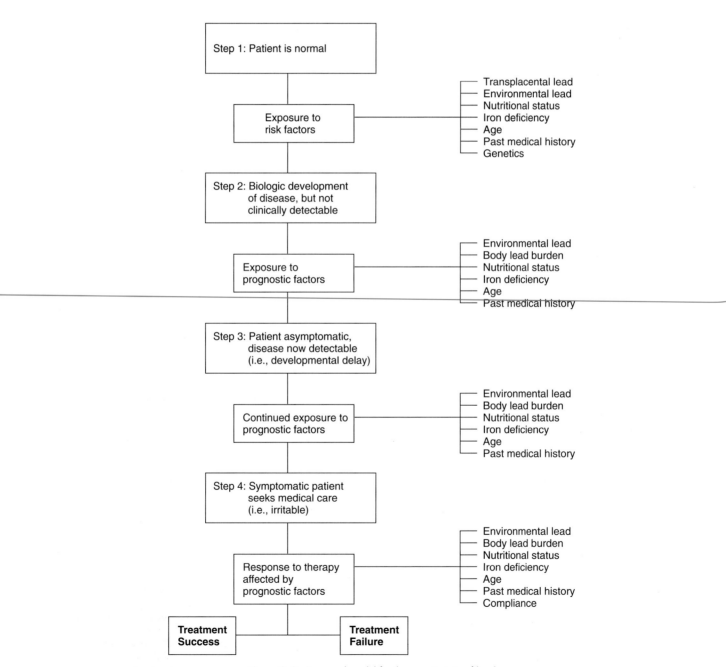

Figure 3–2. Proposed model for the neurotoxicity of lead.

- Determining whether such factors are confounders or causal agents
- The clinical significance of the risk factor

IDENTIFYING RISK FACTORS

The identification of potential risk factors can be difficult. A clinician may not recognize a possible association between plasma lead levels and a child's developmental delay. The barriers to detecting risk factors range from long latency periods to the necessary interaction of multiple factors before a disease can occur.

In risk factors with a *long latency period*, the exposure can occur years before the onset of the disease. If the exposure was transient, it may either be forgotten or go undetected. An example of such a risk factor is asbestos with resulting mesotheliomas. The exposure to asbestos may have occurred decades prior to development of the tumor.

With *frequently occurring* risk factors, the risk factor occurs so commonly that one may assume that it is a normal component of everyday life. Because everyone has been exposed to the factor, there are no unexposed individuals. Without a control group, one cannot appreciate the increased incidence of disease in those with the exposure. This problem occurs when a risk factor is geographically or culturally based. For example, the increased risk of stomach cancer associated with diet in native Japanese was not fully appreciated until they were compared with Americans of Japanese descent who consumed a different diet.

When a *small effect* is associated with a risk factor, its contribution toward causing the disease may go unnoticed. Just as in issues of "power and sample size" with regard to showing small differences, the same holds true for clinical observations. A large number of patients with the disease are needed before the clinician can appreciate that it is a risk factor.

The *incidence* of a disease may also affect the ability to detect a risk factor. If the disease is extremely rare, it would be unlikely that a single clinician would have sufficient experience with the disease to notice any potential risk factors. In contrast, if the disease is common, many risk factors may be identified for this disease. Because these risk factors explain most of the cases, there is little motivation to isolate a new risk factor.

The *interaction* of risk factors may be critical for the development of a disease. Certain risk factors may need to occur in a special sequence or simultaneously before a disease can develop. This may be the case with aspirin and Reye syndrome. For Reye syndrome to develop, three risk factors need to be present simultaneously: aspirin exposure, concurrent viral illness (influenza, varicella), and a susceptible patient.

CAUSATION

The goal of understanding any disease process is to know what actually causes the disease. By understanding this process, one can design more effective interventions. Unfortunately, this process is hampered by false associations and multifactorial causes of disease.

Before a potential risk factor can be considered to be an etiologic agent, its association with the disease must first be examined to determine whether the association is true. The association is examined for (1) the potential for bias, (2) chance, and (3) confounding.

The *potential for bias* is primarily based on the strength of the type of study design employed by the investigator. The strongest design is the randomized clinical trial followed by the cohort and the case-control study. A study must be well designed to minimize the potential for bias.

Once an association is found in a study with a low potential for bias, one then determines whether this association occurred by *chance* alone. Just as a player might be dealt a bridge hand with a predominance of one suit from a shuffled deck, random error or chance can cause the selection of a group of patients having a spurious predominance of that risk factor. The strength of an association is reported as either the *relative risk* (from cohort studies) or the *odds ratio* (from case-control studies) (see Chapter 2). By the rules of probability, the effect of random error is addressed by the 95% confidence interval around the value for relative risk-odds ratio. In interpreting this interval, one is 95% sure that the true value in nature (from an unbiased study) resides somewhere in that interval. If the interval contains 1, no association probably exists. However, the association may still be clinically significant, but the study may have lacked the necessary power to generate a narrow enough confidence interval to exclude 1.

The third problem with associations is the issue of *confounding*. A confounding variable is associated with both the risk factor and the outcome, but it does not take part in causing the disease. An example of confounding is altitude and cholera. It was once a widely accepted fact that cholera was caused by altitude. In sparsely populated mountains, cholera was nonexistent; however, in densely populated cities like London, which is at sea level, cholera was a common endemic disease. Even though altitude was strongly associated with the incidence of cholera, it was also strongly associated with the true risk factor, which was poor sanitation and population density.

Once a factor or association passes the tests for bias, chance, and confounding, one can determine its true role in causing a disease. Because of the interactions of various factors (both beneficial and harmful), the actual causation of a disease is difficult to prove.

A major breakthrough in establishing criteria for causation is the Henle-Koch postulates, which state:

> The parasite occurs in every case of the disease in question and under circumstances which account for the pathological changes and clinical course of the disease.
>
> It occurs in no other disease as a fortuitous and nonpathological parasite.
>
> After being fully isolated from the body and repeatedly grown in pure culture, it can induce disease anew.

These postulates were a major advance in establishing the etiology of disease for single agent causing an infectious disease. However, problems associated with these postulates include long latency periods, asymptomatic infection, carrier states, inability to culture organisms, lack of an animal model, and the multifactorial nature of many disease processes. Nevertheless, these postulates are still useful today and were used to establish the role of Hantavirus in the outbreaks of respiratory failure and death in the rural southwestern United States.

Because of the inability to apply Henle-Koch postulates to multifactorial, noninfectious diseases, guidelines are needed to establish causality for a risk factor. Essential components are:

- Temporality
- Consistency
- Strength of association
- Reversibility
- Dose response
- Biologic plausibility

In regard to *temporality*, the risk factor must occur before the development of the disease. The problem with temporality is establishing when the disease actually developed in relation to the exposure. Did the subclinical state of the disease cause one to experience the risk factor? For example, the treatment of postmenopausal women with dysfunctional uterine bleeding is estrogen replacement therapy. This therapy has been associated with an increased risk of uterine cancer. The debate centers around whether the estrogen therapy caused the cancer or whether the cancer was already present (but not detectable by our diagnostic tests), causing the uterine bleeding that led to the use of estrogen therapy. To satisfy the condition of temporality, the patient must be healthy before exposure and the preclinical state (see Fig. 3–2, Step 2) should not lead to the exposure.

In regard to *consistency*, the association should be reproduced in a variety of clinical settings to enhance the external validity of the finding. If the same methodology is used repetitively, there is the possibility that the same flaw in methodology is being inadvertently reproduced in all the studies. This has occurred in the case-control studies that repetitively showed an increased risk of breast cancer in patients who used reserpine. The flaw in these studies was that only perfectly healthy patients were enrolled as controls. This exclusion criterion was not applied to patients with breast cancer, and hence cancer patients with hypertension (and therefore receiving reserpine) were included. Because of the unequal application of the exclusion criteria, more reserpine users were preferentially recruited into the case group, which biased the results toward a spurious association.

The *strength of the association* is based on both the magnitude of the association and the method by which it was obtained. The larger the association, the less likely that it is secondary to an unrecognized source of bias. In addition, with strong study designs the potential for that bias is less. If an association comes from a randomized controlled trial, in contrast to a case-control study, there is more certainty.

As for *reversibility*, if a risk factor is removed from the environment, the incidence of disease should be reduced concomitantly by the amount of the disease that is caused by that risk factor. For example, in the association of Reye syndrome and aspirin, once aspirin use was curtailed in the management of the febrile child, the incidence of Reye syndrome fell precipitously.

The *dose-response* relationship refers to a greater incidence of disease with either a longer duration of exposure or a higher intensity of that exposure. This relationship occurs with regard to the risk of cigarette smoking and cardiovascular disease. The incidence of disease increases with more cigarettes smoked. For some diseases, a dose-response relationship cannot be established. In teratology, any exposure (e.g., thalidomide with phocomelia) at a critical point in organogenesis results in a malformation.

Biologic plausibility means that the association makes sense because it is consistent with the current understanding of pathophysiology. This criterion is not necessary for causality, but when present, it supports the causal relationship. Many times, the process of how a risk factor causes a disease is unknown. For example, the process of oncogenesis is often undetermined but the associations of the risk factors with cancer have identified various cancer-causing agents (e.g., cigarettes, radiation, diethylstilbestrol).

No statistical test or mathematical model can prove causation. Instead, one must evaluate these six components for causality and make a judgment after evaluating the evidence. The components necessary for causality are (1) a temporal relationship, (2) strength of association, (3) reversibility, and (4) consistency. Factors that are supportive for, but not critical for, a causal model are a dose-response relationship and biologic plausibility.

To address the question raised by a recent television documentary on the effects of low-level lead poisoning on intelligence, the clinician decides to see whether or not the evidence supports a causal relationship.

In building a causal model for the neurotoxic effect of lead poisoning, a clinician decides to critique the research articles on this topic that were published from 1990 to 1994 and adds these findings to the CDC's critique of the studies published before 1990. The literature search uncovers 10 articles published in this time period, of which 8 were actual research studies. The other 2 dealt with methodologic problems, such as the effect of attrition in cohort studies.

In the CDC's critique, 14 case-control or retrospective cohort studies and 7 prospective cohort studies were reviewed. Even though there were inconsistencies among the results, it appeared that the intelligence quotient (IQ) fell from 2 to 10 points as the plasma lead level rose from 5 to 35 μg/dl. The inconsistencies in the results were dependent on the strength of the design, the sources of bias, and the adjustments used for potential confounders.

After reviewing the two sets of articles and after weighing the evidence for each of the 6 points for causality (Table 3–1), the clinician concludes that a mild to moderate causal relationship probably exists. This relationship is strong enough to support the identification of children with mild to moderate lead burdens and to warrant further research on the reversibility of the neurotoxicity through interventions designed to reduce the body's lead burden.

SIGNIFICANCE OF A RISK FACTOR

Once a risk factor has been identified as a significant contributor to the disease process, the next step is to determine its actual importance in relationship to the other risk factors. *Relative risk* (incidence in exposed versus non-exposed) measures only the magnitude of an association. It does not account for the prevalence of the risk factor in the community. For example, the relative risk for uranium mining and lung cancer is 25 times that of cigarette smoking; however, it is such a rare risk factor that it contributes only a few cases of lung cancer in relationship to smoking.

With *attributable risk* (incidence in exposed versus non-exposed), the background rate of disease is subtracted out. This difference represents the increase in disease that is secondary to that risk factor.

Population attributable fraction (attributable risk $\times$ prevalence of risk factor $\div$ the incidence of disease in that population) reports the percentage of disease in a community that is secondary to that risk factor.

Thus, relative risk supports causality, but the population attributable fraction determines which risk factor is responsible for most cases of the disease. This fraction would direct one toward the elimination of the risk factor that would result in the greatest reduction in disease.

THE INTERVENTION

After understanding the natural history of a disease process and identifying important risk factors, the next step is to decide on how to alter this process. The goal of any intervention is the maximal prevention of morbidity. Depending on when an intervention is applied in the disease process, its prevention of disease and/or morbidity may either be primary, secondary, or tertiary.

Primary Prevention

The intervention is instituted prior to the development of the disease process. This intervention consists of the elimination of an important risk factor, hence reducing one's chance for having that disease. Primary prevention can be implemented at an individual level or as part of a public health policy. An example of a primary prevention instituted at the national level with regard to the neurotoxicity of lead is the removal of lead from water pipes, paint, and gasoline.

Table 3–1. Building a Causal Model for Low-Level Lead and Developmental Delay

Factor	Assessment	Rationale
Temporality	Mild to moderate	Some studies measured maternal and cord lead; correlations best with levels from older children
Consistency	Mild	Most studies show a harmful effect but inconsistencies present
Strength	Mild	Possible reduction of 0.2 to 1.0 intelligence quotient (IQ) points for every 3 μg/dl increase in plasma lead
Reversibility	Mild to moderate	One study so far has shown an improvement in IQ with reduction in lead; replication needed
Dose Response	Moderate	The higher the lead level, the worse the impairment
Plausibility	Mild to moderate	There is some biologic evidence that lead inhibits cellular growth and function

Secondary Prevention

The disease has developed, but the patient remains asymptomatic. The premise of a secondary prevention is that an appropriate screening process, coupled with an effective, early intervention, will reduce the morbidity more than just treating patients when they have symptoms. Before a secondary prevention program can be implemented, one needs to consider the type of program to implement, the criteria of an effective screening program, and the bias associated with the program. The two types of screening programs are *mass screening* and a *case-finding* approach.

In a *mass screening* program, everyone in a geographic location, whether it is a community or a school, is offered a test. If the results are abnormal, the patient is encouraged to seek medical care. The advantage of the mass screening strategy is that some individuals who do not undergo routine health maintenance examinations may still be screened. The potential disadvantages of this method are suboptimal testing, poor follow-up, lack of counseling, and cost.

For example, a community agency may decide to screen for lead with a finger stick blood test. If the agency's budget is limited, it may choose to use the zinc protoporphyrin, which has a poor sensitivity for detecting lead levels in the 25 to 40 μg/dl range (sensitivity, 74%). If the finger stick lead test is chosen and the finger is not cleaned properly, the results will be spuriously high from skin contaminated with lead. With the increase in the false-positive and false-negative rates, the cost of medical care will increase either by unnecessary visits to health care providers or by the increased morbidity of a missed diagnosis. In addition, the interpretation and follow-up of an abnormal test result are left to the patient's discretion. Unfortunately, compliance with patient-directed follow-up is suboptimal. For example, only 47% of patients with high blood pressure identified by a mass screening program seek medical care.

In the *case-finding* method, during the health maintenance examination the clinician performs a selective battery of tests in the asymptomatic patient that are tailored to the individual's risk factors. The physician then reviews the results with the patient, and a decision is made about further testing. The type of tests, the performance of the tests, and the follow-up of the results are under the control of the clinician. With the proper choice and the selective use of screening tests, the cost of a case-finding program should be less than a mass screening program. The disadvantages of such a program, however, are the types of patients screened, and the fact that successful implementation of the program is left to the clinician. The patients who are in the most need of that diagnostic test may not seek medical care for routine health maintenance and will not be detected by a case-finding program. In addition, if the clinician chooses a suboptimal test or does not follow up on

abnormal results, this type of program will miss patients with the disease. For example, one case-finding program for detection of lead poisoning used the FEP (a cheaper, but suboptimal test) and obtained plasma lead values in only 43% of the patients with abnormal FEP results.

If the *screening program* has been efficacious in a randomized clinical trial, it should be implemented. Efficacy of a screening program is defined as a reduction in the morbidity of the screened patients that offsets the cost of such a program when compared with the unscreened patient. Unfortunately, there are very few randomized trials documenting the efficacy of screening programs. Instead, the decision is based on the availability of efficacious therapies, morbidity justifying screening, a good screening test, targeting of the proper population, resources available for treatment, and compliant patients. The disease must be severe and prevalent enough to justify the cost of a screening program.

The screening test should be inexpensive and simple to conduct with acceptable test characteristics. These tests usually have high sensitivities (to minimize the chance of missing disease) with acceptable specificities (false-positive rates). Once the disease is diagnosed, an efficacious therapy must be available. To enhance compliance, the patient must agree with the importance of early intervention and the therapy needs to be inexpensive and easy to implement.

The problems of a screening program involve labeling and the special biases associated with early detection. Labeling occurs when a healthy person is told that he or she is sick according to a laboratory test. A truly negative test may be reassuring and hence maintain the patient's sense of well-being. However, a false-negative or false-positive result or a truly positive result when there is no cure (as in Huntington's chorea) could cause detrimental physical and emotional problems.

The biases associated with screening programs are lead-time bias and length-time bias. *Lead-time bias* occurs when early treatment does not improve survival. Because of earlier diagnosis, the knowledge that the patient has had the disease for a longer time gives the false impression of improved survival. With *length-time bias*, patients with highly malignant tumors will die before they can be screened. With slow-growing tumors, the patient will still be alive and screenable, which gives a false impression of efficacy.

After deciding that there may be a causal relationship of lead intoxication and developmental delay, the clinician decides to review the evidence supporting a screening program.

There is no randomized clinical trial to substantiate the efficacy of lead screening. The information supporting such a program are its prevalence, morbidity, and target population. The prevalence of lead levels over 25 μg/dl ranges from 0.12% to 1.6%. There is a probable causal relationship of lead levels and developmental delay. The appropriate population would be reached through a combination of case-finding (health maintenance examinations) and mass screening programs (inner city housing projects). The cost of such a program in the United States is estimated at $352 million or approximately $19,000 per case detected. This cost would be justified if the developmental delay could be reduced by appropriate therapy.

Because of the poor sensitivities and specificities of detecting cases with FEP or questionnaires, plasma lead levels need to be performed. Efficacious treatment programs are available for treating high levels of lead poisoning (≥ 45 μg/dl). This screening program could also be used to assess the effectiveness of public health policies aimed at the reduction of environmental exposure to lead by monitoring the prevalence of lead toxicity. The information against such a program is that there is insufficient evidence documenting that therapy improves the developmental delay secondary to plasma lead levels lower than 45 μg/dl.

Tertiary Prevention

Tertiary prevention refers to the prevention of complications or morbidity once a disease becomes symptomatic. This form of prevention basically takes the form of therapeutic interventions. Once the quality of a clinical trial (minimal bias) and the precision (reproducible) of an intervention have been established, the next step is to compare interventions to choose the best therapy. The tools used to compare interventions are the relative risk reduction (RRR) and the number needed to treat (NNT) to obtain one treatment success. The RRR and the NNT are used in studies that use dichotomous (yes/no) outcomes. These two measures are calculated as follows:

$$RRR = [1 - (\text{relative risk})] \times 100$$

$$\text{relative risk} = \frac{I_{rx}}{I_{con}} = \frac{(\text{incidence of outcome in } \textit{treated} \text{ group})}{(\text{incidene of outcome in } \textit{control} \text{ group})}$$

where NNT = [1/absolute risk reduction] and absolute risk reduction = $[I_{con} - I_{rx}]$.

Just as in relative risk, which is used to show the strength of an association, the RRR reports the magnitude of the success of an intervention. The NNT brings this magnitude of success into perspective by referencing it to the incidence of the outcome. If a hypothetical intervention reduces the incidence of developmental delay secondary to lead poisoning from 10% to 7%, the RRR would be 30%:

$$RRR = [(1 - 0.07/0.10) \times 100]$$

The number of patients needed to be treated in order to have one treatment success is 33 patients:

$$NNT = [1/(0.10 - 0.07)]$$

Statistical significance around RRR and NNT is reported as the 95% confidence interval, which would estimate the upper and lower boundaries of success for that intervention. By comparing the RRR and NNT with the corresponding 95% confidence intervals, the clinician can then decide which intervention has the best success rate. In studies that have interval level outcomes, the effectiveness among therapies can be expressed by the 95% confidence interval around the difference in the values between the treatment group and its corresponding control group.

Most randomized clinical trials are conducted under ideal conditions. These optimal results establish the *efficacy* of an intervention. In contrast, *effectiveness* studies report the success of an intervention conducted under the constraints of a general practice setting.

The difference in the results from these two types of studies deal with the issues of *external validity*.

To determine whether the results of an efficacy study can be generalized to all patients, the following components of external validity need to be evaluated:

- The types of patients studied
- The availability of the intervention
- The ease of implementing the intervention
- The effect of being studied

The types of patients studied should be the same as the practitioner's with regard to diagnosis, severity of illness, and demographic variables. Even though these patients may be similar to the clinician's with regard to the preceding factors, they still may be different because they have volunteered to participate in a research study. Volunteers are more likely to be compliant with instructions and medications than the general population.

The intervention needs to be available and simple to implement (without the support of a research team). In addition, the improved outcome may be secondary to the effect of being included in a study. This observation, called the *Hawthorne effect*, was first noted by an industrial engineer at the Hawthorne Works of the Western Electric Company. This engineer observed that the increase in productivity was not a result of their interventions but of being observed.

The cost of a study must also be factored into the process of choosing the best therapy. Cost must be measured both in monetary terms and in morbidity. The NNT can be used to estimate the cost of a program to generate "one" treatment success. Besides economic cost, morbidity from complications also must be considered. To determine whether the complication has been caused by the intervention, the same process and criteria for causality must be used. Once causality has been shown, the NNT formula can be used to estimate the number of patients needed to be treated to generate one patient with the complication.

For example, if the complication rate for anaphylaxis secondary to penicillamine is 10% versus 0.1% in the control group, the number of patients that need to be treated to generate one patient with such a complication would be

$$10.1 = [1/(0.10 - 0.001)]$$

A risk-benefit ratio can then be computed by dividing the number needed for one success divided by the number needed for one complication. In the above example, this hypothetical ratio for penicillamine and developmental delay would be 3.3 (= 33.3/10.1). Hence, for every 10 treatment successes there would be 33 patients with this complication. The final risk-benefit ratio would be done by assigning patient-derived relative values to the success and to the complication.

Besides integrating efficacy with cost in choosing a therapy, the clinician must also consider the ethical ramifications along with the incorporation of patient and parental beliefs into the decision-making process. Failure to consider these two issues reduces the effectiveness of any intervention. Once a decision is made regarding a therapy, the decision must be re-evaluated at appropriate intervals.

In a review of the literature on the treatment of lead published after 1990, one randomized clinical study was found that involved the effect of home versus home plus soil abatement on plasma lead levels. The authors concluded that the average cost of soil abatement ($9600 per home) did not justify the 0.8 to 1.6 μg/dl reduction in plasma lead levels. The rest of the studies were observational. Two studies on the therapy of lead levels between 25 and 55 μg/dl had promising results. In one small observational study, oral 2,3-dimercaptosuccinic acid (DMSA) reduced plasma lead by 30% one month after therapy in an outpatient setting. The other observational study showed no additional benefit of EDTA chelation therapy in reducing plasma lead, but did show an improvement in IQ following reduction in plasma lead. *Because of the bias in a noncontrolled trial, the results need to be replicated by further studies.*

There is a paucity of evidence in the literature to document the efficacy of treating lead levels in the 25 to 45 µg/dl range with the resulting improvement in IQ. Hence, a risk-benefit equation cannot be accurately constructed.

RECOMMENDATIONS TO THE FAMILY

Lead values in the range of 25 to 45 µg/dl may cause developmental problems. Because of the age of the family's home, the child is at risk for lead poisoning and should be retested using a venipuncture to detect the plasma lead level. If the result is in this range, treatment consists of abatement and frequent monitoring of plasma lead values. Unfortunately, the sparse evidence in the literature is not enough to endorse pharmacologic intervention.

REFERENCES

American Medical Association, Office of Quality Assurance and Healthcare Organizations. *In* Swartwourt JE (ed). Directory of Practice Parameters, 1992. Chicago: American Medical Association, 1991.

Bellinger D, Sloman J, Leviton A, et al. Low-level lead exposure and children's cognitive function in the preschool years. Pediatrics 1991;87:219–227.

Bradford-Hill A. The environment and disease: Association or causation? Proc R Soc Med 1965;58:295–300.

Cadman D, Chambers L, Feldman W, et al. Assessing the effectiveness of community screening programs. JAMA 1984;251:1580–1585.

Centers for Disease Control (CDC). Preventing Lead Poisoning in Young Children: A Statement by the Centers for Disease Control. Atlanta: CDC, 1991.

Cone DC. Lead screening and follow-up in an urban pediatric clinic. NY State Med J 1992;92:338–342.

Dawson NV. Physician judgment in clinical settings: Methodological influences and cognitive performance. Clin Chem 1993;39:1468–1480.

Dietrich KN, Berger OG, Succop PA. Lead exposure and the motor developmental status of urban six-year-old children in the Cincinnati Prospective Study. Pediatrics 1993;91:301–307.

Eddy DM. Designing a practice policy: Standards, guidelines, and options. JAMA 1990;263:3077, 3081, 3084.

Eddy DM. Guidelines for policy statements: The explicit approach. JAMA 1990;263:2239–2240, 2243.

Ellenberg JH, Nelson KB. Sample selection and the natural history of disease: Studies of febrile seizures. JAMA 1980;243:1337–1340.

Ernhart CB, Greene T. Low-level lead exposure in the prenatal and early preschool periods: Language development. Arch Environ Health 1990;45:342–354.

Fergusson DM, Horwood LJ. The effects of lead levels on the growth of word recognition in middle childhood. Int J Epidemiol 1993;22:891–897.

Fletcher RH, Fletcher SW, Wagner EH (eds). Clinical Epidemiology: The Essentials, 2nd ed. Baltimore: Williams & Wilkins, 1988.

Gellert GA, Wagner GA, Maxwell RM, et al. Lead poisoning among low-income children in Orange County, California: A need for regionally differentiated policy. JAMA 1993;270:69–71.

Glotzer DE, Bauchner H. Management of childhood lead poisoning: A survey. Pediatrics 1992;89:614–618.

Goyer RA. Lead toxicity: Current concerns. Environ Health Perspect 1993;100:177–187.

Guyatt GH, Sackett DL, Cook DJ. II. How to use an article about therapy or prevention. B. What were the results and will they help me in caring for my patients? JAMA 1994;271:59–63.

Haynes RB. Determinants of compliance. *In* Haynes RB, Taylor DW, Sackett DL (eds): Compliance in Health Care. Baltimore: Johns Hopkins University Press, 1979:49.

Horwitz RI, Feinstein AR. Methodologic standards and contradictory results in case-control research. Am J Med 1979;66:556–564.

Levine M, Walter S, Lee H, et al. IV. How to use an article about harm. JAMA 1994;271:1615–1619.

Leviton A, Bellinger D, Allred EN, et al. Pre- and postnatal low-level lead exposure and children's dysfunction in school. Environ Res 1993;60:30–43.

Liebelt EL, Shannon M, Graef JW. Efficacy of oral meso-2,3-dimercaptosuccinic acid therapy for low-level childhood plumbism. J Pediatr 1994;124:313–317.

McMahon B, Pugh TF (eds). Epidemiology: Principles and Methods. Boston: Little, Brown & Co, 1970.

McNeil BJ, Pauker SG, Sox HC, et al. On the elicitation of preferences for alternative therapies. N Engl J Med 1982;306:1259–1262.

Oxman AD, Sackett DL, Guyatt GH. User's guides to the medical literature: I. How to get started. JAMA 1993:270;2093–2095.

Rifai N, Cohen G, Wolf M, et al. Incidence of lead poisoning in young children from inner-city, suburban, and rural communities. Ther Drug Monitor 1993;15:71–74.

Rolfe PB, Marcinak JF, Nice AJ, et al. Use of zinc protoporphyrin measured by the Protofluor-z hematofluorometer in screening children for elevated blood lead levels. Am J Dis Child 1993;147:66–68.

Ruff HA, Bijur PE, Markowitz M, et al. Declining blood lead levels and cognitive changes in moderately lead-poisoned children. JAMA 1993;269:1641–1646.

Sackett DL, Haynes RB, Guyatt GH, Tugwell P (eds). Clinical Epidemiology: A Basic Science for Clinical Medicine, 2nd ed. Boston: Little, Brown & Co, 1991.

Schriger DL, Cantrill SV, Greene CS. The origins, benefits, harms, and implications of emergency medicine clinical policies. Ann Emerg Med 1993;22:597–602.

Sciarillo WG, Alexander G, Farrell KP. Lead exposure and child behavior. Am J Public Health 1992;82:1356–1360.

Shannon M, Graef J, Lovejoy FH. Efficacy and toxicity of D-penicillamine in low-level lead poisoning. J Pediatr 1988;112:799–804.

Shen XM, Guo D, Xu JD, et al. The adverse effect of marginally higher lead level on intelligence development of children: A Shanghai study. Indian J Pediatr 1992;59:233–238.

Tversky A, Kahneman D. Judgment under uncertainty: Heuristics and biases. Science 1974;185:1124–1131.

Weitzman M, Aschengrau A, Bellinger D, et al. Lead-contaminated soil abatement and urban children's blood levels. JAMA 1993;269:1647–1654.

Williamson JW, German PS, Weiss R, et al. A survey of U.S. primary care practitioners and their opinion leaders. Ann Intern Med 1989;110:151–160.

4 Understanding the Importance of Cultural Beliefs and Behaviors in Clinical Practice

Jill E. Korbin   Paula Brinkley   Lisa Reebals   Nimi Singh

A caution in Western biomedical training is that the sound of hoofbeats should initiate the search for horses, not zebras. Part of the process of becoming prepared to deal with rare maladies is learning to first rule out the more likely common entities. On the African savannah, however, hoofbeats would be a better indication of zebras, gazelles, or any number of animals other than horses and the caution would be framed in the opposite direction. Much of the literature on culture and health has taken the tack of documenting and understanding how hoofbeats reflect different animals, or realities, in different cultural contexts. It is important to situate culture, often regarded as quite exotic and zebra-like, with the horses.

When confronted with a child needing care, pediatricians are trained to use the whole battery of modern biomedicine at their disposal. Stopping to consider other strategies, often unfamiliar and unproven by Western biomedical standards, goes against that training. It is not suggested that the pediatrician just consider cultural diversity in the case of an acutely ill child needing attention. Rather, it is suggested that the pediatrician can develop a strategy for eliciting information on the influence of culture within the framework of obtaining a medical history, and without adding a burdensome time commitment. The inclusion of culture as a potentially important variable for all patients will enhance the likelihood of patient adherence to medical advice, increase patient satisfaction, and facilitate negotiation and resolution in the event of physician-patient conflict.

In view of the range of cultural diversity and the individual variability within any culture, few pediatricians can be expert on all cultures that they will encounter. A card catalogue of cultural beliefs and behaviors related to health and medicine does not exist. Further, this type of cookbook approach would run the risk of stereotyping patients by ignoring within-culture variability and would promote a focus on the exotic in culturally diverse peoples. Cataloguing would not move us beyond documenting health care practices at odds with the traditional white middle-class United States culture on which most medical assumptions are based.

CULTURE AND MEDICAL CARE

Culture and Ethnicity

Hundreds of definitions have been offered for the concept of culture. In its broadest sense, culture is the acquired and shared knowledge, values, beliefs, symbols, and behaviors that people use to interact with others and to make life meaningful.

Cultural and ethnic groups are not homogeneous, and there is substantial diversity within any group. Culture and ethnicity are too often defined on the basis of large groupings of people based on skin color or geographic area of origin. The commonly used broad classifications of African-American, Asian-American, Native American, Hispanic, and European-American do not necessarily correspond to the reality of day-to-day life or health care. There is as much diversity within these broad groupings as across them. There are many kinds of Hispanics/Latinos (Cubans, Puerto Ricans, Mexicans, Mexican-Americans, Guatemalans), Blacks (African-Americans, Haitians, West Indians, Kenyans), Asians (Chinese, Japanese, Koreans, Thai, Cambodians, Hmong), Pacific Island peoples (Hawaiians, Samoans, Tahitians), Native-Americans (Navajo, Sioux), and European-Americans (Italians, Germans, British).

Furthermore, within any of these cultures there is substantial individual variability. For some individuals, cultural affiliation is intricately and inseparably woven into their lives. This is referred to as *behavioral ethnicity,* or patterns of behavior learned at grandmother's knee. In contrast, *ideological ethnicity* is a more politically based identification with a cultural group. The expression of ethnicity has implications for health behavior. As but one example, behavioral ethnicity might be expressed when a Jewish adult gives chicken soup for a child's flu symptoms, remembering soup received in the adult's childhood. The chicken soup might be given alone or in combination with prescription medicine obtained from a physician. The giving of the soup would be almost automatic, without recourse to some current suggestions that chicken soup might indeed provide comfort and rehydration to an ill child. A Jewish individual with similar socioeconomic status but different childhood socialization experiences, and therefore with a more ideologically based ethnicity might, but would not necessarily, turn to chicken soup. The information that an individual is of Jewish heritage is not sufficient of itself to understand the impact of ethnicity on health and medicine. Traditional remedies among other cultural groups show a similar pattern.

Cross-cultural research has demonstrated substantial within-cultural variability along the lines of generation, acculturation, education, income, gender, age, and past experience. Within-culture variability sometimes exceeds cross-cultural variability.

Disease and Illness

A conceptual distinction has been drawn in medical anthropology between disease, "the malfunctioning of biological and/or psychological processes," and illness, "the psychosocial experience and meaning of perceived disease." This distinction is not one that will be elicited from patients, but it provides an important conceptual framework for the pediatrician. Disease and illness do not necessarily coincide. For example, an individual can be diagnosed with hypertension (disease) without having any perception of ill health (illness). In pediatric practice, otitis media can serve as an example. Otitis media (disease) can be diagnosed by the pediatrician even if the child is experiencing no signs of pain (illness). When a child experiences severe ear pain (illness) that coincides with the pediatrician's diagnosis (disease), a 10-day course of antibiotics is likely to be prescribed. However, the child's pain that defines the illness component may resolve in a few days. Parents may then cease administering the antibiotics, particularly if the antibiotics are then linked to symptoms of another illness, such as antibiotic-associated diarrhea. Although patients will not be explicit in using a disease or illness terminology, in the absence of an experienced illness, compliance with physician advice on curing the disease may seem unnecessary to the patient or family.

ELICITING PATIENT INFORMATION ON CULTURE AND HEALTH

The need for cultural consideration is most obvious among patients who, for example, wear traditional dress or speak another language. In some cases, cultural diversity is easy to spot, although the possible health effects are not always straightforward. For example, the infant of an observant Muslim woman was admitted to a hospital with hypocalcemic seizures and rickets. Retrospectively, several cultural beliefs and practices contributed to putting this child at risk. First, the mother believed that the natural way was always superior. She therefore exclusively breast-fed, declined vitamin supplementation, and distrusted most medical advice. The lack of dietary vitamin D was exacerbated by insufficient sunlight exposure, both to the infant and to the veiled and completely covered breast-feeding mother. This problem could have conceivably been anticipated had the doctor caring for the family realized that the mother's mode of dress implied more than her religious affiliation.

Even if a patient appears to be culturally similar to the physician, congruence in health beliefs and behaviors cannot be assumed. Slightly more than 33% of a national sample in the United States used "unconventional" medicine in the past year, and visits to unconventional practitioners exceeded visits to primary care providers. Use of unconventional therapy may be most frequent among better-educated individuals with higher incomes. Differing views on medical care simply cannot be disregarded.

What might be assumed to be similarities in orientation do not necessarily ensure optimal care. A study of pediatric care of physicians' children found that such children had better access to the pediatrician and more pediatrician visits if the child was hospitalized than other children did. However, these physicians were more likely to delay in seeking pediatric care and to practice self-referral to specialists. Pediatricians provided less detailed instructions to these families and indicated a reluctance to discuss behavior problems that they thought might be intrusive to another physician.

Pediatricians should be familiar with the major cultural groups in the geographic areas that they serve. This familiarity can be developed through multiple pathways. First, there is an existing, and growing, literature on cultural diversity in health and medicine. Examples of cultural diversity in health care beliefs, behaviors, and practices also have been documented in the literature. Second, pediatricians can establish relationships with local community organizations to gain familiarity with cultural beliefs and behaviors concerning childrearing and health beliefs and behaviors. Third, relationships with local departments of anthropology can be established. Colleagues in anthropology may be available to consult in the form of seminars on culture, collaborate on individual cases, or provide guidance to the most relevant literature.

Most importantly, pediatricians must become culturally informed through contact with their patients. Familiarity with culture, based on the literature or on consultations from cultural experts, be they community members or academics, must be validated through knowledge generated from patients. Because of the diversity of cultures and intracultural variability, the pediatrician should approach culture as an interested learner and should regard patients and their families as teachers about that culture.

Because the goal for the pediatrician is to discover what facts about a patient's culture are likely to be important in health care, it is suggested that questioning be directed primarily toward cultural

health beliefs and behaviors grounded in the family's experience. This will seem more appropriate to the patient than general discussions of cultural background and will allow the pediatrician to open the doors to discussing culture without having to expend scarce clinical time on exploring the entirety of cultural affiliation. This line of questioning is best initiated over the process of taking a history during repeated well-child visits. If continuity of care is not possible, such questions can be directed specifically toward the presenting problem. The following suggestions can serve as guidelines:

What did your parents do when you were ill? Do you know why? Do you think it helped (some, most, or all of the time)? Do you do the same with your child?

Do you have any family traditions for preventing or treating health problems (specify, for example, stomach aches, vomiting, colds)?

NATURAL HISTORY OF ILLNESS

The concept of illness as a series of unfolding stages can be usefully employed as an organizing framework for the incorporation of culture into pediatric practice. Knowledge about each stage accrued by the pediatrician can prevent cultural conflict or can resolve it more quickly if it occurs. Components of a natural history of illness might be gathered in the process of medical diagnosis, but we suggest the addition of explicit attention to cultural components as the natural history unfolds.

Translating Signs into Symptoms of Ill Health

What did you notice in your child that let you know that he or she was ill? What worried or concerned you?

The initial point in an illness episode is the identification of a constellation of signs that translate into symptoms of ill health. Whether or not patients and physicians converge on the significance of symptoms is important to the course of subsequent treatment.

Folk diagnoses and medical diagnoses may appear divergent even when they converge in important ways. Among Hispanic farm workers in Florida, mothers traditionally regard *susto* (fright sickness) and *mal de ojo* (evil eye) as untreatable by Western physicians. At the same time, physicians are likely to dismiss these folk classifications in their diagnosis. However, even though the labels for these conditions, and their etiologies, may differ between mothers and physicians, both recognize the presenting symptoms as significant and potentially life-threatening, and this thereby establishes more common ground than at first apparent.

As another example, even though Western biomedicine conceptualizes dehydration as a complication of diarrheal disease, some cultures distinguish between the two. In a community in India, symptoms of diarrhea were thought to result from physiologic disturbance and thus were amenable to treatment at the local clinic. Dehydration, in contrast, was thought to indicate a state of pollution that could be cured only ritually. A therapeutic compromise can be achieved that can meet both the biomedical goal of rehydration and the cultural goal of purification.

Etiology

What do you think caused your child to become ill?

Much of the conflict between patient and physician is thought to result from cultural incongruity in beliefs about illness etiology. Etiologic explanations form the basis for subsequent action. That cultural conflicts in medical care may emanate from disagreement as to the precise etiology is a dominant theme in the literature.

Cultural models of illness and health may include biologic, supernatural, and social causes. One type of cause may predominate for a specific illness, or multiple causes may be employed. In some cultures, a child's disability or chronic illness is viewed as punishment for some social transgression (by the child, family member, or parents) in the past so that collecting a genetic history may be perceived by parents and families as a search for the culprit.

Pediatricians should elicit the parents', the child's, and, if possible and relevant, the extended family members' views of why the child became ill. In well-child visits, the pediatrician may ask whether the family holds any ideas or beliefs about how or why the child or other family members become ill. Even if cultural beliefs are not shared in a non-illness context, the pediatrician has set the stage for later discussion of the causes of specific illnesses. When a child is ill, parents generally attempt to use all possible strategies. If they are in an environment conducive to the presentation of culturally diverse beliefs about etiology, it is more likely that they will do so. For example, if a child has an illness that the parents ascribe to the evil eye, they may be more likely to share this with a pediatrician who previously has sought their views than with one who has not.

If the patient and physician think that the etiology is physical, there may be incompatibility in the precise physical cause. A case of cultural conflict between pediatric hospital personnel and a family from the Caribbean may hinge on the mother's belief that the child's illness has been precipitated by a fall and injury to the child's back and nerves, whereas the pediatric personnel may hypothesize sepsis. The resulting conflict may require a court order because repeated blood tests can draw in Caribbean beliefs about the dangers of blood loss. The child may leave the hospital successfully cured in the eyes of the pediatricans but dangerously ill because of blood loss and with an untreated illness from a fall in the eyes of the mother. Thus, in the short run, the health care providers may have prevailed over parental objections and successfully treated potentially life-threatening sepsis in a young child. In the long run, however, there is a reduced likelihood that the mother will seek out biomedical care for her child's subsequent health problems.

As another example, rural Hawaiian-American-Polynesians diagnose a physical malady called *opu huli*. The symptoms of *opu huli* in infants, who are particularly susceptible to this malady, are similar to colic and are accompanied by inconsolable crying for long periods of time and seeming stomach discomfort. Western biomedicine has offered many hypotheses about the physical origins of colic, but the etiology is not certain. Parents of colicky infants are regarded with sympathy and assured that the condition will pass with time. In contrast, Hawaiian-American-Polynesians view *opu huli* as inflicted by parents or caretakers jiggling and bouncing a baby. If a baby is bounced in the parents' arms or tossed in the air, the still-delicate stomach *(opu)* is thought to turn or become twisted *(huli)*. Hawaiian-American-Polynesians, then, would regard the infant with sympathy for the illness inflicted by parents. Further, the illness requires treatment by a knowledgeable individual who can massage the *opu* back into its proper position. Middle-class parents on the United States' mainland jiggle and bounce infants as a strategy for amusing or calming them, and even purchase devices to perform this function while they are busy.

Even if the cause of illness is spiritual, the physician may be sought to treat the physical symptoms or to monitor the progress of traditional alternative healers in resolving the illness. In Hawaii, a child became seriously injured in an accident. The underlying cause was attributed to retribution for an interpersonal conflict the parents had in the past. This did not preclude medical attention to the injuries. Indeed, the best medical care was sought, but it was widely believed in the community that unless the parents remedied their relations with others, their children, the most vulnerable members of families, would continue to pay the price. Thus, both biomedical practitioners and traditional healers needed to be consulted.

Beliefs set the stage, but people do not always behave consistently with their beliefs and there is no simple one-to-one correspondence between health beliefs and behaviors.

What Came Before the Physician Encounter

What do you do at home when your child becomes ill? Patients try to get better on their own first.

Are there things that your family does to try to help the child feel better before coming to see me?

Have you seen or are you currently seeing any other health care providers?

Knowing what came before physician contact and what components are congruent or discongruent with biomedicine can be invaluable in determining what happens between the child and family and the pediatrician. If, for example, the grandmother was important in seeking a referral to a lay healer, perhaps the pediatrician should ask the parents whether the grandmother should be consulted or included in the discussion about the decision for physical therapy. If, for example, home remedies have been used, just as over-the-counter medicines are an important part of a medical history, so too are cultural remedies that have been administered prior to physician contact.

Patterns of Resort

Health care can be conceptualized as occurring in three overlapping sectors. The *dominant*, or *professional, sector* is composed of biomedically trained physicians and health care providers, such as nurses and paraprofessionals. The *folk*, or *alternative, sector* is composed of practitioners of alternative medicine, including acupucturists, *curanderos* (indigenous healers), and herbalists. The *popular sector* involves health care that occurs within the context of the home and family.

Although most research on health care utilization has focused on professional biomedical health care, most illnesses do not come to the physician's attention. From 60% to 90% of episodes of ill health are handled at home, in the popular sector. Further, when illnesses are taken to a physician, the physician is generally not the first point of resort. If the illness is not perceived as immediately dangerous, home remedies are often the first recourse. Understanding the pre-physician period is an important component of cultural competence. The anticipatory inclusion of culture shows respect for the patient's heritage and indicates that the pediatrician will engage in a collaborative effort with the family to ensure that the child stays or gets well.

Cultures and individuals organize their efforts to seek medical help into what has been termed *patterns of resort*. Practitioners from different sectors of the health care system may be consulted in a hierarchical or simultaneous pattern.

For example, a Chamorro (the indigenous culture on Guam) mother brought an infant with an unusual rash for pediatric care. This was identified by a biomedically trained Chamorro physician as the kind of rash that older Chamorros ascribed to the wrath of spirits, and it therefore was treated by a *suruhano* (healer). The mother then said that the father wanted to consult the *suruhano* first, but she wanted to come to the pediatrician. As they were discussing the case, a call came from the father on the mother's cellular phone to find out the diagnosis. Since the pediatricians could not find a cause and the child appeared basically well, the pediatricians agreed that it would not be a bad idea to also consult the *suruhano* but to let them know what the *suruhano* suggested. Follow-up indicated that the rash had disappeared, as most childhood problems do.

Treatment Actions

If culture is to be included in assessments of all patients, an important step is to delineate those cultural practices that will have an impact on health care. Just as the pediatrician should not ignore the use of over-the-counter remedies in treating a patient, the pediatrician cannot ignore home and alternative remedies, even if one is uncertain about their effects.

Neither best medical practice nor culture is static. Each is a constantly changing system. For example, therapy for a disease as common as otitis media has varied significantly over time, and even now there is no single best "scientific" answer regarding optimal therapy. Although repeated and sometimes prolonged courses of antibiotics are the cornerstone of treatment in the United States, some European physicians have found analgesics alone to be equally effective in treating mild cases. This success is not surprising, given the high frequency with which viruses may be associated with middle ear infections and the high spontaneous cure rate for non-pneumococcal bacterial middle ear disease. However, most American pediatricians would consider failure to treat an acute otitis media with antibiotics, however mild, poor medical practice.

Culture can have a neutral, positive, negative, or mixed impact on health care. For example, Hawaiian massage treatment of *opu huli* may be positive because it comforts the child. It may be neutral because it would not interfere with other treatment, particularly because there is no documented effective treatment for symptoms of colic. And, finally, it may be negative if the child had a more serious illness that went undiagnosed while the family relied on a traditional diagnosis and treatment strategy. Similarly, massage with coconut oil among the Chamorro of Guam is soothing to a child and unlikely to interfere with other biomedical conditions. However, if the child has impetigo, the massage may serve to spread the infection.

Among Hispanics in the southwestern United States, indigenous medications are used to cure *empacho* (a blockage in the stomach that must be purged). Some purgatives are indeed harmless and would not interfere with biomedical care, but others contain high levels of lead. Educational and community awareness efforts in these areas have been successful in diminishing the harmful form of these substances and thus the incidence of lead poisoning while not minimizing the cultural importance or reality of treating *empacho*.

In considering responses to illness and treatment actions, one may find it helpful to recall that health beliefs of both patients and practitioners are embedded in cultural systems that differ to varying degrees from one another. Whereas it would be much simpler if patients and practitioners shared the same beliefs about health, illness, and interventions, this is not reality. The implications of various health beliefs and cultural systems on the perceived need for and acceptability of treatment actions and interventions offered by the practitioner can be enormous. As the health beliefs of practitioners are heavily influenced by Western biomedicine, in addition to their own cultures, attention must be given to individuals who bring different beliefs to the therapeutic encounter—beliefs that influence decisions to seek treatment, the point at which to seek treatment, the source of (lay versus religious versus medical) treatment, and the expectations of what constitutes appropriate treatment.

An awareness of differences in health beliefs that translate into differences in "folk" or lay versus medical diagnosis may facilitate finding a "middle ground" in treatment that optimally accommodates both belief systems in addition to enhancing the provision of care by both the family and the pediatrician. Decisions to seek medical treatment generally indicate that home remedies have not entirely resolved the problem, but the practitioner must keep in mind that this decision does not negate existing beliefs of those seeking care and certainly does not rule out the syncretic use of home remedies or continued seeking of alternative interventions.

Because most illnesses are self-limiting, cultural knowledge is also empirical knowledge. That is, since remedies have worked in the past, it is assumed that they will work in the future. In the United States, middle-class parents routinely accept a physician prescription of a second course of antibiotics if a child's symptoms persist, assuming not that antibiotics are useless but that a different drug, or a longer course of treatment, will resolve the problem. Similarly, a Caribbean mother who has not been able to cure her child's illness with traditional teas will not decrease her belief in those teas. She assumes that the dosage or some other factor needed correcting.

Patient Adherence with Pediatric Advice

An important stage of the health care process is whether or not patients and their families follow a physician's advice. Cultural conflict in medical care often presents itself at this stage and then the search ensues for differences in beliefs or problems in communication style that have contributed to the noncompliance. If cultural factors have been accommodated in the preceding steps of the health-seeking process in an anticipatory fashion, compliance will be much more likely. Noncompliance will then be more likely due to misunderstanding of directions than a harder-to-solve problem of differences in beliefs as to the cause of the problem.

Communication and the Clinical Encounter

Pediatricians should be open to diversity in communication strategies. In the role of a learner, pediatricians should direct their attention toward culturally appropriate verbal and nonverbal communication styles. In many groups, aversion of eye contact, for example, does not mean lack of attention. Failure of a patient or parent to ask questions does not imply disinterest. Responding with only yes or no answers by the patient does not imply the lack of an opinion but perhaps indicates respect for the physician's expertise. Offering an opinion to the expert might be seen as rude and offensive. Language barriers do not necessarily lend themselves to simple solutions. The use of an interpreter, for example, may violate privacy and increase a patient's distress in a small, closely knit community. Further, individuals may regard the assumption of the need for an interpreter as an insult that they have not mastered English.

POVERTY, CULTURE, AND CHILD HEALTH

The impact of poverty on the health of children is significant. That approximately 25% of very young children in the United States live below the poverty line has enormous impact. The United States performs dismally on most measures of young child health. The proportion of children who are without adequate access to health care, who are not monitored to ensure proper growth and development, and who are incompletely immunized stands in stark contrast to the position of the United States as a leader in the industrialized world. "Culture" and "poverty" must be distinguished. Because culturally diverse peoples are disproportionately represented among the poor, and since the poor are more likely to use public clinics, it is easy to confound culture and socioeconomic class. One way to overcome this difficulty is to first rule out more tangible issues that might be interfering with health care. For example:

- Does a mother really disagree with a recommended course of treatment, or does she face the danger of getting a prescription filled in a high-crime neighborhood if the appointment is at the end of the day?
- Does her insurance cover the prescription at any pharmacy?
- If clinic patients are often late, does a family really have a different cultural orientation to time, or are they dependent on unreliable public transportation (often in cold weather with many young children in tow)?
- Is a family inappropriately using the nighttime emergency department for a cold, or is this the only time that a mother can get someone to drive her to the hospital or clinic?

We suggest that physicians explore these possibilities before assuming a cultural discrepancy in health care and beliefs.

REFERENCES

Baer R, Ackerman A. Toxic Mexican folk remedies for the treatment of empacho: The case of *Azarcon, Greta* and *Albayalde.* J Ethnopharmacol 1988;24:31–39.

Baer R, Bustillo M. *Susto* and *mal de ojo* among Florida farmworkers: Emic and etic perspectives. Med Anthropol Q 1993;7:90–100.

Barker J, Clark M (eds). Cross-cultural medicine a decade later. Special issue. West J Med 1992;157.

Chrisman N. The health seeking process: An approach to the natural history of illness. Cult Med Psychiatry 1977;1:351–377.

Clark M (ed). Cross-cultural medicine. Special issue. West J Med 1983;139.

Eisenberg D, Kessler R, Foster C, et al. Unconventional medicine in the United States: Prevalence, costs, and patterns of use. N Engl J Med 1993;328:246–252.

Groce N, Zola I. Multiculturalism, chronic illness, and disability. Pediatrics 1993;91:1048–1055.

Harkness S, Super C, Keefer C. Culture and ethnicity. *In* Levine M, Carey C, Crocker A. (eds). Developmental Behavioral Pediatrics, 2nd ed. Philadelphia: WB Saunders, 1992:103–108.

Harwood A. The hot-cold theory of disease: Implication for treatment of Puerto Rican patients. JAMA 1971;216:1153–1158.

Harwood A (ed). Ethnicity and Medical Care. Cambridge, Mass: Harvard University Press, 1981.

Helman C. Culture, Health and Illness, 2nd ed. London: Wright, 1990.

Korbin J, Johnston M. Steps toward resolving cultural conflict in a pediatric hospital. Clin Pediatr 1982;21:259–263.

Korbin J. *Hana'ino*: Child maltreatment in a Hawaiian-American community. Pacific Studies 1990;13:6–22.

Lozoff B, Kamath KR, Feldman RA. Infection and disease in South Indian families: Beliefs about childhood diarrhea. Hum Organization 1975;34:353–357.

McDermott J. The effects of ethnicity on child and adolescent development. *In* Lewis M. (ed). Child and Adolescent Psychiatry. Baltimore: Williams & Wilkins, 1991:408–412.

Pachter LM. Ethical and cultural issues in pediatric care. *In* Behrman RE (ed). Nelson Textbook of Pediatrics, 14th ed. Philadelphia: WB Saunders, 1992:10–12.

Rosenbaum S. The health consequences of poverty. Am Behav Scientist 1992;35:275–289.

Scott C. Health and healing among five ethnic groups in Miami, Florida. Public Health Rep 89:524–532.

Trotter R, Ackerman A, Rodman D, et al. "Azarcon" and "Greta": Ethnomedical solution to epidemiological mystery. Med Anthropol Q 1983;14:318.

Wasserman R, Hassuk B, Young P, et al. Health care of physicians' children. Pediatrics 1989;83:319.

Young A. When rational men fall sick. Cult Med Psychiatry 1981;5:317–335.

5 Applying Ethical Principles to Clinical Decision Making

Jeffrey R. Botkin

Ethical principles need to be considered in most clinical decision-making circumstances. These principles are quite relevant to pediatric practitioners.

CASE 1

Diane is a 14-month-old child with a 2-day history of upper respiratory infection symptoms and a 1-day history of fever and irritability. Her physical examination is notable for an erythematous, immobile left tympanic membrane. Diane has a history of four previous episodes of otitis media, the last two occurring 5 weeks and 3 weeks prior to the current illness. She has been treated with amoxicillin and trimethoprim/sulfamethoxazole for the last two episodes, respectively. The family has very limited financial resources. They are insured, but their insurance does not cover medications. Which antibiotic should be used in this clinical circumstance?

The choice of antibiotics for otitis media is a common dilemma for practicing pediatricians. The problem in Diane's case can be simply stated: Is it better to use a broad-spectrum agent despite the higher medication costs, or should a cheaper, more narrow-spectrum antibiotic be used? The former choice will burden the family with the costs of the medication; the latter choice involves a risk of inadequate treatment that may entail additional discomfort for the child and perhaps additional costly visits to the office. Although a knowledge of bacteriology, pharmacology, anatomy, and pathophysiology is relevant to this problem, the dilemma is basically an ethical one. Ethical issues are issues of human values, and in the case of Diane, the dilemma can be solved only by considering which is valued more—the costs of the broader-spectrum agents or the risks of inadequate treatment.

Contemporary medicine provides an extraordinary array of diagnostic and therapeutic interventions. A knowledge of what *can* be done in medicine is essential to being a competent clinician. But equally important is the ability to determine what *should* be done given an expanding menu of choices. The discipline of medical ethics assists physicians and other care providers when complex problems arise over what should be done. Clinical choices force us to consider two aspects of each option: the probability that a particular outcome will materialize and the value that is placed on that outcome. Analyzing these values and developing clear justifications for holding certain values constitute the work of medical ethics. Ethical issues are a fundamental part of medicine, whether the case is one of otitis media or of terminal cancer. The challenge is to determine which actions we as individuals, and we as a society, believe are right or wrong, or, more commonly, the best among unattractive options.

The care of children offers a broad range of ethical issues that must be addressed by care providers. The analysis of issues requires both a basic set of "tools" and a body of knowledge. In medical ethics, the tools consist of an analytic approach and the body of knowledge is the literature of concepts and cases involving issues relevant to the dilemma at hand.

There are several misconceptions about medical ethics. First, it is often claimed that ethical analysis cannot provide the "right answer" in clear and unequivocal terms in many cases. This claim may be expressed in the comment that ethics is "just a matter of opinion" and thus not worthy of extended discussion. It must be acknowledged that ethical analysis often does not provide a clear and convincing answer in many cases. Yet such a criticism demands too much of the discipline. Parallels can be drawn with other forms of medical decision making. A large number of issues in pediatric care remain matters of debate. There are respected clinicians who disagree on many questions, yet we should be reluctant to conclude that the debates become just matters of opinion. Because the issues are unsettled, we must carefully assess the data and arguments that underlie the opposing opinions and draw a justification for our own decisions. We may not feel absolute certainty in the answers we derive, but we will have solid justifications for our actions. The same considerations hold true for ethical decision making. Opinions on ethical issues are abundant, but not all opinions are equally valid. Informed, carefully considered opinions are the best guides for action.

Second, some claim that the study of ethics will not make people ethical. Character is largely developed before adulthood, and the study of ethics is not likely to change those who have significant moral deficiencies. But ethical analysis can help only those who are looking for guidance about the best choices. Those who know right from wrong, yet choose to do wrong, are beyond the help of ethics education. The ethical analysis of medical cases only rarely involves an assessment of the moral character of the individuals involved. Care providers and family members should not feel personally threatened by ethics case discussions.

A SYSTEMATIC APPROACH TO ETHICAL PROBLEM SOLVING

There is no uniformly accepted approach to the analysis of ethical problems in medicine. The basic approach is a practical method to organize thinking:

1. Collect the data.
2. Define the ethical issue(s).
3. Outline the choices.
4. Weigh the ethical principles.
5. Develop an action plan with follow-up.

It is usually important to work through this process with all of those who have responsibility for care decisions, including the parents (and patient when appropriate), physicians, nurses, and appropriate others as dictated by the case. An analysis of Case 2 will be used to illustrate this approach.

CASE 2

Alex weighed 2800 g at birth; his mother, a 32-year-old gravida 3 para 3, had had a full-term, uncomplicated pregnancy. Delivery was uncomplicated, with an Apgar score of 6 at 1 minute and 7 at 5 minutes. Alex has the clinical stigmata of trisomy 18—the diagnosis is subsequently confirmed on chromosome analysis. Alex also has esophageal atresia and a large ventricular septal defect. After discussions with the clinician and the consultants, the parents decide not to have Alex's esophageal defect repaired. They request that Alex not be provided artificial nutrition and that he be allowed to die naturally. The attending physician decides to respect the parents' request. However, the medical director of the nursery learns of the care plan and states that to allow this child to die is both illegal and immoral. What should be done?

The management of the infant in Case 2 is complex, but the difficulties presented by the case do not arise primarily from technical challenges in managing the child's care. The problems arise from the ethical dilemmas that are posed: Is esophageal surgery in the best interest of this child? Do parents have full authority to make care decisions? Is it ever appropriate to deny nutrition to an infant? If this infant is allowed to die, is it acceptable to provide pain relief, even though the pain medications may hasten the child's death?

Data Acquisition

Clinical ethics is an exercise in practical problem solving with relatively little need to refer to abstract philosophic theory. As a practical matter, ethical decisions in specific cases frequently hinge on the details of the individual case. These details must be thoroughly explored before the ethical problem can be adequately stated or a solution pursued. Returning to Case 2, a broad range of information must be obtained before the primary ethical issues can be adequately addressed. First, there are medical issues relevant to the case. We need to know the type of esophageal atresia present, the risks of surgical repair for *this* infant, and the prospects for success. Further, we need to know about any other life-threatening medical conditions present for the infant. In sum, we need to know what can be done for this infant and what risks, benefits, and burdens are associated with the treatment modalities.

Second, we must know more generally about the long-term prospects for individuals with trisomy 18. What is their life span? What are their intellectual capabilities? What are their functional capabilities? What new interventions might be on the horizon? How do they relate to family and friends? How do they experience their own lives?

Third, information about the attitudes of those involved in the care of the infant must be explored. What have the parents been told and what do they understand? Why have they made a particular choice? What are the attitudes of the physicians, nurses, and involved family, friends, and clergy toward the care of the infant? It is essential in the ethical analysis that accurate information be pursued in a comprehensive fashion. This aspect of the analysis is analogous to the medical history and physical examination in medical problem solving.

Defining the Ethical Issues

Once the relevant information has been obtained, the ethical issues can be identified. Quite often, the pursuit of information itself resolves the issue when it becomes apparent that the problem was one of misunderstanding; for example, the parents did not understand the medical situation, or the physician did not understand the parents' request. The ethical issues need not be identified through the use of ethics jargon. It is often useful simply to ask what aspects of the situation are creating anxiety.

In Case 2, there are a number of issues, but two major concerns can be briefly stated: Is it right to allow Alex to die when something might be done to sustain his life? Second, do physicians have to do what the parents request? In ethical terms, does allowing the infant to die violate our duty of beneficence to the child, and what are the limits of parental autonomy in making health care decisions for their children?

Once the key problems have been isolated, the subsequent discussion can be focused. Often in the discussion of ethics, when an analytic approach is not used, the conversation ranges back and forth across several issues at once, leading to an unproductive dialogue. When more than one problem is present, it is useful to explore the issues separately at the outset, then subsequently to explore their interactions. This aspect of the analysis is analogous to the problem list in medical decision making.

Outlining the Choices

For each of the ethical issues identified, the available options must be outlined. It is worth noting that when there are no choices available, there are no ethical issues present. For example, if the infant in Case 2 has a fatal and irreparable cardiac malformation, there is no longer an ethical dilemma over whether to make vigorous attempts to sustain the infant's life. Physicians are not required to use interventions that will not work. However, when choices are available, they should be explicitly stated and explored in detail. It is particularly important to explore the possibility of compromise solutions that may not be immediately apparent. In Case 2, for example, if the parents' primary concern is the impact of this infant on the family, the possibility of placing the infant for adoption might be explored. With each of the choices available, it is important to predict the logical consequences of actions to be taken. Both short-term and long-term consequences should be considered.

Balancing the Principles

The best of the available options can be selected only after a careful evaluation of the advantages and disadvantages of each option. In ethical problem solving, this is where a knowledge of and sensitivity to human values are applied. This process can be more fully illustrated when the basic principles of medical ethics have been outlined (see later, ''Ethical Principles''). However, an understanding of the method requires an appreciation of two fundamental aspects of ethical discussion. First is the question,

Whose ethics are to be applied to determine the best option? The second question is, What standard is used to measure which action is best?

Each person has a set of values that will differ in degrees from others. Basic ethical principles in our society are broadly recognized; nevertheless, individual biases and life situations often lead to different perspectives on the more difficult ethical problems. Given the potential diversity of opinions from those involved in the care of a child, whose values should be used to analyze the case? The traditional answer has been to approach the analysis from a neutral or disinterested perspective. The hypothetical ideal for an ethics consultant is someone who is omniscient, wise, and disinterested. ''Disinterested'' does not mean that the ideal consultant doesn't care about the outcome but that the consultant has no personal stake in the outcome that may bias the analysis. The desired outcome is the identification of an action that is the ''best'' action, all facts and perspectives considered. Of course, such an ideal consultant does not exist, yet awareness of the disinterested perspective as an ideal can assist those confronted with ethical problems in recognizing and reducing personal biases. The need for a disinterested perspective also emphasizes the value of including in the discussions an ethicist, an ethics committee, or others who are knowledgeable about the issues but who are not immediately involved in care decisions.

The second set of issues concerns how we measure the value of certain actions. For example, there is a strong tradition in medicine, and society more generally, against lying. This prohibition against lying is a moral rule; however, it is important to consider the foundation of this rule. Why is it wrong to lie?

CASE 3

Ann is a 14-year-old with cystic fibrosis. Her condition was diagnosed at 3 years of age, but her parents have demanded that the diagnosis not be revealed to the child—you have reluctantly agreed. However, in a private moment with Ann, she asks: ''I have something serious, don't I, Doc?'' Should you reveal the truth?

Understanding the justification for the rule against lying is essential in determining whether there are appropriate exceptions to the rule. The philosophic foundation for moral rules or action guides has a rich history and remains the subject of continued scholarly debate. In brief, there are two widely recognized schools of thought: *utilitarianism* (also termed *consequentialism*) and *deontology*. Utilitarians believe that ethically correct actions are those that promote the greatest good for the greatest number of individuals. Because an action may benefit some while harming others, from a utilitarian perspective the action that promotes the most net benefit (or least harm) is preferred. The task in a utilitarian analysis is to predict the significant short-term and long-term benefits and harms from actions and then to choose the correct action based on its consequences.

There are two forms of utilitarian thinking that differ in their approach to specific actions in individual cases. *Act utilitarians* believe that it is appropriate to gauge the consequences of each act in specific cases to determine the ethically preferred action. *Rule utilitarians,* in contrast, believe that it is appropriate to establish moral rules that, if generally followed, will promote the greatest good for the greatest number. The distinction can be illustrated using the example of lying in Case 3. An act utilitarian may argue that a specific act of lying may produce sufficient net benefit to the patient (and perhaps others) that it is ethically justifiable. In the case of Ann, the act utilitarian would balance the potential benefits of Ann's knowing the truth with the harms to her, to her parents, and to the physician-parent relationship potentially created by this disclosure. In contrast, a rule utilitarian might look at the same case and argue that while there may seem to be a benefit to lying in some cases, other individuals in the aggregate would experience the greatest benefit by maintaining a firm rule against lying. Rule utilitarians believe that it is acceptable to forgo maximum benefits in individual cases in order to maximize the long-term benefits overall.

Deontologic theories, in contrast, maintain that qualities of actions may make the actions right or wrong, independent of their consequences. Consequences may still be important, but they are not of exclusive importance. Some actions are held to be intrinsically right or wrong, such as the prohibition against killing or the requirement to respect the dignity of others. In analyzing Case 3, a deontologist might argue that lying or deception is intrinsically wrong, even if the patient is harmed from the truth. Of course, the deontologist also would argue that disclosure of the truth should be done in a fashion that minimizes potential harms. For deontologists, good consequences do not justify wrong actions.

Both theories suffer from significant problems. Utilitarians must specify what the "good" is that is to be maximized—is it human happiness or pleasure or some other aspect of human welfare? Further, how do we compare the magnitude of experiences like pleasure, suffering, or loneliness in order to balance them in an equation? Utilitarians must also have confidence in their ability to predict the future.

Deontologists are challenged to describe the foundation for their claims. Some absolute moral rules may be theologically derived, as with the Ten Commandments, but in a secular society we must argue why it is intrinsically wrong to lie or kill in secular terms. These arguments have proved difficult to develop without reference to consequences. Further, deontologists must determine how to respond when principles are in conflict. If the physician in Case 3 is forced into a choice between lying to the patient or breaking a promise to her parents, a deontologist must decide which principle takes precedence, preferably for reasons other than utility.

This discussion of utilitarian and deontologic theories should provide some insight into how we commonly think about moral decisions. Neither theory alone effectively captures how most of us think about these issues in many cases. Intuitive beliefs in both of these approaches often leave us confused in attempts to resolve problems. For example, we may be attracted to the use of deception if it might benefit the patient, but deception still may seem wrong despite the benefits. Appreciating the distinction between utilitarian and deontologic theories of moral value helps to explain our ambivalent response to such conflicts.

In weighing ethical principles to solve problems, we must consider the criteria by which the best solution will be judged. Because the practice of medicine seeks to maximize the good of individual patients, clinicians often use act utilitarian thinking in analyzing ethical problems in medicine. This is not wrong, but such an analysis is incomplete. Consideration of rule utilitarian and deontologic perspectives is important in providing a comprehensive discussion.

Resolution and Follow-through

Since medical ethics involves practical problem solving, there is not the luxury of extended debate on issues. Choices must be made, sometimes rather quickly. After a careful consideration of the data, the attitudes, and the ethical issues, a choice can be made with explicit justification. The goal cannot be to reach the "right" answer, because this is rarely realistic. The goal is to reach a justifiable decision based on a careful consideration of all the relevant factors.

Once an action has been taken, it is important to follow through on the ethical issues. An action may be heavily dependent on the

clinical circumstances of the case, and as these circumstances change, it is essential to reconsider the ethical issues. There is no need to be faithful to an earlier ethical decision if key aspects of the case have changed.

ETHICAL PRINCIPLES

The principles of *beneficence, autonomy,* and *justice* must be applied to pediatric care. These principles are basic values that are broadly shared in our society as well as in most societies through history. Even though there may be controversy over the meaning of the principles in individual cases or over which principle is most important when they are in conflict, there is no controversy over the importance of these fundamental values in human affairs. In this strong sense, ethics is not just a matter of opinion.

Beneficence

Beneficence is the moral duty to offer benefit to others. This duty is particularly strong in medicine, a field in which physicians are dedicated to the welfare of patients. This duty has many manifestations: the duty to be attentive to the patient's problems, the duty to competently diagnose and treat illness, the duty to prevent future illness, the duty to relieve suffering, and the duty to offer empathy and compassion. These are the benefits that patients seek from a physician and the benefits physicians strive to provide; thus, beneficence lies at the core of the physician-patient relationship.

Closely tied with the concept of beneficence is the principle of *nonmaleficence.* Nonmaleficence is the duty in medicine not to harm patients—a traditional duty captured in the Hippocratic imperative "First, do no harm." For the purpose of simplicity, nonmaleficence will be folded in with our consideration of beneficence, since a responsibility to help patients generally includes a responsibility not to harm them. In some circumstances, however, such as nontherapeutic research, the principle of nonmaleficence must be explicitly considered. In contrast to clinicians, researchers may have no duty to benefit research subjects, yet they have a strong duty to minimize risks of harm.

The duty of beneficence is often more complex in the care of children than in the care of adults. Young children have not autonomously formed their personal values, and therefore patient preferences cannot guide decisions about what is best in specific situations. The adolescent patient is an exception. In addition, children have the bulk of their lives before them, so often hope is fostered that time will permit recovery from serious impairments or that new treatments will become available in the future that will improve the long-term outcome. Families and physicians may be more tempted to hope for miracles for children than for older adults with serious illness. This is appropriate in many circumstances but potentially harmful to the child when no reasonable hope exists. The physician's knowledge of the relevant medical literature is essential in fostering realistic hopes.

In fulfilling the duty of beneficence to a younger child, we generally must ask what action will be in the child's "best interest." Determining the child's best interest is the foremost responsibility in ethical decision making for children. How do we determine a child's best interest? In Case 2, is it in Alex's best interest to have an esophageal repair? Assuming that successful repair is possible, the question becomes whether the burdens of surgery and subsequent care are worth the benefits of longer-term survival. The pain and suffering associated with surgery are easier to gauge for those in medicine because we can directly observe their manifestations in patients. The longer-term benefits and burdens of living with trisomy 18 are less easy to understand without substantial experience with these children. While there is some variability in individuals with trisomy 18, generally they are profoundly developmentally delayed with a life span of less than 1 year. Most infants with trisomy 18 die within the first 6 months of life. A few children with trisomy 18 have lived beyond the toddler years, but their mental development remains that of a young infant.

To explore further whether those with trisomy 18 derive benefit from their lives requires that we step back and look briefly at what it is that makes life valuable in general. Obviously, there will be a range of opinions on this issue. It can be argued that all life is intrinsically valuable and that it is not our prerogative to measure the value of life for others. This is a clear and powerful position, yet it does not capture for many how they feel about their own lives. Unremitting, severe suffering and a persistent vegetative state are conditions for which many believe continued life is not valuable. If we believe this for ourselves, we must admit the possibility that others would agree who cannot speak for themselves.

Another argument claims that life holds value when individuals can be or will be contributing members of society. Care must be taken with this argument. If the claim is that individuals themselves believe that their lives are valuable only when they can provide a tangible contribution to society, this claim is false. If the claim is that people's lives are valuable to *society* when they are contributing members, then we are no longer evaluating the value of life to the individual. The relative value of people's lives to society is a separate question.

A third argument claims that the value of life is, at a minimum, embodied in the ability to have some cognitive interaction with others. If an individual cannot, or will not in the future, experience a relationship with others, including love and companionship, it is claimed that there is no significant value to the individual of continued existence. Such a relationship with others requires only limited mental capabilities. This argument suggests that individuals with even profound mental retardation may experience significant benefit in their lives. However, there are limits to this argument—we cannot know the nature of the experience of those with serious mental disabilities, nor can we judge when the burdens of medical treatments outweigh what limited benefits are experienced in life by such individuals. The "best interest" standard cannot be applied without ambiguity for those with profound mental impairments.

The challenge in determining the best interest of the child is to see life from the perspective of the child. This is conceptually difficult, particularly since there are at least two sources of bias that are prevalent within the medical professions. First, physicians and nurses tend to see children with disabilities most often when the child is ill and is in a structured "foreign" clinical environment. This is a narrow window on the child's life and can lead to underestimates of the child's capabilities and the richness of the child's experiences. Second, we all share a tendency to see the value of life in our own terms. We enjoy the ability to see, to hear, and to experience physical and intellectual pleasures. If these are valuable to us, we may presume that life for others without such pleasures is devoid of value. But those who have not had these experiences might not miss their absence. A full value in life may be felt through a more limited set of pleasures. Care must be taken not to assume that life is of less value if it is not like the life that we enjoy.

With these perspectives in mind, we can return to the question of Alex's best interest. Given the high mortality rate for infants with trisomy 18, their profound developmental delay, and the burdens of a major surgical procedure, it is by no means clear that surgery is in the best interest of this child. If this is so, our duty of beneficence (considered alone) does not require that the physician advocate surgery for this child. If the parents are fully informed of the medical circumstances and they do not believe that surgery is

appropriate for Alex, it is acceptable to withhold such burdensome procedures.

When it is not clear that life-sustaining therapy is in the best interest of the child and if the parents agree with this assessment, then it is morally and legally acceptable to withhold or withdraw life-sustaining measures, including surgical procedures, ventilators, dialysis, and antibiotics. The most important criterion for deciding whether to withhold or withdraw life-sustaining treatments of all types in children is whether the treatments are expected to benefit the child. This approach to decision making has been consistently supported by the courts. There have been no cases in the United States in which a physician has been successfully prosecuted for the appropriate withholding or withdrawal of life-sustaining care from a patient.

Although the duty of beneficence to the child is usually primary, it is not our only duty of beneficence. We have a responsibility to promote the welfare of the family as well. When the duty to the family clearly conflicts with the duty to the child, our responsibility to the child generally takes precedence. When the benefit to the child is small or uncertain and the benefit to the family is potentially large, preference to the family may be justifiable. However, care must be taken not to assume that the birth of a child with moderate disabilities, such as Down syndrome, is necessarily a harm to the family. Care of a child with complex and expensive problems can be devastating to families—emotionally, physically, and financially. But many other parents find the care of a "special" child to be the most rewarding experience of their lives. However, predicting the long-term benefit or harm to families while an impaired infant is still in the nursery is difficult, if not impossible, for both care providers and families.

Finally, it is important to put the duty of beneficence in its larger perspective. We have a responsibility to our patients, but we also have a responsibility to consider the moral rules that are designed to promote the welfare of others. Imagine in Case 2 that the infant is expected to die within a few days. It can be argued that a lethal injection for the infant will prevent needless suffering. If such an injection will benefit the infant, do we have a moral duty to provide it? Of course, providing a lethal injection is illegal, but a narrow moral argument based on the child's welfare alone suggests that it might be ethically acceptable. Moral arguments opposing lethal interventions hinge on the intrinsic wrong of killing or on the potential risks to other children in relaxing the moral (and legal) rules. Concerns are raised that other children who do not have terminal conditions but who are viewed as less desirable to some parents and to some segments of society will be provided the "benefits" of a lethal injection. This type of argument is a "slippery slope" argument; the claim is that if we take a first step in a morally risky direction, the logic of the justification may lead to a progressive slide in our moral standards until tragic consequences develop. Slippery slope arguments are worthy of careful consideration, but they can be challenged if they are not based on a reasonable prediction of future human behavior. The tradition in our society against lethal injections by the medical profession remains intact because of these deontologic and slippery slope concerns.

Autonomy

Autonomy means "self-rule." The ethical principle involves our responsibility to respect the choices of others in governing their own lives. In medicine, promotion of this principle means giving people information about their medical situation and encouraging them to be full participants in health care decisions. Unlike beneficence, patient autonomy has not been a strong traditional value for the medical profession. The predominant tradition through the history of medicine was one of *benevolent paternalism,* whereby physicians gave only limited amounts of information to patients and provided treatments based on their own perception of what was best for their patients. This tradition of paternalism has been under significant criticism by society. The discipline of medical ethics was founded to a large degree on a broad-based desire in society to enhance the autonomy of patients, particularly in decisions around care at the end of life.

Perhaps the most common and significant ethical conflicts in clinical medicine today are between the physician's duty to do what the clinician believes is best for the patient and respecting the wishes of the patient. This conflict was illustrated by one of the first high-profile medical ethics cases, that of Karen Ann Quinlan. This patient was a young woman who was in a persistent vegetative state following a severe neurologic injury. She was thought to be ventilator-dependent. When it became clear that recovery from her injury was not possible, her father asked her physicians, and subsequently the court, to permit withdrawal of the ventilator. In a landmark decision, the court decided it is within the prerogative of the family to make the decision to withdraw ventilator care when the prognosis for any neurologic recovery is extremely poor. This important case was seen both as a confirmation that withdrawal of life support is acceptable in some circumstances and that the family should have the surrogate autonomy to make such decisions for those, like children, who cannot decide for themselves.

Closely allied with the concept of autonomy are competency and decision-making capacity. *Competency* is often considered a legal term. Therefore, many authors refer to *capacity* in the clinical setting as the set of personal characteristics that permit one to make informed, considered choices. Although decision-making capacity is necessary for autonomy, it is not sufficient. Competent individuals can make non-autonomous choices if they have been coerced or manipulated in the decision-making process.

Young children are not competent to make health care decisions, yet teenagers have the capacity for many important decisions about their care. Decision-making capacity and our corresponding respect for autonomy are not all-or-none phenomena, and they emerge in the process of child development. Several key developmental processes underlie decision-making capacity in children.

First, children must be able to understand the medical issues. Understanding in this context requires the develoment of a simple health vocabulary; an understanding of basic biologic concepts of life, death, health, and illness; and sufficient life experiences to appreciate the personal implications of these terms.

Second, children must be able to apply logic and reason to sort through the available choices. It must be understood that there are multiple short-term and long-term consequences for each choice, both for the child and for others.

Third, children must develop a set of values by which to weigh the benefits and the harms. Typical for young children is the focus on immediate pain and separation from family that are part of medical interventions, with little appreciation for the longer-term gains.

Finally, children must develop an independence from parents that enables choice based on personal values and not on the need to please (or punish) parents. Generally, these capacities are not well developed before about 13 to 14 years of age. However, our expectations for these capacities should depend on the magnitude of the decisions. If children are participating in minor treatment decisions, then less than fully developed capacities may be sufficient. If a child is participating in major treatment decisions, these capacities should be well developed before much weight can be given to the child's choices. Even when children are not invited to participate in decision making, they should be informed to the extent possible about their condition and care plan.

Adolescents are in transition to adulthood, and society generally treats them accordingly with respect to medical care. In many circumstances, adolescents need not have the consent of a parent to receive routine care. ''Emancipated minors'' are a class of adolescents who are considered adults in their medical decision-making capacity by virtue of their independence from parents. Emancipated minors include married minors, self-supporting minors living apart from parents, college students, and, in some states, pregnant adolescents. Over the past three decades, many states have passed treatment statutes that permit adolescents over a certain age, generally 16 years old, although in some as young as 14 years, to consent to medical care. Other states that do not have general statutes permit physicians to care for adolescents with venereal disease or alcohol or drug problems without parental consent; indeed, these statutes may prohibit parental notification. Practitioners can provide contraception to adolescents without informing the parents; however, in many states abortion services remain an issue of controversy. In some states, parental notification is required for an abortion, although these states must permit an alternative to parental consent, such as a private hearing by a judge. In general, parents will not be responsible for paying the bills when they have not consented to care. Despite the legislation in this area, a physician's legal liability over consent issues with adolescents is quite low. It does not follow, however, that adolescents have the right to refuse medical care that is requested by parents and is necessary for their welfare.

The freedom of families to make independent decisions for their children is an important issue. Families (parents or guardians) are usually involved in decision making for young children and, in general, consent must be obtained from parents before treatment can be given to a child. Through much of Western history, parents had virtual ownership of their children, including decisions about life and death for neonates. Over the past two centuries, parental control over children has been limited in a number of important ways, including child labor laws and child abuse and neglect statutes. With respect to medical care, parents have broad prerogatives to choose among available alternatives, but they do not have absolute authority.

CASE 4

Chad was a 3-year-old child with a diagnosis of acute lymphocytic leukemia (ALL). Physicians offered a good prognosis for cure using standard chemotherapy. The parents initially gave consent to standard medical care, but they subsequently stopped Chad's chemotherapy and began treatments with laetrile, vitamins, and enzyme enemas. Chad experienced a relapse. The physicians petitioned the court to mandate medical care over the objections of the parents. The parents claimed the right to pursue treatments that they thought best for their child.

In this 1979 case, the ethical and legal dilemma was posed by a conflict between the interests of the child in receiving potentially effective treatment and the freedom of parents to decide about care for their child. The court carefully analyzed this case by seeking testimony on the efficacy of the parents' chosen treatment modalities. No licensed physician was willing to testify that these measures were effective. In contrast, there was abundant evidence that standard care was potentially curative. The court mandated standard care, but the court did not do so simply because it thought this best for the child. In order to override parental autonomy, the court, in this case and others, required that the potential harm to the child by parental choice be serious or life-threatening and that the parent's choice not conform to a medically justifiable option. Given several medical options promoted by legitimate medical authorities, the courts have not been willing to interfere with parental choice. Society has been willing to honor parental decision making unless the decisions of the parents are without reasonable justification and pose risk of serious harm or death for the child.

The professional autonomy of physicians is also an important consideration in many cases. Each professional must establish his or her own ethical and professional standards with respect to patient care. If a family insists on a form of care that violates the physician's standards and no further compromises can be reached, it is the prerogative of the physician to withdraw from the care of the patient. Patients and families must be permitted time to find another physician whose philosophy is consistent with theirs; a 2-week notification may be a reasonable time in most circumstances. Despite disagreements over care, it is never acceptable to abandon a patient.

Informed Consent

Respect for autonomy in health care is most commonly manifested as a respect for the decision-making authority of patients with respect to their own care. Thus, autonomy is at the foundation of the practice of informed consent. Although informed consent has many complexities, the basic idea is that patients should have the opportunity to make informed choices about their health care. In the care of young children, informed consent is obtained from the parents or guardians. The concept of informed consent arose largely through the courts and has been adopted by the medical profession, yet the foundation of informed consent in the law is the ethical principle of autonomy, not abstract legal considerations.

The elements of informed consent are relatively simple:

1. Patients (or their surrogates) should know the diagnosis or the basic diagnostic possibilities.
2. The alternatives for treatment or further evaluation should be outlined.
3. The risks and benefits of the alternatives should be detailed.
4. A recommendation by the physician should be offered.

It should be apparent that these elements of informed consent are basic components of virtually all clinical encounters with patients. Therefore, informed consent is at the foundation of the physician-patient relationship. Too often, informed consent is considered only in the context of getting signatures on forms for invasive procedures. Rather, informed consent is the dialogue that should surround every medical intervention. In both legal and moral terms, consent forms have little value in themselves and should be considered only as documentation that a full discussion has occurred between physician and patient. In some major medical centers, consent forms have been abandoned entirely and the chart notes alone are used to document the relevant discussions and decisions.

An aspect of informed consent that clinicians often find troublesome is the extent of the disclosure of risks associated with treatments or procedures. Treatments and procedures usually have a spectrum of associated risk from the mild and relatively common to the rare and severe. In regard to the child in Case 1 who has otitis media, imagine that the physician and parents decide on amoxicillin/clavulanate as the best antibiotic choice. This antibiotic commonly causes diarrhea (at least 1 in 10 cases) and is rarely associated with life-threatening anaphylaxis (perhaps 1 in 50,000 cases). Should these risks be disclosed to the child's parents?

In the development of the concept of informed consent, three general standards have been used to guide clinicians with respect to disclosure. The first has been termed the *professional practice standard,* by which physicians are required to disclose information that other competent physicians would disclose in similar circumstances. This approach holds physicians to the standard of their peers. The problems with this approach are that we generally do not know what other physicians are doing about disclosure and, more importantly, there is no assurance that what physicians commonly discuss corresponds to what patients want or need to make their own decisions about acceptable risks.

According to a second standard, the *reasonable person standard,* the physician should offer information that a reasonable person would need in the circumstances to make an informed choice. This standard promotes autonomy better than the professional practice standard does because it views disclosure from the perspective of the patient rather than from the physician. However, the standard remains vague because it is unclear in many situations what a hypothetical reasonable person would want. In general, it is safe to conclude that people want to know the common side effects, even if they are mild, and the potentially severe reactions, even if they are rare. It is also safe to conclude that the more ''elective'' the treatment, the more should be disclosed about risks. However, patients need information for reasons other than consent. Patients also need to know how to recognize adverse events and to know how to respond. In the antibiotic example above, the risk of rare but severe reactions is impossible to avoid with any antibiotic choice, yet it is still advisable to discuss potential reactions to antibiotics so that the parents can respond appropriately should one occur.

The third standard of disclosure is the *subjective standard,* by which physicians must disclose that information that is important to an individual patient to make a decision. Because not all patients are ''reasonable'' in some homogeneous way, this standard encourages physicians to explore individual needs with respect to information. Experienced clinicians recognize the large variation between different patients and parents in their needs for information. This standard suggests that physicians need to offer information to all patients but that more detailed information need be given only when it is desired by the patient or family. This standard is most consistent with the principle of autonomy.

There are several clinical circumstances in which informed consent can be delayed or forgone. Physicians need not obtain informed consent in emergency circumstances in which any delay may threaten the welfare of the patient. The justification is simply that there is not time to discuss what the patient or family might want under the circumstances. Of course, the physician must still inform the patient or family about what is being done, but the purpose is not to obtain consent. This exception to informed consent does not apply when the emergency has been anticipated and patients (or family) have made their wishes known in advance about specific interventions. For example, if the parents have made a justified and informed refusal of life-sustaining ventilator support for their child, sudden respiratory failure does not constitute an emergency in which the ventilator can be used without parental consent.

Informed consent can also be delayed or forgone in pediatric care when the parents or guardian is not available for discussion and the child requires care. This exception applies to circumstances that are not true emergencies but in which the medical condition is sufficiently severe that prompt treatment is appropriate. Consider a case in which a 9-year-old child is brought to the emergency department following a bicycle accident with a fracture of the radius, a scalp laceration, and several abrasions. If the parents are not immediately available, care for these problems should proceed without informed consent. Any interventions that entail significant risk that are not immediately necessary should be delayed pending consent.

Two other exceptions to informed consent can be mentioned briefly. Occasionally, parents or patients may be unwilling to listen to information and participate in decisions. If the parents explicitly state that they do not want information and that they wish for the physician to make the decisions, they have waived their right to informed consent. Physicians should be reluctant to accept waivers, and a persistent lack of participation by parents in important decisions may be an indication of psychosocial problems within the family. The physician must document a waiver in detail and should make repeated attempts to re-engage the parents as care proceeds.

A fourth and controversial exception to informed consent is termed *therapeutic privilege.* In some circumstances, revealing the full information about a patient's condition to the patient or the family members is considered so potentially harmful to them that the physician can withhold the information. Therapeutic privilege is controversial for two reasons. First, empirical studies have shown that most people handle difficult information better than physicians often predict; second, this exception is open to abuse by physicians who would prefer to save the time and emotional toll of a full discussion. This exception is only rarely justified.

Justice

CASE 5

The death of a child in an automobile accident has made a heart available for transplantation. Two local children are on the list for a transplant. Child A is 12 years old. She has been waiting for 9 months for a transplant and is now seriously ill. Her family is uninsured and not eligible for Medicaid until they "spend down" their resources. The transplant team has significant concerns about the ability of the family to understand and comply with the complex treatment regimen. Child B is 3 years old. He has been on the list for 1 month and is also seriously ill. His parents are well educated and well insured for the transplant procedure and subsequent care. The transplant team must promptly decide which child should be offered the heart.

Which child deserves to be chosen first? Should the choice be made by need (severity of illness), utility (the best chance of success), ability to pay, age, or time on the waiting list? If we can't decide which child is more deserving, perhaps it would be acceptable to develop a fair procedure to choose, such as a lottery. To approach this dilemma, we must consider the principle of justice.

The first formal principle of justice is attributed to Aristotle. It states that equals should be treated equally and unequals should be treated unequally. This formal principle captures our sense that benefits and harms should not be distributed randomly, but consensus about justice quickly breaks down as we try to decide what equal and unequal mean with respect to benefits, harms, and human attributes. Obviously, people are not all the same with respect to race, age, sex, talents, and wealth, but should these differences count in our decision about health care?

In clinical medicine, issues of justice arise in two general forms. *Microallocation* decisions are decisions about the allocation of available resources to specific patients, such as beds in an intensive care unit (ICU) and organs for transplantation. *Macroallocation* decisions pertain to decisions about how resources should be allocated within the health care system more broadly.

Utilitarian thinking is prevalent in medicine, and this is reflected in the most common approaches to microallocation issues. Utilitarian theory is intended to be broad enough to cover justice concerns with the belief that the distribution of benefits and harms that is the most just is the distribution that will produce the greatest good for the greatest number. If this theory is applied in the context of limited medical resources, it is often justifiable to argue that resources should be directed to those who will benefit the most. Thus, transplantable hearts and ICU beds are preferentially given to those who are the most critically ill, assuming that there is a reasonable chance for benefit. This is a particularly useful approach in medicine because severity of illness can be roughly quantified, and those who are less ill may survive long enough to benefit from the next available resource. In Case 5, because the severity of illness was described as serious for both children, the principle of need is not sufficient to make a decision between the children. In

this case, the current standards call for the organ to be offered to the child who has been on the list the longest, which is perhaps also a measure of need in a different sense.

Macroallocation issues are enormously complex, with decisions to be made about the allocation to health care versus other social needs and decisions about allocations within health care. The important question is the extent to which these issues are relevant to bedside decision making by families and physicians. For example, are the costs to society relevant to decisions about whether to perform additional tests and procedures on a patient? The answer is usually a qualified yes. First, however, clinicians must understand the coverage status of the patient; the physician may be spending the *family's* money, not society's, in which case the family can help decide whether it is worth it. Second, most clinical decisions can be made on the basis of benefit. If an expensive test has a small likelihood of benefit, then, unless the test has a sensitivity and specificity of 100%, the yield of false-positive and false-negative results will be relatively high. The validity of the test then will be poor, and this is a good reason for not performing the test, whatever the costs. Justice considerations are also relevant because the resources for health care are not infinite. If the likely benefit of a test or procedure is small and the costs are great to society, it is reasonable and prudent to consider the costs for the larger benefit of others in society.

The statement is often heard in regard to some critically ill children that the costs are too great and that money should not be wasted on further care. In many of these cases, issues of justice are raised when care providers have not come to understand the more basic issue of the child's best interest. If the child is not benefiting from the medical care, it is justifiable to discontinue the care on that basis alone. Consideration of costs is not necessary. However, if the child is thought to be benefiting from the care, then we must ask if it is the prerogative of care providers to withhold such care in the presumed interest of general social welfare. Such a decision is not consistent with a duty of beneficence to patients. If society chooses, through a democratic process, to limit care for children in some medical circumstances, consideration of justice may override our duty of beneficence. Until society has made such choices, physicians should remain advocates for their own patients. When the benefits of care are unclear, high costs become a more legitimate consideration for clinicians.

Mechanisms for Resolution of Ethical Issues

Most hospitals within the United States have ethics committees that have been organized to offer support for clinicians faced with ethical dilemmas. Ethics committees are usually designed to have three functions: case consultation, policy development, and education for staff and the community. Those serving on ethics committees should be from a variety of disciplines within the hospital community, and they must have made a commitment to study the discipline. In the case consultation function, committees are available to provide guidance to patients, families, and medical staff when ethical issues arise around an active case. The purpose of case consultation is usually to clarify the issues and to offer guidance on appropriate responses. Often physicians and families have a clear idea of what they believe is right but would like support for the difficult decisions.

Ethics committees are usually not decision-making bodies; decision-making authority remains with the patient, family, and physicians. In addition, most ethics committees become involved in a case only at the request of those involved with the case. With education and experience, ethics committees can provide valuable support to providers, patients, and institutions in this complex area of medicine.

REFERENCES

Arras JD. Toward an ethic of ambiguity. Hastings Cent Rep 1984;14:25–33.

Beauchamp T, Childress J. Principles of Biomedical Ethics. New York: Oxford University Press, 1989.

Brock DW. Children's competence for health care decision making. *In* Kopelman LM, Moskop JC (eds). Children and Health Care: Moral and Social Issues. Norwell, Mass: Kluwer Academic Press, 1989.

Fiedler LA. The tyranny of the normal. Hastings Cent Rep 1984;14:40–42.

Holder AR. Minors' right to consent to medical care. JAMA 1987;257:3400–3402.

Katz J. The Silent World of Doctor and Patient. New York: The Free Press, 1984.

Meisel A. Legal myths about terminating life support. Arch Intern Med 1991;151:1497–1502.

Murphy MA. The family with a handicapped child: A review of the literature. Dev Behav Pediatr 1992;3:73–82.

Pelligrino E. Can ethics be taught? An essay. Mt Sinai J Med 1989;56:490–494.

Wolraich ML, Siperstein GN, O'Keefe P. Pediatricians' perceptions of mentally retarded individuals. Pediatrics 1987;80:643–649.

SECTION TWO

PRACTICAL STRATEGIES

Respiratory Disorders

6 Sore Throat

Robert R. Tanz   Stanford T. Shulman

Sore throat is a common complaint that prompts patients to seek medical care. In 1990 it was estimated that nearly 18.9 million patients in the United States visited office-based physicians because of throat complaints. The large majority of these illnesses are nonbacterial and do not require or benefit from antibiotic therapy (Tables 6–1 to 6–3). On the other hand, acute streptococcal pharyngitis warrants accurate diagnosis and therapy to prevent serious suppurative and nonsuppurative complications. Furthermore, life-threatening infectious complications of streptococcal and nonstreptococcal oropharyngeal infections may present with mouth pain, pharyngitis, parapharyngeal space infectious extension, and airway obstruction (Tables 6–4 and 6–5).

VIRAL PHARYNGITIS

Most episodes of pharyngitis are caused by viruses (see Tables 6–2 and 6–3). It is difficult to distinguish clinically between viral and bacterial pharyngitis with a very high degree of precision, but certain clues may help the physician. Accompanying symptoms of conjunctivitis, rhinitis, croup, or laryngitis are common with viral infection but rare in bacterial pharyngitis.

Many viral agents can produce pharyngitis (see Tables 6–2 and 6–3). Some cause distinct clinical syndromes that are readily diagnosed without laboratory testing (Table 6–6). In pharyngitis caused by parainfluenza and influenza viruses, rhinoviruses, coronaviruses and respiratory syncytial virus (RSV), the symptoms of coryza and cough often overshadow sore throat, which is generally mild. Influenza virus may cause high fever, cough, headache, malaise, myalgias, and cervical adenopathy in addition to pharyngitis. In younger children, croup or bronchiolitis may develop. Respiratory syncytial virus is associated with bronchiolitis, pneumonia, and croup in young children. RSV infection in older children is usually indistinguishable from a simple upper respiratory tract infection. Pharyngitis is not a prominent finding of RSV infection in either age group. Parainfluenza viruses are associated with croup and bronchiolitis; minor sore throat and signs of pharyngitis are common at the outset but rapidly resolve. Episodes of infections caused by parainfluenza, influenza, and RSV are often seen in seasonal (winter) epidemics.

Adenoviruses can cause upper and lower respiratory tract disease, ranging from ordinary colds to severe pneumonia. The incubation period of adenovirus infection is 2 to 4 days. Upper respiratory infection typically produces fever, erythema of the pharynx, and follicular hyperplasia of the tonsils together with exudate. Enlargement of the cervical lymph nodes occurs frequently. When conjunctivitis occurs in association with adenoviral pharyngitis, the resulting syndrome is called *pharyngoconjunctival fever.* Pharyngitis may last as long as 7 days and does not respond to antibiotics.

There are many adenovirus serotypes; adenovirus infections may therefore develop in children more than once. Laboratory studies may reveal a leukocytosis and an elevated erythrocyte sedimentation rate. Outbreaks have been associated with swimming pools and contaminated health care workers.

The *enteroviruses* (coxsackievirus and echovirus) can cause sore throat, especially in the summer. High fever is common. The throat is slightly red; tonsillar exudate and cervical adenopathy are unusual. Resolution of symptoms occurs within a few days. Enteroviruses can cause meningitis, rash, and two specific syndromes that involve the oropharynx.

Herpangina is characterized by distinctive discrete, painful, gray-white papulovesicular lesions distributed over the posterior oropharynx (see Table 6–6). The vesicles are 1 to 2 mm in diameter and are initially surrounded by a halo of erythema before they ulcerate. Fever may reach 39.5°C. The illness generally lasts less than 7 days, but severe pain may impair fluid intake and necessitate medical support.

Coxsackievirus A16 causes *hand-foot-mouth disease.* Vesicles can occur throughout the oropharynx; they are painful, and they ulcerate. Vesicles also develop on the palms and soles, less often on the trunk or extremities. Fever is present in most cases, but many children do not appear seriously ill. This disease lasts less than 7 days.

Primary infection caused by herpes simplex virus (HSV) usually produces high fever with acute *gingivostomatitis* involving vesicles (which become ulcers) throughout the anterior portion of the mouth, including the lips. There is sparing of the posterior pharynx in herpes gingivostomatitis; the infection usually occurs in young children. High fever is common, pain is intense, and intake of oral fluids is often impaired, which may lead to dehydration. In addition, HSV may present in adolescents with respiratory complaints, such as pharyngitis. Approximately 35% of new-onset HSV-positive adolescent patients have herpetic lesions; most patients with HSV pharyngitis cannot be distinguished from patients with other causes of their illnesses. The classic syndrome of herpetic gingivostomatitis in infants and toddlers lasts up to 2 weeks; data on the course of more benign HSV pharyngitis are lacking. The differential diagnosis of vesicular-ulcerating oral lesions is noted in Table 6–6. A common cause of a local and large lesion of unknown etiology is aphthous stomatitis (Fig. 6–1). Some children have periodic fever (recurrent), aphthous stomatitis, pharyngitis, and cervical adenitis that is idiopathic and may respond to oral cimetidine (40 mg/kg/day).

Experience with infants and toddlers during a measles epidemic in Chicago emphasizes the prominence of oral findings early in the course of this disease. In addition to high fever, cough, coryza, and conjunctivitis, the pharynx may be intensely and diffusely erythematous, without tonsillar enlargement or exudate. The presence of *Koplik spots*, the pathognomonic white or blue-white enan-

Table 6-1. Etiology of Sore Throat

Infection

Bacterial (see Tables 6–2, 6–3)
Viral (see Tables 6–2, 6–3)
Fungal (see Table 6–3)
Neutropenic mucositis (invasive anaerobic mouth flora)
Tonsillitis
Epiglottitis
Uvulitis
Peritonsillar abscess (quinsy sore throat)
Retropharyngeal abscess (prevertebral space)
Ludwig angina (submandibular space)
Lateral pharyngeal space cellulitis-abscess
Buccal space cellulitis
Suppurative thyroiditis
Lemierre disease (septic jugular thrombophlebitis)
Vincent angina (mixed anaerobic bacteria–gingivitis–pharyngitis)

Irritation

Cigarette smoking
Inhaled irritants
Reflux esophagitis
Chemical toxins (caustic agents)
Paraquat ingestion
Smog
Dry hot air
Hot foods, liquids

Other

Tumor, including Kaposi sarcoma, leukemia
Wegener granulomatosis
Sarcoidosis
Glossopharyngeal neuralgia
Foreign body
Stylohyoid syndrome
Behçet disease
Kawasaki syndrome
Posterior pharyngeal trauma—pseudodiverticulum
Pneumomediastinum
Hematoma
Systemic lupus erythematosus
Bullous pemphigoid
Syndrome of periodic fever, aphthous stomatitis, pharyngitis, cervical adenitis

Table 6-2. Infectious Etiology of Pharyngitis

Definite Causes	**Probable Causes**
Streptococcus pyogenes (Group A streptococci)	Group C streptococci
Corynebacterium diphtheriae	Group G streptococci
Arcanobacterium haemolyticum	*Chlamydia pneumoniae*
Neisseria gonorrhoeae	*Chlamydia trachomatis*
Epstein-Barr virus	*Mycoplasma pneumoniae*
Parainfluenza viruses	
Influenza viruses	
Rhinoviruses	
Coronavirus	
Adenovirus	
Respiratory syncytial virus	
Herpes simplex virus	

Table 6-3. Additional Potential Pathogens Associated with Sore Throat

Bacteria	**Virus**	**Fungus**
Fusobacterium necrophorum (Lemierre disease)	Coxsackievirus A, B	*Candida* species
Neisseria meningitidis	Cytomegalovirus	Histoplasmosis
Yersinia enterocolitica	Viral hemorrhagic fevers	Cryptococcosis
Tularemia (oropharyngeal)	Human immunodeficiency virus (HIV) (primary infection)	
Yersinia pestis	Human herpesvirus 6	
Bacillus anthracis	Measles	
Chlamydia psittaci	Varicella	
Secondary syphilis	Rubella	
Mycobacterium tuberculosis		
Lyme disease		
Corynebacterium ulcerans		
Leptospira		
Mycoplasma hominis		

Table 6–4. Distinguishing Features of Parapharyngeal–Upper Respiratory Tract Infections

	Peritonsillar Abscess	Retropharyngeal Abscess (Cellulitis)	Submandibular Space (Ludwig Angina)†	Lateral Pharyngeal Space†	Masticator Space†	Epiglottitis	Laryngotracheobronchitis (Croup)	Bacterial Tracheitis	Postanginal Sepsis† (Lemierre Disease)
Etiology	Group A streptococci, oral anaerobes*	Staphylococcus aureus, oral anaerobes,* group A streptococci, "suppurative adenitis"	Oral anaerobes*	Oral anaerobes*	Oral anaerobes*	Haemophilus influenzae type b	Parainfluenza virus; influenza virus; adenovirus and respiratory syncytial virus less common	Moraxella catarrhalis, S. aureus, H. influenzae type b	Fusobacterium necrophorum
Age	Teens	Infancy, preteens, occasionally teens	Teens	Teens	Teens	2–5 yrs	3 mo–3 yr	3–10 yr	Teens
Manifestations	Initial episode of pharyngitis, followed by sudden worsening of unilateral odynophagia, trismus, hot potato (muffled) voice, drooling, displacement of uvula	Fever, dyspnea, stridor, dysphagia, drooling, stiff neck, pain, cervical adenopathy, swelling of posterior pharyngeal space Descending mediastinitis (rare) Lateral neck x-ray reveals swollen retropharyngeal prevertebral space: infants > 1 × width of adjacent vertebral body (> 2–7 mm); teens > ⅓ × width of vertebral body (> 1–7 mm) CT distinguishes cellulitis from abscess	Fever, dysphagia, odynophagia, stiff neck, dyspnea; airway obstruction, swollen tongue and floor of mouth (tender) Muffled voice	Severe pain, fever, trismus, dysphagia, edematous appearing, painful lateral facial (jaw) or neck swelling (induration) May lead to Lemierre disease	Pain, prominent trismus, fever Swelling not always evident	Sudden onset high fever, toxic, muffled voice, anxious, pain, retractions, dysphagia, drooling, stridor, sitting up, leaning forward tripod position, cherry red swollen epiglottis Usually not hoarse or coughing Lateral neck x-ray shows "thumb sign" of swollen epiglottis	Low-grade fever, barking cough, hoarse-aphonia, stridor; mild retractions; x-ray shows "steeple sign" of subglottic narrowing on anteroposterior neck view	Prior history of croup with sudden onset of respiratory distress, high fever, toxic, hoarseness, stridor, barking cough, tripod sitting position; x-ray as per croup plus ragged tracheal air column	Prior pharyngitis with sudden onset fever, chills, odynophagia, neck pain, septic thrombophlebitis of internal jugular vein with septic emboli (e.g., lungs, joints)
Treatment	Penicillin for abscess and cellulitis Aspiration for abscess (needle or I and D) Needle is preferred	Airway management, nafcillin, ceftriaxone Surgical drainage if an abscess	Airway management Penicillin, clindamycin Rarely surgical drainage	Penicillin, clindamycin Surgical drainage usually required	Penicillin, clindamycin	Airway management (intubation), ceftriaxone	Airway management (rare) Cool mist, racemic epinephrine, dexamethasone	Airway management (frequent intubation) Ceftriaxone with or without nafcillin	Clindamycin, penicillin, or cefoxitin

*Peptostreptococcus, Fusobacterium, Bacteroides (usually melaninogenicus).
†Often odontogenic; check for tooth abscess, caries, tender teeth.

53

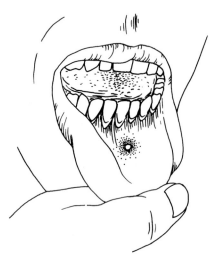

Figure 6–1. Aphthous stomatitis ("canker sore"). (From Reilly BM. Sore throat. In Practical Strategies in Outpatient Medicine, 2nd ed. Philadelphia: WB Saunders, 1991.)

them of measles, on the buccal mucosa near the mandibular molars provides evidence of the correct diagnosis before the rash develops.

INFECTIOUS MONONUCLEOSIS

Pathogenesis

Acute exudative pharyngitis commonly occurs with infectious mononucleosis caused by primary infection with Epstein-Barr virus (EBV) (Table 6–7). Mononucleosis is a febrile, systemic, self-limited lymphoproliferative disorder that is usually associated with hepatosplenomegaly and generalized lymphadenopathy. The pharyngitis associated with infectious mononucleosis may be mild or severe, with significant tonsillar hypertrophy (possibly producing airway obstruction), erythema, and impressive tonsillar exudates. Regional lymph nodes may be particularly enlarged and slightly tender.

Infectious mononucleosis usually occurs in adolescents and young adults; it is also a frequent infection with generally milder clinical manifestations or is subclinical among preadolescent children. In United States high school and college students, attack rates

Table 6–5. "Red Flags" Associated with Sore Throat

Fever > 2 weeks
Duration > 2 weeks
Trismus
Drooling
Cyanosis
Hemorrhage
Asymmetric tonsillar swelling or asymmetric cervical adenopathy
Respiratory distress (airway obstruction)
Suspicion of parapharyngeal space infection
Suspicion of diphtheria (bull neck, uvula paralysis, thick membrane)
Apnea
Severe unremitting pain
"Hot potato" voice
Weight loss

of 200 to 800 per 100,000 population per year have been estimated. Epstein-Barr virus is transmitted primarily by saliva.

Clinical Features

After a 2- to 4-week incubation period, patients with infectious mononucleosis usually experience an abrupt onset of malaise, fatigue, fever, and headache, followed closely by pharyngitis. The tonsils are enlarged with exudates and cervical adenopathy. More generalized adenopathy with hepatosplenomegaly often follows. Fever and pharyngitis typically last 1 to 3 weeks, while lymphadenopathy and hepatosplenomegaly subside over 3 to 6 weeks. Malaise and lethargy can persist for several months, possibly leading to impaired school or work performance.

Diagnosis

Laboratory studies of diagnostic value include atypical lymphocytosis; these lymphocytes are primarily EBV-specific, cytotoxic T lymphocytes that represent a reactive response to EBV-infected B lymphocytes. A modest elevation of the serum transaminase level is common, reflecting EBV hepatitis. Tests useful for diagnosis include detection of heterophile antibodies that react with bovine erythrocytes (most often detected by the monospot test) and specific antibody against EBV viral capsid antigen (VCA), early antigen (EA), and nuclear antigen (EBNA). Acute infectious mononucleosis is usually associated with a positive heterophile test and antibody to VCA and EA (Fig. 6–2).

The findings of acute exudative pharyngitis together with hepatomegaly, splenomegaly, and generalized lymphadenopathy suggest infectious mononucleosis. Early in the disease and in cases without liver or spleen enlargement, differentiation from other causes of pharyngitis, including streptococcal pharyngitis, is difficult. Indeed, a small number of patients with infectious mononucleosis may have a positive throat culture for group A streptococci. Serologic evidence of mononucleosis should be sought when splenomegaly or other features are present or if symptoms persist beyond 7 days.

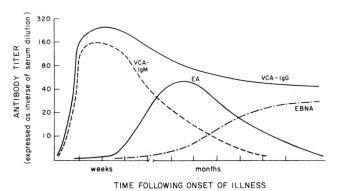

Figure 6–2. Typical human serologic response to Epstein-Barr virus infection. At time of clinical presentation (usually 2 to 7 weeks after exposure), anti-VCA (viral capsid antigen) response may consist of IgM and IgG antibodies; anti-EA (early antigen) response is often present; and anti-EBNA (nuclear antigen) is usually negative. The IgM anti-VCA response usually subsides within 2 to 4 months, and the anti-EA response usually disappears within 2 to 6 months. (Data from Andiman WA, et al. J Pediatr 1981;99:880–886; Fleisher GR, et al. J Infect Dis 1979;139:553–558; Brown NA. The Epstein-Barr virus [infectious mononucleosis, B-lymphoproliferative disorders]. In Feigin RD, Cherry JD [eds]. Textbook of Pediatric Infectious Diseases, 2nd ed. Philadelphia: WB Saunders, 1987.)

Table 6–6. Vesicular-Ulcerating Eruptions of the Mouth and Pharynx

	Gingivostomatitis	Herpangina	Hand-Foot-Mouth Disease	Chickenpox	Systemic Lupus Erythematosus (SLE)	Inflammatory Bowel Disease (IBD)	Aphthous Stomatitis	Behçet Disease	Vincent Stomatitis	Recurrent Scarifying Ulcerative Stomatitis (Sutton Disease)
Etiology	Herpes simplex virus (HSV) I	Coxsackievirus A, B; echovirus or HSV (rarely)	Coxsackievirus A, coxsackievirus B (rarely)	Varicella-zoster virus	Unknown, autoimmune	Unknown, autoimmune	Unknown	Unknown; vasculitis	Unknown or anaerobic bacteria	Unknown
Location	Ulcerative vesicles of pharynx, tongue, palate plus lesions of mucocutaneous (perioral) margin	Anterior fauces (tonsils), soft palate (uvula), less often pharynx	Tongue, buccal mucosa, palate, palms, soles, anterior oral cavity	Tongue, gingiva, buccal mucosa, marked cutaneous lesions; trunk > face	Oral, nasal mucosa; palate, pharynx, buccal mucosa	As in aphthous stomatitis	Lips, tongue, buccal mucosa, oropharynx	Oral (similar to aphthous stomatitis); genital ulcers	Gingiva; ulceration at base of teeth	Tongue; buccal mucosa
Age	Less than 5 yr	3–10 yr	1 yr–teens	Any age	Any age	Any age	Teens and adults	Teens, adults, occasionally < 10 yr	Teens; if younger, consider immunodeficiency and blood dyscrasia	Teens
Manifestations	Fever, mouth pain, toxic, fetid breath, drooling, anorexia, cervical lymphadenopathy; cracked, swollen hemorrhagic gums; second-degree inoculation possible (fingers, eye, skin); reactivation with long latency (any age)	Fever, sore throat, odynophagia; summer outbreaks; 6–12 lesions (2–4 mm) papule → vesicle → ulceration; headache, myalgias	Painful bilateral vesicles, fever	Fever, pruritic cutaneous vesicles, painful oral lesions	Renal, central nervous system, arthritis, cutaneous, hematologic, other organ involvement; ulcers minimally to moderately painful; may be painless	Similar to aphthous stomatitis	Multiple recurrences; painful ulcerations 1–2 mm, but may be 5–15 mm	Painful ulcerations (heal without scarring); uveitis, arthralgia, arthritis, lower gastrointestinal ulceration (similar to IBD); recurrences; spontaneous remissions	Fever, bleeding gums; gray membrane	Deep, large, painful ulcerations; relapsing; scarring with distortion of mucosa
Treatment	Avoid dehydration; acyclovir if immunocompromised	Avoid dehydration; rarely secondary aseptic meningitis or myocarditis	Avoid dehydration	Avoid dehydration, secondary infection; acyclovir if immunocompromised	Specific therapy for SLE	Specific therapy for IBD	Topical corticosteroids; must exclude SLE, IBD, human immunodeficiency virus (HIV), Behçet disease	Topical corticosteroids; oral (viscous) lidocaine	Oral hygiene; tetracycline wash	Topical corticosteroids, analgesics; must rule out malignancy by biopsy

Table 6–7. Manifestations of Infectious Mononucleosis (Epstein-Barr Virus)

Common
  Fever (1–2 weeks)
  Lymphadenopathy (bilateral, minimally tender
    primarily cervical nodes with axillary, inguinal,
    epitrochlear, supraclavicular nodes)
  Tonsillopharyngitis (exudative)
  Splenomegaly
  Hepatomegaly
  Elevated liver enzymes (transaminases)
  Malaise
  Fatigue

Less Common
  Rash (spontaneous or associated with ampicillin or
    allopurinol)
  Oropharyngeal petechiae
  Jaundice
  Eyelid edema
  Abdominal pain
  Thrombocytopenia—purpura
  Hemolytic or aplastic anemia—pallor
  Severe upper airway obstruction
  Meningoencephalitis
  Guillain-Barré syndrome
  Bell's palsy (seventh cranial nerve)
  Hemophagocytic syndrome
  X-linked lymphoproliferative disorder (Duncan
    syndrome)
  Lymphoproliferative disorder in immunocompromised
    hosts
  Splenic rupture
  Glomerulonephritis
  Orchitis

Treatment

Patients with infectious mononucleosis require supportive treatment. Corticosteroids may be indicated for acute life-threatening conditions, such as airway obstruction from enlarged tonsils.

GROUP A STREPTOCOCCAL INFECTION

In the evaluation of a patient with sore throat, the primary concern is accurate diagnosis and treatment of pharyngitis caused by group A streptococci (GAS), which accounts for about 15% of all episodes of pharyngitis. The preoccupation with this pathogen is well deserved: the sequelae of group A streptococcal pharyngitis, especially acute rheumatic fever and acute glomerulonephritis (AGN), at one time resulted in considerable morbidity and mortality in the United States and continue to do so in many parts of the world. Prevention of acute rheumatic fever in particular depends on accurate, timely diagnosis of streptococcal pharyngitis and prompt antibiotic treatment.

Billroth coined the term streptococcus in 1868 (from the Greek *streptos* = chain, *kokkos* = berry). In 1923, Felty and Hodges established the relationship between acute pharyngitis and beta-hemolytic streptococci. About 1930, Rebecca Lancefield identified the serologically distinct cell wall carbohydrates of various beta-hemolytic streptococci and arbitrarily used letters to denote them. Group A streptococci are thus characterized by the presence of group A carbohydrate in the cell wall, and they are further distin-

guished by several kinds of cell wall protein antigens (M, R, T). These protein antigens are useful for studies of epidemiology and pathogenesis.

Clinical Epidemiology

Before World War II, streptococcal pharyngitis was identified mainly in well-defined epidemics. Since then, group A streptococcal pharyngitis has been endemic in the United States and it occurs sporadically. Episodes typically peak in the late winter and early spring; children from 5 to 11 years old have the highest rates of group A streptococcal pharyngitis. This infection is less common before age 3 and after age 11, but it can occur at all ages.

Spread of group A streptococci in classrooms and among family members, especially in crowded living conditions, is common. Transmission occurs primarily by inhalation of organisms in large droplets or by direct contact with respiratory secretions. Pets do not appear to be a frequent reservoir of group A streptococci. Untreated streptococcal pharyngitis is particularly contagious early in the acute illness and for the first 2 weeks after the organism has been acquired. Appropriate antibiotic therapy rapidly eliminates contagiousness. Within 24 hours of institution of therapy with penicillin, it is difficult to isolate group A streptococci from patients with acute streptococcal pharyngitis, and children can return to school.

Clinical Features

The classic patient with acute streptococcal pharyngitis presents with the sudden onset of fever and sore throat. Headache, malaise, abdominal pain, nausea, and vomiting occur frequently. Cough, rhinorrhea, conjunctivitis, stridor, diarrhea, and hoarseness are distinctly unusual and suggest a viral etiology.

Examination of the patient reveals marked pharyngeal erythema. Petechiae may be noted on the palate but also can occur in viral pharyngitis (see Table 6–7). Tonsils are enlarged, symmetric, and red, with patchy exudates on their surfaces. The papillae of the tongue may be red and swollen, leading to the designation ''strawberry tongue.'' Tender, enlarged anterior cervical lymph nodes are often found.

Combinations of these signs can be used to assist in diagnosis; in particular, tonsillar exudates in association with fever, palatal petechiae, and tender anterior cervical adenitis should strongly suggest group A streptococci. However, other diseases can produce this constellation of findings. Some or all of these classic characteristics may be absent in patients with streptococcal pharyngitis. Younger children often have coryza with crusting below the nares, more generalized adenopathy, and a more chronic course, a syndrome called *streptococcosis*.

When rash accompanies the illness, accurate clinical diagnosis is easier. *Scarlet fever*, so-called because of the characteristic fine, diffuse red rash, is essentially pathognomonic for infection with group A streptococci. Scarlet fever is rarely seen in children younger than 3 years old or in adults.

SCARLET FEVER

The rash of scarlet fever is caused by infection with a strain of group A streptococci that contains a bacteriophage encoding for production of an erythrogenic (redness-producing) toxin, usually erythrogenic (or pyrogenic) exotoxin A. Scarlet fever is simply group A streptococcal pharyngitis with a rash and should be explained as such to patients and their families. Although patients with the *streptococcal toxic shock syndrome* also appear to be infected with group A streptococci that produce erythrogenic toxin A, most infections with group A streptococci are not associated with unusual severity (Table 6–8). Streptococcal toxic shock syndrome is usually associated with a primary cutaneous rather than a pharyngeal focus of infection.

The rash of scarlet fever feels like sandpaper and blanches with pressure. It usually begins on the face, but after 24 hours it becomes generalized. The face, especially the cheeks, is red, and the area around the mouth often appears pale in comparison (circumoral pallor). Accentuation of erythema occurs in flexor skin creases, especially in the antecubital fossae (Pastia's lines). The erythema begins to fade within a few days. Desquamation begins within a week of onset on the face and progresses downward, often resembling that seen subsequent to a mild sunburn. Occasionally, sheet-like desquamation occurs around the free margins of the fingernails and is usually more coarse than the desquamation seen with Kawasaki disease. Differential diagnosis of scarlet fever includes Kawasaki disease, measles, and staphylococcal toxic shock syndrome (Table 6–9).

Table 6–8. Characteristics of Severe Invasive-Toxigenic Group A Streptococcal Infection

Positive Culture Sites
Blood
Soft tissue abscess
Synovial fluid
Throat
Peritoneal fluid
Surgical wound
Cellulitis aspirate

Clinical Manifestations	*Laboratory Manifestations*
Fever	Leukocytosis
Toxic shock*	Lymphopenia
Confusion	Thrombocytopenia
Headache	Hyponatremia
Abdominal pain	Hypoalbuminemia
Vomiting	Hyperbilirubinemia
Local extremity pain and	(direct)
swelling	Elevated AST, ALT
Hypesthesia	Renal sediment
Cellulitis	abnormalities
Scarlatiniform rash (40%)	Coagulopathy
Erythroderma (25%)	
Conjunctival injection	
Red pharynx	
Pneumonia with or	
without empyema	
Osteomyelitis	
Vaginitis	
Proctitis	
Desquamation	
Necrotizing fasciitis	
Diarrhea	

*Case definition of streptococcal toxic shock syndrome requires (I) isolation of group A streptococci from: (a) a normally sterile site (blood, synovial or peritoneal fluid) or (b) a nonsterile site (throat, wound). (II) Severity is defined by (a) hypotension and (b) two or more of renal impairment, coagulopathy, liver involvement, adult respiratory distress syndrome, a generalized erythematous macular rash (with or without later desquamation), and soft tissue necrosis (necrotizing fasciitis, myositis, gangrene). The definitive diagnosis requires criteria IA and IIA plus B. Criteria IB and IIA plus B are considered probable if no other identifiable cause is present.

Abbreviations: ALT = alanine aminotransferase; AST = aspartate aminotransferase.

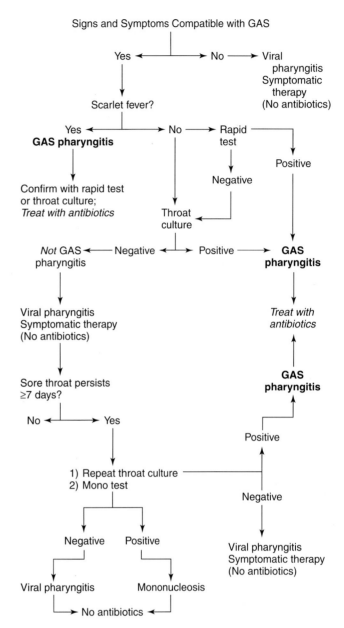

Figure 6–3. Management of patients with sore throat. GAS = group A streptococci.

Diagnosis

Although signs and symptoms may strongly suggest acute streptococcal pharyngitis, laboratory diagnosis is strongly recommended, even for patients with scarlet fever (Fig. 6–3). Scoring systems for diagnosing acute group A streptococcal pharyngitis on clinical grounds have not proved very useful. Using clinical criteria alone, physicians have overestimated the likelihood that patients have streptococcal infection. The throat culture has traditionally been used to diagnose streptococcal pharyngitis. Plating a swab of the posterior pharynx and tonsils on sheep blood agar, identifying beta-hemolytic colonies, and testing them for the presence of sensitivity to a bacitracin-impregnated disc is the "gold standard" diagnostic test, but it takes 24 to 48 hours. A number of rapid diagnostic tests that take less than 30 minutes have been developed. These "rapid strep" antigen detection tests generally use enzyme-linked immunosorbent assay (ELISA) or latex agglutination meth-

Table 6–9. Differential Diagnosis of Scarlet Fever

	Scarlet Fever	Kawasaki Disease	Measles	Staphylococcal Toxic Shock Syndrome	Staphylococcal Scalded Skin Syndrome
Agent	Group A streptococci	Unknown	Measles virus	*Staphylococcus aureus*	*S. aureus*
Age range	All (peak 5–15 yr)	Usually <5 yr	<2 yr, 10–20 yr	All (especially >10 yr)	Usually <5 yr
Prodrome	No	No	Fever, coryza, cough, conjunctivitis	Usually no	No
Enanthem	No	Occasionally	Koplik spots	No	Limited
Mouth	Strawberry tongue, exudative pharyngitis, palatal petechiae	Erythema; red, cracked lips, strawberry tongue	Diffusely red, no cracked lips	Usually normal	Erythema
Rash	Fine, red, "sandpaper," periungual membranous desquamation, circumoral pallor, Pastia lines	Variable polymorphic erythematous face, trunk, and diaper area; tips of fingers and toes desquamate 11–12 days after onset	Maculopapular; progressing from forehead to feet; may desquamate	Diffuse erythroderma; desquamates	Erythema, painful bullous lesions; positive Nikolsky sign; desquamates
Other	Cervical adenitis, gallbladder hydrops, fever	Coronary artery disease; fever >5 days; conjunctival (nonpurulent) injection; tender, swollen hands and feet; cervical adenopathy (size >1.5 cm); thrombocytosis; pyuria (sterile); gallbladder hydrops	"Toxic" looking; dehydration; encephalitis, pneumonia; fever	Shock (hypotension, including orthostatic); encephalopathy; diarrhea; headache	Fever, cracked lips; conjunctivitis

ods to detect the presence of the cell wall group A carbohydrate antigen of group A streptococci following acid extraction of organisms obtained by throat swab. Rapid strep tests are highly *specific* (generally >95%), with the throat culture used as the standard. Specificity reflects the percentage of positive results that come from patients who truly harbor group A streptococci. Unfortunately, the *sensitivity* (the percentage of true-positives identified by antigen detection) of most of these rapid tests is considerably lower. Although the sensitivities of these tests are 80% to 85%, they can be much lower, which results in frequent false negative tests and the correct diagnosis of streptococcal pharyngitis being missed.

The low sensitivity of these tests, coupled with their excellent specificity, has led to the recommendation that two swabs should be obtained from patients with suspected streptococcal pharyngitis. One swab is used for a rapid test. When the rapid antigen detection test is positive, it is highly likely that the patient has group A streptococcal infection, and the extra swab can be discarded. When the rapid test is negative, group A streptococci may still be present; thus, the extra swab should then be processed for culture in routine fashion.

In general, patients with a negative rapid test do not require treatment before culture verification unless there is a particularly high index of suspicion that group A streptococci are involved (e.g., scarlet fever, peritonsillar abscess, or tonsillar exudates plus tender cervical adenopathy plus palatal petechiae plus fever and recent exposure to a person with group A streptococcal pharyngitis).

Rapid tests are designed for the diagnosis of acute streptococcal pharyngitis, and they should not be used to evaluate the effectiveness of therapy, because a positive result in an asymptomatic patient does not distinguish between infection, colonization, or the presence of nonviable organisms. A negative result must be confirmed by throat culture.

Testing patients for serologic evidence of an antibody response to extracellular products of group A streptococci (such as streptolysin O) is not useful to diagnose acute pharyngitis. Because it generally takes several weeks for antibody levels to rise, streptococcal antibody tests are valid only for determining past infection. Specific antibodies include antistreptolysin O (ASO), anti-DNase B, and antihyaluronidase (AHT). When antibody testing is desired to evaluate a possible post-streptococcal illness, more than one of these tests should be performed to improve sensitivity. The Streptozyme test, an assay that uses latex particles coated with group A streptococcal broth culture supernatants, is poorly standardized and therefore cannot be recommended.

Treatment

The primary indication for treating acute streptococcal pharyngitis is to prevent the development of acute rheumatic fever. Treatment begun within 9 days of the onset of group A streptococcal pharyngitis is effective in preventing acute rheumatic fever. Therapy does not appear to affect the risk of the other nonsuppurative sequela, acute post-streptococcal glomerulonephritis. Antibiotic therapy also reduces the incidence of suppurative sequelae of group A streptococcal pharyngitis, such as peritonsillar abscess and cervical adenitis.

In addition, treatment effects a more rapid resolution of signs and symptoms also terminates contagiousness within 24 hours.

For these reasons, antibiotics should be instituted as soon as the diagnosis is supported by laboratory studies.

The drug of choice for treating streptococcal pharyngitis is penicillin. Despite the widespread use of penicillin to treat streptococcal and other infections, penicillin resistance among group A streptococci has not developed. Penicillin can be given by mouth for 10 days (125 to 250 mg of penicillin V, three or four times each day) or intramuscularly as a single injection of benzathine penicillin (600,000 units for patients who weigh under 60 pounds [27 kg], 1.2 million units for those weighing 60 pounds [27 kg] or more). Although it is a painful drug, use of intramuscular benzathine penicillin alleviates concern with patient compliance. A less painful alternative is 900,000 units of benzathine penicillin in combination with 300,000 units of procaine penicillin for all patients. Intramuscular procaine penicillin alone is inadequate for prevention of acute rheumatic fever because adequate levels of penicillin are not present in blood and tissues for a sufficient time. Other beta-lactams, including semisynthetic derivatives of penicillin and the cephalosporins, are at least as effective as penicillin for treating group A streptococcal pharyngitis. Their broader spectrum, their much greater cost, and the lack of formal data concerning prevention of acute rheumatic fever currently relegate them to second-line status. The decreased frequency of dose administration of some of these agents may improve patient compliance, compared with oral penicillin, and makes their use attractive in selected circumstances.

Patients who are allergic to penicillin should receive erythromycin or another non–beta-lactam antibiotic, such as clindamycin. Resistance of group A streptococci to erythromycin has been reported in such areas as Japan, France, Spain, and Finland, where erythromycin is widely used. This has not yet emerged as a problem in the United States. Sulfa drugs, including sulfamethoxazole combined with trimethoprim, tetracyclines, and chloramphenicol should not be used for treatment of acute streptococcal pharyngitis because they do not eradicate group A streptococci.

Complications

SUPPURATIVE COMPLICATIONS

Antibiotic therapy has greatly reduced the likelihood of developing suppurative complications of group A streptococcal infections that are due to spread of group A streptococci from the pharynx or middle ear to adjacent structures. *Peritonsillar abscess* ("quinsy") presents with fever, severe throat pain, dysphagia, "hot potato voice," pain referred to the ear, and bulging of the peritonsillar area with asymmetry of the tonsils and sometimes displacement of the uvula (Fig. 6–4; see Table 6–4). Occasionally, there is peritonsillar cellulitis without a well-defined abscess cavity. Trismus may be present. When an abscess is found clinically or by an imaging study such as a computed tomography (CT) scan, surgical drainage is indicated.

Retropharyngeal abscess represents extension of infection from the pharynx or peritonsillar region into the retropharyngeal (prevertebral) space, which is rich in lymphoid structures (Figs. 6–5 and 6–6; see Table 6–4). Fever, dysphagia, drooling, stridor, extension of the neck, and a mass in the posterior pharyngeal wall may be noted. Surgical drainage is often required if frank suppuration has occurred. Spread of group A streptococci via pharyngeal lymphatics to regional nodes can cause *cervical lymphadenitis*. The markedly swollen and tender anterior cervical nodes that result can suppurate.

Otitis media, mastoiditis, and sinusitis also may occur as complications of group A streptococcal pharyngitis. Additional parapharyngeal suppurative infections which may mimic streptococcal disease are noted in Table 6–4. Furthermore, any pharyngeal infectious process may produce torticollis if there is inflammation that extends to the paraspinal muscles and ligaments, producing pain, spasm, and occasionally rotary subluxation of the cervical spine.

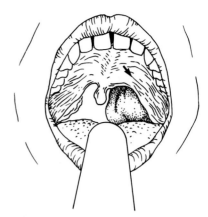

Figure 6–4. Peritonsillar abscess (quinsy, sore throat). The left tonsil is asymmetrically inflamed and swollen; there is displacement of the uvula to the opposite side. The supratonsillar space *(arrow)* is also swollen; here is the usual site of the surgical incision for drainage. Prominent unilateral cervical adenopathy typically coexists. (From Reilly BM. Sore throat. *In* Practical Strategies in Outpatient Medicine, 2nd ed. Philadelphia: WB Saunders, 1991.)

The differential diagnosis of torticollis is presented in Table 6–10. Oropharyngeal torticollis lasts less than 2 weeks and is not associated with abnormal neurologic signs or pain over the spinous process.

NONSUPPURATIVE SEQUELAE

Nonsuppurative complications include acute rheumatic fever (see Chapter 16), acute post-streptococcal glomerulonephritis (see Chapter 29), and possibly reactive arthritis/synovitis. As noted above, prevention of acute rheumatic fever and resultant permanent rheumatic heart disease is the principal reason to treat group A streptococcal pharyngitis. Therapy with an appropriate antibiotic within 9 days of onset of symptoms is highly effective in preventing this complication. In contrast to acute rheumatic fever, acute glomerulonephritis does not appear to be prevented by treatment of the antecedent streptococcal infection. Pharyngitis that is caused by one of the nephritogenic strains of group A streptococci precedes symptoms by about 10 days. Unlike acute rheumatic fever, which occurs only after group A streptococcal pharyngitis, acute glomerulonephritis also can follow group A streptococcal skin infection.

TREATMENT FAILURE AND CHRONIC CARRIAGE

Treatment with penicillin may cure group A streptococcal pharyngitis but may be unable to eradicate group A streptococci from the pharynx in approximately 25% of patients (Fig. 6–7). This causes considerable consternation among patients and their families. Penicillin resistance is not the cause of treatment failure. A small proportion of these patients are symptomatic and are thus characterized as having *clinical treatment failure*. Reinfection with the same or a different strain is possible, as is intercurrent viral pharyngitis. Some of these patients may be chronic pharyngeal carriers of group A streptococci who are suffering from a new superimposed viral infection; others may be noncompliant with therapy. However, patients who are treated with intramuscular benzathine penicillin do not respond to treatment.

Many patients who do not respond to bacteriologic treatment are asymptomatic and are identified when follow-up culture specimens

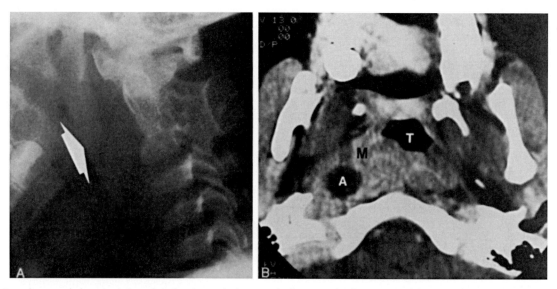

Figure 6–5. Retropharyngeal abscess. *A,* Lateral neck radiograph shows marked increased soft tissue *(arrow)* between the upper airway air and cervical spine. *B,* Axial CT scan shows the lower attenuation center of the abscess (A), the anterior and leftward shift of the trachea (T), and the soft tissue mass (M) of abscess and surrounding edema. (Courtesy of A. Oestreich, M.D., Cincinnati, Ohio.)

are obtained, a practice that is usually unnecessary. If patients are compliant with therapy, they are at minimal risk for acute rheumatic fever. One explanation for asymptomatic persistence of group A streptococci after treatment is that these patients were chronic carriers of group A streptococci who were initially symptomatic because of a concurrent viral pharyngitis and who did not truly have acute streptococcal pharyngitis.

Patients who are chronically colonized with group A streptococci are called *chronic carriers.* Carriers do not appear to be at risk for acute rheumatic fever or for development of suppurative complications, and they are rarely sources of spread of group A streptococci

in the community. There is no reason to exclude these carriers from school.

There is no easy way to identify chronic carriers prospectively among patients with symptoms of acute pharyngitis. Streptococcal antibody titers are often elevated in carriers, and neither they nor

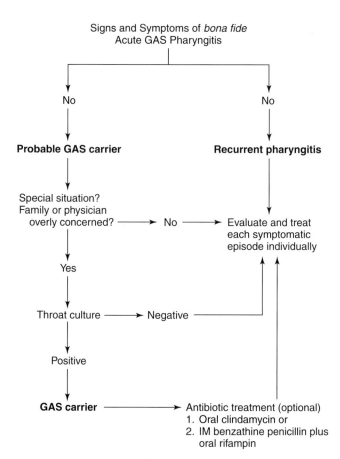

Figure 6–6. Normally, in a teenager the retropharyngeal space does not exceed 7 mm when measured from the anterior aspect of the C-2 vertebral body to the posterior pharynx. In infants the retropharyngeal space is usually less than one width of the adjacent vertebral body. However, with crying this distance may be three widths of the vertebral body. Also, under normal circumstances, the retrotracheal space does not exceed 22 mm in teenagers when measured from the anterior aspect of C-6 to the trachea. *Dotted lines* depict the "thumbprint" sign noted on a lateral neck x-ray made by a swollen epiglottis. (From Reilly BM. Sore throat. *In Practical Strategies in Outpatient Medicine,* 2nd ed. Philadelphia: WB Saunders, 1991.)

Figure 6–7. Management of patients with repeated or frequent positive rapid tests or throat cultures. GAS = group A streptococci; IM = intramuscular.

Table 6-10. Differential Diagnosis of Torticollis (Wryneck)

Congenital
  Muscular torticollis
  Positional deformation
  Hemivertebra (cervicosuperior dorsal spine)
  Unilateral atlanto-occipital fusion
  Klippel-Feil syndrome
  Unilateral absence of sternocleidomastoid
  Pterygium colli

Trauma
  Muscular injury (cervical muscles)
  Atlanto-occipital subluxation
  Atlantoaxial subluxation
  C2–C3 subluxation
  Rotary subluxation
  Fractures

Inflammation
  Cervical lymphadenitis
  Retropharyngeal abscess
  Cervical vertebral osteomyelitis
  Rheumatoid arthritis
  Spontaneous (hyperemia, edema) subluxation with adjacent
    head and neck infection (rotary subluxation syndrome)
  Upper lobe pneumonia

Neurologic
  Visual disturbances (nystagmus, superior oblique paresis)
  Dystonic drug reactions (phenothiazines, haloperidol,
    metoclopramide)
  Cervical cord tumor
  Posterior fossa brain tumor
  Syringomyelia
  Wilson disease
  Dystonia musculorum deformans
  Spasmus nutans

Other
  Acute cervical disk calcification
  Sandifer syndrome (gastroesophageal reflux, hiatal hernia)
  Benign paroxysmal torticollis
  Bone tumors (eosinophilic granuloma)
  Soft-tissue tumor
  Hysteria

From Behrman RE (ed). Nelson Textbook of Pediatrics, 14th ed. Philadelphia: WB Saunders, 1992:1718.

quantitative throat cultures have proved useful. The clinician should consider the possibility of chronic group A streptococcal carriage when a patient or a family member has multiple culture-positive episodes of pharyngitis, especially when symptoms are mild or atypical. A culture specimen that has been obtained when the suspected carrier is symptom-free or is receiving treatment with penicillin (intramuscular benzathine penicillin is recommended) usually is positive for group A streptococci.

Carriers often receive multiple unsuccessful courses of antibiotic therapy in attempts to eliminate group A streptococci. Physician and patient anxiety is common and can develop into "streptophobia." Unproven and ineffective therapies include tonsillectomy, prolonged administration of antibiotics, use of beta-lactamase–resistant antibiotics, and culture or treatment of pets.

Available treatment options for the physician faced with a chronic streptococcal carrier include:

1. Ignoring the problem and stopping throat cultures, even for new symptomatic attacks of pharyngitis.
2. Obtaining a rapid test, throat culture, or both each time the patient has pharyngitis and treating with penicillin each time a test is positive.
3. Treating with one of the effective regimens for terminating chronic carriage.

Of these three options, the first solution is the most risky because a patient may become infected with a new strain of group A streptococci and acute rheumatic fever may develop. The second option is simple, as safe as penicillin, and appropriate for many patients. The third option should be reserved for particularly anxious patients; those with a history of acute rheumatic fever or living with someone who had it; or those living or working in nursing homes, chronic care facilities, hospitals, and perhaps schools.

The two treatment regimens that have been effective are:

- Intramuscular benzathine penicillin plus oral rifampin (10 mg/kg/dose up to 300 mg, given twice daily for 4 days beginning on the day of the penicillin injection)

- Oral clindamycin, given for 10 days (20 mg/kg/day up to 450 mg, divided into three equal doses)

Clindamycin may be preferred because it is easier to use than intramuscular penicillin plus oral rifampin and may be somewhat more effective. No other antibiotic regimens have been demonstrated in controlled, comparative trials to reliably terminate the chronic streptococcal carrier state. Successful eradication of the carrier state makes evaluation of subsequent episodes of pharyngitis much easier, although chronic carriage can recur upon re-exposure to group A streptococci.

RECURRENT ACUTE PHARYNGITIS

Some patients seem remarkably susceptible to group A streptococci. The reasons for frequent *bona fide* acute group A streptococcal pharyngitis are obscure, but appropriate antibiotic treatment results in resolution of symptoms and eradication of group A streptococci.

The role of tonsillectomy in the management of patients with multiple episodes of streptococcal pharyngitis remains controversial. Fewer episodes of sore throat have been reported among patients treated with tonsillectomy (in contrast to patients treated without surgery) during the first 2 years after operation. The patients enrolled in that study had experienced numerous episodes of pharyngitis, but it appears that not all episodes were caused by group A streptococci. Of particular concern is the reported tonsillectomy complication rate of 14% and the improvement over time noted among the non-tonsillectomy patients.

Finally, the presence of tonsils is not necessary for group A streptococci to infect the throat. Tonsillectomy cannot be recommended except in unusual circumstances. It seems preferable to treat most patients with penicillin whenever symptomatic group A streptococcal pharyngitis occurs. Obtaining follow-up throat specimens for culture may be needed to distinguish recurrent pharyngitis from chronic carriage.

NON–GROUP A STREPTOCOCCAL INFECTION

Certain beta-hemolytic streptococci of serogroups other than group A can induce acute pharyngitis. Well-documented epidemics of food-borne group C and group G streptococcal pharyngitis have been reported in young adults. In these situations, a high percentage of individuals who have ingested the contaminated food promptly developed acute pharyngitis, and throat cultures yielded virtually pure growth of the epidemiologically linked organism. There have been outbreaks of group G streptococcal pharyngitis among suburban children. However, the role of these non–group A streptococcal organisms as etiologic agents of acute pharyngitis in endemic circumstances has been difficult to establish. Data suggest that group C and group G beta streptococci may be responsible for acute pharyngitis, particularly in adolescents. However, the exact role of these agents, most of which are carried asymptomatically in the pharynx of some children and young adults, remains to be fully characterized.

When they are implicated as agents of acute pharyngitis, group C and G organisms do not appear to require treatment, since they cause self-limited infections. Acute rheumatic fever is not a sequela to these infections, although post-streptococcal acute glomerulonephritis has been rarely documented following epidemic group C and group G streptococcal pharyngitis.

ARCANOBACTERIUM INFECTION

Arcanobacterium (formerly *Corynebacterium*) *haemolyticum* is a gram-positive rod that has been reported to cause a scarlet fever–like illness with acute pharyngitis and scarlatinal rash, particularly in teenagers and young adults. This agent requires special methods for culture and has not routinely been sought in patients with scarlet fever or pharyngitis.

The clinical features of *A. haemolyticum* pharyngitis are indistinguishable from group A streptococcal pharyngitis; pharyngeal erythema is present in almost all patients, patchy white to gray exudates in about 70%, cervical adenitis in about 50%, and moderate fever in 40%. Palatal petechiae and strawberry tongue may also occur. The scarlatiniform rash rarely involves the face, palms, or soles; blanches; is erythematous; may be pruritic; and may demonstrate minimal desquamation.

Erythromycin appears to be the treatment of choice.

DIPHTHERIA

Diphtheria is a very serious disease that is caused by pharyngeal infection by toxigenic strains of *Corynebacterium diphtheriae*. It has become very rare in the United States and other developed countries. This is a tribute to the success of immunization programs that incorporate diphtheria toxoid. The handful of diphtheria cases recognized annually in the United States usually occur in unimmunized individuals, and the fatality rate is about 5%. A relatively large outbreak of diphtheria in the former Soviet Union has been recorded (1990–1995), and infection has been documented in several travelers from Western Europe.

Pathogenesis

The pathogenesis of diphtheria involves nasopharyngeal mucosal colonization by *C. diphtheriae* and toxin elaboration after a 1- to 5-day incubation period. Toxin leads to local tissue inflammation and necrosis (producing an adherent grayish membrane made up of fibrin, blood, inflammatory cells, and epithelial cells) and to absorption of toxin into the blood stream. Fragment B of the polypeptide toxin binds particularly well to cardiac, neural, and renal cells, and the smaller fragment A enters cells and interferes with protein synthesis. Toxin fixation by tissues may lead to fatal myocarditis (with arrhythmias) within 10 to 14 days and peripheral neuritis within 3 to 7 weeks.

Clinical Features

Acute tonsillar and pharyngeal diphtheria is characterized by anorexia, malaise, low-grade fever, and sore throat. The grayish membrane forms within 1 to 2 days over the tonsils and pharyngeal walls, and occasionally extends into the larynx and trachea. Cervical adenopathy varies but may be associated with development of a "bull neck." In mild cases, the membrane sloughs after 7 to 10 days and the patient recovers. In severe cases, an increasingly toxic appearance can lead to prostration, stupor, coma, and death within 6 to 10 days. Distinctive features include palatal paralysis, laryngeal paralysis, ocular palsies, diaphragmatic palsy, and myocarditis. Airway obstruction (from membrane formation) may complicate the toxigenic manifestations.

Diagnosis and Treatment

Accurate diagnosis requires isolation of *C. diphtheriae* on culture of material from beneath the membrane, with confirmation of toxin production by the organism isolated. Laboratories must be forewarned that diphtheria is suspected. Other tests are of little value.

Treatment includes equine antitoxin to neutralize circulating toxin as well as systemic penicillin or erythromycin.

GONOCOCCAL PHARYNGITIS

Acute symptomatic pharyngitis caused by *Neisseria gonorrhoeae* occurs occasionally in sexually active individuals as a consequence of oral-genital contact. In young children, sexual abuse must be suspected. The infection usually presents as an ulcerative exudative tonsillopharyngitis but may be asymptomatic and resolve spontaneously. Gonococcal pharyngitis occurs in homosexual men and heterosexual women after fellatio and is less readily acquired after cunnilingus. Gonorrhea rarely is transmitted from the pharynx to a sex partner, but pharyngitis can serve as a source for gonococcemia.

Diagnosis requires culture on appropriate selective media (e.g., Thayer-Martin). Recommended therapeutic regimens include a single intramuscular dose of 125 to 250 mg of ceftriaxone, a single 400-mg oral dose of cefixime, a single oral 500-mg dose of ciprofloxacin, or a single oral 400-mg dose of ofloxacin. Spectinomycin is ineffective in gonococcal pharyngitis. Examination and testing for other sexually transmitted diseases and pregnancy are recommended.

CHLAMYDIAL AND MYCOPLASMAL INFECTIONS

Chlamydia species and *Mycoplasma pneumoniae* may cause pharyngitis, although the frequency of these infections is a subject

Table 6-11. Spectrum of *Mycoplasma pneumoniae* Infection

Common
  Primary atypical pneumonia* (with or without pleural effusion)
  Pharyngitis
  Tracheobronchitis

Less Common
  Wheezing
  Rhinitis
  Bullous myringitis
  Otitis media
  Myocarditis
  Pericarditis
  Meningoencephalitis—aseptic meningitis
  Polyneuritis—Guillain-Barré syndrome
  Transverse myelitis
  Sinusitis
  Erythema multiforme—Stevens Johnson syndrome
  Erythema nodosum
  Urticaria
  Intravascular hemolysis (high titer cold agglutinins)
  Arthralgia

*Manifestations during pneumonia include sore throat, hoarseness, malaise, headache, cough, earache, chills, and fever > 102°F (38.9°C). Less often there may be coryza, rash, pleuritis, diarrhea, or leukocytosis > 10,000/mm^3.

of some dispute. *C. trachomatis* has been implicated serologically as a cause of pharyngitis in as many as 20% of adults with pharyngitis, but isolation of the organism from the pharynx has proved more difficult. *C. pneumoniae* (formerly named TWAR) has also been identified as a cause of pharyngitis. Because antibodies to this organism show some cross-reaction with *C. trachomatis*, it is possible that infections formerly attributed to *C. trachomatis* were really caused by *C. pneumoniae*.

Diagnosis of chlamydial pharyngitis is difficult, whether by culture or serologically, and neither method is readily available to the clinician.

M. pneumoniae most likely causes pharyngitis (Table 6–11). Serologic (positive mycoplasma immunoglobulin M [IgM]) or, less often, culture methods can be used to identify this agent, which was found in 33% of college students with pharyngitis in one unconfirmed study.

Currently, there is no need to seek evidence of these organisms routinely in pharyngitis patients in the absence of ongoing research studies of nonstreptococcal pharyngitis. The efficacy of antibiotic treatment for *M. pneumoniae* and chlamydial pharyngitis is not known, but these illnesses appear to be self-limited. Treatment of more complicated *M. pneumoniae* infections, such as pneumonia (see Table 6–10), is indicated with erythromycin (azithromycin, clarithromycin) or doxycycline (if the patient is older than 10 years of age).

REFERENCES

Group A Streptococci

Bisno AL. Group A streptococcal infections and acute rheumatic fever. N Engl J Med 1991;325:783–793.
Chapnick EK, Gradon JD, Lutwick LI, et al. Streptococcal toxic shock syndrome due to noninvasive pharyngitis. Clin Infect Dis 1992;14:1074–1077.
Denny FW. Group A streptococcal infections—1993. Curr Probl Pediatr 1993;23:179–185.
Givner LB, Abramson JS, Wasilauskas B. Apparent increase in the incidence of invasive group A beta-hemolytic streptococcal disease in children. J Pediatr 1991;118:341–346.
Hoge CW, Schwartz B, Talkington DF, et al. The changing epidemiology of invasive group A streptococcal infections and the emergence of streptococcal toxic shock–like syndrome: A retrospective population-based study. JAMA 1993;269:384–389.
Jackson MA, Burry VF, Olson LC. Multisystem group A β-hemolytic streptococcal disease in children. Rev Infect Dis 1991;13:783–788.
Kaplan EL. The group A streptococcal upper respiratory tract carrier state: An enigma. J Pediatr 1980;97:337–345.
Kaplan EL, Huwe BB. The sensitivity and specificity of an agglutination test for antibodies to streptococcal extracellular antigens: A quantitative analysis and comparison of the streptozyme test with the anti-streptolysin O and anti-deoxyribonuclease B tests. J Pediatr 1980;96:367–373.
Poses RM, Cebul RD, Collins M, et al. The accuracy of experienced physicians' probability estimates for patients with sore throats: Implications for decision making. JAMA 1985;254:925–929.
Torres-Martinez C, Mehta D, Butt A, et al. Streptococcus associated toxic shock. Arch Dis Child 1992;67:126–130.
Veasy LG, Tani LY, Hill HR. Persistence of acute rheumatic fever in the intermountain area of the United States. J Pediatr 1994;124:9–16.
Wegner DL, Witte DL, Schrantz RD. Insensitivity of rapid antigen detection methods and single blood agar plate culture for diagnosing streptococcal pharyngitis. JAMA 1992;267:695–697.
Wheeler MC, Roe MH, Kaplan EL, et al. Outbreak of group A streptococcus septicemia in children: Clinical, epidemiologic, and microbiological correlates. JAMA 1991;266:533–537.
Working Group on Severe Streptococcal Infections. Defining the group A streptococcal toxic shock syndrome: Rationale and consensus definition. JAMA 1993;269:390–391.

Other Pathogens

Feder HM. Cimetidine treatment for periodic fever associated with aphthous stomatitis, pharyngitis and cervical adenitis. Pediatr Infect Dis J 1992;11:318–321.
Gerber MA, Randolph MF, Martin NJ, et al. Community-wide outbreak of group G streptococcal pharyngitis. Pediatrics 1991;87:598–603.
Huovinen P, Lahtonen R, Ziegler T, et al. Pharyngitis in adults: The presence and coexistence of viruses and bacterial organisms. Ann Intern Med 1989;110:612–616.
Karpathios T, Drakonaki S, Zervoudaki A, et al. *Arcanobacterium haemolyticum* in children with presumed streptococcal pharyngotonsillitis or scarlet fever. J Pediatr 1992;121:735–737.
Komaroff AL, Branch WT, Aronson MD, et al. Chlamydial pharyngitis. Ann Intern Med 1989;111:537–538.
Lajo A, Borque C, Del Castillo F, et al. Mononucleosis caused by Epstein-Barr virus and cytomegalovirus in children: A comparative study of 124 cases. Pediatr Infect Dis J 1994;13:56–60.
McMillan JA, Weiner LB, Higgins AM, et al. Pharyngitis associated with herpes simplex virus in college students. Pediatr Infect Dis J 1993;12:280–284.
Nakayama M, Miyazaki C, Ueda K, et al. Pharyngoconjunctival fever caused by adenovirus type 11. Pediatr Infect Dis J 1992;11:6–9.
Straus SE, Cohen JI, Tosato G, et al. Epstein-Barr virus infections: Biology, pathogenesis, and management. Ann Intern Med 1993;118:45–58.
Sumaya CV, Ench Y. Epstein-Barr virus infectious mononucleosis in children: I. Clinical and general laboratory findings. Pediatrics 1985;75:1003–1010.
Sumaya CV, Ench Y. Epstein-Barr virus infectious mononucleosis in children: II. Heterophil antibody and viral-specific responses. Pediatrics 1985;75:1011–1019.
Waagner DC. *Arcanobacterium haemolyticum*: Biology of the organism and diseases in man. Pediatr Infect Dis J 1991;10:933–939.

Complications

Blomquist IK, Bayer AS. Life-threatening deep fascial space infections of the head and neck. Infect Dis Clin NA 1988;2:237–264.

Chow AW. Life-threatening infections of the head and neck. Clin Infect Dis 1992;14:991–1004.

de Marie S, Tham RT, van der Mey AGL, et al. Clinical infections and nonsurgical treatment of parapharyngeal space infections complicating throat infection. Rev Infect Dis 1989;11:975–982.

Savolainen S, Jousimies-Somer HR, Makitie AA, et al. Peritonsillar abscess: Clinical and microbiologic aspects and treatment regimens. Arch Otolaryngol Head Neck Surg 1993;119:521–524.

Wald ER, Guerra N, Byers C. Upper respiratory tract infections in young children: Duration of and frequency of complications. Pediatrics 1991;87:129–133.

White B. Deep neck infections and respiratory distress in children. Ear Nose Throat J 1985;64:30–38.

Treatment

El-Daher NT, Hijazi SS, Rawashdeh NM, et al. Immediate vs delayed treatment of group A beta-hemolytic streptococcal pharyngitis with penicillin V. Pediatr Infect Dis J 1991;10:126–130.

Markowitz M, Gerber MA, Kaplan EL. Treatment of streptococcal pharyngotonsillitis: Reports of penicillin's demise are premature. J Pediatr 1993;123:679–685.

Massel BF, Chute CG, Walker AM, et al. Penicillin and the marked decrease in morbidity and mortality from rheumatic fever in the United States. N Engl J Med 1988;318:280–286.

Paradise JL, Bluestone CD, Bachman RZ, et al. Efficacy of tonsillectomy for recurrent throat infection in severely affected children: Results of parallel randomized and nonrandomized clinical trials. N Engl J Med 1984;310:674–683.

Randolph MF, Gerber MA, DeMeo KK, et al. Effect of antibiotic therapy on the clinical course of streptococcal pharyngitis. J Pediatr 1985;106:870–875.

Seppala H, Nissinen A, Jarvinen H, et al. Resistance to erythromycin in group A streptococci. N Engl J Med 1992;326:292–297.

Shulman ST, Gerber MA, Tanz RR, et al. Streptococcal pharyngitis: The case for penicillin therapy. Pediatr Infect Dis J 1994;13:1–7.

Snellman LW, Stang HJ, Stang JM, et al. Duration of positive throat cultures for group A streptococci after initiation of antibiotic therapy. Pediatrics 1993;91:116–117.

Tanz RR, Poncher JR, Corydon KE, et al. Clindamycin treatment of chronic pharyngeal carriers of group A streptococci. J Pediatr 1991;119:123–128.

7 Cough

David M. Orenstein

Cough is an important defense mechanism of the lungs and is a common symptom prompting visits to the physician, particularly during winter months. In most patients, it is self-limited and only a minor nuisance. However, cough can be ominous, indicating serious underlying disease, because of accompanying problems (hemoptysis) or because of serious consequences of the cough itself (e.g., syncope and hemorrhage). Treatment of cough may be unnecessary, or it may be lifesaving, depending on the underlying disorder.

PATHOPHYSIOLOGY OF COUGH

The cough reflex serves to prevent the entry of harmful substances into the tracheobronchial tree and to expel excess secretions and retained material from the tracheobronchial tree. Cough begins with stimulation of cough receptors, located in the upper and lower airways, and in many other sites such as the ear canal, tympanic membrane, sinuses, nose, pericardium, pleura, and diaphragm. Receptors send messages via vagus, phrenic, glossopharyngeal, or trigeminal nerves to the "cough center," which is in the medulla. Because cough is not only an involuntary reflex activity but one that can be initiated or suppressed voluntarily, "higher centers" must also be involved in the afferent limb of the responsible pathway. The neural impulses go from the medulla to the appropriate efferent pathways to the larynx, tracheobronchial tree, and expiratory muscles.

The act of coughing (Fig. 7–1) begins with an inspiration, followed by expiration against a closed glottis (compressive phase), resulting in the buildup of impressive intrathoracic pressures (50–300 cm H_2O). These pressures may be transmitted to vascular, cerebrospinal, and intraocular spaces. Finally, the glottis opens, allowing for explosive expiratory air flow (300 m/second) and expulsion of mucus, particularly from the larger, central airways. The inability to seal the upper airway (tracheostomy) impairs, but does not abolish, the effectiveness of cough. Weak ventilatory muscles (muscular dystrophy) impair both the inspiratory and the compressive phase.

DIAGNOSIS

Using information from the history, physical examination, and laboratory evaluation, one can uncover a specific cause for most instances of cough in children.

History

The history often provides the most important body of information about a child's cough. A diagnosis can often be made with relative certainty from the family history, the environmental and exposure history, and the acuteness and characterization of the cough.

DEMOGRAPHICS

The patient's age (Tables 7–1 and 7–2) helps to focus the diagnostic possibilities. Congenital anatomic abnormalities may be

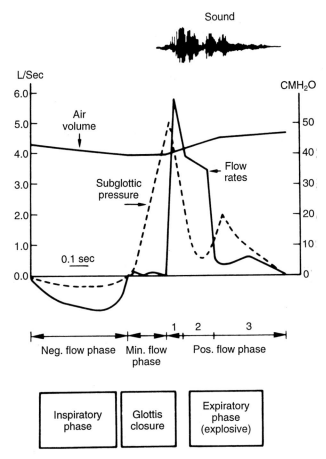

Figure 7–1. Cough mechanics, showing changes in expiratory flow rate, air volume, subglottic pressure, and sound recording during cough. (From Bianco S, Robuschi M. Mechanics of cough. *In* Braga PS, Allegra L [eds]. Cough. New York: Raven Press, 1989.)

symptomatic from birth, whereas toddlers, who may have incomplete neurologic control over swallowing and often put small objects in their mouths, are at risk for foreign body aspiration; adolescents may experiment with smoking or inhaled drugs. Socioeconomic factors must be considered; a family that cannot afford central heating may use a smoky wood-burning stove; spending time at a day care center may expose an infant to respiratory viruses; and several adult smokers in a trailer home expose children to a high concentration of respiratory irritants.

CHARACTERISTICS OF THE COUGH

The various cough characteristics can help to determine their causes. The causes of acute, recurrent, and chronic coughs may be quite different from each other (see Table 7–1). A cough can be paroxysmal, brassy, productive, weak, volitional, and "throat-clearing," or it may occur at different times of the day (Tables 7–3 and 7–4).

RESPONSES TO PREVIOUS TREATMENT: DRUG HISTORY

The previous response or lack of response to some therapies for recurrent and chronic cough can give important information (see

Table 7–4). Furthermore, some coughs may be caused or worsened by medications (Table 7–5).

ASSOCIATED SYMPTOMS

A history of accompanying signs or symptoms, whether localized to the respiratory tract (wheeze, stridor) or elsewhere (failure to thrive, frequent malodorous stools) can give important clues (Tables 7–3, 7–4, and 7–6). It is essential to remember that the daily language of the physician is full of jargon that may be adopted by parents, but with a different meaning from that understood by physicians. If a parent says that a child "wheezes," or "croups," or is "short of breath," it is important to find out what the parent means by that term.

FAMILY AND PAST MEDICAL HISTORY

Since many disorders of childhood have genetic or nongenetic familial components, the family history can provide helpful information:

Are there two older siblings with cystic fibrosis or asthma?

Is there a coughing sibling whose kindergarten class has been closed because of pertussis?

Similarly, the key to today's problems may be found in the past:

Was the child premature, spent a month on the ventilator and now has chronic lung disease (bronchopulmonary dysplasia)?

Did the toddler choke on a carrot 3 months ago?

Did the child receive a bone marrow transplant a year ago?

Is the child immunized?

Did the infant have a tracheoesophageal fistula repaired in the newborn period?

Physical Examination

As with the history, the physical examination may provide the diagnosis. If not absolutely diagnostic, the physical examination often yields important information.

INSPECTION

Initial inspection can often inform the examiner as to the extent of an illness:

Is the child struggling to breathe (dyspnea)?

Does the child have an anxious look?

Can the child be calmed or engaged in play?

Is the child's skin blue (representing cyanosis) or ashen?

The respiratory rate is often elevated with parenchymal lung disease or extrathoracic obstruction. Respiratory rates vary with the age of the child (Table 7–7) and with pulmonary infection, airway obstruction, activity, wakefulness and sleep, fever, metabolic acidosis, and anxiety. Does the child appear wasted, with poor growth that may indicate a chronic illness?

Odors may also give helpful clues. Does the examining room or the clothing smell of stale cigarette smoke, which may indicate that the child is exposed to respiratory irritants? Is there a foul odor from a diaper with a fatty stool, which may suggest pancreatic insufficiency and cystic fibrosis? Is the child's breath malodorous, as can be noticed in sinusitis, nasal foreign body, lung abscess, or bronchiectasis?

Table 7–1. **Causes of Cough**

Age Group	Acute	Recurrent	Chronic (>3 weeks)
Infants	Infection[1]* Aspiration[2] Foreign body[3]	Reactive airways[1] CF[1] GER[1] Aspiration[2] Anatomic abnormality[3]† Passive smoking[3]	Reactive airways[1] CF[1] GER[1] Aspiration[2] Pertussis[2] Anatomic abnormality[3]† Passive smoking[3] Miscellaneous[3] (see Table 7–2)
Toddlers	Infection[1] Foreign body[2] Aspiration[3]	Reactive airways[1] CF[1] GER[1] Aspiration[2] Anatomic abnormality[3] Passive smoking[3]	Reactive airways[1] CF[1] GER[1] Aspiration[2] Pertussis[2] Anatomic abnormality[3] Passive smoking[3] Miscellaneous[3]
Children	Infection[1] Foreign body[3]	Reactive airways[1] CF[1] GER[1] Passive smoking[3]	Reactive airways[1] CF[1] GER[2] Pertussis[2] *Mycoplasma*[3] Psychogenic[3] Anatomic abnormality[3] Passive smoking[3] Miscellaneous[3]
Adolescents	Infection[1]	Reactive airways[1] CF[1] GER[1] Aspiration[2] Anatomic abnormality[3]	Reactive airways[1] CF[1] GER[2] Smoking[2] *Mycoplasma*[2] Psychogenic[2] Pertussis[3] Aspiration[3] Anatomic abnormality[3] Miscellaneous[3]

*Infections include upper (pharyngitis, sinusitis, tracheitis, rhinitis, otitis) and lower (pneumonia, abscess, empyema) respiratory tract disease.
†Anatomic abnormality includes tracheobronchomalacia, tracheoesophageal fistula, vascular ring, abnormal position, or take-off of large bronchi.
Key: 1 = common; 2 = less common; 3 = much less common.
Abbreviations: CF = cystic fibrosis; GER = gastroesophageal reflux.

Table 7–2. **Miscellaneous Causes of Cough in Children**

Postnasal drip (?)	Cerumen impaction
Ciliary dyskinesia syndrome	Irritation of external auditory canal
Interstitial lung disease	Obliterative bronchiolitis
Heart failure/pulmonary edema	Follicular bronchiolitis
Pulmonary hemosiderosis	Mediastinal disease (nodes, pneumomediastinum)
Drug-induced (see Table 7–5)	Nasal polyps
α_1-antitrypsin deficiency	Hypersensitivity pneumonitis (extrinsic allergic alveolitis)
Graft-versus-host disease	Thyroid lesions
Bronchopulmonary dysplasia	Subphrenic abscess
Tumor (bronchial adenoma, carcinoid; mediastinal)	Sarcoidosis
Alveolar proteinosis	Anaphylaxis
Tracheomalacia, bronchomalacia	Pulmonary embolism
Spasmodic croup	Lung contusion

Table 7–3. Clinical Clues About Cough

Characteristic	Think of
Staccato, paroxysmal	Pertussis, cystic fibrosis, foreign body, *Chlamydia, Mycoplasma*
Followed by "whoop"	Pertussis
All day, never during sleep	Psychogenic, habit
Barking, brassy	Croup, psychogenic, tracheomalacia, tracheitis, epiglottitis
Hoarseness	Laryngeal involvement (croup, recurrent laryngeal nerve involvement)
Abrupt onset	Foreign body, pulmonary embolism
Follows exercise	Reactive airways disease
Accompanies eating, drinking	Aspiration, gastroesophageal reflux, tracheoesophageal fistula
Throat clearing	Postnasal drip
Productive (sputum)	Infection
Night cough	Sinusitis, reactive airways disease
Seasonal	Allergic rhinitis, reactive airways disease
Immunosuppressed patient	Bacterial pneumonia, *Pneumocystis carinii, Mycobacterium tuberculosis, Mycobacterium avium–intracellulare*, cytomegalovirus
Dyspnea	Hypoxia, hypercarbia
Animal exposure	*Chlamydia psittaci* (birds), *Yersinia pestis* (rodents), *Francisella tularensis* (rabbits), Q fever (sheep, cattle), hantavirus (rodents), histoplasmosis (pigeons)
Geographic	Histoplasmosis (Mississippi, Missouri, Ohio River Valley), coccidioidomycosis (southwest), blastomycosis (north and midwest)
Weekday with weekend clearing	Occupational exposure

Table 7–4. Cough: Some Aspects of Differential Diagnosis

Cause	Abrupt Onset	Only When Awake	Yellow Sputum	Responds to Inhaled Bronchodilator (by History)	Responds to Antibiotics (by History)	Responds to Steroids (by History)	Failure to Thrive	Wheeze	Digital Clubbing
Reactive airways disease/asthma	+	+ +	+ +	+ + +	+	+ + +	+	+ + +	−
Cystic fibrosis	+	+ +	+ +	+	+ + +	+	+ +	+ +	+ + +
Other infection	+	+	+ +	−	+ +	−	+	+	−
Aspiration	+	+	+	+	+	+	+ +	+ +	+
Gastroesophageal reflux	+	+ +	−	−	−	+	+ +	+ +	−
Foreign body	+ + +	+	+ +	+	+ +	+	+	+ +	+
Habit	−	+ + +	−	+	+	+	−	−	−

Key: + + + = very common and suggests the diagnosis; + + = common; + = uncommon; − = almost never and makes one question the diagnosis.

Table 7–5. Drugs Causing Cough

Drug	Mechanism
Tobacco, marijuana	Direct irritant
Beta-adrenergic blockers	Potentiate reactive airways disease
ACE inhibitors	(?) Possibly potentiate reactive airways disease
Bethanechol	Potentiates reactive airways disease
Nitrofurantoin	(?) Via oxygen radicals versus via autoimmunity
Antineoplastic agents	Various (including pneumonitis/fibrosis, hypersensitivity, noncardiogenic pulmonary edema)
Sulfasalazine	(?) Causes bronchiolitis obliterans
Penicillamine	(?) Causes bronchiolitis obliterans
Diphenylhydantoin	Hypersensitivity pneumonitis
Gold	(?) Causes interstitial fibrosis
Aspirin, NSAIDs	Potentiate reactive airways disease
Nebulized cromolyn	Potentiates reactive airways disease via hypotonicity
Nebulized antibiotics	(?) Direct irritant
Bronchodilators	Indirect, via worsened gastroesophageal reflux (relax lower esophageal sphincter); or via reaction to vehicle; increases bronchial wall instability in bronchomalacia
Metabisulfite	Induces allergic reactive airways disease
Cholinesterase inhibitors	Induce mucus production (bronchorrhea)

Abbreviations: NSAIDs = nonsteroidal anti-inflammatory drugs; ACE = angiotensin-converting enzyme.

NORMAL   CLUBBING

Phalangeal Depth Ratio

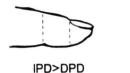 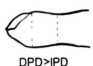

IPD>DPD   DPD>IPD

Hyponychial Angle

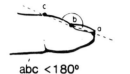 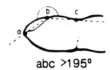

abc <180°   abc >195°

Schamroth's Sign

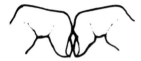 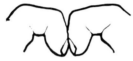

Figure 7–2. Measurement of digital clubbing. The ratio of the distal phalangeal depth (DPD) to the interphalangeal depth (IPD), or the *phalangeal depth ratio*, is normally less than 1 but increases to more than 1 with finger clubbing. The DPD/IPD ratio can be measured with calipers or more accurately with finger casts. The *hyponychial angle* is measured from lateral projections of the finger contour on a magnifying screen and is normally less than 180 degrees but greater than 195 degrees with finger clubbing. *Schamroth's sign* is useful for bedside assessment. The dorsal surfaces of the terminal phalanges of similar fingers are placed together. With clubbing, the normal diamond-shaped aperture or "window" at the bases of the nail beds disappears, and a prominent distal angle forms between the end of the nails. In normal subjects this angle is minimal or nonexistent. (From Pasterkamp H. The history and physical examination. *In* Chernick V [ed]: Kendig's Disorders of the Respiratory Tract in Children, 5th ed. Philadelphia: WB Saunders, 1990.)

Fingers

It has been said that the examination of the lungs begins at the fingertips. Cyanotic nail beds suggest hypoxemia, poor peripheral

Table 7–6. Nonpulmonary History Suggesting Cystic Fibrosis

Maldigestion, malabsorption, steatorrhea in 50% to 85%
Poor weight gain
Family history of cystic fibrosis
Salty taste to skin
Rectal prolapse (up to 20% of patients)
Digital clubbing
Meconium ileus
Intestinal atresia
Neonatal cholestatic jaundice

Table 7–7. Respiratory Rates* of Healthy Children of Both Sexes, Sleeping and Awake

	Sleeping		Awake	
Age	Mean	Range	Mean	Range
6–12 mo	27	22–31	64	58–75
1–2 yr	19	17–23	35	30–40
2–4 yr	19	16–25	31	23–42
4–6 yr	18	14–23	26	19–36
6–8 yr	17	13–23	23	15–30
8–10 yr	18	14–23	21	15–31
10–12 yr	16	13–19	21	15–28
12–14 yr	16	15–18	22	18–26

Data from Waring WW. The history and physical examination. *In* Kendig EL Jr (ed). Pulmonary Disorders. Vol 1. Disorders of the Respiratory Tract in Children, 2nd ed. Philadelphia: WB Saunders, 1972:78.
*In breaths per minute.

circulation, or both. The examiner looks for the presence of digital clubbing (Fig. 7–2), which makes asthma or acute pneumonia extremely unlikely. The absence of clubbing but a history of severe chronic cough makes cystic fibrosis unlikely.

Chest and Abdomen

The shape of the chest gives information. Is the anteroposterior (AP) diameter increased, which indicates hyperinflation of the lungs from obstruction of small airways (asthma, bronchiolitis, cystic fibrosis)? Is this diameter small, as can be seen with some restrictive lung diseases with small lung volumes? The normal infant has a "round" chest configuration, with the AP diameter of the chest about 84% of the transverse (lateral) diameter. With growth, the chest becomes more flattened in the AP dimension, and the AP-to-transverse ratio is closer to 70% to 75%. Although obstetric calipers can be used to give an objective assessment of the AP diameter of the chest, most clinicians rely on their subjective assessment of whether the diameter is increased: Does the patient look "barrel-chested"?

Intercostal, suprasternal, and supraclavicular *retractions* (inspiratory sinking in of the soft tissues) indicate increased effort of breathing and reflect both the contraction of the accessory muscles of respiration and the resulting difference between intrapleural and extrathoracic pressure. Retractions are most commonly seen with obstructed airways (upper or lower), but they may occur with any condition leading to the use of the accessory muscles. Any retractions other than the mild normal depressions seen between an infant's lower ribs indicate a greater-than-normal work of breathing.

Less easy to notice than the in-sinking of the soft tissues between the ribs is their bulging out with expiration in a child with expiratory obstruction (asthma). Contraction of the abdominal muscles with expiration is easier to notice and is another indication that a child is working harder than normal to push air out through obstructed airways.

Spine

Inspection of the spine may reveal kyphosis or scoliosis. There is a risk of restrictive lung disease or static pneumonia if the curvature is severe.

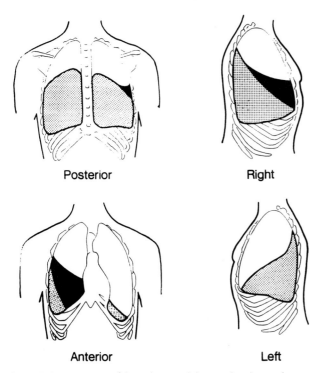

Posterior   Right

Anterior   Left

Figure 7–3. Projections of the pulmonary lobes on the chest surface. The upper lobes are white, the right-middle lobe is black, and the lower lobes are dotted. (From Pasterkamp H. The history and physical examination. *In* Chernick V [ed]. Kendig's Disorders of the Respiratory Tract in Children, 5th ed. Philadelphia: WB Saunders, 1990.)

PALPATION

Palpating the trachea, particularly in infants, may reveal a shift to one side, which suggests loss of volume of the lung on that side or extrapulmonary gas (pneumothorax) on the other side. Placing one hand on each side of the chest while the patient breathes may enable the examiner to detect asymmetry of chest wall movement, either in timing or degree of expansion. The former indicates a partial bronchial obstruction, and the latter suggests a smaller lung volume, voluntary guarding, or diminished muscle function on one side. Palpating the abdomen gently during expiration may allow one to feel the contraction of the abdominal muscles in cases of expiratory obstruction.

Palpation for *tactile fremitus*, the transmitted vibrations of the spoken word ("ninety-nine" is the word often used to accentuate these vibrations), helps to determine areas of increased parenchymal density and hence increased fremitus (pneumonic consolidation, atelectasis) or decreased fremitus (pneumothorax, pleural effusion).

PERCUSSION

The percussion note determined by tapping of one middle finger on the middle finger of the other hand, which is firmly placed over the thorax, may be dull over an area of consolidation or effusion and hyperresonant with air-trapping. Percussion can also be used to determine diaphragmatic excursion. The lowest level of resonance at inspiration and expiration determines diaphragmatic motion.

AUSCULTATION

The stethoscope can give useful information in many children with cough (Table 7–8). Because lung sounds tend to be higher-pitched than heart sounds, the diaphragm of the stethoscope is better suited to pulmonary auscultation than the bell, whose target is primarily the lower-pitched heart sounds. The adult-sized stethoscope generally is far superior to the smaller pediatric or neonatal diaphragms, even for listening to small chests, because its acoustics are better. The two-headed stethoscope enables the user to hear homologous segments of both lungs simultaneously (Fig. 7–3) in order to identify instances in which there is a delay in air entry or exit. The traditional single-headed stethoscope is adequate in most children with cough. The ability to recognize normal breath sounds comes with practice (Fig. 7–4).

Adventitious Sounds

Adventitious sounds come in a few varieties, namely, stridor, crackles, and wheezes. Other sounds should be described in clear everyday language.

Stridor is a continuous musical sound heard on inspiration and is caused by narrowing in the extrathoracic airway, as with croup or laryngomalacia.

Crackles are discontinuous, representing the popping open of air-fluid menisci as the airways dilate with inspiration. Fluid in larger airways makes its crackles early in inspiration (congestive heart failure); crackles that tend to be a bit lower in pitch ("coarse" crackles) than the early, higher-pitched ("fine") crackles are associated with fluid in small airways (pneumonia). Although crackles usually signal the presence of excess airway fluid (pneumonia, pulmonary edema), they may also be produced by the popping open of noninfected fibrotic or atelectatic airways. Fine crackles are not audible at the mouth, while coarse crackles may be. In most cases, crackles is the preferred term rather than the previously popular "rales."

Wheezes are continuous musical sounds (lasting longer than 200 msec), caused by vibration of narrowed airway walls, as with asthma, and perhaps vibration of material within airway lumens. These sounds are much more commonly heard during expiration than inspiration.

Other Sounds

Air moving through bronchi surrounded by consolidated lung may produce a hollow sound, similar to the noise produced by blowing over the mouth of a bottle; hence the adjective "amphoric" (from the Latin and Greek for jar or bottle) is sometimes applied to this sound. Some abnormal respiratory sounds do not fit into the preceding categories and should be described as they sound; "squeaks," "groans," "rubs" (pleural or pericardial), or "creaking sounds" can be meaningful descriptions.

Laboratory Findings

ROENTGENOGRAPHY

The chest radiograph is often the first and sometimes the most useful laboratory test in the evaluation of the child with cough. Table 7–9 highlights some of the roentgenographic features of the most common causes of cough in pediatric patients. Roentgeno-

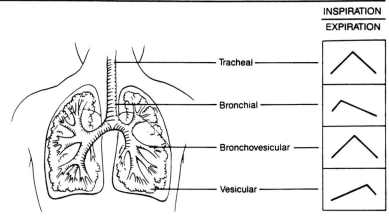

Characteristic	Tracheal	Bronchial	Bronchovesicular	Vesicular
Intensity	Very loud	Loud	Moderate	Soft
Pitch	Very high	High	Moderate	Low
I:E Ratio*	1:1	1:3	1:1	3:1
Description	Harsh	Tubular	Rustling, but tubular	Gentle rustling
Normal locations	Extrathoracic trachea	Manubrium	Over mainstem bronchi	Most of peripheral lung

* Ratio of duration of inspiration to expiration.

Figure 7–4. Characteristics of breath sounds. *Tracheal* breath sounds are very harsh, loud, and high-pitched; they are heard over the extrathoracic portion of the trachea. *Bronchial* breath sounds are loud and high-pitched; normally, they are heard over the lower sternum and sound like air rushing through a tube. The expiratory component is louder and longer than the inspiratory component; a definite pause is heard between the two phases. *Bronchovesicular* breath sounds are a mixture of bronchial and vesicular sounds. The inspiratory and expiratory components are equal in length. They are usually heard only in the first and second interspaces anteriorly and between the scapulae posteriorly, near the carina and mainstem bronchi. *Vesicular* breath sounds are soft and low-pitched; they are heard over most of the lung fields. The inspiratory component is much longer than the expiratory component; the latter is softer and often inaudible. (From Swartz MH. The chest. *In* Textbook of Physical Diagnosis History and Examination. Philadelphia: WB Saunders, 1989.)

graphic findings are often similar for a number of disorders, and thus x-ray studies may not give a definitive diagnosis. Chest films are normal in children with psychogenic (habit) cough and in children with sinusitis or gastroesophageal reflux as the *primary* cause of cough. Gastroesophageal reflux (GER) or sinusitis can occur in someone with an abnormal chest film, but because neither of these disorders should cause an abnormal chest film, finding an x-ray abnormality makes it difficult to attribute the cough solely or primarily to simple GER or sinusitis. A normal chest x-ray makes pneumonia caused by respiratory syncytial virus (RSV), influenza, parainfluenza, adenovirus, *Chlamydia*, or bacteria extremely unlikely. Although children with cough resulting from cystic fibrosis, *Mycoplasma*, tuberculosis, aspiration, a bronchial foreign body, or an anatomic abnormality usually have abnormal chest radiographs, a normal radiograph does not exclude these diagnoses. Hyperinflation of the lungs is commonly seen on chest films of infants with RSV bronchiolitis or *Chlamydia* pneumonia, and a lobar or round (coin lesion) infiltrate is the radiographic hallmark of bacterial pneumonia. The diagnosis of sinusitis cannot be sustained with normal sinuses on x-ray or computed tomography (CT) scan; the same is usually true for the diagnosis of cystic fibrosis.

HEMATOLOGY/IMMUNOLOGY

The white blood cell (WBC) count may help exclude or include certain entities for a differential diagnosis, but, with the possible exception of pertussis, can seldom establish a diagnosis with certainty. A WBC count of 35,000 with 85% lymphocytes strongly suggests pertussis, but not every child with pertussis presents such a clear hematologic picture. The presence of a high number or

large proportions of immature forms of WBCs suggests an acute process, such as a bacterial infection. Immunoglobulins provide supportive evidence for a few diagnoses, such as chlamydial infection, which rarely occurs without elevated serum concentrations of immunoglobulins IgG and IgM.

BACTERIOLOGY/VIROLOGY

Specific bacteriologic or virologic diagnoses can be made in a number of disorders causing cough, including RSV, influenza, adenovirus, and *Chlamydia* pneumonia. In most cases, these diagnoses are based on culturing the organism from nasopharyngeal washings. In some cases, the viruses can be rapidly identified with immunofluorescence or newer molecular techniques, including amplification of viral DNA using polymerase chain reaction (PCR). In bacterial pneumonia, the offending organism can be cultured from the blood in a small portion (10%) of patients. A positive culture provides definitive diagnosis, but a negative culture specimen is not helpful. Throat cultures are seldom helpful (except in cystic fibrosis) in identifying lower respiratory tract organisms. Sputum cultures and Gram stains may help guide initial empirical therapy in older patients with pneumonia or purulent bronchitis, but their ability to identify specific causative organisms with certainty (again excepting cystic fibrosis) has not been shown clearly.

Infants and young children usually do not expectorate but, rather, swallow their sputum. Specimens obtained via bronchoscopy may be contaminated by mouth flora, but heavy growth of a single organism in the presence of polymorphonuclear neutrophils certainly suggests the organism's importance. If pleural fluid or fluid obtained directly from the lung via needle aspiration is cultured,

Table 7-8. Physical Signs of Pulmonary Disease

Disease Process	Mediastinal Deviation	Chest Motion	Fremitus	Percussion	Breath Sounds	Adventitious Sounds	Voice Signs
Consolidation (pneumonia)	No	Reduced over area, splinting	Increased	Dull	Bronchial or reduced	Crackles	Egophony,* whispering pectoriloquy increased†
Bronchospasm	No	Hyperexpansion with limited motion	Normal or decreased	Hyperresonant	Normal to decreased	Wheezes, crackles	Normal to decreased
Atelectasis	Shift toward lesion	Reduced over area	Decreased	Dull	Reduced, absent	None or crackles	None
Pneumothorax	Tension deviates trachea and PMI to opposite side	Reduced over area	None	Resonant, tympanitic	None	None	None
Pleural effusion	Deviation to opposite side	Reduced over area	None	Dull	None	Friction rub; splash, if hemopneumothorax	None
Interstitial process	No	Reduced	Normal to increased	Normal	Normal	Crackles	None

Adapted from Dantzker D, Tobin M, Whatley R. Respiratory diseases. *In* Andreoli TE, Carpenter CJ, Plum F, Smith LH (eds). Cecil Essentials of Medicine. Philadelphia: WB Saunders, 1986:126–180.

*Egophony is present when *e* sounds like *a*.

†Whispering pectoriloquy produces clearer sounding whispered words, e.g., "ninety-nine."

Table 7-9. Cough: Laboratory Evaluation

	Chest Radiograph					Abnl Sinus Chest Radiograph	Complete Blood Count							+NP Cult	Other
	Nl	Hyper	Lobr Infil	Diff Infil	Other		↑WBC	↑LY	↑EOS	↑PMN	↑IgG	↑IgM	↑IgE		
RAD/asthma	+	++	-	-	-	+	+	+	++	-	+	+	++		+bdilator[1]
Cystic fibrosis	+	++	+	+	++	+++	++	+	+	++	++	+	+		See Table 7-10
Other infection															
Croup	++	+	+	+	++[2]	-	-	+	+	-				Paraflu	
Epiglottitis	++	+	+	+	++[3]	+	+++	+	+	+++				+++	Direct look
Sinusitis	+++	-	-	-	-	+++	++	-	+	+++	++		+		
Bronchiolitis	-	+++	+	++	+	-	+	-	+	+	++		+	RSV	
Pneumonia															
Influenza	-	++	+	++	+	-	++	+	+	+				++	
Paraflu	-	-	+	++	+	-	++	+	+	+				++	
Adenovirus	-	-	+	++	+	-	++	+	+	++				++	
Pertussis	++	+	-	+	+	-	+	+++	++		+			+[4]	
Chlamydia	-	+++	-	+	+	-	+	+	++		+++	+++	-	++	
Mycoplasma	+	+	+	+	++[5]	++	+	+	+		-	++	-		+Cold agglutinin
TB	+	-	++	+	++	-	+	+	+						+PPD
Bacterial	-	+	+++	+	++[5]	-	+++	+	+	+++	++	+	+	+	+Bld cult[6]
Foreign body	-	++[7]	++	-	++[7]	-	++	+	-	++					Bronch
GE reflux	+++	+	-	-	+	+	-	-	-	-	-	-	+	-	Esoph pH[8]
Aspiration	+	+	+	+	++[9]	+	+	-	+	+	-	-	+	-	[10]
Anatomic	+	-	+	-	++[11]	-	-	-	-	+	-	-	-	-	[12]
Habit	+++	-	-	-	-	-	-	-	-		-	-	-	-	

[1]Positive response to bronchodilators, either as a home therapeutic trial, or in a pulmonary function test in the laboratory.

[2]"Steeple" sign, of narrowing of upper tracheal air column.

[3]"Swollen thumb," sign of thickened epiglottis.

[4]Low yield on culture in paroxysmal stage.

[5]Pleural effusion relatively common.

[6]Blood culture positive in 10%; needle aspiration of pleural fluid or lung fluid may yield organism; bacterial antigen in urine. In older infants and children, common pathogens include pneumococci, group A streptococci, and *Haemophilus influenzae. Staphylococcus aureus* is rare and may be associated with pneumatoceles or empyema.

[7]Localized hyperinflation is common; localized atelectasis is common; inspiratory-expiratory films may show ball-valve obstruction.

[8]Esophageal biopsy specimen shows esophagitis.

[9]Multilobular or multisegmental, dependent lobes.

[10](?) Lipid-laden macrophages from bronchoscopy or gastric washings; barium swallow or radionuclide study showing aspiration.

[11]Right-sided arch, mass effect on airways, mass identified; magnetic resonance imaging (MRI).

[12]Bronchoscopy: computed tomography: MRI.

Key: +++ = almost always—if not present, must question diagnosis; ++ = common; + = less common; − = seldom—if present, must question diagnosis.

Abbreviations: Nl = normal; Hyper = hyperinflated; Lobr Infil = lobar infiltrates; Diff Infil = diffuse or scattered infiltrates; Abnl = abnormal; ↑WBC = increased white blood cell count; ↑LY = increased lymphocyte count; ↑EOS = increased eosinophil count; ↑PMN = increased polymorphonuclear neutrophil count; +NP Cult = nasopharyngeal culture positive for specific organism; Esoph pH = prolonged esophageal pH probe monitoring; RSV = respiratory syncytial virus; Ig = immunoglobulin; RAD = reactive airways disease; GE = gastroesophageal; TB = tuberculosis; Paraflu = parainfluenza virus; +Bld cult = blood culture may be positive; Bronch = bronchoscopy can reveal the foreign body; PPD = purified protein derivative (TB).

Table 7–10. Laboratory Tests for Cystic Fibrosis

Usefulness	Test	Sensitivity	Specificity	Cost
Definitive	"Sweat test"	.99+	.95+	$175
	DNA analysis	.85–.90	.99	$100–$200
Suggestive	Throat or sputum culture positive for mucoid			$140
	Pseudomonas aeruginosa	.70–.80	.85	
	Sinus x-ray films			$179
	Pansinusitis	.95	.90	
	Positive IRT newborn screen	.98	.25	$1
	Typical histology of appendix	.95	.98	*
Supportive	Absent stool trypsin	.40–.75	.75(?)	$103
	Abnormal Chymex test for pancreatic insufficiency	.70–.90	.90+	$98
	Pulmonary function tests:			$100–800
	Obstructive pattern, especially small airways and especially if patient is poorly responsive to bronchodilator	.70+	?	
	Chest film:			$160
	Hyperinflation, ± other findings; especially with right upper lobe infiltrate/atelectasis	.70+	?	
	Throat or sputum culture*:			$140
	Positive for *Staphylococcus aureus*	.20	.20	
	Positive for *Haemophilus influenzae*	.05–.20	.15	

*Throat is usually deep pharyngeal culture.
Abbreviations: IRT = immunoreactive trypsinogen.

the same rules apply: Positive cultures are definitive, but negative cultures are not. Bacterial antigen detection in serum or urine by various techniques (latex agglutination) can help identify pneumococcus and *Haemophilus influenzae* type b.

OTHER TESTS

A number of specific tests can help to establish diagnoses in a child with cough (see Table 7–9). These include a positive response to bronchodilators in a child with asthma; visualizing the red, swollen epiglottis in epiglottitis (to be done only under very controlled conditions, as described later) or the bronchoscopic visualization of the peanut, plastic toy, or other offender in foreign body aspiration; a positive purified protein derivative (PPD) in tuberculosis; and several studies of the esophagus in GER. Several imaging techniques, such as CT or magnetic resonance imaging (MRI) with or without contrast, can help to delineate various intrathoracic anatomic abnormalities. Finally, multiple tests can be employed to confirm the diagnosis of cystic fibrosis (Table 7–10).

DIFFERENTIAL DIAGNOSIS AND TREATMENT

Infection

Infections are the most common cause of acute cough in all age groups and are responsible for some chronic coughs. The age of the patient has a large impact on the type of infection.

INFANTS

Viral upper respiratory infections (common cold), croup (laryngotracheobronchitis), viral bronchiolitis, particularly with RSV, and viral pneumonia are the most frequently encountered respiratory tract infections and hence the most common causes of cough in infancy. Viral illness may predispose to bacterial superinfection (croup and *Staphylococcus aureus* tracheitis or influenza and *H. influenzae* pneumonia).

Common Cold

Cold symptoms and signs usually include stuffy nose, with nasal discharge (rhinorrhea); sore throat and sneezing frequently occur. There may be fever, constitutional signs (irritability, myalgias, headache), or both. Cough is common and may persist for 5 to 7 days. The mechanism by which upper respiratory infections cause cough in children is undetermined. In adults, it is generally thought that "postnasal drip," that is, nasal or sinus secretions draining into the posterior nasopharynx, causes cough and, in fact, may be one of the most frequent causes of cough. Indeed, sinus CT in older patients with colds often reveals involvement of the sinus mucosa. Whether this is true in children remains undetermined. Others believe that cough in a child with a cold indicates involvement (inflammation or bronchospasm) of the lower respiratory tract. One's bias on this matter will likely influence how to treat the child with cough accompanying a cold. In adults, the cough of the common cold may respond to a combination antihistamine-decongestant preparation, presumably from the decreased postnasal drip. It is uncertain whether such treatment is effective or indicated in children, particularly young infants, in whom toxicity of the drugs may be a greater concern than in adults.

Common viral pathogens include rhinovirus, RSV, and parainfluenza virus. The differential diagnosis includes allergic rhinitis, which often demonstrates clear nasal secretions with eosinophils and pale nasal mucosa, in contrast to mucopurulent nasal secretions with neutrophils and erythematous mucosa.

Croup (Laryngotracheobronchitis)

Infectious croup (see Chapter 10) is a syndrome with peak incidence in the first two years of life. Its most dramatic components are the barking ("croupy") cough and inspiratory stridor, which appear a few days after the onset of a cold. In most cases, the patient has a low-grade fever, and the disease is self-limited within a day or two. In severe cases, the child can be extremely ill and is at risk for complete laryngeal obstruction. There may be marked intercostal and suprasternal retractions and cyanosis. Stridor at rest signifies severe obstruction. Diminishing stridor in a child who is becoming more comfortable is a good sign, but diminishing stridor in and of itself is not necessarily good: If the child becomes fatigued because of the tremendous work of breathing through an obstructed airway and can no longer breathe effectively, smaller than needed tidal volumes will make less noise.

It is important to distinguish croup from epiglottitis in the child with harsh barky cough and inspiratory stridor because the natural history of the two diseases is quite different (see Table 7–10). Epiglottitis occurs more commonly in toddlers than in infants and is discussed below.

Treatment of mild croup is usually not needed. For decades, pediatricians have recommended putting a child with croup in a bath or steamy shower or driving to the office or emergency room with the car windows rolled down. (It is likely that these remedies are effective because of the heat exchange properties of the upper airway; air that is cooler or more humid than the airway mucosa will serve to cool the mucosa, thus causing local vasoconstriction, and probably decreasing local edema.)

In a child who is stridorous at rest, hospitalization is indicated. Symptomatic, often dramatic relief through decreased laryngeal edema can usually be achieved with aerosolized racemic epinephrine. It is essential to remember that the effects of the epinephrine are transient, lasting only a few hours, although the course of the illness is often longer. The result is that when the racemic epinephrine's effect has worn off, the child's cough and stridor will likely be as bad or even worse than before the aerosol was administered. This is *not* a "rebound" effect—the symptoms are not worse because of the treatment but, rather, because of the natural progression of the viral illness. Repeating the aerosol will likely again have a beneficial effect and reduce the likelihood of requiring a tracheotomy or endotracheal intubation. The lesson to be kept in mind is that a child who responds favorably to such an aerosol should not be sent home from the emergency department, since further treatment may be needed again until the disease has run its course. A single dose of dexamethasone (0.6 mg/kg IM or IV) reduces the severity and hastens recovery but does not necessarily reduce the need for racemic epinephrine aerosols. Aerosolized steroids (budesonide) may also be effective in patients with mild to moderately severe croup.

Bronchiolitis

Bronchiolitis is a common and potentially serious lower respiratory tract disorder in infants (see Chapters 8 and 10). It is usually caused by RSV, but on occasion by parainfluenza, influenza, or adenovirus. It occurs in the winter months often in epidemics. RSV bronchiolitis is seen uncommonly after age 4 years. Typically, "cold-like" symptoms of rhinorrhea precede the harsh cough, increased respiratory rate, and retractions. Respiratory distress and cyanosis can be severe. The child's temperature is seldom elevated above 38°C.

The chest is hyperinflated, widespread crackles are audible on inspiration, and wheezing marks expiration. The most striking laboratory abnormalities are in the chest x-ray, which invariably reveals hyperinflation, as depicted by a depressed diaphragm, with an enlarged retrosternal air space in as many as 60% of patients, peribronchial thickening in some 50%, and consolidation and/or atelectasis in 10% to 25%.

The diagnosis is confirmed with demonstration of RSV by immu-

nofluorescent stain of nasopharyngeal washings. In most cases, no treatment is needed because the disease does not interfere with the infant's eating or breathing. In severe cases, however, often those in whom there is underlying chronic heart, lung, or immunodeficiency disease, RSV can be life-threatening. In these cases, hospital care with supplemental oxygen and intravenous fluids is indicated. The effect of aerosolized bronchodilators is not clear but is probably beneficial. The aerosolized antiviral agent ribavirin may be beneficial for the sickest infants. It is expensive and difficult to administer; it needs to be given 12 to 18 hours per day and may block ventilator tubing and valves. Ribavirin may improve oxygenation but should not be used in lieu of mechanical ventilation in severe patients with hypoxia and hypercarbia (respiratory failure).

Viral Pneumonia

Viral pneumonia can be similar to RSV bronchiolitis in its presentation, with cough and tachypnea, following a few days of apparent upper respiratory infection. There can be a variable degree of temperature elevation and of overall illness. Infants and children with viral pneumonia may appear relatively well or, particularly with adenovirus, may have a rapidly progressive course, ending in death within a few days after the onset of illness. Frequent symptoms include poor feeding, cough, cyanosis, fever (some may be afebrile), apnea, and rhinorrhea. Frequent signs include tachypnea, retractions, crackles, and cough. Cyanosis is less common.

The most common agents causing viral pneumonia in infancy and childhood are RSV, influenza, and parainfluenza. Adenovirus is less common, but it is important because it can be lethal and, even if not life-threatening, can leave residua, including bronchiectasis and bronchiolitis obliterans. Adenovirus pneumonia is often accompanied by conjunctivitis and pharyngitis in addition to leukocytosis and an elevated erythrocyte sedimentation rate (ESR); the ESR and leukocyte count are usually not elevated in viral pneumonia. Additional viral agents include enteroviruses and rhinovirus. Roentgenograms most often reveal diffuse peribronchial infiltrates, with a predilection for the perihilar regions, but occasionally lobar infiltrates are present. Pleural effusions are not common. On occasion, if an infant is extremely ill, bronchoscopy with bronchoalveolar lavage may be indicated to isolate the virus responsible for the pneumonia.

Treatment is largely supportive, with oxygen and intravenous fluids. Mechanical ventilation may be necessary in a small minority of infants. In young infants, the *afebrile pneumonia syndrome* may be due to *Chlamydia, Ureaplasma, Mycoplasma,* cytomegalovirus, or *Pneumocystis carinii*. Severe pneumonia may develop in neonates as a result of herpes simplex.

Pertussis (Whooping Cough)

Pertussis is an extremely important cause of lower respiratory tract infection in infants and children. The causative organism, *Bordetella pertussis*, has a tropism for tracheal and bronchial ciliated epithelial cells; thus the disease is primarily bronchitis, but spread of the organism to alveoli, or secondary invasion by other bacteria, can cause pneumonia. The disease can occur at any age, from early infancy onward, although its manifestations in young infants and in those who have been partially immunized may be atypical.

Most commonly, pertussis has three stages:

- Catarrhal, in which symptoms are indistinguishable from the common cold
- Paroxysmal, dominated by as many as 20 forceful, paroxysmal

Table 7-11. **Potential Complications of Cough**

Musculoskeletal	Rib fractures
	Vertebral fractures
	Rupture of rectus abdominis muscle
	Asymptomatic elevation of serum creatine phosphokinase
Pulmonary	Chest wall pain*
	Bronchoconstriction
	Pneumomediastinum
	Pneumothorax
	Mild hemoptysis
	Subcutaneous emphysema
	Irritation of larynx and trachea
Cardiovascular	Rupture of subconjunctival,* nasal,* and anal veins
	Bradycardia, heart block
	Transient hypertension
Central nervous system	Cough syncope
	Headache
	Subarachnoid hemorrhage
Gastrointestinal	Hernias (ventral, inguinal)
	Emesis
	Rectal prolapse
	Pneumoperitoneum
Miscellaneous	Anorexia*
	Malnutrition
	Sleep loss*
	Urinary incontinence
	Disruption of surgical wounds
	Vaginal prolapse
	Displacement of intravenous catheters

*Common.

coughing spells per day; many spells may be punctuated by an inspiratory "whoop," post-tussive emesis, or both
• Convalescent, in which the intensity and frequency of coughing spells gradually diminish

Each stage typically lasts 1 to 2 weeks, except the paroxysmal stage, which last many weeks. The Chinese term for pertussis translates to "100 days of cough." Most children are entirely well between coughing spells, when physical findings are remarkably benign. Infants younger than 3 months of age may have the most severe illness, and in this age group pertussis is a lethal disease, with mortality rates as high as 40%.

Diagnosis can be difficult because the definitive result, namely, culturing the organism from nasopharyngeal secretions, requires special culture medium (Bordet-Gengou, which must be prepared fresh for each collection). Culture specimens are much less likely to be positive during the paroxysmal stage than during the catarrhal stage, when the diagnosis is not being considered. Fluorescent antibody stains (for the antigen) of secretions are also helpful if they are positive, but similarly they are more likely to be positive before the paroxysmal stage. Perhaps the laboratory test that is most helpful is the WBC count, which is typically elevated; values are as high as 20,000 to 50,000, with lymphocytes predominating. Chest radiographic findings are nonspecific. Infants with severe courses may require hospitalization.

Treatment is largely supportive, with oxygen, fluids, and small frequent feeds for those who do not tolerate their normal feedings. Treatment with erythromycin estolate (50 mg/kg/day for 14 days, every 6 hours, p.o.) decreases infectivity and may or may not influence the course of the disease. In some patients, aerosolized

bronchodilators (albuterol) or systemic steroids may help, although such treatment is controversial. Cough suppressants are not helpful, but good hydration, oxygenation, and nutrition—in addition to not disturbing the infant—are important.

Complications include those related to severe coughing (Table 7–11) and those specific to pertussis, such as seizures and encephalopathy. Pertussis is prevented by three primary immunizations (at 2, 4, and 6 months of age) and regular booster immunizations at 15 to 18 months and 4 to 6 years of age. Pertussis infection produces lifelong immunity.

Chlamydial Infection

Chlamydia trachomatis can cause pneumonia in young infants, particularly those from 3 to 12 weeks of age. Cough, nasal congestion, low-grade or no fever, and tachypnea are common. Conjunctivitis is an important clue to chlamydial disease but is present in only 50% of infants with chlamydial pneumonia at the time of presentation. The infant may have a paroxysmal cough similar to that of pertussis, but post-tussive emesis is less common in chlamydial disease. Crackles are commonly heard on auscultation, but wheezing is much less common than the overinflated appearance of the lungs on roentgenograms would suggest. The organism may be recovered from the nasopharynx by culture or antigen testing. The complete blood count (CBC) may reveal eosinophilia. Chlamydial infection responds to oral erythromycin therapy (40 to 50 mg/kg/day, every 6 hours for 7 to 10 days).

Ureaplasmal Infection

Ureaplasma urealyticum pneumonia is difficult to diagnose but causes cough in some infants. There are no particularly outstanding features to distinguish this relatively uncommon infection from viral pneumonias.

Bacterial Pneumonia

Bacterial pneumonia is relatively less common in infants (compared with viral pneumonia) but can cause severe illness, with cough, respiratory distress, and fever. Chest films are strikingly abnormal; the WBC count is elevated.

Treatment is with broad-spectrum intravenous antibiotics effective against *H. influenzae* type b, pneumococci, group A (possibly B) streptococci, and, if illness is severe, *S. aureus*. Cefotaxime with or without nafcillin or erythromycin may be effective choices.

TODDLERS AND CHILDREN

Colds

In early childhood, as children attend day care and nursery schools, they are constantly exposed to respiratory viruses to which they have little or no immunity (e.g., rhinoviruses, adenoviruses, parainfluenza, and coxsackievirus). Such children may have as many as six to eight or even more colds in a year. The remarks concerning colds and cough in infants (above) apply to this older age group. The differential diagnosis of rhinorrhea is noted in Table 7–12.

Sinusitis

The sinuses may become the site for viral and subsequent secondary bacterial infection spreading from the nasopharynx (Fig. 7–5). The signs and symptoms are usually localized, including nasal congestion, a feeling of "fullness" or pain in the face (Fig. 7–6), headache, sinus tenderness, day or night cough, and fever. Maxillary toothache, purulent nasal discharge for more than 10 days, a positive transillumination (opacification), and a poor response to oral antihistamines or nasal decongestants are important clues. Sinus x-rays or (more accurately) CT scan may facilitate the diagnosis of sinusitis by demonstrating opacification of the sinus with mucosal thickening. Sinusitis is thought to be a cause of cough in adults, but it can probably be listed, with lower certainty, as a cause of cough in children.

Sinusitis is frequently seen in other conditions known to cause cough, especially cystic fibrosis (CF), asthma, and ciliary dyskinesia. It may be difficult to ascertain whether the cough is a direct result of the sinus infection or the underlying problem (purulent bronchitis in the child with CF or ciliary dyskinesia, exacerbation of asthma). In the first two situations, it may not matter because treatment will be the same. In the case of the child with asthma, it is important to treat the asthma with bronchodilating and anti-inflammatory agents as well as the infected sinuses with antibiotics.

The treatment of sinusitis involves the use of oral antibiotics active against the common pathogens (*Streptococcus pneumoniae*, nontypable *H. influenzae, Moraxella catarrhalis*, and, rarely, anaerobic bacteria or *S. aureus*). Treatment regimens include the use of amoxicillin, amoxicillin-clavulanate, trimethoprim-sulfamethoxazole, cefaclor, cefixime, cefuroxime, or loracarbef. Amoxicillin is considered the initial agent of choice. Oral (pseudoephedrine, phenylephrine) or topical (phenylephrine, oxymetazoline) decongestants may be of benefit by increasing the patency of the sinus ostia permitting drainage of the infected and obstructed sinuses. Oral antihistamines may benefit patients with an allergic history. Treatment with antimicrobial agents should continue for at least 7 days after the patient has responded. This may require 14 to 21 days of therapy.

Complications of acute sinusitis include orbital cellulitis, abscesses (orbital, cerebral), cranial (frontal) osteomyelitis (Pott puffy tumor), empyema (subdural, epidural), and thrombosis (sagittal or cavernous sinus).

Croup and Epiglottitis

See above text and Chapter 10.

Pneumonia

Viral Pneumonia. The features discussed for viral pneumonia in infants are relevant for viral pneumonia in older children. The

Table 7–12. Differential Diagnosis of Rhinorrhea

Etiology	Frequency	Duration*	Discharge	Comment
Viral	Common	Acute	Purulent	Polymorphonuclear neutrophils in smear
Allergic	Common	Acute/chronic	Clear	Eosinophils in smear, seasonal
Vasomotor	Common	Chronic	Variable	
Sinusitis	Common	Chronic	Purulent	Sinus tenderness
Rhinitis medicamentosus	Common	Chronic	Variable	Medication use
Response to stimuli	Common	Acute	Clear	Odors, exercise, cold air, pollution
Nasal polyps	Uncommon	Chronic	Variable	Consider cystic fibrosis
Granulomatous disease	Uncommon	Chronic	Bloody	Sarcoid, Wegener granulomatosis, midline granuloma
Cerebrospinal fluid fistula	Uncommon	Chronic	Watery	Trauma, encephalocele
Foreign body	Uncommon	Chronic	Purulent	Often malodorous
Tumor	Uncommon	Chronic	Clear to bloody	Angiofibroma, hemangioma, rhabdomyosarcoma, lymphoma, nasopharyngeal carcinoma, neuroblastoma
Choanal atresia, stenosis	Uncommon	Chronic	Clear to purulent	Congenital
Nonallergic eosinophilic rhinitis syndrome	Uncommon	Chronic	Clear	Eosinophils in smear
Septal deviation	Unknown	Chronic	Clear	
Drugs	Uncommon	Chronic	Variable	Cocaine, glue and organic solvents, angiotensin-converting enzyme inhibitors, beta blockers
Hypothyroidism	Uncommon	Chronic	Clear	
Cluster headache	Uncommon	Intermittent	Clear	Associated tearing, headache
Horner syndrome	Uncommon	Chronic	Clear	Ptosis, miosis, anhidrosis

*Less than 1 week is considered acute.

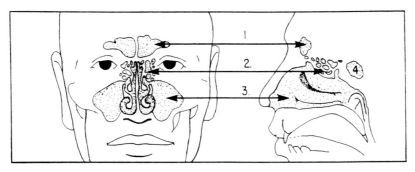

Figure 7–5. The paranasal sinuses. 1, Frontal. 2, Ethmoid. 3, Maxillary. 4, Sphenoid. (From Smith RP. Common upper respiratory tract infections. *In* Reilly B [ed]. Practical Strategies in Outpatient Medicine, 2nd ed. Philadelphia: WB Saunders, 1991.)

differentiation of viral or atypical pneumonia from classical bacterial pneumonia is noted in Table 7–13.

Bacterial Pneumonia. Bacterial pneumonia is more common in toddlers and older children than in infants. Many childhood bacterial pneumonias are pneumococcal, but in addition to *S. pneumoniae*, other bacteria, as noted in Table 7–14, can also cause pneumonia in children. Cough may not be as prominent a presenting symptom or sign as tachypnea and grunting, sometimes (especially in infants) with vomiting. Manifestations are noted in Table 7–13. Raised respiratory rates (≥50 if 2 to 12 months old or ≥40 if 1 to 5 years old) plus retractions and grunting with or without hypoxia (oxygen saturation <90%) have a high specificity and sensitivity for pneumonia. Chest pain, abdominal pain, headache, or any combination of these symptoms may occur. Upper lobe pneumonia may produce meningeal signs, and lower lobe involvement may cause abdominal pain and an ileus.

Examination of the chest shows tachypnea but may be otherwise surprisingly normal. In older children, there may be localized dullness to percussion, with crackles or amphoric breath sounds over a consolidated lobe. The chest film may be normal in the first hours of the illness as the x-ray findings often lag behind the clinical manifestations. Nonetheless, both posteroanterior and lateral views are the main diagnostic tools; lobar consolidation is usual, with *or* without pleural effusion. In infants, the pattern may be more diffuse and extensive.

Some clinical and radiographic features may be suggestive of the bacterial cause of pneumonia. Children (especially infants) with staphylococcal pneumonia are more likely to have a rapid overwhelming course; in one extensive series, however, 40% of children with staphylococcal pneumonia had been mildly ill for many days before presentation. Staphylococcal pneumonia may be accompanied by more extensive roentgenographic abnormalities, including multilobar consolidation, pneumatocele formation, and extensive pleural (empyema) fluid. The presence of a pleural effusion is not helpful in giving the specific bacterial diagnosis because other bacterial pneumonias may be accompanied by pleural effusion. Pleural effusions may represent a reactive parapneumonic effusion or an empyema. Pleural fluid may be characterized as transudate, exudate, and complicated empyema in need of closed chest drainage with a chest tube (Table 7–15). If of sufficient size, as demonstrated by a lateral decubitus film or ultrasonography, a thoracentesis is indicated to differentiate the nature of the effusion and to identify possible pathogens.

Differentiating among the causes of bacterial pneumonia can be done with certainty only with positive cultures from blood, pleural fluid, fluid obtained by direct lung tap, or, rarely, sputum. Current or previous antibiotic treatment diminishes the yield of such cultures. The presence of bacterial antigens in the urine for *S. pneumoniae* or *H. influenzae* provides strong evidence of the causative agent. Bronchoscopy with or without lavage may yield helpful specimens from the progressively ill child or the child who has not responded promptly to empirical antibiotics.

Treatment is with antibiotics. Cefotaxime or ceftriaxone is the drug of choice for the previously healthy child who requires hospitalization with lobar pneumonia. Many children with pneumonia do well with oral antibiotics (amoxicillin, new oral cephalosporins, trimethoprim-sulfamethoxazole) and respond within hours to the first dose. A smaller number may require hospitalization and intravenous antibiotics along with supportive measures (e.g., oxygen and intravenous fluids). Repeated or follow-up chest films may remain abnormal for 4 to 6 weeks following pneumonia and are not indicated for a single episode of uncomplicated pneumonia (i.e., no effusion, no abscess, and good response to treatment). Children with suspected pneumococcal pneumonia must be followed up carefully because of the emergence of penicillin and cephalosporin resistance.

Mycoplasma pneumoniae pneumonia is a common pneumonia among school-aged children. The disease often occurs in community outbreaks in the fall months. Patients typically begin with cold-like symptoms (i.e., sore throat, myalgias, headache, fever), which then progress to include worsening cough, paroxysmal at times. Patients do not often appear acutely ill, but cough may persist for weeks. There may be no specific abnormalities on the

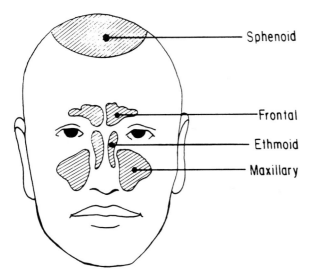

Figure 7–6. Typical pain location among patients with various anatomic sites of acute sinusitis. (From Smith RP. Common upper respiratory tract infections. *In* Reilly B (ed). Practical Strategies in Outpatient Medicine, 2nd ed. Philadelphia: WB Saunders, 1991.)

Table 7-13. Differentiation of Classical Bacterial Pneumonia from Viral and Atypical Pneumonias*

	Bacterial	Viral/Atypical
History	Precedent URI	Headache, malaise, URI, myalgias
Course	Often biphasic illness	Often monophasic
Onset	Sudden	Gradual
Temperature	High fever	Low-grade fever
Rigors	Present	Uncommon
Vital signs	Tachypnea, tachycardia	Less toxic
Pain	Pleuritic	Unusual
Chest examination	Crackles, signs of consolidation	Consolidation unusual
Sign of pleural effusion	Common	Uncommon
Sputum	Productive, purulent, many PMNs, one dominant organism on Gram stain	Scant, no organisms; PMNs or mononuclear cells
ESR	Elevated	Usually normal
WBC count	15,000–25,000; left shift	Often normal
Chest radiography	Lobar consolidation, round infiltrate, parapneumonic effusion; may be ''bronchopneumonia''	Diffuse, bilateral, patchy, interstitial or bronchopneumonia; lower lobe involvement common; chest film may look worse than patient's condition
Progression	May be rapid	Rapid if *Legionella,* hantavirus, herpesvirus, adenovirus
Diagnosis	Blood, sputum, and pleural fluid specimens for culture; antigen detection possible; BAL if progressive	Viral, chlamydial culture or antigen detection; acute and convalescent titers; BAL if progressive

*Atypical pneumonias include *Chlamydia pneumoniae* (formerly TWAR), *Mycoplasma pneumoniae, Legionella* species (*L. pneumophila, L. micdadei*), Q fever, psittacosis.
Abbreviations: URI = upper respiratory tract infection; ESR = erythrocyte sedimentation rate; PMNs = polymorphonuclear neutrophils; WBC = white blood cell; BAL = bronchoalveolar lavage.

chest examination, although a few crackles may be heard, and about one third of younger patients wheeze.

The x-ray findings can mimic almost any intrathoracic disease; scattered infiltrates with nonspecific ''dirty'' lung fields, predominantly perihilar or lower lobes, are common, and lobar infiltrates and pleural effusion are occasionally seen. Laboratory data (CBC, ESR, sputum culture) may not be helpful. A rise in antimycoplasmal IgG over 1 to 2 weeks may be demonstrated but is seldom helpful in guiding therapy. A positive IgM response may be useful. The cold agglutinin test is positive in about 70% of patients with mycoplasmal pneumonia, but is also positive in other conditions, including adenovirus infection. The more severe the illness the greater the frequency of positive cold agglutinins. The diagnosis is often made by the history of an older child who has a lingering coughing illness in the setting of a community outbreak, unresponsive to most (non-erythromycin) antibiotic regimens.

Treatment is with erythromycin (azithromycin or doxycycline is an alternative), which usually shortens the course of the illness. Extrapulmonary complications of mycoplasmal infection include aseptic meningitis, transverse myelitis, peripheral neuropathy, erythema multiforme, myocarditis, pericarditis, hemolytic anemia, and bullous otitis media (myringitis). In patients with sickle cell anemia, severe respiratory failure and acute chest syndrome may develop. Infection with *Chlamydia pneumoniae* (formerly TWAR agent) mimics respiratory disease resulting from *M. pneumoniae,* as it occurs in epidemics, is seen in older children, and produces an atypical pneumonia syndrome and pharyngitis.

Tuberculosis

The incidence of tuberculosis (TB) is increasing as a result of the risks of acquired immunodeficiency syndrome (AIDS), home-lessness, urban poverty, and immigration from endemic countries. TB must be considered seriously in the child with chest disease that is not easily explained by other diagnoses, especially if the child has been exposed to an adult with active TB. Nonetheless, TB is an infrequent cause of cough in children, even in those with active disease.

The diagnosis is made primarily by skin testing (PPD), a history of contact, and recovery of the organism from sputum, bronchoalveolar lavage, pleural fluid or biopsy, or morning gastric aspirates (Table 7–16). The yield from these procedures is relatively low, even from children with active pulmonary TB.

The patterns of disease in normal hosts include primary pulmonary TB, with subsequent inactivation usually noted in young children and reactivation pulmonary disease among adolescents. Primary pulmonary disease is often noted as a lower or middle lobe infiltrate during the period of T-lymphocyte reaction to the initial infection. Prior to resolution the *Mycobacterium tuberculosis* may disseminate to the better-oxygenated upper lobes and extrathoracic sites, such as bone, or the central nervous system (CNS). If the immune response contains the initial infection, the x-ray findings may be indistinguishable from those of any other pneumonic process. With altered immune function, however, there may be progressive local disease, dissemination to miliary pulmonary disease, or early reactivation (months to 5 years) at distal sites producing tuberculous meningitis or osteomyelitis. Reactivation of upper lobe pulmonary disease may produce cavities that are similar to the disease among adults. Cavitary and endobronchial lymph node involvement are highly infectious, in contrast to the much less contagious nature of the hypersensitivity reaction noted in primary pulmonary disease.

Treatment of active disease, especially in regions of multidrug-resistant TB, consists of three or four drug regimens, including

Table 7–14. Etiology of Infectious Pneumonia

Bacterial

Common

Streptococcus pneumoniae	See Table 7–13
Haemophilus influenzae type B	See Table 7–13
Group B streptococci	Neonates
Group A streptococci	See Table 7–13
Mycoplasma pneumoniae*	Adolescents, summer-fall epidemics
Chlamydia pneumoniae*	Adolescents (see Table 7–13)
Chlamydia trachomatis	Infants
Mixed anaerobes	Aspiration pneumonia
Gram-negative enteric	Nosocomial pneumonia

Uncommon

Staphylococcus aureus	Pneumatoceles; infants
Moraxella catarrhalis	
Neisseria meningitides	
Francisella tularensis	Animal, tick, fly contact
Nocardia species	Immunosuppressed
Chlamydia psittaci*	Bird contact
Yersinia pestis	Plague
Legionella species*	Exposure to contaminated water; nosocomial

Viral

Common

Respiratory syncytial virus	See Table 7–13
Parainfluenza types 1–3	Croup
Influenza A, B	High fever; winter months
Adenovirus	Can be severe; often occurs between January–April

Uncommon

Rhinovirus	Rhinorrhea
Enterovirus	Neonates
Herpes simplex	Neonates
Cytomegalovirus	Infants, immunosuppressed
Measles	Rash, coryza, conjunctivitis
Varicella	Adolescents
Hantavirus	Southwestern United States

Fungal

Histoplasma capsulatum	Geographic region; bird, bat contact
Cryptococcus neoformans	Bird contact
Aspergillus species	Immunosuppressed
Mucormycosis	Immunosuppressed
Coccidioides immitis	Geographic region
Blastomyces dermatitides	Geographic region

Rickettsial

Coxiella burnetii*	Q fever, animal (goat, sheep, cattle) exposure
Rickettsia rickettsiae	Tick bite

Mycobacterial

Mycobacterium tuberculosis	See Table 7–16
Mycobacterium avium–intracellulare	Immunosuppressed

Parasitic

Pneumocystis carinii	Immunosuppressed, steroids
Eosinophilic	Various parasites (e.g., *Ascaris, Strongyloides*)

*Atypical pneumonia syndrome (see Table 7–13); atypical in terms of extrapulmonary manifestations, low-grade fever, patchy diffuse infiltrates, poor response to penicillin-type antibiotics, and negative sputum Gram stain.

isoniazid, rifampin, pyrazinamide with or without streptomycin, and ethambutol. Screening protocols are presented in Table 7–16.

Aspiration, Including Foreign Body

Inhaling food, mouth, or gastric secretions, or foreign bodies into the tracheobronchial tree causes acute, recurrent, or chronic cough. Interference with normal swallowing disrupts the coordination of swallowing and breathing that prevents aspiration. Structural causes of disordered swallowing include esophageal atresia (neonates), strictures, webs, or congenital stenoses. Mediastinal lesions (tumors, lymph nodes), including vascular rings, may compromise the esophageal lumen and esophageal peristalsis increasing the likelihood of aspiration. Functional disorders include CNS dysfunction (e.g., coma, myopathy, neuropathy) or immaturity, dysautonomia, achalasia, and diffuse esophageal spasm. Prior neck surgery, including tracheostomy, may alter normal swallowing. Tracheoesophageal fistula and laryngeal clefts are congenital malformations with direct physical connections between the tracheobronchial tree and the upper gastrointestinal tract; oral contents directly enter the lungs.

Making the diagnosis of aspiration as the cause of cough may be difficult. Barium contrast studies during swallowing may help characterize these disorders if barium enters the trachea. Because most patients aspirate sporadically, a normal barium swallow does not rule out aspiration. Radionuclide studies can be helpful if ingested radiolabeled milk or formula fed is demonstrated over the lung fields at several-hour intervals after the meal. Bronchoscopy and bronchoalveolar lavage that recover large numbers of lipid-laden macrophages suggest that milk aspiration has taken place; however, the finding is neither sensitive nor specific for aspiration.

Treatment depends largely on the cause of aspiration. Because many patients who aspirate do so because of lack of neurologic control of swallowing and breathing, it is often difficult to prevent. Even gastrostomy feedings cannot prevent aspiration of oral secretions. In extreme cases, tracheostomy with ligation of the proximal trachea has been employed. This prevents aspiration but also prevents phonation, and it must be considered only in unusual situations. Aspiration pneumonia is often treated with intravenous penicillin or, preferably, clindamycin to cover mouth flora of predominant anaerobes. Additional coverage against gram-negative organisms (ceftazidime, gentamicin) may be indicated if the aspiration is nosocomial.

Foreign Body

Any child with cough of abrupt onset should be suspected of having inhaled a foreign body into the airway. Toddlers, who by nature put all types of things into their mouths and who have incompletely matured swallowing and airway protective mechanisms, are at high risk. Infants with toddlers or young children in the household who may "feed" the new baby are also at risk. In older children, it is usually possible to obtain an accurate history of the aspiration event. These events are described as choking, gagging, and coughing while something (e.g., peanuts, popcorn, small toys, sunflower seeds) is in the mouth. The child may come to the physician with cough and wheeze immediately after the event, with a clear history and a straightforward diagnosis. In many children with a tracheobronchial foreign body, however, the initial episode is not recognized and these children may not come to medical attention for days, weeks, or even months (Fig. 7–7). The initial episode may be followed by a relatively symptomless period lasting days or even weeks, until infection develops behind an

Table 7-15. Differentiation of Pleural Fluid

	Transudate	Exudate	Complicated Empyema
Appearance	Clear	Cloudy	Purulent
Cell count	<1000	>1000	>5000
Cell type	PMNs	PMNs	PMNs
LDH >200 U/L	Uncommon	Common	LDH >1000 U/L
Pleural/serum LDH ratio	<0.6	>0.6	>0.6
Protein >3g	Unusual	Common	Common
Pleural/serum protein ratio	<0.5	>0.5	>0.5
Glucose*	Normal	Low	Very low* <40 mg/dl
pH*	Normal (7.40–7.60)	7.30–7.45	<7.20 requires chest tube placement
Gram stain	Negative	Usually positive	>85% positive unless patient received prior antibiotics

*Low glucose or pH may be seen in malignant effusion, tuberculosis, esophageal rupture, pancreatitis (positive pleural amylase), and rheumatologic diseases (e.g., systemic lupus erythematosus).
Abbreviations: PMNs = polymorphonuclear neutrophils; LDH = lactate dehydrogenase.

obstructed segmental or lobar bronchus. At this point, cough, perhaps with hemoptysis, with or without wheeze will reoccur.

On physical examination early after an aspiration episode, there is cough, wheeze, or both, often with asymmetry of auscultatory findings. There may be locally diminished breath sounds. Later, localized wheeze or crackles may be detected. In some cases, the two-headed stethoscope may permit the examiner to recognize that a lobe or lung has delayed air entry or exit compared with the other side. The triad of wheezing, coughing, and decreased breath sounds is present in less than 50% of patients. Laryngotracheal foreign bodies often present with stridor, retractions, aphonia, cough, and normal x-rays.

Chest radiographs may be normal in 15% of patients with intrathoracic foreign bodies but should be obtained in both inspiration and expiration, for in some cases the only abnormality is unilateral or unilobar air-trapping, which may occasionally be more clearly identified with a view in expiration. In this view, an overdistended lung that had appeared normal on the inspiratory view does not empty but the normal, unobstructed lung empties normally. This phenomenon causes a shift of the mediastinum toward the emptying lung (away from the side with the obstructing foreign body). In other patients, localized infiltrate or atelectasis may be present behind the obstructing object. In a few patients, it may be possible to identify the foreign body itself; nonetheless, most inhaled food particles are not radiopaque and cannot be seen on radiographs. Aspiration is usually unilateral (80%), with 50% to 60% in the right lung (the lobe depends on body position—supine versus standing—but is often the right middle lobe). The definitive diagnostic and therapeutic maneuver is bronchoscopy; either the flexible or rigid open tube bronchoscope permits direct visualization of the object; the rigid instrument also permits its removal. A child known or strongly thought to have aspirated a foreign body should be scheduled for rigid bronchoscopy in the operating room.

Table 7-16. Diagnosis of Tuberculosis (TB) by Positive Mantoux Skin Test (5 TU)

Cutaneous Induration ≥ *5 mm*
Close exposure to known or suspected active TB
Chest x-ray consistent with TB (old or active)
Clinical evidence of TB
Immunosuppressed children (HIV, corticosteroids, lymphoma, Hodgkin's disease)

Cutaneous Induration ≥*10 mm**
Age ≤ 4 yr of age
Medical *high risks* (chronic renal failure, malnutrition, diabetes mellitus)
High-risk social environment (incarcerated youth, homeless, intravenous drug use, medically indigent, migrant workers, nursing homes, immigrants from regions with TB)

Cutaneous Induration ≥*15 mm**
All children ≥ 4 yr of age without any identifiable risk

Data from Pediatrics 1994;93:131–134.
*BCG vaccination status not relevant. Annual screening with purified protein derivative Mantoux may not be indicated for low-risk children. High-risk children require annual testing. Children in high prevalence regions or who have unreliable histories may be tested at 1, 4–6 and 11–16 yr of age.
Abbreviations: HIV = human immunodeficiency virus; BCG = bacille Calmette-Guérin; TU = tuberculin units.

Gastroesophageal Reflux

Gastroesophageal reflux is a common cause of cough in all age groups (see Chapter 20). The typical patient is an infant in the first 6 months of life who spits up small amounts of milk frequently after feedings. This "regurgitant reflux" most commonly resolves by a year of age. However, many toddlers and children will continue to have reflux, although it may be "silent," or nonregurgitant (without spitting up).

In most people with GER, the GER is innocent and is merely a nuisance or not noticed. Most people have occasional episodes of reflux. In some there are sequelae, and this condition is designated GERD (gastroesophageal reflux disease). One manifestation is cough; the mechanisms for cough are not fully understood. Aspiration of refluxed material is one mechanism for cough but is probably not very common in neurologically intact children. A major mechanism for GERD with cough is mediated by vagal esophago-bronchial reflexes (bronchoconstriction), stimulated by acid in the esophagus. Whether acid in the esophagus is sufficient stimulus to cause bronchoconstriction by itself or whether it merely heightens bronchial reactivity to other stimuli is not yet clear (see Chapter 8). Many children with reactive airways disease have cough or wheeze that is difficult to control until their concurrent gastroesoph-

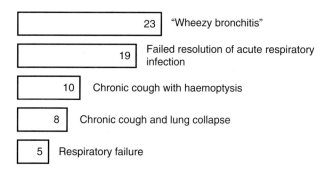

23	"Wheezy bronchitis"
19	Failed resolution of acute respiratory infection
10	Chronic cough with haemoptysis
8	Chronic cough and lung collapse
5	Respiratory failure

Figure 7–7. Presenting problems in children who aspirated foreign bodies in whom diagnosis was delayed over 1 month and the number of children with each problem. (From Phelan PD, Landau LI, Olinsky A. Respiratory Illness in Children. Oxford, England: Blackwell, 1990.)

ageal reflux is also treated. Many episodes of cough caused by GERD occur in children with difficult to control asthma.

The diagnosis of GERD must also be considered in the child with chronic or recurrent cough with no other obvious explanation. The child who coughs after meals or at night, when in the supine position may provoke GER, should be evaluated for GER. If GER is confirmed, the next step is a therapeutic trial of anti-reflux therapy (see Chapter 20). If the results of the therapeutic trial are negative or equivocal, it may make sense to establish a causal relationship between the GER and the cough, by using the modified *Bernstein test*. During this test, hydrochloric acid and saline are alternately infused into the esophagus through a nasoesophageal tube while the child is observed for cough or wheeze or while the older child performs serial pulmonary function tests. If the symptoms occur or if pulmonary function deteriorates during acid but not saline infusion, it is likely that esophageal acidification through GER is the cause of the child's cough or wheeze.

Treatment in a child whose cough is related to GER may be accomplished by treating the reflux (see Chapter 20) or by a combination of anti-reflux and anti-asthma treatment (see Chapter 8). Theophylline may worsen GER by lowering the tone of the lower esophageal sphincter (LES), and some drugs that increase LES tone may cause bronchoconstriction. There is the occasional child whose cough may be abolished by stopping all anti-asthma medications. The cough was a manifestation of reactive airways with esophageal acidification as the trigger for bronchospasm; the esophageal acidification was caused by the bronchodilator effects on the LES. Inhaled bronchodilators are less likely than oral or intravenous drugs to cause GER.

Reactive Airways (Asthma)

Cough is frequently the sole or most prominent manifestation of asthma; wheezing may be entirely absent. In fact, reactive airway disease or asthma (see Chapter 8) is almost certainly the most common cause of recurrent and chronic cough in childhood. Some of the features that characterize the cough of a child with asthma are listed in Table 7–17. Treatment for asthma manifesting as cough is the same as the treatment for asthma (see Chapter 8).

Cystic Fibrosis

Cystic fibrosis is a common cause of recurrent or chronic cough in infancy and childhood. CF occurs in 1 in 2500 live births among Caucasians, is less common in African-Americans (1 in 17,000), and is rare among Native Americans and Asians. Early diagnosis

improves the poor prognosis for untreated CF; if untreated, most patients die by age 1 or 2 years. With current state-of-the-art care, median survival is to age 29.

Cystic fibrosis is a genetic disorder, inherited as an autosomal recessive trait. The CF gene is on the long arm of chromosome 7; there are more than 400 different mutations at the CF locus. Of these mutations, one (Δ F508, indicating a deletion—Δ—of a single phenylalanine—F—at position 508 of the protein product) is the most common, responsible for 70% to 75% of all CF chromosomes. The currently recognized mutations account for approximately 90% of patients. The mutation affects the gene's protein product, termed *cystic fibrosis transmembrane regulator* (CFTR), which acts as a chloride channel and affects other aspects of membrane transport of ions and water. Not all of the consequences of the defective gene and protein have been determined. Most explain the long-observed clinical manifestations of the disease, including thick, viscid mucus in the tracheobronchial tree, leading to purulent bronchiolitis and bronchitis with subsequent bronchiectasis, pulmonary fibrosis, and respiratory failure; pancreatic duct obstruction, leading to pancreatic insufficiency with steatorrhea and failure to thrive; and abnormally high sweat chloride and sodium concentrations. The airway disease in CF is characterized by infection, inflammation, and endobronchial obstruction. The infection begins with *S. aureus, H. influenzae, Escherichia coli, Klebsiella* species, or combinations of these organisms but eventually is dominated by mucoid *Pseudomonas aeruginosa.* Other organisms, such as *Burkholderia cepacia, Xanthomonas maltophilia, Alcaligenes xylosoxidans, Aspergillus fumigatus,* or nontuberculous mycobacteria may also appear; their significance remains undetermined. In some patients, *B. cepacia* has been associated with rapid deterioration and death and in others *Aspergillus* has caused allergic bronchopulmonary aspergillosis. The airway inflammation in all patients with CF appears to be the result of toxic substances, including elastase, released by neutrophils as they respond to the endobronchial infection and by similar enzymes released by the invading organisms.

Cystic fibrosis may present at birth with meconium ileus (10% of patients) or later, with steatorrhea and failure to thrive despite a voracious appetite, in an apparent effort to make up for the calories that are lost in the stool (see Chapter 19). The most common presenting symptom is cough, which may appear within the first weeks of life or may be delayed for decades. The cough can be dry, productive, or paroxysmal. Cough may respond to antibiotics or perhaps steroids, but it is less likely to have improved with bronchodilators (see Tables 7–4 and 7–6). Although CF is a genetic disease, there is often no family history. Furthermore, atypical cases may not have pancreatic insufficiency (usually present in 85% to 90%) and thus not demonstrate steatorrhea and failure to thrive. In addition, malabsorption may not be evident in the neonatal period.

There is no such thing as a child who looks "too good" to have CF; common abnormalities found on physical examination are

Table 7–17. Reactive Airways Disease (Asthma) As a Cause of Cough: History

Any age (even infants)
Coexistence of allergy increases likelihood, *but* absence of allergy does not decrease likelihood
Wheeze need not be present
↑ Cough with upper respiratory infections
↑ Cough with (and especially *after*) exercise
↑ Cough with hard laughing or crying
↑ Cough with exposure to cold
↑ Cough with exposure to cigarette smoke
Usually a history of dramatic response to inhaled beta agonists
May not have responded to oral beta agonists

Table 7–18. Physical Examination Features of Cystic Fibrosis

General
    Low weight for height (>50%)

Head, eyes, ears, nose, and throat
    Nasal polyps (20%)

Chest
    Cough
    Barrel chest (↑ anteroposterior diameter)
    Intercostal, suprasternal retractions
    Crackles, especially right upper lobe
    Wheeze

Abdomen
    Hepatomegaly (10%)
    Right lower quadrant fecal mass (5%–10%)

Extremities
    Digital clubbing (80%)

Table 7–19. Causes of Digital Clubbing in Children

Pulmonary
    Cystic fibrosis[+]
    Non–cystic fibrosis
        bronchiectasis[++]
    Immotile cilia syndrome
    Bronchiolitis obliterans
    Empyema
    Lung abscess
    Malignancy
    Tuberculosis
    Mesothelioma

Cardiac
    Cyanotic congenital
        heart disease[+]
    Subacute bacterial
        endocarditis[++]
    Chronic congestive heart
        disease

Gastrointestinal
    Crohn's disease
    Ulcerative colitis
    Celiac disease[++]
    Severe gastrointestinal
        hemorrhage
    Small bowel lymphoma
    Multiple polyposis

Hepatic
    Biliary cirrhosis
    Chronic active hepatitis

Hematologic
    Thalassemia
    Congenital methemoglobinemia

Miscellaneous
    Familial
    Thyroid deficiency
    Thyrotoxicosis
    Chronic pyelonephritis
    Heavy metal poisoning
    Scleroderma
    Lymphoid granulomatosis
    Hodgkin's disease
    Human immunodeficiency virus

Key: [+] = very common cause of clubbing; [++] = common cause of clubbing.

noted in Table 7–18. One of the most important physical findings is digital clubbing. In most patients with CF, clubbing often develops within the first few years of life. Although the list of conditions associated with clubbing (Table 7–19) is long, they are less common than CF or the incidence of clubbing with these conditions is low. There is some relationship between the degree of pulmonary disease severity and the degree of digital clubbing. Although this relationship is not as clear-cut in the individual patient, a child who has had years of severe respiratory symptoms without clubbing is not likely to have cystic fibrosis.

The diagnosis is confirmed by a positive sweat test, or confirming the presence of two of the recognized CF mutations in DNA, one each on the maternally and paternally derived chromosome 7. The sweat test, if not performed correctly, in a laboratory with extensive experience with the technique (as, for example, in an accredited CF center), yields many false-positive and false-negative results. The proper technique uses the Gibson-Cooke method, with quantitative analysis of the concentration of sodium, chloride, or both, in the sweat produced after pilocarpine iontophoretic stimulation. Chloride (and sodium) concentrations greater than 60 mEq/L are considered positive, and those below 40 mEq/L are negative (normal). Healthy adults have slightly higher sweat chloride concentrations than children, yet the same guidelines hold for positive tests in adults. Other than laboratory error, the non-CF conditions yielding elevated sweat chloride concentrations are listed in Table 7–20. Sweat testing can be performed at any age; newborns within the first few weeks of life may not produce a large enough volume of sweat to analyze, but in those who do (the majority) the results will be accurate. Indications for sweat testing are noted in Table 7–21.

In patients for whom sweat testing is difficult (e.g., because of distance from an experienced laboratory, a small infant who has not produced enough sweat, extreme dermatitis, or a patient with intermediate-range sweat chloride concentrations), DNA testing can be useful. Demonstration of two known CF mutations confirms the diagnosis. Finding one or no known mutation makes the diagnosis less likely but is not exclusive, since there are patients with not-yet-characterized mutations. Further, commercial laboratories do not identify all of the 400-plus mutations.

Recovery of mucoid *P. aeruginosa* from respiratory tract secretions is strongly suggestive of CF. Similarly, pansinusitis is nearly universal among CF patients but is quite uncommon in other children. Some states and some hospitals are using a newborn screen for CF on the dried blood spot used to detect phenylketonuria (PKU) and hypothyroidism. The CF screen is for immunoreac-

tive trypsinogen levels (IRT), which are elevated in most infants with CF for the first several weeks of life. (Some states do genetic testing on DNA.) Because of the very high sensitivity (almost no one with CF has normal IRT levels) and because early institution of treatment is beneficial, this test may come into wider use. Its main drawback is that it has relatively poor specificity; as many as 90% of the positives on the initial screen are false positives. If an infant's IRT screen is positive, the test should be repeated; by the time the test is repeated, at 2 to 3 weeks of age, the false-positive rate has fallen dramatically but is still quite high (25%). Definitive testing needs to be carried out on those infants with two elevated IRT levels. In the unusual older child whose appendix is removed and examined carefully by a knowledgeable pathologist, the diagnosis may be suggested by the typical histologic appearance of the appendix (the mucus-secreting glands are overdistended with eosinophilic material).

Table 7–20. Conditions Other Than Cystic Fibrosis with Elevated Sweat Electrolytes

Adrenal insufficiency (untreated)
Ectodermal dysplasia
Autonomic dysfunction
Hypothyroidism
Malnutrition, including psychosocial dwarfism
Mucopolysaccharidosis
Glycogen storage disease (type I)
Fucosidosis
Hereditary nephrogenic diabetes insipidus
Mauriac syndrome
Pseudohypoaldosteronism
Familial cholestasis
Nephrosis with edema

Table 7-21. Indications for Sweat Testing

Pulmonary Indications
Chronic or recurrent cough
Chronic or recurrent pneumonia
Recurrent bronchiolitis
Atelectasis
Hemoptysis
Staphylococcal pneumonia
Pseudomonas aeruginosa in the respiratory tract (in the absence of such circumstances as tracheostomy or prolonged intubation)
Mucoid *P. aeruginosa* in the respiratory tract
Right upper lobe pneumonia

Gastrointestinal Indications
Meconium ileus
Neonatal intestinal obstruction (meconium plug, atresia)
Steatorrhea, malabsorption
Hepatic cirrhosis in childhood (including any manifestations such as esophageal varices or portal hypertension)
Pancreatitis
Rectal prolapse
Vitamin K deficiency states (hypoprothrombinemia)

Miscellaneous Indications
Digital clubbing
Failure to thrive
Family history of cystic fibrosis (sibling or cousin)
Salty taste when kissed; salt crystals on skin after evaporation of sweat
Heat prostration, especially under seemingly inappropriate circumstances
Hyponatremic hypochloremic alkalosis in infants
Nasal polyps
Pansinusitis
Aspermia

From Kercsmar CM. The respiratory system. *In* Behrman RE, Kliegman RM (eds). Nelson Essentials of Pediatrics, 2nd ed. Philadelphia: WB Saunders, 1994:451.

Laboratory data that may support the diagnosis of CF include absent stool trypsin or chymotrypsin. This suggests pancreatic insufficiency, which occurs most commonly in CF but can be seen in patients who do not have CF. The test is not perfect even for confirming pancreatic insufficiency, since intestinal flora may produce or destroy trypsin. Pulmonary function test findings with an obstructive pattern, incompletely responsive to bronchodilators, are consistent with CF but, of course, can be seen in other conditions. Conversely, some patients with CF also have asthma and may show a marked response to a bronchodilator. Complications of CF that should suggest the diagnosis are noted in Table 7–22.

The treatment of patients with cystic fibrosis requires a comprehensive approach, best performed in, or in conjunction with, an approved cystic fibrosis center. Several studies have shown survival to be significantly better in center-based care than in non–center-based care.

The treatment of the pulmonary aspects of CF involves approaching the obstruction, infection, and inflammation that cause the cough. Cough should be monitored closely, and any increase in frequency, or in the intensity, should be taken as indication that there is worsening endobronchial infection, inflammation, or both. Because active infection and inflammation lead to irreversible lung damage, such changes need to be taken seriously and treated aggressively. This is just as true for the appearance of a mild morning cough in the child who was previously cough-free as it is for severe coughing spells that keep a child awake through the night.

Obstruction is treated with physical means (chest physical therapy, with percussion, vibration, and postural drainage) to dislodge the mucus into the large central airways, where cough can then effectively clear it. Studies have shown this rather crude and time-consuming procedure to be effective in helping to maintain lung function acutely and over a period of years. Variations on the physical maneuvers to help with mucus clearance include forced expiratory technique (FET), positive airway pressure face masks, and masks with expiratory flutter valves. The frequency with which any of these physical means of expelling mucus should be used will vary but should be increased with signs of active infection and obstruction.

Other approaches to relieving obstruction in the bronchial tree include the use of inhaled bronchodilators (despite a paucity of studies showing their long-term efficacy) and mucolytic agents. N-acetylcysteine (Mucomyst) has been available for years, but it may cause tracheobronchial irritation, with bronchorrhea, bronchospasm, or both, in an unacceptably high proportion of patients. An inhaled drug, dornase alpha, or recombinant human DNase (Pulmozyme), is clearly effective in the test tube for liquefying the

Table 7-22. Complications of Cystic Fibrosis

Pulmonary Complications
Bronchiectasis, bronchitis, bronchiolitis, pneumonia
Atelectasis
Hemoptysis
Pneumothorax
Nasal polyps
Sinusitis
Reactive airways disease
Cor pulmonale
Respiratory failure
Mucoid impaction of the bronchi
Allergic bronchopulmonary aspergillosis

Gastrointestinal Complications
Meconium ileus
Meconium peritonitis
Distal intestinal obstruction syndrome (meconium ileus equivalent) (non-neonatal obstruction)
Rectal prolapse
Intussusception
Volvulus
Appendicitis
Intestinal atresia
Pancreatitis
Biliary cirrhosis (portal hypertension: esophageal varices, hypersplenism)
Neonatal obstructive jaundice
Hepatic steatosis
Gastroesophageal reflux
Cholelithiasis
Inguinal hernia
Growth failure
Vitamin deficiency states (vitamins A, K, E, D)
Insulin deficiency, symptomatic hyperglycemia

Other Complications
Infertility
Edema–hypoproteinemia
Dehydration–heat exhaustion
Hypertrophic osteoarthropathy–arthritis
Delayed puberty
Amyloidosis

From Kercsmar CM. The respiratory system. *In* Behrman RE, Kliegman RM (eds). Nelson Essentials of Pediatrics, 2nd ed. Philadelphia: WB Saunders, 1994:451.

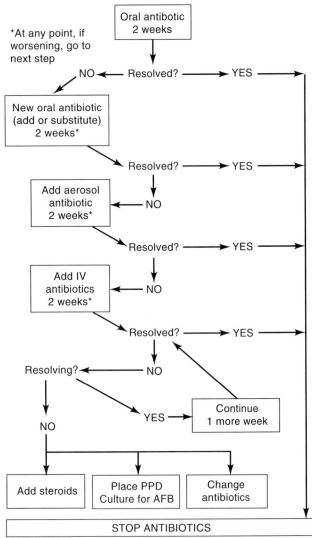

Figure 7–8. Stepwise therapeutic approach to increased cough in patient with cystic fibrosis and airway colonization with *Pseudomonas aeruginosa*. PPD = purified protein derivative; AFB = acid-fast bacillus.

Treatment of infection usually proceeds in a stepwise manner. If colonies of *H. influenzae* or *S. aureus* are present, appropriate antibiotics should be initiated. If no recent throat or sputum specimens for culture are available, and if the patient is young with very mild lung disease, empirical therapy can also be directed at those organisms. In the older or sicker patient who has any sign of chronic pulmonary involvement, such as pulmonary overinflation, infiltrates on a chest film, digital clubbing, or severe coughing spells, it makes sense to include antibiotics effective against *P. aeruginosa*. Figure 7–8 provides one approach to such patients, and Table 7–23 provides more details about individual antibiotics. Progressively more aggressive treatment of cough in CF should not be reserved for the severely ill patient but should be employed in any patient whose cough does not respond to less aggressive treatment.

Treatment of the inflammation associated with CF is evolving. Some patients benefit from short-term oral prednisone. A 4-year study of alternate-day prednisone showed improved pulmonary function but unacceptable side effects (e.g., glucose intolerance, and growth failure) in those taking 2 mg/kg/day and similar side effects (although less severe) in those taking 1 mg/kg/day. The beneficial role of oral nonsteroidal anti-inflammatory agents (NSAIDs) has been demonstrated while the role of inhaled topical steroids and α_1-antitrypsin, is being investigated.

Anatomic Abnormalities

Table 7–24 lists the main anatomic abnormalities (most of them congenital) that cause cough.

VASCULAR RINGS AND SLINGS

Vascular rings and slings are often associated with inspiratory stridor because the abnormal vessels compress central airways, most commonly the trachea (see Chapter 10). The patient may also have difficulty swallowing if the esophagus is compressed.

The diagnosis may be suspected on plain films of the chest, especially with tracheal deviation and a right-sided aortic arch. Further support for the diagnosis can be found at bronchoscopy (which shows extrinsic compression of the trachea or a mainstem bronchus) or barium swallow (which shows esophageal compression), or both. The definitive diagnosis is made with MRI or angiography.

Treatment is surgical.

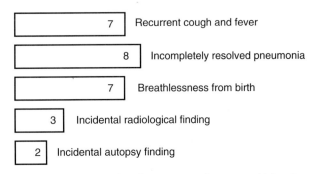

7	Recurrent cough and fever
8	Incompletely resolved pneumonia
7	Breathlessness from birth
3	Incidental radiological finding
2	Incidental autopsy finding

Figure 7–9. Different modes of presentation of sequestered lobe. (From Phelan PD, Landau LI, Olinsky A. Respiratory Illness in Children. Oxford, England: Blackwell, 1990.)

thick mucus associated with CF. This occurs because 40% of the mucus viscosity in CF is attributed to DNA released from dying polymorphonuclear cells. Another drug that appears promising is amiloride. Long available as a diuretic, amiloride can bring about a partial correction of the membrane transport defects in CF. Amiloride aerosols seem to decrease sputum viscosity and increase cough clearance. In a very small 6-month study, aerosolized amiloride appeared to slow the decline in lung function.

The approach to endobronchial infection in children with CF includes prevention and treatment. Prevention involves immunizing patients with CF against preventable respiratory pathogens, particularly influenza (each year), measles, and pertussis. Pneumococcal vaccine is probably not needed. Prevention also means avoiding unnecessary exposure to respiratory viruses (e.g., at day care centers). It should not mean avoiding school or other social functions and settings, since this approach is invariably futile and can cause severe emotional damage.

Table 7–23. Antibiotic Treatment of Cough in Cystic Fibrosis

Route	Organism	Agent	Dosage (mg/kg/24 hr)	Doses Per 24 Hours	Cost* for 2 Weeks	Comments
Oral	*Staphylococcus aureus*	Cloxacillin	50–100	3–4	$ 22	
		Cefaclor	40–60	3	164	
		Clindamycin	20	3–4	93	
		Clarithromycin			77	Less gastrointestinal upset than erythromycin
		Erythromycin	50–100	2–4	12	Gastrointestinal upset common
		Amoxicillin/clavulanate	40	3	105	
	Haemophilus influenzae	Amoxicillin	50–100	3	19	
		Trimethoprim-sulfamethoxazole	20	2–4	29	Dose based on trimethoprim
		Chloramphenicol	50–100	3–4	64	Bone marrow suppression
	Pseudomonas aeruginosa	Ciprofloxacin	15–30	2–3	141	
		Ofloxacin		2–3	98	Also active against *Staphylococcus*
	Empirical	Tetracycline	50–100	3–4	5	Not for children <12 yr
		Vibramycin		2	88	Total dose = 50–100 mg b.i.d.
		Chloramphenicol	50–100	3–4	64	Also active against *Staphylococcus*
Intravenous	*S. aureus*	Oxacillin	150–200	4	665	
	P. aeruginosa	Gentamicin or tobramycin	8–20	1–3	78	Nephrotoxicity, ototoxicity; base doses on serum levels
		Amikacin	15–30	2–3	1380	Nephrotoxicity, ototoxicity; base doses on serum levels
		Netilmicin	6–12	2–3	392	Nephrotoxicity, ototoxicity; base doses on serum levels
		Carbenicillin	250–450	4–6	495	Large sodium load
		Ticarcillin	250–450	4–6	653	Large sodium load
		Piperacillin	250–450	4–6	1171	Sodium < carb, ticar
		Mezlocillin	250–450	4–6	883	
		Azlocillin	250–450	4–6	—	
		Ticarcillin/clavulanate	250–450	4–6	730	Also active against *Staphylococcus*
		Imipenem/cilistatin	45–90	3–4	1881	Nausea with infusion
		Ceftazidime	150	3	1195	
		Aztreonam	200	4	1544	
Aerosol	*P. aeruginosa*	Gentamicin or tobramycin	—	2–4	43–186	80–600 mg/dose
		Colistin	—	2–4	960	1 g in saline
		Carbenicillin	—	2–4	77	500 mg–1 g; strong odor
		Ceftazidime	—	2–4	597	May foam

Modified from Boat TF. Cystic fibrosis. *In* Behrman RE, Kliegman RM, Nelson WE, Vaughn VC (eds). Nelson Textbook of Pediatrics, 14th ed. Philadelphia: WB Saunders, 1992:1113.
*Costs are for an intermediate dose and for drug alone (no delivery devices).

PULMONARY SEQUESTRATION

Pulmonary sequestration is relatively unusual, occurring in one in 60,000 children. It occurs most commonly in the left lower lobe and can present in several different ways (Table 7–24; Fig. 7–9). The chest radiograph usually shows a density in the left lower lobe; this density often appears to contain cysts. The feature distinguishing a sequestered lobe from a complicated pneumonia is that the blood supply arises from the aorta and not the pulmonary circulation. Doppler ultrasound and angiography provide the definitive diagnosis. The treatment is surgical removal.

CYSTADENOMATOID MALFORMATION

Cystadenomatoid malformation is a rare condition. It presents in infancy with respiratory distress in nearly 50% of cases; the other half may manifest as cough with recurrent infection later in childhood or even adulthood. The chest film reveals multiple cysts, separated by dense areas. Chest CT scans can help make the diagnosis with near certainty. Surgical removal is the treatment.

CONGENITAL LOBAR EMPHYSEMA

Congenital lobar emphysema (CLE) occurs in one of 50,000 live births. It can present dramatically in the newborn period with respiratory distress or later (Fig. 7–10), with cough or wheeze, or as an incidental finding on a chest radiograph. Radiography shows localized overinflation, often dramatic, with compression of adjacent lung tissue, and occasionally atelectasis of the contralateral lung because of mediastinal shift away from the involved side. The

Table 7–24. Anatomic Abnormalities Causing Cough

Condition	Other Symptoms	Diagnostic Evidence	Treatment
Vascular ring/sling	Stridor; dysphagia, emesis	X-ray: deviated trachea, right-sided arch Barium swallow: esophageal indentation Bronchoscopy: extrinsic compression MRI/angiography: definitive	Surgical
Pulmonary sequestration	Fever, dyspnea; may be asymptomatic	X-ray: left lower lobe density, usually with cysts Angiography: blood supply from aorta	Surgical
Cystadenomatoid malformation	Respiratory distress; recurrent infection	X-ray: multiple cysts alternating with solid areas CT: typical appearance	Surgical
Congenital lobar emphysema	Respiratory distress; wheeze; may be asymptomatic	X-ray: localized overinflation, other lobes (even other lung) collapsed CT: typical pattern Bronchoscopy in older patients to rule out foreign body	Surgical (if symptomatic)
Tracheoesophageal fistula, cleft	Gagging, choking with feeds; respiratory distress (esp. with esophageal atresia)	Barium swallow: barium in tracheobronchial tree Bronchoscopy: direct visualization	Surgical
Airway hemangioma	Stridor; wheeze; dysphagia; hemoptysis	Bronchoscopy	Steroids; laser; interferon-α
Mediastinal lymph nodes	Stridor	X-ray: hilar nodes; compressed tracheal air column	Treat cause
Bronchial stenosis	Wheeze; recurrent pneumonia	Bronchoscopy	Balloon dilatation; surgery
Bronchogenic cysts	Wheeze, stridor	X-ray: hyperinflation of one lung; ± visible mass (carina, posterior mediastinum) Bronchoscopy: extrinsic compression CT: often definitive	Surgical

Abbreviations: MRI = magnetic resonance imaging; CT = computed tomography.

appearance on chest CT scan is typical, with widely spaced blood vessels (as opposed to congenital cysts, for example, which will have no blood vessels within the overinflated area). Bronchoscopy can document patent bronchi and should probably be carried out in older children, in whom CLE can be confused with acquired overinflation of a lobe as the result of bronchial obstruction, as with a foreign body.

TRACHEOESOPHAGEAL FISTULA

Tracheoesophageal fistula is quite common, with an incidence of about one in 5000 live births. Of these, the large majority (85%) are associated with esophageal atresia; only 3% are the isolated, H-type fistula (a patent esophagus with fistulous tract connecting the esophagus and trachea). A neonate with esophageal atresia experiences respiratory distress, excessive drooling, and choking and gagging with feeding. The H-type fistula will cause more subtle signs and may be undiagnosed for months or even years. The child may have only intermittent feeding trouble, especially with liquids. There may be recurrent lower respiratory tract infection.

The diagnosis is not challenging in the infant with esophageal atresia; a nasogastric tube cannot be passed, and swallowed barium outlines the trachea. In the older child with H-type fistula, a barium esophagram may or may not reveal the fistula. Bronchoscopy and

esophagoscopy should permit direct visualization of the fistula; however, the opening may be hidden in mucosal folds.

Treatment is surgical. Many children born with tracheoesophageal fistula will have recurrent cough and lower respiratory tract infection for many years, even after successful surgical correction. The cough is characteristically the harsh cough of tracheomalacia, which is present at the site of the fistula. The infections result from several causes, including gastroesophageal reflux, with or without aspiration, and altered mucociliary transport. Treatment involves regular chest physical therapy and early and aggressive use of antibiotics whenever there is evidence of increased pulmonary symptoms.

HEMANGIOMAS

Hemangiomas may be present within the airway and can cause cough, rarely with hemoptysis; stridor (if the hemangioma is high in the airway) and respiratory distress (if it is large) may also occur. Rarely, with very large airway hemangiomas, there may even be dysphagia from extrinsic compression. About 50% of children with airway hemangiomas have cutaneous hemangiomas as well.

The diagnosis is made by bronchoscopy. As with cutaneous hemangiomas, these lesions may resolve spontaneously over the first year or so. However, if they cause symptoms, it may not be advisable or possible to wait.

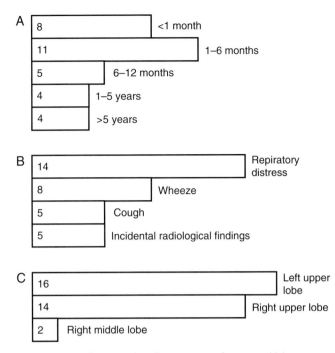

Figure 7–10. Different modes of presentation of congenital lobar emphysema. (From Phelan PD, Landau LI, Olinsky A. Respiratory Illness in Children. Oxford, England: Blackwell, 1990.)

Many airway hemangiomas regress with steroid treatment, although others have been shown to respond to interferon-α. Laser ablation may be indicated in some refractory cases.

ENLARGED LYMPH NODES

Enlarged mediastinal lymph nodes, as from tuberculosis, leukemia, other hematologic malignancies, or other infections, may occasionally be a cause of cough in children (Table 7–25). These nodes are usually seen on plain films of the chest. The x-ray study or bronchoscopy may show extrinsic compression of the trachea. Treatment is directed at the underlying cause of the lymphadenopathy.

BRONCHIAL STENOSIS

Occasionally bronchial stenosis, either congenital or acquired, may cause cough. The diagnosis is made by bronchoscopy, after suspicion has been raised by the child's having recurrent infiltrates in the same lobe, especially with localized wheeze.

Treatment may be difficult. In some cases, endoscopic balloon dilatation is successful; in others, surgical resection of stenotic areas may be necessary.

BRONCHOGENIC CYSTS

Bronchogenic cysts are uncommon, but they can cause cough, wheeze, stridor, or any combination of these. They may also cause recurrent or persistent pneumonia if they block a bronchus sufficiently to interfere with normal drainage of the segment or lobe. Radiography may show localized overinflation if the cyst causes a ball-valve type obstruction. The cyst itself may or may not be seen on plain films. Bronchoscopy reveals extrinsic compression of the airway. CT studies often definitively show the lesion. Surgical removal is indicated.

Habit (Psychogenic) Cough

On occasion, a school-aged child may develop a cough that lasts for weeks, often following a fairly typical cold. This cough occurs only during wakefulness, never during sleep. In many cases the cough is harsh, "foghorn"-like. It often disrupts the classroom, and the child is asked to leave. The child is otherwise well and may seem rather unbothered by the spectacle created. There has been no response to medications. It seems that this type of cough, often termed "psychogenic," or "psychogenic cough tic," but perhaps more accurately and humanely thought of as habit cough, has given the child valuable attention at home and at school. This attention then serves as the sustaining force, and the cough persists beyond the original airway inflammation. In the small minority of cases, there may be deep-seated emotional problems of which the cough is the physical expression.

During the history or physical examination, the child appears completely well and may cough when attention is drawn to the child or when the word "cough" is uttered. The physical examination is otherwise completely normal, as are laboratory values. Because this may occur in any child, evidence of mild reactive airways disease (history or pulmonary function testing) does not rule out the diagnosis. Once one has seen a child with this problem, it is usually possible to make the diagnosis with certainty on entering the examining room or, indeed, from the hallway outside the room.

Treatment can prove more difficult. There are several treatment schools, summarized in Tables 7–26 and 7–27. One approach is "the bed sheet," in which the child is told that he or she coughs

Table 7–25. Intrathoracic Mass Lesions

Anterior Mediastinum
Thymus tumor
T-cell lymphoma
Teratoma
Thyroid lesions
Pericardial cyst
Hemangioma
Lymphangioma

Hilar–Middle Mediastinum
Tuberculosis
Histoplasmosis
Coccidioidomycosis
Acute lymphocytic leukemia–lymphoma
Hodgkin's disease
Sarcoidosis
Hiatal hernia
Pericardial cyst
Bronchogenic or enteric cyst

Posterior Mediastinum
Neuroblastoma-ganglioneuroma
Other neural tumors
Neuroenteric lesions
Esophageal lesions (duplication)
Vertebral osteomyelitis
Diaphragmatic hernia
Meningocele
Aortic aneurysm

Table 7–26. Therapeutic Approaches to Habit Cough

Approach	Advantages	Disadvantages
Perform all possible tests	Can tell patient and family: "We've ruled out all physical problems." In one study, resolution followed bronchoscopy (does this belong under "aversive stimulus"?)	Reinforces the idea of a physical cause
Apply an aversive stimulus (e.g., an electric shock to forearm)	Has worked in some cases	By definition, this treatment is unpleasant
Try the "bed sheet" (see text)	Seems to work in most patients	Demeans the patient
Try placebo drugs	Probably works in some patients	Is a dishonest technique
Give psychotherapy	May work in some patients	Is unnecessary in most patients; labels the patient as having a psychiatric problem
Gently explain that there is no physical cause and this is a habit that the body has sustained	Works in some	Is resented in some families focused on an organic cause or treatment
Prevent mouth breathing by holding a button between the patient's lips	Has worked in some cases	Not known
Apply speech therapy techniques (see Table 7–27)	Works in many; can be presented as specific therapy; nonthreatening	Is resented in some families focused on organic cause or treatment

because of weak chest muscles. A bed sheet is wrapped tightly and uncomfortably around the chest "to serve as added support for the muscles . . . [and] with this support, the muscles would then be able to suppress [the] cough" (Cohlan and Stone, 1984). The child is to go to school wearing the bulky bed sheet under his or her clothes and may not remove the sheet until he or she is certain that the cough will not return. The authors who describe this method call it a "reinforcement suggestion technique." The report of this method brought a flurry of letters to the editor from pediatricians who thought that this approach was demeaning to the child and, in a sense, ridiculed the child. Whatever its mechanism of action, this method is reported to have been successful in 31 of 33 patients.

Other Causes of Cough

Table 7–2 lists several miscellaneous causes of cough in children.

POSTNASAL DRIP

Postnasal drip is thought to be a major cause of cough in adults. The mechanism by which this occurs is unclear, and most pulmonologists believe that this must remain a diagnosis of exclusion for explaining cough in children.

Table 7–27. Speech Therapy Techniques for Treating Habit Cough

Increase abdominal breathing
Reduce muscle tension in neck, chest, and shoulders
Interrupt early cough sensation by swallowing
Substitute gentle cough for racking cough
Interrupt cough sequence with diaphragm breathing and tightly pursed lips
Increase the patient's awareness of initial sensations that would trigger cough

DYSMOTILE CILIA

Conditions in which the cilia do not function properly (dysmotile cilia) lead to cough, usually because infection occurs in the absence of normal mucociliary transport. Treatment is similar to that for cystic fibrosis, with regular chest physical therapy and frequent and aggressive use of antibiotics at the first sign of airways infection, most commonly increased cough.

INTERSTITIAL LUNG DISEASE

Interstitial lung disease (ILD) comes in several varieties: desquamative, lymphoid, and "usual." All are very uncommon in childhood, and little is known about their cause, course, or treatment. One type of pediatric interstitial lung disease, the lymphoid type, is becoming much more common, since it is seen in human immunodeficiency virus (HIV) infection, which itself is increasing in frequency. ILD presents with cough, dyspnea, and crackles on examination. Because the diagnosis is based on histology, it requires lung biopsy. The only exception to this may be in the child with documented AIDS who has new pulmonary infiltrates and symptoms, in whom bronchoscopy and bronchoalveolar lavage are initially used to diagnose infection (*P. carinii*, cytomegalovirus).

ILD in a patient with a chronic seborrhea-like dermatitis should suggest the diagnosis of *histiocytosis X*.

HEART FAILURE

Heart failure can cause cough, but seldom as its sole clinical manifestation.

PULMONARY HEMOSIDEROSIS

Pulmonary hemosiderosis is a rare, and often fatal, condition of bleeding into the lung that can present with cough. If sputum is produced, it is often frothy and blood-tinged. There may be frank hemoptysis. However, the cough may be nonproductive or the sputum may be swallowed. Some cases are associated with milk hypersensitivity (Heiner syndrome), and of these children many have upper airway obstruction. Some cases are associated with collagen vascular disorders. Roentgenograms usually show diffuse fluffy infiltrates, and there is invariably iron deficiency anemia. The diagnosis is based on lung biopsy findings.

Treatment is often unsatisfactory, with mortality as high as 50%. Milk products should be eliminated, and underlying collagen vascular disease should be treated. Some children seem to respond to corticosteroids or cytotoxic drugs (e.g., azathioprine, cyclophosphamide, and chlorambucil), but the episodic nature of the disease, with some clear cases of spontaneous resolution, makes it difficult to evaluate therapies.

BRONCHOPULMONARY DYSPLASIA

See Chapter 8.

TUMORS

Tumors, which fortunately are rare in childhood, can cause cough, usually because of bronchial blockage, either extrinsic or endobronchial (see Table 7–25). The diagnosis is usually made by bronchoscopy, chest CT, or both. Treatment depends on the cell type, but usually involves at least some surgical removal. Chemotherapy or radiation may be used in some.

TRACHEOMALACIA AND BRONCHOMALACIA

Isolated tracheomalacia or bronchomalacia is uncommon but can cause cough in some children. The cough of tracheomalacia is typically harsh and brassy. Treatment is difficult but, fortunately, is seldom needed.

SPASMODIC CROUP

Some children, usually preschoolers, may episodically awaken at night with stridor and a harsh, barking cough indistinguishable from that of viral croup. This entity is termed spasmodic croup and is of unclear etiology. Viral and allergic causes have been postulated. Gastroesophageal reflux may be the cause in some.

Treatment with cool mist or racemic epinephrine is effective in most. If gastroesophageal reflux is the underlying cause, anti-reflux treatment is useful.

OBLITERATIVE BRONCHIOLITIS

Obliterative bronchiolitis is also very rare except in the post–lung transplant patient. In other instances, it may arise following adenovirus, measles, or influenza pneumonia; after exposure to certain toxins; or in other rare circumstances. Children may exhibit cough, respiratory distress, and exercise intolerance.

The diagnosis is suggested by the pulmonary function or radiographic evidence of small airways obstruction; however, these findings are not always present. Not all chest films show overinflated lungs, and not all pulmonary function tests show decreased small airways function.

The definitive diagnosis is histologic via open or transbronchial biopsy. No specific treatment is available. Most children with obliterative bronchiolitis recover, but many progress to chronic disability or death.

Hemoptysis

The child who coughs out blood or bloody mucus presents special diagnostic and therapeutic challenges. Although hemoptysis is relatively uncommon in children, particularly if one excludes cystic fibrosis, many conditions can cause it (Table 7–28). It is important (and not always easy) to distinguish cases in which blood has originated in the tracheobronchial tree (true hemoptysis), the nose *(epistaxis)*, and the gastrointestinal tract *(hematemesis)*. Table 7–29 gives some guidelines to help localize sites of origin of blood that has been reported or suspected as hemoptysis. None of these is foolproof, partly because blood that has originated in one of these sites might well end in another before being expelled from the body; for instance, blood from the nose can be swallowed and vomited or aspirated and coughed out.

Infection is among the most common causes of hemoptysis. Lung abscess and tuberculosis need to be considered. Bronchiectasis, as with cystic fibrosis, can readily cause erosion into bronchial vessels, often made tortuous by years of local inflammation, and produce hemoptysis. Other infectious settings are less common and include necrotizing pneumonias and fungal and parasitic lung invasion.

Foreign bodies in the airway can cause hemoptysis by direct irritation, by erosion of airway mucosa, or by secondary infection.

Pulmonary embolus is uncommon in children and adolescents, but it needs to be considered in the differential diagnosis of an adolescent with hemoptysis of unclear etiology. Clues to the diagnosis of pulmonary embolus include severe dyspnea, chest pain, hypoxia, a normal chest film, an accentuated second heart sound, an abnormal compression ultrasound study of the leg veins, a positive Homan sign, and a high probability lung ventilation perfusion scan.

The diagnosis in several causes of hemoptysis will be straightforward. For example, immediately after a surgical or invasive diagnostic procedure in the chest, hemoptysis should suggest an iatrogenic problem. The chest film can help suggest lung abscess, pulmonary sequestration, bronchogenic cyst, or tumor. Chest CT can help with cases of arteriovenous malformations, and additional laboratory values can support the diagnosis of collagen-vascular disease. Bronchoscopy can sometimes localize a bleeding site, identify a cause (e.g., a foreign body or endobronchial tumor), or recover an offending bacterial, fungal, or parasitic pathogen. In many instances, bronchoscopy does not help except by excluding some possibilities, for either no blood or blood throughout the tracheobronchial tree is found. Bronchial artery angiography may help to identify the involved vessel or vessels.

Treatment of hemoptysis depends on the underlying cause. It can be a terrifying symptom to children and their parents, and a calm, reassuring approach is essential. Because hemoptysis is seldom fatal in children, reassurance is usually warranted. Further, hemoptysis most often resolves and treatment of the bleeding itself is not often needed. What is required is treatment of the underlying cause of the hemoptysis, such as therapy for infection, removal of a foreign body, or control of collagen-vascular disease. When death occurs from hemoptysis, it is more likely to be from suffocation than from exsanguination. In cases of massive bleeding, the open-tube, rigid bronchoscope may help suction large amounts of blood while ventilating and keeping unaffected portions of lung clear of

Table 7–28. Hemoptysis: Differential Diagnosis

Infection	Lung abscess	Pulmonary	Idiopathic or with milk allergy (Heiner's
	Pneumonia*	hemosiderosis	syndrome)
	Tuberculosis	Trauma	Contusion*
	Bronchiectasis* (cystic fibrosis, ciliary dyskinesia)		Fractured trachea, bronchus
	Necrotizing pneumonia	Iatrogenic	Postsurgical
	Fungus (especially allergic		Post–transbronchial lung biopsy*
	bronchopulmonary aspergillosis or		Post–diagnostic lung puncture*
	mucormycosis)	Tumors	Benign (neurogenic, hamartoma,
	Parasite		hemangioma, carcinoid)
	Herpes simplex		Malignant (adenoma, bronchogenic
Foreign body	Retained		carcinoma)
Congenital defect	Heart (various)		Metastatic (Wilms tumor, osteosarcoma,
	Eisenmenger syndrome		sarcoma)
	Abnormal arteriovenous connections	Pulmonary	Cardiogenic
	Arteriovenous malformation	embolus	Deep venous thrombosis
	Telangiectasia (Osler-Weber-Rendu)	Other	Factitious
	Pulmonary sequestration		Endometriosis
	Bronchogenic cyst		Coagulopathy*
Autoimmune-	Henoch-Schönlein purpura		Heart failure
inflammatory	Goodpasture's syndrome		Post-surfactant therapy in neonates
	Wegener's granulomatosis		Kernicterus
	Systemic lupus erythematosus		Hyperammonemia
	Sarcoidosis		Intracranial hemorrhage
			Epistaxis*
			Idiopathic

*A common cause of hemoptysis.

Table 7–29. Hemoptysis: Differentiating Sites of Origin of Blood

	Pulmonary	**Gastrointestinal Tract**	**Nose**
History	Cough; with or without gurgling in lung before episode	Nausea, vomiting, pain	With or without nosebleed dripping in back of throat
Physical	Cough; localized crackles or decreased breath sounds; digital clubbing	↑ Liver, spleen, epigastric tenderness	Blood in nose

Table 7–30. **Cough: Red Flags: When to Refer**

If associated with severe, acute
Hemoptysis
Dyspnea
Hypoxemia

If associated with chronic
Failure to thrive
Steatorrhea
Decreased exercise tolerance
Digital clubbing

Persistence of
Cough for 6 weeks or more
Radiographic abnormality, especially if asymmetric

Failure to respond to empirical therapy
Antibiotics for presumed infection
Bronchodilators for presumed reactive airways

blood. Interventional radiologists treat as well as localize a bleeding site by injecting the offending vessel with occlusive substances, such as Gelfoam or silicone coils. In extremely rare instances, emergency lobectomy may be indicated.

When Cough Itself Is a Problem

Cough is important because it is a symptom and sign of underlying disease that frequently merits treatment. Cough itself seldom deserves specific treatment. Nonetheless, cough is not always completely benign (see Table 7–11). Most of these complications are reasonably uncommon and most accompany only very severe cough, but some are serious enough to justify treatment of the cough itself.

Cough suppressants include codeine and hydrocodone (two narcotics) and dextromethorphan (a non-narcotic *d*-isomer of the codeine analog of levorphanol). Such agents should only be used in severe cough that may produce significant complications (see Table 7–11). For most diseases, suppressing the cough offers no advantage. Disadvantages include narcotic addiction and loss of the protective cough reflex with subsequent mucus retention and possible superinfection. Demulcent preparations (sugar-containing, bland soothing agents) temporarily suppress the cough response from pharyngeal sources, and decongestant-antihistamine combinations may reduce postnasal drip and thus cough in adults.

SUMMARY: RED FLAGS AND WHEN TO REFER

There are instances in which cough merits attention by a specialist. These situations are summarized in Table 7–30. In the acute setting, severe disease, including massive hemoptysis or profound dyspnea or hypoxemia, warrants immediate attention and rapid diagnosis and management. Certain chronic conditions, including those that suggest cystic fibrosis and those in which symptoms have persisted and interfere with a child's daily activities and quality of life, deserve further evaluation and treatment. Finally, a child whose cough fails to respond to what should have been reasonable treatment should be referred to a pulmonary specialist.

An algorithm for the differential diagnosis by category of cough is noted in Figure 7–11.

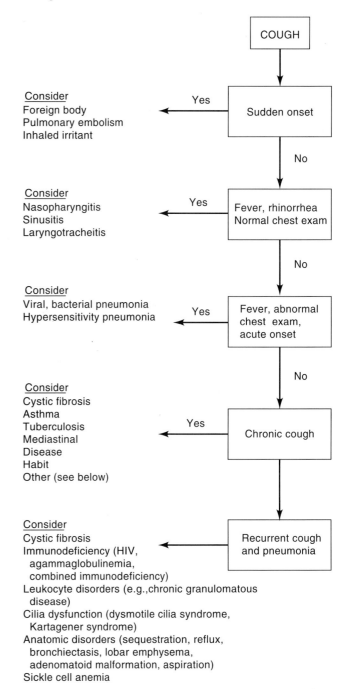

Figure 7–11. Algorithm for differential diagnosis of cough. HIV = human immunodeficiency virus.

REFERENCES

Cough

Black P. Evaluation of chronic or recurrent cough. *In* Hilman BC (ed). Pediatric Respiratory Disease: Diagnosis and Treatment. Philadelphia: WB Saunders, 1993:143–154.

Cohlan S, Stone E. The cough and the bedsheet. Pediatrics 1984;74:11–15.

Irwin RS, Curley FJ. The treatment of cough: A comprehensive review. Chest 1991;99:1477–1484.

Upper Respiratory Infection

Donnelly BW, McMillan JA, Weiner LB. Bacterial tracheitis: Report of eight new cases and review. Rev Infect Dis 1990;12:729–735.

Gwaltney JM, Phillips CD, Miller RD, et al. Computed tomographic study of the common cold. N Engl J Med 1994;330:25–30.

Wald ER. Sinusitis in children. N Engl J Med 1992;326:319–323.

Williams JW, Simel DL. Does this patient have sinusitis? Diagnosing acute sinusitis by history and physical examination. JAMA 1993;270:1242–1246.

Pneumonia

Bourke SJ. Chlamydial respiratory infections. BMJ 1993;306:1219–1220.

Brasfield DM, Stagno S, Whitley RJ, et al. Infant pneumonitis associated with cytomegalovirus, *Chlamydia*, *Pneumocystis*, and *Ureaplasma*: Follow-up. Pediatrics 1987;79:76–83.

Committee on Infectious Diseases. Screening for tuberculosis in infants and children. Pediatrics 1994;93:131–134.

Gibson NA, Hollman AS, Paton JY. Value of radiological follow-up of childhood pneumonia. BMJ 1993;307:117.

McIntosh K, Halonen P, Ruuskanen O. Report of a workshop on respiratory viral infections: Epidemiology, diagnosis, treatment, and prevention. Clin Infect Dis 1993;16:151–164.

Meduri GU, Stein DS. Pulmonary manifestations of acquired immunodeficiency syndrome. Clin Infect Dis 1992;14:98–113.

Mulholland EK, Simoes EAF, Costales MOD, et al. Standardized diagnosis of pneumonia in developing countries. Pediatr Infect Dis 1992;11:77–81.

Nohynek H, Eskola J, Laine E, et al. The causes of hospital-treated acute lower respiratory tract infection in children. Am J Dis Child 1991;145:618–622.

Onyango FE, Steinhoff MC, Wafula EM, et al. Hypoxaemia in young Kenyan children with acute lower respiratory infection. BMJ 1993;306:612–614.

Rubin BK. The evaluation of the child with recurrent chest infections. Pediatr Infect Dis 1985;4:88–98.

Sazawal S, Black RE. Meta-analysis of intervention trials on case-management of pneumonia in community settings. Lancet 1992;340:528–533.

Stark JR, Jacobs RF, Jereb J. Resurgence of tuberculosis in children. Pediatrics 1992;120:839–855.

Foreign Bodies

Black RE, Choi K-J, Syme WC. Bronchoscopic removal of aspirated foreign bodies in children. Am J Surg 1984;148:778–781.

Gay BB, Atkinson GO, Vanderzalm T, et al. Subglottic foreign bodies in pediatric patients. Am J Dis Child 1986;140:165–168.

Puhakka H, Svedstrom E, Kero P, et al. Tracheobronchial foreign bodies. Am J Dis Child 1989;143:543–545.

Cystic Fibrosis

Fiel SB. Clinical management of pulmonary disease in cystic fibrosis. Lancet 1993;341:1070–1074.

Hamos A, Corey M. The cystic fibrosis genotype-phenotype consortium. Correlation between genotype and phenotype in patients with cystic fibrosis. N Engl J Med 1993;329:1308–1316.

Kerem E, Reisman J, Corey M, et al. Prediction of mortality in patients with cystic fibrosis. N Engl J Med 1992;326:1187–1191.

Kerem E, Reisman J, Corey M, et al. Wheezing in infants with cystic fibrosis: Clinical course, pulmonary function, and survival analysis. Pediatrics 1992;90:703–706.

Littlewood JM, Smye SW, Cunliffe H. Aerosol antibiotic treatment in cystic fibrosis. Arch Dis Child 1993;68:788–792.

Ranasinha C, Assoufi B, Shak S, et al. Efficacy and safety of short-term administration of aerosolised recombinant human DNase I in adults with stable stage cystic fibrosis. Lancet 1993;342:199–202.

Taylor RFH, Gaya H, Hodson ME. *Pseudomonas cepacia*: Pulmonary infection in patients with cystic fibrosis. Respir Med 1993;87:187–192.

Tizzano EF, Buchwald M. Recent advances in cystic fibrosis research. J Pediatr 1993;122:985–988.

Asthma

Gustafsson PM, Kjellman N-I M, Tibbling L. Bronchial asthma and acid reflux into the distal and proximal oesophagus. Arch Dis Child 1990;65:1255–1258.

Larsen GL. Asthma in children. N Engl J Med 1992;326:1540–1545.

Warner JO. Asthma: A follow-up statement from an international paediatric asthma consensus group. Arch Dis Child 1992;67:240–248.

Hemoptysis

David M, Andrew M. Venous thromboembolic complications in children. J Pediatr 1993;123:337–346.

Jones DK, Davies RJ. Massive haemoptysis: Medical management will usually arrest the bleeding. BMJ 1990;300:889–890.

Panitch HB, Schidlow DV. Pathogenesis and management of hemoptysis in children. Int Pediatr 1989;4:241–244.

8 Respiratory Distress

Carolyn M. Kercsmar Thomas Ferkol

Respiratory distress occurs for a variety of reasons and with many levels of severity. *Dyspnea,* the sensation of difficult, labored, or uncomfortable breathing, may arise from an increased work of breathing caused by a change in respiratory drive, impaired neuromuscular reserve, or increased ventilatory demand caused by an altered metabolic state. True respiratory distress arises when there is impaired air exchange that leads to decreased ventilation and oxygenation. Physical findings typically associated with respiratory distress include dyspnea, tachypnea, stridor, cough, and wheeze. Respiratory failure ensues if the respiratory efforts and ventilation perfusion ratios are inadequate to maintain arterial oxygen saturation and carbon dioxide (CO_2) clearance necessary to provide appropriate tissue oxygenation and maintenance of blood pH. In general, an arterial PaO_2 of less than 50 mmHg (hypoxemia) while one is breathing room air and a $PaCO_2$ level greater than 45 mmHg (hypercapnia) suggest respiratory failure. The causes of acute respiratory distress are legion, but they often can be identified by considering the associated clinical findings, the history and setting of symptoms, and the age of the patient (Table 8–1).

THE PULMONARY EXAMINATION

History

An appropriate medical history is important in the child with acute respiratory distress (see also Chapter 7). The chief complaint provides insight into the nature of the distress (i.e., cough, wheeze, stridor, dyspnea, or chest pain); some indication of the onset and duration of symptoms should be obtained. Data regarding prodrome, exacerbating or ameliorating factors, history of trauma, previous occurrence of similar symptoms, and response to any therapy should be sought. Past medical history of neonatal events (prematurity), previous endotracheal intubation, recurrent infections, hospitalizations, and gagging or choking episodes may provide valuable information. A family history of asthma and allergies, travel, and environmental exposure (e.g., smoking, pets, or irritants) may uncover etiologic clues. Finally, a review of systems with respect to systemic signs and symptoms associated with respiratory disease, such as fever, weight loss, night sweats, or dysphagia, is useful.

Physical Examination

The physical examination begins with vital signs with attention paid to respiratory rate, heart rate, and blood pressure. Tachypnea often is the most prominent manifestation of respiratory distress caused by airway obstruction or parenchymal lung disease. Age-dependent normal values for resting respiratory rates are listed in Table 7–7. In general, a resting respiratory rate greater than 40 breaths/minute in an infant younger than 1 year of age or greater than 30 breaths/minute for an older child is abnormal.

INSPECTION

Inspection of the patient should focus on skin color, level of consciousness, presence of nasal flaring, grunting, use of accessory muscles of respiration, chest wall symmetry, and respiratory excursion. Altered mental status (either agitation or somnolence) may be indicative of severe respiratory distress, hypoxemia, and/or hypercapnia. The presence of grunting, nasal flaring, chest wall retractions, and the use of accessory muscles of respiration, particularly the strap muscles of the neck, all suggest airway obstruction. Cyanosis suggests severe hypoxemia.

PALPATION

Palpation of the chest wall and cervical region may detect the presence of subcutaneous emphysema indicative of pulmonary air leak. Percussion of the chest wall yielding a hyperresonant note indicates hyperinflation, whereas dullness to percussion suggests atelectasis, pulmonary consolidation, or pleural effusion.

AUSCULTATION

Auscultation of the chest should focus on identifying the degree of air exchange and the presence, timing, and symmetry of adventitious breath sounds. Air entry should be evaluated over all discrete anatomic locations bilaterally. Homologous segments of each lung should be examined sequentially to compare similar areas. The presence of adventitious sounds should be determined next (Table 8–2). The most commonly encountered sounds are wheeze, stridor (a subclass of wheeze), crackle, and rhonchus.

- Crackles (previously called ''rales'') are intermittent, low- or higher-pitched, largely inspiratory noises that are produced by the opening of airways closed during the previous expiration.
- Wheezes are continuous, high-pitched musical noises, similar to a hiss or whistle.
- The rhonchus is also a continuous sound that is lower-pitched and more rumbling or sonorous.
- Stridor, a type of wheeze, is harsher, often localized over the central intrathoracic airways or trachea, and predominates in inspiration.

Determination of the timing (inspiration, expiration, or biphasic) and distribution of the adventitious sounds offers clues as to the site of airway involvement. For example, wheeze that is continuous and heard equally over both lung fields is likely to arise from

Table 8–1. Age-Related Causes of Respiratory Distress

Cause	Preterm Neonate	Term Neonate	Infant–Toddler	Child	Adolescent
Common	RDS Congenital pneumonia[1] Nosocomial pneumonia[2] BPD Congenital heart disease (cyanotic, heart failure, or both) Pneumothorax Transient tachypnea	Meconium aspiration pneumonia Congenital heart disease Transient tachypnea Persistent fetal circulation	Afebrile pneumonia[4] Pneumonia[5] Aspiration[6] Croup (infectious, spasmodic) Bronchiolitis (RSV) Cystic fibrosis Laryngotracheomalacia Asthma	Pneumonia[7] Asthma Cystic fibrosis Sickle cell acute chest crisis Aspiration[6] Tonsillitis	Pneumonia[9] Asthma Sickle cell acute chest crisis Tonsillitis Peritonsillar abscess Hysteria Cystic fibrosis
Uncommon	Congenital anomalies[3] Pulmonary hemorrhage Pneumopericardium Vocal cord paralysis Congenital alveolar proteinosis Pulmonary hypoplasia	Pneumothorax Congenital anomalies[3] Pneumopericardium Polycythemia Vocal cord paralysis Pleural effusions Severe anemia Congenital alveolar proteinosis Pulmonary hypoplasia	Congenital anomalies Epiglottitis Near drowning Pulmonary hemosiderosis Retropharyngeal abscess Trauma Hydrocarbon aspiration Smoke inhalation (burn) Airway hemangioma Papilloma of vocal cords Bacterial tracheitis Heart failure HIV associated[14]	ARDS Anaphylaxis Interstitial lung disease[8] Hemoptysis Retropharyngeal abscess Near drowning Hydrocarbon aspiration Trauma Pulmonary fibrosis Desquamating interstitial pneumonia Pulmonary alveolar proteinosis Smoke inhalation (burn) HIV associated[14]	ARDS Spontaneous pneumothorax Pulmonary embolism Drug-induced[10] Interstitial lung disease[8] Collagen vascular disease[11] Hypersensitivity pneumonitis[12] Allergic bronchopulmonary aspergillosis Trauma Anaphylaxis Smoke inhalation (burn) Scoliosis Bronchiectasis Mediastinal mass[13] Hemoptysis HIV associated[14]

[1]Congenital pneumonia = group B streptococcus, *Escherichia coli, Listeria monocytogenes,* herpes simplex; possible *Ureaplasma urealyticum* and *Mycoplasma hominis.*

[2]Nosocomial pneumonia = *Staphylococcus epidermidis, Staphylococcus aureus, Candida albicans, Klebsiella, Pseudomonas aeruginosa,* adenovirus, RSV.

[3]Congenital anomalies = tracheoesophageal fistula, choanal atresia, tracheal web-stenosis-atresia-cleft, diaphragmatic hernia, eventration of the diaphragm, cystic adenomatoid malformation, lobar emphysema, cleft palate–macroglossia (Pierre Robin syndrome), thyroid goiter, pulmonary hypoplasia including Potter syndrome (renal agenesis, oligohydramnios, pulmonary hypoplasia), lung cysts, chylothorax, pulmonary lymphangiectasia, asphyxiating thoracic dystrophy, vascular rings and slings, arteriovenous malformation, subglottic stenosis.

[4]Afebrile pneumonia = *Chlamydia trachomatis,* cytomegalovirus, RSV, *Pneumocystis carinii, U. urealyticum, M. hominis.*

[5]Pneumonia (infant–toddler) = (see Chapter 7).

[6]Aspiration = gastric fluid or formula aspiration in gastroesophageal reflux (see Chapter 20); foreign body aspiration (see Chapter 7).

[7]Pneumonia (child) = (see Chapter 7).

[8]Interstitial lung disease = (see Tables 8–10 to 8–13) idiopathic, rheumatoid, infection *(P. carinii),* histiocytosis X, hypereosinophilia syndromes, Goodpasture syndrome, LIP, alveolar proteinosis, familial fibrosis, chronic active hepatitis, inflammatory bowel disease, vasculitis (Wegener granulomatosis, Churg-Strauss, hypersensitivity), graft-versus-host disease, pulmonary veno-occlusive disease, sarcoidosis, leukemia, lymphoma, neurofibromatosis, tuberous sclerosis, Gaucher disease, Niemann-Pick disease, Weber Christian disease, organic dusts (e.g., farmer's lung, humidifier/air-conditioner lung, bird feeder, pancreatic extract, rodent handler, cheese worker), inorganic dusts (pneumoconiosis), irradiation.

[9]Pneumonia (adolescent) = (see Chapter 7).

[10]Drugs = azathioprine, bleomycin, cyclophosphamide, methotrexate, nitrosoureas, busulfan, nitrofurantoin, penicillin, sulfonamides, erythromycin, isoniazid, hydralazine, phenytoin, carbamazepine, imipramine, naproxen, penicillamine, cromolyn sodium, mineral oil, paraquat, inhaled drugs (cocaine, hydrocarbons), talc, shoe spray.

[11]Collagen vascular disease = rheumatoid arthritis, progressive systemic sclerosis, systemic lupus erythematosus, dermatomyositis, mixed connective tissue disease.

[12]Hypersensitivity pneumonia (also called *extrinsic allergic alveolitis*) = see No. 8 above for some specific organic dusts (antigens).

[13]Mediastinal masses = *anterior* (teratoma, T-cell lymphoma, thymus, thyroid), *middle* (lymph nodes–infection–tumor–sarcoidosis, cysts), *posterior* (neuroenteric cysts–duplication, meningocele, neural tumors–neuroblastoma, ganglioneuroblastoma, neurofibroma, pheochromocytoma). Parenchymal tumors (hamartoma, arteriovenous malformation, carcinoid, adenoma; metastatic–osteogenic sarcoma, Wilms tumor).

[14]HIV associated = *P. carinii,* LIP, CMV, *Mycobacterium tuberculosis,* atypical mycobacteria, measles, common bacterial pathogens (see Chapter 7).

Abbreviations: RDS = respiratory distress syndrome; BPD = bronchopulmonary dysplasia; RSV = respiratory syncytial virus; ARDS = acute (adult) respiratory distress syndrome; CMV = cytomegalovirus; LIP = lymphocytic interstitial pneumonia.

Table 8–2. Description of Adventitious Lung Sounds

Acoustic Qualities	ATS Nomenclature*	Common Synonyms
Discontinuous, explosive, loud, low-pitched	Coarse crackle	Coarse rale
Softer, higher-pitched than above; shorter duration than coarse crackles	Fine crackle	Fine or crepitant rale
Continuous, high-pitched, hissing or whistling, musical sound†	Wheeze	Sibilant rhonchus or fine wheeze
Longer-duration, lower-pitched than wheeze, continuous, sonorous	Rhonchus	Sonorous rhonchus

Modified from Loudon R and Murphy RLH. Lung sounds. Am Rev Respir Dis 1984;130:663–673.
*American Thoracic Society.
†Also describes stridor, when heard over central extrathoracic airways.

above the tracheal bifurcation, whereas late inspiratory crackles may emanate from the smaller airways. Unilateral or very localized wheeze or decreased breath sounds suggest segmental airway obstruction, such as that found with retained foreign body aspiration, mucus plugging, or atelectasis (Fig. 8–1).

CARDIAC EXAMINATION

Other elements of the physical examination that may have direct bearing on the respiratory system include the cardiac examination and inspection of the distal extremities. Congenital heart disease that results in a large left-to-right shunt, pulmonary hypertension, congestive heart failure, and increased pulmonic blood flow may result in respiratory distress (see Chapter 13). The presence of digital clubbing in the absence of cardiac or gastrointestinal disease usually indicates a significant pulmonary abnormality (see Chapter 7).

DIAGNOSIS

Signs and symptoms of respiratory distress can vary, depending on the severity and cause. Not all causes of respiratory distress

arise within the respiratory tract. Heart failure, pulmonary edema, neuromuscular disorders, toxic ingestion, and central nervous system (CNS) disorders may all present with respiratory signs and symptoms (Table 8–3). The manifestations of respiratory distress include dyspnea, shortness of breath, cough, wheeze, stridor, and chest wall retractions; however, anxiety, pallor, and cyanosis may also herald respiratory embarrassment.

Laboratory Tests

A number of laboratory tests and diagnostic aids can be useful in determining the causes and degree of severity of respiratory distress. The arterial blood gas analysis, obtained while the patient is breathing a known fraction of inspired oxygen (FiO_2), is the "gold standard" for assessing oxygenation, ventilation, and acid-base status. In lieu of an arterial blood gas determination, noninvasive measure of oxygenation by pulse oximetry may provide valuable information. Oximetry measures the degree of hemoglobin saturation with oxygen and should not be confused with partial pressure of oxygen in blood, as measured by blood gas analysis or estimated by transcutaneous measures. A hemoglobin oxygen saturation lower than 93% indicates that significant hypoxemia may be present, and saturations of 90% or lower are clearly abnormal. An arterial blood gas analysis may be necessary to confirm the presence and degree of hypoxemia, as well as information on acid-

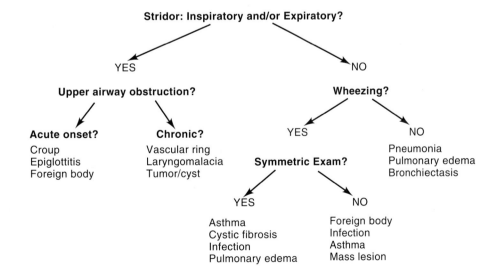

Figure 8–1. Algorithm for a child with respiratory distress.

Table 8–3. Causes of Respiratory Distress

Extrathoracic	Intrathoracic
Nervous System	*Pulmonary*
Intracranial hemorrhage	Airway obstruction
Acidosis	Parenchymal lesions:
Ingestion (aspirin)	pneumonia, hemorrhage,
Ketoacidosis (diabetes)	malformation
Meningitis	Air leaks:
Shock/sepsis	pneumomediastinum,
Neuromuscular disease	pneumothorax
Diaphragmatic paralysis,	Pleural effusion, empyema
paresis	Acute (adult) respiratory
Psychologic (anxiety), vocal	distress syndrome
cord dysfunction	Chest wall trauma
	Pulmonary embolus
	Foreign body (airway or
	esophagus)
	Tumor (cyst, adenoma)
	Cystic fibrosis
Anatomic Lesions of Upper	*Cardiac*
Airway	Myocarditis,
Malacia	cardiomyopathy
Web	Shunt (left to right)
Cyst	Congestive heart failure
Hemangioma	Pulmonary edema
Stenosis (glottic or choanal)	Pericardial effusion
Papillomatosis	
Miscellaneous	
Abdominal masses, distention	
Anemia	

base status (pH) and ventilation ($PaCO_2$). Hemoglobin oxygen saturation, measured by pulse oximetry, *cannot* detect significant hypercapnia; it is relatively accurate ($\pm 3\%$) at oxygen saturations of 70% or more. A variety of conditions can result in inaccurate oximetry measures, such as poor circulation, presence of carboxyhemoglobin or methemoglobin, nail polish, and improper sensor alignment and motion.

Imaging

RADIOGRAPHY

Radiographic imaging of the respiratory tract may be obtained with a variety of techniques and can yield a great deal of insight into the causes of respiratory distress. A plain film of the chest, taken in the posterior-anterior and lateral projections, should be obtained in any patient who presents in respiratory distress. Important information regarding the presence of parenchymal infiltrates, effusion, airway obstruction, cardiac size, pulmonary vascular markings, extrapulmonary air leaks, and presence of radiopaque foreign bodies may be obtained from this test. Plain films of the chest taken during inspiration and expiration may be helpful in identifying the presence of intraluminal bronchial obstruction, such as that seen with a retained endobronchial foreign body. Demonstration of unilateral hyperinflation or a mediastinal shift during expiration suggests localized bronchial obstruction. A lateral decubitus positioning of the patient during the radiographic procedure can identify a pleural effusion in the lower dependent lung. For patients who present with stridor, radiographs of the neck and upper airway should be obtained.

COMPUTED TOMOGRAPHY

Computed tomography (CT) of the upper airway and chest can help to detect the relationship of the vasculature to the airways (trachea and large central airways), pulmonary parenchymal lesions (infiltrates, abscesses, cysts) or masses in the airway, and central airway caliber. The advent of rapid, fine-cut CT makes this technique one of high resolution and short duration, which increases the acceptability for pediatric patients.

MAGNETIC RESONANCE IMAGING

Magnetic resonance imaging (MRI) of the pulmonary system may also be useful in elucidating the relationship of the great vessels to the airways and may be superior to CT for this purpose. MRI is less useful for imaging the lung parenchyma. The need for long imaging times often means sedation for young children and limits the utility of MRI imaging of the chest for some pediatric patients.

FLUOROGRAPHY

Fluoroscopic examination of the chest may be useful in determining the cause of respiratory distress. Real-time visualization of the diaphragm can determine whether paralysis or paresis of this major muscle of respiration is contributing to respiratory embarrassment. Watching for asymmetric chest wall motion or unilateral hyperinflation during the respiratory cycle suggests bronchial obstruction, such as that seen with a retained foreign body in the airways. Likewise, a barium swallow can detect an esophageal foreign body as well as most types of closed vascular rings.

Clinical Observation

Assessing the severity of respiratory distress can be aided by clinical observations. The presence of chest wall retractions signifies airway obstruction. In infants, the particularly compliant chest wall predisposes to intercostal and sternal retractions; in older children, these features may be less prominent. Flaring of the alae nasi also signifies airway obstruction and significant distress in both infants and older children. In addition, infants may grunt during expiration; as fatigue and increased respiratory efforts commence, a head bob may appear. Use of neck strap (accessory) muscles to aid in respiratory efforts is also a harbinger of severe respiratory distress and airway obstruction. Alteration in the child's mental status signifies impending respiratory failure; hypoxemia typically results in agitation and anxiety, whereas hypercapnia can usually produce somnolence and mental confusion.

Pulsus paradoxus, the difference between the systolic blood pressure obtained during inspiration and exhalation, is exaggerated by airway obstruction and pulmonary hyperinflation. As pulmonary overinflation worsens, pulsus paradoxus values increase and correlate well with the degree of airway obstruction. It is difficult to measure pulsus paradoxus in young children with rapid heart rates. A method that allows a reasonable approximation of the pulsus paradoxus can be obtained by using a sphygmomanometer and noting the difference between the pressures at which the first, sporadic faint pulse sounds and the pressure at which all sounds are heard. Values greater than 10 mmHg are abnormal, and values greater than 20 mmHg are consistent with severe airway obstruction.

Although digital clubbing is occasionally seen as a normal and familial variant, its presence in a child who presents with respiratory distress suggests an acute illness superimposed on an underlying chronic condition. The most common pulmonary causes of digital clubbing in pediatric patients are cystic fibrosis, bronchiectasis, and other destructive pulmonary diseases (see Chapter 7). Clubbing is rarely seen in children with asthma.

CAUSES OF RESPIRATORY DISTRESS

Wheezing

Wheezing is best characterized as a continuous, "musical" sound most often heard on expiration, but it may occur in both phases of respiration. The sound is a result of flow limitation in large or medium-sized airways; obstruction of the airways may be due to intraluminal or extraluminal causes.

Intraluminal obstruction is most typically caused by smooth muscle constriction, mucosal edema, hypersecretion of mucus, or cellular infiltrate, most commonly associated with airway inflammation or infection. Other less common sources of intraluminal obstruction include aspirated foreign body and tumors.

Extraluminal obstruction is typically caused by external compression from enlarged lymph nodes, vascular structures, pulmonary cysts, tumors, or intrinsic defects of the airway wall. Because extraluminal obstruction usually involves a fairly localized segment of airway, the wheezing is often restricted to the portion of the chest containing the affected airways. In small infants, however, it may be difficult to define the site of obstruction by physical examination alone because breath sounds are readily transmitted throughout the thorax.

Asthma

The most common cause of intraluminal obstruction is asthma. Asthma is a common disorder that affects nearly 5 million children in the United States; 5% to 10% of children experience symptoms of asthma at some time. The prevalence of asthma in African-American children is significantly higher than in whites; the morbidity and mortality are likewise increased. Asthma is defined as airway obstruction that is reversible either spontaneously or with the use of medication. Additional definitions include the concepts of airway inflammation and bronchial hyperresponsiveness. The airways of patients with even mild asthma demonstrate inflammation, manifested as mucosal edema, hypersecretion of mucus, smooth muscle constriction, and inflammatory cell infiltrate. Even when asthma symptoms are not present, airway inflammation may be demonstrated. Furthermore, bronchial hyperresponsiveness, the tendency of airway smooth muscle to constrict in response to a variety of environmental stimuli, is present in virtually all asthmatics and may be exacerbated by airway inflammation.

DIAGNOSIS

The diagnosis of asthma is made by a combination of clinical observations and laboratory tests (Fig. 8–2). For the child who

Figure 8–2. Diagnostic algorithm for asthma. CVS = cardiovascular system. (From Special Report of the Steering Committee: Asthma: A follow-up statement from an international paediatric asthma consensus group. Arch Dis Child 1992;67:240–248.)

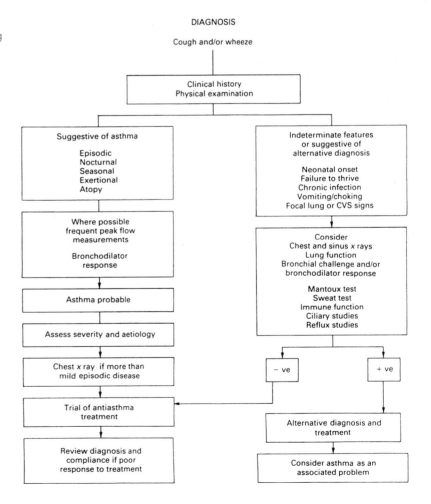

presents with acute wheezing and respiratory distress, a therapeutic trial of an inhaled or less often a subcutaneous adrenergic agonist is also the best "diagnostic test" for reversible airway obstruction. Once the acute symptoms have improved, other diagnostic studies can be undertaken. Spirometry, particularly measurement of the forced expiratory flow rates (FEV_1) and mid-maximal flow rates ($FEF_{25-75\%}$), provides a good indication of air flow obstruction in the larger and smaller airways, respectively. If airway obstruction is detected in the resting state, a bronchodilating aerosol (isoproterenol or albuterol) is administered and spirometry (pulmonary function tests) is repeated. An improvement in flow rates of 15% is considered significant and indicative of reversible airway obstruction. If the baseline spirometry is normal, an inhalation challenge test, with either increasing doses of methacholine or hyperventilation of cold, dry air, can provoke a statistically (but usually not clinically) significant decrease in FEV_1; generally, a fall in FEV_1 of 10% or greater is considered diagnostic of airway hyperresponsiveness and asthma. In children too young to perform spirometry, the repeated nature of wheezing episodes and the improvement in symptoms following treatment with anti-inflammatory agents and bronchodilators are generally sufficient to confirm the diagnosis of asthma. Other diagnostic studies include measurement of total serum IgE levels; this immunoglobulin is often elevated in individuals with asthma and/or allergy as well as in those predisposed to asthma.

Radiographic findings are nonspecific, but they usually show symmetric hyperinflation and increased peribronchial thickening. A chest radiograph may also help to rule out other causes of wheezing, such as foreign body, pneumonia, or atelectasis (Table 8–4). The peripheral white blood cell (WBC) count may reveal eosinophilia; if sputum is available, it may also demonstrate eosinophils.

Patients with acute asthma typically present with shortness of breath, wheeze, cough, and increased work of breathing. However, persistent cough may be the most prominent or even sole feature of acute asthma. Many asthma episodes are misdiagnosed as bronchitis (see Chapter 7). Chest wall and suprasternal notch retractions and nasal flaring may be present. Chest wall retractions and the use of neck strap (accessory) muscles indicate significant airway obstruction. Acute asthma exacerbations that are unresponsive to aggressive bronchodilator administration are termed *status asthmaticus*. The severity of asthma may be assessed with the parameters presented in Tables 8–5 and 8–6. Common triggers of acute episodes include upper respiratory tract infections, exposure to cold air, exercise, allergens, pollutants, strong odors, and cigarette smoke.

A brief but pertinent history should be obtained for every child with acute asthma to determine the duration of symptoms, the character of previous episodes (severity, need for hospitalization, and need for intensive care, including mechanical ventilation), antecedent illness, symptoms, exposures, and both chronic and acute use of medications, including dose and time of last administration.

It is critical to rule out other causes of wheezing that are not asthma and that require different therapy (see Table 8–4). Anatomic

---

Table 8–4. Causes of Wheezing in Childhood

Acute	**Chronic or Recurrent** *Continued*
Reactive Airways Disease	*Aspiration*
Asthma*	Foreign body
Exercise-induced asthma*	Gastroesophageal reflux
Hypersensitivity reactions	Tracheoesophageal fistula (repaired or unrepaired)
Bronchial Edema	*Bronchial Hypersecretion or Failure to Clear Secretions*
Infection* (bronchiolitis, ILD, pneumonia)	Bronchitis, bronchiectasis
Inhalation of irritant gases or particulates	Cystic fibrosis*
Increased pulmonary venous pressure	Immotile cilia syndrome
Bronchial Hypersecretion	Immunodeficiency disorder
Infection	Vasculitis
Inhalation of irritant gases or particulates	Lymphangiectasia
Cholinergic drugs	Alpha$_1$-antitrypsin deficiency
Aspiration	*Intrinsic Airway Lesions*
Foreign body*	Endobronchial tumors
Aspiration of gastric contents (reflux, H-type TEF)	Endobronchial granulation tissue
Chronic or Recurrent	Plastic bronchus syndrome
Reactive Airways Disease (see above)	Bronchial or tracheal stenosis
Hypersensitivity Reactions, Allergic Bronchopulmonary Aspergillosis	Bronchiolitis obliterans
	Sequelae of bronchopulmonary dysplasia
Dynamic Airways Collapse	Sarcoidosis
Bronchomalacia	
Tracheomalacia*	*Congestive Heart Failure*
Vocal cord adduction	
Airway Compression by Mass or Blood Vessel	
Vascular ring/sling	
Anomalous innominate artery	
Pulmonary artery dilation (absent pulmonary valve)	
Bronchial or pulmonary cysts	
Lymph nodes or tumors	

Modified from Kercsmar CM. The respiratory system. *In* Behrman RE, Kliegman RM (eds). Nelson Essentials of Pediatrics, 2nd ed. Philadelphia: WB Saunders, 1994:445.
*Common.
Abbreviations: ILD = interstitial lung disease; TEF = tracheoesophageal fistula.

Table 8-5. Estimation of Severity of Acute Exacerbation in Children with Asthma

Sign/Symptom	Mild	Moderate	Severe
Peak expiratory flow rate	70%–90% predicted or baseline	50%–70% predicted or baseline	<50% predicted or baseline
Respiratory rate	Normal to 30% above mean	30%–50% increase above mean	>50% increase above mean
Alertness	Normal	Normal	May be decreased
Dyspnea	Absent or mild, speaks in complete sentences	Moderate, speaks in phrases or partial sentences	Severe, speaks only in single words or short phrases
Accessory muscle use	No intercostal to mild retractions	Moderate intercostal retractions with tracheosternal retractions, use of sternocleidomastoid muscles, chest hyperinflation	Moderate intercostal retractions, tracheosternal retractions with nasal flaring during inspiration, chest hyperinflation
Color	Good	Pale	Possibly cyanotic
Auscultation	End expiratory wheeze only	Inspiratory and expiratory wheezing	Breath sounds inaudible
Oxygen saturation (opt)*	>95%	90%–95%	<90%
$PCO_{2(opt)}$	<35	<40	>40

From National Asthma Education Program. Guidelines for the Diagnosis and Treatment of Asthma. Office of Prevention, Education and Control, National Heart, Lung, Blood Institute; Bethesda, Md: National Institutes of Health, NIH Publication No. 91–3042, 1991.

*Oxygen saturation values will have to be adjusted for altitude. These values assume that the patient is at sea level.

abnormalities of the airway, such as vascular ring, tracheobronchomalacia, ciliary dyskinesia, and foreign body aspiration, may cause airway obstruction and wheezing, especially in infants and young children. Viral infections, notably respiratory syncytial virus (RSV), adenovirus, parainfluenza, and influenza, are also common causes of wheezing in infants and young children. Infection with *Mycoplasma* may produce airway hyperactivity in older children. Other entities to consider are cystic fibrosis, interstitial lung disease, or a behavioral disorder, such as vocal cord dysfunction. Compared with asthma, the key distinguishing feature of these diagnoses is that the wheezing does not respond to treatment with bronchodilators.

The physical examination should focus on respiratory rate, air exchange, degree and localization of wheezing, other adventitious lung sounds, mental status, presence of cyanosis, and degree of fatigue (see Tables 8–5 and 8–6). An arterial blood gas analysis should be obtained if the clinical evaluation reveals moderate to severe airway obstruction. The presence and degree of hypoxemia and hypoventilation can be determined. Pulse oximetry is a noninvasive means of rapidly assessing oxygenation; when used in conjunction with measurement of the venous PCO_2 or pH it is an acceptable alternative to an arterial blood gas determination in mild to moderately ill patients.

Chest roentgenograms should be obtained for all patients who present with a first episode of wheezing. Patients known to have asthma should have a chest radiogram if there is fever, localized crackles or wheeze, decreased breath sounds, a poor response to therapy, or significant tachypnea.

Spirometry has limited efficacy in the emergency management of status asthmaticus. Although peak expiratory flow meters are

Table 8-6. Factors Associated with Risk of Severe Status Asthmaticus

History
　Chronic steroid-dependent asthma
　Prior intensive care admission
　Prior mechanical ventilation for asthma
　Recurrent visits to emergency unit in past 48 hr
　Sudden onset of severe respiratory distress
　Poor compliance with therapy
　Poor recognition by patient, family, or physician, of severity of attack
　Family dysfunction, crisis
　Respiratory arrest
　Hypoxic seizures, encephalopathy

Physical Examination
　Pulsus paradoxus >20 mmHg
　Hypotension, tachycardia, tachypnea
　Cyanosis
　1–2 word dyspnea
　Lethargy
　Agitation
　Sternocleidomastoid, intercostal, suprasternal retractions
　Poor air exchange (e.g., quiet chest with severe distress)

Laboratory Tests
　Hypercapnia
　Hypoxia with supplemental oxygen
　FEV_1 <30% expected; no improvement 1 hr after aerosol therapy
　Chest x-ray (pneumothorax, pneumomediastinum)

Therapy
　Overreliance on aerosol, inhaler therapy
　Delayed use of systemic corticosteroids
　Sedation
　Delayed admission to hospital or intensive care unit

From Behrman RE: Nelson Textbook of Pediatrics, 14th ed. Philadelphia: WB Saunders, 1992:593.

often available in the emergency department, this test is a measure of large airway function only, is effort-dependent, and may be most unreliable in an anxious, untrained patient. The major value of peak flow measurements in acute asthma is to provide an objective trend indicative of improvement (or lack thereof) in airway caliber.

A complete blood cell count (CBC) is not of use unless other complicating conditions (e.g., infection, anemia, hemoglobinopathy) are suspected. Serum electrolytes are of little value unless dehydration is suspected. Hypokalemia is associated with the frequent administration of beta-adrenergic agonists. Most children cannot produce sputum, but if sputum is available, it should be examined for the presence of bacteria and inflammatory cells.

TREATMENT

Acute Asthma

Treatment of acute asthma should be instituted in any child who presents with wheezing, dyspnea, cough, and no other immediately discernible cause of the symptoms.

Patients with all but the mildest degree of airway obstruction will have significant hypoxemia as a result of ventilation-perfusion mismatch. Consequently, supplemental humidified oxygen, usually 30% by face mask, is of benefit. Oxygen should be used in any child who has significant wheezing, accessory muscle use, or an oxygen saturation of less than 93%.

The mainstay of treatment for status asthmaticus is the administration of an inhaled (or less often subcutaneous) beta-adrenergic agonist. Inhalation of nebulized medication is the route of choice because the onset of action is rapid, sustained, and relatively free of significant side effects even in the most severely affected patients (Table 8–7). Patients who do not respond to initial therapy with aerosolized medication or cannot comply should be given a subcutaneous injection. Although parenteral beta agonists are equally effective, the procedure causes some discomfort and anxiety and may yield a higher incidence of side effects. Administration of beta agonists from metered dose inhalers is effective treatment of acute asthma in adults, but most children cannot successfully use these devices when they are acutely ill.

The role of anticholinergic agents in the treatment of acute asthma remains uncertain. Atropine and its congeners are relatively poor bronchodilators compared with beta-adrenergic agonists. Corticosteroids are potent anti-inflammatory agents that are extremely useful in attenuating acute asthma exacerbations. With few exceptions, any patient who presents with other than mild wheezing responsive to minimal bronchodilator therapy or any patient requiring hospital admission should receive corticosteroids (see Tables

8–7 and 8–8). Although theophylline (or the intravenous formulation aminophylline) is an effective bronchodilator in chronic use, when optimal amounts of inhaled or parenteral beta-adrenergic agonists are administered, the addition of theophylline does not provide further significant improvement. Intravenous fluids should be administered in any patient who has clinical or laboratory signs of dehydration. Fluids above those required for normal homeostasis should not be routinely given. Chest physiotherapy and postural drainage may be useful for the patient who has significant atelectasis or sputum production.

A small percentage of children with acute asthma progress to severe status asthmaticus and respiratory failure. A number of clinical signs and symptoms define respiratory failure in such severely affected patients: a PaO_2 less than 60 mm in room air or cyanosis in 40% FiO_2, a $PaCO_2$ of 40 mm or higher or rising and accompanied by respiratory distress, deterioration in clinical status in spite of aggressive treatment, a change in mental status and fatigue (see Tables 8–5 and 8–6). Patients meeting any of these criteria should be observed in an intensive care unit, and they should receive maximal medical therapy. Algorithmic approaches to the treatment of asthma are presented in Figure 8–3 and Table 8–8.

Chronic Asthma

Treatment of chronic asthma requires careful assessment of the severity of the disease, according to frequency and intensity of symptoms and subsequent grading into mild, moderate, and severe categories (Table 8–9). In general, all patients except those with very mild disease are best managed with chronic administration of an inhaled anti-inflammatory agent (cromolyn or, if the asthma is more severe, corticosteroids) and the intermittent use of an inhaled beta-adrenergic agonist for treatment of acute wheezing episodes. Oral corticosteroids are administered for short intervals to control more severe exacerbations. Avoidance of environmental triggers (allergens, cigarette smoke) is also paramount to successful management.

RESPIRATORY DISTRESS IN INFANTS AND TODDLERS

Viral Bronchiolitis

Bronchiolitis is a frequent manifestation of acute viral infections of the distal lower respiratory tract and a cause of wheezing and

Table 8–7. Drugs for Treatment of Acute Asthma

Drug	Form	Dosage
Albuterol	Nebulizer solution, 0.5% (5 mg/ml)	0.15–0.3 mg/kg/dose every 20 minutes for 1–2 hours; 1.25 mg minimum dose; 5 mg maximum dose
Epinephrine HCl	1:1000 (1 mg/ml)	0.01 mg/kg subcutaneous injection every 20 minutes up to 3 injections; 0.3 mg maximum dose
Terbutaline	0.1% (1 mg/ml)	0.01 mg/kg subcutaneous injection every 2 hours; 0.5 mg maximum dose
Systemic corticosteroid	Oral prednisone or prednisolone Intravenous methylprednisolone	Prednisone, 1–2 mg/kg/day as single dose, 60 mg maximum dose; Prednisolone, 1–2 mg/kg/day; maximum dose 125 mg

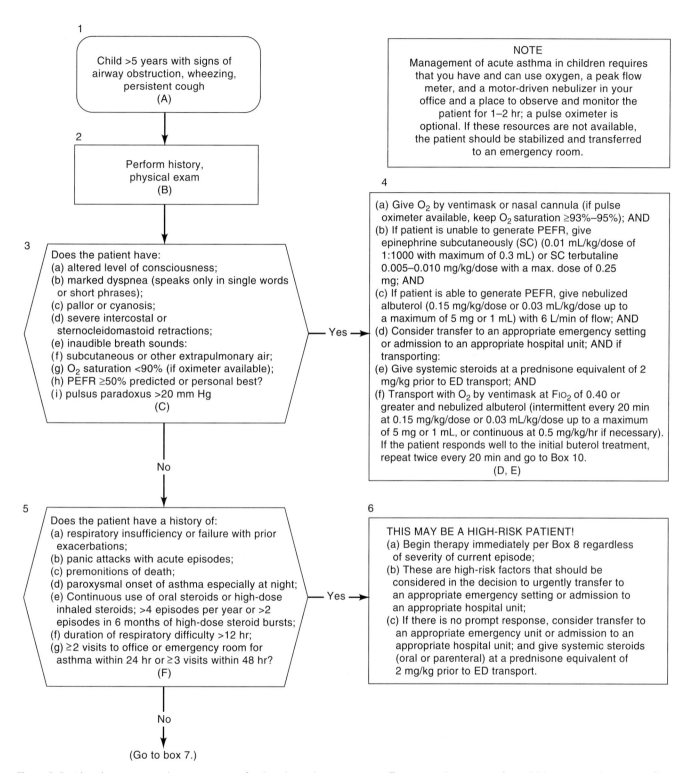

1
Child >5 years with signs of airway obstruction, wheezing, persistent cough
(A)

2
Perform history, physical exam
(B)

NOTE
Management of acute asthma in children requires that you have and can use oxygen, a peak flow meter, and a motor-driven nebulizer in your office and a place to observe and monitor the patient for 1–2 hr; a pulse oximeter is optional. If these resources are not available, the patient should be stabilized and transferred to an emergency room.

3
Does the patient have:
(a) altered level of consciousness;
(b) marked dyspnea (speaks only in single words or short phrases);
(c) pallor or cyanosis;
(d) severe intercostal or sternocleidomastoid retractions;
(e) inaudible breath sounds:
(f) subcutaneous or other extrapulmonary air;
(g) O_2 saturation <90% (if oximeter available);
(h) PEFR ≥50% predicted or personal best?
(i) pulsus paradoxus >20 mm Hg
(C)

— Yes →

4
(a) Give O_2 by ventimask or nasal cannula (if pulse oximeter available, keep O_2 saturation ≥93%–95%); AND
(b) If patient is unable to generate PEFR, give epinephrine subcutaneously (SC) (0.01 mL/kg/dose of 1:1000 with maximum of 0.3 mL) or SC terbutaline 0.005–0.010 mg/kg/dose with a max. dose of 0.25 mg; AND
(c) If patient is able to generate PEFR, give nebulized albuterol (0.15 mg/kg/dose or 0.03 mL/kg/dose up to a maximum of 5 mg or 1 mL) with 6 L/min of flow; AND
(d) Consider transfer to an appropriate emergency setting or admission to an appropriate hospital unit; AND if transporting:
(e) Give systemic steroids at a prednisone equivalent of 2 mg/kg prior to ED transport; AND
(f) Transport with O_2 by ventimask at FIO_2 of 0.40 or greater and nebulized albuterol (intermittent every 20 min at 0.15 mg/kg/dose or 0.03 mL/kg/dose up to a maximum of 5 mg or 1 mL, or continuous at 0.5 mg/kg/hr if necessary). If the patient responds well to the initial buterol treatment, repeat twice every 20 min and go to Box 10.
(D, E)

No

5
Does the patient have a history of:
(a) respiratory insufficiency or failure with prior exacerbations;
(b) panic attacks with acute episodes;
(c) premonitions of death;
(d) paroxysmal onset of asthma especially at night;
(e) Continuous use of oral steroids or high-dose inhaled steroids; >4 episodes per year or >2 episodes in 6 months of high-dose steroid bursts;
(f) duration of respiratory difficulty >12 hr;
(g) ≥2 visits to office or emergency room for asthma within 24 hr or ≥3 visits within 48 hr?
(F)

— Yes →

6
THIS MAY BE A HIGH-RISK PATIENT!
(a) Begin therapy immediately per Box 8 regardless of severity of current episode;
(b) These are high-risk factors that should be considered in the decision to urgently transfer to an appropriate emergency setting or admission to an appropriate hospital unit;
(c) If there is no prompt response, consider transfer to an appropriate emergency unit or admission to an appropriate hospital unit; and give systemic steroids (oral or parenteral) at a prednisone equivalent of 2 mg/kg prior to ED transport.

No

(Go to box 7.)

Figure 8–3. Algorithm presenting the management of asthma by pediatricians in an office setting; this version is for a child using a peak expiratory flow meter. PEFR = peak expiratory flow rate; ED = emergency department; FiO_2 = fraction of inspired oxygen; MDI = metered dose inhaler. (From Provisional Committee on Quality Improvement. Practice parameter: The office management of acute exacerbations of asthma in children. Reproduced by permission of Pediatrics 1994;93:119–126.)

Illustration continued on following page

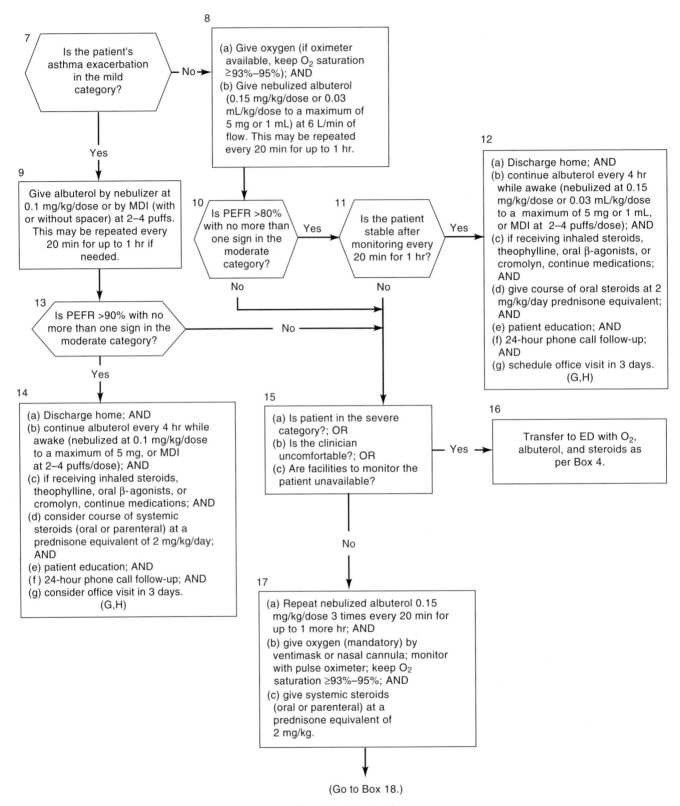

7 Is the patient's asthma exacerbation in the mild category?

— No →

8
(a) Give oxygen (if oximeter available, keep O_2 saturation ≥93%–95%); AND
(b) Give nebulized albuterol (0.15 mg/kg/dose or 0.03 mL/kg/dose to a maximum of 5 mg or 1 mL) at 6 L/min of flow. This may be repeated every 20 min for up to 1 hr.

Yes ↓

9 Give albuterol by nebulizer at 0.1 mg/kg/dose or by MDI (with or without spacer) at 2–4 puffs. This may be repeated every 20 min for up to 1 hr if needed.

10 Is PEFR >80% with no more than one sign in the moderate category? — Yes → **11** Is the patient stable after monitoring every 20 min for 1 hr? — Yes →

12
(a) Discharge home; AND
(b) continue albuterol every 4 hr while awake (nebulized at 0.15 mg/kg/dose or 0.03 mL/kg/dose to a maximum of 5 mg or 1 mL, or MDI at 2–4 puffs/dose); AND
(c) if receiving inhaled steroids, theophylline, oral β-agonists, or cromolyn, continue medications; AND
(d) give course of oral steroids at 2 mg/kg/day prednisone equivalent; AND
(e) patient education; AND
(f) 24-hour phone call follow-up; AND
(g) schedule office visit in 3 days.
(G,H)

13 Is PEFR >90% with no more than one sign in the moderate category? — No →

No (from 10 and 11)

Yes ↓

14
(a) Discharge home; AND
(b) continue albuterol every 4 hr while awake (nebulized at 0.1 mg/kg/dose to a maximum of 5 mg, or MDI at 2–4 puffs/dose); AND
(c) if receiving inhaled steroids, theophylline, oral β-agonists, or cromolyn, continue medications; AND
(d) consider course of systemic steroids (oral or parenteral) at a prednisone equivalent of 2 mg/kg/day; AND
(e) patient education; AND
(f) 24-hour phone call follow-up; AND
(g) consider office visit in 3 days.
(G,H)

15
(a) Is patient in the severe category?; OR
(b) Is the clinician uncomfortable?; OR
(c) Are facilities to monitor the patient unavailable?

— Yes →

16 Transfer to ED with O_2, albuterol, and steroids as per Box 4.

No ↓

17
(a) Repeat nebulized albuterol 0.15 mg/kg/dose 3 times every 20 min for up to 1 more hr; AND
(b) give oxygen (mandatory) by ventimask or nasal cannula; monitor with pulse oximeter; keep O_2 saturation ≥93%–95%; AND
(c) give systemic steroids (oral or parenteral) at a prednisone equivalent of 2 mg/kg.

(Go to Box 18.)

Figure 8–3 *Continued*

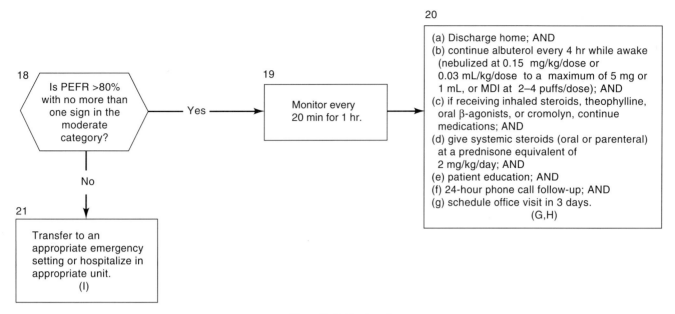

Figure 8-3 *Continued*

respiratory distress. Respiratory syncytial virus is the single most important respiratory pathogen in infants and young children. RSV has been identified as the etiologic agent in 5% to 40% of pneumonias in young children. Although infections with other viruses, such as adenovirus and parainfluenza, can produce inflammation of the bronchioles, RSV causes most cases of bronchiolitis in the first 2 years of life. Furthermore, the most severe disease occurs in infants younger than 6 months of age, although the occurrence of lower respiratory tract disease during the first month of life is uncommon. When RSV infection does occur in neonates, it is often characterized by nonspecific signs, such as poor feeding, lethargy, and apnea. By 5 years of age, 95% of children will have serologic evidence of RSV infection. Furthermore, re-infections are common in older children and adults, since immunity to RSV is short-lived and incomplete. In older children and adolescents, infections with RSV are often limited to the upper respiratory tract; re-infections are common.

In temperate climates, RSV epidemics occur yearly, beginning in mid-winter and persisting through early spring. Intervals between epidemics often alternate between long (13 to 16 months) and short (7 to 12 months) duration; outbreaks may last 1 to 5 months.

Nosocomial acquisition of RSV poses a major and severe threat to hospitalized infants and children. As many as 35% of hospitalized infant contacts may acquire RSV infection, and 40% of the hospital staff caring for infected infants also may become ill. Control of nosocomial spread is particularly difficult. RSV infection is readily spread by contact with contaminated secretions; subsequent self-inoculation via the ocular or nasal routes is common. Moreover, the virus can survive for hours in secretions contaminating surfaces, such as countertops or hands. Masks and gowns are of minimal benefit, but cohorting of patients and staff and good hand washing are the most efficacious control mechanisms.

Infants with congenital heart disease and pulmonary hypertension have a much increased morbidity and somewhat increased mortality from RSV. The course of illness is usually prolonged and frequently entails intensive care and mechanical ventilation. About 40% of infants with RSV and congenital heart disease may have a fatal outcome, in contrast to 1.5% of infected infants who were otherwise normal. Recent reports cite a mortality of less than 4%, presumably due to earlier recognition and modern intensive care. Chronic obstructive pulmonary disease (COPD) and immunodefi-

ciency also increase the risk of severe morbidity or death from RSV infection.

In infected infants, upper respiratory tract symptoms usually precede the lower respiratory tract involvement by 3 to 7 days. Low-grade fever, rhinitis, and pharyngitis are common signs. Cough and wheezing are consistent and prominent features of RSV infection. Chest wall retractions and dyspnea are frequently observed, and adventitious sounds (wheezing, crackles) are appreciated on auscultation of the chest. Most children with bronchiolitis or pneumonia demonstrate clinical improvement after 3 to 4 days, but the duration of illness can be as long as 21 days. Bacterial superinfection of the lower respiratory tract is rare. Approximately 30% of infants with bronchiolitis caused by RSV have recurrent episodes of wheezing caused by bronchial hyperactivity, in part because of persistent inflammation of the distal respiratory tract produced by the viral infection.

Impaired gas exchange can occur as a result of airway obstruction and ventilation-perfusion inequalities. The clinical determination of the severity of the lower respiratory tract involvement in infants infected with RSV can be difficult. Physical findings often associated with respiratory distress, such as tachypnea, intercostal retractions, and wheezing, do not necessarily correlate with the level of hypoxemia. Cyanosis is an insensitive sign of arterial hypoxemia. Carbon dioxide retention secondary to alveolar hypoventilation is not a common finding in otherwise normal children, but hypercapnia and acute respiratory acidosis can be serious problems in infants with chronic pulmonary disease (e.g., bronchopulmonary dysplasia) or heart disease. Roentgenographic findings include a diffuse interstitial pneumonitis and bilateral lung overinflation; alveolar infiltrates or consolidation is present in approximately 20% of children with lower respiratory disease. Roentgenographic abnormalities frequently persist longer than the clinical symptoms, and areas of lung consolidation are often the last to resolve.

The diagnosis of viral bronchiolitis is usually made on clinical grounds. Bronchiolitis is most common in children under 2 years of age and should be suspected in the wheezing child who has current or antecedent upper respiratory tract infection symptoms in the late fall or winter months. The definitive diagnosis of RSV infection is based on the presence of virus or viral antigens in respiratory secretions. Nasopharyngeal washings readily yield the virus when placed into cell culture. Alternatively, fluorescent anti-

Table 8–8. Management of Acute Exacerbations of Asthma in a Child Who Is Capable of Using a Peak Flow Meter

Assessment	Recommended Actions

A. **Initial Assessment and Emergency Treatment**
Does the patient have:
  Altered level of consciousness
  Marked dyspnea, speaks only in single words or short phrases
  Severe intercostal or sternocleidomastoid retractions
  Cyanosis, pallor, or diaphoresis
  Inaudible breath sounds
  Subcutaneous or other extrapulmonary air
  Oxygen saturation <90% if oximeter available
  Peak expiratory flow rate <50% of predicted norm or baseline
  PCO_2 >40 mmHg if arterial blood gases are available
	If any of these conditions exist:
	Give oxygen by ventimask or nasal cannula. If unable to generate PEFR, give epinephrine subcutaneously (SC), 0.01 ml/kg/dose of 1:1000 epinephrine with a maximum dose of 0.3 ml or SC terbutaline 0.005–0.010 mg/kg/dose with a maximum dose of 0.25 mg. If able to generate PEFR, give nebulized albuterol 0.15 mg/kg/dose or 0.03 ml/kg/dose up to a maximum of 5 mg with 6 L/min of O_2 flow. Give systemic steroids at a prednisone equivalent of 2 mg/kg. Consider transfer to an appropriate emergency setting at an FiO_2 of 0.40 or greater and intermittent albuterol treatments every 20 min or continuous albuterol treatments at 0.5 mg/kg/hr if initial response is inadequate. If patient responds well to initial albuterol treatment, repeat twice every 20 min and go to **Follow-up Treatment.**

Does the patient have a history of:
  Steroid-dependent asthma
  Panic attacks with acute exacerbations
  Duration of asthma >12 hr
  History of respiratory failure
  Premonitions of death
  ≥2 visits to office or ED in 24 hr
  >3 visits in 48 hr
  Paroxysmal attacks especially at night
	This is a high-risk patient! Begin therapy immediately as outlined in **Initial Treatment**: moderate or severe exacerbation, regardless of the severity of the current episode. These are high-risk factors that should be considered in the decision to urgently transfer the patient to an appropriate emergency setting. If there is not a prompt clinical response to therapy, consider transfer and give systemic steroids (oral or parenteral) at a prednisone equivalent of 2 mg/kg before transfer.

B. **Initial Treatment** If the exacerbation is in the mild category	Give albuterol by nebulizer at 0.1 mg/kg/dose or 0.02 ml/kg/dose with a minimum dose of 1.25 mg or 2–4 puffs by metered dose inhaler (with or without spacer). This may be repeated every 20 min for up to 1 hr as needed.
If the exacerbation is in the moderate or severe category	Give oxygen. If an oximeter is available, keep O_2 saturation ≥93%–95%. Give nebulized albuterol at 0.15 mg/kg/dose or 0.03 ml/kg/dose up to a maximum of 5 mg or 1 ml at 6 L flow. This may be repeated every 20 min for up to 1 hr
C. **Follow-up Treatment** For patients who were in the mild category, if the PEFR is >80% of predicted norm or baseline with no more than one sign in the moderate category after initial treatment	Discharge home *and* continue albuterol every 4 hr while awake at the same dose previously given. If the patient is receiving inhaled steroids, theophylline, oral β-agonists or cromolyn, continue medications and consider monitoring theophylline levels. Consider systemic steroids (oral or parenteral) at a prednisone equivalent of 2 mg/kg. Give patient education and follow-up with patient in 24 hr by phone call and schedule visit in 3 days to reevaluate need for continuing corticosteroids.
For patients who were in the moderate or severe category, if the PEFR >80% of predicted norm or baseline with no more than one sign in the moderate category after initial treatment	Give systemic steroids (oral or parenteral) at a prednisone equivalent of 2 mg/kg and monitor the patient every 20 min for 1 hr. If stable after this time, discharge home as described above, and if patient is not stable go to **Additional Treatment or Transfer to ED.**
D. **Additional Treatment or Transfer to ED or Direct Admission to Appropriate Hospital Unit** If the patient is in the severe category, *or* if the clinician is uncomfortable with additional treatment *or* if facilities to monitor the patient with pulse oximetry are unavailable	Transfer to ED with O_2, albuterol, and steroids, or direct admission to a hospital unit.
If the patient is in the mild or moderate category with a PEFR <80% of predicted norm or baseline *and* the clinician is comfortable with further treatment *and* facilities are available to monitor the patient with pulse oximetry	Give systemic steroids (oral or parenteral) at a prednisone equivalent of 2 mg/kg. Repeat nebulized albuterol at 0.15 mg/kg/dose or 0.03 ml/kg/dose up to a maximum of 5 mg or 1 ml at 6 L/min of O_2. This may be repeated every 20 min for up to 1 hr *and* give oxygen (mandatory) by ventimask or nasal cannula; monitor with pulse oximeter to keep O_2 saturation ≥93%–95%.
E. **Additional Treatment and/or Hospitalize** If after additional treatment the patient has a PEFR >80% of predicted norm or baseline and no more than one clinical sign in the moderate category and if after monitoring every 20 min for 1 hr the patient remains stable	Discharge home as described above and continue corticosteroids (oral or parenteral) at a prednisone equivalent of 2 mg/kg/d.
If after additional treatment, the PEFR is <80% of predicted norm or baseline	Transfer to an appropriate emergency setting or hospitalize in appropriate unit.

Modified from Provisional Committee on Quality Improvement. Practice parameter: The office management of acute exacerbations of asthma in children. Reproduced by permission of Pediatrics 1994; 93:119–126.
Abbreviations: PEFR = peak expiratory flow rate; FiO_2 = fraction of inspired oxygen; ED = emergency department.

Table 8-9. Pharmacotherapy of Chronic Childhood Asthma*

Disease Severity Before Treatment	Frequency of Symptoms	Treatment†	
		Infants and Young Children	*Children*
Mild	Infrequent, brief	Inhaled β-agonist as needed If inhalation therapy not practical, then oral medication as needed	Inhaled β-agonist as needed
Moderate	>Twice weekly	Cromolyn sodium Theophylline or oral β-agonist	Cromolyn sodium Inhaled corticosteroids Theophylline
Severe	Daily	Inhaled corticosteroids‡ Oral corticosteroids	Oral corticosteroids Oral β-agonists§

Reproduced with permission from Larsen GL. Asthma in children. The New England Journal of Medicine 1992;326:1540–1546.

*Medications are listed in the order in which they are given (alone or in combination) as the severity of disease increases. An extensive summary of guidelines for grading disease severity is included in the National Asthma Education Program Expert Panel report. (See J Allergy Clin Immunol 1991;88:425–534.)

†"As needed" indicates that the drugs are not used routinely, but rather they are used to relieve acute symptoms that occur infrequently.

‡No corticosteroid preparation is approved for nebulized administration in the United States. Preparations available in Europe have been recommended for the treatment of severe asthma in infants and young children. (See Arch Dis Child 1989;64:1065–1079, and 1992;67:240–248.)

§A long-acting oral β-agonist may be helpful in controlling nocturnal asthma in older children with severe chronic asthma, but it is not a substitute for corticosteroids.

body staining of epithelial cells obtained from washing or swabbing the nasopharynx can identify viral infection. When properly performed, the technique is highly sensitive and specific. Moreover, compared with cell culture, fluorescent antibody staining is rapid and readily available. Enzyme-linked immunosorbent assay (ELISA) can also be used to detect RSV in nasopharyngeal secretions.

Unlike asthma, the wheezing accompanying bronchiolitis may be less responsive to bronchodilators. Nonetheless, patients with significant hypoxia and hypercapnia are usually treated with aerosols, as noted in Table 8–7. Infants with bronchiolitis do not usually respond to treatment with anti-inflammatory agents, such as corticosteroids and cromolyn sodium. Although a successful vaccine for RSV remains to be developed, a pharmacologic agent is now available for treatment.

Ribavirin is a synthetic triazole nucleoside that exhibits *in vitro* antiviral activity against a number of RNA and DNA viruses, notably influenza A and B and RSV. Infants treated with ribavirin experience more rapid resolution of lower respiratory tract signs and improvement in oxygenation than do untreated infants; however, the effect is modest at best. The duration of viral shedding may also be reduced by the treatment. Although ribavirin shows some promise for the treatment of RSV bronchiolitis, several limitations prevent its widespread use. The drug must be administered for 12 to 20 hours/day as an aerosol generated by a special delivery system. Treatment is therefore limited to hospitalized patients. Moreover, the small degree of improvement provided by ribavirin probably does not warrant its use in all patients. Because bronchiolitis is typically a self-limited disease, only those infants with underlying cardiopulmonary disorders or those with life-threatening infection should be considered for therapy.

Intravenous gamma globulin containing high titers of RSV-specific neutralizing antibodies has also been reported in pilot studies to ameliorate the course of RSV bronchiolitis. Infants treated with gamma globulin showed increased arterial oxygen saturation and decreased viral shedding compared with controls. The need for intensive care as well as the length of hospital stay may be decreased.

Cystic Fibrosis

Cystic fibrosis (CF) is a multisystem disorder that involves the eccrine and mucous secretory glands (see Chapter 7). Inherited as an autosomal recessive trait, cystic fibrosis is the most common lethal genetic disease in Caucasians and is an important cause of chronic, suppurative pulmonary disease, which ultimately leads to respiratory failure and death. The earliest pulmonary defect exists in the peripheral airways, where viscous, mucopurulent material accumulates in the lumen of the bronchi and bronchioles and obstructs the airways. The involved bronchi become infiltrated with inflammatory cells and infected with *Pseudomonas aeruginosa* and *Staphylococcus aureus,* secondary to impaired mucociliary clearance. Chronic infection and inflammation lead to the weakening and destruction of the airway wall, which results in *bronchiectasis,* the abnormal dilatation of the subsegmental airways, and in pulmonary abscesses.

Dyskinetic Cilia Syndrome

Dyskinetic (immotile) cilia syndrome, an unusual cause of chronic wheezing, occurs in approximately 1 in 16,000 children and is the result of ultrastructural abnormalities of the cilia. The absence of dynein arms (inner and outer) is the most common form of the syndrome, but other structural abnormalities can produce decreased or absent ciliary movement. Acquired ciliary dyskinesia may be caused by a number of different environmental and infectious agents and is usually a temporary condition. The abnormal mucociliary clearance of endobronchial secretions causes a chronic bronchitis; wheezing is a common clinical manifestation resulting from the obstruction of the airways by mucus. Repeated or persistent severe upper respiratory tract infections, usually in the form of chronic pansinusitis or recurrent suppurative otitis media, are typical. Male sterility resulting from the impaired movement of spermatozoa is also present. Although Kartagener initially described several patients who presented with situs inversus totalis, chronic sinusitis, and bronchiectasis, dextrocardia is present in only 50% of patients with this syndrome.

Arriving at a diagnosis necessitates a high index of suspicion and warrants pursuit in the child with recurrent wheeze, bronchitis, sinusitis, and otitis media. Findings on chest roentgenograms are generally nonspecific, but they frequently demonstrate areas of pulmonary consolidation. Extensive atelectasis with significant respiratory distress has been described in neonates with this condition. Bronchiectasis is a late sequela of dyskinetic cilia syndrome. Functional assays for mucociliary clearance or examination of respiratory epithelial cells for ultrastructural ciliary defects using electron microscopy are required to establish a diagnosis.

Gastroesophageal Reflux

Gastroesophageal reflux can be a primary cause or exacerbating factor of wheezing in infants and young children (see Chapters 7 and 20). Direct inhalation of stomach contents into the lungs can produce bronchospasm and a chemical pneumonitis. Gastroesophageal reflux with aspiration has also been implicated in cases of bacterial pneumonia, bronchiectasis, obliterative bronchiolitis, and lung abscesses. Tachypnea, wheezing, and cough are the usual clinical findings, typically occurring within 1 hour of the aspiration event. The signs and symptoms of the pneumonitis, however, can be delayed.

Although pulmonary aspiration of gastric contents was once assumed to be the basis of reflux-induced wheezing, reflex broncho-constriction in response to esophageal acidification can also produce bronchospasm in some patients. Other respiratory symptoms associated with gastroesophageal reflux, such as stridor and obstructive apnea, can present as the result of reflex laryngospasm. Gastroesophageal reflux can also complicate and worsen underlying lung diseases, such as asthma, by provoking bronchospasm and potentiating airway inflammation and possibly bronchial hyperactivity.

Pulmonary Aspiration of Oropharyngeal Contents

Central nervous system or neuromuscular disease in infants and children can result in a dysfunctional swallowing mechanism leading to repeated episodes of pulmonary aspiration. This is the most common cause of respiratory distress in such children and typically presents with intractable wheezing, chronic airway inflammation, and recurrent pneumonias.

Modified barium esophagrams, in which barium-laced foods of a variety of textures and consistencies are fed to a child under direct visualization and fluoroscopy, can be useful in making the diagnosis and establishing that the child has an abnormal swallowing mechanism. In addition, modified barium esophagography can be helpful with regard to therapy and may determine the appropriate feeding techniques, food consistencies, and feeding volumes that are less likely to cause aspiration in a vulnerable child.

Nasogastric tube or gastrostomy tube feedings may be necessary in children who do not respond to conservative management and who continue to have repeated episodes of pulmonary aspiration. Nevertheless, the affected child can continue to have periodic inhalation of oropharyngeal secretions (saliva) despite these interventions.

Anatomic Airway Malformations

Anatomic or structural anomalies of the intrathoracic airways (see Chapter 7) can present as recurrent or persistent wheezing in infants and children (see Table 8–1). Conversely, malformations that obstruct the extrathoracic airway produce predominantly stridor. The lumens of the large proximal airways (trachea and bronchi) are maintained by cartilaginous rings. However, if these support structures are absent, malformed, or excessively pliant, the airways will collapse during expiration, thus producing symptoms of airway obstruction.

Tracheobronchomalacia, excessively collapsible central airways producing wheeze, cough, and tachypnea, is usually generalized throughout the airways and is a congenital anomaly. Acquired bronchomalacia or tracheomegaly has also been described in premature infants following prolonged mechanical ventilatory support, presumably because of barotrauma. Tracheobronchomalacia can be focal, particularly if the malformation is associated with extrinsic compression of the involved airway. Extrinsic compression of the intrathoracic airway by enlarged hilar lymph nodes, mediastinal tumors, and bronchogenic cysts, or vascular rings can produce progressively worsening airway obstruction. Congenital bronchial stenosis and absence of bronchial cartilage are rare conditions that produce fixed obstruction of the involved airway, resulting in persistent, localized wheezing refractory to treatment with bronchodilators. These conditions are all associated with persistent wheeze (which may be localized over the affected segment), recurrent lower respiratory infections, and a chronic, productive cough.

Abnormalities of the lung parenchyma usually present in infants as tachypnea and respiratory distress. Nevertheless, congenital lobar hyperinflation, pulmonary sequestrations, and cystic adenomatoid malformations can cause wheezing secondary to compression of the intrathoracic airways.

Tracheoesophageal fistula, an unusual malformation of the respiratory tract, is a congenital communication between the airways and gastrointestinal tract. The most frequent form of this anomaly —distal tracheoesophageal fistula with esophageal atresia—typically presents early in life (see Chapter 7). Wheezing often persists despite appropriate surgical repair, as gastroesophageal reflux or bronchomalacia may be present.

Vascular Rings

Several types of vascular malformations caused by irregularities in the development of the primitive aortic arches can produce extrinsic compression and narrowing of the intrathoracic trachea (see Chapter 10). The three most common types of complete vascular rings that affect the airway are:

- Double aortic arch
- Right aortic arch with left ligamentum arteriosum
- Anomalous left carotid artery

In the case of the double aortic arch, the right dorsal aorta persists, courses posterior to the esophagus, and joins the left dorsal aorta, which lies anterior to the trachea. This type of malformation produces a complete vascular ring that surrounds both the trachea and esophagus and compresses both structures.

Similarly, a persistent right aortic arch associated with ductus or ligamentum arteriosum completely entraps the trachea and esophagus, thus frequently leading to difficulties in breathing and swallowing. The anomalous left carotid artery anteriorly compresses the trachea and does not represent a complete vascular ring unless it is accompanied by an associated malformation.

An anomalous innominate artery, probably the most common form of this vascular malformation, also is not a complete ring; instead, it produces an anterior compression of the trachea. Consequently, the symptoms associated with this abnormality (i.e., harsh cough, stridor, and wheezing) are usually not as severe.

The clinical presentation of these vascular rings depends on the type of vascular malformation, its relative location in the airway, and the extent of airway compression. The pulmonary signs and symptoms of vascular defects are usually manifested during the first year of life as progressively worsening and ultimately persistent stridor, tachypnea, dyspnea, and respiratory distress. Cough is prominent and is typically harsh and stridulous. A prolonged expiratory phase and wheezing may also be appreciated on auscultation. Most of these conditions in children are mistakenly diagnosed as bronchiolitis or asthma.

Chest roentgenograms usually do not demonstrate parenchymal lesions of the lung, and the airways may appear normal. However, leftward deviation of the trachea by a right aortic arch should alert one of the possibility of a vascular ring, particularly in a patient who has chronic respiratory symptoms. In patients with "complete" vascular rings, posterior compression of the esophagus is evident on contrast esophagram. Bronchoscopy reveals a pulsatile (anterior) compression of the trachea.

Foreign Body Aspiration

Aspiration of a foreign body into the intrathoracic airways must be considered in the differential diagnosis of a child who presents with the *sudden onset* of respiratory distress or wheezing (see Chapter 7). Aspiration of foreign bodies is most common in children between 1 and 4 years of age, particularly in boys. It is rare in children younger than 6 months of age. The most common objects aspirated by children are food products. Endobronchial aspiration of peanuts, raisins, popcorn kernels, or seeds tends to produce more difficulties than other kinds of foreign bodies (metallic or plastic objects), since, in addition to causing physical obstruction of the airway, vegetable matter tends to produce an intense, local inflammatory response secondary to chemical and allergic bronchitis. Larger objects, such as coins, are also frequently aspirated but usually lodge in the esophagus. Nevertheless, esophageal foreign bodies can produce significant respiratory symptoms as a result of extrinsic compression of the posterior trachea.

The typical clinical presentation following the acute event in most of the children is abrupt respiratory distress, characterized by choking, gagging, cyanosis, and a harsh, paroxysmal cough. However, because many aspiration events occur while the child is unsupervised, the history of foreign body ingestion or aspiration is frequently not elicited. Chronic cough, dyspnea, hemoptysis, and wheezing may develop. Because the object is most frequently aspirated into mainstem or segmental bronchus, the wheezing is typically unilateral. Physical examination may also reveal a decrease in breath sounds on the obstructed side, prolongation of the expiratory phase, and a tracheal shift.

In some instances, retained foreign bodies in the airways can produce a persistent pneumonitis, and the chronic inflammatory response can result in bronchiectasis or lung abscess. If both mainstem bronchi or the trachea are obstructed, the patient may have asphyxia; inhalation of foreign bodies is a leading cause of accidental death in children younger than 6 years of age. Large foreign bodies in the proximal esophagus can also produce respiratory distress, stridor, and wheezing by the extrinsic compression of the posterior wall of the trachea, especially in infants and young children. Dysphagia and vomiting can be late symptoms associated with an esophageal foreign body.

The diagnosis of foreign body aspiration can be difficult and necessitates a combination of clinical examination, radiographic studies, and ultimately endoscopic visualization. Because most inhaled objects are not radiopaque, chest roentgenograms frequently do not demonstrate the foreign body. In a clinical series, chest roentgenographs were interpreted as normal in 25% of patients with foreign bodies and did not contribute to the diagnosis. However, the abrupt interruption of a bronchus (air bronchograms), persistent pulmonary infiltrates, and lobar or segmental atelectasis may be evidence of the presence of a retained, radiolucent foreign body. Unilateral hyperaeration on expiratory plain films or fluoroscopy indicates a check-valve obstruction of the airway. Nevertheless, the fluoroscopic evaluation is negative in approximately 10% of patients with a retained endobronchial foreign body.

The definitive diagnostic procedure for foreign body aspiration is bronchoscopy. Obviously, an unambiguous history of foreign body aspiration is a clear indication for bronchoscopy. However, bronchoscopic evaluation of the airways should also be considered in a child who has a history of recurrent or persistent atelectasis or pneumonia in a single lobe, particularly if the pneumonia is refractory to treatment.

Bronchopulmonary Dysplasia

Bronchopulmonary dysplasia is a chronic pulmonary disorder that is a sequela of mechanical ventilation and supplemental oxygen therapy for neonatal respiratory distress syndrome. It is most likely the response of an immature lung to oxygen toxicity, barotrauma, and the resultant inflammation. The histologic features of the pulmonary disease include squamous metaplasia of the airways, peribronchial smooth muscle hypertrophy, alveolar septal fibrosis, and hyperinflation. The risk for development of bronchopulmonary dysplasia increases with decreasing gestational age and birth weight and with the duration of oxygen and ventilator therapy.

Bronchopulmonary dysplasia is clinically characterized by prolonged oxygen requirements (either more than 1 month or beyond 36 weeks of gestational age), tachypnea, wheezing, scattered rhonchi, and increased respiratory effort. Chest roentgenograms typically show alternating areas of subsegmental atelectasis and hyperinflation. Persistent hypoxemia, secondary to abnormal lung mechanics and ventilation-perfusion inequalities, is common, especially in patients with severe lung injury. Patients with bronchopulmonary dysplasia have an increased susceptibility to viral infections of the lower respiratory tract, and exacerbations caused by infections with RSV are particularly troublesome. Airway hyperactivity resulting in episodes of acute bronchospasm is common in infants with bronchopulmonary dysplasia and often persists into adolescence. However, clinical symptoms abate in most children after 3 years of age. Pulmonary function studies in older children may show improvement, but elevated residual lung volumes, decreased lung compliance, decreased expiratory air flows, and bronchial hyperresponsiveness can persist into adulthood.

The diagnosis of bronchopulmonary dysplasia is made on the basis of clinical history and typical radiographic findings. The best treatment of bronchopulmonary dysplasia is prevention. However, acute exacerbations are generally treated in much the same fashion as asthma, with inhaled bronchodilators and corticosteroids. Theophylline and inhaled anti-inflammatory and anticholinergic agents may also be of benefit.

RESPIRATORY DISTRESS IN CHILDREN AND ADOLESCENTS

Asthma is the most common cause of respiratory distress in children and adolescents, although infectious agents (e.g., viruses) may produce wheezing in children. Furthermore, persistent bronchial hyperactivity following acute lower respiratory tract infections can also result in recurrent episodes of wheezing. Nevertheless, other less common causes of persistent wheezing and respiratory distress should be sought, particularly if therapeutic interventions do not affect the patient's clinical condition.

Hypersensitivity Pneumonitis

Hypersensitivity pneumonitis, or extrinsic allergic alveolitis, results from the inhalation of organic dust particles. Although numerous causes have been identified, the clinical features of the various types of hypersensitivity pneumonitis are similar. The clinical manifestations of hypersensitivity pneumonitis depend on the intensity and frequency of exposure to the allergen; both acute and chronic forms have been described.

In the acute form of the disease, the patient typically has fever, rigors, cough, and dyspnea several hours after exposure. The symptoms usually resolve within 24 hours of the onset once the offending material is removed. In the chronic or subacute forms of hypersensitivity pneumonitis, the affected individual may have exercise intolerance, anorexia, weight loss, and a productive cough. Diffuse crackles (rales) are the prominent finding on physical examination, although the patient may be cyanotic if gas exchange is significantly impaired. Digital clubbing is an unusual finding. In acute cases, inflammation of the alveoli and pulmonary interstitium are common reactions, whereas the chronic form can result in interstitial fibrosis and noncaseating granulomas. Chronic hypersensitivity pneumonitis can insidiously lead to respiratory failure and cor pulmonale.

A number of laboratory studies may be helpful in confirming the diagnosis of hypersensitivity pneumonitis. Chest roentgenograms demonstrate diffuse reticulonodular infiltrates, and lung hyperinflation is atypical. Pulmonary function studies characteristically show a restrictive defect, and the carbon monoxide diffusion capacity (D_LCO) is reduced. During the acute phase of the disease, the patient may have a peripheral leukocytosis and eosinophilia. Serologic studies for precipitating immunoglobulin G antibodies to specific antigens are useful in identifying the offending agent. However, these antibodies may be found in asymptomatic individuals exposed to the allergen and thus do not necessarily correlate with severity of pulmonary disease. Percutaneous or intradermal tests may also be useful, particularly if an avian hypersensitivity pneumonitis is suspected.

Removal of the specific organic dust from the patient's environment is critical. Mild episodes of hypersensitivity pneumonitis may resolve spontaneously once the offending allergen is eliminated. Severe exacerbations often necessitate treatment with systemic cor-

---

Table 8-10. Known Causes of Interstitial Lung Disease in Children

Infectious or Postinfectious
  Viral
    Cytomegalovirus
    Human immunodeficiency virus (HIV)
    Respiratory syncytial virus
    Adenovirus
    Influenza virus
    Parainfluenza viruses
    Mycoplasma
    Measles
  Mycobacterial
  Fungal
    *Pneumocystis carinii**
    Aspergillus species
  Bacterial
    Legionella pneumophila
    Bordetella pertussis

Environmental Inhalants, Toxic Substances, Foreign Materials, or Antigenic Dusts
  Inorganic Dusts
    Silica
    Asbestos
    Talcum powder
    Zinc stearate
  Organic Dusts
    Hypersensitivity pneumonitis
    Bird-fancier's lung
    Farmer's lung
  Fumes
    Sulfuric acid
    Hydrochloric acid
  Gases
    Chlorine
    Nitrogen dioxide
    Ammonia

Drug-Induced Disorders
  Antineoplastic Drugs
    Cyclophosphamide
    Nitrosoureas (carmustine, lomustine)
    Azathioprine
    Cytosine arabinoside
    6-Mercaptopurine
    Vinblastine
    Bleomycin
    Methotrexate

  Miscellaneous Drugs
    Nitrofurantoin
    Penicillamine
    Gold salts

Neoplastic Diseases
  Leukemia
  Hodgkin's disease
  Non-Hodgkin's lymphoma
  Letterer-Siwe disease
  Hand-Schüller-Christian disease
  Eosinophilic granuloma
  Histiocytosis X

Lymphoproliferative Disorders
  Familial erythrophagocytic lymphohistiocytosis
  Angioimmunoblastic lymphadenopathy
  Lymphoid interstitial pneumonitis
  Pseudolymphomas of the lung

Metabolic
  Storage Disorders
    Hermansky-Pudlak syndrome
  Pulmonary Lipidosis
    Gaucher's disease
    Niemann-Pick disease
  Disorders of Ion Transport
    Cystic fibrosis
  Other
    Cardiac failure
    Renal disease

Degenerative Disorders
  Idiopathic pulmonary alveolar microlithiasis

Neurocutaneous Syndromes with Interstitial Lung Disease
  Tuberous sclerosis
  Neurofibromatosis
  Ataxia-telangiectasia

Adapted from Hilman BC. Interstitial lung disease in children. *In* Hilman BC (ed). Pediatric Respiratory Disease: Diagnosis and Treatment. Philadelphia: WB Saunders, 1993:362.
**P. carinii*, previously considered a protozoan, is now classified as a fungus.

Table 8–11. Interstitial Lung Disease in Children with Unknown Causes

Usual interstitial pneumonitis	Pulmonary alveolar
Idiopathic pulmonary fibrosis	proteinosis
and familial idiopathic	Pulmonary infiltrates with
pulmonary fibrosis	eosinophilia
Sarcoidosis	Chronic eosinophilic
Pulmonary hemosiderosis	pneumonia
Idiopathic pulmonary	
hemosiderosis	

From Hilman BC. Interstitial lung disease in children. *In* Hilman BC (ed). Pediatric Respiratory Disease: Diagnosis and Treatment. Philadelphia: WB Saunders, 1993:363.

ticosteroids, and bronchodilators may be beneficial if the patient is experiencing symptoms of bronchospasm.

Hypersensitivity pneumonitis must be differentiated from other causes of interstitial lung disease (Tables 8–10 to 8–12). A diagnostic approach to interstitial lung disease is presented in Table 8–13.

Allergic Bronchopulmonary Aspergillosis

Allergic bronchopulmonary aspergillosis (ABPA) is an immunologic disorder identified in patients with chronic lung disease, in which airway colonization (but not invasive infection) with *Aspergillus fumigatus* causes chronic antigen exposure and increased bronchial hyperactivity. This condition can lead to pulmonary fibrosis, bronchiectasis, and progressive respiratory insufficiency. Hypersensitivity to other fungal species that produces a clinical picture similar to ABPA has been reported.

It is important that the diagnosis of ABPA be made and appro-

priate therapy with systemic corticosteroids be instituted, since this condition can result in irreversible lung damage. ABPA is characterized by fever, weight loss, wheezing, and productive cough yielding purulent or rust-colored sputum. This condition should be considered in patients with chronic or atypical and progressive or frequently relapsing lung diseases (e.g., asthma) who have undergone clinical deterioration. ABPA is associated with peripheral eosinophilia and markedly elevated serum immunoglobulin E (IgE) levels. Although these laboratory findings are not pathognomonic for this condition, the presence of a normal serum IgE makes the diagnosis of active disease unlikely. Affected individuals have evidence of hypersensitivity to *A. fumigatus,* and sputum evaluation may demonstrate *Aspergillus* hyphal elements. Elevated levels of specific IgE and IgG antibodies to *A. fumigatus* can be useful in establishing the diagnosis.

The typical radiographic findings include increased bronchopulmonary markings, opacification of the affected area, and localized pulmonary consolidation. Linear radiolucencies and parallel markings radiating from the hilum ("tram lines") caused by dilated, thickened bronchi may also be present. Chest CT may demonstrate a localized (central) saccular bronchiectasis.

The treatment of choice is systemic corticosteroids administered for weeks to months. Antifungal agents, such as itraconazole and amphotericin B, alone are not effective in this disorder but may be a useful adjunct to corticosteroid therapy.

Mycoplasmal Infections

One of the basic tenets regarding respiratory infections in children is, "bacteria do not make you wheeze." *Mycoplasma pneumoniae* is an exception to that rule and should be considered in an older child who presents with new-onset wheezing (see Chapter 7). In addition, infections with *M. pneumoniae* can precipitate exacerbations in patients with asthma. The peak incidence of *M.*

Table 8–12. Interstitial Lung Disease in Children Associated with Other Conditions

Interstitial Lung Disease Associated with Collagen Vascular Disease	*Interstitial Lung Disease Associated with Liver Disease*
Juvenile rheumatoid arthritis	Chronic active hepatitis
Dermatomyositis/polymyositis	Primary biliary cirrhosis
Scleroderma	
Progressive systemic sclerosis	*Interstitial Lung Disease Associated with Bowel Disease*
Ankylosing spondylitis	Ulcerative colitis
Sjögren's syndrome	Crohn's disease
Behçet's syndrome	
	Interstitial Lung Disease Caused by Failure of Other Organs
Interstitial Lung Disease Associated with Pulmonary Vasculitides	Chronic left ventricular failure
Polyarteritis	Chronic left-to-right intracardiac shunt
Wegener's granulomatosis	Chronic renal disease with uremia
Churg-Strauss syndrome	
Lymphomatoid granulomatosis	*Amyloidosis*
Hypersensitivity vasculitis	
Systemic necrotizing vasculitides	*Graft-Versus-Host Disease*
"Overlap" vasculitis	
	Recovering Phase of Adult Respiratory Distress Syndrome
	Goodpasture's Syndrome
	Hypereosinophilic Syndrome
	Pulmonary Veno-occlusive Disease

From Hilman BC. Interstitial lung disease in children. *In* Hilman BC (ed). Pediatric Respiratory Disease: Diagnosis and Treatment. Philadelphia: WB Saunders, 1993:362.

Table 8-13. Investigations for Interstitial Lung Disease in Children

Pediatric Acquired Immunodeficiency Syndrome (AIDS) Testing for HIV antibodies or antigen ELISA or Western blot for HIV antibodies Polymerase chain reaction (PCR) for HIV antigen	*Collagen-Vascular Disorders* Antinuclear antibody (ANA) Rheumatoid factor (RF) Antineutrophil cytoplasmic antibodies (ANCA)
Cystic Fibrosis Quantitative analysis of sweat electrolytes Genetic (DNA) testing	*Infectious Disease* Viral cultures/serology/viral probe studies, ELISA for respiratory syncytial virus Cultures/serology tests for *Mycoplasma* Culture for bacterial pathogens/Gram's stain
Gastroesophageal Reflux/Chronic Aspiration Barium swallow pH probe BAL for lipid-laden macrophages	Fungal cultures/smears Mycobacterial cultures/smear for acid-fast bacilli; PPD Silver stains *(Pneumocystis carinii)* Fluorescent antibodies for *Chlamydia, Legionella* Immunofluorescence for *Pneumocystis carinii*

Immunodeficiency
Quantitative immunoglobulins
Immunoglobulin G subclasses
Assay of antibody response to tetanus, diphtheria,
   Pneumovax, *Haemophilus influenzae* type b
T and B lymphocyte subset quantitation
Anergy panel
	Hypersensitivity Pneumonitis
	Serum precipitins
	
	Pulmonary Hemosiderosis
	Cytology (gastric lavage, BAL fluid, lung biopsy) for hemosiderin-
	   laden macrophages

Ciliary Disorders Electron microscopy of nasal scrapings or tracheal biopsy for ciliary morphology	

Adapted from Hilman BC. Interstitial lung disease in children. *In* Hilman BC (ed). Pediatric Respiratory Disease: Diagnosis and Treatment. Philadelphia: WB Saunders, 1993:361.
Abbreviations: HIV = human immunodeficiency virus, ELISA = enzyme-linked immunosorbent assay, BAL = bronchoalveolar lavage; PPD = purified protein derivative of *Mycobacterium tuberculosis.*

pneumoniae infection is between the ages of 5 and 19 years; it usually does not produce disease in children younger than age 2. Infections with *M. pneumoniae* tend to be seasonal, occurring most frequently during autumn and early winter.

The findings during *M. pneumoniae* infection on chest roentgenographs are variable. A diffuse, bilateral, reticular infiltrate is the classic roentgenographic appearance of mycoplasmal pneumonia. However, lobar, alveolar, and interstitial infiltrates have also been described. Enlargement of hilar or peritracheal lymph nodes may also be evident. Pleural effusions (usually small) are found in 14% of patients with *M. pneumoniae* pneumonia. *M. pneumoniae* tracheobronchitis may produce only subtle roentgenographic changes.

Vocal Cord Dysfunction

A functional disorder that mimics asthma, vocal cord dysfunction is typically manifested as wheezing, dyspnea, and shortness of breath refractory to treatment with inhaled bronchodilators. The wheezing is produced by the adduction of the vocal cords during inspiration and expiration, and the resultant high-pitched inspiratory and expiratory noises are transmitted to the chest, although the sounds are best appreciated over the larynx. Despite the patient's apparent dyspnea, pulmonary gas exchange is unaffected. Pulmonary function studies may demonstrate variable extrathoracic airway obstruction, but only during an "attack." The diagnosis is established by direct laryngoscopy, which demonstrates paradoxical motion of the vocal cords.

Pneumothorax

A pneumothorax occurs when air leaks from the alveoli or airways into the pleural space. The most common cause of pneumo-

thorax in children is chest wall trauma. However, spontaneous pneumothorax can occur in otherwise healthy children with no antecedent illness or injury. This most likely affects adolescent or young adult males who are typically tall, thin, and athletic; Marfan syndrome should be considered. Clinical presentation usually includes acute onset of dyspnea and chest or shoulder pain.

The physical examination shows hyperresonance to percussion over the ipsilateral chest, with decreased breath sounds auscultated on the affected side. If the air dissects up through the mediastinum, it may escape into the subcutaneous tissues producing subcutaneous emphysema. Progressive air leak without air escape can lead to a tension pneumothorax. With increasing pressure, there is mediastinal shift, airway compression, and a decrease in cardiac output. Tension pneumothorax can be life-threatening if it is not recognized and treated rapidly.

The treatment of choice for a pneumothorax greater than 20% volume is drainage with needle aspiration or indwelling chest tube.

Nonpulmonary Causes of Respiratory Distress

Cardiac disease is probably the most important and common nonpulmonary cause of respiratory distress. Increased work of breathing and respiratory distress most commonly occur in cardiac diseases caused by large left to right shunts, dysfunction of the systemic ventricle, and vascular lesions which obstruct the airway (see above). Cardiac failure from any cause is often manifested as respiratory distress. Infants with congenital heart defects producing a large left to right shunt resulting in pulmonary vascular engorgement, edema formation, and reduced lung compliance demonstrate tachypnea, dyspnea, and grunting. Wheezing or "cardiac asthma" can occur when there is compression of intrathoracic airways by vascular engorgement and edema. With most congenital heart defects with left to right shunts, an abnormal heart murmur and cardiomegaly are prominent clues to diagnosis (see Chapters 13 and 16). Acute myocarditis, usually of viral etiology, can present with tachypnea, dyspnea, grunting, and diaphoresis.

The physical examination reveals tachycardia and decreased heart sounds, and chest radiography shows a massively enlarged heart. Cardiomyopathy may be congenital, may have a metabolic or toxic cause, may be familial, or may be idiopathic. Other causes of cardiac failure, such as severe hypertension, renal failure, and severe anemia, should also be sought. Systemic ventricular failure caused by obstructing lesions, such as aortic stenosis, coarctation of the aorta, or mitral stenosis, also causes increased pulmonary vascular engorgement and edema, resulting in the same symptoms as those for a large left to right shunt. Depending on the severity of the left ventricular outflow obstruction, systemic blood flow may be decreased, resulting in poor perfusion and metabolic acidosis. If blood flow into the systemic ventricle from the pulmonary veins or left atrium is decreased or obstructed, as in total anomalous pulmonary venous return or mitral stenosis, severe pulmonary edema, hypoxemia, and respiratory distress ensues. Many of these lesions present early in infancy. Tachypnea, wheezing, cyanosis, and metabolic acidosis are typical presenting signs. Accurate diagnosis depends on echocardiography; cardiac catheterization may be needed in complex cases.

Children with certain primary neurologic disorders (e.g., increased intracranial pressure or neuromyopathic weakness) may present in respiratory distress. Common symptoms include irregular respirations, hypoventilation, or hyperventilation. These symptoms, accompanied by an altered mental status, should prompt an evaluation of the CNS for problems such as meningitis, cerebritis or encephalitis, intracranial hemorrhage, mass lesion, or toxic ingestion. Metabolic derangement that results in acidosis produces tachypnea and possible dyspnea. Common causes of acidosis include diabetic ketoacidosis, sepsis, and ingestions (aspirin). The presence of multisystem involvement in addition to respiratory distress should lead to arterial blood gas determination, urinalysis, and possibly a toxicologic screen.

RESPIRATORY DISTRESS IN THE NEONATAL PERIOD

Preterm and full-term infants can have respiratory distress for several reasons (Table 8–14; see also Table 8–1), many of which do not directly involve the respiratory system (e.g., hypoglycemia, sepsis, anemia, intracranial hemorrhage, and necrotizing enterocolitis). Respiratory distress in the neonate is usually characterized by cyanosis, tachypnea, grunting, chest wall retractions, and nasal flaring. Cyanosis is common and may be caused by congenital heart disease with right to left shunt, severe pulmonary disease, methemoglobinemia, CNS depression, shock, or sepsis.

In the preterm infant, *respiratory distress syndrome* (RDS), caused by surfactant deficiency, alveolar collapse, and hyaline membrane formation, is the most common cause of respiratory distress. Although it can be recognized on the basis of diffuse bilateral atelectasis (ground-glass appearance with air bronchograms) on chest radiography, hypoxemia, and late-onset hypercapnia, bacterial pneumonia and sepsis can present in an almost identical fashion (see Tables 8–1 and 8–14).

Meconium aspiration at the time of delivery can cause severe respiratory distress and pneumonia in full-term infants. *Persistent fetal circulation* (PFC), persistent pulmonary hypertension of the newborn, can also accompany meconium aspiration, pneumonia, and sepsis. Profound but fluctuating hypoxemia refractory to treatment with supplemental oxygen and occurring in the absence of cyanotic congenital heart disease helps confirm the diagnosis of PFC.

Other pulmonary causes of respiratory distress in the newborn include *spontaneous pneumothorax*, which can occur in up to 2% of all live births (see Table 8–1). Most pneumothoraces are small (<20%) and resolve spontaneously or with only the administration of supplemental oxygen.

Pulmonary hypoplasia is a rare condition that generally occurs in infants with oligohydramnios with or without renal dysgenesis or agenesis and abnormal facies *(Potter syndrome)*. In these infants, bilateral pneumothoraces may develop, particularly following resuscitative efforts in the delivery room.

Transient tachypnea of the newborn is a relatively benign condition most often seen in more mature preterm and some term infants delivered by cesarean section following an uneventful pregnancy. The disorder is characterized by tachypnea without significant distress and usually normal arterial blood gas values (an FiO_2 of 40% may be needed to treat mild hypoxemia). Although grunting may occur, other signs of dyspnea are not present and the infant is otherwise well. Chest radiography may demonstrate central perihilar streaking. The condition is self-limited and usually resolves within 2 to 3 days.

Hematologic abnormalities resulting in profound anemia (erythroblastosis, nonimmune hydrops) or polycythemia can also result in respiratory distress. These conditions are often recognized prenatally or in the immediate newborn period because of the significant pallor or plethora exhibited, respectively.

A newborn who presents with severe respiratory distress, absent left-sided breath sounds, bowel sounds in the chest, and a scaphoid abdomen should be suspected of having a *congenital diaphragmatic hernia* (CDH). This lesion occurs five times more frequently on the left than the right and is identified when loops of bowel are seen within the thoracic cavity on a chest radiograph. In many cases, the lung on the affected side is hypoplastic and accounts for the residual pulmonary symptoms seen following surgical repair of the defect. Diaphragmatic hernias are often detected on prenatal ultrasound examination and are operated on immediately after delivery or following stabilization on extracorporeal membrane oxygenation (ECMO). Survival remains approximately 60%. Extracorporeal membrane oxygenation is beneficial to patients with CDH, both preoperatively and in the immediate postoperative period. Although infants affected with CDH are usually profoundly ill in the immediate newborn period, an occasional patient may present later in infancy or even childhood and with milder symptoms. These patients tend to do quite well and have few, if any, long-term sequelae.

The diagnostic, therapeutic, and preventive approaches to common disorders associated with neonatal respiratory distress are noted in Table 8–14. The hyperoxia test is another diagnostic test used to attempt to differentiate cyanotic congenital heart disease from pulmonary diseases, such as respiratory distress syndrome. If the response to breathing 100% oxygen, often with continuous positive airway pressure (CPAP + 4 to 6 cm H_2O), does not improve the umbilical arterial oxygenation to greater than 150 mmHg, cyanotic heart disease may be considered. However, this test may not produce a hyperoxic response if the patient has persistent fetal circulation or may produce a hyperoxic response if the umbilical arterial catheter is misplaced. Therefore immediate evaluation with echocardiography is indicated if the differential diagnosis includes cyanotic heart disease or persistent fetal circulation (see Chapter 15).

RED FLAGS AND THINGS NOT TO MISS

Respiratory distress may be a result of disorders of the extrathoracic or intrathoracic airways (intrinsic or extrinsic compression-obstruction), the alveolus, pulmonary vasculature (pulmonary emboli), pleural space, or thorax. The distress may be secondary to

Table 8-14. Differentiation of Respiratory Distress in the Neonatal Period

	Respiratory Distress Syndrome	Transient Tachypnea of Newborn	Congenital Pneumonia	Persistent Fetal Circulation	MAS	Congenital Heart Disease*
Gestational age	Preterm	Preterm, full term	Preterm, full term	Full term	Full term; postdates (>40 wk)	Preterm, full term
Perinatal history	Preterm labor, no antenatal corticosteroids; Vaginal bleeding; Fetal distress; Second twin; IDM	Cesarean section; No labor; CNS depressant drugs; IDM	PROM; Maternal fever and leukocytosis; Group B streptococcal cervical colonization; Uterine tenderness; Fetal tachycardia; Amnionitis; May be negative	Fetal distress; MSAF; Low Apgar score; Amnionitis; Oligohydramnios (if pulmonary hypoplasia)	MSAF; Fetal distress	Family history; Abnormal fetal echocardiography; Fetal nonimmune hydrops; Fetal arrhythmia; IDM syndrome—malformation complex
Onset	Birth–12 hr	Birth–12 hr	Birth–1 wk	Birth–6 hr	Birth–6 hr	Birth–1 wk
Neonatal history	Grunting, flaring, retractions, cyanosis, tachypnea, borderline hypotension, edema, oliguria	Tachypnea, flaring, minimal cyanosis or retractions; Hypotonia; Lasts 2–3 days	As per RDS plus hypotension, mottling, cold extremities, apnea, bradycardia; Multiorgan system dysfunction secondary to sepsis–shock†	Tachypnea, cyanosis; Minimal retraction; Multiorgan system dysfunction from perinatal asphyxia†	Meconium below vocal cords; Meconium-stained umbilical cord and fingernails; Failure to suction trachea at birth	Heart murmur; Cyanosis; Minimal flaring, grunting, retraction unless pulmonary edema–heart failure; Poor pulses, active precordium
Arterial blood gas analysis	Progressive but varying hypoxia; Hypercapnia as the disease progresses; Acidosis is mixed respiratory and metabolic	Mild hypoxia (requires ≤50% FiO_2)	Profound often fixed hypoxia, poorly responsive to therapy; Severe metabolic acidosis secondary to sepsis syndrome–shock	Profound but fluctuating—labile hypoxia; at times therapy-responsive hyperoxia; may have minimal or no hypercapnia or therapy induced hypocapnia; Arterial oxygen gradient between right radial and umbilical arteries secondary to intracardiac shunts (RRA > UA)	As per PFC	Fixed profound hypoxia especially if ductus arteriosus is closed; Minimal or no hypercapnia; Profound metabolic acidosis secondary to hypoxia or left-sided heart failure

	RDS	TTN	Pneumonia–sepsis	PFC (PPHN)	MAS	CHD
Chest x-ray	Air bronchogram; Ground glass–bilateral white-out; Atelectasis	Normal, hyperinflated; Perihilar edema	As per RDS; Often bilateral white-out; Focal infiltrates	Normal	Normal or meconium-induced pneumothorax-pneumo-mediastinum, atelectasis, marked hyperinflation	Unusual heart shape or location; Right-sided aortic arch; Decreased or increased pulmonary vascular markings
Laboratory findings	Immature amniotic fluid, tracheal or gastric aspirate L/S ratio; Hypoalbuminemia	None	Neutropenia, leukocytosis, or high band count; Positive Gram stain of tracheal aspirate or buffy coat; Positive blood culture; Positive latex agglutination for GBS; Elevated CRP	Occasionally polycythemia (Hct >65%)	None	Abnormal ECG; Echocardiogram is definitive test; Cardiac catheterization for complex lesions
Treatment	Oxygen, CPAP mechanical ventilation, exogenous intratracheal surfactant; Because congenital pneumonia–sepsis can be indistinguishable, add IV ampicillin and gentamicin	Oxygen	Oxygen, mechanical ventilation,‡ broad spectrum antibiotics (ampicillin and gentamicin); Blood pressure support (IV fluids, dopamine, epinephrine); Possibly hyperimmune globulin for GBS; ECMO	Oxygen, mechanical ventilation,‡ INO, ECMO	As per PFC	Initial palliation with prostaglandins, then surgery; Digoxin, inotropic agents (dopamine, dobutamine, amrinone)
Prevention	Antenatal dexamethasone or betamethasone; Exogenous surfactant; Prevent preterm birth	Avoid unnecessary cesarean section	Intrapartum ampicillin for GBS	Prevent and treat fetal distress and neonatal hypoxia	Suction (DeLee) oropharynx after delivery of head; Suction trachea after birth if born through thick meconium, if signs of fetal or neonatal distress, or if no DeLee suctioning of oropharynx on perineum	Avoid teratogenic drugs or chromosomal syndromes

*See Chapters 15 and 16.

†Multisystem organ dysfunction includes myocardial depression (shock, heart failure, tricuspid regurgitation), pulmonary hypertension (hypoxia), acute tubular necrosis (oliguria-anuria, renal failure), hepatic abnormalities (direct reacting jaundice, elevated liver enzymes, prolonged prothrombin time), hematologic abnormalities (disseminated intravascular coagulation, neutropenia, anemia, thrombocytopenia), and CNS dysfunction (coma, seizures).

‡Mechanical ventilation includes conventional rate, flow or pressure-regulated ventilators, or high-frequency jet or oscillator ventilators.

Abbreviations: RDS = respiratory distress syndrome; PFC = persistent fetal circulation—also known as persistent pulmonary hypertension of the newborn; MAS = meconium aspiration syndrome (pneumonia); CHD = congenital heart disease; CNS = central nervous system; PROM = premature, prolonged rupture of the fetal membranes (>18–24 hr); MSAF = meconium-stained amniotic fluid; GBS = group B streptococci; RRA = right radial artery (preductal blood); UA = umbilical artery (postductal blood); CRP = "C" reactive protein–acute phase reactant; INO = inhaled nitric oxide; ECMO = extracorporeal membrane oxygenation (heart-lung or lung bypass); Hct = hematocrit; ECG = electrocardiogram; L/S = lecithin-sphingomyelin ratio: determines active surfactant maturity and reduced risk for RDS; CPAP = continuous positive airway pressure; IDM = infant of diabetic mother; IV = intravenous.

respiratory, cardiovascular, hematologic, or central nervous system diseases. Red flags include sudden onset of distress (pulmonary embolism, foreign body aspiration), chronicity (asthma, mass, immune deficiency, anomaly, cystic fibrosis), clubbing (see Chapter 7), weight loss, fever, hemoptysis (see Chapter 7), focal physical findings, pleural effusions, positive family history, dyspnea, and cyanosis. Hypoxia in the presence of a normal chest film should suggest a pulmonary embolism.

In the neonatal period, respiratory distress syndrome must be differentiated from infections, meconium aspiration, persistent fetal circulation, and congenital respiratory, hematologic, or cardiovascular anomalies.

REFERENCES

Overview

Bailey PV, Tracy T, Connors RH, et al. Congenital bronchopulmonary malformations: Diagnostic and therapeutic considerations. J Thorac Cardiovasc Surg 1990;99:597–603.

Bokulic RE, Hilman BC. Interstitial lung disease in children. Pediatr Clin North Am 1994;41:543–569.

Brasfield DM, Stagno S, Whitley RJ, et al. Infant pneumonitis associated with cytomegalovirus, Chlamydia, Pneumocystis, and Ureaplasma: Follow-up. Pediatrics 1987;79:76–83.

Cressman WR, Myer CM. Diagnosis and management of croup and epiglottitis. Pediatr Clin North Am 1994;41:265–277.

Davis SL, Furman DP, Costarino AT. Adult respiratory distress syndrome in children: Associated disease, clinical course, and predictors of death. J Pediatr 1993;123:35–45.

deMello DE, Nogee LM, Heyman S, et al. Molecular and phenotypic variability in the congenital alveolar proteinosis syndrome associated with inherited surfactant protein B deficiency. J Pediatr 1994;125:43–50.

Dumez Y, Mandelbrot L, Radunovic N, et al. Prenatal management of congenital cystic adenomatoid malformation of the lung. J Pediatr Surg 1993;28:36–41.

Evans DA, Wilmott RW. Pulmonary embolism in children. Pediatr Clin North Am 1994;41:569–585.

Kramer SS, Wehunt WD, Stocker JT, et al. Pulmonary manifestations of juvenile laryngotracheal papillomatosis. AJR 1985;144:687–694.

Kravitz RM. Congenital malformations of the lung. Pediatr Clin North Am 1994;41:453–473.

McIntosh K, Halonen P, Ruuskanen O. Report of a workshop on respiratory viral infections: Epidemiology, diagnosis, treatment, and prevention. Clin Infect Dis 1993;16:151–164.

Moler FW, Custer JR, Bartlett RH, et al. Extracorporeal life support for severe pediatric respiratory failure: An updated experience 1991–1993. J Pediatr 1994;124:875–880.

Mulholland EK, Simoes EAF, Costales MOD, et al. Standardized diagnosis of pneumonia in developing countries. Pediatr Infect Dis J 1992;11:77–81.

Nikolaizik WH, Warner JO. Aetiology of chronic suppurative lung disease. Arch Dis Child 1994;70:141–142.

Nohynek H, Eskola J, Laine E, et al. The causes of hospital-treated acute lower respiratory tract infection in children. Am J Dis Child 1991;145:618–622.

Ruddy RM. Smoke inhalation injury. Pediatr Clin North Am 1994;41:317–337.

Sarniak AP, Lieh-Lai M. Adult respiratory distress syndrome in children. Pediatr Clin North Am 1994;41:337–365.

Singhi S, Dhawan A, Kataria S, et al. Clinical signs of pneumonia in infants under 2 months. Arch Dis Child 1994;70:413–417.

Stigers KB, Woodring JH, Kanga JF. The clinical and imaging spectrum of findings in patients with congenital lobar emphysema. Pediatr Pulmonol 1992;14:160–170.

The Pulmonary Examination

Accurso FJ, Eigen H, Loughlin GM. History and physical examination. In Loughlin GM, Eigen H (eds). Respiratory Disease in Children: Diagnosis and Management. Baltimore: Williams & Wilkins, 1994.

Loudon R, Murphy RLH. Lung sounds. Am Rev Respir Dis 1984;130:663–673.

Schapp LM, Cohen NH. Pulse oximetry, uses and abuses. Chest 1990;98:1244.

Causes of Respiratory Distress

Guidelines for the Diagnosis and Management of Asthma. Expert Panel Report: Bethesda, Md: National Heart, Lung, and Blood Institute. National Institutes of Health. Pub No. 91-3042, 1991.

McFadden ER, Gilbert IA. Asthma. N Engl J Med 1992;327:1928–1937.

Rubin BK, Marcushamer S, Priel I, et al. Emergency management of the child with asthma. Pediatr Pulmonol 1990;8:45–57.

Scarfone RJ, Fuchs SM, Nager AL, et al. Controlled trial of oral prednisone in the emergency department treatment of children with acute asthma. Pediatrics 1993;92:513.

Respiratory Distress in Infants and Toddlers

Antó JM, Sunyer J, Reed CE, et al. Preventing asthma epidemics due to soybeans by dust-control measures. N Engl J Med 1993;329:1760–1763.

Aronson JK, Hardman M, Reynolds DJM. Theophylline. BMJ 1992;305:1355–1358.

Carter E, Cruz M, Chesrown S, et al. Efficacy of intravenously administered theophylline in children hospitalized with severe asthma. J Pediatr 1993;122:470–476.

Committee on Infectious Diseases, American Academy of Pediatrics. Use of ribavirin in the treatment of respiratory syncytial virus infection. Pediatrics 1993;92:501–504.

Connett GJ, Warde C, Wooler E, et al. Prednisolone and salbutamol in the hospital treatment of acute asthma. Arch Dis Child 1994;70:170–173.

DiGiulio GA, Kercsmar CM, Krug SE, et al. Hospital treatment of asthma: Lack of benefit from theophylline given in addition to nebulized albuterol and intravenously administered corticosteroid. J Pediatr 1993;122:464–469.

Editorial. Steroids in acute severe asthma. Lancet 1992;340:1384–1386.

Groothuis JR, Simoes EAF, Levin MJ, et al. Prophylactic administration of respiratory syncytial virus immune globulin to high-risk infants and young children. N Engl J Med 1993;329:1524–1530.

Gustafsson PM, Kjellman N-IM, Tibbling L. Bronchial asthma and acid reflux into the distal and proximal oesophagus. Arch Dis Child 1990;65:1255–1258.

Kamada AK, Leung DYM, Szefler SJ. Steroid resistance in asthma: Our current understanding. Pediatr Pulmonol 1992;14:180–186.

Katz RW, Kelly HW, Crowley MR, et al. Safety of continuous nebulized albuterol for bronchospasm in infants and children. Pediatrics 1993;92:666–669.

Larsen GL. Asthma in children. N Engl J Med 1992;326:1540–1546.

McFadden ER, Gilbert IA. Exercise-induced asthma. N Engl J Med 1994;330:1362–1366.

McWilliams B, Kelly HW, Murphy S. Management of acute severe asthma. Pediatr Ann 1989;18:774–783.

Provisional Committee on Quality Improvement. Practice parameter: The office management of acute exacerbations of asthma in children. Pediatrics 1994;93:119–126.

Sanchez I, De Koster J, Powell RE, et al. Effect of racemic epinephrine and salbutamol on clinical score and pulmonary mechanics in infants with bronchiolitis. J Pediatr 1993;122:145–151.

Special Report of the Steering Committee. Asthma: A follow-up statement from an international paediatric asthma consensus group. Arch Dis Child 1992;67:240–248.

Strauss RE, Wertheim DL, Bonagura VR, et al. Aminophylline therapy does not improve outcome and increases adverse effects in children hospitalized with acute asthmatic exacerbations. Pediatrics 1994;93:205–210.

Weinberger M. Theophylline: When should it be used? J Pediatr 1993;122:403–405.

Wiener C. Ventilatory management of respiratory failure in asthma. JAMA 1993;269:2128–2132.

Wohl MEB, Chernick V. Bronchiolitis. Am Rev Respir Dis 1978;118:759–781.

Cystic Fibrosis

Birnkrant DJ, Stern RC. Sweat testing in the 90s: Am J Asthma Allergy Pediatricians 1991;4:194–198.

Davis PB. Cystic Fibrosis: Lung Biology in Health and Disease. New York: Marcel Dekker, 1993:64.

Schidlow DV, Taussig LM, Knowles MR. Cystic fibrosis foundation consensus conference report on pulmonary complications of cystic fibrosis. Pediatr Pulmonol 1993;15:187–198.

Dyskinetic Cilia Syndrome

Palmblad J, Mossberg B, Afzelius BA. Ultrastructural, cellular, and clinical features of the immotile-cilia syndrome. Ann Rev Med 1984;35:481–492.

Pulmonary Aspiration of Oropharyngeal Contents

Epstein P. Aspiration diseases of the lungs. *In* Fishman A (ed). Pulmonary Diseases and Disorders. New York: McGraw-Hill, 1988.

Orenstein SR, Orenstein DM. Gastroesophageal reflux and respiratory disease in children. J Pediatr 1988;112:847–858.

Vascular Rings

Backer CL, Ilbawi MN, Idriss FAS, et al. Vascular anomalies causing tracheoesophageal compression. J Thorac Cardiovasc Surg 1989;97:725–731.

Burch M, Balaji S, Deanfield JE, et al. Investigation of vascular compression of the trachea: The complementary roles of barium swallow and echocardiography. Arch Dis Child 1993;68:171–176.

Kravitz RM. Congenital malformations of the lung. Pediatr Clin North Am 1994;41:453–472.

Foreign Body Aspiration

Wagner MH. Foreign body aspiration. *In* Loughlin GM, Eigen H (eds). Respiratory Disease in Children: Diagnosis and Management. Baltimore: Williams & Wilkins, 1994.

Weisberg D, Schwartz I. Foreign bodies in the tracheobronchial tree. Chest 1988;91:730.

Respiratory Distress in Children and Adolescents

Cunningham CK, McMilan JA, Gross SJ. Rehospitalization for respiratory illness in infants of less than 32 weeks gestation. Pediatrics 1991;88:527–532.

O'Brodovich HM, Mellins RB. Bronchopulmonary dysplasia. Am Rev Respir Dis 1985;132:694–709.

Interstitial Lung Disease

du Bois RM. Diffuse lung disease: An approach to management. BMJ 1994;309:175–179.

Fan LL, Mullen ALW, Brugman SM, et al. Clinical spectrum of chronic interstitial lung disease in children. J Pediatr 1992;121:867–872.

Smyth RL, Carty H, Thomas H, et al. Diagnosis of interstitial lung disease by a percutaneous lung biopsy sample. Arch Dis Child 1994;70:143–144.

Allergic Bronchopulmonary Aspergillosis

Greenberger PA. Allergic bronchopulmonary aspergillosis and fungoses. Clin Chest Med 1988;9:599–608.

Mycoplasmal Infections

Sabato AR, Martin AJ, Marmion BP, et al. *Mycoplasma pneumoniae*: Acute illness, antibiotics, and subsequent pulmonary function. Arch Dis Child 1984;59:1034–1037.

Vocal Cord Dysfunction

Alpert SE, Dearborn DG, Kercsmar CM. Vocal cord dysfunction in wheezy children. Pediatr Pulmonol 1991;19:142–143.

Pneumothorax

Lichter I, Gwynne JF. Spontaneous pneumothorax in young adults: A clinical and pathological study. Thorax 1971;26:409–417.

Respiratory Distress in the Neonatal Period

Abman SH, Griebel JL, Parker DK, et al. Acute effects of inhaled nitric oxide in children with severe hypoxemic respiratory failure. J Pediatr 1994;124:881–888.

Beca J, Butt W. Extracorporeal membrane oxygenation for refractory septic shock in children. Pediatrics 1994;93:726–729.

Clark RH, Yoder BA, Sell MS. Prospective, randomized comparison of high-frequency oscillation and conventional ventilation in candidates for extracorporeal membrane oxygenation. J Pediatr 1994;124:447–454.

Cunniff C, Jones KL, Jones MC. Patterns of malformation in children with congenital diaphragmatic defects. J Pediatr 1990;116:258–261.

Evans NJ, Archer LNJ. Doppler assessment of pulmonary artery pressure and extrapulmonary shunting in the acute phase of hyaline membrane disease. Arch Dis Child 1991;66:6–11.

Faix RG, Viscardi RM, DiPietro MA, et al. Adult respiratory distress syndrome in full-term newborns. Pediatrics 1989;83:971–976.

Fleischer A, Anyaegbunam A, Guidetti D, et al. A persistent clinical problem: Profile of the term infant with significant respiratory complications. Obstet Gynecol 1992;79:185–190.

Kari MA, Hallman M, Eronen M, et al. Prenatal dexamethasone treatment in conjunction with rescue therapy of human surfactant: A randomized placebo-controlled multicenter study. Pediatrics 1994;93:730–736.

Lister G, Fontan JJP. Congenital heart disease. *In* Loughlin GM, Eigen H (eds). Respiratory Disease in Children: Diagnosis and Management. Baltimore: Williams & Wilkins, 1994.

Miller OI, Celermajer DS, Deanfield JE, et al. Guidelines for the safe administration of inhaled nitric oxide. Arch Dis Child 1994;70:F47–F49.

Rouse DJ, Goldenberg RL, Cliver SP, et al. Strategies for the prevention of early-onset neonatal group B streptococcal sepsis: A decision analysis. Obstet Gynecol 1994;83:483–494.

Schwartz RM, Luby AM, Scanlon JW, et al. Effect of surfactant on morbidity, mortality, and resource use in newborn infants weighing 500 to 1500 g. N Engl J Med 1994;330:1476–1480.

Walsh-Sukys M, Stork EK, Martin RJ. Neonatal ECMO: Iron lung of the 1990s? J Pediatr 1994;124:427–430.

Weisman LE, Stoll BJ, Cruess DF, et al. Early-onset group B streptococcal sepsis: A current assessment. J Pediatr 1992;121:428–433.

9 Earache

Colin D. Marchant

Earache (otalgia) is pain that arises from a pathologic process in the external, middle, or inner ear or that is referred to the ear from another structure. The most common cause of ear pain in children is acute otitis media. By age 7 years, 90% of all children have had at least one episode of acute otitis media. The second most common cause of ear pain is otitis externa, followed by dermatitis and infections of the pinna. All other causes are rare (Tables 9–1 and 9–2). A careful examination of the pinna, external auditory canal, and tympanic membrane can identify most causes of ear pain. When the findings are normal, the clinician should consider referred pain from another source (Table 9–3).

DIAGNOSTIC APPROACH

History

Verbal children with ear pain are usually able to localize and accurately describe their symptoms. Infants and younger children often cannot localize their pain and may present with a variety of nonspecific symptoms. These include fever, irritability, rhinorrhea (from an associated upper respiratory tract infection), and ear pulling. Even though ear pulling is associated with ear pain, it is neither specific nor sensitive in the diagnosis of ear pathology. Many infants with acute otitis media are afebrile and present with various degrees of irritability. Parents often cannot tell whether the irritability is due to ear pain or to some other cause (e.g., teething). These symptoms may be neither specific nor severe enough for the parent to seek medical attention. Indeed, 50% of the first episodes of acute otitis media during the first year of life present during a routine health maintenance examination without a chief complaint, suggesting ear pain. The clinician should have a high index of suspicion of ear pathology during the first year of life or in any preschool child with fever, irritability, or an upper respiratory tract infection.

Risk factors for acute otitis media include a sibling history of recurrent acute otitis media, household cigarette smoke, bottle feeding, Native American or Eskimo heritage, cleft palate, acquired

Table 9–1. Differential Diagnoses of Painful Disorders of the External Ear and Auditory Canal

Disorder	Clinical Features
Acute otitis externa	Diffuse redness, swelling, and pain of the canal with greenish to whitish exudate, often very tender pinna
Malignant otitis externa	In immunocompromised hosts and poorly controlled diabetics; rapidly progressive, severe swelling and redness of pinna; pinna may be laterally displaced
Dermatitis	
Eczema	History of atopy, presence of lesions elsewhere; lesions are scaly, red, pruritic, and weeping
Contact	History of cosmetic use or irritant exposure; lesions are scaly, red, pruritic, and weeping
Seborrhea	Scaly, red, papular dermatitis; scalp may have thick, yellow scales
Psoriasis	History or presence of psoriasis elsewhere; erythematous papules that coalesce into thick, white plaques
Cellulitis	Diffuse redness, tenderness, and swelling of the pinna
Furuncles	Red, tender papules in areas with hair follicles (distal third of the ear canal)
Infected periauricular cyst	Discrete, palpable lesion; history of previous swelling at same site; cellulitis may develop, obscuring cystic structure
Insect bites	History of exposure; lesions are red, tender papules
Herpes zoster	Painful, vesicular lesions in the ear canal and tympanic membrane in the distribution of cranial nerves V and VII
Perichondritis	Inflammation of the cartilage usually secondary to cellulitis
Tumors	Very rare, palpable mass, destruction of surrounding structures
Foreign body	Almost any type of foreign body is possible; the foreign body may cause secondary trauma to the ear canal or become a nidus for an infection of the ear canal
Trauma	Bruising and swelling of external ear; there may be signs of basilar skull fracture (cerebrospinal fluid otorrhea, hemotympanum)
Myringitis bullosa	Presumably viral vesicles and bullae often with hemorrhage on the tympanic membrane; illness may also be caused by the same bacterial pathogens of acute otitis media

Table 9–2. Differential Diagnosis of Painful Middle Ear Disorders

Disorder	Clinical Features
Acute otitis media	Immobile tympanic membrane that may appear bulging, red, and/or opaque
Myringitis bullosa	Presumably viral vesicles and bullae often with hemorrhage on the tympanic membrane; illness may also be caused by the same bacterial pathogens of acute otitis media
Acute mastoiditis with periostitis	Tenderness and erythema over mastoid process; no destruction of bony trabeculae
Acute mastoid osteitis	Destruction of bony trabeculae; tenderness and erythema over mastoid process coupled with outward displacement of pinna
Wegener's granulomatosis	Severe necrotizing vasculitis; ulcerative and destructive granulomatous lesions of upper and lower respiratory tract
Histiocytosis	Pituitary dysfunction, exophthalmos, seborrheic dermatitis, and bony lesions; if bony lesions involve the ear, patient will present with mastoid tenderness and otorrhea

immunodeficiency syndrome (AIDS), and group day care attendance. Because of the high incidence of acute otitis media coupled with the low negative predictive value of these risk factors, the clinician should still consider this diagnosis in the absence of these risk factors.

Children with pathology of the external auditory canal or the pinna present with a history of redness, tenderness, and/or purulent otorrhea. With otitis externa (''swimmer's ear''), the patient may complain of redness and swelling of the pinna, tenderness with manipulation of the pinna and tragus, extreme pain, and drainage from the external ear canal. Relapsing polychondritis also involves swelling and redness of the pinna; however, this condition is usually bilateral and recurrent and other cartilaginous structures are affected.

With referred ear pain, there are often additional symptoms associated with the respective head and neck structures (see Table 9–3). For example, patients with referred ear pain secondary to maxillary sinusitis may also complain of headaches and purulent rhinorrhea.

Examination of the Ear

The examination begins by inspection of the pinna and adjacent tissues for dermatitis, redness, and edema. In mastoiditis, the redness is over the mastoid process; in otitis externa, it is localized to the external auditory canal and the pinna. In both conditions, the swelling may be so severe that the pinna is laterally displaced. The opening of the external ear canal is also examined for the presence of discharge or exudate. The pinna, including the cartilaginous portions, and the mastoid process are palpated for any tenderness. Most disorders of the external ear can be detected through this examination (see Table 9–1).

Otoscopy provides an opportunity to indirectly view the middle ear through the tympanic membrane. The middle ear is normally an air-filled cavity that transmits sound from the eardrum to the bony ossicle and then into the internal ear (Fig. 9–1). Otoscopy

begins by properly positioning and, if necessary, restraining the patient. Infants are best examined on an examining table in the prone position, with a parent or an attendant firmly holding the patient's arms and preventing the patient from moving. Toddlers should sit on the parent's lap, with the examiner sitting in a chair opposite them. The parent holds the child against his or her chest, with one hand and arm holding the child's arms and the other around the child's head so that one ear is exposed.

The eardrum is often obscured by cerumen (ear wax). Failure to remove the debris is the major reason for diagnostic errors. To view the eardrum properly, the examiner first removes the wax either by irrigating the ear canal gently with lukewarm water or by lifting the wax out with a blunt curet. Contraindications for irrigation are a tympanostomy tube, perforated tympanic membrane, or an organic foreign body (e.g., legumes swell in contact with water). To minimize the risk of damaging the tympanic membrane or scratching the external auditory canal, the examiner should remove wax with a curet under direct observation using an operating otoscopic head.

During the insertion of the speculum, the clinician should note any redness, edema, tenderness, exudate, furuncles, or vesicles that may be present in the external auditory canal. In some illnesses (otitis externa), the ear canal may be so edematous that the speculum cannot be inserted and the eardrum cannot be seen.

Because pneumatic otoscopy is more accurate than otoscopy in detecting middle ear effusion, it should be part of every ear examination. In performing pneumatic otoscopy, the examiner first selects a speculum that will fit snugly in the external auditory canal. The examiner partially depresses the rubber bulb of the pneumatic otoscope and inserts the otoscope into the ear canal (Fig. 9–2). Once the eardrum is seen, the examiner should observe the color, appearance, position, and mobility of the tympanic membrane (Table 9–4). If the eardrum is not perforated, the clinician observes its mobility by alternating positive and negative pressure by gently depressing and releasing the bulb of the pneumatic otoscope. A poorly mobile eardrum may be secondary to middle ear effusion, a perforated tympanic membrane, or lack of an airtight seal.

In neonates and young infants, the eardrum is less perpendicular to the observer, the bony landmarks are less distinct, and the eardrum is less mobile than in older infants and children. Failure to appreciate these normal otoscopic findings may lead to the overdiagnosis of middle ear effusion in young infants.

In the first few hours of acute otitis media, the inflamed and

Table 9–3. Causes of Referred Ear Pain

Neck
Cervical lymphadenitis
Infected cervical cysts
Subluxation of the atlantoaxial joint (torticollis and otalgia)

Salivary Glands
Parotitis

Thyroid
Thyroiditis

Teeth and Gums
Dental abscess
Impacted teeth
Gingivitis

Temporomandibular Joint
Arthritis, juvenile rheumatoid arthritis
Spasm from bruxism or dental malocclusion

Tonsils
Tonsillitis
Peritonsillar abscess
Post-tonsillectomy neuralgia

Pharynx
Pharyngitis

Paranasal Sinuses
Maxillary sinusitis

Other
Herpes zoster (Ramsey-Hunt syndrome: postherpetic neuralgia, migraine, Bell's palsy)
Tumors (e.g., facial nerve)

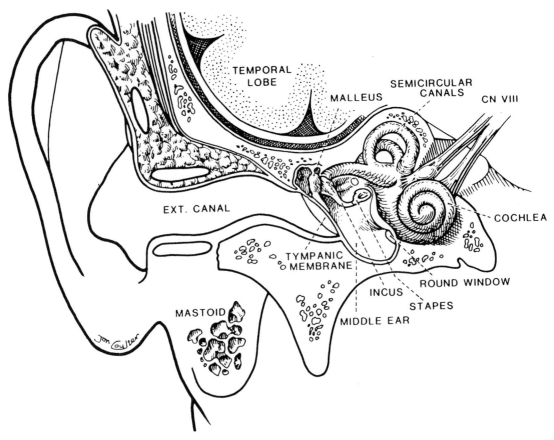

Figure 9–1. Anatomy of the ear. (From Bluestone CD, Klein JO. Otitis Media in Infants and Children. Philadelphia: WB Saunders, 1995:11.)

painful middle ear cavity may not yet be filled with fluid. At this early stage of the illness, the mobility may be normal. By the time the patient is usually examined, however, the middle ear cavity is filled with fluid. At this point, the eardrum is opaque and bulging

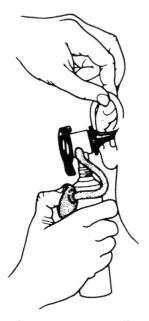

Figure 9–2. Technique for pneumatic otoscopy. (From Bluestone CD, Klein JO. Otitis Media in Infants and Children. Philadelphia: WB Saunders, 1988:72.)

and has decreased mobility. Even though a reddened eardrum may be from inflammation of the tympanic membrane, the specificity of this physical finding is reduced because crying alone induces diffuse redness of the eardrum. In addition, the interobserver variability of differentiating color is high and may in part be due to the intensity and type of light source used in otoscopy.

Otitis media with effusion (OME) is also called *serous otitis media* and *mucoid otitis media.* The cardinal sign is decreased mobility of the eardrum. The eardrum may also be opaque, but it should not be bulging or grossly inflamed. Patients are asymptomatic except for decreased hearing acuity. A challenge for the clinician is the child with symptoms consistent with acute otitis media (ear pain) but with the physical findings of OME. In such cases, it is difficult to decide whether there is an acute infection of the middle ear or whether it is OME with an illness at another site causing the symptoms.

When the external ear and tympanic membrane are normal in a child with an earache, the clinician must consider the possibility of referred pain (see Table 9–3). Innervation of the external and middle ear includes pain fibers of the trigeminal, glossopharyngeal, and vagus nerves and, to a lesser extent, the facial nerve and upper cervical nerves. The clinician should examine the neck, parotid gland, thyroid, mouth, tongue, teeth, temporomandibular joint, tonsils, and throat. In children, the cause of referred pain is usually infectious rather than noninfectious (e.g., a tumor).

Diagnostic Tests

BACTERIAL CULTURES

Routine microbial cultures of middle or external ear fluid are not required because most infections of the ear are self-limited and

Table 9–4. The Tympanic Membrane in Acute Otitis Media and Otitis Media with Effusion

Characteristic	Normal Findings	Acute Otitis Media	Otitis Media with Effusion	Comments
Color	Gray to pink	Often red from inflammation; yellow to white from purulent fluid behind eardrum	Usually gray to pink, but may still be yellow or white; should not be red (inflamed)	Interobserver variation of color is high; redness occurs from crying alone
Appearance	Translucent	Opaque	Translucent or opaque	Opacity is due to opaque fluid or to scarring of eardrum
Position	Neutral	Fluid under pressure produces bulging of eardrum; bony landmarks may be distorted and the light reflex lost	Should not be bulging; may be retracted by negative middle pressure (caused by eustachian tube obstruction)	
Mobility (to positive and negative pressure)	Tympanic membrane moves freely	Mobility to positive and negative pressure reduced	Mobility to positive and negative pressure reduced	
Other findings		Perforation with otorrhea		

readily respond to empirical antimicrobial therapy. In selected instances (e.g., multiple treatment failures, an immunocompromised host), bacterial or fungal culture of otorrhea from the external auditory canal or cultures of middle ear fluid by tympanocentesis may guide therapy. In a child with acute otitis media, the offending pathogen is usually present in the nasopharynx, but other bacterial species or strains may also colonize this area. Nasopharyngeal cultures are not helpful in directing therapy because it is not known which organism is actually causing the middle ear infection. With the emergence of strains of *Streptococcus pneumoniae* that are resistant to all commonly used antibiotics, the incidence of treatment failures may increase. This may necessitate a greater reliance on tympanocentesis for culture of middle ear fluid to determine the appropriate antimicrobial agent.

Tympanocentesis is performed with a spinal (20-gauge) needle attached to either a sterile syringe or an Alden-Senturia sterile suction trap (Fig. 9–3). After the stylet is removed from the spinal needle, the needle is bent near the needle hub to a convenient angle and the syringe or suction trap is attached. The patient is then immobilized (on a papoose board), and the cerumen is removed. The discomfort of the procedure may be reduced by ionophoresis of lidocaine applied directly to the tympanic membrane or through other protocols for conscious sedation (intranasal midazolam). Under direct observation through the use of an operating head of an otoscope, the needle is inserted through the anterior-inferior quadrant of the tympanic membrane. The middle ear fluid is aspirated by drawing on the syringe or by applying suction through the suction trap. A specimen of middle ear exudate is then obtained for culture on chocolate and blood agar plates or other appropriate culture media. If no fluid is obtained, the tip is cultured by drawing sterile broth through the needle. In most patients, the perforation is healed in 3 to 5 days. Persistent perforations from this procedure are rare.

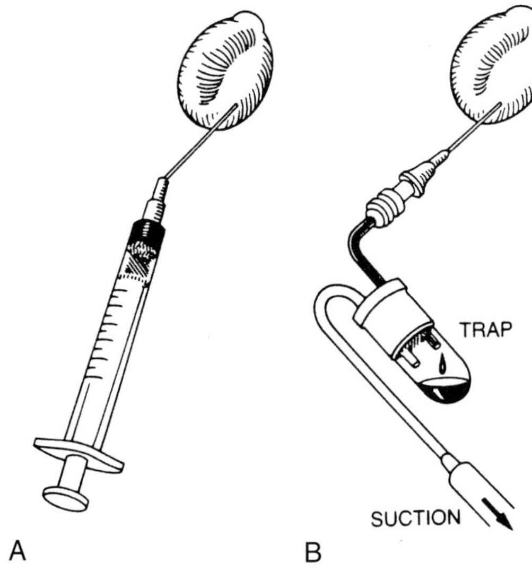

AUDIOMETRY

Even though testing hearing acuity in the initial evaluation of otalgia is not often useful, it becomes important in deciding when to refer for tympanostomy tube placement in the management of persistent otitis media with effusion (Fig. 9–4). Hearing acuity should be assessed in a quiet room by pure tone threshold audiometry, and both air and bone conduction are measured at 500, 1000, 2000, and 4000 hertz (Hz). Behavioral observation audiometry by a certified audiologist conducted in a sound-proof room may be needed to assess hearing acuity in children under 4 years of age.

TYMPANOMETRY

Tympanometry is an objective method for detecting the presence of middle ear effusion. A soft plastic probe is inserted into the opening of the external auditory canal in order to obtain an airtight seal. The tympanometer measures the flow of sound energy into the middle ear under conditions of changing air pressure. When the air pressure is equal on both sides of an intact eardrum, with the drum in neutral position, the transmission of sound energy through the tympanic membrane is at its maximum. The peak on

TRAP

SUCTION

A   B

Figure 9–3. Tympanocentesis using a sterile spinal needle attached to a tuberculin syringe *(A)*, or an Alden-Senturia suction trap *(B)*. (From Bluestone CD, Klein JO. Otitis Media in Infants and Children. Philadelphia: WB Saunders, 1995:127.)

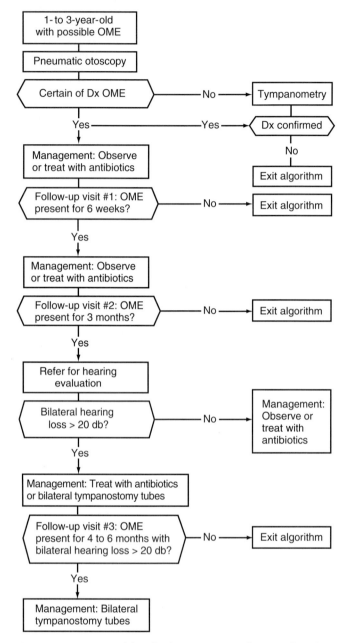

Figure 9–4. Practice guidelines for the management of otitis media with effusion (OME) in children from 1 to 3 years old. Dx = diagnosis; db = decibels. (Adapted from recommendations of the Otitis Media Guideline Panel, Agency for Health Care Policy and Research, Pub. No. 94–0622. Rockville, Md: July 1994.)

edly elevated baseline. This method can also be used for confirming the patency of a tympanostomy tube.

The sensitivity and specificity of tympanometry depend on the patient population, the instrument, and the criteria for interpretation. In expert hands, tympanometry and pneumatic otoscopy have equivalent sensitivity (approximately 90%) and specificity (70% to 80%). Tympanometry is neither more accurate nor more convenient than properly performed pneumatic otoscopy. Some tympanometers do not perform well in infants younger than 6 months of age. Tympanometry is advantageous if the clinician is unsure of the otoscopic findings, and it provides an objective and printed record documenting the status of the middle ear effusion.

ACOUSTIC REFLECTOMETRY

Acoustic reflectometry detects middle ear effusion by directing a sound of varying frequency toward the tympanic membrane and measuring the intensity of reflected sound. This hand-held instrument is similar in size to that of an otoscope. The tip of the reflectometer is inserted in the external opening of the ear canal.

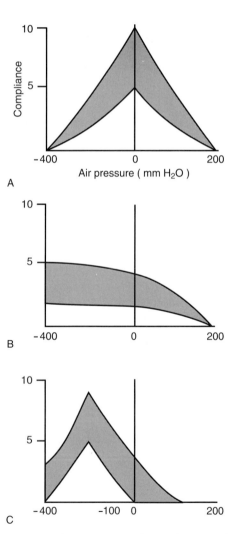

Figure 9–5. *A,* A normal tympanogram with a peak at atmospheric pressure indicating an air-filled middle ear with normal (atmospheric) pressure. *B,* A "flat" tympanogram indicating middle ear effusion. *C,* A tympanogram with a negative peak pressure, indicating eustachian tube obstruction.

the tympanogram represents the pressure in which the flow of sound energy is maximal. For example, in a normal air-filled middle ear cavity, the peak occurs at ambient atmospheric pressure (type A curve, Fig. 9–5). With eustachian tube dysfunction (a retracted eardrum but no middle ear effusion), the peak occurs in the negative pressure range on the recording (type C curve, Fig. 9–5). With middle ear effusion, the sound energy flow into the middle ear is reduced, which produces a flat tympanogram (type B curve, Fig. 9–5). A flat tympanogram may also result from cerumen or the wall of the external auditory canal occluding the opening of the probe. In a perforated eardrum, the sound energy is readily transmitted through the hole in the drum throughout the entire pressure range, which results in a flat tympanogram with a mark-

In contrast to tympanometry, an airtight seal is not required. The frequency of maximal reflected sound depends on the arbitrary distance of the probe from the eardrum. Middle ear effusion is detected not by the frequency but by the magnitude of maximal reflected sound. When middle ear effusion is present, reflectance is increased compared with the air-filled ear.

Reflectometry is easily learned, quick, convenient, and useful in a crying child. With a sensitivity of 80% to 87% and a specificity of 54% to 70%, reflectometry is less accurate than properly performed pneumatic otoscopy in detecting middle ear effusion. Because the accuracy of current models decreases in infants under 1 year old, this technique should not be used in infants younger than 6 months of age. Like tympanometry, reflectometry can reveal only whether middle ear effusion is present and cannot tell whether the effusion is secondary to acute otitis media or otitis media with effusion. Reflectometry is useful if otoscopic findings are indefinite.

DIAGNOSTIC IMAGING

Radiologic techniques are rarely required in the evaluation of external or middle ear disease, but they may be useful in the assessment of intratemporal and intracranial complications of otitis media. Roentgenograms of the mastoid are helpful in the diagnosis of acute and chronic mastoiditis. Opacification of the normally aerated mastoid air cells is usually seen in acute otitis media because the mastoid air cells communicate with the middle ear space. By definition, this is acute *mastoiditis*; however, this opaci-

fication resolves concomitantly with the successful treatment of acute otitis media. In contrast, in *acute mastoid osteitis,* also called *acute coalescent mastoiditis,* there is destruction of bony trabeculations in the mastoid air cells.

Computed tomographic (CT) scans of the mastoid yield clearer images of the destructive process in the bony trabeculations. Other imaging studies that may be useful in evaluating a patient for complications of acute otitis media include CT scans of the head for suspected cholesteatomas and intracranial mass lesions (brain abscess) and magnetic resonance venography for sinus thrombosis.

Differential Diagnosis

Most disorders of the external and middle ear are readily apparent following the examination of the ear (see Tables 9–1 and 9–2). If examination findings are unremarkable, the clinician should consider referred pain to be the cause for the otalgia (see Table 9–3). The clinician must be careful in attributing the child's fever and irritability solely to acute otitis media because some other illness (bacterial meningitis) might be present simultaneously and may be causing these symptoms. Most cases of otitis media are uncomplicated; however, the clinician should be alert to the complications and sequelae of acute otitis media (Table 9–5).

SPECIFIC ILLNESSES
Otitis Externa

Otitis externa, an infection of the external ear canal, is associated with warm humid weather and swimming. The moisture may cause

Table 9–5. Sequelae and Complications of Otitis Media

Complications	Clinical Features
Acute	
Perforation with otorrhea	Immobile tympanic membrane secondary to visible perforation, exudate in ear canal
Acute mastoiditis with periostitis	Tenderness and erythema over mastoid process, no destruction of bony trabeculae
Acute mastoid osteitis	Destruction of bony trabeculae; tenderness and erythema over mastoid process coupled with outward displacement of pinna
Petrositis	Infection of perilabyrinthine cells; may present with otitis, paralysis of lateral rectus, and headache (Gradenigo syndrome)
Facial nerve palsy	Peripheral cranial nerve VII paralysis
Labyrinthitis	Vertigo, fever, ear pain, nystagmus, hearing loss, tinnitus, nausea and vomiting
Lateral sinus thrombophlebitis	Headache, fever, seizures, altered states of consciousness, septic emboli
Meningitis	Fever, headache, nuchal rigidity, seizures, altered states of consciousness
Extradural abscess	Fever, headache, seizures, altered states of consciousness
Subdural empyema	Fever, headache, seizures, altered state of consciousness
Brain abscess	Fever, headache, seizures, altered state of consciousness, focal neurologic examination
Non-acute	
Indolent infections as above	
Chronic perforation	Immobile tympanic membrane secondary to perforation
Otitis media with effusion (OME)	Immobile, opaque tympanic membrane
Adhesive otitis	Irreversible conductive hearing loss secondary to chronic OME
Tympanosclerosis	Thickened white plaques, may cause conductive hearing loss
Chronic suppurative otitis media	Following acute otitis media with perforation, secondary infection with *Staphylococcus aureus, Pseudomonas aeruginosa,* or anaerobes develops, causing chronic otorrhea
Cholesteatoma	White, pearl-like destructive tumor with otorrhea arising near or within tympanic membrane; may be secondary to chronic negative middle ear pressure
Otitic hydrocephalus	Increased intracranial pressure secondary to AOM; signs and symptoms include severe headaches, blurred vision, nausea, vomiting, papilledema, diplopia (abducens paralysis)

small abrasions in the protective lipid layer of skin of the ear canal. These abrasions become infected on exposure to pathogenic bacteria, especially *Pseudomonas aeruginosa* and other gram-negative bacteria. Saprophytic fungi may also play a role in this infection. Less commonly, otorrhea draining from a perforated tympanic membrane secondary to otitis media may cause otitis externa. The patient may complain of pain (especially with manipulation of the pinna), redness, and otorrhea. On physical examination, the ear canal is red, edematous, and tender.

Treatment consists of a topical suspension containing both antibiotics (polymyxin b sulfate/neomycin) and corticosteroids. Most patients quickly respond in a few days to a regimen of four to five drops applied to the affected canal three to four times per day for 5 to 7 days. If there is marked edema of the canal, antibiotics may not reach the site of infection. In this case, the canal should be cleaned with gentle suction and a cotton wick should be inserted into the auditory canal. Antibiotic suspension is then dripped into the wick, which allows the medication to diffuse further into the ear canal. In some cases, daily cleaning and replacement of the wick are necessary. Most cases of otitis externa respond to the above therapy. If the infection should progress, the patient may need parenteral antibiotics and a consultation with an otolaryngologist.

Chondritis is a potential complication of severe otitis externa. It occurs when the infection progresses into the cartilaginous structures of the ear. This complication is rare without a history of previous trauma or surgery.

Malignant Otitis Externa

Malignant otitis externa is a fulminant condition that causes extensive tissue destruction. The illness may result in chondritis and osteitis of both the middle and inner ear. This condition occurs primarily in patients with poorly controlled diabetes and those who are immunocompromised. The pinna is markedly swollen and laterally displaced. Aggressive treatment with broad-spectrum parenteral antibiotics, including antibiotics directed against *P. aeruginosa* and *Staphylococcus aureus* is indicated.

Acute Otitis Media

Acute otitis media is usually a bacterial complication of a viral respiratory illness. It usually occurs several days after the onset of a viral upper respiratory infection. The viral infection enables pathogenic bacteria in the nasopharynx to ascend the eustachian tube into the middle ear either by impairing local host defenses or by eustachian tube dysfunction. The bacterial pathogens then cause a secondary infection, which consists of fever, irritability, and/or ear pain coupled with otoscopic findings of decreased mobility, opacity, and bulging tympanic membrane (see Table 9–4).

BACTERIOLOGY

The leading bacterial pathogens isolated from the middle ear fluid in acute otitis media are *S. pneumoniae* (30% to 35%), nontypable *Haemophilus influenzae* (20% to 25%), and *Moraxella catarrhalis* (15% to 20%); group A streptococci cause 1% to 2% of cases. Staphylococci are rare pathogens. In the first month of life (especially the first 2 weeks), gram-negative enteric bacteria (e.g., *Escherichia coli, Klebsiella pneumoniae*) may also be isolated from the middle ear in hospitalized neonates. After discharge from the hospital, the bacterial pathogens are the same as in older infants

and children. When *P. aeruginosa* is isolated from middle ear fluid, there is usually a prior history of a perforated eardrum with otorrhea. Otitis media with ipsilateral conjunctivitis is often due to nontypable *H. influenzae*.

For many years, the major pathogens were sensitive to amoxicillin. Increasing bacterial resistance has gradually lessened the role of amoxicillin as the drug of choice. Currently, 30% to 40% of *H. influenzae* strains and 90% of *M. catarrhalis* strains produce beta lactamase enzymes, which hydrolyze penicillins and some cephalosporins. In addition, strains of *S. pneumoniae* have emerged with altered penicillin-binding proteins on the bacterial cell wall, which makes them less susceptible to beta lactam drugs (penicillins and cephalosporins). Some of these strains may also be resistant to erythromycin and trimethoprim-sulfamethoxazole by other resistance mechanisms. Beta lactam susceptibility of *S. pneumoniae* may be classified as follows:

- Susceptible
- Relatively resistant
- Highly resistant

Susceptible strains are inhibited by less than 0.1 μg/ml of penicillin (minimal inhibitory concentration [MIC] ≤ 0.1). The MICs of relatively resistant and highly resistant strains are 0.1 to 1.0 μg/ml and greater than 1.0 μg/ml, respectively.

Relatively resistant strains may be inhibited by amoxicillin because peak concentrations of amoxicillin in middle ear fluid exceed 1.0 μg/ml. However, amoxicillin concentrations in the middle ear may not be sufficient to inhibit highly resistant strains.

The incidence of *highly resistant* strains remains low in the United States. If the incidence of these highly resistant strains increases, the treatment for otitis media may need to be revised; these strains may be sensitive only to rifampin, clindamycin, and vancomycin.

TREATMENT OF THE INITIAL EPISODE

The goals of treatment in acute otitis media are to relieve discomfort, prevent infectious complications, and reduce the time spent with middle ear effusion and the accompanying conductive hearing loss. Acute otitis media (especially due to *M. catarrhalis* or *H. influenzae*) usually resolves without antibiotic treatment.

In placebo-controlled studies, antibiotic therapy results in a quicker resolution of ear pain, a lower symptomatic failure rate in the first 48 hours of treatment, and a greater reduction in the rate of middle ear effusion at the end of therapy. Antibiotics do not reduce the recurrence rate of acute otitis media once the medications are stopped. Without antibiotics, the incidence of acute mastoid osteitis complicating acute otitis media is less than 1:1000. Since the introduction of antibiotics, the incidence has been much less, which suggests that the prevention of mastoid osteitis is an additional benefit of therapy. Despite the modest effect of antibiotics, they are indicated for the treatment of all symptomatic cases of acute otitis media.

In choosing an antibiotic, the clinician must consider the efficacy, safety, convenience, palatability, and costs of therapy. Comparative clinical trials of sufficient rigor and size have not been performed to enable direct comparison of the relative clinical effectiveness of available drugs. Efficacy must be inferred from the comparative *in vitro* antimicrobial activity of drugs against the major pathogens, and the results of clinical trials in which *in vivo* antibacterial efficacy has been determined by performing tympanocentesis and culture during therapy (Table 9–6). On the basis of cost, safety, and antimicrobial coverage, amoxicillin is the appropriate initial therapy for most cases of acute otitis media. Since otitis media is usually a self-limited illness, the use of broad-spectrum antibiotics for the initial treatment should be discouraged

Table 9–6. Antibiotic Regimens for Treatment of Acute Otitis Media

Antibiotic	Dosage/Regimen	Efficacy/Antibacterial Spectrum	Comments
Amoxicillin	40 mg/kg/day p.o., divided t.i.d. for 10 days	Hydrolyzed by beta lactamases of *Haemophilus influenzae* and *Moraxella catarrhalis;* probably effective against relatively resistant (but not highly resistant) *Streptococcus pneumoniae*	Has an established safety record; is inexpensive
Amoxicillin plus clavulanate	40 mg/kg/day p.o., divided t.i.d. for 10 days	Active against beta lactamase–producing *H. influenzae* and *M. catarrhalis;* probably effective against relatively resistant (but not highly resistant) *S. pneumoniae*	Causes more diarrhea than do most other drugs
Cefaclor	40 mg/kg/day p.o., divided t.i.d. for 10 days	Bacteriologic efficacy less than that of other drugs; some strains of *H. influenzae* and *M. catarrhalis* hydrolyze cefaclor	Is associated with increased urticaria, erythema multiforme, and serum sickness–like reactions compared with amoxicillin
Cefixime	8 mg/kg/day p.o., single daily dose for 10 days	Effective against beta lactamase–producing strains of *H. influenzae* and *M. catarrhalis;* eliminates most strains of *S. pneumoniae,* but *in vivo* efficacy lower than amoxicillin	Once-daily dosing
Cefpodoxime	10 mg/kg/day p.o., divided b.i.d. for 10 days	*In vivo* efficacy against major pathogens	
Cefprozil	30 mg/kg/day p.o., divided q12h for 10 days	Poor *in vivo* activity against *H. influenzae*	Is associated with reported serum sickness–like reactions
Ceftriaxone	50 mg/kg IM, single dose	Single dose may be effective bacteriologically	IM injections are painful, often given with lidocaine for local anesthesia. Single dose efficacy not yet confirmed
Cefuroxime	250 mg tablets only, p.o., b.i.d. for 10 days	*In vivo* activity against major pathogens	Crushed tablets have a bitter taste; oral suspension not available
Clarithromycin	15 mg/kg/day, divided b.i.d. for 10 days	Poor *in vivo* activity against *H. influenzae*	
Erythromycin plus sulfisoxazole	50 mg/kg/day erythromycin plus 150 mg/kg/day sulfisoxazole p.o., divided q.i.d. for 10 days	Effective against major pathogens; some strains of *S. pneumoniae* may now be resistant to erythromycin	Rarely causes Stevens-Johnson syndrome
Loracarbef	30 mg/kg/day p.o., divided b.i.d. for 10 days	*In vitro* antibacterial activity similar to cefaclor; *in vivo* antibacterial efficacy not known	
Trimethoprim-sulfamethoxazole	8 mg/kg/day TMP plus 40 mg/kg/day SMX, divided b.i.d. for 10 days	Resistant *S. pneumoniae* increasing in prevalence	Rarely causes Stevens-Johnson syndrome, but fatalities have occurred

because of their high cost, the increased risk for adverse reactions, and the potential for the development of resistant strains.

Special circumstances that may necessitate the use of extended spectrum antibiotics (beta lactamase stable) for the initial treatment include an immunocompromised patient, a neonate, an infant with presumed sepsis or occult bacteremia, and acute otitis media coupled with purulent conjunctivitis. In all of these cases, there may be an increased risk of a gram-negative organism (*H. influenzae, E. coli*) causing the infection that may be resistant to amoxicillin. For example, 70% of the cases of acute otitis media coupled with purulent conjunctivitis are caused by *H. influenzae.*

PATIENTS WITH PERSISTENT SYMPTOMS

After 48 to 72 hours of antibiotic therapy, most patients are either asymptomatic or are improving. After tympanocentesis is performed and a specimen of the middle ear is analyzed in patients with persistent symptoms, bacterial cultures are sterile in more than 50% of cases. Many of these cases involve an active viral infection, whereas others may involve a persistent inflammatory reaction despite elimination of viable bacteria. Other cases involve bacterial species that are sensitive to the prescribed antibiotic, which suggests noncompliance or failure of the prescribed drug to achieve adequate concentrations in middle ear fluid. Some patients have resistant bacteria, such as beta lactamase–producing organisms or resistant *S. pneumoniae*. To address the causes of persistent symptoms, the clinician should:

1. Prescribe analgesic-antipyretic medications (e.g., acetaminophen, ibuprofen, or a topical analgesic with antipyrine and benzocaine) for relief of symptoms.

2. Discuss the issues of compliance, including palatability and dosing interval.

3. Prescribe an alternative antibiotic effective against probable resistant bacterial strains, such as amoxicillin-clavulanic acid, cefixime, erythromycin-sulfamethoxazole, or trimethoprim-sulfamethoxazole.

The above approach is reasonable when beta lactamase–producing *H. influenzae* and *M. catarrhalis* are the major bacterial causes of persistent symptoms. With the emergence of *S. pneumoniae* resistant to beta lactam antibiotics, erythromycin, and trimethoprim-sulfamethoxazole, it may become necessary to perform tympanocentesis and to obtain specimens of the middle ear for culture in patients with persistent symptoms to guide antibiotic therapy.

EARLY RECURRENCES OF ACUTE OTITIS MEDIA

Up to 30% of patients who respond to initial antibiotic treatment of acute otitis media will have a recurrent infection within a few weeks after discontinuing therapy. In only 20% of these cases is the organism the same. Thus, most recurrences are not a result of failure of the previous antibiotic regimen. However, if the first episode is treated with amoxicillin, there is an increased chance that the second episode may be caused by a beta lactamase–producing organism. Therefore, a beta lactamase stable drug should be used for treatment of the second episode. If a broad-spectrum agent is used initially, it is reasonable to prescribe the same drug for the second episode.

RECURRENT ACUTE OTITIS MEDIA

Thirty-five percent of children experience six or more episodes of acute otitis media by 7 years of age. Risk factors for recurrent acute otitis media include:

- Onset of acute otitis media in the first year of life
- Male gender
- A sibling history of recurrent acute otitis media
- Craniofacial anomalies
- Trisomy 21
- Cleft palate
- Day care attendance
- Household cigarette smoke
- Human immunodeficiency virus (HIV) infection
- The absence of breast milk in the diet

Measures that may prevent acute otitis media and recurrent acute otitis media include promotion of breast feeding, reduction or elimination of household smoking, and child care in the home rather than in large group day care settings. Although the polyvalent pneumococcal vaccine is partially effective in the prevention of pneumococcal acute otitis media, it does not reduce the overall attack rate of acute otitis media in high-risk children. In addition, this vaccine induces only limited immune responses in children younger than 2 years of age.

Recurrent acute otitis media is defined as three or more episodes in the past 6 months or four or more episodes during the past year. Most children with recurrent acute otitis media will have subsequent ear infections. Antimicrobial chemoprophylaxis may prevent the subsequent infections and reduce the time spent with middle ear effusion. A single daily dose of antibiotics at half the daily therapeutic dose reduces the attack rate in high-risk children.

Amoxicillin (20 mg/kg/day), sulfisoxazole (75 mg/kg/day), or erythromycin (20 mg/kg/day) is a suitable agent for chemoprophylaxis. More expensive, broad-spectrum agents have no proven advantages as prophylactic agents. Although trimethoprim-sulfamethoxazole is effective as a prophylactic agent, it is associated with an increased risk for Stevens-Johnson syndrome and should be used only when other agents are not available (as with a penicillin allergy and a non-response to sulfisoxazole).

The optimal duration of chemoprophylaxis is not known. Two options are to prescribe prophylactic antibiotics throughout the autumn, winter, and spring when risk of acute otitis media is higher and to treat for shorter periods, such as 3 months. The major problems of chemoprophylaxis are noncompliance, which may lead to breakthrough episodes and selection of resistant pathogens.

When two or more episodes of acute otitis media occur despite chemoprophylaxis, myringotomy and tympanostomy tube placement should be considered. Tympanostomy tubes reduce the number of attacks of acute otitis media and prevent recurrences of otitis media with effusion. Tympanostomy tubes are eventually extruded from the eardrum by the normal process of epithelial growth. Recurrent episodes of otitis media may then resume. Adenoidectomy coupled with tympanostomy is partially effective and may be considered when both chemoprophylaxis and tympanostomy tubes have not been successful.

OTITIS MEDIA WITH EFFUSION

After the acute earache and fever have subsided, middle ear fluid can persist for weeks. For example, after 3 months, the effusion is still present in 10% to 15% of patients. Since most cases resolve without treatment, a period of observation is the most appropriate initial strategy.

One potential complication is the effect of persistent middle ear effusion, which usually produces a 20- to 30-db conductive hearing loss, on language development and cognitive abilities. There is a weak association between prolonged middle ear effusion and abnormal speech and language development in children younger than 4 years of age and expressive language and attention deficits in children over 4 years of age. Despite this association, there is limited information showing that treatment of effusion can reduce these abnormalities. Until such data become available, the goal of therapy is to remove the effusion and improve hearing acuity in order to optimize language acquisition with the least morbidity.

Medical therapy of otitis media with effusion has not been consistently successful. Antihistamines, decongestants, and nonsteroidal anti-inflammatory agents (NSAIDs) do not promote the resolution of middle ear effusion. With systemic corticosteroids (prednisone), the effusion may resolve in up to 50% of the cases, but it recurs within a few weeks on stopping the steroids. Although bacterial specimens can be obtained for culture from up to 30% of cases, antibiotic therapy has only a minimal effect on the resolution of effusion. A period of observation for 4 to 6 months is recommended before surgical intervention is considered.

Surgical therapy for persistent OME consists of myringotomy, tympanostomy tubes, adenoidectomy, and adenotonsillectomy. Because of the high recurrence rate of OME following myringotomy, this procedure should not be performed alone. Instead, a tympanostomy tube should be inserted at the time of myringotomy to maintain patency. Tympanostomy tube placement improves hearing and usually maintains aeration of the middle ear. The median patency of tympanostomy tubes is approximately 10 to 12 months. Because of the recurrence of persistent OME following extrusion of the tubes, approximately 30% of patients will require a second insertion of tympanostomy tubes.

The complication rates of tympanostomy tubes include tympanosclerosis (51%; 95% confidence interval: 43, 58%) and postoperative otorrhea (13%; 95% confidence interval: 5.5, 21%). Less frequent complications include intrusion of tube into the middle ear cavity, chronic perforation, cholesteatoma, and granuloma formation at the myringotomy site. In children over 4 years of age, adenoidectomy reduces the recurrence of middle ear effusion. The benefit of adenoidectomy in children younger than age 4 or of adenotonsillectomy has not been established.

To assist the clinician in the management of persistent middle ear effusion, the Otitis Media Guideline Panel from the Agency for Health Care Policy and Research (AHCPR) has developed a set of practice guidelines for affected children between 1 and 3 years (see Fig. 9–4). The panel recommends documentation of effusion with pneumatic otoscopy, confirmation of effusion by tympanometry when pneumatic otoscopy is inconclusive, reduction of risk factors for otitis media (smoking), and myringotomy with tympanostomy tube placement in children with bilateral effusion lasting longer than 3 months coupled with bilateral hearing loss. In addition, a course of antibiotics may be tried before one decides to place tympanostomy tubes. The panel does not recommend decongestants, steroids, antihistamines, tonsillectomy, or adenoidectomy in the management of persistent OME. The panel also recommends against tympanostomy tube placement with unilateral hearing loss secondary to OME unless the patient has an underlying sensorineural hearing loss or has only one functional ear. As with any set of guidelines, the clinician needs to individualize these recommendations and discuss the treatment options with the parents.

SUMMARY AND RED FLAGS

A careful examination of the pinna, external auditory canal and the tympanic membrane can identify most causes of ear pain. If findings are normal, one should consider referred pain from another source. Because young children may have trouble localizing their pain, clinicians should have a high index of suspicion of ear pathology in any health maintenance examination conducted during the 1st year of life or in any preschool child with fever, irritability, or upper respiratory tract infection.

Even though most conditions causing ear pain respond readily to therapy, the clinician must be aware of the following red flags associated with the complications of these conditions:

- Laterally displaced pinna (malignant otitis externa, mastoid osteitis)
- Mastoid tenderness (mastoid osteitis)
- Persistently immobile tympanic membrane with an associated hearing loss
- Perforated tympanic membrane
- A pearl-like tumor in the tympanic membrane (cholesteatoma)

Although meningitis and otitis media may be present simultaneously, otitis media alone is not a common site for the onset of meningitis. Nonetheless, a high index of suspicion is needed to determine that the patient's manifestations are a result of both otitis media and meningitis (see Chapter 53).

SELECTED BIBLIOGRAPHY

Arola M, Ziegler T, Ruuskanen O. Respiratory virus infection as a cause of prolonged symptoms in acute otitis media. J Pediatr 1990;116:697–701.

Carlin SA, Marchant CD, Shurin PA, et al. Early recurrences of otitis media: Reinfection or relapse? J Pediatr 1987;110:20–25.

Carlin SA, Marchant CD, Shurin PA, et al. Host factors and early therapeutic response in acute otitis media: Does symptomatic response correlate with bacterial outcome? J Pediatr 1991;118:178–183.

Gates GA, Avery CA, Prihoda TJ, et al. Effectiveness of adenoidectomy and tympanostomy tubes in the treatment of chronic otitis media with effusion. N Engl J Med 1987;317:1444–1451.

Henderson FW, Collier AM, Sanyal MA, et al. A longitudinal study of respiratory viruses and bacteria in the etiology of acute otitis media with effusion. N Engl J Med 1982;306:1377–1383.

Kaleida PH, Casselbrant ML, Rockette HE, et al. Amoxicillin or myringotomy or both for acute otitis media: Results of a randomized clinical trial. Pediatrics 1991;87:466–474.

Klein JO. Microbiologic efficacy of antibacterial drugs for acute otitis media. Pediatr Infect Dis J 1993;12:973–975.

Marchant CD, Carlin SA, Johnson CE, et al. Measuring the comparative efficacy of antibacterial agents for acute otitis media: "The Pollyanna Phenomenon." J Pediatr 1992;120:72–77.

Otitis Media Guideline Panel. Clinical Practice Guideline Number 12: Otitis Media with Effusion in Young Children. Rockville, Md: U.S. Department of Health and Human Services, Agency for Health Care Policy and Research, Pub. No. 94–0622, July 1994. (Summary published in Pediatrics 1994;94:766–773.)

Paradise JL, Bluestone CD, Rogers KD, et al. Efficacy of adenoidectomy for recurrent otitis media in children previously treated with tympanostomy–tube placement: Results of parallel randomized and nonrandomized trials. JAMA 1990;263:2066–2073.

Perrin JJM, Charney E, MacWhinney JB, et al. Sulfisoxazole as chemoprophylaxis for recurrent otitis media. N Engl J Med 1974;291:664–667.

Teele DW, Klein JO, Chase C, et al. Otitis media in infancy and intellectual ability, school achievement, speech, and language at age seven years. J Infect Dis 1990;162:685–694.

Teele DW, Klein JO, Rosner B. Epidemiology of otitis media during the first seven years of life in children in greater Boston: A prospective, cohort study. J Infect Dis 1989;160:83–94.

Teele DW, Pelton SI, Klein JO. Bacteriology of acute otitis media unresponsive to initial therapy. J Pediatr 1981;98:537–539.

10 Airway Obstruction in Children

James E. Arnold

A child with an upper airway obstruction may require immediate life-saving intervention or simply extended observation and various diagnostic studies to determine the site and cause of obstruction before treatment is begun. In the absence of an imminent respiratory arrest, a brief directed history should be obtained. The time of onset and rapidity of progression of the obstruction should be noted along with possible previous episodes of airway compromise, their therapy, and outcome. A review of the birth and neonatal history is important to determine a prior need for airway intervention, such as aggressive suctioning or endotracheal intubation. Questions should be directed toward any change in voice or cry as well as feeding problems. Although a foreign body is not always observed, its possibility should be raised and, of course, a short review of any underlying medical problems and their therapy should be briefly determined. Most cases (~80%) of upper airway obstruction (with or without stridor) are acute infections (Table 10–1). An age-related differential diagnosis is noted in Table 10–2.

PHYSICAL EXAMINATION

The physical examination is most important and should be performed in a warm, well-lit room, preferably with the child in the parent's lap and the child's chest exposed. An examination of the oropharynx or auscultation of the lungs is not as important as taking a few seconds to note the child's general appearance, sense of well-being, degree of dyspnea, and respiratory pattern. The respiratory rate (see Chapter 8) as well as the presence of cyanosis, degree of anxiety, and any posture assumed in an effort to minimize the airway difficulties should be determined (see Table 10–1).

Stridor is noise generated by the flow of air through the large airways and should be categorized as inspiratory, expiratory, or biphasic. Nasal flaring, the use of accessory muscles of respiration (neck), and the degree of retractions, which may vary from a slight sternal tug, to intercostal, and significant deep sternal, should be observed. The patient's cry or voice, and difficulty in a child's ability to handle oral secretions should be noted. A feeding trial should not be attempted because some children may require control of their airway (endotracheal intubation) or other diagnostic or therapeutic procedures in the operating room with anesthesia; feeding may increase the risk of aspiration or further airway compromise.

Radiologic evaluations are needed *only* if the diagnosis is not clear on the basis of history and physical examination; if there is concern for the degree of the acute respiratory distress, that patient should be accompanied to the radiology suite by a person able to evaluate and control any airway problems. Physical restraints are sometimes needed to limit a child's motion, but in general these should be avoided because they often are more upsetting and may precipitate airway problems. Anterior-posterior and lateral soft tissue x-ray studies of the neck and chest are frequently needed. Neck films should be obtained during inspiration, since the soft tissues of the pharynx may bulge with expiration, causing a false-

positive finding of a soft tissue mass that may mimic a retropharyngeal infection. Radiopaque foreign bodies are generally easily seen on a radiograph. If there is a possibility of a radiolucent foreign body, inspiratory and expiratory chest x-ray studies are performed. These identify air trapping distal to a foreign body, which acts as a ball valve with airway obstruction on expiration as the bronchial diameter decreases. Hyperinflation causes a mediastinal shift away from the obstructed side.

Similar information may be obtained with lateral decubitus films or fluoroscopy, which can be particularly helpful with the child who will not hold still. A barium swallow, either directed to assess any associated abnormalities in swallowing or tracheoesophageal problems, such as a vascular ring, may also be obtained. In unusual or complicated cases, the use of computed tomography (CT) or magnetic resonance image (MRI) scanning provides excellent soft tissue definition. These studies usually require a very cooperative patient or sedation. Sedatives must be used very carefully and only in monitored situations with the availability of personnel and equipment to provide possible resuscitation. The developmental relative anatomy of the upper airway is shown in Figure 10–1.

Once the clinical and radiologic examinations have been completed, the examiner determines the site of the airway obstruction, its likely cause, and type of treatment needed (see Tables 10–1 and 10–2). The key physical findings (see Table 10–1) in determining the site of obstruction are:

- The character of the stridor
- Retractions
- The voice
- The ability to handle secretions

Inspiratory stridor is characteristic of airway obstruction at or above the vocal cords and is caused by collapse of the soft tissues with the negative pressure generated by inspiration; it is usually soft and muffled.

Biphasic (inspiratory and expiratory) stridor indicates little change in airway size with respiration caused by a fixed obstruction. One phase may necessitate a stethoscope, whereas the other may require no assistance to be heard. The cricoid cartilage immediately below the vocal cords is the only rigid circumferential structure in the upper airway; narrowing in this site (as in subglottic stenosis or croup) is a common cause of biphasic stridor.

Obstruction within the larger portions of the intrathoracic tracheobronchial tree causes *expiratory stridor* because there is a decrease in airway diameter with expiration. This is a similar mechanism to the generation of the typical expiratory wheeze heard from the smaller airways in a patient with reactive airway disease (see Chapter 8).

The degree of retractions varies greatly and depends on the site of obstruction. Pharyngeal or supraglottic (above the vocal cords) laryngeal obstructions often produce minimal retractions, as the patients may sense that increased respiratory effort actually increases the amount of soft tissue obstruction and collapse. These patients may have very shallow respirations with no retractions until the airway obstruction is severe. At the level of the vocal

Table 10–1. Differential Diagnosis of Upper Airway Obstruction*

	Laryngotracheo-bronchitis (Croup)	Laryngitis	Spasmodic Croup	Epiglottitis	Membranous Croup (Bacterial Tracheitis)	Retropharyngeal Abscess‡	Foreign Body	Angioedema	Peritonsillar Abscess†	Laryngeal Papillomatosis
Age Location	3 mo-3 yr Subglottic	5 yr-teens Subglottic	3 mo-3 yr Subglottic	2-6 yr Supraglottic	Any age (3–10 yr) Trachea	<6 yr Posterior pharynx	6 mo-5 yr Supraglottic, subglottic, variable	All ages Variable	>10 yr Oropharynx	3 mo-3 yr Larynx—vocal cords—trachea
Etiology	Parainfluenza virus; influenza virus, RSV; rarely Mycoplasma, measles, adenovirus	As per croup	Unknown	Haemophilus influenzae b	Prior croup or influenza virus with secondary bacterial infection by Staphylococcus aureus, Moraxella catarrhalis, H. influenzae	S. aureus, anaerobes	Small objects, vegetable, toys, coins	Congenital C-1 esterase deficiency; acquired anaphylaxis	Group A streptococci, anaerobes	HPV
Prodrome onset	Insidious, URI	As per croup	Sudden onset at night; prior episodes	Rapid, short prodrome	Biphasic illness with sudden deterioration	Insidious to sudden	Sudden	Sudden	Biphasic with sudden worsening	Chronic
Stridor	Yes—biphasic	None	Yes	Yes—soft inspiratory	Yes	None	Yes	Yes	No	Possible
Retractions	Yes	None	Rare	Yes	Yes	Yes	Yes—variable	Yes	No	No
Voice	Hoarse	Hoarse; whispered	Hoarse	Muffled	Normal or hoarse	Muffled	Complete obstruction—aphonic; other variable	Hoarse, may be normal	"Hot potato," muffled	Hoarse
Position and appearance	Normal	Normal	Normal	Tripod sitting leaning forward; agitation	Normal	Arching of neck or normal	Normal	Normal; may have facial edema	Normal	Normal
Swallowing (dysphagia)	Normal	Normal	Normal	Drooling	Normal	Drooling	Variable, usually normal	Normal	Drooling, trismus	Normal
Barking cough	Yes	Rare	Yes	No	Yes	No	Variable; brassy if tracheal	Possible	None	Variable
Toxicity	Rare	No	No	Severe	Severe	Severe	No, but dyspnea	No unless anaphylactic shock or severe anoxia	Dyspnea	None
Fever	<101°F	<101°F	None	>102°F	>102°F	>101°F	None	None	>101°F	None
X-ray	Subglottic narrowing; steeple sign	Normal	Subglottic narrowing	Thumb sign of thickened epiglottis	Ragged irregular tracheal border; as per croup	Thickened retropharyngeal space	Radiopaque object may be seen	As per croup	None needed	May be normal
WBC count	Normal	Normal	Normal	Leukocytosis with left shift	Leukocytosis with left shift	Leukocytosis with left shift	Normal	Normal	Leukocytosis with left shift	Normal
Therapy	Racemic epinephrine aerosol, systemic steroids, aerosolized steroids, cool mist	None	Cool mist; occasionally as for croup	Endotracheal intubation, ceftriaxone	Ceftriaxone; intubation if needed	Nafcillin; ampicillin-sulbactam; ceftriaxone; surgical drainage if abscess	Endoscopic removal	Anaphylaxis; epinephrine, IV fluids, steroids; C-1 esterase deficiency; replacement infusion therapy	Penicillin; aspiration	Laser therapy, repeated excision, interferon
Prevention	None	None	None	H. influenzae b conjugated vaccine	None	None	Avoid small objects; supervision	Avoid allergens; FFP for congenital angioedema	Treat group A streptococci early	Treat maternal genitourinary lesions; possible cesarean section?

*See also Table 6-4.
†See Figure 6-4.
‡See Figures 6-5 and 6-6.
Abbreviations: FFP = fresh frozen plasma; HPV = human papillomavirus; RSV = respiratory syncytial virus; URI = upper respiratory tract infection, coryza, sneezing; WBC = white blood cell.

127

Table 10–2. Age-Related Differential Diagnosis of Airway Obstruction

Newborn
  Foreign material (meconium, amniotic fluid)
  Congenital subglottic stenosis (uncommon)
  Choanal atresia
  Micrognathia (Pierre Robin syndrome, Treacher Collins
    syndrome, DiGeorge syndrome)
  Macroglossia (Beckwith-Wiedemann syndrome,
    hypothyroidism, Pompe disease, trisomy 21, hemangioma)
  Laryngeal web, clefts, atresia
  Laryngospasm (intubation, aspiration, transient)
  Vocal cord paralysis (weak cry; unilateral or bilateral, with or
    without increased intracranial pressure from Arnold-Chiari
    malformation or other CNS pathology; birth trauma)
  Tracheal web, stenosis, malacia, atresia
  Pharyngeal collapse (cause of apnea in preterm infant)

Infancy
  Laryngomalacia (most common etiology)
  Subglottic stenosis (congenital; acquired after intubation)
  Hemangioma
  Tongue tumor (dermoid, teratoma, ectopic thyroid)
  Laryngeal papillomatosis
  Vascular rings

Toddlers
  Viral croup (most common etiology in children 3 mo–4 yr
    of age)
  Bacterial tracheitis (toxic, high fever)
  Foreign body (sudden cough; airway or esophageal)
  Spasmodic (recurrent) croup
  Laryngeal papillomatosis
  Retropharyngeal abscess
  Diphtheria (uncommon)

Over 2–3 Yr Old
  Epiglottitis (epiglottis, aryepiglottic folds)
  Inhalation injury (burns, toxic gas, hydrocarbons)
  Foreign bodies
  Angioedema (familial history, cutaneous angioedema)
  Anaphylaxis (allergic history, wheezing, hypotension)
  Trauma (tracheal or larynx fracture)
  Peritonsillar abscess (adolescents)
  Ludwig angina
  Diphtheria

Abbreviations: CNS = central nervous system.
Modified from Kercsmar C. The respiratory system. *In* Behrman RE, Kliegman RM (eds). Nelson Essentials of Pediatrics, 2nd ed. Philadelphia: WB Saunders, 1994:444.

cords or subglottic larynx, the degree of retractions generally correlates with the degree of obstruction. If the obstruction is in the trachea, retractions are not present unless the obstruction is severe, since the tracheobronchial diameter increases with inspiration. A muffled "hot potato" voice is typical of pharyngeal obstruction caused by inflammation or mass effect. *Hoarseness* is seen with involvement of the vocal cords, usually by an inflammatory process. Tracheal obstructions generally produce a normal voice.

Neonates are predominantly nasal breathers, and nasal obstruction usually interferes greatly with their ability to feed. Most neonates can switch to oral respirations either spontaneously or with crying, but while feeding they may be unable to swallow before stopping to breathe. Obstruction in the pharynx and larynx

above the vocal cords often makes feeding and swallowing difficult; these children often present with drooling. If the site of obstruction is at or below the vocal cords or in the trachea, feedings are usually normal except as determined by the degree of respiratory obstruction unless an esophageal foreign body is narrowing the trachea by compressing the soft tracheoesophageal wall.

Endoscopy can provide direct visualization of the cause of the airway obstruction; however, its use involves manipulation of the airway, which should not be undertaken unless the personnel and equipment are present to manage possible worsening airway compromise. Short flexible fiberoptic nasopharyngolaryngoscopes are widely used to visualize the upper airway. Flexible pediatric bronchoscopy provides visualization of both the upper and lower air-

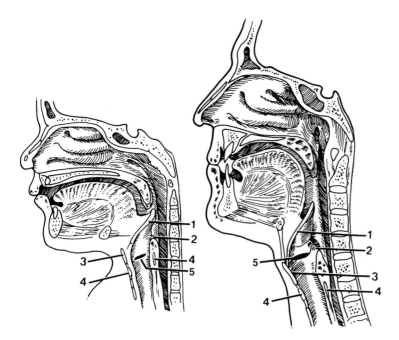

Figure 10–1. Relative comparative anatomy of the larynx in an infant *(left)* and an adult *(right)*. Specific landmarks: 1, epiglottis; 2, arytenoid cartilages; 3, thyroid cartilage; 4, cricoid cartilage; 5, laryngeal ventricle, the airspace below the false vocal cords and above the true vocal cords. Its radiolucency is an excellent landmark on lateral x-ray. The infant larynx is situated relatively high in the cervical region. Additionally, the base of the infant's tongue is close to the larynx and the epiglottis is located near the palate. These anatomic differences partially explain the predominantly obligate nose breathing of the young infant as well as the relative ease with which upper airway obstructions develop in infants. (From Grad R, Taussig LM. Acute infections producing upper airway obstruction. *In* Chernick V, Kendig EL [eds]. Kendig's Disorders of the Respiratory Tract in Children, 5th ed. Philadelphia: WB Saunders, 1990.)

way, and cardiopulmonary monitoring and intravenous access for sedation are required. In cases of significant upper airway obstruction requiring intervention, or if there is any likelihood of a foreign body, direct laryngoscopy and rigid bronchoscopy in the operating room are the safest procedures that can secure the airway, provide a diagnosis, and accomplish treatment, such as extraction of the foreign body.

CONGENITAL CAUSES OF AIRWAY OBSTRUCTION

Nasal Obstruction

Nasal obstruction is often an uncomfortable nuisance for the older child. It may sometimes contribute to sinusitis (by obstructing the sinus ostia) and may be exacerbated by allergic inflammation. Obstruction in the neonate who is a predominant nasal breather is very significant; it can cause respiratory distress and, by interfering with feeding, can cause a delay in growth and development.

Choanal atresia (Fig. 10–2) is a lack of the opening of the posterior nasal airway. In approximately 66% of the cases, it is unilateral; in 90%, there is a bony obstruction between the posterolateral wall of the nose and the nasal septum. In the remaining 10%, the obstruction is membranous. In *unilateral* cases, there is usually no respiratory distress but a constant, persistent unilateral nasal drainage. This is usually diagnosed in an older child, and it is important to be sure that obstruction is not caused by a foreign body. *Bilateral* choanal atresia may cause severe neonatal respiratory distress that is often relieved by crying; a pattern of cyclic cyanosis may develop in which infants become cyanotic while trying to breathe through the nose and then recover as they begin to cry.

The diagnosis is suspected on the basis of the clinical presentation and is confirmed by the inability to pass a small catheter or feeding tube through the nose into the pharynx. Care must be taken to ensure that a small catheter has not curled in the nose and seemingly passed further than choanal atresia would allow; this is best done by being able to visualize the catheter in the oropharynx.

Approximately 50% of children with choanal atresia have other congenital anomalies (such as the CHARGE* association); initial

---

*Coloboma (iris, retina), *h*eart disease (tetralogy of Fallot, patent ductus arteriosus, ventricular septal defect, atrial septal defect), *a*tresia choanae, *r*etarded growth and mental deficiency, *g*enital hypoplasia (males), and *e*ar anomalies (external ear plus deafness).

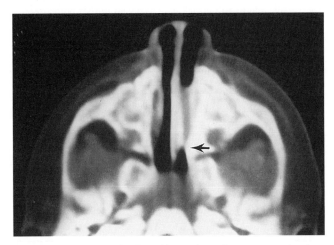

Figure 10–2. CT scan of unilateral bony choanal atresia *(arrow)* with mucus collected within left nasal cavity.

management is directed toward maintaining the airway, often with a McGovern nipple (a modified baby bottle nipple used as an oral airway) and tube feedings, while an evaluation for other congenital anomalies is being performed.

Surgical correction of choanal atresia is usually performed through either a transnasal or a transpalatal route. The operative timing depends on the severity and in unilateral cases can be delayed until the child is several years of age. Because the repaired choanae often scar, form contractures, and restenose, long-term follow-up is needed. Patients with the CHARGE association often have associated feeding problems over and above that caused by their nasal obstruction; management often needs a tracheotomy and gastrostomy tube with delayed repair of the choanal atresia when the child's nasal structures are larger and less likely to have postoperative problems.

Deviated Septum

Passage through the birth canal may cause a neonatal septal deviation, which can often be corrected with minor manipulation immediately after delivery. This problem manifests with asymmetric nares, is often asymptomatic, and is less common in Asian-American and African-American children who have a lower nasal profile. Other causes of nasal obstruction include intranasal cysts, bony narrowing of the anterior portion of the nose, and a reactive nasal mucosa secondary to vigorous suctioning or other manipulation. Evaluation with flexible nasal endoscopy and the use of CT scanning give the best analysis of any abnormal anatomy.

Laryngomalacia

Laryngomalacia is the most common cause of inspiratory stridor and noisy respirations in neonates and infants. It is caused by the inspiratory collapse of the laryngeal cartilages, with the epiglottis or arytenoid cartilages prolapsing into the airway with inspiration. This may occur at birth, but it often has a delayed onset at 2 to 4 weeks of age. It is usually self-limited and resolves with time, often by 8 to 12 months but occasionally not until 18 to 24 months of age.

The diagnosis is made on the basis of the clinical presentation (stridor is worse when supine or during activity and exacerbations occur with upper respiratory tract infections) and outpatient flexible laryngoscopy, which can generally be safely performed with topical anesthesia. Recommendations have been made for a complete airway evaluation in children with laryngomalacia, because 15% to 25% have other airway lesions. This approach has been used on selected referral patient populations and should be considered if the stridor of laryngomalacia does not follow the typical course of being mild and resolving spontaneously. Laryngomalacia may be accompanied by *tracheomalacia,* a partial collapse of the tracheal cartilages with respiration. This rarely occurs alone in the absence of extrinsic compression, such as may be caused by a vascular ring that can be identified on barium swallow. Unusually severe cases of laryngomalacia may require operative intervention, such as an epiglottiplasty to trim redundant soft tissue or even a temporary tracheotomy.

Vocal Cord Paralysis

Vocal cord paralysis is the second most common cause of congenital neonatal laryngeal obstruction. It is usually bilateral and associated with neurologic syndromes, such as the Arnold-Chiari malformation. Traction on the brain stem or increased intracranial pressure and herniation puts pressure on the vagus nerve. Tracheotomy may be required to maintain the airway, and neurologic and MRI evaluation should be performed to identify any central causes. Children with Arnold-Chiari malformation who have had a ventriculoperitoneal (VP) shunt may present with airway obstruction secondary to increased intracranial pressure if their VP shunt is obstructed. Vocal cord paralysis may also be a result of traction on the recurrent laryngeal nerve secondary to a difficult delivery; it is usually unilateral, resolves with time, and causes few airway problems. Vocal cord paralysis also occurs in older children and may be due to a polyneuropathy (Guillain-Barré syndrome), brain stem encephalitis, neck or thoracic surgery, or compression by local masses.

Other Lesions

The cricoid cartilage immediately below the vocal cords and above the trachea is the only circumferential rigid structure of the upper airway. Occasionally, a child is born with a smaller than normal cricoid cartilage that may have an elliptical shape. These children may present at birth with airway obstruction or within the first year of life with recurrent atypical croup-like episodes that may not completely clear. Laryngoscopy and bronchoscopy can assess the airway size, and if the stenosis is only minimal, the child may be watched with nighttime cardiorespiratory monitors, with the expectation of improvement as growth occurs. Most often, surgical correction is required. *Acquired subglottic stenosis* may develop secondary to endotracheal intubation, particularly if the intubation has been prolonged for several months, if an oversized tube was used, or if multiple intubations were required. Subglottic stenosis should be suspected in any child with these risk factors who does not respond to extubation because of upper airway obstruction. Laryngoscopy and bronchoscopy are required for evaluation. A cricoid split operation, tracheotomy, or laryngotracheal reconstruction may be needed. Serial dilations are no longer commonly used because they may continue to injure the cartilage and its overlying mucosa. Apparently successful dilations have probably been used for mild stenotic areas and have allowed time for growth of the airway.

A variety of other lesions may cause laryngotracheal obstruction in children. *Laryngeal cysts* may occur as mucoceles from minor salivary glands that are present within the laryngeal mucosa whose secretions do not drain externally. Similar *subglottic cysts* have been reported in children who have undergone prolonged endotracheal intubation; it is thought that a soft tissue reaction secondary to the intubation has obstructed the drainage of these glands into the airway, causing the cyst fluid to accumulate. Cysts may occur deeper within the laryngeal tissue when the saccule, an air-containing appendage of the laryngeal ventricle, becomes blocked and fills with mucus. Excision, either endoscopically or with an external neck incision, is necessary.

Laryngeal webs may form as a result of the incomplete canalization of the laryngeal airway. These usually present soon after birth with an absent or very weak cry. Webs may be thick, and complex surgical reconstruction with a tracheotomy to maintain the airway is often required.

Complete tracheal rings, which may not increase in size with growth, are another source of airway obstruction. Rarely, the failure of separation between the esophagus and larynx and trachea may occur, resulting in a posterior *laryngeal cleft* causing both feeding and airway difficulties. The cleft may involve only part of the larynx, or it may extend to the carina.

A *subglottic hemangioma* is a vascular tumor occurring just below the vocal cords. It usually presents a few weeks to a few months after birth. As with all hemangiomas, there is a postnatal proliferative phase with increase in size and, therefore, an increase in obstruction followed by a plateau phase and then a spontaneous resolution phase (1 to 5 years of age). Airway obstruction is usually severe, and treatment with carbon dioxide (CO_2) laser vaporization of the tumor often supplemented by intermittent use of steroids and interferon (IFN-α_{2a}) may help avoid a tracheotomy. Care must be used to avoid aggressive intervention because increased scarring may occur, causing long-term subglottic stenosis.

The differential diagnosis of congenital anomalies of the pharynx and tracheobronchial tree that may produce airway obstruction is noted in Tables 10–3 and 10–4.

INFLAMMATORY DISORDERS OF THE UPPER AIRWAY

Mononucleosis and Retropharyngeal Abscess

Infections that cause significant airway obstruction in children are considered according to their site of involvement (see Table 10–1). Oropharyngeal obstruction may occur in severe cases of mononucleosis (tonsil, adenoid hypertrophy) or with a retropharyngeal abscess. Children with mononucleosis (see Chapter 48) and upper airway obstruction usually respond to steroid therapy, although intubation is sometimes needed. Tonsillar and adenoid hypertrophy from mononucleosis or other causes may obstruct the airway and produce acute pulmonary edema or cor pulmonale (see Chapters 11 and 13). With resolution of the infection, the tonsil size usually returns to normal and causes no further problems.

A retropharyngeal abscess causes a child to have difficulty swallowing, and because of inflammation of the prevertebral muscle,

Table 10–3. Anomalies of the Pharynx

Supraglottic	Glottic	Subglottic
Congenital flaccid larynx	Vocal cord paralysis	Subglottic hemangioma
Supraglottic atresia	Laryngeal web	Subglottic web
Supraglottic hemangioma	Cri du chat syndrome	Subglottic atresia
Laryngocele	Laryngeal atresia	Subglottic stenosis
Bifid epiglottis	Anterior laryngeal cleft	Posterior laryngeal cleft
Anomalous cuneiform cartilage	Duplication of vocal folds	G syndrome
Absent epiglottis	Neurofibroma of larynx	
Supraglottic web	Plott syndrome	
Lymphangioma of vallecula	Arthrogryposis multiplex	
	Laryngoptosis	

From Cotton RT, Reilly JS. Congenital malformations of the larynx. *In* Bluestone CD, Stool SE, Scheetz MD (eds). Pediatric Otolaryngology, 2nd ed. Philadelphia: WB Saunders, 1990:1122.

Table 10–4. **Classification of Congenital Anomalies of the Tracheobronchial Tree**

I. *Anomalies of the Trachea*
  A. Agenesis or atresia
  B. Constriction
    1. Fibrous strictures
      a. Webs
      b. Fibrous stenosis of tracheal segments
    2. Absence or deformity of tracheal cartilages
      a. Tracheomalacia
      b. Deformity due to vascular anomalies
      c. Individual cartilage deformity
  C. Tracheal enlargement (congenital trachiectasis)
  D. Tracheal evaginations or outgrowths
    1. Tracheoceles, cysts
    2. Fistulas
  E. Abnormal bifurcation
    1. Tracheal bronchus
    2. Other anomalies of gross morphology

II. *Anomalies of Bronchi and Lungs*
  A. Agenesis or atresia
  B. Constriction
    1. Fibrous strictures
      a. Webs
      b. Fibrous stenosis of bronchial segments
    2. Absence or deformity of bronchial cartilages
      a. Bronchomalacia
      b. Bronchial hypoplasia
  C. Bronchial enlargements
    1. Congenital bronchiectasis
    2. Kartagener syndrome
  D. Bronchial evaginations
    1. Bronchoceles, cysts
    2. Fistulas
  E. Abnormal bifurcation
  F. Anomalous attachments
    1. Sequestered lung
    2. Lung tissue attached to the gastrointestinal tract

Adapted from Hollinger PH, Zimmerman AA, Schild JA. Tracheobronchial tree malformations. *In* Ferguson CF, Kendig EL Jr (eds). Pediatric Otolaryngology, 2nd ed. Vol. 2. Philadelphia: WB Saunders, 1972:1286. Reprinted from Bluestone CD, Stool SE, Scheetz MD (eds). Pediatric Otolaryngology, 2nd ed. Philadelphia: WB Saunders, 1990:1129.

there is usually limitation of neck motion and sometimes a slight torticollis.

The diagnosis of either enlarged tonsils or a retropharyngeal abscess can be made by direct inspection or with a lateral soft tissue x-ray of the neck (see Chapter 6). Cases that are difficult to visualize are best evaluated with a contrast-enhanced CT scan, which shows the exact location of the infection and permits its separation from other deep neck infections (see Chapter 6). A retropharyngeal abscess may not always cause severe respiratory compromise.

Treatment of retropharyngeal abscesses consists of intravenous antibiotics directed at anaerobes and gram-positive bacteria plus incision and drainage. Following surgical drainage, the patient needs continued observation because of the rare possibility of edema formation. Rare causes of oropharyngeal airway obstruction include tonsillitis, not associated with mononucleosis; this usually responds to antibiotics. A peritonsillar abscess, which normally presents with trismus, uvular deviation, and fullness to the superior pole of the tonsil, is usually not associated with airway obstruction unless the abscess is particularly large. It will respond to intravenous antibiotics, to incision and drainage, or, less often, to an immediate tonsillectomy (see Table 10–1).

Epiglottitis

Epiglottitis, sometimes called *supraglottitis* because it involves the larynx above the vocal cords, is the most serious life-threaten-ing infection in this area. Croup involves the subglottic larynx and trachea, while bacterial tracheitis is usually a secondary bacterial infection following a viral prodrome (see Table 10–1).

Epiglottitis is an acute, rapidly progressive, potentially lethal infection of the epiglottis, aryepiglottic folds, and false vocal cord area. It is a surgical emergency because of the potential for rapid airway obstruction; evaluation and treatment are directed toward establishing an airway while the physician is confirming the diagnosis and treating the infection. In the past, pediatric epiglottitis has been due to *Haemophilus influenzae* type b nearly 100% of the time. Blood cultures are positive in 90% of the cases and are used to confirm the diagnosis. Epiglottic or throat cultures are unreliable, with only approximately 50% being positive.

Since the introduction of the polysaccharide conjugated *H. influenzae* type b vaccine, there has been a dramatic fall in the incidence of acute epiglottitis in the United States. However, in an internationally mobile world, patients who have not been vaccinated may acquire epiglottitis and can be seen in any country. Because the new generation of pediatricians and otolaryngologists are not familiar with epiglottitis, it may actually become a more dangerous disease on a case-by-case basis. Unusual presentations will also become more common, with children presenting at a younger age range and immunosuppressive diseases having atypical organisms.

Typically, there is an abrupt onset, usually without an obvious prodrome, with rapid progression toward airway compromise. Initially, complaints of sore throat and odynophagia are common. Patients are usually febrile, and drooling is present. The typical presentation is an ill-appearing child sitting forward with her or his head hyperextended who does not want to lie down (Fig. 10–3). There is a "hot potato" voice and drooling, the mouth is open, and the tongue is protruding. Mild inspiratory stridor and retractions may be present, but these are usually not obvious, since the patient generally takes short, shallow breaths. An intraoral examination is contraindicated because it may predispose to laryngospasm and airway obstruction.

If there is any question as to the diagnosis, a lateral soft tissue

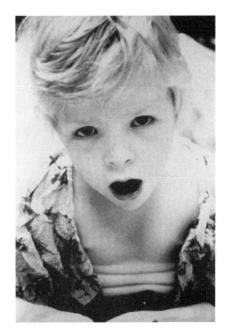

Figure 10–3. Characteristic posture in a patient with epiglottitis. The child is leaning forward and drooling, and the neck is hyperextended. (From Grad R, Taussig LM. Acute infections producing upper airway obstruction. *In* Chernick V, Kendig EL [eds]. Kendig's Disorders of the Respiratory Tract in Children, 5th ed. Philadelphia: WB Saunders, 1990.)

radiograph of the neck can be confirmatory (Fig. 10–4). The patient should be accompanied to the radiologic suite by someone who has the expertise and equipment to handle sudden airway decompensation. When a clinical diagnosis of epiglottitis is at all likely, the patient should be taken immediately to the operating room and cared for by experienced pediatric anesthesiology and otolaryngology personnel.

Once the airway is secured and the diagnosis confirmed, blood specimens are obtained for culture and treatment is begun with a ceftriaxone or cefotaxime. Patients usually require 36 to 48 hours of endotracheal intubation, with observation in the pediatric intensive care unit (PICU). A nasotracheal tube is easier to secure and is more comfortable for the patient. Development of an air leak and the patient's clinical improvement can be used as indicators for extubation, which is generally done in the PICU. If a patient self-extubates prematurely, there is not an immediate loss of airway because the previously placed endotracheal tube has acted as a stent. It takes a few minutes for the inflammatory edema to reaccumulate. Depending on the time of self-extubation and the presence of airway obstruction, some patients may be managed with observation in the PICU to avoid reintubation. If there is a question of safety of extubation, a second laryngoscopy, either in the PICU or operating room, is indicated.

Croup

Laryngotracheal bronchitis (croup) is generally a slowly progressive, mild, self-limited viral inflammation of the subglottic larynx occurring in infants and young children (see Table 10–1). The most common causes are parainfluenza, virus types 1 and 3, influenza A, respiratory syncytial virus (RSV), and adenovirus. The circumferential cricoid cartilage, which comprises the subglottic

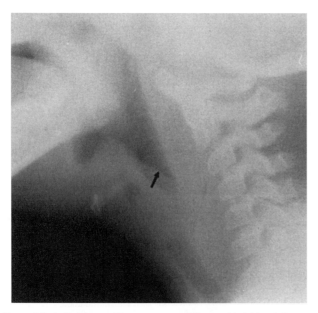

Figure 10–4. Epiglottitis. The patient is a 3½-year-old child with fever and sudden onset of stridor. A lateral radiograph shows an enlarged epiglottis ("thumb-print" sign) and aryepiglottic folds *(arrow)* and distention of the pharynx. Such films are unnecessary if the clinical manifestations are classic for epiglottitis. The patient should be taken immediately to the operating room for intubation. If the diagnosis is uncertain, a physician accompanies the patient to the radiology department. (From Effmann EL. Pediatric chest diseases. *In* Putman CE, Ravin CE [eds]. Textbook of Diagnostic Imaging. Philadelphia: WB Saunders, 1988.)

airway just below the vocal cords, is the narrowest part of the upper airway in a child. The inflammation associated with a viral infection in this location causes airway obstruction as edema develops within the confines of the cricoid cartilage (Fig. 10–5). The cry or voice is usually normal, though occasionally hoarse. There is biphasic stridor with retractions. Unless the airway obstruction is severe, the child generally has no trouble handling saliva; the typical barking cough of croup is present.

Management varies from outpatient observation with parent education to possible endotracheal intubation. For mild cases, the patient must be well hydrated; the use of extra humidity is soothing to the airways and helps to keep secretions from being tenacious so that they are less likely to become obstructive. In more severe cases (stridor at rest, retractions), nebulized epinephrine used as a mucosal vasoconstrictor may provide relief. Usually, patients being treated in this manner are observed in the hospital for a possible rebound effect that may occur 2 to 6 hours after treatment. Parenteral dexamethasone is a safe and effective additional therapy for moderate to severe croup. Aerosolized steroids may be beneficial in mild to moderate croup. Patients with severe croup are usually admitted to the hospital for observation; steroid use has decreased the number of patients requiring endotracheal intubation. If intubation is needed, an endotracheal tube one-half to one size smaller than that used for a child with a normal airway of the same age and size is chosen. A nasotracheal tube is more comfortable, and guidelines for extubation are similar to those for patients who have epiglottitis. In atypical cases of recurrent croup or in those patients who are difficult to extubate, an endoscopic evaluation of the airway with laryngoscopy and bronchoscopy is required to exclude an anatomical abnormality (see Tables 10–2 and 10–3).

Spasmatic croup is a poorly defined process that is generally self-limited with a very short course. It may be related to allergic tendencies (see Table 10–1).

Bacterial Tracheitis

Bacterial tracheitis is a bacterial superinfection of a previous tracheal (croup, influenza virus) viral process and is usually caused by *Staphylococcus aureus*. A variety of other organisms, including *Moraxella catarrhalis*, *Streptococcus pneumoniae*, and *H. influenzae* (nontypable) have also been identified as being occasionally involved. There is generally a viral-like mild phase followed by a rapid deterioration of the airway as the patient clinically appears more ill with an elevated temperature and white blood cell (WBC) count. Neck and chest films often show irregular scalloping of the trachea. Radiopaque densities from inspissated mucus may be seen. Close monitoring and intensive intravenous antibiotic treatment (ceftriaxone, nafcillin), directed toward the likely causative organisms, are required. Endotracheal intubation for control of the airway is usually necessary, particularly in younger patients. Extubation is based on the clinical improvement and a resolution of excessive amounts of purulent secretions. Sometimes the exudate secondary to the tracheitis is thick and can cause airway obstruction similar to that from a foreign body; bronchoscopy is needed. Extubation is based on the clinical improvement and a resolution of purulent secretions.

OTHER CAUSES OF PEDIATRIC AIRWAY OBSTRUCTION

Foreign Body

Whenever a child presents with airway obstruction, the possibility of a foreign body should be considered (see Chapters 7 and 8).

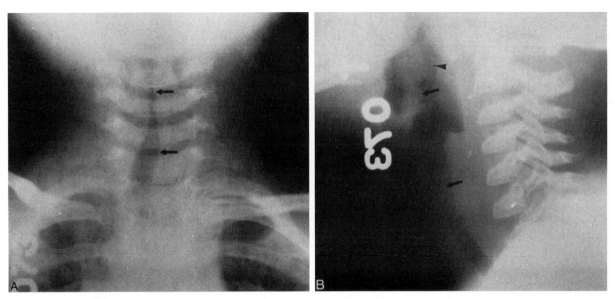

Figure 10–5. Croup in a 1-year-old infant with stridor. *A,* Frontal radiograph of the neck shows a tapered reduction of the subglottic trachea caliber from the level of the vocal cords *(upper arrow)* to the normal caliber trachea below *(lower arrow)*. The right mild tracheal deviation is a normal sign due to the left aortic arch. *B,* Lateral view shows a normal epiglottis *(upper arrow)*, distention of the pharynx, normal palatine tonsils *(arrowhead)*, and increased density in the subglottic trachea *(lower arrow)*. (From Effmann EL: Pediatric chest diseases. *In* Putman CE, Ravin CE [eds]. Textbook of Diagnostic Imaging. Philadelphia: WB Saunders, 1988.)

Table 10–5. **Vascular Rings**

Lesion	Symptoms	Plain Film	Barium Swallow	Bronchoscopy	Angiography	Treatment
Double arch	Stridor Respiratory distress Swallowing dysfunction Reflex apnea	AP—wider base of heart Lat.—Narrowed trachea displaced forward at C3–C4	Bilateral indentation of esophagus	Bilateral tracheal compression— both pulsatile	Diagnostic but often unnecessary	Ligate and divide smaller arch (usually left)
Right arch and ligamentum/ductus	Respiratory distress Swallowing dysfunction	AP—Tracheal deviation to left (right arch)	Bilateral indentation of esophagus R > L	Bilateral tracheal compression— r. pulsatile	Usually unnecessary	Ligate ligamentum or ductus
Anomalous innominate	Cough Stridor Reflex apnea	AP—Normal Lat.—Anterior tracheal compression	Normal	Pulsatile anterior tracheal compression	Unnecessary	Conservative Apnea then suspend
Aberrant right subclavian	Occasional swallowing dysfunction	Normal	AP—Oblique defect upward to right Lat.—Small defect on right posterior wall	Usually normal	Diagnostic but often unnecessary	Ligate artery
Pulmonary sling	Expiratory stridor Respiratory distress	AP—Low l. hilum, r. emphysema/ atelectasis Lat.—Anterior bowing of right bronchus and trachea	± Anterior indentation above carina between esophagus and trachea	Tracheal displacement to left Compression of right main bronchus	Diagnostic	Detach and reanastomose to main pulmonary artery in front of trachea

From Keith HH. Vascular rings and tracheobronchial compression in infants. Pediatr Ann 1977;6:540–549.

Approximately 90% of foreign body ingestions or aspirations are witnessed; it is important to question the adult who accompanies a child with airway obstruction. Radiopaque foreign bodies are generally easily visualized by x-ray studies. Radiolucent foreign bodies may become apparent with the use of inspiratory or expiratory chest x-rays, lateral decubitus films, fluoroscopy, or barium swallows when an esophageal foreign body could be compressing the posterior tracheal wall. Because an occasional foreign body may not lodge in a bronchus, typical radiologic findings may not be seen. If a foreign body is likely, rigid bronchoscopy for examination of the lower airway and foreign body removal is indicated. Flexible bronchoscopy provides an excellent look at the airway and should be reserved when other diagnoses appear to be much more likely. A typical clinical course for an aspirated foreign body is for there to be an *immediate* onset of coughing, often followed by a day or two of minimal symptoms, then recurrence of paroxysms of coughing and sometimes localized physical diagnostic (wheezing) and radiographic findings.

Foreign bodies remain a cause of significant morbidity and mortality and must be looked for in an atypical presentation of airway obstruction. With significant recent improvements in pediatric anesthesia techniques as well as instrumentation for removal of foreign bodies, rigid bronchoscopy is indicated in their management, and maneuvers such as bronchodilators and percussion and postural drainage used in the hope of the patient coughing out a foreign body have no place in the management of this problem.

Recurrent Respiratory Papilloma

Recurrent respiratory papillomas are exophytic, wart-like growths caused by human papillomaviruses (HPV 6 and 11) and may occur anywhere in a child's airway (see Table 10–1). The most common location for their involvement is the larynx, followed by the uvula, tonsillar area, nose, and nasopharynx. The virus is acquired by passage through a birth canal infected with condyloma acuminata (also HPV 6 and 11). The papilloma may appear shortly after birth, but more commonly it occurs when the child is several years of age. Lesions have previously been called ''laryngeal papillomas,'' but because they can occur anywhere in the respiratory tract and have a high likelihood of recurrence, the name has been changed. Although the natural history has not been well studied, there is a tendency toward spontaneous regression. As the child's airway enlarges with growth, the papillomas also become less obstructing.

Treatment is directed toward conservative removal of the papillomatous lesions to allow maintenance of an airway that will allow full activities and a normally functioning voice. CO_2 laser vaporization is most commonly used. It is not unusual for some children to require dozens of procedures, as the viral genome has been found to persist in the airway epithelium and total removal is impossible. Tracheotomies are avoided, unless upper airway obstruction is severe, because the placement of a tracheotomy predisposes to distal pulmonary parenchymal involvement. Interferon has been used for refractory cases with mixed results. Radiation therapy is avoided to lower the risk of malignant degeneration or secondary (thyroid) malignancies.

RED FLAGS AND THINGS NOT TO MISS

The most important aspect of the evaluation of a child with airway obstruction is the observation of the child's breathing pattern and a brief, directed history. Supplemental radiologic studies may be needed, and once the site of the obstruction and likely cause are identified, treatment is instituted. Because patients with airway obstruction may require operative intervention, these patients should not receive feedings during the evaluation period.

Red flags include sudden onset (epiglottitis, foreign body), lack of resolution with normal therapy (foreign body, anatomic narrowing), chronic noisy respiration from birth (anatomic-laryngomalacia), positional worsening (epiglottitis—acute, laryngomalacia—chronic), and exacerbations by upper respiratory tract infections. Feeding difficulties (emesis, dysphagia) combined with respiratory manifestations (cough, stridor, noisy respiration) should suggest an esophageal foreign body, a vascular ring (Table 10–5), or other connecting congenital anomalies (e.g., clefts). Additional danger signs include cyanosis, sitting up-leaning forward posture, dysphagia-drooling, aphonia, severe retractions, dyspnea, and lethargy (possibly CO_2 narcosis). It is imperative not to miss epiglottitis and delay endotracheal intubation with unnecessary clinical or radiologic studies. It is also important not to miss a foreign body, which with time may produce chronic respiratory disease that is often confused with pneumonia or asthma.

REFERENCES

Anatomic Abnormalities

Burch M, Balaji S, Deanfield JE, et al. Investigation of vascular compression of the trachea: The complementary roles of barium swallow and echocardiography. Arch Dis Child 1993;68:171–176.

Cozzi F, Steiner M, Rosati D, et al. Clinical manifestations of choanal atresia in infancy. J Pediatr Surg 1988;23:203–206.

Ezekowitz RAB, Mulliken JG, Folkman J. Interferon Alfa-2a therapy for life-threatening hemangiomas of infancy. N Engl J Med 1992;326:1456–1463.

Holinger PH, Brown WT: Congenital webs, cysts, laryngoceles and other anomalies of the larynx. Ann Otol Rhinol Laryngol 1967;76:744–752.

Kaplan LC: The CHARGE association: Choanal atresia and multiple congenital anomalies. Otolaryngol Clin North Am 1989;22:661–672.

Thomson AH, Beardsmore CS, Firmin R, et al. Airway function in infants with vascular rings: Preoperative and postoperative assessment. Arch Dis Child 1990;65:171–174.

Zalzal GH. Stridor and airway compromise. Pulmonary Clin North Am 1989;36:1389–1402.

Infectious Etiologies

Brook I. Microbiology of retropharyngeal abscesses in children. Am J Dis Child 1987;141:202–204.

Coulthard M, Isaacs D. Retropharyngeal abscess. Arch Dis Child 1991;66:1227–1230.

Cressman WR, Myer CM. Diagnosis and management of croup and epiglottitis. Pediatr Clin North Am 1994;41:265–276.

Donnelly BW, McMillan JA, Weiner LB. Bacterial tracheitis: Report of eight new cases and review. Rev Infect Dis 1990;12:729–735.

Gorelick MH, Baker MD. Epiglottitis in children, 1979 through 1992: Effects of *Haemophilus influenzae* type b immunization. Arch Pediatr Adolesc Med 1994;148:47–50.

Klassen TP, Feldman ME, Watters LK, et al. Nebulized budesonide for children with mild-to-moderate croup. N Engl J Med 1994;331:285–289.

Leventhal BG, Kashima HK, Mounts P, et al. Long-term response of recurrent respiratory papillomatosis to treatment with lymphoblastoid interferon Alfa-n1. N Engl J Med 1991;325:613–617.

Mauro RD, Poole SR, Lockhart CH. Differentiation of epiglottitis from laryngotracheitis in the child with stridor. Am J Dis Child 1988;142:679–682.

Saipe C. Respiratory emergencies in children. Pediatr Ann 1990;19:637–646.

Super DM, Cartelli NA, Brooks LJ, et al. A prospective randomized double-blind study to evaluate the effect of dexamethasone in acute laryngotracheitis. J Pediatr 1989;115:323–329.

11 Apnea and Sudden Infant Death Syndrome

Carl E. Hunt

Apnea (from the Greek, without breath) is the cessation of breathing for greater than 20 seconds or a shorter duration in the presence of pallor, cyanosis, or bradycardia. *Periodic breathing* includes three or more episodes of respiratory pauses of greater than 3 seconds; the duration of respirations interrupting the apnea is 20 seconds or less. *Cheyne-Stokes respiration*, a form of periodic breathing, is characterized by cycles of increasing rate and amplitude of respirations, followed by progressive diminution until the cycle ends in apnea. Cheyne-Stokes respiration is noted in heart failure, increased intracranial pressure, narcotic use, and high altitude.

Apnea, by definition, is caused by a neural arrest of respiration, which may be initiated by central, obstructive, or a combination of both factors (mixed apnea). Nonetheless, this neural arrest of respiration with subsequent absent air flow may be primary (resulting from central nervous system mechanisms) or secondary (resulting from systemic disorders). The cause of apnea varies with the age of the patient and the presence of other identifiable demographic, biologic, or environmental risk factors (Tables 11–1 through 11–4). The most common causes of primary apnea include apnea of prematurity, sudden infant death syndrome (SIDS), and breath-holding spells. Infections, central nervous system diseases, trauma, and poisonings are common secondary causes of apnea.

APNEA OF PREMATURITY

Apnea of prematurity (AOP) is caused by a maturational delay in brainstem function. The frequency and severity of AOP are inversely related to gestational age. AOP is defined by central apnea (no ventilatory effort, no respiratory muscle activity) of greater than 15 to 20 seconds or obstructive apnea associated with bradycardia (<100 beats per minute) with or without cyanosis. Apnea of prematurity is a diagnosis of exclusion after other potential common causes of apnea have been eliminated (see Table 11–2). Preterm infants with AOP have partial deficits in respiratory center output, as manifested by decreased ventilatory responsiveness to hypercarbia, compared with matched preterm infants without AOP. In addition, in affected infants, resting PCO_2 levels are higher, and resting minute ventilation is decreased.

Apnea spells in the preterm infant can be central (10% to 25%), obstructive (12% to 20%), or mixed (53% to 71%). Obstruction is usually in the pharynx and is rarely in the larynx. Because many electronic surveillance monitors detect only central apnea (respiratory pauses), obstructive apnea is recognized if it is associated with a significant central component (mixed apnea), or with bradycardia, or cyanosis, or both. Color changes (erythema, plethora) other than cyanosis are uncommon. AOP with or without bradycardia and cyanosis is typically, but not exclusively, sleep related.

History

The initial presentation of apnea of prematurity includes episodes of apnea with bradycardia (heart rate <100) and cyanosis. If the apneic spells are predominately obstructive, the initial clinical presentation may be limited to the bradycardia, cyanosis, or both. The onset of symptoms is unusual in the first day of life, or after a postconceptional age of 34 weeks, and by definition the condition does not begin after 37 weeks. AOP can become evident any time after spontaneous respirations have been established, even as early as 1 to 2 days of age. AOP does not present in the delivery room (see Table 11–3).

Physical Examination

The physical examination is noncontributory except as related to the gestational age. Any other physical findings are pertinent only as associated with a specific cause of apnea other than AOP (see Table 11–2). Particular attention must be directed at signs of cardiovascular compromise from sepsis, necrotizing enterocolitis, heart failure, intraventricular hemorrhage, or other acute life-threatening disorders.

Diagnostic Evaluation

The diagnosis of AOP is one of exclusion, based on the clinical symptoms and the absence of specific medical causes (see Table 11–2). Laboratory evaluation includes an arterial blood gas (or capillary blood gas plus pulse oximetry) to determine hypoxia or acidosis, serum electrolyte level (Na^+, K^+, Cl^-, HCO_3^-), serum glucose and calcium levels, a complete blood count (to detect anemia, leukocytosis or leukopenia for infection), a head ultrasonographic study (to detect intracranial hemorrhage), and other diagnostic studies based on the history or physical examination (abdominal radiograph for necrotizing enterocolitis, chest radiograph for pneumonia or postextubation atelectasis). Multichannel cardiorespiratory recordings may document the extent of periodic breathing, hypercarbia, oxygen desaturation, and relative distribution of central, obstructive, and mixed apneas. Such recordings are usually unnecessary for clinical care. *Severity* is defined by the frequency of spells and the extent of any necessary intervention. Resolution is best determined by clinical observation.

Differential Diagnosis

In preterm infants weighing less than 1500 g at birth, symptomatic apnea occurs at least once in approximately 70% of appropriate-for-gestational-age infants. Even though approximately 80% (57% in total) have apnea of prematurity, the diagnosis of AOP is one of exclusion (see Table 11–2). Severe hypoxemia from any cause can cause apnea. Apnea may be the first clinical indication of hypoglycemia, hypocalcemia, or of sepsis and/or meningitis.

Table 11-1. Categories of Apnea

Disease	Example	Mechanism	Signs	Treatment
Apnea of prematurity	Premature baby (<36 wk)	Central control, airway obstruction	Apnea, bradycardia	Theophylline, caffeine, nasal CPAP, intubation
Congenital central hypoventilation	Previously called Ondine curse	Central control	Apnea, hypoventilation	Mechanical ventilation
SIDS	Previously normal child; increased incidence with prematurity, SIDS in sibling, maternal drug abuse, cigarette smoking, males; may have preceding minor URI	Central respiratory control?	Child (2–3 mo) found cyanotic, apneic, and pulseless in bed	No treatment; prevention with home apnea monitor unproved, and supine or side sleep position suggestive
Cyanotic "breath-holding spells"	Breath holder < 3 yr old	Prolonged expiratory apnea, hyper-ventilation, cerebral anoxia	Cyanosis, syncope, brief tonic-clonic movements	Reassurance that the condition is self-limiting, must exclude seizure disorder
Pallid "breath-holding spells"	Breath holder	Asystole, reflex anoxic seizures	Rapid onset, with or without crying; pallor; bradycardia; opisthotonus; seizures; follows painful stimuli	Atropine?, must exclude seizure disorder, less benign than cyanotic breath holding
Obstructive sleep apnea (OSA)	Obesity, chronic tonsil hypertrophy, Pierre Robin syndrome, Down syndrome, cerebral palsy, myotonic dystrophy, myopathy	Airway obstruction by enlarged tonsils and/or adenoids, choanal stenosis and/or atresia, large tongue, temporomandibular joint dysfunction, micrognathia, velopharyngeal incompetence Also may be central	Daytime sleepiness, loud snoring, nighttime insomnia and enuresis, hyperactivity, poor school performance, behavior problems, mouth breathing, inspiratory stridor, hypertension	Tonsillectomy, adenoidectomy, nasal trumpets, nasal CPAP, uvuloveloplasty
Obesity (subcategory of OSA) (pickwickian syndrome)	Obesity, Prader-Willi syndrome	Airway obstruction, central control	Obesity, nocturnal wakefulness, daytime somnolence, hypoxia, hypercarbia, polycythemia, cor pulmonale (see obstructive sleep apnea)	Theophylline, weight loss
Narcolepsy	Sleep apnea (variable), onset 10–20 yr of age	Familial sleep disturbance	Daytime drowsiness, cataplexy (induced by stress, anger, surprise), hypnagogic (onset or end of sleep) hallucinations, sleep paralysis	Methylphenidate for sleep attacks, drowsiness; imipramine for cataplexy; γ-hydroxybutyrate(?) for sleep paralysis, hallucinations, narcolepsy

Abbreviations: CPAP = continuous positive airway pressure; SIDS = sudden infant death syndrome; URI = upper respiratory infection.
? = unproven questionable effects.

Patients with seizures may present with apnea-related symptoms. Although patients with AOP are generally not anemic, hematocrit levels are lower in preterm infants with AOP than in matched infants without AOP; symptoms often improve after transfusion or erythropoietin therapy. Thermal stress (fever or overheating) can cause apnea. In premature infants, especially those weighing less than 1000 g, apnea-bradycardia-cyanosis spells may be related to feeding and not necessarily to AOP. Gastroesophageal reflux is common in preterm infants and is sometimes associated with significant awake-related apnea-bradycardia-cyanosis symptoms; although infants with AOP with sleep-related symptoms may also have evidence of gastroesophageal reflux, the AOP and gastroesophageal reflux episodes are not temporally related. A sudden increase or new onset of apnea in a preterm infant over 2 to 3 weeks of age is not AOP and warrants an evaluation to exclude more serious diseases (see Table 11–2). Similarly, apnea at birth is always caused by a more serious disorder (see Table 11–3).

usu resolve by 34–36 wks post-conceptual age

Treatment

Mild episodes of apnea that resolve spontaneously and are unassociated with cyanosis do not require treatment. Contributing acid-base imbalance, hypoxemia, or anemia, however, should be corrected. Tactile stimuli that nonspecifically increase central adrenergic input may be helpful, including mild shaking or stroking (massage) or the use of an air mattress with low-frequency intermittent inflation or a water mattress. If multiple episodes occur daily and require vigorous stimulation, or if any episodes require bag-and-mask ventilation with supplemental oxygen, more aggressive treatment is indicated. Although no consensus exists as to when a methylxanthine should be used, both theophylline (loading dose, 5 to 6 mg/kg; maintenance dose, 1 to 2 mg/kg every 8 hours;

Table 11–2. Etiology of Apnea-Related Spells in Preterm Infants

Cause	Comment
Idiopathic*	Apnea of prematurity with immaturity of respiratory center; modified by sleep state, position, upper airway collapse
CNS	IVH,† seizures,† depressant drugs, hypoxic injury
Respiratory	Pneumonia, obstructive airway lesions, atelectasis,† severe RDS, laryngeal reflex, phrenic or vocal cord paralysis, pneumothorax, hypoxia, hypercarbia, nasal occlusion caused by phototherapy eye patches, tracheal occlusion caused by neck position
Cardiovascular	Heart failure, hypotension, hypertension, hypovolemia, increased vagal tone
Gastrointestinal	Nasogastric tube feedings,† gastroesophageal reflux, esophagitis, necrotizing enterocolitis, intestinal perforation, bowel movement
Infection	Sepsis, meningitis: bacterial, viral, fungal
Metabolic	Hypoglycemia, hypocalcemia, hyponatremia, hypernatremia, hyperammonemia, elevated organic acid levels, fluctuations of ambient temperature, hypothermia, hyperthermia
Hematologic	Anemia†

*Most common cause, with onset in first week of life (not in first day) and generally resolution by 34–36 weeks' postconceptional age.
†Common.
Abbreviations: CNS = central nervous system; IVH = intraventricular hemorrhage; RDS = respiratory distress syndrome.

Table 11–3. Etiology of Apnea at Birth

Cause	Comment
Intrauterine asphyxia*	Antenatal, intrapartum, postnatal
Placental transfer of CNS-depressant drugs*	Narcotics, magnesium sulfate
Airway obstruction	Choanal atresia, macroglossia—mandibular hypoplasia (Pierre Robin syndrome), tracheal web or stenosis, airway mass lesions
Neuromuscular disorders	Congenital myotonic dystrophy, congenital myopathies or neuropathies
Trauma*	Cranial hemorrhage, spinal cord transection, phrenic nerve palsy
Infection*	Consolidated congenital pneumonia
Severe immaturity*	Weight <1000 g
CNS lesions	Infantile thalamic degeneration, familial multisystem atrophy, infantile neuroaxonal dystrophy, Pena-Shokeier syndrome, CNS brainstem tumor, Arnold-Chiari malformation, Dandy-Walker malformation, Joubert syndrome, lissencephaly, Miller-Dieker syndrome, medullary hypoplasia, Möbius syndrome, congenital central hypoventilation
Skeletal lesions	Osteogenesis imperfecta, camptomelic dysplasia, achondroplasia, asphyxiating thoracic dystrophies, short-rib polydactyl syndromes, chondroectodermal dysplasia (Ellis–van Creveld syndrome)

Data from Brazy JE, Kinny HC, Oakes WJ. Central nervous system structural lesions causing apnea at birth. J Pediatr 1987;111:163–175.
*Common.
Abbreviations: CNS = central nervous system.

serum level, 5 to 10 μg/ml) and caffeine (loading dose, 10 mg/kg; maintenance dose, 2.5 mg/kg every day; serum level, 8 to 20 μg/ml) are effective treatments. For the same extent of central respiratory stimulation, caffeine appears to be associated with fewer systemic side effects (tachycardia), and fewer doses per day are necessary. Both agents are central respiratory stimulants and increase diaphragmatic contraction, decrease muscle fatigue, and increase metabolic rate and catecholamine activity. Treatment with methylxanthines results in rapid and significant clinical improvement and eliminates symptoms in 50% or more of preterm patients. Whether administered parenterally or orally, methylxanthines appear to be effective for mixed, obstructive, and central apnea. Doxapram is a potent central stimulant, but experience with the agent is limited. It should be considered when intubation and assisted ventilation appear necessary. Nonetheless, if the patient requires intubation, endotracheal tube placement and mechanical ventilation should not be delayed while waiting for a drug to start to work.

Nasal continuous positive airway pressure (NCPAP) is usually started after methylxanthine administration or simultaneously with these agents in severe AOP. NCPAP is generally effective in improving and often eliminating clinical symptoms of AOP. In addition to reducing hypoxia and splinting the upper airway, thus reducing upper airway resistance, this therapy may also have some effect related to increased sensory input and secondary changes in sleep state. Since the advent of NCPAP (+2 to +5 cm H_2O), assisted ventilation has seldom been required for uncomplicated AOP.

Outcome

Most symptoms of apnea of prematurity resolve by a postconceptional age of 35 to 37 weeks. Symptoms occasionally persist until

40 weeks or rarely longer. Infants should be symptom-free for at least 3 days before they are discharged from the hospital. If a methylxanthine is used, the drug should be discontinued in symptom-free infants at least 3 days and preferably 4 to 5 days before discharge.

There is no increased risk of a subsequent cardiorespiratory control deficit, such as sudden infant death syndrome (SIDS), as a consequence of AOP. The incidence of SIDS is increased in preterm infants; this risk is related to gestational age and is unrelated to presence or severity of AOP. Neurodevelopmental sequelae in preterm infants correlate with low gestational age and low birth weight and are unaffected by the presence of appropriately treated AOP.

Prevention

The only definitive prevention of AOP is to prevent prematurity. To the extent that this goal cannot be achieved, the risk for symptoms can be minimized by maintaining optimal acid-base balance, oxygenation, and hemoglobin level (thus oxygen-carrying capacity and oxygen delivery). Because frequent blood transfusions to treat anemia of prematurity have other potential risks, the use of recombinant erythropoietin may be a useful adjunctive treatment.

APPARENT LIFE-THREATENING EVENT

"Apparent life-threatening event" (ALTE) is a clinical label for any acute episode of apnea that was thought to be potentially life-threatening. An ALTE has some combination of apnea, bradycardia, cyanosis, and loss of tone or consciousness. An ALTE may necessitate cardiopulmonary resuscitation. Apnea of infancy (AOI), the major subcategory of ALTE, can be diagnosed only after the exclusion of all other diagnoses that could explain the acute episode (Fig. 11-1; see Table 11-4). AOI is an idiopathic sleep state–dependent episode associated with bradycardia, cyanosis, and hypotonia; AOI and ALTE were formerly called "aborted" or "near-miss" SIDS.

History

The typical history is that of a previously normal infant in whom an acute sleep-related episode of color change, hypotonia, and apnea occurs at home. The history needs to include a number of specific questions to focus the differential diagnosis and diagnostic

Table 11-4. Conditions That May Cause Apparent Life-Threatening Events or Sudden Death

Cause	Comment
CNS	Arteriovenous malformation, seizures, congenital central hypoventilation (see also Table 11-1), neuromuscular disorders (Werdnig-Hoffmann disease), Arnold-Chiari crisis, Leigh syndrome
CVS	Subendocardial fibroelastosis, aortic stenosis, anomalous coronary artery, myocarditis, myocardiopathy, arrhythmias (prolonged QT syndromes, Wolff-Parkinson-White syndrome, congenital heart block)
Pulmonary	Idiopathic pulmonary hypertension, vocal cord paralysis
Gastrointestinal	Pancreatitis, diarrhea and/or dehydration, gastroesophageal reflux
Endocrine-metabolic	Congenital adrenal hyperplasia, malignant hyperpyrexia, long- or medium-chain acyl coenzyme A deficiency, hyperammonemias (urea cycle enzyme deficiencies), glutaricaciduria, carnitine deficiency (systemic or secondary), glycogen storage disease type I, maple syrup urine disease, congenital lactic acidosis, biotinidase deficiency
Infection	Sepsis, meningitis, encephalitis, hepatitis, pyelonephritis, bronchiolitis (RSV), infant botulism, brain abscess
Trauma	Child abuse (see Chapter 37), suffocation, physical trauma, Munchausen syndrome by proxy
Poisoning	Boric acid, carbon monoxide salicylates, barbiturates, ipecac, cocaine, insulin

Abbreviations: CNS = central nervous system; CVS = cardiovascular system; RSV = respiratory syncytial virus.

evaluation (Table 11-5) and to determine the severity of the episode. Risk factors may be similar to those of SIDS (Table 11-6). Conditions that may cause sudden death or an ALTE are noted in Table 11-4.

Physical Examination

The role of the physical examination is to identify any specific abnormality that is sufficient to explain the ALTE (see Fig. 11-1; see also Table 11-4). Abnormal results of a neurologic examination

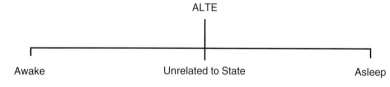

ALTE

Awake	Unrelated to State	Asleep
Gastroesophageal reflux	Airway obstruction (severe)	Obstructive sleep apnea
Breath-holding spells	Neurologic dysfunction	Suffocation
Airway obstruction	Infection	Idiopathic (apnea of infancy)
	Cardiac disturbance	Alveolar hypoventilation
	Metabolic error	
	Toxic–poisoning	
	Autonomic dysfunction	
	Child abuse, including Munchausen syndrome by proxy	

Figure 11-1. Possible causes of an apparent life-threatening event (ALTE) in infancy and their relationship to sleep state. Causes classified as "variable" have no specificity related to state and can occur while the child is awake or asleep.

Table 11–5. Questions That Guide the Evaluation of Apparent Life-Threatening Events*

1. Who discovered the infant?
2. Was the infant awake or asleep?
3. Where was the infant sleeping, and what were the circumstances related to sleeping surface, bedding, and covering (swaddling)?
4. In what sleep position was the infant found? If the position was prone, what was the position of the face?
5. What were the specific observations in regard to color, muscle tone, pulse, and respiratory effort?
6. What was the timing and the sequence of intervention, and what was required for a response?
7. When was the last feeding?
8. Has there been a recent febrile illness?
9. Have any other spells occurred?
10. How long did it take the infant to fully recover after the episode?
11. If available, what were the objective findings of the Emergency Medical Service or ambulance personnel?

*Responses to all of these questions are necessary as part of the assessment of an apparent life-threatening event.

might suggest the presence of a neurodegenerative disease, trauma, or a seizure-related cause, an especially likely consideration if multiple episodes have occurred. If the infant is lethargic or unresponsive, intoxication, inborn errors of metabolism, hypoglycemia, and meningitis are prominent considerations. Severe hypoxia due to ALTE also produces a hypoxic-ischemic encephalopathy. The presence of midfacial hypoplasia, or micrognathia, or both, suggests obstructive sleep apnea. A cardiac cause for the episode is not common and is usually evident from the examination. Evidence of neglect or unexplained bruising requires consideration of child abuse. Delay in seeking care, a physical finding unexplained by the history, and inconsistent historical information from the same or multiple family members should raise suspicions for abuse (see Chapter 37). Depending on parental behavior and consistency of

Table 11–6. Epidemiologic Risk Factors for Sudden Infant Death Syndrome

Low birth weight (<2500 g)
Very low birth weight (<1500 g)
Male sex
Black race
Winter months
Formula (versus breast) feeding
Prone sleeping position*
Prior ALTE
Co-sleeping
Natural fiber mattress use*†
Swaddling*†
Recent respiratory illness*†
Thermal stress*†
Poor or no prenatal care
Previous sibling with SIDS
Maternal urinary tract infection
Maternal cigarette smoking
Maternal illicit drug use
Low socioeconomic status
Maternal age <19 yr

* = The combination of these factors may impose the greatest and most significant risk.
† = If sleeping prone.
Abbreviation: ALTE = apparent life-threatening event.

the history and clinical findings, Munchausen syndrome by proxy with intentional suffocation may also need to be considered.

Diagnostic Evaluation

If the examination findings are normal and the history is consistent with an idiopathic ALTE (apnea of infancy), the laboratory evaluation can be very limited. If seen within 2 to 4 hours of the episode, a serum bicarbonate level might show evidence of hypoxia-induced metabolic acidosis if the episode was of significant severity and duration. A urine toxicology screen should be obtained; 10% to 15% of screens demonstrate a drug that can explain the ALTE, related to either well-intentioned but overzealous parents or to intent to do harm. Tests such as electroencephalography, chest roentgenography, electrocardiography, complete blood count, evaluation for gastroesophageal reflux, or lumbar puncture should be performed only if indicated by the history and physical examination. The diagnosis of AOI is suggested by the history and is confirmed by normal results of the physical examination.

No specific diagnostic evaluation can provide positive confirmation that the ALTE is idiopathic and is thus appropriately labeled as AOI. A partial deficit in central inspiratory drive, as indicated by blunted ventilatory or arousal responsiveness to hypercarbia or hypoxemia and perhaps mild alveolar hypoventilation, occurs in approximately 30% to 40% of infants with AOI. Pneumograms have often been performed, but results are abnormal in no more than 50% of infants with AOI. The respiratory pattern abnormalities that can be observed include prolonged apnea, excessive respiratory pauses, and excess periodic breathing. Further, the pneumographic results do not predict risk for recurrence and do not correlate with the potential future risk for SIDS. Polysomnograms (PSGs) may be obtained in patients with AOI, but results in as many as 90% have been normal; a normal result does not contradict the diagnosis of AOI. An interval of documented monitoring can be a useful diagnostic test to better characterize the diagnosis by recording any alterations in cardiorespiratory pattern that occur during a clinical event that are sufficient to exceed the record or alarm thresholds.

Differential Diagnosis

In a large series of infants with ALTE, 62% had a known cause; among these, the diagnoses included 47% digestive, 29% neurologic, 15% respiratory, 3.5% cardiovascular, 2.5% endocrine-metabolic, and 3% miscellaneous (see Table 11–4). The other 38% had apnea of infancy: 61% of these infants had mild AOI, and 39% had severe AOI requiring vigorous stimulation or cardiopulmonary resuscitation for recovery.

The ALTE should first be classified as awake-related or sleep-related or unrelated to sleep (see Fig. 11–1). If the ALTE is exclusively awake-related, the possible diagnoses are limited; if postprandial and especially if associated with regurgitation or vomiting, gastroesophageal reflux is a likely consideration. If the ALTE is associated with behavioral or vagally induced antecedents, a breath-holding spell is the likely diagnosis. There is a continuum between breath-holding spells and autonomic spells, the latter being generally unassociated with any behavioral antecedents; autonomic spells (familial dysautonomia, autoimmune neuropathy) are not common but need to be considered when predominately or exclusively awake spells are severe and recurrent, and especially if the severity seems to be increasing after the initial presentation. Acute upper airway obstruction can also cause an ALTE (see Chapter 10).

If the cause of the ALTE is a respiratory control abnormality, such as obstructive sleep apnea or central hypoventilation syndrome, then the symptoms are sleep related and extend into awake periods only in the most severe instances. If the cause for the ALTE is related to infection, metabolic, neurologic, cardiac, or toxic causes, there is generally no clear relationship to sleep state. Child abuse by suffocation has to be considered; in most instances, the child abuse is related to Munchausen syndrome by proxy, in which the infant is a victim of imposed illness for the psychological benefit of a parent, generally the mother. Although this syndrome is an uncommon cause of an ALTE, presentation as an ALTE may account for 40% to 50% of Munchausen syndrome by proxy in infancy. If a careful history and counseling do not reveal this diagnosis, and whenever the suspicion for Munchausen syndrome by proxy seems warranted, covert video surveillance may be necessary (see Chapter 37).

Treatment

If the ALTE is attributed to a specific cause, the appropriate treatment should then be apparent. If the final diagnosis by exclusion is apnea of infancy, then the predominant treatment strategy has been the use of a home monitor until the infant is free of recurrent symptoms for at least 2 to 3 months and often until 5 or 6 months of age. Although there are no data to indicate that home monitoring for AOI reduces the risk for SIDS, home monitors are indicated to alert the family to any potentially life-threatening recurrences and thus permit timely intervention and prevention of serious morbidity. The availability of documented monitoring with stored events and respiratory patterns in computerized memory permits a more objective use of the home monitor. These event recordings permit characterization of any clinically significant events that recur and establish whether any of the alarms occurring at home are of clinical or physiologic significance.

In patients with AOI with an abnormal respiratory pattern, a methylxanthine has also been recommended. As with apnea of prematurity (see earlier), the respiratory pattern abnormalities generally resolve with such treatment, and the clinical symptoms also tend to resolve. Although methylxanthines have been used as an adjunct or even as an alternative to home monitoring in patients with AOI, only anecdotal data are available regarding their efficacy. All families of infants with AOI should be taught basic cardiopulmonary life support.

Outcome

The outcome of an ALTE depends on the identified medical cause. If the cause is idiopathic (apnea of infancy) 40% to 50% of affected infants are likely to have no further life-threatening episodes, and those having recurrences generally show progressive improvement over the ensuing months. Of patients with AOI, 90% or more have at least one apnea ($\geq$20 seconds) at home as determined by monitor alarms. Most infants triggering alarms receive stimulation, divided approximately equally between gentle stimulation, vigorous stimulation, and resuscitation. Although not necessary for routine clinical care, hypoxic arousal responses do help to identify patients with AOI who are at highest risk for severe recurrent ALTE; patients with deficient hypoxic arousal responsiveness have a higher incidence of subsequent apneas than do those with normal arousal responsiveness. Although most true alarm signals occurring at home are due to apnea, about 15% are associated with bradycardia and about 15% are isolated bradycardia. These outcome data are based on undocumented home monitoring. More detailed studies have demonstrated that parental observations and home monitor logs significantly overstate the occurrence of events; that is, approximately 90% of home alarms are not caused by a clinically significant event. Loose monitor leads and movement artifact alarms account for 65% to 70%, and false alarms account for the remaining 20% to 25% of nonphysiologic alarms.

Follow-up studies have not been performed with sufficient frequency to clarify the extent to which immature or abnormal brainstem respiratory output later improves. Infants with AOI may have a small but increased risk for respiratory control disorders in later years, such as alveolar hypoventilation or obstructive sleep apnea. Previous reports in patients with AOI indicate a risk of SIDS as low as zero and as high as 5% to 6%. The natural risk is likely closer to the 5%, and the extent to which home monitoring may reduce this risk is unknown.

Follow-up studies of patients with AOI to 7 to 10 years of age reveal no neurodevelopmental differences between affected and normal children. Nevertheless, a small number of children in whom the ALTE was of sufficient severity to cause a hypoxic-ischemic event have significant neurobehavioral sequelae. Children with AOI do have a higher frequency of breath-holding spells and minimal behavioral problems.

Prevention

It is not possible to prevent an ALTE except when an identifiable abnormality did not receive appropriate and timely medical attention. It is not possible to prevent the first episode of apnea of infancy, because there is no way to predict which infants will develop the condition. There may be an increased incidence of AOI in families with a prior history of SIDS or AOI, but 95% or more of subsequent siblings are normal, and there is no accurate means of prospectively identifying the few who might be at an increased risk for developing AOI.

SUDDEN INFANT DEATH SYNDROME

Sudden infant death syndrome is the most common cause of sudden and unexpected death in infants (Fig. 11–2); 40% to 50% of postneonatal infant mortality is caused by SIDS. The peak incidence is at 2 to 4 months of postconceptional age; 95% of all SIDS has occurred by age 6 months. SIDS is the sudden death of an infant that remains unexplained despite a complete autopsy, examination of the death scene, and review of the history. An autopsy is thus required in all instances of sudden infant death because the history and death scene investigation are not sufficient to exclude most congenital or acquired causes (Table 11–7; see also Table 11–4).

History

The location, time, and circumstances of the death need to be ascertained as soon as possible. If the infant was asleep, which is usually the case, the position in which he or she was found and the nature of the sleeping surface (hard or soft mattress, pillow, blanket) also need to be documented. Approximately 50% of SIDS victims have a history of a recent or intercurrent minor upper respiratory or other febrile illness, such as gastroenteritis. Decreased activity or listless appearance in the last day is also common but an autopsy is needed to exclude severe infection. Many epidemiologic risk factors are associated with SIDS (see Table 11–6); absence of risk factors does not eliminate the risk for SIDS. Because most SIDS infants have not been identified in advance, most of the assessments of biologic risk factors have been evaluated in surviving infants who presented with apnea of infancy.

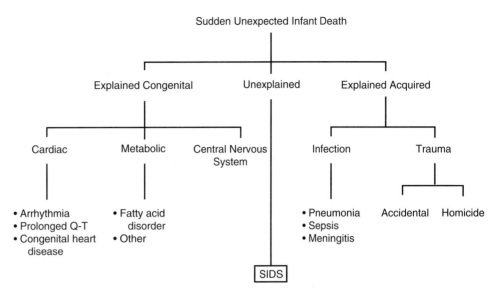

Figure 11-2. Differential diagnosis of sudden unexpected death in infancy (see Table 11–4).

Physical Examination

The examination begins with the death scene investigation and ends with the autopsy. The body needs to be examined for any evidence of trauma. Even in the absence of any external evidence, the presence of internal hemorrhage or fracture needs to be ascertained. It is necessary to rule out unsuspected congenital defects, such as cardiac defects (e.g., critical aortic stenosis), or central nervous system anomalies. Blood and urine need to be examined for toxic substances and for medium-chain fatty acid metabolism defects. The presence of a significant infection, such as meningitis, sepsis, or overwhelming pneumonia, needs to be determined.

Minimal pulmonary edema and diffuse intrathoracic petechiae are commonly observed in SIDS; they are associated and not diagnostic findings, because neither has been of sufficient specificity and sensitivity to prove or explain SIDS. Numerous other findings suggestive of chronic prenatal or postnatal asphyxia have been reported. Detailed examination of the brain has also revealed other subtle findings that suggest delayed maturational changes that may contribute to the causation of SIDS.

Table 11-7. Differential Diagnosis of Recurrent Sudden Infant Death in a Sibship

Idiopathic	Recurrent true sudden infant death syndrome
CNS	Congenital central hypoventilation, neuromuscular disorders, Leigh syndrome
CVS	Endocardial fibroelastosis, Wolff-Parkinson-White syndrome, prolonged QT syndrome, congenital heart block
Pulmonary	Pulmonary hypertension
Endocrine-metabolic	See Table 11–4
Infection	Disorders of immune host defense (see Chapter 52)
Child abuse	Filicide, infanticide, Munchausen syndrome by proxy

Abbreviations: CNS = central nervous system; CVS = cardiovascular system.

Differential Diagnosis

The diagnosis of SIDS is based on exclusion of all known causes of sudden infant death (see Fig. 11–2 and Tables 11–4 and 11–7) by the history, death scene, and pathologic investigations. Episodes of recurrent ALTE in a patient or of SIDS in a sibship may be clues to other identifiable disorders (Table 11–7). Perhaps as many as 10% of deaths consistent with SIDS are in fact explained by child abuse (filicide).

Inborn errors of metabolism may present as an ALTE or SIDS. Hepatomegaly (glycogen storage disease), hypoglycemia (glycogen storage disease, disorders of fat metabolism: carnitine deficiency, medium acyl coenzyme A dehydrogenase deficiency), absence of fasting ketosis (disorders of fat metabolism), hypotonia (carnitine deficiency), cardiomyopathy (glycogen storage disease, carnitine deficiency) and reoccurrences of SIDS in a family increase the possibility of an inborn error of metabolism.

Treatment

The only available "treatment" strategy pertains to the surviving family. Local SIDS support groups are available to provide information and support to the family. The recent increased focus on filicide is justified, but a negative consequence has been delayed implementation of the support process, even when SIDS is the correct final diagnosis. A primary forensic approach to all sudden and unexpected deaths can thus unduly delay the support process for the 90% or more of such deaths that are indeed SIDS.

Prevention

It is not possible to prospectively identify those infants who, in the absence of effective intervention, will die of SIDS. Therefore, preventive measures have been suggested for all infants.

Public education campaigns in numerous countries have advocated large-scale efforts to reduce SIDS rates by interventions such as supine or lateral position for sleep, breast-feeding, parental smoking cessation, solitary sleeping, avoidance of overheating, and early evaluation of any febrile illness. Although these educational interventions, such as the focus on infant sleep position, are promising, the hypothesis of prone position as the dominant risk factor for SIDS has not yet been validated in an appropriately designed prospective study. Nonetheless, the American Academy of Pediatrics recommends placing all infants in the supine or side position prior to sleep, to reduce the risk of SIDS. The epidemiology of SIDS is complex, the mechanism is unknown, the determination of position at death has been imprecise and generally retrospective, and the interaction of prone (face down) sleeping with other biologic and epidemiologic risk factors is unknown but causally suggestive (see Table 11–6).

OBSTRUCTIVE SLEEP APNEA

Obstructive sleep apnea (OSA), a common disorder in adults (affecting 1% to 2%), is also a significant clinical entity in children (see Table 11–1). OSA is a sleep-related airway obstruction associated with severe, prolonged, partial airway obstruction, intermittent episodes of reversible complete obstruction, or both. In children, this condition is usually a result of adenoidal-tonsillar hypertrophy–induced upper airway obstruction. Obesity is another risk factor. The peak incidence in childhood is at 2 to 5 years of age, but the specific age at presentation depends on the underlying mechanism (see Table 11–1). Brainstem respiratory center output is generally normal to increased in response to obstruction in patients with OSA. Especially in obese children, however, OSA may indeed be associated with diminished central respiratory drive and thus with alveolar hypoventilation that may remain if the obstructive problem is treated. Additional causes include micrognathia, midfacial hypoplasia, extrinsic or intrinsic anatomic lesions obstructing the airway, and functional obstruction from pharyngeal muscle dysfunction (see Table 11–1).

History

A careful delineation of awake (daytime sleepiness) and asleep (snoring, night wakefulness, unrestful sleep) symptoms is essential. Snoring is loud and harsh and persists through most or all of sleep. Brief episodes of respiratory silence indicate episodic complete obstruction. Sleep disturbances are related to the severity of obstruction-related sleep asphyxia and the resultant repetitive arousals leading to sleep deprivation.

The occurrence of daytime symptoms is a direct consequence of chronic sleep deprivation. Depending on the patient's age and the severity of the sleep disturbance, the history may reveal hypersomnolence, behavioral changes, morning headache, or decreased school performance.

Physical Examination

The physical examination performed while the patient is awake is generally not helpful in diagnosing obstructive sleep apnea. However, mouth breathing suggests significant nasal obstruction (adenoids), and the presence of midfacial underdevelopment indicates an anatomic predisposition. Evidence of marked adenoidal hypertrophy, tonsillar hypertrophy, or both, confirms the most likely cause for OSA; the absence of significant adenotonsillar hypertrophy does not exclude such hypertrophy as the cause because the adenotonsillar contribution to nasopharyngeal airway narrowing may be present only during sleep.

When the history is suggestive of OSA, the physical examination is incomplete until the child has also been examined while asleep. Heavy and persistent snoring strongly suggests significant partial upper airway obstruction, especially if the snoring is associated with color change or bradycardia, or with cor pulmonale. The occurrence of episodes of complete obstruction is indicated by intervals of silent breathing despite severe retractions.

Diagnostic Evaluation

To determine the severity and to clarify the underlying mechanism, polysomnography is necessary. This assessment requires referral to a sleep laboratory experienced in the evaluation of infants and young children. The diagnosis of obstructive sleep apnea in children is confirmed by (1) episodes of partial or complete airway obstruction during sleep that result in an oxygen saturation of less than 90% and an end-tidal PCO_2 of greater than 45 mmHg or (2) sleep-related asphyxia and sleep deprivation resulting in clinically significant effects, such as failure to thrive, cor pulmonale, or neurobehavioral disturbance.

The presence of polycythemia is consistent with a greater severity of chronic sleep-related asphyxia. Radiographic examination of the sinuses and nasopharynx may be helpful in some children, but lateral neck radiography performed during wakefulness may significantly underrepresent the degree of sleep-related nasopharyngeal collapse that would be evident by airway fluoroscopy performed while asleep. The presence and severity of any cor pulmonale (cardiomegaly, hepatomegaly, hypoxia, right ventricular hypertrophy on electrocardiography, accentuated P_2 sound on cardiac auscultation, and narrow splitting of the second heart sound) also need to be evaluated.

Differential Diagnosis

Other airway conditions can potentially be confused with obstructive sleep apnea. Any condition causing stenosis or collapse of the airway can secondarily be associated with snoring and partial airway obstruction asleep; the absence of significant awake symptoms, however, indicates OSA (see Chapter 10). Reactive airway disease should be distinguished by the history and the results of the physical examination. Gastroesophageal reflux can cause stridor and coughing and can certainly be present as an additional finding, but the history and polysomnographic results distinguish between OSA and gastroesophageal reflux as the primary diagnosis (see Chapter 20).

Narcolepsy is manifested by daytime sleepiness and cataplexy, sleep paralysis, or hypnagogic hallucinations (see Table 11–1). It begins before the age of 20 years and has a hereditary component. Narcolepsy is a severely disabling sleep disorder that may or may not be associated with apnea.

Treatment

In most children, obstructive sleep apnea can be cured by both tonsillectomy and adenoidectomy. If the history and physical examination results indicate the presence of severe sleep-related OSA and the absence of any craniofacial abnormality, polysomnography can be deferred until 4 to 6 weeks after the tonsillectomy and adenoidectomy are performed and should then be performed only if significant symptoms have persisted. If any discrete anatomic airway obstruction is present, surgical correction may be possible. OSA that is unresponsive to surgery or for which no surgery is possible may benefit from NCPAP. Acting as a splint to maintain higher end-expiratory nasopharyngeal cross-sectional area, NCPAP has been a very successful treatment strategy in adults and, more recently, in older children. Tracheostomy is seldom necessary in

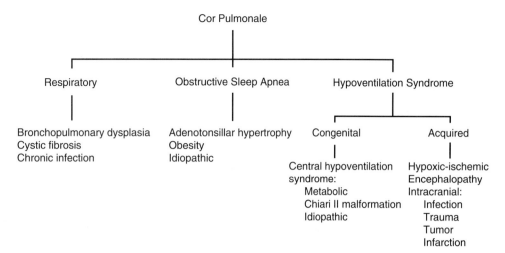

Figure 11-3. Causes of cor pulmonale in infants and children.

children. Patients with obesity or pickwickian syndrome usually improve after significant weight reduction (see Table 11–1).

Outcome

The outcome for children with obstructive sleep apnea is generally excellent. Because most cases are related to adenotonsillar hypertrophy, tonsillectomy and adenoidectomy should be curative. Chronic problems generally occur only if permanent consequences of severe sleep-related asphyxia occurred before diagnosis and treatment (Fig. 11–3); hypoxic-ischemic encephalopathy is rare, but it does occur. In children with midfacial hypoplasia or other discrete causes of airway obstruction, the outcome depends on the specific problem.

Prevention

The occurrence of severe long-term sequelae can be prevented by an awareness of the presenting symptoms in children and by a timely response to early symptoms.

HYPOVENTILATION SYNDROMES

History

Alveolar hypoventilation encompasses all respiratory control deficits associated with decreased central respiratory drive and resultant deficiency of autonomic control of ventilation. Alveolar hypoventilation is also a descriptive label for the milder form of hypoventilation syndromes. *Central hypoventilation syndrome* (CHS) represents the severe end of the respiratory control spectrum, in which output of the brainstem respiratory centers is not sufficient to sustain spontaneous ventilation (Table 11–8). The range of severity encompasses milder forms that are evident only during quiet sleep; ventilation may be sufficient to avoid acute symptoms but insufficient to prevent progressive cor pulmonale. In severe cases, spontaneous sleep ventilation is inadequate for survival. In the most severe cases, the deficient respiratory center output extends to variable degrees into wakefulness. Patients with CHS

typically have normal respiratory rates associated with shallow breathing (hypopnea). These rates do not increase in response to progressive asphyxia due to the underlying deficiency in automatic control of respiration. Voluntary ventilation is normal but cannot be adequately regulated. Overt apnea is uncommon.

Infants with a severe congenital disorder present with persistent hypopnea that requires ventilatory support. If the extent of hypoventilation is not severe, the diagnosis may not be clinically evident until cor pulmonale develops or an acute respiratory infection occurs. In children with alveolar hypoventilation, the extent of sleep-related asphyxia may thus be minimal, so that diagnosis does not occur until adolescence. As with any respiratory control deficit, the history is not complete until sleep-related symptoms have been evaluated in a sleep lab.

Physical Examination

The physical findings in the patient with mild alveolar hypoventilation are unremarkable while the patient is awake unless the presentation was precipitated by acute respiratory infection or cor pulmonale. Examination during the patient's sleep reveals hypopnea, a normal respiratory rate, mild cyanosis or pallor, and perhaps sweating. Obesity may be an associated finding.

Table 11–8. Respiratory Control Abnormalities Characteristic of Central Hypoventilation Syndrome

1. Hypoventilation (hypopnea) during quiet sleep, all sleep, or all states, depending on severity of the condition, leading to progressive hypercarbia and hypoxemia
2. Absent or negligible ventilatory and arousal sensitivity to hypercarbia during sleep
3. Absent or negligible hypercarbic ventilatory responsiveness awake, regardless of the adequacy of awake ventilation
4. Variable deficiency in hypoxic ventilatory responsiveness in all states, being absent in the most severe cases
5. Absent or negligible hypoxic arousal responsiveness during sleep
6. General unresponsiveness to respiratory stimulants, especially during sleep
7. Absence of autoresuscitation or gasping (asleep) and inability to perceive asphyxia or to experience dyspnea during wakefulness

The physical examination results of a patient with CHS depend on the severity of the hypoventilation and the patient's age. Infants with severe congenital CHS are likely to be symptomatic in the delivery room or within the first 12 to 24 hours, with marked hypopnea, secondary bradycardia, and cyanosis requiring assisted ventilation.

The physical examination needs to include a search for associated congenital or acquired abnormalities. In the newborn, hypoventilation may be associated with a myelomeningocele and Chiari II malformation. Patients with CHS generally have mild hypotonia, but more substantial degrees of hypotonia might indicate a specific metabolic or neuromuscular disorder. If the deficit is acquired, the physical examination should suggest the underlying cause, such as severe central nervous system infection, trauma, or brain tumor.

Differential Diagnosis

Regardless of the patient's age at presentation, the differential diagnosis of CHS includes acute cardiac and respiratory conditions capable of causing cardiorespiratory failure. If the extent of hypopnea is not sufficiently severe to cause acute cardiorespiratory failure, the sleep-related hypopnea and secondary asphyxia result in cor pulmonale, and the differential diagnosis for cor pulmonale (see Fig. 11–3) then needs to be considered.

Treatment

Drug therapy is effective in the milder degrees of alveolar hypoventilation. Theophylline or caffeine may be sufficient to normalize sleep ventilation, and progesterone has sometimes been effective. Intravenous doxapram improves ventilation in most CHS patients, but seldom to the extent that ventilatory support can be withdrawn. Long-term treatment with doxapram is not realistic because of its generalized adrenergic side effects.

Mechanical ventilatory support is an essential component of the treatment for CHS. The options include positive- and negative-pressure ventilation and diaphragm pacing. In infants and young children, negative-pressure methods are generally not practical and chronic tracheostomy is usually necessary. Positive-pressure ventilation has been the most commonly used long-term treatment for CHS. Home ventilators are most practical and least intrusive when children require support only during sleep. As an alternative to chronic tracheostomy, limited success with positive-pressure ventilation delivered by nasal mask has been achieved in a few older children. Negative-pressure ventilation has been successful in some older children who require mechanical assistance only during sleep. A chest shell (cuirass) and a jump suit (wrap ventilator) have both been advocated. The primary advantage of negative-pressure over positive-pressure ventilators is that the children may then successfully receive ventilation without a tracheostomy.

Substantial clinical experience with diaphragm pacing is now available in infants and children. The pacer system includes an external transmitter and a loop antenna as well as three internal components: a receiver, unipolar phrenic nerve electrodes, and an indifferent electrode (anode). A radiofrequency signal is emitted from the antenna, converted by the receiver to an electrical impulse, and transmitted to the phrenic nerve. To be eligible for diaphragm pacing, the child must have intact phrenic motoneurons and must not have any significant reduction in lung compliance. If awake pacing is being contemplated, age-appropriate activities are fully achievable if supplemental oxygen is not required. The primary complication of pacing is periodic failure of an implanted pacemaker component, generally a receiver and, less commonly, an electrode wire. Chronic phrenic nerve or diaphragm damage ("burnout") has not occurred in children enrolled in a recommended clinical pacing regimen. The relative advantages of diaphragm pacing may be further enhanced with a pacer system that relies on rotation of three phrenic nerve stimulation sites within each electrode and thus reduces the risk for diaphragm fatigue.

Outcome

Except for congenital patients with CHS with associated abnormalities, optimal long-term outcome appears to be primarily related to the avoidance of cor pulmonale. Timely diagnosis, establishment of an effective home ventilation program, and effective long-term surveillance combining noninvasive blood gas monitoring with periodic sleep laboratory evaluations should be sufficient to prevent cor pulmonale.

The neurodevelopmental outcome should be normal for patients with alveolar hypoventilation who respond to drug therapy. Although neurodevelopmental data are limited and variable in CHS patients, full-scale intelligence quotient (IQ) scores are typically above 70. Although results of extensive neuropsychologic assessments suggest that CHS may actually be a more generalized central nervous system process than previously thought, in individual cases severe pretreatment asphyxia or subsequent chronic or recurrent asphyxia caused by the deficient perception of asphyxia may also be a cause of sequelae.

There is no evidence that children with congenital CHS later outgrow the central respiratory control deficiency. There is a tendency for such children to later demonstrate some stabilization and amelioration of symptoms, but not to the extent that ventilatory support becomes unnecessary. In acquired deficiencies, later normalization should not be anticipated if the ventilatory control deficit has been stable for 3 to 6 months.

Prevention

There is no way to prevent congenital hypoventilation syndromes. The ultrastructural or biochemical abnormality is unknown, as is the molecular genetics. Periconceptional folic acid does reduce the occurrence of myelomeningocele, however, and congenital CHS associated with Chiari II malformation thus does have a potential for prevention. To the extent that clinical entities causing CHS can be prevented or treated more effectively, of course, acquired CHS is at least theoretically amenable to prevention.

SUDDEN UNEXPECTED DEATH

Sudden unexpected death is much less common in older children and adolescents than in adults. Respiratory, cardiac, vascular, or neurologic disorders may be identified at postmortem examination or by history. The causes of sudden unexpected death in children are listed in Table 11–9.

SUMMARY AND RED FLAGS

An algorithm for the differential diagnosis of apnea is noted in Figure 11–4. "Red flags" for apnea and SIDS are noted in Table 11–10.

Table 11-9. Etiology of Sudden Unexpected Death in Children, Adolescents, and Young Adults

Cause	Comment
Drug abuse*	Cocaine, amphetamines, and inhalants (freon, cleaning fluid [trichloroethylene], gasoline, glue, typewriter correction fluid, nitrites [amyl, butyryl]), emetine
Foreign body aspiration	Sudden onset—cough, gagging
Severe asthma*	Sudden onset, often at night
Spontaneous pneumothorax	Tension pneumothorax
Suicide*	Poisoning (carbon monoxide), firearms
Sickle cell anemia	Risk is also increased in sickle cell trait with intense exercise and/or high altitude (hypoxia)
Anaphylaxis*	Drug or food induced
Anorexia nervosa, severe starvation	Electrolyte disturbance, emetine abuse, arrhythmia
Heat stroke	Risk increased with exercise and high humidity
Pericardial tamponade	Pericardial effusion, trauma
Myocarditis*	Kawasaki disease, viral, rheumatic fever
Cardiomyopathy	Hypertrophic, familial, dilated, metabolic
Right ventricular cardiomyopathy*	Also known as right ventricular dysplasia (arrhythmogenic right ventricle)
Mitral valve prolapse	Arrhythmia, embolism, uncertain as a cause of sudden death
Marfan syndrome	Aortic dissection, mitral valve prolapse
Pulmonary embolism	Chest pain, hypoxia, normal chest radiograph
Blunt chest trauma	Commotio cordis, cardiac contusion, concussion
Coronary arteritis	Kawasaki disease, Takayasu disease, periarteritis nodosa
Anomalous position of coronary artery*	Anomalous origin of ostia (right artery from left sinus or vice versa or from pulmonary artery), anomalous deep intramyocardial course
Idiopathic coronary artery dissection	More common in women
Coronary ostia obstruction	Congenital webs
Atherosclerotic coronary artery disease	Idiopathic or familial hyperlipidemia
Aortic valve stenosis	Congenital
Shone syndrome	Parachute mitral valve and subaortic stenosis
Conduction system pathway	Fibrosis, congenital heart block, tumor
Sinus node disturbance	Idiopathic, after atrial surgery, sick sinus syndrome
Preexcitation-induced arrhythmia	Wolff-Parkinson-White or other accessory pathways
Prolonged QT syndrome	Familial; risk of ventricular arrhythmia
Recent cardiac surgery	Sinus node, atrioventricular node (heart block) or ventricular arrhythmia, obstructed baffle
Ruptured berry aneurysm	Severe headache, meningismus, coma
Cerebrovascular accident	Paradoxical embolism through patent foramen ovale; carotid or left side cardiac source; spontaneous thrombosis (hypercoagulable state secondary to hereditary [protein C, protein S, antithrombin III deficiency] or acquired [antiphospholipid antibodies])

Data from Am J Dis Child 1991;145:177–183; Br Heart J 1992;68:601–607; Am J Med 1990;89:588–596.
*Common cause of unexplained death.
  For cardiac pathology, the cause may be myocardial infarction or fatal ventricular arrhythmia (ventricular fibrillation—tachycardia rarely asystole or bradyarrhythmia). In many cardiac related deaths there is often a history of chest pain (see Chapter 14), palpitations (see Chapter 12), or syncope (see Chapter 43). Exertion is often a preceding event for cardiac-based sudden death. Sudden cardiac death occurs within 1 hour of the onset of acute symptoms and is unexpected even in the presence of existing disease.

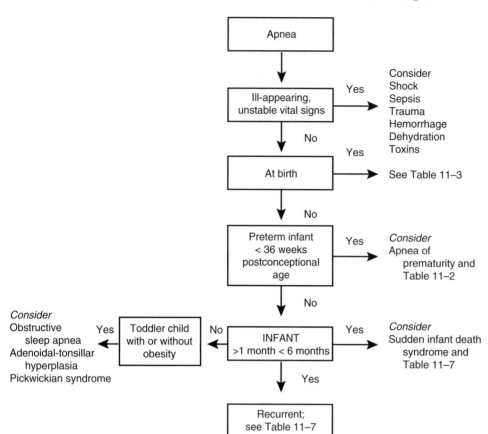

Figure 11–4. Algorithm for evaluation and differential diagnosis of apnea.

Table 11–10. Red Flags for Apnea and Sudden Unexpected Death

Problem	Suspect
Repeated episodes in patient or family	Child abuse or neglect, inborn errors of metabolism, carbon monoxide or other poisoning (see Table 11–7)
Retinal hemorrhages	Child abuse
Hypotension, fever, poor capillary perfusion, persistent tachycardia	Sepsis, shock, hemorrhage, dehydration, myocarditis
Onset at birth	Asphyxia, birth trauma (see Table 11–3)
Onset ≥ 6 mo of age	Primary CNS pathology (seizure, increased intracranial pressure, drug overdose, trauma), primary cardiovascular disorder, obstructive apnea, systemic infection, shock (see Table 11–4)
Obesity	Obstructive sleep apnea
Daytime drowsiness, nighttime wakefulness	Obstructive sleep apnea, narcolepsy
Syncope	See Chapter 43
Chest pain	See Chapter 14
Palpitations	See Chapter 12

Abbreviation: CNS = central nervous system.

REFERENCES

Apnea

Bechensteen AG, Hågå P, Halvorsen S, et al. Erythropoietin, protein, and iron supplementation and the prevention of anemia of prematurity. Arch Dis Child 1993;69:19–23.

Brazy JE, Kinney HC, Oakes WJ. Central nervous system structural lesions causing apnea at birth. J Pediatr 1987;111:163–175.

Brouard C, Moriette G, Murat I, et al. Comparative efficacy of theophylline and caffeine in the treatment of idiopathic apnea in premature infants. Am J Dis Child 1985;139:698–700.

Finer NN, Barrington KJ, Hayes BJ, et al. Obstructive, mixed, and central apnea in the neonate: Physiologic correlates. J Pediatr 1992;121:943–950.

Hunt C. Apnea and SIDS. Clin Perinatol 1992;19:701–961.

Joshi A, Gerhardt T, Shandloff P, et al. Blood transfusion effect on the respiratory pattern of preterm infants. Pediatrics 1987;80:79–84.

Peliowski A, Finer NN. A blinded, randomized, placebo-controlled trial to compare theophylline and doxapram for the treatment of apnea of prematurity. J Pediatr 1990;116:648–653.

Ruggins NR. Pathophysiology of apnoea in preterm infants. Arch Dis Child 1991;66:70–73.

Apparent Life-Threatening Event

Arens R, Gozal D, Williams JC, et al. Recurrent apparent life-threatening events during infancy: A manifestation of inborn errors of metabolism. J Pediatr 1993;123:415–418.

Berger D. Child abuse simulating ''near-miss'' sudden infant death syndrome. J Pediatr 1979;95:554–556.

Dunne K, Matthews T. Near-miss sudden infant death syndrome: Clinical findings and management. Pediatrics 1987;79:889–893.

Editorial. Gastro-oesophageal reflux and apparent life-threatening events in infancy. Lancet 1988;11:261–262.

Hickson GB, Altemeier WA, Martin ED, et al. Parental administration of chemical agents: A cause of apparent life-threatening events. Pediatrics 1989;83:772–776.

Kahn A, Rebuffat E, Sottiaux M, et al. Sleep apneas and acid esophageal reflux in control infants and in infants with an apparent life-threatening event. Biol Neonate 1990;57:144–149.

Lewis JM, Ganick DJ. Initial laboratory evaluation of infants with ''presumed near-miss'' sudden infant death syndrome. Am J Dis Child 1986;140:484–486.

Samuels MP, McClaughlin W, Jacobson RR, et al. Fourteen cases of imposed upper airway obstruction. Arch Dis Child 1992;67:162–170.

Steinschneider A, Santos V. Parental reports of apnea and bradycardia: Temporal characteristics and accuracy. Pediatrics 1991;88:1100–1105.

Weese-Mayer DE, Brouillette RT, Morrow AS, et al. Assessing validity of infant monitor alarms with event recording. J Pediatr 1989;115:702–708.

Sudden Infant Death Syndrome

American Academy of Pediatrics Task Force on Infant Positioning and SIDS. Positioning and SIDS. Pediatrics 1992;89:1120–1126.

Arnon SS, Midura TF, Damus K, et al. Intestinal infection and toxin production by *Clostridium botulinum* as one cause of sudden infant death syndrome. Lancet 1978;1:1273–1278.

Chiodini BA, Thach BT. Impaired ventilation in infants sleeping facedown: Potential significance for sudden infant death syndrome. J Pediatr 1993;123:686–692.

Committee on Child Abuse and Neglect and Committee on Community Health Services. Investigation and review of unexpected infant and child deaths. Pediatrics 1993;92:734–735.

Denborough MA, Galloway GJ, Hopkinson KC. Malignant hyperpyrexia and sudden infant death. Lancet 1982;2:1068–1070.

Emery JL. Child abuse, sudden infant death syndrome, and unexpected infant death. Am J Dis Child 1993;147:1097–1100.

Holton JB, Allen JT, Green CA, et al. Inherited metabolic diseases in the sudden infant death syndrome. Arch Dis Child 1991;66:1315–1317.

Lemieux B, Giguere R, Cyr D, et al. Screening urine of 3-week-old newborns: Lack of association between sudden infant death syndrome and some metabolic disorders. Pediatrics 1993;91:986–988.

Ponsonby AL, Dwyer T, Gibbons LE, et al. Factors potentiating the risk of sudden infant death syndrome associated with the prone position. N Engl J Med 1993;329:377–382.

Taylor J, Sanderson M. A reexamination of the risk factors of the sudden infant death syndrome. J Pediatr 1995;126:887–891.

Willinger M. Sleep position and sudden infant death syndrome. JAMA 1995;273:818–819.

Obstructive Sleep Apnea

Carroll JL, Loughlin GM. Diagnostic criteria for obstructive sleep apnea syndrome in children. Pediatr Pulmonol 1992;14:71–74.

Douglas NJ. The sleep apnoea/hypopnoea syndrome and snoring. BMJ 1993;306:1057–1060.

Gaultier C. Clinical and therapeutic aspects of obstructive sleep apnea syndrome in infants and children. Sleep 1992;15:S36–S38.

Kales A, Vela-Bueno A, Kales JD. Sleep disorders: Sleep apnea and narcolepsy. Ann Intern Med 1987;106:434–443.

Hypoventilation Syndromes

DiMario FJ. Breath-holding spells in childhood. Am J Dis Child 1992;146:125–131.

Gozal D, Marcus CL, Shoseyov D, et al. Peripheral chemoreceptor function in children with the congenital central hypoventilation syndrome. J Appl Physiol 1993;74:379–387.

Hunt CE. Hypoventilation syndromes. *In* Burg FD, Ingelfinger JR, Polin RA, Wald ER (eds). Gellis and Kagen's Current Pediatric Therapy 15. Philadelphia: WB Saunders, 1994.

Keens TG, Davidson Ward SL. Ventilatory treatment at home. *In* Beckerman RC, Brouillette RT, Hunt CE (eds). Respiratory Control Disorders in Infants and Children, Baltimore: Williams & Wilkins, 1992:371–385.

Marcus CL, Jansen MT, Poulsen MK, et al. Medical and psychosocial outcome of children with congenital central hypoventilation syndrome. J Pediatr 1991;119:888–895.

Silvestri JM, Weese-Mayer DE, Nelson MN. Neuropsychologic abnormalities in children with congenital central hypoventilation syndrome. J Pediatr 1992;120:388–393.

Weese-Mayer DE, Hunt CE, Brouillette RT, et al. Diaphragm pacing in infants and children. J Pediatr 1992;120:1–8.

Cor Pulmonale

Hunt CE, Brouillette RT. Abnormalities of breathing control and airway maintenance in infants and children as a cause of cor pulmonale. Pediatr Cardiol 1982;3:249–256.

Sofer S, Weinhouse E, Tal A, et al. Cor pulmonale due to adenoidal or tonsillar hypertrophy or both in children. Chest 1988;93:119–122.

Cardiac Disorders

12 Palpitations and Arrhythmias

George F. Van Hare

Palpitation refers to a patient's conscious and often uncomfortable or frightening awareness of the heart's actions. Palpitations may be slow or fast, regular or irregular. The sensation is described as pounding, fluttering, flopping, skipping or missing of beats, stopping, or jumping. Some patients report feeling that the heart has turned over. Palpitations are often due to a change in the rate, rhythm, or contractibility of the heart. Although arrhythmias may cause palpitations, many arrhythmias are imperceptible by the patient. A broad overview of factors associated with palpitations is presented in Table 12–1. Common arrhythmias based on the patient's age are noted in Table 12–2, and arrhythmias associated with congenital heart disease are noted in Table 12–3.

Because palpitations raise the possibility of cardiac disease, their occurrence is frequently associated with anxiety. However, most patients with palpitations do not have a serious cardiac condition. Although evaluation and occasionally invasive testing are required for some patients, most can be safely reassured. The goal is to identify patients in whom the symptom of palpitations is a manifestation of a life-threatening arrhythmia and to evaluate them appropriately.

DIAGNOSTIC METHODS

History

The only definitive way to diagnose the cause of the palpitations is to record an electrocardiogram during the symptom. Nonetheless, information from the patient's history may be helpful in diagnosing the problem and in assessing the urgency of reaching a diagnosis.

The patient's description of the sensation is important. Sustained tachycardia is usually described as a "racing" heartbeat, whereas premature beats and second-degree atrioventricular block are usually described as skipping of a beat. For the latter symptom, the sensation of the heart stopping is likely caused by the pause that follows a premature beat. Rapid abrupt onset of palpitations, with equally abrupt spontaneous termination, especially if paroxysmal, suggests supraventricular tachycardia and not sinus tachycardia. The duration and rate of the symptoms should be noted; for sustained fast rhythms, some assessment of likely rate may be obtained by asking the patient or parent to imitate the rhythm by tapping it out. Parents or patients may be taught to take the pulse during such episodes. Patients can usually tell whether the fast rhythm is regular or irregular. Fast rhythms, such as atrial fibrillation and often atrial flutter (with block), are irregular, whereas supraventricular tachycardia and ventricular tachycardia are usually regular.

Symptoms associated with palpitations give clues to the severity of the problem. The most ominous sign is *syncope,* defined as a sudden loss of consciousness with inability to maintain posture. Syncope occurs as a result of hemodynamic compromise caused by the arrhythmia (rapid supraventricular tachycardia, ventricular tachycardia, atrioventricular block) (see Chapter 43). Patients with syncope associated with possible arrhythmia require full cardiac evaluation because of the possibility that future episodes may result in sudden death. Patients may complain of transient dizziness or lightheadedness, which also suggests hemodynamic compromise of a lesser degree. Chest pain is occasionally reported but is often due to the strong rapid heartbeat rather than to any coronary artery abnormality. Sensation of the palpitation in the neck may signify atrioventricular nodal reentrant tachycardia or ventricular tachycardia and is caused by contraction of the atria against closed atrioventricular valves, resulting in jugular venous regurgitation (cannon a waves).

Factors that elicit the symptom are important to note. For example, certain forms of ventricular tachycardia are elicited only by exercise. These causes of arrhythmia may depend on sympathetic activity, and "stress" is frequently reported as an eliciting factor. Such patients may respond best to beta-adrenergic receptor–blocking agents.

Factors that terminate the episodes help in the diagnosis as does the manner of termination. Sustained fast heart rhythms that end suddenly are more likely to have reentrant causes, whereas those that slow gradually are more likely to be have an automatic focus. Termination by the Valsalva maneuver, gagging, or facial immersion in cold water suggests reentrant supraventricular tachycardia, although atrial flutter may also terminate with these maneuvers.

The past medical history and review of systems are important, primarily for identifying structural cardiac disease (Table 12–3), which may affect the prognosis and therefore the urgency of evaluation, and any possible noncardiac causes of palpitations. The most important example of the latter is hyperthyroidism, which may manifest as sinus tachycardia or as atrial fibrillation (Table 12–1). A history of deafness (some cases of prolonged QT syndrome), ocular disease (Kearns-Sayre syndrome: progressive ophthalmoplegia, pigmentary retinal degeneration, AV block), or muscle weakness (Kearns-Sayre syndrome, myotonic dystrophy: AV block) may suggest specific disorders.

Physical Examination

Few specific physical findings aid in the diagnosis. However, any signs of structural cardiac disease (see Chapter 16) are important because patients with serious structural cardiac disease are likely to tolerate arrhythmias more poorly and are likely to have more complex and dangerous cardiac rhythms than are those without heart disease. Several specific cardiac abnormalities are strongly

Table 12-1. **Possible Etiologic Factors in Palpitations***

Sinus tachycardia†	Proarrhythmia agents§
Arrhythmias	Erythromycin lactobionate
Paroxysmal atrial or ventricular tachycardia	Terfenadine (± ketoconazole)
Paroxysmal atrial flutter or fibrillation	Astemizole
Sinus bradycardia.	Quinidine (and other class Ia agents)
Junctional rhythm	Amiodarone
Complete heart block	Flecainide
Premature atrial or ventricular beats‡	Encainide
Drugs‡	Endocrine
Tobacco	Hyperthyroidism†
Tea	Pheochromocytoma
Coffee	Insulin excess (hypoglycemia)
Colas	Others
Cocaine	Anemia†
Amphetamines	Panic-anxiety syndrome (panic attacks)‡
Atropine	Epilepsy
Tricyclic antidepressant agents	Arteriovenous malformation†
Amyl nitrate	Fever†
Epinephrine	Porphyria
Ephedrine	Guillain-Barré syndrome (autonomic neuropathy)
Aminophylline	Myocarditis
Albuterol	Lyme disease
Terbutaline	Mitral valve prolapse
Carbon monoxide	Arrhythmogenic right ventricle
Digitalis	

*Many of these etiologic factors are interrelated; e.g., anemia produces sinus tachycardia, as do various drugs (e.g., caffeine, cocaine).
†High cardiac output states.
‡Common.
§Proarrhythmic agents induce arrhythmias by prolonging the QT interval, resulting in ventricular tachycardia, often of the torsades de pointes type.

Table 12-2. **Common Arrhythmias by Patient Age**

Age	Arrhythmia	Comment
Fetal	Sinus bradycardia (<100 bpm)	Fetal hypoxic stress
	Complete heart block (<60 bpm)	Isolated, or associated with maternal SLE or fetal congenital heart disease. May cause hydrops
	Sinus tachycardia (>180 bpm)	Maternal fever, drugs, fetal stress, anemia
	Supraventricular tachycardia (>200 bpm)	Causes hydrops if sustained
	Atrial flutter (280–450 bpm ± conduction delay, 2:1)	Causes hydrops if sustained
	Ventricular tachycardia (>120 bpm)	Rare
Neonate	Often a continuation of fetal arrhythmia	
	Sinus bradycardia	Associated with apnea of prematurity as primary event
Infant	Sinus tachycardia (<250 bpm)	Fever, anxiety, shock, dehydration, heart failure, pain
	Supraventricular tachycardia	Primary or sympathomimetic drug administration, fever, myocarditis, trauma
Older child and adolescent	Premature atrial beats	
	Premature ventricular beats	
	Paroxysmal atrial tachycardia	Thyrotoxicosis, idiopathic, atrial enlargement, mitral stenosis, sympathomimetic drugs
	Sinus bradycardia	Trained athlete, vasodepressor syncope
	Sinus tachycardia	As for infant (see above) plus drug abuse (cocaine, amphetamine)
	Various post–cardiac surgery arrhythmias	See Table 12-3

Abbreviations: bpm = beats per minute; SLE = systemic lupus erythematosus.

Table 12–3. Arrhythmias Associated with Congenital Heart Disease

Anomaly	Arrhythmia		
	Preoperative	*Postoperative*	*Delayed-Late Onset*
Ostium secundum ASD	Mild prolonged PR interval Occasional atrial tachyarrhythmias	Atrial tachycardia Junctional tachycardia Atrial fibrillation Atrial flutter Sinus bradycardia	Atrial tachycardia Sinus bradycardia

Ostium primum ASD	Prolonged PR interval	As in ostium secundum
		    ASD plus AV block
			As in ostium secundum
			    ASD

Complete AV canal	Prolonged PR interval	Atrial tachycardia Junctional tachycardia Transient complete AV block	Complete AV block
Total anomalous venous return	As in ASD	As in ASD	As in ASD

Transposition of great arteries:
    Mustard or Senning repair
		Sinus bradycardia
		Atrial flutter
		Accelerated junctional
		    tachycardia
		AV block
			Sinus bradycardia
			Atrial tachycardia

Arterial switch repair		Premature atrial contractions	
Tricuspid atresia Fontan repair	Atrial fibrillation Preexcitation	Junctional tachycardia Atrial fibrillation Atrial flutter Complete AV block Sinus bradycardia	Supraventricular tachycardia
VSD		Right bundle branch block Bifascicular block Transient complete AV block	Complete AV block Right bundle branch block

Tetralogy of Fallot	Ventricular tachycardia (rare)
	Supraventricular tachycardia
	    (rare)
		As in VSD, plus
		    ventricular premature
		    contractions
			As in VSD, plus sustained
			    ventricular tachycardia

Ebstein anomaly	Wolff-Parkinson-White
	    preexcitation
	Atrial flutter or fibrillation
	Supraventricular tachycardia
		Transient AV block
		Atrial flutter or fibrillation
		Premature ventricular
		    contractions
			Complete AV block

Corrected transposition (L-transposition)	Complete AV block	As in VSD if present AV block	As in VSD if present AV block

Abbreviations: ASD = atrial septal defect; AV = atrioventricular; VSD = ventricular septal defect.

associated with arrhythmias. Patients with *dilated cardiomyopathy* may have ventricular arrhythmias, including ventricular fibrillation, and often have a gallop rhythm or signs of heart failure (see Chapter 13). Those with *hypertrophic cardiomyopathy* may have nonspecific ejection murmurs and may also have an increased apical impulse; these patients are at risk for ventricular arrhythmias. Arrhythmias are often noted in patients with congenital heart disease both before and after corrective or palliative surgery (Table 12–3).

During the episode, the rate, rhythm, blood pressure, and arterial and venous (cannon a jugular waves) pulsations should be determined.

Electrocardiographic Monitoring

RESTING

The resting 15-lead electrocardiogram (ECG), which is obtained when the patient is asymptomatic, can be valuable in indicating a specific diagnosis associated with arrhythmias, but unfortunately it is not useful in ruling out arrhythmias *per se*. Electrocardiography should always be performed in any patient presenting with such symptoms.

For reference, a standard cardiac cycle as noted on the ECG is noted in Figure 12–1; the corresponding conduction systems are noted in Figure 12–2. The *P wave* represents atrial depolarization, and the *PR interval* represents the time for the signal to travel from the sinus node to the ventricles, with most time spent in the atrioventricular node. The PR interval increases with age. Conduction time is shortened when an accessory pathway (Wolff-Parkinson-White) bypasses the atrioventricular node. A prolonged PR interval indicates prolonged conduction anywhere between the sinus node and the myocardium but usually indicates atrioventricular node block.

The *QRS complex* represents ventricular depolarization, and the *QT interval* represents ventricular repolarization. Examples of diagnoses that may be evident on the ECG include the Wolff-Parkinson-

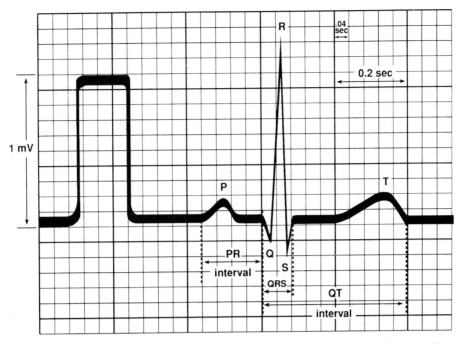

Figure 12–1. Waves and intervals in a P-QRS-T complex. Standard calibration is 1 mV = 10 mm; paper speed is 25 mm/second. (From Victorica BE. Electrocardiogram interpretation and diagnostic value. *In* Gessner IH, Victorica BE [eds]. Pediatric Cardiology: A Problem Oriented Approach. Philadelphia: WB Saunders, 1993.)

White syndrome (Fig. 12–3), the long QT syndrome, and conduction abnormalities, such as second-degree and third-degree atrioventricular block. In addition, patients who are symptomatic as a result of premature beats (atrial, Fig. 12–4; or ventricular, Fig. 12–5) may have these on the resting ECG. Nonspecific changes, such as T-wave abnormalities, may suggest the presence of a myocardial problem, and specific findings, such as left ventricular hypertrophy, may not provide a diagnosis but may suggest the presence of hypertrophic cardiomyopathy.

If the ECG captures the arrhythmia, it may reveal supraventricular tachycardia (Fig. 12–6), atrial flutter (Fig. 12–7), ventricular tachycardia (Figs. 12–8 and 12–9), polymorphous ventricular tachycardia—torsades de pointes (Fig. 12–10), or, rarely, ventricular fibrillation (Fig. 12–11).

AMBULATORY ELECTROCARDIOGRAPHIC MONITORING

Twenty-four-hour ambulatory monitoring *(Holter monitoring)* is commonly used to attempt to capture the abnormality on the ECG when symptoms occur. With Holter monitoring, the ECG is continuously recorded onto magnetic tape for 24 hours, capturing two separate leads simultaneously, for later playback and analysis. The patient keeps a diary of events and symptoms, and the Holter tape may be examined at these times to determine the existing heart rhythm during the symptom. If symptoms are a daily occurrence, Holter monitoring is probably the most efficient method of diagnosis. It is particularly valuable in patients with very frequent symp-

Figure 12–2. Cardiac conduction system. (From Epstein ML. Disturbances of cardiac rhythm. *In* Gessner IH, Victorica BE [eds]. Pediatric Cardiology: A Problem Oriented Approach. Philadelphia: WB Saunders, 1993.)

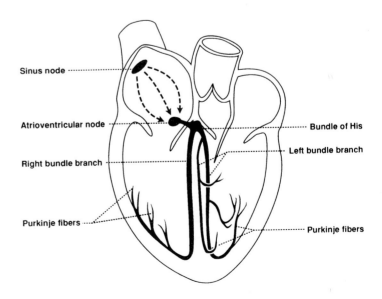

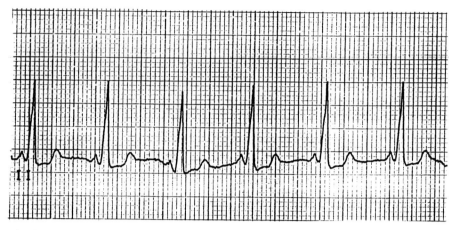

Figure 12–3. Rhythm strip, lead II, in a patient with Wolff-Parkinson-White syndrome. Note the lack of an isoelectric interval between the end of the P wave and the start of the QRS complex as well as the slurred QRS upstroke.

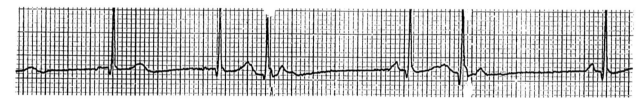

Figure 12–4. Rhythm strip, lead AVF, in a patient with premature atrial contractions. The clear deformation of the T wave prior to the premature beat indicates the presence of a premature P wave.

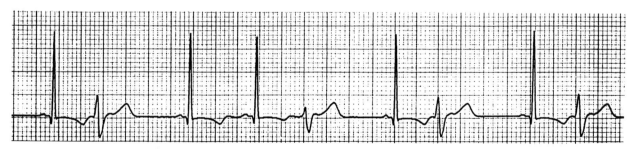

Figure 12–5. Rhythm strip, lead V5, in a patient with frequent premature ventricular contractions. Note the lack of clear deformation of the T wave preceding the premature beat, the prolonged QRS duration of the premature beat, and the full compensatory pause.

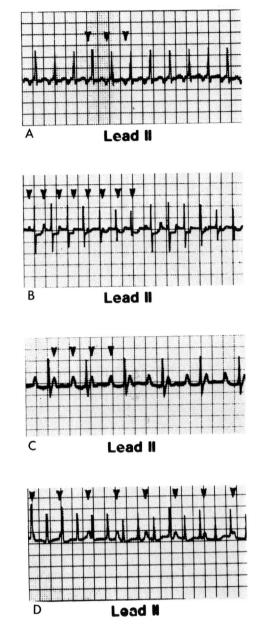

Figure 12–6. P-QRS relationship in supraventricular tachycardia. P waves are marked by *arrowheads. A,* There is a 1:1 relationship between P waves and QRS complexes. *B,* Supraventricular tachycardia with type II second-degree atrioventricular (AV) block. *C,* Supraventricular tachycardia with 2:1 AV block. *D,* Rare supraventricular tachycardia with AV dissociation. (From Garson A. Arrhythmias in pediatric patients. Med Clin North Am 1984;68:1171–1208.)

toms (many times per day) that are not clearly a result of an arrhythmia. In such patients, the recording of many episodes that turn out to be normal electrocardiographically provides strong and reassuring evidence against a dangerous cardiac arrhythmia. In addition, information about cardiac conduction, average heart rates, response of sinus rates to normal daily exertion, and the prominence of atrial ectopy, ventricular ectopy (premature beats), or both is also available and may be useful if an episode of palpitations is not captured.

Echocardiography

Echocardiography is usually helpful in diagnosing structural cardiac disease. Because many of the structural abnormalities (congenital heart disease, rhabdomyoma, endocarditis) associated with arrhythmias are difficult to diagnose on the basis of the physical examination and electrocardiographic results, certain patients re-

quire echocardiography. Patients whose symptoms are very worrisome (syncope, chest pain, dyspnea, prolonged duration) and who may have life-threatening episodes of tachycardia should undergo echocardiography. In most cases, the echocardiogram is normal.

Transtelephonic Incident Monitoring

When symptoms are not a daily occurrence, Holter monitoring is inefficient, because several consecutive Holter recordings may need to be made to capture a single episode. Such an approach frequently fails altogether. Transtelephonic incident recorders are small, battery-powered devices that the patient carries for 1 month or more. When the symptom occurs, the patient makes a recording by placing the device on the chest or connecting it to wrist electrodes. A single ECG lead is recorded into the device's memory for 60 to 90 seconds. The patient then plays the recording back over the telephone to the clinician's office or monitoring center.

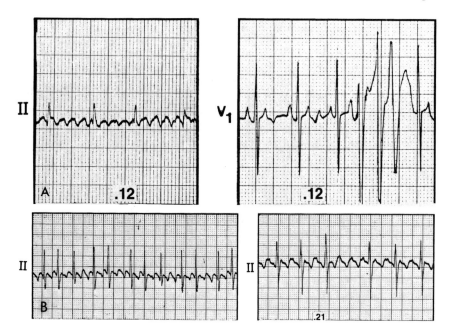

Figure 12–7. *A,* Atrial flutter in infants. In the left tracing, classic flutter waves (sawtooth waves) are seen at an atrial rate of 500 per minute with 4:1 and 5:1 atrioventricular (AV) conduction. In the right tracing, blocked premature atrial contractions follow the first two QRS complexes. Then there are two beats of atrial flutter. The rapid wide QRS rhythm on the right results from 1:1 AV conduction of atrial flutter at a ventricular rate of 460 per minute. *B,* The tracing on the left is taken from a 3-month-old child. The atrial rate is 375 per minute with 2:1 and 3:1 conduction. The tracing on the right is taken from a 16-year-old. The atrial rate is 285 per minute with varying 4:1 and 2:1 AV conduction. (From Garson A. Arrhythmias in pediatric patients. Med Clin North Am 1984;68:1171–1208.)

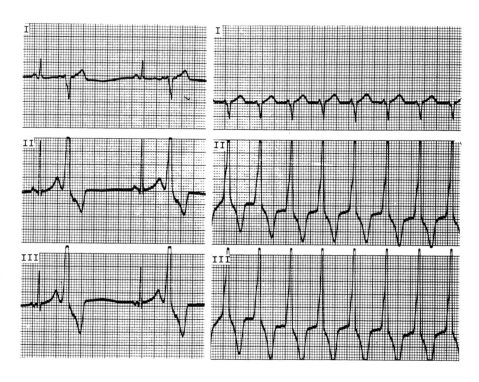

Figure 12–8. Paroxysmal ventricular tachycardia in a 14-year-old boy with no other evidence of organic heart disease. The ectopic ventricular beats are probably left ventricular in origin. Retrograde atrial capture is present. (From Chou T-C. Sinus rhythms. In Chou T-C [ed]. Electrocardiography in Clinical Practice, 3rd ed. Philadelphia: WB Saunders, 1991:395.

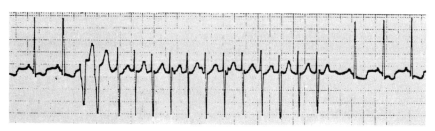

Figure 12–9. Tracing from a newborn infant with ventricular tachycardia and a "narrow" QRS complex. After two sinus beats, there are two obviously wide premature ventricular contractions. This initiates ventricular tachycardia. There is atrioventricular dissociation. The QRS complexes are narrow but have a completely different morphology from that of the sinus QRS. (From Garson A. Arrhythmias in pediatric patients. Med Clin North Am 1984;68:1171–1208.)

Figure 12–10. Torsades de pointes resulting from quinidine administration. The tracing shows a basic sinus rhythm. There is a marked prolongation of the QT interval, measuring 0.56 second. In the bottom strip, there is an ectopic ventricular beat falling on the T wave of the preceding sinus beat. The ectopic beat initiates an episode of ventricular tachyarrhythmia. The tachycardia has a rate of about 200 beats per minute. The RR interval is irregular. The QRS complexes have a negative polarity in the first part of the episode and an upright polarity in the second part. (From Chou T-C. Sinus rhythms. *In* Chou T-C [ed]. Electrocardiography in Clinical Practice, 3rd ed. Philadelphia: WB Saunders, 1991:399.)

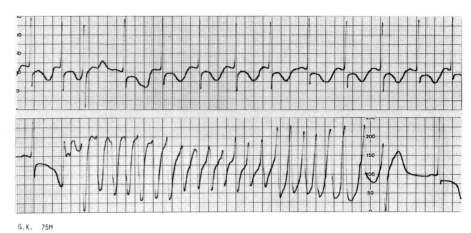

The unit generates a series of signals that are decoded by the monitoring center into the ECG. For very transient symptoms, devices are available that are connected to the patient like a Holter monitor that continuously record the heart rhythm in a memory loop. When the patient experiences a symptom, he or she presses a button, which causes the device to store the ECG for the 30 to 45 seconds before as well as for a short period after the button was pushed.

Exercise Testing

In some patients, an exercise test helps to elicit an episode of tachycardia or irregular heart rhythm and is recommended when symptoms are primarily exercise-related. The patient's ECG and blood pressure are monitored while the patient runs on a treadmill or rides a stationary bicycle. During the test, the work load is increased in discrete steps. The ECG is monitored both during exercise and in the recovery phase.

Electrophysiologic Study

For carefully selected patients, the definitive method of diagnosing the mechanism of an arrhythmia is the invasive electrophysiologic study (EPS), which is a form of cardiac catheterization. Two to four electrode catheters are inserted into the cardiac chambers via the veins or arteries and are positioned in various sites for pacing and for recording of intracardiac conduction signals. Atrioventricular conduction may be carefully studied, and sustained tachycardias may be induced and diagnosed by programmed stimulation of the heart. Such testing is also useful in determining appropriate drug treatment of the arrhythmia.

MECHANISMS OF TACHYCARDIAS

Reentrant versus Automatic Tachycardias

Two common mechanisms for the tachyarrhythmias are seen in clinical practice: those caused by *reentry* and those caused by *increased automaticity*. The term reentry refers to the circular movement of impulses within the myocardium or conduction system. The term increased automaticity refers to the abnormal state in which specific localized cardiac cells display automatic repetitive depolarization at a rate faster than normal.

For a tachycardia to be termed reentrant, three conditions must be met. First, an anatomically distinct reentrant circuit must be present, allowing for the circular movement of excitation conduction. Second, an area of this potential reentrant circuit must be subject to delay in conduction. Third, unidirectional conduction block must occur, allowing subsequent reversed conduction in that segment (Fig. 12–12).

An example of a reentrant supraventricular tachyarrhythmia is the reciprocating atrioventricular reentrant tachycardia seen in patients with the Wolff-Parkinson-White syndrome (Figs. 12–3 and 12–13). A premature atrial contraction may block in the accessory pathway but be conducted down the atrioventricular node and the His-Purkinje system, but with significant delay. Impulses arriving in the ventricle are then conducted retrograde in the accessory pathway back to the atrium. The conduction delay in the atrioventricular node allows the accessory pathway and atrium sufficient time to recover and thus allows establishment of the tachycardia.

The *reentrant* tachycardias include sinoatrial and intra-atrial reentry, atrioventricular node reentry, atrioventricular reciprocating tachycardia involving an accessory pathway, atrial flutter, the permanent form of junctional reciprocating tachycardia, atrial fibrillation, and the reentrant form of ventricular tachycardia. Tachycardias caused by increased *automaticity* include sinus tachycardia, atrial ectopic tachycardia, junctional ectopic tachycardia, and (automatic focus) ventricular tachycardia.

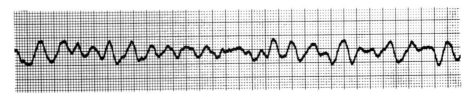

Figure 12–11. This tracing of ventricular fibrillation with no distinct QRS complex or T waves demonstrates irregular undulations with varied amplitude and contour and shows no palpable pulse. (From Chou T-C. Sinus rhythms. *In* Chou T-C [ed]. Electrocardiography in Clinical Practice, 3rd ed. Philadelphia: WB Saunders, 1991:403.)

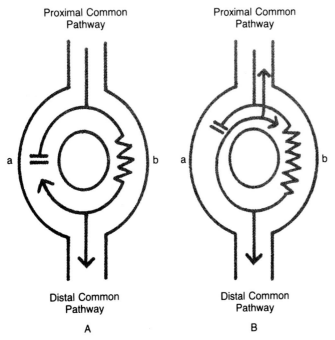

Figure 12–12. *Mechanism of reentry. Reentry requires the presence of two separate pathways that join proximally and distally. A, A premature impulse blocks antegradely in pathway "a" (double bars) but conducts down pathway "b," albeit with a moderate conduction delay (serpentine arrow). The impulse attempts to return up pathway "a" but meets refractory tissue. B, A more premature impulse blocks earlier in pathway "a" and experiences more conduction delay in pathway "b." This impulse finds pathway "a" recovered from its previous activation and returns retrogradely to the proximal common pathway. If able to again travel antegradely over pathway "b," it would activate the distal common pathway prematurely. If this cycle were to continue, a circus movement or reentrant tachycardia would result. For example, in atrioventricular (AV) nodal reentrant tachycardia, the atrium represents the proximal common pathway and the His bundle represents the distal common pathway, with the reentrant circuit located within the AV node. (From Andreoli TE, Bennett JC, Carpenter CCJ, et al [eds]. Cecil Essentials of Medicine, 2nd ed. Philadelphia: WB Saunders, 1990:82.)*

A major characteristic of the reentrant tachycardias that allows differentiation from the automatic tachycardias is their tendency to start and stop suddenly. Premature atrial and ventricular contractions may initiate or terminate these rhythms. Direct-current cardioversion is usually successful in terminating reentrant tachycardias but not automatic focus tachycardias.

Sinus Tachycardia

Sinus tachycardia may masquerade as paroxysmal supraventricular tachycardia in children and is usually secondary to some other problem; a careful search for such problems may allow the diagnosis of sinus tachycardia (see Table 12–2). The gradual slowing of a narrow QRS tachycardia after an intravenous fluid bolus in a patient thought to have intravascular depletion provides strong evidence for sinus tachycardia and against other forms of paroxysmal supraventricular tachycardia. Other causes of sinus tachycardia include high fever, pain, hypoxia, hyperthyroidism, seizures, chronotropic agents (isoproterenol or dobutamine), and sedation in paralyzed, patients undergoing ventilation.

The criteria for *sinus tachycardia* are:

- Normal P-wave axis
- Gradual onset and termination
- Heart rates below 250 beats per minute (bpm)

Rates above 250 bpm rule out sinus tachycardia, whereas narrow complex tachycardias below 250 bpm are often sinus tachycardias.

Sinus tachycardia must be ruled out, if possible, before antiarrhythmic therapy is instituted. The diagnosis may be quite difficult in children because the P wave may be hidden on the preceding T wave. Several leads should be carefully analyzed for deformation of the T wave by a P wave. Vagal maneuvers and other methods for converting supraventricular tachycardia do not terminate sinus tachycardia. Vagal maneuvers may briefly slow the rhythm, but because the underlying cause of sinus tachycardia is unaffected by such maneuvers, the rhythm resumes immediately. Therapy should be directed to the likely underlying causes of the sinus tachycardia. The response to such measures may well be diagnostic.

MECHANISMS OF BRADYCARDIA

Sinus Bradycardia

Sinus bradycardia is recognized as a regular, slow atrial rate with normal P waves and 1:1 conduction. Causes include hypoxia, acidosis, increased intracranial pressure, abdominal distention, and hypoglycemia. Agents such as digoxin, organophosphate pesticides, and propranolol may cause sinus bradycardia. Mild heart rate slowing may also be due to increased vagal tone or cardiac conditioning in a trained athlete.

Atrioventricular Block

Complete atrioventricular block may be congenital, may be surgically induced, or may occur suddenly as a result of myocarditis. It is recognized as atrioventricular dissociation and regular RR intervals, regular PP intervals, an atrial rate greater than the ventricular rate, and the absence of capture beats. Associated features of congenital AV block include maternal systemic lupus erythemato-

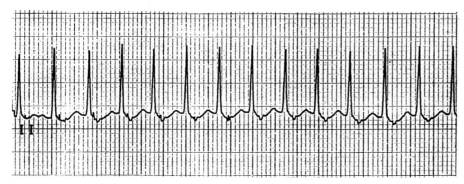

Figure 12–13. *Rhythm strip, lead II, in a patient with supraventricular tachycardia caused by an accessory pathway (same patient as in Fig. 12–3). Note the normalization of QRS duration in tachycardia versus the prolonged QRS duration in sinus rhythm (see Fig. 12–3) as a result of the loss of antegrade accessory pathway conduction in favor of retrograde accessory pathway conduction during tachycardia as well as the clear P wave seen on the upstroke of the T wave, closest to the previous QRS complex.*

sus (diagnosed or asymptomatic; anti-Ro antibody positive), while associated features of acquired heart block may include those of Lyme disease, Kearns-Sayre syndrome (mitochondrial inheritance, weakness, progressive external ophthalmoplegia, pigmentary retinal degeneration), or myotonic dystrophy (myotonia, weakness).

Second-degree atrioventricular block should be classified as *Mobitz type 1 (Wenckebach)* or *Mobitz type 2.* Wenckebach conduction is characterized by progressive PR interval prolongation followed by a blocked beat, followed by recovery of conduction. Type 2 block lacks this characteristic PR prolongation with shortening after the blocked beat. Type 1 generally carries a better prognosis than does type 2 and readily responds to medication.

Other causes of bradycardia are (1) sinus exit block, in which sinus P waves intermittently disappear as a result of block of impulses leaving the region of the sinus node, and (2) frequent premature atrial contractions, which occur too early to be conducted to the ventricles and which therefore slow the resulting ventricular rate.

MECHANISMS OF PREMATURE BEATS

Supraventricular Premature Contractions

Supraventricular premature contractions are narrow and early QRS beats. They occasionally may also have wide QRS complexes as a result of an associated bundle branch aberration. Those that originate in the atrium (*premature atrial contractions* [PACs]) may be recognizable by the finding of a premature P wave superimposed on the previous T wave, deforming it (see Fig. 12–4). This sign may be subtle, requiring the examination of multiple leads.

Ventricular Premature Complexes

Ventricular premature complexes (PVCs) are recognizable as wide, often bizarre early beats, generally without preceding P waves. The differentiation between ventricular contractions and aberrantly conducted supraventricular contractions is sometimes difficult or impossible from the surface ECG. Although traditionally, premature ventricular beats may be differentiated from supraventricular beats by the presence of a full compensatory pause (see Fig. 12–5), this sign is unreliable. The identification of fusion beats, in which a sinus beat occurs simultaneously with a premature beat, thus creating an intermediate morphology, is helpful and establishes the premature beat as ventricular in origin.

DIAGNOSTIC EVALUATION OF PALPITATIONS

The starting point in the diagnostic evaluation of palpitations is a careful history and physical examination and the recording of a baseline ECG (i.e., while the patient is not having the symptom). The approach is summarized in the flow diagram in Figure 12–14. In obtaining the patient's history, one is attempting to determine (1) whether the rhythm abnormality might be caused by a life-threatening problem; (2) whether it is likely that the patient is experiencing episodes of tachycardia, premature beats, or bradycardia; (3) whether the symptoms are exercise related; and (4) whether there is structural cardiac disease.

During the physical examination, one is looking for evidence of structural heart disease. On the ECG, one is looking for obvious evidence of a problem, such as a prolonged QT interval or the Wolff-Parkinson-White syndrome. The QT interval varies with the heart rate. A corrected QTc interval may be determined by dividing the QT interval by the square root of the RR interval. The normal QTc interval should be less than 0.44 second.

One may suspect a life-threatening problem if the episodes of palpitations are associated with near-syncope, syncope, severe chest pain, or aborted sudden death or if there is a family history of the long QT syndrome or unexplained sudden death. Patients with a long QT interval are treated with beta-adrenergic receptor blocking agents and avoidance of proarrhythmia drugs, which prolong the QT interval (see Table 12–1). Patients with normal QT intervals but who may have a life-threatening problem are referred for invasive electrophysiologic evaluation, to avoid delay in capturing an episode and to initiate appropriate and early treatment of a dangerous arrhythmia.

Patients who do not have obvious evidence of a life-threatening arrhythmia are then differentiated by whether they are likely to be experiencing episodes of tachycardia versus premature beats or bradycardia. Those with tachycardia proceed to a noninvasive evaluation (discussed later), with the goal of capturing an episode electrocardiographically for the purpose of diagnosis. If there is evidence of structural cardiac disease, an echocardiogram is obtained. Likewise, if there is electrocardiographic evidence of Wolff-Parkinson-White syndrome, an echocardiogram is obtained, primarily to rule out the possibility of an associated Ebstein anomaly of the tricuspid valve. In patients who are likely to have premature beats or bradycardia with no evidence of structural cardiac disease or an abnormal ECG, noninvasive evaluation is considered optional and is performed according to the severity of the symptoms. If there is structural cardiac disease or an abnormal ECG (e.g., complete atrioventricular block), an echocardiogram is obtained, followed by a noninvasive evaluation. An invasive electrophysiologic study may be recommended, depending on the results of the noninvasive evaluation and the severity of the symptoms.

Noninvasive evaluation involves the use of any of the modalities for diagnosis that do not involve intracardiac electrophysiologic study. The goal is to capture an episode of the patient's symptom electrocardiographically. The approach is summarized in the flow diagram shown in Figure 12–15. Patients whose symptoms are brought on by exercise may be referred for exercise testing in hopes that the test will reproduce the abnormal rhythm. If the results of the exercise test are negative or if the symptoms are unrelated to exercise, consideration of the frequency of symptoms leads to use of either a Holter monitor, for those with daily symptoms, or transtelephonic incident recording, for those with less frequent symptoms. If incident recording is used, it is important to choose the correct mode for recording. In general, if the episodes last less than 30 seconds, it is difficult for the patient or parent to produce the monitor, connect it, and make a recording before the symptom resolves. In such patients, the use of a continuous memory-loop recorder is recommended.

When a symptomatic episode is recorded, it is important to determine, by discussion with the patient, whether the symptom was in fact typical, because benign arrhythmias may coexist with more serious conditions. Recording of multiple episodes may increase the reliability of the diagnosis, particularly in patients who do not have a cardiac arrhythmia when they are symptomatic.

Electrocardiographic Diagnosis

The electrocardiographic diagnosis of the arrhythmia's mechanism is vital for determining the best treatment, particularly when antiarrhythmic medications are contemplated. Failure to document the tachycardia can often lead to inappropriate treatment of patients experiencing sinus tachycardia or benign premature contractions.

An initial determination is made as to whether the QRS duration

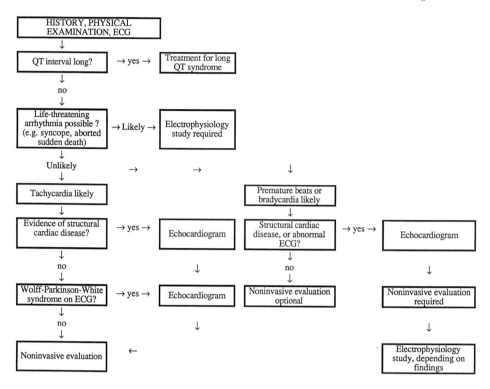

Figure 12–14. Flow diagram for evaluation of palpitations.

and morphology during tachycardia are normal or increased. The "narrow" QRS tachycardias are usually caused by supraventricular tachycardia (Table 12–4). The "wide" QRS tachycardias may be caused by either ventricular tachycardia or supraventricular tachycardia with sustained aberration conduction or bundle branch block; in children, most wide complex tachycardias are ventricular tachycardias (Table 12–5).

Next, the relationship between P waves and QRS complexes is determined, if possible; this relationship is often diagnostic (see Table 12–4). For example, a narrow QRS tachycardia with atrioventricular dissociation and an atrial rate lower than the ventricular

rate may be diagnosed as junctional ectopic tachycardia. For rhythms with a 1:1 relationship between P waves and QRS complexes, the relative timing of the respective waves is often helpful (i.e., P waves close to preceding QRS, close to following QRS, or on top of QRS). These characteristics help to differentiate between accessory pathway tachycardia, atrial tachycardia, and atrioventricular node reentry. These observations are not completely reliable, but an exact electrophysiologic diagnosis may not be necessary for initial decisions concerning treatment.

TREATMENT

Tachycardia

Immediate treatment of patients with sustained symptomatic tachycardia starts with an assessment of the patient's hemodynamic status. Patients with signs of shock require immediate cardioversion, whatever the mechanism of tachycardia. Other modalities may be tried first in patients who are less symptomatic. Patients with prolonged QRS durations should probably undergo electrical cardioversion because of the high likelihood that the prolonged durations are caused by ventricular tachycardia. Intravenous lidocaine may be used alternatively, provided that the diagnosis of ventricular tachycardia is certain and the hemodynamic status is stable. In uncertain cases, intravenous procainamide may be used because it is effective in ventricular tachycardia as well as in most forms of supraventricular tachycardia.

Patients with normal QRS durations should initially be approached with several maneuvers designed to increase vagal tone. Older children may be coached through a Valsalva maneuver or facial immersion in ice water, whereas younger children may have gagging induced, have rectal stimulation, or, more often, have an ice bag applied to the face. Although these measures often work, a time limit should be placed on them, so that the patient's hemodynamic status does not deteriorate during prolonged unsuccessful

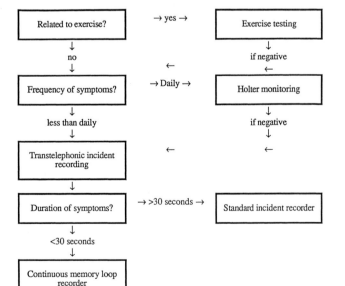

Figure 12–15. Flow diagram for noninvasive evaluation of palpitations.

Table 12–4. Mechanisms of Tachycardia with Normal QRS Duration

Diagnosis	Electrocardiographic Findings
Reentrant Tachycardias	
Atrial and sinoatrial reentry	P waves present, precede next QRS complex Terminates with QRS rather than P wave Variable AV conduction possible—AV block does not terminate atrial rhythm P-wave axis may be superior or inferior, depending on origin
Atrial flutter	Sawtooth flutter waves AV block does not terminate atrial rhythm Atrial rate 300 in older children, up to 500 in newborns

Accessory pathway–mediated tachycardia (Wolff-Parkinson-White syndrome and concealed accessory pathway)	P waves follow QRS, typically on upstroke of T wave
	Superior or rightward
	  P-wave axis
	AV block always terminates tachycardia
	Typically terminates with
	  P wave
	After termination, those with Wolff-Parkinson-White have preexcitation

Permanent form of junctional reciprocating tachycardia	Incessant P waves precede QRS Inverted P waves in II, III, AVF AV block always terminates tachycardia May terminate with QRS or with P wave No preexcitation after termination
Atrioventricular node reentry	P waves usually not visible, are superimposed on QRS AV block usually terminates tachycardia
Atrial fibrillation (probably reentrant)	"Irregularly irregular"—no two RR intervals exactly the same P waves difficult to see, or bizarre and chaotic
Increased Automaticity	
Sinus tachycardia	Normal P-wave axis P waves precede QRS Caused by extrinsic factor, e.g., heart failure, fever, anemia, catecholamine, or theophylline infusion Continues in presence of AV block
Atrial ectopic tachycardia	Incessant Abnormal P-wave axis, which predicts location of focus P waves precede QRS Continues in presence of AV block
Junctional ectopic tachycardia	Incessant Usually with AV dissociation and slower atrial than ventricular rate Capture beats with no fusion

Abbreviation: AV = atrioventricular.

attempts. If maneuvers fail, the administration of adenosine intravenously is the preferred approach (Table 12–6), with continuous electrocardiographic monitoring in a room with a cardioverter-defibrillator available. The agent is given by very rapid intravenous injection at an initial dose of 0.05 mg/kg, and the ECG is observed for 10 to 15 seconds. If there is no effect, the dose is repeatedly doubled until a dose of 0.40 mg/kg is reached (24 mg in adolescents and adults). In patients with tachycardia involving the atrioventricular node (accessory pathway tachycardia, atrioventricular node reentry), adenosine should bring about termination by its effect of stopping atrioventricular conduction for 1 to 2 seconds. In patients with sinus or atrial tachycardia or atrial flutter, adenosine causes a short episode of atrioventricular block, and the underlying atrial rhythm is revealed on the continuous electrocardiographic recording. If the diagnosis is shown to be atrial tachycardia or flutter, patients older than 6 months may receive intravenous verapamil.

Those younger than 6 months should never receive verapamil; instead, they may undergo pace conversion using esophageal pacing or cardioversion or may receive intravenous procainamide.

Many patients may not require long-term treatment if the episodes are not severely symptomatic and are either self-limited or easily converted with vagal maneuvers. If suppressive drug therapy is indicated, depending on the likely diagnosis, various medications may be used, including digoxin, beta blockers, verapamil, flecainide, sotalol, and amiodarone. The last three agents are more potent antiarrhythmic agents than the former and are also associated with increased risk of side effects.

Finally, intracardiac catheter ablation techniques during cardiac catheterization using radiofrequency energy are available for pediatric patients with nearly all forms of abnormal tachycardia and may be offered to ease life-threatening tachycardia. In older children, this treatment may be used as an alternative to long-term

Table 12–5. Mechanisms of Tachycardia with Prolonged QRS Duration

Diagnosis	Findings on Electrocardiogram
Ventricular tachycardia	Often with AV dissociation Capture beats with narrower QRS than on other beats Fusion beats
Supraventricular tachycardia with preexisting bundle branch block	QRS morphology similar to that in sinus rhythm QRS morphology is that of right or left bundle branch block
Supraventricular tachycardia with rate-dependent bundle branch block	QRS morphology usually similar to that of right or left bundle branch block Rare in small children Difficult to distinguish from ventricular tachycardia in children
Antidromic supraventricular tachycardia in Wolff-Parkinson-White syndrome	QRS morphology similar to preexcited sinus rhythm, but wider Never with AV dissociation
Atrial fibrillation with Wolff-Parkinson-White syndrome	"Irregularly irregular"—wide QRS tachycardia

Abbreviation: AV = atrioventricular.

medication therapy, or in younger children, it may be used when medication fails to control the tachycardia.

Bradycardia

The hemodynamic effect of a slow heart rate depends on how different it is from the patient's usual heart rate. Sudden decreases in rate may be poorly compensated by increases in stroke volume, particularly in those with preexisting poor cardiac function. Moderate sinus bradycardia in normal children rarely necessitates treatment. Underlying causes, such as hypothyroidism, should be corrected. Patients with third-degree atrioventricular block and those with severe sinus node dysfunction may require permanent artificial cardiac pacing. In all cases, the occurrence of symptoms (over and above the symptom of palpitations) such as syncope, exercise intolerance, or dizziness prompts pacing. With severe sinus node dysfunction, pacing may be required if the patient is to be given antiarrhythmic agents to suppress episodes of tachycardia because of the danger that such medications will worsen sinus node dysfunction. Patients with persisting complete atrioventricular block as a result of cardiac surgery generally require pacing, even in the absence of symptoms. Prophylactic cardiac pacing may be recommended in completely asymptomatic patients with complete congenital atrioventricular block if daytime average heart rates fall below 50, if nighttime rates are below 30, or if long pauses (>3 seconds) are recorded on Holter monitoring. This is because patients with these findings are at greater risk for progressing to syncope or sudden death.

Premature Beats

In the absence of tachycardia, patients only rarely need to be treated for premature beats of any kind. Patients with supraventricular premature contractions virtually never require treatment; those with ventricular premature contractions may require treatment in a few situations:

1. When the contractions are multiform.
2. When the contractions occur in couplets or in short runs of ventricular tachycardia.
3. When the contractions are seen in association with a recently converted ventricular tachycardia.

Table 12–6. Intravenous Antiarrhythmic Agents

Agent	Dosage	Comments
Verapamil	0.1–0.2 mg/kg IV, 5–10 mg maximum	Beware of hypotension. Definitely contraindicated under 6 months of age, probably under 12 months of age. Do *not* give with beta blockers.
Propranolol (beta blocker)	0.02 mg/kg IV every 5 minutes, to 0.1 mg/kg	Monitor pulse, blood pressure. Contraindicated in those with asthma and those with congestive heart failure. Do *not* give with verapamil.
Procainamide	15 mg/kg IV over 30 minutes	May cause hypotension; continuous monitoring is essential. Cardiology guidance is recommended.
Digoxin	10 μg/kg IV as initial load Second dose in 6 hr, third at 24 hr	Do not use in hypokalemia or if digoxin toxicity is suspected
Lidocaine	1–2 mg/kg IV over 15 minutes Continuous infusion 30–50 μg/kg/minute	
Phenylephrine	0.02 mg/kg IV slowly	Used for raising blood pressure and eliciting a baroreceptor vagal reflex.
Adenosine	Starting IV dose: 0.05 mg/kg; increment by 0.05 mg/kg repeatedly until effect is seen, to maximum of 0.4 mg/kg	Contraindicated in preexisting second- or third-degree AV block without pacemaker. Use with caution in severe asthma; half-life is 10 seconds in serum.

Abbreviations: AV = atrioventricular; IV = intravenously.

Table 12–7. Red Flags: Palpitations

Family history of sudden death
Syncope
Heart failure
Chest pain
Stroke
Prior cardiac surgery
Structural congenital heart surgery
Drug overdose
Hypotension
Exercise-induced
Prolonged duration
Exercise intolerance
Suicide attempt (drug overdose)

4. When the contractions exhibit the "R on T" phenomenon (i.e. they fall repeatedly on the early part of the T wave of the preceding beat).

Decisions concerning treatment of premature beats are difficult and should be made in consultation with a cardiologist. Possible inciting factors, such as drugs, hypoxia, and acidosis, should be corrected. If ventricular premature contractions require emergency treatment, the agent of choice is lidocaine, given by a continuous intravenous infusion. Bretylium has been used by some cardiologists to terminate ventricular tachycardia.

RED FLAGS

Table 12–7 lists the red flags associated with palpitations that warrant immediate attention and evaluation.

REFERENCES

Etiology

Brugada P, Gursoy S, Brugada J, et al. Investigation of palpitations. Lancet 1993;341:1254–1258.
Dungan WT, Garson A, Gillette PC. Arrhythmogenic right ventricular dysplasia: A cause of ventricular tachycardia in children with apparently normal hearts. Am Heart J 1981;102:745–750.
Frustaci A, Caldarulo M, Buffon A, et al. Cardiac biopsy in patients with "primary" atrial fibrillation. Histologic evidence of occult myocardial diseases. Chest 1991;100:303–306.
Klitzner TS. Arrhythmias in the general pediatric population: An overview. Pediatr Ann 1991;20:347–349.
Lambert EC, Menon R, Wagner HR, et al. Sudden unexpected death from cardiovascular disease in children. Am J Cardiol 1974;34:89–96.
Mendelsohn A, Dick M, Serwer GA. Natural history of isolated atrial flutter in infancy. J Pediatr 1991;119:386–391.
Murgatroyd FD, Camm AJ. Atrial arrhythmias. Lancet 1993;341:1317–1322.
O'Connor BK, Dick M. What every pediatrician should know about supraventricular tachycardia. Pediatr Ann 1991;20:368–377.
Schmidt KG, Ulmer HE, Silverman NH, et al. Perinatal outcome of fetal complete atrioventricular block: A multicenter experience. J Am Coll Cardiol 1991;17:1360–1366.

Scott WA. Evaluating the child with syncope. Pediatr Ann 1991;20:350–359.
Silka MJ. Sudden death due to cardiovascular disease during childhood. Pediatr Ann 1991;20:360–367.
Vetter VL. What every pediatrician needs to know about arrhythmias in children who have had cardiac surgery. Pediatr Ann 1991;20:378–385.
Yabek SM. Ventricular arrhythmias in children with an apparently normal heart. J Pediatr 1991;119:1–11.

Pathogenesis

Ben-David J, Zipes DP. Torsades de pointes and proarrhythmia. Lancet 1993;341:1578–1582.
Campbell RWF. Ventricular ectopic beats and non-sustained ventricular tachycardia. Lancet 1993;341:1454–1458.
Shenasa M, Borggrefe M, Haverkamp W, et al. Ventricular tachycardia. Lancet 1993;341:1512–1518.
Waldo AL, Wit AL. Mechanisms of cardiac arrhythmias. Lancet 1993;341:1189–1194.

Treatment

Azancot-Benistry A, Jacqz-Aigrain E, Guirgis NM, et al. Clinical and pharmacologic study of fetal supraventricular tachyarrhythmias. J Pediatr 1992;121:608–613.
Deal BJ, Keane JF, Gillette PC, et al. Wolff-Parkinson-White syndrome and supraventricular tachycardia during infancy: Management and follow-up. J Am Coll Cardiol 1985;5:130–135.
Funck-Brentano C, Kroemer HK, Lee JT, et al. Propafenone. N Engl J Med 1990;322:518–525.
Garratt CJ, Malcolm AD, Camm AJ. Adenosine and cardiac arrhythmias: The preferred treatment for supraventricular tachycardia. BMJ 1992;305:3–4.
Garson A Jr, Gillette PC, McVey P, et al. Amiodarone treatment of critical arrhythmias in children and young adults. J Am Coll Cardiol 1984;4:749–755.
Garson A Jr, Randall DC, Gillette PC, et al. Prevention of sudden death after repair of tetralogy of Fallot: Treatment of ventricular arrhythmias. J Am Coll Cardiol 1985;6:221–227.
Jackman WM, Beckman KJ, McClelland JH, et al. Treatment of supraventricular tachycardia due to atrioventricular nodal reentry by radiofrequency catheter ablation of slow-pathway conduction. N Engl J Med 1992;327:313–318.
Klitzner TS, Wetzel GT, Saxon LA, et al. Radiofrequency ablation: A new era in the treatment of pediatric arrhythmias. Am J Dis Child 1993;147:769–771.
Kugler JD, Danford DA. Pacemakers in children: An update. Am Heart J 1989;117:665–679.
Moak JP, Smith RT, Garson A Jr. Newer antiarrhythmic drugs in children. Am Heart J 1987;113:179–185.
Perry JC, Garson A. Diagnosis and treatment of arrhythmias. Adv Pediatr 1989;36:177–200.
Perry JC, McQuinn RL, Smith RT, et al. Flecainide acetate for resistant arrhythmias in the young: Efficacy and pharmacokinetics. J Am Coll Cardiol 1989;14:185–191.
Pritchett ELC. Management of atrial fibrillation. N Engl J Med 1992;326:1264–1271.
Ralston MA, Knilans, TK, Hannon DW, et al. Use of adenosine for diagnosis and treatment of tachyarrhythmias in pediatric patients. J Pediatr 1994;124:139–143.
Sreeram N, Wren C. Supraventricular tachycardia in infants: Response to initial treatment. Arch Dis Child 1990;65:127–129.
Van Hare GF, Lesh MD, Scheinman MM, et al. Percutaneous radiofrequency catheter ablation for supraventricular arrhythmias in children. J Am Coll Cardiol 1991;17:1613–1620.

13 Heart Failure

Dennis P. Ruggerie

HEART FAILURE PARADIGMS

Our understanding of heart failure involves various clinical and basic science concepts. Clinically, organ failure describes heart failure as altered pump function and abnormal hemodynamic responses. Governed by Starling's law, cardiac performance is viewed in terms of impaired ejection and filling volumes and low cardiac output. Circulatory consequences rest in the balance between the neurohumoral adaptive mechanisms of peripheral vascular constriction (afterload) with salt and water retention (preload) versus vasodilation and salt excretion.

A second paradigm describes heart failure in terms of cell biochemistry. For example, the clinical manifestations of heart failure would be viewed in terms of altered diastolic as well as systolic intracellular Ca^{+2} fluxes.

Another developing paradigm suggests that altered myocardial gene expression may play an important role in determining the physiologic adjustments to acute and chronic changes affecting the individual cells of the heart and circulation. This paradigm provides a cellular and molecular understanding of the long-term adaptive cellular processes produced by congenital malformations and acquired diseases, such as pulmonary vascular obstructive disease, myocardial hypertrophy, and irreversible heart failure.

WHAT IS HEART FAILURE?

To meet systemic aerobic metabolic requirements, the supply and transport of oxygen to growing and developing tissues require integration and regulation of the lungs, heart and circulation, and blood. Oxygen participates in the cellular production of adenosine (ATP), which supports cellular processes such as tissue growth and development and maintenance (e.g., electromechanical work). The heart is vital in coordinating the peripheral tissue delivery of oxygen at rest or during periods of increased oxygen consumption (infection, inflammation, fever, exercise). Cardiac performance can be altered by ventricular myocardial stresses. A ventricular stress

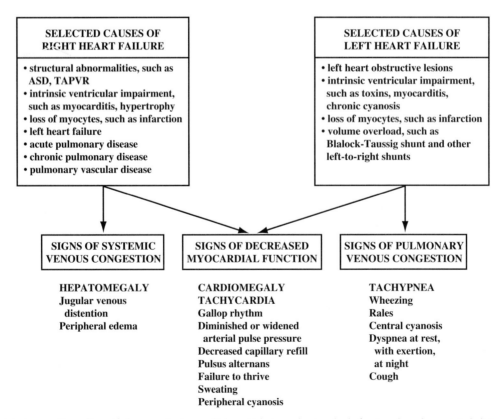

Figure 13–1. Physiologic paradigm of heart failure, emphasizing which ventricle is predominantly dysfunctional, and associated clinical signs and symptoms. ASD = atrial septal defect; TAPVR = total anomalous pulmonary venous return. (From Ruggerie, DP: Congestive heart failure. *In* Blumer J [ed]. Practical Guide to Pediatric Intensive Care, 3rd ed. St. Louis: Mosby Year Book, 1990.)

Table 13–1. Signs and Symptoms of Heart Failure by Age

Fetus	Premature Infant	Full-Term Neonate–Infant	Child	Adolescent
Hydrops fetalis*	Tachycardia*	Tachycardia*	Breathlessness*	Same as child*
Polyhydramnios	Cardiomegaly*	Tachypnea*	Tachycardia*	Delayed sexual maturity*
	Pallor*	Feeding difficulties*	Tachypnea*	Orthopnea
	Peripheral vasoconstriction*	Excessive perspiration*	Cardiomegaly*	Syncope
		Cardiomegaly*		
	Wide pulse pressure*	Gallop rhythm*	Hepatomegaly*	Peripheral edema
	Increased oxygen requirement	Hepatomegaly*	Peripheral edema	Rales
	Hepatomegaly	Failure to thrive*	Eyelid puffiness	Gallop rhythm
			Rales, wheezes cough	
		Shock*	Neck vein distention	
		Hepatic dysfunction	Fatigue, weakness	
		Wheezing	Ascites, effusion	
		Rales		
		Cough		

Adapted from Ruggerie DP. Congestive heart failure. *In* Blumer J (ed). Practical Guide to Pediatric Intensive Care, 3rd ed. St. Louis: Mosby–Year Book, 1990.
*Common findings.

due to pressure or volume overload, depressed contractility, or myocyte loss produces a cellular and molecular response characterized by reactive hypertrophy with the potential for subsequent further decrease in contractility and diastolic function. This response is mediated through hemodynamic factors as well as neurohumoral activation. The clinical manifestations of heart failure are the result of these hemodynamic alterations, myocardial remodeling, and neurohumoral responses.

Heart failure is a symptom complex that includes tachypnea, tachycardia, systemic venous congestion (hepatomegaly), and cardiomegaly (Fig. 13–1 and Table 13–1). Heart failure may be considered a relatively stable altered perfusion state in which compensatory mechanisms support vital organ functions but may result in symptoms. Shock is an unstable cardiac state in which compensatory mechanisms become exhausted and tissue hypoxia ensues. Untreated shock leads to death.

AGE-RELATED AND DEVELOPMENTAL ISSUES

The age of onset of heart failure serves as a guide to differential diagnosis of the underlying etiology (Table 13–2). The most common cause of heart failure in the fetus is nonimmune hydrops (Table 13–3). Patent ductus arteriosus (PDA) is the most common cause of heart failure in premature infants with respiratory distress

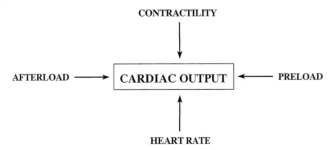

Figure 13–2. The determinants of cardiac output. (From Ruggerie DP. Congestive heart failure. *In* Blumer J [ed]. Practical Guide to Pediatric Intensive Care, 3rd ed. St. Louis: Mosby Year Book, 1990.)

syndrome (RDS). Delayed closure of the ductus arteriosus and rapidly falling pulmonary vascular resistance in infants younger than 32 weeks of gestation recovering from RDS lead to early and hemodynamically significant left-to-right shunting through a ductus arteriosus or, less often, a ventricular septal defect (VSD).

Cardiac muscle dysfunction is a common cause of heart failure during the first day of life in full-term newborns and is usually due to perinatal hypoxic-ischemic events at times complicated by hypoglycemia. Heart failure caused by structural lesions typically manifests shortly after closure of the ductus arteriosus and subsequent acute increase in left ventricular afterload. Frequently, the clinical presentation is shock. The most common lesions that produce heart failure and that are ductal-dependent are coarctation of the aorta and hypoplastic left heart syndrome. Right-sided obstructive lesions also present at this time because of a reduction in total pulmonary blood flow secondary to ductal closure. Tetralogy of Fallot, hypoplastic right heart syndrome (tricuspid atresia, pulmonary atresia), and critical pulmonary stenosis are common lesions. However, the initial clinical symptom in these infants is cyanosis (see Chapter 15).

As transitional circulatory changes, including a significant reduction of pulmonary vascular resistance, continue through the first 4 to 8 weeks of life, structural heart defects associated with left-to-right shunts typically are present. Onset of heart failure relates to the rapidity of the postnatal fall of pulmonary vascular resistance. The most common lesion in this group is a ventricular septal defect (see Table 13–2) (see Chapter 16).

In older infants, children, and adolescents acquired heart disease plays a more common etiologic role. Myocarditis and cardiomyopathy are common causes of acquired heart disease at this age (Table 13–4; see Table 13–2).

An important concept is that myocardial contractility increases with age. The basic processes that control cardiac output appear to be the same in the fetal, neonatal, and adolescent heart (Fig. 13–2). At all ages, heart rate is the dominant mechanism augmenting cardiac output. The newborn heart functions at a high diastolic volume, which limits preload reserve. This has clinical importance when presented with an increased volume load, such as a left-to-right shunt or hypervolemia. Fetal myocardial contraction is weaker than adult sarcomere contraction. This assumes clinical importance in adaptation to acute increases in afterload, as might be encountered with coarctation of the aorta or hypertension. Maturation enhances the contractile ability of the heart, and the clinical expres-

Table 13–2. Age-Based Approach to the Etiology of Heart Failure*

Fetus
  Severe anemia
  Supraventricular tachycardia
  Congenital heart block
  Ventricular tachycardia
  Complex congenital anomalies
  Myocarditis-cardiomyopathy
  Nonimmune hydrops (see Table 13–3)

Premature Infant
  Fluid overload
  Patent ductus arteriosus
  Ventricular septal defect
  Bronchopulmonary dysplasia (cor pulmonale)
  Hypertension (aortic-renal artery thrombosis)

First Week of Life
  Left heart obstructive defects
    Hypoplastic left heart syndrome
    Coarctation of aorta
    Interrupted aortic arch
    Aortic stenosis
    Mitral valve stenosis, atresia
    Total anomalous pulmonary venous return (obstructed)
  Left-to-right shunt
    PDA
    Arteriovenous malformations
    Aortopulmonary window
    Total anomalous venous return (unobstructed)
  Mixing lesions
    Truncus arteriosus
    Single ventricle
    Transposition of great arteries with ventricular septal defect
  Other
    Hypoxic-ischemic cardiomyopathy (asphyxia)
    Anemia
    Arrhythmias
    Sepsis
    Myocarditis
    Transposition of great arteries with intact ventricular septum
    Hypoglycemia
    Hypocalcemia

Older Neonate, Infant, or Toddler
  Left-to-right shunts
    Ventricular septal defect
    Patent ductus arteriosus
    Atrial septal defect (rare)
    Endocardial cushion defect
    Tricuspid atresia
  Other congenital heart defects
    Coarctation of the aorta
    Aortic stenosis
    Anomalous left coronary artery from the pulmonary artery
    Ebstein anomaly
    Absent pulmonary valve
    Critical pulmonary stenosis
  Acquired
    Arrhythmia (tachyarrhythmia, bradyarrhythmia)
    Anemia
    Myocarditis (see Table 13–4)
    Cardiomyopathy (see Table 13–4)
    Hypertension (see Tables 13–9, 13–10)
    Endocarditis
    Airway obstruction (acute, chronic, see Chapter 10)
    Arteriovenous malformation
    Kawasaki disease

School-Aged Child or Adolescent
  Myocarditis (see Table 13–4)
  Cardiomyopathy (see Table 13–4)
  Rheumatic fever
  Endocarditis
  Hypertension (see Tables 13–9, 13–10)
  Thyrotoxicosis
  Hemochromatosis
  Cancer therapy (radiation, adriamycin)
  Cor pulmonale (cystic fibrosis, chronic airway obstruction—sleep apnea syndrome)

*Following corrective or palliative heart surgery, ventricular failure may occur acutely in the postoperative period or may develop 1 to 20 years later. It may be due to prosthetic valve malfunction, progressive valve insufficiencies, endocarditis, ischemia, intrinsic myocardial failure resulting from cardiopulmonary bypass, surgical shunts, or natural progression of disease (i.e., single-ventricle, right pump failure after a Mustard operation, long-term cyanosis).

sion of the developmental differences results in the immature myocardium, demonstrating:

1. A decreased responsiveness to preload, hence the belief that the neonatal cardiac output is more heart rate dependent with less contractility reserve.
2. Greater ventricular stiffness.
3. A decreased inotropic responsive to catecholamines; that is, dose-response curves for dopamine and dobutamine are shifted to the right as higher dosages may be needed to achieve identical effects on cardiac output compared with the mature myocardial pharmacodynamic response.

EXAMINATION

The history and physical examinations remain essential methods both in the detection of heart disease and in the evaluation of its

severity. Achieving a calm patient in a quiet room speaks directly to the value of initial examination by observation of appearance and respiration. Spending a few minutes talking with the family may allow the patient to become familiarized with the physician. A good stethoscope is essential as auscultation is the primary test for assessing the heart (see Chapter 16). Because inflation of the blood pressure cuff may induce anxiety in the infant or child, it is often best to leave this part of the examination until the end.

A systemic head-to-toe inspection should be performed. Most major congenital anomalies recognizable at birth have an increased incidence of associated structural heart disease. Some syndromes may not become apparent until later infancy or childhood (such as Noonan and Williams syndromes) or adolescence (Marfan syndrome).

In the newborn, complete history taking often follows stabilization efforts as the presentation of heart failure is often acute, severe, and life-threatening. Nonetheless, a brief birth history should be obtained, including gestational age, Apgar scores, and any diffi-

Table 13–3. Selected Causes of Heart Failure in the Fetus

I. *Nonimmune Hydrops Fetalis**
  A. Cardiovascular
    1. Congenital heart disease
    2. Dysrhythmias (supraventricular tachycardia, congenital heart block)
    3. Myocarditis
    4. Complicated congenital heart disease
    5. Rhabdomyoma
  B. Hematologic
    1. Twin-twin transfusion, fetomaternal hemorrhage
    2. Arteriovenous malformation
    3. Alpha thalassemia
  C. Chromosomal
    1. Turner syndrome
    2. Trisomies 13, 18, 21
  D. Metabolic diseases
    1. Maternal diabetes (poor control)
    2. Gaucher and other storage diseases
  E. Infection
    1. Syphilis
    2. Cytomegalovirus
    3. Parvovirus (anemia)
    4. Chagas disease
    5. Toxoplasmosis
  F. Pulmonary
    1. Cystic adenomatoid malformation
    2. Diaphragmatic hernia
    3. Lymphangiectasia
  G. Hepatic-gastrointestinal
    1. Hepatitis
    2. Hepatic fibrosis
    3. Atresia
    4. Volvulus
    5. Chylous ascites
    6. Cystic fibrosis
  H. Renal
    1. Nephrosis
    2. Prune belly syndrome
  I. Tumor
    1. Neuroblastoma
    2. Placental chorioangioma
  J. Malformation complex
    1. Arthrogryposis
    2. Thanatophoric dysplasia
    3. Noonan syndrome

II. *Erythroblastosis Fetalis (Immune Hydrops Fetalis)*

*Group I represents the most common etiologic factors.

culties with pregnancy, labor, and delivery. Details of the prenatal course, delivery, maternal history (i.e., maternal diabetes, systemic lupus erythematosus, and drug usage), and further information about difficulties should be obtained after the newborn has been stabilized.

The infant with heart failure usually has a history of feeding difficulties. Normal infant feeding times are 10 to 20 minutes regardless of the age. Feeding duration with heart failure is generally 30 to 60 minutes with frequent interruptions due to dyspnea. Increased oxygen demand with feeding leads to increased work of breathing, which results in excessive perspiration, prolonged feeding duration, inadequate caloric intake, and possibly failure to thrive.

Children and adolescents in whom heart failure develops may have a history of known congenital or acquired heart disease or surgical interventions for congenital heart disease. Midline sternotomy and lateral thoracotomy incisional scars provide clear evidence of likely previous cardiac surgery. Others may have a history of general malaise; weight loss over several weeks; increasing respiratory effort with activity; difficulty with everyday activities, such as walking up stairs; breathlessness; palpitations; or possible delayed sexual maturation. A history of recurrent lower respiratory tract infections should prompt an investigation of possible underlying heart disease. In other children, the onset of febrile illness may "unmask" symptoms of heart failure that have previously been compensated.

PATTERN RECOGNITION

The key to the diagnosis of heart failure is the pattern recognition of signs and symptoms as manifestations of physiologic events. Although the physiology may be similar, the clinical manifestations of heart failure differ in the fetus through infancy, childhood, and adolescence (see Table 13–1).

The hallmarks (pattern recognition) of heart failure are:

- Tachypnea
- Tachycardia
- Cardiomegaly
- Hepatomegaly

Tachycardia and cardiomegaly are early signs of heart failure, followed by tachypnea. Hepatomegaly is a late sign. Splenomegaly is rarely associated with heart failure, and its presence suggests inferior vena cava obstruction, portal hypertension, anemia, infectious processes, or a myeloproliferative disorder (see Chapter 23). Despite compensatory mechanisms, heart failure may progress to shock.

Heart failure often leads to perturbations in respiratory function. Ventilation is assessed by auscultation of breath sounds and observation of respiratory effort; oxygenation is assessed by the absence of cyanosis. Respiratory distress is a clinical state of increased respiratory rate and work of breathing (intercostal-supraclavicular-subcostal retractions, nasal flaring, grunting) developed in an effort to maintain minute ventilation. Respiratory failure is a clinical state characterized by inadequate ventilation and/or inadequate oxygenation manifested by pallor or central cyanosis, labored respiratory effort, irregular or apneic respiratory pattern, and altered mental status (see Chapter 8).

Tachycardia, a sensitive but nonspecific sign of heart failure, is due to increased circulating endogenous catecholamines that augment cardiac output by increasing myocardial contractility and heart rate. The heart rate is increased and often fixed without respiratory variation. Sustained resting tachycardia greater than 160 beats per minute (BPM) in infants and greater than 100 BPM in children is common. Sustained heart rates greater than 220 BPM in infants and 150 BPM in children should prompt the possibility of supraventricular tachycardia, which may be the etiologic feature of the heart failure (see Chapter 12).

Tachypnea is due to increased pulmonary artery flow (left-to-right shunt), obstruction to pulmonary venous return (left heart obstructive defects or ventricular failure), or pulmonary edema and on occasion compensation for poor perfusion associated with metabolic acidosis. Mild to moderate degrees of hypoxemia or decreased cardiac output usually do not cause tachypnea; respiratory distress develops when either hypoxemia or cardiac output is severely diminished. When heart failure progresses and tachypnea alone cannot maintain minute ventilation, further signs of increased work of breathing develop. Rales, uncommon in infancy, are common in children and adolescents and represent pulmonary edema from advanced myocardial failure. Wheezing is more likely a result of intercurrent bronchiolitis, pneumonitis, or asthma but may be

Table 13–4. Etiology of Myocardial Disease

Familial-Hereditary
  Carnitine deficiency syndromes*
  Mitochondrial myopathy syndromes*
  Hypertrophic cardiomyopathy*
  Duchenne muscular dystrophy*
  Other muscular dystrophies (Becker, limb girdle)
  Myotonic dystrophy
  Kearns-Sayre (progressive external
    ophthalmoplegia)
  Friedreich ataxia
  Mucopolysaccharidosis
  Hemochromatosis
  Fabry disease
  Pompe disease (glycogen storage disease)
  Primary endocardial fibroelastosis
  Mucopolysaccharidosis (Hurler, Hunter, others)

Infection
  Viruses: coxsackievirus A and B,* human
    immunodeficiency virus (AIDS), echovirus,
    rubella, varicella, influenza, mumps, Epstein-
    Barr, measles, poliomyelitis
  Rickettsiae: Coxiella, Rocky Mountain spotted
    fever, typhus
  Bacteria: diphtheria, *Mycoplasma,*
    meningococcus, leptospirosis, Lyme disease,
    typhoid fever, tuberculosis, *Streptococcus,*
    listeriosis, psittacosis
  Parasites: Chagas disease, toxoplasmosis, *Loa
    loa, Toxocara canis,* schistosomiasis,
    cysticercosis, *Echinococcus,* trichinosis
  Fungi: histoplasmosis, coccidioidomycosis,
    actinomycosis

Metabolic, Nutritional, Endocrine
  Beriberi (thiamine deficiency)
  Keshan disease (selenium deficiency)
  Kwashiorkor
  Hypothyroidism
  Hyperthyroidism
  Carcinoid
  Pheochromocytoma
  Hypercholesterolemia
  Infant of diabetic mother*
  Hypoglycemia
  Hypocalcemia

Connective Tissue-Granulomatous Disease
  Systemic lupus erythematosus
  Scleroderma
  Churg-Strauss vasculitis
  Rheumatoid arthritis
  Rheumatic fever*
  Sarcoidosis
  Amyloidosis
  Dermatomyositis
  Periarteritis nodosa

Drugs-Toxins
  Doxorubicin*
  Cyclophosphamide
  Chloroquine
  Ipecac (emetine)
  Iron overload (hemosiderosis)
  Sulfonamides
  Mesalezine
  Chloramphenicol
  Hypersensitivity reaction (penicillin)
  Alcohol
  Irradiation
  Envenomations (snake, scorpion)

Coronary Arteries
  Kawasaki disease*
  Medial necrosis
  Anomalous left coronary artery

Other
  Anemia*
  Sickle cell anemia (sickling)*
  Hypertension*
  Cor pulmonale*
  Hypereosinophilic syndrome (Loeffler syndrome)
  Tachyarrhythmias*
  Endomyocardial fibrosis
  Ischemia-hypoxia
  Peripartum cardiomyopathy
  Idiopathic dilated cardiomyopathy (familial, enteroviral,
    autoimmune)
  Arrhythmogenic right ventricular dysplasia (familial and
    nonfamilial)
  Uhl right ventricular anomaly
  Histiocytoid (oncocytic, lipidosis) cardiomyopathy
  Acute eosinophilic necrotizing myocarditis
  Rhabdomyoma

Adapted from Behrman RE (ed). Nelson Textbook of Pediatrics, 14th ed. Philadelphia: WB Saunders, 1992.
*Relatively common causes of myocarditis-cardiomyopathy.

due to large airway compression by enlarged pulmonary arteries or a dilated left atrium and bronchial edema associated with interstitial pulmonary edema.

In addition to hepatomegaly, evidence of systemic venous congestion can be seen in older children and adolescents by the presence of distention of the neck veins. In children 6 years of age or older who are sitting upright, jugular venous distention should not be visible above the clavicle unless central venous pressure is elevated. If the patient is supine at 45°, jugular venous pulsations should not rise above an imaginary straight line from the clavicle across to the manubrium of the sternum. In the supine position, venous pulsations are always present unless the superior vena cava is not connected to the right atrium, as with Glenn or Fontan palliative cardiac operations.

Cardiac examination invariably reveals *cardiomegaly.* Inspection of the precordium may reveal a prominent precordium due to an enlarged heart. Nearly all shunt lesions are associated with increased palpable precordial activity, whereas heart failure from cardiomyopathy may have a relatively quiet precordium. The asymmetric precordium noted in infants and children with prolonged cardiomegaly is uncommon in the neonate. When present, a precordial prominence in the neonate is associated with lesions with altered prenatal hemodynamics, including arteriovenous malformations, tetralogy of Fallot with absent pulmonary valve, Ebstein's anomaly with severe tricuspid insufficiency, fetal dysrhythmias, and myocarditis. A visible precordial impulse is a normal finding frequently present in the term newborn and may be due to transient patency of a ductus arteriosus. In the absence of cardiopulmonary disease, this sign frequently disappears by 12 hours of age. A visible precordial impulse in the absence of ventricular overload is frequent in premature infants in whom there is less development of anterior thoracic and abdominal musculature. Premature infants who subsequently develop left-to-right shunts through a PDA may have visible and marked precordial activity.

A third heart sound may be a common and normal auscultatory finding in children, but a fourth heart sound is never normal and is limited to advanced cardiomyopathy. Frequently, a gallop rhythm is present in infants with heart failure. Additional auscultatory findings, such as first and second heart sounds, clicks, rubs, and murmurs, vary, depending on the underlying reason for the heart failure (see Chapter 16).

At all ages, the physical examination also defines the adequacy of the cardiac output. This is best accomplished by measuring heart rate and blood pressure and evaluating the adequacy of end-organ perfusion. Perfusion is best evaluated by cutaneous blood flow, central nervous system function and urine output. A rule for minimally acceptable systolic blood pressure over the age of 2 years has been approximated by the formula $70 + (2 \times$ age in years). Decreases in cardiac output are balanced by increases in heart rate and systemic vascular resistance aimed at maintaining blood pressure. Initial increases in systemic vascular resistance are clinically manifested in the extremities as prolonged capillary refill (normal < 2 to 3 seconds), cool temperature to touch, mottling or paleness of the skin, and weaker peripheral pulses compared to central pulses. Altered brain perfusion may be characterized by irritability, inconsolability, lethargy, unresponsiveness to voice or pain, and decreased muscle tone from decreased oxygen delivery. Urine output is usually maintained at 1 to 3 ml/kg/hour; oliguria indicates poor renal perfusion, hypovolemia, or acute tubular necrosis. Signs and symptoms of altered perfusion with normal blood pressure define compensated heart failure, and the same signs and symptoms with hypotension define decompensated shock.

Figure 13–3 presents a critical pathway utilizing pattern recognition of the symptoms of heart failure, a rapid cardiopulmonary assessment based on simple physiologic relationships of cardiac output and minute ventilation, leading one to subsequent physiologic diagnoses, etiologic diagnosis, and therapies. Table 13–5 presents normal age-related heart and respiratory rates.

DIFFERENTIAL DIAGNOSIS

Age of heart failure presentation is an initial guide to identifying common causes. Table 13–2 provides expanded etiologic features, including common and uncommon causes; Tables 13–6 and 13–7 present more in-depth comparisons.

Congenital Heart Disease

Congenital heart defects are the most common cause of heart failure in infancy and childhood. Of infants with significant struc-

Table 13–5. Age-Related Normal Respiratory and Heart Rates

Age	Respiratory Rate	Heart Rate (Mean)
Premature	<60	110–180 (150)
Newborn	40–60	85–205 (140)
Infant to 2 years old	24–40	100–190 (130)
2 to 10 years old	20–24	60–140 (80)
Over 10 years old	18–20	60–100 (75)

tural heart disease, 80% manifest heart failure. Approximately 50% of critically ill infants have one of the following five high-risk cardiac defects which manifest as heart failure, cyanosis, or both:

- Hypoplastic left heart syndrome
- Coarctation of the aorta
- Transposition of the great vessels
- Hypoplastic right heart syndrome
- Tetralogy of Fallot

Low-risk lesions are the simple left-to-right shunt lesions. Ventricular septal defect and PDA are the two most frequent defects (left to right shunts) presenting with heart failure in infancy. Although frequently diagnosed in the young child or adolescent, 10% of symptomatic atrial septal defects present under 1 year of age.

The signs and symptoms of newborn heart disease are:

- Central cyanosis
- Respiratory distress
- Systemic venous congestion
- Low cardiac output

Heart murmurs are not consistently the presenting sign; murmurs are usually soft in the sickest neonates (see Chapter 16).

Central cyanosis due to cardiac disease is the result of right-to-left shunting in which systemic venous (blue) blood does not enter the lungs but is shunted to the left heart and into the systemic circulation (see Chapter 15). As a result of right-to-left shunting, cyanosis occurs in structural defects associated with right heart obstruction, resulting in decreased total pulmonary blood flow, sometimes referred to as "tetralogy" physiology. *Heart failure is unusual with tetralogy physiology.* Central cyanosis may also occur in those complex cardiac defects in which fully oxygenated (red) blood mixes at the ventricular level with systemic venous (blue) blood via a large VSD resulting in recirculation of a mixture of oxygenated and unoxygenated blood into the pulmonary and systemic circulations (see Table 13–2). This type of cardiac shunting, in which fully oxygenated blood recirculates to the lungs and does not reach the systemic circulation, which instead receives mainly unoxygenated blood returning from the body resulting in central cyanosis, is known as *"transposition" physiology.* In these lesions, as pulmonary vascular resistance falls, and in the absence of pulmonary obstruction, total pulmonary blood flow increases, resulting in heart failure with cyanosis.

An approach to differentiate causes of heart failure in the high-risk neonate is noted in Figure 13–4.

Diagnoses of Increasing Importance: Heart Failure Without a Significant Murmur (Table 13–8)

Cardiomyopathy is widely used for diseases of the myocardium of both known and unknown causes (see Table 13–4). Specific causes have been identified with several cardiomyopathies, such as doxorubicin (Adriamycin) myopathy and primary or secondary carnitine deficiency. Although 80% to 90% of all children presenting with cardiomyopathy will have no identifiable cause, known causes must be vigorously investigated to identify treatable diseases (see Table 13–4; Fig. 13–5). Myopathies of increasing importance include:

- Myocarditis
- Disorders of mitochondrial fatty acid beta-oxidation
- Cardiotoxicity of anticancer agents

MYOCARDITIS

Myocarditis remains an enigmatic disease. Presentation is variable, ranging from an early presentation with fever, malaise, heart

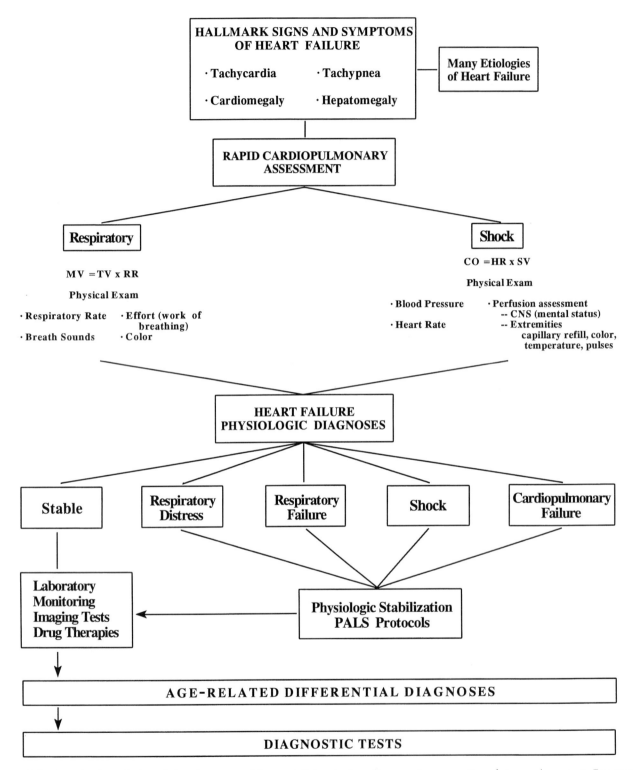

Figure 13–3. Critical pathway for heart failure diagnosis and therapy. Initial evaluation relies on pattern recognition of signs and symptoms. Transition from physiologic assessment through stabilization and onto diagnosis relies on laboratory findings, monitoring, imaging tests, and drug therapies. These objective data are used to assess response to stabilization interventions, anticipate changing physiology, and, ultimately, make an etiologic diagnosis. MV = minute ventilation; TV = tidal volume; RR = respiratory rate; CO = cardiac output; HR = heart rate; SV = stroke volume; PALS = pediatric advanced life support.

failure, and dysrhythmia or late in the course of the disease with end-stage dilated cardiomyopathy.

Diagnosis relies on clinical suspicion. The gold standard for diagnosis is evidence of myocardial inflammation by endomyocardial biopsy and, less persuasively, by nuclear scintigraphy. Newer molecular techniques (polymerase chain reaction amplification of viral genomes in myocardial biopsy specimens) are being developed to increase the sensitivity and specificity of diagnostic criteria and to target new therapy.

Treatment involves supportive efforts (e.g., diuretics, digoxin, captopril), rest, anticoagulation if indicated, and evaluation for cardiac transplantation for some patients. Immunosuppression (prednisone and/or cyclosporine) is controversial but may be useful as a short-term measure for the sickest of patients. Newer treatment modalities are rapidly being developed, such as antiviral agents and immune modulation. Considerable evidence suggests a link between acute viral myocarditis and the later onset of idiopathic dilated cardiomyopathy.

METABOLIC CARDIOMYOPATHY

Metabolic cardiomyopathies affect a small number of children; nonetheless, their importance rests in the fact that some are preventable with genetic counseling while others are treatable. Those disorders associated with heart disease involve defects in energy production and utilization (i.e., glycogenoses, fatty acid beta oxidation, and oxidative phosphorylation-respiratory chain defects). Clinical manifestations vary and include failure to thrive, hypoglycemia with hypoketonuria (fatty acid oxidation defects), lactic acidosis, coma, heart failure, hypotonia if skeletal muscle is involved, hepatic encephalopathy if the liver is involved, and sudden death.

Impaired glycogen degradation (*glycogen storage disease*) results in massive glycogen accumulation in organs lacking the specific enzyme. Muscle or generalized enzyme deficiencies result in muscle weakness or rhabdomyolysis. Because energy needs cannot be met solely through gluconeogenic pathways and beta oxidation of fatty acids, chronic protein wasting and episodes of ketotic hypoglycemia occur. Although frequent high-protein feeds may allow short term benefits, no effective therapies are presently available. *Pompe (cardiac-muscle) disease* is the classic disorder of this group.

Free fatty acids are the predominant energy substrate for the myocardium. Multiple inborn errors of beta oxidation have been reported. *Primary carnitine deficiency* is caused by a defective carnitine transport protein in fibroblasts, kidney, and muscle; decreased plasma carnitine levels are the result of large urine losses from impaired renal reabsorption of filtered carnitine. Fortunately, partial repletion therapy can result in excellent clinical responses. Other mitochondrial beta-oxidation defects have been identified. Therapy varies according to the specific defect and may include avoiding prolonged fasting, use of a low-fat, high-carbohydrate diet, L-carnitine replacement therapy, or all three interventions. Other cardiomyopathies (familial, hypertrophic) have been recently elucidated and may be due to genetic defects of myosin, dystrophin, or other cardiac muscle components. Some forms of familial (hypertrophic) cardiomyopathy respond to therapy with beta-adrenergic receptor blocking agents.

CARDIOTOXICITY OF ANTICANCER AGENTS

Approximately one in a thousand young adults at age 20 will be a childhood cancer survivor. These patients are at risk for multiple

Table 13-6. Comparison of Clinically Similar Causes of Heart Failure

Etiology	History	Age of Onset	Examination Results	Laboratory Findings	Electro-cardiography	Echo-cardiography	Diagnosis
Myocarditis	Variable, ± recent viral illness	Any age	Heart failure	IgM-specific antibodies and CPK generally not helpful	Tachycardia, low voltage, diffuse ST-T wave changes, generally no LVH	Profound ventricular dilatation and decreased systolic function, ± effusion	Endomyocardial biopsy, PCR
Idiopathic dilated myopathy	Variable, 6%–20% familial occurrence	50% are younger than 2 years	Heart failure, often pulsus alternans	Not specific	Diffuse ST-T wave changes, 70% with LVH	Dilated ventricles, decreased systolic function	Endomyocardial biopsy, PCR
Doxorubicin myopathy	Doxorubicin therapy	Within 24 hr to years after chemotherapy	Heart failure	Not specific	Dysrhythmias, ST-T wave changes, low voltages	Dilated ventricles, decreased systolic function	By history and endomyocardial biopsy
Rheumatic fever	± recent scarlet fever, streptococcal infection	Young school-aged child	Heart failure plus murmur of mitral and/or aortic regurgitation	+ strep throat culture, + rapid strep antigens, ASO > 500	Prolonged PR interval	Dilated ventricles, decreased systolic function, mitral and/or aortic regurgitation	Jones criteria, on occasion endomyocardial biopsy
Anomalous left coronary artery	Variable	Most are younger than 6 months; present in few adolescents	Heart failure	Not specific	Myocardial infarction, ST-T wave changes	Dilated ventricles, decreased systolic function, anomalous origin of left coronary artery	Delineation of coronary artery anatomy by angiography
AIDS	Risk factors; blood transfusion, hemophilia, perinatal (maternal drug use, multiple sexual partners)	Any age, usually younger than 2 years	Heart failure, chronic pneumonitis, splenomegaly, lymphadenopathy	Inverted CD4/CD8 ratio, + HIV serology	LVH, right bundle branch block	Dilated ventricles, decreased systolic function, ± effusion	HIV serology

Abbreviations: AIDS = acquired immunodeficiency syndrome; ASO = antistreptolysin O; CD = cluster designation; CPK = creatine phosphokinase; HIV = human immunodeficiency virus; Ig = immunoglobulin; LVH = left ventricular hypertrophy; PCR = polymerase chain reaction for virus, aberrant familial genes.
Key: ± = with or without.

Table 13–7. Heart Failure with Cardiomegaly in Newborns, Infants, and Children, Excluding Unoperated and Postoperative Congenital Heart Defects

Etiology	History	ECG Findings	Imaging (Echocardiography)	Diagnostic Test	Clinical Commentary
Hypoxic-ischemic injury	Perinatal history consistent with such an event, low Apgar, fetal distress	± ST-T wave changes	Depressed systolic function, ± dilated ventricles	By history	Frequently associated with tricuspid insufficiency (± murmur) and hypotension
Patent ductus arteriosus	Typically a premature infant during first week of life	± ST-T wave changes with significant L→R shunt	PDA with L→R shunt, LA/Ao ratio >1.2, reverse diastolic flow in descending aorta	Echocardiography	Pulse palpation is the most sensitive clinical sign of a large PDA with L→R shunt; UAC may render femoral artery palpation unreliable
Primary pulmonary hypertension not specified	Risk factors may or may not be identified	If abnormal, suspect congenital heart disease	R→L shunt in a structurally normal heart	Echocardiographic evidence of R→L shunt at ductal, atrial level, or both	Loud P_2 by auscultation; although highly specific, differential cyanosis rare; preductal and postductal TcO_2 monitors helpful for continuous monitoring of shunt
Gestational diabetes	Maternal history consistent with diabetes	50% LVH, 50% RVH	Ventricular hypertrophy with LVOT obstruction	By history	Positive inotropic agents worsen heart failure; symptoms may occur at rest or with feedings; tachypnea may be due to heart failure or respiratory disease
Premature closure PDA	History of maternal prostaglandin synthetase inhibitors	± RVH	Dilated right ventricle	Clinical suspicion	Controversial; suspect in cases of unexplained right heart failure and closed ductus on day 1 of life
Sepsis	Maternal risk factors for sepsis may or may not be identifed	Normal	May be normal, with or without depressed ventricular systolic function	Positive blood or placental cultures	Initiation of antibiotics depends on clinical judgement; the placenta is the record of prenatal life; its culture, inspection, and histology are valuable
Myocarditis	Variable: acute febrile illness, prolonged viral symptoms, palpitations, resting tachycardia, or unexpected cardiomegaly	Low-voltage, ST-T wave abnormality, resting tachycardia, abnormal QRS complexes herald poor acute outcome	Dilated (often profound) ventricles with decreased systolic function; ± pericardial effusion	Problematic, endomyocardial biopsy "gold standard"	Varied clinical presentation; suggested by tachycardia out of proportion to systemic illness or fever
Pericardial effusion	Febrile illness with or without chest pain; recent cardiothoracic surgery (post pericardiotomy syndrome)	Generalized ST elevation and T-wave abnormality	Cardiomegaly by chest x-ray with normal pulmonary vascularity	Echocardiography	Friction rub may be heard, often associated with chest pain; if cardiac compromise occurs, signs are those of shock
Carnitine deficiency	Failure to thrive, hypoglycemia, coma, or skeletal myopathy, no ketonuria	Hypertrophy	Dilated or hypertrophic cardiomyopathy	Tissue and/or blood carnitine levels, specific enzyme deficiencies	Much less common than previously believed; more and more specific enzyme deficiencies are being identified
Pompe disease	Autosomal recessive inheritance	Short PR interval; marked hypertrophy	Ventricular hypertrophy with LVOT obstruction	WBC assays, fibroblast culture, skeletal muscle biopsy	Associated clinical findings include macroglossia and diffuse weakness; classic ECG, short PR interval, and marked hypertrophy

Abbreviations: ECG = electrocardiogram; LVH = left ventricular hypertrophy; LVOT = left ventricular outflow tract; PDA = patent ductus arteriosus; RVH = right ventricular hypertrophy; WBC = white blood cell count; LA/Ao = left atrial-aortic root ratio; UAC = umbilical artery catheter; TcO_2 = transcutaneous oxygen.

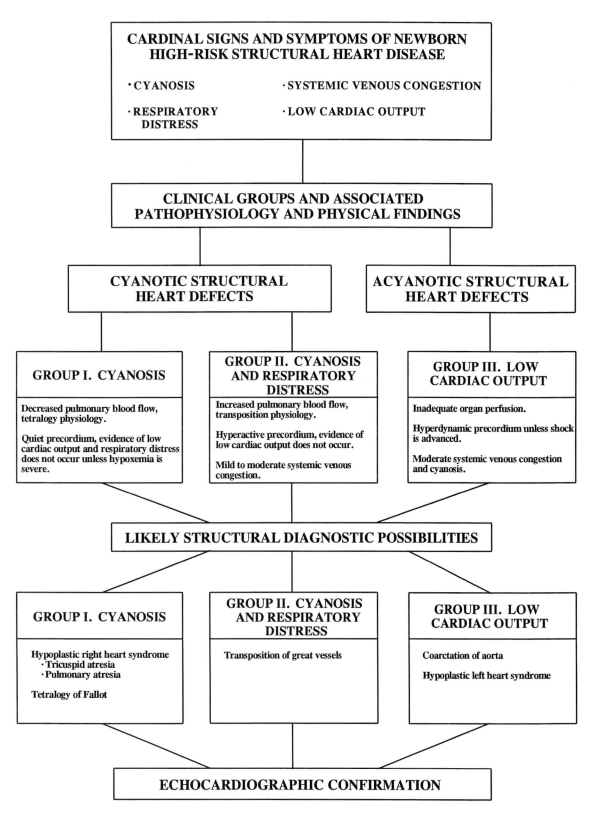

Figure 13–4. Critical pathway approach to the infant with high-risk structural heart disease.

Table 13-8. Heart Failure Without a Significant Murmur

   I. *Myocarditis** (see Table 13–4)

  II. *Cardiomyopathy** (see Table 13–4)

 III. *Arrhythmias** (see Chapter 12)

 IV. *Severe Anemia** (see Chapter 49)
    A. Sickle cell anemia
    B. Hemorrhage
    C. Fetal maternal hemorrhage
    D. Hemolytic anemias
    E. Nonproductive anemia (bone marrow hypoplasia-aplasia)

  V. *Coronary Artery Lesions*
    A. Kawasaki disease—aneurysms*
    B. Anomalous origin
    C. Anomalous intramyocardial course
    D. Periarteritis nodosa
    E. Spontaneous dissection
    F. Medial necrosis
    G. Idiopathic calcification
    H. Premature arteriosclerosis (familial hyperlipidemia, after heart transplantation)
    I. Embolization-thrombosis

 VI. *Congenital Heart Disease*
    A. Coarctation of aorta
    B. Critical aortic stenosis (neonate)
    C. Ebstein anomaly

 VII. *Cor Pulmonale*

VIII. *Catecholamine Excess*
    A. Pheochromocytoma
    B. Drugs of abuse (e.g., cocaine, amphetamine)
    C. Hyperthyroidism

 IX. *Hypertension* (see Tables 13–9 and 13–10)

  X. *Arteriovenous Malformation*
    A. Intracranial
    B. Hepatic
    C. Extremity
    D. Pulmonary

*Potentially common causes of heart failure without a significant heart murmur.

organ toxicity as a result of their multimodal chemotherapeutic and/or radiation therapies. The acute and chronic clinical impact on the cardiovascular system includes pericarditis, myocarditis, ventricular dysfunction, dysrhythmias, coronary artery disease, and myocardial infarction. The most well-known cardiotoxins are doxorubicin and daunorubicin (Daunomycin). Long-term surveillance studies indicate that an increasing number of patients are experiencing late-onset cardiovascular disease.

Diagnoses Not to Miss

The clinician cannot exclude a diagnosis that has not been considered. Rushing too eagerly to accept a diagnosis or narrowing diagnostic possibilities without adequate consideration may harm the patient. Patent ductus arteriosus, obstructed total anomalous pulmonary venous return (TAPVR), cor triatriatum, endocarditis, anomalous origin of the left coronary artery from the pulmonary artery (ALCA), Kawasaki disease, hypertension, and bacterial sepsis are examples of "diagnoses not to miss."

PATENT DUCTUS ARTERIOSUS

PDA, a common cause of heart failure, and TAPVR, an uncommon congenital defect, may mimic the "ground glass" radiographic description resulting from atelectasis of hyaline membrane disease in the premature infant. Diffuse alveolar collapse or pulmonary venous congestion may obscure radiographic evidence of cardiomegaly. Such a radiograph in an infant with a $PaCO_2$ lower than 40 mmHg after endotracheal intubation and positive ventilation suggests the possibility that cardiac, rather than pulmonary, disease is the primary pathophysiologic abnormality.

Prompt echocardiographic evaluation can achieve the following:

1. Confirm the presence of a large PDA with a left-to-right shunt.
2. Rule out PDA-dependent structural heart defects.
3. Allow early intravenous indomethacin therapy (80% ductal closure success rate in premature infants).
4. Accurately assess the need for surfactant replacement therapy.

TOTAL ANOMALOUS PULMONARY VENOUS RETURN

TAPVR with obstruction should be suspected in any infant with radiographic pulmonary "ground glass" appearance, and severe and fixed hypoxemia unresponsive to 100% oxygen, positive end expiratory pressure and surfactant replacement therapy, with or without hepatomegaly. The diagnosis is initiated by clinical suspicion and confirmed by echocardiography.

ANOMALOUS LEFT CORONARY ARTERY

Nearly 75% of infants with ALCA present with heart failure in early infancy because of declining antegrade coronary artery perfusion, once pulmonary vascular resistance falls, leading to myocardial ischemia. Chest radiography shows cardiomegaly, and an electrocardiogram (ECG) may demonstrate an anterolateral infarction pattern. Despite echocardiographic evaluation, coronary angiography is often necessary to delineate the coronary artery anatomy. With early diagnosis, infants and children with ALCA may benefit from medical management, surgical revascularization, or cardiac transplantation.

ENDOCARDITIS

Endocarditis is a potential cause of heart failure by causing valve dysfunction, myocarditis, or dysrhythmias (see Tables 16–8 and 16–9). Endocarditis may be seen on a previously normal native valve, one damaged due to congenital anomaly or prior endocarditis, or a prosthetic valve. The agents causing endocarditis are noted in Table 16–9; *S. aureus, Streptococcus viridans* group, and enterococcus are the more common pathogens.

HYPERTENSION

Acute or chronic hypertension, by increasing afterload, is an important cause of heart failure that may initially be overlooked. The cause of acute hypertension (Table 13–9) varies, but poststreptococcal glomerulonephritis and hemolytic uremic syndrome

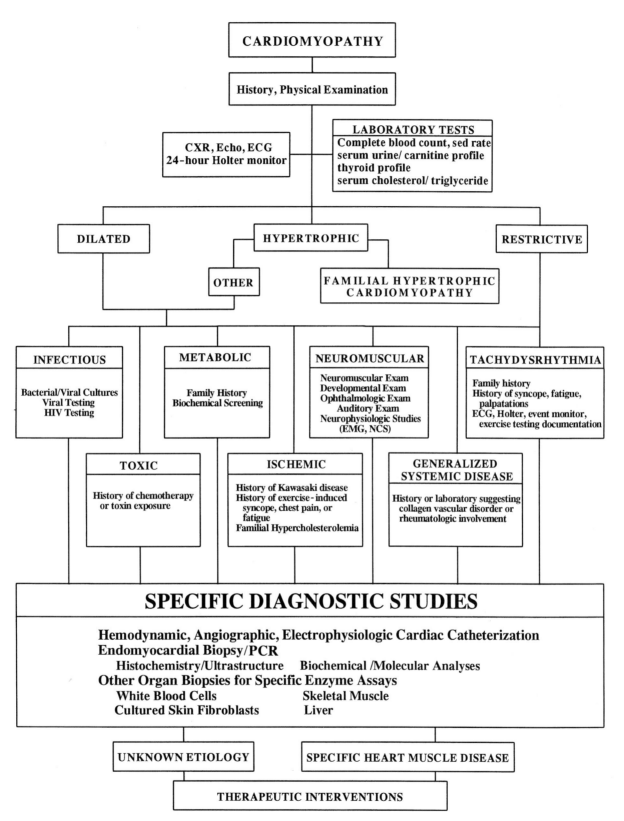

Figure 13–5. Cardiomyopathy critical pathway. Unknown versus specific heart muscle disorders. Metabolic category includes endocrine causes. CXR = Chest roentgenogram; ECG = electrocardiogram; Echo = echocardiogram; EMG = electromyography; HIV = human immunodeficiency virus; NCS = nerve conduction studies; PCR = polymerase chain reaction.

Table 13–9. Conditions Associated with Acute Transient or Intermittent Hypertension in Children

Renal
    Acute postinfectious glomerulonephritis
    Anaphylactoid (Henoch-Schönlein) purpura with nephritis
    Hemolytic-uremic syndrome
    Acute tubular necrosis
    After renal transplant (immediate and during episodes of
        rejection)
    After blood transfusion in patients with azotemia
    Hypervolemia
    After surgical procedures on genitourinary tract
    Pyelonephritis
    Renal trauma
    Leukemic infiltration of kidney
    Obstructive uropathy associated with Crohn disease

Drugs and Poisons
    Cocaine
    Oral contraceptives
    Sympathomimetic agents
    Amphetamines
    Phencyclidine
    Corticosteroids and adrenocorticotropic hormone (ACTH)
    Cyclosporine treatment
    Licorice (glycyrrhizic acid)
    Lead, mercury, cadmium, thallium
    Antihypertensive withdrawal (clonidine, methyldopa,
        propranolol)
    Vitamin D intoxication

Central and Autonomic Nervous System
    Increased intracranial pressure
    Guillain-Barré syndrome
    Burns
    Familial dysautonomia
    Stevens-Johnson syndrome
    Posterior fossa lesions
    Porphyria
    Poliomyelitis
    Encephalitis

Miscellaneous
    Pre-eclampsia
    Fractures of long bones
    Hypercalcemia
    Postcoarctation repair
    White cell transfusion
    Extracorporeal membrane oxygenation (ECMO)
    Chronic upper airway obstruction

Modified from Behrman RE (ed). Nelson Textbook of Pediatrics, 14th ed. Philadelphia: WB Saunders, 1992:1223.

are two common causes whereas chronic hypertension (Table 13–10) is often a result of structural renal disease, such as anomalies, reflux nephritis, or infection.

Treatment consists of antihypertensive agents, and specific approaches to the underlying disorder, including surgery for coarctation, prednisone, or other immunosuppressive agents for systemic lupus erythematosus. Commonly used antihypertensive agents (Table 13–11) include furosemide, hydralazine, and captopril (angiotensin-converting enzyme inhibitors).

BACTERIAL SEPSIS

Sepsis may present at any age with signs and symptoms of heart failure. Bacterial organisms such as group A streptococci and *S.*

aureus may present as toxic shock syndrome. If the history and physical examination leave any doubt about the diagnosis, blood specimens for culture should be obtained and antibiotics should be administered. Certain patients with congenital heart disease may be at an increased risk for sepsis; asplenia, cyanotic infants, DiGeorge–interrupted aortic arch, or transposition of the great vessels.

Avoid "Forcing a Diagnosis"

The increased prevalence of rheumatic fever in the United States has been associated with a change in severity, presentation, epide-

Table 13–10. Conditions Associated with Chronic Hypertension in Children

Renal
    Chronic pyelonephritis
    Chronic glomerulonephritis
    Hydronephrosis
    Congenital dysplastic kidney
    Multicystic kidney
    Solitary renal cyst
    Vesicoureteral reflux nephropathy
    Segmental hypoplasia (Ask-Upmark kidney)
    Ureteral obstruction
    Renal tumors (Wilms tumor)
    Renal trauma
    Rejection damage following transplantation
    Postirradiation damage
    Systemic lupus erythematosus (other connective tissue diseases)

Vascular
    Coarctation of thoracic or abdominal aorta
    Renal artery lesions (stenosis, fibromuscular dysplasia,
        thrombosis, aneurysm)
    Umbilical artery catheterization with thrombus formation
    Neurofibromatosis (intrinsic or extrinsic narrowing of vascular
        lumen)
    Renal vein thrombosis
    Vasculitis
    Arteriovenous shunt
    Williams Beuren syndrome

Endocrine
    Hyperthyroidism
    Hyperparathyroidism
    Congenital adrenal hyperplasia (11β-hydroxylase and
        17-hydroxylase defect)
    Cushing syndrome
    Primary aldosteronism
    Dexamethasone-suppressible hyperaldosteronism
    Pheochromocytoma
    Other neural crest tumors (neuroblastoma,
        ganglioneuroblastoma, ganglioneuroma)
    Diabetic nephropathy

Central Nervous System
    Intracranial mass
    Hemorrhage
    Residual following brain injury
    Quadriplegia

Essential Hypertension
    Low renin
    Normal renin
    High renin

From Behrman RE (ed). Nelson Textbook of Pediatrics, 14th ed. Philadelphia: WB Saunders, 1992.

Table 13–11. Antihypertensive Drugs

Drug	Mechanism of Action	Dosage Range	Route	Duration	Side Effects
Vasodilators					
Hydralazine	Relax arteriolar smooth muscle	0.4–0.8 mg/kg/dose	IV	2–4 hr	Tachycardia, nausea
		0.5–2 mg/kg and increase to max 200 mg/24 hr	p.o.	6–8 hr	Drug-induced lupus
Diazoxide	Relax smooth muscle	2–5 mg/kg/dose, max 100 mg	IV	6–24 hr	Tachycardia, hypotension, hyperglycemia
Nitroprusside	Dilatation of arterioles and venules	0.5–8.0 μg/kg/min	IV	With infusion	Thiocyanate production, rarely hypothyroidism
Minoxidil	Arteriolar dilatation	0.2–1.0 mg/kg/24 hr, max 50 mg/24 hr	p.o.	12–24 hr	Hypertrichosis, fluid retention
Adrenergic blockade					
Phentolamine	α-Receptor blockade	0.1 mg/kg/dose, max 5 mg	IV	1 hr	Reflex tachycardia
Phenoxybenzamine	α-Receptor blockade	2–5 mg/24 hr	p.o.	6–12 hr	Tachycardia may progress to arrhythmia
Prazosin	α-Receptor blockade	1-mg initial dose, may increase to 15 mg/24 hr	p.o.	8–12 hr	First-dose orthostatic hypotension
Propranolol	β-Receptor blockade Reduces renin release	0.025–0.1 mg/kg/dose 0.25–1.0 mg/kg/dose	IV p.o.	6–8 hr	Bronchospasm, bradycardia, vivid dreams
Labetalol	α-β Blockade	Titrate 0.2–2 mg/kg/hr (based on adult dose) 100–400 mg (adult)	IV p.o.	With infusion 12 hr	Orthostasis, dizziness, bronchospasm
Sympatholytic agents					
α-Methyldopa	Decrease sympathetic tone	10 mg/kg/24 hr and increase	p.o.	6–8 hr	Sedation, hepatic dysfunction, positive Coombs reaction
Clonidine	α Agonist in CNS	3–5 μg/kg/dose	p.o.	6–8 hr	Sedation, constipation, rebound withdrawal, hypertension
Renin-angiotensin enzyme inhibition					
Captopril	Converting-enzyme inhibition of angiotensin II synthesis	0.1–0.3 mg/kg/dose and increase to max 2 mg/kg/dose	p.o.	8 hr	Proteinuria, neutropenia, rash, dysgeusia
Enalaprilat	Same as captopril	0.005–0.010 mg/kg/dose	IV	8–12 hr	Transient hypotension
Calcium channel blocker					
Nifedipine	Calcium channel blocker	0.2–0.5 mg/kg, max 10–20 mg	p.o. Sublingual	Repeat q 30–60 min	Facial flushing, tachycardia
Verapamil	Calcium channel blocker	120–240 mg (adults)	p.o.	12–24 hr	Limited pediatric experience
Diuretic agents					
Hydrochlorothiazide	Diuresis	1–2 mg/kg/24 hr	p.o.	12–24 hr	Hypokalemia, hyperuricemia, hypercalcemia
Furosemide	Diuresis	1 mg/kg/dose 2 mg/kg/dose	IV p.o.	4–6 hr 4–6 hr	Hypokalemia, alkalosis

Adapted from Med Lett Drug Ther 1989;1:25 and 1989; 31:31. Reprinted in Behrman RE (ed). Nelson Textbook of Pediatrics, 14th ed. Philadelphia: WB Saunders, 1992:1223.

miology, age range, and clinical manifestation. Heart failure resulting from rheumatic carditis is predominantly associated with a murmur of the mitral valve (and, if severe, aortic valve) insufficiency.

Myocarditis in the absence of valvulitis by auscultation is not likely rheumatic in origin and one should avoid forcing the diagnosis of acute rheumatic fever in such cases. Rarely, myocarditis may be difficult to differentiate from rheumatic fever in the absence of classic clinical manifestations. Endomyocardial biopsy may be helpful (see Chapter 16).

The hypoglycemic infant of a diabetic mother presents another situation of potential forcing the diagnosis (see Chapter 63). The infant of a diabetic mother is large for gestational age, shows an exaggerated fall in blood glucose and an attenuated rise in free fatty acids due to hyperinsulinemia, and may present with heart failure from a transient hypertrophic (septal hypertrophy) cardiomyopathy. Alternately, heart failure may be due to hypocalcemia, asphyxia, or congenital heart disease—all of which are more common among infants of diabetic mothers. Heart failure in the infant that is caused by hypertrophic cardiomyopathy is reversible with appropriate diagnosis and beta-adrenergic receptor blocking agents.

PHYSIOLOGY OF HEART FAILURE: THE BASIS FOR THERAPY

It is clinically useful to distinguish left-sided from right-sided heart failure and biventricular failure (see Fig. 13–1). Failure of one ventricle may produce hemodynamic, cellular, and biochemical abnormalities of the other ventricle. Physical findings are dominated by signs and symptoms of right-sided or left-sided heart failure, or both.

The second paradigm recognizes two fundamental hemodynamic states underlying the clinical picture of heart failure. High-output failure is often due to volume overloading conditions primarily due to left-to-right shunts (Fig. 13–6). Low-output failure is primarily due to left-sided obstructive lesions, cardiomyopathies, and tachydysrhythmias (Fig. 13–7). Myocardial contractility is usually, though not always, preserved in high-output failure and the principal signs and symptoms of heart failure are due to pulmonary vascular congestion and the increased work of breathing. Myocardial contractility is diminished in patients with low-output states in which principal signs and symptoms are those of markedly decreased systemic perfusion with altered vital organ function.

The third paradigm describes the relationship between ventricular pressure and volume, stroke volume, and the Frank-Starling law of the heart. This paradigm is the most therapeutically useful (Fig. 13–8). Pressure-volume diagrams relate cardiac output (stroke volume), preload, afterload, and contractility with the two phases of the cardiac cycle: systole and diastole (Figs. 13–8 and 13–9). The end-systolic pressure-volume curve represents an index of contractility. Pressure-volume loops can then be used to conceptualize a family of loops representing various contractility states (Fig. 13–10).

In a normal heart, the stroke volume increases with increasing left ventricular volume (or pressure), as noted in Fig. 13–8, curve C. Heart failure, represented by the lowest curve, is due to decreased contractility and myocardial dysfunction. Digitalis or arterial vasodilating agents moves the curve upward (e.g., to A). Venodilation and diuretic agents move function to a safer (e.g., from A to B) position on the same curve, thus reducing the risk of pulmonary edema.

ASSESSMENT AND DIAGNOSIS
Laboratory Data

Laboratory tests (i.e., glucose, serum electrolytes, complete blood count, and blood gas analysis) help to assess the severity of heart failure on the body's normal function but rarely provide a diagnosis. Exceptions include heart failure caused by hypoglycemia, endocrine disorders, poisoning, anemia, or electrolyte disturbances. Markers of inflammation (i.e., leukocytosis, C-reactive protein, elevated sedimentation rate, and other acute-phase reactants) are helpful indicators of systemic illness but lack diagnostic specificity. The value of laboratory data includes the ability to:

- Serve as a marker of specific physiologic perturbations (i.e., anemia, acidosis, hypoglycemia, hypoxemia, renal and liver dysfunction)
- Guide therapeutic decisions and interventions (airway management, drug administration, transfusion therapies)
- Provide a yardstick against which therapies and interventions are monitored (improved acidosis, oxygenation, blood glucose, and hypokalemia as well as hypomagnesemia due to diuretic therapy and resolving inflammation)
- Allow ongoing monitoring of anticipated perturbations due to the disease process (oxygen delivery, vital organ function, and nutritional support)

Cardiopulmonary Monitoring

Cardiopulmonary monitoring provides continuous heart rate, respiratory rate, and rhythm surveillance. Continuous pulse oximetry identifies oxygen needs and helps to direct oxygen therapy. Blood pressure should be assessed initially and frequently thereafter in acutely ill hospitalized patients. Certain clinical conditions may demand more frequent and invasive monitoring. Cardiac output may be clinically assessed at the bedside or may be directly measured by echocardiographic techniques. Placement of a central venous catheter at the level of the right atrium and an arterial catheter permits cardiac output determination by Fick principle or indicator dye technique. Pulmonary artery catheterization allows for thermodilution cardiac output determination.

Chest Roentgenography

If heart failure is present, chest radiography will show an enlarged cardiac silhouette; if not, the diagnosis of heart failure should be questioned. Cardiomegaly on a chest x-ray film more reliably reflects volume overload than pressure overload. Pressure overload is more reliably represented by ECG evidence of ventricular hypertrophy and by echocardiography. Pulmonary venous congestion on chest radiography suggests left-sided obstructive lesions or left ventricular failure; increased pulmonary arterial markings suggest left-to-right shunt. Cardiomegaly ("boggy water bottle heart") with normal vascular patterns suggests pericardial effusion. Pleural effusions should prompt the possibility of superior vena cava obstruction, right-sided or left-sided heart failure, or noncardiac pathology.

Electrocardiography

The ECG is helpful in identifying ventricular hypertrophy, atrial enlargement, and changes in ST-T wave segments. Although lacking diagnostic specificity, the ECG is helpful in the diagnosis of heart failure due to myocarditis (ST-T wave changes, decreased QRS voltage), dysrhythmia (i.e., supraventricular tachycardia, complete heart block, sick sinus syndrome), or myocardial infarction (Q-wave pattern). When ischemic ECG findings are present, one must consider the diagnoses of anomalous origin of the left coro-

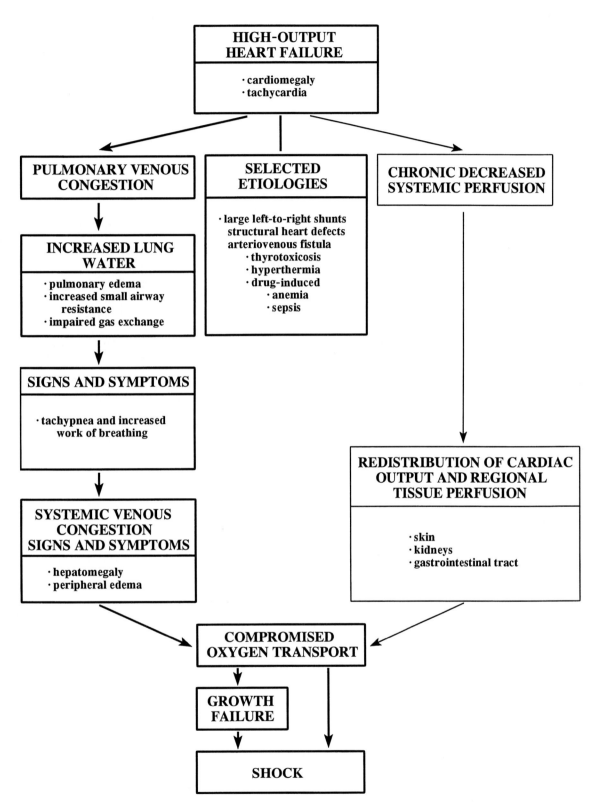

Figure 13–6. Hemodynamic classification of heart failure based on increased cardiac output. Physiologic emphasis is on abnormalities of pulmonary function, both circulatory and gas exchange, as a result of increased pulmonary blood flow. Regional circulations are compromised but to a lesser extent than in low cardiac output states. Outstanding signs and symptoms are those due to pulmonary dysfunction. Once oxygen delivery can no longer meet metabolic demands, growth failure ensues.

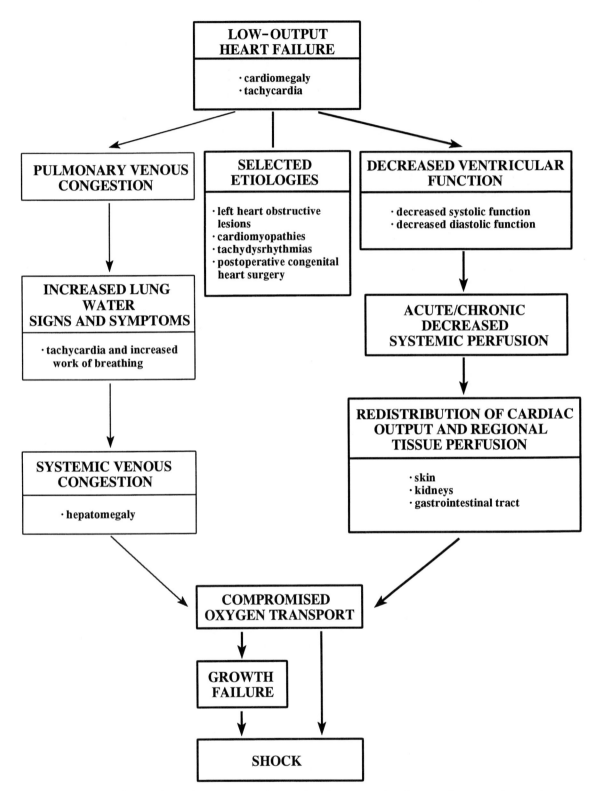

Figure 13–7. Hemodynamic classification of heart failure based on decreased cardiac output. Physiologic emphasis is on decreased systemic perfusion and redistribution of cardiac output. Once oxygen delivery can no longer meet metabolic demands, growth failure or shock ensues. Outstanding signs and symptoms are those due to decreased system perfusion.

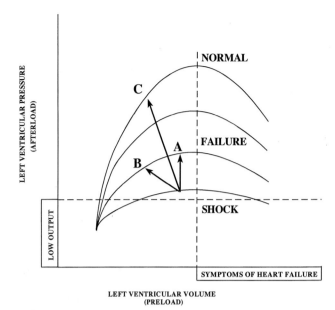

Figure 13–8. Effects of inotropic and afterload reducing agents on ventricular function curve. Beginning on the shock curve, positive inotropic stimulation improves cardiac performance to point A, afterload reduction to point B. Combination therapy (point C) enhances cardiac performance to a greater degree than therapy focused on a single determinant of cardiac output. (Adapted from Friedman WF, George BL. Treatment of congestive heart failure by altering loading conditions of the heart. J Pediatr 1985;106:704.)

nary artery, Kawasaki disease (acute or long-term sequelae), myopericarditis, cocaine ingestion, and, in the premature infant, a PDA.

Rare causes of ECG ischemia include coronary obstruction due to metabolic heart disease, familial hypercholesterolemia, and coronary stenosis in William syndrome. Long-term survivors of Kawasaki disease, cardiac transplantation, and Jatene arterial switch operation for transposition of the great vessels are potential at-risk populations for myocardial ischemia.

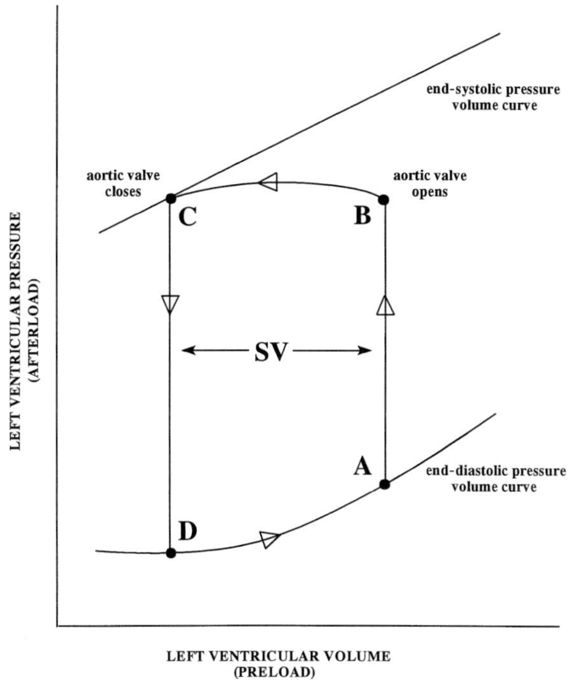

Echocardiography

Echocardiography is the most applicable, cost-effective imaging modality to identify the cause of heart failure and to monitor therapeutic interventions as well as long-term sequelae. Echocardi-

Figure 13–9. Pressure-volume loop. Contraction begins at point A, representing end-diastolic volume preload. Isovolumetric contraction occurs along line A to B. At point B, the aortic valve opens and ejection begins. Ejection ends at point C, where the aortic valve closes. Isovolumetric relaxation occurs along line C to D, with a fall in ventricular pressure. At point D, the mitral valve opens to fill the left ventricle, generating the preload for the next cardiac cycle. Stroke volume (SV) is represented by the distance from line CD to AB. A similar curve can be drawn for the right ventricle. The end-systolic pressure-volume curve is a measure of contractility. The end-diastolic pressure-volume curve represents the Frank-Starling relationship.

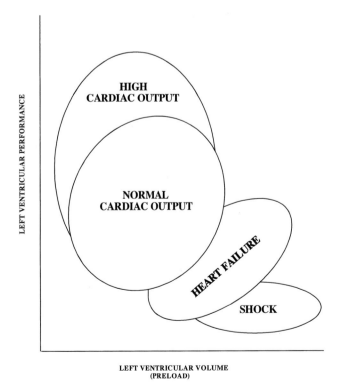

Figure 13–10. A family of pressure-volume loops representing various contractility states.

ography significantly narrows the field of potential causes and usually identifies a specific diagnosis. Images may be obtained with the conventional transthoracic approach or by transesophageal technique. Complete echocardiographic evaluation permits rapid, simultaneous acquisition of anatomic detail, blood flow analysis, and hemodynamic data. Echocardiographic indices of left ventricular function include shortening fraction (normal 30% to 40%), ejection fraction (normal 67% ± 8%), cardiac output, and velocity of circumferential shortening (contractility index).

Cardiac Catheterization

Diagnostic catheterization is beneficial when questions regarding anatomy or hemodynamics (i.e., shunt quantification, magnitude of pulmonary hypertension, degree of ventricular dysfunction) remain unanswered following echocardiographic imaging or when a discrepancy exists between clinical presentation and noninvasive diagnostic findings. Certain circumstances may require diagnostic or therapeutic catheterization. Examples include complex heart defects requiring surgical repair, balloon valvuloplasty, blade atrial septostomy to decompress the left atrium (thereby relieving pulmonary venous congestion in severe mitral stenosis), endomyocardial biopsy in a patient with cardiomyopathy or suspected cardiac transplant rejection, and electrophysiologic catheterization with or without ablation therapy in a patient presenting with heart failure due to a dysrhythmia (see Chapter 12).

Radionuclide Imaging

Radionuclide angiography and myocardial perfusion imaging (^{201}Tl, ^{99m}Tc-sestamibi) are useful in assessing myocardial blood flow and function in response to exercise. As a part of long-term management, nuclear cardiac imaging may help to assess the sequelae and efficacy of therapeutic interventions when combined with exercise (bicycle or treadmill) or pharmacologic stress exercise protocols (dipyridamole, dobutamine, or adenosine). For myocardial inflammation, ^{67}Ga has shown adequate specificity but lacks sensitivity to be clinically useful. ^{111}In-labeled antimyosin antibody has shown high sensitivity (80% to 100%) but low specificity (<60%). Therefore, myocardial biopsy remains the diagnostic procedure of choice for cardiac inflammation.

TREATMENT

Treatment includes supportive, symptomatic, pharmacologic, mechanical, and surgical approaches (Table 13–12). The goals of therapy are to restore the balance between sodium and free water, to optimize vascular tone (preload and afterload), to improve myocardial performance (heart rate and contractility), and to accomplish these goals in a cost-effective manner.

Symptomatic Treatment

Symptomatic measures address oxygen needs and correction of metabolic, hematologic, and endocrine abnormalities adversely affecting cardiac performance. This may involve positioning the patient to maintain minute ventilation, maintaining normothermia, and administering supplemental oxygen, glucose, calcium, or magnesium. Patients with anemia may require a transfusion, and those with polycythemia may require partial exchange transfusion or

phlebotomy, thereby reducing viscosity and enhancing oxygen delivery. Specific management of systemic illness, such as sepsis, Kawasaki disease, collagen vascular disease, trauma, or envenomation, is indicated with antibiotics, aspirin and gamma globulin, steroids, neurocardiopulmonary resuscitation, and antivenin, respectively.

Drug Therapy

Drug therapy is the cornerstone of management (Tables 13–12 and 13–13). The initial pharmacologic approach is directed by physiologic assessment and stabilization. Drug therapy targets the determinants of cardiac output (see Fig. 13–2) as well as alterations in salt and water balance.

Multiple Therapies

Multiple drug therapies improve ventricular function to a greater extent than therapy focused upon a single determinant of cardiac output (see Fig. 13–8). This is because the failing circulation typically has multiple hemodynamic abnormalities. Multimodal pharmacodynamic effects may be obtained by combining agents such as digoxin and a diuretic, digoxin and captopril, or in more severe life-threatening disease, epinephrine and nitroprusside, or using single agents with multiple effects, such as dobutamine and amrinone. Preload is the most commonly manipulated determinant of stroke volume. The right ventricle appears to be more readily responsive to afterload reduction than inotropic stimulation, whereas the left ventricle appears equally responsive to modulation of either determinant. If there is biventricular failure, positive inotropic agents may improve right ventricular performance by reducing that portion of right-sided heart dysfunction attributable to impaired left-sided heart function.

INOTROPIC AGENTS

There are three classes of inotropic agents:

- Cardiac glycosides
- Catecholamines
- Phosphodiesterase inhibitors

Cardiac Glycosides. Digoxin is the most important agent for initial and long-term management of heart failure outside the intensive care unit. Its advantages include (1) oral preparation, (2) lack of induction of beta-adrenergic receptor desensitization, (3) no increase in heart rate, and (4) availability of a specific antidote, Digibind, for acute toxicity. A low toxic-therapeutic index, slow onset of action, long half-life, and increased arrhythmogenesis are substantial drug efficacy and safety issues in patients with rapidly changing physiology associated with respiratory failure or abnormal perfusion (shock), altered or uncertain renal function, and electrolyte abnormalities.

Catecholamines. The catecholamines remain the mainstay of acute positive inotropic intervention for the critically ill patient. This role is related to several factors, including a favorable pharmacokinetic profile for each, a relatively predictable pharmacodynamic response, and a wide range of hemodynamic effects. Side effects include tachycardia, arrhythmogenicity, excess vasoconstric-

Table 13-12. Treatment of Heart Failure

Therapy	Mechanism
General Care	
Rest	Reduces cardiac output
Oxygen	Improves oxygenation in presence of pulmonary edema
Sodium, fluid restrictions	Decreases vascular congestion; decreases preload
Diuretics	
Furosemide	Salt excretion by ascending loop of Henle; reduces preload; afterload reduced if hypertension improves; also may cause venodilation
Combination of distal tubule and loop diuretics	Greater sodium excretion
Inotropic Agents	
Digitalis	Inhibits membrane Na^+, K^+-ATPase and increases intracellular Ca^{2+}, improves cardiac contractility, increases myocardial oxygen consumption
Dopamine	Releases myocardial norepinephrine plus direct effect on beta receptor, may increase systemic blood pressure; at low infusion rates, dilates renal artery, facilitating diuresis
Dobutamine	Beta (β_1)-receptor agent; often combined with dopamine
Amrinone	Nonsympathomimetic, noncardiac glycosides with inotropic effects; also may produce vasodilation
Afterload Reduction	
Hydralazine	Arteriolar vasodilator
Nitroprusside	Arterial and venous relaxation; venodilation reduces preload
Prazosin	Oral alpha-adrenergic blocking agent; arterial and venous dilator; venodilation reduces preload
Captopril/enalapril	Inhibition of angiotensin-converting enzyme; reduces angiotensin II production

From Behrman RE, Kliegman RM (eds). Nelson Essentials of Pediatrics, 2nd ed. Philadelphia: WB Saunders, 1994.

tion or vasodilation, increased myocardial oxygen consumption, receptor down-regulation, and catecholamine-induced hypertrophic cardiomyopathy. Predominant vasopressor effects are achieved with norepinephrine, combined vasopressor-inotropism with epinephrine and dopamine, and vasodilator inotropic effects with dobutamine and isoproterenol. Furthermore, catecholamines can be used in any combination to minimize unwanted side effects and to achieve an even wider spectrum of hemodynamic effects.

Because there is no consensus on drug selection, it is important to remember the goals of initial therapy:

- Restoration of adequate blood pressure
- Effective perfusion
- Correction of hypoxia and acidosis

Figure 13–11 illustrates an approach to catecholamine selection.

Phosphodiesterase Inhibitors. The bipyridine phosphodiesterase III inhibitors form the third class of inotropic agents, which are also peripheral vasodilators. Amrinone is the most commonly employed of these compounds. Advantages include nonadrenergic-mediated, combined inotropic, and afterload reduction effects unaffected by beta-adrenoreceptor down-regulation. Disadvantages include hypotension, thrombocytopenia, and short duration of benefit. Because dysrhythmias are uncommon with amrinone, it may be a potential first-line agent in heart failure management associated with myocardial irritability, such as the child with myocarditis or the acute postoperative cardiac patient with a dysrhythmia. However, it is premature to assign amrinone a major role in the management of critically ill children with heart failure from a noncardiac cause, such as septic shock, adult respiratory distress syndrome, or trauma.

Table 13-13. Dosage of Drugs Commonly Used for the Treatment of Congestive Heart Failure

Drug	Dosage
Digoxin	
Digitalization (p.o.) (3 doses q 8 hr)	Premature 0.02–0.025 mg/kg Neonate ($\leq$ 1 mo) 0.03–0.04 mg/kg Infant or child 0.04–0.06 mg/kg Adolescent or adult 1.0–1.5 mg in divided doses
Digitalization (IV) (Timing of dosage variable, depending on clinical indications)	75% of p.o. dose
Maintenance	$\frac{1}{4}$–$\frac{1}{3}$ of digitalizing dose, divided q 12 hr
Furosemide	
IV	1–2 mg/dose, p.r.n.
p.o.	1–4 mg/kg/24 hr, q.d., b.i.d., or q.i.d.
Bumetanide	
IV	0.01–0.2 mg/kg/dose
p.o.	0.04–0.8 mg/kg/24 hr q 6–8 hr
Chlorothiazide (p.o.)	20–50 mg/kg/24 hr, b.i.d. or q.i.d.
Spironolactone (p.o.)	2–3 mg/kg/24 hr, b.i.d.
β Agonists (IV)	
Isoproterenol	0.01–0.5 μg/kg/min
Dopamine	2–20 μg/kg/min
Dobutamine	2–20 μg/kg/min
Amrinone (IV)	0.75 mg/kg bolus 5–10 μg/kg
Afterload-reducing agents	
Nitroprusside (IV)	0.5–8 μg/kg/min
Hydralazine	
IV	0.5 mg/kg
p.o.	0.5–7.5 mg/kg/24 hr, t.i.d.
Captopril (p.o.)	0.5–6 mg/kg/24 hr, q.i.d.

From Behrman RE (ed). Nelson Textbook of Pediatrics, 14th ed. Philadelphia: WB Saunders, 1992:1214.

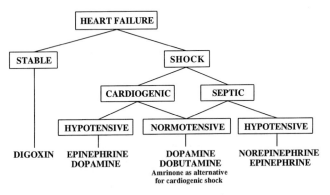

Figure 13–11. Suggested initial selection of inotropic agents.

VASODILATORS

There are three classes of vasodilators:

- Venous (e.g., nitroglycerin)—reduce preload
- Arteriolar—reduce afterload
- Mixed (nitroprusside, captopril, enalapril, prazosin)—reduce both preload and afterload

Arteriolar vasodilators may be further categorized into those commonly used to reduce left ventricular afterload (nifedipine, hydralazine) and right ventricular afterload (oxygen, prostaglandin E_1, nifedipine, adenosine, nitric oxide).

DIURETICS

Diuretics (e.g., hydrochlorothiazide, furosemide, bumetamide, metolazone) are used to correct the positive balance of salt and water perturbations; their actions affect preload, pulmonary function, and renal excretion.

Mechanical Methods

Mechanical interventions include mechanical ventilation (positive end-expiratory pressure), pacemakers, and mechanical assist devices, such as a cardiopulmonary bypass, extracorporeal membrane oxidation (ECMO), and an intra-aortic balloon pump. These interventions are reserved for critically ill patients and are often coupled with corrective surgical interventions for those with congenital heart disease, end-stage heart failure awaiting transplantation, multiple trauma, or severely poisoning. Congenital heart defects and cardiomyopathy represent the most common indications for pediatric cardiac transplantation. Expanding clinical experience coupled with improved immunopharmacology and myocardial preservation techniques provides encouraging 1-year (81%) and 5-year (78%) survival rates for the general cardiac transplant population.

REFERENCES

Pathophysiology

Bonow RO, Udelson JE. Left ventricular diastolic dysfunction as a cause of congestive heart failure. Ann Intern Med 1992;117:502–510.
Goldsmith SR, Dick C. Differentiating systolic from diastolic heart failure: Pathophysiologic and therapeutic considerations. Am J Med 1993; 95:645–655.
Haworth SG, Bull C. Physiology of congenital heart disease. Arch Dis Child 1993;68:707–711.
Muntoni F, Cau M, Ganau A, et al. Brief report: Deletion of the dystrophin muscle-promoter region associated with X-linked dilated cardiomyopathy. N Engl J Med 1993;329:921–925.
Packer M. Pathophysiology of chronic heart failure. Lancet 1992;340:88–92.
Watkins H, Rosenzweig A, Hwang D-S, et al. Characteristics and prognostic implications of myosin missense mutations in familial hypertrophic cardiomyopathy. N Engl J Med 1992;326:1108–1114.

Differential Diagnosis

Artman M, Parrish MD. Congestive heart failure in infancy: Recognition and management. Am Heart J 1982;103:1040–1046.
Artman M, Parrish MD. Congestive heart failure in childhood and adolescence: Recognition and management. Am Heart J 1983;105:471–478.
Anonymous. Dilated cardiomyopathy and enteroviruses. Lancet 1990; 336:971–972.
Awadallah SM, Kavey REW, Byrum CJ, et al. The changing pattern of infective endocarditis in childhood. Am J Cardiol 1991;68:90–94.
Baltimore RS. Infective endocarditis in children. Pediatr Infect Dis J 1992;11:907–913.
Baughman KL. Hypertrophic cardiomyopathy. JAMA 1992;267:846–849.
Chow LC, Dittrich HC, Shabetai R. Endomyocardial biopsy in patients with unexplained congestive heart failure. Ann Intern Med 1988;109:535–539.
Clark AL, Coats AJS. Screening for hypertrophic cardiomyopathy. BMJ 1993;306:409–410.
Frontera-Izquierdo P, Cabezuelo-Huerta G. Natural and modified history of isolated ventricular septal defect: A 17-year study. Pediatr Cardiol 1992;13:193–197.
Lie JT. Myocarditis and endomyocardial biopsy in unexplained heart failure: A diagnosis in search of a disease. Ann Intern Med 1988;109:525–528.
Michels VV. Progress in defining the causes of idiopathic dilated cardiomyopathy. N Engl J Med 1993;329:960–961.
Michels VV, Moll PP, Miller FA, et al. The frequency of familial dilated cardiomyopathy in a series of patients with idiopathic dilated cardiomyopathy. N Engl J Med 1992;326:77–82.
Saiman L, Prince A, Gersony WM. Pediatric infective endocarditis in the modern era. J Pediatr 1993;122:847–853.
See DM, Tilles JG. Viral myocarditis. Rev Infect Dis 1991;13:951–956.
Shaddy RE, Bullock EA. Efficacy of 100 consecutive right ventricular endomyocardial biopsies in pediatric patients using the right internal jugular venous approach. Pediatr Cardiol 1993;14:5–8.
Sugrue DD, Rodeheffer RJ, Codd MB, et al. The clinical course of idiopathic dilated cardiomyopathy. A population-based study. Ann Intern Med 1992;117:117–123.
Tunkel AR, Kaye D. Endocarditis with negative blood cultures. N Engl J Med 1992;326:1215–1217.
Watanakunakorn C, Burkert T. Infective endocarditis at a large community teaching hospital, 1980–1990: A review of 210 episodes. Medicine 1993;72:90–102.

Treatment

Aronson JK, Hardman M. Digoxin. BMJ 1992;305:1149–1152.
Chan KY, Iwahara M, Benson LN, et al. Immunosuppressive therapy in the management of acute myocarditis in children: A clinical trial. J Am Coll Cardiol 1991;17:458–460.
Cohn JN, Johnson G, Ziesche S, et al. A comparison of enalapril with hydralazine-isosorbide dinitrate in the treatment of chronic congestive heart failure. N Engl J Med 1991;325:303–310.
Dajani AS, Bison AL, Chung KJ, et al. Prevention of bacterial endocarditis. Recommendations by the American Heart Association. JAMA 1990;264:2919–2922.
Dargie HJ, McMurray JJV. Diagnosis and management of heart failure. BMJ 1994;308:321–328.
Feldman AM. Can we alter survival in patients with congestive heart failure? JAMA 1992;267:1956–1961.

Frenneaux M, Stewart RAH, Newman CMH, et al. Enalapril for severe heart failure in infancy. Arch Dis Child 1989;64:219–223.

Friedman WF, George BL. Treatment of congestive heart failure by altering loading conditions of the heart. J Pediatr 1985;106:697–706.

Gilbert EM, Anderson JL, Deitchman D, et al. Long-term β-blocker vasodilator therapy improves cardiac function in idiopathic dilated cardiomyopathy: A double-blind, randomized study of bucindolol versus placebo. Am J Med 1990;88:223–229.

Jaeschke R, Guyatt GH. Medical therapy for chronic congestive heart failure. Ann Intern Med 1989;110:758–760.

Kulick DL, Rahimtoola SH. Current role of digitalis therapy in patients with congestive heart failure. JAMA 1991;265:2995–2997.

Lewis AB, Chabot M. The effect of treatment with angiotensin-converting enzyme inhibitors on survival of pediatric patients with dilated cardiomyopathy. Pediatr Cardiol 1993;14:9–12.

O'Connell JB. Immunosuppression for dilated cardiomyopathy. N Engl J Med 1989;321:1119–1121.

Packer M, Gheorghiade M, Young JB, et al. Withdrawal of digoxin from patients with chronic heart failure treated with angiotensin-converting-enzyme inhibitors. N Engl J Med 1993;329:1–7.

Packer M. Treatment of chronic heart failure. Lancet 1992;340:92–95.

Parrillo JE, Cunnion RE, Epstein SE, et al. A prospective, randomized, controlled trial of prednisone for dilated cardiomyopathy. N Engl J Med 1989;321:1061–1068.

Tolan RW, Kleiman MB, Frank M, et al. Operative intervention in active endocarditis in children: Report of a series of cases and review. Clin Infect Dis 1992;14:852–862.

Waagstein F, Bristow MR, Swedberg K, et al. Beneficial effects of metoprolol in idiopathic dilated cardiomyopathy. Lancet 1993;342:1441–1446.

14 Chest Pain

Garry Sigman

Chest pain in children and adolescents is a common phenomenon, although not as common as headache and abdominal pain. It is responsible for 650,000 physician visits annually in patients between the ages of 10 and 21 years. Chest pain is a major cause of referral to pediatric cardiology clinics, second only to heart murmur.

Chest pain affects males and females with equal frequency, and as many preadolescents as adolescents present with chest pain. The average age of presentation is between 12 and 14 years of age.

These basic facts have emerged from the empirical studies that have been completed:

1. Chest pain in children and adolescents is rarely associated with serious illness.

2. Chest pain is often chronic and an ongoing source of concern and morbidity.

3. The precise diagnosis is not made in a high percentage of cases.

4. The complaint of chest pain is of significant concern to children, adolescents, and their parents.

The importance of chest pain derives not from its mortality rates but from diagnostic difficulties and the tendency for chronicity. The possible causes of the pain are extensive (Table 14–1); clinical acumen is required to make the diagnosis (Table 14–2). The chronic nature of the problem in a high percentage of patients compels the physician to focus on symptom treatment and on minimizing disability. Because precise diagnosis is not always possible, the physician must deal with uncertainty, must not over-test or over-refer, and must provide ongoing care that minimizes disability. Finally, because the complaint is one that engenders fear in patients and in parents, the physician must be reassuring and must help patients who have psychosocial contributions to their chest pain receive the care that is needed to help them resolve the pain.

COMMON CAUSES OF CHEST PAIN

The most common diagnostic categories for chest pain are listed in Table 14–1. The diagnoses that are responsible for the highest percentage of cases that present in a primary care setting include:

- Pain from chest wall–musculoskeletal causes (Table 14–3)
- Psychological causes (anxiety, somatoform disorder, hyperventilation)
- Respiratory causes (cough, asthma, pneumonia, pleural effusion, pneumothorax)

Overall, the etiologic features of chest pain in children and adolescents in primary care settings vary in different studies and are idiopathic or undiagnosed in 23% to 45%, are of musculoskeletal origin in 18% to 32%, are respiratory in 12% to 21%, are psychological in 7% to 20%, are gastrointestinal in 2% to 9%, are cardiac in 1% to 8%, and have other causes in 4% to 21%. A large category is idiopathic, signifying that (1) many cases of chest pain are undiagnosed, and that with better diagnostic acumen other categories would contain higher percentages, or that (2) many cases of chest pain are unable to be diagnosed, and the idiopathic category remains common, independent of what other diagnostic strategies are adopted. The former implication would compel us to develop better diagnostic methods: taking better histories and performing further diagnostic tests, such as studies seeking evidence of bronchospasm or esophageal disease, or performing more detailed psychiatric assessments.

Red flags suggesting a significant disease are noted in Table 14–4. The implication for the second concept challenges us to develop approaches to help control the symptoms and to achieve optimal function despite the pain.

Chest Wall and Musculoskeletal Pain

Discomfort emanating from the chest wall is the most common identifiable cause of chest pain in children and adolescents. Pain can involve the ribs, costochondral junctions, costal cartilages, intercostal muscles, sternum, clavicle, and spine. Figure 14–1 illustrates the anatomic structures on the chest wall important in the etiology of chest pain. Musculoskeletal causes are characterized by an insidious onset (except for trauma or overuse injuries) and the demonstration of localized tenderness over specific areas of the

Table 14–1. Differential Diagnosis of Pediatric Chest Pain

Musculoskeletal (common) (see Table 14–3)
    Trauma (accidental, abuse)
    Exercise, overuse injury (strain, bursitis)
    Tietze syndrome
    Costochondritis
    Herpes zoster (cutaneous)
    Pleurodynia
    Sickle cell anemia vaso-occlusive crisis
    Osteomyelitis (rare)
    Primary or metastatic tumor (rare)
    Fibrositis
    Slipping rib

Pulmonary (common)
    Pneumonia
    Pleurisy
    Asthma
    Chronic cough
    Pneumothorax, pneumomediastinum
    Infarction (sickle cell anemia)
    Foreign body
    Embolism (rare)
    Pulmonary hypertension (rare)
    Tumor (rare)

Gastrointestinal (rare)
    Esophagitis (gastroesophageal reflux)
    Esophageal foreign body
    Esophageal spasm

Esophageal rupture
Cholecystitis
Subdiaphragmatic abscess
Perihepatitis (Fitz-Hugh–Curtis syndrome)
Peptic ulcer disease
Pancreatitis
Cardiac (rare)
    Pericarditis (see Table 14–8)
    Postpericardiotomy syndrome
    Endocarditis
    Mitral valve prolapse (uncertain cause)
    Aortic stenosis (angina)
    Arrhythmias
    Hypertrophic cardiomyopathy
    Marfan syndrome (dissecting aortic aneurysm)
    Anomalous coronary artery (angina)
    Kawasaki disease (angina)
    Cocaine, sympathomimetic ingestion (angina)
    Familial hypercholesterolemia (angina)
Idiopathic (common)
    Anxiety, hyperventilation
    Panic disorder
Other (rare)
    Spinal cord or nerve root compression
    Breast-related pathology
    Castleman disease (lymph node neoplasm)

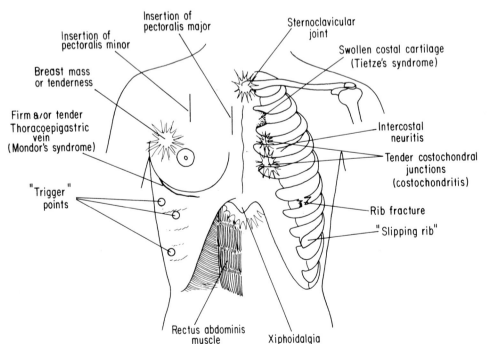

Figure 14–1. Palpable and/or visible abnormalities of the chest wall that may be found in different "chest wall syndromes." In addition, various proximal abdominal causes of chest pain, such as disease of the gallbladder, liver, stomach, pancreas, or subdiaphragmatic space, must be considered. (From Reilly BM. Chest pain. *In* Practical Strategies in Outpatient Medicine, 2nd ed. Philadelphia: WB Saunders, 1991.)

Table 14–2. Differentiation of Chest Pain

Cause	Example	Pleuritic*	Clinical Characteristic	Laboratory Data	Comments
Angina	Anomalous left coronary artery from pulmonary artery	No	Infant with poor feeding, diaphoresis, tachycardia, irritability.	Q-wave infarction pattern or ST-segment changes, echo demonstrates anomalous vessels	Difficult diagnosis, may demonstrate heart failure, cyanosis.
	Anomalous origin (ostia) or course of coronary artery	No	Adolescent with exercise-induced, oppressive, constricting, retrosternal anterior pain. Episodic, brief duration, radiation to neck, shoulder interscapular area.	ST-segment depression	Infarction demonstrates Q-wave pattern, more prolonged pain (>30 min), elevated CPK (MB), history of prior angina, sudden death.
Reactive airway disease	Asthma	No	Exercise-induced dyspnea, dull or sharp pain lasting 1–5 min, may occur at rest.	Pulmonary function tests with response to beta-agonist aerosols	Very common. Cough or wheeze may be absent.
Chest wall syndrome (see Table 14–3)	Tietze syndrome, pleurodynia, overuse exercise	Yes	Pain and palpable local tenderness or swelling. Pain with chest movement.	CXR may demonstrate rib fracture or rarely other pathology	Exclude trauma, pneumonia, pleural effusion.
Pericarditis (see Table 14–8)	Viral, SLE	Possibly	Sharp pain worse while recumbent, better while sitting up leaning forward, 3-component pericardial friction rub: atrial systole, ventricular systole, diastolic filling. Tachycardia.	ECG: ST-segment elevation, T-wave flattening, electrical alternans. Echo: pericardial fluid CXR: large heart, normal pulmonary vasculature	If severe dyspnea, fever, suspect purulent bacterial pericarditis and tamponade.
Pulmonary embolism	Hypercoagulable state, deep venous thrombosis, central catheter related	Possibly	Sudden pain, dyspnea, hypoxia, apprehension, palpitation. Pain is pressurelike or pleuritic. Hemoptysis rare.	CXR: normal or small pleural effusion or atelectasis. ECG: RV strain. Positive (high probability) ventilation-perfusion scan.	Pulmonary angiography is gold standard.
Pneumonia	Viral, bacterial	Usually	Cough, fever, dyspnea, crackles.	CXR: infiltrate. CBC: leukocytosis. Positive sputum or blood culture.	See Chapter 7.
Pleural effusion	Viral, bacterial, parapneumonic; SLE	Yes	Sudden onset, dullness to chest percussion, diminished breath sounds.	CXR: effusion	See Chapter 7.
Pneumothorax	Secondary to asthma, trauma, cystic fibrosis, severe cough, idiopathic, Valsalva maneuver	Possibly	Sudden onset dyspnea, pain, cough, cyanosis (if tension pneumothorax), hyperresonant to chest percussion.	CXR: pneumothorax	Treat with chest tube if patient is symptomatic.
Trauma (nonpenetrating)	Pneumothorax, rib fracture, hemothorax, pulmonary contusion	Yes	As per specific diagnosis.	As per specific diagnosis	
Esophagitis	Reflux, hiatal hernia, chalasia	No	Heartburn, worse if bending over.	Endoscopy, upper GI study, pH probe study	See Chapter 20.
Peptic ulcer disease	Gastric, duodenal ulcer	No	Epigastric, preprandial, nighttime sharp pain. Relief with food, antacids.	Endoscopy	See Chapters 18 and 21.

*Pleuritic chest pain results from stimulation of pain receptors of the parietal pleura (inner chest wall, diaphragm, mediastinum, hilum), the inferior pericardium, and the bone and soft tissue of the chest wall.

Abbreviations: CBC = complete blood count; GI = gastrointestinal; CPK = creatine phosphokinase; CXR = chest x-ray study; ECG = electrocardiogram; echo = echocardiogram; RV = right ventricular; SLE = systemic lupus erythematosus.

Table 14–3. Chest Wall Syndromes

Syndrome	Manifestation
Female breast	Fibroadenoma, hypertrophy, cystic disease, menstrual swelling, pregnancy, panniculitis, malignancy (rare).
Male breast	Gynecomastia.
Pleurodynia	Intercostal muscle infection with coxsackievirus (group B), rarely other enteroviruses. Epidemics. Sudden onset of spasmodic, paroxysmal, stitchlike chest and abdominal pain. Lasts 4–6 days.
Rib fractures	Traumatic, pathologic (tumor, rickets), cough induced. Localized tenderness with local crepitus.
Xiphoidalgia	Idiopathic or traumatic. Sternal tenderness rarely caused by hematologic malignancy.
Costochondritis	Idiopathic, traumatic, or rheumatologic. Tenderness over costochondral junction.
Myodynia	Idiopathic, sickle cell anemia. Tenderness of intercostal or pectoralis muscles.
Fibrositis	Fibromyalgia. Point tenderness in parasternal-intercostal area.
Herpes zoster	Vesicular rash over unilateral dermatome.
Tietze syndrome	Idiopathic—must consider osteomyelitis, tumor, rheumatoid arthritis, fracture in differential diagnosis. Characterized by painful, tender bulbous or fusiform swelling of costal cartilages with or without warmth, erythema.
Slipping rib syndrome	Recurrent subluxation of usually the eighth, ninth, or tenth costal cartilage.
Pectoralis major syndrome	Exertional overuse. Pain in parasternal area or with contraction of the muscle.
Thoracic outlet syndrome	Multiple causes. Suspect if pain and dysesthesia are predominantly in arm, forearm, or hand.

chest wall or of pain elicited by specific manipulation of the thorax. The pain is nagging and localized to the affected area but might radiate; in more severe cases, there is pain on deep breathing. General features of musculoskeletal chest wall pain are listed in Tables 14–2 and 14–3. Most causes are generally benign conditions but can be slow to resolve.

EXERTION

Various forms of physical exertion, especially some athletic pursuits, can readily strain chest wall muscles. New activities tend to stress chest muscles that have not been used; it is important to determine whether the patient has recently started training for a sport. Weight lifting has a particular predilection for causing postexercise chest wall pain. Coughing for a prolonged duration may strain chest muscles and cause pain (see Chapter 7).

TRAUMA

Direct trauma to the thoracic cavity may also cause chest wall pain. Contusion or rib fracture causes a particularly painful syndrome with pain on inspiration and exquisite tenderness on palpation. Palpable crepitus may be present along the rib. Trauma to the intercostal muscles and the chondrosternal areas is common.

Trauma or strain to specific muscles on the chest wall may be recognized as painful syndromes that are recognized by distribution:

In *pectoral syndrome,* the pain is in a band across the anterior parasternal chest wall on the right or left. On the left, this ache may be mistaken for angina or cardiac-related pain.

The *coracoid syndrome* is characterized by a strain of pectoralis minor muscle and tenderness at its insertion into the coracoid process.

The *xiphoid process syndrome* results in pain in the anterior chest and epigastrium and tenderness over the xiphoid process. Pain in the lateral upper back is caused by strain of the *trapezius muscle.* Pain in the anterior lateral chest wall can be caused by strain of the *serratus anterior muscle.*

Strain of the *deltoid* and other muscles of the shoulder girdle may cause chest pain.

The diagnosis of specific injured muscle groups can be aided by the chest wall maneuvers described in Figure 14–2.

Table 14–4. Red Flags Associated with Serious Causes of Chest Pain

Sudden onset of severe crushing pain with exercise
Syncope
Palpitations and/or dysrhythmias
Family history of sudden death
High fever
Severe dyspnea
Cyanosis
Tachycardia
Hypotension
Congenital heart disease (unoperated or repaired)
Family history of DVT or PTE
Significant other disease (SLE, Kawasaki disease, sickle cell anemia, Marfan syndrome, cystic fibrosis, pneumonia)
Previous esophageal surgery (esophageal rupture)
Night pain

Abbreviations: DVT = deep venous thrombosis; PTE = pulmonary thromboembolism; SLE = systemic lupus erythematosus.

Figure 14–2. Chest wall maneuvers.

A, B, The "scissors" maneuver. The patient's arm is adducted across the anterior chest, and the examiner pulls the patient's hand beyond the contralateral shoulder *(A).* When both arms are tested together, traction is applied to both *(B)* and the patient turns the head to either side—the arms form a "scissors." Pain originating in the scapula, thoracic spine, pectoral muscles, or ribs and intercostal structures will often be precipitated by the scissors maneuver.

C, The "hedge clipper" maneuver. The pectoralis major muscles are stressed by asking the patient to "press" the palms forcefully together with the elbows flexed anterior to the chest. The pectorals are thus more clearly defined, and pain is often appreciated within the muscles or at their insertion in the upper parasternal area (see Fig. 14–1).

D, The "racing dive" maneuver. The pectoralis minor muscles are stressed by forcefully resisting the patient's attempt to throw forward the shoulder and upper arm from an initial position behind (dorsal to) the chest wall. The attempted arm motion is that of flinging the arm and hand forward, as a swim racer would when beginning a racing dive. The examiner resists this forward arm and shoulder motion.

E, The "crowing rooster" maneuver. The patient hyperextends the neck while the examiner lifts both of the patient's arms backward and superiorly. Pain originating in the cervical spine or anterior chest wall or both will often thus be reproduced.

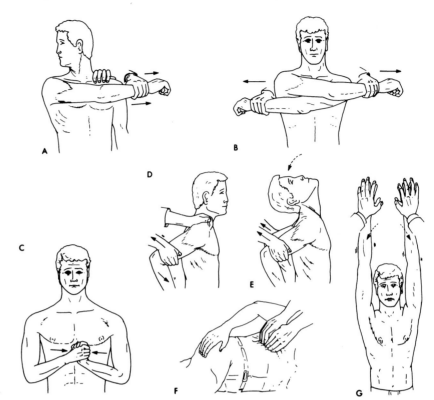

F, The "hooking" maneuver. With the patient supine, the examiner stands at the patient's side, facing the patient's feet. The examiner then "hooks" his or her fingers around the lower costal margin of the rib cage and pulls anteriorly (ventrally) and superiorly (cephalad). This maneuver may elicit pain when costochondritis or traumatic rib injuries involve the lower rib cage, when the upper rectus abdominis muscle is torn, or when a "slipping rib" is the problem.

G, The "high ten" maneuver. The patient raises both hands overhead, elbows extended, and then presses forward with the hands against resistance offered by the examiner. Pain originating in the anterior rib cage, thoracic spine, or pectoral muscles may be elicited here.

(A–G, From Reilly BM. Chest pain. *In* Practical Strategies in Outpatient Medicine, 2nd ed. Philadelphia: WB Saunders, 1991.)

PRECORDIAL CATCH SYNDROME

Episodes of very brief (30 seconds to 3 minutes), sharp pains in the left parasternal area or near the cardiac apex may be caused by the precordial catch syndrome. This syndrome occurs more commonly in the slouched or bent over posture, is completely benign, and responds to reassurance and attention to posture.

TIETZE'S SYNDROME

Pain emanating from the costal cartilages, *costochondritis,* is a common cause of chest pain. Tietze's syndrome, a rare condition, causes visible swelling in that location with pain. In contrast, costochondritis is more common and demonstrates pain and tenderness in the costal cartilage without visible swelling. The pain is often unilateral (left-sided more than right-sided) and affects females more than males. The fourth left sternocostal cartilage is most frequently involved.

SLIPPING RIB SYNDROME

Another cause of mechanical rib pain is the slipping rib syndrome, which causes pain at the lower costal margin and is associated with increased mobility of the tenth rib (less commonly the eighth or ninth). The pain can be duplicated by hooking the fingers under the anterior costal margins and pulling the ribs anteriorly.

PUBERTY

Chest discomfort may be caused by breast budding. Occasionally, adolescents and their parents are not aware of normal early pubertal development. The small breast nodule that normally develops in females and some males can produce discomfort, especially if it is palpated by the patient repeatedly. Other breast abnormalities in females may present with pain and include fibroadenoma, cystosarcoma phylloides, breast infections, and other breast tumors.

DISEASE OF THE SPINE

Diseases of the lower cervical or upper thoracic spine can cause chest pain. *Cervical spinal root compression* causes referred pain in the region of the serratus anterior and pectoral muscles. Thoracic root disease causes pain in the skin of the chest wall and intercostal muscles. Spinal root pain, when sharp, may radiate widely and lead to spasm in the muscles innervated by the nerve root. Pain and tenderness over the anterior chest wall therefore may indicate spinal disease. Clues to the correct diagnosis include history of back pain in addition to anterior pain, a history of vertigo, headache or pain after prolonged recumbency or straining, tenderness over the spine, and elicitation of pain with maneuvers that stress the cervical and thoracic spine.

Ankylosing spondylitis causes disease of the sacroiliac joints and variable involvement in the thoracic and cervical spine. Although typically a disease of young adults, it may occur in childhood in males older than age 8 years. Chest pain may be present before the onset of lower spinal symptoms. Other disease processes of the spine may cause back and radiating chest pain in children; these include trauma, transverse myelitis, kyphosis, spondylolysis, spondylolisthesis, disk herniation, Scheuermann disease, neoplasms, diskitis, epidural abscess, and osteomyelitis (see Chapter 47). Cervical ribs may rarely cause chest pain. These ribs arise from C7 (less commonly C5 or C6). Pain involves the shoulder girdle, extremities, and upper chest; pain may radiate down the arms and cause paresthesia of the fingers. The cervical ribs may impinge on the brachial plexus or subclavian artery. The symptoms and signs of nerve or vascular compression at the thoracic outlet may be caused by supernumerary scalene muscles in addition to cervical ribs. The costoclavicular angle between the first rib and the clavicle may compress the brachial plexus or the subclavian artery. Patients may have chest pain in addition to paresthesia, muscle weakness, or vascular signs of blanching, cyanosis, or edema of the upper extremity.

FIBROMYALGIA SYNDROME

Fibromyalgia syndrome is a common cause of musculoskeletal pain in adults and possibly in children. The pain syndrome, in addition to other systemic symptoms, causes areas of point tenderness of muscle. The most common areas of tenderness are on the trapezius muscle and at the costochondral junction areas.

Psychologic Causes of Pain

Studies of chest pain in primary care settings indicate that psychological causes are common (Table 14–5).

Two basic precepts for recognizing these disorders are as follows:

1. Patients are usually not classifiable into purely (solely) the psychologic designation. Most have biomedical or physiologic causes of pain, usually of a benign nature, in addition to psychological factors that exacerbate the clinical presentation.

2. Patients with chest pain may have more than one psychologic phenomenon (see Table 14–5). Anxiety, depression, and psychosomatic features often coexist and are not often extricable in the primary care setting.

The functional effects of the pain might be considerable because adolescents with chest pain, compared with a pain free control group, may demonstrate more bodily worries, more limitation of general activity, and more school absence. The symptom of acute or chronic chest pain causes concern in children and their parents because most adolescents with chest pain associate their pain with heart disease. This concern is so pervasive that reassurance by physicians is not always simple. The effectiveness of physicians in reassuring a patient and family has significant implications for the chronicity of the pain and the functional outcome. Effectiveness depends on awareness of anxiety levels, awareness of cognitive

Table 14–5. Psychologic Causes of Chest Pain in Children and Adolescents

Functional effects of nonspecific chest pain
Hyperventilation syndrome
Anxiety and Panic Disorder
Depression
Somatization Disorder

Table 14–6. Type and Incidence of System Involvement During Hyperventilation in Children

System	Percent of Cases
Cardiovascular	
Chest pain	86
Palpitation	74
Pallor	72
Cold extremities	42
Respiratory	
Deep-sighing respirations	100
Dyspnea, breathlessness	68
Neurologic	
Numbness	66
Dizziness	58
Tingling	34
Loss of consciousness	22
Musculoskeletal	
Aches and pains	38
Limping	20
Tetany	10
Gastrointestinal	
Dry mouth	52
Abdominal bloating and pain	40
Belching	26

developmental factors, and proper use of tests and consultants (see Treatment).

SYNDROME OF HYPERVENTILATION

Patients who have significant psychological factors associated with chest pain may also have other somatic symptoms, including breathlessness, fatigue, nervousness, faintness, near-syncope, and palpitation. The syndrome of hyperventilation is defined as overbreathing accompanied by dyspnea and anxiety to a degree that results in systemic symptoms, including paresthesia and lightheadedness. It may also be accompanied by palpitation, confusion, and chest pain. Symptoms of hyperventilation syndrome are physiologic phenomena caused by hypocapnia, respiratory alkalosis, and chest muscle strain (Table 14–6; Fig. 14–3). Hyperventilation should also be thought of as a symptom of underlying acute or chronic psychiatric problems. Occasionally, hyperventilation might present as an acute, nonrecurrent event; however, it often indicates a long-term disorder that requires psychiatric management. If chronic and recurrent, hyperventilation most commonly represents a panic disorder. Forty percent of children who hyperventilate continue to do so as adults.

ANXIETY

Anxiety disorders are common in children of all ages. Many children with anxiety disorder or panic disorder have episodic chest pain. Anxiety symptoms might cause chest pain without hyperventilation. Children and adolescents with anxiety conditions manifest the same spectrum of symptoms as adults with panic disorders (see Chapter 36). Many of the acute symptoms are related temporally to stressful situations, such as death, divorce, separation from friends, school failure, pregnancy, or physical illness. Stressors also include a family member with chest pain because psy-

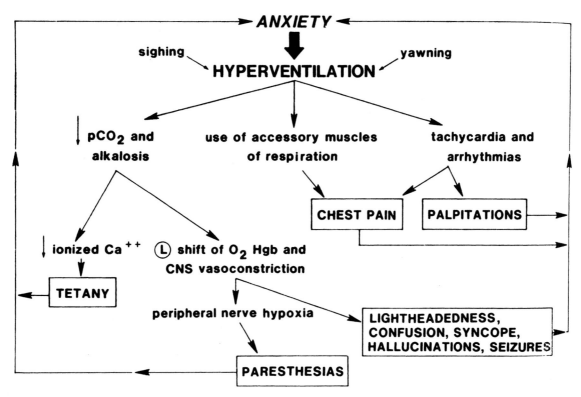

Figure 14–3. Pathophysiologic mechanisms of hyperventilation. (From Herman SP, Stickler GB, Lucas AR. Hyperventilation syndrome in children and adolescents: Long-term follow-up. Pediatrics 1981;67:183–187.)

chogenic pain is four times as likely with a family history of chest pain. Children with anxiety disorders also manage everyday common stresses with difficulty, so their history does not always indicate a significant identifiable life event. School or athletic activities might be initiating events. Athletes with chest pain and psychological causes might be a difficult group to treat because of the necessary concerns about the cardiovascular system in athletes.

DEPRESSION

Depression in children and adolescents has become increasingly recognized (see Chapter 46). Chest pain is an associated symptom in some patients; depression is demonstrated in approximately 10% of children with chest pain. Multiple studies have reported the common association of depression in children with somatic complaints. Depression may be a primary etiologic factor in chest pain, or it might be related to a reaction to an identified physical illness or to chronic undiagnosed and potentially serious symptoms.

SOMATOFORM DISORDER

Another common psychological cause of chest pain in children and adolescents is somatoform disorder, formerly known as psychosomatic illness. Somatoform disorders fall along a spectrum that includes severe problems, like conversion hysteria, to more mild forms of bodily concerns. Anxiety and depressive symptoms might be present but are not uniformly present. The chest is included in the many bodily concerns of these patients, along with headaches, abdominal symptoms, dizziness, and other sensory-related symptoms. The diagnosis of a somatoform disorder demands a complete history that identifies many factors often present

in a child or adolescent with a psychosomatic disorder (see Chapter 46).

Respiratory Causes of Pain

Respiratory causes of chest pain are common.

ASTHMA AND RESPIRATORY INFECTION

Bronchial asthma and acute respiratory infections are common entities that cause cough and respiratory distress (see Chapter 8). Prolonged symptoms are likely to stress chest wall muscles, causing pain. Pain from prolonged cough or respiratory distress might be a constant ache or pain with respiratory excursions; the pain might be localized to a specific area of the chest wall, or it may be a diffuse discomfort. Pain recedes with the cessation of cough and with improvement in tachypnea and in labored respirations.

Bronchial asthma causes chest pain with or without significant respiratory distress. Patients with chest pain associated with exercise often have bronchospasm provoked by exercise and no cardiac abnormalities. The location of the pain is mostly midsternal but is also parasternal, left or right sided, or diffuse. The character of the pain is mostly sharp but also is tight, stabbing, or dull. Patients with undiagnosed chest pain have a greater likelihood than normal control subjects to have abnormal results on methacholine challenges, providing further support for the association of bronchial hyperactivity with chest pain. For some patients with asthma, the chest pain may result from esophageal pathology (reflux esophagitis). Many patients have resolution of chest pain with treatment for esophagitis.

PNEUMONIA AND PLEURISY

Chest pain can be caused by pneumonia and pleurisy (see Table 14–2) (see Chapter 7). These illnesses are the most common identifiable causes of acute chest pain with fever. Inflammation of the pleural surface of the lung causes chest discomfort during inspiration as the pleural surfaces rub together. Bacterial pneumonia (*Haemophilus influenzae,* pneumococcus, *Mycoplasma pneumoniae,* group A streptococcus, less often *Staphylococcus aureus*) is the most common cause of pleuritis in children. Pain is exaggerated by deep breathing, coughing, or straining. It might be sharp and stabbing or dull. Localization may be over the anterior chest wall but may radiate to the back or shoulder. Characteristic physical and radiographic findings are usually present (see Table 14–2).

PNEUMOTHORAX

Pneumothorax may cause acute chest pain along with dyspnea. The severity of the pain does not correlate with the degree of the pneumothorax. It may accompany a known pulmonary disease, such as acute asthma, pneumonia with empyema, trauma, or cystic fibrosis, but it may also occur spontaneously in a previously healthy male adolescent (suspect Marfan disease). A tympanitic percussion note over decreased breath sounds is the characteristic physical finding. Chest x-ray study confirms the diagnosis.

LESS COMMON CAUSES OF CHEST PAIN

Cardiac Causes

HEART DISEASE

Heart disease is one of the less common, but clinically important, causes of chest pain. Its clinical importance derives from the likelihood of providing efficacious treatment and severity of prognosis.

The presence or absence of heart disease must be carefully evaluated to detect a causative lesion or to reassure the patient and family that such a lesion does not exist. This is necessary because of the general belief that chest pain indicates heart disease. A more complicated matter is how this evaluation and management should occur when the diagnostic work-up indicates a noncausally related heart abnormality. Discovery of any cardiac abnormality, no matter how benign, is often difficult for the patient and family to cope with. Apprehension already precedes the cardiac examination, so that the added realization of an abnormality might be construed by patient or family as a serious problem. This concern might contribute to a cycle of chest pain and anxiety that is related to the perception that serious organic disease exists.

Evidence-based data are limited for the prevalence of the various cardiac causes of chest pain in children and adolescents (see Table 14–1). Cardiac causes of chest pain include:

- Aortic stenosis
- Pulmonary hypertension
- Pericarditis
- Postpericardiotomy syndrome
- Arrhythmia
- Dilated cardiomyopathy
- Myocarditis
- Kawasaki disease–related coronary ischemia
- Hypertrophic cardiomyopathy
- Myocardial infarction

Structural abnormalities of the heart that produce ischemic chest pain might also produce altered cardiac output, leading to syncope or sudden death. In this group, *hypertrophic obstructive cardiomyopathy* and *aortic valve* or *subvalvular stenosis* are most common and therefore the most important to recognize in the assessment of patients with chest pain. If these structural disorders are severe, increased systolic wall stress and shortening of the diastolic period of perfusion can compromise blood flow to the myocardium. Exercise would be expected to provide the hemodynamic stress that worsens chest discomfort in these patients; a history of chest pain with exercise is a significant finding. A family history of recurrent syncope or premature sudden death is significant because hypertrophic obstructive cardiomyopathy is inherited in an autosomal dominant pattern.

Pulmonic stenosis of a significant degree may also cause ischemic-type chest pain. Children with pulmonic stenosis or pulmonary vascular obstructive disease (Eisenmenger complex) are at risk for ischemia, arrhythmia, and sudden death. Pulmonary hypertension, whether it be primary or secondary, may present with chest pain.

Ischemic chest pain, although a common phenomenon in adults, is not common in children and adolescents. If present, it should invoke the possibility of the obstructive lesions mentioned earlier, or various anomalies of the coronary arteries. The characteristic pain gradually increases during physical exertion or other stress. It usually persists for a short time (1 to 5 minutes) and is relieved by rest (see Table 14–2). The pain is typically diffuse, not easily localized but characteristically retrosternal, and occasionally epigastric, with radiation to the neck, jaw, arms, or interscapular area. It is a constricting, choking, tight feeling. If the history indicates previous episodes of chest discomfort similar to this description that is now persistent and associated with syncope, diaphoresis, tachycardia, tachypnea, and hypotension, myocardial infarction must be considered (see Table 14–2). It is important to recognize that this classic presentation may be absent, especially in infants and small children who cannot verbalize the experience of pain.

Physical findings in these patients might allow recognition of left ventricular outflow tract obstruction (Table 14–7). The fixed obstruction of aortic stenosis results in a harsh ejection murmur heard best at the upper right sternal border, radiating to the carotids, and sometimes associated with a thrill. Many children and adolescents with high-output states (fever, anemia, hyperthyroidism, pregnancy) have basilar ejection murmurs, but the relative harshness of the murmur and the presence of a thrill would be important clues of an anatomic valve abnormality. Table 14–7 reviews various systolic murmurs and their relation to patients with chest pain. Laboratory studies in this group of patients are necessary to determine the anatomic diagnosis and severity. The sensitivity of the chest film and ECG in this group of patients is low. Patients with these lesions do not always demonstrate left ventricular hypertrophy. The presence of a prominent septal Q wave strongly suggests hypertrophic cardiomyopathy. Echocardiography is the most important test because it determines the nature and the degree of outflow obstruction, as well as the degree of ventricular hypertrophy. Exercise electrocardiography may also be useful in the functional assessment of a child or adolescent with left-sided outflow obstruction.

MITRAL VALVE PROLAPSE

Mitral valve prolapse (MVP) is an important consideration in the search for the cause of chest pain. Its prevalence is higher than all of the cardiac disorders heretofore discussed. It is not a simple matter to determine whether discomfort arises biologically or functionally (psychologically), as a result of an awareness that a cardiac abnormality is present. It is important to consider which patients

Table 14-7. Systolic Murmurs Important in the Diagnosis of Chest Pain*

Cardiac Diagnosis	Physical Findings	Maneuvers
Innocent ejection murmur	Loudest left sternal border at base, 1 to 3 intensity, peaks early in systole, no click, gallop, heave, or diastolic murmur	Diminishes with standing and Valsalva

Valvular aortic stenosis	Mild
	  Similar to innocent murmur but can have ejection click
	Severe
	  Loudest right second intercostal space, peaks late in systole, delayed carotid upstroke, thrill present, left ventricular heave, audible S_4 gallop, may also have aortic insufficiency murmur	

Hypertrophic cardiomyopathy	Loudest left second intercostal space, peaks in mid systole, carotid upstroke brisk or bisferiens, no diastolic murmur	Increases with standing or Valsalva; decreases on squatting

Pulmonic stenosis	Mild
	  Similar to innocent murmur but ejection click is possible
	Severe
	  Loudest left second intercostal space; loud, widely split S_2; thrill present, right ventricular heave, ejection click at left second intercostal space	

Mitral valve prolapse	Loudest at left sternal border and apex; mid- to late-systolic murmur; click precedes murmur	Increases with patient standing after squatting and during expiration

Modified from Reilly BM. Practical Strategies in Outpatient Medicine, 2nd ed. Philadelphia: WB Saunders, 1991:458.
*See Chapter 16, Heart Murmur.

have hemodynamically important lesions, which are at risk for life-threatening arrhythmia, and which have coincident anxiety disorders that demand treatment.

Mitral valve prolapse describes a phenomenon in which the mitral valve leaflets protrude during ventricular systole beyond the boundary of the mitral ring, toward the left atrium. There are varying degrees of redundancy of the valve leaflets, a lengthening of the chordae, and a dilated valvular ring. When the ventricle contracts, the abnormal leaflets balloon into the left atrium, resulting in a variable degree of mitral insufficiency.

Prolapse of the mitral valve seems to be more clinically significant with increasing age (beyond 30 to 40 years); there appears to be an age-dependent expression of the syndrome. Among young adults, the prevalence has been reported to be between 4% and 20%, whereas studies in children have described lower rates. MVP may be seen in conjunction with an atrial septal defect (secundum type) and with generalized connective disease disorders, such as Marfan syndrome, osteogenesis imperfecta, pseudoxanthoma elasticum, and Ehlers-Danlos syndrome. Isolated MVP has a familial incidence, with a probable dominant inheritance pattern. All studies report that the syndrome is more common in females than in males.

Most pediatric patients with MVP are asymptomatic; chest pain does not occur in most patients, even in those with thickened and furled mitral valve leaflets. In some young patients with chest pain, the only clinical finding is MVP. In adult samples, 40% to 50% of patients with MVP complain of chest pain. Some children with prolapsing mitral valves may have vague, nonexertional chest discomfort. Possible pain mechanisms include papillary muscle or endocardial ischemia as well as discomfort from supraventricular and ventricular dysrhythmia. It is not known why some children and adolescents with MVP have chest discomfort but most do not.

Cardiac examination should be performed with the patient supine, sitting, standing, squatting, and standing after squatting. Findings are accentuated when the patient stands after squatting, which leads to less ventricular filling. Characteristically, any maneuver that decreases left ventricular volume (e.g., standing, Valsalva maneuver), accentuates the posterior protrusion of the leaflets and makes the auscultatory findings more prominent. The ECG may be normal or may demonstrate T-wave abnormalities or prominent U waves. Echocardiography is highly specific and permits exclusion of other cardiac defects. Patients with thoracoskeletal deformity should be carefully examined to rule out MVP. The association of MVP with mitral insufficiency, bacterial endocarditis, stroke, and arrhythmia indicates that MVP may not always be benign. Nonetheless, the prognosis of MVP in children is usually excellent.

Recognition of MVP provides a challenge because it may not necessarily be the cause of the chest pain. There is a lack of empirical evidence that chest pain is caused by the prolapsing mitral valve. Chest pain has no prognostic significance in a patient with no family history and with an isolated mid-systolic click. Noncardiac causes of chest pain might be present in children with benign forms of MVP. For example, esophagitis may be the cause of chest pain in some patients with MVP. Anxiety is a common noncardiac cause of chest pain in young people with MVP that bears closer investigation. There may be an association of panic disorder and MVP.

ACUTE PERICARDITIS

Acute pericarditis of a viral, bacterial, autoimmune, rheumatic, or traumatic cause must be considered when a child presents with chest pain (Table 14-8). Patients with idiopathic or viral pericarditis often have a preceding or accompanying flu-like illness with myalgias, arthralgias, and fever. Most commonly, the pain is sharp and is aggravated by deep inspiration, coughing, or straining. The patient with a large pericardial effusion may feel less pain while leaning forward in the sitting position. Dysphagia, dyspnea, or hiccup may accompany the pain. Pain is typically in the substernal area, but it may refer elsewhere. Pain may be intermittent or constant. A pericardial rub with three components (one systolic and two diastolic) may be present and if so greatly aids in the diagnosis (see Table 14-2). Electrocardiography might reveal a diffuse ST elevation and a low QRS voltage (Fig. 14-4). The chest x-ray study, if positive, may show a globe-shaped, enlarged cardiac

Table 14–8. Etiology of Pericarditis and Pericardial Effusion

Idiopathic (Presumed Viral)

Infectious Agents

Bacteria: group A streptococcus, *Staphylococcus aureus,* pneumococcus, meningococcus,* *Haemophilus influenzae,** *Salmonella* species, *Mycoplasma pneumoniae, Borrelia burgdorferi, Mycobacterium tuberculosis,* rickettsia, tularemia

Viral:† coxsackievirus (group A, B), echovirus, mumps, influenza, Epstein-Barr, cytomegalovirus, herpes simplex, herpes zoster, hepatitis B

Fungal: *Histoplasma capsulatum, Coccidioides immitis, Blastomyces dermatitidis, Cryptococcus neoformans, Candida* species, *Aspergillus* species

Parasitic: *Toxoplasma gondii, Entamoeba histolytica,* schistosomes

Collagen Vascular–Inflammatory and Granulomatous Diseases
Rheumatic fever
Systemic lupus erythematosus (idiopathic and drug induced)
Rheumatoid arthritis
Kawasaki disease
Scleroderma
Mixed connective tissue disease
Reiter syndrome
Inflammatory bowel disease
Wegener granulomatosus
Dermatomyositis
Behçet syndrome
Sarcoidosis
Vasculitis
Familial Mediterranean fever
Serum sickness
Stevens-Johnson syndrome

Traumatic
Cardiac contusion (blunt trauma)
Penetrating trauma
Postpericardiotomy syndrome
Radiation

Contiguous Spread
Pleural disease
Pneumonia
Aortic aneurysm (dissecting)

Metabolic
Hypothyroidism
Uremia
Gaucher disease
Fabry disease
Chylopericardium

Neoplastic
Primary
Contiguous (lymphoma)
Metastatic
Infiltrative (leukemia)

Others
Drug reaction
Pancreatitis
After myocardial infarction
Thalassemia
Central venous catheter perforation
Heart failure
Hemorrhage (coagulopathy)
Biliary-pericardial fistula

*Infectious or immune complex.
†Common (viral pericarditis or myopericarditis is probably the most common cause of acute pericarditis in a previously normal host).

shadow. Echocardiography is the definitive test for diagnosis to quantify the amount of pericardial fluid and the degree of ventricular dysfunction.

RHYTHM DISTURBANCES

Chest pain may be caused by various rhythm disturbances (see Chapter 12). This pain may be caused by an imbalance of myocardial oxygen supply and demand, subendocardial wall stress, and diminished diastolic coronary perfusion. Any of the tachyarrhythmias, ventricular or supraventricular, may bring about these events. Many of these abnormalities have a paroxysmal nature, so that intermittent symptoms are expected. The pain is not classically related to exercise. Chest pain associated with dizziness, palpitations, or syncope may be the presenting complaint and should prompt the physician to perform electrocardiography.

ACUTE AORTIC DISSECTION, ACUTE PULMONARY EMBOLISM

Two acute, potentially catastrophic cardiovascular events, acute aortic dissection and acute pulmonary embolism, deserve mention when one is considering acute chest pain. In patients with Marfan syndrome, Ehlers-Danlos syndrome, and Erdheim's familial cystic necrosis, acute aortic dissection may occur. In addition, there have been case reports of aortic dissection in otherwise well, recreational

weight-lifting athletes. Dissection causes acute, tearing chest pain in the anterior or posterior chest that migrates to the arms, abdomen, and legs. Clinical clues include pulse deficits, an aortic insufficiency murmur, and a normal ECG.

Pulmonary embolism may occur in adolescents (see Chapter 8). This condition presents with acute, pleuritic-type pain, dyspnea, cough, and occasionally hemoptysis. Usually, factors that might predispose to venous thrombosis are present and include oral contraceptive use; recent elective abortion; the early postoperative period; protein C, S, or antithrombin III deficiency; the antiphospholipid antibody syndrome (anticardiolipin, lupus anticoagulant); and immobilization (see Chapter 51). An abnormal ventilation perfusion scan confirms the diagnosis.

Gastrointestinal Causes

Esophagitis (acid reflux, infectious) and *esophageal motility disorders* (diffuse esophageal spasm, achalasia) can cause chest pain in adults and children (see Chapter 20).

If esophageal manometry or esophagoscopy is performed on children and adolescents with chest pain, abnormal findings are occasionally discovered. It is possible that some of the patients in the large idiopathic group in empirical studies have esophageal disease. Furthermore, esophageal disease may be associated with asthma and MVP.

PEPTIC ESOPHAGITIS

Peptic esophagitis occurs in infants, children, and adolescents when gastric contents reflux to the esophagus. Typical "heart-

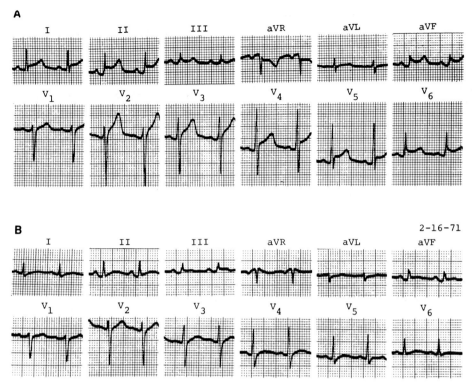

Figure 14–4. Serial changes of acute idiopathic pericarditis. *A,* Diffuse ST segment elevation involving all the leads except aVR and aVL. In lead aVR, the ST segment is depressed. The QRS complex is normal. *B,* The ST segment is almost isoelectric, and the T waves are flattened or notched. (From Chou T-C. Pericarditis. *In* Electrocardiography in Clinical Practice, 3rd ed. Philadelphia: WB Saunders, 1991.)

burn,'' a substernal burning sensation, occurs in children and adolescents but less so than in adults. Indwelling esophageal pH probe studies, barium swallows, scintigraphy, or esophagoscopy are used to diagnose the condition unequivocally. Unfortunately, the percentage of patients with reflux esophagitis who present primarily with chest pain is not known because most patients have not been evaluated with these investigations.

ESOPHAGEAL MOTILITY DISORDERS

Motility disorders of the esophagus are probably less common than reflux esophagitis. Chest pain from a motility disorder may last only for a few seconds, or it may continue for several hours. The pain is nonexertional but may be exacerbated by bending forward. This type of pain is typically substernal but may radiate to the infrascapular area and into the neck. It may therefore resemble the pain of coronary obstruction. Motility disorders have been classified on the basis of manometry studies into nutcracker esophagus, diffuse esophageal spasm, achalasia, and nonspecific motility disorder.

Achalasia is a condition that classically causes dysphagia, nocturnal regurgitation, and chest pain. The symptoms may not be dramatic, and the diagnosis may be elusive. Achalasia may occur at any age. Chest pain occurs in 19% to 95% of patients with achalasia.

ESOPHAGEAL RUPTURE

Acute rupture of the esophagus may occur rarely. It has been described in patients with bulimia nervosa, a condition that is prevalent in the adolescent age range, or after surgery for a tracheoesophageal fistula.

OTHER GASTROINTESTINAL PROBLEMS

Any of the gastrointestinal disorders that affect organs in the upper aspect of the abdominal cavity may cause pain that is sensed in the chest. Disorders such as gastric and duodenal ulcers, cholecystitis, pancreatitis, hepatitis, and infections of the subdiaphragmatic space can cause chest discomfort in addition to their presenting symptomatology.

Other Causes of Chest Pain

SUBSTANCE ABUSE

Adolescent substance use or abuse can cause chest pain. Cigarette smokers complain more often of chest pain than do nonsmokers. Smoking also appears to be a factor in the development of acute chest syndrome in adolescents with sickle cell anemia. Cocaine has also been implicated as a cause of chest pain in adolescents. Chest pain in acute cocaine intoxication frequently resembles myocardial infarction. Abnormal ST-segment and T-wave changes and the quality of the pain contribute to the diagnostic difficulty. Nonetheless, the incidence of myocardial infarction in young patients presenting with acute chest pain after cocaine use is low. The incidence may be increased in cocaine-using patients who also smoke cigarettes.

FOREIGN BODIES

Foreign bodies in the airways and esophagus might be unusual causes of chest discomfort in younger children. Usually, there are other symptoms that suggest the diagnosis, including dysphagia, drooling, choking, wheezing, stridor, and dyspnea. Both solid bodies like coins or caustic substances like acid or alkaline liquid cleaners, which damage the esophagus, can cause chest pain.

NEOPLASTIC DISEASES

Neoplastic diseases may be characterized by chest pain. A mediastinal tumor may cause a constant boring pain that may be associated with cough or dysphagia. Hodgkin's disease, non-Hodgkin's lymphoma, neural-derived neoplasms, and other tumors may present in this fashion.

THE APPROACH TO THE PATIENT WITH CHEST PAIN

The practical approach to chest pain requires a detailed history and physical examination. The process not only is necessary to make a diagnosis but also can serve as a therapeutic intervention. A deliberate, orderly, and complete approach to the clinical evaluation can do much to calm an anxious child and parent. Physicians must not forget that chest pain is, in the mind of many, an ominous symptom that needs immediate attention.

Because the most common causes of chest pain are discernible by history and physical examination, there is a high likelihood that the diagnosis can be made solely on the merits of this clinical evaluation, without other testing (see Tables 14–1 through 14–3). However, identifying one diagnostic cause does not eliminate others. The diagnosis of psychogenic chest pain should not be made as a diagnosis of exclusion. One should set out to discover the positive features that support the psychogenic diagnosis along with the features that suggest a bio-organic cause.

History

Much can be learned by the way the symptoms are reported by patient and parent, together and separately. The parental response to the child's symptoms and the intensity of the parents' concern are important to observe. It is always helpful to elicit beliefs about the symptom from the parent and child. Asking "What are you concerned that this pain is caused by?" can give much information about previous communications between parent and child and about overriding fears. In assessing the severity of pain, it is useful to ask a parent about how the symptom is being expressed by the child. Asking "Would you know that she has pain if she didn't tell you?" is a good way of obtaining this information.

For older children and adolescents, it is necessary to interview the patient alone, without the parent in the room. This measure allows the practitioner to assess the child's level of concern, to clarify the nature of the symptoms in the words of the patient, and to explore areas that might be easier to talk about in private. It is hard for children to discuss areas of difficulty in their family life or school or concern about physical changes (like breast development) until they are given some degree of confidentiality.

Table 14–9 reviews the appropriate historical features to explore. Duration of pain is first. Acute pain that has not previously occurred suggests acute chest wall injury or strain or the onset of a chest

Table 14–9. Historical Features of Chest Pain That Are Essential to Its Assessment

Duration of pain (how long present but also duration of each episode)
Acuteness of onset
Severity of pain (use scale of 1 to 10)
Associated symptoms
Precipitating and ameliorating factors
Quality of pain (pleuritic, sharp, dull)
Location of pain
Limitation of activities by pain
Radiation of pain
Time of day that pain occurs
Recent activity, injury, and stresses
Full psychosocial review, including behaviors
Past medical history
Family medical history

infection. Sudden, significant pain in a patient who appears ill suggests acute pneumothorax, pericarditis, pulmonary embolism, or dissecting aneurysm. Longer-term pain or recurrent pain suggests a psychological cause, a dysrhythmia, or a gastrointestinal problem. Pain that has persisted for months rarely has a serious organic cause. However, if long-term pain persists and increases in severity or is associated with night sweats, fever, or weight loss, a malignancy should be considered.

Determination of associated symptoms is helpful. Fever suggests an acute infectious process; cough, dyspnea, or wheezing suggests a bronchospasmic condition or acute infection. Vomiting, postprandial fullness, or abdominal pain suggests a gastrointestinal cause. Tachypnea is consistent with pneumonia, asthma, and hyperventilation. Tingling in the extremities suggests hyperventilation. Multisystemic complaints are evocative of psychogenic causes, unless they include weight loss, intermittent chronic fevers, or syncope.

The character of pain is not always useful in sorting out its cause. Children are often vague in their description of chest pain. Pain that is "sharp" or "achy" may suggests a chest wall pain or pleural irritation, whereas pain that is "burning" or "gnawing" suggests a thoracic or abdominal visceral origin. Pain that is associated with respiration suggests chest wall discomfort or pleural irritation.

It is helpful to determine factors that exacerbate or reduce pain. Pain that is worse when the patient is lying down or after a large meal or after the consumption of particular foods is consistent with reflux esophagitis. This pain is often relieved by antacids, which patients may take empirically. Pain that is relieved by sitting up and leaning forward might be caused by pericarditis. Pain that is worsened by any movement or sneezing might be related to pleuritic irritation. Pain that is present only during intense exercise must be thought of as consistent with myocardial ischemia and must be actively explored. Pain that is temporally related to perceived stress and is relieved by relaxation is an important historical feature for anxiety-related chest pain. Pain that awakens a patient at night is more likely to have an organic cause.

Localization of the pain is useful. Noncardiac pain is often diffuse and radiates to the abdomen. However, in children, pain may also be noncardiac when it is substernal. When pain radiates to the left shoulder, a cardiac origin is more common. Chest wall syndromes have specific locations (see Table 14–3 and Figs. 14–1 and 14–2).

Information about the recent past can be helpful. Paroxysmal, chronic coughing causes chest wall pain. If the child or adolescent has recently begun to participate in a new sporting activity, especially weight lifting or football, the chest wall may be strained. Recent trauma to the chest is sometimes remembered only with direct questioning.

A full psychosocial review should be performed in each patient. This action ensures that details regarding personal stressors and behaviors will emerge. Asking about school attendance, family relationships, and recent personal and family stressors is necessary. Children with somatoform disorders might have a history of school absences out of proportion to their degree of illness. It is helpful to ask older children whether anyone close to them has had an illness recently. Occasionally, this question yields information that might determine that there is an adult with chest pain and an anxious reaction in the young person.

Review of symptoms and past medical history is sought for specific features. A history of unexplained syncope might suggest a psychogenic condition, a left-sided cardiac obstruction, or a recurrent arrhythmia (see Chapter 43). One should always elicit the past history of recognized or unrecognized Kawasaki disease. The history of sickle cell anemia is usually known. Previous history of vague, recurrent symptoms for which no specific diagnosis has been made might indicate that the child has a psychosomatic disorder.

A family medical history should be sought. Not only does the history of chest disease or heart disease in adults put families at risk for anxiety, but it is possible that some diseases are genetically transmitted. Idiopathic hypertrophic subaortic stenosis (hypertrophic cardiomyopathy) and familial hypercholesterolemia might have caused premature death in a parent or relative. Other inherited conditions that may cause chest pain include asthma, sickle cell disease, Marfan syndrome, other forms of myocardiopathy, peptic ulcer disease, and reflux esophagitis.

Physical Examination

One should start by observing the child for general states of distress, respirations, splinting, and interaction with parents. Does this child look distressed or ill? Who looks worse, the child or the parent? Vital signs should be checked next. Catastrophic causes of chest pain increase the resting heart rate and increase or decrease the blood pressure. Increased body temperature suggests an acute infectious or inflammatory-rheumatic cause of chest pain.

One should observe the chest wall for signs of trauma, for abnormal breathing patterns, and for deformity. Dilated jugular venous pulsations consistent with heart failure should be sought. The single most helpful physical finding is the elicitation of chest wall tenderness. This is the most common physical finding in patients who have no cardiac diseases. Palpation and percussion over the chest should be performed, including the ribs, intercostal areas, sternum, xiphoid, manubrium, axilla, clavicles, epigastric area, spinous processes, and paraspinal areas. Tenderness is pathognomonic for chest wall pain. Pain over the breasts helps diagnose chest pain due to gynecomastia. Dullness over the thorax suggests consolidation, effusion, or atelectasis. Hyperresonance suggests pneumothorax or asthma. Palpation should also detect evidence of a cardiac heave or cardiac thrill as well as determine the point of maximal intensity and peripheral pulses.

Auscultation of the lungs and heart is next. Presence of a friction rub or gallop rhythm helps to make an immediate cardiac diagnosis. Systolic heart murmurs provide the clinical evidence of a cardiac cause of the chest pain (see Table 14–7).

Palpation of the abdomen should be performed for tenderness and the presence of organomegaly.

Laboratory Testing

The physician should be certain whether the testing is being performed for the purpose of diagnosis or reassurance. Testing is of little usefulness if the history is unrevealing and the results of the physical examination are normal. Testing might be helpful in confirming a positive physical finding. Laboratory tests that may be helpful, depending the patient's clinical findings, include the results of the chest x-ray study, ECG, and echocardiogram. None of these should be ordered routinely.

Results of chest x-ray studies are seldom abnormal when physical examination findings are negative. Radiographic studies are indicated if there is a history of trauma, if there is pleuritic chest pain and fever, and if history and physical findings give positive evidence of heart disease. The likelihood of finding bony or intrathoracic abnormalities in the absence of these factors is extremely low.

Electrocardiography should not be thought of as routine but is useful if the history and physical examination indicate the possibility of arrhythmia, pericarditis, myocardial ischemia, or MVP. Obtaining an ECG as a "baseline" measurement but for no other reason is not necessary.

Other testing is indicated based on the hypothesis derived from the assessment. Echocardiography is helpful if MVP, valvular heart disease, hypertrophic cardiomyopathy or pericarditis is suspected. Exercise testing with the ECG is useful if the history suggests angina-type pain and the rest of the testing results are normal. A 24-hour Holter monitor is indicated if arrhythmia is suspected but the resting ECG is normal.

Testing might be indicated to determine whether or not bronchospasm is present. Exercise testing and methacholine challenge testing with concurrent monitoring of pulmonary function are the most sensitive methods. If exercise-induced asthma is suspected, the testing protocol should include an exercise stimulus. A decrease in forced expiratory volume in 1 second (FEV_1) of 10% to 15% is indicative of exercise-induced asthma.

For a complaint like chest pain, over-testing and over-referring to subspecialists can cause harm to the patient. Because the prevalence of chest pain caused by heart disease is low, the physician should avoid reinforcing this association. Patients may experience increased anxiety after their medical encounter.

The patient and family need the physician to make a resolute, clear diagnosis. If heart disease is strongly suspected from a carefully taken history and carefully performed physical examination, it is unreasonable to equate negative results on chest film and electrocardiography with the absence of heart disease. Therefore, it is better to refer the patient to a qualified pediatric cardiologist who should choose the best diagnostic tests. The flow charts that are depicted in the Figure 14–5 provide some general guidelines for appropriate assessment and treatment of patients with chest pain.

TREATMENT

For patients who have pain at rest and no abnormal physical finding or unusual historical clues, reassurance is the most important treatment. As simple as this sounds, physicians are not uniformly successful at implementing it, especially in just one visit. Successful reassurance demands trust, a symptomatic treatment approach, and a follow-up plan. Successful reassurance occasionally helps the patient recognize that the acute chest pain is benign and does not merit concern. Performing this step successfully can help the patient avoid a chronic course with possible disability. It is not normal to have pain, so the persistence of chest pain indicates that the diagnosis has not yet been adequately made or that the treatment is either ineffective or has not had sufficient time to help the patient.

All patients with chest pain should be given follow-up appointments. At the follow-up visit, the physician should determine whether the patient's symptoms have responded to the prescribed approach. Because chest pain has a predilection to chronicity and can cause disability in young people, the physician's role is to help

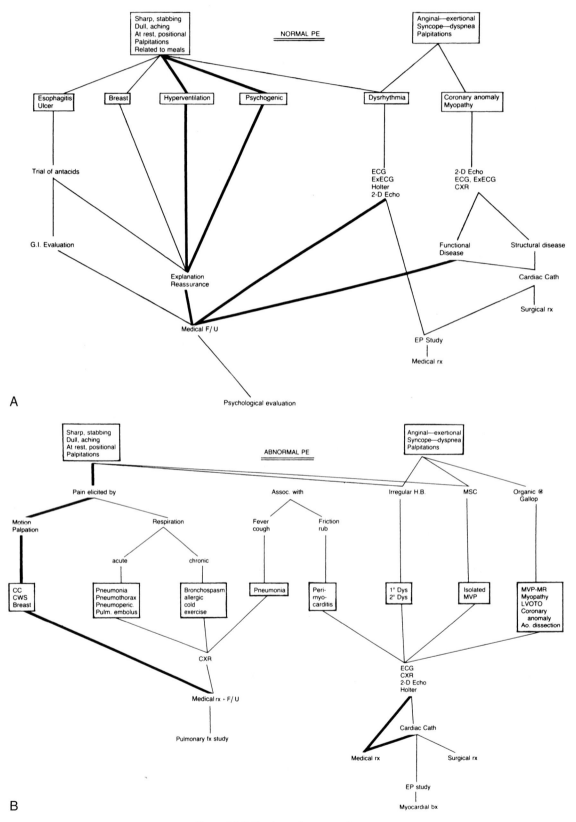

A

B

Figure 14–5 *See legend on opposite page*

patients resolve the complaint. This is especially important if the evaluation for chest pain has revealed a cardiac lesion that is not thought to cause the chest pain. For these patients, exploration of the patient and family's beliefs and attitudes about the diagnosis are necessary to correct misconceptions, to reassure, and to help the patient cope with the stress of having a cardiac diagnosis.

A symptomatic treatment plan is needed so that patients go home with specific directions as to how they can help themselves. If musculoskeletal pain is thought to be present, application of heat, administration of anti-inflammatory medication, or specific exercises may be helpful.

Psychogenic pain calls for an active treatment plan that can be developed by the primary care physician. Emergency department settings are not conducive to the effective diagnosis or treatment of these disorders. Making the diagnosis of hyperventilation syndrome in an emergency department or office setting does not help the patient deal with the causative psychiatric illness. Similarly, prescribing rebreathing into a paper bag is not an adequate treatment without more specific treatment for the psychiatric disorder. Referral from the emergency department to the primary care physician is warranted to gather more history and to plan an approach.

It is not appropriate to make a diagnosis of psychological causes of chest pain without developing a plan for treatment. Such an approach gives the patient the unfortunate message that the physician is interested in helping him or her only with bio-organic illness but is not interested in the patient's problem. Specific treatments have been shown to be successful for chest pain that is primarily of psychogenic origin. Treatments for hyperventilation have been developed, including breathing retraining, behavioral treatment, and group treatment. Specific treatments for anxiety disorders, depression, and somatoform disorders are warranted if they cause chest pain. These treatments include behavioral techniques for relaxation, guided imagery, individual or group psychotherapy, and/or the use of psychotropic medications.

A pain diary, in which frequency, severity, and circumstances are charted by the patient, is a useful device for follow-up discussion of how the patient can learn to reduce the symptoms. If the physician is not equipped to work with patients in this way, or if the patient is not responding to treatment, a referral should be made to a behavioral pediatrician, an adolescent medicine specialist, or a mental health professional with experience in somatoform disorders in children. Referral to mental health professionals may be warranted but requires that the physician stay actively involved and instrumental in the treatment plan. This involvement is important to provide ongoing treatment of symptoms of pain and to verify that the patient and family are following through with the mental health treatment plan.

If gastroesophageal reflux is thought to be present, a trial of antacids or H_2-blocking agents seems reasonable as well as education regarding limiting foods that seem to worsen the condition, not eating at a time close to bedtime, and raising the head of the bed at night. If the patient does not respond to this approach, or if other gastrointestinal pathology is suspected, referral to a pediatric gastroenterologist is indicated.

Because many patients have more than one interacting influence that results in chest pain, the primary care physician must stay involved even if referrals are made. Patients and families are not always sure who is "in charge" of the plan. A complaint like chest pain, which, if chronic, can have a complex variety of causes, requires a primary physician to coordinate consultations and to interpret the specialist's recommendations to the patient.

REFERENCES

General

Bass C. Unexplained chest pain and breathlessness. Med Clin North Am 1991;75:1059–1173.

Coleman WL. Recurrent chest pain in children. Pediatr Clin North Am 1984;31:1007–1027.

Diehl AM. Chest pain in children. Pediatr Chest Pain 1983;73: 335–342.

Goodman-Kaden G, Shenker R, Gootman N. Chest pain in adolescents. J Adolesc Health 1991;12:251–255.

Pantell RH, Goodman BW. Adolescent chest pain: A prospective study. Pediatrics 1983;71:881–887.

Perry LW. Pinpointing the cause of pediatric chest pain. Contemp Pediatr February 1985, pp 71–76.

Selbst SM. Adolescent chest pain and cardiac emergencies. Adolesc Med 1993;4:23–33.

Selbst SM. Chest pain in children. Pediatrics 1985;75:1068–1070.

Selbst SM. Pediatric chest pain: A prospective study. Pediatrics 1988;82:319–323.

Selbst SM, Ruddy R, Clark BJ. Chest pain in children (follow-up of patients previously reported). Clin Pediatr 1990;29:374–377.

Zavaras-Angelidou KA, Weinhouse E, Nelson DB. Review of 180 episodes of chest pain in 134 children. Pediatr Emerg Care 1992;8:189–192.

Cardiac Disorders

Alpert MA. Mitral valve prolapse, panic disorder, and chest pain. Med Clin North Am 1991;75:1119–1133.

Figure 14–5. *A, B,* These flow diagrams are designed to differentiate the types of chest pain likely to be encountered, with management options based on whether the physical examination (PE) is normal or abnormal. The *heavy lines* indicate the pathway that would be most commonly encountered. Diagnostic possibilities are listed across the page; pertinent laboratory evaluation and further therapy (rx) are suggested. In patients with normal physical findings, unless the pain is anginal or associated with syncope, progressive dyspnea, or suspected rhythm disturbance, laboratory evaluation is rarely necessary. Cardiac disease is divided into structural abnormalities (coronary lesions), functional disease (myopathy), or dysrhythmia. ECG = electrocardiogram; ExECG = exercise electrocardiogram; Holter = 24-hour ambulatory ECG monitor; 2-D Echo = two-dimensional echocardiogram or color Doppler echocardiogram; CXR = chest x-ray; EP study = intracardiac electrophysiologic study; G.I. = gastrointestinal.

In patients with chest pain and abnormal physical findings, the diagnostic pathway will be determined by the physical examination. If pain is produced by palpation or trunk motion or is associated with gynecomastia or breast nodule, a chest x-ray study is only occasionally needed. Acute or chronic respiratory disorders generally require radiographic assessment. An irregular rhythm may be a primary problem or may be secondary to myocardial inflammation or mitral valve prolapse (MVP). Chest pain associated with fever and cough may be due to bronchopneumonitis. The addition of pericardial friction rub with a history of fever and cough raises concern about perimyocarditis and should prompt specific cardiac studies. Isolated MVP may be confirmed by two-dimensional echo or color Doppler echocardiography, but when it is associated with mitral regurgitation or if other structural cardiac disease is suspected, a more detailed evaluation is suggested. CC = costochondritis; CWS = chest wall syndrome (rib, vertebral, muscle abnormalities); pneumoperic. = pneumopericardium; pulm. embolus = pulmonary embolus; $1°$ = primary; $2°$ = secondary; Dys = dysrhythmia; MSC = mid-systolic click; MR = mitral regurgitation; LVOTO = left ventricular outflow obstruction; Ao = aortic; bx = myocardial biopsy; fx = function; H.B. = heart beat. (*A* and *B,* From Brenner JI, Ringel RE, Berman MA. Cardiologic perspectives of chest pain in childhood: A referral problem? To whom? Pediatr Clin North Am 1984;31:1241–1258.)

Arfken CL, Schulman P, McLaren MJ, et al. Mitral valve prolapse: Associations with symptoms and anxiety. Pediatrics 1990;85:311–315.

Benjamin SB, Goff JS, Hackshaw BT. Chest pain: Cardiac or esophageal. Patient Care July 15 1987, pp 116–132.

Bor I. Myocardial infarction and ischemic heart disease in infants and children. Arch Dis Child 1969;44:268–281.

Bowen RC, D'Arcy C, Orchard RC. The prevalence of anxiety disorders among patients with mitral valve prolapse syndrome and chest pain. Psychomatics 1991;32:400–406.

Brenner JD, Ringel RE, Berman MA. Cardiologic perspectives of chest pain in childhood: A referral problem? To whom? Pediatr Clin North Am 1984;31:1241–1258.

Declue JJ, Malone JI, Root AW. Coronary artery disease in diabetic adolescents. Clin Pediatr 1988;27:587–590.

Fyfe, DA, Moodle DS. Chest pain in pediatric patients presenting to a cardiac clinic. Clin Pediatr 1984;23:321–324.

Gitter MJ, Goldsmith SR, Dunbar DN, et al. Cocaine and chest pain: Clinical features and outcome of patients hospitalized to rule out myocardial infarction. Ann Intern Med 1991;115:277–282.

Schaffer MS, Nouri S, Chen SC, et al. Fatal aortic rupture presenting as chest pain in an adolescent. Clin Pediatr 1985;24:216–217.

Schor JS, Horowitz MD, Livingstone AS. Recreational weight lifting and aortic dissection: Case report. J Vasc Surg 1993;17:774–776.

Woodward GA, Selbst SM. Chest pain secondary to cocaine use. Pediatr Emerg Care 1987;3:153–154.

Noncardiac Causes

Berezin S, Medow MS. Esophageal chest pain in children with asthma. J Pediatr Gastroenterol Nutr 1991;52–55.

Bernstein DS, Schonberg SK. Pulmonary embolism in adolescents. Am J Dis Child 1986;140:667–671.

Brown RT. Costochondritis in adolescents. J Adolesc Health 1981;1:198–201.

Buskila D, Press J, Gedalia A, et al. Assessment of nonarticular tenderness and prevalence of fibromyalgia in children. J Rheumatol 1993;20:368–370.

Fam AG, Smythe HA. Musculoskeletal chest wall pain. Can Med Assoc J 1985;133:379–389.

Fisher RZ. Masked depression: Its interference with somatization, hypochondriasis and conversion. Int J Psychiatry Med 1987;17:367–379.

Gedalia A, Press J, Klein M, et al. Joint hypermobility and fibromyalgia in schoolchildren. Ann Rheum Dis 1993;52:494–496.

Gelfand MJ, Daya SA, Rucknagel DL, et al. Simultaneous occurrence of rib infarction and pulmonary infiltrates in sickle cell disease patients with acute chest syndrome. J Nucl Med 1993;4:614–618.

Glassman MS, Medow MS, Berezin S, et al. Spectrum of esophageal disorders in children with chest pain. Dig Dis Sci 1992;37:663–666.

Greydanus DE, Parks DS, Farrell EG. Breast disorders in children and adolescents. Pediatr Clin North Am 1989;36:601–638.

Hayward C, Killen JD, Taylor CB. Panic attacks in young adolescents. Am J Psychiatry 1989;146:1061–1062.

Hegel MT, Abel GG, Etscheidt M, et al. Behavioral treatment of angina-like chest pain in patients with hyperventilation syndrome. J Behav Ther Exp Psychiatry 1989;20:1–9.

Heinz GJ, Zavala DC. Slipping rib syndrome. Diagnosis using the "hooking maneuver." JAMA 1977;237:794–795.

Key JD, Hammill WW, Everett L. Pulmonary embolus in an adolescent on oral contraceptives. J Adolesc Health 1992;13:713–715.

Klimes I, Mayou RA, Pearce MJ, et al. Psychological treatment for atypical non-cardiac chest pain: A controlled evaluation. Psychiatr Med 1990;20:605–611.

Koren A, Wald I, Halevi R, et al. Acute chest syndrome in children with sickle cell anemia. Pediatr Hemat Oncol 1990;7:99–107.

Langevin S, Castell DO. Esophageal motility disorders and chest pain. Med Clin North Am 1991;75:1045–1063.

Leffert RD. Thoracic outlet syndromes. Hand Clin 1992;8:285–297.

Ley R. The efficacy of breathing retraining and the centrality of hyperventilation in panic disorder: A reinterpretation of experimental findings. Behav Res Ther 1991;29:301–304.

Makhoul RG, Machleder HI. Developmental anomalies at the thoracic outlet: An analysis of 200 consecutive cases. J Vasc Surg 1992;10:534–542.

Malleson PN, al-Mater M, Petty RE. Idopathic musculoskeletal pain syndromes in children. J Rheumatol 1992;19:1786–1789.

Medow S, Glassman MS, Newman LJ. Esophageal chest pain in children with asthma. J Pediatr Gastroenterol Nutr 1991;12:52–55.

Orenstein SR. Controversies in pediatric gastroesophageal reflux. J Pediatr Gastroenterol Nutr 1992;14:338–348.

Prazar G. Conversion reactions in adolescents. Pediatr Rev 1987;8:279–286.

Richter JE. Gastroesophageal reflux disease as a cause of chest pain. Med Clin North Am 1991;785:1065–1080.

Wiens L, Sabath R, Ewing L, et al. Chest pain in otherwise healthy children and adolescents is frequently caused by exercise-induced asthma. Pediatrics 1992;90:350–353.

15 Cyanosis

Frank Smith

CYANOSIS

Cyanosis is one of the most dramatic and challenging emergencies in pediatric practice. Detection of cyanosis, understanding the physiology of oxygenation, and differentiating the causes of cyanosis are important for the successful treatment of the child.

Definition

True or *central cyanosis* is a bluish discoloration of the skin, mucous membranes, lips, and conjunctiva and indicates significant arterial oxygen desaturation. Central cyanosis should be distinguished from *acrocyanosis*, a bluish discoloration of the hands and feet only. Acrocyanosis indicates the presence of peripheral vasoconstriction rather than arterial oxygen desaturation. Peripheral vasoconstriction causes decreased peripheral perfusion and increased oxygen extraction from peripheral capillary blood. This results in a decreased oxygen content of venous return, which produces the peripheral bluish discoloration. Acrocyanosis can be associated with fever, hypovolemia, exposure to cold temperatures, sympathomimetic agents, sepsis, congestive heart failure, or shock. Acrocyanosis in an otherwise healthy 1- to 2-day-old infant is probably physiologic and is relatively common.

Differential cyanosis and *reverse differential cyanosis* are special variants of central cyanosis that may occur in the newborn and are very rare in older children. Differential cyanosis is defined as relative cyanosis in the postductal circulation: the circulation supplied by the aorta distal to the origin of the patent ductus. In this case, the lower abdomen, legs, and feet are diffusely cyanotic but the right arm, face, and often the left arm appear less cyanotic or even normal in color. Reverse differential cyanosis indicates relative cyanosis in the right arm, face, and sometimes the left arm compared with the lower abdomen and legs. Either condition may be clinically inapparent and may need to be confirmed by comparing pulse oximetry or arterial blood gas PO_2 from sites representing preductal circulation (usually the right arm or hand) and postductal circulation (usually the umbilical artery or feet). The detection of differential or reverse differential cyanosis significantly streamlines the differential diagnosis of cyanosis.

Detection and Confirmation of Cyanosis

Prior to the use of pulse oximetry, cyanosis was first noted by parents, nurses, or a physician. Pulse oximetry has improved the detection of cyanosis and a low "pulse-ox" reading may often be the "chief complaint." The detection of cyanosis by physical examination requires an absolute amount of at least 3 to 4 g/dl of deoxygenated or desaturated hemoglobin. Clinical cyanosis is therefore directly related to the degree of oxygen saturation (or desaturation) and to the total hemoglobin.

Oxygen saturation is the percentage of hemoglobin molecules bound to oxygen within the circulation. This percentage is determined by the arterial partial pressure of oxygen (PO_2) and the hemoglobin-oxygen dissociation curve (Fig. 15–1). This curve represents a sigmoidal rather than a linear relationship. When the arterial PO_2 is ≥ 60 mmHg, the arterial oxygen saturation is usually above 90%. As the PO_2 falls below 60 mmHg, there is a precipitous

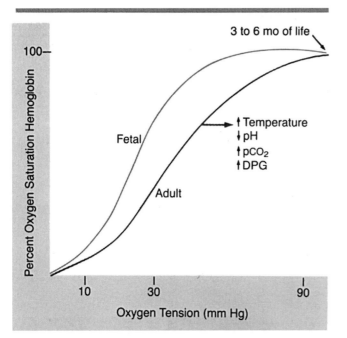

Figure 15–1. Hemoglobin-oxygen dissociation curves. The position of the adult curve depends on the binding of adult hemoglobin to 2,3-diphosphoglycerate (DPG), temperature, carbon dioxide tension (pCO₂), and hydrogen ion concentration (pH). (From Behrman RE, Kliegman RM [eds]. Nelson's Essentials of Pediatrics, 2nd ed. Philadelphia: WB Saunders, 1994:166.)

decrease in oxygen saturation to a level of 50% at a PO_2 of 27 (the P_{50} for adult hemoglobin).

The dissociation curve shifts rightward or leftward under various conditions. For example, the fetal hemoglobin curve is shifted to the left because this hemoglobin has a higher affinity for oxygen (oxygen is released less easily to the tissues). Thus, a given PO_2 produces a higher oxygen saturation of fetal hemoglobin than of adult hemoglobin. Acidosis, carbon dioxide (CO_2) retention, hyperthermia, or elevated levels of erythrocyte 2,3-DPG (diphosphoglycerate) will shift the curve to the right (oxygen is released more easily to the tissues). Under these conditions, the oxygen saturation will be lower than normal for any given PO_2. Some abnormal hemoglobins have altered affinity for oxygen and functionally shift the curve to the right.

Methemoglobinemia occurs when ferric (Fe^{+3}) rather than ferrous (Fe^{+2}) ion is bound to the hemoglobin molecule. The Fe^{+3} ion has a poor affinity for oxygen at any given PO_2. In this case, the hemoglobin oxygen desaturation can be severely depressed even though arterial PO_2 is normal. Thus, with the exception of methemoglobinemia, arterial oxygen desaturation implies arterial hypoxemia (a depression of arterial PO_2).

The detection of cyanosis requires the presence of an absolute amount of 3 to 4 g/dl desaturated hemoglobin. Therefore, the total hemoglobin also affects the examiner's ability to detect cyanosis. When the hemoglobin value is normal, detection of cyanosis is easier. When the total hemoglobin is low, the detection is more difficult. Normally, cyanosis is evident at an arterial oxygen saturation below 78% to 80%.

When a newborn has a normal hemoglobin count of 18 g/dl, cyanosis can be detected more easily. Since 3 g/dl hemoglobin must be desaturated to detect cyanosis, $18 - 3 = 15$ g/dl is the amount of hemoglobin that is saturated with oxygen. Dividing 15 g/dl (amount saturated) by 18 g/dl (total hemoglobin), 83% of the hemoglobin is saturated (oxygen saturation is 83%). Thus, an oxygen saturation of 83% or less produces detectable cyanosis in a neonate or child with a hemoglobin of 18 g/dl.

If the child is anemic with a hemoglobin count of 9 g/dl, detection of cyanosis may be more challenging. Because 3 g/dl hemoglobin must be desaturated before cyanosis can be detected, only 6 g/dl is saturated. Dividing saturated hemoglobin (6 g/dl) by total hemoglobin (9 g/dl) reveals that the child must have 67% or less oxygen saturation for cyanosis to be detected.

The arterial blood gas provides the clinician with additional information about the patient's acid-base status as well as the arterial PO_2. *Hypoxemia* is defined as a PO_2 below 60 mmHg [8kPa] during the first day of life and below 80 mmHg thereafter. Because [10.6kPa] the arterial saturation reported on an arterial blood gas analysis is not measured directly with a cooximeter (it is calculated from the measured PO_2 and the hemoglobin-oxygen dissociation curve for adult hemoglobin), this calculated value may be inaccurate. This value may not correlate with pulse oximetry in neonates and young infants, who have high levels of fetal rather than of adult hemoglobinemia, or in patients with methemoglobinemia.

PHYSIOLOGY OF OXYGENATION

Oxygenation requires adequate ambient oxygen, an intact central nervous system, normal hemoglobin, and normal respiratory and cardiac systems. Mechanisms of cyanosis (hypoxemia) include alveolar hypoventilation, abnormalities of hemoglobin oxygen affinity, ventilation-perfusion imbalance, oxygen diffusion defects (rare), and shunts (intrapulmonary or cardiac right-to-left shunts), respectively. The role of the circulation in the oxygenation of the fetus and newborn is noted in Figure 15–2.

The significance of differential and reverse differential cyanosis can now be explained (Fig. 15–3). *Differential cyanosis* (implying

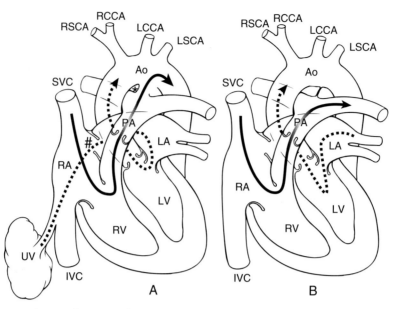

Figure 15–2. Prenatal *(A)* and postnatal *(B)* circulation. *A,* Relatively oxygenated blood *(dashed line* with *arrow)* from the placenta returns to the umbilical vein, coursing through the foramen ovale to the left heart and ascending aorta. Deoxygenated blood *(unbroken line* with *arrow)* returns to the right heart, pulmonary artery, and then mainly to the descending aorta through the patent ductus arteriosus since pulmonary vascular resistance is very high *in utero. B,* Oxygenated blood *(dashed line* with *arrow)* from the lungs returns to the left heart and aorta. Deoxygenated blood *(unbroken line* with *arrow)* returns to the right heart, pulmonary artery, and lungs. RA = right atrium; LA = left atrium; RV = right ventricle; LV = left ventricle; PA = pulmonary artery; Ao = aorta; RSCA = right subclavian artery; RCCA = right common carotid artery; LCCA = left common carotid artery; LSCA = left subclavian artery; SVC = superior vena cava; IVC = inferior vena cava; UV = umbilical vein; asterisk (*) = patent ductus arteriosus; # = patent foramen ovale.

relatively more cyanosis in the postductal circulation) occurs when pulmonary vascular resistance remains abnormally high after birth. Flow into the pulmonary artery avoids the pulmonary vascular bed and passes across the patent ductus into the descending aorta, similar to the fetal circulation. This condition is known as *persistent fetal circulation.* A right-to-left ductal shunt may also occur when descending aortic flow is dependent on the patent ductus because

of obstruction of flow upstream, as in critical coarctation of the aorta or interrupted aortic arch.

Reverse differential cyanosis (implying relatively more cyanosis in the preductal circulation) occurs when pulmonary vascular resistance remains abnormally high after birth *and* there is transposition of the great vessels. In this case, the pulmonary artery arises from the oxygenated left ventricle. If pulmonary vascular resistance is

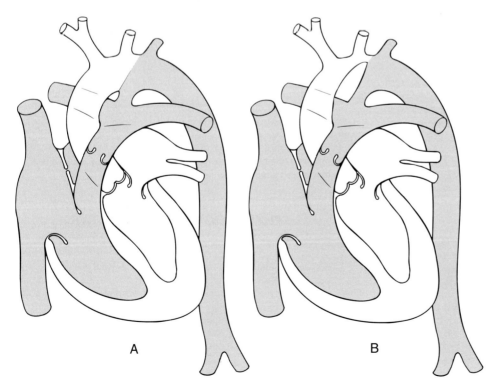

Figure 15–3. Differential cyanosis. *A,* Differential cyanosis occurs when pulmonary vascular resistance remains abnormally high after birth. Flow into the pulmonary artery avoids the pulmonary vascular bed and passes across the patent ductus into the descending aorta. *B,* Critical coarctation of the aorta with dependence on a patent ductus arteriosus.

abnormally high, this oxygenated blood passes from the pulmonary artery into the descending aorta via the patent ductus arteriosus. The ascending aorta, however, arises from the deoxygenated right ventricle, and thus the preductal aortic circulation receives desaturated blood. Reverse differential cyanosis occurs with transposition of the great vessels and patent ductus arteriosus with persistent fetal circulation or with transposition, critical coarctation of the aorta, or interrupted aortic arch.

THE NEWBORN

Determining the underlying etiology of cyanosis requires different approaches for the neonate, infant, and older child.

History

A history of fetal distress, difficult delivery, low Apgar scores, excessive maternal sedation, intracranial hemorrhage, seizures, or neuromuscular disease may implicate central nervous system depression or disease that has resulted in *central hypoventilation.* *Respiratory disease* can be suspected as the cause of cyanosis when there is a history of prematurity (respiratory distress syndrome), prolonged rupture of membranes or maternal fever (neonatal sepsis or pneumonia), a history of meconium-stained amniotic fluid (meconium aspiration, persistent fetal circulation), respiratory distress with cyanosis in the delivery room (severe pulmonary compromise, i.e., pneumothorax, diaphragmatic hernia), or cyanosis, particularly with feeds (choanal stenosis or atresia, Pierre Robin syndrome).

Methemoglobinemia is rarely a cause of cyanosis in a newborn, but a family history should be elicited when the baby is blue for seemingly unexplained reasons. A history of exposure to oxidizing agents, including drugs or nitrate-rich well water, may be obtained in infants or children.

Cardiac disease is an important cause of cyanosis in the neonate. The history may be remarkable for the absence of findings of central nervous system or pulmonary disease. The newborn with cyanotic heart disease is usually full term with a normal labor and delivery history. The Apgar score is often 8 and 8 at 1 and 5 minutes because of central cyanosis. Often this initial cyanosis improves enough so that many infants with cyanotic congenital heart disease are transferred unnoticed to the normal nursery. However, they are soon found to be cyanotic as gradual closure of the foramen ovale and ductus arteriosus occurs. Even if cyanosis is observed within hours after delivery, a significant history of respiratory distress is usually absent.

Physical Examination

In the infant, central nervous system depression or disease that results in hypoventilation can be noted by observing an abnormally low respiratory rate or diminished air entry over the lung fields, hypotonia, flaccid posture, weak cry, poor response to stimuli, obvious abnormalities of size, shape, or transillumination of the head, brachial plexus palsy, or shoulder dystocia (possibly associated phrenic palsy and secondary unilateral hypoventilation).

The signs of neonatal respiratory distress (pulmonary disease) include tachypnea, dyspnea with intercostal, subcostal, or suprasternal retractions, nasal flaring, stridor, grunting, wheezes, or rales. Severe respiratory distress with cyanosis and a scaphoid abdomen shortly after birth are the classic signs of a diaphragmatic hernia. Unilateral breath sounds suggest this diagnosis but may also be consistent with a pleural effusion, pneumothorax, or hemidiaphragm palsy. Transillumination of the thorax may confirm the presence of a pneumothorax. Inability to pass a feeding tube through each nostril to the stomach indicates the presence of airway obstruction from choanal stenosis or atresia.

A neonate with a slate-gray appearance who has brown-red "chocolate" discoloration of the blood that fails to become bright-red when exposed to oxygen in room air may have methemoglobinemia.

A remarkable absence of signs of respiratory distress or central nervous system disease may be seen in neonates with congenital cardiac defects. The infant with cardiac cyanosis is remarkably alert and comfortable for the degree of cyanosis. The typical child has normal tone and usually has no abnormal respiratory signs other than mild tachypnea. Exceptions include cyanotic heart lesions associated with pulmonary edema or with severe congestive heart failure. Pulmonary edema may occur early with lesions that cause severe pulmonary venous obstruction (total anomalous pulmonary venous return with obstruction). Congestive heart failure can occur precipitously with the *hypoplastic left heart syndrome,* in which ductal closure leads to circulatory collapse as well as commitment of all the cardiac output to the pulmonary artery.

Although the cardiac examination may be deceptively normal in newborns with cyanotic heart disease, the presence of cardiac abnormalities on cardiac examination increases the likelihood of a cardiac cause for cyanosis: abnormal visible or palpable parasternal precordial activity (right ventricular enlargement/hypertrophy or left ventricular hypoplasia), abnormal apical activity (right ventricular hypoplasia), single S_2 (pulmonary hypertension, transposition of the great vessels, atretic pulmonic or aortic valve, truncus arteriosus), systolic or diastolic murmurs, a systolic ejection click (pulmonic stenosis, truncus arteriosus), gallop rhythm (hypoplastic left heart syndrome), hepatomegaly (heart failure), or diminished or unequal pulses (coarctation of the aorta or interrupted aortic arch) (see Chapter 16).

Stigmata of certain genetic syndromes suggest particular cyanotic heart defects (Table 15–1).

Differential Diagnosis

The neonate requires adequate ambient oxygen to breathe, an intact central nervous system to control the rate and depth of

Table 15–1. Syndromes Associated with Cyanotic Heart Disease

Down syndrome	Endocardial cushion defects (including complete atrioventricular septal defect with or without pulmonic stenosis)
DiGeorge syndrome	Interrupted aortic arch, conotruncal defects (tetralogy of Fallot, truncus arteriosus)
CHARGE syndrome	Conotruncal defects
Turner syndrome	Hypoplastic left heart syndrome, coarctation
Asplenia and polysplenia syndromes (see Chapter 16)	Complex cyanotic heart disease with multiple lesions: endocardial cushion defect, pulmonic stenosis or atresia, transposition, anomalous pulmonary venous return

Abbreviation: CHARGE = coloboma, heart disease, atresia choanae, retarded growth, ears (deafness). (The Shprintzen syndrome [velocardiofacial] is also related.)

respiration, a normal upper airway to allow air to pass to the lungs, normal lungs to allow adequate oxygenation of pulmonary capillary blood, normal hemoglobin to bind oxygen at the alveolar capillary membrane, and a normal heart to deliver deoxygenated systemic venous return to the pulmonary artery and deliver oxygenated pulmonary venous return to the aorta. The causes of cyanosis are categorized in Table 15–2.

The general causes of cyanosis in the neonate can often be identified or excluded within minutes by means of a complete history and physical examination in combination with a chest radiograph, an electrocardiogram (ECG), and an arterial blood gas analysis on room air and maximum ($\sim$100%) FiO_2 (hyperoxia test).

CHEST RADIOGRAPHY

The chest radiograph in the newborn with apparent respiratory disease may show abnormalities of the upper airway or tracheal air column or tracheal bifurcation. There may be a reticulogranular appearance consistent with respiratory distress syndrome or sepsis, infiltrates or interstitial densities (pneumonia, hemorrhage), pneumothorax, pleural effusion, or air-filled densities consistent with a diaphragmatic hernia or cystic adenomatoid malformation. With partial airway obstruction, there may be air-trapping with hyperaeration of one or both lungs and flattening of the hemidiaphragms.

Table 15–2. Differential Diagnosis of Cyanosis in the Newborn

Inadequate ambient O_2 or less O_2 delivered than expected (rare)
  Incubator malfunction
  Disconnection of oxygen supply to nasal cannula, head hood
  Connection of air, rather than oxygen, to a mechanical ventilator

Central or peripheral nervous system hypoventilation
  Birth asphyxia
  Intracranial hypertension, hemorrhage
  Oversedation (direct or through maternal route)
  Diaphragm palsy
  Neuromuscular diseases
  Seizures

Respiratory disease
  Upper airway
    Choanal atresia/stenosis
    Pierre Robin syndrome
    Intrinsic airway obstruction (laryngeal/bronchial/tracheal stenosis)
    Extrinsic airway obstruction (bronchogenic cyst, duplication cyst, vascular compression)

  Lower airway
    Respiratory distress syndrome
    Transient tachypnea
    Meconium aspiration
    Pneumonia/pneumonitis
    Pneumothorax
    Congenital diaphragmatic hernia
    Pulmonary hypoplasia
    Persistent fetal circulation (persistent pulmonary hypertension of newborn)

Cardiac right-to-left shunt
  Abnormal connections (pulmonary blood flow normal or increased)
    Transposition of the great vessels
    Total anomalous pulmonary venous return
    Truncus arteriosus
    Hypoplastic left heart syndrome
    Single ventricle or tricuspid atresia with large ventricular septal defect without pulmonic stenosis
  Obstructed pulmonary blood flow (pulmonary blood flow decreased)
    Pulmonic atresia with intact ventricular septum
    Tetralogy of Fallot
    Critical pulmonic stenosis with patent foramen ovale or atrial septal defect
    Tricuspid atresia
    Single ventricle with pulmonic stenosis
    Ebstein malformation of the tricuspid valve
    Persistent fetal circulation (persistent pulmonary hypertension of newborn)

Methemoglobinemia
  Congenital (hemoglobin M, methemoglobin reductase deficiency)
  Acquired (e.g., nitrates, nitrites)

Spurious/artifactual
  Oximeter artifact (poor contact between probe and skin, poor pulse searching)
  Arterial blood gas artifact (contamination with venous blood)

Other
  Hypoglycemia
  Adrenogenital syndrome
  Polycythemia
  Blood loss

Table 15–3. Differentiating Cardiac Cyanosis by X-ray

Normal or increased pulmonary vascular markings
    Transposition of the great vessels
    Total anomalous pulmonary venous return
    Truncus arteriosus
    Single ventricle without pulmonic stenosis
    Tricuspid atresia with ventricular septal defect and mild/no
        pulmonic stenosis

Decreased pulmonary vascular markings
    Pulmonary atresia with intact ventricular septum
    Tetralogy of Fallot
    Tricuspid atresia with small ventricular septal defect/
        pulmonic stenosis
    Ebstein malformation of the tricuspid valve
    Single ventricle with pulmonic stenosis

Right aortic arch
    Truncus arteriosus
    Tetralogy of Fallot/pulmonic atresia
    Transposition complex

Discordant situs of heart and stomach
    Complex cardiac disease (polysplenia and asplenia
        syndrome)

Cardiomegaly
    Total anomalous pulmonary venous return
    Truncus arteriosus
    Single ventricle with mild or no pulmonic stenosis
    Ebstein malformation of the tricuspid valve

Abnormal cardiac shape
    Transposition of the great vessels ("egg on a string")
    Total anomalous pulmonary venous return ("snowman")
    Tetralogy of Fallot ("wooden shoe," "boot-shaped")

The chest radiograph in the newborn with cyanotic heart disease usually lacks findings of parenchymal lung disease and may lack abnormalities of the cardiac silhouette and pulmonary vascular markings as well. Evidence of abnormal cardiac size and shape, and especially abnormal pulmonary vascular markings, may help to identify the newborn with heart disease and to determine which cardiac defect is present (Table 15–3). A large right atrial shadow suggests the presence of tricuspid incompetence. The "wooden shoe"–shaped cardiac silhouette resulting from an upturned apex (right ventricular dominance) and an absent main pulmonary segment may be seen with tetralogy of Fallot. Other shapes ("egg on a string," "snowman," "globular heart") may be seen with transposition, total anomalous venous return, and tricuspid atresia, respectively, but they are inconsistent findings and their absence does not exclude these diagnoses. Aneurysmal dilatation of the proximal pulmonary artery branches, which may cause air trapping by compression of mainstem bronchi, is seen with tetralogy of Fallot with absent pulmonary valve.

The location of the stomach, if visualized on the chest or abdominal film, may provide an important clue to the presence of significant cyanotic heart disease. The cardiac apex and stomach are normally both left-sided (*situs solitus*). When both structures are right-sided, *situs inversus totalis* is present. In this case, there is a slightly higher risk of congenital heart disease. When the cardiac apex and the stomach bubble are on opposite sides, *situs ambiguus* is likely. This often occurs with asplenia and polysplenia syndromes, which are both associated with complex heart disease (see Chapter 16). The presence of a right aortic arch is suggested by a round density at the upper right border of the cardiac silhouette, displacing the distal trachea to the left. This is frequently seen

with truncus arteriosus and tetralogy of Fallot with or without pulmonary atresia.

Detection of increased or decreased pulmonary vascular markings not only suggests congenital heart disease but also helps to determine which particular defects are present (see Table 15–3).

ELECTROCARDIOGRAM

The ECG is usually within normal limits in newborns with neurologic disease, although nonspecific T-wave or ST-segment changes may occur. The ECG is usually normal with respiratory disease.

Although the ECG may be normal in newborns with cyanotic congenital heart disease, certain ECG abnormalities suggest particular cardiac defects (Table 15–4). Abnormally peaked P waves (>2.5 mm) may be seen with lesions associated with right atrial enlargement (tricuspid atresia, pulmonic stenosis or atresia with intact ventricular septum, *Ebstein's malformation* of the tricuspid valve). Pre-excitation, a short PR interval with wide QRS complex consisting of an initial slurred "delta wave" (otherwise known as *Wolff-Parkinson-White syndrome* when associated with tachycardia), is seen with Ebstein's malformation of the tricuspid valve and less commonly with complex transposition. An abnormal left axis deviation for age (<30 degrees) is associated with diminished right ventricular forces (tricuspid atresia). Severe left axis deviation (<−60 degrees) is seen with an endocardial cushion defect, such as atrioventricular septal defect or "atrioventricular canal." Simple or complex canal defects are associated with trisomy 21. Complex forms of atrioventricular septal defect may occur with asplenia or polysplenia syndromes (see Chapter 16).

ARTERIAL BLOOD GAS ANALYSIS AND PULSE OXIMETRY

Pulse oximetry now provides a noninvasive alternative to arterial blood gas measurement in many questionable cases. It provides an accurate, quick, and easy estimate of oxygen saturation and has become a routine part of the diagnostic evaluation of any acutely ill infant or child. The pulse oximeter can estimate the oxygen saturation with reasonable accuracy for an oxygen saturation of 60% or greater.

Table 15–4. Differential Cardiac Cyanosis by Electrocardiographic Abnormalities

Peaked P wave lead II (right atrial enlargement)	Pulmonary atresia with intact ventricular septum, tricuspid atresia
Inverted P waves lead I, II (atrial situs inversus)	Situs inversus, complex cyanotic heart disease, lead malposition
Wolff-Parkinson-White syndrome	Ebstein malformation of the tricuspid valve, complex transposition
Prolonged PR interval, heart block	Complex transposition, asplenia and polysplenia syndromes
Severe left axis deviation (superior axis)	Endocardial cushion defects with or without pulmonic stenosis
Mild left axis deviation	Tricuspid or pulmonic atresia
Absent right ventricular forces	Tricuspid or pulmonary atresia
Absent left ventricular forces	Hypoplastic left heart syndrome

The accuracy of pulse oximetry is limited when oxygen saturation is less than 60%. Pulse oximetry may not estimate the true oxygen saturation when methemoglobinemia is present. In this case, the estimated oxygen saturation is usually low (~85%). If an abnormally low oxygen saturation is detected when cyanosis appears unlikely, another sensor should be used and different extremities sampled. Finally, pulse oximetry cannot detect hyperoxemia. A pulse oximetry saturation of ≥95% could correspond to an arterial PO_2 of 80 or 380. This is a particularly important limitation in the management of the premature infant in whom inadvertent hyperoxemia must be avoided to prevent the development of retinopathy of prematurity.

Transcutaneous oxygen monitors require placement of a heated probe on the infant's skin. These monitors estimate arterial PCO_2 as well as PO_2 and are particularly useful for management of the premature infant, since PO_2 can be monitored and hyperoxemia can be avoided. The pulse oximeter is currently preferred for most other noninvasive oxygen monitoring.

When significant desaturation (<80%) is detected by pulse oximetry, an arterial blood gas analysis should be performed to confirm hypoxemia. The arterial PO_2 may be artifactually depressed if the arterial specimen is contaminated with venous blood or if the child is sufficiently agitated to produce a transient right-to-left shunt across the patent foramen ovale.

The arterial blood gas measurement confirms arterial hypoxemia, and the pH and PCO_2 help to differentiate respiratory (may see hypercarbia) from cardiac causes of hypoxemia. An arterial blood gas analysis that is repeated while the infant breathes maximum (~100%) FiO_2 (the *hyperoxia test*) may further differentiate respiratory from cardiac cyanosis (see later).

With respiratory disease, the elimination of CO_2 is often impaired and there is respiratory acidosis. With compensated cyanotic heart disease, however, the PCO_2 is either normal or slightly lower than normal as a result of mild hyperventilation. Carbon dioxide retention occurs only with cyanotic heart disease when pulmonary blood flow is extremely limited or if there is concomitant pulmonary disease. If arterial hypoxemia is significant enough to depress oxygen delivery to the tissues (in spite of a relatively high hemoglobin and the presence of fetal hemoglobin), a metabolic (lactic) acidosis will develop with respiratory compensation.

If a low arterial PO_2 is originally obtained from the postductal circulation (usually the umbilical artery), differential cyanosis or differential hypoxemia should be considered and excluded. Pulse oximetry, transcutaneous oximetry, or an arterial blood gas measurement performed in the right radial artery should be taken to exclude or confirm this. If the preductal PO_2 is 20 mmHg greater than the postductal valve, differential cyanosis is present.

For the hyperoxia test, an arterial blood gas analysis is performed after the child inhales maximum (~100%) FiO_2 for at least 10 to 15 minutes. If the hypoxemia is due to respiratory disease, the arterial PO_2 often rises significantly unless respiratory disease is severe or unless there is concomitant persistent fetal circulation. If the PO_2 is less than 50, respiratory disease is still possible, particularly in association with persistent fetal circulation, but cyanotic heart disease should be seriously considered. The two most common cyanotic heart defects in the newborn (transposition, pulmonic atresia) are characteristically associated with an arterial PO_2 below 50 mmHg on room air and with hyperoxia in the absence of respiratory acidosis or clinical respiratory distress.

When the PO_2 is above 200 mmHg with hyperoxia, primary respiratory disease is much more likely. Only cyanotic heart defects with torrential pulmonary blood flow (truncus arteriosus, unobstructed anomalous venous return, or variants of single ventricle with minimal pulmonic stenosis) may be associated with an arterial PO_2 above 200 mmHg. In these cases, cyanosis in room air is usually mild but abnormal cardiac or chest findings often suggest a cardiac cause.

When the arterial PO_2 remains low during the hyperoxia test and the differential diagnosis is practically limited to cyanotic heart disease or persistent fetal circulation, an additional maneuver—intubation and mechanical hyperventilation—can be performed. If persistent fetal circulation of the newborn is present, hyperventilation may cause pulmonary vasodilation, a reduction in right-to-left shunting at the atrial or ductal levels, and a dramatic increase in arterial PO_2. If cyanotic heart disease is present, the arterial PO_2 remains low. A response to inhaled nitric oxide (NO) will occur in patients with pulmonary hypertension (persistent fetal circulation) but not in most cases of cyanotic congenital heart disease.

Initial Approach to the Cyanotic Newborn

A stepwise approach to the newborn with cyanosis is presented in Figure 15–4. First, the airway, breathing, and circulation must be assessed and stabilized. Hypoglycemia should be excluded. Pulse oximetry of the right hand and foot can be performed while an arterial blood gas value is obtained from the right radial artery; if this is unsuccessful, another site can be used. A history and physical examination should focus on the predisposing factors and manifestations of neurologic, pulmonary, or cardiac disease. A chest radiograph, the ECG, detection of differential cyanosis, and the hyperoxia test help to establish the diagnosis.

Establishing the Cause of Cardiac Cyanosis in the Newborn

Once the diagnosis of cyanotic congenital heart disease is suspected, a pediatric cardiologist should be consulted and transfer to a tertiary care nursery should be considered. The diagnosis of congenital heart defects must be established quickly by echocardiography.

Certain cyanotic heart defects present earlier than others. Those defects that depend on ductal patency usually produce significant cyanosis within the first 3 days of life. Because of this ductal dependency, neonates with suspected cyanotic heart disease may benefit from intravenous (IV) prostaglandin E_1 to maintain patency of the ductus arteriosus. Age of presentation may help to focus the differential diagnosis (Table 15–5).

CYANOTIC LESIONS WITH NORMAL OR INCREASED PULMONARY BLOOD FLOW

Transposition of the Great Vessels

Transposition of the great vessels (Fig. 15–5) is the most common cause of cyanotic heart disease in the neonate. The aorta arises from the right ventricle, and the pulmonary artery arises from the left ventricle. Venous desaturated blood returns to the right ventricle and is recirculated to the aorta. Oxygenated blood from the lungs returns to the left ventricle and is immediately recirculated to the lungs. Survival after birth depends on the presence of bidirectional shunts through a patent foramen ovale, a ventricular septal defect, or a patent ductus arteriosus. Infants with transposition of the great vessels and no ventricular septal defect thus rely on patency of the foramen ovale or patent ductus arteriosus.

Cyanosis usually appears in the first day of life. Cardiac findings may be otherwise normal, although often a single S_2 will be heard because of the anterior placement of the aorta, which leads to a louder aortic closure sound that obscures the closure sound of the posteriorly placed pulmonary valve. The chest radiograph may be

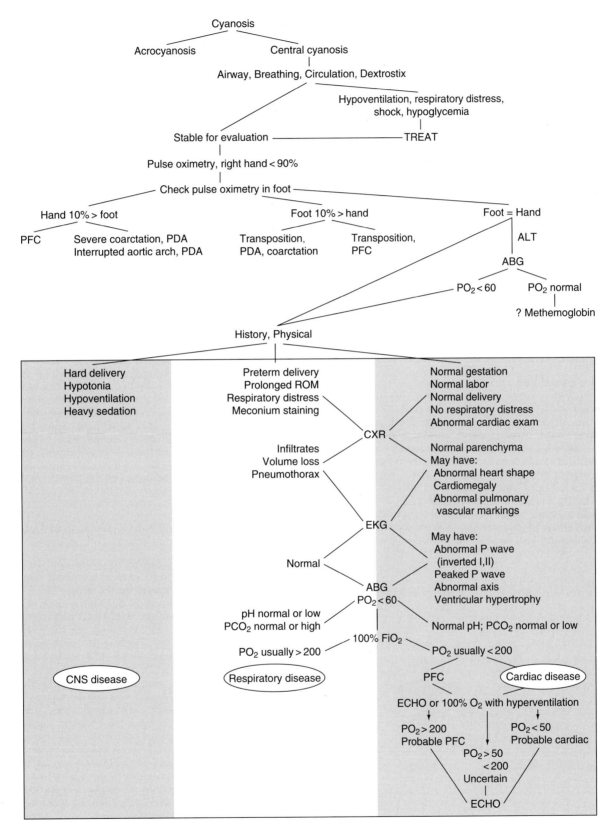

Figure 15–4. Approach to neonatal cyanosis. PFC = persistent fetal circulation; ABG = arterial blood gas; ECG = electrocardiogram; ECHO = echocardiogram; PDA = patent ductus arteriosus; nl = normal; CXR = chest x-ray; ROM = rupture of membranes.

Table 15–5. **Presentation of Cyanotic Heart Disease by Age**

Newborn–1 day
Transposition of the great vessels with intact ventricular
    septum
Pulmonic atresia
Tricuspid atresia with small ventricular septal defect or intact
    ventricular septum and pulmonic stenosis
Hypoplastic left heart syndrome
Ebstein malformation
Total anomalous venous return (obstructed)

1–7 days
Transposition of the great vessels with or without ventricular
    septal defect
Tetralogy of Fallot
Hypoplastic left heart syndrome
Tricuspid atresia with or without ventricular septal defect
Truncus arteriosus
Ebstein malformation of the tricuspid valve
Total anomalous venous return (obstructed)

>7 days
Tetralogy of Fallot
Transposition of the great vessels with ventricular septal
    defect
Tricuspid atresia with ventricular septal defect
Single ventricle with or without pulmonary stenosis
Total anomalous pulmonary venous return (unobstructed)

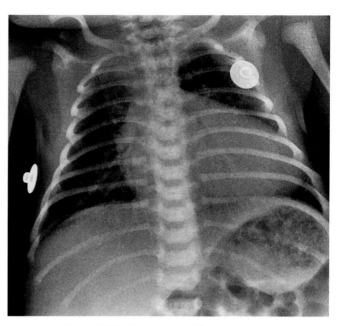

Figure 15–6. Transposition of the great vessels.

normal, although the cardiac shape may occasionally resemble an egg on a string (Fig. 15–6). This is a result of the right ventricular predominance of the silhouette and a narrow superior mediastinum due to the anterior-posterior position of the great vessels at the base of the heart. Pulmonary vascular markings appear normal or slightly increased. The ECG is often normal but may show right ventricular hypertrophy. The arterial blood gas PO_2 is usually below 50 mmHg on room air and with hyperoxia.

The initial treatment of this lesion may include cardiac catheterization with balloon atrial septostomy to encourage interatrial mixing. Prostaglandin E may be instituted to encourage mixing at the ductal level. The surgical treatment is the arterial switch procedure, which is usually performed in the first 10 days of life.

Transposition with a moderate to large ventricular septal defect may not be diagnosed in the first days of life. In this case, interventricular mixing leads to minimal systemic desaturation and cyanosis. As pulmonary vascular resistance falls during the first weeks of life, however, findings of a left-to-right shunt (murmur) and fluid congestion (tachypnea, poor feeding) develop. The degree of cyanosis usually depends on the severity of pulmonic stenosis. The presence of a systolic murmur of pulmonic stenosis with cyanosis usually leads to cardiac diagnosis.

Total Anomalous Pulmonary Venous Return

In the case of total anomalous pulmonary venous return (TAPVR), the pulmonary veins return to a systemic vein or directly to the right atrium rather than to the left atrium. Thus, all systemic and pulmonary veins return to the right atrium, right ventricle, and pulmonary artery, which causes right ventricular volume overload and pulmonary overcirculation. Left atrial and left ventricular flow depend on the presence of a right-to-left shunt across a patent foramen ovale or atrial septal defect. If the atrial septal defect is restrictive, systemic output is reduced as well.

The pulmonary veins most often connect to a vertical vein, which enters the left innominate vein and the superior vena cava; alternate connections include the coronary sinus, which empties into the right atrium just above the tricuspid annulus, or to a descending vein, which passes behind the heart, through the diaphragm, and into the hepatic or portal venous system. This last type is most often associated with pulmonary venous obstruction.

Less commonly, the pulmonary veins may all enter the right atrium directly or there may be mixed points of entry. In the latter case, the diagnosis of asplenia or polysplenia syndrome should be considered. TAPVR without pulmonary venous obstruction may present with milder cyanosis because pulmonary blood flow is excessive. The cardiac examination reveals an abnormally strong parasternal (or right ventricular) impulse. A fixed split S_2 may be detected as a result of torrential pulmonary blood flow and delayed pulmonic valve closure regardless of respiratory variations. There

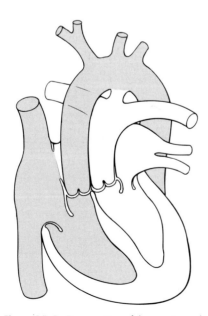

Figure 15–5. Transposition of the great vessels.

is often a systolic ejection murmur at the middle and upper left sternal border, representing a pulmonary flow murmur. Usually, the chest radiograph reveals cardiomegaly with increased pulmonary vascular markings and the ECG shows right ventricular hypertrophy. Since pulmonary blood flow is increased, the amount of oxygenated blood returning from the lungs to mix with systemic venous blood is high. The arterial PO_2 may be only mildly diminished and may increase significantly with the hyperoxia test. Nonetheless, with severe obstruction the PO_2 is low and fixed.

If the anomalous pulmonary venous connection is *obstructed,* there will be pulmonary venous hypertension and pulmonary edema. In this case, combined cyanosis and marked respiratory distress are present. The chest radiograph is distinctive; there is a normal or small cardiac silhouette and evidence of pulmonary venous congestion and pulmonary edema (Fig. 15–7). The lung fields may be misinterpreted as "diffuse interstitial pneumonia." TAPVR with or without obstruction may also be associated with reflex elevation of pulmonary vascular resistance and findings of persistent fetal circulation (PFC). In this case, differentiation of TAPVR with PFC versus PFC alone may be difficult. Color Doppler echocardiography, fortunately, has improved the ability to differentiate the two conditions. The usual surgical treatment includes reanastomosis of the pulmonary venous confluence to the posterior wall of the left atrium.

Truncus Arteriosus

In truncus arteriosus (Fig. 15–8), a common arterial trunk arises from the heart, which gives rise to the aorta and the pulmonary artery. In most cases, the common trunk overrides a large ventricular septal defect and receives outflow from both ventricles, which otherwise have no egress. The classification of truncus is made according to the location of the pulmonary artery or branches as they arise from the trunk.

Generally, there is excessive pulmonary flow because of shunting

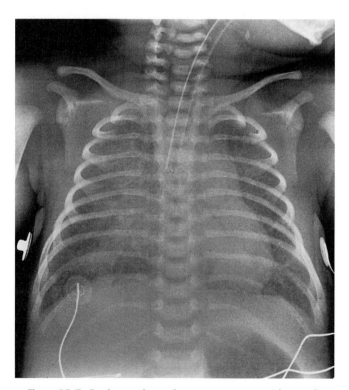

Figure 15–7. Total anomalous pulmonary venous return (obstructed).

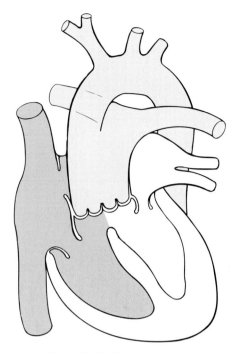

Figure 15–8. Truncus arteriosus.

from the main truncus to the pulmonary artery during both systole and diastole. The findings of a left-to-right shunt may be minimal at birth because of persistent elevation of pulmonary vascular resistance, but signs of a significant shunt usually occur within 2 to 4 weeks of age as pulmonary vascular resistance falls. The truncal valve consists of two to six cusps, and there is often truncal valve stenosis or incompetence. The cardiac examination often reveals a hyperdynamic precordium with systolic or continuous murmurs over both lung fields. There is often a loud, single S_2 resulting from closure of the single truncal valve and a systolic ejection click heard at the apex related to valve opening. There may be a systolic murmur of truncal stenosis or a diastolic decrescendo murmur of truncal incompetence similar to the murmur of aortic incompetence. Because there is runoff of flow from the aorta to the pulmonary arteries during diastole, the aortic diastolic pressure is decreased, the pulse pressure is increased, and the pulses may be bounding.

The chest radiograph reveals a normal or increased cardiac size. Pulmonary vascular markings are usually increased. There may be a right aortic arch in 33% of cases. The ECG often reveals biventricular hypertrophy. Since pulmonary blood flow is usually elevated, the PO_2 is mildly decreased and may approach 200 with hyperoxia. Surgical treatment includes closing the ventricular septal defect and partitioning the truncus in such a way so that the pulmonary artery and branches are excluded from the remaining truncal root and are connected to the right ventricle by way of a patch.

Hypoplastic Left Heart Syndrome

Hypoplastic left heart syndrome (Fig. 15–9) is associated with arterial hypoxemia, although the presentation is usually that of diminished cardiac output, shock, and pallor rather than just cyanosis. This diagnosis includes multiple left heart anomalies in which systemic cardiac output cannot be supplied by the hypoplastic, small left ventricle and ascending aorta and is thus supplied by the right ventricle and pulmonary artery via the patent ductus arterio-

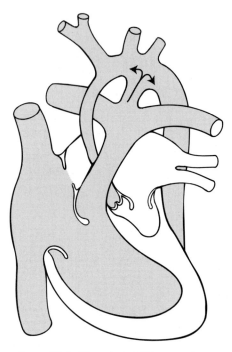

Figure 15–9. Hypoplastic left heart syndrome.

sus. Because ascending and descending aorta depend on the pulmonary artery for circulation, there is generalized rather than differential cyanosis. This contrasts with the findings of differential cyanosis in the case of interrupted aortic arch or severe coarctation of the aorta, which is also ductal-dependent.

The cardiac findings in an infant with hypoplastic left heart syndrome depend on the patency of the ductus arteriosus. If the ductus is restrictive, findings of significant systemic circulatory collapse are present. If the ductus is patent, findings may be more subtle.

Precordial palpation usually reveals an active precordium with an increased parasternal (right ventricular) impulse; this may be the most impressive cardiac finding; S_2 will be single and loud, reflecting pulmonary valve closure at an increased pressure. There may be a soft systolic murmur of tricuspid incompetence and hepatomegaly. Peripheral pulses may be diminished, and they become weaker as ductal constriction progresses. The chest radiograph initially may appear normal. As aortic outflow becomes limited, the heart enlarges and pulmonary vascular markings increase. Intravenous prostaglandin E_1 maintains ductal patency and temporarily ensures adequate systemic circulation in infants with hypoplastic left heart syndrome, interrupted aortic arch, or duct-dependent coarctation until further treatment is considered.

Surgical options include a Norwood procedure or heart transplantation.

LESIONS WITH DIMINISHED PULMONARY BLOOD FLOW

Lesions with diminished pulmonary blood flow involve obstruction of flow to the pulmonary artery. If pulmonary flow is obstructed, systemic venous flow must reach the left heart by means of a right-to-left shunt at the atrial, ventricular, or arterial levels.

Pulmonary Atresia with Intact Ventricular Septum or with Ventricular Septal Defect (Tetralogy of Fallot with Pulmonary Atresia)

Pulmonary atresia constitutes the second most common form of cyanotic heart disease in the neonate next to transposition of the great vessels. There is complete atresia of the pulmonic valve and no antegrade pulmonary blood flow. Pulmonary artery perfusion depends completely on the presence of a patent ductus arteriosus. Systemic venous return to the right atrium cannot enter the right ventricle and be adequately ejected into the pulmonary artery. Instead, it must pass from right to left across an atrial or a ventricular septal defect to reach the aortic circulation.

Since there is no antegrade flow across the pulmonic valve, there is no associated murmur except for the murmur of a patent ductus arteriosus. Infants with pulmonary atresia usually become severely cyanotic during the first day of life as the patent ductus closes. The chest radiograph usually shows markedly diminished pulmonary vascular markings (Fig. 15–10). The ECG often shows a mild left axis deviation because of the relative absence of right ventricular forces and peaked P waves in lead II because of right atrial enlargement. The arterial PO_2 is usually below 50 mmHg on room air and with 100% O_2.

Initial stabilization includes institution of prostaglandin E_1 to maintain ductal patency. If the foramen ovale is restrictive, catheterization and balloon atrial septostomy are performed. Initial surgical treatment depends on the size of the tricuspid valve, the right ventricle, and the pulmonary arteries and may include pulmonary valvotomy, a Blalock-Taussig shunt, or both. The latter shunt is an anastomosis of a graft between the subclavian artery and the ipsilateral (usually right) pulmonary artery.

Tetralogy of Fallot

Tetralogy of Fallot (Fig. 15–11) consists of a large ventricular septal defect, overriding aorta, pulmonic stenosis, and right ventricular hypertrophy. The pulmonic stenosis may occur at the subvalvar (infundibular), valvar, or pulmonary arterial level. This is the most

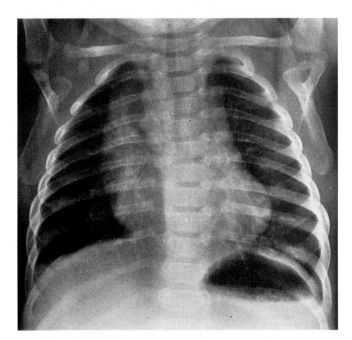

Figure 15–10. Pulmonary atresia with intact ventricular septum.

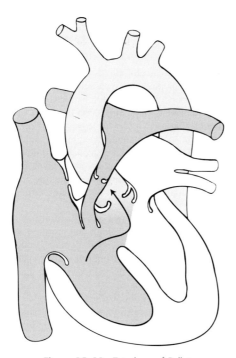

Figure 15–11. Tetralogy of Fallot.

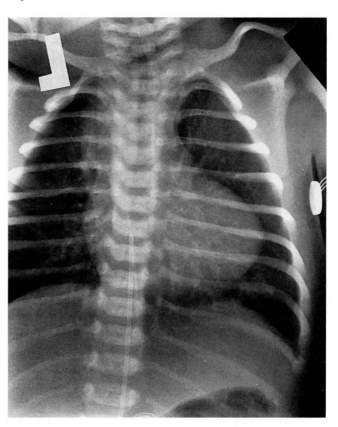

Figure 15–12. Tetralogy of Fallot. Also note that the x-ray is misplaced or reversed, since there is also dextrocardia as determined by the "L," which is correctly placed over the patient but reversed on the view box.

common cyanotic heart defect in children of all ages. Because there is some antegrade flow across the pulmonary outflow tract, a systolic ejection murmur is heard over the upper left sternal border and over both sides of the chest and back. The degree of cyanosis is directly related to the degree of pulmonic stenosis. The greater the pulmonic stenosis, the more right-to-left shunting of deoxygenated systemic venous return to the overriding aorta and the greater the cyanosis. This diagnosis may present at birth with severe cyanosis or may go undetected for several months, when it may present with an asymptomatic murmur and minimal cyanosis (see later). There may be an ejection click of pulmonic stenosis. The chest radiograph reveals diminished pulmonary blood flow, a normal-sized heart with a right ventricular configuration, and a right aortic arch in 25% of cases (Fig. 15–12). The ECG usually reveals right ventricular hypertrophy. The arterial PO_2 demonstrates hypoxemia, which is also a reflection of the severity of pulmonic stenosis.

Tricuspid Atresia

The presentation of tricuspid atresia, absence of a communication between right atrium and ventricle (Fig. 15–13), depends on the presence of a ventricular septal defect. In the absence of a ventricular septal defect, it is usually associated with severe right ventricular hypoplasia and often pulmonic valve atresia. In this case, systemic venous return must pass from right to left across a foramen ovale or an atrial septal defect. The findings may be very similar to pulmonic atresia.

The cardiac examination may reveal no murmur other than that of a patent ductus arteriosus. The chest radiograph demonstrates diminished pulmonary blood flow and may show absence of the main pulmonary artery segment. The cardiac shape may have a "left ventricular" configuration, and the heart may appear round or bullet-shaped on the posteroanterior film as a result of diminished right ventricular mass. The ECG usually reveals left axis deviation due to virtual absence of right ventricular forces and peaked P waves due to right atrial enlargement. The degree of

cyanosis and hypoxemia depends on the patency of the ductus arteriosus. Lesions with ductal-dependent pulmonary blood flow require intravenous prostaglandin E_1 to maintain ductal patency. Balloon atrial septostomy may be necessary to ensure adequate

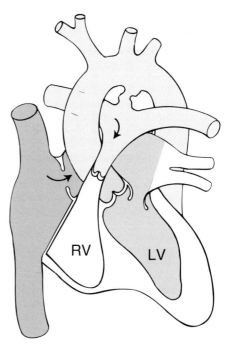

Figure 15–13. Tricuspid atresia.

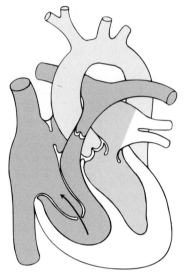

Figure 15–14. Ebstein's malformation of the tricuspid valve.

decompression of the right atrium. Initial surgical therapy is usually a Blalock-Taussig shunt placement.

With tricuspid atresia and moderate to large ventricular septal defect and minimal pulmonic stenosis, the pulmonary blood flow is excessive and cyanosis may not be noticed initially. In these cases, the child may present weeks later with a murmur and signs of pulmonary overcirculation, congestive heart failure, and only mild cyanosis. If the ventricular septal defect becomes restrictive, as it may close with time, the cyanosis may become more severe.

Ebstein's Malformation of the Tricuspid Valve

Ebstein's malformation (Fig. 15–14) is unusual and has many presentations, including cyanosis. There is redundancy of the tricuspid leaflets and adherence of the leaflets to the walls of the right ventricle, so that the valve apparatus is "drawn downward" into the right ventricular cavity. There is usually significant tricuspid regurgitation, and when this is severe, there may be limited antegrade flow across the right ventricular outflow tract to the pulmonary artery, especially during the first days of life when pulmonary vascular resistance is still elevated. In extreme cases, there is complete atresia of the pulmonic valve. The concomitant elevation of right atrial pressure from impaired right ventricular filling and significant tricuspid incompetence leads to right-to-left shunting across the patent foramen ovale and cyanosis. The cyanosis in neonates with Ebstein's malformation often improves during the first weeks of life. As pulmonary vascular resistance falls, tricuspid incompetence improves somewhat and antegrade pulmonary blood flow improves. Right-to-left atrial shunting diminishes, and cyanosis improves. A pansystolic murmur of tricuspid incompetence is often heard at the lower left sternal border and a diastolic rumble is present because of turbulent flow across the tricuspid valve during diastole. There may also be multiple clicks related to opening or closure of the redundant valve leaflets.

The chest radiograph typically shows an enlarged heart with a particularly large right heart border caused by right atrial enlargement. The mediastinum is usually narrow, since output from neither great vessel is significantly increased. Pulmonary vascular markings are diminished. This is the most common congenital heart defect associated with preexcitation and the Wolff-Parkinson-White syndrome, and this ECG finding should suggest this cardiac diagnosis in the cyanotic infant.

Only medical management in infancy is often required.

Persistent Fetal Circulation or Persistent Pulmonary Hypertension of the Neonate

PFC is due to the presence of significant hypoxemia secondary to aggravated elevation of pulmonary vascular resistance with secondary right-to-left shunting across the foramen ovale or patent ductus arteriosus and diminished pulmonary blood flow. It is usually associated with pulmonary disease, asphyxia, sepsis, metabolic (hypoglycemia) or hematologic (polycythemia) derangements, although it may be idiopathic or may occur with a congenital heart defect (TAPVR). When right-to-left shunting occurs at the atrial level, there is cyanosis of both preductal and postductal circulations. If right-to-left shunting occurs predominantly at the ductal level, differential cyanosis is present.

Differentiation of PFC with generalized cyanosis from cyanotic heart disease may be clinically difficult and requires color Doppler echocardiography. PFC with differential cyanosis may be difficult to distinguish from a coarctation or interrupted aortic arch, although the cardiac lesions are not usually associated with underlying pulmonary disease or predisposing factors for PFC. Echocardiography, again, is helpful in revealing the distinction.

Treatment includes mechanical ventilation with or without hyperventilation, prevention of acidosis, hypoxemia, hypothermia or other external stresses, inotropic support, and, when necessary, inhaled nitric oxide or extracorporeal membrane oxygenation (ECMO).

Management of the Neonate with Cyanotic Heart Disease

Treatment should be arranged in conjunction with a pediatric cardiologist. If possible, echocardiography should be performed to confirm the cardiac defect, the presence of myocardial dysfunction, and the status of dependent shunting (e.g., patent foramen ovale or patent ductus arteriosus). After the airway, breathing, and circulation are stabilized, serum glucose, electrolytes, calcium, and complete blood count are assessed, the decision to institute prostaglandin therapy should be made. Prostaglandins may be administered intravenously or, if venous access is lacking, within an umbilical arterial catheter.

The usual starting dose of prostaglandin E_1 is 0.05 μg/kg/minute. The dosage range varies from 0.01 to 0.15 μg/kg/minute. Side effects include jitteriness, hyperthermia, hypoventilation, and apnea. For this reason, respiratory status should be monitored particularly well in the neonate who is not mechanically ventilated.

Coexisting respiratory, metabolic, or infectious disease should be considered and excluded or treated. The clinician should maintain a high index of suspicion for noncardiac anomalies and syndromes associated with congenital heart disease. The early diagnosis of a syndrome may be helpful in assessing general prognosis, in prioritizing management of congenital defects, and in preventing further morbidity. The diagnosis of trisomy 13, 18, or 21 helps to establish a long-term prognosis and to prepare the family for a suspected outcome. The diagnosis of certain syndromes, such as asplenia, would increase the likelihood of infection, or DiGeorge syndrome would require the use of irradiated blood products to avoid graft-versus-host disease.

THE OLDER INFANT AND TODDLER

Cyanosis in infancy may be caused by pulmonary, hematologic, or cardiac disease. As in the neonatal period, the general cause of cyanosis may often be discerned by history, physical examination, and chest radiograph. Pulmonary causes are quite common and include apnea, bronchiolitis, pneumonia, croup, aspiration, drowning, sepsis, and asthma.

Any infectious, inflammatory, obstructive, or infiltrative pulmonary disease may result in cyanosis. In almost all cases, respiratory distress with CO_2 retention can be documented. The chest radiograph (lung fields) is usually abnormal (see Chapter 8).

Certain cardiac diseases may present with cyanosis several weeks or months after birth. In most cases, the lesions involve abnormal connections with significant mixing of saturated and desaturated blood within the heart or obstructive lesions with milder pulmonary outflow obstruction.

The most common cyanotic heart defect to present after 1 month of age is tetralogy of Fallot. The degree of cyanosis depends on the degree of subvalvar, valvar, and supravalvar pulmonic stenosis. Because the severity of the pulmonic stenosis progresses with age, the child may initially have little pulmonic stenosis and thus no right-to-left shunting across the ventricular septal defect. In this case, there may be findings of pulmonary overcirculation. As the child grows and pulmonary stenosis progresses, the obstruction to flow across the right ventricular outflow tract increases and gradually more deoxygenated blood from the right ventricle will shunt from right to left across the ventricular septal defect and return to the aorta.

The physical findings of tetralogy of Fallot include a systolic ejection murmur at the upper left sternal border that radiates to the back. There may be an associated systolic thrill. As the pulmonic stenosis worsens, there is less pulmonary outflow and the systolic murmur becomes softer rather than louder. The hypoxic "tetralogy spell" occurs when desaturated blood transiently shunts to the aorta to a greater degree than usual. This may occur when the child becomes irritable, tachycardic, dehydrated, or hypotensive. The child with a "tet spell" usually first demonstrates irritability and progressive cyanosis with hyperpnea. If cyanosis progresses, the child may lose consciousness momentarily. The "tet spell" generally resolves spontaneously, but the child with a more severe case requires analgesic (morphine sulfate), beta blockade (propranolol), IV bicarbonate, or phenylephrine. Phenylephrine increases systemic vascular resistance and discourages right to left shunting across the ventricular septal defect. Similarly, placement of the infant in the knee-chest position may help to reverse a spell by increasing systemic vascular resistance and thus reduce the degree of right-to-left shunting across the ventricular septal defect.

Other congenital heart defects that may present with cyanosis after several weeks include the rare Ebstein's malformation of the tricuspid valve or, more likely, a variation of the tetralogy of Fallot physiology: double-outlet right ventricle with pulmonic stenosis, transposition of the great vessels with ventricular septal defect with or without pulmonic stenosis, tricuspid atresia with ventricular septal defect with or without pulmonic stenosis, or single ventricle with or without pulmonic stenosis. In each case, there is usually a systolic ejection murmur of pulmonic stenosis at the mid or upper left sternal border or a pansystolic murmur at the lower left sternal border reflecting a left-to-right shunt at the ventricular level. The chest radiograph usually reveals normal or diminished pulmonary vascular markings. The ECG often reveals right ventricular hypertrophy or combined ventricular hypertrophy.

Unusual congenital heart defects that cause cyanosis include *cor triatriatum dexter*. In this case, there is persistence of a valve of the sinus venosus that diverts inferior or superior vena caval return to the foramen ovale and the left atrium. There is usually no associated murmur, and the diagnosis can usually be made by contrast or color Doppler echocardiography. A similar obstruction to tricuspid and right ventricular inflow can occur with tumors of the heart that obstruct vena caval return or filling and output of the right ventricle. In infants, this rarely occurs with cardiac rhabdomyoma (associated with tuberous sclerosis); in older children, it occurs extremely rarely with metastatic renal tumors.

Multiple pulmonary venous malformations may cause a significant right-to-left shunt at the pulmonary level. In contrast to systemic venous malformations, the pulmonary arteriovenous malformation (AVM) is often not associated with a bruit or murmur. When the pulmonary AVM is solitary, large, and in a lower lobe of the lung, the degree of right-to-left shunting through the lesion may vary with body position, particularly when the child is standing or reclining. Increased cyanosis while the child is supine is referred to as *orthodeoxia* or *orthocyanosis*. The diagnosis may be suggested by a parenchymal opacification on the chest radiograph. A contrast echocardiogram may demonstrate the presence of an intrapulmonary right-to-left shunt. Saline injected quickly into a peripheral vein produces microcavitations on the echocardiogram within the right atrium, right ventricle, and pulmonary artery. If there is an intrapulmonary right-to-left shunt, there is return of microcavitations to the pulmonary veins and left atrium after several cardiac cycles. Pulmonary AVMs may be associated with similar malformations of the skin or intestinal tract (*Osler-Weber-Rendu syndrome*). They may also occur in the presence of long-standing hepatic cirrhosis.

CYANOSIS IN LATER CHILDHOOD

In childhood and adolescence, cyanosis is rarely an isolated clinical symptom or sign. Chronic cyanosis is often associated with digital clubbing. Clubbing is an abnormal widening and thickening of the nail, with loss of concavity at the nail bed. Chronic cyanosis in childhood is almost always associated with longstanding respiratory disease (e.g., cystic fibrosis). Hematologic or cardiac causes of cyanosis presenting in childhood are rare.

Methemoglobinemia

Although rare, congenital or acquired methemoglobinemia may present at any time during infancy and childhood. Mild forms of congenital methemoglobinemia may present with cyanosis and symptoms of inadequate oxygen delivery during infections or with exposures to precipitating agents. The most common congenital forms of methemoglobinemia are abnormalities of hemoglobin (hemoglobin M), which preferentially bind the ferric ion (Fe^{+3}) or abnormalities of enzymes (e.g., methemoglobin reductase deficiency), which otherwise keep the iron bound to hemoglobin in the ferrous (Fe^{+2}) state. Hemoglobin M is an autosomal dominant disorder in which hemoglobin is more easily oxidized to methemoglobin. This may present at birth, but therapy is rarely required. Methemoglobin reductase deficiency is an autosomal recessive disorder. Patients are susceptible to precipitous drops in O_2 saturation and increases in methemoglobinemia resulting from various drugs and agents (Table 15–6). Treatment is IV methylene blue.

Acquired methemoglobinemia may occur as a result of intestinal infection with certain bacteria, exposure to nitrates and nitrites in well water, or oxidizing agents in dyes and medications.

The diagnosis of methemoglobinemia is suspected in cyanotic patients with no predisposing pulmonary or cardiac disease who present acutely with cyanosis and metabolic acidosis. The cyanosis often appears slate-gray. The blood is more brown than burgundy and does not become redder when exposed to oxygen in room air. The PaO_2 is normal or high if the patient is receiving oxygen; the saturation is low—hence, the cyanosis with a normal PO_2.

The diagnosis is confirmed by obtaining a methemoglobin level. The normal level is 1% to 3%, and a level above 15% is usually associated with symptoms. Since pulse oximetry does not correlate closely with the actual saturation of oxygen in the blood, the oxygen saturation should be measured directly by cooximetry. The oxygen saturation reported on the blood gas analysis will be

Table 15–6. Agents That Oxidize Hemoglobin

I. Direct oxidation
　Ferricyanide
　Copper
　Hydrogen peroxide
　Hydroxylamine
　Others: Chromate, chlorate, nitrogen trifluoride,
　　　　tetranitromethane, quinones, dyes

II. Interaction with oxygen
　Nitrites, nitroglycerin
　Hydrazines
　Thiols
　Others: Arsine, aminophenols, arylhydroxylamines,
　　　　N-hydroxyurethane, phenylenediamines

III. Requiring biochemical transformation
　Aniline, dyes (diaper and laundry inks, red wax crayons)
　Sulfonamides
　Procaine derivatives
　4,4'-Diaminodiphenylsulfone (dapsone)
　8-Aminoquinolines: primaquine and pamaquine
　N-Acylarylamines: acetanilid, phenacetin

Adapted from Kiese M. Methemoglobinemia: A Comprehensive Treatise. Boca Raton, Fla: CRC Press, 1974.

factitiously high because this value is simply calculated from the measured PO_2 using an algorithm that applies only to normal hemoglobin.

Eisenmenger Syndrome

The cardiac causes of cyanosis in childhood have usually been diagnosed in early infancy. Cardiac defects that may present with cyanosis after 2 years of age are untreated large left-to-right shunts with pulmonary hypertension and *Eisenmenger syndrome*. This situation occurs less frequently now, thanks to earlier detection of these lesions and early surgical intervention to prevent longstanding complications from pulmonary hypertension. Large ventricular or arterial communications are associated with pulmonary hypertension at systemic level as well as with pulmonary overcirculation. After several years (and probably sooner in children with trisomy 21) the unrepaired left-to-right shunt and associated pulmonary hypertension lead to irreversible pulmonary vascular disease, demonstrated microscopically by intimal hyperplasia and medial hypertrophy of the small pulmonary arteries.

Clinically, there is an increase in pulmonary vascular resistance and a decrease in the left-to-right shunt. With time, pulmonary vascular resistance increases inexorably and eventually surpasses systemic vascular resistance. This leads to right-to-left shunting across the defect and progressive cyanosis. If the cardiac defect is at the ventricular level (large ventricular septal defect, atrioventricular canal, single ventricle) or ascending aortic level (truncus arteriosus or aortopulmonary window), the right-to-left shunt will occur at the ventricular or proximal aortic level and general cyanosis will be observed. In the rare case of a large patent ductus arteriosus with Eisenmenger syndrome, the right-to-left shunt will occur from the pulmonary artery to the descending aorta through the ductus, similar to the newborn with persistent fetal circulation. In this case, differential cyanosis and even differential clubbing may be present. The lower extremities will demonstrate clubbing and cyanosis in comparison to the right arm and hand.

The diagnosis of Eisenmenger syndrome is usually made in children with previously diagnosed or treated congenital heart dis-

ease. The physical findings include clubbing of the digits from longstanding cyanosis; an active parasternal impulse from right ventricular hyperactivity; and a single, loud S_2 from early and loud closure of the pulmonic valve simultaneously with the aortic valve. A high-pitched diastolic murmur of pulmonic regurgitation *(Graham-Steele murmur)* may be heard at the upper left sternal edge. The chest radiograph shows a normal heart size or a prominent right ventricular shadow. The main pulmonary artery segment and proximal branches are prominent, but there is abrupt tapering of the more distal vascular markings. The ECG usually reveals right ventricular hypertrophy. In advanced stages, chronic hypoxemia leads to progressive polycythemia. In the second and third decades of life, signs and symptoms of hyperviscosity, hemoptysis, gout, and right-sided heart failure ensue.

The treatment of Eisenmenger syndrome includes symptomatic therapy for hemoptysis and congestive heart failure and avoidance of relative iron deficiency, dehydration, and hypotension. The only theoretical surgical treatment is heart-lung or lung transplantation with correction of the underlying cardiac defect.

RED FLAGS

The initial presentation of cyanosis usually constitutes a diagnostic emergency. In the neonate, congenital heart disease or a pulmonary disorder is the most likely lesion. A normal chest radiograph may suggest a cardiac cause of the cyanosis. Acrocyanosis must be distinguished from generalized cyanosis. Asymmetric or absent pulses must be noted. Noncardiac anomalies need to be recognized so that a syndrome might be considered. In older infants and children, noncardiac causes become more common, and lung disease, infection, and methemoglobinemia must be considered. In the older child, clubbing should strongly suggest a chronic cardiac or pulmonary disorder. The sudden onset of cyanosis in an older child might suggest pulmonary disease or acquired methemoglobinemia.

REFERENCES

Cyanosis in the Newborn

DiMaio AM, Singh J. The infant with cyanosis in the emergency room. Pediatr Clin North Am 1992;39:987.

Driscoll DJ. Evaluation of the cyanotic newborn. Pediatr Clin North Am 1990;37:1.

Franklin RCG, Spiegelhalter DJ, Macartney FJ, et al. Evaluation of a diagnostic algorithm for heart disease in neonates. BMJ 1991;302:935.

Gersony WM, Duc GV, Sinclair JC. ''PFC'' syndrome (persistence of the fetal circulation). Circulation 1969;40:III.

Lees MH, King DK. Cyanosis in the newborn. Pediatr Rev 1987;9:36.

Lewis AB, Takahashi M, Lurie PL. Administration of prostaglandin E1 in neonates with critical congenital cardiac defects. J Pediatr 1978;93:481.

Linday LA, Ehlers KH, O'Loughlin, et al. Noninvasive diagnosis of persistent fetal circulation versus congenital cardiovascular defects. Am J Cardiol 1983;52:847.

Rudolph AM. Congenital Diseases of the Heart. Chicago. Year Book Medical Publishers, 1974.

Siassi B, Goldberg SJ, Emmanouilides GC, et al. Persistent pulmonary vascular obstruction in newborn infants. J Pediatr 1971;78:610.

Stevenson DK, Benitz WE. A practical approach to diagnosis and immediate care of the cyanotic neonate. Clin Pediatr 1987;26:325.

Yabek S. Neonatal cyanosis. Am J Dis Child 1984;138:880.

Cyanosis in the Older Infant and Child

Emmanouilides GC, Riemenschneider TA, Allen HD, et al (eds). Moss and Adams Heart Disease in Infants, Children and Adolescents Including the Fetus and Young Adult, 5th ed. Baltimore: Williams & Wilkins, 1995.

Margolis PA, Ferkol TW, Marsocci S, et al. Accuracy of the clinical examination in detecting hypoxemia in infants with respiratory illness. J Pediatr 1994;124:552.

Nadas AS. Hypoxemia. *In* Fyler DC (ed). Nadas' Pediatric Cardiology. Philadelphia: Hanley and Belfus, 1992.

Watcha MF, Connor MT, Hing AV. Pulse oximetry in methemoglobinemia. Am J Dis Child 1989;143:845.

Pulse Oximetry

Hay WW Jr, Brockway JM, Eyzaquirre M. Neonatal pulse oximetry: Accuracy and reliability. Pediatrics 1989;83:717.

Meier-Strauss P, Bucher HU, Hurlimann R, et al. Pulse oximetry used for documenting oxygen saturation and right-to-left shunting immediately after birth. Eur J Pediatr 1990;149:851.

Methemoglobinemia

Jaffe ER. Methemoglobinemia in the differential diagnosis of cyanosis. Hosp Pract 1985;20:92.

16 Heart Murmur

Jerome Liebman

Heart murmurs are quite common in neonates and children. Many heart murmurs are normal ejection murmurs or are physiologic (e.g., secondary to anemia), whereas others represent congenital or acquired heart disease (Table 16–1). The cause of congenital heart disease is often unknown, but genetic (gene or chromosomal) disorders, syndrome complexes, metabolic disorders, or teratogenesis may be responsible. Acquired heart diseases include rheumatic fever, endocarditis, and diseases caused by systemic illnesses, such as systemic lupus erythematosus (SLE) (see Table 16–1). Murmurs may not originate in the heart and may represent arteriovenous malformations of the central nervous system, lung, liver, or extremities. Such extracardiac sounds may be secondary to an innocent jugular venous hum or a carotid or abdominal vessel bruit. The relationship between the normal heart cycle and that of potentially abnormal heart sounds is noted in Figure 16–1.

When a phonocatheter is passed into the heart, vibrations are recorded that can be transmitted directly to the ear and recorded on paper. An external phonocardiogram can also be recorded simultaneously with direct auscultation of the chest. Simultaneous listening and recording from within the heart and great arteries have taught us about auscultation of the heart in children and young adults, especially those with congenital heart disease.

The intracavitary phonocardiogram has documented that normal people rarely have a murmur within the four cardiac chambers. However, in all people, there is a murmur in the root of the pulmonary artery and the root of the aorta (Fig. 16–2). These murmurs are present because each great artery comes off at an angle from the ventricle and because the origin of each great artery is narrower than the ventricle, which ejects blood. The length and intensity of these normal murmurs as recorded by the intracavitary phonocatheter appear to be the same in all normal people, but transmission to the outside of the chest varies greatly (Fig. 16–3). Transmission depends on how close the chest wall is to the areas where the murmur is generated and on the frequency of the murmur itself. When a murmur is able to be recorded within the four cardiac chambers, an abnormality is usually found, but there are exceptions (Fig. 16–4).

For an understanding of the meaning of a particular heart murmur, the following are needed:

1. A minimum of two different types of stethoscopes must be available, one that allows the full appreciation of low-frequency sounds and one that allows high-frequency sounds to be as clear as possible. Whether the stethoscope is light and comfortable is not important; a loud diaphragm may be a detriment.

2. There must be an understanding as to what these two different types of stethoscopes do and why.

3. There must be an understanding of the mechanisms that create the normal and abnormal sounds and murmurs generated by the heart (see Fig. 16–1).

4. There must be an understanding of normal cardiovascular hemodynamics, as well as specific abnormal cardiovascular hemodynamics.

5. There must be a knowledge of common cardiac lesions and their resulting hemodynamics (see Table 16–1).

6. There must be a knowledge of the changes in heart sounds and murmurs caused by the specific hemodynamic abnormalities that result from common cardiac lesions.

7. There must be the discipline necessary to concentrate on one sound at a time as part of auscultation (e.g., the ability to dissect the sounds).

8. There must be the ability to understand and perform the nonauscultative portions of the cardiac examination and to integrate these findings with those found at auscultation.

STETHOSCOPE

The heart sounds are transmitted in many different directions through many kinds of tissues before they reach the surface of the chest. Thus, the sounds are complex and modified. The frequencies generated vary from 650 cycles per second (cps) to 5 to 10 cps, although the ear cannot hear below 30 to 40 cps. Importantly, the human auditory system needs greater intensity to hear lower-frequency sounds than it does to hear higher-frequency sounds. As a complex sound becomes more intense, the low-frequency (or low-pitch) sounds become more prominent because the higher-frequency components are masked. In practical terms, a 10-inch

Table 16–1. Etiology of Heart Murmurs

Neonate*	Infant	Older Child
Transient patency of ductus arteriosus	Congenital heart disease (L→R shunt or R→L shunt)†	Congenital valvular obstruction Ejection murmurs (normal)
Peripheral pulmonic stenosis	Ejection murmurs (normal)	Repaired congenital heart disease
Cyanotic congenital heart disease	Anemia	Anemia Mitral valve prolapse Venous hum
Congenital valvular obstruction	Arteriovenous malformation	Bacterial endocarditis
Arteriovenous malformation (CNS, hepatic, pulmonary) Anemia	Infective endocarditis	Rheumatic fever
		Marfan syndrome Prosthetic valves
	Kawasaki disease	Obstructive (hypertrophic) cardiomyopathy (subaortic stenosis)
Asphyxia myocardial ischemia (transient TI or MI)	Hunter-Hurler syndrome Fabry syndrome	Carotid or abdominal bruit Tumor (atrial myxoma) Thyrotoxicosis Systemic lupus erythematosus Pericardial friction rub

*Common causes of congenital heart disease in low-birth-weight infants include PDA, VSD, tetralogy of Fallot, coarctation of the aorta—interrupted aortic arch, hypoplastic left heart syndrome, heterotaxias, and D-transposition of the great arteries, in that order. Common causes of congenital heart disease in term infants include VSD, D-transposition of the great arteries, tetralogy of Fallot, coarctation of the aorta, pulmonary stenosis, hypoplastic left heart syndrome, and PDA; other causes represent a smaller percentage.

†The relative percentages of congenital heart lesions are VSD (25%–30%), ASD (6%–8%), PDA (6%–8%), coarctation of aorta (5%–7%), tetralogy of Fallot (5%–7%), pulmonary valve stenosis (5%–7%), aortic valve stenosis (5%–7%), D-transposition of great arteries (3%–5%) and hypoplastic left ventricle, truncus arteriosus, total anomalous venous return, tricuspid atresia, single ventricle, and double-outlet right ventricle representing 1%–3% each. Other and more complex lesions (heterotaxias) together represent 5%–10% of all lesions.

Abbreviations: ASD = atrial septal defect; CNS = central nervous system; L = left; MI = mitral insufficiency; PDA = patent ductus arteriosus; R = right; TI = tricuspid insufficiency; VSD = ventricular septal defect.

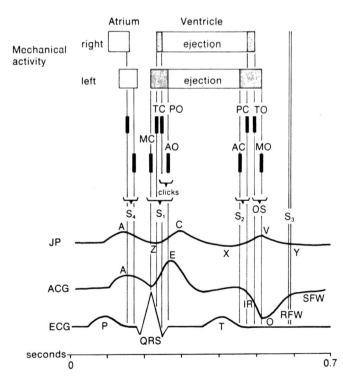

Figure 16–1. The cardiac cycle. Relationship among electrical and mechanical events, valvular motion, heart sounds, the jugular pulse wave (JP), and the apexcardiogram (ACG). MC and MO = mitral component and opening; TC and TO = tricuspid component and opening; AC and AO = aortic component and opening; PC and PO = pulmonic component and opening; OS = opening snap of atrioventricular valves; IC = isovolumic (isochronic) contraction wave; IR = isovolumic (isochronic) relaxation wave; O = opening of mitral valve; RFW = rapid-filling wave; SFW = slow-filling wave. (From Tilkian AG, Conover MB. Understanding Heart Sounds and Murmurs: With an Introduction to Lung Sounds, 3rd ed. Philadelphia: WB Saunders, 1993.)

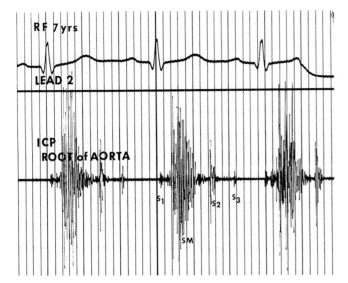

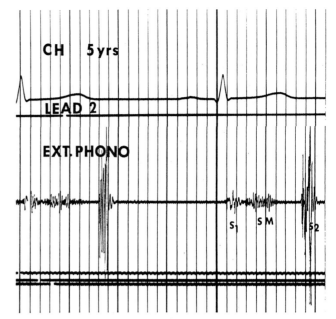

Figure 16–2. An intracavitary phonocardiogram (ICP) in the root of the aorta of a normal 7-year-old child. Note the ejection murmur. S_1 begins just after the QRS of the electrocardiogram. There is a sound-free period, followed by a diamond-shaped, high-frequency murmur, which ends well before A_2. S_2 has been recorded. This is a typical normal aortic ejection murmur, which was audible on the surface of the chest at the fourth left interspace at the left sternal edge. (A similar murmur was recorded from the root of the pulmonary artery.) (From Liebman J, et al. Diastolic murmurs in normal children. Circulation 1968; 38:755–762. Reprinted with permission by the American Heart Association.)

Figure 16–3. External phonocardiogram (Ext. phono.) of a normal 5-year-old child recorded at the fourth left interspace at the left sternal edge. The murmur starts after S_1 and stops well before S_2. The length of the murmur is approximately two-thirds systole. This is a medium-frequency murmur, which sounded "vibratory." There was no transmission to the back, and transmission to the neck was excellent. (The intracavitary phonocardiogram was similar to that shown in Figure 16–2.) This is a normal murmur and is believed most likely to represent a normal aortic ejection murmur. (From Liebman J, et al. Diastolic murmurs in normal children. Circulation 1968; 38:755–762. Reprinted with permission by the American Heart Association.)

length of tubing is considered optimal for auscultation, although a significant decrease in efficiency may not develop until the tubing is greater than 12 inches.

For sounds on the higher side of the frequency spectrum, a taut stethoscope diaphragm is optimal because the diaphragm's natural frequency of oscillation is higher when it is taut. When the natural frequency of a diaphragm is increased, the upper-frequency range to which the diaphragm is capable of responding is increased. This effect cannot be attained without a decrease in the diaphragm's sensitivity throughout the entire lower-frequency range. This decrease would be good because the higher-frequency sounds would be clearer. But, the larger diameter of the diaphragm, the lower its natural frequency. Therefore, if a large diaphragm is used to make sounds loud, the size may defeat the purpose of the taut diaphragm in that it may make all sounds appear to be of lower

frequency. The author uses the stethoscope developed by Rappaport and Sprague, which comes with two diaphragms, 3 and 4.5 cm in diameter; almost always use the smaller one, reserving the larger one only for very large adults, in whom sound transmission from the heart to the outside is reduced.

A misconception about the open bell of the stethoscope is that it accentuates low-frequency sounds and attenuates high-frequency sounds. All sounds heard on the chest appear louder with the bell, which must be applied gently to not create the effect of a diaphragm by tensing the skin. Because low-frequency sounds are inherently soft and more difficult to hear than are high-frequency sounds, a

Figure 16–4. Intracavitary phonocardiogram (ICP) from the body of the left ventricle of the same 7-year-old child as in Figure 16–2. The gain has not been changed. The ejection murmur is much decreased in intensity from that in the root of the aorta and is believed to be transmitted. There is an additional murmur, early in diastole, which is diamond-shaped, and of medium to high frequency. A short grade II diastolic medium- to high-frequency murmur was heard at the fourth left interspace at the left sternal edge only while the patient was lying down. The cardiac catheterization was normal. This is believed to be a normal diastolic murmur. (From Liebman J, et al. Diastolic murmurs in normal children. Circulation 1968; 38: 755–762. Reprinted with permission by the American Heart Association.)

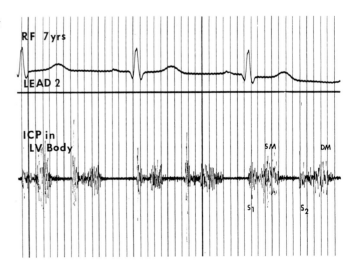

lightly applied bell is essential. The bell should be shallow to be most efficient but not so shallow that the patient's tissues interfere with the volume of air. The larger the diameter of this bell, the more efficient the stethoscope, particularly below 200 cps, although the smaller bell has its major effect below 100 cps. The stethoscope the author uses comes with three bells. The largest one allows sounds to be so loud for most children that it is often difficult to delineate the low-frequency sounds. The smallest one is useful mainly for newborn babies. The middle sized open bell, lightly applied, allows selective listening to the lowest-frequency sounds without making higher-frequency sounds too loud.

To our knowledge, a scientific study of the exact frequencies of the various normal and abnormal heart sounds has never been published. However, the third and fourth sounds and the low-velocity murmurs associated with flow across the tricuspid and mitral valves are the lowest frequency, between 30 and 115 cps. The higher frequencies (approximately 600 cps) are related to regurgitation from the aorta to the left ventricle and from the pulmonary artery to the right ventricle (in the presence of systemic level pulmonary hypertension).

METHOD OF AUSCULTATION

Because the right ventricle is in front of the left ventricle, sounds originating from the right side are generally better heard than those of equal intensity originating from the left. However, once the pulmonary vascular resistance has decreased (from the high-resistance fetal state to the low-resistance state in infancy and childhood), the left ventricular and aortic pressures are so much higher than the right ventricular and pulmonary artery pressures that the intensity of heart sounds and murmurs originating on the left side is usually greater than the intensity of those originating from the right side. Another difference between the two sides of the heart is that because the left ventricle is further away from the chest than the right, its transmission is over a wider area than is transmission from the right side.

There is a widely used concept that we must think of "listening areas" (Fig. 16–5), which include (1) the apex, which for many auscultors includes not only the apex but also the interspaces at the lower left sternal border (LLSB); (2) the pulmonary area, the interspaces at the upper left sternal border, (ULSB); and (3) the aortic area, the interspaces at the upper right sternal border (URSB). Some do not use these terms, preferring to describe more exactly where sounds are heard. Sounds heard at the apex are likely to originate at the mitral valve, or left ventricle, or both. However,

sounds at the fourth or fifth left interspace at the left sternal edge are likely to originate from the tricuspid valve, or right ventricle, or both. At the first, second, or third left interspace at the left sternal edge, the pulmonary closure sound and pulmonary ejection murmurs are usually best heard. However, murmurs from infundibular pulmonic stenosis may be better heard at lower interspaces.

Furthermore, the aortic closure sound is usually best analyzed in terms of timing at the second left interspace at the left sternal edge. Aortic valvular stenosis murmurs, although the sound is usually best heard at the second right interspace at the right sternal edge, may be best heard over the sternum or at the left sternal edge. In addition, the murmurs of subaortic stenosis can be best heard from the URSB at the second interspace to the third, fourth, or fifth interspace at the left sternal edge. Finally, in rare cases of ventricular inversion with L transposition, the URSB would have to become the pulmonary listening area, and the upper left sternal border would have to become the aortic listening area. Obviously, in light of this information, it is preferred to describe exactly where the sounds and murmurs are best heard, describe their best transmission, and then make the judgment as to their origin.

For auscultation and full appreciation of what is being heard, the technique of *dissection* is essential. First, one listens to the entire cardiac cycle to get an appreciation of the cadence and to differentiate between systole and diastole. After some practice, it is usually not necessary to feel the carotid pulse to determine the first sound (S_1) and to determine systole. After that, the auscultor then listens to each possible sound and murmur everywhere with discipline. In so doing, the auscultor listening to S_1, for example, listens everywhere with such concentration that he or she does not really hear anything else except S_1. After listening in the same manner for pulmonic and aortic ejection clicks, mid-systolic non-ejection clicks, the second sound (S_2), the opening snap, the third sound (S_3), and the fourth sound (S_4), the auscultor finally listens to systole for systolic murmurs and diastole (with both the diaphragm and the bell) for early, mid- and late diastolic murmurs. All of this process appears to require a tremendous effort, but once it is performed enough to become routine, it becomes automatic and fast, as well as thorough.

HEART SOUNDS

First Sound (S₁)

Figure 16–1 illustrates the genesis and timing of each heart sound. Four major components make up S_1, usually a broad sound

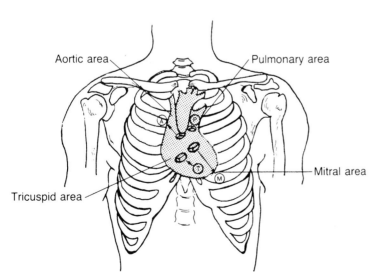

Figure 16–5. Traditional areas of auscultation. (From Tilkian AG, Conover MB. Understanding Heart Sounds and Murmurs: With an Introduction to Lung Sounds, 3rd ed. Philadelphia: WB Saunders, 1993.)

Aortic area

Pulmonary area

Mitral area

Tricuspid area

of 10 to 12 milliseconds. The first and fourth components are inaudible and of no apparent significance. The second component, the first sound heard, is caused mainly by mitral valve closure and is thus called M_1, but the rapid rise of left ventricular pressure may contribute to this sound. The third component, the second sound heard, is most likely caused by tricuspid valve closure and is thus called T_1, although some believe it is a muscular sound associated with left ventricular, not right ventricular, ejection. Occasionally, a normally split S_1 is present when the patient has mitral or tricuspid valve atresia, giving credence to the theory that the second component of S_1 is a muscular sound related to the sharp rise in left ventricular pressure at the beginning of ejection. M_1 and T_1 are of relatively high frequency. Usually, only one sound is heard, but frequently, a split of perhaps 20 to 30 milliseconds is best appreciated at the fourth or fifth left interspace at the left sternal edge. In the normal child, S_1 is usually best heard at the apex, although if right ventricular pressure is high, it may be better heard at the LLSB (fourth or fifth left interspace at the left sternal edge). When an S_1 split is heard, the second component usually sounds very thin and is better heard on inspiration than on expiration. (The duration of the split does not change with respiration.) This second component is usually weaker at the apex and is weaker or absent at the axillary line. To be confident of the normally split S_1, the observer should ensure that the patient does not have a fourth sound (S_4) followed by an S_1, or an S_1 followed by a pulmonic or aortic ejection click. It is unusual to have difficulty in determining that there is not an S_4 followed by an S_1, or an S_1 followed by a pulmonary ejection click. However, occasionally, it is difficult to separate the normally split S_1 from an S_1 followed by an aortic ejection click. This is because the second component of S_1 is occasionally loud and broad and because the aortic ejection click is occasionally louder at the LLSB than at the apex.

Ejection Click

An audible ejection click is always abnormal and is related to the hemodynamics associated with a dilated root of the aorta (aortic ejection click) or a dilated root of the pulmonary artery (pulmonary ejection click). The sound is sharp and of very high frequency. The pulmonary ejection click is best heard at the ULSB (Fig. 16–6), whereas the aortic ejection click is usually best heard at the apex, occasionally at the LLSB, where it is slightly louder than at the apex. It may be heard at the URSB, but if so, it is always louder at the apex or the LLSB. The click arises either from sudden tension of the semilunar valve or from sudden distention with lateral pressure at the root of the aorta or pulmonary artery (Fig. 16–7). The sound is almost always present in aortic or pulmonic valvular stenosis. In such cases, the rapid movement of the stenotic valve is suddenly checked. In simultaneous intracavitary phonocardiography-cineangiography studies, the ejection click and the sudden valve tensing were found to be simultaneous. However, the sudden jet of blood into the root of the aorta or pulmonary artery with lateral pressure also occurs at exactly the same time. Furthermore, an aortic ejection click may be heard in the presence of a normal aortic valve (severe tetralogy of Fallot with a large aortic root); a pulmonary ejection click may be heard with a normal pulmonic valve (Eisenmenger syndrome with a large pulmonary root).

The aortic ejection click, best heard at the apex, does not vary with respirations. However, the pulmonary ejection click, best heard at the ULSB, is better heard on expiration than inspiration. The explanation for this apparently paradoxical phenomenon does not require an abnormality of the pulmonic valve. With inspiration, the increased negative intrathoracic pressure causes more flow into the right ventricle and pulmonary artery, causing the pulmonary valve to be maximally open and the root of the pulmonary artery

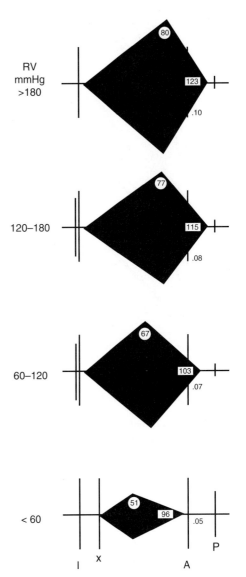

Figure 16–6. Diagrammatic descriptions of the phonocardiogram at the upper left sternal border of patients with varying severity of valvular pulmonic stenosis. There is a sharp sound after S_1 (x), which is closer to S_1 with increasing severity. In the most severe case (RV pressure > 180 mmHg), the sound (pulmonary ejection click) is either not heard or is at the same time as S_1. The more severe the case, the longer the murmur, the more widely separated is P_2 from A_2 and the softer is P_2. RV = right ventricular. (From Vogelpoel L, Schrire V. Auscultatory and phonocardiographic assessment of pulmonary stenosis with intact ventricular septum. Circulation 1960; 22:55–72. Reprinted with permission by the American Heart Association.)

to be maximally dilated when each jet of blood is ejected through the pulmonary valve. During expiration, there is less negative intrathoracic pressure, so that the pulmonary valve is less open and the root of the pulmonary artery is less distended when the jet of blood is ejected through the pulmonary valve. Thus, during expiration, there is maximal excursion of the pulmonary valve and maximal lateral pressure to suddenly dilate the root of the pulmonary artery, and this is when the pulmonary ejection click is heard.

In the case of the aortic ejection click, the sound is usually very well separated from S_1. However, the pulmonary ejection click is usually closer to S_1 than an aortic click. In fact, in some moderate to severe cases, the pulmonary ejection click occurs at the same

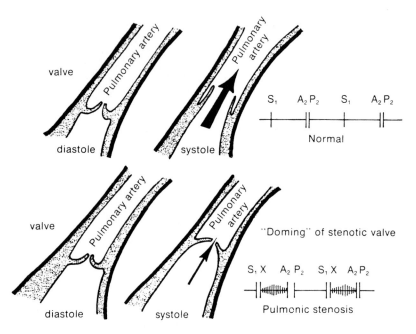

Figure 16–7. Comparison of the ejection of blood through the normal and abnormal pulmonary valves and the resultant auscultatory events. The abrupt arrest of the domed stenosed pulmonary valve coincides with the ejection sound (X). Systolic sounds are heard. (From Tilkian AG, Conover MB. Understanding Heart Sounds and Murmurs: With an Introduction to Lung Sounds, 3rd ed. Philadelphia: WB Saunders, 1993.)

time as S_1. The intensity of S_1 is normally very low at the ULSB. When a loud S_1 appears to be present there, a careful analysis may reveal that this loud S_1 is maximal on expiration, indicating that the loudness is because of a prominent pulmonary ejection click occurring at the same time as a normally soft S_1. This latter phenomenon may explain some cases of severe valvular pulmonic stenosis in which the pulmonary ejection click is not recognized.

Non-ejection Click

Non-ejection clicks are heard at the apex and occur a third to a half of the way between S_1 and S_2. Thus, they are commonly called mid-systolic clicks. The sounds are of medium to high frequency. The sound is caused by the sudden tensing of the posterior mitral valve leaflet as it prolapses into the left atrium; rarely, there may

be multiple mid-systolic clicks. The click may be loud, but it may also be soft and easily missed.

Second Sound (S₂)

The second sound is made up mainly of aortic and pulmonic valve closures and is normally best appreciated at the ULSB (Fig. 16–8). The sounds are of high frequency. The split of S_2, with aortic closure (A_2) preceding pulmonary closure (P_2) is of greater duration (40 to 50 msec) on inspiration than on expiration (0 to 30 msec). The reason for the wider split on inspiration is that with inspiration, there is an increase in negative intrathoracic pressure, resulting in increased systemic venous blood returned into the right ventricle. The result is that more blood goes through the pulmonic valve on inspiration than on expiration, keeping the valve open

Figure 16–8. The normal respiratory splitting of S_2 and where it is best heard. A, P = aortic and pulmonic components of S_2. The second heart sound (S_2). Note that on inspiration P_2 is delayed and A_2 is a little early. (From Tilkian AG, Conover MB. Understanding Heart Sounds and Murmurs: With an Introduction to Lung Sounds, 3rd ed. Philadelphia: WB Saunders, 1993.)

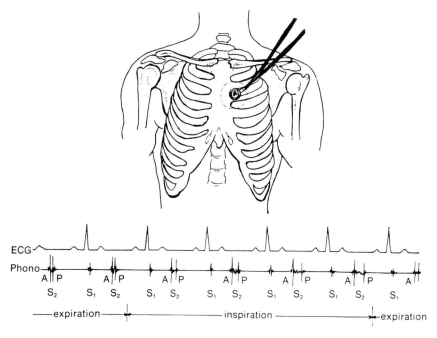

longer. On inspiration, pulmonic venous blood pools, resulting in less filling of the left ventricle. Thus, on inspiration, the A_2 is earlier than on expiration, but the change in A_2 is much less than the change in P_2. The semilunar valves are closed by the aortic or pulmonary diastolic pressure. Thus, the *higher* the pulmonary artery diastolic pressure, the earlier the pulmonary valve closure. In adults but not in children, if P_2 is heard at the apex, pulmonary hypertension is likely. Pulmonary hypertension in children is suggested when P_2 is loud and narrowly split or not separated from A_2. In the presence of pulmonic stenosis, there is low pulmonary artery diastolic pressure. The pulmonary valve closure is therefore delayed and of decreased intensity.

Single or narrow splitting is noted in pulmonary hypertension, severe pulmonic or aortic valve stenosis, tetralogy of Fallot, truncus arteriosus, pulmonary atresia, hypoplastic left heart syndrome, tricuspid atresia, and Eisenmenger syndrome with a ventricular septal defect (VSD).

Wide splitting, fixed splitting, or both, are noted in atrial septal defects (ASDs), partial anomalous venous return, right bundle branch block, mitral regurgitation, VSDs, left ventricular ectopic beats, and right ventricular outflow obstruction.

Opening Snap

The opening snap, present only in rheumatic mitral stenosis when the anteromedial leaflet is mobile, is heard early in diastole, usually above the apex, and is of medium frequency. Because the leaflets are fused, the downward movement of the valve that is trying to open is suddenly checked, resulting in the opening snap. This sound is often confused with an S_3. The frequency is somewhat higher, and the timing is earlier.

Third Sound (S_3) (Fig. 16–9)

The third sound, which is of very low frequency, occurs about a third of the way into diastole, at the time of the most rapid filling of the ventricles. It is caused most likely by sudden tension of the

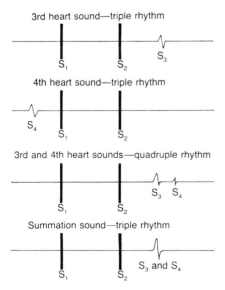

Figure 16–9. The third and fourth heart sounds. Four possible rhythms due to the presence of S_3, S_4, or both. (From Tilkian AG, Conover MB. *Understanding Heart Sounds and Murmurs: With an Introduction to Lung Sounds*, 3rd ed. Philadelphia: WB Saunders, 1993.)

ventricles, enough to produce sound vibrations within the myocardial wall. Vibrations in the atrioventricular valve itself as well as chordae may also contribute to the sound. The amplitude of S_3 increases with increased ventricular filling rate, but also the frequency of the sound increases with increased end-diastolic pressure (which perhaps makes the sound easier to hear). When heard at the apex, S_3 is considered to be left ventricular in origin, and when heard at the LLSB, S_3 is likely to be right ventricular in origin. An apical S_3 of soft to moderate intensity, is readily heard in virtually all children and young adults. An S_3 gallop may also be caused by lesions associated with left or right ventricular diastolic overload or diminished ventricular compliance.

Fourth Sound (S_4) (Fig. 16–9)

The fourth sound (S_4) is also of low frequency and can be both left sided and right sided in origin. It occurs with atrial contraction against a high resistance and is therefore heard just before S_1. It is a more difficult sound to hear than is S_3, particularly in children whose PR interval is usually shorter than that in the adult. The accepted explanation for the genesis of the S_4 is that of forceful atrial contraction against a poorly compliant left ventricle (e.g., as in diastolic overload). Indeed, the sound is readily heard in adults with significant chronic hypertension or left ventricular cardiomyopathy and, except for its timing, sounds much like an S_3. In children, the sound sometimes sounds like a sigh just before S_1 and is very difficult to appreciate. However, in a young baby with total anomalous pulmonary venous return, low pulmonary vascular resistance, and huge right ventricular and pulmonary blood flow, a very loud right ventricular S_4 (as well as S_3) is heard as part of a quadruple rhythm at the LLSB (see Fig. 16–9). Belying the concept that the only explanation for an audible S_4 is atrial contraction against a poorly compliant ventricle is the common physical finding of an intermittent loud S_4 in children with complete atrioventricular block. The S_4 is intermittent because it is generated when the atrium contracts against a closed atrioventricular valve. When the atrium contracts against an open atrioventricular valve, there is no S_4. Thus, the sound cannot be arising solely in the ventricle. The explanation for an audible S_4 is therefore forceful atrial contraction against a high resistance. It is generally accepted that an audible S_4 is abnormal.

MURMURS

Six grades are utilized for systolic murmurs, and four grades for diastolic murmurs. This grading is, of course, subjective in many aspects.

Grading of Murmurs

1. Systolic Murmur Grades
    I. Barely audible
    II. Soft, but easily heard
    III. Moderately loud, no thrill
    IV. Loud, associated with a thrill
    V. Loud, audible with the stethoscope barely off the chest
    VI. Loud, audible with the stethoscope off the chest

    Murmurs of grades V and VI are not commonly recognized and are of little use diagnostically. Having a thrill felt in the chest is of no more importance than being able to describe a grade IV murmur, but suprasternal notch and carotid thrills are diagnostic.

2. Diastolic Murmur Grades
   I–IV. Same as systolic murmur grading description.
      In addition to describing intensity, one must also describe many other aspects involving timing and frequency.
3. Timing
   a. Systolic or diastolic
   b. Early, mid, or late
   c. Relationship of murmur to S_1 and A_2 or P_2
   d. Length of murmur
   e. If full length, does murmur peak early or late?
4. Frequency
   a. Low, medium, or high
   b. Degree of harshness (a nonspecific term separate from frequency)
   c. Vibratory (like pulling a cello string)
5. If systolic, is murmur ejection or regurgitant? Ejection murmurs start clearly after S_1 and are diamond-shape (crescendo-decrescendo) but have varying lengths. Regurgitant murmurs tend to be long and closer to S_1 and plateau-shaped, but whether they peak early or peak late is very important.
6. If diastolic, decrescendo or not?
7. Exact localization of maximal intensity
8. Best transmission
9. Change with respiration
10. Continuous murmur (extends across A_2 at least part way into diastole)

GENERAL EXAMINATION

Obviously, the general examination is important in the evaluation of the cardiovascular system, but key aspects of the rest of the examination of the body are as follows:

- *Pulses.* The brachial and femoral pulses should be felt together for delay, and both brachial pulses should be felt together. An estimate must be made of the pulse pressure (e.g., average, wide, or narrow).
- *Skin color.* Fingernails and conjunctivae are good indicators for mild cyanosis, clubbing (fingers), or petechiae.
- *Palpation of the liver.* Palpation is best performed by feeling lightly from above in order not to cause guarding and loss of the edge. Thus, a 4-cm soft liver not felt across the midline may be normal, but a tense 3-cm liver well felt across the midline may be part of congestive heart failure. The left lobe is the ''failure lobe.'' A transverse liver is suggestive of *heterotaxia syndromes* (Table 16–2).
- Rales in the lungs in infants and even young children usually indicate infection; pulmonary edema must be a consideration.
- Red fingers, well demarcated above the nail, are common in patients with valvular pulmonic stenosis and atrial septal defect for reasons not clear, but especially if they are shiny, red fingers and toes may be a precursor to clubbing and cyanosis.
- Evaluation of the chest for evidence of cardiomegaly does not include percussion, which is bothersome and of little use in infancy but occasionally helpful in adolescents. Feeling the chest for left chest prominence may give a clue to cardiac enlargement, and palpation may demonstrate activity of the heart well past the nipple line.
- The type of impulse (right ventricular versus left ventricular) is readily appreciated. When the chest is felt, it is mainly the right ventricle that is under the hand. In normal newborns, the impulse is felt closer to the sternum, and in systole, the impulse pushes the hand up in that area. This is the normal right ventricular impulse. An impulse felt like this later in life than the newborn period is an abnormal right ventricular impulse. After early infancy, the normal pulse is left ventricular where the heart pushes the hand up at or outside the apex.

Table 16–2. Comparison of Cardiosplenic Heterotaxia Syndromes

	Asplenia	Polysplenia
Spleen	Absent	Multiple
Sidedness (isomerism)	Bilateral right	Bilateral left
Lungs	Bilateral trilobar with eparterial bronchi	Bilateral bilobar with hyparterial bronchi
Sex	Male (65%)	Female ≥ male
Right-sided stomach	Yes	Less common
Symmetric transverse liver	Yes	Yes
Partial intestinal rotation	Yes	Yes
Dextrocardia (%)	30–40	30–40
Pulmonary blood flow	Decreased	Increased
Severe cyanosis	Yes	No
Transposition of great arteries (%)	60–75	15
Total anomalous pulmonary venous return (%)	70–80	Rare
Common atrioventricular valve (%)	80–90	20–40
Single ventricle (%)	40–50	10–15
Absent inferior vena cava with azygos continuation	No	Characteristic
Bilateral superior vena cava	Yes	Yes
Other common defects	PA, PS	Partial anomalous pulmonary venous return, ventricular septal defect, double-outlet right ventricle
Risk of sepsis	Yes	No
Howell-Jolly and Heinz bodies, pitted erythrocytes	Yes	No
Absent gallbladder; biliary atresia	No	Yes
Mortality	High	Moderately high if symptomatic

Modified from Behrman RE (ed). Nelson Textbook of Pediatrics, 14th ed. Philadelphia: WB Saunders, 1992.

The normal left ventricular impulse is gentle, and the abnormal left ventricular impulse is more forceful.

- The hyperdynamic heart occurs in various forms. For example, a forceful and sustained left ventricular impulse is consistent with significant aortic stenosis. If the area of the apex or outside it has great excursions, then there is a hyperdynamic apex, as occurs in mitral regurgitation. If the left sternal edge has great excursion, then there is a hyperdynamic left sternal edge, usually indicating a large left-to-right shunt. The latter finding is best appreciated in infants and young children and can be correlated with the main pulmonary artery and perhaps the right ventricular outflow tract being very active. In mitral regurgitation, the hyperactivity occurs because with each beat, the left ventricle sends increased volume to the left atrium as well as to the aorta; in large left-to-right shunts increased volume must enter the pulmonary artery with each beat.

- *Thrills.* On the chest, thrills indicate only that the murmur is loud, that is, at least a grade IV; elsewhere, however, thrills are diagnostic. Suprasternal notch thrills almost always indicate aortic or pulmonic stenosis, but an associated carotid systolic thrill indicates aortic stenosis. Occasionally at the suprasternal notch there may be an active thrust, probably not with a thrill, in the presence of coarctation of the aorta. Occasionally, while the patient is sitting up, a systolic or even continuous thrill may be appreciated in the suprasternal notch, despite a normal heart and a prominent venous hum.

MURMURS IN CHILDREN WITH NORMAL HEARTS

All normal people have murmurs in the root of the pulmonary artery and aorta. Particularly when the heart is close to the chest, as in the preschool-aged child, these normal murmurs are often well heard on the outside of the anterior chest (see Fig. 16–3). During the preschool years, the normal murmur is usually maximal at the LLSB, usually at the fourth left intercostal space at the left sternal edge, but it can be at the third or fifth left intercostal space. The murmur is always ejection, starts after S₁, ends well before S₂, and is diamond-shaped. Its duration is usually about two-thirds the length of systole, and its intensity is no greater than grade III. Transmission is to the apex, the anterior axillary line and neck, and rarely to the back. Sometimes this murmur is very vibratory (commonly called *Still's murmur*), like the pulling of a cello string. Why this murmur sounds this way is not known. The normal LLSB ejection murmur is very rarely heard in the newborn period and begins to be heard after a few months of age, becoming increasingly common up to the preschool period, when its prevalence begins to decrease. The major differential diagnosis to consider is that of mild subaortic stenosis. It is very rarely heard in teenagers. Conversely, normal pulmonary ejection murmurs are uncommon prior to adolescence. The normal pulmonary ejection murmur—the normal murmur most commonly heard in teenagers and young adults—is usually best heard at the second left intercostal space at the left sternal edge. Best transmission is to the neck, apex, and left shoulder, but not to the back. The murmur is ejection, starts well after S₁, stops well before S₂, and is diamond-shaped. It is usually one-half to two-thirds the length of systole, and its intensity is no greater than grade III. Obviously, for a diagnosis of normality, all other parameters of the cardiac examination must be normal. The differential diagnosis includes mild valvular pulmonic stenosis and ASD.

These are normal murmurs. As described earlier, they are found within the heart of all normal people and are easy to describe to families with a diagram. In addition, parents appreciate hearing the word "normal," and there is no need to use other expressions. Until now, the phrase "flow murmur" has not been mentioned, because indeed, there is no such thing as a murmur not caused by flow! The expression "innocent murmur" obviously has merit because families understand the word innocent, but many abnormal murmurs are innocent as well, such as those caused by trivial valvular pulmonic stenosis and tiny VSDs. A very poor expression is "functional murmur," for various reasons, the most important of which is perhaps that most families have no idea as to the meaning of the word functional, and because truly functional murmurs are not normal. For example, in an ASD with a pulmonary blood flow three times that of normal, there is three times the normal flow going through the tricuspid and pulmonary valves. The murmurs are caused by this large flow through normal valves. They are functional murmurs, but they are far from normal.

When the patient sits up, it is very common to hear a medium-frequency continuous murmur at the URSB. This murmur is called a *venous hum* and may be prominent enough to even cause a systolic or continuous suprasternal notch thrill. It usually decreases markedly with the patient's head sharply turned to the left and disappears with the patient lying down, at which time, of course, the suprasternal thrill is no longer felt. The murmur is believed to be caused by the sharp angle made by the right subclavian vein as it enters the superior vena cava. Having the patient turn his or her head to the left and lie down opens up the angle.

It has been accepted that diastolic murmurs are always abnormal, an appropriate assumption. However, we have recognized and documented a soft, high-frequency diastolic murmur that begins right after S₂ but is diamond-shaped, and maximal at the LLSB. This murmur is usually absent when the patient sits up, which makes the murmur very easy to differentiate from mild aortic regurgitation. We hypothesize that we are hearing normal coronary flow because of its timing and character, but the cause is truly not known.

The newborn period is special for various reasons. The circulation is complex and changing as the infant changes from its prenatal to its postnatal circulation. There is continued change in the first weeks of life that is related to pulmonary resistance vessels and ventricular muscle. On hearing murmurs in apparently normal newborns, many pediatric residents state, "it is just the ductus," but there really is no evidence that this is the case. There is some evidence that at approximately 24 hours, a soft, continuous murmur may occur briefly at the ULSB in some normal, full-term babies. That this murmur is indeed caused by the closing ductus is reasonable. Ejection murmurs at the ULSB and the URSB are commonly heard with best transmission to each axilla and back. These murmurs are almost certainly related to the sharp angle between the main pulmonary artery and each branch as well as to immature size development of the pulmonary arteries in the periphery. The diagnosis is *peripheral pulmonic stenosis*, which should disappear within a few months. If still present at 6 months of age, the peripheral pulmonic stenosis is likely to be pathologic. With other normal infants, LLSB ejection murmurs eventually disappear. The origin of these ejection murmurs is not known.

CHANGES IN CIRCULATION: FETUS TO NEWBORN TO EARLY WEEKS

The pediatrician must have an excellent understanding of the changes in the circulation from fetal life to the early weeks of life because these changes determine how infants with left-to-right shunt lesions act, both in the early weeks and in the future. Some particularly important aspects of this transition follow:

- The pulmonary vascular resistance is very high *in utero*, with the arterioles and small muscular arteries having extensive medial muscle. This muscle is also vasoconstricted because of the newborn's normal but low PaO₂. After birth, at the first breath, the vasoconstriction is relieved, and in the next few days the pulmonary artery muscle rapidly diminishes. Although it takes many weeks before these resistance vessels mature to the adult type of thin-walled vessels, the pulmonary artery pressure in the normal newborn is probably normal by 5 days of life. The fetal resistance vessels cannot dilate very much, whereas the mature adult-type vessels can dilate a great deal. In fact, there can be an increase of three to four times the normal flow (thus decreasing pulmonary vascular resistance three to four times) without causing an increase in pulmonary artery pressure. The muscle in the pulmonary resistance vessels is not very extensive at 24 weeks of gestation, but it increases rapidly thereafter, so that usually by 36 weeks gestation, there is as much or more muscle than in the systemic resistance vessels. By 40 weeks gestation, the difference may be considerable, and because the placenta has a very low vascular resistance, the effective total pulmonary vascular resistance before birth is much greater than is the systemic vascular resistance.

- Because of the vascular difference described earlier, the right and left ventricular muscle thickness appears to follow the changes in pulmonary and systemic vascular resistance. At 24 weeks gestation, the left ventricle thickness is considerably more than that of the right ventricle, but after 30 to 32 weeks gestation, they approach each other, and by 36 weeks gestation, the right ventricle is at least as thick as the left ventricle. At 40 weeks gestation, the right ventricle is as thick or up to a third thicker than the left ventricle.

- After birth, with the placenta out of the circuit and the pulmonary vascular resistance rapidly decreasing, the systemic vascular resistance becomes much higher than the pulmonary vascular resistance, resulting in a very rapid relative increase in left ventricular muscle. By one month of age, the left ventricle is approximately twice as thick as the right ventricle (already approaching the adult ratio of three to one).

- In specific abnormal situations, the above changes after birth described earlier may be modified. The most important aspect is the slowing up of the maturation of the pulmonary vascular resistance vessels from the very muscular, thick-walled, high-resistance vessel to the nonmuscular, thin-walled, low-resistance vessel. Hemodynamics that slow this maturation are (1) an increase in pulmonary venous pressure, (2) a persistently high pulmonary artery pressure, (3) a high pulmonary blood flow, and (4) a very low PO_2, or pH, or both.

OTHER IMPORTANT HEMODYNAMIC ASPECTS

Vascular resistance is measured in terms of a ratio of pressure to flow. One good way to think about resistance is that flow goes where resistance is least. With this in mind, it is easy to understand not just that more flow will go into a dilated vessel than into a very muscular constricted vessel, but that a small intracardiac opening provides more resistance than does a wide-open one; a narrowed valve provides more resistance than does a wide-open valve; and a thick-walled, less compliant ventricle provides more resistance than does a thinner-walled, compliant ventricle.

Figure 16–10 illustrates an important concept regarding cardiac lesions. In the fluid-filled barrel with two spigots, the pressure on each side of the barrel is the same, no matter which spigot is more open than the other. If a board separating the two sides is placed in the barrel but there is a large (nonrestrictive) opening in that board, the same dynamics hold, with the pressure on each side of the barrel being the same. If instead of a fluid-filled barrel there is a larger, nonrestrictive VSD between the right and left ventricles, exactly the same situation exists. The right and left ventricles

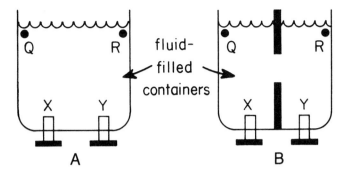

Figure 16–10. A nonrestrictive defect. The pressure on each side of the fluid-filled container (Q and R) is equal. Resistances at the X and Y spigots determine the fluid flow, but no matter how the resistances vary, the pressures at Q and R always remain the same. X and Y are valves. (From Liebman J, Borkat G, Hirschfeld S. The heart. *In* Klaus MH, Fanaroff AA [eds]. Care of the High-Risk Neonate, 2nd ed. Philadelphia: WB Saunders, 1979;297.)

always have the same pressure, no matter what the status of the pulmonary or aortic spigot. The right ventricle will then have systemic level pressure, no matter what the pulmonary blood flow is (high, normal, or low). If there is pulmonic stenosis, of course, the pulmonary artery pressure is lower than the right ventricular pressure; if there is no pulmonic stenosis, the pulmonary artery pressure is also at the systemic level. The status of the pulmonary and aortic spigots determines the ratio of pulmonary to systemic flow. If the pulmonary spigot resistance is higher than the systemic spigot resistance, there will be a right-to-left shunt. If the pulmonary resistance spigot is lower than the systemic spigot resistance, there will be a left-to-right shunt. If both resistances are the same, there will be no shunt.

PHYSICAL EXAMINATION OF COMMON LESIONS WITH LEFT-TO-RIGHT SHUNT

Atrial Septal Defect

As with all cardiac lesions, the hemodynamics can be explained by a simple line diagram, the same diagram used in explaining diagnoses to parents (Fig. 16–11). For example, systemic cardiac output is described not as 4 L/minute/m², but as one unit of cardiac output. Thus, each chamber of the normal heart has a flow of one. In an ASD with a left-to-right shunt, there may be twice as much flow in the pulmonary artery than in the aorta, a 2:1 pulmonary-to-systemic flow ratio. As can be seen in Figure 16–12, there is one unit of systemic output, resulting in the return of one unit to the heart via systemic veins. One unit enters the right atrium. Two units are in the pulmonary veins, and two units enter the left atrium. One of the two units crosses the atrial septal opening into the right atrium, making two units in the right atrium. These two units of flow then go through the normal tricuspid valve into the right ventricle, whereas just one goes through the mitral valve into the left ventricle and then through the aortic valve into the aorta. (One always presumes a systemic output of one unit.) The two units in the right ventricle go through the pulmonic valve into the pulmonary artery.

This simple approach allows an understanding of the hemodynamic load in each area of the heart; in addition, in an ASD with a large left-to-right shunt, there is usually very little increase in right ventricular and pulmonary artery pressure. This approach also allows an understanding of the cardiac examination. There is a pure right ventricular impulse, the left sternal edge is hyperdy-

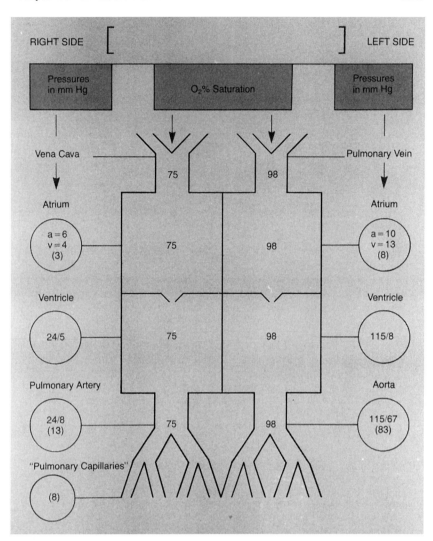

Figure 16–11. Box diagram of normal data from cardiac catheterization. (From Behrman RE, Kliegman RM [eds]. Nelson Essentials of Pediatrics, 2nd ed. Philadelphia: WB Saunders, 1994:478.)

namic, and, because murmurs are not loud, there are no thrills. Intracavitary phonocardiographic studies have shown that there is no murmur of blood flowing across the ASD in systole or in diastole. The only murmurs in ASD are functional murmurs caused by high flow across normal valves. Thus, the flow is twice that of normal and moves at low pressure across the tricuspid valve, resulting in a mid-diastolic rumbling murmur of low frequency (Fig. 16–13). Because there is so much flow to go through the tricuspid valve, it must go through very rapidly so that the murmur is initiated by a loud right ventricular S_3 (of the same low frequency as the murmur) (see Fig. 16–13).

Diastole is silent until the period of the most rapid filling across the tricuspid valve, and because no true stenosis exists, the right ventricle can accept the flow rapidly. Therefore, late diastole is also silent. The loud S_3 and mid-diastolic rumble are best heard at the LLSB, where sounds and murmurs of tricuspid valve and right ventricular origin are best heard. The intensity of the diastolic rumble vary between grades I and III, depending on the magnitude of the left-to-right shunt. In general, a 2:1 pulmonary-to-systemic flow ratio is necessary to hear a mid-diastolic rumble whether through the tricuspid or the mitral valve. There is then twice the normal flow through a normal pulmonary valve, resulting in a pulmonary ejection murmur (Fig. 16–14), which is usually about two-thirds the length of systole and no more than grade III in intensity (often less). In an ASD with a large left-to-right shunt, there is a specific characteristic of the second sounds, which are widely split and vary little or not at all with respiration. Because

an ASD with a left-to-right shunt is a pure right ventricular volume overload with lower than normal pulmonary vascular resistance, the pulmonary closure sound is delayed. There is usually little or no increase in the pulmonary closure delay on inspiration, mainly because the right ventricle is fully loaded by the shunt. In addition, if the ASD is nonrestrictive, there may be an expiratory increase in pulmonary vein flow, which is reflected on the right side. The intensity of the pulmonary closure sound may be normal or increased, the latter occurring because the pulmonary valve leaflets are fully open until it is time to close and therefore close rapidly from a long distance. Thus, we have an example of a loud pulmonary closure sound in the presence of a lower than normal pulmonary vascular resistance and pulmonary artery pressure that is normal or minimally elevated. The wide split of S_2 indicates that pulmonary hypertension is not present.

Palpation reveals no thrills, an abnormal right ventricular impulse, and a hyperdynamic left sternal edge. Patients with an ASD usually are asymptomatic and present with a murmur. If the left-to-right shunt is large, heart failure may develop at any age. In the third to fourth decade, irreversible pulmonary hypertension may develop.

Patent Ductus Arteriosus

The patent ductus arteriosus (PDA) with a left-to-right shunt provides an example of a pure left ventricular volume overloading

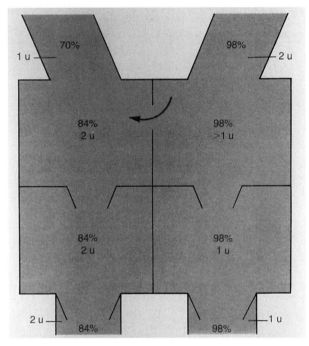

Figure 16–12. Box diagram of an atrial septal defect with a 2:1 pulmonary to systemic (P/S) flow ratio. One unit (u) of cardiac output is 4 L/minute/m². % is percent saturation. (From Behrman RE, Kliegman RM [eds]. Nelson Essentials of Pediatrics, 2nd ed. Philadelphia: WB Saunders, 1994:486.)

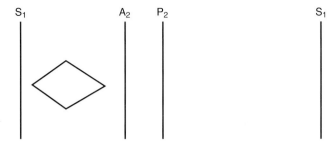

Figure 16–14. Diagram of systolic ejection murmur and widely split S_2 in an atrial septal defect (ASD) with left-to-right shunt. These sounds are maximal at the upper left sternal border.

There is twice the normal flow through a normal mitral valve, and the flow goes through the valve very quickly. Consequently, there is a prominent S_3 followed by a mid-diastolic rumble beginning with S_3. Diastole is silent until the period of most rapid filling across the mitral valve (S_3), and because no true stenosis exists, late diastole is also silent. The loud S_3 and mid-diastolic rumble are best heard at the apex, where sounds and murmurs of mitral valve and left ventricular origin are best heard. The intensity of the diastolic rumble varies, depending on the magnitude of the left-to-right shunt. There is then twice the normal flow through a normal aortic valve, causing an aortic ejection murmur (at the URSB) that is grade III at its maximal intensity and is about two-thirds the length of systole. This latter murmur is usually unappreciated because the murmur of blood flowing through the ductus is usually loud and is best heard high in the left side of the chest. It is often well transmitted to the high right side of the chest near the sternal

lesion, unless the communication is large enough to allow higher than normal pulmonary artery pressure. Because the ductal opening is a long narrow tube, there is, in the congenital ductus after early infancy, enough ductal resistance that the pulmonary artery pressure is normal or only minimally elevated. However, considerable variation exists. The wider the bore of the ductus and the shorter the ductus, the higher the pulmonary artery pressure. Fortunately, after the newborn period, a large congenital ductus is not common.

With the presumption that there is a high pulmonary blood flow PDA (2:1 pulmonary-to-systemic flow ratio) with normal pulmonary artery pressures, Figure 16–15 shows that there is pure left ventricular volume overload. As always, one unit of cardiac output returns to the heart via the systemic veins and one unit enters the right atrium, then the right ventricle and pulmonary artery. However, two units of flow enter the pulmonary vein, the left atrium, and the left ventricle. Then, after the two units pass through the aortic valve, one unit goes through the PDA into the pulmonary artery. Because of the marked left ventricular volume overloading, A_2 may be so delayed that it may be recorded and heard after P_2.

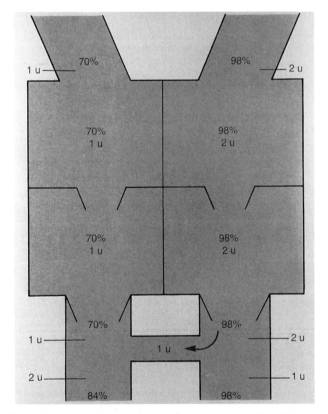

Figure 16–15. Box diagram of patent ductus arteriosus with a 2:1 pulmonary to systemic (P/S) flow ratio. (From Behrman RE, Kliegman RM [eds]. Nelson Essentials of Pediatrics, 2nd ed. Philadelphia: WB Saunders, 1994:486.)

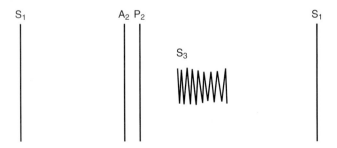

Figure 16–13. Diagram of S_3 and mid-diastolic rumble in an atrial septal defect with left-to-right shunt. These sounds are maximal at the lower left sternal border.

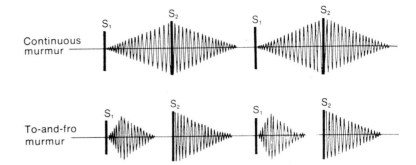

Figure 16–16. A comparison between a continuous murmur and a to-and-fro murmur. (Adapted from Leonard JJ, Kroetz FW, Shaver JA. Examination of the Heart: Auscultation. Dallas, Texas: American Heart Association, 1990.)

edge. Because the communication is after the aortic valve, there is continued run-off in systole and diastole. There is thus a wide pulse pressure with low diastolic pressure, but if pulmonary hypertension is not present, a constant gradient exists in both systole and diastole. Therefore, a continuous murmur is present that becomes audible in systole and continues through aortic valve closure, ending in diastole (Fig. 16–16).

As aortic flow makes the sharp angle into the pulmonary artery, the turbulence is considerable, so that, particularly in systole, the murmur may have a remarkable harsh characteristic that we have termed ''like water going through the Colorado rapids.'' With large PDAs (larger bore and shorter length), the pulmonary artery pressure is higher. The consequence may be pressures such as 110/40 mmHg in the aorta and 70/40 mmHg in the pulmonary artery. There is thus a gradient only in systole. This systolic murmur may be short and high in frequency, but most commonly it is still unusually harsh, except that there is little or no extension into diastole. Thus, if there is evidence from the examination and electrocardiogram of left ventricular volume overload and there is a wide pulse pressure, the diagnosis is readily made without an audible continuous murmur. (The PDA murmur in newborns is often different and is discussed later.) The second sounds are of interest, although because of the continuous murmur, they may be difficult to appreciate. Because pure left ventricular volume overload exists, left ventricular systole is prolonged, resulting in delayed aortic closure. If there is a large left-to-right shunt, the aortic closure may be so delayed that the S_2 split may be paradoxical. Thus, on inspiration there may be little or no split, and on expiration there may be a wider split. On expiration, aortic closure would occur after pulmonary closure.

Palpation reveals a thrill in systole at the upper left sternal edge (when the murmur is grade IV); an abnormal left ventricular impulse; and, if the left-to-right shunt is large, a hyperdynamic left sternal edge. Patients with a PDA may have an asymptomatic murmur, or if the left-to-right shunt is large, they may have heart failure (see Chapter 13). Treatment is surgical ligation and division.

The premature infant should be considered separately. If the ductus arteriosus occurs with a significant left-to-right shunt, the most important aspect of the examination is not the murmur but the easily palpable and recognizable wide pulse pressure, which is best appreciated by placing the thumb lightly over the brachial artery. Obviously, to appreciate the wide pulse pressure, the physician or nurse clinician must practice on infants known not to have a ductus arteriosus with a left-to-right shunt. (With right-to-left ductal shunts, there is no murmur.)

Many prematurely born infants who do not have severe lung disease have PDAs, which often close at a total (gestation plus life) of 40 weeks. However, most of the PDAs of concern are in the premature infant who has severe respiratory distress syndrome. In some of these babies, the PDA murmur is just like that of the older child; in many cases, however, the murmur is not continuous, not uneven, and, in fact, nondescript. Perhaps this is because these PDAs are not ''real'' PDAs, in that they are not congenital and would not be there unless the baby was born prematurely and ill. It is not because the PDAs are always large and nonrestrictive, for

they vary in size and amount of left-to-right shunt. The important lesson is that if the pulse pressure is not wide, the nondescript murmur is not likely to be caused by a significant PDA, and if the pulse pressure is wide, the murmur is likely to be due to a PDA with a significant left-to-right shunt. Preterm infants with a PDA show heart failure, pulmonary edema, a hyperdynamic precordium, and difficulty in weaning from the respirator. Treatment in preterm infants includes indomethacin and fluid restriction; if these measures are unsuccessful, surgery is indicated.

Ventricular Septal Defect

Figure 16–17 shows a patient with VSD and a 2:1 pulmonary-to-systemic flow ratio. The one unit of cardiac output returns via systemic veins into the right atrium and enters the right ventricle. Two units of flow come from the pulmonary veins to enter the left atrium and then the left ventricle. Thus, twice the normal flow goes through a normal mitral valve, resulting, as in PDA with a large left-to-right shunt, a loud S_3 and a mid-diastolic rumble. Then, one of the two units goes through the VSD to enter the right ventricle, although some of this VSD flow may enter the pulmonary artery

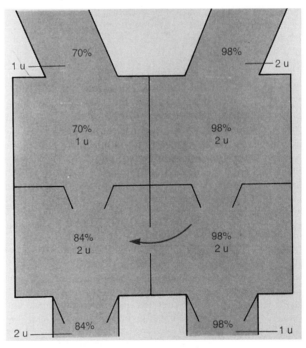

Figure 16–17. Box diagram of a ventricular septal defect with a 2:1 pulmonary-to-systemic (P/S) flow ratio. (From Behrman RE, Kliegman RM [eds]. Nelson Essentials of Pediatrics, 2nd ed. Philadelphia: WB Saunders, 1994:487.)

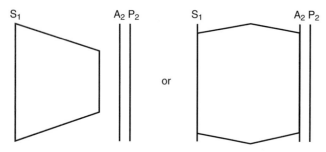

Figure 16–18. Typical heart murmurs (maximal lower left sternal border) in a ventricular septal defect with left-to-right shunt. There may be many variations, but the murmur always starts early and usually obscures S_1. There are very few true holosystolic murmurs in which S_1 is obscured and the murmur continues into aortic closure.

directly. The two units of flow going into the pulmonary artery by way of the pulmonary valve cause a pulmonary ejection murmur as occurs in ASD with a left-to-right shunt (see Fig. 16–14). However, the VSD with left-to-right shunt causes a loud murmur, which may make it difficult to appreciate the pulmonary ejection murmur. *The most important thing about the VSD murmur is that it starts very early* (Fig. 16–18). The left ventricular pressure curve begins to upstroke before the right ventricular pressure curve. Therefore, there may be some left-to-right shunt before mitral valve closure. Consequently, the VSD murmur usually obscures or partially obscures S_1. Occasionally, S_1 is not obscured, but the murmur comes off S_1. Because blood frequently is ejected from the left ventricle to the right ventricle throughout systole, the murmur may be heard throughout systole. A murmur heard throughout systole is called "holosystolic," but the true definition of the word includes obscuring of S_1 and at least partially obscuring of aortic closure (A_2). It is no more difficult to say "full length" than "holosystolic"; in addition, it is more useful to state that the murmur is full length (obscuring, partially obscuring, or not obscuring) S_1 and is obscuring or not obscuring A_2.

VSD murmurs do not have to be full length. They are often shorter and in the presence of heart failure may be much shorter; it is the early part of systole that is important. In Doppler echocardiographic studies, the larger the defect, the lower the velocity of the blood being ejected from left to right; in more restrictive defects, the velocity may be very high. In the larger defects, the murmur on the chest tends to be closer to plateau or may be decrescendo; in the more restrictive defects, the murmur tends to be more diamond-shaped, expressing the obstructive nature of the opening. Very small defects with small left-to-right shunts have soft murmurs. In children whose defects spontaneously close, softer and softer murmurs are commonly heard with time until after closure, when there is no murmur at all. The old misconception that larger nonrestrictive defects have no murmur comes from the era when many patients with an untreated VSD, high pulmonary vascular resistance, and right-to-left shunt (Eisenmenger's syndrome) were available to be examined. In these cases, the only shunt through the VSD is right to left, at low velocity and of small volume. Such shunts are not audible.

Analysis of the second sound in VSD is particularly useful. In the presence of a left-to-right shunt through a VSD, left ventricular systole is shortened. Thus, A_2 is heard early. If there is a large pulmonary blood flow, P_2 is delayed, resulting in a well-split S_2. The larger the defect and thus the higher the pulmonary artery pressure, the earlier the pulmonary closure. Thus, the split of S_2 may become very narrow or even single, a finding of great concern. In large defects, a balance exists between delayed P_2, caused by large pulmonary blood flow, and early P_2 caused by high pulmonary artery pressure. The wider the split of S_2, the less the concern because pulmonary vascular resistance is likely to be low.

Palpation reveals a thrill in systole, usually at the LLSB if the systolic murmur is grade IV, a usually diffuse cardiac impulse, and, if the shunt is large, a hyperdynamic left sternal edge. Patients with a small VSD usually manifest an asymptomatic murmur; the VSD usually closes spontaneously. A patient with VSD with a significant left-to-right shunt manifests heart failure (see Chapter 13). Treatment is surgical.

Complete Atrioventricular Canal

There is great variation in the anatomy of endocardial cushion defects. In the complete atrioventricular canal, where chordae do not close up the ventricular opening between the left and right ventricles and there is a common atrioventricular valve, nonrestrictive communications (Fig. 16–19) exist between the left and right ventricles, the left ventricle and the right atrium, and the right ventricle and the left atrium. In addition, there may be considerable mitral regurgitation (sometimes tricuspid as well). For various reasons, the maturation of the pulmonary arteries and small muscular arteries is slowed, and elevated pulmonary vascular resistance early in life is common. Therefore, the lesion must not be missed early in life. About two thirds of children with complete atrioventricular canal as described have Down syndrome. Therefore, in children born with Down syndrome, at least 40% of whom have congenital heart disease, a cardiac evaluation must be performed. If an endocardial cushion defect is present, by far the most common lesion, the electrocardiogram usually demonstrates an abnormally superior vector (usually called "left axis deviation"). If this finding is present, an echocardiogram should be performed. In the presence of less complete endocardial cushion defects, few patients have Down syndrome.

After the newborn period, when pulmonary vascular resistance decreases as much as it is going to, the examination is usually similar to that for a nonrestrictive VSD. In some cases, cardiac output is quite low, and the systolic and diastolic murmurs may be quite soft. In some cases, a murmur of mitral or tricuspid regurgitation may be present, making the examination more complex.

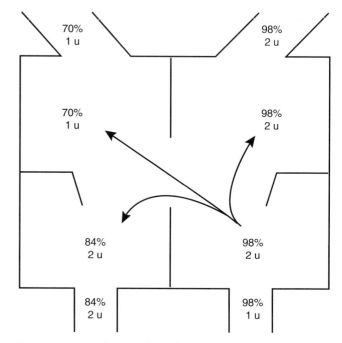

Figure 16–19. Box diagram of complete atrioventricular (AV) canal with 2:1 pulmonary-to-systemic (P/S) flow ratio.

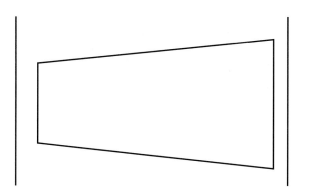

Figure 16–20. Typical heart murmur, maximal at the apex, in a patient with mitral regurgitation. The murmur peaks late. If the mitral regurgitation is considerable, a loud S_3 and mid-diastolic rumble would also be present at the apex, as in Figure 16–13, because of increased volume across a normal mitral valve from the left atrium to the left ventricle.

In the simplest form of endocardial cushion defect, there may be just an ostium primum ASD with left-to-right shunt. In such an examination, the findings are the same as those described for ASD of the secundum type. Usually, however, additional mitral regurgitation is present, making the examination more complex. Mitral regurgitation murmurs tend to be full length but do not obscure S_1. The murmurs may be very prominent late in systole as papillary muscle dysfunction comes into play, so that the murmur usually peaks late in systole (Fig. 16–20). If the volume of mitral regurgitation is large, for example, twice as much going from the left atrium to the left ventricle as from left ventricle to the aorta, then the flow will be three times that of normal (see Fig. 16–17) going from the left atrium to the left ventricle. Thus there will be the same type of loud S_3 and mid-diastolic rumble as heard in VSD with a 3:1 pulmonary-to-systemic flow ratio.

In endocardial cushion defects, palpation varies from one child to the next because the anatomy and pathophysiology vary so much. With significant mitral regurgitation, there is an abnormal left ventricular impulse and a very hyperdynamic apex. With a large left-to-right shunt, the left sternal edge is hyperdynamic. The cardiac impulse is both right ventricular and left ventricular in complete atrioventricular canal and is purely right ventricular if there is a mostly an atrial shunt without mitral regurgitation. Patients with an atrioventricular canal often manifest heart failure very early in infancy (see Chapter 13).

PHYSICAL EXAMINATION OF COMMON LESIONS WITH SIMPLE OBSTRUCTION

Valvular Pulmonic Stenosis

The only hemodynamic abnormality in valvular pulmonic stenosis is increased pressure in the right ventricle. The more severe the stenosis, the higher the pressure. The pulmonary closure sound (P_2) is very helpful because the more severe the pulmonary valve stenosis, the more delayed the P_2; in mild cases, P_2 may actually be of increased intensity because the valve is good, and when it closes, it does so from a longer distance than normal. As the stenosis increases, the intensity of the pulmonary closure decreases. The more dysplastic the valve, the lower the intensity of the P_2 sound. As the stenosis increases, the murmur is louder, but much more importantly, the murmur is longer. In general, a murmur that stops far short of A_2 is associated with only minimally elevated right ventricular pressure, but a murmur that extends up to A_2 is likely to be near the systemic level. If the murmur goes well across

A_2, then there may be suprasystemic right ventricular pressure. In such cases, P_2 is very delayed and very soft, so that often it is difficult to appreciate any S_2.

Finally, a pulmonary ejection click is almost always present, associated with the hemodynamics that cause a dilated root of the pulmonary artery. It can be generalized that the more severe the valvular pulmonary stenosis, the earlier and softer the pulmonary ejection click, but that observation is not reliable. Frequently, a clearly audible pulmonary ejection click is not appreciated because it occurs at the same time as S_1, which is best heard at the LLSB or apex and should be soft at the ULSB. Pulmonary ejection clicks are best heard at the ULSB. Thus, if it is interpreted that there is a loud S_1 at the ULSB (and especially if this sound is louder on expiration than on inspiration), what is being heard is a loud pulmonary ejection click coming at about the same time as S_1 (see Fig 16–6).

In newborns with very severe critical pulmonic stenosis and low cardiac output, the examination may be quite different. There may be no pulmonary ejection click, and the murmur may be very short, or soft, or both.

In *infundibular pulmonic stenosis,* there is no pulmonary ejection click. Pure infundibular stenosis is exquisitely rare in the unoperated state and can occur only if a VSD was present that closed spontaneously.

Palpation in pulmonic valve stenosis reveals a suprasternal notch thrill in systole (except in mild cases), a thrill at the ULSB in many moderate to severe cases, and an abnormal right ventricular impulse (except in mild cases). The heart is usually quiet, but in some cases, the post-stenotic dilatation is so striking that there may be a localized hyperdynamic ULSB. Treatment includes balloon valve dilatation or surgical valvotomy.

Table 16–3 describes the differential diagnosis among the three situations in which there is a grade III (maximum) ejection systolic murmur at the ULSB.

Valvular Aortic Stenosis

The only hemodynamic abnormality of valvular aortic stenosis is an increased pressure in the left ventricle. Obviously, the more severe the stenosis, the higher the left ventricular pressure. The aortic closure sound (A_2) is helpful, but not as helpful as is P_2 in valvular pulmonic stenosis. Firstly, the intensity is almost invariably normal because there is systemic pressure distal to the valve. However, the more severe the stenosis, the more it is delayed, but again, the correlation is not as evident as in pulmonic stenosis. When there is very little delay of A_2, resulting in a normally split S_2, then almost invariably the AS is mild. When there is significant delay in A_2 so that the split of S_2 is narrow or not present, there is usually significant stenosis (Fig. 16–21). The paradoxical split, occurring when there is a large delay of A_2, is quite rare in children and young adults, and is seen mainly in older people with calcific aortic stenosis. The length of the murmur is particularly valuable in determining whether the valvular aortic stenosis is significant or not. The aortic stenosis associated with a full-length murmur should be considered as being much more significant and much more likely to increase in severity in childhood than would be a ½- to ⅔-length murmur. An aortic ejection click is usually present in valvular aortic stenosis and is not related to the severity of the stenosis (Fig. 16–22).

In newborns, with severe or *critical aortic stenosis* with low cardiac output, the examination may be different. Firstly, there is often no aortic ejection click, and strikingly, the murmur may be short, soft, or both. Significant heart failure and poor perfusion are present.

Palpation, except in very mild cases, reveals a suprasternal notch thrill and a carotid systolic thrill. (In childhood, the presence of suprasternal notch and carotid thrills is diagnostic of aortic steno-

Table 16–3. Differential Diagnosis of a Systolic Ejection Murmur at the Upper Left Sternal Border

	Normal Pulmonary Ejection	Mild Pulmonary Stenosis	Atrial Septal Defect—Secundum
Murmur	Maximal grade III	Maximal grade III	Maximal grade III
Impulses	Normal	± RV	RV +
Left sternal edge	Normal	Normal	Hyperdynamic
Left chest bulge	None	±	+
Thrill	None	± SSN	None
S_1	Normal	Normal	Normal or ↑ LLSB
S_2 split	Normal	Slightly ↑ intensity	Wide and persistent
S_2 intensity	Normal	P_2 normal or slightly ↓ intensity	P_2 normal or ↑
S_3	Normal	Norm? at LLSB	Loud at LLSB
Diastolic murmur	None	None–occ diastolic decrescendo of mild pulmonary regurgitation	Mid-diastolic low-frequency at LLSB
Pulmonary ejection click	None	Usually ULSB	None

Abbreviations: ULSB = upper left sternal border; LLSB = lower left sternal border; RV = right ventricle; SSN = suprasternal notch; + = present and abnormal; occ = occasionally; Norm = normal = no murmur.

sis.) There is also a systolic thrill at the URSB if the murmur is grade IV or greater. The murmur (and thus the thrill, if present) does not have to be maximal at the URSB; it can be at the upper sternum or even at the ULSB.

Two other major types of aortic stenosis exist: subvalvular and supravalvular. Neither is associated with post-stenotic dilatation; therefore, neither has an aortic ejection click. In *supravalvular aortic stenosis* (the major cardiac lesion associated with Williams syndrome), the murmur is usually at the URSB, whereas in subvalvular aortic stenosis, the murmur position is variable. It is commonly maximal at the LLSB, but the murmur can be maximal anywhere between the LLSB and URSB. The examinations are otherwise the same except that in supravalvular aortic stenosis, because the narrowing is after the aortic valve, there is no delay in A_2.

In both valvular and *subvalvular aortic stenosis,* there may be an additional early high-frequency, short diastolic decrescendo murmur of mild aortic regurgitation. In neither case is the aortic regurgitation significant in the unoperated state. However, there may be primary congenital aortic regurgitation of various causes. When a bicuspid aortic valve is present, an aortic ejection click is present, but in the other cases, it is variably present, especially in more severe cases. In rheumatic aortic regurgitation, even in severe cases, an aortic ejection click is unusual, even when there is some associated aortic stenosis.

Importantly, a bicuspid aortic valve is commonly present without either stenosis or regurgitation. This anomaly is recognized by noting the aortic ejection click, which must not be missed, because an isolated bicuspid aortic valve is prone to endocarditis. Treatment of valvular aortic stenosis includes surgical valvotomy or valve replacement; some respond to balloon dilatation.

Coarctation of the Aorta

The only hemodynamic abnormality due to a coarctation of the aorta is a high systolic pressure proximal to the area of narrowing, in the ascending and transverse aorta and in the left ventricle. Because the aortic valve is proximal to the coarctation, there is no delay in A_2. The diastolic pressure may not be elevated, so that an early A_2 may not be present either. The murmur is of the ejection type, is rarely louder than grades III or III +, starts well after S_1, and may peak late. The point of maximal intensity is very variable and is often maximal on the anterior chest, but it is often maximal outside the apex, with excellent transmission to the anterior axillary line and left side of the back.

In approximately 40% to 50% of patients with simple coarctation of the aorta, there is an associated bicuspid aortic valve, usually without stenosis. In these cases, there is an aortic ejection click, but there is no ejection click in the absence of the bicuspid aortic valve.

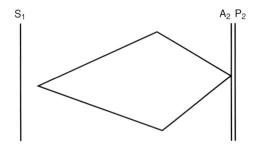

Figure 16–21. Long ejection murmur at the upper right sternal border of significant aortic stenosis. The S_2 is narrowly split as a result of delayed aortic closure.

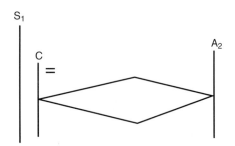

Figure 16–22. Aortic ejection click (C), well separated from S_1 at the apex in valvular aortic stenosis.

The key to the diagnosis of simple coarctation of the aorta is recognition of systemic hypertension in the right arm and decreased arterial pulsation in the femoral arteries and the dorsalis pedis compared with that in the brachial arteries. The femoral pulses may be absent, or they may be diminished and delayed. Importantly, the coarctation is usually in the same place, near the left subclavian artery and opposite the ductus arteriosus (ligamentum after the ductus has closed). The left subclavian may be hypoplastic, it may come off the coarctation itself, or it may come off below the coarctation. In each case, the left brachial pulse may be diminished or absent. Therefore, brachial pulses must be felt on both sides for the most information to be obtained, and the blood pressure must be obtained in both arms as well as in one leg. If only one arm pressure is obtained, it must be the right arm. Rarely, an anomalous right subclavian artery originates below the coarctation so that the right brachial pulse and blood pressure are decreased rather than increased. The diagnosis of coarctation of the aorta is more challenging in these cases. All other aspects of the examination are the same, including very strong pulsation in the suprasternal notch and the carotid arteries.

The examination of the newborn with simple pure coarctation of the aorta has created anxiety among pediatricians who cannot understand how they may miss the diagnosis. The problem is that while the ductus arteriosus is open, there may be no obstruction, no significant murmur, and good femoral pulses. This is because the posterior ledge of the coarctation is just opposite the insertion of the ductus, allowing an unobstructed pathway of blood to go from proximal to distal of the coarctation. Once the ductus closes, however, the tissue contracts, and a circumferential obstruction occurs. Fortunately, pure coarctation of the aorta usually causes no trouble in infancy, and if it does, it usually occurs after the 2-week check-up. Treatment is surgery.

Mitral Stenosis

Rheumatic mitral stenosis remains very common in many areas of the world, but in this country, it is no longer very common. The physical examination is striking. If the stenosis is severe, left atrial and pulmonary vein pressures are elevated so that there is reflex pulmonary hypertension associated with very muscular pulmonary arterioles and the small muscular pulmonary arteries (the resistance vessels). Thus, there is a quiet heart with an abnormal right ventricular impulse, usually a loud S_1, and a loud narrowly split or single S_2. Above the apex, an opening snap is heard if the anterior leaflet is mobile. Systole is silent, or mild mitral regurgitation may be present. There is no left ventricular S_3, because filling of the left ventricle is not rapid, but there may be a right ventricular S_3 that is best heard at the LLSB. The diastolic murmur is at the apex, is low in frequency, begins about one third into diastole, and is very long. There is frequently presystolic accentuation that ends in the loud S_1 if there is sinus rhythm, as the atrial ''kick'' sends blood through the stenotic valve (Fig. 16–23).

Congenital mitral stenosis is uncommon. It can be mild and nonprogressive; it is more often significant and progressive. A common type of significant stenosis, caused by a parachute mitral valve, is associated with just one papillary muscle. The physical findings are atypical. There is no opening snap, because the anterior leaflet is not mobile enough, and presystolic accentuation is usually not present. Congenital mitral stenosis can be seen by itself, or it can be part of a complex of left-sided obstructions, particularly with coarctation of the aorta. In its most severe form, it is part of the hypoplastic left ventricle syndrome, in which the valve is small, very stenotic, or atretic. In these patients, cyanosis, heart failure, and poor perfusion are evident within the first few days after birth.

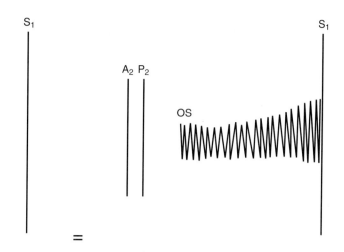

Figure 16–23. An opening snap (OS), closer to S_2 than is an S_3; no S_3; and a long diastolic rumbling murmur with presystolic accentuation, maximal at the apex. This is typical of rheumatic mitral stenosis. Note the narrowly split S_2 caused by early pulmonary closure, associated with pulmonary hypertension.

PHYSICAL EXAMINATION OF ATRIOVENTRICULAR VALVE AND SEMILUNAR VALVE REGURGITATION

Tricuspid Valve Regurgitation

Tricuspid regurgitation is often secondary to another primary problem. For example, pulmonary hypertension is often present secondary to left-sided disease or to lung disease. If the pulmonary hypertension is acute, there may be secondary right ventricular dilatation and dilatation of the tricuspid valve. If left ventricular disease is present, the cardiac impulse is expected to be biventricular, but if lung disease (cor pulmonale) is present, then a pure right ventricular impulse is present. The pulmonary closure sound is loud, and in lung disease the split of S_2 is narrow; but if left ventricular disease is present, the auscultatory findings depend on the specific left ventricular disease's effect on the aortic valve closure.

The murmur of tricuspid regurgitation is usually maximal at the LLSB, especially at the fourth interspace. It is usually relatively high in frequency (it starts close to, but doesn't obscure, S_1), and it continues through most of systole. The intensity is usually no more than grade III or IV. If the heart rate is slow enough, one can usually appreciate that the murmur is louder on inspiration than on expiration, a finding consistent with the increased volume of blood entering the right ventricle on inspiration. In older children, a prolonged V wave in the neck veins may be appreciated.

Congenital tricuspid regurgitation is uncommon. It is often recognized in the newborn period because high pulmonary vascular resistance may make the regurgitation worse. As the resistance decreases, the tricuspid regurgitation decreases. Newborns with asphyxia are known also to frequently have dilatation of the right ventricle and thus tricuspid regurgitation. This regurgitation eventually disappears as the baby recovers but in congenital tricuspid regurgitation the murmur remains.

Ebstein anomaly is also often associated with considerable tricuspid regurgitation, which, in the newborn period, may decrease as the pulmonary vascular resistance decreases. Ebstein anomaly is an extremely variable abnormality. There may be a tricuspid valve that is so far displaced into the right ventricle that it obstructs flow into the pulmonary artery; alternately there may be a valve that is minimally displaced into the ventricle, where there is little or no regurgitation. The condition is also complicated in that many children have considerable right-to-left atrial shunting, which may not correlate with the amount of tricuspid regurgitation. In a newborn with considerable tricuspid regurgitation, the distinction between Ebstein anomaly and congenital tricuspid regurgitation is usually not difficult in that in the former, there is usually advanced right bundle branch block. Echocardiographic results are often diagnostic. After infancy, the clinical diagnosis is usually not difficult, but the clinical picture is variable. The patient may be cyanotic. If there is no tricuspid regurgitation, the clinical picture is striking; a quiet heart, a loud right ventricular S_3 at the LLSB, a loud right ventricular S_4 at the LLSB (because the small functioning right ventricle is poorly compliant), and a well-split S_2 because of right bundle branch block. There is a quadruple rhythm, but five sounds may be heard. Sometimes, after infancy, there is considerable tricuspid regurgitation that is not well appreciated by murmur. The left sternal edge is very hyperdynamic.

Mitral Valve Regurgitation

It is important to stress the differences in the examination of mitral regurgitation versus VSD with a left-to-right shunt because each is often mistaken for the other. Both disorders have been described as causing full-length murmurs, but they may sound very different. The mitral regurgitation murmur is usually maximal at the apex, with best transmission to the left axilla and the back because the left atrium is posterior to the left ventricle. The regurgitant jet can even be directed posteriorly so that the murmur is heard in the left back. If the mitral regurgitation is caused by an endocardial cushion defect, the cause of the flow is deficiency of tissue in the anteromedial leaflet, so that sometimes the jet is more to the right, causing the murmur to be maximal at the LLSB.

The first sound is usually of normal to increased intensity, but if the valve abnormality is rheumatic in origin, it may be deformed enough so that S_1 is quite soft. The murmur is usually high in frequency, and because the papillary muscle is involved late in systole, the murmur often peaks late, extending up to aortic closure (see Fig 16–20). In *mitral valve prolapse,* in which the murmur begins with the mid-systolic click, the murmur is usually only late

systolic. Thus, in VSD with left-to-right shunt, the early part of systole is the most important, whereas in mitral regurgitation, the end of systole is the most important.

If the mitral regurgitation is quite significant, the physical findings are straightforward. There is an abnormal left ventricular impulse with a very hyperdynamic apex. For every unit of systemic output from the left ventricle, the left ventricle may send two units back to the atria. If that is the case, three units must go forward through the valve very rapidly. The rapid filling of the left ventricle causes a loud S_3, and if three times the normal flow goes across the non-stenotic valve, there is relative mitral stenosis. Thus, a mid-diastolic, low-frequency, rumbling murmur is present at the apex that is identical in sound and etiology to the apical mid-diastolic rumble associated with a VSD and a 3:1 pulmonary-to-systemic flow ratio. In the presence of significant mitral stenosis, there is no apical S_3, because filling of the left ventricle is not rapid.

Mitral valve prolapse is a diagnosis that depends on an accurate physical examination. Classical mitral valve prolapse in childhood usually occurs in girls and in women who have asthenic bodies and an asymptomatic murmur. A mid-systolic sound is correlated with prolapse of the posterior leaflet, after which there is frequently, but not necessarily, regurgitation that causes a late systolic murmur (Fig. 16–24). When the patient is sitting up (and even more so during standing), the murmur gets louder or may be heard when no murmur had been present when the patient was lying down. This is because the left ventricular architecture changes in the upright position. Rarely, the position change may result in a late systolic murmur's becoming full length, although still accentuated late. The electrocardiogram often shows unusually anterior and superior T waves with prominent U waves, leading many to believe that papillary muscle dysfunction is at the root of the problem. Mitral valve prolapse does not usually progress in childhood, but it may rarely be associated with supraventricular tachycardia, chest pain, and, even less often, endocarditis or cerebrovascular embolism. Ventricular tachycardia and fibrillation may occur in adults, but sudden death is unusual during childhood and adolescence.

Pulmonary Valve Regurgitation

Congenital regurgitation of the pulmonic valve is quite rare and when present is usually associated with a pulmonary ejection click

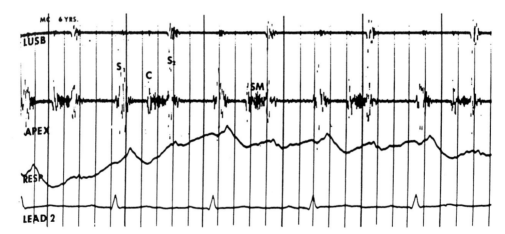

Figure 16–24. External phonocardiogram of a 16-year-old girl with classical mitral valve prolapse and trivial mitral regurgitation. There are simultaneous phonocardiographic registrations at the left upper sternal border (LUSB) and the apex as well as a respiration marker (inspiration is higher on trace) and lead 2 electrocardiogram. An intracavitary recording had also been made in the left atrium, where it is almost identical to that seen at the apex. There is a sound-free space slightly more than halfway into systole, at which time there is a sharp sound. This sharp sound (C) is a non-ejection click, which does not vary with respiration. Following the click is a late systolic murmur that ends at S_2. Aortic ejection clicks do not vary with respiration but are close to the first sound. Pulmonary ejection clicks are louder on expiration and are usually closer to S_1. (From Sreenivasan VV, Liebman J, Linton D. Posterior mitral regurgitation in girls possibly due to posterior papillary muscle dysfunction. Pediatrics 1968; 42:276–290.)

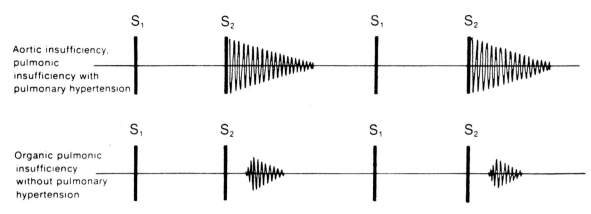

Figure 16–25. The murmurs of aortic insufficiency and pulmonic insufficiency with pulmonary hypertension compared with those of pulmonic insufficiency without pulmonary hypertension. (Adapted from Leonard JJ, Kroetz FW, Shaver JA. Examination of the Heart: Auscultation. Dallas, Texas: American Heart Association, 1990.)

as described for valvular pulmonary stenosis. The murmur is diastolic and begins with closure of the pulmonic valve. It is almost always decrescendo at the second through fourth interspaces at the left sternal edge, and because the pressure is low, it is usually of medium to low frequency.

The most common types of pulmonary regurgitation are acquired. Pulmonary hypertension, particularly when associated with a high pulmonary vascular resistance, is a common cause (Fig. 16–25). Often, but not always, a pulmonary ejection click is present, and S_2 is narrowly split or single because the high pulmonary artery diastolic pressure closes the valve early. A diastolic decrescendo murmur then begins with pulmonary valve closure and is high in frequency because the pulmonary artery pressure is high.

Pulmonary regurgitation commonly occurs after surgery for severe pulmonic stenosis, as occurs with tetralogy of Fallot, when the pulmonary valve is virtually ablated and an outflow tract patch has been placed. The murmur is maximal in the same area, is decrescendo, and is low to medium in frequency. Because no pulmonary valve closure sound exists, the murmur often appears to start significantly after S_2. Because most of those patients have surgically acquired right bundle branch block (from a right ventriculotomy), the pulmonary closure would be well separated from aortic closure if the sound could be heard. The diastolic decrescendo murmur begins at that time.

Aortic Valve Regurgitation

Congenital regurgitation of the aortic valve is more common than that of the pulmonic valve and is usually mild. The valve may or may not be bicuspid. There is usually an aortic ejection click that is well separated from S_1, does not vary with respiration, and is usually best heard at the apex. The S_2 split is normal, although A_2 may be loud. The decrescendo diastolic murmur is usually best heard at the third through fifth intercostal spaces at the left sternal edge and is high in frequency because aortic pressure is high (Fig. 16–26). The pulse pressure is normal if the leak is mild, so that on the basis of murmur alone, it cannot be distinguished from the pulmonary regurgitation associated with high pulmonary artery pressure. A rare form of congenital aortic regurgitation results from a tunnel between the aorta just distal to the valve and the left ventricle just proximal to the valve. This type of aortic regurgitation is usually not associated with an aortic ejection click and is likely to be very severe and have a very wide pulse pressure.

The most common acquired aortic regurgitation is rheumatic in origin and can be present in both acute rheumatic fever and chronic rheumatic heart disease. In acute rheumatic fever, there is usually no aortic ejection click. The left ventricular impulse is abnormal, and a wide pulse pressure is present, depending on the severity of the regurgitation, which varies from very mild to very severe. Aortic regurgitation may be inaudible even in cases which are not mild.

A long, low-frequency diastolic rumble beginning one third into diastole, sometimes with presystolic accentuation, especially in the left lateral decubitus, may be heard in the presence of aortic regurgitation and in the absence of mitral stenosis. This is called the *Austin Flint murmur*. It is generally associated with more severe cases of aortic regurgitation and is related to increased velocity of mitral valve inflow.

Aortic Valve Regurgitation in the Presence of Aortic Stenosis

Mild aortic regurgitation in the presence of mild, moderate, and severe congenital aortic stenosis is very common and does not indicate progression of the disease. After surgery for valvular aortic stenosis, however, the regurgitation may be more severe. After

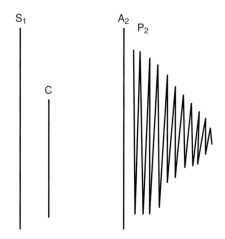

Figure 16–26. Diagram of heart sounds and murmurs in congenital aortic regurgitation. The sharp sound after S_1 is an aortic ejection click maximal at the apex, and there is a high-frequency diastolic decrescendo murmur heard along the left sternal edge. This murmur begins before P_2. C = click.

balloon dilatation for aortic stenosis, regurgitation may occur, but it is usually of mild to moderate severity.

In congenital subaortic stenosis, about half of cases have mild aortic regurgitation, the valve being distorted by an abnormal flow pattern through the subaortic area. Progressive aortic regurgitation has not been a problem.

COMMON LESIONS ASSOCIATED WITH CYANOSIS

Tetralogy of Fallot (see Chapter 15)

Tetralogy of Fallot can be defined in two different ways. The first is pathophysiologic and is that of a nonrestrictive VSD with severe pulmonic stenosis that is severe enough so that there is right-to-left shunt through the VSD. In some patients, the pulmonic stenosis is sometimes not severe at first, so that there is only a left-to-right shunt through the VSD. Later, as the pulmonic stenosis progresses, there is bidirectional flow and, finally, just a right-to-left shunt. The other definition is embryologic, in which there is hypoplasia of the conus, resulting in infundibular stenosis. Because conal tissue is needed for closure of the membranous ventricular septum, the hypoplasia of the conus results in a VSD, which is in this case nonrestrictive. Because of the conal hypoplasia, the aorta extends more to the right, resulting in overriding of the aorta. Thus, the diagnosis can be made echographically, even when pulmonary stenosis is not yet so severe and there is a left-to-right shunt through the VSD. In cases in which there is only a left-to-right shunt, the murmur may be full length at the LLSB, obscuring or partially obscuring S_1, but it is likely also to be harsh and diamond-shaped because of the pulmonic stenosis. The pulmonary stenosis murmur extends up the left sternal border. Because right ventricular pressure is at the systemic level, the intensity of S_1 may be increased at the LLSB. S_2 is located at the LLSB and is loud and single because aortic closure (A_2) is being heard.

In cases in which there is a left-to-right shunt, there may be a very wide split of S_2 and a soft pulmonary closure sound (P_2). There is usually a right ventricular S_3, heard best at the LLSB. On palpation, there is a right ventricular impulse. Usually, the left-to-right shunt is not severe, so that there is usually not an additional

left ventricular impulse and the left sternal edge is not usually hyperdynamic.

In standard cases of tetralogy of Fallot, in which there is mainly a right-to-left shunt and the patient is cyanotic, there is usually a loud S_1 at the LLSB and always a loud S_2 at the LLSB (A_2), but the P_2 is very soft and is thus not audible at the chest. The P_2 is delayed very far, often 14 to 16 milliseconds. There may be a right ventricular S_3 at the LLSB. The systolic murmur is harsh and diamond-shaped and is variable in position. Usually, the murmur is maximal at the LLSB, but it may be maximal higher, even at the ULSB. In tetralogy of Fallot with a right-to-left shunt, there is no murmur of blood flowing from right to left through the VSD, and the only murmur is that of the pulmonic stenosis. Therefore, the more severe the tetralogy of Fallot, the softer and shorter the murmur. In maximal tetralogy of Fallot, such as that with pulmonary atresia, there is no murmur, because all the blood is flowing from right to left through the VSD. Treatment of tetralogy of Fallot is surgical.

Infants with tetralogy of Fallot may develop *cyanotic spells* possibly caused by infundibular spasm or increased pulmonary vascular resistance with or without systemic arterial hypotension. During a spell, flow through the pulmonic valve is reduced, and thus the murmur is reduced in intensity or is absent. Treatment of this condition includes placing the child in a knee-chest position to increase venous return and to increase systemic vascular resistance; administration of oxygen, sodium bicarbonate, morphine, and propranolol; and administration of alpha-adrenergic agonists (phenylephrine or methoxamine) to increase systemic vascular resistance without increasing inotropy. Inotropic agents are contraindicated as they cause contraction of the infundibulum, thus worsening outflow obstruction of the right ventricle.

The differential diagnosis of cyanotic congenital heart disease is noted in Table 16–4.

Hypoplastic Right Ventricle with Tricuspid Atresia (see Chapter 15)

Since the right ventricle is very small and the left ventricle is large in this lesion, the cardiac impulse should be left ventricular. However, the left ventricle is more medial than normal, and in the newborn period, when these children are often first seen for cyano-

Table 16–4. Categories of Cyanotic Heart Lesions in the Neonate

Group	Heart Size	Pulmonary Blood Flow	Low Cardiac Output	Respiratory Distress	Examples
I	Small	Reduced	No	None	Hypoplastic RV with pulmonary atresia Hypoplastic RV with tricuspid atresia Tetralogy of Fallot (severe)
II	Small or slight cardiomegaly	Increased	No	Moderate	Transposition of great arteries with intact ventricular septum
III	Large	Increased	Yes	Yes	Complicated coarctation of aorta with VSD, hypoplastic LV
IV	Small	Pulmonary venous congestion	Yes	Yes	Obstructed total anomalous pulmonary veins

Modified from Gillette PC. *In* Behrman RE, Kliegman RM (eds). Nelson Essentials of Pediatrics, 2nd ed. Philadelphia: WB Saunders, 1994:503.
Abbreviations: LV = left ventricle; RV = right ventricle; VSD = ventricular septal defect.

sis, the impulse appears to be right ventricular. However, with aging, the overloaded left ventricle becomes clearly dominant, and there is usually an abnormal left ventricular impulse. All right atrial blood must enter the left atrium and the left ventricle, so that even when pulmonary blood flow is deficient, the left ventricle has an increased volume load. Patients with tricuspid atresia always have a VSD, which is the source of the pulmonary blood flow. This VSD is in the endocardial cushion position, so that the electrocardiogram reveals an abnormally superior vector. On the examination, there is a VSD murmur. Importantly, the softer and shorter the murmur, the less the pulmonary blood flow, so that just as in tetralogy of Fallot, the softer the murmur, the more severe the case. If there is enough pulmonary blood flow, P_2 may be heard as well as A_2.

Hypoplastic Right Ventricle with Pulmonary Atresia (see Chapter 15)

Just as in hypoplastic right ventricle with tricuspid atresia, the cardiac impulse in hypoplastic right ventricle with pulmonary atresia may be right ventricular even though the dominant ventricle is the left. Unlike in tricuspid atresia, a VSD is not part of the lesion. The source of the pulmonary blood flow is a ductus arteriosus with left-to-right shunt. A murmur from this ductus is usually not audible. There is a single S_2 (aortic closure) and usually no murmur. However, occasionally, there is tricuspid regurgitation, which may be confused with a VSD murmur. The electrocardiogram helps differentiate tricuspid and pulmonary atresia. Both disorders have left ventricular hypertrophy, but in pulmonary atresia, there is a normal inferior vector. Echocardiography confirms the diagnosis. Patients with pulmonary atresia are cyanotic; the hypoxia becomes most profound if the ductus arteriosus closes.

As in all lesions that are ductus dependent, intravenous prostaglandin therapy temporarily enhances ductal patency, and in pulmonary atresia such therapy provides a right-to-left shunt to improve pulmonary blood flow. In other circumstances (coarctation, interrupted aortic arch, or hypoplastic left heart syndrome) prostaglandin therapy temporarily improves cardiac function by enhancing ductal patency, creating systemic blood flow with a right-to-left shunt. If a ductus-dependent lesion is suspected, prostaglandins should be started immediately, even before an accurate diagnosis is made. Complications of prostaglandin therapy include apnea and fever; rarer complications include seizures, bone changes, and pyloric obstruction.

Transposition of the Great Arteries (see Chapter 15)

The presentation of transposition of the great arteries is usually in the newborn period if there is no VSD. In this condition, the pulmonary artery arises from the left ventricle, and the aorta from the right ventricle. The anatomy of the systemic and pulmonary venous return is normal. The child presents with hypoxia, probably with some tachypnea, but not grunting. There may be a soft short ejection murmur that is varied in position along the left sternal border, as a result of increased pulmonary blood flow. Heart failure is not expected. The right ventricular impulse is abnormal, and aortic closure is loud because it is anterior. Pulmonary closure may be heard, but because the pulmonary artery is posterior and the pressure is less than systemic, P_2 is often not heard. Sometimes there is a small VSD, which effectively causes little improvement in the patient's cyanosis. There is a right-to-left shunt through the VSD, causing no murmur, but there may also be some left-to-right shunt, resulting in a soft VSD murmur.

If there is a large VSD, patients usually do not present in the newborn period. Their minimal cyanosis may be difficult to detect. They usually become ill at 2 to 3 weeks of age as a result of congestive heart failure rather than hypoxia. There is a much different cardiac examination for those with transposition and no VSD, because the impulse is biventricular, there is a large heart, and there may be a systolic thrill at the LLSB. A VSD murmur is usually present, together with a loud aortic closure sound. Pulmonary closure is usually also present since there is systemic level pulmonary hypertension, and the split of S_2 is narrow. Treatment consists of surgical switching of the great vessels.

Hypoplastic Left Ventricle Syndrome (see Chapter 15)

In the first day or two of life, the baby may not be recognized as being ill if the ductus arteriosus remains wide open, allowing adequate systemic output with a right-to-left shunt. After the ductus closes, however, perfusion deteriorates, and the pulses are poor everywhere. There is considerable pulmonary blood flow, leaving the heart hyperdynamic, and there may be an ejection murmur at the ULSB. In addition, particularly if the atrial opening is restrictive, the pulmonary venous pressure is very high, and there is pulmonary venous congestion. Thus, the baby is tachypneic. After intravenous prostaglandin E_1 has been given, causing opening of the ductus arteriosus, there is again a reasonable systemic output and decent pulses. Treatment includes heart transplantation; Norwood two-stage operations; or, because of the poor prognosis, comfort care.

Complicated Coarctation of the Aorta (see Chapter 15)

Patients with severe congestive heart failure usually present at 1 to 2 weeks of age, but they could present earlier or later. The most common form of complicated coarctation is that of coarctation of the aorta plus a VSD. Unlike that of a simple VSD, in this disorder, the left ventricle works against the high systemic resistance of the coarctation and must drive blood through the VSD. Thus, there is obligatory high pulmonary blood flow, plus high pulmonary venous pressure, resulting in pulmonary hypertension, even if the VSD is not large. Thus, the baby is usually tachypneic, sometimes with grunting, and is often very diaphoretic. Importantly, when the congestive heart failure is severe, all pulses may be poor, although usually the right brachial pulse is stronger. The heart is hyperdynamic, especially at the left sternal edge, but the VSD murmur, because of the severe congestive heart failure, is usually not as loud as one would expect, nor is the coarctation murmur. Treatment consists of corrective surgery.

Approach to Congenital Heart Disease (see Chapter 15)

Congenital heart disease may produce an asymptomatic murmur, heart failure, cyanosis, cyanosis with heart failure, or severe cardiogenic shock (Fig. 16–27, see also Table 16–4). Lesions associated with profound and fixed cyanosis without heart failure are usually associated with right-sided obstructive lesions and a right-to-left shunt (pulmonary atresia, tetralogy of Fallot). Transposition of the great arteries with intact ventricular septum also presents with profound and fixed hypoxia, with mild tachypnea and no heart failure. Lesions associated with cyanosis and heart failure have a large mixing lesion (single ventricle, truncus arteriosus, transposi-

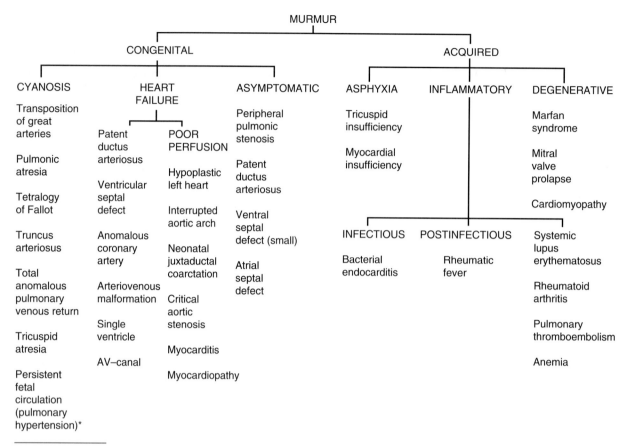

*Murmur represents tricuspid insufficiency (usually no murmur in persistent fetal circulation).

Figure 16–27. Algorithmic approach to the child with a heart murmur.

tion plus a VSD), where pulmonary oxygenated venous return mixes with desaturated systemic venous return before ejection to the systemic arterial circulation. In addition, obstructed total anomalous pulmonary veins may produce severe cyanosis, pulmonary venous engorgement, and pulmonary hypertension. Lesions associated with left-sided obstruction (critical aortic stenosis, interrupted aortic arch, hypoplastic left heart syndrome) produce significant cardiogenic shock, poor perfusion, and profound lactic acidosis.

The chest roentgenogram may provide helpful clues to the cause of the lesion, depending on the paucity (pulmonary atresia) or plethora (obstructed total anomalous pulmonary venous return) of the pulmonary vascular markings; the left- or right (tetralogy of Fallot, truncus arteriosus)-sided position of the aorta; the configuration of the heart (boot-shaped, as in tetralogy of Fallot; egg-shaped, as in transposition of the great arteries; or massive enlargement, as in Ebstein anomaly); or the side of the chest (higher risk of heart disease with dextrocardia, especially if the stomach bubble is on the left side of the abdomen or if the liver is midline). The chest roentgenogram is some help in distinguishing heart disease from congenital pneumonia, respiratory distress syndrome, pneumothorax, or congenital diaphragmatic hernia. No chest roentgenogram is pathognomonic for a specific congenital heart lesion.

The electrocardiogram in infancy is of help in discriminating atrial and ventricular enlargement or hypertrophy and very helpful when there is an abnormal superior vector (complete atrioventricular canal, tricuspid atresia).

Two-dimensional real-time color Doppler echocardiography is most useful in identifying the anatomy of congenital heart lesions. The echocardiogram can determine the four chambers, the intercon-

necting valves, the great arteries, the pulmonary venous return (the most difficult to visualize), and the anatomic relationships between these structures. Furthermore, color Doppler flow studies can determine the presence, direction, and magnitude of right-to-left or left-to-right shunts. Echocardiography has replaced cardiac catheterization for all but the most complex congenital heart lesions.

The therapy of congenital heart disease depends on the specific nature of the congenital anomaly (Tables 16–5 and 16–6). Certain lesions require immediate palliative therapy (see Table 16–5) with subsequent complete repair when the neonate becomes older and bigger (see Table 16–6). Other lesions require complete repair in the neonatal period (see Table 16–6).

ACUTE RHEUMATIC FEVER AND RHEUMATIC HEART DISEASE

The incidence of acute rheumatic fever is increasing in the United States; it remains very common in many areas of the world. Rheumatic fever is a post-infectious immunologically mediated inflammatory disease (caused by group A streptococcus) of the heart, joints, brain, and skin. Valvulitis, as manifested by specific and new heart murmurs, is often part of the initial clinical picture. The specific heart murmurs are three: mitral regurgitation, aortic regurgitation, and the Carey-Coombs murmur, a mid-diastolic rumble at the apex. No other murmur occurs as part of acute rheumatic fever, although pericarditis may produce a friction rub. Pericarditis is usually associated with valvulitis.

After the acute rheumatic fever has run its course, any remaining

Table 16–5. Palliative Therapy for Congenital Heart Disease

Procedure	Lesion	Comments
Blalock-Taussig Teflon tube graft or shunt (subclavian artery to ipsilateral pulmonary artery, usually right-sided)	TOF, pulmonary valve atresia	Improves pulmonary blood flow; most common shunting procedure
Waterston shunt (aorta to right pulmonary artery)	TOF, pulmonary valve atresia, tricuspid atresia	Improves pulmonary blood flow
Balloon atrial septostomy (Rashkind procedure)	TGA, tricuspid atresia	Improves oxygenation with increased atrial mixing
Operative atrial septostomy (Blalock-Hanlon operation)	TGA	
Catheter balloon–dilating valvotomy (balloon angioplasty)	Pulmonary valve stenosis; aortic valve stenosis	Increases valve patency
Operative valvotomy	As above for balloon plus pulmonary atresia	Increases valve patency; resultant pulmonary valve insufficiency enhances RV growth
Prostaglandin E$_1$ infusion	Pulmonary atresia, tricuspid atresia, TOF, coarctation of aorta, interrupted aortic arch	Maintains pulmonary blood flow via PDA
Pulmonary artery banding	Single ventricle	Decreases pulmonary blood flow, prevents heart failure
Device occlusion (embolization, umbrella); correction/closure	PDA, VSD, ASD, arteriovenous malformations	New and experimental

From Gillette PC. The cardiovascular system. *In* Behrman RE, Kliegman RM (eds). Nelson Essentials of Pediatrics, 2nd ed. Philadelphia: WB Saunders, 1994.
Abbreviations: ASD = atrial septal defect; PDA = patent ductus arteriosus; RV = right ventricular; TGA = transposition of great arteries; TOF = tetralogy of Fallot; VSD = ventricular septal defect.

Table 16–6. Corrective Procedures for Congenital Heart Disease

Procedure	Lesion	Effect
Repair of septal defects (patching)	ASD, VSD, endocardial cushion defects	Complete repair
Valve replacement, repair	Aortic, mitral, pulmonic stenosis; Ebstein anomaly	Repair but prosthetic valve complications
Aortic graft or subclavian flap angioplasty	Interrupted arch, coarctation of aorta	Repair but possible late recoarctation
Total correction possible	TOF, anomalous venous return, PDA	Complete repair
Mustard or Senning procedure (atrial switch by an intra-atrial baffle)	TGA	RV remains systemic ventricle
Jatene procedure (arterial switch)*	TGA	Anatomic correction
Fontan procedure (right atrium to pulmonary artery anastomosis)	Tricuspid atresia, single ventricle, pulmonary atresia	Alleviates shunting, enhances pulmonary blood flow; atrium functions as right ventricle
Norwood procedure	Hypoplastic left heart	Two-stage procedure with variable success
Heart transplant	Hypoplastic left heart	Normal heart with risk of immune rejection, premature atherosclerosis
Heart-lung transplant	Eisenmenger syndrome; cor pulmonale?	Normal organs with risk of rejection

Modified from Gillette PC. The cardiovascular system. *In* Behrman RE, Kliegman RM (eds). Nelson Essentials of Pediatrics, 2nd ed. Philadelphia: WB Saunders, 1994.
*Preferred procedure.
Abbreviations: ASD = atrial septal defect; PDA = patent ductus arteriosus; RV = right ventricle; TGA = transposition of great arteries; TOF = tetralogy of Fallot; VSD = ventricular septal defect.

Table 16–7. Major Criteria in the Jones System for Acute Rheumatic Fever*†

Sign	Comments
Polyarthritis	Most common. Swelling, limited motion, very tender, erythema; migratory (may be aborted by anti-inflammatory agents): involves large joints (knees, ankles, wrists, elbows) but rarely small or unusual joints, such as vertebrae. Universally benign long-term joint prognosis. Robust response to salicylate within 48 hr.
Carditis	Common. Pancarditis, valvulitis, pericarditis, myocarditis; tachycardia greater than that explained by fever; new murmur of mitral or aortic insufficiency; Carey-Coombs mid-diastolic murmur; heart failure. Echocardiographic findings without auscultatory findings do not count as a major criterion.
Chorea (Sydenham disease)	Uncommon. Presents long after infection has resolved; may be associated with antineuronal antibody.
Erythema marginatum	Uncommon. Evanescent pink macules on trunk and proximal extremities, evolving to serpiginous border with central clearing; elicited by application of local heat; nonpruritic.
Subcutaneous nodules	Uncommon. Associated with repeated episodes and severe carditis; present over extensor surface of elbows, knees, knuckles, and ankles or scalp and spine; firm, nontender, painless.

*Minor criteria include fever (101°–102°F [38.2°–38.9°C]), arthralgias, previous rheumatic fever, leukocytosis, elevated erythrocyte sedimentation rate/C-reactive protein, prolonged P-R interval.

†One major plus two minor criteria, or two major criteria with evidence of recent group A streptococcal disease (scarlet fever, positive throat culture, or elevated antistreptolysin O or other antistreptococcal antibodies), strongly suggest the diagnosis of acute rheumatic fever.

Exceptions to these recommendations include chorea (which may occur too late after other signs or laboratory tests are not useful), some cases of recurrent carditis that may not fulfill the criteria, indolent carditis or late stenotic or regurgitant murmurs far removed in time from the original episode of rheumatic fever. Isolated reactive post-streptococcal arthritis has been considered by some authorities to be in the spectrum of rheumatic fever. Nonetheless, this has not been met with uniform agreement.

murmurs become part of chronic rheumatic heart disease. Assuming that the patient has remained on permanent reliable penicillin prophylaxis, the severity of the mitral regurgitation often disappears, which is less common in aortic regurgitation. It has been accepted that the development of mitral stenosis is part of the natural history of severe repeated episodes of acute rheumatic fever. Pure aortic stenosis does not develop, although in the presence of long-standing rheumatic heart disease with severe aortic regurgitation, some aortic stenosis may be present. In some very severe cases, tricuspid regurgitation has been documented, but it is rare.

The diagnosis of acute rheumatic fever is suggested (although not definitively confirmed) by application of the modified Jones criteria last edited in 1992 (Table 16–7). The differential diagnosis is limited in the presence of carditis and arthritis (see Chapter 45) but includes systemic lupus erythematosus.

Treatment of acute carditis includes salicylate if mild and steroids if severe carditis is present and standard therapy for heart failure (see Chapter 13). Valvular scarring and progression of carditis can be avoided by prevention of repeated episodes of group A streptococcal infections. Daily penicillin V, 250 mg taken orally twice a day (or, if patient is allergic to penicillin, sulfisoxazole, 1 g taken orally once a day if patient weighs > 60 pounds, or 0.5 g if patient weighs < 60 pounds) or long-acting penicillin, 1,200,000 U injected intramuscularly every 28 days, prevents most cases of new group A streptococcal diseases and recurrent rheumatic fever. Prophylaxis is continued for at least 5 years and at least until age 21 years (some believe prophylaxis should be for life); prophylaxis is lifelong in patients with documented rheumatic heart disease.

INFECTIVE ENDOCARDITIS

An acute or subacute infection of the cardiac valves produces infective endocarditis. Infection may involve a native, previously normal heart valve, a valve or structure (e.g., PDA, VSD opposite an endocardial wall that is subjected to a jet stream) which is anomalous secondary to congenital heart disease (most common sites), or a prosthetic device (e.g., valve, conduit, patch, graft, shunt, or pacemaker).

Endocarditis may affect congenital heart lesions (most commonly, tetralogy of Fallot, VSD, aortic stenosis, patent ductus arteriosus, transposition of the great arteries), valves affected by rheumatic heart disease, and mitral valve prolapse. Endocarditis may develop in congenital heart anomalies in the unoperated and the postoperative state. Furthermore, 10% to 30% of cases of infective endocarditis occur on previously normal native valves.

Endocarditis is the result of a bacteremia, which in a normal host is usually transient, asymptomatic, and without sequelae. The presence of a damaged valve, a jet stream–injured endocardium, or a foreign body (e.g., central catheter, graft, shunt, or patch) creates a nidus of infection that permits the bacteria to bind, proliferate, and remain sequestered from normal host defense mechanisms. Transient and predisposing bacteremias occur during dental procedures that induce bleeding (even dental cleaning); tonsillectomy or adenoidectomy; intestinal (e.g., gall bladder), urinary (e.g., catheterization, dilatation), prostatic (e.g., cystoscopy), or respiratory surgery; esophageal manipulation (e.g., sclerotherapy, dilatation), incision and drainage of infected tissue; and gynecologic procedures (e.g., vaginal hysterectomy, vaginal delivery).

Bacterial vegetations grow and produce cardiovascular, embolic, or immune complex–mediated signs and symptoms (Table 16–8). Responsible bacteria are noted in Table 16–9; *Staphylococcus aureus,* α-hemolytic oral mucosa–derived streptococci, and enterococcus are the dominant pathogens in native normal and unoperated anomalous valves. *Staphylococcus epidermidis* and *S. aureus* are common pathogens in the postoperative patient and in patients with prosthetic devices.

The definitive diagnosis of infective endocarditis includes recovery of a microorganism from culture or histology of a heart or embolized vegetation or intracardiac abscess. Vegetations are best demonstrated by transesophageal echocardiography because transthoracic echo cardiography may not demonstrate as many as 30% to 60% of vegetations. In the absence of direct definitive evidence, the following are important diagnostic factors: persistently positive blood cultures with a compatible pathogen (see Table 16–9); echocardiographic evidence of an intracardiac mass, vegetations, perivalvular abscess, or new partial dehiscence of a prosthetic valve; and a new valvular murmur (regurgitation, or worsening of changing of a preexisting murmur). Blood cultures are helpful if two or

Table 16–8. Manifestations of Infective Endocarditis

History
   Prior congenital or rheumatic heart disease
   Preceding dental, urinary, or intestinal procedure
   Intravenous drug use
   Central venous catheter
   Prosthetic heart valve

Symptoms
   Fever
   Chills
   Chest and back pain
   Arthralgia/myalgia
   Dyspnea
   Malaise
   Night sweats
   Weight loss
   CNS manifestations (stroke, seizures, headache, confusion)

Signs
   Elevated temperature
   Tachycardia
   Embolic phenomena (Roth spots, petechiae, splinter nailbed
      hemorrhages, Osler nodes, CNS or ocular lesions)
   Janeway lesions
   New or changing murmur
   Splenomegaly
   Arthritis
   Heart failure
   Arrhythmias, heart block, conduction disturbances
   Metastatic infection (arthritis, meningitis, mycotic arterial
      aneurysm, pericarditis, abscesses, septic pulmonary emboli)
   Clubbing

Laboratory
   Positive blood culture
   Elevated erythrocyte sedimentation rate; may be low with heart
      or renal failure
   Elevated C-reactive protein level
   Anemia
   Leukocytosis
   Immune complexes
   Hypergammaglobulinemia
   Hypocomplementemia
   Cryoglobulinemia
   Rheumatoid factor
   Hematuria
   Azotemia, high creatinine level (glomerulonephritis)
   Echocardiographic evidence of valve vegetations, prosthetic
      valve dysfunction or leak, or myocardial abscess

Modified from Behrman RE (ed). Nelson Textbook of Pediatrics, 14th ed. Philadelphia: WB Saunders, 1992.
Abbreviations: CNS = central nervous system.

more drawn 12 hours apart are positive or if a majority (e.g., three of four) of separate cultures drawn in 1 hour are positive. Over 85% of first blood cultures are positive; the yield approaches 95% with the second blood culture. Sufficient blood must be inoculated into the media to detect the low-grade bacteremia of infective endocarditis; excessive blood inoculation may inhibit bacterial growth by continued activity of leukocytes unless the technique uses centrifugation lysis. The cultures should be incubated for more than the routine 72 hours (often 1 to 2 weeks), and the laboratory should be notified of the possible diagnosis so that laboratory personnel can enrich the media to encourage the growth of fastidious nutrient-dependent organisms.

Less important criteria for infective endocarditis include fever;

predisposing heart lesions and procedures (many patients have no identifiable procedure); vascular phenomenon (embolism, Janeway lesions, petechiae, septic pulmonary infarcts, intracranial hemorrhage); immune lesions (glomerulonephritis, Roth spots, Osler nodes); a suggestive but not definitive echocardiogram; and microbiologic criteria (positive blood culture but not as defined earlier, serologic evidence of active infection).

The treatment of presumed infective endocarditis with no known cause and the treatment of bacteriologic-proven infective endocarditis are noted in Table 16–10. With appropriate therapy, the blood should be culture-negative within 72 to 96 hours, and fever should subside by 1 to 2 weeks. Persistent fever should suggest the presence of resistant organisms, metastatic foci of infection, an infected clot, a myocardial abscess, pulmonary emboli, a nosocomial infection, and drug fever. Persistent infection, severe refractory heart failure, intracardiac abscess, recurrent emboli, and possible fungal infective endocarditis are indications for surgical intervention.

To prevent infective endocarditis, high-risk patients and factors that predispose to bacteremia need to be identified (Table 16–11).

Table 16–9. Bacterial Agents in Pediatric Infective Endocarditis

Common: Native Valve
   Streptococcus viridans group (e.g., *S. mutans, S. sanguis, S. mitis*)
   Staphylococcus aureus
   Group D streptococcus (enterococcus) *(S. bovis, S. faecalis)*

Uncommon: Native Valve
   Streptococcus pneumoniae
   Haemophilus influenzae
   Group A or B streptococci
   Staphylococcus epidermidis
   Coxiella burnetii (Q fever)
   Neisseria gonorrhoeae
   Brucella species*
   *Chlamydia psittaci**
   *Chlamydia trachomatis**
   *Chlamydia pneumoniae**
   HACEK group†
   *Streptobacillus moniliformis**
   *Pasteurella multocida**
   Campylobacter fetus
   Polymicrobial
   Fungal
   Culture negative (5% of cases)

Prosthetic Valve
   Staphylococcus epidermidis
   S. aureus
   S. viridans
   Pseudomonas aeruginosa
   Serratia marcescens
   Diphtheroids
   Legionella species*
   HACEK group†
   Fungi‡

Modified from Behrman RE (ed). Nelson Textbook of Pediatrics, 14th ed. Philadelphia: WB Saunders, 1992.
*These fastidious bacteria plus some fungi and pretreatment with antibiotics may produce culture-negative endocarditis. Detection may require special media, incubation for more than 7 days, or serology.
†HACEK group includes *Haemophilus* species (*H. paraphrophilus, H. parainfluenzae, H. aphrophilus*), *Actinobacillus actinomycetemcomitans, Cardiobacterium hominis, Eikenella corrodens, Kingella* species.
‡*Candida* species, *Aspergillus* species, *Pseudallescheria boydii, Histoplasma capsulatum.*

Table 16–10. **Treatment of Infective Endocarditis**

Etiologic Agent	Drug	Dose	Route	Duration of Therapy (Weeks)
Streptococcus viridans, S. bovis (Minimal inhibitory concentration [MIC] ≤0.1 μg/ml)	1. Penicillin G *or*	200,000–300,000 U/kg/24 hr q 4 hr, not to exceed 20 million U/24 hr	IV	4–6
	2. Penicillin G plus	As in No. 1 under drug column	IV	2–4
	gentamicin	2–4 mg/kg/24 hr q 8 hr, not to exceed 80 mg/24 hr	IV	2
S. viridans, S. bovis (MIC ≥0.1 μg/ml)	3. Penicillin G plus	As in No. 2	IV	4–6
	gentamicin	As in No. 2	IV	2
S. viridans or enterococcus (*S. bovis* or *S. faecalis*) (MIC >0.5 μg/ml)	4. Penicillin G *or*	As in No. 2	IV	4–6
	ampicillin	300 mg/kg/24 hr q 4–6 hr, not to exceed 12 g/24 hr	IV	4–6
	plus gentamicin	As in No. 2	IV	4–6
*S. viridans, S. bovis** (penicillin allergy†)	5. Vancomycin	40–60 mg/kg/24 hr q 8–12 hr, not to exceed 2 g/24 hr*	IV	4–6
	plus 6. Gentamicin if resistant*	As in No. 2	IV	4–6
Staphylococcus aureus	7. Nafcillin *or* oxacillin	200 mg/kg/24 hr q 4–6 hr, not to exceed 12 g/24 hr	IV	6–8
	plus optional gentamicin	As in No. 2	IV	1–2
S. aureus (methicillin resistant; penicillin allergy)	8. Vancomycin plus optional trimethoprim-sulfamethoxazole	As in No. 5

12 mg/kg/24 hr of trimethoprim q 8 hr, not to exceed 1 g/24 hr | IV

IV, p.o. | 6–8

4–8 |
S. aureus (with prosthetic device; methicillin sensitive)‡	9. Nafcillin plus gentamicin plus optional rifampin	As in No. 7 As in No. 2 15–30 mg/kg/24 hr q 12 hr, not to exceed 600 mg/24 hr	IV IV p.o.	6–8 2 ≥6
S. aureus (with prosthetic device; methicillin resistant)	10. Vancomycin plus gentamicin plus optional rifampin	As in No. 5 As in No. 9 As in No. 9	IV IV p.o.	6–8 2 ≥6
S. epidermidis	11. Vancomycin plus optional rifampin	As in No. 5 As in No. 9	IV p.o.	6–8 6–8
Haemophilus species	12. Ampicillin plus optional gentamicin	As in No. 4 As in No. 2	IV IV	4–6 2–4
Unknown Postoperative Nonoperative	13. Vancomycin plus gentamicin 14. Nafcillin *or* vancomycin plus gentamicin plus optional ampicillin	As in No. 5 As in No. 2 As in No. 7 As in No. 5 As in No. 2 As in No. 4	IV IV IV IV IV IV	6–8 2–4 6–8 6–8 2–4 6–8

Modified from Behrman RE (ed). Nelson Textbook of Pediatrics, 14th ed. Philadelphia: WB Saunders, 1992.

*Add gentamicin for relatively resistant organisms. Monitor vancomycin peaks 1 hour after infusion (30–45 μg/ml). Adjust dose according to vancomycin levels.

†Desensitization should be considered for patients who are allergic to penicillin. Cephalosporins are not recommended.

‡May require valve (device) replacement.

Abbreviations: IV = intravenously; p.o. = orally; q = every.

Table 16–11. Recommendations for Prevention of Infective Endocarditis*

Dental Procedures and Surgery of Upper Respiratory Tract

1. Most patients:
   Oral amoxicillin

   Adults: 3 g 1 hr before a procedure and 1.5 g 6 hr after the initial dose
   Children: 50 mg/kg 1 hr before a procedure and 25 mg/kg 6 hr after the initial dose†

2. Patients with penicillin allergy:
   Oral erythromycin

   Adults: 1 g 2 hr before a procedure and 500 mg 6 hr after the initial dose
   Children: 20 mg/kg 2 hr before a procedure and 10 mg/kg 6 hr after the initial dose†

   or

   Oral clindamycin

   Adults: 300 mg 1 hr before a procedure and 150 mg 6 hr after the initial dose
   Children: 10 mg/kg 1 hr before a procedure and 5 mg/kg 6 hr after the initial dose†

3. High-risk patients‡
   Parenteral ampicillin plus
   gentamicin (IV or IM)

   Adults: Ampicillin, 2 g 30 min before a procedure§
   Gentamicin, 1.5 mg/kg 30 min before a procedure§
   Children: Ampicillin, 50 mg/kg 30 min before a procedure†§
   Gentamicin, 2 mg/kg 30 min before a procedure§

4. High-risk, penicillin-allergic patients:
   Vancomycin (IV)

   Adults: 1 g infused slowly in 1 hr, initiated 1 hr before a procedure, no repeat dose needed
   Children: 20 mg/kg infused as adults; no repeat dose needed†

Gastrointestinal and Genitourinary Tract Surgery and Instrumentation

1. Most patients:
   Parenteral ampicillin plus
   gentamicin (IV or IM)

   Adults: Ampicillin, 2 g 30 min before a procedure§
   Gentamicin, 1.5 mg/kg 30 min before a procedure§
   Children: Ampicillin, 50 mg/kg 30 min before a procedure†§
   Gentamicin, 2 mg/kg 30 min before a procedure

2. Patients with penicillin allergy:
   Parenteral vancomycin plus
   gentamicin

   Adults: Vancomycin, 1 g infused slowly over 1 hr before a procedure‖
   Gentamicin, 1.5 mg/kg 30 min before a procedure‖
   Children: Vancomycin, 20 mg/kg infused slowly over 1 hr before a procedure†
   Gentamicin, 2 mg/kg 30 min before a procedure‖

3. Low-risk patients:
   Oral amoxicillin

   Adults: 3 g 1 hr before a procedure and 1.5 g 6 hr later
   Children: 50 mg/kg 1 hr before a procedure and 25 mg 6 hr later†

From Recommendations for prevention of bacterial endocarditis. The cardiovascular system: Infective endocarditis. *In* Nelson Textbook of Pediatrics, 14th ed. Behrman RE (ed). Philadelphia: WB Saunders, 1992. Adapted from JAMA 264:2919, 1990, Copyright 1990, American Medical Association; Med Lett Drug Ther 31:112, 1989; and 1994 Red Book Report of the Committee on Infectious Diseases. American Academy of Pediatrics.

Oral regimens are less expensive, more convenient, and safer than parenteral routes. Amoxicillin is recommended because of excellent bioavailability and good activity against streptococci and enterococci. Parenteral routes are more effective and are recommended by some authorities for high-risk patients.

*Prophylaxis is recommended for patients with previous endocarditis, valvular heart disease, prosthetic heart devices, idiopathic hypertrophic subaortic stenosis, mitral valve prolapse with regurgitation, cardiac transplantation (possibly), and congenital heart disease except for patients with an isolated secundum atrial septal defect and for those who have recovered at least 6 mo from surgery for a patent ductus arteriosus or simple atrial septal defect without a patch.

†Maximal doses for children should not exceed adult doses.

‡High risk includes prosthetic valves, previous endocarditis, continuous penicillin prophylaxis for rheumatic fever, surgically constructed systemic-pulmonary shunts or conduits.

§Additional parenteral (ampicillin and gentamicin), or, more often, oral dose (amoxicillin) should be given 6–8 hr after the initial dose in high-risk patients. The dose of gentamicin should not exceed 80 mg.

‖Additional dose may be repeated 8 hr after the initial dose.

Abbreviations: IV = intravenously; IM = intramuscularly.

Patients needing infective endocarditis prophylaxis include those with intracardiac foreign bodies (prosthetic valve, grafts), prior episodes of infective endocarditis, most congenital heart defects (except isolated secundum ASD, a repaired secundum ASD, VSD, or patent ductus arteriosus after 6 months of operation, and valvular pulmonic stenosis), hypertrophic cardiomyopathy, rheumatic or other acquired valve disease, and mitral valve prolapse with regurgitation.

RED FLAGS AND THINGS NOT TO MISS

Murmurs may be caused by cardiac or noncardiac lesions and may be congenital or acquired. Murmurs in the newborn period are often transient, as a result of the changing hemodynamics of the transitional circulation between fetal and neonatal life, or as a result of the common occurrence of a small VSD, which usually closes in the first 1 to 5 years of life. Most murmurs at all ages are not due to cardiac pathology and are not associated with symptoms or increased risk for disease.

Red flags in the neonatal period include cyanosis, fixed profound hypoxia, heart failure, and other congenital anomalies or syndromes, such as trisomy 21. Such anomalies often manifest with multiple congenital anomalies, including those involving the cardiovascular, gastrointestinal, and central nervous systems. In the neonatal period, things not to miss include ductus-dependent lesions, in which systemic blood flow (as in interrupted aortic arch, hypoplastic left heart) or pulmonary blood flow (as in pulmonary atresia) is through the patent ductus arteriosus. Sudden deterioration, cyanosis, or heart failure with increasing metabolic acidosis and a reduction in the murmur suggests closure of the ductus arteriosus. Another thing not to miss is the murmur associated with an arteriovenous malformation, such as the cerebral vein of Galen malformation, which presents with heart failure and a cranial bruit transmitted to the thorax. Finally, obstructed total anomalous venous return is a difficult diagnosis that may be confused with persistent fetal circulation. Total anomalous venous return is associated with fixed and profound cyanosis ($PaO_2 < 35$ mmHg), severe pulmonary venous congestion, and a small heart.

Acquired murmurs or symptomatic murmurs that change in quality should suggest acute (recurrent) rheumatic fever or infective endocarditis. Systemic symptoms and peripheral signs associated with these disorders are suggestive of the diagnosis. Arthritis (associated with rheumatic fever or endocarditis-induced immune complexes), fever, anemia, leukocytosis, cutaneous manifestations (in rheumatic fever—erythema marginatum, subcutaneous nodules; in infective endocarditis—Osler nodes, Janeway lesions, petechiae, splinter hemorrhages), and evidence of prior (streptococcal antibodies) or current (positive blood cultures) infection help identify the nature of the acquired heart disease. Finally, heart murmurs in a normal heart may be caused by hemodynamic factors, such as severe anemia or thyrotoxicosis.

REFERENCES

Basic Principles: Heart Sounds and Murmurs

American Heart Association. Physiologic Principles of Heart Sounds and Murmurs. Monograph No. 46. New York: American Heart Association, 1975.

Ongley PA, Sprague HB, Rappaport MB, et al. Heart Sounds and Murmurs: A Clinical and Phonocardiographic Study. New York: Grune & Stratton, 1960.

Segal BL, Novack P, Kasparian H. Intracardiac phonocardiography. Am J Cardiol 1964;83:188–197.

Sreenivasan VV, Liebman J, Linton D. Posterior mitral regurgitation in girls possibly due to posterior papillary muscle dysfunction. Pediatrics 1968;42:276–290.

Stethoscope

Luisada AA. The Heart Beat: Graphic Methods in the Study of the Cardiac Patient. New York: Paul B. Hoeber, 1953.

Rappaport MB, Sprague HB. Physiologic and physical laws that govern auscultation and their clinical application: The acoustic stethoscope and the electrical amplifying stethoscope and stethograph. Am Heart J 1941;21:257–318.

Rappaport MB, Sprague HB. The effects of tubing bore on stethoscope efficiency. Am Heart J 1951;42:605–609.

Method of Auscultation

Gessner IH. Evaluation of the infant and child with a heart murmur. In Gessner IH, Victoria BE (eds). Pediatric Cardiology: A Problem Oriented Approach. Philadelphia: WB Saunders, 1993.

Liebman J. Diagnosis and management of heart murmurs in children. Pediatr Rev 1982;321–329.

McNamara DG. Value and limitations of auscultation in the management of congenital heart disease. Pediatr Clin North Am 1990;37:93–113.

Perloff JK. The Clinical Recognition of Congenital Heart Disease, 2nd ed. Philadelphia: WB Saunders, 1978.

Ravin A. Auscultation of the Heart, 2nd ed. Chicago: Year Book Medical Publishers, 1967.

Heart Sounds

Glover DD, Murrah RL, Olsen CO, et al. Mechanical correlates of the third heart sound. J Am Coll Cardiol 1992;19:450–457.

Hultgren HN, Reeve R, Cohn K, et al. The ejection click of valvular pulmonic stenosis. Circulation 1969;40:631–640.

Nitta M, Ihenacho D, Hultgren HN. Prevalence and characteristics of the aortic ejection sound in adults. Am J Cardiol 1988;61:142–145.

Ozawa Y, Smith D, Craige E. Origin of the third heart sound: I. Studies in dogs. Circulation 1983;67:393–398.

Ozawa Y, Smith D, Craige E. Origin of the third heart sound: II. Studies in human subjects. Circulation 1983;67:399–404.

Shaver JA, Nadolny RA, O'Toole JD. Sound pressure correlates of the second heart sound: An intracardiac sound study. Circulation 1974;49:316–325.

Shaver JA, O'Toole JD. The second heart sound: Newer concepts, Part I: Normal and wide physiological splitting. Mod Concepts Cardiovasc Dis 1977;46:7–12, and 1977;46:13–17.

Tilkian AG, Conover MB. Understanding Heart Sounds and Murmurs, With an Introduction to Lung Sounds, 3rd ed. Philadelphia: WB Saunders, 1993.

Vancheri F, Gibson D. Relation of third and fourth heart sounds to blood velocity during left ventricular filling. Br Heart J 1989;61:144–145.

Zoneraich S. Evaluation of century-old physical signs, S_3 and S_4, by modern technology. J Am Coll Cardiol 1992;19:458–459.

Murmurs

Levine SA, Harvey WP. Clinical Auscultation of the Heart, 2nd ed. Philadelphia: WB Saunders, 1959.

Shabetai R. Classification of systolic murmurs. Am Heart J 1960;59:637–638.

Murmurs in Children with Normal Hearts

Lembo N, Dell'Italia L, Crawford M, et al. Bedside diagnosis of systolic murmurs. N Engl J Med 1988;318:1572–1578.

Luisada AA, Haring OM, Aravanis, et al. Murmurs in children: A clinical and graphic study in 500 children of school age. Ann Intern Med 1958;48:597–615.

Rosenthal A. How to distinguish between innocent and pathologic murmurs in childhood. Pediatr Clin North Am 1984;31:1229–1240.

Shiekh MV, Lee WR, Mills RJ, et al. Musical murmurs: Clinical implications, long term prognosis, and echo-phonocardiographic features. Am Heart J 1984;108:377–386.

Stein PD, Sabbah HN. Aortic origin of innocent murmurs. Am J Cardiol 1977;39:665–671.

Wennevold A. The origin of the innocent "vibratory" murmur studied with intracardiac phonocardiography. Acta Med Scand 1973;181:679–684.

Changes in Circulation: Fetus to Newborn to Early Weeks

Dawes G. Physiologic changes in the circulation after birth. In Fishman A, Richards D (eds). Circulation of the Blood: Men and Ideas. Oxford University Press, 1964.

Emmanouillides G, Moss A, Duffie E, et al. Pulmonary arterial pressure changes in human newborn infants from birth to 3 days of age. J Pediatr 1964;65:327–333.

Physical Examination of Common Lesions with Left-to-Right Shunt

Haworth SG, Bull C. Physiology of congenital heart disease. Arch Dis Child 1993;68:707–711.

Liebman J, Freed MD. The cardiovascular system. In Behrman RE, Kliegman RM (eds). Nelson's Essentials of Pediatrics. Philadelphia: WB Saunders, 1990.

Poskitt EME. Failure to thrive in congenital heart disease. Arch Dis Child 1993;68:158–160.

Rudolph A. The changes in the circulation after birth: The importance in congenital heart disease. Circulation 1970;41:343–349.

Silove ED. Assessment and management of congenital heart disease in the newborn by the district paediatrician. Arch Dis Child 1994;70:F71–F74.

Physical Examination of Common Lesions with Simple Obstruction

Fyler DC. Nadas' Pediatric Cardiology. St. Louis: Mosby–Year Book, 1992.

Harvey WP. Auscultatory features of congenital heart disease. Cardiovasc Clin 1979;10:53.

Vogelpoel L, Schrire V. Auscultatory and phonocardiographic assessment of pulmonary stenosis with intact ventricular septum. Circulation 1960;22:55–72.

Physical Examination of Atrioventricular Valve and Semilunar Valve Regurgitation

Alpert MA. Mitral valve prolapse. Mostly benign. BMJ 1993;306:943–944.

Bisset GS, Schwartz DC, Meyer RA, et al. Clinical spectrum and long-term follow-up of isolated mitral valve prolapse in 119 children. Circulation 1980;62:423–429.

Devereux RB, Kramer-Fox R, Kligfield P. Mitral valve prolapse: Causes, clinical manifestations, and management. Ann Intern Med 1989;111:305–317.

Emi S, Fukuda N, Oki T, et al. Genesis of the Austin Flint murmur: Relation to mitral inflow and aortic regurgitant flow dynamics. J Am Coll Cardiol 1993;21:1399–1405.

Mair DD. Ebstein's anomaly: Natural history and management. J Am Coll Cardiol 1992;19:1047–1048.

Common Lesions Associated with Cyanosis

Celermajer DS. Adults with congenital heart disease: A comprehensive specialist service is needed. BMJ 1991;303:1413–1414.

Karr SS, Brenner JI, Loffredo C, et al. Tetralogy of Fallot. The spectrum of severity in a regional study, 1981–1985. Am J Dis Child 1992;146:121–124.

Kopf GS, Hellenbrand W, Kleinman C, et al. Repair of aortic coarctation in the first three months of life: Immediate and long-term results. Ann Thorac Surg 1986;41:425–430.

Madan A, Parisi M, Wood BP. Radiological case of the month. Am J Dis Child 1992;146:113–114.

Acute Rheumatic Fever and Rheumatic Heart Disease

Bland EF, Jones TD. Rheumatic fever and rheumatic heart disease: A twenty year report on 1000 patients followed since childhood. Circulation 1991;4:836–843.

Marcus RH, Sareli P, Pocock WA, et al. The spectrum of severe rheumatic mitral valve disease in a developing country. Correlations among clinical presentation, surgical pathologic findings, and hemodynamic sequelae. Ann Intern Med 1994;120:177–183.

Special Writing Group of the Committee on Rheumatic Fever, Endocarditis, and Kawasaki Disease of the Council on Cardiovascular Disease in the Young of the American Heart Association: Guidelines for the diagnosis of rheumatic fever. Jones criteria, 1992 update. JAMA 1992;268:2069–2073.

Stollerman GH. Variation in Group A streptococci and the prevalence of rheumatic fever: A half-century vigil. Ann Intern Med 1993;118:467–469.

Taquini AC, Massell BF, Walsh BJ. Phonocardiographic studies of early mitral disease. Am Heart J 1940;20:295–303.

Veasy LG, Tani LY, Hill HR. Persistence of acute rheumatic fever in the intermountain area of the United States. J Pediatr 1994;124:9–16.

Wald ER. Acute rheumatic fever. Curr Probl Pediatr 1993;23:264–270.

Wu M, Lue H, Wang J, et al. Implications of mitral valve prolapse in children with rheumatic mitral regurgitation. J Am Coll Cardiol 1994;23:1199–1203.

Infective Endocarditis

Awadallah SM, Kavey REW, Byrum CJ, et al. The changing pattern of infective endocarditis in childhood. Am J Cardiol 1991;68:90–94.

Baltimore RS. Infective endocarditis in children. Pediatr Infect Dis J 1992;11:907–913.

Bayer AS. Infective endocarditis. Clin Infect Dis 1993;17:313–322.

Bayer AS, Ward JI, Ginzton LE, et al. Evaluation of new clinical criteria for the diagnosis of infective endocarditis. Am J Med 1994;96:211–218.

Blumberg EA, Robbins N, Adimora A, et al. Persistent fever in association with infective endocarditis. Clin Infect Dis 1992;15:983–990.

Carpenter JL. Perivalvular extension of infection in patients with infectious endocarditis. Rev Infect Dis 1991;13:127–138.

Dajani AS, Bisno AL, Chung KJ, et al. Prevention of bacterial endocarditis. Recommendations by the American Heart Association. JAMA 1990;264:2919–2922.

Fang G, Keys TF, Gentry LO, et al. Prosthetic valve endocarditis resulting from nosocomial bacteremia. A prospective, multicenter study. Ann Intern Med 1993;119:560–567.

Freedman LR. Editorial response: To prevent or not to prevent bacterial endocarditis—that is the question! Clin Infect Dis 1993;17:195–197.

Hansen D, Schmiegelow K, Jacobsen JR. Bacterial endocarditis in children: Trends in its diagnosis, course, and prognosis. Pediatr Cardiol 1992;13:198–203.

Saiman L, Prince A, Gersony WM. Pediatric infective endocarditis in the modern era. J Pediatr 1993;122:847–853.

Tolan RW, Kleiman MB, Frank M, et al. Operative intervention in active endocarditis in children: Report of a series of cases and review. Clin Infect Dis 1992;14:852–862.

Watanakunakorn C, Burkert T. Infective endocarditis at a large community teaching hospital, 1980–1990: A review of 210 episodes. Medicine 1993;72:90–102.

Gastrointestinal Disorders

17 Failure to Thrive and Malnutrition

Douglas S. Kerr

DILEMMAS IN UNDERSTANDING FAILURE TO THRIVE

Organic versus Non-organic Failure to Thrive

There are few greater challenges in pediatrics than that of evaluating and successfully intervening in the development of an infant who has "fallen off" the growth chart. The informed diagnostician knows that most of these infants generally have nothing intrinsically wrong with them. This is a most unwelcome thought because it may implicate the caretaker, who is apparently looking for help. At the same time, the physician realizes that there could be something seriously wrong with the infant (Tables 17–1 and 17–2). The chances are that this possible organic problem is not going to be obvious.

The physician must keep an open mind, be patient, remain nonjudgmental, and recognize his or her own responsibility and limitations. It is also important to realize that combinations of organic and non-organic failure to thrive may occur. In addition, a nonjudgmental approach will help in engaging the parents in a treatment plan. Parents may have lifelong personality disorders that include deep feelings of inadequacy, even though they may present themselves in an aggressive manner. Finally, the physician should not back out if the problem appears to be psychosocial or expect to resolve these dilemmas alone; various health professions should be involved in the diagnosis and treatment, including nursing, nutrition, social work, and behavioral pediatrics. Although initial improvement may come relatively rapidly, long-term resolution is likely to require prolonged multiprofessional involvement.

Failure to Thrive versus Infant Malnutrition

What is commonly called "failure to thrive" in more advantaged environments is no different than what is called "infant malnutrition" (or some variation thereof) in severely impoverished populations. The frequency and the probability of organic versus non-organic causes vary, but both possibilities must be kept in mind in any medical setting. In impoverished settings, physicians may assume that weight loss or growth failure is due to inadequate infant

Table 17–1. Etiology of Failure to Thrive

Mechanism	Disorders
Nonorganic	
Psychosocial	Poor maternal-child interaction, poor feeding technique, psychologically disturbed mother, unusual maternal nutritional beliefs, errors in formula preparation, emotional deprivation, dwarfism, child neglect
Organic	
Inability to suck, swallow, or masticate	CNS pathology (psychomotor retardation), neuromuscular disease (Werdnig-Hoffmann, myotonia congenita, dysautonomia)
Maldigestion, malabsorption	Cystic fibrosis, celiac disease, Schwachman-Diamond syndrome, chronic diarrhea, HIV
Poor nutrient utilization	Renal failure, renal tubular acidosis, inborn errors of metabolism
Vomiting	CNS abnormality (tumor, infection, increased pressure), metabolic toxin (inborn errors of amino or organic acid metabolism), intestinal obstruction (pyloric stenosis, malrotation), renal tubular disease
Regurgitation	Gastroesophageal reflux, hiatal hernia, rumination syndrome
Elevated metabolic rate	Thyrotoxicosis, chronic disease (bronchopulmonary dysplasia, heart failure), cancer, inflammatory lesions (SLE, inflammatory bowel disease, chronic infection), immunodeficiency diseases, burns
Reduced growth potential	Chromosomal disorders, primordial dwarfism, skeletal dysplasia, specific syndromes (fetal alcohol)

From Foye HR Jr, Sulkes SB. Developmental and behavioral pediatrics. *In* Behrman RE, Kliegman RM (eds). Nelson Essentials of Pediatrics, 2nd ed. Philadelphia: WB Saunders, 1994:37.
Abbreviations: CNS = central nervous system; SLE = systemic lupus erythematosus; HIV = human immunodeficiency virus.

Table 17–2. Some Causes of Failure to Thrive and Screening Tests

Cause	Screening Tests
Environmental and Psychosocial*	
Inadequate caloric intake	History; observation in hospital
Emotional deprivation and disruptions	History; observation in hospital
Rumination; chronic diarrhea, gastroesophageal reflux	History; observation in hospital
Anorexia nervosa and bulimia	History; examination
Secondary to impact of organic disease	History and observation
Organic	
Central nervous system abnormalities, infection	Neurodevelopmental assessment; transillumination of skull; brain CT or MRI
Gastrointestinal system	
Malabsorption, cystic fibrosis, inflammatory bowel disease, parasites, aganglionic megacolon; liver disease; food intolerance; celiac disease; gastroesophageal reflux	Examination of stools: stool fat, sweat test, stool ova and parasites; liver function tests; barium swallow, sedimentation rate, food challenge, intestinal biopsy
Partial cleft palate	Physical examination; observation of feeding
Chronic heart failure	Physical examination; chest roentgenography; echocardiography
Endocrine disorders	Growth chart; thyroid function tests; bone age, cortisol
Pulmonary disease	
Bronchopulmonary dysplasia; bronchiectasis; cystic fibrosis	Physical examination; chest roentgenography; tuberculin test, pulmonary function tests, sweat test
Renal disease	
Anomalies; infection; renal failure; renal tubular disorder	Urinalysis; blood urea nitrogen; ultrasound; urinary amino acid screen; urine pH
Chromosomal disorders or syndromes	
Turner syndrome	Chromosomal analysis; identification of peculiar facies or multisystem defects, skeletal x-rays
Skeletal dysplasias	
Other metabolic or inborn errors	Urine amino and organic acid screen
Chronic infection	
Tuberculosis, mycotic, congenital, AIDS	Tuberculin test; appropriate laboratory identification of infectious agent
Chronic inflammation	
Juvenile rheumatoid arthritis, SLE	Physical examination; sedimentation rate; CBC, ANA
Immunodeficiency disease	
DiGeorge syndrome; combined immunodeficiency	History of rash and diarrhea; thymus size; tonsil size; skin tests; complete blood count
AIDS or AIDS-related complex	HIV test
Malignancies (kidney, hematologic, adrenal, brain)	Roentgenography of abdomen, chest; ultrasonography; brain CT or MRI, bone marrow
Congenital syndromes caused by alcohol, Dilantin, drugs, infection	Physical examination; history, TORCH evaluation

Modified from Barbero GJ. Failure to thrive. *In* Behrman RE (ed). Nelson Textbook of Pediatrics, 14th ed. Philadelphia: WB Saunders, 1992:215.
*Nonorganic may also be combined with organic.
Abbreviations: AIDS = acquired immunodeficiency syndrome; CBC = complete blood count; CT = computed tomography; HIV = human immunodeficiency virus; MRI = magnetic resonance imaging; SLE = systemic lupus erythematosus; ANA = antinuclear antibodies; TORCH = toxoplasmosis, other, rubella, cytomegalovirus, herpes simplex.

feeding. Nonetheless, many of these infants in developing countries also have associated respiratory or, more often, gastrointestinal infections or infestations; some have less common underlying systemic problems. *Parenting disorders occur at all income levels.* One cannot assume that nutrition is adequate for an infant raised in a wealthy home, nor should one attribute lack of adequate infant nutrition to poverty. Most infants reared under conditions of severe poverty do not become malnourished unless there is widespread famine or a disaster. The psychosocial profiles that have emerged from studies in more affluent settings of parents whose infants have non-organic failure to thrive and from studies of parents of malnourished infants in impoverished settings are similar. Therefore, the principles guiding diagnostic and intervention strategies for infants in either environment should be the same.

INTERPRETATION OF GROWTH CHARTS

The definition of failure to thrive starts with analysis of growth charts. The more data one has, the better; however, this information may not be available because of lack of prior medical care or change of medical setting. The accuracy of the data should be questioned and confirmed. Measurements of length are the most susceptible to error. Possible errors in weight, head circumference, date of birth, or plotting on the growth chart should all be considered. Once one has the correct data, the charts should be examined to answer the following questions:

- Are the measurements of length, weight, and head circumference proportionate? Is this a proportionately small infant? Is this a thin infant? Has the head grown proportionately?
- How severe are the deficits of each measurement, relative to what is expected (in units of normal developmental age, standard deviation, or percentile)?
- What is the chronology of development of deficits? When did the problem start and progress? Is this an acute or chronic problem?

It is useful to look at the growth chart even before one obtains a history or examines the infant because one then has a sense of how serious the problem is, which questions to ask, and which of the various diagnostic categories are most probable.

Although weight is usually the most readily available measurement in various pediatric settings, measurement of length is particularly critical, since it serves as the point of reference for other measurements. For accurate measurement of an infant's length the following are required:

1. A hard surface, such as an examining table (without a mattress) or a special measuring table or board.
2. A stable, fixed upright square (90°) end against which to place the top of the head.
3. A movable, sliding upright square (90°) end to press against the feet.
4. A nonstretchable, straight, accurate measuring tape.
5. Two people to assist in obtaining the measurement—one to hold the infant's head against the head board and straighten the neck and shoulders and the other to hold down the knees and press the sliding foot board firmly up against the infant's feet while measuring or noting the exact position of the slider.

The best way to obtain accurate length measurements is to use a specially constructed device designed with these features (e.g., a reclining stadiometer). In the absence of such a device, one can use a table or desk with the infant's head pressed against the wall and a firm square box or thick textbook for the sliding footer. Measurements obtained with the infant lying on a mattress and marked with a pen on the sheet are not accurate. As a result of the difficulty of inexperienced personnel in obtaining accurate length

measurements, it is highly recommended that the measurements be taken again and confirmed.

The choice of growth curves is important; reliable age and sex-specific growth charts based on data from the National Center for Health Statistics are widely available, and more sensitive weight and height increment standards for various ages of infancy have been established. Measurements for infants (ages 0 to 36 months) are all in length (recumbent), and measurements for children (ages 2 to 18 years) are all in height (standing). Although it is optimal to have population-specific growth charts, these are less important for infants younger than 2 years of age, since there is little difference between populations at this young age (population and genetic differences become increasingly important for older children). Conventions differ in whether to plot age in relation to actual birth date or to use corrected gestational age. The difference, of course, is greatest for very young infants. Beyond the equivalent of 40 weeks of gestation, it really does not matter which method is used, as long as it is used consistently and as long as the interpretation takes into account the method used.

Because infants with failure to thrive will, by definition, have fallen off their growth charts, the usual convention of expressing growth measurements in relation to normal percentiles is not likely to be very useful. The first step in interpretation should be to look at the length. What percentile (or how many standard deviations below or above the median—50%) does the length fall, and what is the age at which the infant's actual length corresponds to the median (the "length age")?

Next, the actual weight should be related to the expected-weight-for-length. The expected-weight-for-length can be determined by either of two methods: on the weight/age graph, this is the median (50%) of weight for the length age; on the direct graph of length and weight independent of age (which is included with most current versions of infant growth charts), this is the median weight for length. The difference of actual weight and expected-weight-for-length can then be expressed as a percentage (or percentile, if within two standard deviations). A ±10% variation of weight-for-length is within the normal range for infants. Some conventions classify the severity of wasting or "malnutrition" by the weight deficit. If this is done, it should be clear whether one is comparing actual weight with expected-weight-for-age or expected-weight-for-length (the latter is recommended). Loss of about 40% of expected-weight-for-length (actual weight/expected-weight-for-length = 60%) is the extreme of wasting compatible with survival. Therefore, 80% to 90% actual weight/expected-weight-for-length corresponds to mild wasting, 70% to 80% is moderate, and 60% to 70% is severe. These calculations are critical to planning nutritional rehabilitation and therefore essential to the overall diagnostic and treatment processes.

Measurements of head circumference can also be best interpreted if the measurements are expressed in relation to length age. In other words, it makes sense to express the actual head circumference as a "head-circumference-age," which can then be compared with the length age. If a child's head has grown proportionately with length, these developmental "ages" will be the same. It is important to note the following points:

1. *Infants who are small but have grown proportionately should be considered to have primary growth problems, including various endocrine and skeletal disorders* (see Chapter 62).
2. *Infants who have had inadequate feeding or assimilation or chronic illness are likely, at some point, to be abnormally thin.* If the problem developed at some time after birth, one would expect weight to drop off before growth in length or head circumference.
3. *Infants with disproportionately small heads may have primary neurologic problems affecting brain growth,* since head growth is the last to be affected by primary malnutrition and is not characteristic of primary skeletal growth problems.

Several examples of how one might interpret these patterns are presented in Figures 17–1 to 17–4.

Text continued on page 250

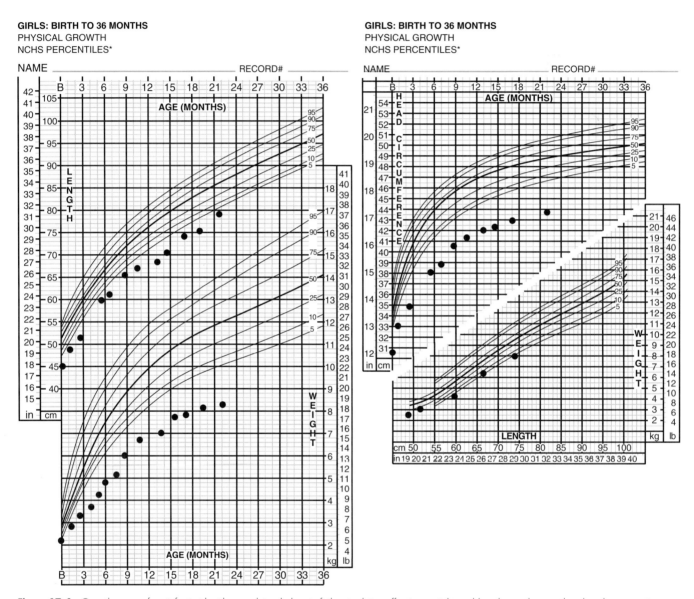

Figure 17–1. Growth curve of an infant girl with unexplained chronic failure to thrive affecting weight and head growth more than length, suggesting an organic disorder. Intrauterine growth retardation without postnatal catch-up growth is demonstrated (see Chapter 62). (Adapted from National Center for Health Statistics: NCHS Growth Charts, 1976. Monthly Vital Statistics Report. Vol 25, No. 3, Suppl (HRA) 76-1120. Health Resources Administration, Rockville, Md, June 1976. Data from The Fels Research Institute, Yellow Springs, Ohio. © 1976, Ross Laboratories.)

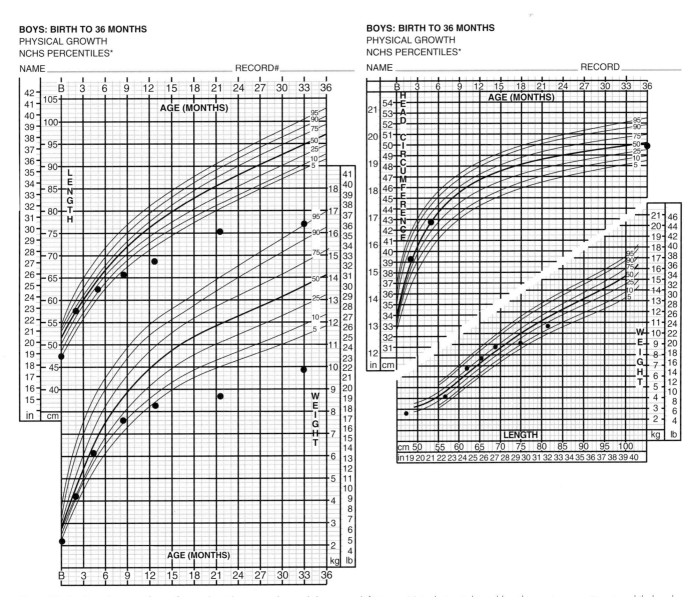

Figure 17–2. Growth curve of an infant male with untreated growth hormone deficiency. Note that weight and length remain proportionate, while head growth is less affected. (Adapted from National Center for Health Statistics: NCHS Growth Charts, 1976. Monthly Vital Statistics Report. Vol 25, No. 3, Suppl (HRA) 76-1120. Health Resources Administration, Rockville, Md, June 1976. Data from The Fels Research Institute, Yellow Springs, Ohio. © 1976, Ross Laboratories.)

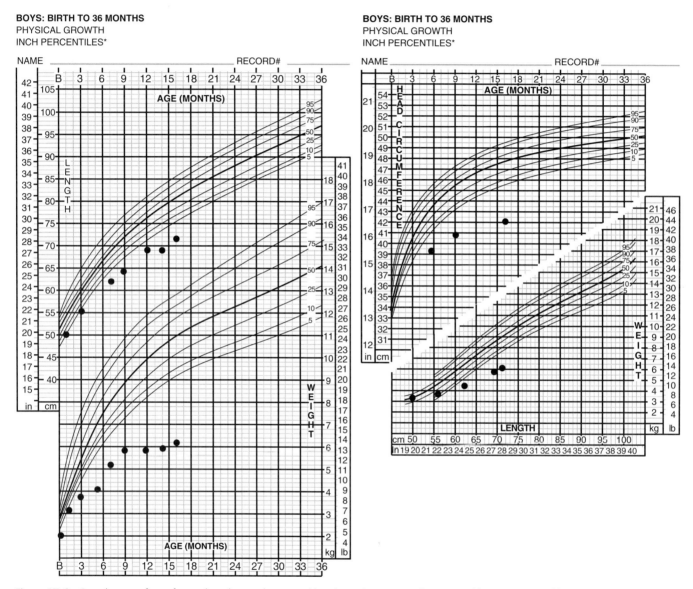

Figure 17–3. Growth curve of an infant male with severely impaired head growth, poor weight gain, and less impairment of length. Most obvious is the marked microcephaly associated with developmental delay suggestive of an underlying neurologic disorder. (Adapted from National Center for Health Statistics: NCHS Growth Charts, 1976, Monthly Vital Statistics Report. Vol 25, No. 3, Suppl (HRA) 76-1120. Health Resources Administration, Rockville, Md, June 1976. Data from The Fels Research Institute, Yellow Springs, Ohio. © 1976, Ross Laboratories.)

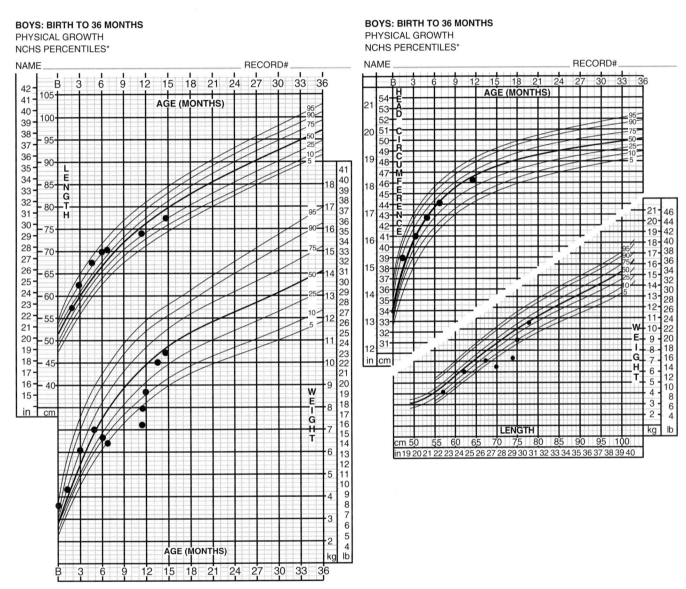

Figure 17–4. Growth curve of an infant male with acute weight loss and catch-up weight gain. Prior to 4½ months, there was normal growth while breast-feeding. After a change to an inadequate weaning diet, severe weight loss developed but less impairment of length occurred. Head size was not affected. An acute episode of diarrhea led to multiple dietary changes that resulted in further weight loss. With a proper diet history, nutritional rehabilitation with a balanced diet resolved this child's problem. (Adapted from National Center for Health Statistics: NCHS Growth Charts, 1976. Monthly Vital Statistics Report. Vol 25, No. 3, Suppl (HRA) 76-1120. Health Resources Administration, Rockville, Md, June 1976. Data from The Fels Research Institute, Yellow Springs, Ohio. © 1976, Ross Laboratories.)

GENERAL DIAGNOSTIC CONSIDERATIONS
(see Table 17–1)

Environmental (Non-organic) Disorders

INADEQUATE FEEDING OR NUTRITION

The most common form of failure to thrive is usually called infant malnutrition. Although this phenomenon is much more frequent in impoverished societies or in environments disrupted by war, famine, or other disasters, infant malnutrition occurs in all countries and at all socioeconomic levels. This possibility, however unlikely as it may seem, should be the first consideration in evaluation of any infant with failure to thrive, because the diagnostic and therapeutic interventions that will be beneficial should be provided early rather than late in the evaluation. Social and dietary histories can be misleading in these situations because of parental denial, which makes the physician reluctant to consider what is most likely. The presence of an associated chronic illness does not necessarily preclude the possibility that the infant's lack of weight gain may in part be due to inadequate nutrition. This may even happen within hospitals, where routine nutritional support may be overlooked as a result of preoccupation of the professional staff with complex medical and surgical problems.

In a retrospective review of medical records of 185 infants hospitalized for failure to thrive at a large metropolitan children's hospital, organic causes were proven in only 18% of the cases. In 58%, the final diagnosis was non-organic. In 24% of cases, no diagnosis was made but non-organic causes were suspected. In another review of 82 infants hospitalized for failure to thrive, non-organic causes were noted in 39%, organic causes in 26%, and both organic and non-organic causes in 23%. In rural primary care settings or environments where primary infant malnutrition is prevalent, the percentage of patients who respond to nutritional rehabilitation without evidence of a significant chronic underlying organic illness may exceed 95%.

DISTURBED PARENTING RELATIONSHIP

It is difficult to separate the nurturing of infants from their nutrition. Even in impoverished populations, most infants do not become malnourished, but parents of the affected infants are more likely to have limited coping skills. Therefore, regardless of socioeconomic status, one should always be sensitive to the importance of evaluating the adequacy of parenting in these cases. In some cases, parental neglect may be initially obvious. More commonly, parental concern at first may seem adequate, but after one becomes more familiar with the case and has made more direct observations, serious problems become apparent. The reverse error of initially assuming that parents are failing to provide for their infant may interfere with appropriate diagnostic recognition of an underlying disease. Therefore, *the evaluation of all cases of failure to thrive should include a thorough, nonjudgmental, psychosocial assessment.* This component of the evaluation should be started as soon as possible and continued through the diagnostic and treatment phases, since it usually takes time to obtain the full picture. Direct observations of parent-infant interactions and reactions of parents to evaluation and treatment can provide useful clues.

Specific Organic Disorders

There are so many possible diseases of infants that may be associated with failure to thrive that a thorough description of

alternatives constitutes an exhausting list (see Tables 17–1 and 17–2). Because almost any serious chronic illness may result in failure to thrive in an infant, one must keep in mind a broad diagnostic screening approach (directed by the history and physical findings) to these disorders while simultaneously considering the more likely possibility that there is nothing primarily wrong with the infant (see Table 17–2).

Frustrating as this approach may appear, *in most cases of chronic illness, there is likely to be some clue provided in the history or physical examination, supplemented with selected standard diagnostic laboratory screening tests.* The few rare cases of organic failure to thrive that pass through these early detection nets become evident once one discovers that the infant does not respond to nutritional rehabilitation. If, however, one attempts to pursue every conceivable diagnostic test for organic causes of failure to thrive before implementing vigorous nutritional rehabilitation, one is likely to run out of time, patience, and resources and to come to no conclusion. Some unusual cases may take months or years to unravel while they are under the scrutiny of the best of physicians.

Combined Non-organic and Organic Disorders

It is not uncommon for failure to thrive to result from a combination of several causes. For example, a severely malnourished child is likely to have had recurrent infections as well as inadequate nutritional support. A developmentally delayed child born to young parents who are overwhelmed may not receive optimal nurturing. Therefore, even after reaching a presumptive diagnostic conclusion in a particular case, the physician must keep open diagnostic alternatives until the child is fully recovered and thriving in the original environment.

Disorders of Undetermined or Unresolved Etiology

Finally, in a significant number of cases, one never identifies the cause or is never quite sure that the tentative diagnosis is the correct one. As with other types of chronic disabilities, such as mental retardation, these are the most frustrating experiences to deal with and the hardest in which to successfully maintain a physician-parent relationship. The only solution is to make every effort to stay involved, to maintain a relationship, and to keep an open mind to all possibilities not yet considered or to re-examine the previous assumptions and data that may have interfered with discovery of the actual diagnosis.

INITIAL EVALUATION

The initial diagnosis of failure to thrive is based largely on measurements of length and weight, but much can be learned from the first visit, which serves as a tentative guide to the longer evaluation that follows.

History and Observation

A comprehensive detailed history is essential, including the story of pregnancy and delivery, newborn course, subsequent illnesses, review of systems, and family and social histories. It is worth emphasizing a few questions that may be particularly useful for developing clues to the parent-infant relationship. These questions are designed to determine the initial acceptance and attachment of the parents to the child, the parental perception of seriousness of the child's condition and beliefs about cause, their description of feeding behavior and development, and the parents' relationship with each other (Table 17–3). These questions need to be asked in a nonjudgmental, nonthreatening manner. Some physicians may feel reluctant to ask these questions because they believe that parents will perceive them as intrusive or accusatory. However, most parents of children with organic causes of failure to thrive have little difficulty responding; a hostile or defensive response should be noted as cause for concern.

Further questions about the time course of diet changes, illnesses, and changes in the family situation (especially changes of caretakers or separations) subsequently can be related to the infant's growth curve (see Figs. 17–1 to 17–4). Has the child had appropriate routine pediatric care, including immunizations? A detailed nutritional history is very important, but caution is needed as to the quantitative accuracy of how much infants eat. This is particularly true if other health professionals have already questioned the adequacy of nutritional support. An exaggerated description of quantity consumed or introduction of inappropriate foods into the infant's diet (e.g., fruit juices) may increase a physician's suspicion. Assessment of parental perceptions of developmental progress subsequently can be related to one's own assessment. A thorough review of systems is essential for detection of unusual causes of failure to thrive; the physician must be attentive to descriptions of unexplained details, which initially may not make much sense but later may turn out to be valuable clues. Finally, extra time is needed for the family medical and social histories, since in most cases this is the information on which the answers and opportunities for intervention will depend.

While this interview is being conducted, the physician should observe how the parent interacts with the child and other individuals. Are emotions expressed appropriately? How comfortably is the infant held? This may be an excellent opportunity to have the responsible parent feed the infant and note whether or not the feeding techniques are age-appropriate and supportive. Does the baby seem hungry, suck appropriately, and keep the milk down?

Physical Examination

The general appearance of the infant is likely to be the most useful part of the physical examination.

Is the infant alert and appropriately developed for age?

Does he or she establish eye contact, show normal anxiety during separation from the parent or reactive passively without crying?

Table 17–3. Questions to Include in the Initial Interview with Parents of Infants with Failure to Thrive

---

1. How did you feel when you first learned that you were pregnant? Was it a difficult pregnancy?

2. How did your baby look to you right after birth? Was your baby difficult to take care of then? Since then?

3. How do you feel your child is doing? Are you concerned that there might be something wrong? If so, do you have an opinion as to what is causing this problem?

4. Who helps you in the care of your child? What is their opinion as to how he or she is developing? Do you and your spouse or partner share responsibility? Do you agree?

Is there wasting (indicating more recent weight loss) or is the infant proportionately small (indicating chronic growth failure)?

Does the infant appear well-cared for?

Has the hair grown properly, and is the skin and hair pigmentation and texture appropriate, as further evidence of nutritional status?

Are there any scars, bruises, or unexplained marks suggestive of child abuse? (See Chapter 37).

Are there signs of specific vitamin or mineral deficiencies (Tables 17–4 and 17–5)?

A thorough general examination that involves looking for dysmorphic features and specific system abnormalities may provide additional clues to organic causes. An accurate evaluation of the child's development should be planned, probably as a separate procedure but, in any case, as soon as possible.

Laboratory Screening Tests

A plan for choosing an appropriate initial battery of laboratory tests should include several general screening tests (complete blood count, urinalysis, serum electrolyte levels, blood urea nitrogen level) to detect treatable conditions that one would not want to miss and, in addition, specific tests that may have been suggested by the particular child's history and physical findings (see Table 17–2). Most tests can be done on a single outpatient visit with one blood sample, a urine sample, and if indicated, a trip to the radiology department. Additional specific tests need to be tailored to fit the situation, or they may be added later. For example, a child with developmental delay and failure to thrive may deserve a blood lead test, metabolic screening tests, a karyotype, imaging of the head, or a lumbar puncture, whereas a child with apparent malabsorption is evaluated completely differently.

Criteria for Hospitalization

Decisions about when to hospitalize an infant with failure to thrive are inevitably influenced by practical considerations of the available and quality of hospital services, cost, and distance from the family. The medical issues are whether hospitalization will facilitate further diagnostic steps and whether the affected child is severely enough malnourished to create a sense of urgency about nutritional rehabilitation. Loss of more than 30% of the average weight for length (to less than 70% of expected weight for length) constitutes severe malnutrition, which most physicians would be reluctant to treat on an outpatient basis unless there is no satisfactory alternative.

Sufficient time must be anticipated in the hospital for substantial recovery; in severe cases, full recovery requires about 6 weeks. After initial stabilization and reassurance that the infant is doing well, the child can spend much of this recovery period in a less expensive, non-intensive supervised medical care facility that emphasizes nutritional support and psychosocial stimulation. Hospitals located in environments with extremely limited resources may be overcrowded with children who have severe contagious diseases; such an environment is usually disastrous for vulnerable, malnourished infants. Creative approaches to well-organized outpatient day programs or frequent home visiting by properly trained health care workers may provide an attractive alternative.

COMPLETE HOSPITAL EVALUATION AND TREATMENT

Management of Acute Needs

The first priority in the care of these vulnerable infants is to look after their most acute needs, which frequently may be precipitating

Table 17–4. Characteristics of Vitamin Deficiencies

Vitamin	Purpose	Deficiency	Comments	Source
Water-Soluble				
Thiamine (B_1)	Coenzyme in ketoacid decarboxylation (e.g., pyruvate → acetyl-CoA transketolase reaction)	*Beri-beri:* polyneuropathy, calf tenderness, heart failure, edema, ophthalmoplegia	Inborn errors of lactate metabolism; boiling milk destroys B_1	Liver, meat, milk, cereals, nuts, legumes
Riboflavin (B_2)	FAD coenzyme in oxidation-reduction reactions	Anorexia, mucositis, anemia, cheilosis, nasolabial seborrhea	Photosensitizer	Milk, cheese, liver, meat, eggs, whole grains, green leafy vegetables
Niacin (B_3)	NAD coenzyme in oxidation-reduction reactions	*Pellagra:* photosensitivity, dermatitis, dementia, diarrhea, death	Tryptophan is a precursor	Meat, fish, liver, whole grains, green leafy vegetables
Pyridoxine (B_6)	Cofactor in amino acid metabolism	Seizures, hyperacusis, microcytic anemia, nasolabial seborrhea, neuropathy	Dependency state; deficiency secondary to drugs	Meat, liver, whole grains, peanuts, soybeans
Pantothenic acid	Coenzyme A in Krebs cycle	None reported	—	Meat, vegetables
Biotin	Cofactor in carboxylase reactions of amino acids	Alopecia, dermatitis, hypotonia, death	Bowel resection, inborn errors of metabolism and ingestion of raw eggs	Yeast, meats; made by intestinal flora
B_{12}	Coenzyme for 5-methyl-tetrahydrofolate formation; DNA synthesis	Megaloblastic anemia, peripheral neuropathy, posterior lateral column disease, vitiligo	Vegans; fish tapeworm; transcobalamin or intrinsic factor deficiencies	Meat, fish, cheese, eggs
Folate	DNA synthesis	Megaloblastic anemia	Goat milk deficient; drug antagonists; heat inactivates	Liver, greens, vegetables, cereals, cheese
Ascorbic acid (C)	Reducing agent; collagen metabolism	*Scurvy:* irritability, purpura, bleeding gums, periosteal hemorrhage, aching bones	May improve tyrosine metabolism in preterm infants	Citrus fruits, green vegetables; cooking destroys it
Fat-Soluble				
A	Epithelial cell integrity; vision	Night blindness, xerophthalmia, Bitot spots, follicular hyperkeratosis	Common with protein-calorie malnutrition; malabsorption	Liver, milk, eggs, green and yellow vegetables, fruits
D	Maintain serum calcium, phosphorus levels	*Rickets:* reduced bone mineralization	Prohormone of 25- and 1,25-vitamin D	Fortified milk, cheese, liver
E	Antioxidant	Hemolysis in preterm infants; areflexia, ataxia, ophthalmoplegia	May benefit patients with G6PD deficiency	Seeds, vegetables, germ oils, green leafy vegetables
K	Post-translation carboxylation of clotting factors II, VII, IX, X and proteins C, S	Prolonged prothrombin time; hemorrhage; elevated PIVKA (protein induced in vitamin K absence)	Malabsorption; breast-fed infants	Liver, green vegetables; made by intestinal flora

Modified from Tershakovec A, Stallings VA. Pediatric nutrition and nutritional disorders. *In* Behrman RE, Kliegman RM (eds). Nelson Essentials of Pediatrics, 2nd ed. Philadelphia: WB Saunders, 1994:74.

Abbreviations: FAD = flavin adenine dinucleotide; G6PD = glucose-6-phosphate dehydrogenase; NAD = nicotinamide adenine dinucleotide.

Table 17–5. Characteristics of Mineral Deficiencies

Mineral	Function	Manifestations of Deficiency	Comments	Sources
Iron	Heme-containing macromolecules (e.g., hemoglobin, cytochrome, myoglobin)	Anemia, spoon nails, reduced muscle and mental performance	History of pica, cow's milk, gastrointestinal bleeding	Liver, eggs, grains
Copper	Redox reactions (e.g., cytochrome oxidase)	Hypochromic anemia, neutropenia, osteoporosis, hypotonia, hypoproteinemia	Inborn error, Menkes kinky hair syndrome	Liver, oysters, meat, nuts, grains, legumes, chocolate
Zinc	Metalloenzymes (e.g., alkaline phosphatase, carbonic anhydrase, DNA polymerase; wound healing)	*Acrodermatitis enteropathica;* poor growth, acro-orificial rash, alopecia, delayed sexual development, hypogeusia, infection	Protein–calorie malnutrition; weaning; malabsorption syndrome	Meat, grains, cheese, nuts
Selenium	Antioxidant Glutathione peroxidase	Keshan cardiomyopathy in China	Endemic areas; long-term TPN	Meat, vegetables
Chromium	Insulin cofactor	Poor weight gain, glucose intolerance, neuropathy	Protein–calorie malnutrition, long-term TPN	Yeast, breads
Fluoride	Strengthen dental enamel	Caries	Supplementation during tooth growth, narrow therapeutic range, fluorosis may cause staining of the teeth	Seafood, water
Iodine	Thyroxine, tri-iodothyronine production	Simple endemic goiter *Myxedematous cretinism:* congenital hypothyroidism *Neurologic cretinism:* mental retardation, deafness, spasticity, normal T_4 level at birth	Endemic in New Guinea, the Congo; endemic in Great Lakes area prior to iodized salt	Seafood, iodized salt, most food in nonendemic areas

From Tershakovec AM, Stallings VA. Pediatric nutrition and nutritional disorders. *In* Behrman RE, Kliegman RM (eds). Nelson Essentials of Pediatrics, 2nd ed. Philadelphia: WB Saunders, 1994:81.
Abbreviation: TPN = total parenteral nutrition.

factors leading to hospitalization. This includes acute infections (especially respiratory, gastrointestinal, skin, and systemic sepsis), dehydration (usually secondary to diarrhea), acute electrolyte disturbances, and anemia. Because typical signs of infection, such as fever and leukocytosis, may not be present, one should not rely on clinical evaluation of altered physiologic homeostasis, behavior, or appetite. When there is doubt, appropriate treatment for suspected sepsis after obtaining blood, urine, and possibly CSF specimens for culture may be indicated. Severely malnourished infants are likely to be moderately volume-depleted, but they probably will avidly retain sodium and water and may easily become edematous if they are rehydrated too vigorously. Potassium depletion is likely to be significant, and the electrolytes must be replaced, either parenterally or orally. In most cases, oral rehydration and initiation of feeding will be possible shortly after admission, but if diarrhea or other factors prevent enteral support, intravenous fluids and possibly parenteral nutrition need to be considered.

Nutritional Strategy and Methods

The goal of nutritional intervention for infants with failure to thrive is to attempt to make them thrive. In most cases, this means short-term rapid, substantial weight gain. If this goal is achieved in an unequivocal way, the benefit is both diagnostic and therapeutic.

If not, the benefit is to turn attention to organic disorders that may be interfering with nutritional assimilation and weight gain.

The potential for deficit replacement can be measured as the difference between weight and expected-weight-for-length (after correction of acute dehydration or edema). This difference is a simple, albeit indirect, measure of depletion of stored energy reserves. The major form of stored body energy is fat, for both infants and adults. Stored carbohydrate, in the form of glycogen, is relatively trivial, accounting for not more than one day's energy reserves. About half of total body protein, primarily skeletal muscle, can be sacrificed to meet energy requirements during starvation. In a healthy adult, these energy reserves can provide maintenance requirement for 3 months (longer in an obese person), provided that there is an adequate intake of water. By contrast, in a typical 1-year-old infant, stored energy reserves are depleted within 3 weeks because of the much greater rate of required energy utilization relative to body weight in the infant. This difference accounts for the more rapid dramatic effects of starvation on infants than adults in acute famine situations or, more commonly, in response to recurrent acute infections in environments with endemic malnutrition. Rapid replenishment of this deficit is the objective of nutritional rehabilitation. In practice, it is realistic to attempt to replace this deficit in a controlled environment as rapidly as this deficit would have developed had the infant not eaten at all.

To help the infant achieve such rapid weight gain and rehabilitation, one must provide an intake that dramatically exceeds the

$$\text{weight change (kg)} = \frac{\text{total energy intake} - \text{maintenance utilization (kcal)}}{\text{energy value of weight change (kcal/kg)}} \quad (1)$$

$$\text{energy value (``cost'') of weight change} = (\sim) \ 6000 \text{ kcal/kg or 6 kcal/g} \quad (2)$$

infant's "normal" nutritional needs. Most of normal nutritional requirements are utilized to meet maintenance requirements; for a typical 1-year-old infant, about 95% of the total energy consumed is required to maintain constant body weight and only about 5% is utilized for growth. Therefore, *if one doubles the infant's total energy intake, so as to provide every day for that day's requirements plus making-up for one day when the infant was not eating, one effectively is increasing the amount of energy available for weight gain 20-fold, and very rapid weight gain will occur.*

These considerations are based on actual clinical practice and illustrate the quantitative relationship between energy intake and weight gain in a variety of clinical situations, ranging from small infants to obese adults. The amount of weight gain or loss can be predicted from measurements of intake by the equations above.

Although this estimate of the energy value or "cost" of weight change is derived from actual clinical experience, in principle this value is between the values that would be predicted for pure fat or pure protein. The "cost" of 6 kcal/g corresponds to a theoretical estimate of the composition of weight change, which is about 50% fat (4.5 kcal/g), 25% protein (1.0 kcal/g), and 25% water, with the difference (0.5 kcal/g) accounted for by the biosynthetic or catabolic cost of metabolic energy converted to heat. Differences between observed weight gain and predicted weight gain are to be expected in the short term and are largely due to changes in body water.

These calculations can be used to determine how much total amount of formula or food intake will be required for full recovery and to determine how rapidly weight gain can be expected to occur at different levels of intake (Table 17–6). In this example, the maximum rate of recovery shown corresponds to a reversal of the body weight (energy) deficit within the same amount of time that this might have developed if the infant had not been fed at all, that is, each day the infant is fed enough to meet the current day's requirement plus enough extra to replace the equivalent of one previous day's requirement (when the infant had not eaten).

This example has been somewhat simplified. In reality, the infant's daily energy requirements will gradually increase in relation to increased weight and activity; therefore, the total intake actually needs to be increased somewhat more than that shown.

The outdated belief that malnourished infants have higher than normal maintenance energy requirements in relation to body weight has proved to be incorrect by careful indirect calorimetry measurements.

For rapid recovery to happen, two considerations are critical. One is the composition of the formula utilized, which must be significantly enriched to achieve intakes in the range of twice normal maintenance. Second, intake and assimilation of nutrients depend on an infection-free status, which is the most common interfering factor in nutritional rehabilitation; even infants who are initially infection-free may acquire acute respiratory or gastrointestinal infections while they are in the hospital.

There is a misconception that severely malnourished individuals, particularly infants, are too delicate and cannot or should not be fed ordinary formulas or foods by mouth. Acute precipitating complications are common in this population and require prompt attention. However, the concept is misguided, in that a severely malnourished infant without a complicating acute infection or gastroenteritis is likely to be very hungry and is quite capable of consuming and assimilating most standard nutritional products efficiently. Since one does not know initially how much an infant may or may not tolerate, it is reasonable to start with a standard infant formula or whatever formula the infant reportedly tolerated best at home. If there is evidence for gastroenteritis, it would be prudent to dilute this formula initially to lower the osmolality. However, use of diluted formulas should be considered *transitional* only and should be advanced as rapidly as possible to initiate effective rehabilitation.

To provide a very high energy intake, it is necessary to utilize techniques that increase caloric density without excessively increasing osmolality. The major solute in milk or various infant formulas is carbohydrate (lactose, sucrose, maltose, or glucose). If the formula is concentrated by adding less water to the starting powder or concentrate, high osmolality becomes the limiting factor. A standard formula (20 kcal/ounce) has an osmolality of approximately 270 mOsm/l (Table 17–7); a typical concentrated version of 27 kcal/ounce has an osmolality of 360 mOsm/l, which is about the maximum that can be tolerated without diarrhea. On the other hand, changes in the fat content of formulas do not alter their osmolality, since fat is not a solute. Manufacturers preparing standard infant formulas start with cow's milk powder or concentrate, usually after removing the butterfat, and then add vegetable oil and lactose to end up with a formula that is more like human milk than cow's milk. This is possible because cow's milk contains about three times as much protein in relation to energy as human milk; human milk is relatively higher in fat than cow's milk (see Table 17–7).

With these concepts in mind, a tolerable very-high-energy infant formula can be prepared by adding emulsified vegetable oil and a little carbohydrate (as lower osmolality dextrins) to fat-free or whole-fat cow's milk (Table 17–8). Because this formulation is based on dilution of excess high-quality protein with fat and carbohydrate, the protein-to-energy ratio (9%) remains equivalent to that recommended for infants. This should not be done starting with a standard infant milk or soy protein–based formula because the final protein content or quality would be too low. Since this enriched formula will be deficient in iron, supplementation with an iron source is essential; use of a complete multivitamin and mineral mixture suitable for infants is recommended.

Use of this type of formula, which provides twice the energy

Table 17–6. Relationship of Energy Intake to Recovery of Weight Deficit

Example:	Infant with failure to thrive, age 1 yr		
	Expected weight for length	=	10 kg
	Actual weight	=	7 kg
	Weight deficit	=	3 kg
	Energy deficit (6000 × 3)	=	18,000 kcal
	Maintenance energy (100 × 7)	=	700 kcal/day

Total Intake (kcal/day)	Excess Intake (kcal/day)	Weight Gain (g/day)	Recovery Time (Days)
700	0	0	∞
760	60	10	300
940	240	40	75
1660	960	160	18

Table 17–7. Comparison of Human Milk and Some Commonly Used Infant Formulas

Milk or Formula*	Energy (kcal/L)	Distribution (% kcal)			Sodium (mEq/L)	Potassium (mEq/L)	Potential Renal Solute Load (mOsm/L)	Osmolality (mOsm/L)
		Protein	*Fat*	*CHO*				
Human	740	6	56	38	7	14	79	273
Cow	670	21	50	29	22	35	230	260
Similac	670	9	48	43	8	18	108	270
Enfamil	670	9	50	41	8	18	97	270
SMA	670	9	48	43	7	14	91	270
Isomil	670	10	49	41	13	19	126	230
ProSobee	670	12	48	40	10	21	127	170
Nursoy	670	12	48	40	9	19	121	266

*Formula names and data are from Ross, Mead Johnson, and Wyeth Laboratories, respectively.
Abbreviation: CHO = carbohydrate.

density of a standard infant formula (40 kcal/ounce) without excessive osmolality (330 mOsm/l), makes it possible to provide in the same volume ordinarily consumed by an infant sufficient energy to ensure rapid weight gain if the infant is capable of responding. Practical use of such a nutritional rehabilitation scheme has been extensive with very positive results. Commercial products are now available that are intended to be used for the same purpose (e.g., Pediasure, Ross).

Some practical considerations in feeding these infants are as follows:

1. Start out gradually, but advance the volume of the feeds as rapidly as tolerated, *ad libitum*;
2. Give smaller, frequent feedings initially to prevent vomiting (every 3 hours);
3. Feed at least once during the night to significantly add to the total intake and shorten recovery.
4. Older infants can usually drink very efficiently from a cup.
5. Avoid giving significant amounts of "solid" food until after the child is approaching full recovery; the high-energy formula has a higher-energy density than do most infant foods, such as fruit and cereal.

500 g in a week ($7 \times 7 \times 60/6$). The responses observed are frequently dramatic and gratifying to both the professional staff and to the family. Doubts as to whether some obscure organic cause of failure to thrive has been overlooked will rapidly disappear. That is why this approach to rapid rehabilitation is important diagnostically. Given all the impediments to successful rapid rehabilitation, especially intercurrent infections, full recovery should be expected to require as long as 6 weeks for infants.

Failure to gain weight under these circumstances becomes a *red flag* and should be investigated. Is the intake as great as planned? Is the formula being properly prepared? Continued failure to take in an adequate amount of formula could be secondary to lack of appetite (because of an underlying illness), or due to impaired neurologic development. This type of observation should stimulate further diagnostic evaluation, since it is likely that there will be an organic component. Losses of intake from vomiting, diarrhea, or urinary excretion (diabetes mellitus) should be quite obvious; significant malabsorption is not associated with normal-appearing stools. Excessive energy utilization without weight gain is exceedingly rare but can be associated with hyperthyroidism or certain forms of mitochondrial dysfunction with uncoupled oxidative phosphorylation.

Evaluation of the Response to Nutritional Therapy

If the infant achieves an energy intake of at least 150 kcal/kg/day and, optimally, closer to 200 kcal/kg/day, there will be no question after a week as to whether or not the infant is responding. For example, a 7-kg infant fed 160 kcal/kg/day should gain nearly

Observations of the Parents and Infant

If an adequate nutritional rehabilitation program is successfully established, the priority must soon be turned during the recovery period from medical diagnosis to dealing with the underlying psychosocial issues. Continued evaluation of parental visiting and interactions with the infant and professional staff as well as periodic

Table 17–8. High-Energy Formula for Treatment of Infants with Failure to Thrive

Ingredient	Amount	Carbohydrate (g)	Protein (g)	Fat (g)	Energy (kcal)	Osmolality (mOsm)
Whole cow milk*	900 ml	44	32	33	603	234
Oil (emulsified)†	100 ml			50	450	32
Dextrins‡	75 g	71			284	75
TOTAL§	1000 ml	115	32	83	1337	341
% Total energy		34	10	56		

*Reconstituted whole dry milk or evaporated milk can be used; if low-fat milk is used, additional vegetable oil should be added.
†Calculations shown are for Microlipid (Sherwood), a safflower oil emulsion; other vegetable oils (50 g) can be used if the formula is homogenized vigorously in a blender.
‡Calculations shown are for Polycose (Ross); higher-molecular-weight dextrins are preferable to reduce osmolality.
§The total caloric density of this formula is 40 kcal/ounce.

re-evaluation of the infant's development should be documented. Intensive stimulation of the infant is likely to be rewarded with rapidly improving social and motor skills. The parents should be included as much as possible in feeding and stimulation of the infant so that they will become more sensitive to the infant's needs and will feel responsible for the progress made. The parent's own needs must be attended to, including repeated sessions with a medical social worker to review family relationships, their own childhood experiences, and identification of family and community resources that may be helpful in the care of the infant. Parents who do not visit regularly or who are critical of the staff and insensitive to their infant are likely to quickly antagonize those who are presiding over the infant's recovery. These are the most challenging and difficult cases, and extra effort is required. *Nonjudgmental encouragement of positive parental involvement requires the time of experienced, mature professional staff who are not preoccupied with more urgent medical crises.*

Transfer to a special setting where these priorities can be supportively attended to is usually beneficial. Following hospitalization, close outpatient monitoring and reassurance that the child is continuing to grow and develop normally are essential. This may involve home visiting and interaction of several different type of health care professionals.

EVALUATION OF ENVIRONMENTAL FACTORS

An understanding of some of the contributing environmental factors to non-organic failure to thrive helps one to recognize relevant evidence earlier and provides a more effective, nonjudgmental approach to the parents.

Infant Malnutrition in Impoverished Populations

Although infant malnutrition (failure to thrive) is common in impoverished nations, it is remarkable that only a minority of infants become malnourished under situations of extreme poverty. Even the most extreme estimates of severe malnutrition in these situations indicate fewer than 10% of all infants, and usually the problem is much less frequent. Malnutrition and potentially preventable infections account for most infant deaths and morbidity in poor, underdeveloped countries and are major correlates of impaired mental development.

Breast-feeding is probably the most frequently cited protective influence against infant malnutrition. Infants who breast-feed are much less likely to become malnourished than bottle-fed infants. Socioeconomic changes and cultural practices play a major role in whether a mother chooses breast-feeding. In developed countries, there has been a historical shift from breast-feeding to bottle-feeding and back to breast-feeding among the more advantaged populations, but this has not held true in underdeveloped countries. If bottle-fed infants are exposed to potentially contaminated water sources, acquired and recurrent gastroenteritis will contribute to malnutrition.

Common Personality Characteristics of Parents

Data are available to a limited extent from impoverished populations and more so from developed countries to indicate significant personality differences between parents of infants with non-organic failure to thrive and parents from similar socioeconomic status whose children have thrived. Mothers of infants hospitalized with malnutrition in Jamaica showed an increased probability of preoccupation with their own needs instead of the child's needs; frequent separation from their children and use of unreliable caretakers, transient relationships with men, difficulty keeping jobs, and dysfunctional enmeshment with their own families were observed. These findings are characteristic of "borderline personalities" and are remarkably similar to what has been described for mothers of failure to thrive infants in the United States and the United Kingdom. Such mothers have been described as depressed, deprived, hostile, blaming, overburdened, young, isolated, and ill. Infants of mothers with acute depression resulting from a recent loss or with postpartum depression appear to have a better prognosis for infant rehabilitation than do infants of angry, hostile mothers or mothers with chronic psychiatric disorders. Frequently, evidence of abnormal behavior is evident at the time of the first contact.

Relatively little is known about the fathers of infants with failure to thrive. Families in which infants develop failure to thrive more often have less adaptive relationships than in other families.

History of Nurturing and Support of the Parents

It seems highly probable, although it is difficult to document, that the parents of many infants with failure to thrive were themselves victims of deprivation during infancy and childhood. In some intensively evaluated parents of such infants, it is possible to determine that they themselves were separated from their own parents, that they recall exceptional family conflict, that they have difficulty in feeling close to their own parents, or that they may have even had a feeding problem in early childhood. Indeed, infants with failure to thrive who were observed prospectively and retested at age 3 showed significant deficits in behavioral organization and ego control. Although it may be impossible to document this type of information in most cases, it is important for health care professionals to recognize that behaviors that may seem incomprehensible or maddening are likely to be lifelong in origin and very difficult for the parents to change. This consideration, it is hoped, should make health professionals more tolerant and supportive of such parents who need support and who do not respond as one might prefer to negative judgments. Because parents may be very vulnerable to criticism, suggestions about how they should handle the infant are often interpreted as evidence of their inadequacy and may result in further detachment. On the other hand, consistent support of the parents' importance to the child and pointing out the infant's special attachment to them promote self-esteem and awareness that they are essential to their infant's well-being.

In some cases, the parents may be continuing to live under dysfunctional circumstances or may themselves be a victim of continuing abuse. It is valuable to inquire with questions such as:

Whom can they depend on?

What are current personal and financial stresses in their lives?

How is the parents' relationship working out?

Are there conflicts with the extended family?

Are there problems with alcohol or drugs?

Who is available among their friends or communities?

Where do the parents turn for health care or for emotional support?

Long-Term Developmental Outcome

There is considerable reason to be concerned about the long-term effects of severe failure to thrive on subsequent growth and mental development. Many, but not all, infants with severe malnutrition or failure to thrive do not perform as well as their peers when they reach school age. However, because sometimes it is impossible to distinguish nutrition from other forms of parental nurturing of these infants, the mechanisms of how mental development is impaired and exactly which infants are at greatest risk are not clear.

A study of school-age developmental outcome of siblings who were or were not malnourished as infants showed that infants who became malnourished in a household that was considered socially "favorable" (evidence of infant stimulation in the home, including available toys, and evidence of parental playing and talking with the children) did better than infants who had been equally malnourished but had lived in a socially "unfavorable" home. Some pediatricians who have followed up children who had severe organic failure to thrive caused by treatable organic disorders as infants find that future mental development may be normal or well above average; this suggests that nutritional insufficiency alone does not necessarily impair mental development. Unfortunately, because most infants who have "environmental" failure to thrive or malnutrition are likely to suffer both nutritional and parental deprivation, the outcome usually is not favorable.

EARLY RECOGNITION OF RISK AND INTERVENTION

Identification of Parents or Infants at Risk

If families in which infants are likely to be at greater risk could be identified, limited resources for intervention or prevention could be focused more efficiently. Various intervention or follow-up programs are based on this premise, i.e., providing special help for very young mothers, parents of infants with disabilities, or "high-risk" parents of low-birth-weight infants. For the average provider of infant health care, identification of risk is based on routine child care, including prospective nutritional counseling and frequent monitoring of growth and development. Missed appointments, lack of immunizations, inappropriate diet choices, observations of parent-child interaction during the visit, and evidence of less than expected weight gain should all increase concern about the adequacy of parenting.

Intervention Techniques

Appropriate intervention with the goal of prevention or early identification of failure to thrive should start during pregnancy and should be intensified during the newborn period. Early home visiting after discharge of high-risk newborns should be part of this routine. Efficient implementation of home-visiting programs on a routine basis depends on an infrastructure of support for preventive health care, which is more highly developed in some countries than others. The model most commonly followed is that a parent must bring the infant to the health care provider's office or clinic, which assumes a level of responsibility that may not be realistic for some parents.

Optimally, all infants within a community can be identified on a centralized basis, providers correctly identified, and routine health care monitored in such a way that infants who do not show up for appointments, receive their immunizations, or gain and grow normally would be identified. Such infants are then flagged as "high-risk" and receive special attention.

Intervention after identification of failure to thrive may be possible on an outpatient basis, provided that the necessary resources are available. Again, this can involve home visiting or a day care program or a combination of the two. Very inexpensive models tested in rural areas of Third World countries involves bringing malnourished infants and their mothers to a daytime "nutrition center," where mothers receive instruction about the nutritional needs of their children and participate in the actual preparation of low-cost foods prepared from ingredients obtained at the local market place. The benefit of such an experience is that it serves the needs of the mothers as well as the infants, providing education and socialization along with nutrition. Similar arrangements can be made for younger infants that support breast-feeding, appropriate weaning foods, and models of infant stimulation.

Certainly, there are some parents who are ultimately unable to provide satisfactory child care despite every effort to intervene and support them. Under these conditions, it may be necessary to place the child in a different home. Issues involved in placement of children are complex and controversial, and frequently none of the alternatives available in the community are very satisfactory. Regardless of the outcome of these difficult decisions, practical and legal considerations require that a thorough evaluation and attempted intervention must precede placement, except in extreme situations in which the child's life and health are considered acutely endangered if the child returns to the parent's home. These circumstances involve social work intervention and legal notification of the appropriate government agency.

SUMMARY AND RED FLAGS

Failure to thrive in the United States is more often non-organic and is associated with various psychosocial attributes of the parents, family, or child. Such infants rapidly gain weight under close nutritional supervision in the hospital. In addition, weight is most severely affected. Length reduction comes next, whereas head growth is rarely affected, and most certainly head circumference is never the first affected growth parameter. Clues to organic causes are often evident from the history, physical and a limited selection of screening tests. Signs and symptoms of organic diseases that are red flags are in Tables 17–1 and 17–2. Additional red flags include refusal to eat, poor response to feedings, an inappropriately small head size, and physical signs incompatible with malnutrition. Precipitating factors (acute gastroenteritis or pneumonia) should be separated from more chronic causes, such as malabsorption (celiac disease, cystic fibrosis, giardiasis) and chronic heart, neurologic or lung disease (cystic fibrosis, immune deficiency).

REFERENCES

Casey PH, Kelleher KJ, Bradley RH, et al. A multifaceted intervention for infants with failure to thrive: A prospective study. Arch Pediatr Adolesc Med 1994;148:1071–1077.

Drotar D, Sturm L. Personality development, problem solving, and behavior problems among preschool children with early histories of nonorganic failure-to-thrive: A controlled study. J Dev Behav Pediatr 1992;13:266–273.

Drotar D, Pallotta J, Eckerle D. A prospective study of family environments of children hospitalized for nonorganic failure-to-thrive. J Dev Behav Pediatr 1994;15:78–85.

Evans SL, Reinhart JB, Succop RA. Failure to thrive: A study of 45 children and their families. J Am Acad Child Psychiatry 1972;11:440–457.

Fishhoff J, Whitten CF, Pettit MG. A psychiatric study of mothers of infants with failure to thrive secondary to maternal deprivation. J Pediatr 1971;79:209–215.

Frank DA, Zeisel SH. Failure to thrive. Pediatr Clin North Am 1988;35:1187–1206.

Grantham-McGregor S, Schofield W, Powell C. Development of severely malnourished children who received psychosocial stimulation: six-year follow-up. Pediatrics 1987;79:247–254.

Guo SM, Roche AF, Fomon SJ, et al. Reference data on gains in weight and length during the first two years of life. J Pediatr 1991;119:355–362.

Homer C, Ludwig S. Categorization of etiology of failure to thrive. Am J Dis Child 1981;135:848–851.

Kelleher KJ, Casey PH, Bradley RH, et al. Risk factors and outcomes for failure to thrive in low birth weight preterm infants. Pediatrics 1993;91:941–948.

Kerr MAD, Bogues JL, Kerr DS. Psychosocial functioning of mothers of malnourished children. Pediatrics 1978;62:778–784.

Marcovitch H. Failure to thrive. BMJ 1994;308:35–38.

Mitchell WG, Gorrell RW, Greenberg RA. Failure to thrive: A study in a primary care setting; Epidemiology and follow-up. Pediatrics 1980;65:971–977.

National Center for Health Statistics. NCHS growth curves for children, birth–18 years, United States. Series 11, No. 165, Vital and Health Statistics. Hyattsville, Md: Health Resources Administration, 1977.

Polansky NA, DeSaix C, Sharlin SA. Child Neglect: Understanding and Reaching the Parent. New York: Child Welfare League of America, Inc, 1973.

Richardson SA. The relation of severe malnutrition in infancy to the intelligence of school children with differing life histories. Pediatr Res 1976;10:57–61.

Sills RH. Failure to thrive: The role of clinical and laboratory evaluation. Am J Dis Child 1978;132:967–969.

Smith MM, Lifshitz F. Excess fruit juice consumption as a contributing factor in nonorganic failure to thrive. Pediatrics 1994;93:438–443.

Stier DM, Leventhal JM, Berg AT, et al. Are children born to young mothers at increased risk of maltreatment? Pediatrics 1993;91:642–648.

Wright JA, Ashenburg CA, Whitaker RC. Comparison of methods to categorize undernutrition in children. J Pediatr 1994;124:944–946.

18 Acute and Chronic Abdominal Pain

Ellen Hrabovsky

Abdominal pain in children is a common and challenging complaint. Approximately 20% of children will see a physician for abdominal pain by the age of 15 years. Only 5% will require hospitalization or surgical intervention. The primary care physician, pediatrician, emergency physician, and surgeon must be able to distinguish serious and potentially life-threatening diseases from more benign or trivial problems (Table 18–1). Complicating this task is the fact that abdominal pain may be a single acute event (Tables 18–2 and 18–3), a recurring acute problem, or a chronic problem (Table 18–4). The differential diagnosis is lengthy, differs from that in adults, and varies by age group. Although some disorders occur throughout childhood (constipation, gastroenteritis, pneumonia, urinary tract infections), others are common only in a specific age group (e.g., intussusception in infancy) (see Table 18–2).

The clinician must develop an organized approach to the evaluation of the child with abdominal pain, and the history and physical examination are the keys to an accurate diagnosis. Laboratory and radiologic tests are at best supportive and usually do not change the clinical diagnosis. The child with acute abdominal pain is frequently seen in the emergency department and requires a different approach from that required for the child with chronic complaints of pain, who most often is seen in an ambulatory care setting.

PATHOPHYSIOLOGY OF ABDOMINAL PAIN

Abdominal pain results from stimulation of nociceptic receptors (nociceptors) and afferent sympathetic stretch receptors. The pain is classified as *visceral* or *parietal* (somatic).

Visceral Pain

Visceral pain is initiated when nociceptors are triggered by excessive contraction, stretching, or tension of the walls of a hollow viscera (intestinal obstruction, appendiceal inflammation or fecalith, biliary or urinary stone), or of the capsule of a solid organ (liver, spleen, kidney), or of the mesentery. In addition, extremes of temperature or tissue release of inflammatory mediators (cytokines, histamine, prostaglandins) may trigger visceral pain. Increased contraction of the smooth muscle of a hollow viscera may be due to infection, toxins (bacterial or chemical agents), ulceration, inflammation, or ischemia. Increased hepatic capsule tension may be secondary to passive congestion (heart failure, pericarditis) or inflammation (hepatitis).

Visceral pain is often of gradual onset; is poorly localized relative to the internal anatomy as a result of multisegmental and bilateral innervation of the viscera; is generally of a dull, cramping, burning, gnawing, or sickening quality; and often has secondary manifestations, such as pallor, perspiration, emesis, nausea, and restlessness. Although localization may be imprecise with visceral pain, some general rules may be helpful (Fig. 18–1)

Parietal Pain

Parietal pain arises from direct noxious (usually inflammation) stimulation of the contiguous parietal peritoneum (e.g., right lower quadrant—McBurney's point and appendicitis) or the diaphragm (splenic rupture, subdiaphragmatic abscess). Parietal pain is usually sharp, exacerbated by movement or cough, is accompanied by tenderness over the sight of irritation, and lateralizes to one of four quadrants (Fig. 18–2). Because of the relative localization of the noxious stimulation to the underlying peritoneum and the more

Table 18-1. **Distinguishing Features of Abdominal Pain in Children**

Disease	Onset	Location	Referral	Quality	Comments
Functional: irritable bowel syndrome	Recurrent	Periumbilical	None	Dull, crampy, intermittent, duration 2 hr	Family stress, school phobia, diarrhea/constipation
Gastroenteritis	Acute–gradual	Periumbilical, rectal, tenesmus	None	Crampy, dull, intermittent	Emesis, fever, watery diarrhea or dysentery (mucus and blood)
Esophageal reflux	Recurrent, after meals, bedtime	Substernal	Chest	Burning	Sour taste in mouth, Sandifer syndrome
Duodenal ulcer	Recurrent, before meals, at night	Epigastric	Back	Severe burning, gnawing	Relieved by food, milk, antacids, family history
Pancreatitis	Acute	Epigastric/hypogastric	Back	Constant, sharp, boring	Nausea, emesis, marked tenderness
Intestinal obstruction	Acute or gradual	Periumbilical—lower abdomen	Back	Alternating cramping (colic) and painless periods	Distention, obstipation, bilious emesis, increased bowel sounds
Appendicitis	Acute or gradual (1–2 days)	Initially periumbilical or epigastric; later localized to right lower quadrant	Back or pelvis if retrocecal	Sharp, steady	Nausea, emesis, local tenderness ± fever, patient is motionless
Meckel diverticulitis (mimics appendicitis)	Recurrent or constant	Generalized diffuse with perforation: periumbilical—lower abdomen	None	Sharp	Hematochezia; painless unless intussusception, diverticulitis, or perforation
Inflammatory bowel disease	Recurrent	Depends on site of involvement		Dull cramping, tenesmus	Fever, weight loss, ± hematochezia
Intussusception	Acute	Periumbilical—lower abdomen	None	Cramping, with painless periods	Guarded position with knees pulled up, "currant jelly" stools
Lactose intolerance	Recurrent with milk products	Lower abdomen	None	Cramping	Distention, gaseousness, diarrhea
Urolithiasis	Acute, sudden	Back	Groin	Severe colicky pain	Hematuria, calcification on KUB x-ray study
Pyelonephritis	Acute, sudden	Back	None	Dull to sharp	Fever, costochondral tenderness, dysuria, pyuria, urinary frequency
Cholecystitis/cholelithiasis	Acute	Right upper quadrant	Right shoulder, scapula	Severe colicky pain	Hemolysis ± jaundice

Adapted from Andreoli TE, Carpenter CJ, Plum F, et al. Cecil Essentials of Medicine. Philadelphia: WB Saunders, 1994:326.
Reprinted and modified from Behrman R, Kliegman R. Nelson Essentials of Pediatrics, 2nd ed. Philadelphia: WB Saunders, 1994:396.
Abbreviation: KUB = kidney, ureter, and bladder.

Table 18–2. Causes of Acute Abdominal Pain by Age Group

Neonate	*Child (2–11 yr)*	*Adolescent (12–19 yr)*
Necrotizing enterocolitis*	Appendicitis*	Appendicitis*
Obstruction*	Gastroenteritis*†	Pelvic inflammatory disease*
Malrotation with volvulus*	Trauma*	Trauma*
Idiopathic or drug (indomethacin,	Henoch-Schönlein purpura	Tubo-ovarian abscess
steroid)–induced intestinal	Hepatitis	Fitz-Hugh–Curtis syndrome
perforation	Peptic ulcer disease	Labor (pregnancy)
	Sickle cell anemia—vaso-occlusive crisis	Hepatitis
Infant (<2 yr)	Pancreatitis	Pancreatitis (any cause)
Intussusception*	Pneumonia (lower lobe)	Ectopic pregnancy
Incarcerated hernia*	Abdominal tumors	Crohn's disease
Urinary tract infection*	Pyelonephritis/cystitis	Ovarian cyst/mittelschmerz*
Gastroenteritis*†	Testicular torsion	Sickle cell crisis
Intestinal obstruction	Torsed cryptorchid testis	Peptic ulcer disease
Malrotation with volvulus	Incarcerated hernia	Omental torsion
Trauma (e.g., abuse)	Typhlitis	Mesenteric adenitis
Pneumonitis (lower lobe)	Pharyngitis/tonsillitis	Urinary tract infection
Hirschsprung disease	Meckel diverticulitis	Muscle strain (exercise, coughing)
Aerophagia	Mesenteric adenitis	Idiopathic*
Spontaneous bacterial peritonitis	Spontaneous bacterial peritonitis	
	Idiopathic*	

*Most commonly seen problems.

†Gastroenteritis indicates intestinal infection with viral, bacterial, protozoal, or parasitic agents. Giardiasis and cryptosporidiosis are particularly common and may produce acute or chronic pain.

anatomically specific and unilateral innervation (peripheral–non-autonomic nerves) of the peritoneum, it is usually easier to identify the precise anatomic location that is producing parietal pain (Fig. 18–2).

ACUTE ABDOMINAL PAIN

The clinician evaluating the child with abdominal pain of acute onset must decide in an expeditious manner whether the child has a "surgical abdomen," a serious medical problem requiring admission, or a process that can be managed on an outpatient basis. Even though surgical diagnoses represent slightly fewer than 10% of all causes of abdominal pain in children, untreated, they can be life-threatening. Approximately 55% of children evaluated for acute abdominal pain have a specific medical diagnosis, and another 35% never have a defined cause.

History

Obtaining an accurate history is paramount to arriving at an accurate diagnosis but is dependent on both the ability and willing-

Table 18–3. Sudden Acute Excruciating Abdominal Pain (Within Minutes)

Intestinal Perforation	*Luminal Occlusion*
Peptic ulcer disease	Urolithiasis
Appendicitis	Cholelithiasis
Diverticula	Strangulated hernia
Vascular Occlusion	*Intra-abdominal Hemorrhage*
Midgut volvulus	Ectopic pregnancy
Emboli	Ruptured aortic aneurysm
Endocarditis	Ruptured spleen
Strangulated hernia	
Ovarian torsion	

ness of the child to communicate and on the skill of the parent or guardian as an observer. In infants, the person providing the infant's care is the best source of information about the current illness. Children 4 years of age and older may contribute to the history. Some small children can give a remarkably clear and accurate account of their own illness. On the other hand, some older children may be totally unwilling to communicate or may be completely silenced by a talkative parent. The examining physician should try to elicit as much information from the child as possible.

Some children can give a good account of the current problem when they are simply asked to describe it; however, most children must be asked specific nonleading questions. For example, to determine the presence of anorexia, the physician must ask questions about food intake, the time the food was eaten, and how that behavior compares to the child's normal intake. The answers are often quite different from the responses to the more general questions "Are you hungry?" or "Have you eaten today?" The child's (and parents') vocabulary, especially of body parts and functions, is not a medical vocabulary. The clinician should use terms the child understands and should not be reluctant to ask what terms the child does know.

The history is obtained in as relaxed and nonthreatening a setting as is possible. During the history taking, the child should remain in the parent's arms, at play, or comfortably seated beside the parent, as appropriate for the child's age. Many children become quite upset by being made to remove their clothes. While the history is obtained, there is no particular reason why the child should be undressed. The clinician must resist distraction or the urge to speed things up by examining the child while taking the history. Occasionally, when seeing a seriously ill child, the physician may need to abbreviate the diagnostic process, but taking short cuts may lead to inaccurate conclusions.

ESSENTIAL COMPONENTS OF THE HISTORY

Time of Onset of Pain. The time of onset of the pain is important. Pain of less than 6 hours' duration is accompanied by nonspecific

Table 18–4. Causes of Chronic and Recurrent Abdominal Pain by Age Group*

Infant (<2 Yr)	Child (2–11 Yr)	Adolescent (12–19 Yr)
Colic†	Constipation†	Irritable bowel syndrome†
Inguinal hernia	Functional pain†	Psychogenic†
Malabsorption‡	Giardiasis†	Dysmenorrhea†
Milk allergy	Peptic ulcer disease	Mittelschmerz†
Hirschsprung disease	Toxins (lead)	Peptic ulcer disease
Cystic fibrosis	Pancreatitis	Gallbladder disease
Rotational defects	Parasites	Pelvic inflammatory disease
Malformations	Tumors/masses	Ovarian cysts
Esophagitis	Discitis/osteomyelitis	Diabetes mellitus
	Abdominal migraine	Inflammatory bowel disease
	Diabetes mellitus	Malignancy
	Volvulus	Giardiasis
	Intra-abdominal abscess§	Serositis (e.g., SLE, familial Mediterranean fever)
	Choledochal cyst	Intra-abdominal abscess§

*See also Table 18–6.
†Most common diagnoses.
‡Includes lactose and sorbitol (and other fruit juice polyalcohols) intolerance.
§Hepatic, pancreatic, subphrenic, psoas, perinephric, renal, pelvic.
Abbreviation: SLE = systemic lupus erythematosus.

findings, and observation is often needed to determine the nature of the illness. Pain lasting from 6 to 48 hours is more apt to have a "surgical" cause, although delays in presentation and diagnosis in children are not unusual. Timing of the progression of symptoms must be detailed.

Location of Pain. The location of the pain at its onset and any change in location are very important (Table 18–5, see also Table 18–1). As stated by Apley (1975), "the further the pain from the umbilicus the more likely there is to be an underlying organ disorder."

Most intraperitoneal visceral pain is a response to stimulation of stretch fibers in the bowel wall and is mediated through the spinal nerves at T-10. This pain is sensed as a deep, aching periumbilical pain. Pain caused by inflammation of the parietal peritoneum (acute appendicitis) is localized to the area of the inflamed organ or is diffuse if the inflammation is extensive and involves the peritoneal cavity. Pain resulting from an obstructed organ is localized to the area of that organ and radiates to the commonly innervated region

(stones in the ureter cause intense flank pain with radiation into the groin.) Pain that is migratory or fleeting in location is rarely suggestive of a surgical problem requiring operative intervention. It is more likely to accompany gastroenteritis, constipation, or colic.

Character of Pain. The character of the pain is often difficult for the child to describe. The older child may be able to differentiate cramping, aching, and burning sensations, but most children do not do this well. The child can relate whether the pain comes and goes or is unrelenting. The character of the pain is usually unknown in the toddler and infant, although the parent can determine whether the discomfort is constant, cramping, or intermittent. If the child intermittently draws the legs up in a flexed position and cries, one can assume that intermittent pain is present, as in intussusception.

Child's Activity Level. The effect of the pain on the child's activities is an important indicator of the severity of the underlying disease. If the pain is sufficiently severe to awaken the child from

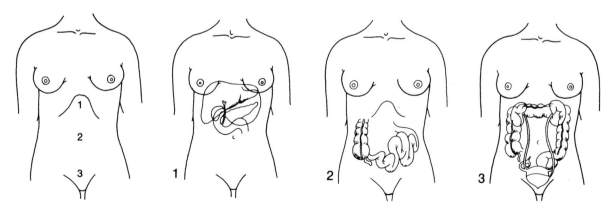

Figure 18–1. "Visceral" abdominal pain: deep, dull, diffuse. The three general localizations of midline "visceral" abdominal pain: epigastric, periumbilical, and hypogastric. *1*, Epigastric pain usually suggests disease of the thorax, stomach, duodenum, pancreas, liver, or gallbladder. *2*, Periumbilical pain usually implies disease of the small intestine, cecum or both. *3*, Hypogastric pain usually implicates the large intestine, pelvic organs, or urinary system. (From Reilly BM. Abdominal pain. *In* Practical Strategies in Outpatient Medicine, 2nd ed. Philadelphia: WB Saunders, 1991:702.)

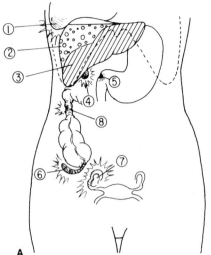

A

1. Pleurisy
2. Subdiaphragmatic abscess
3. (Peri) hepatitis
4. Cholecystitis
5. Perforated duodenal ulcer
6. Appendicitis
7. Ectopic pregnancy, tuboovarian hemorrhage, abscess, or rupture
8. Perforated colon (cancer or diverticulum)

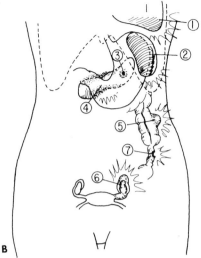

B

1. Pleurisy
2. Splenic rupture or infarct
3. Perforated gastric ulcer
4. Pancreatitis
5. Diverticulitis (splenic flexure)
6. Ectopic pregnancy, tuboovarian hemorrhage, abscess, or rupture
7. Perforated colon (carcinoma)

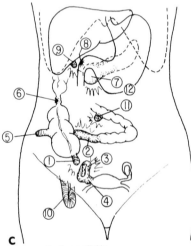

C

1. Appendicitis
2. Acute Crohn's disease
3. Ectopic pregnancy, tuboovarian abscess, or ovarian torsion/hemorrhage
4. Pelvic inflammatory disease
5. Cecal diverticulitis
6. Colon cancer (perforation)
7. Acute pancreatitis and/or pseudocyst
8. Perforated duodenal ulcer
9. Acute cholecystitis
10. Incarcerated inguinal hernia
11. Meckel's diverticulitis
12. Leaking aortic aneurysm

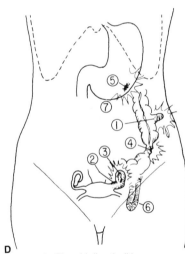

D

1. Sigmoid diverticulitis
2. Pelvic inflammatory disease
3. Ectopic pregnancy, tuboovarian abscess, or ovarian torsion / hemorrhage
4. Perforated sigmoid carcinoma
5. Perforated gastric ulcer
6. Incarcerated inguinal hernia
7. Leaking aortic aneurysm

Figure 18–2. Common and uncommon conditions that may cause "parietal" pain and localized peritonitis in the various quadrants of the abdomen: A, Right upper quadrant. B, Left upper quadrant. C, Right lower quadrant. D, Left lower quadrant. (From Reilly BM. Abdominal pain. In Practical Strategies in Outpatient Medicine, 2nd ed. Philadelphia: WB Saunders, 1991:703.)

Table 18–5. Localization of Abdominal Pain: Referred or Radiated

Referred	
Extra-abdominal lesion pain referred to abdomen	Intra-abdominal extraperitoneal origin
Thorax	Pancreas
Spine	Kidney
Hips	Ureters
Pelvis	Great vessels
	Pelvic organs
	Retroperitoneal space

Radiated
Origin is primary site with simultaneously perceived pain in a secondary site
Cholecystitis radiates to subscapular area
Splenic injury radiates to shoulder
Ureteral colic (stones) radiates to testis, upper leg or groin
Pancreatitis radiates to back

a sound sleep, it is of much more significance than pain that occurs only at school and never on weekends. If a child has had to avoid a favorite activity, the pain is more apt to have a defined organic cause. Asking whether motion worsens the pain helps to differentiate peritoneal irritation from more nonspecific problems. The child with acute appendicitis lies motionless, whereas the child with a renal stone or gallstone or gastroenteritis may toss and turn and writhe in discomfort.

Gastrointestinal Symptoms. The presence or absence of gastrointestinal symptoms differentiates intestinal problems (acute appendicitis, gastroenteritis, acute cholecystitis) from those arising from other intra-abdominal organs (urinary tract infection, ovarian disease, abdominal wall pain).

Anorexia and nausea are difficult symptoms for a small child to describe. Often, if simply asked about hunger, the child will respond in the affirmative. This may be partly because mild nausea is difficult to differentiate from hunger. Questions about recent food intake, normal eating habits, the last normal meal, and the current desirability of a favorite food often provide more accurate information about the presence or absence of anorexia and nausea than direct questions about appetite or nausea.

Vomiting is usually associated with intestinal disease, such as ileus, gastroenteritis, or acute surgical problems of the gastrointestinal tract (see Chapter 20). However, vomiting may occur as a response to severe non-intestinal pain such as in testicular torsion; this vomiting is not recurring and is not a prominent feature. Care should be taken to determine whether the pain occurs before or after the onset of the vomiting. In acute surgical lesions (those caused by intestinal obstruction, acute appendicitis, acute cholecystitis), the pain always occurs before or during the vomiting. If vomiting occurred *before* the onset of pain, one should suspect gastroenteritis or another nonspecific problem. The appearance of the vomited material is also important. Feculent or dark green material always suggests intestinal obstruction. Dark brown or frankly bloody material indicates a gastritis, Mallory-Weiss gastric tears, or peptic ulcer disease as the source of pain.

Diarrhea occurs commonly in intestinal diseases of viral and bacterial origin (see Chapter 19). The stool volume is large, and defecation is usually preceded by cramping pain that is alleviated by the passage of the diarrheal stool. Diarrhea may also occur in the presence of acute appendicitis or other pelvic infections (such as those resulting from pelvic inflammatory disease, tubo-ovarian

abscess) caused by inflammation and irritation of an area of colon adjacent to an inflammatory mass. The diarrhea in this instance is of small volume and frequent. It is important to obtain an estimate of the volume of stool passed. Diarrhea may also occur in lesions that cause partial obstruction of the bowel, such as strictures, adhesions, and Hirschsprung disease. In this situation, the patient also has some degree of abdominal distention. *Diarrhea with abdominal distention suggests intestinal obstruction.*

Constipation alone can cause acute abdominal pain, low-grade fever, and possibly mild elevation of the white blood cell count (see Chapter 25). Constipation may also indicate other gastrointestinal dysfunction. Some children present with a picture very similar to that seen in acute appendicitis but have a large amount of stool filling the entire colon. The pain often disappears after enemas and a brief period of bowel rest. The "gas-stoppage sign" describes a sensation of fullness that suggests the need for a bowel movement in patients with appendicitis. However, attempts at defecation provide no relief.

Systemic Symptoms. The presence of headache, sore throat, and other generalized aches and pains moves the examiner away from a diagnosis of an acute surgical problem and strongly suggests a viral flu-like syndrome. Asking the child where the worst pain is sometimes results in the child's pointing a finger to the head or throat. One must be careful to remember the whole child and not to focus on the abdomen just because that is the area of the presenting complaint. Many systemic diseases directly or indirectly produce abdominal pain and must be considered in the differential diagnosis (Table 18–6).

Family History and Past Medical History. Viral gastroenteritis, other viral syndromes, or food poisoning may affect the family or schoolmates; it is important to ask whether other family members, classmates, or playmates have recently had similar symptoms. Certain systemic and inherited diseases, such as sickle cell anemia, diabetes mellitus, spherocytosis, and porphyria, are associated with episodes of abdominal pain. The family must be asked about familial diseases and any previous episodes of pain that the child has suffered (see Table 18–6). Previous intra-abdominal operations may result in adhesions that can cause pain, or intestinal obstruction, or both. A history of such procedures alerts the examiner to the possibility of bowel obstruction. Some specific medical illnesses result in identifiable or predictable causes of abdominal pain (Table 18–7).

Physical Examination

The physical examination begins when the clinician enters the room. Observing the child's activity and demeanor while obtaining the history is the first step of the physical examination.

Does the child appear ill?

Is the patient lethargic, rolling about in discomfort, alert but lying very still, or bouncing all over the room?

Each of these activities conveys a message. The listless, lethargic child is most likely in shock, dehydrated, and quite ill. The child who is crying out loudly and generally dominating the scene does not have a surgical problem and most likely has gastroenteritis with cramping abdominal pain. The child who seems only mildly ill but moves with great care, if at all, most likely has an inflammatory process, such as acute appendicitis or an incarcerated hernia.

Once the history is satisfactorily completed, the child should be asked to get onto the examination table with as little assistance as possible. If the child does this easily, the probability of an intra-abdominal inflammatory process is quite low. Outer bulky clothing

Table 18–6. Systemic Causes of Acute Abdominal Pain

Metabolic, Hematologic	*Neurologic*	*Infectious, Inflammatory*
Acute porphyria	Abdominal epilepsy	Acute rheumatic fever
Familial Mediterranean fever	Abdominal migraine	Infectious mononucleosis
Hereditary angioneurotic edema	Brain tumor	Rocky Mountain spotted fever
Sickle cell crisis	Multiple sclerosis	Measles
Leukemia	Radiculopathy	Mumps
Acute hemolytic states	Neuropathy	Pneumonia
Diabetic ketoacidosis	Herpes zoster	Pericarditis
Hemolytic uremic syndrome	Dysautonomia (Riley-Day syndrome)	Pharyngitis
Addison disease		Epididymitis/orchitis
Uremia	*Drugs, Toxins*	Henoch-Schönlein purpura
Electrolyte disturbances	Heavy metal poisoning	Systemic lupus erythematosus
Hyperparathyroidism-hypercalcemia	Lead	Endocarditis
(urolithiasis, pancreatitis)	Arsenic	Anaphylaxis
Hypertriglyceridemia (pancreatitis)	Mercury	
	Mushroom ingestion	*Other*
Musculoskeletal	Narcotic withdrawal	Pneumothorax
Arthritis/discitis	Black widow spider bite	Pulmonary embolism
Osteomyelitis		Functional
Thoracic nerve root dysfunction		Aerophagia
Trauma/child abuse		
Hernia		

should be removed, but the child does not need to be completely undressed, especially if being undressed seems distressing to the child. Clothing can be rearranged to allow good exposure of the abdomen without the child's having to feel completely vulnerable.

The examination must be performed in a relaxed, friendly manner with attention fully focused on the child. An accurate examination depends on the child's trust and cooperation. A conversation with the child about family, friends, pets, school, sports, music, or other specific interests of that child diverts attention from the examination and increases cooperation. The examiner should never

surprise the child and should never lie. The first surprise or untruth "this won't hurt" destroys any trust that has developed. The examination then becomes very difficult.

Low-grade fever (<101°F) is seen in early appendicitis but is also common in many other diseases. The absence of fever does not exclude the diagnosis of acute appendicitis or other problems requiring surgical intervention. If the parent has given an antipyretic just before the visit, the temperature will be suppressed and will be an inaccurate measure of illness. Tachycardia may reflect only anxiety or may be due to dehydration, shock, or fever. Tachy-

Table 18–7. Present or Past Medical History That May Suggest Cause of Abdominal Pain

Historical Factor	Cause of Pain
Cystic fibrosis	Pancreatitis, diabetes mellitus, meconium ileus equivalent, appendicitis, intussusception, biliary or urinary stones
Sickle cell anemia	Vaso-occlusive crisis, cholelithiasis, hepatitis, hemolytic crisis, renal infarction, splenic sequestration
Diabetes mellitus	Pancreatitis, gastric neuropathy
Cirrhosis, nephrotic syndrome	Primary bacterial peritonitis
SLE, other autoimmune disorders	Vasculitis, pancreatitis, serositis, infarction
Corticosteroids	Gastric ulceration, pancreatitis
NSAID	Ileal perforation, gastric ulceration, renal-papillary necrosis
HIV	Gastroenteritis, hepatitis, pancreatitis, esophagitis, lymphoma
Mononucleosis	Hepatitis, splenic rupture
Henoch-Schönlein purpura	Mucosal hemorrhage, intussusception
Hemolytic-uremic syndrome	Colitis
Upper respiratory tract infection	Pneumonia, mesenteric adenitis
Prior surgery	Abscess, adhesions, obstruction, stricture, pancreatitis, ectopic pregnancy
Inborn errors of metabolism, hypertriglyceridemia, hypercalcemia	Pancreatitis

Abbreviations: HIV = human immunodeficiency virus; NSAID = nonsteroidal anti-inflammatory drug; SLE = systemic lupus erythematosus.

pnea suggests a metabolic acidosis, an intrapulmonary process, sepsis, or fever. The vital signs must be viewed in context but may be the first clue to a serious illness.

Examination of the head, neck, chest, and extremities should precede the abdominal examination, and any uncomfortable parts should be deferred. In infants, otitis media is sufficiently painful to cause striking restlessness and may be confused with abdominal pain. In children too young to describe the location of the pain, a careful examination of the ears is very important but can be performed after the rest of the examination. Streptococcal pharyngitis or mononucleosis is sometimes accompanied by severe abdominal pain. Affected children have a significant fever, appear ill, and have tender cervical adenopathy and an obvious tonsillitis, pharyngitis, or both.

Decreased breath sounds and/or rales in a lower lobe, especially on the right side, may indicate pneumonia. Children with bacterial pneumonia present with severe abdominal pain, high fever, tachypnea, and occasionally vomiting. Such children appear quite ill. This presentation may mimic that of a child with peritonitis from a perforated acute appendicitis. However, the abdominal findings are not consistent with the diagnosis of an acute intra-abdominal process, and examination of the lungs should demonstrate the pneumonia.

The *abdominal examination* should be performed systematically and with the child as comfortable as possible. Before the examiner actually touches the abdomen, he or she should observe it, looking for distention, inguinal masses, peristaltic waves, scars from old injuries, or surgical incisions. Inguinal and femoral hernias are an often-forgotten and all too common cause of abdominal pain. Next, the child should be asked to indicate with one finger the point of greatest pain. The point may be a vague circle in the area of the umbilicus, but if the child specifies a defined spot, the examiner should avoid that area until the remainder of the abdomen has been palpated.

Gentleness is essential to successful palpation of the abdomen. It should not be necessary to remind the examiner to warm both hands and stethoscope before touching the patient with either. The stethoscope is a wonderful tool for palpation of the abdomen. Auscultation of the chest can simply be extended to the abdomen, with the examiner assuring the child that the stethoscope did not hurt on the chest. The initial examination of the abdomen with the stethoscope should be just for listening, with no pressure exerted so that no discomfort results.

Bowel sounds are usually nonspecific in most children with abdominal pain; however, in certain processes, they are helpful. High-pitched tinkles or rushes are usually associated with an obstructive process. Bowel sounds in gastroenteritis are ordinarily very active and loud but may be normal. Acute appendicitis is accompanied by normal sounds in the early stages, but absent bowel sounds develop with diffuse peritonitis.

Watching the child's reaction to the auscultation may be a valuable clue to areas of true tenderness. Most children do not expect the auscultation to be uncomfortable, so they are not guarding in anticipation of pain. As the examiner continues to listen over the entire anterior abdomen, the pressure on the head of the stethoscope increases until the examiner is, in fact, palpating with the stethoscope. This often is a much more reliable method of eliciting true tenderness and guarding than is the palpating hand. If the child is cooperative, stethoscope palpation may not be needed and the examiner can proceed to manual palpation of the abdomen.

Palpation is begun as *far away* from the area of pain identified by the child as possible. The hand should be softly placed flat (in parallel) on the abdomen. Directing fingers into the abdomen (perpendicular) as a method of palpation is unnecessary and is often frightening. The clinician should watch the child's face, not the abdomen, during the palpation. Some children are extremely stoic, and only the slightest grimace betrays the discomfort they are experiencing. Attention is paid during palpation to the presence

of masses or feces in a full colon. Voluntary guarding usually starts before the palpation starts and can be overcome by asking the child to take deep breaths or using other distractions appropriate to the child's age and temperament. Involuntary guarding occurs when the examiner's hand encounters an area of tenderness. When encountering tenderness, the examiner should palpate only deeply enough to elicit the complaint of pain and some guarding. There is no need to bring on unnecessary pain by rough or deep palpation. A rigid or board-like abdomen is the result of involuntary guarding of the entire anterior abdominal wall because of diffuse intraperitoneal inflammation.

Rebound pain is an indicator of peritoneal irritation and is elicited during examination of the anterior abdominal wall. It occurs when an inflamed focus within the abdomen is compressed and the pressure is then quickly released, resulting in sudden and sometimes severe pain. The standard method to elicit rebound is to palpate deeply, then suddenly remove the palpating hand. Although this sign aids in the determination of the presence of an intraperitoneal inflammatory process, it is often not necessary to cause the child this extra discomfort. If one feels the need to assess the presence or absence of rebound pain, the child should be told what is happening before the examining hand is removed. The suddenness of the maneuver alone frightens the unsuspecting child and renders the remainder of the examination difficult for all concerned.

Other areas of inflammation can be detected by maneuvers that move muscles adjacent to the inflammation. The *psoas sign* occurs when elevation and extension of the leg against the pressure of the examiner's hand causes pain. An inflammatory mass, such as an inflamed appendix, a psoas abscess, or a perinephric abscess, in contact with the psoas muscle is the cause for this pain (Fig. 18–3). Likewise, the *obturator sign* is pain with flexion of the thigh at right angles to the trunk and external rotation of the same leg while the patient is in the supine position. This sign results from contact of an inflammatory mass with the obturator muscle (Fig. 18–3).

The flanks and back must be inspected and palpated. Percussion at the costovertebral angle elicits pain in the presence of renal or perinephric inflammation. The perineum and genitalia must be inspected and palpated as needed. External examination of the genitalia in prepubertal girls is adequate. If a more thorough examination or an intravaginal examination is needed in prepubertal females it should generally be performed with the patient under anesthesia. In postpuberal females, a pelvic examination may be valuable, regardless of the patient's sexual activity history.

A complete abdominal examination includes a rectal examination. If a diagnosis is already obvious, the rectal examination may be eliminated, but this should not be a common practice. The rectal examination should be the last part of the physical and should be performed only once if at all possible. The child should be relaxed and should be given an honest explanation of the procedure. The examiner should use plenty of lubricant and should perform the rectal examination very gently. If the child is fighting, it is pointless to perform a forceful exam. This is when the rectal examination may truly be deferred for a while. Lateralizing pain, masses, and the presence and character of stool in the rectum are assessed. The stool should always be tested for blood.

Clues to an organic and at times more serious cause of abdominal pain are noted in Table 18–8. Furthermore, peritoneal signs, which suggest a surgical abdomen most often caused by peritonitis, are noted in Table 18–9. In addition, the presence of shock suggests other serious diseases (Table 18–9).

Laboratory Evaluation

After completion of a careful history and thorough physical examination, the diagnosis or a short list of possible diagnoses

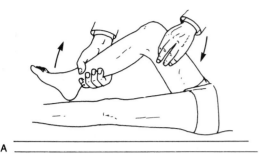

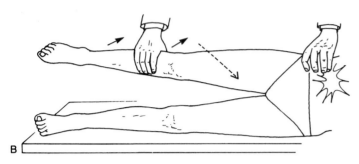

Figure 18–3. A, The obturator sign. Pain occurs when the hip is flexed and rotated. Internal rotation is most likely to cause pain as a result of pelvic or retroperitoneal disease or both. B, The psoas sign may be performed passively or actively. The hip is passively extended, thus stretching the psoas muscle (solid arrow). The hip is actively flexed usually against resistance, thus tensing the psoas muscle (dotted arrow). (From Reilly BM. Abdominal pain. In Practical Strategies in Outpatient Medicine, 2nd ed. Philadelphia: WB Saunders, 1991:714.)

should be apparent. Laboratory data are supportive in confirming or ruling out suspected disease.

COMPLETE BLOOD COUNT

The hemoglobin and hematocrit levels can reveal anemia caused by acute or chronic blood loss (such as that caused by ulcers, inflammatory bowel disease, Meckel diverticula) or the anemia of chronic disease (systemic lupus erythematosus, inflammatory bowel disease). The white blood cell count indicates the possibility of infection or blood dyscrasias. In uncomplicated acute appendicitis, the white blood cell count ranges from normal values to 15,000 to 16,000. A very high white blood cell count (>18,000) indicates intestinal gangrene, perforation, or abscess formation but may also be high in acute gastroenteritis, streptococcal diseases, pyelonephritis, pelvic inflammatory disease, and pneumonia.

The differential cell count may be helpful in the evaluation of the neutrophil count. In studies of children with acute appendicitis, 95% had neutrophilia, but only half had leukocytosis in the first 24 hours. If the child's history and physical examination are highly

---

Table 18–8. Red Flags and Clues to an Organic Cause of Abdominal Pain

Localized pain in nonperiumbilical site
Referred pain
Pain awakes child from sleep
Sudden onset of excruciating pain
Crescendo nature of pain
Sudden worsening of pain
Fever (high fever >39.4°C suggests pneumonia, pyelonephritis, dysentery, cholangitis, more than perforation or abscess)
Jaundice
Distention*
Dysuria
Emesis (especially bilious)
Anorexia
Weight loss
Positive family history (metabolic disorders, peptic ulcer disease)†
Change in urine or stool color (blood, acholic)
Vaginal discharge
Sexual activity
Delayed sexual development (chronic pain)
Anemia
Elevated erythrocyte sedimentation rate
Specific physical findings (hepatomegaly, absent bowel sounds, adnexal tenderness, involuntary guarding, focal or diffuse tenderness, positive rectal examination results, perianal disease)

*Consider 5 Fs (fat, feces, flatus [aerophagia, obstruction], fluid [ascites, hydrone-phrosis, cysts], fetus [pregnancy, or fetal-like abnormal growth, e.g., tumors]).
†Family history is also positive for dysfunctional pain syndromes (constipation, irritable bowel, dysmenorrhea, and lactase deficiency).

Table 18–9. Peritoneal Signs of a Surgical Abdomen

Severe pain
Patient's eyes anxiously open during examiner's palpation
Patient is motionless
Absent bowel sounds
Extreme tenderness to palpation or percussion
Voluntary guarding with gentle palpation
Involuntary guarding—boardlike rigidity
Rebound tenderness (do not intentionally elicit)
Pain with movement or cough

If shock is present, consider:
Severe pancreatitis
Trauma—intra-abdominal hemorrhage
Ruptured spleen (trauma, mononucleosis)
Spontaneous peritonitis
Secondary peritonitis (appendicitis, intussusception, perforated ulcer)
Urosepsis
Associated severe gastrointestinal bleeding
Ruptured ectopic pregnancy
Pulmonary embolism
Aortic dissection
Volvulus
Child abuse
Addisonian crisis

suggestive of appendicitis, a normal or mildly elevated white blood cell count should not dissuade the clinician from that diagnosis. On the other hand, a striking lymphocytosis may suggest a viral gastroenteritis or other viral illness. Over reliance on the complete blood count can cause delay in reaching the correct diagnosis.

The *urinalysis* is an important and useful laboratory test in the evaluation of abdominal pain. The presence of ketones and a high specific gravity suggest poor food intake and dehydration. Large amounts of glucose and ketones in the urine indicate diabetic ketoacidosis. A pregnancy test should be performed on postpuberal girls, regardless of sexual activity history. The presence of both white cells *and* bacteria indicate a urinary tract infection. Either finding alone is not sufficient for that diagnosis. White blood cells and red blood cells may be present in the urine from irritation caused by an inflammatory mass adjacent to the bladder or ureter.

Other laboratory tests, such as measurement of serum electrolytes, amylase, and lipase; liver function studies; and arterial blood gases should be ordered based on the differential diagnosis after a thorough history and physical examination are completed.

Radiologic Evaluation

A multitude of imaging studies are available; none should be obtained until the patient has been examined.

PLAIN RADIOGRAPHY

Plain radiographs, especially kidney-ureter-bladder (KUB) with or without upright, lateral views, of the chest and abdomen are routinely obtained in most emergency departments as part of the evaluation of acute abdominal pain. The chest film helps to assess the presence of a lower-lobe pneumonia, which often causes severe abdominal pain, especially in small children. However, early in the disease, the physical examination may be more helpful. Often, if the KUB–abdominal x-ray study includes the lower lobes, the chest x-ray study can be deferred and performed only if the KUB demonstrates lung abnormalities.

Only approximately 10% of abdominal radiographic results are positive when they are obtained as part of the routine work-up for abdominal pain. When they are limited to patients with serious illness, 46% of the results may be positive. Used to confirm the presence of intestinal obstruction, renal or biliary tract calculi, calcified fecaliths, or intestinal perforation (pneumoperitoneum—free air), plain abdominal radiographs may be helpful. These studies detect bowel distention (air fluid levels on upright views), calcification, free air, and large masses but are not helpful in detecting most other diseases. If free air or intestinal obstruction is suspected, the abdominal films must include a flat and upright or decubitus view of the abdomen to demonstrate the air-fluid interface.

In acute appendicitis, a calcified appendicolith may be seen (Fig. 18–4). This finding automatically makes the diagnosis of appendiceal dysfunction and confirms the need for appendectomy. The absence of an appendicolith (fecalith) does not rule out appendicitis. More often, the noncalcified appendicolith may obstruct the appendix; ultrasonographic imaging is necessary to visualize this lesion. If an inflammatory mass lies near the iliopsoas muscle, a mild lumbar scoliosis may be present as a result of spasm of the muscle.

Radiographic studies are not always necessary. If the diagnosis is already obvious, specific therapy is indicated. In some situations, other types of imaging studies are more useful, and plain radiographs are not prerequisite.

ULTRASONOGRAPHY

Ultrasound examination is ideal for children. It is usually painless, emits no radiation, requires no intravenous contrast material, and can be performed without sedation. It is usually readily available and in selected patients can be extremely helpful.

Lower abdominal gynecologic pain in girls, especially in adolescent girls, can be confused with appendicitis. Pelvic ultrasonography demonstrates pathology of the ovaries and fallopian tubes, the size of the uterus, and the presence of free fluid in the pelvis. An enlarged, inflamed appendix can be visualized (Fig. 18–5). Any girl with abdominal pain in whom the diagnosis is not obvious should undergo an ultrasonographic examination.

Figure 18–4. The patient described the gradual onset of anorexia, nausea, and vague periumbilical abdominal pain. Twenty-four hours later, the pain was much more severe in the right lower quadrant, where localized peritoneal signs were apparent. The x-ray film of the abdomen reveals a huge calcified density in the right lower quadrant; it proved to be an appendiceal fecalith at surgery. (From Reilly BM. Abdominal pain. *In* Practical Strategies in Outpatient Medicine, 2nd ed. Philadelphia: WB Saunders, 1991:16.)

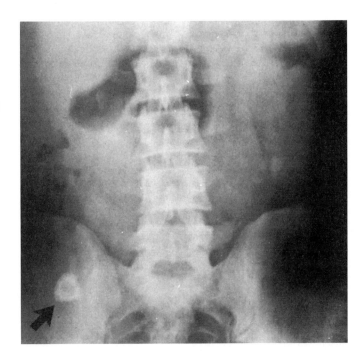

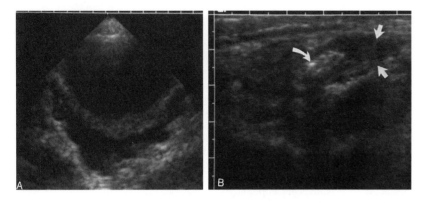

Figure 18–5. A transverse scan of the pelvis shows free fluid pooling behind the bladder *(A)*. The longitudinal scan of the right lower quadrant *(B)* shows a shadowing appendicolith *(curved arrow)* in a thick-walled appendix, typical of appendicitis. *Straight arrows* outline the appendiceal tip, which looks ready to perforate. Free fluid in the pelvis always increases the suspicion of appendicitis. (From Teele R, Share J. Appendicitis and other causes of intra-abdominal inflammation. *In* Ultrasonography of Infants and Children. Philadelphia: WB Saunders, 1991:349.)

Gallstones, a dilated thick-walled gallbladder, or a dilated common bile duct can be visualized by ultrasonography and support the diagnosis of biliary disease. Edema of the pancreas is seen in acute pancreatitis. Ultrasonography also details the character of abdominal masses, differentiating cystic from solid masses, and can be helpful in demonstrating free fluid or abscesses. The anatomy of the urinary tract is also well defined by ultrasonography. If an ileus or intestinal obstruction is present, interpretation of the ultrasound examination becomes difficult because of the multiple air-filled loops of intestine.

CONTRAST STUDIES

In certain situations, the examination and plain radiographs may suggest bowel lesions, which are best delineated with a contrast medium placed in the bowel either in an upper gastrointestinal series or by enema. If a colonic obstruction is suspected, such as in Hirschsprung disease, the appropriate contrast study is a barium enema. If the presence of a perforation is possible, as in a perforated duodenal ulcer, a water-soluble agent is the contrast medium of choice.

Malrotation of the midgut in both infants and older children is best diagnosed by an upper gastrointestinal study. In the past, the barium enema was the favored study, but confusion about the position of the cecum, as a result of either reflux of barium into the ileum or the mobile nature of the cecum in infants, led to inaccurate conclusions. In both the infant who presents with an acute abdomen and bilious vomiting and the older child who manifests chronic abdominal pain and intermittent vomiting, the oral barium contrast study is highly reliable. The significant findings include incomplete obstruction of the duodenum caused by compression or volvulus of the intestine and abnormal position of the duodenojejunal junction (position of the ligament of Trietz).

Intussusception is both diagnosed and treated by means of barium enema. A previously well young child who presents with the sudden onset of severe, diffuse pain, evidence of blood in the stool, and the suggestion of a soft, nontender mass in the right upper quadrant of the abdomen classically has intussusception. The plain films may be nonspecific, may show evidence of intestinal obstruction, or may show a mass. A high index of suspicion is all that is needed to obtain the barium enema; some centers now use air rather than barium. Sedation with morphine is helpful to comfort the child and to perform a useful study. The weight of the barium column (elevated a *maximum* of 36 inches above the table) often completely reduces the intussusception, eliminating the need for surgical intervention. Brisk reflux of contrast into the terminal ileum signifies a complete reduction. This study should always be performed in consultation with a surgeon and with the child prepared to go to the operating room in case of failure of reduction or perforation of the colon. Successful hydrostatic reduction of the intussusception is accomplished in 50% to 75% of cases. Contraindications for reduction enemas include perforation and signs of peritonitis. Patients beyond the normal age range (3 months to 6 years) for intussusception often have an anatomic lead point (polyp, Meckel diverticulum, lymphoma); successful hydrostatic reduction may not be possible in these situations. In the presence of pneumoperitoneum, peritonitis, or unsuccessful hydrostatic reduction, surgical intervention is indicated. Recurrences occur in 5% of those treated with reduction enemas.

The barium enema has been used to identify acute appendicitis, especially when the signs and symptoms are atypical. A mass pressing against the cecum or thickening of the cecal wall may be seen on the barium enema, but ultrasonography and computed tomography (CT) with oral contrast are much more reliable. Contrast studies of the bowel are quite useful in the patient with suspected *inflammatory bowel disease* or *polypoid lesions* of the colon and small intestine.

COMPUTED TOMOGRAPHY

CT scanning is expensive and has limited value in the evaluation of acute-onset abdominal pain. CT is very useful in the initial evaluation of abdominal trauma and in the detailing of the extent of abdominal masses. The paucity of body fat in infants reduces its utility in that age group. Intravenous and gastrointestinal contrast must be used in CT of the abdomen to obtain the most information. CT is much more useful in the evaluation of chronic pain or persistent undefined inflammatory processes.

Management

Numerous diseases can cause acute abdominal pain (see Tables 18–1 and 18–2). It is necessary to be aware of the multiple etiologic factors; however, many are rare "zebras" and deserve little initial attention unless there is a family history or other specific clues (see Tables 18–6 and 18–7). The immediate concern in the child with the acute onset of abdominal pain is the differentiation of serious surgical and medical problems from the more common nonspecific causes of abdominal pain (see Tables 18–1, 18–3, 18–8, and 18–9). In fact, nonspecific findings and no specific diagnosis are what are usually found. A guide to the treatment of the child with acute-onset abdominal pain is noted in Figure 18–6.

An obvious diagnosis leads promptly to appropriate consultation and management. Mild, nonspecific illness is easily treated on an outpatient basis, with follow-up by telephone or in the office. However, the child who appears ill but in whom a specific diagnosis is not apparent presents a problem. That child should have an examination by a surgeon to be sure that no correctable intra-

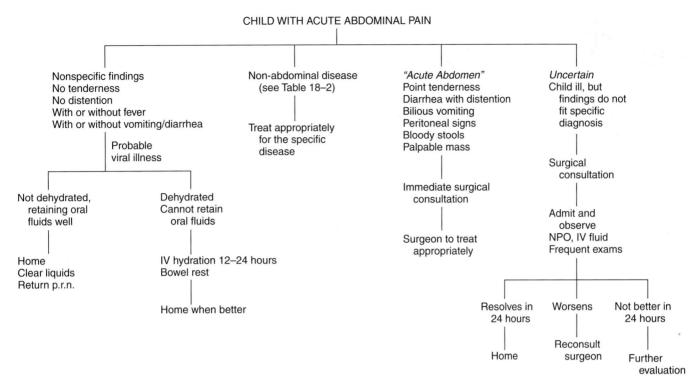

CHILD WITH ACUTE ABDOMINAL PAIN

Nonspecific findings
No tenderness
No distention
With or without fever
With or without vomiting/diarrhea

Probable
viral illness

Not dehydrated,
retaining oral
fluids well

Home
Clear liquids
Return p.r.n.

Dehydrated
Cannot retain
oral fluids

IV hydration 12–24 hours
Bowel rest

Home when better

Non-abdominal disease
(see Table 18–2)

Treat appropriately
for the specific
disease

"Acute Abdomen"
Point tenderness
Diarrhea with distention
Bilious vomiting
Peritoneal signs
Bloody stools
Palpable mass

Immediate surgical
consultation

Surgeon to treat
appropriately

Uncertain
Child ill, but
findings do not
fit specific
diagnosis

Surgical
consultation

Admit and
observe
NPO, IV fluid
Frequent exams

Resolves in
24 hours

Home

Worsens

Reconsult
surgeon

Not better in
24 hours

Further
evaluation

Figure 18–6. Algorithm to evaluate acute abdominal pain. NPO = *nil per os* (no oral intake); IV = intravenous.

abdominal disease is present. If the diagnosis is still not apparent, the child should be admitted for active observation, which includes no oral food or liquid, appropriate intravenous fluids, hourly vital signs, and frequent examinations. If the abdominal examination is difficult because of poor cooperation, sedation is appropriate but often not needed. The sedative should be a short-acting non-analgesic agent. Such an agent permits an adequate abdominal examination but does not eliminate the tenderness caused by an inflammatory process. The examination should be repeated 2 to 3 hours later. About 10% of children admitted for observation go on to show obvious signs of a surgical process in the first few hours. In approximately 50% of the observed children, a specific diagnosis, such as constipation or gastroenteritis, becomes apparent. The other patients improve with this management and are discharged with no specific cause being found for the pain.

Specific Causes of Acute Abdominal Pain

APPENDICITIS

Appendicitis is an acute inflammation of the appendix, which may be initiated by luminal obstruction by a fecalith, lymphoid hyperplasia (secondary to viral infections), or rarely, parasites (pinworm, *Ascaris*). Obstruction with ongoing distal secretion of mucus causes distention of the appendix, increased luminal pressure, and subsequent arterial obstruction and ischemia. Mucosal ulceration, fibropurulent serosal exudates, and bacterial infection lead to gangrene (from arterial obstruction) and rupture. Occasionally, the greater omentum may seal over a ruptured appendix, producing a right lower quadrant mass and periappendiceal abscess.

Appendicitis may be *simple* (focal inflammation, no serosal exudate), *suppurative* (obstructed, inflamed, edematous, increased local peritoneal fluid, with omental and mesenteric containment, or walled off), *gangrenous* (as in suppurative, plus gray-green or red-black areas of gangrene, with or without microperforations, purulent peritoneal fluid), *ruptured* (gross perforation, usually on antimesenteric side; peritonitis present) and *abscessed* (development of pus from rupture into right ileal fossa, lateral to cecum or retrocecal, subcecal, or pelvic). The bacteriology of appendicitis includes normal intestinal flora, such as enterococci, *Escherichia coli, Pseudomonas, Klebsiella* species, and anaerobic bacteria, such as *Clostridium* and *Bacteroides* species.

Appendicitis affects approximately 60,000 children each year in the United States; it primarily affects adolescents and young adults but may develop at any age, even in neonates. The disease is particularly severe in young children, often because of a delay in diagnosis with subsequent perforation. Appendicitis in young children is difficult to diagnose because of atypical presentations and the clinician's inability to obtain an accurate history. The thinness of the appendix and the paucity of the omentum in younger children may result in rapid unimpeded spread of intra-abdominal infection after rupture.

Diagnosis

An accurate and early diagnosis is critical to avoid rupture and peritonitis and to exclude other causes of abdominal pain. Appendicitis usually presents initially with a gradual onset of periumbilical (occasionally epigastric) pain, which may begin as a dull ache but becomes constant (or less often colicky) and of mild to moderate intensity. This is then followed by anorexia, nausea, and occasionally a few episodes of emesis. There may be constipation and the sensation that a bowel movement will improve the condition ("gas-stoppage sensation"). Occasionally, an inflamed appendix irritates the colon, producing diarrhea. Furthermore, the appendix may irritate the bladder, causing urinary frequency and dysuria. Pain may transiently stop, or, as local peritonitis develops, the pain may continue and shift to the right lower quadrant. (McBurney's point is defined by placing the little finger of one

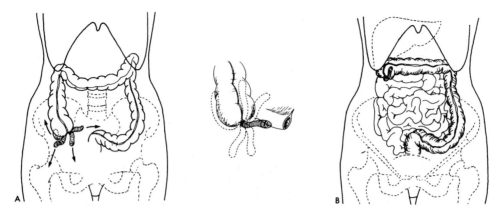

Figure 18–7. The appendix. A, The appendix may be located anteriorly, medially, or retrocecally or in the pelvis. B, The location of the appendix depends on the location of the cecum. Because the bowel may be quite mobile in some patients, the appendix may be located in many different sites in the abdomen. In this figure, the appendix is in the right upper quadrant. (From Reilly BM. Abdominal pain. In Practical Strategies in Outpatient Medicine, 2nd ed. Philadelphia: WB Saunders, 1991:728.)

hand in the umbilicus and the thumb on the anterior superior ileal spine. The index finger, if extended perpendicularly to the abdominal wall, identifies McBurney's point). The shifting of pain from the periumbilical to the right lower quadrant area may take 12 to 36 hours but usually occurs in 2 to 8 hours, and may not yet be evident in an acute onset of less than 4 to 6 hours. Unfortunately, the appendix is not always in its classic position; thus, appendicitis may produce pain in the pelvis, in the retrocecal area (back or flank pain, psoas muscle spasm with limp), or elsewhere (Fig. 18–7). With these locations, the psoas or obturator sign may be positive (see Fig. 18–3).

Patients with unperforated appendicitis have a low-grade fever (<38.5°C), are anxious while watching where examiners place their hands, are motionless, walk slowly, get on the examining table with difficulty, and exhibit a non-distended but tender abdomen with voluntary guarding, reduced bowel sounds, and point tenderness in any area overlying the appendix. Rectal examination may reveal right-sided or diffuse tenderness and a mass.

Perforation (rupture) or extensive gangrene should be suspected in the presence of progression for more than 36 to 48 hours, high fever, diffuse abdominal pain and tenderness, a rigid board-like abdomen, leukocytosis, a right lower-quadrant mass, and other signs of generalized peritonitis (see Table 18–9).

Laboratory and Radiographic Testing

The use of laboratory and radiographic tests in determining the differential diagnosis of acute abdominal pain has been discussed previously. Ultrasonography has been of benefit in the diagnosis of appendicitis and in excluding other important disease processes (Table 18–10). Helpful ultrasonographic features suggestive of appendicitis include a noncompressible appendix, an inability to visualize an appendix (ruptured), the presence of periappendiceal fluid, and the presence of an appendicolith (Figs. 18–8 and 18–9). Ultra-

sonography helps to define other disease processes, such as mesenteric adenitis (Fig. 18–10) and gynecologic processes. The latter conditions must be considered in all female patients. Ectopic pregnancy is a particularly serious condition, not to be missed (Fig. 18–11). Nonetheless, gastroenteritis is one of the more common conditions to be considered in the differential diagnosis (Table 18–11).

Treatment

The treatment of appendicitis is by surgical appendectomy and ligation of the stump by open or laparoscopic methods. If an abscess mass is present in the right lower quadrant and the patient demonstrates few signs of toxicity, elective nonurgent appendectomy may be delayed for 4 to 8 weeks to permit pre-operative rehydration and antibiotic therapy. In appendicitis, parenteral antibiotics (usually ampicillin, gentamicin, and clindamycin) are given before surgery and are continued postoperatively only in the presence of frank contamination (gangrenous or perforated appendicitis). The duration of antibiotic therapy is determined by the presence of infectious complications. If the appendix appears normal, other intra-abdominal sources of pain, such as Meckel's diverticulitis, should be sought during the surgery.

Complications of appendicitis are uncommon but include bacteremia-sepsis, intra-abdominal abscess formation, wound infections, ileus, peritoneal adhesion formation, and subsequent risk for intestinal obstruction and tubal infertility in female patients.

PANCREATITIS

Pancreatitis is an acute inflammatory condition of the pancreas and is often a result of obstruction of the pancreatic duct. Release and activation of pancreatic digestive enzymes subsequently result in extensive destruction (autodigestion) of pancreatic and, if severe, adjacent tissue. Proteolysis, fat necrosis, and hemorrhage are noted in severe or fatal cases of pancreatitis, which is often complicated by multiorgan dysfunction syndrome (e.g., hypotension, adult respiratory distress syndrome, acute tubular necrosis, cardiogenic shock).

Pancreatitis is less common in children than in adults, in whom the cause is often alcohol ingestion or gallstones. The etiology in childhood encompasses a broad differential diagnosis (Table 18–12) but often includes passage of biliary sludge (microlithiasis), drugs, multisystem diseases (Reye syndrome, hemolytic uremic syndrome, cystic fibrosis), trauma (including abuse), biliary or pancreatic anatomic anomalies, infections, and metabolic conditions (hypercalcemia, hypertriglyceridemia).

Table 18–10. Final Diagnoses in Cases of Clinically Suspected Appendicitis

Appendicitis	Gastroenteritis
Pelvic inflammatory disease	Urinary tract infection
Ovarian cyst—torsion	Meckel diverticulitis
Ectopic pregnancy	Pancreatitis
Mesenteric adenitis	Primary peritonitis
Perforated peptic ulcer	Cholecystitis

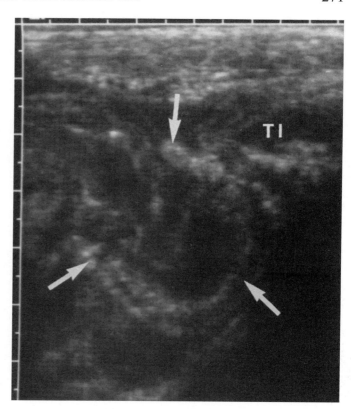

Figure 18–8. An ultrasound scan of the right lower quadrant in a 6-year-old girl, demonstrating a thick-walled cecum *(arrows)* outlined by echogenic fluid. No appendix was found in spite of careful ultrasonographic searching. During surgery, the patient was found to have a perforated appendix and early periappendiceal abscess. TI = terminal ileum. (From Teele R, Share J. Appendicitis and other causes of intra-abdominal inflammation. *In* Ultrasonography of Infants and Children. Philadelphia: WB Saunders, 1991.)

Manifestations

Manifestations of acute pancreatitis include intense epigastric abdominal pain that is steady, boring, constant, ache-like, knife-like, exacerbated by recumbency, and may radiate to the back, the upper abdominal quadrants, or the scapula. Emesis is common, often protracted, and occasionally bilious. Fever is usually low to moderate grade; high fever (>39 to 40°C) suggests the presence of a primary infectious process with or without secondary pancreatitis or bacterial superinfection. The patient often assumes a hunched over or knee-chest lateral fetal posture and may manifest epigastric tenderness and reduced or absent bowel sounds. Signs of peritonitis suggest more extensive necrosis, as do signs of spreading hemorrhage, such as blue-green discoloration of the flanks (Grey Turner sign) or of the periumbilical region (Cullen sign). Intravascular fluid depletion, cardiogenic shock, hemorrhagic shock, hypocalcemic tetany, or systemic inflammatory response syndrome with multiorgan system failure may ensue. Pain may last for 3 to 10 days.

The diagnosis is confirmed by an elevated serum amylase and/

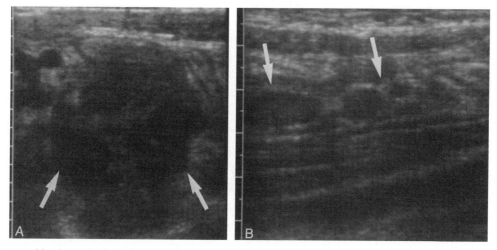

Figure 18–9. An 11-year-old girl presented with fever, diarrhea, and vomiting. Ten days before admission to the hospital, she was seen by a physician because of abdominal pain. She had been partially treated with antibiotics for a presumed "strep throat" in the interim. When she presented to the hospital, she again had pain in the right lower quadrant, especially when the ultrasound transducer was pressed over the area. *A,* The right lower quadrant abscess *(arrows)* was quickly identified. The appendix could not be visualized. In scans along the psoas *(B),* multiple lymph nodes *(arrows)* were apparent. The child's appendix had ruptured 1 week before admission, but her symptoms had been masked by the antibiotics that she had been given. (From Teele R, Share J. Appendicitis and other causes of intra-abdominal inflammation. *In* Ultrasonography of Infants and Children. Philadelphia: WB Saunders, 1991:348.)

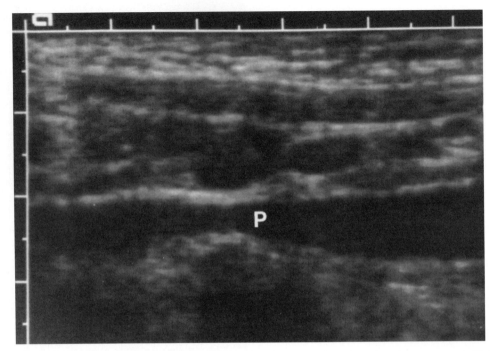

Figure 18–10. This longitudinal scan of the right lower quadrant shows lymph nodes arranged in a line along the psoas muscle (P). These are nodes enlarged from mesenteric adenitis. The patient did not have appendicitis. (From Teele R, Share J. Appendicitis and other causes of intra-abdominal inflammation. *In* Ultrasonography of Infants and Children. Philadelphia: WB Saunders, 1991.)

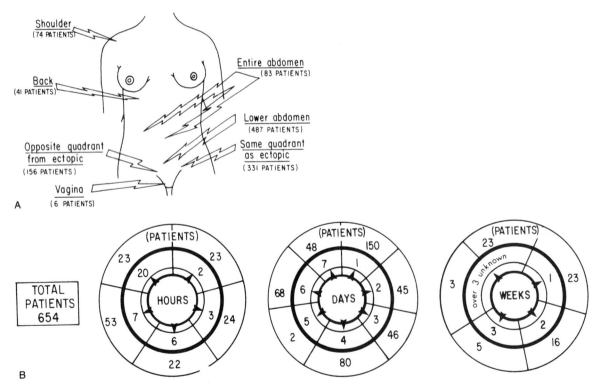

Figure 18–11. Ectopic pregnancy. *A,* Anatomic location of pain in 654 patients with ectopic pregnancy. *B,* Duration of abdominal pain before the diagnosis of ectopic pregnancy was confirmed among 654 patients. (Adapted from Breen JL. A 21-year survey of 654 ectopic pregnancies. Am J Obstet Gynecol 1970;106:1004–1019.)

Table 18–11. Comparison of Gastroenteritis and Appendicitis

	Gastroenteritis	Appendicitis
Pain	Diffuse, cramps, intermittent	Periumbilical shifting to RLQ; constant. Exacerbated by movement, coughing.
Vomiting	With or before pain	Follows pain
Diarrhea	Frequent, large volume	Can occur, small volume (from irritation of bowel)
Fever	Variable	Low grade, goes up with gangrene or perforation
Course	Intermittently improves	Worsens with time
Systemic symptoms	Variable: headache, malaise, myalgia, arthralgia, sore throat	Rare
Physical examination	General: fussy, restless, frequent motion	Quiet, discomfort with movement
	Abdomen: soft, mild, diffuse tenderness, hyperactive bowel sounds	Abdomen: RLQ tenderness, guarding peritoneal signs, ± rectal tenderness/mass, absent bowel sounds
Laboratory values	WBC: variable, may be quite high	WBC: mild elevation, early left shift. Becomes high only with gangrene or perforation
	Urine: nonspecific	Urine: may have WBCs and/or RBCs if bladder irritated, ketosis if prolonged vomiting
Imaging studies	Abdominal films: nonspecific ileus	Abdominal films: often nonspecific, ± fecalith, ± loss of psoas definition, ± scoliosis due to inflammation in RLQ.
	Ultrasonography: not indicated	Ultrasonography: enlarged appendix, peritoneal fluid, RLQ abscess, absent appendix, fecalith

Abbreviations: RBC = red blood cell; RLQ = right lower quadrant; WBC = white blood cell.

Table 18–12. Etiology of Acute Pancreatitis in Children

Drugs and Toxins	*Infections*	*Systemic Disease*
Alcohol	Coxsackie B virus	α_1-Antitrypsin deficiency
Acetaminophen	Epstein-Barr virus	Cystic fibrosis
Azathioprine	Hepatitis A, B	Diabetes mellitus
L-Asparaginase	HIV	Henoch-Schönlein purpura
Cimetidine	Influenza A	Hemochromatosis
Corticosteroids	Leptospirosis	Hemolytic uremic syndrome
Didanosine	Measles	Hyperlipidemia types I, IV, and V
Estrogens	Mumps	Hyperparathyroidism
Furosemide	Mycoplasma	Kawasaki syndrome
6-Mercaptopurine	Rubella	Systemic lupus erythematosus
Methyldopa	Reye syndrome	Malnutrition
Organophosphates		Organic acidemias
Pentamidine	*Obstructive*	Periarteritis nodosa
Scorpion bites	Ascariasis	Peptic ulcer
Sulfonamides	Biliary sludge	Postpancreatic transplantation
Tetracycline	Biliary tract malformation	Refeeding after malnutrition
Thiazides	Cholelithiasis	Reye syndrome
Valproic acid	Crohn disease	Uremia
	Duplication cyst	
Hereditary Pancreatitis	Pancreatic pseudocyst	*Traumatic*
Idiopathic	Pancreas divisum	Blunt injury
	Postoperative	Child abuse
	Sphincter of Oddi dysfunction	Surgical trauma
	Tumor	Total body cast

Adapted from Behrman RE (ed). Nelson Textbook of Pediatrics, 14th ed. Philadelphia: WB Saunders, 1992:999.
Abbreviation: HIV = human immunodeficiency virus.

Table 18–13. Differential Diagnosis of Hyperamylasemia

Pancreatic Pathology
  Acute or chronic pancreatitis
  Complications of pancreatitis (pseudocyst, ascites, abscess)
  Factitious pancreatitis
  Complication of ERCP

Salivary Gland Pathology
  Parotitis (mumps, *Staphylococcus aureus,* CMV, HIV, EBV)
  Sialadenitis (calculus, radiation)
  Eating disorders (anorexia nervosa, bulimia)

Intra-abdominal Pathology
  Biliary tract disease (cholelithiasis)
  Peptic ulcer perforation
  Peritonitis
  Intestinal obstruction
  Appendicitis

Systemic Diseases
  Metabolic acidosis (diabetes mellitus, shock)
  Renal insufficiency, transplantation
  Burns
  Anorexia–bulimia
  Pregnancy
  Drugs (morphine)
  Head injury
  Cardiopulmonary bypass

Adapted from Behrman RE (ed). Nelson Textbook of Pediatrics, 14th ed. Philadelphia: WB Saunders, 1992:999.
Abbreviations: CMV = cytomegalovirus; HIV = human immunodeficiency virus; EBV = Epstein-Barr virus; ERCP = endoscopic retrograde cholangiopancreatography.

or lipase level (lipase levels may be elevated initially with normal amylase values) (Table 18–13). In addition, ultrasonography and CT are helpful in identifying the acutely inflamed pancreas (Fig. 18–12) or the later development of a pancreatic pseudocyst (Fig. 18–13).

Adverse prognostic factors in severe acute pancreatitis include the presence of leukocytosis (white blood count > 16,000/mm³), hyperglycemia (glucose level > 200 mg/dl), a high lactic dehydrogenase level (>350 U/L), and a high aspartate aminotransferase level (>250 U/L) on admission, a decrease in hematocrit value (>10%), an increase in blood urea nitrogen level (>5 mg/dl), a low calcium level (<8 mg/dl), hypoxia (<60 mmHg), acidosis (base deficit >4 mmol/L), or severe dehydration (>6 L in adults) by 48 hours of hospitalization.

Complications

Complications of pancreatitis include local tissue necrosis with or without superinfection (pancreatic abscess), fistulization (to colon), left-sided pleural effusion, gastrointestinal hemorrhage (ulceration, vascular rupture, splenic rupture), shock, coagulopathy, acute tubular necrosis, myocardial depression, adult respiratory distress syndrome, hyperglycemia, hypocalcemia, subcutaneous nodules (fat necrosis), hypoalbuminemia, psychosis, and retinopathy.

Management

The management of acute pancreatitis consists of supportive care, such as nasogastric tube decompression for patients with an ileus or severe emesis, administration of intravenous fluids, administration of narcotics (meperidine) for pain, and therapy for accompanying complications (e.g., shock, adult respiratory distress syndrome, and acute tubular necrosis). Endoscopic sphincterotomy by endoscopic retrograde cholangiopancreoscopy (ERCP) is of benefit if gallstones and possibly if microlithiasis may be present. Nonetheless, this procedure has its own risks, which include the induction of pancreatitis.

Additional, but incompletely tested (i.e., efficacy unproven), therapies include peritoneal lavage; somatostatin, cimetidine, or glucagon administration; antiprotease (aprotinin) therapy; and acute surgical debridement or resection of sterile necrotic tissue. Nonetheless, infected necrotic tissue must be removed surgically; large persistent pseudocysts must also be managed by surgical drainage.

CHOLELITHIASIS

Gallstones (see Chapter 24) are uncommon in children and frequently complicate other chronic diseases, such as hemolytic anemia (sickle cell anemia, spherocytosis), cholestatic jaundice in which total parenteral nutrition is given, and other cholestatic diseases; it may result from prematurity or drug intake (furosemide, ceftriaxone), or it may be idiopathic. Biliary obstruction (stone in cystic or common bile duct) often results in jaundice, sudden onset of severe, sharp right upper quadrant pain, localized deep tenderness in the right upper quadrant (superficial tenderness suggests an associated cholecystitis) and emesis. The pain is episodic, colicky (but often constant, superimposed with waves of more intense pain), and may radiate to the angle of the scapula, the back, or other areas of the abdomen or chest. Patients frequently move about to find a comfortable position. There is associated diaphoresis, pallor, tachycardia, weakness, nausea, and lightheadedness. There may be a round or pear-shaped slightly tender mass palpated in the right upper quadrant of the abdomen if the gallbladder is distended. The pain may be diurnal, with increased intensity at night. Many patients with single or multiple gallstones (without obstruction) are asymptomatic.

Acute cholecystitis is due to inflammation of the gallbladder wall (as a result of duct obstruction [calculus] or nonobstructing [acalculus] conditions) and is manifested by fever, mild jaundice, severe abdominal pain, emesis, nausea, and leukocytosis. Pain may be similar to that in cholelithiasis and radiates to the right scapula, shoulder, or chest. *Murphy's sign* is demonstrated by palpating an acutely inflamed gallbladder, which causes the patient to halt respiration and feel the pain. Fever of greater than 39.5°C suggests perforation or gallbladder gangrene, whereas a high direct bilirubin level (>4 mg/dl) suggests a common duct stone. Pain may last for 5 to 10 days. Passage of stones or microlithiasis (sludge) may also produce acute pancreatitis. Intolerance (pain) to fatty foods is unfortunately a nonspecific observation.

Diagnosis

The diagnosis is confirmed by ultrasonography demonstrating acalculus or calculus-induced cholecystitis or acute duct obstruction by a stone (Fig. 18–14).

Treatment

Treatment of obstructing stones often includes open or laparoscopic cholecystectomy. However, medical management may include ERCP (for common duct stones); ursodeoxycholic acid stone

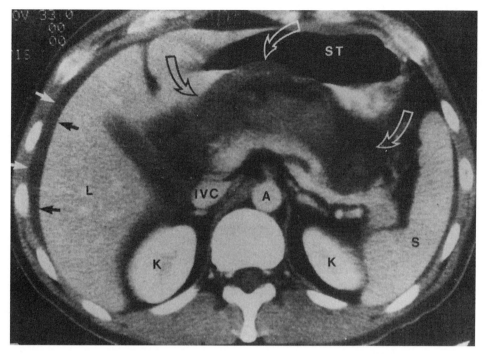

Figure 18–12. Acute pancreatitis. Computed tomography (CT) through the body of the pancreas demonstrates a halo of decreased attenuation around the pancreas that represents a peripancreatic zone of edema and fluid *(curved arrows).* Note the pancreatic ascites, most obvious lateral to the liver *(small arrows).* If intravenous contrast was administered before the CT scan, the inflamed pancreas would appear more dense (whiter). L = liver; A = aorta; K = kidney; PV = portal vein; S = spleen; IVC = inferior vena cava; ST = stomach. (From Freeny P, Lawson T. *In* Putman CE, Ravin CE [eds]. Textbook of Diagnostic Imaging. Philadelphia: WB Saunders, 1988.)

dissolution, and rarely extracorporeal gallstone lithotripsy. Meperidine is used for pain relief, and broad-spectrum antibiotics are indicated for cholecystitis or cholangitis.

PEPTIC ULCER DISEASE

Peptic ulceration is becoming recognized in children with increasing frequency. Risk factors for peptic ulcer disease (see Chapter 21), including gastritis, include a positive family history of ulcer disease, presence of *Helicobacter pylori,* treatment with nonsteroidal anti-inflammatory agents and possibly corticosteroids, cigarette smoking, and severe illness (burns, head injury, shock). Manifestations include pain, gastrointestinal bleeding (melena, hematemesis, anemia), emesis, and rarely perforation. Nocturnal pain, pain relieved by food, and a positive family history for peptic ulcer disease are often present. The pain is often chronic, recurrent, and located in the epigastrium; tenderness may be localized to the epigastric region but is an inconsistent finding.

Acute perforation is characterized by sudden worsening of pain or a new abrupt onset of severe excruciating epigastric pain. There

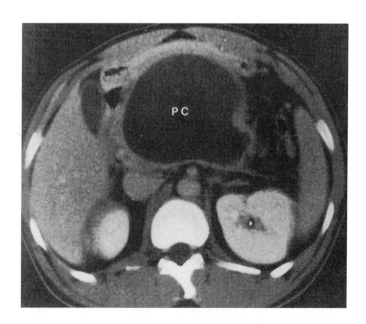

Figure 18–13. Pseudocyst. Follow-up CT scan (same patient as in Fig. 18–12) 5 months after the episode of acute pancreatitis demonstrates a large pseudocyst (PC). This large pseudocyst will probably not resolve spontaneously and may need drainage. (From Freeny P, Lawson T: *In* Putman CE, Ravin CE [eds]. Textbook of Diagnostic Imaging. Philadelphia: WB Saunders, 1988.)

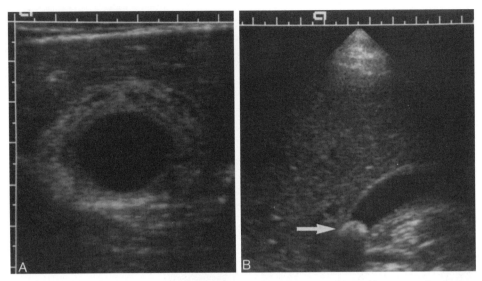

Figure 18-14. Transverse scan with linear array transducer shows pericholic edema in a teenaged boy, who presented with severe pain in the right upper quadrant from acute cholecystitis (A). A longitudinal scan of the right upper quadrant (B) shows a stone (arrow) that was thought to be impacted in the neck of the gallbladder because it did not change at all with position. The patient had severe pain with palpation over the gallbladder. (From Teele R, Share J. The liver. *In* Ultrasonography of Infants and Children. Philadelphia: W.B. Saunders, 1991.)

is associated pallor, faintness, weakness, syncope, diaphoresis, and a rigid abdomen. Corticosteroids may mask some of the signs of perforation.

CHRONIC AND RECURRENT ABDOMINAL PAIN

Chronic abdominal pain refers to recurrent or persistent bouts of pain that occur over a minimum of 3 months and may or may not compromise normal daily activities. An estimated 10% to 15% of school-aged children will experience recurring abdominal pain at some point (see Table 18–4). This general category of disease is often referred to as recurrent abdominal pain. The "functional" nature of this pain does not mean that the pain is imaginary or that it may not interfere with the child's daily activities.

Organic pain originates from a specific organ, which may be intra-abdominal or extra-abdominal in location. The cause of organic abdominal pain may be inflammation, obstruction, the presence of masses, or peritoneal irritation.

Dysfunctional pain is real and quite perceivable and arises from normal physiologic processes that become uncomfortable, such as alteration of bowel motility, excessive luminal pressure (distention) or muscle (muscularis) contraction (spasms), colic, and *mittelschmerz*. A very high percentage of children with chronic or recurrent abdominal pain have dysfunctional pain. The pain is real, but a specific diagnosis (e.g., ulcer) may not be identifiable.

Psychogenic pain is pain experienced in the absence of physical stimuli.

Chronic or recurring abdominal pain may begin with an acute episode, which is evaluated in the manner already described. The initial episode may be attributed to gastroenteritis, or no diagnosis may be made. Diseases not to be missed include peptic ulcer disease, inflammatory bowel disease, recurrent intestinal obstruction, biliary or urinary stones, esophagitis, carbohydrate intolerance, giardiasis and infection with other parasites, and genitourinary tract disease. Helpful clues to identify organic conditions are noted in Tables 18–7 and 18–8. Nevertheless, patients with recurrent abdominal pain experience real pain and should not be considered to be faking it or to be not experiencing it at all.

If the evaluation has been thorough and no cause for the complaints have been found, referral to a specialist, such as a pediatric gastroenterologist or pediatric surgeon, may be necessary to provide reassurance to both the family and the clinician that nothing has been missed. The person seeing the child in referral must be careful to support the conclusions of the primary care clinician if the workup has been appropriate and no organic cause for the pain can be found. Reassurance that the primary care physician has done a fine job is often enough to permit the family to work together with their doctor to monitor and support the child.

On the other hand, if the original complaints of pain were not completely investigated, now might be time to start again and search for possible organic or non-organic causes of the pain. If the history includes any aberration in bowel function, upper and/or lower gastrointestinal radiologic studies followed by upper or lower endoscopy (if indicated by radiologic studies) should be pursued. Evidence of malabsorption syndromes (e.g., lactase deficiency, celiac disease) would be suggested by cramping pain, weight loss, and diarrhea.

Complaints of abdominal pain with absolutely no gastrointestinal symptoms should lead to a thorough evaluation of the urinary tract, a search for inguinal or femoral hernias, and rarely a neurologic evaluation, including electroencephalogram (EEG). Abdominal migraines and abdominal epilepsy are unusual causes of recurring pain. Musculoskeletal problems, such as costochondritis, muscle sprain, or nerve root irritation, may cause abdominal wall pain.

The evaluation of the child with chronic or recurring abdominal pain requires the integration of history, objective findings, and laboratory data. The history should be detailed and, in most instances, obtained separately from the parents and the child. A private conversation with each often provides better insight into all factors affecting the child. In addition to covering the historical information already detailed, the clinician should pay attention to factors in the child's environment, family, school, and social interactions that may be sources of undue stress. Stress has been an inconsistent cause of recurrent abdominal pain. Furthermore, little convincing evidence suggests that patients with recurrent abdominal pain have specific or generalized psychologic disturbances. In addition, patients with recurrent abdominal pain do not have a lower pain threshold than unaffected patients. Just because stress exists (e.g., marital discord, school problems) does not mean that stress is the cause of the pain until all other reasonable diagnoses have been investigated. The incidence of life stresses is relatively high among children, and the clinician must not assume that chronic pain is not organic on the basis of poor school performance or perceived psychologic dysfunction.

Functional abdominal pain (non-organic, recurrent abdominal pain) is described as dull and in the periumbilical area, but, it may be colicky or burning. Onset often begins between 4 and 14 years of age. There may be a family history of irritable bowel disease and a personal history of sleepwalking, infant colic, enuresis, or nightmares. There is no consistent duration, frequency, or periodicity. The pain is usually brief (<1 hour); pain-free intervals range from days to weeks. When asked to point to the site of pain, the child may place the entire hand over the umbilicus or, less often, the epigastrium. There is usually no radiation to other sites.

Laboratory studies may not be specific but should include a complete blood count, erythrocyte sedimentation rate, urinalysis, stool assessment for ova and parasites and for occult blood, and if indicated, a breath hydrogen test (for lactose malabsorption) and stool assessment for α_1-antitrypsin (for inflammatory bowel disease). Anemia, leukocytosis, an elevated sedimentation rate, and abnormal serum protein levels are some of the data that may indicate organic disease.

Once the evaluation, including the history, physical examination, and appropriate screening laboratory tests has been completed and is normal, a search for non-organic sources of pain is appropriate. Many disorders can cause chronic abdominal pain, but only 10% or fewer of all children with chronic complaints of abdominal pain have an organic cause as the source of the pain. Other systemic symptoms, such as headache, nausea, pallor, sleepiness, diarrhea, and dizziness, may be present in patients with functional abdominal pain. In patients with functional recurrent abdominal pain, alterations in bowel habits are common. Growth and development are normal in patients with functional pain.

The child with functional pain may improve once the child and the family understands the nature of the pain. Knowing that there is no serious organic disease and that the sensations are not imaginary is usually welcome information to the family. Simple treatment strategies, such as stool softeners for the constipated child or dietary manipulation for the child who seems to have a lactose (or sorbitol) intolerance, often provide sufficient relief that the child can resume a more normal life.

When there is neither an organic source nor a dysfunctional origin for the pain, a more in-depth examination of psychologic factors is needed. Referral to a mental health professional may trigger more anxiety than it relieves in many families. One must gather positive evidence of emotional maladaptation, such as symptoms of depression, recent academic deterioration, maladaptive coping, or serious family discord, before referring for mental health evaluation. When a child is responding to environmental stresses, the primary physician is usually in the best position to evaluate and counsel.

Occasionally, specific medical (organic) conditions may mimic recurrent abdominal pain of functional etiology.

Peptic ulcer disease (see Chapter 21), often presents with abdominal pain that may be atypical from the classic description given by adults. Peptic ulcer disease should be considered if there is chronic pain that is present at night (awakens the patient) or in the morning or before meals (and is relieved by food). There may be recurrent emesis after meals and a positive family history of ulcers. Anemia and occult or gross gastrointestinal blood loss (hematochezia, melena, or hematemesis) may also be present.

Gastroesophageal reflux and peptic esophagitis may present with recurrent abdominal pain in the epigastric or substernal area (see Chapter 20). Classic signs of retrosternal pain (odynophagia) or discomfort (dysphagia) and water brash (dyspepsia) are often absent. Patients may respond to antireflux precautions and antacids or H_2-receptor blocking agents.

Carbohydrate malabsorption or intolerance from lactose or sorbitol or related polyalcohol sugars (fruit juices) may produce ingestion-related pain that responds to dietary elimination of the offending sugar (see Chapter 19). Additional conditions to consider include inflammatory bowel disease (see Chapter 19), pancreatitis, intestinal obstruction (see Chapter 20), and genitourinary tract diseases (see Chapters 27 to 31). Persistent, unrelieved, escalating, debilitating pain with associated fever, night sweats, and weight loss should suggest more serious disorders, such as a malignancy (lymphoma, hepatoblastoma, neuroblastoma) or infection (abscesses).

Sometimes, despite diligent evaluation by the most skilled and patient clinician, symptoms persist. In such cases, the following guidelines can help:

1. Assure the parents and the child that no major illnesses are present.
2. Identify any "red flags" that might arise and pursue an appropriate investigation (see Table 18–8).
3. Avoid emotional or psychologic labels arrived at by a process of elimination.
4. Assure the child and the family that the pain is real and not imaginary.
5. See the child regularly to monitor the symptom or symptoms.
6. Have the family document the episodes of pain and review this diary at the patient's regular office visit.
7. Do not feel pressured to make a specific diagnosis before the situation is clarified.
8. Avoid making a pseudo-diagnosis, such as "allergy" or "virus" or "nervous bowel."
9. During return office visits, allow time to speak with the child alone and the parents alone.
10. Obtain consultation, especially when the family does not seem completely satisfied with the current situation.
11. Try to normalize the child's life by encouraging school attendance and participation in all other regular activities.

Pharmacologic therapy with antispasmodic, anticholinergic, anticonvulsant, or antidepressant agents has not proved effective in children with functional recurrent abdominal pain. Such therapy has sometimes been effective in young adults with irritable bowel syndrome but is not recommended for younger children. If reassurance and time do not result in improvement in children with recurrent abdominal pain, a high-fiber diet may be effective therapy. Ten grams of corn fiber each day, introduced slowly, may benefit as many as 50% of patients.

Managing recurring abdominal pain can be a severe test of the physician's endurance, tenacity, and patience, but in most circumstances, the long-term support of these children and their families can be most satisfying. In as many at 30% to 50% of appropriately diagnosed cases, improvement may be seen within 2 to 6 weeks. An undetermined number of children continue to have abdominal or other pain syndromes (headache) into adulthood. Poor prognostic features include coming from a "pain-identifying" family, male gender, onset of pain before 6 years of age, and duration of pain for more than 6 months before therapy.

REFERENCES

Apley J. The Child with Abdominal Pains, 2nd ed. Oxford: Blackwell Scientific Publications, 1975.
Hatch EI. The acute abdomen in children. Pediatr Clin North Am 1985;32:1151–1164.
Harberg FJ. The acute abdomen in childhood. Pediatr Ann 1989;18:169–178.

Purcell TB. Nonsurgical and extraperitoneal causes of abdominal pain. Emerg Med Clin North Am 1989;7:721–740.

Reynolds S, Jaffe D, Lavigne J. Abdominal pain in a pediatric emergency department. Pediatr Emerg Care 1988;4:297–301.

Acute Abdominal Pain

Alford BA, McIlhenny J. The child with acute abdominal pain and vomiting. Radiol Clin North Am 1992;30:441–453.

Ashorn M, Maki M, Ruuska T, et al. Upper gastrointestinal endoscopy in recurrent abdominal pain of childhood. J Pediatr Gastroenterol Nutr 1993;16:273–277.

Barr RG, Levine MD, Watkins JB. Recurrent abdominal pain of childhood due to lactose intolerance. N Engl J Med 1979;300:1449–1451.

Bonadio WA. Clinical features of abdominal painful crisis in sickle cell anemia. J Pediatr Surg 1990;25:301–302.

Brewer RJ, Golden GT, Hitch DC, et al. Abdominal pain: An analysis of 1000 consecutive cases in a university hospital emergency room. Am J Surg 1976;131:219–223.

Buchert GS. Abdominal pain in children: An emergency practitioner's guide. Emerg Med Clin North Am 1989;7:497–517.

Byrne WJ, Arnold WC, Stannard MW, et al. Ureteropelvic junction obstruction presenting with recurrent abdominal pain: Diagnosis by ultrasound. Pediatrics 1985;76:934–937.

Franken EA, Kao SCS, Smith WL, et al. Imaging of the acute abdomen in infants and children. AJR Am J Roentgenol 1989;153:921–928.

Gallegos NC, Hobsley M. Abdominal wall pain: An alternative diagnosis. Br J Surg 1990;77:1167–1170.

Grey DWR, Dixon MD, Collin J. The closed eye sign: An aid to diagnosing non-specific abdominal pain. BMJ 1988;297:836–837.

Jeddy TA, Vowles RH, Southam JA. "Cough sign": A reliable test in the diagnosis of intra-abdominal inflammation. Br J Surg 1994;81:279–281.

Katz JA, Wagner ML, Gresik MV, et al. Typhlitis: An 18-year experience and postmortem review. Cancer 1990;65:1041–1047.

Leahy AL, Fogarty EE, Fitzgerald RJ, et al. Discitis as a cause of abdominal pain in children. Surgery 1984;95:412–414.

Lebenthal E, Rossi TM, Nord KS, et al. Recurrent abdominal pain and lactose absorption in children. Pediatrics 1981;67:828–832.

Paterson-Brown S. Emergency laparoscopic surgery. Br J Surg 1993;80:279–283.

Schaller RT, Schaller SF. The acute abdomen in the immunologically compromised child. J Pediatr Surg 1983;18:937–944.

Siegel MJ, Carel C, Surratt S. Ultrasonography of acute abdominal pain in children. JAMA 1991;266:1987–1989.

Soltero MJ, Bill AH. The natural history of Meckel's diverticulum and its relation to incidental removal. Am J Surg 1976;132:168–173.

Towne BH, Mahour GH, Woolley MM, et al. Ovarian cysts and tumors in infancy and childhood. J Pediatr Surg 1975;10:311–320.

Peptic Ulcer Disease

Chiang B-L, Chang M-H, Lin M-I, et al. Chronic duodenal ulcer in children: Clinical observation and response to treatment. J Pediatr Gastroenterol Nutr 1989;8:161–165.

Colin-Jones DG. Acid suppression: How much is needed? Adjust it to suit the condition. BMJ 1990;301:564–565.

Drumm B, Rhoads JM, Stringer DA, et al. Peptic ulcer disease in children: Etiology, clinical findings, and clinical course. Pediatrics 1988;82:410–414.

Feldman M, Burton ME. Histamine$_2$-receptor antagonists: I. Standard therapy for acid-peptic diseases. Part 1. N Engl J Med 1990;323:1672–1680.

Feldman M, Burton ME. Histamine$_2$-receptor antagonists: II. Standard therapy for acid-peptic diseases. Part 2. N Engl J Med 1990;323:1749–1755.

Gormally S, Drumm B. *Helicobacter pylori* and gastrointestinal symptoms. Arch Dis Child 1994;70:165–166.

Hosking SW, Ling TKW, Chung SCS, et al. Duodenal ulcer healing by eradication of *Helicobacter pylori* without anti-acid treatment: Randomised controlled trial. Lancet 1994;343:508–510.

Murphy MS, Eastham EJ, Jimenez M, et al. Duodenal ulceration: Review of 110 cases. Arch Dis Child 1987;62:554–558.

Appendicitis

Alvarado A. A practical score for the early diagnosis of acute appendicitis. Ann Emerg Med 1986;15:557–564.

Andersson R, Hugander A, Thulin A, et al. Indications for operation in suspected appendicitis and incidence of perforation. BMJ 1994;308:107–110.

Dickson AP, MacKinley GA. Rectal examination and acute appendicitis. Arch Dis Child 1985;60:666–667.

Doraiswamy NV. Progress of acute appendicitis: A study in children. Br J Surg 1978;65:877–879.

Doraiswamy NV. Leukocyte counts in the diagnosis and prognosis of acute appendicitis in children. Br J Surg 1979;66:782–784.

Jones DJ. Appendicitis. BMJ 1992;305:44–48.

Knight PJ, Vassy LE. Specific diseases mimicking appendicitis in childhood. Arch Surg 1981;116:744–746.

Neilson IR, Laberge J-M, Nguyen C. Appendicitis in children: Current therapeutic recommendations. J Pediatr Surg 1990:25:1113–1116.

Oestreich AE, Adelstein EH. Appendicitis as the presenting complaint in cystic fibrosis. J Pediatr Surg 1982;17:191–194.

Puylaert JBCM, Rutgers PH, Lalisang RI, et al. A prospective study of ultrasonography in the diagnosis of appendicitis. N Engl J Med 1987;317:666–669.

Tate JJT, Dawson JW, Chung SCS, et al. Laparoscopic versus open appendicectomy: Prospective randomised trial. Lancet 1993;342:633–637.

Wade DS, Morrow SE, Balsara ZN, et al. Accuracy of ultrasound in the diagnosis of acute appendicitis compared with the surgeon's clinical impression. Arch Surg 1993;128:1039–1046.

Walker DH, Henderson FW, Hutchins GM. Rocky Mountain Spotted Fever: Mimicry of appendicitis or acute surgical abdomen? Am J Dis Child 1986;140:742–744.

Pancreatitis

Buntain WL, Wood JIS, Woolley MM. Pancreatitis in childhood. J Pediatr Surg 1978;13:143.

Dugernier TH, Reynaert MS, Kesterns PJ. Severe acute pancreatitis the therapeutic dilemma: Medical or surgical intensive care? Intens Crit Care Dig 1991;10:47–50.

Fernandez-del Castillo C, Rattner DW, Warsha AL. Acute pancreatitis. Lancet 1993;342:475–479.

Kahler SG, Sherwood WG, Woolf D, et al. Pancreatitis in patients with organic acidemias. J Pediatr 1994;124:239–243.

Lee SP, Nicholls JF, Park HZ. Biliary sludge as a cause of acute pancreatitis. N Engl J Med 1992;326:589–593.

Rabeneck L, Feinstein AR, Horwitz RI, et al. A new clinical prognostic staging system for acute pancreatitis. Am J Med 1993;95:61–70.

Ranson JHC, Rifkind KM, Roses DF, et al. Prognostic signs and the role of operative management in acute pancreatitis. Surg Gynecol Obstet 1974;138:69–81.

Steinberg W, Tenner S. Acute pancreatitis. N Engl J Med 1994;330:1198–1210.

Weizman Z, Durie PR. Acute pancreatitis in childhood. Pediatrics 1988;113:24–29.

Williamson RCN. Endoscopic sphincterotomy in the early treatment of acute pancreatitis. N Engl J Med 1993;328:279–280.

Hepatobiliary Tract Disease

Debray D, Pariente D, Gauthier F, et al. Cholelithiasis in infancy: A study of 40 cases. J Pediatr 1993;122:385–391.

Goodman DB. Cholelithiasis in persons under 25 years old. JAMA 1976;236:1731–1734.

Johnston DE, Kaplan MM. Pathogenesis and treatment of gallstones. N Engl J Med 1993;328:412–421.

Kim SH. Choledochal cyst: Survey by the surgical section of the American Academy of Pediatrics. J Pediatr Surg 1981;16:402–407.

Reif S, Sloven DG, Lebenthal E. Gallstones in children. Am J Dis Child 1991;145:105–108.

Chronic Abdominal Pain

Camilleri M, Prather CM. The irritable bowel syndrome: Mechanisms and a practical approach to management. Ann Intern Med 1992;116:1001–1008.

Castile RG, Telander RL, Cooney DR, et al. Crohn's disease in children: Assessment of the progression of disease, growth and prognosis. J Pediatr Surg 1980;15:462–469.

Goldstein DP, deCholnoky C, Leventhal JM, et al. New insights into the old problem of chronic pelvic pain. J Pediatr Surg 1979;14:675–680.

Janik JS, Ein SH. Normal intestinal rotation with non-fixation: A cause of chronic abdominal pain. J Pediatr Surg 1979;14:670–674.

Levine MD, Rappaport LA. Recurrent abdominal pain in school children: The loneliness of the long distance physician. Pediatr Clin North Am 1984;31:969–991.

Liebman WM. Recurrent abdominal pain in children: A retrospective survey of 119 patients. Clin Pediatr 1978;17:149–153.

Murphy MS. Management of recurrent abdominal pain. Arch Dis Child 1993;69:409–415.

Silverberg M. Chronic abdominal pain in adolescents. Pediatr Ann 1991;20:179–185.

19 Diarrhea

Jonathan Flick

The word diarrhea is derived from the Greek *diárrhoia,* meaning "a flowing through." The adult human intestine handles 7 L per 24 hours of endogenous secretions (salivary, gastric, intestinal, pancreatic, biliary) and 2 L of ingested fluids. Three to 5 L are absorbed by the jejunum, 2 to 4 L by the ileum, and 1 to 2 L by the colon, resulting in 100 to 200 ml of daily stool output. In simple pathophysiologic terms, diarrhea results from a relative increase in secretion or a decrease in intestinal absorption, or both (Tables 19–1 and 19–2).

Diarrhea in adults is usually defined as a stool volume output of more than 200 ml each day. In children, a stool output that exceeds 10 ml/kg/day is considered to be diarrhea. A more practical definition is that diarrhea is present when stools increase in frequency, fluidity (water content), or volume, as compared with the previously established "normal" pattern. Wide variability exists in normal bowel patterns from child to child, and age-related changes also can occur. Breast-fed infants may pass a loose or seedy stool with each nursing. In older infants or children, stool frequency may vary from several times each day to once every several days.

Diarrhea in children is frequently accompanied by abdominal pain, defecatory urgency, fecal incontinence, vomiting, or some combination of these.

Acute-onset diarrhea is one of the most common presenting complaints during childhood and is usually a self-limited illness. Causes of acute and chronic childhood diarrhea are listed in Tables 19–3 and 19–4. Chronic diarrhea is defined as that which persists for more than 2 or 3 weeks.

ACUTE DIARRHEA

Viral Gastroenteritis

Viral agents account for most cases of acute gastroenteritis in childhood (Tables 19–4 and 19–5). Viruses cause diarrhea by localizing to the surface absorptive cells of the small intestine and

Table 19–1. Mechanisms of Diarrhea

Primary Mechanism	Defect	Stool Examination	Examples	Comment
Secretory	Decreased absorption, increased secretion	Watery, normal osmolality; osmols = $2 \times (Na^+ + K^+)$	Cholera, toxigenic *Escherichia coli,* carcinoid, VIP, neuroblastoma, congenital chloride diarrhea, *Clostridium difficile,* cryptosporidiosis (AIDS)	Persists during fasting; bile salt malabsorption also may increase intestinal water secretion; no stool leukocytes
Osmotic	Maldigestion, transport defects, ingestion of unabsorbable solute	Watery, acidic, + reducing substances; increased osmolality; osmols $>2 \times (Na^+ + K^+)$	Lactase deficiency, glucose-galactose malabsorption, lactulose, laxative abuse	Stops with fasting, increased breath hydrogen with carbohydrate malabsorption, no stool leukocytes
Increased motility	Decreased transit time or stasis (bacterial overgrowth)	Fecal-like, stimulated by gastrocolic reflex	Irritable bowel syndrome, thyrotoxicosis, postvagotomy dumping syndrome	Infection also may contribute to increased motility
Decreased surface area	Decreased functional capacity	Watery	Short bowel syndrome, celiac disease, rotavirus enteritis	May require elemental diet plus parenteral alimentation
Mucosal invasion (motile or secretory)	Inflammation, decreased colonic reabsorption, increased motility	Blood and increased WBCs in stool	*Salmonella, Shigella,* amebiasis, *Yersinia, Campylobacter*	Dysentery = bloody mucus, and WBCs

From Kirschner BS, Black DD. The gastrointestinal tract. *In* Behrman RE, Kliegman RM (eds). Nelson Essentials of Pediatrics, 2nd ed. Philadelphia: WB Saunders, 1994:398.
Abbreviations: AIDS = acquired immunodeficiency syndrome; VIP = vasoactive intestinal peptide; WBC = white blood cell.

Table 19–2. Causes of Osmotic Diarrhea

Ingestion of Poorly Absorbable Solutes
  Magnesium sulfate, sodium sulfate, citrate-containing laxatives
  Some antacids—Mg(OH)$_2$
  Mannitol, sorbitol (chewing gum, diet candy)

Maldigestion
  Disaccharidase deficiencies (lactose, sucrose-isomaltose, trehalose
    intolerance)
  Gastrocolic fistula, jejunoileal bypass, short-bowel syndrome
  Lactulose therapy

Mucosal Transport Defects
  Glucose-galactose malabsorption
  Chloridorrhea
  Congenital sodium diarrhea
  General malabsorption in diffuse disease of small-bowel mucosa

Adapted from Krejs GJ. Diarrhea. *In* Wyngaarden JB, Smith LH, Bennett JC (eds). Cecil Textbook of Medicine, 19th ed. Philadelphia: WB Saunders, 1992:682.

inducing a noninflammatory enteritis. Stools are typically watery and do not contain white or red blood cells. Systemic features, such as low-grade fever, vomiting, and respiratory symptoms, often accompany the diarrhea (Table 19–6). Infants in particular are prone towards dehydration.

Rotavirus is the most common cause of diarrhea in childhood. Person-to-person transmission of this ribonucleic acid (RNA) virus occurs by the fecal-oral route, although respiratory transmission has also been suggested. Household spread, transmission at day care centers and schools, and nosocomial infection are common. Children younger than 2 years of age are most susceptible, although infection occurs in all age groups. In temperate climates, the disease displays seasonal distribution, with infection being most common during the cooler months (November through May). Affected children are usually ill for 2 to 8 days, following a 1- to 3-day incubation period. Asymptomatic infections are common in newborns and older individuals. Acute diarrhea in the young child, occurring during winter and associated with vomiting, low-grade fever, and dehydration, most likely represents rotavirus infection. Confirmation may be obtained with enzyme-linked immunosorbent assay (ELISA) and latex agglutination assays for rotavirus detection in stool. Chronic infection does not occur in immune-competent hosts, but after severe infection, the small intestinal mucosa may take 3 to 8 weeks to fully recover its absorptive ability, leading to a chronic, postinfectious enteropathy in some individuals. Rotaviral vaccines are under active development.

Norwalk agent, also an RNA virus, is the second most common cause of viral gastroenteritis in children. Affected children are older than those seen with rotavirus infection, and a seasonal pattern of infection is not consistently recognized. In addition to diarrhea and

Table 19–3. Differential Diagnosis of Diarrhea

	Infant	Child	Adolescent
Acute			
Common	Gastroenteritis	Gastroenteritis	Gastroenteritis
	Systemic infection	Food poisoning	Food poisoning
	Antibiotic associated	Systemic infection	Antibiotic associated
	Overfeeding	Antibiotic associated	
Rare	Primary disaccharidase deficiency	Toxic ingestion	Hyperthyroidism
	Hirschsprung toxic colitis		
	Adrenogenital syndrome		
	Neonatal opiate withdrawal		
Chronic			
Common	Postinfectious secondary lactase deficiency	Postinfectious secondary lactase deficiency	Irritable bowel syndrome
	Cow's milk/soy protein intolerance	Irritable bowel syndrome	Inflammatory bowel disease
	Chronic nonspecific diarrhea of infancy	Celiac disease	Lactose intolerance
	Excessive fruit juice (sorbitol) ingestion	Lactose intolerance	Giardiasis
	Celiac disease	Excessive fruit juice (sorbitol) ingestion	Laxative abuse (anorexia nervosa)
	Cystic fibrosis	Giardiasis	Constipation with encopresis
	AIDS enteropathy	Inflammatory bowel disease	
		AIDS enteropathy	
Rare	Primary immune defects	Acquired immune defects	Secretory tumor
	Glucose-galactose malabsorption	Secretory tumors	Primary bowel tumor
	Microvillus inclusion disease (microvillus atrophy)	Pseudo-obstruction	Gay bowel disease
	Congenital transport defects (chloride, sodium)	Sucrase-isomaltase deficiency	Appendiceal abscess
	Primary bile acid malabsorption	Eosinophilic gastroenteritis	Addison disease
	Münchausen by proxy		
	Hirschsprung disease		
	Shwachman syndrome		
	Secretory tumors		
	Acrodermatitis enteropathica		
	Lymphangiectasia		
	Abetalipoproteinemia		
	Eosinophilic gastroenteritis		
	Short bowel syndrome		
	Intractable diarrhea syndrome		
	Autoimmune enteropathy		

Adapted from Kirschner BS, Black DD. The gastrointestinal tract. *In* Behrman RE, Kliegman RM (eds). Nelson Essentials of Pediatrics, 2nd ed. Philadelphia: WB Saunders, 1994:399.
Abbreviations: AIDS = acquired immunodeficiency syndrome.

Table 19–4. Epidemiology of Infectious Agents Causing Diarrhea in the United States

	Percentage of Cases of Diarrhea	Epidemiology
Viruses		
Rotavirus	15–35	Person-to-person spread; winter months; infants
Enteric adenovirus	5–15	Types 40, 41. Person-to-person spread; all ages
Norwalk-like viruses (Snow Mountain, Hawaii, Ditchling)	5–15	Food- and water-borne common source, person-to-person spread; all ages
Astrovirus (Marin County agent)	1–5	Nosocomial, food-, water-borne; epidemics; all ages
Calicivirus	1–2	Year round, sporadic and epidemic cases; infants
Coronavirus	<1	Pathogenicity uncertain
Bacteria		
Campylobacter jejuni	5–15	Source: wild and domestic animals, poultry, water, raw milk; fecal-oral spread; infants and adolescents
Salmonella enteritidis	3–5	May be underreported. Source: poultry, meat, eggs, milk, pigs, turtles; fecal-oral spread; infants, young children
*Shigella (sonnei, flexneri)**	3–5	Person-to-person transmission, summer-fall season, dysentery; young children (1–3 yr)
Escherichia coli 0157:H7*	1–3	Person-to-person spread, food-borne, milk, meat; all ages
Enterotoxigenic *E. coli*	1–3	Most common cause of traveler's diarrhea
Yersinia enterocolitica	1–3	Source: animals, raw milk, tofu, bean sprouts, chitterlings, diarrhea in infants, mesenteric adenitis in adolescents
Clostridium difficile	1–2	Antibiotic associated: person-to-person nosocomial spread
Staphylococcus aureus	1	Toxin-mediated food poisoning, common source
Clostridium perfringens	1	Toxin-mediated food poisoning, common source
Aeromonas hydrophila	<1	Water-borne: shellfish, sewage, vegetables
Plesiomonas shigelloides	<1	Shellfish, foreign travel
Vibrio cholerae	<1	Gulf of Mexico, shellfish, water
Vibrio parahaemolyticus	<1	Gulf of Mexico, shellfish
Bacillus cereus	<1	Toxin-mediated food poisoning, common source
Parasites		
Giardia lamblia	High incidence in day care centers, residential facilities	Most common parasitic cause of diarrhea, person-to-person, fecal-oral, water-borne spread; all ages
Cryptosporidium	Unknown, common in day care centers	Water-borne, animal-human, person-to-person, AIDS spread; infants, older if AIDS is a factor
Entamoeba histolytica	<1	Person-to-person spread, southwestern United States
Balantidium coli	<1	Pig contact, contaminated water
Strongyloides stercoralis	<1	Eosinophilia, urticaria

Modified from Behrman RE (ed). Nelson Textbook of Pediatrics, 14th ed. Philadelphia: WB Saunders, 1992:664.
Abbreviations: AIDS = acquired immunodeficiency syndrome.
**E. coli* 0157:H7 and less often *Shigella* are associated with the hemolytic-uremic syndrome.

vomiting, headache, myalgia, and malaise are common. Epidemic outbreaks of infection are common, although sporadic cases also occur. Diagnostic tests for the Norwalk virus are not commercially available. Numerous other viruses are associated with childhood diarrhea (see Tables 19–4 and 19–5), the clinical features of which may be indistinguishable from those of the more common viral agents.

Viral gastroenteritis is best managed with oral electrolyte-carbo-hydrate (glucose and starch) rehydration solutions. In the absence of severe dehydration (shock, tachycardia, hypotension [Table 19–7]), most infants can be treated with 24 to 48 hours of oral rehydration therapy, followed by re-initiation of standard formula. If unstable vital signs or refractory emesis is present, intravenous fluid therapy is indicated to correct shock, re-establish perfusion, correct past fluid losses, and replace ongoing losses in addition to providing daily maintenance fluid and electrolyte needs. Nonethe-

Table 19–5. Viral Enteric Pathogens

	Predominant Age Group Affected	Seasonality	Duration of Symptoms
Rotavirus	6–24 months	↑ in winter months	2–8 days
Norwalk virus	Older children, adults	Winter and summer	12–48 hours
Enteric adenovirus	<2 years	↑ in summer months	Up to 14 days
Calicivirus	3 months–6 years	Unknown	2–8 days
Astrovirus	1–3 years	Unknown	1–4 days

From Laney DW Jr, Cohen MB. Infectious diarrhea. *In* Wylie R, Hyams JS (eds). Pediatric Gastrointestinal Diseases: Pathophysiology, Diagnosis, Management. Philadelphia: WB Saunders, 1993:613.

Table 19–6. Differentiation of Bacterial and Viral Causes of Gastroenteritis

Variable	Bacterial	Viral
Temperature >38.5°C	Yes	Unusual
Abdominal pain, tenesmus	Yes	Unusual
>8 bowel movements/24 hr	Yes	Unusual
Emesis	Unusual	Yes
Duration >5 days	Yes	No
Erythrocyte sedimentation rate	Elevated	Normal
Leukocytosis	Yes	No
Stool leukocytes and mucus present	Yes (*Shigella, Salmonella, Yersinia, Campylobacter,* invasive *Escherichia coli, Plesiomonas*)	
Stool leukocytes absent: secretory diarrhea	Yes (*Vibrio cholerae,* toxigenic *E. coli, Aeromonas*)	No
Hematochezia	Yes (*Shigella, Salmonella, Yersinia, Campylobacter,* enterohemorrhagic *E. coli,* pseudomembranous colitis due to *Clostridium difficile, Plesiomonas*)	No, except rotavirus in preterm infants
History of shellfish consumption	Yes (*E. coli, Vibrio cholerae, Vibrio parahaemolyticus, Campylobacter*)	Yes (Norwalk agent)
Traveler's diarrhea	Yes (toxigenic *E. coli, Salmonella, Shigella*)	Unusual (Norwalk agent and rotavirus)
Single-source outbreak	Yes (*Salmonella, Shigella, Staphylococcus aureus, Bacillus cereus, Clostridium perfringens, Yersinia, E. coli*)	Yes (Norwalk agent)
Seasonal epidemics	Unusual (*Campylobacter*)	Yes (rotavirus)

From Behrman RE (ed). Nelson Textbook of Pediatrics, 14th ed. Philadelphia: WB Saunders, 1992:665.

less, most infants with emesis can be treated with small-volume frequent oral rehydration feeding, and those in shock can be resuscitated parenterally and then given oral rehydration solutions.

Bacterial Diarrhea

Bacterial infections of the intestine cause diarrhea through one or more mechanisms (Tables 19–8 and 19–9). Direct invasion of intestinal epithelial cells leads to mucosal inflammation and cell necrosis and is responsible for the clinical features of dysentery, which include blood and mucus (fecal leukocytes), fever, and abdominal pain. *Salmonella, Shigella, Campylobacter,* and *Yersinia* species as well as enteroinvasive *Escherichia coli,* act through this mechanism. *Vibrio cholerae,* noncholera vibrios, enterotoxigenic *E. coli, Aeromonas* species, and *Plesiomonas* species elaborate *enterotoxins* that alter the mucosal transport of water and electrolytes. Infected individuals develop watery diarrhea that contains neither red nor white blood cells. *Cytotoxins,* in contrast, cause mucosal cell necrosis and an inflammatory diarrhea. Examples of cytotoxins include enterohemorrhagic *E. coli* and *Clostridium dif-*

Table 19–7. Assessment of Degree of Dehydration

	Mild	Moderate	Severe
Infant	5%	10%	15%
Adolescent	3%	6%	9%
Signs and Symptoms			
General appearance and condition			
Infants/young children	Thirsty; alert; restless	Thirsty; restless or lethargic but irritable or drowsy	Drowsy; limp, cold, sweaty, cyanotic extremities; may be comatose
Older children	Thirsty; alert; restless	Thirsty; alert (usually)	Usually conscious (but at reduced level), apprehensive; cold, sweaty, cyanotic extremities; wrinkled skin on fingers/toes; muscle cramps
Tachycardia	Absent	Present	Present
Palpable pulses	Present	Present (weak)	Decreased
Blood pressure	Normal	Orthostatic hypotension	Hypotension
Cutaneous perfusion	Normal	Normal	Reduced/mottled
Skin turgor	Normal	Slight reduction	Reduced
Fontanel	Normal	Slightly depressed	Sunken
Mucous membrane	Moist	Dry	Very dry
Tears	Present	Present/absent	Absent
Respirations	Normal	Deep, may be rapid	Deep and rapid
Urine output	Normal	Oliguria	Anuria/severe oliguria

From Lewy JE. Nephrology: fluids and electrolytes. (Adapted from World Health Organization Guide.) *In* Behrman RE, Kliegman RM (eds). Nelson Essentials of Pediatrics, 2nd ed. Philadelphia: WB Saunders, 1994:582.

Table 19–8. Enteric *Escherichia coli* Infections

Type	Mechanism	Clinical Syndrome	Stools
Enterotoxigenic	Enterotoxin(s); adherence	Traveler's diarrhea; nursery outbreaks	Watery; no blood or polys
Enteropathogenic	Adherence; Shiga-like toxin	Infantile diarrhea; asymptomatic carriage	Watery ± blood; no polys
Enterohemorrhagic*	Shiga-like toxin	Hemorrhagic colitis	Bloody; rare polys
Enteroadherent	Adherence	Chronic childhood diarrhea; traveler's diarrhea	Chronic watery; no blood or mucus
Enteroinvasive	Shiga-like toxin	Dysentery	Blood, polys, mucus in stools
Enteroaggregative	? Toxin	Persistent diarrhea in developing countries	Watery with or without blood

*Associated with hemolytic-uremic syndrome.
Abbreviation: polys = polymorphonuclear leukocytes.

ficile. Enteropathogenic *E. coli,* as well as the protozoal organisms *Cryptosporidium* and *Giardia,* adhere closely to the surface of the intestinal absorptive cell, causing damage to the brush border of the enterocyte and interference with normal digestion.

The epidemiology of common bacterial pathogens is noted in Table 19–4. Differentiation from viral pathogens is noted in Table 19–6.

SPECIFIC BACTERIAL PATHOGENS

Salmonella

Salmonellae are gram-negative rods that may cause an asymptomatic intestinal carrier state, enterocolitis with diarrhea, or bacteremia without gastrointestinal manifestations but with subsequent local infections (meningitis, osteomyelitis). Serotyping of lipopolysaccharide cell wall antigens allows salmonellae to be divided into five major groups, A through E. Important serotypes include *Salmonella typhi* (group D), *Salmonella choleraesuis* (group C), *Salmonella typhimurium* (group B), and *Salmonella enteritidis* (group D).

Epidemiology. With the exception of *S. thyphi* infection, which occurs only in humans, most *Salmonella* infections are acquired through ingestion of food products derived from infected animals (eggs, poultry, raw milk). Most infections in the United States are sporadic rather than epidemic. Outbreaks may occur among institutionalized children, although outbreaks in day care are rare. Infants and children under 5 years of age are particularly susceptible. Infections are most common during the summer months.

Clinical Features. Symptomatic intestinal damage may follow clinical illness or may result in a carrier state with inapparent infection. Most carriers spontaneously clear their infection within weeks to months but remain infectious as long as fecal excretion of the organism occurs. Chronic carriage (defined as >1 year duration) in children is uncommon.

Enterocolitis. After a 12- to 48-hour incubation period, gastroenteritis develops. It is characterized by the sudden onset of diarrhea, abdominal cramps and tenderness, and fever. The diarrhea is watery, with stools containing polymorphonuclear leukocytes and occasionally blood (Fig. 19–1). Symptoms slowly and spontaneously resolve within 3 to 5 days.

Diagnosis. The peripheral blood white blood cell count is usually normal in *Salmonella* gastroenteritis. The organism is readily isolated from stool culture or rectal swab. The differential diagnosis includes all causes of acute diarrhea.

Table 19–9. Gastrointestinal Infections: Mechanisms of Diarrhea

Agent	Location	Mechanism	White Blood Cells in Stool
Rotavirus	Small intestine	Villous injury	No
Norwalk agent	Small intestine	Villous injury	No
Salmonella sp.	Ileum-colon	Mucosal ulceration	Yes—variable
Shigella sp.	Ileum-colon	Toxin; mucosal ulceration	Yes
Campylobacter sp.	Ileum-colon	Ulceration; toxin (?)	Yes
Yersinia sp.	Ileum-colon	Toxin; mucosal ulceration	Yes—variable
Escherichia coli	See Table 19–8	—	—
Clostridium difficile	Colon	Toxin	Yes—variable
Aeromonas sp.	Small intestine; colon	Toxin	No
Giardia sp.	Small intestine	Villous injury	No
Ameba	Colon	Mucosal ulceration	Yes
Cryptosporidium sp.	Small intestine, colon	Mucosal injury	No
Vibrio sp.	Small intestine	Toxin	No

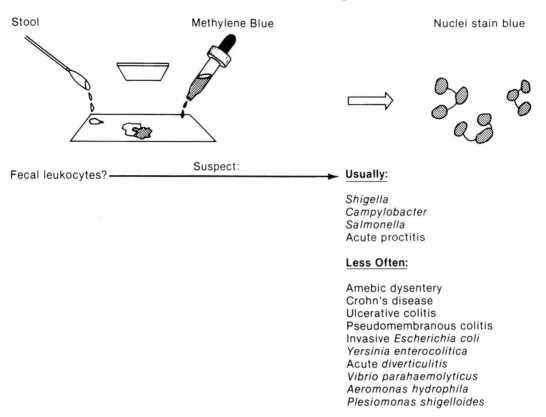

Figure 19–1. Staining for fecal leukocytes. Fecal leukocytes are detected by placing a small fleck of fecal mucus on a microscopic slide, mixing it thoroughly with 2 drops of *methylene blue,* and then examining the cover-slipped slide under high-power microscopy (after 2 or 3 minutes to allow adequate "staining" of the cellular nuclei with the blue dye). (From Reilly BM. Diarrhea. *In* Practical Strategies in Outpatient Medicine, 2nd ed. Philadelphia: WB Saunders, 1991:853.)

Treatment. *Salmonella* enterocolitis is generally a self-limited illness. Antibiotic therapy is not indicated for uncomplicated infections, because it may prolong the period of fecal excretion while having no effect on the clinical course. Treatment is indicated in those at increased risk for bacteremia and invasive disease, including infants younger than 3 months of age and immunocompromised patients (Table 19–10). For others, treatment is directed at maintaining adequate hydration. Treatment with antiperistaltic drugs is contraindicated in cases of invasive bacterial dysentery because it may lead to more severe symptoms or intestinal perforation.

Shigella

Shigella organisms are gram-negative rods. Four species are recognized, with *Shigella sonnei* and *Shigella flexneri* accounting for most infections in the United States; *Shigella dysenteriae* is extremely rare in the United States.

Epidemiology. Most *Shigella* infections in the United States occur in young children, 1 to 4 years of age, with a peak incidence in late summer and early autumn. The organism is transmitted by the fecal-oral route, most often by hands. Outbreaks in day care centers and institutions for the developmentally disabled are common. Chronic carriage does not occur, but organisms may be excreted in the feces for up to 6 weeks after clinical symptoms have resolved.

Clinical Features. During a 12- to 72-hour incubation period,

patients may develop a nonspecific prodrome characterized by fever, chills, nausea, and vomiting. A colitis affecting predominately the rectosigmoid region develops and results in abdominal cramps and watery diarrhea. In more severe infections (bacillary dysentery), blood and mucus are passed in small, very frequent stools. High fever in young infants may induce a febrile seizure (see Chapter 40).

Diagnosis. Stools may test positive for leukocytes and blood, but this result is not helpful in distinguishing shigellosis from acute diarrhea caused by other invasive enteric pathogens (*Salmonella, Campylobacter, Yersinia*) (see Table 19–9). Specimens of feces or rectal swab specimens should be obtained for culture.

Treatment. Unlike *Salmonella* gastroenteritis, antibiotic treatment is indicated in shigellosis because it shortens the duration of diarrhea and prevents further spread of the organism (see Table 19–10). Trimethoprim-sulfamethoxazole (TMP-SMZ) is usually effective, but because plasma-mediated antimicrobial resistance is common, drug susceptibility testing should be performed. Attention should be given to fluid and electrolyte replacement.

Campylobacter

Campylobacter is a curved or spiral gram-negative rod. *Campylobacter jejuni* is the most important species in human infection. Other species occasionally causing diarrhea include *Campylobacter fetus* and *Campylobacter laridis.*

Table 19–10. Antibiotic Therapy for Diarrhea

Organism	Treatment*	Comment
Salmonella typhi	Ampicillin†, chloramphenicol†, trimethoprim-sulfamethoxazole, cefotaxime, ciprofloxacin‡	Invasive, bacteremic disease
Other *Salmonella*	Usually none; amoxicillin, ampicillin, trimethoprim-sulfamethoxazole, cefotaxime, ceftriaxone if susceptible	Treatment indicated if less than 3 mo of age, or if malignancy, sickle cell anemia, AIDS, evidence of nongastrointestinal foci of infection are present
Shigella	Trimethoprim-sulfamethoxazole, ampicillin, cefixime, cefotaxime, ciprofloxacin‡	Amoxicillin is not recommended; treatment reduces infectivity and improves outcome
E. coli Toxigenic	Usually none if endemic; trimethoprim-sulfamethoxazole or ciprofloxacin for traveler's diarrhea	Prevention of traveler's diarrhea with bismuth subsalicylate, doxycycline, or ciprofloxacin‡
Invasive or pathogenic	Trimethoprim-sulfamethoxazole, neomycin, gentamicin (oral)	
Campylobacter	Mild disease needs no treatment; erythromycin for diarrhea, gentamicin for systemic illness; ciprofloxacin‡	If started early (days 1–3), treatment reduces symptoms and fecal organisms
Yersinia	None for diarrhea; gentamicin, chloramphenicol, trimethoprim-sulfamethoxazole for systemic illness	Value of treatment of mesenteric adenitis with antibiotics is not established
Vibrio cholerae	Tetracycline, trimethoprim-sulfamethoxazole	Fluid maintenance is critical
Clostridium difficile	Oral vancomycin, metronidazole§	*C. difficile* is an agent of antibiotic-associated diarrhea and pseudomembranous colitis
Giardia lamblia	Quinacrine, furazolidone, metronidazole§	Furazolidone only preparation available in liquid form
Cryptosporidium	None; azithromycin or paromomycin + octreotide in AIDS	A serious infection in immunocompromised patients (AIDS)
Entamoeba histolytica	Metronidazole§, tinidazole followed by iodoquinol	

Adapted from Kirschner BS, Black DD. The gastrointestinal tract. *In* Behrman RE, Kliegman RM (eds). Nelson Essentials of Pediatrics, 2nd ed. Philadelphia: WB Saunders, 1994:400.
*All treatment is predicated on knowledge of antimicrobial sensitivities.
†Often resistant.
‡Ciprofloxacin is not indicated for children with growing bones (less than 17 yr).
§The safety of metronidazole in children is unknown.
Abbreviation: AIDS = acquired immunodeficiency syndrome.

Epidemiology. Many animal species, including poultry, farm animals, and household pets, serve as reservoirs of *C. jejuni.* Transmission occurs through ingestion of contaminated food and through person-to-person spread via the fecal-oral route. Perinatal transmission from an infected mother to her newborn infant can result in neonatal gastroenteritis or sepsis. The disease is common in infants and adolescents. Day care outbreaks have been reported. Asymptomatic carriage is uncommon.

Clinical Features. Incubation period is from 1 to 7 days. The organism causes a diffuse, invasive enteritis that includes the ileum and colon. Fever, cramping, abdominal pain, and bloody diarrhea are characteristic symptoms and occasionally mimic those of acute appendicitis. Fever and diarrhea usually resolve after 5 to 7 days; prolonged illness or relapse occasionally occur. Symmetric peripheral neuropathy (Guillain-Barré syndrome) may follow *Campylobacter* infection.

Diagnosis. Gram stain of the stool may reveal characteristic organisms to the trained observer but is relatively insensitive. Culture of the organism from fecal specimens requires special techniques; the clinician should specifically indicate to the lab that *Campylobacter* infection is suspected.

Treatment. Most *C. jejuni* strains are sensitive to erythromycin but resistant to penicillin, ampicillin, cephalosporins, and TMP-SMZ. Although antibiotic treatment eradicates the organism from the stool and may, therefore, prevent person-to-person spread, it may also shorten the period of clinical illness only if it is started early in the disease process.

Yersinia

Yersinia organisms are gram-negative rods; important species include *Yersinia pseudotuberculosis* and *Yersinia enterocolitica.* They may cause various clinical syndromes, including gastroenteritis, mesenteric adenitis, pseudoappendicitis, and postinfectious reactive arthritis.

Epidemiology. The organism is present in animals and may be spread to humans by consumption of undercooked meat (especially pork), unpasteurized milk, and other contaminated foods. Person-to-person spread also occurs. Young children are particularly susceptible to disease, and the frequency of infections is increased during the summer months.

Clinical Features. Enterocolitis with fever, abdominal pain, and bloody, mucoid diarrhea are the most common manifestations. Symptoms usually resolve after 1 or 2 weeks but rarely persist longer. Nonspecific abdominal pain and an appendicitis-like illness may occur in older children. Less common manifestations include bacteremia with septic complications, such as osteomyelitis, meningitis, or reactive arthritis.

Diagnosis. The organisms may be cultured from rectal swab or stool specimens, but selective media are required and the organism may not be identified for several weeks. The microbiology laboratory should be notified if *Yersinia* infection is suspected.

Treatment. The benefit of antibiotic treatment of uncomplicated intestinal disease has not been established. Patients with extraintestinal infection should receive therapy (see Table 19–10). Most *Yersinia* organisms are susceptible to aminoglycosides, third-generation cephalosporins, chloramphenicol, and TMP-SMZ.

Escherichia coli

Although *E. coli* is the predominant aerobic species in the normal colon, it can also be a cause of diarrheal illness. Diarrhea caused by *E. coli* can be watery, inflammatory, or bloody, depending on the strain of organism involved (see Table 19–8).

Epidemiology and Treatment. *Enteric* infections with *E. coli* are acquired by the fecal-oral route. The highest age-specific attack rates for enterotoxigenic and enteropathogenic *E. coli* infections are in infants and young children; such infections are uncommon in the United States. Enterohemorrhagic strains are the only diarrhea-producing *E. coli* that are common in the United States and have been associated with food-borne epidemic outbreaks transmitted by undercooked meat. Some cases of enterohemorrhagic-associated diarrhea evolve into the hemolytic-uremic syndrome (HUS).

Enterotoxigenic infection with *E. coli* is the major cause of traveler's diarrhea; occasional nosocomial outbreaks have also occurred in hospitalized infants. After *E. coli* is ingested in contaminated food or water, the organism colonizes the upper small intestine. Following a 2- to 7-day incubation period, a syndrome of nausea, vomiting, low-grade fever, abdominal cramps, and watery diarrhea develops. The illness resembles mild cholera but occasionally can be severe. It usually abates in 1 to 5 days and rarely persists beyond 2 weeks. At least three different types of *E. coli* enterotoxins (heat-labile, heat-stable toxin A, heat-stable toxin B) have been identified. Definitive diagnosis requires enterotoxin identification and is not widely available. A presumptive diagnosis is made in a compatible clinical setting (e.g., the abrupt onset of large volume, watery, non-bloody diarrhea in a recent traveler to an endemic area).

Prophylactic antibiotics are effective in reducing the incidence of traveler's diarrhea but are not recommended for use in children. Empiric treatment with TMP-SMZ at the time of onset of symptoms may reduce the duration of illness from 3 to 5 days to 1 to 2 days. Replacement and maintenance of fluid and electrolytes is a more important measure.

Enteropathogenic infection with *E. coli* is a well-established cause of infantile diarrhea, especially in underdeveloped countries. Asymptomatic carriage is common. At least two separate mechanisms are responsible for diarrhea: adherence to intestinal epithelial cells, leading to villous injury and mucosal inflammation, and production of a toxin similar to that of *Shigella*. Clinically, enteropathogenic *E. coli* infections cause a moderate volume, clear to bloody diarrhea that can rapidly lead to dehydration in neonates. Chronic infection with failure to thrive may also occur. Diagnosis requires serotyping of fecal *E. coli* isolates but is not recommended in sporadic disease because of the high carrier rate and the uncertain pathogenic role of these organisms. Antimicrobial treatment of older children or adults with enteropathogenic *E. coli* diarrhea is unnecessary because of the self-limited nature of the illness. Neonates with documented enteropathogenic *E. coli* infection and diarrhea may be treated with nonabsorbable antibiotics, such as neomycin (100 mg/kg/day three times daily, for 5 days). For more severe disease, TMP-SMZ may be useful.

Enterohemorrhagic infection with *E. coli* produces a Shiga-like cytotoxin and cause diarrhea, hemorrhagic colitis, and the hemolytic-uremic syndrome. Both epidemic and sporadic cases have been recognized. Infection is more common in the summer and fall. A particular serotype, *E. coli* 0157:H7, has been isolated in several outbreaks associated with undercooked beef from fast food restaurants and has been linked to the development of HUS in young children. The most common presentation of enterohemorrhagic *E. coli* infection begins with severe abdominal cramps and watery diarrhea, followed by grossly bloody stools and emesis. Fever is uncommon. Fecal leukocytes are absent or few.

Other presentations include asymptomatic infection and watery diarrhea without progression to hemorrhagic colitis. *E. coli* 0157:H7 is rapidly cleared from the stool in 5 to 12 days. HUS develops in a small number of children in the week after the onset of diarrhea. HUS manifests with renal failure (high BUN, creatinine and oliguria-anuria), microangiopathic hemolytic anemia (anemia, reticulocytosis, abnormal-shaped erythrocytes on blood smear, and thrombocytopenia), and diarrhea. Specialized microbiologic techniques are required for identification of enterohemorrhagic *E. coli* but are indicated in cases of hemorrhagic colitis, HUS, diarrhea in HUS contacts, and epidemic, severe diarrhea. The role of antimicrobial therapy in enterohemorrhagic *E. coli* disease is uncertain. Antibiotics neither shorten the duration of disease nor prevent progression to HUS.

The *enteroadherent* forms of *E. coli* attach to the small intestinal mucosal surface and damage microvilli. They have been observed in children with chronic, mild diarrhea, resulting in failure to thrive, and in some cases of traveler's diarrhea. Antibiotic treatment has not proved to be effective.

Enteroinvasive infection with *E. coli* is a rare cause of epidemic dysentery.

Clostridium Difficile

Epidemiology. *Clostridium difficile* is an anaerobic, spore-forming, gram-positive rod. *C. difficile* can be recovered from stool samples in 2% to 5% of healthy adults in the community and from as many as 20% of asymptomatic hospitalized patients. The organism flourishes when other intestinal pathogens are suppressed by antibiotic therapy, and once present in the stool, it can be spread rapidly from patient to patient.

Transmission occurs through person-to-person contact and environmental contamination. Environmental contamination occurs through the spores formed by *C. difficile,* which can retain their viability for up to 1 week on dry surfaces. *C. difficile* and its toxin have been identified in the feces of up to 70% of healthy neonates and infants in concentrations similar to those found in adults with pseudomembranous colitis. The apparent resistance of newborns to *C. difficile* and its toxin is caused by a developmental absence of the toxin-binding site in the newborn intestine.

The isolation frequency of *C. difficile* declines with increasing age: the organism is present in the stool of about 3% of asymptomatic children older than 1 year, and in only 2% or fewer of healthy adults.

Clinical Features. *C. difficile* infection is highly associated with recent antibiotic exposure (ampicillin, amoxicillin, cephalosporins, clindamycin, erythromycin). These drugs disrupt the endogenous colonic flora that inhibit the growth of *C. difficile*. Other risk factors for *C. difficile* diarrhea include gastrointestinal medications (laxatives, stimulants), gastrointestinal surgery or procedures, and cancer chemotherapy.

C. difficile–associated colitis is caused by the potent toxins that this organism produces: toxin A, a lethal enterotoxin that causes hemorrhage and fluid secretion in the intestines, and toxin B, a cytotoxin detectable by its cytopathic effects in tissue culture. Both toxins seem to play an important role in disease production, although toxin A is more important initially.

C. difficile infection should be considered in patients who develop diarrhea during or within several weeks of antibiotic therapy. Pseudomembranous colitis, the most severe form of antibiotic-associated diarrhea, is usually secondary to *C. difficile,* whereas antibiotic-associated diarrhea without colitis commonly occurs in the absence of *C. difficile*. Rare presentations of *C. difficile* infection include fever or abdominal pain without diarrhea, or diarrhea in the absence of recent antibiotic use. *C. difficile* diarrhea may be mild and self-limited or may be associated with high fever, profound leukocytosis, and systemic toxicity. Life-threatening or fatal complications, such as toxic megacolon and colonic perforation, occur rarely.

Diagnosis. Diagnostic evaluation for *C. difficile* infection is performed by identification of the organism and its cytotoxin or by endoscopic examination of colonic mucosa. Sigmoidoscopy or colonoscopy reveal pseudomembranes in 30% to 50% of cases, typically in association with more severe disease.

Treatment. Table 19–10 outlines treatment of *C. difficile*–induced diarrhea and colitis. The offending antibiotic is discontinued, and oral vancomycin or metronidazole therapy is initiated. Parenteral metronidazole therapy is used for severe ileus, toxic megacolon, or impending intestinal perforation.

Aeromonas

Aeromonas species are gram-negative organisms that may cause a mild, self-limited diarrheal illness in children. The most common manifestation is a watery, non-bloody, non-mucoid diarrhea seen during the late spring, summer, and early fall. More severe infections may resemble ulcerative colitis, with chronic bloody diarrhea and abdominal pain. Treatment with TMP-SMZ is indicated in these cases.

Plesiomonas

Plesiomonas shigelloides is a vibrio-like organism that is sometimes implicated in childhood diarrhea. It has been linked to consumption of shellfish and travel to Mexico and Asia.

PROTOZOAN DIARRHEA

Giardia

Epidemiology. *Giardia lamblia* is a flagellated protozoan that can cause diarrhea, malabsorption, abdominal pain, and weight loss. It spreads through contaminated food and water as well as through person-to-person contact by the fecal-oral route. The latter mode of transmission is responsible for outbreaks of diarrhea in day care centers and residential facilities.

Clinical Features. Infection is frequently asymptomatic. Symptomatic illness usually develops 1 to 3 weeks after exposure and may mimic acute gastroenteritis with fever, nausea, vomiting, and watery diarrhea. In some patients, a chronic illness develops, characterized by intermittent, foul-smelling diarrhea, abdominal bloating, nausea, abdominal pain, and weight loss.

Diagnosis. The stool should be examined for cysts or trophozoites on at least three fresh specimens, owing to the intermittent excretion of the organism in feces. An ELISA-based *Giardia* antigen test is a more sensitive means of detecting infection and should be performed, if available.

Treatment. All infected persons should be treated. Many agents are available. Metronidazole (20 mg/kg/day for 5 days) is highly effective, but the drug is not available in liquid form and may cause gastrointestinal upset. Furazolidone (1.25 mg/kg four times a day for 7 days) is less effective but is better tolerated and is available in liquid form.

Other Protozoa

Entamoeba histolytica is an organism acquired in warm climates (Mexico, southwestern United States) by ingestion of cysts in fecally contaminated material. Infected individuals are often asymptomatic. Amebic dysentery may occur but hepatic abscess and other remote infections are uncommon. Because cysts are shed in the stool on an intermittent basis, examination of several fecal specimens may be required for identification of infected individuals. Asymptomatic or mild infections may be treated with a luminal amebicide, such as diiodohydroxyquin; more severe infections (invasive intestinal or extraintestinal) are treated with metronidazole.

Cryptosporidium is a coccidian protozoan that causes watery diarrhea in both immunocompetent and immunocompromised hosts. It is an important cause of diarrhea in individuals infected with the human immunodeficiency virus (HIV). It has also been recognized as an occasional cause of self-limited diarrhea in travelers as well as in children in day care centers and persons in residential institutions.

The mechanisms by which these organisms cause diarrhea are unknown. Special techniques are required for identifying the oocysts in fecal specimens and should be requested if *Cryptosporidium* is suspected. Antimicrobial therapy is not indicated in immune-competent hosts and is ineffective in immunocompromised infected individuals.

Blastocystis hominis is an anaerobic organism of uncertain taxonomy that appears to be an occasional cause of abdominal pain, diarrhea, and vomiting in infected children.

OTHER CAUSES OF ACUTE DIARRHEA

Parenteral Secondary Diarrhea

Acute diarrhea may accompany infection outside of the gastrointestinal tract (so-called parenteral diarrhea). Thus, upper respiratory tract and urinary tract infections may be associated with increased bowel movement frequency or stool water. The mechanism is unclear but may involve alterations in bowel motility, changes in diet, or effects of antibiotic treatment.

Drugs

Various prescription and over-the-counter drugs may cause acute diarrhea. The most commonly implicated agents are antibiotics, acting through mechanisms other than *C. difficile*. Other medications sometimes associated with diarrhea in children are shown in Table 19–11.

Food Poisoning (Table 19–12)

Staphylococcal food poisoning results from ingestion of preformed enterotoxin, produced in contaminated food that has incubated at or above room temperature for a suitable period. Staphylococcal food intoxication is suggested by the sudden onset of vomiting followed by explosive diarrhea, usually within 4 to 6 hours after ingestion of the contaminated food. The illness is self-limited and usually resolves within 12 to 24 hours. The diagnosis is made on the basis of a characteristic clinical picture. Treatment is supportive (fluid and electrolyte replacement); antibiotics are not indicated.

Bacillus cereus, a gram-positive, spore-forming organism found in soil, is usually associated with contaminated refried rice or vegetables. Two food poisoning syndromes can occur. A short-incubation disease (1 to 6 hours) results from ingestion of preformed toxin and is characterized by nausea, vomiting, and diarrhea, similar symptoms to those of staphylococcal food poisoning. A long-incubation period disease (8 to 16 hours) is caused by *in vivo* production of an enterotoxin and is characterized by abdominal pain, tenesmus, and profuse watery diarrhea. Vomiting is usually absent. Both syndromes resolve spontaneously within 24 hours and are managed with supportive care.

Clostridium perfringens food poisoning has been associated with ingestion of contaminated beef and poultry. The disease results from production and release into the lower bowel of an enterotoxin 8 to 24 hours after ingestion of the vegetative form of the organism. Onset is sudden, with abdominal pain and watery diarrhea. Fever and vomiting are absent.

Other causes of food poisoning are noted in Table 19–12.

CHRONIC DIARRHEA

The causes of chronic diarrhea (defined as diarrhea of greater than 2 or 3 weeks in duration) are numerous (see Table 19–3). Certain etiologic features are seen more frequently in specific age groups.

Chronic diarrhea needs to be distinguished from various malabsorption states, which may be classified by the nutrient that is malabsorbed (Table 19–13) or by the site of the malabsorptive defect (Table 19–14). Manifestations of malabsorption are noted in Table 19–15. Initial screening and stepwise testing for malabsorption are noted in Table 19–16, and a more detailed explanation is noted in Table 19–17. Common causes of malabsorption are noted in Table 19–18. Therapy depends on the primary disease and includes therapy of that process plus replacement of the malabsorbed nutrient by parenteral or higher-dose enteral routes.

Chronic Diarrhea in Infancy

PROLONGED INFECTION AND POSTINFECTIOUS ENTEROPATHY

Chronic intestinal infections are uncommon but occur occasionally, particularly in infants with preexisting malnutrition and in those with immunologic deficiencies. More commonly, persistent diarrhea following an acute enteritis is due to a postinfectious enteropathy. Predisposing factors include age of less than 6 months, malnutrition, formula feeding rather than breast milk feeding, and poverty. Pathophysiologic mechanisms include damage to the small intestinal villi with loss of disaccharidase activity and reduction in the mucosal surface absorptive area. Small-bowel bacterial overgrowth and absorption of potentially antigenic proteins may aggravate the malabsorptive state. Patients with mild involvement may do well on a non–lactose-containing formula. More severely affected infants may require a semi-elemental formula (Pregestimil), whereas the most severe cases may not tolerate any enteral feedings and must be placed on parenteral nutrition. Recovery usually occurs over 4 to 6 weeks, provided that the child is supplied with adequate nutrition.

FORMULA PROTEIN INTOLERANCE

Formula protein (cow's milk and/or soy protein) intolerance is caused by sensitization to dietary proteins that are absorbed intact through the intestinal mucosa. Two syndromes are most commonly seen: an *enterocolitis,* with inflammatory changes in the small bowel and colon, usually presenting with bloody diarrhea in the first 3 months of life; and a *protein-losing enteropathy,* associated with diarrhea, occult intestinal blood loss, and hypoproteinemia, most often seen after the age of 6 months.

Table 19–11. Medications Associated with Diarrhea in Children

Agent	Mechanism
Stimulant laxatives (senna, phenolphthalein, bisacodyl)	Increased intestinal secretion
Antacids	Osmotic effect (Mg^{2+})
Pro-kinetic agents (metoclopramide, bethanechol, cisapride)	Increased peristalsis
Measles-mumps-rubella vaccine	Unknown
Thyroid hormone	Increased peristalsis
Monosodium glutamate	Unknown
Chemotherapeutics	Intestinal mucosal injury
Mushrooms	Multiple mechanisms
Heavy metals	Toxic effect
Organophosphates	Cholinergic effects
Diuretics	Unknown
Digitalis	Unknown
Colchicine	Unknown
Indomethacin	Prostaglandin synthesis inhibition
Theophylline	Increased peristalsis

Table 19–12. Food-Borne Gastrointestinal Illnesses

Cause	Incubation Period	Clinical Clues	Common Vehicle	Diagnosis
Monosodium glutamate	Minutes to 2 hours	Chinese restaurant syndrome Burning in abdomen, neck, chest, extremities Lightheadedness, chest pain	Chinese food	Large amount of monosodium glutamate found in incriminated food
Heavy metals (copper, zinc, cadmium, tin)	Minutes to 2 hours	Metallic taste, diarrhea Vomiting prominent No fever	Carbonated or acidic beverages in metal containers	Chemical study of incriminated beverage
Mushroom toxin*	Minutes to 2 hours	Altered mental status with visual disturbance (encephalopathy) Hepatitis	Non-commercially obtained mushrooms	Identify mushroom and/or toxic chemical (e.g., muscarine, psilocybin)
Fish/shellfish* Scombrotoxin	Minutes to 2 hours	Histamine reaction: flushing, headache, dizziness, burning of throat and mouth	Tuna, mackerel, bonito, skipjack, mahi-mahi	Identify fish and/or chemical toxin (ciguatoxin, tetrodotoxin, histamine, etc.)
Paralytic shellfish toxin	Minutes to 2 hours	Paresthesias, dizziness Sometimes paralysis "Red tide" in incriminated water	Mussels, clams, oysters, scallops	
Puffer fish toxin Ciguatoxin	Minutes to 2 hours 2–24 hours	Paresthesias Paresthesias, cramps Itching, arthralgias, metallic taste, visual disturbances "Loose" painful teeth	Puffer fish Barracuda, red snapper, grouper, amberjack, mackerel	
Norwalk virus	24–48 hours	Epidemic watery diarrhea	Clams, oysters	Radioimmunoassay
Staphylococcus aureus†	2–8 hours	Prominent vomiting No fever Duration less than 24 hours	Ham, poultry, pastries (cream-filled), mixed salads, egg salad	Isolate 10^5 organisms from food Preformed toxin
Bacillus cereus Emetic form—short incubation	2–8 hours	Prominent vomiting No fever Duration less than 48 hours	Fried rice Macaroni/cheese	Isolate 10^5 organisms from food Preformed toxin
Diarrhea form—long incubation	8–14 hours	Abdominal cramps Severe diarrhea No fever Duration less than 48 hours	Fried rice, vegetables Macaroni/cheese	Isolate 10^5 organisms from food and/or stool *In vivo* toxin production
Clostridium perfringens†	8–14 hours	Abdominal cramps Severe diarrhea No fever Duration less than 48 hours	Meat, poultry, gravy	Isolate 10^5 organisms from food and/or stool *In vivo* toxin production
Enterotoxigenic Escherichia coli	12 hours to several days	Abdominal cramps, watery diarrhea May be prolonged (up to 1 week)	Incomplete data (rarely reported)	Isolate organism and test for enterotoxin production
Vibrio cholerae	12 hours to days	Abdominal cramps, watery diarrhea May be prolonged (up to 1 week)	Incomplete data (very rare in United States)	Isolate organism in stool and/or food
Invasive E. coli	12 hours to days	Prolonged febrile diarrhea and/or dysentery	Incomplete data	Isolate organism in stool and test for enteroinvasiveness
Shigella	12 hours to days	Prolonged febrile diarrhea and/or dysentery	Fish, mixed salads	Stool culture (or food culture)
Salmonella†	12 hours to days	Prolonged febrile diarrhea and/or dysentery, emesis	Meat, poultry, dairy products, eggs, various salads	Stool culture (or food culture)
Vibrio parahaemolyticus	12 hours to days	Prolonged febrile diarrhea and/or dysentery	Seafood	Stool culture (or food culture)
Campylobacter	12 hours to days	Prolonged febrile diarrhea and/or dysentery	Unpasteurized milk Poultry, meat	Stool culture (or food culture)
Clostridium botulinum†	12 hours to days	Diarrhea, constipation Cranial nerve palsies, paralysis, ventilatory failure	Home-canned foods, fish, honey	Botulinum toxin in food, stool, and serum
Yersinia enterocolitica	Uncertain	Prolonged diarrhea and/or dysentery	Milk, pig intestine	Stool culture

Adapted from Reilly BM. Practical Strategies in Outpatient Medicine, 2nd ed. Philadelphia: WB Saunders, 1991:888.
*Potentially dangerous—observation in hospital often required.
†*Salmonella* (23%), *S. aureus* (18%), *C. perfringens* (8%), and *C. botulinum* (8%) are the most common causes of food poisoning.

Table 19-13. Specific Defects of Digestive-Absorptive Function Occurring in Children

	Disease
Intestinal	
Fat	Abetalipoproteinemia
Protein	Enterokinase deficiency
	Amino acid transport defects (cystinuria, Hartnup disease, methionine malabsorption, blue diaper syndrome)
Carbohydrate	Disaccharidase deficiencies (congenital: sucrase-isomaltase, lactase; developmental: lactase, acquired)
	Glucose—galactose malabsorption (congenital, acquired)
Vitamin	Vitamin B_{12} malabsorption (juvenile pernicious anemia, transcobalamin II deficiency, Immerslund syndrome)
Ions, trace elements	Chloride-losing diarrhea
	Congenital sodium diarrhea
	Acrodermatitis enteropathica (zinc)
	Menkes syndrome (copper)
	Vitamin D–dependent rickets
	Primary hypomagnesemia
Drug-induced	Sulfasalazine (folic acid malabsorption)
	Cholestyramine (Ca, fat malabsorption)
	Phenytoin (Dilantin) (Ca malabsorption)
Pancreatic	Specific enzyme deficiencies
	Lipase
	Trypsinogen

From Behrman RE (ed). Nelson Textbook of Pediatrics, 14th ed. Philadelphia: WB Saunders, 1992:974.
Abbreviation: Ca = calcium.

The diagnosis of formula protein intolerance is based on exclusion of infectious causes and on response to withdrawal and later re-challenge with the suspected antigen. Skin and radioallergosorbent test results are usually negative. There is a significant cross-reactivity between cow's milk and soy protein allergy (20% to 40%); therefore, use of a protein-hydrolysate formula (e.g., Nutramigen, Alimentum) is indicated in the treatment of affected infants.

CYSTIC FIBROSIS

The diagnosis of cystic fibrosis must be considered in any infant with chronic diarrhea and failure to thrive (see Chapters 7 and 17). Rarer forms of exocrine pancreatic insufficiency include that seen in Shwachman-Diamond syndrome and those noted in Tables 19–13, 19–14, and 19–18.

Chronic Diarrhea in Toddlers

CHRONIC NONSPECIFIC DIARRHEA

Chronic nonspecific diarrhea, also known as "toddler's diarrhea," typically affects children between 1 and 2 years of age and is characterized by the passage of several watery and unformed stools each day. Frequently, the stools are relatively well formed in the morning but become looser as the day progresses. The stool often appears to contain undigested vegetable matter but is without blood, mucus, or excessive fat. Chronic nonspecific diarrhea is characterized by continuing normal weight gain, provided that the child is offered a normal diet. In an attempt to treat the diarrhea, however, many children are placed on diets restricted of milk, other fats, and occasionally starches (wheat), leading to iatrogenic failure to thrive.

The pathophysiology of chronic nonspecific diarrhea, although not completely understood, may involve abnormal intestinal motility with decreased mouth-to-anus transit time. Excessive fruit juice intake, which is common among affected children, may also contribute to the diarrhea by overwhelming the carbohydrate absorptive capacity of the gut. Nonabsorbable sugar-alcohols (sorbitol) present in fruit juices often contribute to the diarrhea. Psychologic factors are suggested by the finding that functional bowel complaints are common in other family members (see Chapter 18).

Because chronic nonspecific diarrhea is a benign and self-limited condition, usually resolving by age 3 to 4 years, drug therapy is neither indicated nor effective. Parents should be encouraged to place the child on a regular, unrestricted diet to provide adequate calories for normal growth and development. The diarrhea often improves with removal of prior dietary restrictions.

CELIAC DISEASE

Celiac disease, also known as *gluten-sensitive enteropathy* or *sprue,* results from immune-mediated damage to the small intestine after ingestion of gluten contained in wheat, oat, barley, and rye. Intestinal villous injury leads to malabsorption and failure to thrive. Symptoms often develop between 6 months to 3 years of age following introduction of cereal grains into the diet and after enough time has elapsed for the injury to become clinically significant.

Genetic factors are important in the development of celiac disease. The condition is most common among those of Irish origin. There is a 10% incidence of latent celiac disease in first-order relatives of affected individuals. Many human leukocyte antigen (HLA) haplotypes, including HLA-B8, -DR3, and -DQW2, are overrepresented in affected patients compared with normal individuals. However, not all individuals with these histocompatibility markers develop the disease, nor do all patients with celiac disease carry one or more of these genetic markers.

Celiac disease manifests as failure to thrive, frequent fatty stools, anorexia, digital clubbing, marked abdominal distention, apathy, and occasionally signs of deficiency states resulting from malabsorbed macronutrients and micronutrients. Some patients develop cutaneous bullous eruptions of dermatitis herpetiformis. The diagnosis depends on demonstrating a small-intestinal biopsy specimen with villous atrophy and intraepithelial lymphocytes and then clinical and histologic resolution after initiation of a gluten-free diet. Serologic testing, which relies on the detection of antigliadin, antiendomysium, and other antibodies, has not replaced intestinal biopsy because of significant false-positive and false-negative rates, but such testing might be useful in following up a child's adherence to a gluten-free diet.

Treatment involves the lifelong adherence to a gluten-free diet. Failure to adhere to a diet does not always reproduce symptoms but places the patient at long-term risk for intestinal lymphoma.

Chronic Diarrhea in Older Children and Adolescents (Inflammatory Bowel Disease)

Epidemiology. The chronic idiopathic inflammatory bowel diseases (IBDs) comprise two principal categories. Ulcerative colitis

Text continued on page 295

Table 19-14. Gastrointestinal Diseases Associated with Maldigestion and Malabsorption

Disease/Condition	Pathophysiology
Intraluminal Digestion	
Stomach	
Protein-calorie malnutrition	Decreased acid production, hypochlorhydria
Zollinger-Ellison syndrome	Inactivation of pancreatic enzymes at a low duodenal pH, and decreased ionization of conjugated bile salts
Pernicious anemia	Decreased intrinsic factor secretion, vitamin B_{12} malabsorption
Dumping syndrome	Rapid emptying of stomach contents into the small intestine, dilution of enzymes
Pancreas	
Cystic fibrosis	Impaired secretion of enzymes and bicarbonate
Shwachman-Diamond syndrome	Impaired secretion of enzymes
Acute/chronic pancreatitis	Impaired secretion of enzymes and bicarbonate
Protein-calorie malnutrition	Impaired secretion of enzymes
Trypsinogen deficiency	Impaired secretion of enzymes
Lipase deficiency	Impaired secretion of enzymes
Amylase deficiency	Impaired secretion of enzymes
Liver	
Cholestasis syndromes	Impaired secretion of bile salts with deficient micelle formation
Ileal disease or surgery	Intestinal malabsorption of bile salts, deficient bile salt pool
Intestine	
Enterokinase deficiency	Impaired activation of luminal pancreatic enzymes
Protein-calorie malnutrition	Bacterial overgrowth with consumption of nutrients, toxin production, and deconjugation of bile acids
Anatomic duplication	Bacterial overgrowth with consumption of nutrients; altered mucosal blood flow
Blind loop syndrome	
Short bowel syndrome	
Pseudo-obstruction	
Digestion at the Enterocyte Membrane	
Congenital disaccharidase deficiency	Impaired digestion of a specific disaccharide leading to bacterial fermentation in the colon
Lactase	
Sucrase-isomaltase	
Trehalase	
Acquired/late-onset disaccharidase deficiency	Loss of enzyme activity due to mucosal injury or loss of activity with age
Lactase	
Sucrase-isomaltase	
Glucoamylase	

Table continued on following page

Table 19–14. Gastrointestinal Diseases Associated with Maldigestion and Malabsorption *Continued*

Disease/Condition	Pathophysiology
Enterocyte Absorption	
Protein-calorie malnutrition	"Damage" versus "adaptive regulation" altered mucosal architecture
Hartnup disease	Transport defect of neutral amino acids
Lysinuric protein intolerance	Transport defect of dibasic amino acids in intestine and kidney
Blue diaper syndrome	Isolated transport defect of tryptophan
Oast-house syndrome	Isolated transport defect of methionine in intestine and kidney
Lowe's syndrome	X-linked trait with defect in transport of lysine and arginine
Glucose-galactose malabsorption	Selective defect in glucose and galactose sodium cotransport system
Congenital chloride diarrhea	Selective defect in chloride transport by the intestine
Abetalipoproteinemia	Absent production of apolipoprotein B, lipoproteins, and chylomicrons absent
Hypobetalipoproteinemia	Impaired production of apolipoprotein B
Celiac disease	Damage to absorptive/digestive surface
Short bowel syndrome	Loss of absorptive/digestive surface, abnormal transit
Mucosal injury syndromes	Damage to digestive/absorptive surface
Milk/soy protein intolerance	
Postenteritis syndrome	
Tropical sprue	Damage to digestive/absorptive surface
Whipple's disease	Lymphatic obstruction, impaired lipid transport(?), patchy enteropathy
Bacterial infection	Damage to digestive/absorptive surface, abnormal motility
Shigella	
Salmonella	
Campylobacter	
Cholera	Secretory water and electrolyte loss
Giardia	Disruption of epithelial function secondary to adhesion or toxin(?)
Crohn disease/regional enteritis	Damage to digestive/absorptive surface, chronic gastrointestinal blood loss
Acrodermatitis enteropathica	Impaired absorption of zinc
Uptake into Blood and Lymph	
Congestive heart failure	Venous distention, bowel wall edema
Intestinal lymphangiectasia	Obstructed lymphatic transport of lipid and fat-soluble vitamins, intestinal protein loss
Intestinal lymphoma	Obstructed lymphatic transport of lipid and fat-soluble vitamins
Carcinoid syndrome	Obstructed lymphatic transport of lipid and fat-soluble vitamins
Miscellaneous Disorders	
Immune deficiency syndromes	Altered bacterial flora
Allergic gastroenteropathy	Unknown immune mechanism
Eosinophilic gastroenteropathy	Unknown immune mechanism
Drugs	
Methotrexate	Damage to mucosal surface by interfering with enterocyte replication
Cholestyramine	Blocked reabsorption of bile salts in the ileum by drug; malabsorption of calcium, fat, bile acids, and fat-soluble vitamins
Phenytoin	Calcium, folic acid malabsorption
Sulfasalazine	Folic acid malabsorption
H_2-receptor antagonists	Impair the acid/proteolytic liberation of vitamin B_{12}

Adapted from Erdman SH, Udall JN. Maldigestion and malabsorption. *In* Wyllie R, Hyams JS (eds). Pediatric Gastrointestinal Diseases. Pathophysiology, Diagnosis, Management. Philadelphia: WB Saunders, 1993:515–516.

Table 19–15. Symptoms and Signs of Malabsorption

History	Pathophysiology	Physical Examination	Pathophysiology
Diarrhea	Increased secretion and impaired absorption of water and electrolytes, unabsorbed dihydroxy bile acids, unabsorbed fatty acids	Pallor	Anemia secondary to iron, folate, or cobalamin deficiency
		Glossitis, stomatitis, cheilosis	Iron, folate, cobalamin, and other vitamin deficiencies
Greasy, bulky, malodorous stools that are difficult to flush	Increased fat in stool		
Oil seeping from rectum	Unabsorbed triglyceride (pancreatic insufficiency)	Ecchymosis, purpura	Vitamin K malabsorption
		Acrodermatitis	Zinc and fatty acid deficiency
Weight loss despite good appetite	Loss of calories from malabsorption	Dehydration, hypotension	Water and electrolyte malabsorption
Excessive flatus	Fermentation of unabsorbed carbohydrates by colonic bacteria	Edema	Protein malabsorption (decreased serum albumin)
Diffuse abdominal pain	Inflammation or infiltration of tissue (pancreatic insufficiency, Crohn disease, lymphoma)	Peripheral neuropathy	Cobalamin, thiamine, vitamin E and B_6 deficiencies
Postprandial (30 minutes after eating) midabdominal pain	Intestinal ischemia		
Abnormal bruisability	Vitamin K malabsorption		
Weakness and fatigue	Protein, electrolyte, fat, iron, folate, cobalamin malabsorption		
Milk intolerance	Lactase deficiency		
Bone pain	Calcium and protein malabsorption		
Tetany, paresthesias	Calcium and magnesium malabsorption, cobalamin deficiency (paresthesias only)		
Night blindness	Vitamin A malabsorption		
Nocturia	Delayed absorption of water, hypokalemia		
Amenorrhea	Protein malabsorption		

Modified from Toskes PP. Malabsorption. *In* Wyngaarden JB, Smith LH, Bennett JC (eds). Cecil Textbook of Medicine, 19th ed. Philadelphia: WB Saunders, 1992:691.

Table 19–16. Diagnostic Studies in the Evaluation of Maldigestion and Malabsorption

Initial Studies

Stool examination for blood, leukocytes, reducing substances, and *Clostridium difficile* toxin. Stool examination for ova and parasites and cultures for infectious bacterial pathogens.
Complete blood count
Serum electrolytes, blood urea nitrogen, creatinine, calcium, phosphorus, albumin, total protein
Urinalysis and culture

Second-Phase Studies

Sweat chloride test—cystic fibrosis
Breath analysis—lactose-induced hydrogen excretion
D-Xylose test—celiac disease
Serum carotene, folate, B_{12}, and iron levels
Fecal alpha$_1$-antitrypsin level—protein-losing enteropathy
Fecal fat studies or coefficient of fat absorption studies
Fatty test meal, Lundh test meal
Antigliadin, antiendomysium antibody—celiac disease

Third-Phase Studies

Fat-soluble vitamin levels: A, 25-hydroxy D, and E, prothrombin time
Contrast radiographic studies: upper gastrointestinal series, or barium enema
Small intestinal biopsy for histology, and mucosal enzyme determination

Specialized Studies

Bentiromide excretion test
Schilling test
Serum/urine bile acid determination
Endoscopic retrograde pancreatography
Provocative pancreatic secretion testing

Adapted from Erdman SH, Udall JN. Maldigestion and malabsorption. *In* Wyllie R, Hyams JS (eds). Pediatric Gastrointestinal Diseases. Pathophysiology, Diagnosis, Management. Philadelphia: WB Saunders, 1993:524.

Table 19–17. Tests for Malabsorption

Test	Normal Values	Comments Relevant to Patients with Malabsorption
Screening Tests		
Serum carotene	>0.06 mg/dl	Decreased, very good test if poor oral intake has been excluded
Serum calcium	9.0 to 10.5 mg/dl	Decreased, not very sensitive
Serum cholesterol	150 to 250 mg/dl	Decreased, not very sensitive
Serum albumin	4.0 to 5.2 mg/dl	Decreased, not very sensitive
Serum magnesium	1.7 to 2.0 mEq/L	Decreased, not very sensitive
Prothrombin time	Control value	Increased, not very sensitive
Qualitative stool fat	No fat globules per hpf	Numerous fat globules per hpf; part 1 for neutral fats, part 2 for split fats
Specific Tests		
Serum iron	80–150 μg/dl	Malabsorbed in proximal small-bowel disease
Serum folate	5–21 ng/ml	Decreased in proximal small-bowel disease, may be increased in bacterial overgrowth
Serum cobalamin (vitamin B_{12})	200–900 pg/ml	Malabsorbed in distal small-bowel disease, pernicious anemia, bacterial overgrowth, chronic pancreatitis
Urinary D-xylose	>5 g/5 hr	Decreased in small-bowel disease and bacterial overgrowth, normal in pancreatic disease
Bentiromide test	Arylamine excretion >57% in 6 hr	A value of <50% is diagnostic of pancreatic insufficiency
Serum trypsin–like immunoreactivity	29–80 ng/ml	A value of <20 ng/ml is specific for pancreatic insufficiency
Secretin test	HCO_3^- concentration >80 mEq/L Volume >1.8 ml/kg/hr	Most sensitive test of pancreatic function
^{57}Cyanocobalamin urinary excretion test	>8%/24 hr	Decreased in pernicious anemia, chronic pancreatitis, bacterial overgrowth, ileal disease
Urine 5-HIAA	1.7–8.0 mg/24 hr	Markedly elevated in carcinoid syndrome, minimally elevated in any kind of malabsorption
Breath tests		
^{14}C-xylose	<0.0013% of administered dose as breath $^{14}CO_2$ at 30 min	Elevated in bacterial overgrowth
Cholyl-l-^{14}C-glycine	<1% of administered dose as breath $^{14}CO_2$ at any interval over 4 hr	Elevated in bacterial overgrowth or bile acid malabsorption
Lactulose H_2	<10 ppm rise in breath H_2 over baseline at any interval for 120 min	Elevated in bacterial overgrowth; increase in fasting breath H_2 suggests bacterial overgrowth; up to 27% of subjects may not have flora that produces H_2
Lactose-H_2	<20 ppm rise in breath H_2 over baseline at any interval for 180 min	Elevated in lactase deficiency
Small intestinal culture	$\leq 10^5$ organisms per ml jejunal secretions	>10^5 organisms per ml jejunal secretions indicates bacterial overgrowth
Small intestinal biopsy		Morphology re: villus atrophy; bacteriology; enzyme assays

Adapted from Toskes PP. Malabsorption. *In* Wyngaarden JB, Smith LH, Bennett JC (eds). Cecil Textbook of Medicine, 19th ed. Philadelphia: WB Saunders, 1992:691.
Abbreviations: hpf = high-power field; 5-HIAA = 5-hydroxyindoleacetic acid; ppm = parts per million.

Table 19–18. Generalized Malabsorptive States in Childhood

Site	More Common	Less Common
Exocrine pancreas	Cystic fibrosis Chronic protein-calorie malnutrition	Shwachman-Diamond syndrome Chronic pancreatitis
Liver, biliary tree	Biliary atresia	Other cholestatic states
Intestine Anatomic defects	Massive resection Stagnant loop syndrome	Congenitally short gut
Chronic infection	Giardiasis	Immune deficiency
Others	Celiac disease	Dietary protein intolerance (milk, soy) Tropical sprue Idiopathic diffuse mucosal lesions

From Behrman RE (ed). Nelson Textbook of Pediatrics, 14th ed. Philadelphia: WB Saunders, 1992:973.

is a diffuse mucosal inflammation limited to the colon; it invariably affects the rectum and may extend proximally in a symmetric, uninterrupted pattern to involve part or all of the large intestine. Crohn disease, by contrast, is a patchy transmural inflammation that may affect any part of the gastrointestinal tract from the mouth to the anus. Its most common distributions are either small bowel alone, colon alone, or both large and small bowel simultaneously.

The incidence of Crohn disease and, to a lesser extent, that of ulcerative colitis has been rising over the past 50 years, for unknown reasons. There is a peak in the age-related incidence of Crohn disease in adolescence and young adulthood. Of new cases of Crohn disease, 25% present in patients younger than age 20 years. Of new cases of ulcerative colitis, 15% are diagnosed before the age 20. An increased frequency of IBD in families of patients with the disease has been well documented.

Signs and Symptoms. The presenting signs and symptoms of IBD fall into two large categories: enteric manifestations and extraintestinal manifestations. The intestinal, or enteric manifestations include diarrhea, abdominal pain, intestinal obstruction, rectal bleeding, perforation, perianal disease, and malabsorption (Table 19–19). Extraintestinal manifestations are numerous and include fever, oral aphthous ulceration, uveitis, arthralgias, arthritis, and hepatobiliary disorders (Table 19–20). Growth failure is a unique and significant feature of pediatric IBD.

Table 19–19. Comparison of Clinical and Pathologic Features of Crohn Colitis and Ulcerative Colitis

Feature	Crohn Colitis	Ulcerative Colitis
Clinical		
Smoker	+ +	+ / −
Malaise, fever	+ +	+
Rectal bleeding	+ +	+ + +
Abdominal tenderness	+ + +	+
Abdominal mass	+ +	−
Abdominal pain	+ + +	+
Perianal disease	+ + +	−
Risk of cancer	+	+ +
Endoscopic		
Rectal disease	+	+ + +
Diffuse, continuous symmetric involvement	+	+ + +
Aphthous or linear ulcers	+ + +	−
Cobblestoning	+ +	−
Friability	+ +	+ + +
Radiologic		
Continuous disease	+	+ + +
Ileal involvement	+ +	−
Asymmetry	+ + +	−
Strictures	+ +	+
Fistulas	+ +	−
Tone dilatation	−	+
Pathologic		
Discontinuity	+ +	−
Transmural involvement	+ + +	+ / −
Lymphoid aggregates	+ + +	−
Crypt abscesses	+ + +	+ + +
Granulomas	+ +	−
Sinus tract/fistula	+ + +	−

Adapted from Hanauer SB. Inflammatory bowel disease. *In* Wyngaarden JB, Smith LH, Bennett JC (eds). Cecil Textbook of Medicine, 19th ed. Philadelphia: WB Saunders, 1992:705.
+ + + = always; + + = common; + = occasional; − = never.

Table 19–20. Extraintestinal Manifestations of the Inflammatory Bowel Diseases

Nutritional and Metabolic Abnormalities
  Weight loss, growth retardation
  Hypoalbuminemia—nutritional, protein-losing enteropathy
  Vitamin deficiencies*
  Deficiencies of calcium, magnesium, or zinc*

Hematologic Abnormalities
  Anemia—iron, folate, B_{12}* deficiency
  Leukocytosis, thrombocytosis
  Venous thrombosis

Skin and Mucous Membranes
  Pyoderma gangrenosum
  Erythema nodosum
  Stomatitis with multiple aphthous ulcers

Musculoskeletal
  Ankylosing spondylitis, sacroiliitis (HLA-B27 associated)
  Peripheral arthritis of large joints
  Osteoporosis
  Osteomalacia*
  Clubbing

Hepatic and Biliary Manifestations
  Fatty liver
  Pericholangitis
  Sclerosing cholangitis
  Gallstones*
  Carcinoma of the bile ducts

Renal Complications
  Kidney stones
    Uric acid
    Calcium oxalate*
  Obstructive uropathy*
  Fistulas to urinary tract*
  Amyloidosis (rare)

Eye Complications
  Conjunctivitis, episcleritis, iritis
  Uveitis (HLA-B27)

Adapted from Hanauer SB. Inflammatory bowel disease. *In* Wyngaarden JB, Smith LH, Bennett JC (eds). Cecil Textbook of Medicine, 19th ed. Philadelphia: WB Saunders, 1992:703.
*Crohn disease.

Diarrhea, with or without blood and often associated with tenesmus, low-grade fever, weight loss, and mild anemia, is a very common presenting picture of ulcerative colitis. In Crohn disease, periumbilical abdominal pain, often colicky in nature and worse after meals; diarrhea; fever; and weight loss are the most common symptoms. Bleeding is less often seen. These two clinical patterns relate to the predilection for the site of involvement of each disease: ulcerative colitis is limited to the colon, whereas Crohn disease involves the small intestine, with or without colonic involvement, in more than 75% of cases. A differential diagnosis is shown in Tables 19–21 and 19–22. Additional conditions to consider in patients with a subacute presentation include Henoch-Schönlein purpura, hemolytic-uremic syndrome, and lead poisoning.

Laboratory Findings. Anemia, an elevated sedimentation rate, and leukocytosis are common in Crohn disease and ulcerative colitis. The degree of hypoalbuminemia and thrombocytosis, or the plasma levels of acute phase reactive proteins, may correlate with disease activity (Table 19–23). Altered absorptive and secretory functions

Table 19–21. Infectious Agents Mimicking Inflammatory Bowel Disease

Agent	Manifestations	Diagnosis	Comments
Bacterial			
Campylobacter jejuni	Acute diarrhea, fever, fecal blood and leukocytes	Culture	Common in adolescents, may relapse
Yersinia enterocolitica	Acute→ chronic diarrhea, right lower quadrant pain, mesenteric adenitis—pseudoappendicitis, fecal blood and leukocytes	Culture	Common in adolescents as FUO, weight loss, abdominal pain
	Extraintestinal manifestations, mimics Crohn disease		
Clostridium difficile	Postantibiotic onset, watery diarrhea, pseudomembrane on sigmoidoscopy	Culture and cytotoxin	May be nosocomial Toxic megacolon possible
Escherichia coli 0157:H7	Colitis, fecal blood, abdominal pain	Culture and typing	Hemolytic-uremic syndrome
Salmonella	Watery→ bloody diarrhea, food-borne, fecal leukocytes, cramps	Culture	Usually acute
Shigella	Watery→ bloody diarrhea, fecal leukocytes, fever, pain, cramps	Culture	Dysentery symptoms
Edwardsiella tarda	Bloody diarrhea, cramps	Culture	Ulceration on endoscopy
Aeromonas hydrophila	Cramps, diarrhea, fecal blood	Culture	May be chronic Contaminated drinking water
Plesiomonas	Diarrhea, cramps	Culture	Shellfish source
Tuberculosis	Rarely bovine, now Mycobacterium tuberculosis	Culture, PPD, biopsy	May mimic Crohn disease
	Ileocecal area, fistula formulation		
Parasites			
Entamoeba histolytica	Acute bloody diarrhea and liver abscess, colic	Trophozoite in stool, colonic mucosal flask ulceration, serology	Travel to endemic area
Giardia lamblia	Foul-smelling, watery diarrhea, cramps, flatulence, weight loss. No colonic involvement	"Owl"-like trophozoite and cysts in stool; rarely duodenal intubation	May be chronic
AIDS-Associated Enteropathy			
Cryptosporidium	Chronic diarrhea, weight loss	Stool microscopy	Mucosal findings not like IBD
Isospora belli	As in Cryptosporidium		Tropical location
Cytomegalovirus	Colonic ulceration, pain, bloody diarrhea	Culture, biopsy	

From Behrman RE (ed). Nelson Textbook of Pediatrics, 14th ed. Philadelphia: WB Saunders, 1992:968.
Abbreviations: FUO = fever of unknown origin; PPD = purified protein derivative; AIDS = acquired immunodeficiency syndrome; IBD = inflammatory bowel disease.

of the gut are reflected in decreased levels of serum total proteins, albumin, immunoglobulins, folate, iron, and zinc.

Radiologic studies (barium enema, upper gastrointestinal series) are an essential part of the evaluation to determine the nature and the extent of the disease. When colitis develops, a granular mucosa appears, with punctate collection of contrast material lodged in small ulcers. In more advanced cases, the colon develops irregular margins with spiculations and deeper ulcers. In Crohn disease, transmural inflammation and lymphoid proliferation, characteristically affecting the terminal ileum, account for the typical radiologic features of nodularity, ulceration, and narrowing and irregularity of the lumen, sometimes progressing to the classic string sign in the terminal ileum. However, any segment of the intestine may be affected.

Sigmoidoscopic and colonoscopic examination with mucosal biopsies are essential for the diagnosis and management of IBD. In active ulcerative colitis, hyperemia, edematous mucosa with spontaneous, and induced friability are seen; ulcerations or a granular appearance may be present, and the vascular pattern is diminished. Lesions tend to be diffuse and continuous from the rectum proximally. The endoscopic appearance of Crohn disease may be similar to that of ulcerative colitis, it may be normal if the colon is not involved, or it may show rectal sparing or aphthous ulcerations with skip areas and a cobblestone appearance.

Treatment. Steroids are the mainstay of therapy in IBD, especially in patients with active disease, and may be used in either oral or parenteral form, the latter for those with more severe disease. Unfortunately, the relapse rate after discontinuation of steroids may be as high as 70% within 1 year's time. In addition to the oral or parenteral forms of steroids, steroid enemas have been used with some success in patients with distal disease. Many new steroid enema preparations are under investigation; these have lower systemic absorption and less bioavailability and thus allow a larger dose to be used without systemic complications.

Sulfasalazine (Azulfidine) is the most widely used of the aminosalicylate preparations and is used to treat both Crohn colitis and ulcerative colitis. Mild cases may be controlled with this drug alone, which also appears to reduce the frequency of relapses once remission is achieved.

Sulfasalazine analogs have been designed to deliver the aminosalicylate (ASA) to the colon without using the toxic sulfa moiety. These include olsalazine sodium (Dipentum), which is a dimer of

Table 19–22. Differential Diagnosis of Presenting Symptoms of Crohn's Disease

Primary Presenting Symptom	Diagnostic Considerations
Right lower quadrant abdominal pain, with or without mass	Appendicitis, infection (e.g., *Campylobacter, Yersinia*), lymphoma, intussusception, mesenteric adenitis, Meckel's diverticulum, ovarian cyst
Chronic periumbilical or epigastric abdominal pain	Irritable bowel syndrome, constipation, lactose intolerance, peptic disease
Rectal bleeding, no diarrhea	Fissure, polyp, Meckel's diverticulum, rectal ulcer syndrome
Bloody diarrhea	Infection, hemolytic-uremic syndrome, Henoch-Schönlein purpura, ischemic bowel, radiation colitis
Watery diarrhea	Irritable bowel syndrome, lactose intolerance, giardiasis, *Cryptosporidium,* sorbitol, laxatives
Perirectal disease	Fissure, hemorrhoid (rare), streptococcal infection, condyloma (rare)
Growth delay	Endocrinopathy
Anorexia, weight loss	Anorexia nervosa
Arthritis	Collagen vascular disease, infection
Liver abnormalities	Chronic hepatitis

From Hyams JS. Crohn's disease. *In* Wyllie R, Hyams JS (eds). Pediatric Gastrointestinal Diseases. Pathophysiology, Diagnosis, Management. Philadelphia: WB Saunders, 1993:754.

Table 19–23. Inflammatory Bowel Disease: Severity Criteria*

	Mild	Severe	Fulminant/Toxic
Bowel frequency	<4/day	>6/day	>10/day
Blood in stool	+/−	+ +	Continuous
Fever	Normal	>37.5°C	>37.5°C
Pulse	Normal	>90/min	>90/min
Hemoglobin	Normal	<75% of normal	Transfusion required
Erythrocyte sedimentation rate	<30 mm/hr	>30 mm/hr	>30 mm/hr
Abdominal radiograph	Normal	Colonic edema, thumb-printing, air-fluid levels	Dilated colon or small bowel
Clinical sign		Abdominal tenderness	Rebound tenderness, distention, diminished bowel sounds

From Hanauer SB. Inflammatory bowel disease. *In* Wyngaarden JB, Smith LH, Bennett JC (eds). Cecil Textbook of Medicine, 19th ed. Philadelphia: WB Saunders, 1992:705.
*Criteria are based on adolescent and adult norms (e.g., pulse).

Table 19–24. Indications for Surgery in Crohn's Disease

Failure of medical therapy
  Intractable symptoms
  Corticosteroid toxicity
  Social invalidism

Obstruction—acute or chronic
  Gastroduodenal
  Small bowel
  Large bowel

Hemorrhage
  Small bowel lesion
  Large bowel lesion
  Fulminant colitis, with or without toxic megacolon

Perforation
  Free
  Closed, with abscess

Fistula
  Intractable perirectal disease
  Enteroenteric
  Enterocutaneous
  Enterovesical
  Enterovaginal

Growth retardation

Carcinoma

Obstructive uropathy

From Hyams JS. Crohn's disease. *In* Wyllie R, Hyams JS (eds). Pediatric Gastrointestinal Diseases. Pathophysiology, Diagnosis, Management, Philadelphia: WB Saunders, 1993:757.

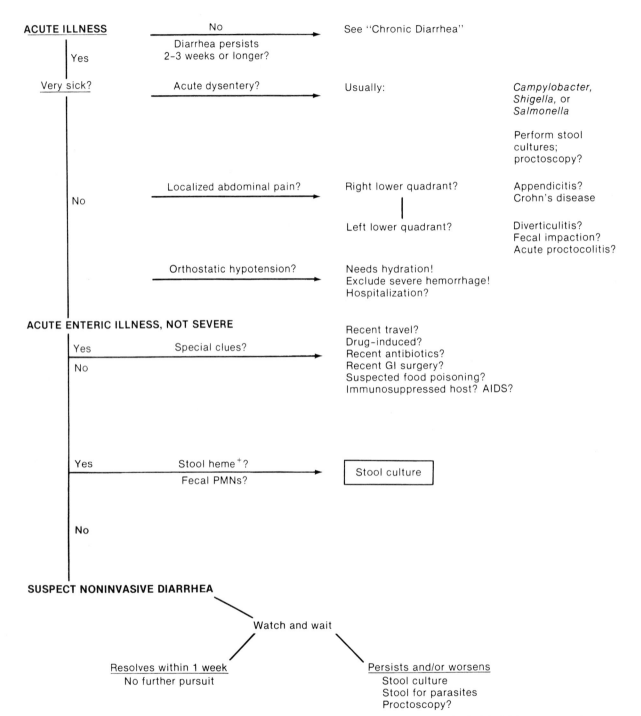

Figure 19–2. Acute diarrhea. (From Reilly BM. Diarrhea. *In* Practical Strategies in Outpatient Medicine, 2nd ed. Philadelphia: WB Saunders, 1991:854.)

5-ASA, and Asacol, which is 5-ASA coated with an acrylic resin designed to break down when the tablet reaches the terminal ileum. These drugs are of potential usefulness in the 30% of patients who do not tolerate sulfasalazine because of side effects that include headache, nausea, hemolytic anemia, or rashes. 5-ASA enemas (mesalamine [Rowasa]) are useful for treating patients with left-sided colitis; this treatment has allowed many such patients to discontinue taking systemic steroids.

Despite the efficacy of salicylate preparations, many children cannot be maintained in remission without the use of steroids. Because long-term use can lead to numerous complications, alternative immunosuppressive agents may be useful. The two most commonly agents used are azathioprine (Imuran) and 6-mercaptopurine. Both appear to maintain remission while allowing reduction in steroid dosage. In addition, 6-mercaptopurine is effective in the healing of perineal fistulas. These drugs are best used when the patient is in a state of relative remission, because there is a lag period of 3 to 4 months before the drugs work. There may be associated side effects, but judicious use of these immunosuppressive drugs can offer an alternative to long-term steroid therapy. Cyclosporine is the newest immunosuppressive drug being studied for the treatment of severe, refractory disease. Antibiotics, particularly metronidazole (Flagyl), are effective in healing certain perineal lesions in Crohn disease and are beneficial in the general management of Crohn colitis and ileocolitis.

Nutrition is among the most valuable therapies for IBD in children, particularly for those with Crohn disease. Nutritional therapy can serve both as primary treatment and as adjunctive support for drug treatment. Weight loss occurs in 87% of children presenting with Crohn disease and is often accompanied by impaired linear growth, decreased bone mineralization and delayed sexual maturation. Undernutrition is multifactorial, including poor intake caused by anorexia, meal-related cramping, and diarrhea as well as malabsorption from small-bowel involvement and increased metabolic demands from the chronic inflammatory process. Nutritional support can be provided by either the enteral or parenteral routes. If possible, use of the patient's intestine is optimal. Even patients with severe inflammation can often tolerate an enteral, elemental formula. However, because of the poor taste and the large volumes required, nasogastric tube infusions are frequently used. Some patients do not tolerate enteral nutrition because of severe abdominal symptoms, and therefore parenteral hyperalimentation may be required.

Surgery. Crohn disease cannot be cured by surgery, because there is a high postoperative recurrence rate of up to 50% at 10 years. Surgery in Crohn disease is therefore reserved for the management of certain complications of the disease, such as intestinal perforation, obstruction, bleeding, and abscess, and occasionally for growth failure in the prepubertal child with a delayed bone age in whom all macroscopically abnormal bowel can be resected (Table19–24). In contrast, surgical resection can cure ulcerative colitis but in most patients is reserved for those with severe, acute complications; colonic cytologic dysplasia (precursor of carcinoma); or persistent disease that is unresponsive to medical therapy. Numerous surgical procedures are available, including total colectomy with standard ileostomy or with continent ileostomy. More acceptable to patients are sphincter-sparing operations in which the colon is resected, and then, often at a later date, the terminal ileum is placed inside the retained muscular wall of the rectum and is anastomosed to the anus. Satisfactory continence is achieved in 70% to 90% of patients.

SUMMARY AND RED FLAGS

Acute diarrhea is a common childhood illness, and every child probably experiences more than one episode of infectious gastroen-

teritis. For most children, the etiologic agent is of no therapeutic significance unless there are signs of giardiasis, HIV, pseudomembranous colitis, or dysentery suggestive of *Shigella* infection, amebiasis, or *Campylobacter* infection (Fig. 19–2). Of greater importance are the secondary complications associated with gastrointestinal fluid and electrolyte losses resulting from emesis and diarrhea and the reduced oral fluid intake resulting from emesis, anorexia, or crampy abdominal pain.

Red flags for acute diarrhea are associated with manifestations of dehydration and include decreased urine output, altered mental status, absent tearing, sunken eyes or fontanel, tachycardia, tachypnea (from acidosis), hypotension, poorly palpable pulses, prolonged capillary refill time, cold extremities, metabolic acidosis, and azotemia. Young age (<6 months) is associated with a greater risk of dehydration, as are 10 or more stools a day and frequent emesis.

Chronic diarrhea may be benign (toddler's diarrhea) or may signify a more serious illness associated with malabsorption, inflammation, or congenital defects. *Red flags* include a positive family history, onset in the neonatal period or with dietary changes, travel to high-risk countries, weight loss, growth stunting, digital clubbing, ravenous appetite but poor growth, anorexia, fever, fatty stools, blood in stools, extraintestinal manifestations associated with intestinal disease, and specific nutritional deficiencies associated with malabsorption.

REFERENCES

Gastroenteritis

General, Bacterial, Parasitic

Baird-Parker AC. Foodborne illness: Foodborne salmonellosis. Lancet 1990;336:1231–1235.

Blake PA, Ramos S, MacDonald KL, et al. Pathogen-specific risk factors and protective factors for acute diarrheal disease in urban Brazilian infants. J Infect Dis 1993;167:627–632.

Cohen JI, Bartlett JA, Corey R, et al. Extra-intestinal manifestations of salmonella infections. Medicine 1987;66:349–388.

de la Morena ML, Van R, Singh K, et al. Diarrhea associated with *Aeromonas* species in children in day care centers. J Infect Dis 1993;168:215–218.

Doyle MP. Foodborne illness. Pathogenic *Escherichia coli, Yersinia enterocolitica* and *Vibrio parahaemolyticus.* Lancet 1990;336:1111–1115.

Goldberg MB, Rubin RH. The spectrum of *Salmonella* infection. Infect Dis Clin North Am 1988;2:571–598.

Guerrant RL. Lessons from diarrheal diseases: Demography to molecular pharmacology. J Infect Dis 1994;169:1206–1218.

Guerrant RL, Lohr JA, Williams EK. Acute infectious diarrhea: I. Epidemiology, etiology and pathogenesis. Pediatr Infect Dis 1986;5:353–359.

Huskins WC, Griffiths JK, Faruque ASG, et al. Shigellosis in neonates and young infants. J Pediatr 1994;125:14–22.

Lee LA, Shapiro CN, Hargrett-Bean N, et al. Hyperendemic shigellosis in the United States: a review of surveillance data for 1967–1988. J Infect Dis 1991;164:894–900.

Lengerich EJ, Addiss DG, Juranek DD. Severe giardiasis in the United States. Clin Infect Dis 1994;18:760–763.

MacKenzie WR, Hoxie NJ, Proctor ME, et al. A massive outbreak in Milwaukee of cryptosporidium infection transmitted through the public water supply. N Engl J Med 1994;331:161–167.

Murphy GS, Bodhidatta L, Echeverria P, et al. Ciprofloxacin and loperamide in the treatment of bacillary dysentery. Ann Intern Med 1993;118:582–586.

Naqvi SH, Swierkosz EM, Gerard J, et al. Presentation of *Yersinia enterocolitica* enteritis in children. Pediatr Infect Dis J 1993;12:386–389.

Taylor JL, Tuttle J, Pramukul T, et al. An outbreak of cholera in Maryland associated with imported commercial frozen fresh coconut milk. J Infect Dis 1993;167:1330–1335.

Waites WM, Arbuthnott JP. Foodborne illness: An overview. Lancet 1990;336:722–725.

Wood RC, MacDonald KL, Osterholm MT. *Campylobacter* enteritis outbreaks associated with drinking raw milk during youth activities: A 10-year review of outbreaks in the United States. JAMA 1992;268:3228–3230.

Wurtz R. *Cyclospora:* A newly identified intestinal pathogen of humans. Clin Infect Dis 1994;18:620–623.

Viral

Graham DY, Jiang X, Tanaka T, et al. Norwalk virus infection of volunteers: New insights based on improved assays. J Infect Dis 1994;170:34–43.

Haffejee IE. Neonatal rotavirus infections. Rev Infect Dis 1991;13:957–962.

Kapikian AZ. Viral gastroenteritis. JAMA 1993;269:627–630.

Kotloff KL, Losonsky GA, Morris JG, et al. Enteric adenovirus infection and childhood diarrhea: An epidemiologic study in three clinical settings. Pediatrics 1989;84:219–225.

Mitchell DK, Van R, Morrow AL, et al. Outbreaks of astrovirus gastroenteritis in day care centers. J Pediatr 1993;123:725–732.

Uhnoo I, Olding-Stenkvist E, Krueger A. Clinical features of acute gastroenteritis associated with rotavirus, enteric adenoviruses, and bacteria. Arch Dis Child 1986;61:732–738.

Wilde J, Van R, Pickering L, et al. Detection of rotaviruses in the day care environment by reverse transcriptase polymerase chain reaction. J Infect Dis 1992;166:507–511.

Treatment

Bang A. Towards better oral rehydration. Lancet 1993;342:755–756.

Fayad IM, Hashem M, Duggan C, et al. Comparative efficacy of rice-based and glucose-based oral rehydration salts plus early reintroduction of food. Lancet 1993;342:772–775.

Islam A, Molla AM, Ahmed MA, et al. Is rice based oral rehydration therapy effective in young infants? Arch Dis Child 1994;71:19–23.

Maulén-Radován I, Brown KH, Acosta MA, et al. Comparison of a rice-based, mixed diet versus a lactose-free, soy protein isolate formula for young children with acute diarrhea. J Pediatr 1994;125:699–706.

Celiac Disease

Catassi C, Ratsch I-M, Fabiani E, et al. Coeliac disease in the year 2000: exploring the iceberg. Lancet 1994;343:200–203.

Challacombe D. When is a coeliac? [comment]. Lancet 1994;343:188.

McMillan SA, Haughton DJ, Biggart JD, et al. Predictive value for coeliac disease of antibodies to gliadin, endomysium, and jejunum in patients attending for jejunal biopsy. BMJ 1991;303:1163–1165.

Rossi TM, Albini CH, Kumar V. Incidence of celiac disease identified by the presence of serum endomysial antibodies in children with chronic diarrhea, short stature, or insulin-dependent diabetes mellitus. J Pediatr 1993;123:262–264.

Valletta EA, Trevisiol D, Mastella G. IgA anti-gliadin antibodies in the monitoring of gluten challenge in celiac disease. J Pediatr Gastroenterol Nutr 1990;10:169–173.

Inflammatory Bowel Disease

Greenberg GR, Feagan BG, Martin F, et al. Oral budesonide for active Crohn's disease. N Engl J Med 1994;331:836–841.

Greenberger NJ, Miner PB. Is maintenance therapy effective in Crohn's disease? Lancet 1994;344:900–901.

Hanauer SB. Medical therapy of ulcerative colitis. Lancet 1993;342:412–417.

Langholz E, Munkholm P, Davidsen M, et al. Course of ulcerative colitis: Analysis of changes in disease activity over years. Gastroenterology 1994;107:3–11.

Lichtiger S, Present DH, Kornbluth A, et al. Cyclosporine in severe ulcerative colitis refractory to steroid therapy. N Engl J Med 1994;330:1841–1845.

Shanahan F. Pathogenesis of ulcerative colitis. Lancet 1993;342:407–411.

Treem WR, Hyams JS. Cyclosporine therapy for gastrointestinal disease. J Pediatr Gastroenterol Nutr 1994;18:270–278.

Chronic Diarrhea

Bisset WM, Stapleford P, Long S, et al. Home parenteral nutrition in chronic intestinal failure. Arch Dis Child 1992;67:109–114.

Drossman DA, Grant Thompson W. The irritable bowel syndrome: Review and a graduated multicomponent treatment approach. Ann Intern Med 1992;116:1009–1016.

Fell JM, Miller MP, Finkel Y, et al. Congenital sodium diarrhea with a partial defect in jejunal brush border membrane sodium transport, normal rectal transport, and resolving diarrhea. J Pediatr Gastroenterol Nutr 1992;15:112–116.

Girault D, Goulet O, Le Deist F, et al. Intractable infant diarrhea associated with phenotypic abnormalities and immunodeficiency. J Pediatr 1994;125:36–42.

Johnston KR, Govel LA, Andritz MH. Gastrointestinal effects of sorbitol as an additive in liquid medications. Am J Med 1994;97:185–191.

Orenstein SR. Enteral versus parenteral therapy for intractable diarrhea of infancy: A prospective randomized trail. J Pediatr 1986;109:277–286.

Phillips AD, Schmitz J. Familial microvillous atrophy: A clinicopathological survey of 23 cases. J Pediatr Gastroenterol Nutr 1992;14:380–396.

Sanderson IR, Risdon RA, Walker-Smith JA. Intractable ulcerating enterocolitis of infancy. Arch Dis Child 1990;65:295–299.

Smith LJ, Szymanski W, Foulston C, et al. Familial enteropathy with villous edema and immunoglobulin G2 subclass deficiency. J Pediatr 1994;125:541–548.

Thomas AG, Phillips AD, Walker-Smith JA. The value of proximal small intestinal biopsy in the differential diagnosis of chronic diarrhoea. Arch Dis Child 1992;67:741–744.

Treem WR. Chronic nonspecific diarrhea of childhood. Clin Pediatr 1992;31:413–420.

20 Vomiting and Regurgitation

Susan R. Orenstein

Vomiting in its most ominous forms accompanies catastrophic, life-threatening disorders; in contrast, vomiting can also be a physiologic behavior in young infants. Determining the cause of vomiting in a child, and treating it appropriately, is thus of major importance. It is critical to remember that vomiting may be due to gastrointestinal disease or to more systemic disturbances, including inborn errors of metabolism, intracranial pathology, nongastrointestinal infection, or systemic poisoning.

PATHOPHYSIOLOGY

Definitions

Vomiting is a protective reflex that removes toxic material from the body or relieves pressure in hollow organs distended by distal obstruction. In this context, the term vomiting encompasses all retrograde ejection of gastrointestinal (or esophageal) contents from the mouth. Strictly speaking, however, vomiting is subdivided according to its forcefulness, such that effortless, or nearly effortless, regurgitation is distinguished from true vomiting, which is propelled both by forceful abdominal wall contractions and by retrograde intestinal peristalsis (Table 20–1).

True vomiting is often accompanied by nausea and retching. *Nausea* is an unpleasant, vaguely epigastric or abdominal sensation accompanied by a variety of autonomic changes: decreases in gastric tone, contractions, secretion, and mucosal blood flow; increases in salivation, sweating, pupil diameter, and heart rate; and changes in respiratory rhythm. During nausea, retrograde peristalsis from the small intestine to the gastric antrum or generalized simultaneous contractions of antrum and duodenum may produce duodenogastric reflux.

Retching is defined as strong, involuntary efforts to vomit, which may be seen as preparatory maneuvers to vomiting. These efforts consist of spasmodic contractions of the diaphragm and abdominal wall at the same time that the lower esophageal sphincter relaxes. This sphincter is also pulled cephalad by contraction of the longitudinal muscles of the upper esophagus and may herniate through the diaphragmatic hiatus, preventing the increased intra-abdominal pressure from augmenting the sphincter pressure. During retching, gastric material is moved into the esophagus by the combination of increased abdominal pressure and decreased intrathoracic pressure, but this material may be returned to the stomach by secondary (non-swallow) esophageal peristalsis.

Vomiting (emesis) differs from retching in that material is expelled from the mouth. This is fostered by relaxation of the diaphragm and reversal of intrathoracic pressure from negative to positive. The upper esophageal sphincter also relaxes, perhaps in response to the increase of intraluminal pressure in the esophagus.

Regurgitation is considered a form of gastroesophageal reflux and, as such, is predominantly due to lower esophageal sphincter dysfunction. Although apparently effortless, it may be propelled by contraction of abdominal wall musculature; this propulsion perhaps distinguishes regurgitant from nonregurgitant reflux, which remains in the esophagus.

Rumination is similar to regurgitation in its effortless appearance and its probable propulsion by somatic muscle contraction. However, ruminated material is usually reswallowed rather than ejected from the mouth, and psychologic or behavioral problems are considered the cause.

Neuroanatomy of Vomiting

The stereotypic motor response of vomiting is mediated by efferents in the vagal, phrenic, and spinal nerves. Input to these nerves arise from the brainstem "vomiting center." There is probably not a single anatomic structure identifiable as the vomiting center, but the final common pathway for this centrally programmed complex reflex is through medullary interneurons in the solitary tract nucleus and a variety of sites in the nearby reticular formation. These interneurons receive input from the cortex, the vagus, the vestibular system, and the area postrema. The area postrema, the "chemoreceptive trigger zone," is located on the dorsal surface of the floor of the fourth ventricle, outside the blood-brain barrier, and has been identified as a crucial source for neural input causing vomiting, particularly as a response to circulating drugs and toxins. Brain tumors, other central nervous system disease, and emotional stress, on the other hand, cause vomiting via cortical afferents, whereas intra-abdominal pathology, such as luminal obstruction or distention, causes vomiting via vagal afferents. Vomiting may be classified by the origin of the afferents (Table 20–2).

When vomiting is a result of intra-abdominal pathology, it is useful to define whether obstruction, dysmotility, inflammation, or ischemia is the mechanism.

DATA TO GUIDE THE DIAGNOSIS

History

DEMOGRAPHICS

The child's age is a major determinant of the diagnostic possibilities (Table 20–3). Neonates present with congenital disorders—

Table 20–1. Force of Vomiting

Force	Cause	Example
None	Esophageal emptying	Achalasia; some reflux
Minimal	Regurgitation	Regurgitant reflux; rumination
Moderate	Vomiting	Most vomiting diseases
Severe	Projectile vomiting with retching	Obstructions; metabolic; poisons

Table 20-2. Differential Diagnosis of Vomiting by Anatomic Locus of Stimulus

I. Stimulation of supramedullary receptors:
   A. Psychogenic vomiting
   B. Increased intracerebral pressure (subdural effusion or hematoma, cerebral edema or tumor, hydrocephalus, meningoencephalitis, Reye's syndrome)
   C. Vascular (migraine, severe hypertension)
   D. Seizures
   E. Vestibular disease, "motion sickness"
II. Stimulation of chemoceptive trigger zone:
   A. Drugs: opiates, ipecac, digoxin, anticonvulsants
   B. Toxins
   C. Metabolic products (acidemia, ketonemia, hyperammonemia, uremia, etc.):
      Acidemia, ketonemia (diabetic ketoacidosis, lactic acidosis, phenylketonuria, renal tubular acidosis)
      Aminoacidemia (tyrosinemia, hypervalinemia, hyperglycinemia, lysinuria, maple syrup urine disease)
      Organic acidemia (methylmalonic acidemia, proprionic acidemia, isovaleric acidemia)
      Hyperammonemia (Reye's syndrome, urea cycle defects)
      Uremia (renal failure)
      Other (hereditary fructose intolerance, galactosemia, fatty acid oxidation disorders, diabetes insipidus, adrenal insufficiency, hypercalcemia, hypervitaminosis A)
III. Stimulation of peripheral receptors and/or obstruction of the gastrointestinal tract:
   A. Pharyngeal: gag reflex (sinusitis secretions, post-tussive, self-induced, rumination)
   B. Esophageal:
      Functional: reflux, achalasia, other esophageal dysmotility
      Structural: stricture, ring, atresia, etc.
   C. Gastric:
      Peptic ulcer disease (incl. Zollinger-Ellison syndrome), infection, dysmotility/gastroparesis
      Obstruction (e.g., bezoar, pyloric stenosis, web, chronic granulomatous disease, eosinophilic gastroenteritis)
   D. Intestinal:
      Infection, enteritis, enterotoxin, appendicitis
      Dysmotility (e.g., metabolic or diabetic neuropathy; intestinal pseudo-obstruction)
      Nutrient intolerance (e.g., cow's milk, soy, gluten, eosinophilic enteropathy)
      Obstruction (e.g., atresia, web, stenosis, adhesions, bands, volvulus, intussusception, superior mesenteric artery syndrome, duplication, meconium plug, meconium ileus, Hirschsprung's disease, distal intestinal obstruction syndrome in cystic fibrosis)
   E. Hepatobiliary, pancreatic: hepatitis, cholecystitis, pancreatitis, cholelithiasis
   F. Cardiac: intestinal ischemia
   G. Renal: pyelonephritis, hydronephrosis, renal calculi, glomerulonephritis
   H. Respiratory: pneumonia, otitis, pharyngitis, sinusitis, common cold
   I. Miscellaneous: peritonitis, sepsis, pregnancy; improper feeding techniques

Modified from Orenstein SR. Dysphagia and vomiting. *In* Wyllie R, Hyams JS (eds). Pediatric Gastrointestinal Disease: Pathophysiology, Diagnosis, Management. Philadelphia: WB Saunders, 1983:147.

particularly structural abnormalities of the gastrointestinal tract or severe metabolic diseases. Sepsis is also an important neonatal consideration.

Older infants with vomiting may have less severe structural or metabolic disorders, or they may have common and acquired disorders such as gastroenteritis, mild systemic infections, gastroesophageal reflux, or allergies. Some metabolic disorders first manifest in older infants when dietary changes expose them to provocative foods for the first time, while gastroenteritis (especially rotavirus and Norwalk virus) and sepsis are important considerations in these relatively immunocompromised younger patients.

Toddlers frequently experience gastroenteritis, as they are repeatedly exposed to organisms that they have no immunity to; this age group also presents with acquired obstructive gastrointestinal disorders such as intussusception or volvulus or with vomiting due to ingested poisons.

Throughout childhood and adolescence, a wide variety of acquired disorders become symptomatic, and some subtle congenital malformations may also first become evident at these older ages. Metabolic disorders continue to be an important but infrequent cause of recurrent vomiting throughout childhood. In adolescents, pregnancy, drug ingestion, and eating disorders (anorexia nervosa or bulimia) are added to the diagnostic considerations.

CHARACTERISTICS OF THE VOMITING

The contents (Table 20–4) and forcefulness (see Table 20–1) of the vomitus narrow the diagnostic possibilities. Hematemesis and bilious vomiting, in particular, are approached in a manner very different from that of vomiting without these characteristics, and they represent more serious underlying disorders.

ASSOCIATED SYMPTOMS

Vomiting must be characterized as acute, chronic, or recurrent. Temporal associations of chronic or recurrent vomiting are important (Table 20–5). Associated symptoms must be elicited (Table 20–6); they are crucial, for example, in distinguishing life-threatening intracranial and metabolic disorders (Table 20–7). Abdominal pain is a central symptom that, if present, narrows the diagnosis. Vomiting associated with neurologic symptoms requires very careful evaluation. Post-tussive emesis is not usually confused with vomiting of other causes; it should direct diagnostic attention to the cause of the cough itself (see Chapter 7). Regurgitation in an infant with apnea may signal reflux-associated apnea, although

Table 20–3. Differential Diagnosis of Vomiting: Suggestions Provided by Age

I. Newborn
   A. Congenital obstructive gastrointestinal malformations:
      Atresias or webs of esophagus or intestine
      Meconium ileus or plug; Hirschsprung disease
   B. Inborn errors of metabolism:
      Organic acidemias, amino acidemias, hyperammonemias
      (urea cycle), adrenogenital syndromes

II. Infant
   A. Acquired or milder obstructive lesions:
      Pyloric stenosis, malrotation and volvulus,
      intussusception
   B. Metabolic diseases, inborn errors of metabolism
   C. Nutrient intolerances
   D. Functional disorders:
      Gastroesophageal reflux
   E. Psychosocial disorders:
      Rumination, injury due to child abuse

III. Child
   Most causes in Table 20–6
IV. Adolescent
   Most childhood causes, plus pregnancy, drugs (of abuse,
      suicide), eating disorders

Modified from Orenstein SR. Dysphagia and vomiting. *In* Wyllie R, Hyams JS (eds). Pediatric Gastrointestinal Disease: Pathophysiology, Diagnosis, Management. Philadelphia: WB Saunders, 1993:147.

many infants with reflux-associated apnea have minimal regurgitation (see Chapter 11).

MEDICAL, FAMILY, AND SOCIAL HISTORY

Previous surgery, hospitalizations, and medications may provide important clues. A family history of fetal or neonatal deaths suggests a genetic or metabolic cause; similar illness in family or other contacts may suggest infections or common toxic exposures. Psychosocial stressors may be found in adolescents with bulimia, peptic ulcer disease, or intentional self-poisonings representing suicide attempts.

Physical Examination

Although vomiting is a ''gastrointestinal'' symptom, it can be a manifestation of disease in multiple systems of the body. A complete physical examination is thus critical. Vital signs identify fever, which is important in narrowing the differential diagnosis, and shock (tachycardia, hypotension), which is important in determining the urgency of evaluation. Kussmaul breathing (deep, slow respirations with a prolonged expiratory phase) represents respiratory compensation for metabolic acidosis. It is an important clue in vomiting illness because acidosis is seen only with vomiting from metabolic causes or poisoning or with vomiting associated with marked diarrhea or shock. Examination of the fundi is often inappropriately neglected. The absence of venous pulsations or sharp discs may be the only evidence for a brain tumor or other intracranial lesion causing vomiting.

ABDOMINAL EXAMINATION

Simple observation of scars may suggest the possibility of obstruction from adhesions, and visible distention may represent ascites due to liver disease or intraluminal distention due to intestinal obstruction or ileus. The order of the examination is important because auscultation performed after stimulation of intestinal motility by palpation may artifactually change the auscultatory findings. An important distinction in the vomiting child is whether bowel sounds are increased, as in gastroenteritis or in bowel obstructions, or absent, as in ileus due to peritonitis or in pseudo-obstruction. Increased bowel sounds due to luminal obstruction are often characterized by intermittent ''rushes'' of high-pitched sounds that are coordinated with episodes of colicky pain.

Abdominal pain and tenderness associated with vomiting often represent disorders requiring surgery (see Chapter 18). Vague periumbilical pain is quite nonspecific, but the localized, very sharp pain signifying inflammation of the peritoneum requires immediate attention. Initial luminal obstruction may progress to later ileus as peritonitis intervenes. Localization of non-periumbilical pain or tenderness helps a great deal in determining the diseased intraabdominal organ (see Table 20–6).

Abdominal pain often represents luminal obstruction, ischemia, or perforation (surgical disease), but nonsurgical diseases must also be considered (see Chapter 18). These disorders include nonobstructive inflammatory diseases (infectious gastroenteritis, pancreatitis), metabolic crises (e.g., adrenal crisis), and poisonings (e.g., lead, narcotics, insecticides).

RECTAL EXAMINATION

There must be a very good reason for not performing a rectal examination in the vomiting child. Because this examination is so often inappropriately neglected in children, some hints as to its performance and utility are provided here.

Table 20–4. Contents of Emesis

Material	Source	Examples
Undigested food	Esophageal	Stricture, achalasia
Digested food—curds	Gastroduodenal	Pyloric stenosis, bezoar
Bile—green/yellow	Postampullary	Small bowel obstruction
Blood—red/brown	Lesion above ligament of Treitz	See Tables 20–11 and 20–12
Feculent—malodorous	Bacterial overgrowth	Stasis syndrome
	Colon	Gastrocolic fistula
	Necrotic bowel	Ischemic injury, peritonitis
Acid—clear (voluminous)	Gastric outlet obstruction	Pyloric stenosis
	Increased gastric secretion	Zollinger-Ellison syndrome
Mucus	Gastric, respiratory mucus	Sinusitis

Table 20–5. Temporal Associations of Chronic or Recurrent Vomiting

Temporal Associations	Diagnosis	Other Clues
Time of day: early A.M.	Increased intracranial pressure	Headache, fundi
	Sinusitis with postnasal mucus	Sinus tenderness
	Pregnancy	Secondary amenorrhea
	Uremia	
During or after meals		
Any meals	Peptic ulcer disease, reflux	Epigastric pain, heartburn
Specific foods		See Tables 20–7, 20–14, 20–15
Fructose	Hereditary fructose intolerance	
Galactose	Galactosemia	
High protein	Metabolic inborn error	Hyperammonemia, acidosis
Specific protein		
Cow, soy	Cow's or soy milk intolerance	
Gluten	Gluten-sensitive enteropathy (celiac)	Irish: celiac disease
Various (esp. egg, wheat, fish, nut, chocolate, strawberry	Miscellaneous allergic, eosinophilic gastroenteropathies	History of asthma, hives, ↑ eosinophils, family history of allergies
After fasting		
Food vomited	Gastric stasis/obstruction	Distention, tympany
Food not vomited	Metabolic disease	See Tables 20–7, 20–14, and 20–15
Other precipitants		
Cough	Post-tussive	Respiratory disease
Infections	Metabolic	See Tables 20–7, 20–14, and 20–15
	Recurrent gastroenteritis	
Vestibular stimulation	Motion sickness	Nystagmus
	Ménétrier's disease	Vertigo
Hyperhydration	Ureteropelvic junction obstruction ("beer-drinker's kidney")	Spontaneous resolution with normal hydration
Menses	Dysmenorrhea-associated vomiting	Relief with NSAIDs
	Acute intermittent porphyria	Non-peritonitis pain, distention, tachycardia, constipation
	Pelvic inflammatory disease	Vaginal discharge
Medications, toxins	Med side effect: pancreatitis, hepatitis	Look up meds taken
	Acute intermittent porphyria	
	Steroid withdrawal: Addison's disease	
	Poisonings; NSAID stricture; laxative, etc.	
	Ipecac abuse in anorexia nervosa	
Episodic/cyclic	Abdominal migraine, abdominal epilepsy	
	Pheochromocytoma	
	Porphyria	
	Familial dysautonomia	
	Metabolic inborn error	
	Familial Mediterranean fever	
	Malrotation and intermittent volvulus	
	Intermittent intussusception	
	Self-induced	
	Cyclic vomiting	

Abbreviation: NSAIDs = nonsteroidal anti-inflammatory drugs.

Table 20–6. Clues to the Diagnosis and Localization of the Cause of Emesis

Associated Symptoms	Diagnoses to Consider
Local abdominal pain	See Chapter 18
Epigastric	Peptic ulcer disease, reflux, pancreatitis
Periumbilical	Nonspecific or small intestinal obstruction
Pelvic	Cystitis, pelvic inflammatory disease
Right upper quadrant	Hepatitis, pancreatitis, cholecystitis, biliary colic, duodenal hematoma/ulcer, right pyelonephritis, pneumonia
Left upper quadrant	Peptic ulcer disease, pancreatitis, splenic torsion, left pyelonephritis
Right lower quadrant	Appendicitis, right tubo-ovarian disease
Left lower quadrant	Left tubo-ovarian disease, sigmoid disease
Right flank	UPJ/renal, biliary obstruction, adrenal hemorrhage
Left flank	UPJ/renal obstruction, adrenal hemorrhage
Other pain	
Headache	Increased intracranial pressure
	Sinusitis with postnasal mucus
	Migraine
Chest pain, dysphagia	Esophagitis, achalasia
	Pneumonia
Joint pain	SLE, FMF, IBD
Diarrhea	Partial intestinal obstruction
	Infectious enteritis
	Poison, metabolic inborn error
Constipation	Intestinal obstruction or dysmotility (pseudo-obstruction)
	Hypercalcemia, hypokalemia, porphyria, lead
Jaundice	Hepatitis, cholecystitis
	Hepatobiliary obstruction
	Metabolic disease
	Urinary obstruction or pyloric stenosis (neonate)
Neurologic	Metabolic, toxic (lead), central nervous system disease, porphyria, hepatic failure
Vertigo	
Visual changes	
Abnormal tone, seizure	
Full fontanelle	
Cardiac	
Valvular disease	Mesenteric arterial thrombosis (or embolism)
Hypotension	Mesenteric thrombosis, intestinal ischemia
Hypertension	Pheochromocytoma
Respiratory	Pneumonia, otitis, aspiration of vomitus
Urinary	Pyelonephritis, hydronephrosis, calculi, renal hypertension, cholestasis, porphyria
Gynecologic	
Menstrual irregularity	Pregnancy, ectopic pregnancy
Vaginal discharge	Pelvic inflammatory disease
Menses-associated	Porphyria, endometriosis, dysmenorrhea

Abbreviations: UPJ = ureteropelvic junction; SLE = systemic lupus erythematosus; FMF = familial Mediterranean fever; IBD = inflammatory bowel disease.

Preparation of the child depends on the age, but all verbal children benefit from a description of the examination. Even preschool children can usually be examined without discomfort or crying if they are properly prepared. The physician should ascertain from them or the parent if they have ever had a rectal examination. Even if they have had one that hurt or frightened them, they can be reassured and examined atraumatically. For young children, the description can be something like: "I will put this glove on my hand and some of this goo on my finger, and then I will put my finger in your bottom—where your poops come from. It doesn't hurt. The only time it would hurt is if you get scared and squeeze your muscles back there, so if you feel that happening you just say 'stop' and I will stop right away. When your muscles get soft again, you can say 'go' and we'll go further. You're in charge." Children between about 12 and 24 months generally object to the examination in any case; with them, one can briefly describe it but proceed gently but firmly. Infants are easiest, and adolescents respond much as adults if their sensitivity and privacy are respected.

The rectal examination is simpler to perform with the patient recumbent rather than standing. Patients are placed with their head toward the examiner's left; most children are examined lying on their left side, but the infant may be easiest to examine prone or supine. Children older than 2 years of age are appropriately draped. Before starting, it is important to get the child's hips and knees flexed maximally, thus preventing gluteal contraction from interfering with the examination. ("Curl up in a ball—try to touch your knees to your chin.") The buttocks are spread, and the anus is carefully observed for presence and patency in the newborn and for tags or fistulas suggesting inflammatory bowel disease in the

Table 20–7. When to Consider Metabolic Work-up*

Nutritional abnormalities	Failure to thrive, anorexia
Dietary provocations	Fructose, galactose, protein, fasting
Neurologic abnormalities	Lethargy, coma Tone ↑ ↓, developmental delay Seizures
Liver abnormalities	Hepatosplenomegaly Jaundice
Respiratory abnormalities	Apnea Respiratory distress Hyperpnea (due to metabolic acidosis)

Odd odors (breath, urine, ear wax)	Maple syrup: maple syrup urine disease
	Cabbage: tyrosinemia
	Sweaty feet: isovaleric acidemia
	Musty: phenylketonuria, hepatic coma
	  (fetor hepaticus)
	Fruity: ketones—many, nonspecific
	Other: 3-methylcrotonyl-CoA
	    carboxylase deficiency
	  Multiple carboxylase deficiency
	  Acyl-CoA dehydrogenase deficiency
	Putrid: sinusitis
	Alcohol: alcohol ingestion

Miscellaneous abnormalities	Eye abnormalities (cataracts) Hair abnormalities (fragile) Pigmentation of skin ("tan") and mucosa Adrenal calcifications Ambiguous genitalia Cardiomyopathy Family history of fetal or neonatal deaths; consanguinity
Screening study abnormalities	Metabolic acidosis Hypoglycemia (hyper- or hypoketonuric) Hyperkalemia (with hyponatremia) Hyperammonemia Hypertransaminasemia Anemia, leukocytopenia, thrombocytopenia Urinary non–glucose-reducing substance Urinary Fanconi's syndrome

*See also Tables 20–14 and 20–15.

older child. The lubricated finger is inserted with gentle, persistent pressure into the anus. (The index finger is the most sensitive and may be used by many examiners in most children—one can mentally compare the size of the finger to the usual diameter of the child's stools.)

A common mistake is to hurry the examination, thus causing spasm of the external anal sphincter and associated discomfort. The child's trust that one will stop when he or she says "stop" helps the sphincter to relax receptively; if the sphincter is tightening but the child does not say "stop," it is useful to stop anyway and allow the sphincter to relax. The examiner should not withdraw the finger but, rather, simply wait until the child consents to continuing. In young children, the sensation of losing control of feces, often provoked by the examination, produces anxiety; it helps to reassure them that although it feels as though they are going to defecate, they will not. The finger is inserted to the metacarpal joint, the walls of the rectum are explored by rotating the hand, and then the finger is withdrawn. In adolescents, a gynecologic examination and bimanual examination may be useful.

The presence and consistency of rectal stool are determined. Simple fecal impaction occasionally causes vomiting in children, while liquid stools may suggest gastroenteritis as the cause for vomiting. Pelvic masses and tenderness identified rectally may represent pelvic appendicitis, ovarian torsion, or pelvic inflammatory disease. Stool may be obtained on the glove, by spontaneous evacuation after stimulation by the examination, or found on the diaper. The stool should always be tested for blood and should be considered for testing for pH, reducing substances, fat, leukocytes, and infectious organisms, depending on the situation.

Laboratory Data

Well-appearing infants with typical regurgitant reflux usually require no laboratory evaluation, except probably an upper gastrointestinal study if they do not respond readily to conservative therapy (see later). Similarly, a single, brief episode of mild vomiting with a clear etiology and no suggestion of dehydration or other complications may require no laboratory studies. Most other children, those with severe acute vomiting or with chronic or recurrent vomiting, should have screening studies of blood or urine (Table 20–8).

Radiographic and Procedure Data

If the history and physical examination suggest the possibility of abdominal pathology, endoscopic evaluation or abdominal (flat plate–supine) plain films (including a second image such as an upright film) are usually warranted (Table 20–9). Endoscopy is particularly useful in hematemesis, in suspected peptic ulcer disease, or when tissue is needed for histology. Radiographic testing is useful in most other situations. Further evaluation, such as contrast studies, ultrasonography, computed tomography (CT), or magnetic resonance imaging (MRI), is tailored to the suspected diagnoses. Rarely, manometric evaluation is prompted by the suggestion of motor dysfunctions, such as achalasia and chronic intestinal pseudo-obstruction. A pH probe study is not useful in infants in whom regurgitation is the symptom suggesting reflux disease.

Consultation

Consultation is particularly important when specialized diagnostic procedures (endoscopy or radiography) or therapeutic procedures (surgery or endoscopy) may be needed.

DIFFERENTIAL DIAGNOSIS

Emergencies

Symptoms suggesting vomiting emergencies are listed in Table 20–10. These are generally diseases that are surgical, metabolic, or due to poisoning, but liver failure and neurologic disorders are also included.

General Approach

Cardinal symptoms or signs accompanying the vomiting direct the differential diagnosis. Abdominal pain, which frequently ac-

Table 20–8. Diagnostic Tests: Blood and Urine

	Findings	Possible Significance
Blood Test		
CBC		
Hct/Hb	↑	Dehydration—general vomiting
	↓	Hematemesis; metabolic; chronic—malnutrition; hypersplenism; hemolysis (e.g., sickle cell)
WBC (PMN, bands)	↑	Sepsis; inflammatory/ischemic lesions
	↓	Metabolic; sepsis; viral; hypersplenism; malnutrition
Eosinophils	↑	Allergic (eosinophilic gastroenteropathy), parasitic
Platelets	↑	Inflammatory (e.g., inflammatory bowel disease)
	↓	Hematemesis; metabolic; hypersplenism
Electrolytes		
NA	↓ (↓)	Adrenal insufficiency; general vomiting
	↑	Salt poisoning, dehydration
K	↓	General vomiting
	↑	Adrenal insufficiency; uremia; bleeding; digitalis; diuretics (e.g., spironolactone)
Cl	↓ (↓)	Adrenal insufficiency; general vomiting
	↑	Salt poisoning, hypernatremic dehydration
Bicarbonate	↑ (pH ↑)	General vomiting, pyloric stenosis
	↓ (pH ↓)	Metabolic; adrenal insufficiency; poison; renal tubular acidosis; severe diarrhea; shock
Glucose	↑	Metabolic—diabetic ketoacidosis
	↓	Metabolic, toxins
BUN	↑	Dehydration, hematemesis
Creatinine	↑	Dehydration, renal failure
Calcium	↑	Hypercalcemia
Blood gas	↓ pH, ↓ P_{CO_2}	Metabolic disease; adrenal insufficiency; poison; severe diarrhea; shock
ALT, AST	↑	Hepatitis; metabolic
GGT, ALP	↑	Biliary obstruction
Bilirubin	↑	Hepatitis; metabolic; hemolysis (e.g., sickle cell)
Conjugated	↑	Biliary obstruction
Amylase, lipase	↑	Pancreatitis
NH₄	↑	Metabolic, liver failure, *Proteus* urinary infection
Ketones	↑	Metabolic, fasting/starvation
Amino acids	↑	Metabolic
Organic acids	↑	Metabolic
IgE, RAST (esp. foods)	↑	Allergic enteropathies
PT, PTT	↑	Hematemesis
Toxicology	+	Drug; poison
Culture	+	Sepsis; ischemic/perforated bowel
Urine Test		
pH	↑	General vomiting
WBC	+	Urinary tract infection
Protein, casts	+	Renal disease
Blood	+	Urinary tract infection or bleeding
Bilirubin	+	Liver disease, hemolysis
Electrolytes		
Na	↓	General vomiting
K	↑	General vomiting
Cl	↓	General vomiting
Bicarbonate	↑	General vomiting
Ketones	+	Metabolic, fasting/starvation
Reducing substance		
Glucose	+	Diabetic ketoacidosis
Non-glucose	+	Galactosemia
Fanconi	+	Metabolic
FeCl	+	Metabolic
Amino acids	↑	Metabolic
Organic acids	↑	Metabolic
Toxicology	+	Drug; poison
Culture	+	Urinary tract infection; sepsis

Abbreviations: CBC = complete blood count; Hct/Hb = hematocrit/hemoglobin; WBC = white blood cell count; PMN = polymorphonuclear neutrophils; Na = sodium; K = potassium; Cl = chloride; BUN = blood urea nitrogen; ALT = alanine aminotransferase; AST = aspartate aminotransferase; GGT = γ-glutamyltransferase; ALP = alkaline phosphatase; NH₄ = ammonium; IgE = immunoglobulin E; RAST = radioallergosorbent test; PT = prothrombin time; PTT = partial thromboplastin time; FeCl = iron chloride; metabolic = inborn errors of metabolism.

Table 20–9. Diagnostic Tests: Other

Test	Findings	Possible Significance
Radiography		
Routine		
Plain abdomen	Isolated/distended loops	Obstruction, ischemia
	"Ladder" pattern	Small-bowel obstruction
	"Inverted U" pattern	Distal colon obstruction
	Double bubble	Duodenal atresia
	Calcifications	Biliary, renal stones
	Free air	Intestinal perforation
	Free fluid	Ascites
	Foreign bodies	Foreign body
	Organomegaly, masses	Organomegaly, masses
Upright abdomen	Air-fluid levels	↑ Secretion—gastroenteritis
		Obstruction
Laterals, decubitus	Free air	Perforation
Chest film	Heart or lung disease; free air	Heart or lung disease; perforation
Barium		
Upper fluoroscopy	Malrotation; obstructions	Volvulus; obstructing lesions
Enteroclysis	Distal obstructions	Distal small bowel lesions
Lower fluoroscopy	Mass, obstruction, intussusception	Rx: intussusception
Gastrografin		
Upper fluoroscopy		
Lower fluoroscopy		Rx: meconium ileus, DIOS
Ultrasound	Mass, cyst, abscess; pyloric stenosis; hepatobiliary, pancreatic, urinary, gynecologic lesions; blood flow in vessels	
CT/MRI abdomen	Mass, cyst, inflammatory lesions; hepatobiliary, pancreatic, urinary, gynecologic lesions	
MRI/CT head	CNS lesions	Neurogenic vomiting
Endoscopy		
Upper		
Diagnostic	Dx: obstruction, hemorrhage, *Giardia or Helicobacter pylori* infection	Obstruction, hemorrhage
Therapeutic		Rx: hematemesis
Lower		
Diagnostic	Dx: distal obstruction, infection	Obstruction, infection
Therapeutic		Rx: sigmoid volvulus
Manometry		
Esophagus	Failure sphincter relaxation	Achalasia
	Dysmotility	Pseudo-obstruction
Small bowel	Dysmotility	Pseudo-obstruction
Rectum/colon	Failure sphincter relaxation	Hirschsprung disease
	Dysmotility	Pseudo-obstruction

Abbreviations: DIOS = distal intestinal obstruction syndrome—cystic fibrosis; CT = computed tomography; MRI = magnetic resonance imaging; CNS = central nervous system; Rx = therapeutic.

Table 20–10. Vomiting Emergencies*

Emergent Symptoms	Drug/Poison†	Metabolic‡	Surgical	Neurologic	Liver Failure	Further Laboratory Studies
Shock	+	+	+			
Mental status change lethargy, coma, seizure, psychosis	+ +	+ +		+ + +	+ + +	NH₃, head CT/ MRI, glucose
Severe abdominal pain/ distention	+ +	+	+ + +		+	Abdominal films
Acute liver dysfunction Jaundice Anicteric	+ +	+ +	+	+	+ + +	NH₃, PT
Respiratory Apnea, Kussmaul's breathing	+ +	+ +	+	+ +	+ +	Blood gas; electro- lytes; urinalysis, glucose
Other Bilious emesis Silent abdomen Hematemesis		+	+ + + + + + +		+ + +	Abdominal films Endoscopy

*An acutely ill child with vomiting needs:
  Physical examination: esp. vital signs, neurologic, funduscopic, abdominal (auscultation, peritoneal signs), rectal.
  Laboratory tests: complete blood count, differential white blood cell count, platelets; sodium, potassium, chloride, carbon dioxide; glucose (Dextrostix); blood urea nitrogen, creatinine; liver function tests; amylase, lipase; blood gas; urinalysis.
  If fever, also needs: Cultures of blood, urine, cerebrospinal fluid (if mentation change), and stool (if diarrhea or hematochezia).
  If hematemesis, also needs: platelets, prothrombin time, partial thromboplastin time.
†See Tables 20–16 and 20–17.
‡See Tables 20–14 and 20–15.
Abbreviations: NH₃ = ammonia; CT = computed tomography; MRI = magnetic resonance imaging; PT = prothrombin time; + = suggestive; + + = moderately suggestive; + + + = highly suggestive.

companies vomiting, can suggest both the type of disorder (luminal obstruction, inflammation, ischemia, or peritonitis) and the organ involved, as suggested previously under Physical Examination. Hematemesis leads to the considerations indicated in Tables 20–11 and Table 20–12 (see Chapter 21). Symptoms referable to nongastrointestinal organ systems direct attention to those systems. For example, accompanying neurologic symptoms direct attention to central nervous system disorders, metabolic disease, poisonings, or psychobehavioral disease. Vomiting due to food poisoning or, more commonly, gastroenteritis is discussed in Chapter 19.

Gastrointestinal Obstruction (Table 20–13)

ESOPHAGEAL OBSTRUCTION

Esophageal lesions produce welling up or drooling of oropharyngeal secretions or esophageal contents rather than actual vomiting; the material is, of course, undigested. Respiratory symptoms from aspiration may be prominent.

Esophageal Atresia. Infants with esophageal atresia present at birth with a history of polyhydramnios and intolerance of even the initial feeding. The esophageal atresia is accompanied by a distal tracheoesophageal fistula in 85% of cases, by a proximal fistula in a few percent, and by no fistula in the remainder (Fig. 20–1). Esophageal atresia is associated with other anomalies 15% to 50% of the time; cardiac, anorectal, and genitourinary defects most commonly occur. Ten percent of all esophageal atresia patients, and a quarter of those without a fistula, have the VATER or VACTERL (*v*ertebral, *a*norectal, *c*ardiac, *t*racheo*e*sophageal, *r*enal,

*r*adial, *l*imb) association. As many as a third of the infants are premature. Diagnosis can usually be made by plain films after passing an opaque rubber catheter, which coils in the upper pouch (Fig. 20–2). Treatment is surgical. Many infants experience reflux and reactive airway disease in the postoperative period.

Esophageal Stenosis. Infants with esophageal stenoses present in later infancy and occasionally as late as adulthood. Stenoses are divided into tracheobronchial rings, often containing cartilage, fibromuscular stenoses, and membranous webs. Diagnosis is by contrast radiography and may require pressure injections of contrast material if the stenosis is not tight. Tracheobronchial rings generally require surgery, membranous webs can be treated with endoscopic dilation, and muscular stenoses may respond to dilation or may require operation.

Esophageal Strictures. Esophageal strictures are acquired lesions that are usually due to reflux esophagitis but are sometimes due to caustic ingestions (acid, alkali) or other causes (Fig. 20–3). The strictures are best demonstrated with contrast radiography; endoscopic biopsies are used to diagnose the cause as reflux. Adequate treatment of the gastroesophageal reflux that has produced a stricture generally requires fundoplication; endoscopic dilation of the strictures is performed repeatedly with balloons or bougies until the strictured site remains patent.

PYLORIC STENOSIS

Pyloric stenosis presents with nonbilious projectile vomiting beginning at 2 to 3 weeks of age and increasing during the next

Table 20–11. Hematemesis

Source of Blood	Lesion	Clues Regarding Source
Nasopharynx, respiratory	Epistaxis	Nosebleed history
	Hemoptysis	Cough, other respiratory symptoms
Esophageal	Varices	Copious; splenomegaly
	Esophagitis, Barrett ulcer	Heartburn
	Foreign body erosion	Foreign body history
	Aortoesophageal fistula	Copious; esophageal intubation
	Duplication	
Gastroduodenal	Mallory-Weiss tear	Emesis before hematemesis
	Peptic ulcer disease	History: smoking, alcohol, NSAIDs, pain, relation to meals
	Gastritis, ulcer	
	Duodenitis, ulcer	
	Stress ulcer	
	Dieulafoy's ulcer	
	Vascular malformation	Recurrent (may have negative endoscopy)
	Aortoenteric fistula	"Herald bleed," arterial graft or aneurysm
	Duplication	
	Pyloric stenosis, web	
	Hemobilia	Trauma, gallstones, pain, jaundice
Extrinsic		
Maternal	Intrapartum	Apt test*
	Mastitis, cracked nipples	Maternal history, Apt test*
Factitious	Psychologic	Affect, secondary gain
Non-blood	Red or brown food or medicine	Guaiac-negative

*See Chapter 21.
Abbreviations: URI = upper respiratory infection; NSAIDs = nonsteroidal anti-inflammatory drugs.

month or so, usually in a firstborn male child. The vomitus may later contain some blood, and propulsive gastric waves can be seen on the abdominal wall. Dehydration, poor weight gain, metabolic alkalosis, and mild jaundice (indirect reacting hyperbilirubinemia) are sometimes evident. A palpable "olive" in the epigastrium (felt best after a feeding) represents the hypertrophied pyloric muscle.

Gastric distention is seen on the plain film, and a contrast study shows the "string sign" of contrast passing through the narrowed pyloric channel. Ultrasound diagnosis is helpful and less invasive (Fig. 20–4). Eosinophilia, eosinophilic infiltration of endoscopic antral biopsies, and an excellent response to nonoperative treatment with a casein hydrolysate "hypoallergenic" formula should suggest an allergic or idiopathic eosinophilic gastroenteropathy and not pyloric stenosis.

Table 20–12. Hematemesis: Causes Not to Miss and Red Flags

Finding	Etiology	Physical Examination and Laboratory Studies: Clues Regarding Source
Coagulopathy (PT ↑, PTT ↑)	Vitamin K deficiency	Newborn, antibiotics, fat malabsorption
	Genetic coagulopathies	Specific factor deficiencies
	Liver failure	Liver disease, Factor VIII normal
	DIC	Sepsis, Factor VIII ↓
	Drug	Drug history
	Warfarin (Coumadin)	
	Heparin	
Thrombocytopenia (platelets ↓)	Hypersplenism	Splenomegaly (Hct ↓, WBC ↓)
	Chemotherapy	Chemotherapy history (Hct ↓, WBC ↓)
	DIC	Sepsis (PT ↑, PTT ↑)
Platelet dysfunction (bleeding time ↑)	Drug	Drug history
	Salicylates/NSAIDs	
	Antibiotics	
Portal hypertension	Varices; gastritis	Splenomegaly
		Abdominal veins; angiomas
		Ascites
		Clubbing; palmar erythema

Abbreviations: PT = prothrombin time; PTT = partial thromboplastin time; DIC = disseminated intravascular coagulation; Hct = hematocrit; WBC = white blood cell count; NSAIDs = nonsteroidal anti-inflammatory drugs.

Table 20–13. Causes of Gastrointestinal Obstruction

Esophagus

Congenital	Esophageal atresia (with or without fistula)
	Isolated esophageal stenosis
Acquired	Caustic agent esophageal stricture
	Peptic stricture
	Chagas disease
	Collagen-vascular disease

Stomach

Congenital	Antral webs
Acquired	Pyloric atresia*
	Bezoars/foreign body
	Pyloric stenosis
	Pyloric stricture (ulcer)
	Crohn disease
	Eosinophilic gastroenteropathy
	Prostaglandin induced pyloric stenosis
	Chronic granulomatous disease

Small Intestine

Congenital	Duodenal atresia
	Annular pancreas
	Malrotation/volvulus
	Malrotation/Ladd bands
	Ileal atresia, stenosis
	Duplications
	Meconium ileus
	Inguinal hernia
Acquired	Postsurgical adhesions, or strictures
	Crohn disease (stricture)
	Intussusception
	Duodenal hematoma (abuse, trauma)
	Meconium ileus equivalent

Colon

Congenital	Meconium plug
	Hirschsprung disease
	Colonic atresia, stenosis
	Imperforate rectum-anus
	Rectal stenosis
	Malrotation/volvulus
	Small left colon syndrome (IDM)
Acquired	Ulcerative colitis (toxic megacolon)†
	Crohn disease (stricture)
	Chagas disease
	Stricture post-NEC

From Behrman R, Kliegman R. Nelson Essentials of Pediatrics, 2nd ed. Philadelphia: WB Saunders, 1944:407.
*Often associated with epidermolysis bullosa.
†Produces an ileus.
Abbreviation: IDM = infant of diabetic mother; NEC = necrotizing enterocolitis.

In older children gastric outlet obstruction may be due to ulceration, chronic granulomatous disease, foreign bodies and bezoars. The latter may be due to hair, vegetable matter, milk curds, or medications. Long-acting formulated oral medications may also become bezoars in the distal intestine and cause obstruction.

INTESTINAL OBSTRUCTIONS

Rushes of bowel sounds associated with cramping and colic often indicate intestinal obstruction. Vomiting is a cardinal sign of intestinal obstruction, being more prominent in high small-bowel obstruction than in low small-bowel or colon obstruction. In high obstructions, vomiting is not feculent, the onset is often acute, and crampy pain may occur at frequent intervals; abdominal distention is minimal. In contrast, the vomiting in low obstructions may be feculent and less acute in onset and the interval between cramping is longer; distention, on the other hand, is more notable. Identification of the site of obstruction is aided by the plain film and by other radiographic studies (see Table 20–9).

Obstructions may be categorized as to their type as well as their site. Intraluminal lesions (such as tumors, intussusceptions, or extrinsic material—feces, foreign bodies, bezoars, gallstones) can be differentiated from bowel wall lesions (strictures, stenoses, atresias) and from extraluminal lesions (adhesions, congenital bands, tumors, volvulus). Again, radiographic studies are useful, beginning with the plain film and progressing to ultrasound or CT. Fluoroscopy using contrast material such as barium or Gastrografin is very helpful in identifying both the site and the type of obstruction, but the decision to introduce such contrast into an intestine that may perforate or be operated on must be made with surgical and radiologic consultation. Often the decision to operate can be made without certain identification of the lesion, and contrast studies are forgone.

Infantile bilious vomiting is an important symptom of intestinal obstruction, which often signals a congenital gastrointestinal anomaly, particularly intestinal obstruction below the ampulla of Vater. Surgical consultation is needed early in the evaluation of an infant with bilious vomiting, which often requires life-saving emergent therapy (see Table 20–13).

Duodenal Atresia, Stenosis, Web; Annular Pancreas. The juxta-ampullary duodenum is susceptible to a cluster of obstructing congenital anomalies. Infants with complete duodenal obstruction, most commonly atresia, present with bilious vomiting and a radiographic "double-bubble" sign (Fig. 20–5). Associated prematurity (and polyhydramnios) or anomalies, including renal, cardiac, and vertebral defects, occur in approximately 75% of infants; trisomy 21 is seen in about 50%. Double atresias, duplications, and malrotations are frequently seen.

Infants with a partial duodenal obstruction due to a stenosis or web may have such mild symptoms that they are not diagnosed until regurgitation produces esophagitis or until a foreign body or bezoar is trapped at the obstruction. Treatment is surgery.

Duodenal Hematoma. Blunt abdominal trauma (seat belt injury, child abuse), or even endoscopic biopsies in the context of a coagulopathy, can produce an obstructing duodenal hematoma. Although this is an uncommon lesion, it is a cause of acquired duodenal obstruction.

Therapy is symptomatic; parenteral nutrition may be required as it resolves.

Jejunal Atresia, Ileal Atresia, Ileal Stenosis. Patients with these congenital lesions present with bilious vomiting and more abdominal distention than those with duodenal lesions.

The atresias are readily suspected and diagnosed in the neonatal period. Stenotic lesions may require radiography for diagnosis. Treatment is surgical.

Intestinal Strictures. Strictures produce partial obstruction of the luminal gastrointestinal tract and may be located from the esophagus to the anus. They may occur postsurgically (anastomotic), following necrotizing enterocolitis, due to Crohn's disease, or due to ingestion of nonsteroidal anti-inflammatory medications or high-dose pancreatic enzymes.

Some patients may be treated with endoscopic dilation, but many require surgical stricturoplasty (opening the bowel longitudinally and closing it transversely) or resection.

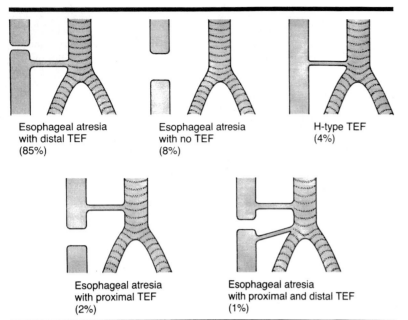

Esophageal atresia
with distal TEF
(85%)

Esophageal atresia
with no TEF
(8%)

H-type TEF
(4%)

Esophageal atresia
with proximal TEF
(2%)

Esophageal atresia
with proximal and distal TEF
(1%)

Figure 20–1. Various types of tracheoesophageal fistulas (TEF) with relative frequency (%). (From Kirschner BS, Black DD. The gastrointestinal tract. *In* Behrman RE, Kliegman RM [eds]. Nelson Essentials of Pediatrics, 2nd ed. Philadelphia: WB Saunders, 1994:413.)

Figure 20–2. Tracheoesophageal fistula (TEF). Coiled radiopaque nasogastric tube in blind upper pouch. Note the air in the gastrointestinal tract, indicating a distal TEF. Rarely, the TEF is so big that a large amount of air enters the stomach and preliminary gastrostomy is necessary to avoid gastric perforation. (From Ein SH. Esophageal atresia and tracheoesophageal fistula. *In* Wyllie R, Hyams JS [eds]. Pediatric Gastrointestinal Disease: Pathophysiology, Diagnosis, Management. Philadelphia: WB Saunders, 1993:320.)

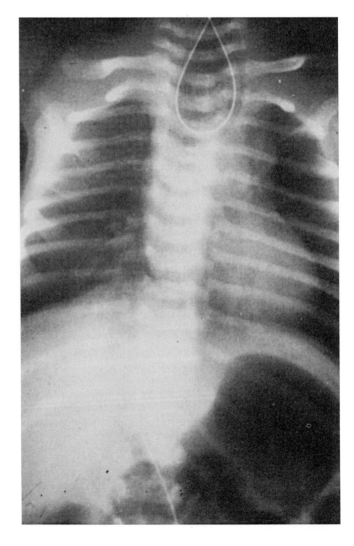

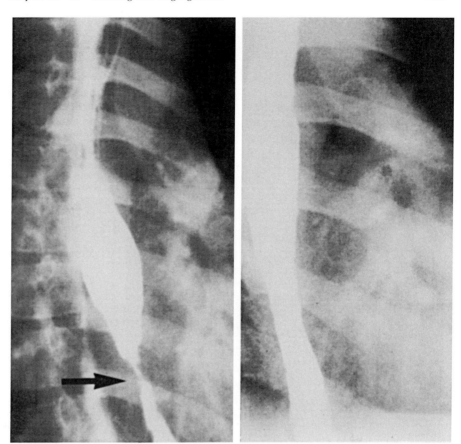

Figure 20–3. Esophageal stricture. Radiograph of a peptic esophageal stricture before and after treatment with dilatations. This 10-year-old boy had a 6-month history of dysphagia before his stricture *(arrow)* was demonstrated by barium esophagram *(left)*. His weight had dropped to the 10th percentile, but his height was at the 50th percentile. The stricture was improved symptomatically and radiographically *(right)* by a series of bougienage dilatations, and subsequent fundoplication allowed the underlying peptic esophagitis to heal. (From Orenstein SR. Dysphagia and vomiting. *In* Wyllie R, Hyams JS [eds]. Pediatric Gastrointestinal Disease: Pathophysiology, Diagnosis, Management. Philadelphia: WB Saunders, 1993:137.)

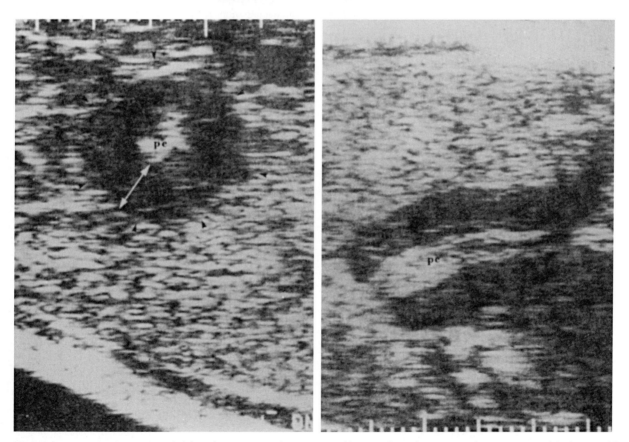

Figure 20–4. Pyloric stenosis. Cross-sectional *(left)* and transverse *(right)* sonogram of hypertrophic pyloric stenosis showing increased thickness and length of pyloric muscle. pc = pyloric channel. (From Alexander F. Pyloric stenosis and congenital anomalies of the stomach and duodenum. *In* Wyllie R, Hyams JS [eds]. Pediatric Gastrointestinal Disease: Pathophysiology, Diagnosis, Management. Philadelphia: WB Saunders, 1993:416.)

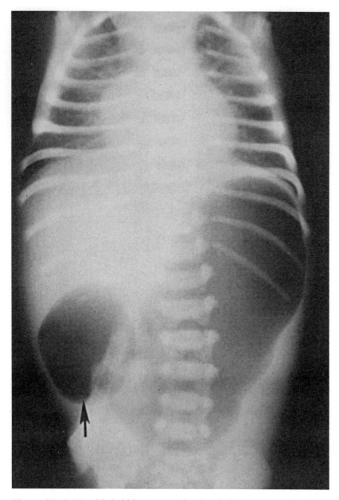

Figure 20–5. "Double-bubble" sign in duodenal obstruction. Swallowed air fills the stomach and obstructed duodenum (arrow). Usually accompanied by bilious vomiting, the double-bubble sign is not specific for any of the duodenal obstructions but implies a need for surgery. (From Teplick SK, Glick SN, Keller MS. The duodenum. In Putman CE, Ravin CE [eds]. Textbook of Diagnostic Imaging. Philadelphia: WB Saunders, 1988:815.)

Adhesions. Obstructive symptoms in the child with a history of prior abdominal surgery may be due to adhesive bands.

Duplications. These uncommon lesions may cause vomiting by extrinsic obstruction of the intestine or by intussuscepting. An abdominal mass may be palpable.

Meconium Ileus, Meconium Ileus Equivalent. Ten percent of infants with cystic fibrosis present in the newborn period with failure to pass meconium—meconium ileus (Fig. 20–6). The inspissated meconium may be treated by Gastrografin enema, but some infants require surgery, particularly if they have perforated, which occurs prenatally in 10% and produces a calcified meconium peritonitis. Virtually all infants with meconium ileus have cystic fibrosis; the diagnosis should be confirmed by sweat test or DNA analysis. Older children with cystic fibrosis who stop stooling and have abdominal pain and occasionally vomiting are said to have distal intestinal obstruction syndrome (DIOS), formerly termed meconium ileus equivalent.

The sticky, poorly hydrated intestinal mucus plays a role. Initial

treatment with intestinal lavage and enemas may be successful, but, if not, Gastrografin enemas (at times mixed with N-acetylcysteine) are nearly always successful. Surgery is rarely required.

Incarcerated Hernia. Whenever vomiting is accompanied by signs of obstruction, sites of potential herniation should be examined for incarceration of a loop of bowel (Fig. 20–7). Inguinal incarceration is most common, but other types of hernias are femoral, obturator, spigelian, umbilical (1 in 1500 incarcerate), epigastric, and postoperative incisional hernias.

Inguinal hernias (nonstrangulated) may often be reduced by gentle, firm, constant pressure directed through the scrotum toward the inguinal canal. Sedation and the Trendelenburg position may facilitate reduction (see Chapter 30).

Malrotation, Volvulus. Volvulus is the twisting of a loop of bowel on the mesentery. Midgut volvulus occurs most often in the context of congenital intestinal malrotation, in which the small intestine is not normally fastened in place (Fig. 20–8). More than half of patients found to have malrotation present symptomatically (the rest being discovered incidentally), and about half of the symptomatic patients present with bilious vomiting due to volvulus in the newborn period. Those presenting later often do not have bilious vomiting; the vomiting may be intermittent for years.

Volvulus is an extremely hazardous obstructing lesion. The luminal obstruction is closed at both ends, causing sepsis from rapidly proliferating and translocating bacteria. There is also vascular obstruction where the root of the mesentery is twisted, quickly producing ischemia of the small intestine. Death occurs rapidly if the symptoms are ignored; even if volvulus is diagnosed and operated on relatively promptly, it may require massive intestinal resection (producing short bowel syndrome), with lifelong dependency on parenteral nutrition. Because volvulus may be intermittent, it may produce episodic or chronic intermittent vomiting or nonspecific abdominal pain prior to a lethal event.

There should be a low threshold for obtaining upper intestinal contrast radiography in the intermittently regurgitating infant and for performing surgery if a malrotation is found (i.e., if the ligament of Treitz is not to the left of the spine), even if volvulus is not

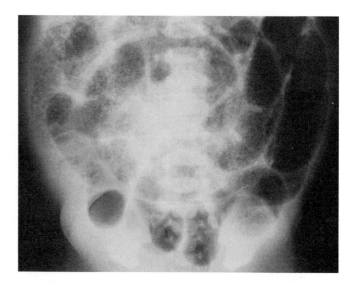

Figure 20–6. Meconium ileus. Supine radiograph shows gas-distended small bowel and mottled appearance of inspissated meconium in this newborn. (From Lappas JC, Maglinte DDT. The small bowel. In Putman CE, Ravin CE [eds]. Textbook of Diagnostic Imaging. Philadelphia: WB Saunders, 1988:859.)

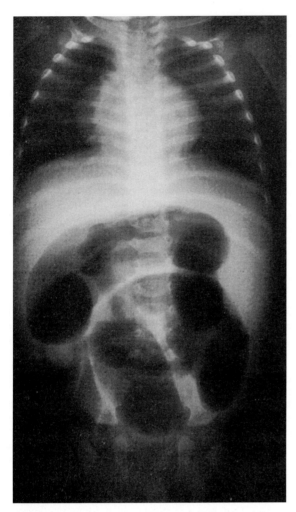

Figure 20–7. Intestinal obstruction. Plain radiograph of the abdomen reveals massive intestinal dilatation in a 4-month-old child with abdominal distention and vomiting secondary to intestinal obstruction from inguinal hernias. Note the presence of gas within the scrotum. (From Markowitz JF. Intestinal obstruction and ileus. *In* Wyllie R, Hyams JS [eds]. Pediatric Gastrointestinal Disease: Pathophysiology, Diagnosis, Management. Philadelphia: WB Saunders, 1993:246.)

present at the time of the examination. In an infant in whom an ongoing volvulus is suspected, an abdominal flat plate may show a "double bubble with distal air" or a "volvulus/corkscrew" pattern. In the sick infant or child in whom volvulus seems likely, surgery without contrast studies may be preferred. Surgery deals both with the malrotation and with the often-accompanying, potentially obstructing Ladd bands.

Other types of volvulus not associated with malrotation include cecal, sigmoid, and transverse colonic volvulus. They are less common in children and less apt to produce short bowel syndrome, but they, too, may present with vomiting and result in death if unrecognized. Sigmoid volvulus is sometimes treated nonoperatively.

Meckel's Diverticulum. Meckel's diverticuli may cause obstructive vomiting by intussusception or by intestinal volvulus around a fibrous band (Fig. 20–9). (They may also cause vomiting by inflammatory changes [see later] and they may bleed.) This fibrous remnant of the omphalomesenteric duct is a small intestinal diverticulum. The "rule of 2s" identifies characteristic findings: 2% of

the population, males 2:1, within 2 feet of the ileocecal valve, 2 inches long, two types of heterotopic mucosa (50% have gastric, a few percent have pancreatic; rarely, colonic mucosa is present), confused with two diseases (appendicitis and peptic ulcer), and has two complications (hemorrhage and perforation—or intussusception and volvulus).

Diagnosis of the ectopic gastric mucosa is by Meckel's scan (^{99m}Tc-pertechnetate); it has imperfect sensitivity, which may be improved by pentagastrin, glucagon, and cimetidine. Treatment is surgical.

Intussusception. The normal function of the intestine is to constrict above and relax below an intraluminal bolus. When such a bolus (a "lead point") is attached to the intestinal wall, the propulsive activity of the intestine produces telescoping of proximal intestine (intussusceptum) into distal intestine (intussuscipiens), causing both luminal obstruction and mesenteric vascular compromise. Abdominal pain occurs in nearly all children with intussusception, whereas vomiting results in about 65% and "currant-jelly stools" (from mucosal hemorrhage) occur in fewer than 20%. The pain is severe, crampy, and often contemporaneous with the vomiting. Between cramps, the child may be listless, may sleep, or may even play. Vomiting and bloody stools are more common in younger infants and in those with longer duration of symptoms. An abdominal mass is palpable in about 25%.

The lead point of the intussusception is usually ileal, with the intussusception ileocecal or ileocolonic. It is probable that prominent ileal lymphoid nodules provide the lead point for most young children presenting with intussusception, 66% of whom are younger than 2 years of age, with a peak late in the first year of life. Other lead points (Meckel's diverticulum [see Fig. 20–9], appendix, duplication, polyp, lymphoma, hematoma—from trauma or from Henoch-Schönlein purpura) or disorders (cystic fibrosis) must be

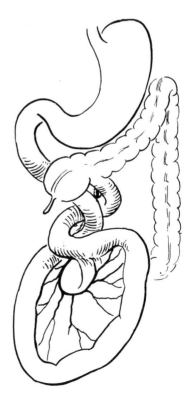

Figure 20–8. Malrotation with the mesentery twisted on its pedicle. (From Wang C, Welch CE. Anomalies of intestinal rotation in adolescents and adults. Surgery 1963;54:839–855; with permission.)

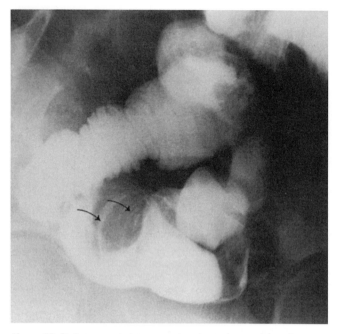

Figure 20–9. Enteroenteric intussusception. Luminal mass defect due to intussusception of Meckel's diverticulum. A coil-spring appearance has been created around the intussusceptum *(arrows)*. (From Lappas JC, Maglinte DDT. The small bowel. *In* Putman CE, Ravin CE [eds]. Textbook of Diagnostic Imaging. Philadelphia: WB Saunders, 1988:858.)

considered in the very young or older child presenting with intussusception (see Chapter 18).

Visualization may be by ultrasonography if the diagnosis is uncertain, but is more often by x-ray studies, as radiologic reduction enemas are usually curative in most infants.

Treatment is by hydrostatic reduction using barium; rectal insufflation of air has also been used but may be less able to document a lead point requiring surgical resection. Contraindications to reduction by hydrostatic enemas include peritonitis and intestinal perforation. Approximately 10% of patients experience recurrences.

Superior Mesenteric Artery (SMA) Syndrome. SMA syndrome is caused by extrinsic compression of the duodenum, which is trapped between the SMA anteriorly and the aorta posteriorly as the SMA crosses over the duodenum in the root of the mesentery. The compression is usually just to the right of midline, where it produces a cutoff of the duodenum radiographically, often with proximal dilation. Synonyms include Wilkie syndrome, arteriomesenteric duodenal compression, and cast syndrome.

SMA syndrome may be suspected when bilious emesis and epigastric discomfort relieved by vomiting occur in the context of weight loss, lordosis, body casts, lengthy bed rest, or prior abdominal surgery, particularly when crampy pain is relieved by prone or knee-chest positions. Adolescents and young adults are most often affected.

Nutritional rehabilitation, either intravenously or by the enteral route (if possible), is important in SMA syndrome. Prone position may improve duodenal emptying. Surgery may be needed if there are chronic symptoms despite nutritional rehabilitation.

Constipation, Meconium Plug, Anal Stenosis. These distal colonic problems produce obstipation primarily, but if they are severe and persistent, vomiting may result. Rectal examination provides the diagnosis.

Enemas, laxatives, dietary changes, and behavioral modification are useful in constipation, whereas surgery is usually required to treat anal atresia or stenosis (see Chapter 25).

Gastrointestinal Dysmotility

ACHALASIA

Achalasia, like esophageal stenoses and strictures, produces effortless emptying of undigested food from the esophagus.

Contrast radiography and esophageal manometry are needed for diagnosis. Calcium channel blockers such as nifedipine produce at least temporary clinical benefit in many patients with achalasia. Balloon dilation or surgical myotomy produce more sustained benefit more reliably but with a somewhat higher complication rate.

GASTROESOPHAGEAL REFLUX

The apparently effortless regurgitation that represents gastroesophageal reflux in infants is of particular importance because (1) it is the most common cause of "vomiting" in infants; (2) physiologic reflux must be distinguished from reflux requiring evaluation and therapy; and (3) the practitioner must be vigilant to avoid misdiagnosing other infantile vomiting diseases as reflux. Lethal malrotation with volvulus, partially obstructing duodenal web, and metabolic disorders are three examples of such misdiagnoses. Children with primary neurologic disease may be more likely to regurgitate and suffer from reflux disease; it must be remembered that many metabolic disorders manifest both as neurologic dysfunction and as regurgitation.

Infants with apparent regurgitant reflux who come to medical attention because of poor weight gain, irritability, and so forth, should have upper gastrointestinal radiography documenting the ligament of Treitz to be to the left of the spine to eliminate the possibility of malrotation. Reflux may cause weight deficit (due to regurgitation or to odynophagia from esophagitis), apnea, chronic respiratory disease, hoarseness or stridor, abdominal or chest pain, infantile irritability, or *Sandifer syndrome* (arching of the spine and turning of the neck). Diagnostic evaluation should be tailored to the presentation: regurgitation prompts barium contrast radiography with fluoroscopy; anorexia or infantile irritability prompts evaluation for esophagitis (by esophageal biopsy and possibly endoscopy); apnea prompts pH probe with pneumogram (especially if the apnea is repetitive); hoarseness or stridor prompts laryngoscopy, endoscopy for esophageal histology, a modified Bernstein test (acid infusion test to reproduce symptoms), or possibly a trial of aggressive therapy; heartburn prompts endoscopy or a single trial of antacid or histamine blocking agent therapy; and Sandifer syndrome prompts endoscopy and pH probe or modified Bernstein test.

Treatment of regurgitant reflux in infants is initiated with avoidance of seated or supine positioning (particularly postprandially) and with thickening of the feedings with 1 tablespoon of dry rice cereal per ounce of formula. In many infants, this reduces regurgitation remarkably, although some have problems with constipation from the rice cereal. If this occurs, the concentration may be reduced, another less constipating cereal may be tried (although no studies have evaluated their efficacy), or juices or other treatment of the constipation may be initiated. Problematic regurgitation persisting during this treatment, particularly if associated with poor weight gain or other signs of illness, requires upper gastrointestinal fluoroscopy and consideration of other causes for the vomiting, such as metabolic or allergic disease. A 2-week trial of a protein hydrolysate formula as empiric therapy for allergic vomiting (formula protein intolerance) may be helpful, particularly if there is a family history of allergy or if there is peripheral eosinophilia. If the diagnosis remains reflux, a prokinetic agent, such as cisapride, is added and consideration is given to addition of an oral H₂-receptor blocker (cimetidine, ranitidine) if esophagitis is suspected or documented.

This management is re-evaluated at least every 2 months for the need to increase doses, to discontinue medications, or to re-evaluate the diagnosis. Infants with reflux usually improve on this management, which can usually be discontinued between 8 and 18 months of age, as symptoms resolve. The rare infant who does not improve is evaluated for surgical fundoplication (Fig. 20–10).

GASTRIC STASIS, GASTROPARESIS

Gastric stasis is suggested by vomiting of food eaten hours earlier and by the presence of food in the stomach of a fasting patient having an upper gastrointestinal series. If the contrast study excludes gastric outlet obstruction, gastroparesis is likely. Diabetic gastroparesis, in which autonomic neuropathy due to diabetes causes gastric atony, is the classic example of this disorder but is rare in childhood. Surgical vagotomy produces similar symptoms, which is the reason surgeons include pyloroplasty when performing a vagotomy. Other causes of generalized ileus or pseudo-obstruction can involve the stomach primarily. Viral infections, perhaps including gastric cytomegalovirus, and drugs such as anticholinergics may also produce gastric stasis.

Gastric stasis may respond to cisapride, erythromycin, or metoclopramide, particularly if the cause is neurogenic. These medications may have additive effects.

ILEUS

Paralytic ileus, typified by the postoperative ileus that follows most abdominal surgery, is very common. Intestinal contents fail to progress, as in intestinal obstruction, causing abdominal pain and vomiting; the cause is failure of normal intestinal peristalsis rather than obstruction. Typically, the bowel sounds are decreased or absent; there may be abdominal distention. Other causes of ileus include unrelieved intestinal obstruction, peritonitis, intestinal ischemia, and sepsis. Signs of ileus may follow signs of intestinal obstruction; in this context ileus is an ominous sign. Other causes of paralytic ileus are drugs (phenothiazines, narcotics, laxative abuse, atropine), electrolyte disturbances (hypokalemia, hypercalcemia), endocrinopathies (hypothyroidism), or injuries (spinal fractures). Both chemotherapy and radiation therapy can produce reversible acute symptoms of vomiting, abdominal pain, and diarrhea within a few days to several weeks of the insult, with intestinal motor disturbances as the suggested cause.

Treatment of ileus requires correction of any correctable provocative abnormalities and nasogastric tube decompression until normal peristalsis begins.

PSEUDO-OBSTRUCTION

Like ileus, intestinal pseudo-obstruction represents intestinal dysmotility rather than obstruction. Pseudo-obstruction, however, is a chronic illness, sometimes with remissions and relapses, and is far rarer than acute ileus. Enteroclysis radiographic studies may be necessary to confirm the absence of partial obstruction. There is a family history in 20% to 30%, and nearly 50% of children with the disorder are symptomatic in the first month of life, although diagnosis is often quite delayed. The disorder may involve any or all of the luminal gastrointestinal tract—esophagus, stomach, small intestine, or colon—and occasionally (in up to 10%) involves the urinary tract. A relatively quiet abdomen or prominent borborygmi may be present, and abdominal distention (in 70%) is often associated with succussion splashes when the patient moves. Vomiting occurs in 50%, and constipation may be prominent (in >50%). Weight loss is caused by both vomiting of nutrients and by bacterial overgrowth-induced malabsorption.

Several causes for pseudo-obstruction have been identified; they are generally classified as either neuropathic or myopathic. Familial versus nonfamilial and primary versus secondary are two other classifications. Differentiation between neuropathic and myopathic types is best made by small intestinal manometry; esophageal manometry may contribute as well. Full-thickness intestinal biopsy is sometimes useful to distinguish specific entities causing the disorder; special silver stains of the myenteric plexus are particularly helpful. The myopathic causes (10%—a much lower proportion than in adults) include collagen-vascular causes of myositis or muscle fibrosis (progressive systemic sclerosis), various muscular dystrophies, megacystis-microcolon, and "familial visceral myopathies"; the neuropathic causes (90%) include Hirschsprung disease, Chagas disease, diabetic and other autonomic neuropathies, autoimmune disorders producing inflammatory neurodegeneration, multiple endocrine neoplasia, and "familial visceral neuropathies." Both types of pseudo-obstruction are difficult to manage; the myopathic form, representing dysfunction of the "end organ," particularly so.

A third category that is sometimes included under the myopathic type is fibrotic involvement of the muscularis propria. It may follow collagen-vascular diseases, radiation (>6 months after), or chemotherapy by months or years, causing either myopathic pseudo-obstruction or obstruction due to inflammatory strictures.

Functional failure of intestinal propulsion can be treated with cisapride, erythromycin, or metoclopramide. These medications are more apt to be useful in neurogenic disorders than in myogenic ones. Because of their different sites of action, they may have

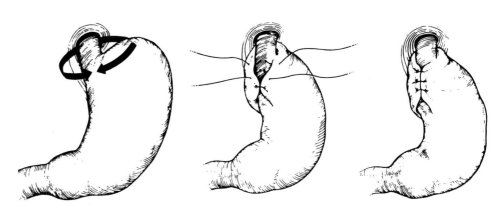

Figure 20–10. Diagram of a Nissen fundoplication. (From Schatzlein MH, Ballantine TVN, Thirunavukkarasu S, et al. Gastroesophageal reflux in infants and children. Arch Surg 1979;114: 505–510. Copyright 1979, American Medical Association; with permission.)

additive effects. Patients with pseudo-obstruction also benefit from antibiotic treatment of bacterial overgrowth syndrome, when present, or from nutritional rehabilitation with total parenteral nutrition. Collagen-vascular or autoimmune causes of pseudo-obstruction may respond to steroids. Cautious surgery is occasionally beneficial.

Gastrointestinal Inflammation

ESOPHAGITIS

Although esophagitis is often associated with vomiting, it is usually not the cause of vomiting. It is due to gastroesophageal reflux or to vomiting from various other causes.

GASTROENTERITIS

Gastroenteritis is a frequent cause of acute vomiting illness in childhood. The vomiting is often associated with diarrhea and sometimes with crampy abdominal pain or fever (see Chapter 19). Rotavirus, especially in infants, is notable for its prominent vomiting, which often precedes the diarrhea. "Food poisoning" also produces vomiting and diarrhea, often via bacterially derived toxin. The time course and symptoms suggest the organism. Gastroenteritis, like regurgitant reflux, is common and often requires minimal diagnosis and therapy; however, one must constantly guard against making this diagnosis in a child who might have metabolic or surgical disease (see Table 20–10).

Treatment of acute gastroenteritis demands attention to hydration. Oral rehydration is feasible in many children with gastroenteritis, but prominent vomiting may make intravenous rehydration necessary. A common error is to use clear liquids longer than 24 hours, thus disregarding nutritional needs. Early refeeding in gastroenteritis is most successful when it is low in fat and lactose and high in complex carbohydrates. No antibiotic therapy is warranted for most infectious causes of gastroenteritis (see Chapter 19).

PEPTIC ULCER DISEASE

The term peptic ulcer disease includes gastritis, gastric ulcer, duodenitis, and duodenal ulcer (see Chapters 18 and 21). In children, in contrast to adults, these disorders frequently cause vomiting. Defined causes for peptic ulcer disease include *Helicobacter pylori* (formerly *Campylobacter pylori*) infections, bile reflux gastritis, nonsteroidal anti-inflammatory agents, and rare gastrin-secreting tumors (Zollinger-Ellison syndrome). Stress ulcers occur in the context of sepsis, burns, surgery, head trauma, and severe acute illness.

Optimal diagnosis is endoscopic, with evaluation for *H. pylori* or elevated gastrin in appropriate cases. H$_2$-receptor blockade is the main treatment, with supplementary antacids sometimes useful and omeprazole beneficial in the intractable patient. Discontinuation of tobacco smoke exposure is important. *H. pylori* infections are less apt to recur if treated with triple antibiotics, such as bismuth, amoxicillin, and metronidazole. Zollinger-Ellison syndrome is optimally treated by tumor resection and evaluation for related endocrine tumors; H$_2$-receptor blockade is helpful if complete tumor resection is impossible.

MECKEL'S DIVERTICULITIS

In addition to presenting as gastrointestinal obstruction, via volvulus or intussusception, Meckel's diverticuli may become inflamed and mimic appendicitis.

Treatment is surgical, so preoperative distinction of Meckel's diverticulitis from other causes of an acute abdomen is not crucial (see Chapter 18).

MESENTERIC ADENITIS

Inflammation of lymph nodes in the mesentery is probably caused by viral (adenovirus, measles) or bacterial *(Yersinia enterocolitica)* infection, but the symptoms are similar enough to appendicitis that the diagnosis is usually not made until surgery for appendicitis.

Ultrasonography can readily distinguish mesenteric adenitis from appendicitis, thus obviating surgery (see Chapter 18).

APPENDICITIS

When vomiting occurs in appendicitis, it *follows* the periumbilical pain but may precede the localization of the pain to McBurney's point, two thirds of the way between the umbilicus and the right anterior iliac spine. Prior to perforation, there is only occasional vomiting. Following perforation, the fever may be higher, the child lies still with the right hip flexed, and vomiting may be more frequent and more feculent. In appendicitis, there is later vomiting, less diarrhea, less bowel sounds, and more rectal or rebound tenderness than in gastroenteritis. It is also associated with less diarrhea, less fever, and less leukocytosis than bacterial enteritis, although *Yersinia* in particular has caused right lower quadrant pain mimicking appendicitis. Crohn disease is usually more chronic than appendicitis.

Treatment of appendicitis is discussed in Chapter 18.

INFLAMMATORY BOWEL DISEASE

Crohn's disease, in particular, may produce vomiting on occasion, particularly when obstructing intestinal strictures develop. Other extraintestinal manifestations of Crohn's disease also rarely produce vomiting (see Chapter 19).

ALLERGIC ENTEROPATHY, EOSINOPHILIC GASTROENTEROPATHY

Vomiting is a frequent response to ingestion of allergens and may be seen as early as the first weeks of life in infants with allergy to cow's milk or soy and in older children as potentially allergenic foods are introduced. There may be associated diarrhea and hematochezia and, in the older child, urticaria or other systemic signs of allergy. A strong family history for allergic diathesis is very suggestive. Laboratory studies may show peripheral blood eosinophilia or an elevated serum immunoglobulin E (IgE); positive radioallergosorbent test (RAST) results to individual foods are helpful if present.

In infants, the simplest diagnostic test is a change to a protein hydrolysate formula for at least 2 weeks. If the vomiting (and other symptoms) resolve, it is generally not necessary to re-challenge for diagnosis, but empiric treatment can be continued for several months. Since infants usually outgrow these "formula protein intolerances" at between 10 and 24 months of age, a normal diet can later be gradually introduced as tolerated. Older children with vomiting that represents eosinophilic gastroenteropathy or other IgE-mediated food allergy are not likely to lose their allergy over time. If particular foods are identified, the diet can be modified. Rarely, systemic treatment, for example with steroids, is required.

Gastrointestinal Ischemia, Vascular Insufficiency

Some of the causes of gastrointestinal ischemia can produce perforation, peritonitis, and death quite rapidly. A high degree of suspicion is useful, since the signs are nonspecific.

ABDOMINAL MIGRAINE

In this periodic syndrome of abdominal symptoms, epigastric or periumbilical pain may accompany nausea and vomiting. Diarrhea, fever, chills, vertigo, irritability, and polyuria have also been reported. The symptoms are likely to be a result of muscular constriction of the mesenteric arteries, causing ischemia. When these abdominal symptoms coexist with head pain, which occurs in 30% to 40% of patients with migrainous headaches, the diagnosis is simpler than when they occur in isolation, which happens in about 3% of patients who later experience typical migrainous headaches. Usually, isolated abdominal migrainous attacks occur suddenly, last an hour to days, and are consistent in character within the same individual. There is usually a family history of migraine, and patients are asymptomatic between attacks.

Symptoms of abdominal migraine respond to prophylactic propranolol; ergotamine may abort an episode.

VASCULITIS

Inflammation of the mesenteric vessels is uncommon but may cause gastrointestinal complaints, including vomiting, abdominal pain, diarrhea, and gastrointestinal bleeding. Henoch-Schönlein purpura is the most common pediatric vasculitis; systemic lupus erthematosus, dermatomyositis, polyarteritis nodosa, and other hypersensitivity vasculitides are occasional causes.

HENOCH-SCHÖNLEIN PURPURA

One reason a complete skin examination is important in the vomiting child is that the most diagnostic sign of Henoch-Schönlein purpura is the palpable purpuric rash, typically found on the buttocks, posterior legs, and feet in 97% of patients. However, since the vomiting or hematemesis and the nonspecific abdominal pain (found in nearly 90%) may precede the rash, the diagnosis may initially be obscure. Repeated re-examination of the skin of a child with persistent vomiting and pain is therefore useful, particularly when the gastrointestinal symptoms are accompanied by polyarthritis, which occurs in 65%.

Platelet function and coagulation studies are normal; hematuria is often present. Steroids may reduce the abdominal pain.

VOLVULUS, INTUSSUSCEPTION

Volvulus and intussusception have been discussed earlier, but, as noted, some of the symptoms and complications result from vascular obstruction and ischemia.

MESENTERIC ISCHEMIA

The mesenteric arteries may be occluded by emboli from a diseased heart or from thrombi formed locally. Nonocclusive ischemia is perhaps due to poor cardiac output, hypotension, dehydration, or endotoxemia. Mesenteric venous occlusion is very rare. Severe, crampy, diffuse abdominal pain may be accompanied by vomiting, diarrhea, or constipation. The crampy pain becomes continuous, and gangrene, peritonitis, sepsis, and shock supervene.

In a suggestive setting (e.g., heart disease), vomiting accompanied by diffuse severe abdominal pain should suggest the possible need for mesenteric and celiac angiography and emergent surgery. Acute arterial insufficiency may be preceded by chronic symptoms of "abdominal angina"—episodes of several hours of crampy pain beginning about 20 minutes following meals. Such premonitory symptoms in suggestive settings should receive serious attention.

Gastrointestinal Perforation, Peritonitis

Gastrointestinal perforation is often the end stage of obstructing, inflammatory, or ischemic disorders. Perforation is heralded by sudden abdominal pain, with subsequent signs of peritonitis (see Chapter 18). Perforated peptic ulcer pain may track to the right lower quadrant and mimic appendicitis, but the onset is more sudden and the child is sicker than with appendicitis. Shock, metabolic acidosis, sepsis, and disseminated intravascular coagulopathy may ensue. Vomiting is not prominent.

When luminal obstruction leads to perforation and peritonitis, the abdominal findings change in characteristic ways. Vague, crampy, periumbilical pain becomes sharp, continuous, and localized. Rushes of increased, high-pitched bowel sounds become the silent abdomen. The active, sometimes writhing child becomes still and avoids movement. Vomiting previously associated with cramping pain is no longer present. The physical examination discloses point tenderness, abdominal rigidity, involuntary guarding, and rebound tenderness.

Hepatobiliary Disorders

HEPATITIS (see Chapter 24)

The presence of acute viral hepatitis is usually suspected in patients who have jaundice, but up to 50% of patients with hepatitis A are anicteric, and even those in whom jaundice develops have a preicteric prodrome lasting up to a week. In children with acute hepatitis, therefore, the presenting symptom may be vomiting, another reason for including liver enzymes in the screening evaluation of the ill-appearing vomiting child. The vomiting is often accompanied by flu-like symptoms—fatigue, fever, headache, rhinorrhea, sore throat, and cough.

Serum antigens and antibodies to hepatitis viruses establish the diagnosis. Acute hepatitis with vomiting is treated symptomatically, with intravenous hydration if needed. Management also includes watching for the ominous findings of progressive encephalopathy, ascites, and coagulopathy, which mandate specific therapy and consideration of fulminant hepatic failure.

BILIARY COLIC, CHOLECYSTITIS
(see Chapters 18 and 24)

Biliary obstruction also produces vomiting and abdominal pain in children, although the vomiting is usually less severe and later than that in pancreatitis. Biliary colic is visceral pain resulting from transient obstruction of the cystic duct, usually by a stone. Occasional patients have biliary dyskinesia causing their symptoms. Biliary colic produces several hours of steady, vaguely localized pain, often in the right upper quadrant; most patients also have vomiting. Episodes of biliary colic commonly recur at unpredictable intervals, from weeks to years. Acute cholecystitis may ensue if the obstruction persists and leads to inflammation of the gallbladder. The pain may localize more clearly to the right upper quadrant and may radiate to the back or shoulder. There may be fever or mild jaundice.

Serum alanine aminotransferase, aspartate aminotransferase, gamma-glutamyl transpeptidase, and alkaline phosphatase may be elevated. In both biliary colic and acute cholecystitis, abdominal films and ultrasonography may disclose stones or gallbladder thickening. Common duct stones may produce concurrent elevations of liver enzymes and pancreatic enzymes.

Recurrent biliary colic and cholecystitis are managed by cholecystectomy, which can now be performed laparoscopically in many children. Endoscopic removal of common duct stones is also possible, although it does not prevent recurrence.

Pancreatic Disorders

PANCREATITIS

Pancreatitis is usually associated with epigastric abdominal pain, which may radiate to the back. If vomiting children with abdominal pain have serum amylase and lipase performed as part of their screening evaluation, pancreatitis will be diagnosed. (Pancreatitis with normal amylase but elevated lipase is not rare.) Important causes of pancreatitis to distinguish are noted in Chapter 18.

Adrenal Disorders: Hemorrhage

Overwhelming sepsis, particularly with meningococcemia (or pneumococcus, *Staphylococcus*, or *Haemophilus influenzae* type b) is the most common cause of adrenal hemorrhage. The precipitous onset is manifested by vomiting accompanying a shaking chill, headache, vertigo, petechial to purpuric rash, and very high or subnormal temperature. Prostration, shock, and death occur quickly. Shock and fulminant sepsis can coexist without adrenal insufficiency. Adrenal hemorrhage may be identified by abdominal ultrasonography. Treatment includes appropriate antibiotics, intensive supportive care, and stress doses of steroids.

Other causes for adrenal hemorrhage are birth or other trauma, adrenal vein thrombosis, seizures, or after excessive anticoagulation. In these settings, vomiting associated with flank or epigastric pain and hypotension should suggest acute adrenal insufficiency due to hemorrhage and the need for steroid support.

Adrenal insufficiency is discussed later.

Gynecologic and Urologic Disorders

PYELONEPHRITIS

High fever, chills, nausea, vomiting, and less often diarrhea develop rapidly. There may be symptoms of cystitis with dysuria, frequency, urgency, and suprapubic pain (see Chapter 27). Costovertebral angle tenderness on either or both sides focuses the diagnosis on the urinary tract.

The urinalysis shows pyuria and bacteriuria, and the hemogram shows leukocytosis. Treatment is with antibiotics.

URETEROPELVIC JUNCTION OBSTRUCTION, HYDRONEPHROSIS

Ureteropelvic junction (UPJ) obstruction, or "beer-drinker's kidney," is due to partial obstruction at the UPJ and resulting hydronephrosis during fluid loading and diuresis. Congenital cases are usually diagnosed in the first year of life (usually on the basis of a renal hydronephrotic mass or urinary tract infection); 10% to 30% of older children present with flank or periumbilical pain, frequently accompanied by vomiting. Involvement of the left side is twice that of the right, but bilateral disease is found in 10% to 40% of children. Males are affected 2:1.

Typically, the symptoms commence in the evening after an increased fluid intake, although the hyperhydration history is often unclear. The child's pain and vomiting usually remit spontaneously in several hours, as dehydration gradually relieves the renal pelvic distention. An aberrant renal vessel or kinked ureter (25%) or intrinsic ureteral lesions (75%) are the cause of this partial obstruction at the UPJ. Superimposed unilateral urinary tract infection may cause additional findings of fever, failure to thrive, and pyuria.

Ultrasonography at the time of an episode or after furosemide, or an intravenous pyelogram, provides the diagnosis; the treatment is surgical.

RENAL COLIC

Passage of a renal stone usually causes more pain than vomiting. Lateralizing colicky pain, hematuria, and confirmatory radiologic studies assist the diagnosis.

DYSMENORRHEA, ENDOMETRIOSIS, PELVIC INFLAMMATORY DISEASE

These gynecologic disorders manifest lower abdominal pain but only occasionally present with vomiting. Association with menses or vaginal discharge aids the diagnosis. Motion of the cervix exacerbates the pain in pelvic inflammatory disease (see Chapter 31).

OVARIAN TORSION

Torsion of a normal ovary occasionally occurs in school-age girls, probably due to laxity of adnexal supports. Repeated attacks of crampy lower abdominal pain culminates in a final acute episode with severe retching and vomiting, an enlarged ovarian mass, and eventual signs of peritonitis. Leukocytosis may be accompanied by fever.

The location of the pain suggests the diagnosis, and the treatment is surgical.

HYPEREMESIS GRAVIDARUM

Although this is generally a problem of adults, the occasional pregnant pediatric patient may suffer from it. In parallel to the experience with ruminating infants, esophagitis has been suggested to play a role in prolonging vomiting during pregnancy.

TESTICULAR TORSION

Testicular torsion is a vascular emergency. It is readily diagnosed by the site of pain, and surgical treatment is required (see Chapter 30).

Respiratory Disorders

SINUSITIS, PHARYNGITIS, OTITIS

Sinusitis in particular may induce chronic, unexplained vomiting in children. The vomiting is more apt to occur in the morning and must be differentiated from serious intracranial processes. Sinus tenderness and sinus radiographs (or CT scans) make the diagnosis, and a successful trial of antibiotic therapy confirms it. Less often, pharyngitis or otitis media may present acutely with nonspecific vomiting.

PNEUMONIA

Pneumonia can cause vomiting in the pediatric patient. Since pneumonia can also be caused by vomiting, on the basis of aspiration it is important to consider the direction of causality in children with pneumonia and vomiting. Aspiration of vomitus is particularly likely in the context of obtundation or other neurologic dysfunction.

Central Nervous System Disorders

INCREASED INTRACRANIAL PRESSURE

Various causes of increased intracranial pressure (e.g., tumors) induce vomiting, typically described as projectile but without retching. This description may be an oversimplification, but the occurrence on awakening and prior to eating is important information.

A careful neurologic and funduscopic examination and relevant radiologic studies (CT or MRI scans) should help make the diagnosis (see Chapter 41).

ABDOMINAL EPILEPSY

The diagnosis of abdominal epilepsy is suggested by recurrent episodes of nausea or vomiting, usually accompanied by abdominal pain and by symptoms suggesting its central nervous system origin,

such as headache, dizziness, confusion, or temporary blindness. Patients may sleep after an episode.

The diagnosis is aided by neurologic consultation, electroencephalography during an episode, and response to anticonvulsant therapy.

VESTIBULAR DISORDERS, MOTION SICKNESS (see Chapter 43)

Motion sickness is a nearly universal experience in some situations. Vestibular disorders produce similar symptoms. Because of the symptoms of nausea, nystagmus, vertigo, and dizziness, the diagnosis is usually obvious. Antihistamines and anticholinergics are particularly useful for motion sickness.

ABDOMINAL MIGRAINE

See earlier discussion under Gastrointestinal Ischemia, Vascular Insufficiency.

VENTRICULOPERITONEAL SHUNT COMPLICATIONS

Occlusion or infection of a shunt may produce vomiting on a neurologic basis, whereas the intra-abdominal end of the shunt may provoke intestinal obstruction by volvulus, adhesions, or loculations. These possibilities must be kept in mind in the vomiting patient with a shunt.

Psychobehavioral Disorders

PSYCHOGENIC VOMITING

The syndrome of vomiting without organic cause illustrates the prominent influence that cortical and psychologic inputs may have in stimulating nausea and vomiting. Characteristic features of psychogenic vomiting include chronicity, association with stress and with meals, suppressibility by distracting the patient, *la belle indifférence* regarding the symptom itself, and relief by hospitalization. There may be no nausea or anorexia, and the vomiting may be self-induced.

RUMINATION

In the process of rumination, food is regurgitated, then mouthed or chewed and reswallowed, apparently voluntarily and pleasurably. Adults and older children may regurgitate by contracting abdominal muscles; infants may put their fingers or fists deep in their mouths in an apparent attempt to stimulate regurgitation. Whereas such apparent self-stimulation probably has a psychogenic etiology in many cases, some infants cease ruminating when their esophagitis is treated, suggesting that in some cases what appears to be an attempt to stimulate the gag reflex may actually be a response to pain in the throat. Thus, diagnosis of, and treatment for, both psychogenic causes and esophagitis should be considered.

Two types of rumination, psychogenic and self-stimulating, have been described. The former tends to occur in normal infants with a disturbed parent-child relationship; the latter occurs in mentally retarded individuals of any age and without regard to nurturing. Both positive and negative reinforcement has been utilized in behavioral therapy.

EATING DISORDERS

Anorexia nervosa and bulimia are considered to be eating disorders primarily of psychogenic origin. However, symptoms of disordered upper gastrointestinal motility, including esophageal dysmotility, may present similarly to these eating disorders and patients with primary anorexia nervosa often manifest delayed gastric emptying, which may benefit from therapy with prokinetic agents.

MANAGEMENT

Psychiatric consultation and therapy are often needed for eating disorders, rumination, and psychogenic vomiting. Principles of behavior modification help to eliminate secondary gain from the vomiting. Nasograstric or nasojejunal feedings can be used to guarantee nutritional rehabilitation if voluntary oral nutrition is not readily re-established; such tube feedings also provide the older child with incentive to return to oral nutrition. A prokinetic agent and H_2-receptor blocker therapy are often useful initially, both to treat esophagitis and to maximize forward movement of enteral nutrients through the gastrointestinal tract.

Metabolic Disorders

Metabolic diseases that cause vomiting are difficult to diagnose because they are both rare and diverse. Their diagnosis and treatment, however, are crucial because of the death and severe morbidity they can cause and their amenability to treatment. They are also important because of their relevance to genetic counseling, since most metabolic disorders are hereditary, on an autosomal recessive basis. Situations that should prompt consideration of metabolic diseases are listed in Table 20–7.

The history and physical examination (Table 20–14) and screening studies (Table 20–15) that help to distinguish among many of the specific metabolic disorders provide useful clues. Laboratory studies should be done while the child is symptomatic. Vomiting accompanied by hyperammonemia is a particular diagnostic problem, for which a schematic is presented in Figure 20–11.

Poisonings, Drugs

Most ingested poisons, and some absorbed by inhalation, skin contact, or intravenous administration, induce vomiting, which can be seen as a physiologic protection against harmful substances. Symptoms and signs of some of the most common pediatric poisonings causing vomiting are indicated in Table 20–16. Acute known poisonings, either accidental (in toddlers) or intentional (in adolescents), are a management problem rather than a diagnostic one. A Poison Control Center phone number or instruction card and more complete references on poisoning (see References) should be consulted for more detail. When an acute poisoning is suspected but the agent is unknown, these resources are also useful.

Initial diagnostic evaluation can be directed by a careful search of the environment for poisonous items and by toxicology screens on blood, urine, vomitus, and stool—these materials should not be discarded (Table 20–17). A few agents, such as lead poisoning, cause chronic poisoning manifested by vomiting, among other symptoms. Because these poisonings may be particularly difficult to suspect and treat, an index of suspicion of poisoning is important in the chronically vomiting child. Useful laboratory studies in addition to toxicology are presented in Table 20–17.

Hematemesis (see Chapter 21)

Endoscopic evaluation (and therapy) is often needed for children with hematemesis. Prior to such evaluation, however, it is important to know the most likely causes (see Table 20–11). The physician should also have determined that there is no underlying coagulopathy requiring correction (Table 20–12) and that hematemesis is a primary symptom, not a secondary one caused by a Mallory-Weiss tear.

Peptic ulcer disease, particularly duodenal ulcer, is the most common cause of hematemesis in children; in newborns, swallowed maternal blood (uterine, breast milk), esophagitis, gastritis, and duodenal ulcers are most common; in preschool children, gastric ulcers predominate; and in older children and adolescents, duodenal ulcers are most common. Esophagitis is occasionally severe enough to cause hematemesis, as is Barrett's ulcer, a premalignant lesion superimposed on chronic esophagitis. Obstructive lesions such as pyloric stenosis and antral webs may occasionally be associated with hematemesis.

Variceal bleeding is uncommon but serious. Gastric vascular malformations are rare, serious, and may be difficult to diagnose. Duplications are lined by gastric mucosa 30% of the time; if they are located above the ligament of Treitz, they may cause hematemesis. The metabolic and toxic (iron, salicylates, theophylline, corrosives, isopropyl alcohol, mushroom poisoning) causes of hematemesis should be kept in mind.

Therapy of hematemesis includes, as needed, correction of any abnormalities of coagulation-hemostasis, stabilization of hemodynamic status, and direct attention to the bleeding site endoscopically (e.g., heater probe, injection therapy) or surgically. Reduction of gastric acid secretion with an H_2-receptor blocking agent is useful in virtually all cases of hematemesis and has minimal risk.

Other Causes of Vomiting

CHEMOTHERAPY

Chemotherapy causes predictable vomiting, which is usually not a diagnostic but a management problem. It may be complicated by anticipatory vomiting. Ondansetron, high-dose metoclopramide (accompanied by diphenhydramine for prophylaxis of extrapyramidal side effects), dexamethasone, and the marijuana-related nabilone have all shown some effectiveness against chemotherapy-induced vomiting. Anxiolytics may also be beneficial as a component of combination antiemetic therapy.

RADIATION THERAPY

Like chemotherapy, radiation therapy may cause acute vomiting, apparently by stimulating giant retrograde peristaltic waves. Subacutely, diarrhea predominates as a complication of radiation therapy. Months to years later, vomiting may again be a result of radiation therapy, often caused by inflammatory ulcers and strictures. These lesions are difficult to treat without surgery.

Table 20–14. Metabolic Disease: History and Physical Examination

	Neurologic			Liver		Gastrointestinal	Respiratory		
	Lethargy, Coma	Hypo-hypertonicity	Seizure	Jaundice	Hepatomegaly	Diarrhea	Tachypnea Apnea	Precipitants/Aversions	Other
Galactosemia	+			+	+	+	(+)	Galactose	Eye: cataracts (use slit lamp)
Fructose-1-phosphate aldolase ↓: HFI	+		+	+	+	+	(+)	Fructose	Absent caries (older child)
Tyrosinemia				+	(+)	+			Odor: cabbage; Quebec native; ↑ AFP; hepatoma
Maple syrup urine disease	+	+	+				+	Protein; infections	Odor: maple syrup
Hypervalinemia*	+	+	+						
HHH syndrome*	+	+			(+)			Protein	Occasional bleeding tendency
Lysinuric protein intolerance	+	+			+/spl	+		Protein; fasting; infections	Hair fragile; Finnish native; ↑; ferritin ↑
Methylmalonic acidemia	+	+	(+)		(+)		+	Protein	Vitamin B$_{12}$ responsive or not?
Propionic acidemia*	+	(+)	(+)		(+)		+	Protein; infections	Osteoporosis
Isovaleric acidemia*	+	+	+			(+)	+	Protein; infections	Odor: sweaty feet
3-Methylcrotonyl-CoA carboxylase ↓*	(+)	+					+	Protein; infections	Odor: cat urine; biotin unresponsive
Multiple carboxylase ↓*	+	+	+				+		Odor: cat urine; biotin responsive; rash
Glutaric acidemia I	+	+	(+)		+		(+)	Infections	Fevers
Glutaric acidemia II	+	+			(+)		(+)	?Fasting	Odor: sweaty feet; heart; renal
Acyl-CoA dehydrogenase ↓: MCAD, etc.	+		(+)		(+)		(+)	Fasting; infections	
HMG-CoA lyase ↓*	+	+	(+)		(+)		+	Protein; fasting	

Table continued on following page

323

Table 20–14. Metabolic Disease: History and Physical Examination *Continued*

	Neurologic			Liver		Gastrointestinal	Respiratory	Precipitants/ Aversions	Other
	Lethargy, Coma	*Hypo-hypertonicity*	*Seizure*	*Jaundice*	*Hepatomegaly*	*Diarrhea*	*Tachypnea Apnea*		
Wolman's disease*				(+)	+/spl	+			Adrenal calcifications; foam cells
Farber's disease*	(+)	(+)			(+)				Skin nodules; arthritis; hoarseness
Urea cycle (AL, AS, CPS, OTC)	+	+	+		+		+	Protein; infections	Respiratory alkalosis; trichorrhexis (AL)
Reye's syndrome ?Misc. fatty acid oxidation ↓	+	+	+	No	+				Prior virus (flu, varicella); salicylates
Diabetic ketoacidosis	+						+		Odor: ketones
Adrenal insufficiency Chronic, primary—Addison's disease	+					(+)			Pigment: skin, mucosa (80%–98%); salt craving (20%)
Acute—adrenal crisis								Sepsis; steroid DC	Shock; abdominal pain (34%); K↑; Na↓
Congenital adrenal hyperplasia	+								M or virile F neonate; salt-losing
RTA, Fanconi's syndrome							(+)		Acidosis and urine findings
Nephrogenic diabetes insipidus								Water deprivation	Polyuria; polydipsia; dehydration
Uremia	(+)		(+)		/spl			Protein	Odor: uremic fetor; BUN↑; BP↑
Glucose-6-phosphatase ↓ (GSD I)			+		+		+	Fasting	Doll face; TG-xanthomas; epistaxis

*Fewer than 100 patients with each of these disorders have been reported. Incidences of the other 11 diseases listed above Reye's are 1/20,000 to 1/200,000. Glycogen storage disease type I (GSD I) is ~1/200,000; diabetes is acquired in ~1/400 children; adrenal insufficiency of all causes is relatively frequent; congenital adrenal hyperplasia with salt-losing 21-hydroxylase deficiency is ~1/5000.

Abbreviations: RR = respiratory rate; HFI = hereditary fructose intolerance; AFP = alpha-fetoprotein; HHH = hyperornithinemia-hyperammonemia-homocitrullinemia syndrome; spl = splenomegaly; MCAD = medium chain acyl-CoA dehydrogenase deficiency; HMG = 3-hydroxy-3methylglutaric acidemia; AL = arginosuccinic acid lyase deficiency; AS = arginosuccinic acid synthase deficiency; CPS = carbamyl phosphate synthase deficiency; OTC = ornithine transcarbamylase deficiency; DC = discontinuation; K = potassium; Na = sodium; M = male; F = female; RTA = renal tubular acidosis; BUN = blood urea nitrogen; BP = blood pressure; TG = triglycerides.

+ = common; (+) = may occur; ↓ = deficiency.

Table 20–15. Metabolic Disease: Laboratory Studies

	Blood							Urine†					
	pH↓	Glucose↓	NH₃*↑	LFTs↑	CBC (Hct↓ WBC↓ Plt↓)	Amino Acids	Ketones	Red. Subs.	FeCl +	Fanconi†	Amino Acids	Organic Acids	Orotate
Galactosemia	+	+		+	Lysis			+Non-glucose	?	+			
Fructose-1-phosphate aldolase↓: HFI	+	+		+	+	+		+Non-glucose	?	+	+		
Tyrosinemia				+	(↑)	+	Suc-ace	+phppa	+Green	+	+	+phppa	
Maple syrup urine disease	(+)	+		+	(↑)	+	+	+glucose	+Gray		+		
Hypervalinemia						+					+		
HHH syndrome			+			+					+	+	
Lysinuric protein intolerance			+	(+)	+	+					+	+	
Methylmalonic acidemia	+	+	+		+	(+)	+				(+)	+	
Propionic acidemia	+	+	+		+	+	+				+	+	
Isovaleric acidemia	+	No:↑	+		+	+	+				+	+	
3-Methylcrotonyl-CoA carboxylase↓	+	+											
Multiple carboxylase↓	+	+	+				+				+	+	
Glutaric acidemia type I	+	+	(+)	+			No				+	+	
Ethylmalonic-adipic aciduria, etc.	+	+	(+)	(+)			No				+	+	
Acyl-CoA dehydrogenase↓: MCAD, etc.	+	+	(+)	(+)			No (↓)				+		
HMG-CoA lyase↓	+	+	(+)	(+)			No				+		
Wolman's disease				+	Vacuoles								
Farber's disease													
Urea cycle defects	+	No	+			+					+	+	
Reye's syndrome	+	+	+	+		+					+	+	+
?Misc. fatty acid oxidation↓		No:↑											
Diabetic ketoacidosis	+	No:↑					+	+ Glucose	+ Red				
Adrenal insufficiency Chronic, primary—Addison's disease													
Acute—adrenal crisis													
Congenital adrenal hyperplasia													
Renal tubular acidosis; Fanconi's syndrome	(+)							(Glucose)		+			
Nephrogenic diabetes insipidus													
Uremia					(+)								
Glycogen storage disease type I	+	+											

*See Figure 20–11.

†Glucose, amino acids, phosphate, bicarbonate.

Abbreviations: NH₃ = ammonia; LFTs = liver function tests; CBC = complete blood count; Hct = hematocrit; WBC = white blood cell count; Plt = platelets; Red. Subs. = reducing substances; FeCl = iron chloride; HFI = hereditary fructose intolerance; Suc-ace = succinylacetone; phppa = p-OH-phenylpyruvate; HHH = hyperornithinemia-hyperammonemia-homocitrullinemia syndrome; MCAD = medium chain acyl-CoA dehydrogenase deficiency; HMG = 3-hydroxy-3methylglutaric acidemia.

(+) = may occur; + = common.

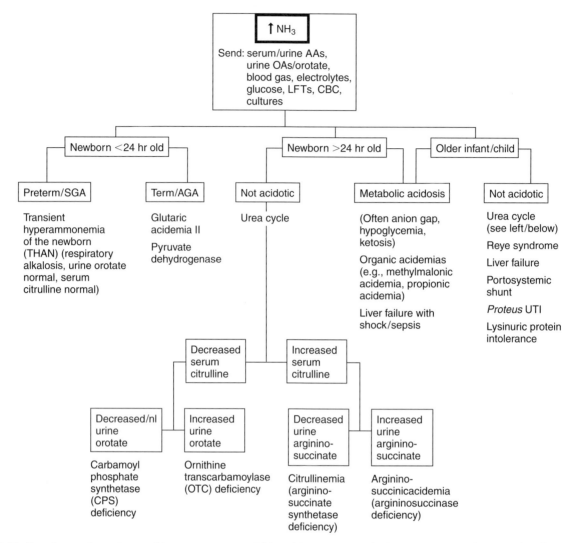

Figure 20–11. Flow diagram for evaluation of hyperammonemia in children. AAs = amino acids; OAs = organic acids; LFTs = liver function tests; CBC = complete blood count; SGA = small for gestational age; AGA = appropriate for gestational age; NL = normal; UTI = urinary tract infection.

CYCLIC VOMITING

Episodes (average 12 per year) of severe vomiting beginning at age 7 years (range 6 months to 18 years), are interspersed between intervals of normal health in this syndrome of unknown cause, which is diagnosed by exclusion, managed symptomatically (including antiemetic agents), and of unknown prognosis. It probably includes children with migrainous, eliptogenic, and psychogenic vomiting; the only advantage of considering it a diagnosis is the mollification provided by diagnostic labeling. Such labeling should not deter the physician from being certain that treatable organic disease is not present. Reported cases of organic disease mislabeled "cyclic vomiting" have included intermittent intussusception or volvulus due to enteric duplication, diverticulum, or malrotation; increased intracranial pressure in shunted patients with slit ventricles; and toxic or metabolic disease. Additional considerations in the differential diagnosis include brainstem glioma, obstructive uropathy, porphyria and familial dysautonomia.

In cyclic vomiting the patient experiences nausea and pallor during the stereotypic and characteristic episodes but is symptom-free between episodes.

PORPHYRIA

Acute intermittent porphyria is an autosomal dominant disorder of episodic abdominal pain (85% to 95% of patients); 40% to 90% of patients have associated vomiting. The association of neurologic symptoms such as mental symptoms (50%), muscle weakness (50%), sensory loss (20%), and convulsions (15%); the onset after puberty; and the frequent association with menses or provocative drugs (phenobarbitol) are suggestive. Elevated levels of porphobilinogen and aminolevulinic acid in urine are suggestive, and decreased red blood cell porphobilinogen deaminase is diagnostic.

FAMILIAL MEDITERRANEAN FEVER (BENIGN PAROXYSMAL PERITONITIS, PERIODIC PERITONITIS, POLYSEROSITIS)

Episodic attacks of abdominal pain with rapid development and resolution (within 48 hours) of peritoneal signs (fever, vomiting, absent bowel sounds) occurring in a child of Israeli or North

Table 20–16. Poisoning: History and Physical Examination

	Vital Signs				Neurologic					Pupils					
	P ↑↓	R ↑↓	BP ↑↓	T ↑↓	Coma	Ψ	Paralysis	Ataxia	Sz	↑	↓	Nystagmus	Skin	Odor	Other
Ipecac			↑•												EKG changes
Salicylates	↑•	↑•		↑•	•				•				Cyanotic	Acetone	Metabolic acidosis; tinnitus; uremia; bleeding
Acetaminophen													Jaundiced		Ill 24 hr→better × 48 hr→liver failure
Digitalis	↓•		↑•		•	•									CNS and arrhythmias; vision changes
Theophylline	↑•	↑•	↓•	↑•	•	•			•						Hematemesis/pain; arrhythmia
Fe (Iron)	↑•	↑•	↓•	↑•	•				•				Jaundiced		Hematemesis/pain→liver failure; pyloric stenosis
Pb (Lead)			↑•		•	•		•	•						Constipation; HA; abdominal pain; renal
Misc. (Sb, As, Cd, Cr, Hg, Zn)					•	•	•	•	•				Jaundiced	Garlic	Diarrhea; LFTs↑; Hct↓; nephritis; neuritis
Metal fume fever (oxides)				↑•											Muscle pain/HA; WBC↑; respiratory distress
Opiates/ narcotics		↓•	↓•	↓•	•	•			•		•		Cyanotic		Abdominal cramping
Opiate withdrawal	↑•	↑•	↑•	↑•						•					Irritable; BS↑/pain; reflexes↑; sweat; tear
Insecticides (misc.)		↑•	↑•		•	•		•	•		•		Misc.		Wheeze; salivation; sweat; tear
Esp. organophosphates	↓•	↓•			•	•			•		•			Garlic	Diarrhea/abdominal pain; vision impaired
Corrosives			↓•		•										Pain; hematemesis; respiratory distress
Methanol		↑•	↓•		•	•				•			Cyanotic	Acetone	Blindness; metabolic acidosis
Ethanol	↓•	↓•	↓•	↓•	•	•		•			•	•	Pink	Alcohol	Vision impaired; hypoglycemia
Isopropyl alcohol					•			•						Acetone	Hematemesis/pain; oliguria
Ethylene glycol			↑•		•				•		•	•	Cyanotic		Anuria
"Food poisoning"															See Chapter 19
Fish poisoning									•						Some seasonally poisonous; paresthesia
Shellfish—summer ingestion							•		•						Respiratory paralysis; paresthesia
Plants (akee, hemlock)	↓•		↑•		•	•	•		•						Respiratory: renal; shock; liver
Mushroom poisoning	↑•								•				Jaundiced		Respiratory: hepatic failure; hematemesis
Venomous bites (see Chapter 54)													Lesion		Bite history

Abbreviations: P = pulse; R = respiration; BP = blood pressure; T = temperature; Ψ = psychologic manifestations; Sz = seizure; CNS = central nervous system; HA = headache; Sb = antimony; As = arsenic; Cd = cadmium; Cr = chromium; Hg = mercury; Zn = zinc; LFTs = liver function tests; Hct = hematocrit; WBC = white blood count; BS = bowel sounds.

327

Table 20–17. Poisoning: Laboratory Studies and Treatment

	Laboratory Studies										Treatment*			
	CBC	Electrolytes	Ca, Mg, Phos.	BUN, Cr	Glucose	LFTs, Coag.	ABG	UA	Other	Level	Emesis (ipecac, 1 mg/kg) and/or Lavage	Charcoal and 70% Sorbitol	Diuresis? Dialysis? Other?	Specific
Ipecac														
Salicylates		•	•	•	•	•	•	•	EKG FeCl	•	•	•	•	Fluids, electrolytes HCO₃, vitamin K
Acetaminophen						•			Purple	•	•	•		N-acetylcysteine
Digitalis		•	•	•					EKG	•	• (Vagal hazard)	•		Digibind, antiarrhythmics
Theophylline		•	•				•		EKG	•		•		Antiarrhythmics, antiseizure
Fe (Iron)	•	•				•			KUB	•	•	No		Deferoxamine, fluids
Pb (Lead)	•								KUB Bones	• δALA FEP				BAL-CaEDTA, fluids, antiseizure
Others (Sb, As, Cd, Cr, Hg, Zn, P)	•	•							KUB	•	•			
Metal fume fever (oxides)														
Opiates/ Narcotics													•	Narcan (0.01 mg/kg)
Opiate withdrawal														Methadone, paregoric, diazepam, phenobarbital
Organophosphate cholinesterase														Atropine
Corrosives									CXR		No	No		Antibiotics, endoscopy
Methanol		•			•		•			•		No	•	Ethanol
Ethanol		•		•	•	•	•		EKG			No	•	Glucose/bicarbonate
Isopropyl alcohol							•					No		Glucose/bicarbonate
Ethylene glycol				•			•					?No		Ethanol, ?Ca gluconate
"Food poisoning"														
Fish poisoning														
Shellfish—summer ingestion														
Plants (akee, castor, hemlock)		•				•		•						
Mushroom poisoning		•				•		•				•		Atropine? cimetidine
Venomous bites	•							•						Antiserum

*The utility of emesis/lavage varies with the poison, the amount ingested, and the duration since ingestion. Use lavage rather than emesis if obtunded or if poisoned by ipecac; lavage in such cases requires endotracheal tube airway protection. Avoid charcoal/sorbitol in recent bowel surgery or ileus.

Abbreviations: CBC = complete blood count; Ca = calcium; Mg = magnesium; Phos. = phosphate; BUN = blood urea nitrogen; Cr = creatinine; LFTs = liver function tests; Coag. = coagulation studies; ABG = arterial blood gases; UA = urinalysis; FeCl = iron chloride; HCO₃ = bicarbonate; KUB = kidney, ureter, and bladder; δALA = δ-aminolevulinic acid; FEP = free erythrocyte protoporphyrin; BAL-CaEDTA = dimercaprol—calcium ethylenediaminetetraacetic acid; Sb = antimony; As = arsenic; Cd = cadmium; Cr = chromium; Hg = mercury; Zn = zinc; P = phosphorus; CXR = chest x-ray.

African descent should suggest this autosomal recessive diagnosis. Synovitis, pleuritis, and an erysipelas-like skin lesion are also characteristic. The sedimentation rate is raised. Fifty percent of patients have their first attack between 1 and 10 years of age; 90% by age 20. Amyloidosis, a possible etiologic role for C5a inhibitor deficiency, and probable response to colchicine have been described.

FAMILIAL DYSAUTONOMIA

Familial dysautonomia may present with episodic vomiting. It is a genetic disorder of the sensory and autonomic nervous systems affecting Askenazi Jewish children. Associated symptoms include disturbed swallowing, drooling, frequent pneumonias, absence of overflow tearing, erratic temperature control, skin blotching, postural hypotension, relative indifference to pain, corneal anesthesia, breath-holding spells, motor incoordination, spinal curvature, and growth retardation. It is diagnosed with the intradermal histamine test, the conjunctival methacholine (or pilocarpine) test. Patients also have absent glossal fungiform papillae.

Management is complex and requires a multidisciplinary team.

Complications of Vomiting

The complications of vomiting are shown in Table 20–18. Their importance is twofold. First, these complications, particularly the metabolic, nutritional, esophagitis, and hemodynamic ones, must be treated. Second, there may be diagnostic importance. Hematemesis resulting from Mallory-Weiss tear should be distinguished from primary hematemesis due to some other lesion, and metabolic acidosis or hyperkalemia should be recognized as atypical for vomiting illnesses and possible crucial signs of metablic disease or severe intra-abdominal pathology.

METABOLIC COMPLICATIONS

Dehydration results from the inability to ingest fluid effectively, because of anorexia or nausea, as well as from the loss of secretions in the emesis. Alkalosis due to loss of gastric hydrogen chloride in the vomitus is exacerbated by a shift of H^+ into cells because of potassium deficiency and by contraction of the extracellular fluid because of sodium deficiency. Potassium and sodium are lost in the vomitus, and are also wasted by the kidneys, when they accompany the renal excretion of bicarbonate due to the alkalosis. In states of marked alkalosis, urine pH is 7 or 8 and urinary sodium and potassium are high despite sodium and potassium depletion. Urine chloride, however, remains low, reflecting the nonrenal losses of sodium chloride and potassium chloride.

If intravenous fluid therapy is required, it must be designed with understanding of the sodium and potassium deficits. The usual metabolic alkalosis will be adequately compensated by the patient's spontaneous hyperpnea and will respond to fluid and electrolyte therapy.

NUTRITIONAL COMPLICATIONS

The nutritional deficits due to chronic vomiting and associated anorexia are obvious. Their correction must be included in the treatment plan for chronic vomiting. No more than a day or so of fluid therapy should take place without attention to nutritional needs. Frequent, small high-carbohydrate feedings may minimize the stimulation to vomit, but continuous nasogastric feedings are sometimes needed for vomiting that has been chronic. Metabolic or allergic disease should be considered when the reintroduction of protein leads to relapse of symptoms.

MALLORY-WEISS TEAR

This linear mucosal laceration in the juxtaesophageal gastric mucosa usually follows prolonged forceful retching or vomiting,

Table 20–18. Complications of Vomiting

Complication	Pathophysiology	History, Physical Examination, and Laboratory Studies
Metabolic	Fluid loss in emesis	Dehydration
	HCl loss in emesis	Alkalosis*; hypochloremia
	Na, K loss in emesis	Hyponatremia; hypokalemia*
	Alkalosis →	
	Na into cells	
	HCO₃ loss in urine	Urine pH 7–8
	Na and K loss in urine	Urine Na ↑, K ↑
	Hypochloremia →	
	Cl conserved by kidneys	Urine Cl ↓
Nutritional	Emesis of calories and nutrients	Malnutrition; "failure to thrive"
	Anorexia for calories and nutrients	
Mallory-Weiss tear	Retching → tear at lesser curve of gastroesophageal junction	Forceful emesis → hematemesis
Esophagitis	Chronic vomiting → esophageal acid exposure	Heartburn; Hemoccult + stool
Aspiration	Aspiration of vomitus, esp. in context of obtundation	Pneumonia; neurologic dysfunction
Shock*	Severe fluid loss in emesis or in accompanying diarrhea	Dehydration (accompanying diarrhea can explain acidosis?)
	Severe blood loss in hematemesis	Blood volume depletion

*If patient is acidotic, hyperkalemic, or in shock, see Table 20–10.
Abbreviations: HCl = hydrogen chloride; Na = sodium; K = potassium; HCO₃ = bicarbonate; Cl = chloride.

but it occasionally produces blood in the initial vomitus. Invisible radiographically, it is diagnosed endoscopically (if necessary) and is often best seen at withdrawal of the instrument or during retroflexion. The tear is initially seen as a red rent oriented parallel to the esophageal length; a day later, while healing, it may appear as a white streak with surrounding erythema.

Mallory-Weiss tears usually require no treatment but occasionally transfusion is necessary. Intractable cases are quite rare and may be treated with vasopressin infusion, balloon tamponade, angiographic embolization, or surgery.

PEPTIC ESOPHAGITIS

Esophagitis similar to that resulting from gastroesophageal reflux may be caused by chronic vomiting from many causes. Diagnosed endoscopically or histologically, it should be treated. The treatment of esophagitis usually includes a prokinetic agent and H_2-receptor blockade, but the use of antacids should be tempered by knowledge of the acid-base status of the patient.

THERAPY

Therapy of vomiting starts with treatment of the cause, treatment of complications, and treatment of behavioral aspects that may perpetuate the vomiting (noted next). Prokinetic and antiemetic drugs are indicated in Table 20–19. One should be very careful about treating the vomiting symptom without diagnosing and treating its cause. In several situations, diagnostic procedures are also therapeutic, such as in meglumine diatrizoate (Gastrografin) enema for fecal obstructions in cystic fibrosis, barium enema for intussusception, and endoscopy with sclerotherapy for variceal hematemesis.

Treatment of Behavioral Aspects

Treatment of psychobehavioral aspects of vomiting may also be important because of the cortical influences on emesis. Such treatment may include eliminating secondary gain for vomiting and reducing anxiety about the vomiting through a confident approach to the child.

Table 20–19. Therapy for Vomiting*

Disease	Therapy—Class: Agent (Dose)
All	Rx Cause: obstruction→operate; allergy→change diet (± steroid); metabolic→Rx defect; peptic ulcer disease→H_2-receptor block; etc.
Complications	(NPO)
Dehydration	IV fluids, electrolytes
Hematemesis	Transfuse, correct coagulopathy
Esophagitis	H_2 blocker
Malnutrition	NG or NJ drip feeding useful for many chronic conditions
Meconium ileus; DIOS	Gastrografin enema
Intussusception	Barium enema
Hematemesis	Endoscopic injection therapy of varices and other lesions
Sigmoid volvulus	Colonoscopic decompression
Reflux	Positioning, dietary measures (infants: rice cereal 1 T/oz formula)
Reflux (avoid in asthma)	Cholinergic: bethanechol (Urecholine) (0.1–0.2 mg/kg q.i.d. p.o. [or SQ])
Reflux†; gastroparesis†; pseudo-obstruction†; chemotherapy† (side effect: extrapyramidal)	Dopamine antagonist: metoclopramide (Reglan) (0.1 mg/kg q.i.d. p.o. [or IV]) (For chemotherapy: ?0.5–1.0 mg/kg with antihistamine prophylaxis)
Reflux; gastroparesis; pseudo-obstruction (?)	Dopamine antagonist (periph.): domperidone (0.2–0.6 mg/kg t.i.d. or q.i.d. p.o.)
Reflux‡; gastroparesis‡; pseudo-obstruction‡	Cholinergic enhancer: cisapride (0.3 mg/kg t.i.d. or q.i.d. p.o.)
Gastroparesis‡; pseudo-obstruction‡	Motilin releaser: erythromycin (2–4 mg/kg t.i.d. or q.i.d. p.o. [or IV])
Motion sickness; vestibular disorders	Antihistamine: dimenhydrinate (Dramamine) (1 mg/kg t.i.d. or q.i.d. p.o. [OTC]) Anticholinergic (CNS): scopolamine (Transderm Scōp) (adult: 1 patch/3 days)
Radiation, chemotherapy, postop (side effects: blood dyscrasias, extrapyramidal)	Phenothiazines: Prochlorperazine (Compazine) (~0.3 mg/kg b.i.d. or t.i.d. p.o.) Chlorpromazine (Thorazine) Butyrophenones: Haloperidol (Haldol)
Chemotherapy‡	Cannabinoids: nabilone (0.05–0.1 mg/kg b.i.d. or t.i.d. p.o.) (tetrahydrocannabinol)
Chemotherapy‡	Serotonin (5HT3) block: ondansetron (Zofran) (0.15 mg/kg t.i.d. IV)
Adrenal crisis (chemotherapy‡)	Steroids: cortisol (~2 mg/kg IV bolus → 0.2–0.4 mg/kg/hr [± 1 mg/kg IM]) (Dexamethasone, 0.1 mg/kg t.i.d. p.o.)
Migraine	Beta-adrenergic blocking agents: propranolol (Inderal) (0.5–2 mg/kg b.i.d.)
Psychogenic component	Psychotherapy; consider NG/NJ drip feedings and prokinetic (cisapride, etc.) Anxiolytic: diazepam (Valium) (~0.1 mg/kg t.i.d. or q.i.d. p.o.) Tricyclic antidepressant: various

*If acidotic, hyperkalemic, or in shock, see Table 20–10 and adrenal crisis (above).
†Acceptable Rx.
‡Preferred Rx.
Abbreviations: NPO = nothing by mouth; IV = intravenous; NG = nasogastric; NJ = nasojejunal; q.i.d. = four times a day; p.o. = orally; SQ = subcutaneous; t.i.d. = three times a day; OTC = over the counter; b.i.d. = twice a day; IM = intramuscular.

Antiemetic Drugs

In situations of persistent vomiting, antiemetic drugs are useful to reduce the metabolic and nutritional consequences and perhaps to interrupt vicious circles in which psychogenic factors may also participate. Antiemetic drugs include the prokinetic agents cisapride, metoclopramide, erythromycin, domperidone, and bethanechol and the other agents listed in Table 20–19. These drugs function at many sites by:

- Modifying central cortical input (anxiolytic agents)
- Depressing the chemoreceptor trigger zone
- Reducing vestibular input
- Blocking serotonin
- Enhancing the secretion or effects of acetylcholine from the motor neuron (cisapride)
- Blocking serotonin receptors, which inhibit the function of the acetylcholine-secreting motor neuron (ondansetron)
- Blocking dopamine's inhibitory effect at the neuromuscular junction (domperidone, metoclopramide)
- Stimulating the motilin receptor on the muscle (possibly erythromycin)
- Substituting for acetylcholine's stimulatory effect at the neuromuscular junction (bethanechol)

The diverse sites of action account for the useful additive effects of these drugs in some settings. Optimal therapy for vomiting due to chemotherapy, for example, may include several agents in order to provide blockade of the multiple receptor types in the chemoreceptive trigger zone and elsewhere. Metoclopramide and ondansetron have been the most widely used general antiemetic agents; however, experience with the newer agent cisapride is encouraging and erythromycin in low doses has recently demonstrated benefit in gastrointestinal dysmotility.

REFERENCES

General

Rowe M, O'Neill J, Grosfeld J, et al. Essentials of Pediatric Surgery. St. Louis: Mosby–Year Book, 1994.

Dreisbach RH. Handbook of Poisoning: Diagnosis and Treatment, 12th ed. Los Altos, Calif: Lange Medical Publishers, 1987.

Lilien LD, Srinivasan G, Pyati SP, et al. Green vomiting in the first 72 hours in normal infants. Am J Dis Child 1986;140:662–664.

Rollins MD, Shields MD, Quinn RJM, et al. Value of ultrasound in differentiating causes of persistent vomiting in infants. Gut 1991;32:612–614.

Scriver CR, Beaudet AL, Sly WS, et al. The Metabolic Basis of Inherited Disease, 6th ed. New York: McGraw-Hill Information Services, 1989.

Gastrointestinal Obstruction

Caniano DA, Beaver BL. Meconium ileus: A fifteen year experience with forty-two neonates. Surgery 1987;102:699–703.

Champoux A, Del Beccaro M, Nazar-Stewart V. Recurrent intussusception: Risk features. Arch Pediatr Adolesc Med 1994;148:474–478.

Depaepe A, Dolk H, Lechat MF, et al. The epidemiology of tracheo-oesophageal fistula and oesophageal atresia in Europe. Arch Dis Child 1993;68:743–748.

Devane SP, Coombes R, Smith VV, et al. Persistent gastrointestinal symptoms after correction of malrotation. Arch Dis Child 1992;67:218–221.

Ford EG, Senac MO, Srikanth MS, et al. Malrotation of the intestine in children. Ann Surg 1992;215:172–178.

Macdessi J, Oates RK. Clinical diagnosis of pyloric stenosis: A declining art. BMJ 1993;306:553–555.

Mitchell LE, Risch N. The genetics of infantile hypertrophic pyloric stenosis. A reanalysis. Am J Dis Child 1993;147:1203–1210.

Rescorla FJ, Shedd FJ, Grosfeld JL, et al. Anomalies of intestinal rotation in childhood: Analysis of 447 cases. Surgery 1990;108:710–716.

Seashore JH, Touloukian RJ. Midgut volvulus. An ever-present threat. Arch Pediatr Adolesc Med 1994;148:43–46.

Gastroesophageal Reflux

Albanese CT, Towbin RB, Ullman I, et al. Percutaneous gastrojejunostomy versus Nissen fundoplication for enteral feeding of the neurologically impaired child with gastroesophageal reflux. J Pediatr 1993;123:371–375.

Booth IW. Silent gastro-oesophageal reflux: How much do we miss? Arch Dis Child 1992;67:1325–1326.

Chidiac P, Alexander IS. Head retraction and respiratory disorders in infancy. Arch Dis Child 1990;65:567.

Grill BB. Twenty-four-hour esophageal pH monitoring: What's the score? J Pediatr Gastroenterol Nutr 1992;14:249–251.

Hoeffel JC, Nihoul-Fekete C, Schmitt M. Esophageal adenocarcinoma after gastroesophageal reflux in children. J Pediatr 1989;115:259–261.

Kiely EM. Surgery for gastro-oesophageal reflux. Arch Dis Child 1990;65:1291–1292.

Orenstein SR. Controversies in pediatric gastroesophageal reflux. J Pediatr Gastroenterol Nutr 1992;14:338–348.

Orenstein SR. Gastroesophageal reflux. In Stockman J, Winter R, (eds). Current Problems in Pediatrics. Chicago: Mosby–Year Book, 1991;193–241.

Orenstein SR. Prone positioning in infant gastroesophageal reflux: Is elevation of the head worth the trouble? J Pediatr 1990;117:184–187.

Simpson H, Hampton F. Gastro-oesophageal reflux and the lung. Arch Dis Child 1991;66:277–283.

Vandenplas Y, Deneyer M, Verlinden M, et al. Gastroesophageal reflux incidence and respiratory dysfunction during sleep in infants: Treatment with cisapride. J Pediatr Gastroenterol Nutr 1989;8:31–36.

Vigneri S, Termini R, Leandro G, et al. A comparison of five maintenance therapies for reflux esophagitis. N Engl J Med 1995;333:1106–1110.

Other Etiologies

Barkin RM. Toxicologic emergencies. Pediatr Ann 1990;19:629–633.

Bray GP. Liver failure induced by paracetamol. Br Med J 1993;306:157–158.

Buck ML, Grebe TA, Bond GR. Toxic reaction to salicylate in a newborn infant: Similarities to neonatal sepsis. J Pediatr 1993;122:955–958.

Duane PD, Magee TM, Alexander MS, et al. Oesophageal achalasia in adolescent women mistaken for anorexia nervosa. Br Med J 1992;305:43.

Fleisher D, Matar M. Cyclic vomiting syndrome: A report of 71 cases and literature review. J Pediatr Gastroenterol Nutr 1993;17:361–369.

Therapy

Grunberg SM, Hesketh PJ. Control of chemotherapy-induced emesis. N Engl J Med 1993;329:1790–1796.

Kulig K. Initial management of ingestions of toxic substances. N Engl J Med 326;25:1677–1681.

Pinkerton CR, Williams D, Wootton C, et al. 5-HT$_3$ antagonist ondansetron—an effective outpatient antiemetic in cancer treatment. Arch Dis Child 1990;65:822–825.

21 Gastrointestinal Bleeding

Vera F. Hupertz   Steven J. Czinn

Gastrointestinal (GI) bleeding constitutes alarming symptoms when brought to the physician's attention. Children with these symptoms should be seen as soon as possible in an effort to institute proper management and make an acute diagnosis. Because treatment is often required before the precise origin of bleeding is identified, a systematic approach together with the knowledge of the most common causes of bleeding in each age group is essential (Tables 21–1 and 21–2).

DEFINITIONS

Children with gastrointestinal bleeding generally present with hematemesis, hematochezia, or melena, although the clinical presentation can be as subtle as a child with evidence of occult blood loss (Table 21–3). The initial diagnostic evaluation should focus on determining whether the source of the bleeding is from the upper or the lower gastrointestinal tract (Tables 21–1 and 21–2). A site of bleeding proximal to the ligament of Treitz or the second portion of the duodenum is considered to be an *upper gastrointestinal bleed*. A *lower gastrointestinal bleed* is defined as a site of bleeding distal to the ligament of Treitz or from those structures supplied by the mesenteric vessels. Distinguishing between upper and lower gastrointestinal sites of bleeding affects not only the differential diagnosis but also therapeutic interventions.

Hematemesis. Vomiting of blood can be either red or like the color of coffee grounds. This is most commonly associated with an upper gastrointestinal bleed. Bright-red hematemesis suggests active bleeding that has not come in contact with gastric secretions. When gastric secretions have had a chance to interact with the blood, "coffee ground" emesis results.

Hematochezia. Maroon stools from the rectum are generally associated with a lower gastrointestinal bleed. The presence of melena or black, tarry stools generally results from significant blood loss proximal to the ileocecal valve. The black color results from bacterial breakdown of the hemoglobin. The presence of hematochezia is generally associated with colonic bleeding.

DIAGNOSTIC STRATEGIES

The first step is to determine whether or not one is actually dealing with gastrointestinal bleeding. Many foodstuffs and other substances can cause vomitus or feces to have the appearance of blood. Punch (Kool-Aid), gelatin, food coloring, and antibiotic syrups can mimic bright-red blood. Other substances, such as iron, bismuth, beets, licorice, spinach, and blueberries, can simulate melena. Other nongastrointestinal sources of bleeding, such as epistaxis, hemoptysis, recent dental work, sore throat, recent tonsillectomy, or menses, can confuse the diagnosis.

Tests for Blood

Stool guaiac and the modified guaiac (Gastroccult) for emeses are the most commonly used tests to determine the presence of blood. These tests are readily available, inexpensive, and easy to perform. They can identify small amounts of heme in the tested material. Red meat (beef, lamb), vegetables, fruit high in vitamin C or rich in peroxidases, supplemental vitamin C in excess of 250 mg/day, aspirin, and anti-inflammatory drugs (steroids and nonsteroidal anti-inflammatory drugs [NSAIDS]) should be avoided for 3 days prior to testing. Although iron preparations may blacken stools, they do not give false-positive tests. Female patients should be told not to collect samples for 3 days after a menstrual period. To avoid potential false-positive or false-negative results, stool should be collected from diapers or from disposable collection devices rather than directly from toilet water.

Table 21–1. Upper Gastrointestinal Bleeding

Age Group	Common	Less Common
Neonates (0–30 days)	Swallowed maternal blood Gastritis Duodenitis	Coagulopathy Vascular malformations Gastric/esophageal duplication Leiomyoma
Infants (30 days–1 yr)	Gastritis and gastric ulcer Esophagitis Duodenitis	Esophageal varices Foreign body Aortoesophageal fistula
Children (1–12 yrs)	Esophagitis Esophageal varices Gastritis and gastric ulcer Duodenal ulcer Mallory-Weiss tear Nasopharyngeal bleeding	Leiomyoma Salicylates Vascular malformation Hematobilia
Adolescents (12 yr–adult)	Duodenal ulcer Esophagitis Esophageal varices Gastritis Mallory-Weiss tear	Thrombocytopenia Dieulafoy's ulcer Hematobilia

Modified from Olson AD, Hillemeier AC. Gastrointestinal hemorrhage. *In* Wyllie R, Hyams JS (eds). Pediatric Gastrointestinal Disease. Philadelphia: WB Saunders, 1993:259.

Table 21–2. **Lower Gastrointestinal Bleeding**

Age Group	Common	Less Common
Neonates (0–30 days)	Anorectal lesions Swallowed maternal blood Milk allergy Necrotizing enterocolitis Mid-gut volvulus	Vascular malformations Hirschsprung's enterocolitis Intestinal duplication Coagulopathy
Infants (30 days–1 yr)	Anorectal lesions Mid-gut volvulus Intussusception (<3 yr) Meckel's diverticulum Infectious diarrhea Milk allergy (<4 yr)	Vascular malformations Intestinal duplication Acquired thrombocytopenia Eosinophilic colitis
Children (1–12 yr)	Juvenile polyps Meckel's diverticulum Intussusception (<3 yr) Infectious diarrhea Anal fissure Nodular lymphoid hyperplasia	Henoch-Schönlein purpura Hemolytic-uremic syndrome Vasculitis (systemic lupus erythematosus) Inflammatory bowel disease Polyps
Adolescents (12 yr–adult)	Inflammatory bowel disease Polyps Hemorrhoids Anal fissure Infectious diarrhea	Arteriovascular malformation Adenocarcinomas Henoch-Schönlein purpura Pseudomembranous colitis

Modified from Olson AD, Hillemeier AC. Gastrointestinal hemorrhage. *In* Wyllie R, Hyams JS (eds). Pediatric Gastrointestinal Disease. Philadelphia: WB Saunders, 1993:259.

Finally, an Apt-Downey test should be done on the breast-fed infant who may vomit bright-red blood or may pass bloody (red) stools, to distinguish whether maternal or fetal hemoglobin is the cause. To perform the Apt test, one takes a grossly (red) bloody sample and adds enough water to obtain a pink supernatant. The mixture is centrifuged. To 5 parts of the supernatant solution, 1 part 0.25 N (1%) sodium hydroxide is added. A yellow-brown color change (within minutes) indicates maternal hemoglobin; infant hemoglobin will stay pink.

History

Historical information can be extremely important and should be obtained as quickly as possible. A history of vomiting, regurgitation, or abdominal pain may suggest a mucosal lesion. Forceful vomiting may result in a Mallory-Weiss tear. Severe acute abdominal pain occurs in patients with vascular compromise, such as in intussusception and mid-gut volvulus. The presence of large amounts of blood from the mouth without the presence of significant gastric fluid suggests variceal bleeding until proven otherwise.

A previous history of jaundice, hepatitis, or blood transfusion should be obtained (see Chapter 24). Sepsis, shock, neonatal exchange transfusions, neonatal umbilical vein catheterization, and neonatal omphalitis are risk factors for portal vein thrombosis and should be questioned. Painless rectal bleeding suggests a Meckel diverticulum, duplication, polyp, or angiodysplasia. On rare occasions, painless rectal bleeding may be secondary to a deep ulcer-

ation of the right colon or terminal ileum, as in *Crohn disease*. Bloody diarrhea, which may or may not be associated with tenesmus, is typical of an inflammatory colitis (see Chapter 19). Infectious causes of bleeding should also be sought (see Chapter 19). Information regarding travel (either the patient or visitors), sick contacts, day care exposure, camping, and antibiotic exposure should also be obtained. Rectal bleeding in infants may be due to milk or soy protein intolerance, and a careful dietary history is mandatory. A history of severe constipation can indicate enterocolitis, such as in Hirschsprung disease. Constipation in a well-appearing child may suggest a rectal fissure as the source of bleeding (see Chapter 25). Often there is a history of perianal pain or discomfort with bowel movements. The blood is often bright-red and coats the stool rather than being mixed throughout. This can also be seen in cases of proctitis or cryptitis. In patients older than 2 years of age, bloody diarrhea in the absence of an infectious etiology suggests inflammatory bowel disease (see Chapter 19).

Information regarding chronic pulmonary disease, renal disease, bleeding disorders, and liver disease should be obtained. Patients with cystic fibrosis are at risk not only for the development of esophageal varices due to biliary cirrhosis but also for coagulopathies from vitamin K deficiency. In patients with renal disease, uremia causes platelet dysfunction, which may manifest as a gastrointestinal bleed. Current medications are important not only as a possible source of bleeding but also for further historical information; a family history of peptic ulcer disease, polyps, or inflammatory bowel disease may also help in determining the underlying cause of bleeding.

Physical Examination

A careful physical examination is mandatory and aids in the differential diagnosis and management (Table 21–4). Immediate attention must be given to signs of hypovolemia, anemia, or shock. An orthostatic change, such as a pulse rate increase of 20 beats/

Table 21–3. **Causes of Occult Gastrointestinal Bleeding**

Inflammatory Causes	*Tumors and Neoplastic Causes*
Peptic esophagitis	Polyps
Crohn's disease	Lymphoma
Chronic ulcerative colitis	Leiomyoma
Mild enterocolitis	Lipoma
Celiac disease	Carcinoma
Eosinophilic gastroenteritis	*Drugs*
Meckel's diverticulum	Nonsteroidal anti-inflammatory drugs
Solitary colon ulcer	
Infectious Causes	*Extragastrointestinal Causes*
Hookworm	Hemoptysis
Strongyloidiasis	Epistaxis
Ascariasis	Oropharyngeal bleeding
Tuberculous enterocolitis	*Artifactual Causes*
Amebiasis	Hematuria
Vascular Causes	Menstrual bleeding
Angiodysplasia and vascular ectasias	Nonspecific test positivity
Gastroesophageal varices	*Miscellaneous Causes*
Congestive gastropathy	Long-distance running
Hemangiomas	Coagulopathies
	Factitial

Modified from Ahlquist DA. Approach to the patient with occult gastrointestinal bleeding. *In* Yamada T (ed). Textbook of Gastroenterology. Philadelphia: JB Lippincott, 1991:620.

Table 21–4. Signs and Symptoms in Gastrointestinal (GI) Hemorrhage

Sign	Indication	Site of Bleeding
Splenomegaly Caput medusae Jaundice	Portal hypertension	Esophageal varices Portal gastropathy
Hemangioma Telangiectasia	Multiple hemangioma syndrome	Vascular malformation of GI tract
Hematemesis	Bleeding from above the ligament of Treitz	Upper GI tract
Melena	Bleeding from above the ileocecal valve	Upper GI tract or small intestine
Hematochezia	Colonic bleeding, massive upper GI bleeding	GI tract
Nasogastric aspirate: gross blood	Bleeding from above the ligament of Treitz	Upper GI tract
Palpable purpura	Henoch-Schönlein purpura	GI tract
Mouth ulcers, perianal fistula, or skin tags; erythema nodosum, arthritis, uveitis	Inflammatory bowel disease	Lower GI tract

Modified from Olson AD, Hillemeier AC. Gastrointestinal hemorrhage. *In* Wyllie R, Hyams JS (eds). Pediatric Gastrointestinal Disease. Philadelphia: WB Saunders, 1993:251.

minute or a drop in systolic blood pressure of greater than 10 mmHg when going from the supine to standing position, is a sensitive index of a significant volume depletion, usually greater than 20%. (Blood pressure may remain normal up to the point of circulatory collapse in children.)

Growth parameters should be checked closely. Both weight and height should be obtained and plotted on the appropriate growth curve. These may be indicators of a chronic disease such as inflammatory bowel disease. Cutaneous lesions should be evaluated. Hyperpigmented lesions of the oral or anal mucosa may indicate Peutz-Jeghers disease. Petechiae can indicate disseminated intravascular coagulation (DIC) or another bleeding abnormality. Henoch-Schönlein purpura and hemolytic uremic syndrome may present with purpura. Cutaneous telangiectasia and hemangiomas may indicate such diseases as Osler-Weber-Rendu syndrome and ataxia-telangiectasia or may simply suggest a predisposition for vascular malformations. Jaundice or spider nevi suggest underlying liver disease; subcutaneous nodules or masses may be part of an underlying polyposis syndrome.

The abdomen is examined closely for bowel sounds and bruits before any palpation of the abdomen is performed, since palpation may induce gas movement in an otherwise silent abdomen. A prominent venous pattern and an enlarged spleen or ascites suggest portal hypertension (see Chapter 23). Tenderness and guarding indicate a significant inflammatory process.

During the rectal examination, which is necessary in the work-up of all new, acute gastrointestinal bleeding presentations, the anus needs to be examined closely for any evidence of fissures or fistulas. During the digital examination, tenderness indicates the presence of inflammation. Stool should be checked for occult blood

by a rectal examination. This procedure should be done even if a bloody specimen is brought directly to the emergency department.

If the history suggests copious rectal bleeding and the Hemoccult is negative on rectal examination, Munchausen's syndrome should be considered (see Chapter 37). Finally, stool should be checked for the presence of white blood cells. If the stool smear shows large numbers of white blood cells, a stool culture for enteric infections, such as *Salmonella*, *Shigella*, *Yersinia*, and *Campylobacter*, is warranted (see Chapter 19).

Laboratory and Diagnostic Evaluation

Laboratory studies to be performed include a complete blood cell count with differential. The hemoglobin and hematocrit indicate signs of anemia, but if the bleeding has been very recent, it may take time for the blood count to equilibrate to a new lower number. The mean corpuscular volume is normal in acute bleeding but is commonly low in chronic, low-grade bleeding. An abnormal differential white blood cell count suggests acute inflammation. An elevated eosinophil count may signify a hypersensitivity or allergic process or eosinophilic gastroenteritis. Thrombocytopenia may indicate hemolytic uremic syndrome, another consumptive process, or failure of bone marrow production. Prothrombin time and a partial thromboplastin time should be done to rule out a bleeding diathesis. Serum, creatinine, electrolytes, and blood urea nitrogen should be obtained to rule out an acidosis, metabolic disturbances, and renal disease. Normal liver enzymes make the diagnosis of liver disease less likely, and normal total protein and albumin levels suggest adequate liver function and rule out a protein-losing enteropathy.

A nasogastric tube should be placed in any child with gastrointestinal bleeding whether it is hematemesis or rectal. Lavage with room temperature saline solution should be carried out to evaluate for ongoing bleeding and to determine whether the source is the upper gastrointestinal tract. In cases of pyloric channel or duodenal bulb lesions, the gastric lavage may be non-bloody as a result of edema and partial obstruction at the level of the lesion. The clinical history of significant vomiting and persistent high volume drainage from the nasogastric tube should make one suspect these lesions. Frequently, there is a question as to whether the bright-red blood retrieved on initial nasogastric intubation is secondary to nasopharyngeal trauma. A simple solution would be to leave the nasogastric tube in place for an additional few hours, and if the gastric fluid remains clear after initial lavage, the blood produced on initial passage of the nasogastric tube was likely due to trauma. Concern regarding the possibility of bleeding varices should not be a contraindication to placement of a nasogastric tube.

Esophagogastroduodenoscopy (EGD) can identify the site of upper gastrointestinal bleeding in more than 80% of patients, but radiologic contrast studies are less accurate (only 50%). EGD can also allow direct intervention at the bleeding site, as in the case of esophageal varices or a visible vessel in an ulcer crater. Endoscopic visualization of the stomach and duodenum should be done even if the bleeding is thought to originate from esophageal varices. Of patients with proven esophageal varices, 50% may be bleeding from gastritis or peptic ulcer disease rather than the varices.

Upper endoscopy is safe, and the complication rate is less than 1%. Complications can be related to sedation or general anesthesia or to the procedure itself. Procedure-associated complications include sore throat, bleeding, aspiration, and, rarely, perforation. Endoscopy should not be performed until the patient is as hemodynamically stable as possible. The hematocrit at that time should be close to 25%.

Lower gastrointestinal tract bleeding can also be evaluated endoscopically. Procedures frequently used in children include proctosigmoidoscopy and flexible colonoscopy. Rigid proctoscopy is associated with significant discomfort and therefore rarely indicated in children. Under appropriate sedation, exploration of the distal colon to the level of the splenic flexure can be achieved with a 60-cm flexible proctoscope, and the entire colon to the terminal ileum can be explored using the flexible colonoscope. Therefore, lower gastrointestinal endoscopy allows for full exploration of the colon, identifies the presence of multiple lesions, allows for therapeutic intervention to bleeding lesions through electrocoagulation, laser therapy, or thermocoagulation, and allows for removal of bleeding lesions, such as polyps. Colonoscopy is indicated when there is melena or severe bleeding with no evidence of upper gastrointestinal lesions, when stools are guaiac-positive over a long time, and when examination of the terminal ileum is indicated to rule out Crohn disease. One disadvantage is that large amounts of luminal blood will obscure visualization of a lesion. Prior to lower gastrointestinal colonoscopy, intestinal lavage with oral administration of polyethylene glycol should be used to remove as much of the luminal blood and stool as possible.

Differential Diagnosis

See also Common Causes of Gastrointestinal Bleeding below.

In the newborn period, esophagitis, gastritis, and peptic ulcers seem to be the most common causes of upper gastrointestinal bleeding. Esophagitis is usually peptic in origin and may be associated with dysphagia, irritability, and arching with feeds (see Chapter 20). Clinical signs of gastroesophageal reflux may be absent. Diagnosis would be made by EGD, and treatment would consist of acid suppression. In children with forceful emesis, hematemesis may be the presenting feature of pyloric stenosis or other causes of gastric outlet obstruction.

Swallowed maternal blood is frequently misinterpreted as upper gastrointestinal bleeding in neonates or breast-fed infants. The blood may have been swallowed during delivery or through cracked, irritated nipples in breast-fed infants. Diagnosis is based on obtaining an Apt test on bloody (red) fluid to confirm the presence of maternal blood. ''Bleeding'' does not recur once the source is eliminated or the initial swallowed blood is passed.

Mallory-Weiss tears occur frequently in infancy. They are most commonly associated with acute gastroenteritis but may be associated with intestinal obstruction. The forcefulness of the vomiting causes a tear in the distal esophagus at the level of the lower esophageal sphincter. The clinical history is generally one of frequent non-bloody vomiting that then becomes hematemesis. Diagnosis can commonly be made on a clinical basis; if not, the diagnosis can be made by esophagoscopy. Treatment is of the underlying cause of vomiting and, if necessary, with blood replacement.

Causes of lower gastrointestinal bleeding in the neonate and infant are also numerous. *Anal fissures* are probably the most frequent cause of streaks of bright-red blood and, occasionally, mucus in the stools of infants. The bleeding may or may not be associated with hard bowel movements. There is an association with group A streptococcal perianal cellulitis and bleeding; if the perianal area is erythematous, this pathogen should be looked for and treated appropriately with antibiotics. If streptococci are not present, healing generally occurs with 24 to 48 hours. Local treatment with zinc oxide and air drying is helpful.

Infectious colitis causes infants to have frequent, often watery, bloody bowel movements (see Chapter 19). The patient feels crampy pain before and during the bowel movement as a result of the colitis. Common pathogens include *Salmonella* and *Shigella*, especially with dysentery type stools, but *Escherichia coli* (hemolytic uremic syndrome), *Campylobacter,* and *Yersinia* should also be considered. A culture specimen obtained by rectal swab is the quickest means to the diagnosis. The specimen is obtained prior to

a rectal examination with lubricant because of the presence of bacteriostatic agents in the lubricants. Antibiotic treatment depends on the specific organism and the status of the patient with regard to age and immunocompetence (see Chapter 19).

Milk protein intolerance may present with bloody stools. There may be a history of increasing frequency along with blood and mucus in the stool. The infant may exhibit cramping with the bowel movements; this needs to be distinguished from infectious colitis. Generally, the patients appear well but may also have vomiting as part of their presentation. Blood studies may show peripheral eosinophilia along with mild anemia. There may be a few white blood cells in the stool and, occasionally, eosinophils. Often there is a family history of food allergies. Milk protein allergy classically occurs in cow's milk–based formulas, but is probably just as common in soy formula-fed infants. Breast-fed infants appear to be most protected; however, cow's milk proteins have been found in breast milk, and milk protein colitis has been diagnosed in breast-fed infants. Diagnosis is often made by a therapeutic trial with a hypoallergenic formula or by flexible sigmoidoscopy with biopsy. Treatment involves the frequent removal of the specific antigen through the change to a hypoallergenic formula.

Meckel's diverticulum occurs in 1% to 3% of the population (Fig. 21–1). Typically, there is gastrointestinal bleeding that may be massive. Bleeding results from mucosal ulceration secondary to secretion of gastric acid or pepsin from ectopic gastric or pancreatic tissue, respectively, in the tip of the diverticulum. Rectal bleeding is painless unless diverticulitis or intussusception develop (rare) (see Chapter 18). The blood is usually dark-red but may be bright-red if there is brisk bleeding. Stool is generally not present.

Diagnosis is made by a Meckel scan (^{99m}Tc) (Fig. 21–2). A positive scan has a high correlation with finding a diverticulum at the time of surgery. There have been reports of negative scans in patients with a documented Meckel diverticulum. In the presence of a negative scan and repeated bleeding episodes, a repeat technetium scan should be done. Treatment is by surgical removal.

Necrotizing enterocolitis is associated with rectal bleeding in sick-appearing low-birth-weight neonates. It is associated with several risk factors, such as prematurity, cyanotic heart disease, polycythemia, chronic diarrhea, and gastrointestinal malformations. The rectal bleeding may be preceded by or accompanied by signs of illness, such as apnea, lethargy, cyanosis, bradycardia, and temperature instability. Diagnosis is confirmed by the presence of pneumoperitoneum, pneumatosis intestinalis, or hepatic portal vein gas on radiologic examination of the abdomen. Treatment is via bowel rest, broad-spectrum antibiotics, and surgery if intestinal perforation is present.

IMAGING

Radiography

Radiographic studies are useful in identifying mass lesions or mucosal ulcerations. A simple flat plate of the abdomen helps to rule out large abdominal masses and may indicate intestinal obstruction. Upper intestinal radiographic studies can discern anatomic lesions, such as strictures, stenoses, atresias, errors in rotation, large ulcerations, and masses. Most mucosal lesions in children are best evaluated with endoscopy because children cannot comply with the procedures necessary for air-contrast examination of the gastrointestinal tract. Small-bowel follow-through examination allows evaluation of the small bowel from the ligament of Treitz to the ileocecal valve. Areas of ulceration, mucosal thickening, and narrowing can also be appreciated.

A barium enema should be performed in neonates and infants in

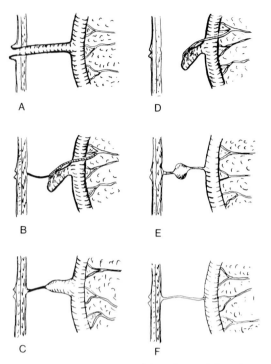

Figure 21-1. Some commoner abnormalities that result from the embryonic yolk sac. A, Patent omphalomesenteric duct representing a communication from the terminal ileum to the umbilicus. B, Meckel's diverticulum with a patent right vitelline artery as blood supply to the Meckel's diverticulum and a residual of the vitelline artery illustrated as a cord to the undersurface of the umbilicus. C, Meckel's diverticulum with a cord connecting the tip of the Meckel's diverticulum to the undersurface of the umbilicus. The cord (band) represents the distal residual of the omphalomesenteric duct. D, Typical appearance of a Meckel's diverticulum with persistence of the vitelline artery. E, Involution of the proximal and distal ends of the omphalomesenteric duct with residual cord or band and central preservation of the omphalomesenteric duct, resulting in a mucosa-lined cyst. F, Intraperitoneal band from the ileum to the undersurface of the umbilicus, representing involution without resolution of the omphalomesenteric duct. (From Schwartz MZ, Smolens I. Meckel's diverticulum and other omphalomesenteric duct remnants. In Wyllie R, Hyams JS [eds]. Pediatric Gastrointestinal Disease. Philadelphia: WB Saunders, 1993:671.)

whom there is a concern of distal intestinal obstruction, such as intussusception. In cases of intussusception, the barium enema not only is diagnostic but also may be therapeutic. The presence of polyps can also be documented. To visualize mucosal lesions of the colon, an air-contrast barium enema is required but can be done in only very cooperative children. Crohn disease and ulcerative colitis may be suggested by this test, but direct visualization of the colon with endoscopy allows for histologic confirmation of this diagnosis. Barium enemas are frequently used as a way to evaluate areas of the colon that could not be examined by endoscopy.

Angiography

Angiography should be considered in a child who is actively bleeding if fiberoptic endoscopy is inconclusive or could not be performed. Angiography is useful in determining the extent of varices, the etiology of portal hypertension, and in excluding other sources of bleeding other than varices in upper gastrointestinal bleeding. In lower intestinal bleeding, angiography's usefulness is limited by the need of the bleeding to be very brisk. A rate of 0.5 ml/minute at the time of contrast injection is required to identify the source of bleeding. Nevertheless, angiography can identify extravasation of contrast in a Meckel diverticulum or the presence of vascular malformations of the bowel, which may be acquired or congenital.

Therapeutic angiography is frequently used to control gastrointestinal bleeding. Vasopressin infusion or transcatheter embolization may directly control bleeding. The complication rate of angiography is 2%, whether diagnostic or therapeutic. Deep sedation or general anesthesia is required.

Nuclear Imaging

Nuclear medicine has markedly improved our ability to determine the site of bleeding with minimal complication, has allowed low radiation exposure, and has been associated with very little need for heavy sedation. ^{99m}Tc-pertechnetate is an agent that is rapidly taken up by gastric mucosa, and it can be useful in identifying sites of bleeding secondary to ectopic gastric mucosa. Gastric mucosa is found in 90% of bleeding Meckel diverticula, which makes this a useful test (see Fig. 21–2). The radioisotope has a short half-life, and the test itself can be done without significant preparation. False-negative results have been reported frequently because of insufficient gastric tissue mass, downstream washout of isotope, impaired blood supply, or suboptimal techniques. Repeated

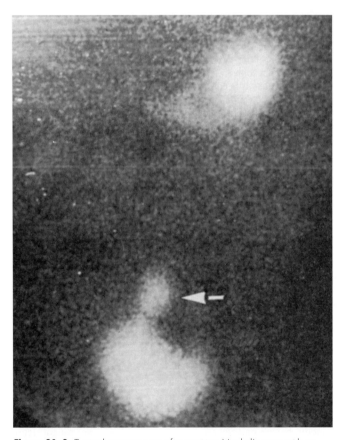

Figure 21-2. Typical appearance of a positive Meckel's scan with an area of increased uptake above the area of the bladder in the lower midabdomen. (From Schwartz MZ, Smolens I. Meckel's diverticulum and other omphalomesenteric duct remnants. In Wyllie R, Hyams JS [eds]. Pediatric Gastrointestinal Disease. Philadelphia: WB Saunders, 1993:674.)

Meckel scans may be necessary to identify ectopic gastric tissue. Positive identification on initial or subsequent study may be improved by the administration of pentagastrin or cimetidine to prevent excretion of pertechnetate from gastric tissue. A ^{99m}Tc-pertechnetate scan does not interfere with subsequent bleeding scans. A recent stannous pyrophosphate red blood cell bleeding scan may interfere with the distribution of ^{99m}Tc-pertechnetate so that gastric tissue is not visualized. With this concern in mind, if a patient requires evaluation of significant gastrointestinal bleeding, a Meckel scan should be performed first.

Bleeding scans are performed by injecting technetium sulfur colloid intravenously. The agent is distributed quickly and is rapidly taken up by the reticuloendothelial system. It can detect a rate of bleeding of 0.1 ml/minute. However, because the technetium is taken up by the reticuloendothelial system, this may hinder finding bleeding sites that may lie behind the liver or spleen. Finally, the clearance is very rapid, with a half-time of 2 minutes, which means that bleeding needs to be occurring at the time of the scan.

The ^{99m}Tc-pertechnetate labeled red blood cell scan is both a sensitive and accurate test for the localization of active bleeding. It can be repeated readily in cases of intermittent bleeding for up to 24 hours and can detect as little blood as 0.5 ml/minute.

TREATMENT

The general guidelines for the treatment of gastrointestinal bleeding are determined by the severity of bleeding (Table 21–5). These include re-establishing and maintaining the intravascular volume and then the oxygen-carrying capacity (transfusion) of packed red blood cells. Subsequently, the site of blood loss must be determined and attempts made to stop the hemorrhage. Therefore, a history and physical examination should be performed, with particular attention paid to vital signs and blood pressure.

Although parents tend to overestimate the amount of blood lost by their child, a major error in the management of gastrointestinal bleeding is underestimating blood loss. The hematocrit value may remain unchanged initially, despite a significant blood loss, and therefore is not a good indicator of significant bleeding. If or-

Table 21–5. Treatment of Patients with Hypovolemic Shock Secondary to Gastrointestinal Hemorrhage

Establish adequate intravenous (IV) access by placing IV catheters: for mild shock, one IV catheter; for moderate or severe shock, two IV catheters.

Recommended catheter size:
Infant: 20 gauge
Child: 18 gauge
Adolescent: 16 gauge

Rapidly infuse saline, lactated Ringer's solution, or Plasmanate (10 ml/kg/10 min until vital signs normalized).

Carefully monitor pulse, blood pressure, central venous pressure to avoid fluid overload.

Monitor urine output and skin perfusion and orthostatic changes in pulse and blood pressure for early recognition of shock.

Transfuse with packed red blood cells to return oxygen-carrying capacity to normal.

Carefully record all fluids transfused, and estimate and record all recognized fluids lost.

Modified from Olson AD, Hillemeier AC. Gastrointestinal hemorrhage. *In* Wyllie R, Hyams JS (eds). Pediatric Gastrointestinal Disease. Philadelphia: WB Saunders, 1993:253.

thostatic blood pressure changes are present, the initial goal of treatment should be to hemodynamically stabilize the patient, maintain the intravascular volume, and protect the oxygen carrying capacity. To do this, large-bore IV lines must be started.

A second potential error is the failure to establish adequate IV access. The largest possible IV line must be rapidly placed in a child with active bleeding. If the blood loss is thought to be 20% or more of the intravascular volume, suggesting hypovolemic shock, two IV lines should be placed. The size of the IV line inserted depends on the child's age and size (Table 21–5). Blood loss should be replaced immediately with a crystalloid solution, such as normal saline or lactated Ringer's. Initially, a fluid push of 20 ml/kg should be given. As this is being done, a second line should be in place and coagulation studies, platelet count, and a type and cross-match should be done. If blood loss continues and the patient appears to be at risk for hypovolemic shock, one can also use colloid solutions (hetastarch or albumin). Plasma is indicated if coagulation factors are depleted. Once bleeding has stopped, transfusions of packed red blood cells should continue to slowly raise the hematocrit to 30%. If bleeding continues, fresh frozen plasma and calcium should be given in addition to packed red blood cells. The platelet count in such patients must be monitored as thrombocytopenia may develop.

Nasogastric lavage can be used to confirm an upper gastrointestinal bleed as well as to treat this bleed. The tube size depends on the child's age and size. A 12 Fr. tube can be used in infants and preschool children; a 14 or 16 Fr. tube is appropriate for children of school age or older. Once the tube is in place, gastric lavage should be undertaken. Although the most appropriate lavage solution has been debated, there does not appear to be any significant advantage to iced normal saline versus room temperature normal saline. In pediatric patients, a theoretic advantage of using normal saline at room temperature is to avoid the possibility of hypothermia. The quantity of normal saline to be used for lavaging a child depends on the patient's age and size:

- 10 ml of normal saline is sufficient to lavage an infant with an upper gastrointestinal bleed
- 100 to 200 ml of normal saline can be used in school-aged and older children

The color of the gastric lavage fluid that is recovered from the stomach gives the physician an indication of the rate of bleeding. Lavage returns that are bright-red indicate significant ongoing bleeding; pink-tinged or brown flecks in the solution indicate less significant or minimal bleeding. Gastric lavage should be continued for 15 minutes. If active bleeding continues, there is no benefit to continuing lavage for a longer period of time; if the gastric aspirate is clear within 15 minutes, the nasogastric tube should be left in for 48 hours. During the first hour, the nasogastric tube should be irrigated every 15 minutes with normal saline. Following that time, antacids should be instilled into the stomach via the nasogastric tube every 2 to 3 hours. The gastric pH must be maintained above 3.5. This can be done by instilling 0.5 ml of antacids every 3 hours into infants, 30 ml in preschoolers, and 60 ml in school-aged children. Maintaining the gastric pH above 3.5 should limit the ability of gastric acid to cause additional erosions as well as enhance the formation of blood clots.

Intravenous H_2 receptor antagonists may also be helpful in stress ulcerations (Table 21–6). However, the IV administration of such agents have not been shown to be beneficial in the presence of ongoing bleeding, and these agents are less reliable than antacids in consistently raising the gastric pH. However, it is reasonable to begin IV administration of H_2 receptor antagonists with a documented upper gastrointestinal bleed and to titrate the dose to ensure the gastric pH is above 3.5.

Vasoactive Agents

If bleeding persists, vasoactive agents, such as vasopressin, can be used to try to control the bleeding. In particular, vasopressin

Table 21–6. Peptic Ulcer Therapy: Selected Agents and Suggested Oral Doses

Medication	Adult Dose	Pediatric Dose
Antacids	30 ml (regular strength) 1 and 3 hr after meals and at bedtime	0.5–1 ml/kg/dose 1 and 3 hr after meals and at bedtime
Cimetidine	300 mg q.i.d. or 400 mg b.i.d.	20–40 mg/kg/day divided into q.i.d. or b.i.d. doses*

Ranitidine	150 mg b.i.d.	2–3 mg/kg/dose
		   b.i.d. (children)†
		   t.i.d. (infants)‡

Omeprazole	20–40 mg daily	No guidelines established
Sucralfate	1 g q.i.d.	250 mg q.i.d. (infants)§ 0.5–1 g q.i.d. (children)

*Efficacy of the b.i.d. dose has not been established in pediatric patients.
†May require t.i.d. dosing.
‡Neonates should be started on the lower dose.
§No pharmacokinetic studies in pediatric patients available.
Data from DeGiacumo et al, 1990; Feldman et al, 1990; Sutphen et al, 1989; Chuing et al, 1989; Tan and Saing 1989; Shaw-Stiffel and Roberts, 1991. Reprinted from Gryboski JD, Moyer MS. Peptic ulcer in children. *In* Wyllie R, Hyams JS (eds). Pediatric Gastrointestinal Disease. Philadelphia: WB Saunders, 1993:459.

has been useful in controlling variceal bleeding. The IV use of vasopressin is as effective as selective arterial installation and appears to produce fewer side effects than arterial use. Side effects include ischemia, fluid and electrolyte imbalances, and arrhythmias.

The infusion begins at a rate of 0.1 units/minute and increases to a maximum of 0.5 units/minute by doubling the dose hourly.

- The maximum dose for children under age 5 is 0.2 units/minute.
- For children between the ages of 5 and 12 years, up to 0.3 units/minute can be used.
- For children above age 12, the maximum dose is 0.4 units/minute.

Vasopressin acts by decreasing splanchnic blood flow, thereby lowering portal venous pressure. If bleeding is successfully controlled, vasopressin should be continued at the dose required for controlling the bleeding for 24 hours and slowly tapered over the next 48 hours. Although there is little evidence to suggest that vasopressin is effective in nonvariceal-related bleeds, it is reasonable to consider a trial of vasopressin if there is significant uncontrolled bleeding.

Somatostatin is another vasoactive agent that may be useful in controlling upper gastrointestinal bleeds.

Balloon-tamponade using a Sengstaken-Blakemore tube is another method for controlling esophageal or gastric varices that is seldom needed. If variceal bleeding continues, despite the use of vasopressin, the Sengstaken-Blakemore or Linton tube may be useful. To use these double-balloon systems, the patient is first intubated. After intubation, the balloon is inflated for 24 hours at a time to tamponade the bleeding. The tube is maintained in this position by taping the tube to an external support, such as a football helmet. An x-ray is obtained to confirm the proper location of the tube. Generally, inflating the gastric balloon is sufficient to control most variceal bleeding in children. The major complication is perforation or aspiration. Because of the relatively high complication rate associated with balloon tamponade, endoscopic sclerotherapy has become the mainstay for the treatment of uncontrollable variceal bleeding.

Endoscopic Modalities

Sclerotherapy is effective in controlling the acute bleeding from esophageal varices. Once bleeding has been controlled, sclerotherapy should be repeated at monthly intervals until the varices are

totally obliterated. Complications include esophageal ulceration and esophageal stricture. A number of sclerosing agents are available (sodium morrhuate, ethanol, tetradecylsulfate) and all such agents appear efficacious in sclerosing varices. Endoscopic ligation may also be effective in controlling variceal bleeding.

One can directly visualize the cause of an upper gastrointestinal bleed through the endoscope. Thermal coagulation or laser photocoagulation can be used to stop active gastric bleeding. The bleeding site must be adequately visualized through the upper endoscope. Complications include perforation.

COMMON CAUSES OF GASTROINTESTINAL BLEEDING

Intussusception

Intussusception is a common cause of lower gastrointestinal bleeding during the first 2 years of life (see Chapter 18). The hallmark of intussusception is the presence of ''currant jelly'' stools associated with colicky abdominal pain, lethargy, or irritability. The physical examination generally reveals a palpable abdominal mass in the right lower quadrant. Generally, a barium enema is not only useful as a diagnostic modality but also therapeutic, in that the intussusception is generally reduced by the hydrostatic pressure. If the barium enema does not reduce the intussusception, surgery may be required.

Esophageal Variceal Bleeding

Esophageal variceal bleeding in association with portal hypertension is a common cause of upper gastrointestinal bleeding in preschool and school-aged children (see Chapter 22 to 24). With the advent of liver transplantation programs nationwide, the incidence of significant liver disease resulting in portal hypertension and esophageal variceal bleeding has declined dramatically. Endoscopy is the test of choice for diagnosing variceal bleeding, and sclerotherapy is the modality best suited for treating variceal bleeding.

Inflammatory Bowel Disease

Inflammatory bowel disease is generally accompanied by fever, weight loss, and rectal bleeding (see Chapter 19). The rectal bleeding can vary from occult positive stools to frank blood in the bowel movements. Generally, the patient is anemic, and the erythrocyte sedimentation rate is elevated. Definitive diagnosis can be made by performing a colonoscopy and obtaining a colonic or terminal ilium biopsy.

Henoch-Schönlein Purpura

Henoch-Schönlein purpura is a syndrome with the following clinical features: purpuric rash, nephritis, and GI symptoms (see Chapters 28 and 29). Gastrointestinal manifestations include abdominal pain and GI bleeding in up to 10% of cases.

Treatment is generally supportive, and patients recover with no significant morbidity. Steroids have been used for children with significant abdominal pain and appear to cause a more rapid resolution of symptoms; however, the use of steroids remains controversial.

Hemolytic-Uremic Syndrome

Hemolytic-uremic syndrome is an acute disorder resulting in renal failure (see Chapters 28 and 29). The vasculitis associated with hemolytic-uremic syndrome can also present as gastrointestinal bleeding. Classically, a radiograph demonstrates mucosal irregularities described as "thumbprinting." Generally, endoscopy is not indicated in patients with hemolytic uremic syndrome. As with Henoch-Schönlein purpura, the treatment for hemolytic-uremic syndrome is supportive, and GI symptoms resolve with no specific therapy.

Peptic Ulcer Disease

Peptic ulcer disease does occur in children (see Chapter 18). A child who presents with epigastric abdominal pain, early satiety, and vomiting with evidence of an upper gastrointestinal bleed should be evaluated for peptic ulcer disease. The presenting manifestations may be age-dependent (Table 21–7).

The diagnosis can most effectively be made by upper endoscopy. *Helicobacter pylori* is a significant risk factor for development of peptic ulcer disease. The discovery of *H. pylori*, a gram-positive

microaerophilic spiral organism, has changed the approach to treating peptic ulcer disease. If a child is to be evaluated for peptic ulcer disease, it is imperative to rule out the presence of *H. pylori* infection. Children with peptic ulcer disease who are infected with *H. pylori* should be treated with antimicrobial agents (Pepto-Bismol, metronidazole, amoxicillin) rather than just with antacids or acid-suppressing agents. The child is treated for 2 weeks. With good compliance, eradication rates of greater than 90% can be achieved with this combination.

Polyps

The hallmark of juvenile polyps is the presence of painless rectal bleeding. Juvenile polyps are uncommon in children under 1 year of age, with a peak incidence between ages 5 and 7 years. Most juvenile polyps are found in the distal colon, and up to 50% of polyps can be palpated on a rectal examination. If there is significant bleeding, a colonoscopy and polypectomy should be performed to remove the polyp.

RED FLAGS

Gastrointestinal bleeding should be viewed in two stages and as an emergent problem. First, signs of hypovolemia and anemia must be determined; if detected, they must be aggressively treated. Blood loss can be gravely underestimated. The amount of bleeding may also go undetected, as a liter of blood can remain unobserved within the gastrointestinal tract. Second, the site of bleeding must be determined. Third, specific therapy must be instituted if possible.

Red flags include signs of prior liver disease or chronic illnesses, such as cystic fibrosis or inflammatory bowel disease. In contrast to the adult situation, tumors are unusual causes of gastrointestinal bleeding in children; however, ulcer disease (e.g., primary or secondary to stress, NSAIDS, burns, increased intracranial pressure) is probably more common than previously thought. Night pain, a family history, and pain relieved by food are clues to peptic ulcer disease.

REFERENCES

Etiology

Ballesteros J, Company J, Gaya J, et al. Mallory-Weiss syndrome: Review of 25 cases. Rev Clin Esp 1985;176:72–73.

Brown C, Olshaker J. Meckel's diverticulum. Am J Emerg Med 1988;6:157–164.

Cox K, Ament M. Upper gastrointestinal bleeding in children and adolescents. Pediatrics 1979;63:408–413.

Halpin T, Byrne W, Ament M. Colitis, persistent diarrhea and soy protein intolerance. J Pediatr 1977;91:404–407.

Hillemeier C, Gryboski JD. Gastrointestinal bleeding in the pediatric patient. Yale J Biol Med 1984;57:135.

Homan W, Tang C, Thorbjarnarson B. Acute massive hemorrhage from intestinal Crohn's disease: Report of seven cases and review of the literature. Arch Surg 1976;111:901–905.

Kaplan B, Benson J, Rothstein F, et al. Lymphonodular hyperplasia of the colon as a pathologic finding in children with lower gastrointestinal bleeding. J Pediatr Gastroenterol Nutr 1984;3:704–708.

Kliegman R, Fanaroff A. Necrotizing enterocolitis. N Engl J Med 1984;310:1093–1103.

Nader P, Margolin F. Hemangioma causing gastrointestinal bleeding: Case report and review of the literature. Am J Dis Child 1966;111:215–222.

Table 21–7. Major Symptoms of Peptic Ulcer Disease in Children According to Age

	Neonatal Period	Infancy	Early Childhood	Late Childhood
Hematemesis	+	+	+	+
Melena	+	+	+	+
Vomiting	+	+	+	
Abdominal pain			+	+
Failure to thrive		+		
Anorexia		+	+	

Modified from Gryboski JD, Moyer MS. Peptic ulcer in children. *In* Wyllie R, Hyams JS (eds). Pediatric Gastrointestinal Disease. Philadelphia: WB Saunders, 1993:453.

Nord KS. Peptic ulcer disease in the pediatric population. Pediatr Clin North Am 1988;35:117.

St Vil D, Brandt ML, Panic S, et al. Meckel's diverticulum in children: A 20-year review. J Pediatr Surg 1991;26:1289–1292.

Diagnosis

Ahlquist D, McGill D, Schwarts S, et al. HemoQuant, a new quantitative assay for fecal hemoglobin: Comparison with Hemoccult. Ann Intern Med 1984;101:297–302.

Cadranel S, Rodesch P, Peters J, et al. Fiberendoscopy of the gastrointestinal tract in children: A series of 100 examinations. Am J Dis Child 1977;131:41–45.

Hassall E, Barclay G, Ament M: Colonoscopy in childhood. Pediatrics 1984;73:594–599.

Hyams JS, Leichtner AM, Schwartz AN. Recent advances in diagnosis and treatment of gastrointestinal hemorrhage in infants and children. J Pediatr 1985;106:1.

Keller F, Rosch J. Value of angiography in diagnosis and therapy of acute upper gastrointestinal hemorrhage. Dig Dis Sci 1981;26:78S–89S.

Kleber G, Sauerbruch T, Ansari H, et al. Prediction of variceal hemorrhage in cirrhosis: A prospective follow-up study. Gastroenterology 1991;100:1332–1337.

McGinn FP, Guyer PB, Wilken BJ, et al. A prospective comparative trial between early endoscopy and radiology in acute upper gastrointestinal hemorrhage. Gut 1975;16:707.

Parikh N, Sebring E, Polesky H. Evaluation of bloody gastric fluid from newborn infants. J Pediatr 1979;94:967–969.

Rex D, Weddle R, Lehman G, et al. Flexible sigmoidoscopy plus air contrast barium enema versus colonoscopy for suspected lower gastrointestinal bleeding. Gastroenterology 1990;98:855–861.

Rosenthal P, Thompson J, Singh M. Detection of occult blood in gastric juice. J Clin Gastroenterol 1984;6:119–121.

Sfakianakis G, Hasse G. Abdominal scintigraphy for ectopic gastric mucosa: A retrospective analysis of 143 studies. Am J Roentgenol 1982;138:7–12.

Wizelberg BG, Froelich JW, McKusick KA, et al. Radionuclide localization of lower gastrointestinal hemorrhage. Radiol Scintigr 1981;139:465.

Treatment

Ament M. Diagnosis and management of upper gastrointestinal tract bleeding in the pediatric patient. Pediatr Rev 1990;12:107–116.

Bryant L, Mobin-Uddin K, Dillon M. Comparison of ice water with iced saline solution for gastric lavage in gastroduodenal hemorrhage. Am J Surg 1972;124:570.

Burroughs A, McCormick P, Hughes M, et al. Randomized, double-blind, placebo-controlled trial of somatostatin for variceal bleeding: Emergency control and prevention of early variceal rebleeding. Gastroenterology 1990;99:1388–1395.

Carey WD: Pharmacological management of portal hypertensive upper intestinal hemorrhage. Semin Gastrointest Dis 1992;3:75–82.

Garden O, Millis P, Birnie G, et al. Propranolol in the prevention of recurrent variceal hemorrhage in cirrhotic patients: A controlled trial. Gastroenterology 1990;98:185–190.

Leitman I, Paull D, Shires G. Evaluation and management of massive lower gastrointestinal hemorrhage. Ann Surg 1989;209:175–180.

Lilly J, Stellin G. Variceal hemorrhage in biliary atresia. J Pediatr Surg 1984;19:476–479.

Maksoud JG, Goncalves ME, Porta G, et al. The endoscopic and surgical management of portal hypertension in children: Analysis of 123 cases. J Pediatr Surg 1991;26:178–181.

Ostro MJ, Russell JA, Soldin SJ, et al. Control of gastric pH with cimetidine boluses versus primed infusions. Gastroenterology 1985;89:532.

Priebe H, Skillman J, Bushnell L, et al. Antacid versus cimetidine in preventing acute gastrointestinal bleeding: A randomized trial in 75 critically ill patients. N Engl J Med 1980;302:426–430.

Protell R, Rubin C, Auth D, et al. The heater probe: A new endoscopic method for stopping massive gastrointestinal bleeding. Gastroenterology 1978;74:257–262.

Ready J, Robertson A, Rector W. Effects of vasopressin on portal pressure during hemorrhage from esophageal varices. Gastroenterology 1991;100:1411–1416.

Williams R. Management of Meckel's diverticulum. Br J Surg 1981;68:477–480.

22 Hepatomegaly

J. Timothy Boyle

Hepatomegaly refers to an enlargement of the liver. Careful examination of the abdomen should be routine in all well-child check-ups, in school and sport physicals, and in the physical evaluation of acute illness. Processes that affect the liver are often insidious in their evolution. Causes of hepatomegaly associated with jaundice are discussed in Chapter 24.

HISTORY

Hepatomegaly can be classified by one of six presenting features:

- Associated jaundice
- Prominent or relapsing vomiting or central nervous system (CNS) deterioration
- Symptoms of progressive neurologic deterioration
- Prominent elevation of aminotransferases
- Signs and symptoms of systemic disease
- Isolated hepatomegaly

Historical information should consider this classification along with the age of the child. Table 22–1 describes disorders that may present with hepatomegaly in infancy, and Table 22–2 lists causes of hepatomegaly in older children and adolescents.

Infants or young children who present with failure to thrive (see Chapter 17) and hepatomegaly usually have a serious underlying disorder. Glycogen storage disease (types I, III, IV, IX, and X) and other metabolic disorders, such as hereditary fructose intolerance, galactosemia, and cystic fibrosis, demonstrate hepatomegaly. Table 22–3 links specific diagnoses with historical clues, such as failure

Table 22-1. Hepatomegaly in Infancy

Disorders of carbohydrate metabolism
    Glycogen storage disease
    Hereditary fructose intolerance
    Galactosemia
    Infants of diabetic mothers
    Beckwith-Wiedemann syndrome
Congenital lactic acidemias
Organic acidemias
Urea cycle defects
Disorders of fatty acid oxidation
Peroxisomal disorders
Lysosomal storage disease
Mucopolysaccharidosis
Wolman disease
Alpha$_1$-antitrypsin deficiency
Cystic fibrosis
Hemophagocytic lymphohistiocytosis
Histiocytosis
Chronic hepatitis B, B and D, neonatal hepatitis, TORCH*
Tumors
    Intrinsic (hepatoblastoma, hemangioendothelioma)
    Extrinsic (neuroblastoma, Wilms tumor)
Hepatomegaly associated with cardiovascular disorder, hemolysis, excess vitamin A
Neonatal iron storage (hemochromatosis)
Fatty liver (obesity)
Biliary tract disease (hepatic fibrosis, Caroli disease, biliary atresia)

*Toxoplasmosis, *other* infections, *rubella, *cytomegalovirus infection, and *herpes simplex.

to thrive, fever, diarrhea, peculiar odor, and neurologic or psychiatric symptoms.

Other important information to consider is a history of prolonged hyperbilirubinemia of infancy (cystic fibrosis, alpha$_1$-antitrypsin deficiency), a family history of hepatic, neurologic or psychiatric disease (metabolic diseases), previous blood transfusions or intrave-

Table 22-2. Hepatomegaly in Older Children and Adolescents

Acute viral hepatitis (hepatitis virus A, B, C, D, E; Epstein-Barr virus)
Chronic viral hepatitis (B, B and D, C)
Autoimmune hepatitis
Drug-induced hepatitis
Wilson disease
Alpha$_1$-antitrypsin deficiency
Sclerosing cholangitis
Steatohepatitis, fatty liver (obesity)
Gaucher (adult form)
Tyrosinemia (chronic form)
Niemann-Pick disease type B
Cholesterol ester storage disease
Hepatomegaly associated with cardiovascular disease, hematologic disorder, diabetes, systemic infection, sarcoidosis, cystic fibrosis
Congenital hepatic fibrosis
Choledochal cyst
Tumor (hepatocellular carcinoma, lymphoma)
Hepatic abscess (bacterial, amebic)
Hepatic venous disorders (veno-occlusive disease, Budd-Chiari syndrome, webs)

Table 22-3. Historical Features in the Diagnostic Evaluation of Hepatomegaly or Hepatosplenomegaly

Symptom	Diagnosis
Failure to thrive (infancy)	Glycogen storage disease I, III, IV, IX, X
	Hereditary fructose intolerance
	Organic acidemias
	Wolman disease
	Cystic fibrosis
	Hemophagocytic lymphohistiocytosis
Fever	Acute and chronic hepatitis
	Systemic illness
	Hepatic abscess
	Hemophagocytic lymphohistiocytosis
	Viral infection
Diarrhea	Wolman disease
Peculiar odor	Organic acidemias
	Hepatic failure
Neurologic/psychiatric symptoms in older child	Wilson disease
	Porphyria
	Urea cycle disorders
	Drug intoxication-toxicity

nous drug abuse in the mother or older child (infections), a past history of hepatitis (chronic hepatitis), protracted vomiting in infancy and childhood (metabolic disease), and a delay in puberty (chronic disease).

Hepatomegaly in an infant or young child with *prominent or recurrent vomiting and CNS deterioration* suggests a metabolic disorder, Reye syndrome, or fulminant hepatic failure. Emesis is forceful and protracted. Signs of acute CNS deterioration include lethargy, hyperventilation, combativeness, disorientation, seizures, and coma. A family history of early infant death is also important. Concern about the presence of sepsis or hypoxia should not dissuade the examiner from embarking on an early metabolic work-up.

Hepatomegaly or hepatosplenomegaly in an infant with *progressive neurological deterioration* suggests a disorder of peroxisomal metabolism or metabolic storage disease. Symptoms of progressive neurologic deterioration include severe hypotonia, poor feeding, drooling, complex seizure disorder, profound psychomotor retardation, or loss of neurologic milestones. In a child older than 5 years of age, neurologic manifestations of Wilson disease may antedate hepatic manifestations in rare circumstances.

In the absence of altered sensorium, hepatomegaly or hepatosplenomegaly with *evidence of hepatocellular injury or dysfunction* suggests either acute or chronic hepatitis. In the absence of jaundice and pruritus, symptoms of both acute and chronic hepatic disease are nonspecific. They include malaise, fatigability, anorexia, weight loss, nausea, episodic vomiting, abdominal enlargement, peripheral edema, amenorrhea, and gastrointestinal bleeding. A specific history suggestive of an acute hepatitis includes exposure to jaundiced or ill individuals within the right incubation time for the viral hepitides, intravenous drug use, or exposure, or exposure to shellfish, potentially toxic drugs, or environmental toxins.

PHYSICAL EXAMINATION

Although a palpable liver below the right costal margin is a *red flag* for suspecting hepatomegaly, liver size can be accurately determined only by percussion, palpation, and auscultation. Liver span is determined in the right midclavicular line with the patient supine and breathing quietly. The dullness of the upper border is easily distinguished by percussion because of the different density of the lung and liver. The lower border may be determined by percussion or palpation. Estimation of span will be more accurate if palpation is used to determine the lower border. Palpation should be gentle, with the examiner's finger slowly moving up from the right lower quadrant. Forceful palpation may miss or push the liver higher into the right upper quadrant.

Table 22–4 lists range of liver span in infants and children at various ages when palpation is used to determine the lower border. The average span may be approximately 2 cm less if the lower border is determined by percussion. The lower border may also be auscultated by placing the bell of a stethoscope just below the xiphoid, and gently scratching the right abdomen from the right lower quadrant upward toward the right costal margin. The auscultation of the scratch is audibly enhanced as the finger passes over the lower border of the liver. Conditions that may displace a normal liver downward include pulmonary hyperinflation, pneumothorax, retroperitoneal mass, and subdiaphragmatic abscess.

Liver span increases with age in children with normal growth patterns. Span seems to correlate more with weight than height. Boys at a given age tend to have a larger mean span than girls. In newborns, liver span also correlates with birth weight to a greater degree than does gestational age. Liver span is usually not affected by minor systemic illnesses or localized trauma. Repeated evaluation of liver span by the same observer applying similar techniques of percussion and auscultation gives the most reliable and clinically revealing information.

Factors that affect accurate measurement of liver span include

- A narrow costal angle
- Wide costal margins
- Pectus excavatum
- Body habitus
- Accessory lobes
- Reidel lobe (a normal elongation of the right lobe)
- Choledochal cyst

In addition to the careful evaluation of the liver size, the nodularity and firmness of the liver must also be assessed. Signs of systemic disease must be searched for, and these include the hard or nodular liver, firm splenomegaly, ascites, a prominent abdominal venous pattern, growth retardation, muscle wasting, clubbing, palmar erythema, spider angiomata, arthritis and papular acrodermatitis. Table 22–5 lists some key findings that should not be missed.

Splenomegaly associated with hepatomegaly may be secondary to portal hypertension or the result of infiltration or storage of the same material or cells affecting the liver (see Chapter 23). Splenomegaly does not distinguish acute from chronic processes. Massive enlargement of the spleen is usually not seen with portal hypertension; it is more characteristic of storage diseases, such as Gaucher disease, Niemann-Pick disease, Wolman disease, the histiocytosis diseases, and malignancies of blood elements.

Table 22–4. Physical Assessment of Hepatomegaly in Children*

Age	Acceptable Span (cm)
Pre-term infants	4–5
Healthy term infants	5–6.5
1–5 years	6–7
5–10 years	7–9
10–16 years	8–10

Liver span is obtained by palpating the lower border and percussing the upper border in the right mid-clavicular line.

Table 22–5. Helpful Physical Signs in the Evaluation of Hepatomegaly

Asymmetric liver	Intrinsic space occupying lesion (hepatic tumor, cyst, abscess)
Firm hepatomegaly	Cirrhosis
	Congenital hepatic fibrosis
	Infiltrative tumors (neuroblastoma, leukemia, lymphoma)
	Histiocytic syndromes
	Congestion (hepatic outflow obstruction, right-sided heart failure)
Rock-hard hepatomegaly	Cirrhosis
	Hepatic tumor
Diffuse liver tenderness	Acute and chronic hepatitis
	Ischemia (left-sided heart failure)
	Congestion (hepatic outflow obstruction, right-sided heart failure)
	Space-occupying lesion (tumor, cyst, abscess)
Hepatic bruit	Hemangioendothelioma
Skin hemangioma	Hemangioendothelioma
Papular acrodermatitis	Hepatitis B
Coarse facial features	Mucopolysaccharidosis
	GM$_1$ gangliosidosis
Mongoloid facies	Zellweger syndrome
Macroglossia	GM$_1$ gangliosidosis
Cataract	Wilson disease
Kayser-Fleischer ring	Wilson disease
Severe hypotonia	Zellweger syndrome
Precocious puberty (boys)	Hepatoblastoma

LABORATORY EVALUATION

Hepatomegaly with jaundice and hyperbilirubinemia are discussed in Chapter 24. In the patient with hepatomegaly, routine laboratory studies should include a complete blood count, serum chemistry profiles, and a urinalysis. Table 22–6 correlates laboratory abnormalities with specific diagnoses.

Hepatic injury or dysfunction is confirmed by a liver profile that includes total and direct levels of bilirubin, serum transaminases (alanine aminotransferase [ALT] and aspartate aminotransferase [AST]), γ-glutamyltransferase (GGT), alkaline phosphatase, serum total protein, and serum albumin. Levels of the transaminases are the most common serum tests to assess hepatocellular injury. Abnormal results of these enzymes are of little specific diagnostic help other than initiating further diagnostic evaluation. Their degree of elevation usually has no correlation with clinical prognosis. Prominent increases of serum alkaline phosphatase and γ-glutamyltransferase activity occur primarily in intrahepatic and extrahepatic cholestatic conditions that are commonly associated with jaundice. None of the above enzymes measures *liver function*.

The serum albumin level and prothrombin time (PT) are measures of hepatic synthetic function. Albumin is the principal serum protein, and it has a half-life of 21 days. Because of albumin's prolonged half-life, a low serum albumin level indicates chronic rather than acute liver disease. Nonhepatic causes of hypoalbuminemia include chronic inadequate protein intake, losses from the urine or gut, or a systemic capillary leak. In a patient with ascites,

Table 22-6. Helpful Laboratory Abnormalities in the Evaluation of Hepatomegaly

Vacuolated white blood cells in peripheral smear	Wolman disease GM$_1$ gangliosidosis
Neutropenia	Glycogen storage disease type 1 Organic acidurias Shwachman syndrome Hemophagocytic lymphohistiocytosis Leukemia, neuroblastoma
Hemolytic anemia	Wilson disease, autoimmune, hemoglobinopathy
Hypophosphatemia	Glycogen storage disease type 1 Hereditary fructose intolerance
Hypertriglyceridemia	Glycogen storage disease type 1 Hemophagocytic lymphohistiocytosis
Elevated creatine phosphokinase level	Disorders of fatty acid oxidation Reye syndrome
Renal tubular dysfunction	Tyrosinemia Glycogen storage disease type 1 Hereditary fructose intolerance Wilson disease Lactic acidurias Galactosemia

decreased albumin levels may be due largely to an increase in the volume of distribution rather than to decreased synthesis.

Because the plasma half-life of the clotting factors is short, the PT rapidly reflects changes in hepatic synthetic function. In a patient with enzymatic evidence of liver injury and a normal serum albumin level, an elevated PT greater than 2 seconds above control may be prognostic indicator of impending fulminant hepatic failure. A prolonged PT also suggests a poor prognosis in chronic liver disease and together with a decreasing serum albumin is one of the most important parameters to consider in deciding to list a patient for liver transplant. Caution should be used in ascribing an abnormal PT to liver dysfunction without first giving parenteral vitamin K to rule out vitamin K deficiency from malabsorption. Because factor VIII is made extensively in nonhepatic sites, including vascular endothelium, plasma levels of this factor can be used to distinguish between hepatic dysfunction (normal levels) and disseminated intravascular coagulation, if the latter is suspected by platelet count or blood smear (see Chapter 51).

If the patient presents with *vomiting,* a number of other laboratory studies should be ordered to identify a metabolic cause for the hepatomegaly (Table 22–7). A blood glucose level of less than 50 mg/dl suggests a defect in energy metabolism, whereas a blood glucose level greater than 100 mg/dl tends to rule out such a defect.

When a child is hypoglycemic, trace or absent ketones in the urine are not an adequate adaptive response, and a disorder in enzymatic or mitochondrial fatty acid oxidation or in hyperinsulinism is possible. Fatty acid oxidation disorders include defects of mitochondrial membrane-bound enzymes and defects of mitochondrial matrix enzymes. Carnitine determination (total and esterified/free ratio) and metabolite analysis (organic acids, acylcarnitines, and acylglycines) are used to establish a diagnosis and localize the defect. Medium-chain acyl dehydrogenase deficiency is a common cause of hypoglycemia without ketonuria.

The presence of large ketones in the urine when the blood glucose level is less than 50 mg/dl is evidence of normal fatty acid mobilization and oxidation and suggests the possibility of an organic aciduria, a defect in gluconeogenesis, liver failure, glycogen storage disease (GSD), or hereditary fructose intolerance (HFI). The combination of hypoglycemia, ketonuria, hepatomegaly, neurologic distress, and marked elevation of blood lactic levels suggests a primary lactic acidosis. The congenital lactic acidemias include disorders of gluconeogenesis, disorders of pyruvate metabolism, Krebs cycle disorders, and respiratory chain defects. Amino acid analysis and organic acid analysis may provide precise laboratory information for diagnosis of the lactic acidemias. The combination of prominent liver enlargement, hypoglycemia, elevated lactate levels, marked hypertriglyceridemia, and hyperuricemia suggests type I or type III glycogen storage disease. Cultured lymphocytes may be used to demonstrate the specific enzyme that is deficient. Clinical presentation of HFI depends entirely on exposure to fructose and sucrose. The younger the child and the higher the load, the more severe the reaction. Besides hypoglycemia, other major metabolic consequences of HFI are hyperuricemia, hypophosphatemia, and lactic acidosis.

Causes of elevated blood ammonia levels include inherited defects of urea cycle enzymes, disorders of organic acid metabolism, defects of mitochondrial fatty acid oxidation, liver failure, portosystemic shunting, and Reye syndrome. In urea cycle disorders, the routine laboratory analysis is dominated by the presence of hyperammonemia and respiratory alkalosis. Inherited defects in ureagenesis will be diagnosed from abnormal patterns of plasma amino acids and urinary orotic acid. Hyperammonemia and severe and persistent metabolic acidosis (associated with an elevated anion gap) suggest an organic acidemia. Most organic acidemias affect the intermediate metabolism of essential branch-chain amino acids isoleucine, leucine, and valine. A positive diagnosis of these disorders ultimately relies on urine organic acid analysis.

Fulminant hepatic failure is unlikely in the absence of jaundice. Portosystemic shunting would be suspected only in a patient with known chronic liver disease, prominent splenomegaly, and hematologic evidence of hypersplenism (see Chapter 23). Reye syndrome is suggested by the clinical presentation. The history is of a recent, usually febrile, illness (influenza, chickenpox) that is waning or has resolved. Aspirin therapy should be a *red flag* to consider Reye syndrome. Patients may experience an abrupt onset of vomiting that usually starts within 1 week following the prodromal illness. Coincident with the onset of vomiting, or shortly thereafter, signs of encephalopathy appear. There may be rapid sequential progression from malaise or lethargy to irritability, combativeness, confu-

Table 22–7. Laboratory Investigation of Patients with Hepatomegaly Associated with Prominent Vomiting and Altered Sensorium

> *Blood*
>   Electrolytes
>   Serum transaminases
>   Glucose
>   Ammonia
>   Lactic acid, pyruvate acid, lactate/pyruvate ratio
>   Uric acid
>   Ketone bodies
>   Carnitine (total, esterified/free ratio)
>   Acylcarnitine (esterified fraction of carnitine)
>   Amino acids
> *Urine* (first voided urine at time of presentation)
>   Ketone bodies and/or reducing substances
>   Organic acids
>   Amino acids
>   Acylcarnitine
>   Acylglycine
>   Drug screen

sion, disorientation, delirium, stupor, and coma (see Chapter 41). Although transaminases and ammonia levels are elevated, hypoglycemia and hyperbilirubinemia are not always noted in Reye syndrome. Ketonuria is classically present.

A liver biopsy may be necessary to diagnose various forms of chronic hepatitis or metabolic disease. Liver biopsy is necessary to diagnose chronic viral, drug-induced, or autoimmune hepatitis; steatonecrosis in cystic fibrosis or obesity; glycogen storage disease type IV; and hereditary fructose intolerance. Liver biopsy of patients with Wilson disease and alpha₁-antitrypsin deficiency may be employed to stage the degree of liver injury. Small duct primary sclerosing cholangitis may be suggested by liver biopsy (bile duct proliferation, fibrosis surrounding the bile ducts, and portal inflammation), but the findings are nonspecific.

USS - CT
Isotope

IMAGING STUDIES

A screening sonogram of the liver and abdomen is often the most readily available diagnostic imaging study that can be performed in patients with hepatomegaly. Careful attention to splenic size, renal size and character, gallbladder abnormalities, the presence of tumors, and liver character are crucial. Table 22–8 presents some imaging findings that correlate to systemic diseases.

Real-time ultrasound with pulsed Doppler sonography of the hepatic vessels is the initial modality of choice for evaluating hepatomegaly in the absence of laboratory evidence of hepatic injury or dysfunction. Liver masses, including neoplasms, abscesses, cysts, and hematomas, can be delineated by ultrasonography. Diffuse parenchymal liver disease, such as fatty infiltration or fibrosis, may be suspected by coarse increased parenchymal echogenicity, often associated with decreased visualization of hepatic vasculature and decreased through transmission. Phased blood flow in the hepatic veins is absent or reversed in hepatic venous outflow obstruction. Computed tomography (CT), angiography, or a liver-spleen scan is reserved for cases in which clearer anatomic delineation is needed.

DIAGNOSTIC CONSIDERATIONS

Table 22–9 summarizes an approach to the patient with an enlarged liver.

Hepatomegaly or hepatosplenomegaly may be associated with systemic disease that includes liver involvement. Systemic disorders in which the liver may be involved include cardiovascular disease, inflammatory bowel disease, collagen-vascular disorders, hematologic disorders, diabetes mellitus, systemic infection, and sarcoidosis. The degree of liver involvement associated with these disorders is highly variable, related to duration of hepatic process as well as to the underlying disorder. In general, the prognosis depends on the response of the underlying disorder to therapy.

Isolated hepatomegaly or hepatosplenomegaly may be caused by

Table 22–8. Helpful Radiologic Signs in the Evaluation of Hepatomegaly

Calcified adrenal glands	Wolman disease
Stippled epiphyses	GM₁ gangliosidosis
Calcified patella	Zellweger syndrome
Rickets	Tyrosinemia
Polycystic kidneys	Congenital hepatic fibrosis, Zellweger syndrome
Microgallbladder	Cystic fibrosis

a heterogeneous group of disorders that may include benign and malignant intrinsic liver tumors, congenital hepatic fibrosis, fatty liver, and chronic variants of certain storage diseases. Transaminase, alkaline phosphatase, and γ-glutamyltransferase levels may be mildly elevated but are rarely greater than three times normal. Regardless of cell type, most hepatic tumors are first detected as a mass or abdominal swelling on routine physical examination or during evaluation of common nonspecific gastrointestinal complaints, including upper abdominal pain, vomiting, diarrhea, anorexia, and weight loss.

Age at presentation of hepatomegaly definitely affects ranking of a differential diagnosis (see Tables 22–1 and 22–2). Acute or chronic viral hepatitis is in the differential at all ages beyond the neonatal period. In infants younger than 2 years of age, it is particularly important to consider metabolic disease, cystic fibrosis, infiltrative processes, and metastatic tumors. In older children and adolescents, autoimmune chronic hepatitis, alpha₁-antitrypsin deficiency, Wilson disease, congenital hepatic fibrosis, and hepatomegaly associated with systemic illness are common.

The combination of hypotonia, neurologic deterioration, and hepatomegaly in an infant should trigger an evaluation for disorders of peroxisomal metabolism or metabolic storage disease. Of the disorders of peroxisomal metabolism, only *Zellweger syndrome* (cerebrohepatorenal syndrome) is associated with hepatomegaly. Most patients with Zellweger syndrome are given a diagnosis as newborns or young infants based on a stereotypical phenotype, including severe hypotonia, mongoloid facies, high arched forehead, large fontanels, cryptorchidism, hypospadias, and hepatomegaly. Other important clues to the diagnosis are abnormal calcification of the patella, glomerulocystic kidney disease, and pigmented retinopathy.

Laboratory tests for diagnosis of defective peroxisomal metabolism include increased plasma levels of very-long-chain fatty acids, phytanic acid, and pipecolic acid and increased levels of urinary pipecolic acid and dicarboxylic and epoxydicarboxylic acids. Lethal or potentially lethal liver disease is almost universal in patients with Zellweger who survive the neonatal period. Liver biopsy reveals portal fibrosis or cirrhosis, abnormally shaped mitochondria, and absent peroxisomes on electron microscopy.

Niemann-Pick disease is an eponymic term that describes a group of sphingomyelin lipidoses. Type A is characterized by the involvement of both viscera and the CNS in infancy, rapid and fatal progression, and severe deficiency of sphingomyelinase. Before 6 months of age, patients with type A disease usually have an enlarged liver and spleen and failure to thrive, often associated with poor feeding patterns and emesis. By age 1 year, gross retardation of development of the CNS is evident.

The next most common phenotype is type C. In patients with type C disease, there is less obvious enlargement of the liver and spleen and the onset of neurologic abnormalities may be delayed until 2 to 6 years of age. The diagnosis of sphingomyelin lipidosis is suggested by cherry-red spots of the macula (see Chapter 44), vacuolation of leukocytes on peripheral smear, and foam cells in a bone marrow aspirate that are distinguishable from Gaucher cells (wrinkled tissue-paper appearance of cytoplasm) by phase microscopy. The definitive diagnosis is established by sphingomyelinase assay of cultured lymphocytes.

Gaucher disease applies to hereditary disorders in the metabolism of glucocerebrosides. The underlying defect appears to be deficient activity of β-glucosidase. Type 2 is the acute neuropathic form, characterized by the involvement of both viscera and CNS in infancy. The infant is usually normal at birth. By 3 months of age, hepatosplenomegaly is usually evident and is associated with difficulty in swallowing and feeding, chronic cough, and failure to thrive. Neurologic deficits are usually evident by 6 months of age; they tend to be stereotyped and feature cranial nerve and extrapyramidal tract involvement. The appearance of a child with hepatosplenomegaly who also has ocular palsy, retracted lips, the

Table 22–9. Evaluation of Patients with Hepatomegaly

Jaundice ─────────────────→ (+)   See Chapter 24

│
↓
(−)

│
↓

Prominent vomiting ─────────────→ (+)   Disorders of mitochondrial fatty acid oxidation
  or altered sensorium   Reye syndrome
                                         Congenital lactic acidemias
│   Disorders of gluconeogenesis
↓   Respiratory chain defects
(−)   Organic acidemias
                                         Urea cycle defects
│   Disorders of carbohydrate metabolism
↓   Glycogen storage disease I and III
                                           Hereditary fructose intolerance*
                                         Fulminant hepatic failure

Progressive neurologic ─────────────→ (+)   Peroxisomal disorders
  deterioration   Zellweger syndrome*
(−)   Lysosomal storage disease
                                             Niemann-Pick disease, Gaucher disease
│   GM$_1$ gangliosidosis
↓   Mucopolysaccharidosis
                                             Wilson disease*

Prominent elevation of ─────────────→ (+)   Acute hepatitis
  serum transaminase levels   Chronic hepatitis B, C, and D
(−)   Chronic drug-induced hepatitis*
                                             Autoimmune hepatitis*
│   Wilson disease*
↓   Alpha$_1$-antitrypsin deficiency*
                                             Sclerosing cholangitis*

Evidence of associated ─────────────→ (+)   Cardiovascular disease, right-sided heart failure*
  systemic disease   Inflammatory bowel disease
                                             Collagen vascular disease
│   Hematologic disorders
│   Leukemia
│   Familial erythrophagocytic lymphohistiocytosis*
│   Sickle cell disease
↓   Post–bone marrow transplant
(−)   Diabetes mellitus
                                             Systemic infection (see text)
│   Cystic fibrosis*
↓   Sarcoidosis

Isolated hepatomegaly ─────────────→ (+)   Hepatic tumors
  (with or without splenomegaly)   Fatty liver*
                                             Hepatic cysts
                                             Hepatic abscess
                                             Congenital hepatic fibrosis*
                                             Choledochal cyst
                                             Hepatic outflow obstruction*
                                             Glycogen storage disease type IV*
                                             Wolman disease*
                                             Cholesterol ester storage disease
                                             Niemann-Pick type B
                                             Gaucher disease (adult form)*
                                             Tyrosinemia*

*Diseases that may result in cirrhosis.

head held in hyperextension, and arms in a flexion position is suggests type 2 Gaucher disease. The diagnosis is established by the unique appearance of Gaucher cells on bone marrow aspirate.

GM₁ gangliosidosis presents as severe progressive cerebral degeneration within the first 2 years. It is associated with accumulation of a specific ganglioside in brain and of ganglioside and mucopolysaccharide in the viscera. The affected infant is severely retarded from birth. Hepatosplenomegaly is invariably present after 6 months of age. Bone deformities resembling *Hurler syndrome* (hypoplastic lumbar vertebral bodies, midshaft widening, periosteal "cloaking," pinching off of the ends of the humerus) are characteristic. Lymphocytes in the peripheral smear are vacuolated. The diagnosis is established by urinary assay for β-galactosidase.

The term *mucopolysaccharidosis* is used for a group of heritable diseases characterized by abnormal deposition in tissues and excretion in urine of acid mucopolysaccharides. The most prominent features are moderate dwarfism, striking facial appearance, hepatosplenomegaly (rarely isolated hepatomegaly), joint contractures, and mental retardation. The patient characteristically has a large head, hypertelorism, thick lips, a large tongue, and a prominent forehead covered by an abnormal amount of dark, coarse hair. The diagnosis is established by qualitative and quantitative determination of urinary mucopolysaccharides.

In about 40% of patients with *Wilson's disease,* neurologic or psychiatric symptoms are the first indication of illness. Neurologic onset has been reported in children as young as 6 years of age. The two major neurologic features of Wilson disease are a movement disorder and dystonia. Movement disorders include intention and resting tremors, titubation, dysmetria, scanning speech, illegible handwriting, and, rarely, choreiform movements. Dystonic symptoms include facial grimaces, cog wheel rigidity, drooling, dysphagia, and contractures. Sensory function and intelligence remain normal. Psychiatric symptoms include neuroses, schizophrenia, antisocial behavior, and manic-depressive psychosis. All patients with neurologic symptoms of Wilson disease should have corneal Kayser-Fleischer rings.

If the child with hepatomegaly or hepatosplenomegaly is accompanied by hepatocellular injury or dysfunction, *acute hepatitis* should be suspected. An acute process is suggested by recent onset of symptoms of fever, anorexia, malaise, nausea, vomiting, or pharyngitis; a history of exposure to a person with jaundice or known viral hepatitis; a history of drug or toxin exposure; and a normal serum albumin level. Most childhood cases of acute hepatitis produce minimal symptoms, are anicteric, and are suspected only by palpation of tender hepatomegaly in the context of a gastrointestinal flu-like illness. Mild splenomegaly may be present in 25% to 50% of patients. Hepatitis is confirmed by elevation of AST and ALT. Alkaline phosphatase levels are usually less than two times the upper limit of normal for age. Levels greater than three times normal should raise suspicion of biliary tract disease; in patients with high fever and adenopathy, cytomegalovirus (CMV) and Epstein-Barr virus (EBV) may be suspected. A decreased serum albumin or increased globulin level should raise suspicion of an acute flare of chronic liver disease. In the absence of a hepatitis A epidemic, serodiagnosis of acute hepatitis is best approached by testing for the major viral etiologic factors: hepatitis A virus (HAV), hepatitis B virus (HBV), hepatitis C virus (HCV), CMV, and EBV. The work-up includes anti-HAV IgM, hepatitis B surface antigen (HBsAg), anti-HB core antibody, anti-HCV (by second-generation enzyme-linked immunosorbent assay [ELISA] or second-generation recombinant immunoblot assay [RIBA-2]), anti-CMV IgM, and EBV serology. The finding of serum IgM anti-HAV is diagnostic of acute HAV infection because antibody is present at the time of clinical symptoms. A positive HBsAg suggests the diagnosis of HBV in a symptomatic patient. Anti-HCV does not appear in the circulation until 1 to 3 months after onset of acute illness and may not be demonstrated for up to 1 year.

Thus, unless the acute presentation is actually an acute flare of chronic HCV, serodiagnosis will await long-term follow-up.

All patients with suspected acute hepatitis should be questioned regarding recent medications, environmental exposure, or hepatic trauma. A serum and urine toxicology screen should be performed in cases of suspected overdose of hepatotoxic drugs or exposure to environmental toxins. A serum ceruloplasmin level should be obtained in all patients over 5 years of age to rule out Wilson disease, which may present with signs and symptoms indistinguishable from acute hepatitis. A chest radiograph and electrocardiogram (ECG) should be performed if there is any suspicion of low cardiac output states (i.e., acute myocarditis).

If a patient presents with hypoalbuminemia and hepatomegaly, an evaluation for suspected *chronic hepatitis* (Table 22–10) is warranted. Chronic hepatitis should be suspected in:

1. Patients with acute hepatomegaly with biochemical evidence of hypoalbuminemia.

2. Patients with prominent elevation of transaminase levels and biochemical evidence of liver dysfunction of 4 weeks' duration (indicating probable subacute hepatic necrosis).

3. Patients with persistent hepatomegaly or an elevated transaminase level of more than 3 months' duration. The typical symptoms of this presentation are nonspecific and include the insidious onset of fatigue, malaise, anorexia, arthralgias, or amenorrhea. The elevated transaminase level is generally more than three times normal.

The major causes of *chronic hepatitis* are infections with hepatitis viruses (B, C, and D). Initial studies, therefore, should look for serologic markers of chronic HBV infection (HBsAg, HBeAg, anti-HBc IgM and IgG, and anti-HDV), and HCV infection (anti-HCV, ELISA 2.0, RIBA-2). Other chronic systemic infections, such as EBV (persistent EBNA) and CMV (urine and blood CMV by PCR), may rarely be causes of chronic liver injury. The possibility of human immunodeficiency virus (HIV) infection should also be considered and pursued during initial evaluation if indicated.

Elevated levels of serum gamma globulin together with evidence of non–organ-specific autoantibodies, including antinuclear antibody (ANA), anti–smooth muscle antibody (SMA), and liver-kidney microsomal antibody (anti-LKM1), suggest autoimmune chronic hepatitis.

Classic autoimmune hepatitis is characterized by hyperglobulinemia, positive ANA and/or SMA. Females are predominantly affected. Chronic inflammatory disorders of other organs are not unusual, such as chronic ulcerative colitis, glomerulonephritis, thyroiditis, arthritis, scleroderma, and Sjogren's syndrome. All of these extrahepatic manifestations may precede the onset of the hepatic disease.

A less common presentation of autoimmune hepatitis is characterized by the absence of ANA and SMA and the presence of anti-LKM1. This presentation may also be associated with other autoimmune diseases. The specific diagnosis of chronic hepatitis depends on fulfilling time criteria for chronicity, ruling out other causes of chronic liver injury, and liver biopsy. Histologic findings include a lymphoplasmocytic portal infiltrate, extension of the inflammatory infiltrate beyond the limiting portal plate with piecemeal necrosis of periportal hepatocytes, and variable bridging necrosis and fibrosis between neighboring portal triads or portal triads and central veins. Even in the absence of anti-HCV, it is reasonable to evaluate biopsy specimens for evidence of hepatitis C using polymerase chain reaction (PCR) methods, especially in patients with anti-LKM.

Clinical manifestations of *Wilson disease* are rare before 5 years of age. Above this age, a work-up of chronic liver disease should always rule out this treatable disorder by measuring serum ceruloplasmin and 24-hour urinary copper excretion. Slit-lamp examination of the eyes for Kayser-Fleischer rings and sunflower cataracts should also be performed.

Type IV GSD (branching enzyme deficiency) presents with failure to thrive, hepatosplenomegaly, variable cardiac and neuromus-

Table 22–10. **Investigation of Suspected Chronic Hepatitis**

Cause	Diagnosis
Chronic hepatitis B	HB$_s$Ag, (−)IgM, anti-HBc, anti-HBe, HBeAg, HBV DNA
Chronic hepatitis C	Anti-HCV (ELISA 2.0 RIBA-2)
Chronic hepatitis D	HBsAg, Anti-HDV
Autoimmune hepatitis	1. Hyperglobulinemia, ANA, anti-SMA 2. (−) ANA, (−) anti-SMA, anti-LKM1 3. Anti-ANA, anti-SLA, anti-LP 4. Hyperglobulinemia alone
Wilson disease	Kayser-Fleischer rings, ceruloplasmin (<20 mg/dl) 24-hour urine copper (>100 mg/24 hr) Hepatic copper concentration (>250 mg/g dry weight)
Alpha$_1$-antitrypsin deficiency	Serum alpha$_1$-antitrypsin, alpha$_1$-antitrypsin phenotype
Sclerosing cholangitis	Direct visualization of abnormal biliary tree by cholangiography (ERCP, PTL, intraoperative cholangiography)
Chronic drug-induced hepatitis	Intake of drug associated with hepatotoxicity
Type IV glycogen storage disease	Characteristic abnormality on liver biopsy Verification of branching enzyme deficiency in cultured fibroblasts or leukocytes

Abbreviations: ANA = antinuclear antibody; DNA = deoxyribonucleic acid; ELISA = enzyme-linked immunosorbent assay; ERCP = endoscopic retrograde cholangiography; HBe = hepatitis Be antigen; HBcAg = hepatitis B core antigen; HBsAg = hepatitis B surface antigen; HBV = hepatitis B virus; HCV = hepatitis C virus; HDV = hepatitis D virus; Ig = immunoglobulin; LKM1 = liver-kidney microsomal antibody; SMA = smooth muscle antibody; RIBA = recombinant immunoblot assay; PTL = percutaneous transabdominal liver cholangiogram.

cular symptoms, and moderate elevations in serum transaminase and alkaline phosphatase levels between the ages of 3 and 15 months. Hypoglycemia is uncommon. The diagnosis is confirmed by identification of structurally abnormal deposits of glycogen in hepatocytes in liver biopsy and by verification of branching enzyme deficiency in cultured fibroblasts or leukocytes.

The chronic phase of *hereditary tyrosinemia* may also present in a similar fashion to type IV GSD. The diagnosis is suspected by a generalized amino aciduria, tyrosinemia and methioninemia, and is confirmed by an elevated urinary succinylacetone level.

Fructose-1-phosphate aldolase deficiency is suspected in young infants with intake of fructose-containing foods, failure to thrive, poor feeding, vomiting, and hepatomegaly. Suspicion is fostered by the presence of hypophosphatemia, hyperuricemia, transient hypoglycemia, and reducing substances in the urine. The diagnosis is confirmed by direct measure of fructose-1-phosphate in hepatic tissue samples.

Primary sclerosing cholangitis (PSC) is a chronic cholestatic liver disorder characterized by progressive obliterative fibrosing inflammation of extrahepatic, large intrahepatic, or small intrahepatic bile ducts or any combination of these. Although PSC most commonly presents with a cholestatic picture (characterized by jaundice and pruritus), patients may be asymptomatic with hepatomegaly as the only physical manifestation. Transaminase levels may be normal or only mildly elevated, but the serum alkaline phosphatase level is characteristically elevated. Most patients with primary sclerosing cholangitis have chronic inflammatory bowel disease. Antineutrophil cytoplasmic antibodies (ANCAs) are present in many of these patients. A suspicion of primary sclerosing cholangitis is an indication to perform endoscopic retrograde cholangiography (ERCP), which can confirm abnormalities in large bile ducts. The results may be normal in isolated small duct disease, which may be suggested only by liver biopsy or by a poor response of chronic active hepatitis to medical therapy.

Hepatic involvement is common in both *acute lymphocytic and acute myelogenous leukemia*. The symptoms of acute leukemia are the symptoms of acute marrow failure, which leads to anemia and thrombocytopenia. Diagnostic evaluation is triggered by abnormal leukocytosis. The liver is also involved in a variety of reactive histiocytic diseases.

Familial erythrophagocytic lymphohistiocytosis (FELS) is an autosomal recessive genetic disorder characterized by fever, failure to thrive, anemia, hypertriglyceridemia, and marked hepatosplenomegaly. Onset is usually within the first 3 months of life. Multiple organ involvement, including lymph nodes, lungs, the CNS, pericardium, bone, and soft tissue, should suggest FELS. Nonfamilial virus-associated hemophagocytic syndrome is a similar disorder that has been reported to follow a number of systemic infections, most commonly EBV. Clinical features in addition to hepatosplenomegaly include fever, myalgia, malaise, and lymphadenopathy.

Langerhans cell histiocytosis syndromes also produce variable hepatic, cutaneous, pulmonary and splenic infiltration by histiocytes, lymphocytes, and eosinophils. Again, generalized lymphadenopathy should be a diagnostic trigger. Liver biopsy reveals infiltration with histiocytes in all the histiocytic diseases.

Virtually all children with *sickle cell anemia* have hepatomegaly and elevated transaminase levels with or without hyperbilirubinemia. The liver disease is a result of a variety of factors, including focal parenchymal necrosis from intrahepatic sickling, congestion from myocardial dysfunction caused by iron overload or anemia, acquired hemachromatosis of the liver, and the high incidence of *post-transfusion chronic viral hepatitis*. The latter complication is also common in patients with hemophilia. Wilson disease should be considered in any patient with hepatomegaly and hemolysis. Hepatomegaly with signs of hepatic injury are also common following bone marrow transplantation. Causes include the chemotherapeutic induction regimen, various infections, parenteral nutrition, veno-occlusive disease, and graft-versus-host disease

Table 22–11 lists red flags in the history, physical examination, laboratory evaluation, and radiologic evaluation the may help the clinician in prioritizing a differential diagnosis.

Cirrhosis refers to the end-stage of virtually any liver disease. Cirrhosis results from a dynamic process that includes hepatocellular injury, fibrosis as a response to injury, and nodule formation as

Table 22–11. "Red Flags" Suggesting Chronic Liver Disease in a Patient with Hepatomegaly

History
  History of prolonged hyperbilirubinemia in infancy
  Family history of liver, neurologic, or psychiatric disease
  Previous blood transfusion, intravenous drug use
  Past history of hepatitis
  Delayed puberty

Physical Examination
  Hard or nodular liver
  Firm splenomegaly
  Ascites
  Prominent abdominal venous pattern
  Growth retardation
  Muscle wasting
  Clubbing
  Palmar erythema
  Spider angiomata
  Arthritis
  Papular acrodermatitis
  Presence of Kayser-Fleischer rings

Laboratory
  Decreased serum albumin

cells are replaced. As cirrhosis advances, liver architecture becomes more distorted, resulting in an uneven delivery of nutrients, oxygen, and metabolites to various segments of the liver. Portal hypertension, ascites, hepatic encephalopathy, and hepatorenal syndrome are complications of cirrhosis. Clinical manifestations of portal hypertension, in addition to splenomegaly, include variceal hemorrhage, ascites, and laboratory signs of hypersplenism (thrombocytopenia, leukopenia, and anemia). In early ascites, the only physical abnormality may be flank dullness that shifts when the patient changes position.

Endocrine Disorders

Hepatomegaly and mild elevations of transaminase levels and bilirubin are common in hypothyroidism and are occasionally observed in hyperthyroidism. Clinically, an enlarged liver is often found in patients with diabetes mellitus, particularly those with severe or poorly controlled diabetes, mainly as a result of excessive glycogen deposition. An extreme, rare case of this process is represented by *Mauriac syndrome,* which is characterized by dwarfism, obesity, moon faces, hypercholesterolemia, and marked hepatomegaly. Patients with *acromegaly* can also have mild to severe hepatomegaly as part of a generalized visceromegaly associated with the disease.

Systemic Infection

Hepatobiliary manifestations are protean in patients with *acquired immunodeficiency syndrome* (AIDS). Hepatomegaly may be present from a heterogeneous group of problems including viral hepatitis, opportunistic infections, drug-induced hepatic injury, malnutrition, peliosis hepatitis, AIDS cholangiopathy, and neoplasm. Pathologic features that are most typical of pediatric AIDS include giant cell transformation and diffuse parenchymal lymphoplasmocytic infiltrate, with the latter being associated with lymphoid interstitial pneumonitis. Hepatosplenomegaly and anicteric hepatitis

have been reported with cat-scratch disease, typhoid, brucellosis, tularemia, syphilis, Lyme disease, leptospirosis, Rocky Mountain spotted fever, Q fever, tuberculosis, and actinomycosis.

Fitz-Hugh-Curtis syndrome is a perihepatitis associated with acute salpingitis. Symptoms and signs include acute onset of severe right upper quadrant abdominal pain, friction rub over the anterior liver surface, and physical signs of pelvic inflammatory disease on pelvic examination. The diagnosis is confirmed by isolation of *Neisseria gonorrhoeae* or *Chlamydia trachomatis* from the cervix, urethra, or rectum.

Hepatic Abscess

A pyogenic, fungal, or parasitic hepatic abscess is an unusual infection in children. Common clinical findings are fever, abdominal pain, and hepatomegaly, with or without tenderness, and physical and x-ray evidence of ileus. Symptoms of respiratory infection are not uncommon, and chest radiography often reveals evidence of lower-lobe pneumonia.

Pyogenic abscesses occur most frequently in infants who have had sepsis or umbilical infections. Cases in older children are usually associated with underlying host defense defects, particularly HIV, chronic granulomatous disease and leukemia, or occurrence of previous blunt trauma to the liver. Pyogenic abscess may follow an episode of appendicitis. Liver abscess occurring in previously well children may also occur. *Staphylococcus aureus* and enteric and anaerobic bacteria are common etiologic agents. Liver function tests are commonly normal. Ultrasound or CT scan confirms the presence and number of lesions. Echogenic debris or gas may be seen. Distal acoustic enhancement is often present, suggesting a cystic origin.

Epidemiologically, *amebiasis* occurs in clusters in the southern United States, with person to person transmission associated with poor sanitation and crowding. Amebic abscess follows portal invasion of the parasite. The diagnosis is established by demonstrating a positive ELISA test for antibody to *Entamoeba histolytica,* or finding trophozoites or cysts in the stool. Toxocariasis and echinococcosis are caused by abortive infection of the liver in humans with the natural parasite of dogs or cats. The diagnosis is confirmed by specific serology.

Fatty Liver

Fatty infiltration, a nonspecific response to hepatocyte injury or metabolic derangement, should be suspected in patients with malnutrition, obesity, diabetes, cystic fibrosis, metabolic disorders, and chemotherapy; those who have received certain drugs (e.g., corticosteroids, methotrexate, tetracycline, valproic acid, salicylates), or those who have been exposed to a toxins (e.g., phosphorus or carbon tetrachloride). Fatty liver is commonly associated with inflammatory bowel disease, parenteral alimentation, HIV infection, Weber-Christian disease, fructose intolerance, abetalipoproteinemia, Wolman disease, and cholesterol ester storage disease. Hepatomegaly caused by fatty infiltration is reported to occur in 15% to 30% of obese subjects. It is important to remember that particularly in chronic obesity, steatosis may be associated with laboratory evidence of hepatic injury. Steatosis in adolescents may be accompanied by biopsy evidence of hepatic necrosis with Mallory bodies (steatohepatitis); in adults it has been reported to progress to cirrhosis.

Hepatic Tumors (see Chapter 26)

Overall, hepatic neoplasms are the third most common cause of solid non-brain tumors, after neuroblastoma and Wilms tumor.

Hepatic metastases can also occur with many childhood neoplasms, most frequently neuroblastoma, leukemia, and lymphoma. Fortunately, the primary tumor is almost always known. An exception is stage IV-S neuroblastoma, which may present as hepatomegaly in an otherwise normal-appearing infant in the first few months of life. Because stage IV-S metastasizes to skin and bone marrow, skin nodules should be a red flag. All patients with suspected neuroblastoma should undergo quantitative evaluation of serum ferritin and urinary catecholamine levels, including levels of homovanillic acid and vanillylmandelic acid (see Chapter 26).

Of primary hepatic tumors, benign liver tumors account for 33% of cases. Benign liver tumors include hemangioendotheliomas, mesenchymal hamartomas, focal nodular hyperplasia, and adenomas. Malignant tumors include hepatoblastoma, hepatocellular carcinoma, and undifferentiated embryonal cell sarcoma. Of all hepatic neoplasms, hepatoblastomas, hepatocellular carcinomas, and infantile hemangioendothelioma are the three most common, accounting for 65% of cases. Most hepatic tumors are asymptomatic or may present with abdominal distention, abdominal pain, weight loss, vomiting or diarrhea. A given lesion may present with acute abdominal pain due to hemorrhage into the tumor or peritoneal cavity.

Hemangioendotheliomas are the most common benign hepatic tumors. Nearly 95% of all hemangioendotheliomas present in the first year of life. Congestive heart failure may be present in 10% to 15% of cases. Hemangiomas of the skin, lungs, lymph nodes, pancreas, retroperitoneum, intestine, or bone as well as anemia suggest hemangioendothelioma. Diagnostic imaging is helpful in evaluation. Following the administration of intravenous contrast, intense peripheral or diffuse enhancement of the tumor becomes evident on CT scans. Delayed CT scans may show a gradual filling of the hypodense central portion over time.

Of mesenchymal hamartomas, 70% present in the first 2 years. Typically, a mesenchymal hamartoma, which consists of multiple cysts filled with serous fluid separated by myxomatous stroma, has no capsule. *Hepatic adenoma* is a rarely occurring benign tumor seen primarily in teenaged girls taking oral contraceptives, in children with diabetes mellitus or glycogen storage disease, and in patients receiving androgen therapy for Fanconi's anemia.

Focal nodular hyperplasia (FNH) is also seen predominantly in females and may occur at all ages. Both adenomas and FNH consist primarily of well-differentiated hepatocytes arranged in cords and plates but with normal lobular pattern. Serum alpha-fetoprotein (AFP) is normal in mesenchymal hamartoma, FNH, and adenoma. The diagnosis is confirmed by needle biopsy, usually with CT guidance.

Of malignant hepatic neoplasms, 68% of *hepatoblastomas* present before age 2 years and 90% by age 4. *Hepatocellular carcinoma*, which is associated with hepatitis B or hepatitis C infections of a chronic nature, and the less commonly seen undifferentiated embryonal sarcoma occur primarily in older children. Serum AFP measurement is the most useful marker of malignant liver tumors; 80% to 90% of hepatoblastomas and 60% to 90% of hepatocellular carcinoma are positive. Hepatoblastoma is distinguished from mesenchymal hamartoma by elevation of the AFP level, calcification on CT scans, and absence of prominent cystic component on sonograms. However, the diagnosis is usually established by biopsy before results of such testing can be completed. Hepatocellular carcinoma is associated with hereditary tyrosinemia, ataxia-telangiectasia, glycogenosis type I, chronic hepatitis B or C, and familial cholestatic cirrhosis, thus justifying screening these patients with serial AFP levels.

Hepatic Cysts

Solitary and traumatic cysts are uncommon. The origin of solitary cysts is unknown. Traumatic cysts are probably the sequelae of intrahepatic hemorrhage. *Peliosis hepatitis,* characterized by blood-filled spaces of varying sizes within the liver parenchyma, can be a complication of long-term treatment with anabolic steroids. Hepatomegaly, often tender, may be present before any evidence of liver biochemical abnormality is evident.

Congenital Hepatic Fibrosis

Congenital hepatic fibrosis is an autosomal recessive disorder characterized by hepatosplenomegaly, normal liver function tests, hypersplenism with thrombocytopenia, and kidney abnormalities. The latter consists either of renal tubular ectasia or polycystic kidney disease ("infantile type"). The liver is divided by bands of fibrous tissue, with multiple dysmorphic bile ducts of various sizes often located at the edge of the fibrous strands. The enlarged liver is firm or "hard" in all patients.

The normality of liver function tests is striking and should suggest the possibility of congenital hepatic fibrosis. For all practical purposes, the physical and biochemical findings together with a general increase in hepatic echogenicity and marked abnormal enlargement and echogenicity of the kidneys are diagnostic of congenital hepatic fibrosis. The diagnosis can be made unequivocally from a liver biopsy specimen but biopsy is indicated only in cases of equivocal renal findings.

Hepatic Venous Outflow Obstruction

Hepatic venous outflow obstruction is classified into three categories based on the level of obstruction:

- Intrahepatic (veno-occlusive disease [VOD])
- Hepatic veins
- Suprahepatic vena cava

Hepatic venous outflow obstruction presents with acute ascites and tender hepatomegaly. Abdominal pain, distention, and splenic enlargement may be prominent. Minimal elevations of the transaminase or serum bilirubin level are present in the acute stage.

The pathologic hallmark of veno-occlusive disease is occlusion of central and sublobular hepatic veins by intimal edema and fibrosis. The illness classically follows ingestion of plants that contain a toxic pyrrolizidine alkaloid *(Senecio, Crotalaria, Heliotropium)*, the leaves of which are used in bush teas, herbal medicines, or may contaminate poorly winnowed wheat. Veno-occlusive disease may also occur as a hepatic response to irradiation and chemotherapy for bone marrow transplantation. A familial form of veno-occlusive disease associated with immunodeficiency has also been reported.

Budd-Chiari syndrome is defined as a noncardiogenic hepatic venous outflow obstruction. It develops in a variety of conditions that predispose to thrombosis, including intake of oral contraceptives, pregnancy, previous trauma, tumor invasion, cirrhosis, inflammatory bowel disease, collagen-vascular disease, protein C deficiency, sickle cell anemia, polycythemia vera, and lymphoproliferative disorders. Membranous obstruction of the suprahepatic vena cava is the most common cause of suprahepatic outflow obstruction. However, thrombosis of the suprahepatic vena cava can occur in any condition that may precipitate Budd-Chiari syndrome. Diagnostic evaluation begins with pulsed Doppler sonography of the hepatic vessels. Liver-spleen scintigraphy may be helpful if it reveals diminished uptake in the right and left lobes and increased uptake in the caudate lobe that drains directly into the vena cava. Liver biopsy in hepatic outflow obstruction reveals a characteristic pattern of sinusoidal dilatation with centrilobular congestion. Cirrhosis is a poor prognostic sign.

THERAPEUTIC CONSIDERATIONS

See also Chapter 24.

Acute Viral Hepatitis

There is no specific treatment for acute viral hepatitis. Most can be managed at home. No restrictions of diet or ambulation are required. The traditional recommendations of bed rest and a high-carbohydrate, low-fat diet have been shown to have no effect on symptoms or duration of disease. Small, frequent feedings may be helpful. The key for both the patient and household contacts is personal hygiene. Siblings should avoid contact with the patient even after they have received immunoprophylaxis. In HAV, shedding of the virus may occur for up to 2 weeks after onset of jaundice. Patients should be kept at home during this time, after which they may return to school even if still with residual icterus. The major complications of acute hepatitis are dehydration and fulminant hepatitis. A prolonged PT, severe emesis, dehydration, or altered mental status are indications for hospitalization.

Drug-Induced Hepatitis

Most drug-induced liver disease resolves spontaneously when the offending drug is withdrawn. The use of steroids in drug-induced liver disease remains controversial. Steroid therapy should be considered when severe acute hepatitis dominates a multisystem hypersensitivity reaction. Acetylcysteine should be given for significant acetaminophen ingestions, preferably by the oral route and within 18 to 24 hours of ingestion.

Autoimmune Chronic Hepatitis

In most children with autoimmune chronic hepatitis, immunosuppressive therapy with corticosteroids, with or without azathioprine, can prevent further deterioration of liver function. The goal of treatment is remission, as defined by a decline in transaminase levels to less than twice the upper limit of the normal range and by a reduction in hepatic inflammation to normal or minimal portal hepatitis. Remission can be achieved in more than 65% of patients. Children with LKM antibodies tend to have more severe liver disease at presentation and to respond less satisfactorily to immunosuppression than the more classic presentation. Enrichment of bile with the oral administration of ursodeoxycholic acid is effective in improving biochemical markers of liver function in patients with chronic active hepatitis.

Chronic Hepatitis Due to Hepatitis B Virus

Treatment of biopsy-proven chronic hepatitis B is indicated in patients with replicating virus as shown by positive HBeAg or HBV DNA. Treatment is indicated because of the natural history of the infection, the risk of hepatocellular carcinoma in those chronically infected, and the infectivity of those patients in the high replicative phase of infection. The only agent shown to be effective in treating chronic hepatitis B viral infection is interferon-α. The goal of treatment should be to move the patient to a low replicative phase of infection (loss of HBeAg and formation of anti-HBe). Loss of HBV replication occurs in approximately 50% of treated patients (loss of HBV-DNA and HBsAg). Several factors, including histologic evidence of inflammation extending beyond the portal area, a serum ALT level greater than 100 IU/L, HBV-DNA level less than 100 pg/ml, female sex, and contraction of the disease in adulthood, are predictive variables of a likely response to interferon. Inflammation confined to the portal area, HBV-DNA greater than 200 pg/ml, serum ALT less than 100 IU/L, acquisition of the disease in childhood, and co-infection with either HIV or hepatitis D virus (HDV) are associated with a poor response to therapy.

Chronic hepatitis due to hepatitis B virus must be distinguished from chronic carriers with hepatitis B surface antigen (in the latter case, there is no treatment and no evidence of hepatic inflammation).

Chronic Hepatitis C

Because symptoms and biochemical liver tests do not correlate with histologic findings, serial liver biopsies are necessary to assess progression of disease. Patients with chronic inflammation extending beyond the portal area or cirrhosis should be considered for treatment. The current recommendation for treatment of chronic active hepatitis C is recombinant interferon-α_{2b}. The goal of treatment should be to eliminate the virus, improve liver tests, and reduce hepatic inflammation. The high relapse rate observed after interferon treatment of chronic hepatitis C suggests that the antiviral properties of the drug act to control the deleterious effects of HCV infection but do not eradicate the virus or cure the disease.

Congenital Hepatic Fibrosis

The mains risks of congenital hepatic fibrosis are gastrointestinal bleeding complicating portal hypertension and cholangitis related to bacterial infection of dilated intrahepatic bile ducts. Hypersplenism is not an indication for splenectomy. Portosystemic shunting has been the treatment of choice following significant episodes of gastrointestinal bleeding. Alternatively, sclerotherapy or pharmacologic management of varices may be attempted in younger patients on the chance that spontaneous portosystemic shunts will develop later in childhood. Unexplained fever or serologic evidence of inflammation (elevated white blood cell count, sedimentation rate, or serum total globulin level) warrants a diagnostic liver biopsy to culture for cholangitis. Any manipulation of the extrahepatic biliary tree in patients with congenital hepatic fibrosis carries an increased risk for development of cholangitis.

Liver Abscess

Surgical drainage and appropriate antibiotic therapy remain the mainstay of therapy for liver abscess. There are now several methods of drainage available. In addition to transperitoneal open drainage and extraserous drainage, which avoids exposing the peritoneal cavity to possible contamination with infected material, it is now possible to perform percutaneous aspiration and placement of drains under ultrasonic or CT guidance. Multiple abscesses that are not amenable to complete surgical drainage have also been successfully cured with prolonged antibiotic therapy alone. Uncomplicated deep amebic liver abscesses are best managed conservatively with oral metronidazole and observation. For the refractory case or for active subcapsular subphrenic abscesses, percutaneous aspiration or open drainage should be performed. Toxocariasis and echinococcosis are treated by careful surgical removal of the cysts.

Hepatic Outflow Obstruction

For patients with hepatic outflow obstruction, efforts should be focused on treatment of the underlying predisposing factors. Medical therapy of thrombotic occlusion has not been successful. Percutaneous transhepatic angioplasty and venous stent placement has been successful in a small number of patients. Surgical therapy is directed at excision of obstruction or portosystemic decompression. Patients with evidence of cirrhosis should be considered candidates for liver transplantation.

Liver Tumors

For benign tumors, such as mesenchymal hamartomas, focal nodular hyperplasia, adenomas, and hemangioendotheliomas, surgery may be unnecessary. Mesenchymal hamartomas, focal nodular hypoplasia, and adenomas that are asymptomatic can be followed with ultrasonography and resected if symptoms develop or progressive enlargement occurs. Some adenomas may regress after contraceptive steroids are discontinued. Hemangioendothelioma may regress following steroid or interferon therapy. The primary goal in treating malignant liver neoplasms is complete surgical removal, followed by postsurgical chemotherapy. When surgery for malignancy is deemed too risky, preoperative chemotherapy has proved effective in shrinking some hepatoblastomas and sarcomas to the point of resectability.

Alpha₁-Antitrypsin Deficiency

There is no specific medical therapy for alpha₁-antitrypsin deficiency. Liver transplantation is indicated for patients with progressive liver disease.

Wilson Disease

Wilson disease is a rare autosomal recessive disorder of copper metabolism. Although the basic biochemical defect is unknown, it appears to be localized within the liver. Treatment includes dietary copper restriction and copper chelation with D-penicillamine or, alternatively, triethylene tetramine dihydrochloride for those with penicillamine toxicity. The role of zinc as an alternative to D-penicillamine for producing negative copper balance is being explored. Liver transplantation cures Wilson disease but is reserved for patients who present with a clinical picture of fulminant hepatitis, patients with severe liver dysfunction that does not improve after 2 to 3 months of adequate chelation therapy, or patients who have been effectively treated but who have severe progressive liver dysfunction after they stop taking D-penicillamine.

Glycogen Storage Disease

Treatment of type I GSD is aimed at providing exogenous glucose at rates that slightly exceed those of normal hepatic glucose production. This includes frequent carbohydrate feedings during the day and continuous overnight intragastric infusions of glucose or glucose polymers. In some patients, feeding of 1 to 2 g/kg of uncooked corn starch suspensions every 6 hours has been effective as a slowly absorbed form of carbohydrate. Most patients require treatment with allopurinol to prevent hyperuricemia and renal stone formation. Liver transplant, which cures GSD type I, is usually only considered in patients with enlarging adenomas raising concern of evolution to hepatocellular carcinoma.

In type III GSD, use of high-protein, low-carbohydrate diet blunts the tendency toward postprandial hypoglycemia. The diet differs from that used for type I GSD because gluconeogenesis is not compromised.

Patients with type II GSD also commonly require overnight continuous intragastric feedings. Hypoglycemia may occur in type IV GSD and type XI GSD but is usually not a problem. Treatment of type XI GSD is directed at correcting the renal tubular disturbances with phosphate and alkali supplements.

Patients with type IV GSD in most cases require liver transplantation because of progressive liver dysfunction. Types VI and IX disease are usually benign, and little or no treatment is required.

Defects of Fatty Acid Oxidation

Management of acute crises warrants institution of intravenous dextrose, even if the blood glucose level is only mildly reduced. The goal of glucose infusion is to raise insulin levels sufficiently to inhibit the need for fatty acid oxidation. Reversal of neurologic symptoms may take several days in severely ill patients. During the recovery phase, intravenous fat emulsions should be avoided. In light of the high risk of mortality during episodes of fasting-induced coma, avoidance of fasting is the mainstay of chronic therapy. The level of nutritional intervention is based on the specific defect. The role of I-carnitine supplementation in both acute and chronic management remains controversial in all defects of fatty acid oxidation except carnitine transport defects.

SUMMARY AND RED FLAGS

Hepatomegaly that is persistent suggests a chronic illness, which with time may produce serious morbidity or mortality, despite an initially well-appearing patient. It is important to determine whether the hepatomegaly is isolated as a result of a specific liver disease or whether it is part of a generalized systemic illness affecting other organs. *Red flags* include signs of acute hepatic failure (coma, hemorrhage), developmental delay, failure to thrive, and those noted in Table 22–11.

REFERENCES

Definition of Hepatomegaly

Lawson EE, Grand RJ, Neff RK, Cohen LF. Clinical estimation of liver span in infants and children. Am J Dis Child 1978;132:474.
Younoszai MK, Mueller S. Clinical assessment of liver size in normal children. Clin Pediatr 1975;14:378.

Assessment of Liver Function and Injury in Children

Malle ES. Laboratory assessment of liver function and injury in children. *In* Suchy FJ (ed). Liver Disease in Children. St. Louis: CV Mosby, 1994:269.

Hepatomegaly with Prominent or Relapsing Vomiting or Acute Central Nervous System Deterioration

Coates PM, Hale DE. Inherited abnormalities in mitochondrial fatty acid oxidation. *In* Walker WA, Durie PR, Hamilton JR, et al (eds). Pediatric Gastrointestinal Disease: Pathophysiology • Diagnosis • Management. Philadelphia: BC Decker, 1991:965.

Huebi JE, Partin JC, Partin JS, et al. Reye's syndrome: Current concepts. Hepatology 1987;7:155.

Hers H, VanHoff F, deBarsy T. Glycogen storage disease *In* Stanbury JB, Wyngarden JB, Frederikson DS (eds). The Metabolic Basis of Inherited Disease, 6th ed. New York: McGraw-Hill, 1989:425.

Hepatomegaly with Progressive Neurological Deterioration

Beutler E. Modern diagnosis and treatment of Gaucher's disease. Am J Dis Child 1993;147:1175.

Hardikar W, Suchy FJ. Lysosomal storage disorder. *In* Suchy FJ (ed). Liver Disease in Children. St. Louis, CV Mosby, 1994:819.

Kelly D, Portmann B, Mowart A, et al. Niemann-Pick disease type C: Diagnosis and outcome in children, with particular reference to liver disease. J Pediatr 1993;123:242.

Hepatomegaly with Prominent Evidence of Liver Injury

Balistreri WF. Viral hepatitis. Pediatr Clin North Am 1988;35:375.

Crosignani A, Battezzati PM, Setchell DDR, et al. Effects of ursodeoxycholic acid on serum liver enzymes and bile acid metabolism in chronic active hepatitis: A dose response study. Hepatology 1991;13:339.

Debray D, Pariente D, Urvoas E, et al. Sclerosing cholangitis in children. J Pediatr 1994;124:49.

Hoofnagle JH, DiBisceglie AM. Serologic diagnosis of acute and chronic viral hepatitis. Semin Liver Dis 1991;11:73.

Ibarquen E, Gross CR, Savik SK, et al. Liver disease in alpha₁-antitrypsin deficiency: Prognostic indicators. J Pediatr 1990;117:864.

Isenberg JN. Cystic fibrosis: Its influence on the liver, biliary tree, and bile salt metabolism. Semin Liver Dis 1982;2:302.

Lee WM. Review article: Drug induced hepatotoxicity. Aliment Pharmacol Ther 1993;7:477.

Maddrey WC, Combs B. Therapeutic concepts for the management of idiopathic autoimmune chronic hepatitis. Semin Liver Dis 1991;11:248.

Stemlieb I. Perspectives on Wilson's disease. Hepatology 1990;12:1234.

Walshe JM. Wilson's disease presenting with features of hepatic dysfunction: A clinical analysis of eighty-seven patients. Q J Med 1989;70:253.

Hepatomegaly As a Manifestation of Systemic Disease

Kastenberg DM, Friedman LS. Hepatobiliary complications of inflammatory bowel disease. *In* Rustgi UK, VanThiel DH (eds). The Liver in System Disease. New York: Raven Press, 1993:61.

Mace S, Borkat G, Liebman J. Hepatic dysfunction and cardiovascular abnormalities. Am J Dis Child 1985;139:60.

Schaller J, Beckwith B, Wedgewood RJ. Hepatic involvement in juvenile rheumatoid arthritis. J Pediatr 1970;77:203.

Schubert TT. Hepatobiliary system in sickle cell disease. Gastroenterology 1986;90:2013.

Hepatomegaly without Prominent Evidence of Hepatocellular Injury and Dysfunction

Bennett WF, Bova JG. Review of hepatic imaging and a problem-oriented approach to liver masses. Hepatology 1990;12:761.

Gentil-Kocher S, Bernard O, Bruneile F, et al. Budd-Chiari syndrome in children: Report of 22 cases. J Pediatr 1988;113:30.

Stocker JT. Hepatic tumors in children. *In* Suchy FJ (ed). Liver Disease in Children. St. Louis, CV Mosby 1994:901.

23 Splenomegaly

Susan B. Shurin

Enlargement of the spleen, or splenomegaly, is usually defined by physical examination. In adults, the most dependable sign of enlargement is that the spleen is palpable below the left costal margin. In children, palpable spleens may not actually be enlarged because of the relatively larger volume of the spleen compared with the size of the abdomen. Splenomegaly may be isolated or combined with hepatomegaly (hepatosplenomegaly or visceromegaly) (see Chapter 22).

Proper attention must be paid to techniques of the physical examination because an enlarged spleen may be missed, particularly in a struggling child who will not quietly lie down. Careful physical assessment requires that the patient be *supine* or in the *right recumbent position,* that the examiner be on the patient's

right side (Fig. 23–1). Creative play is sometimes necessary, with the use of pacifiers or bottles; a child is frequently more relaxed on the mother's lap than on the examining table. A very enlarged spleen is frequently visibly enlarged, with fullness of the left side of the abdomen.

Beginning in the right iliac fossa (to avoid missing a grossly enlarged spleen or liver with extension of the left hepatic lobe into the splenic area in the left upper quadrant), the right hand should move toward the left upper quadrant to find the spleen's lower pole or medial border. The examiner's left hand is placed in the patient's left flank, and gentle displacement of the thoracic cage toward the examiner's right hand often displaces the spleen forward enough to make it appreciable. The spleen should move downward with

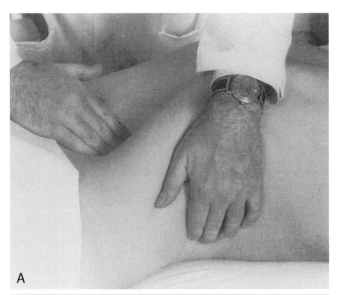

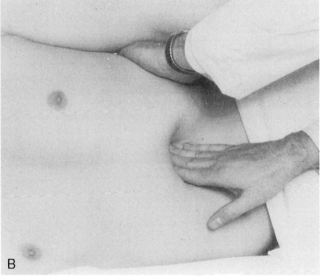

Figure 23–1. *A, B,* Techniques for splenic palpation. (From Swartz MH. Textbook of Physical Diagnosis: History and Examination. Philadelphia: WB Saunders, 1989:345.)

inspiration. It is equally important for the examiner to touch the spleen as it is for the spleen to ''touch'' the examiner during its descent with inspiration. Too aggressive palpation may push the spleen away, whereas gentle or light palpation permits the examiner to feel the spleen's edge passively. The characteristic notch in the medial or inferior border may not be palpable when the spleen is enlarged only a few centimeters, but it usually clearly distinguishes an enlarged spleen from other abdominal masses on the examination alone. Because the extent to which the spleen extends below the costal margin depends heavily on the patient's position, the extent of the spleen below the costal margin should be measured with the patient supine. Measurement from the left costal margin to the lower pole of the spleen defines the splenic axis. Ordinarily, the long axis of the spleen is along the length of the tenth rib. As it enlarges, it extends medially and downwards along the rib.

Percussion over the lower ribs may detect splenomegaly that is not evident on palpation, especially if splenic dullness extends medially beyond the left anterior axillary line.

Masses in the left upper quadrant, especially left renal masses, may be difficult to distinguish from an enlarged spleen (see Chapter 26). Generally, the presence of the splenic notch helps to identify the mass as a spleen, but nodular masses, such as Wilms tumor of the kidney, neuroblastoma, and retroperitoneal teratomas may masquerade as splenomegaly. Imaging studies, such as ultrasonography and computed tomography (CT), usually resolve such questions.

The spleen contains large amounts of lymphoid tissue and normally atrophies as the patient ages, reducing in weight from about 280 g to 35 g. Up to 30% of full-term neonates, 5% to 15% of children, and 3% of college freshmen have palpable spleens.

Many enlarged spleens are not palpable on physical examination because of their relationship to other organs and the thoracic cage. Hyperinflation of lungs (caused by asthma, bronchiolitis, ipsilateral pneumothorax) may make a normal-sized liver and spleen palpable. Some spleens that are repeatedly palpable are not affected by any pathology. Nonetheless, a persistently enlarged spleen should be considered to be potentially affected with significant pathology.

It is important to keep the anatomy of the spleen in mind when considering the disease processes that may lead to splenic enlargement. The spleen consists of red pulp and white pulp, contains large amounts of lymphoid tissue and macrophages, and is heavily involved in immunologic reactions. It is the graveyard of senescent blood cells; red blood cell destruction is a normal function of the spleen. Sensory innervation of the spleen is limited to the capsule; pain with enlargement of the spleen is characteristic of rapid enlargement with stretching of the capsule, or inflammatory processes generating cytokines that cause pain. The splenic blood supply is closely linked to the portal system, and increased pressure in the portal system is transmitted to the spleen.

DIFFERENTIAL DIAGNOSIS (Table 23–1)

History

Historical Features. Many of the common causes of splenomegaly in children are greatly elucidated by the personal and family histories. Key elements to determine are exposure to drugs and infectious agents, results of previous physical examinations and laboratory tests, and ethnic background of the family.

Chief Complaint. It is crucial to determine whether the enlargement of the spleen is *acute* or *chronic*, and whether it is directly related to the child's symptoms. Incidental splenic enlargement is much more likely to represent a more chronic process than is splenomegaly noted as part of evaluation of an acute illness. Symptoms referable to the left upper quadrant, such as fullness or pain (even referred to the left shoulder), indicate that the splenic capsule is being stretched and is causing symptoms that the patient or parent is able to appreciate as different from the baseline. Asymptomatic splenic enlargement noted at a well-child examination in a 5-year-old child is more likely to be due to a *storage disease* than to acute leukemia; *pain on palpation* of a spleen implies that the capsule has been stretched acutely and suggests the presence of acute infection or hemolysis rather than a chronic process, such as a storage disease.

Nonspecific symptoms, or symptoms referable to other organ systems, suggest diagnoses in which the splenomegaly is a secondary, rather than a primary, process. Bone pain, fevers, lethargy, and bruising suggest bone marrow infiltration (acute leukemia); jaundice and ascites suggest primary liver disease.

Past Medical History. In the neonatal period, placement of umbili-

Table 23–1. Differential Diagnosis of Splenomegaly by Pathophysiology

Anatomic Lesions
Cysts, pseudocysts (see Fig. 23–2)
Hamartomas
Polysplenia syndrome
Hemangiomas and lymphangiomas
Hematoma or rupture (traumatic) (see Fig. 23–3)

Hyperplasia Due to Hematologic Disorders

Acute and Chronic Hemolysis*
    Hemoglobinopathies (sickle cell disease in infancy with or without sequestration crisis and sickle variants, thalassemia
        major, unstable hemoglobins)
    Erythrocyte membrane disorders (hereditary spherocytosis, elliptocytosis, pyropoikilocytosis)
    Erythrocyte enzyme deficiencies (severe G6PD deficiency, pyruvate kinase deficiency)
    Immune hemolysis (autoimmune and isoimmune hemolysis)
    Paroxysmal nocturnal hemoglobinuria
Chronic Iron Deficiency

Extramedullary Hematopoiesis
    Severe hemolytic anemias
    Myeloproliferative diseases: chronic myelogenous leukemia (CML), juvenile CML, myelofibrosis with myeloid metaplasia
    Osteopetrosis
    Patients receiving granulocyte and granulocyte-macrophage colony-stimulating factors

Infections†

Bacterial
    Acute sepsis: *Salmonella typhi, Streptococcus pneumoniae, Haemophilus influenzae* type b, *Staphylococcus aureus*
    Chronic infections: infective endocarditis, chronic meningococcemia, brucellosis, tularemia, cat-scratch disease
    Local infections: splenic abscess (*S. aureus,* streptococci, less often *Salmonella,* polymicrobial), pyogenic liver abscess
        (anaerobic bacteria, gram-negative enteric bacteria), cholangitis
Viral*
    Acute viral infections, especially in children
    Congenital cytomegalovirus (CMV), *Herpes simplex,* rubella
    Hepatitis A, B, and C, CMV
    Epstein-Barr virus (EBV)
    Psittacosis
    Viral hemophagocytic syndromes: CMV, EBV, HHV-6
    Human immunodeficiency virus (HIV)
Spirochetal
    Syphilis, especially congenital syphilis
    Lyme disease
    Leptospirosis
Rickettsial
    Rocky Mountain spotted fever
    Q fever
    Typhus
Fungal/Mycobacterial
    Miliary tuberculosis
    Disseminated histoplasmosis
    South American blastomycosis
    Systemic candidiasis (in immunosuppressed patients) (see Fig. 23–4)
Parasitic
    Malaria
    Toxoplasmosis, especially congenital
    Toxocara canis, Toxocara cati (visceral larva migrans)
    Leishmaniasis (kala-azar)
    Schistosomiasis (hepatic-portal involvement)
    Trypanosomiasis
    Fascioliasis

Table 23–1. Differential Diagnosis of Splenomegaly by Pathophysiology *Continued*

Immunologic and Inflammatory Processes*

Collagen vascular diseases
    Systemic lupus erythematosus
    Rheumatoid arthritis
    Mixed connective tissue disease
    Systemic vasculitis
    Serum sickness
    Drug hypersensitivity, especially to phenytoin
    Graft-versus-host disease
    Sjögren syndrome
    Cryoglobulinemia
    Amyloidosis
    Inflammatory bowel disease
    Myasthenia gravis
    Sarcoidosis
    Large granular lymphocytosis and neutropenia
    Histiocytosis syndromes
    Hemophagocytic syndromes (nonviral, familial)
    Graves disease
    Hashimoto thyroiditis

Malignancies

Primary: leukemia (acute, chronic), lymphoma, angiosarcoma, Hodgkin disease
Metastatic

Storage Diseases

Lipidosis (Gaucher disease, Niemann-Pick disease, infantile GM_1 gangliosidosis)
Mucopolysaccharidoses (Hurler, Hunter-type)
Mucolipidosis (I-cell disease, sialidosis, multiple sulfatase deficiency, fucosidosis)
Defects in carbohydrate metabolism: galactosemia, fructose intolerance
Sea-blue histiocyte syndrome
Amyloidosis

Congestive*

Congestive heart failure
Intrahepatic cirrhosis
Extrahepatic portal (thrombosis), splenic, and hepatic vein obstruction (thrombosis, Budd-Chiari syndrome)

*Common.
†Chronic or recurrent infection suggests underlying immunodeficiency.
Abbreviations: G6PD = glucose-6-phosphate dehydrogenase; HHV = human herpes virus-6.

cal catheters may induce thrombosis and persistent obstruction in a number of blood vessels, particularly the extrahepatic portal vein, which may lead to congestive splenomegaly. Exchange transfusion not only requires an umbilical catheter but is usually performed for hematologic indications (hemolysis) that may independently lead to splenomegaly (hereditary spherocytosis).

Certain previous infections may be followed by splenomegaly. These infections include hepatitis, mononucleosis, and malaria. Drugs that may cause liver disease may lead to portal hypertension, which may in turn lead to splenomegaly.

Past surgeries that may provide clues to the cause of splenomegaly include abdominal procedures, especially in the upper abdomen, or any hepatic procedures, and cardiac surgery, which may be followed by blood-borne infections (hepatitis, CMV), thrombosis, portal hypertension, or congestive heart failure.

Abdominal trauma acutely may produce a splenic hematoma (Fig. 23–3) or chronically may be followed by development of a splenic pseudocyst.

Family History. Both ethnic background and medical histories of specific family members must be elicited to identify potential patterns of inheritance. Frequently, family members may not be aware of the specific diagnosis, and a history of anemia, cholecystectomy (for hemolytic anemia–associated bilirubin biliary stones), and splenectomy (for hemolytic anemia) may be known instead. Identification of Mediterranean (thalassemia, glucose-6-phosphate dehydrogenase [G6PD] deficiency), African (sickle cell anemia, G6PD deficiency), southern Asian (thalassemia, G6PD deficiency), or Ashkenazi Jewish (storage disease) ancestry in patients with splenomegaly is helpful in identifying an inherited process.

Red cell membrane disorders, such as hereditary spherocytosis, may occur in any ethnic group, whereas hereditary elliptocytosis and hereditary pyropoikilocytosis occur in persons of African descent. *Red cell enzyme disorders* are associated with splenomegaly only when hemolysis is chronic. Pyruvate kinase deficiency is found primarily in persons of northern European descent (Irish, English, German). It is an autosomal recessive disorder; parental consanguinity greatly increases the probability. Severe G6PD deficiency is associated with chronic hemolysis and splenomegaly in persons of Mediterranean and southern Asian descent. G6PD deficiency is X-linked so males are more often affected.

Hemoglobinopathies frequently have associated splenomegaly. β-*Thalassemia intermedia* and *major* occur in persons of Mediterranean, Middle Eastern, southern Asian, and African extraction. Hemoglobin E occurs with a gene frequency of up to 50% in some areas of southeast Asia. Sickle cell variants—especially hemoglobin SC and S-thalassemia—are seen primarily in persons of African descent but may occur in Mediterranean populations as well. The spleen is usually palpable in young infants with sickle cell disease but the spleen autoinfarcts by 12 to 15 months of age. Sudden onset of splenomegaly should suggest acute splenic sequestration crisis (see Chapter 49).

Ashkenazi Jewish heritage raises the question of Gaucher disease and other storage diseases. Osteopetrosis is an autosomal recessive disorder without ethnic patterns of inheritance.

Review of Systems

Systemic symptoms, such as fever and weight loss, are seen in many disorders that manifest splenomegaly, particularly infections, malignancies, and inflammatory or granulomatous processes, such as histiocytosis and sarcoid. A careful drug history is also important. Exposure to infectious agents, or travel history that might result in exposure to infectious agents unusual for the present community (malaria, leishmaniasis, schistosomiasis, trypanosomiasis) should be determined. Social and behavioral issues of parents, children, and adolescents heavily affect certain risks and exposures. Chief among these issues are homosexual or promiscuous sexual behavior, regardless of sexual orientation, or intravenous and illicit drug exposure, all of which may expose patients to hepatitis, cytomegalovirus, and human immunodeficiency virus (HIV). Sexual abuse may place even young children at risk, and accurate histories may be extremely difficult to elicit (see Chapter 37).

Specific information related to systems may help focus further evaluation.

Skin. Pallor suggests anemia (hemolysis, bone marrow infiltration, hypersplenism); purpura and petechiae suggest thrombocytopenia (bone marrow failure, autoimmune disorder, hypersplenism); and jaundice suggests hemolytic anemia, or liver dysfunction, or both. Itching may also suggest liver disease. Rashes caused by a variety of acute and chronic infections, systemic lupus erythematosus (SLE), rheumatoid arthritis, infective endocarditis, histiocytosis, and hemangiomata that are part of a systemic process involving the spleen may provide cutaneous clues to splenic pathology.

Head, Eyes, Ears, Nose, and Throat. Conjunctival icterus may be easier to appreciate than cutaneous jaundice. Cherry red retinal spots or cloudy corneas suggest storage diseases (see Chapter 44).

Cardiovascular. Dyspnea, orthopnea, and fatigue suggest anemia or congestive heart failure. A previously identified murmur or a changing murmur raises the suspicion of infective endocarditis (see Chapter 16).

Respiratory. Dyspnea, cough, and tachypnea suggest associated respiratory disease, such as infection, Langerhans cell histiocytosis, and sarcoid.

Gastrointestinal. Diarrhea due to *Salmonella* infection or inflammatory bowel disease may be accompanied by splenic enlargement. Abdominal pain may be due to gallstones, hepatitis, trauma,

or acute splenomegaly. A past history of hepatitis raises the question of portal hypertension.

Genitourinary. Sexually transmitted diseases in patients and transplacentally transmitted infections, especially congenital syphilis, are often associated with splenic enlargement.

Extremities. Arthritis resulting from SLE, rheumatoid arthritis, septic arthritis, and other autoimmune inflammatory diseases may also cause splenomegaly.

Neurologic. Poor vision in an infant with splenomegaly suggests osteopetrosis (with deafness) or uveitis-iritis (sarcoidosis, rheumatoid arthritis) (see Chapter 44). Loss of developmental milestones occurs with storage diseases (see Chapter 34). Myasthenia gravis may rarely be accompanied by splenomegaly.

Physical Examination

Isolated splenomegaly has very different implications from splenomegaly when evidence of systemic disease is present.

General. Nutritional status and growth provide clues to disorders that affect the patient's metabolic state and tissue oxygenation. Poor nutrition (as evidenced by such problems as weight loss and failure to thrive) in a child with splenomegaly suggests malignancy, chronic hemolysis, chronic infection, metabolic, or liver disease.

Skin. Pallor, petechiae, purpura, icterus, hemangiomata, septic emboli to the skin, infiltrative lesions (leukemia cutis, solid tumors), seborrhea, or eczema (histiocytosis, immunodeficiency) should be noted.

Head, Eyes, Ears, Nose, and Throat. Conjunctival pallor, cloudy corneas, scleral icterus, fundal hemorrhages or cherry red spots, evidence of sinus infection or otitis media, condition of gingivae, and evidence of salivary gland enlargement should be noted.

Cardiovascular. The clinician should look for signs of heart failure or murmurs, which suggest valvular or other structural heart disease or endocarditis.

Respiratory. Any distress, rales, rhonchi, or suggestions of pneumonia or asthma should be noted.

Abdomen. Distention, prominent veins on the abdomen, hepatomegaly, fluid wave, tenderness, or rebound should be noted, as should specific characteristics of the spleen itself: texture (hard or soft), nodularity, and the size of the spleen in centimeters.

Extremities. Arthritis, poor bone growth (storage diseases, osteopetrosis) should be noted.

Lymph nodes. Size, texture, mobility, tenderness, and distribution (see Chapter 48) should be noted.

Neurologic. Poor development suggests chronic infection, immunodeficiency, or storage diseases.

APPROACH TO THE CHILD WITH SPLENOMEGALY

The most common cause of splenomegaly in childhood is viral infection, which should induce only moderate splenomegaly (<5 cm below the left costal margin) that is transient, lasting less than 4 to 6 weeks. The approach to the child with splenomegaly is affected by several key factors, each of which indicates the probability of significant pathology requiring diagnosis and intervention.

Age

A palpable spleen (≤2 cm below the left costal margin) is a normal finding in a child below 3 years of age and may be a normal finding in an older child. Combinations of the following other factors are necessary to determine whether any evaluation other than repeat examination is indicated.

Ethnicity

Significant splenomegaly may reflect genetic disorders, which vary with ethnic group. Some historical features and physical findings particularly suggest these causes.

In persons of African ancestry, hemoglobinopathies, especially sickle syndromes, are suggested by historical features of pain, swelling of hands and feet (dactylitis), and physical findings of poor physical growth, pallor, and jaundice. Splenic sequestration crisis should be considered in a child with sickle cell disease or S-thalassemia under the age of 4 years who has a spleen that is palpable more than 2 cm below the left costal margin. This manifestation is important to identify, because it is a cause of preventable death in young children with sickle cell disease. Close observation, red cell transfusion, and splenectomy (if recurrent) are often indicated (see Chapter 49).

In persons of Mediterranean (including North Africa, middle East), Indian, and southeast Asian ancestry, hemoglobinopathies, especially thalassemia and hemoglobin E, are suggested by historical features of prominent abdomen or poor exercise tolerance and physical findings of failure to thrive, abdominal distention, characteristic facial features, pallor, and jaundice. In persons of Ashkenazi Jewish ancestry, storage diseases, especially Gaucher disease and Neimann-Pick disease, should be considered.

Fever

Fever suggests three processes: infection, inflammation, and malignancy. When fever is acute in onset, infection is most likely. Chronic fever, often gradual in onset and not associated with chills, is more likely to be due to inflammatory processes (SLE, juvenile rheumatoid arthritis, sarcoid, Langerhans cell histiocytosis) or tumors (lymphomas, especially Hodgkin disease, or leukemia).

Other Systemic Symptoms

Symptoms such as weight loss, lethargy, easy bruising, adenopathy, diarrhea, respiratory difficulties, jaundice, and skin rashes should direct evaluation to specific organ systems or processes involving those organs.

Degree of Splenomegaly

A spleen that is more than 5 cm below the left costal margin is usually not transient and represents significant pathology. A hard or nodular spleen suggests malignancy or chronic hemolysis. A tender spleen suggests either acute enlargement or infection, or both.

Duration of Splenomegaly

Acute onset of splenomegaly is most characteristic of an acute infection or a rapidly progressive malignancy (acute leukemia, lymphoma). Chronic splenomegaly (present for ≥1 month) is much more likely to represent a chronic process, such as storage diseases, congestive processes (portal hypertension, congestive heart failure), hemolysis, chronic infection, or inflammation.

Laboratory Investigation

Laboratory studies should be obtained to answer specific questions and to suggest or exclude certain diagnoses. Once a list of probable processes has been derived from the history and physical examination, laboratory investigation is directed by the processes or diagnoses that are suspected.

Complete Blood Count

A complete blood count (CBC) (differential, examination of the smear, platelet count, reticulocyte count, and erythrocyte sedimentation rate, as indicated) is the first test indicated in all patients with undiagnosed splenomegaly. The CBC provides extensive information about hematologic, infectious, and inflammatory processes and may be abnormal in patients with hypersplenism caused by portal hypertension. Specific features to look for are noted below.

Leukocyte Count and Differential. Elevation or decrease in the number of total white blood cells (WBCs), the neutrophil or lymphocyte count, and the presence of abnormal cells (atypical lymphocytes, blasts) should be noted. Viral infection is the most common cause of splenomegaly in children, and atypical lymphocytosis may be a clue. Most significant bacterial infections produce neutrophilia and reactive changes in the neutrophils. Infections due to intracellular bacteria or some viruses may produce neutropenia.

Hemoglobin, Erythrocyte Morphology, and Reticulocyte Count. Hemolytic anemia may be unsuspected without examination of the smear and the reticulocyte count. Malarial parasites may be seen on smear but may be missed unless a thick preparation is examined.

Platelet Count. Thrombocytopenia (<150,000 platelets/mm³) may be caused by decreased platelet production or increased platelet destruction. Production is diminished in conditions characterized by bone marrow infiltration (leukemia, neuroblastoma). Increased destruction accompanies immunologic processes, drug reactions, histiocytoses, and viral infections. Thrombocytosis (>400,000 platelets/mm³) often accompanies iron deficiency or acute infection as an acute phase reactant.

Pancytopenia. Pancytopenia implies bone marrow dysfunction or portal hypertension with hypersplenic destruction of all of the formed elements of the blood. A bone marrow aspiration and biopsy should be performed in any child with splenomegaly and pancytopenia. Tests of liver function, including prothrombin time and albumin, are indicated.

Erythrocyte Sedimentation Rate. Elevation of erythrocyte sedimentation rate (ESR) is nonspecific but suggests infection, especially bacterial, mycobacterial, or fungal infection, or inflammatory process, such as rheumatoid arthritis or SLE. The ESR may be normal despite significant inflammation.

Liver Function Tests

Liver function tests are indicated if splenomegaly is significant (>2 cm) or persists for over 1 month. Portal hypertension is often

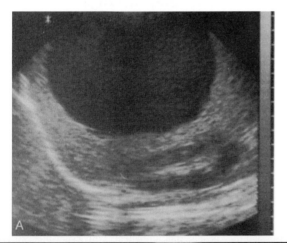

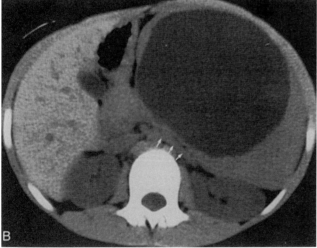

Figure 23–2. The large epidermoid cyst of the spleen in a boy *(A)* is shown by CT scan *(B)* to compress the left renal vein *(arrows).* The boy presented with varicocele. (From Teele RL, Chrestman JS. Ultrasonography of Infants and Children. Philadelphia: WB Saunders, 1991:412.)

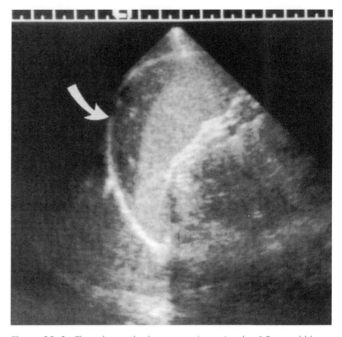

Figure 23–3. The subcapsular hematoma *(arrow)* in this 15-year-old boy, who had been in an automobile accident, was best seen on coronal scans through the left intercostal spaces. (From Teele RL, Chrestman JS. Ultrasonography of Infants and Children. Philadelphia: WB Saunders, 1991:406.)

asymptomatic until hepatic fibrosis is far advanced. Liver synthetic function (albumin, prothrombin time, fibrinogen, direct bilirubin) as well as transaminase enzyme levels should be assessed.

Immunologic Evaluation

Immunologic evaluation is needed when autoimmune disorders (rheumatoid arthritis, SLE) or immunodeficiency disorders (inherited or acquired) are suspected. This assessment includes antinuclear antibody titer, immunoglobulin levels and subclasses, tests of neutrophil function, and measurements of T-cell subclasses. Repeated infections stimulate the immune system and cause splenomegaly.

Viral Antibody Titers

Viral antibody titers should be obtained when a mononucleosis syndrome is present, especially when splenomegaly persists. The results of these tests rarely affect management but may permit a presumptive diagnosis of a self-limited process to be made, and they may prevent more invasive tests (imaging, bone marrow examination) and allay both parental and physician anxiety. Epstein-Barr viral antibody panels may need to include more than antibody to viral capsid antigen (EBV-VCA) alone if persistent Epstein-Barr virus infection is suspected. Cytomegalovirus and toxoplasmosis may also cause a mononucleosis syndrome. Primary infection with HIV frequently causes splenomegaly. It is important to make this diagnosis, since it does affect management; because acute infection may not be accompanied by positive antibody titers, follow-up titers 3 to 6 months after the initial evaluation may be needed.

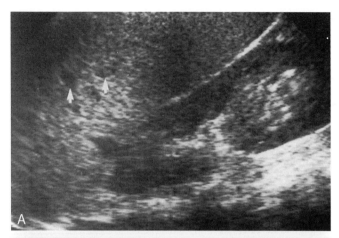

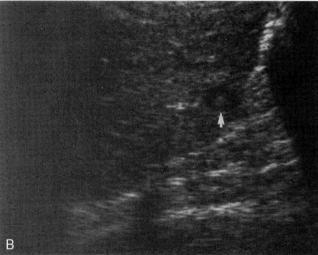

Figure 23–4. A 10-year-old girl had been treated for acute myelogenous leukemia. She had taken multiple antibiotics for recurrent infections. Unremitting fevers then developed. Candidiasis was strongly suspected, and ultrasonography was requested. Two weeks after the clinical suspicion of candidiasis was raised, obvious focal defects (arrows) could be seen within the spleen (A) and liver (B). (From Teele RL, Chrestman JS. *Ultrasonography of Infants and Children*. Philadelphia: WB Saunders, 1991:408.)

Cultures

Bacterial, fungal, and other cultures may be necessary and are dictated by the suspected infection.

Bone Marrow Examination

Bone marrow examination is appropriate to diagnose infiltrative processes (acute leukemia, histiocytosis); storage disorders (Gaucher disease, Neimann-Pick disease, sea-blue histiocyte syndrome); viral-associated hemophagocytic syndromes; and some infections that may be difficult to diagnose from other tissues (disseminated histoplasmosis, miliary tuberculosis, bacterial endo-

carditis, other chronic infections, especially in immunocompromised patients).

Imaging

Imaging of the spleen needs to be performed selectively and is definitely required when two questions are unanswered:

Are there other masses (e.g., hepatic, lymph node) that suggest more widespread involvement by tumor?

Is there silent portal hypertension?

The choice of imaging depends on which of these questions is more probable because Doppler flow ultrasonography is better for portal hypertension, and CT scanning is better for masses. Dynamic liver-spleen scans may also be needed to accurately identify portal hypertension.

Less commonly in children than in adults, splenic cysts and pseudocysts may present with palpable spleens (Fig. 23–2). CT and ultrasonography both identify such cysts well, and they image the pancreas as well. Pancreatitis is a common cause of splenic cysts. Subcapsular hematoma can also be visualized by ultrasonography (Fig. 23–3).

Persistent splenomegaly following systemic infections may be due to splenic abscesses which are visualized with ultrasonography (Fig. 23–4). CT is an alternate imaging procedure for each of these problems.

SUMMARY AND RED FLAGS

Splenomegaly is often a manifestation of acute and benign common viral infections in children. *Red flags* include chronicity, a positive family history, signs of disease in addition to splenomegaly (weight loss, pallor, petechiae), which may or may not be due to hypersplenism or another primary disease and trauma.

REFERENCES

Bohnsack JF, Brown EJ. The role of the spleen in resistance to infection. Annu Rev Med 1986;37:49–98.

Bowdler AJ. Dilution anemia corrected by splenectomy in Gaucher's disease. Ann Intern Med 1963;58:664–669.

DeLand FH. Normal spleen size. Radiology 1970;97:589–595.

Emond AM, et al. Acute splenic sequestration in homozygous sickle cell disease: Natural history and management. J Pediatr 1985;107:201–208.

Jandl JH, Files NM, et al. Proliferative response of the spleen and liver to hemolysis. J Exp Med 1965;122:299–307.

McIntyre OR, Ebaugh FG. Palpable spleens in college freshmen. Arch Intern Med 1967;66:301–305.

McNamara JJ, Murphy LJ, et al. Splenic cysts in children. Surgery 1968;64:487–498.

Munolini F, Merlob J, Ashkenazi S, et al. Palpable spleens in newborn term infants. Clin Pediatr 1985;24:197–198.

Ozsuylu S, Hosain F, McIntyre PA. Functional development of phagocytic activity of the spleen. J Pediatr 1977;90:560–562.

Oclan LF, Tubergen DG. Splenomegaly in children. Identifying the cause. Postgrad Med 1979;64:191–199.

Rogers DW, Vaidya S, Sergeant GR. Early splenomegaly in homozygous sickle cell disease: An indicator of susceptibility to infection. Lancet 1978;ii:963–965.

24 Jaundice

Jane P. Balint   William F. Balistreri

Jaundice, the yellow discoloration of skin and sclerae, results when the serum level of bilirubin, a pigmented compound, is elevated. Jaundice is not evident until the total serum bilirubin is at least 2 to 2.5 mg/dl.

Bilirubin is formed from the degradation of heme-containing compounds, particularly hemoglobin (Fig. 24–1). Microsomal heme oxygenase, located principally in the reticuloendothelial system, catabolizes heme to biliverdin, which is then reduced to bilirubin by biliverdin reductase. This *unconjugated bilirubin* (UCB) is a nonpolar, lipid-soluble compound. It cannot be eliminated via the kidney because of its insolubility in water. UCB is transported in the plasma, bound primarily to albumin, to the liver for metabolism and excretion. A receptor on the hepatocyte surface facilitates bilirubin uptake. A binding protein (Y protein or ligandin) may be involved in intracellular transport to the endoplasmic reticulum, where conjugation with glucuronic acid by bilirubin uridine diphosphate glucuronosyl transferase (UDPGT) occurs. UDPGT can be induced by a variety of drugs (e.g., narcotics, anticonvulsants, and contraceptive steroids) and by bilirubin itself. Enzyme activity is decreased by restriction of calorie and protein intake.

Conjugated bilirubin (CB) is a polar, water-soluble compound that exists primarily as a diglucuronide. It is excreted from the hepatocyte to the bile canaliculi, through the biliary tree, and into the duodenum. Once CB reaches the colon, hydrolysis by bacterial β-glucuronidase converts CB to urobilinogen. A small amount of urobilinogen is reabsorbed and returned to the liver (i.e., enterohepatic circulation) or excreted by the kidneys. The remainder is converted to stercobilin and excreted in feces. In neonates, β-glucuronidase in the intestinal lumen hydrolyzes CB to UCB, which is then absorbed and returned to the liver via the enterohepatic circulation.

Hyperbilirubinemia (an elevation of the serum bilirubin level), and thus jaundice, can result from alteration of any step in this process. Hyperbilirubinemia can be classified as conjugated *(direct)* or unconjugated *(indirect)*, depending on the concentration of CB in the serum. ''Conjugated'' and ''unconjugated'' are more accurate terms, as ''direct'' and ''indirect'' refer to the *van den Bergh reaction*, which is used for measuring bilirubin.

In this assay, the direct (conjugated) fraction is determined first by colorimetric analysis in an aqueous medium. Methanol is then added; it breaks intramolecular hydrogen bonds, converting UCB to CB. The result is a measurement of total bilirubin. The unconjugated fraction is determined by subtracting CB from the total and, therefore, is an indirect measurement. Normal bilirubin values vary by laboratory; however, the total serum bilirubin concentration is generally less than 1.5 mg/dl. Conjugated hyperbilirubinemia exists when more than 20% of the total bilirubin or more than 2 mg/dl is conjugated. If neither criterion is met, the hyperbilirubinemia is classified as unconjugated.

Unconjugated hyperbilirubinemia can be caused by any process that results in increased production, decreased delivery to the liver, decreased hepatic uptake, decreased storage, decreased conjugation, or increased enterohepatic circulation of bilirubin. The primary concern in patients with high levels of unconjugated hyperbiliru-

binemia is *kernicterus*, the neurotoxicity that results from diffusion of UCB across the blood-brain barrier and deposition in the basal ganglia, pons, or cerebellum.

Conjugated hyperbilirubinemia *(cholestasis)* can occur with either hepatocellular or cholestatic disease that causes decreased secretion into the canaliculi or decreased drainage through the biliary tree. In cholestatic disease, there is an impairment of bile flow from either a mechanical or a functional block in any one of the steps involved in the secretion and drainage of bile into the duodenum.

DIAGNOSTIC STRATEGIES

The causes of jaundice in the neonate and infant are not the same as the causes of jaundice in the older child or adolescent (Figs. 24–2 and 24–3). The approach to the problem, including the history, physical examination, and laboratory studies, varies with age.

Bilirubin

In any patient with jaundice, the total serum bilirubin should be fractionated, as the differential diagnosis of unconjugated hyperbilirubinemia is distinct from that of conjugated hyperbilirubinemia (Figs. 24–2 and 24–3). Occasionally, hemolysis interferes with some assays and may result in a falsely elevated conjugated fraction. This can be problematic with specimens obtained by heel stick or finger stick. If the clinical picture is consistent with unconjugated hyperbilirubinemia, the assay should be repeated with a specimen obtained by venipuncture.

Transaminases

The serum levels of aspartate aminotransferase/glutamate oxaloacetate transaminase (AST/SGOT) and alanine aminotransferase/glutamate pyruvate transaminase (ALT/SGPT) are increased to varying degrees in the presence of liver injury. Levels of both are markedly elevated (>5- to 10-fold normal) with hepatocellular injury due to viral hepatitis, toxin- or drug-induced injury, or ischemia. Because AST also resides in muscle tissue, AST levels are increased with cardiac or skeletal muscle damage, and because ALT is less abundant in nonhepatic tissue, an increased ALT level is more suggestive of liver disease. If AST levels are elevated in excess of ALT, a source of injury outside the hepatobiliary system should be sought. AST and ALT levels are only mildly elevated with intrahepatic or extrahepatic obstruction. With acute biliary obstruction, however, there can be an initial sharp increase in ALT and AST levels with a rapid decline in 12 to 72 hours. With

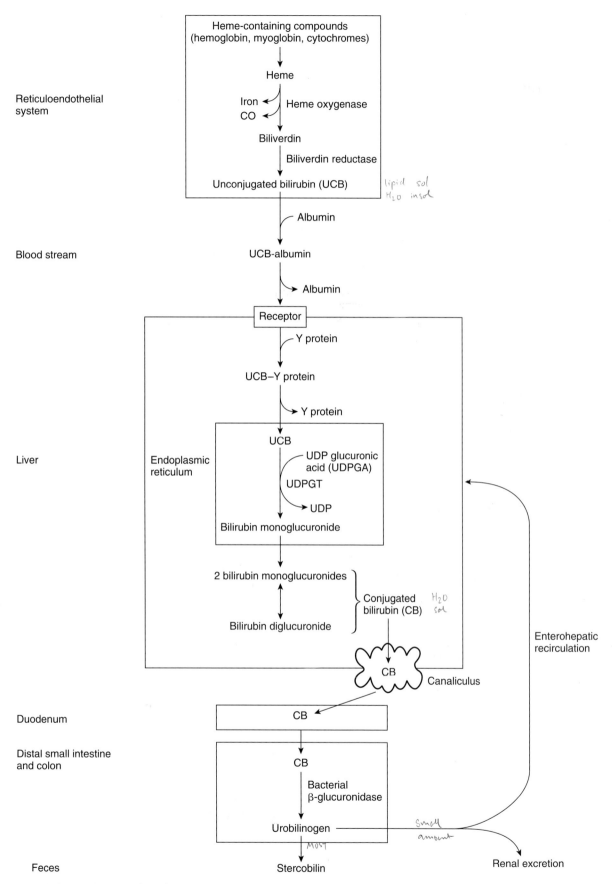

Figure 24–1. Bilirubin production and metabolism. CO = carbon monoxide; UDPGA = uridine diphosphate glucuronic acid; UDPGT = UDP glucuronyl transferase; UCB = unconjugated bilirubin; CB = conjugated bilirubin; UDP = uridine diphosphate. (Modified from Gourley GR. Jaundice. *In* Wyllie R, Hyams JS [eds]. Pediatric Gastrointestinal Disease: Pathophysiology, Diagnosis, Management. Philadelphia: WB Saunders, 1993.)

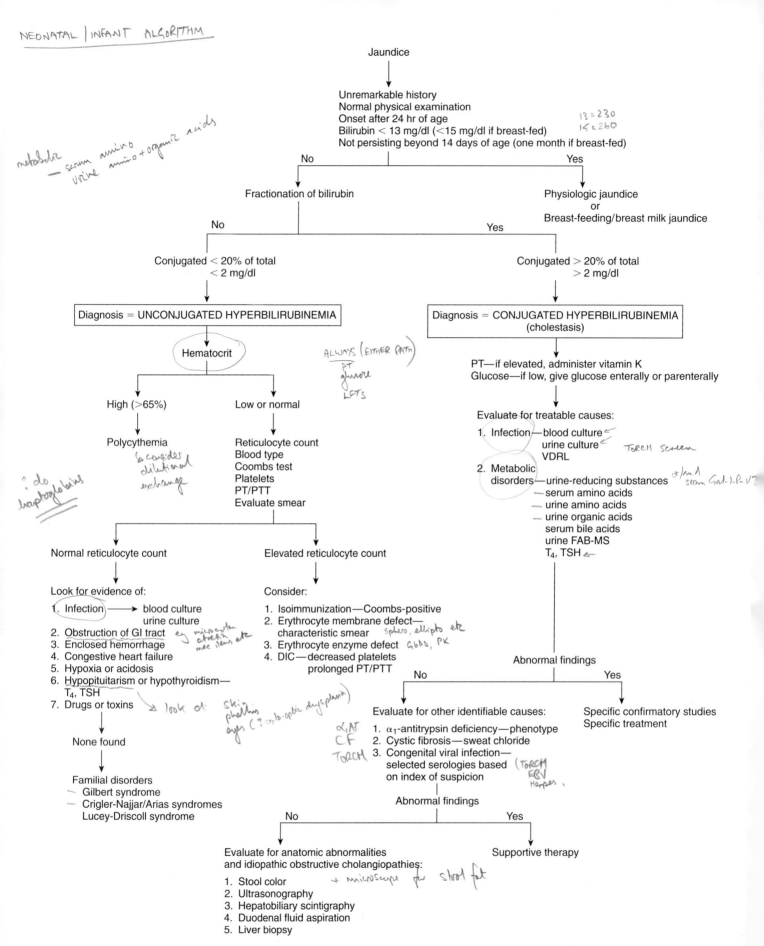

Figure 24–2. Diagnostic approach to the neonate or infant with hyperbilirubinemia. PT = prothrombin time; PTT = partial thromboplastin time; GI = gastrointestinal; T₄ = thyroxine; TSH = thyroid-stimulating hormone; VDRL = Venereal Disease Research Laboratory; FAB-MS = fast atom bombardment/mass spectrometry.

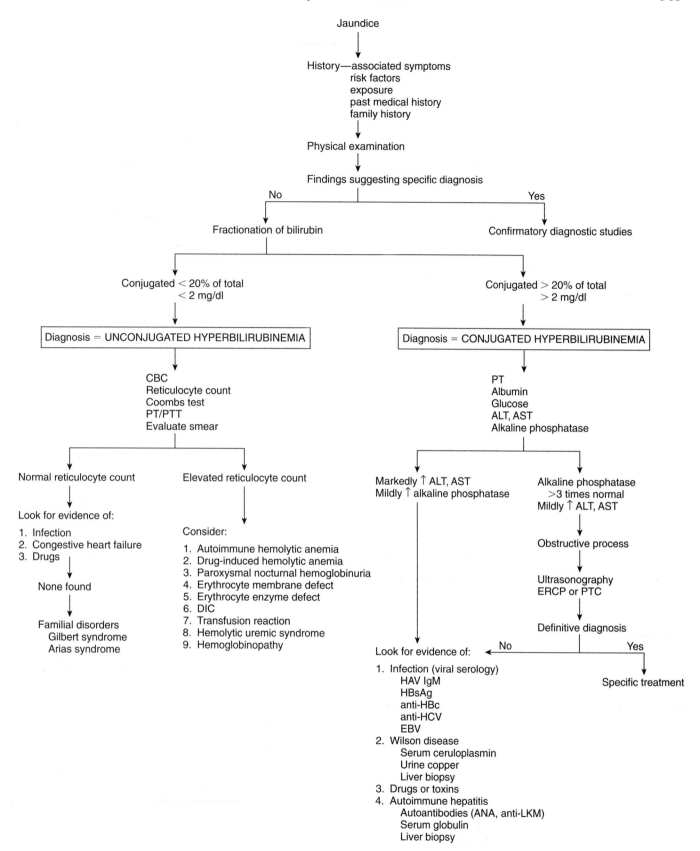

Figure 24–3. Diagnostic approach to the child or adolescent with hyperbilirubinemia. CBC = complete blood count; PT = prothrombin time; PTT = partial thromboplastin time; ALT = alanine aminotransferase; AST = aspartate transaminase; ERCP = endoscopic retrograde cholangiopancreatography; PTC = percutaneous transhepatic cholangiography; HAV = hepatitis A virus; IgM = immunoglobulin M; HBc = hepatitis B core (antigen); HBsAg = hepatitis B surface (antigen); HCV = hepatitis C virus; EBV = Epstein-Barr virus; ANA = antinuclear antibody; LKM = liver/kidney microsomal.

hepatocellular injury, ALT and AST levels tend to remain elevated longer, except in hepatic failure. A rapid decline in ALT and AST levels, with worsening coagulopathy and a decrease in liver size following hepatocellular injury, suggests severe liver failure and poor resolution of the disease process; treatment should be sought promptly.

There is usually no correlation between the severity of the liver disease and the degree of elevation of ALT and AST levels. However, relative changes in serum levels are useful in monitoring disease activity for chronic problems such as chronic viral and autoimmune hepatitis.

Alkaline Phosphatase

ALP > 3x n̄ ⇒ cholestasis. Milder elev in hepatocellular dis

Alkaline phosphatase is an enzyme that can be found in liver, bone, intestine, placenta, and tumors. Thus, elevations in the serum alkaline phosphatase level occur with normal growth, healing fractures, bone disease, pregnancy, malignancy, and hepatobiliary disease. Fractionation of the enzyme sample can help to determine its site of origin. A mild increase can be seen transiently in normal individuals. In the evaluation of conjugated hyperbilirubinemia, an alkaline phosphatase level of greater than three times normal indicates cholestasis; a milder elevation is more consistent with hepatocellular disease.

GGT Levels

The gamma glutamyl transferase (GGT) level is more specific for biliary tract disease than are ALT and AST levels. GGT is inducible by alcohol and anticonvulsants, such as phenytoin and phenobarbital, and levels may be increased in chronic pulmonary disease, renal failure, and diabetes mellitus. Therefore, the GGT level can be elevated in the absence of any hepatobiliary disease. The GGT concentration is most helpful in confirming that an elevated alkaline phosphatase level is a result of liver disease rather than bone disease.

Bile Acids

V. high c̄ obstn
— sl. high (eg x2) = hepatocellular

Bile acids in the serum are a very sensitive measure of cholestatic disease. Bile acid levels may be elevated prior to an increase in bilirubin. Levels are generally very high with obstructive disease but only mildly increased (< twice normal) in hepatocellular disease.

Albumin

Albumin is produced in the liver, and therefore albumin levels can reflect hepatic synthetic function. Serum albumin levels can be useful in monitoring progression of chronic liver disease and in discriminating an acute illness from a previously unrecognized chronic disorder. *Hypoalbuminemia (a low serum albumin level) can also be secondary to poor nutrition, renal disease, or a protein-losing enteropathy* (see Chapter 22).

Prothrombin Time

Prothrombin time (PT) is a useful marker of hepatic synthetic function, as the vitamin K–dependent clotting factors are produced in the liver. It is important not only to measure the PT but also to document the response to parenteral administration of vitamin K. In hepatocellular disease, there is no improvement in the PT. In cholestatic disease, the PT should improve because the coagulopathy is secondary to inadequate enteral absorption of this fat-soluble vitamin.

Ultrasonography

Ultrasound studies are useful, noninvasive, relatively inexpensive diagnostic tools for the evaluation of cholestatic liver disease. Specifically, ultrasonography is used to identify dilatation of the biliary tree, gallstones, and hepatic masses, such as cysts, tumors, or abscesses. Dilated intrahepatic ducts indicate extrahepatic obstruction; however, the absence of dilatation on ultrasound cannot exclude obstruction and further studies are required for definitive diagnosis. The utility of ultrasound is also limited in obese patients and in patients with excessive bowel gas. Ultrasound is preferred over computed tomography (CT) and magnetic resonance imaging (MRI) because it is less expensive and does not involve radiation. Doppler ultrasonography may also demonstrate dynamic flow in hepatic blood vessels.

CT and MRI

While CT scan and MRI are sensitive methods for detecting dilated intrahepatic ducts and mass lesions, ultrasound remains the best initial imaging study in the evaluation of the patient with cholestatic liver disease. The use of CT scan should be reserved for when there are technical problems with ultrasound, when dilated intrahepatic ducts have not been identified on ultrasound but obstruction is suspected, or when further definition of a lesion is required prior to treatment.

MRI is rarely indicated in the evaluation of cholestatic liver disease. MRI can be helpful preoperatively in delineating the vasculature around a mass lesion.

Scintigraphy

Hepatobiliary scintigraphy, which uses a radiolabeled iminodiacetic acid compound, can be helpful in discriminating primarily hepatocellular damage from biliary obstruction. The radionuclide is administered intravenously. In the normal person, hepatic uptake and excretion of the radionuclide via the biliary system are prompt. When there is injury to the hepatocyte, the uptake of radionuclide by the liver is diminished; however, the tracer should eventually be visualized in the intestinal tract. With obstructive processes, such as biliary atresia, uptake should be relatively normal unless the problem has been present long enough to have caused hepatocellular injury, however, there is no excretion into the intestinal tract. Administration of phenobarbital (5 mg/kg/day) for 5 days before the study may increase bile flow and thus can increase the specificity of hepatobiliary scintigraphy in distinguishing bile duct obstruction from other causes of neonatal cholestasis.

Liver Biopsy

Liver biopsy is often required to determine the cause of conjugated hyperbilirubinemia. In some instances, a specific pattern of injury, such as paucity of bile ducts or bile duct proliferation, may be evident. In other cases, specific markers of disease may be identified (the distinctive inclusions in alpha₁-antitrypsin deficiency) or measured (enzyme levels). There can be sampling error with a percutaneous biopsy if a relatively small amount of tissue has been provided. An open biopsy may be necessary when a large sample of tissue is needed or when there are contraindications to the percutaneous approach, such as ascites or coagulopathy. The complications of liver biopsy include bleeding, pneumothorax, infection, and bile leakage.

ERCP

Endoscopic retrograde cholangiopancreatography (ERCP) is performed for evaluation of biliary anatomy. ERCP is both diagnostic and potentially therapeutic for common duct stones and for strictures. It can be used to define the anatomy of the biliary tree in sclerosing cholangitis. Complications of the procedure include cholangitis and pancreatitis.

PTC

Percutaneous transhepatic cholangiography (PTC) can be used as an alternative to ERCP to define the biliary tract. PTC has little value in infants and young children, but it may be helpful in the older child or adolescent. Under ultrasound guidance, a needle is passed through the liver and into the biliary tree and contrast material is injected. If obstruction is identified and biliary drainage is required, this can be performed at the same time. PTC is contraindicated if there is marked ascites or irreversible coagulopathy. The complications are the same as those for liver biopsy.

JAUNDICE IN THE NEONATE AND INFANT

History

The approach to the infant with jaundice is outlined in Figure 24–2. The first step is a careful history, including age at onset and duration of jaundice. In the neonate, the causes of jaundice range from a benign, self-limited process associated with immaturity of hepatic excretory function (*physiologic jaundice*) to life-threatening metabolic (*galactosemia, tyrosinemia*) or anatomic disorders (*biliary atresia*). As the infant gets older, there are fewer benign explanations for jaundice. For example, physiologic jaundice generally resolves by the time the infant is 1 to 2 weeks of age and jaundice associated with breast milk usually resolves by the time the infant is 1 month old.

Clues to the diagnosis of both conjugated and unconjugated hyperbilirubinemia are often found in the prenatal and perinatal history (Table 24–1). Maternal infections that can be transmitted to the fetus or neonate, such as syphilis, toxoplasmosis, cytomegalovirus (CMV), hepatitis B, enterovirus, herpes simplex, and human immunodeficiency virus (HIV), are rare causes of cholestatic liver disease in the neonate. Intrauterine growth retardation is a manifestation of some congenital infections, such as CMV, rubella, and toxoplasmosis. Premature infants are prone to higher bilirubin levels and more prolonged hyperbilirubinemia; they are also more likely to have delayed enteral feedings, require parenteral nutrition, and have perinatal insults with hypoxia and acidosis. Delay of feeding can contribute to both conjugated and unconjugated hyperbilirubinemia. Breast-feeding is associated with higher levels of unconjugated bilirubin and a longer duration of

Table 24–1. Diagnostic Clues in the Evaluation of the Infant with Jaundice

Clue	Possible Diagnosis
Maternal infection	
Syphilis	Syphilis
Toxoplasmosis	Toxoplasmosis
Cytomegalovirus	Cytomegalovirus
Hepatitis B	Hepatitis B
Herpes simplex	Herpes simplex
Enterovirus	Enterovirus
Polyhydramnios	Intestinal atresia
In utero growth retardation	Cytomegalovirus; rubella; toxoplasmosis
Vomiting/poor feeding	Metabolic disorders
Delayed passage of meconium	Cystic fibrosis; Hirschsprung disease
Constipation, hypotonia, hypothermia	Hypothyroidism
Characteristic facies	
Narrow cranium, prominent forehead, hypertelorism, epicanthic folds	Zellweger syndrome
Triangular face with broad forehead, hypertelorism, deep-set eyes, long nose, pointed mandible	Alagille syndrome
Microcephaly	Congenital viral infections
Ophthalmologic findings	
Cataracts	Galactosemia; rubella
Chorioretinitis	Congenital infections
Nystagmus with hypoplasia of optic nerve	Hypopituitarism with septo-optic dysplasia
Posterior embryotoxon	Alagille syndrome
Microphallus	Hypopituitarism

jaundice compared with formula feeding. Galactosemia does not present in the infant who receives a lactose-free formula. Hereditary fructose intolerance is not clinically apparent until the infant ingests formula or solids containing fructose or sucrose. Infants with metabolic disorders often present with a history of vomiting, lethargy, and poor feeding. Vomiting may also be a symptom of intestinal obstruction.

Acholic stools are never normal, usually indicating obstruction of the biliary tree; however, nonpigmented stools can be seen with severe hepatocellular injury. The center of the stool should be examined, as the outside may be lightly pigmented from sloughed jaundiced cells of the intestinal tract. Delayed passage of meconium may be secondary to cystic fibrosis or Hirschsprung disease. Delayed passage of stools, by itself, can lead to increased enterohepatic circulation of bilirubin.

The family history can often provide direction to the evaluation, particularly with some of the less common hereditary disorders. This can include most of the metabolic disorders, hemolytic diseases, and disorders associated with intrahepatic cholestasis listed in Tables 24–2 and 24–3.

Physical Examination

With increasing levels of bilirubin, neonatal icterus becomes more extensive, spreading in a cephalopedal direction. When the

[handwritten top margin: May get L atrial isomerism in polysplenia]

Table 24–2. Differential Diagnosis of Unconjugated Hyperbilirubinemia in Neonates and Infants

(A) **Physiologic Jaundice** *[handwritten: <230. Well. <14/7 (1/12 if br fed)]*

Breast Milk Jaundice

(B) **Polycythemia**
Diabetic mother
Fetal transfusion (maternal, twin)
Intrauterine hypoxemia
Delayed cord clamping
Adrenogenital syndrome
Fetal thyrotoxicosis *[handwritten: TFT]*

(C) **Hemolytic Disease** *[handwritten: FILM]*
Isoimmune
Rh incompatibility *[handwritten: DCT]*
ABO incompatibility
Other (M, S, Kidd, Kell, Duffy)
Erythrocyte membrane defects
Hereditary spherocytosis *[handwritten: FILM / osm fragility]*
Hereditary elliptocytosis
Infantile pyknocytosis
Erythrocyte enzyme defects
Glucose-6-phosphate dehydrogenase *[handwritten: Assay]*
Pyruvate kinase
Hexokinase
Other

(D) **Infection (?)** *[handwritten: Blood, urine culture]*

(E) **Intestinal Obstruction**
Pyloric stenosis
Intestinal atresia *[handwritten: U4 Sweat test]*
Hirschsprung disease
Cystic fibrosis

(F) **Enclosed Hematoma (Cephalohematoma,** *[handwritten: O/E /U4]*
Ecchymoses)

(G) **Congestive Heart Failure** *[handwritten: O/E]*

(H) **Hypoxia**

(I) **Acidosis**

(J) **Hypothyroidism or Hypopituitarism** *[handwritten: TFT / glsse / look so nystagmus i SOD.]*

(K) **Drugs**
Maternal oxytocin
Vitamin K
Antibiotics
Phenol disinfectants

(L) **Familial Disorders of Bilirubin Uptake, Storage,**
or Metabolism
Gilbert syndrome
Crigler-Najjar (I) or Arias (II) syndrome *[handwritten: FH Assay]*
Lucey-Driscoll syndrome

Modified from Balistreri WF, Schubert WK. Liver disease in infancy and childhood. *In* Schiff L, Schiff ER (eds). Diseases of the Liver, 7th ed. Philadelphia: JB Lippincott, 1993:1104.

serum bilirubin level is approximately 5 mg/dl, only the head and neck are icteric. With an increase to 10 mg/dl, jaundice extends to the trunk. When the level reaches 15 mg/dl, the lower extremities become involved. Pallor may indicate hemolytic disease. Petechiae alert the clinician to possible sepsis, congenital infections, or severe hemolytic disease.

The facies can provide clues to chromosomal disorders or inherited disorders, such as Zellweger syndrome or Alagille syndrome (see Table 24–1). The characteristic facies of Alagille syndrome

may not be recognizable until later in childhood. Microcephaly is associated with congenital viral infections.

An ophthalmologic examination can demonstrate a variety of abnormalities associated with diseases causing jaundice. Cataracts are seen in galactosemia and rubella. Chorioretinitis accompanies congenital infections (toxoplasmosis, syphilis, rubella, CMV, HSV). Nystagmus with hypoplasia of the optic nerve suggests hypopituitarism associated with septo-optic dysplasia. Posterior embryotoxon is found in Alagille syndrome.

A heart murmur may be due to underlying congenital heart disease, which may be associated with Alagille syndrome, trisomy 21, trisomy E, and some forms of biliary atresia (polysplenia syndrome). Heart disease that results in ischemia or congestion can be a cause of conjugated or unconjugated hyperbilirubinemia.

Hepatomegaly, splenomegaly, and ascites are nonspecific findings but are not associated with physiologic or breast milk jaundice.

Microphallus is associated with septo-optic dysplasia and hypopituitarism.

Differential Diagnosis

When a neonate has jaundice, a careful history and physical examination should provide most of the information necessary to determine whether this represents physiologic jaundice or breast milk jaundice or whether further investigation, as outlined in figure 24–2, is needed. A total and fractionated bilirubin may help in this decision.

PHYSIOLOGIC AND BREAST MILK JAUNDICE

A number of factors are responsible for production of jaundice in the normal neonate. Increased bilirubin production is due to the normally increased neonatal red blood cell mass and the decreased life span of the red blood cell (80 versus 120 days). Albumin binding is decreased because of lower albumin concentrations and diminished binding capacity, resulting in decreased transport of UCB to the liver with increased deposition in tissues. Uptake of bilirubin by the hepatocyte is defective. Low levels of Y protein decrease intracellular binding, which may impede transport of UCB to the endoplasmic reticulum for further processing. Conjugation is impaired by decreased activity of UDPGT. Secretion into the canaliculi is impaired. There is increased enterohepatic circulation of unconjugated bilirubin as a result of the presence of β-glucuronidase in the intestinal lumen, which hydrolyzes conjugated bilirubin to the unconjugated lipid-soluble, more easily absorbed form and as a result of decreased intestinal bacterial flora, leading to diminished urobilinogen formation.

These features contribute in varying degrees to cause physiologic jaundice in the neonate that is characterized by a peak bilirubin level of less than 13 mg/dl on postnatal days 3 to 5, a decrease to normal by 2 weeks of age, and a conjugated fraction less than 20%. In premature and breast-fed infants, the peak is higher and lasts longer.

Breast-feeding has been associated with an increased incidence of unconjugated hyperbilirubinemia outside the expected range (>13 mg/dl). Jaundice of this level may occur in 10% to 25% of breast-fed infants, in contrast to 4% to 7% of formula-fed infants. This can occur within the first 5 days of life and is referred to as "early" or "breast-feeding" jaundice. In a second group of breast-fed infants, the jaundice develops slowly, occurring after the first week of life, and peaks between the second and third weeks of life at 10 to 20 mg/dl. This is referred to as "late" or "breast milk" jaundice. The precise cause of increased bilirubin in this latter

[handwritten bottom margin: 175 → 350]
[handwritten: • Early - "breast feeding jaundice"]
[handwritten: • Late = "breast milk jaundice"]

Table 24–3. Differential Diagnosis of Conjugated Hyperbilirubinemia in Infants

Heart Disease

Toxin- or Drug-Related
Cholestasis associated with total parenteral nutrition
Chloral hydrate
Sepsis with possible endotoxemia (urinary tract
infection, gastroenteritis)

Treatable Infections
Bacterial sepsis
Urinary tract infection
Syphilis
Toxoplasmosis
Tuberculosis

Treatable Metabolic Disorders
Disorders of carbohydrate metabolism
Galactosemia
Hereditary fructose intolerance (Fructosemia)
Disorders of amino acid metabolism
Tyrosinemia
Disorders of bile acid synthesis and metabolism
Primary enzyme deficiencies
3β-Hydroxysteroid Δ^5-C_{27}steroid dehydrogenase/
isomerase
Δ4-3-oxosteroid 5β-reductase
Endocrine disorders
Idiopathic hypopituitarism
Hypothyroidism

Other Metabolic Disorders
Metabolic diseases in which the defect is not well
characterized:
α_1-Antitrypsin deficiency
Cystic fibrosis
Familial erythrophagocytic lymphohistiocytosis
Neonatal iron storage disease (perinatal
hemochromatosis)
Infantile copper overload
Disorders of carbohydrate metabolism
Glycogen storage disease type IV
Disorders of bile acid synthesis and metabolism
Secondary (peroxisomal disorders)
Zellweger syndrome (cerebrohepatorenal
syndrome)
Specific peroxisomal enzymopathies
Disorders of lipid metabolism
Wolman disease
Cholesterol ester storage disease
Niemann-Pick disease
Gaucher disease

Congenital Viral Infections
Cytomegalovirus
Herpesvirus
Rubella virus
Hepatitis B virus (?hepatitis C and other non-A,non-B
viruses)
Human immunodeficiency virus (HIV)
Coxsackievirus
Echovirus
Parvovirus B19

Idiopathic Obstructive Cholangiopathies
Extrahepatic biliary atresia*
Idiopathic neonatal hepatitis
Intrahepatic cholestasis
Persistent
With intrahepatic bile duct paucity
Arteriohepatic dysplasia (Alagille syndrome)
Nonsyndromic paucity
Progressive familial intrahepatic cholestasis
Byler disease
Nielsen syndrome (Greenland Eskimo)
Microfilament dysfunction (North American Indian)
Benign familial chronic intrahepatic cholestasis
Recurrent
Familial benign recurrent cholestasis
Hereditary cholestasis with lymphedema (Aagenaes)

Anatomic Disorders
Choledochal cyst
Spontaneous bile duct perforation
Obstruction associated with cholelithiasis, bile or mucous
plug, or mass or neoplasia
Neonatal sclerosing cholangitis
Bile duct stenosis
Anomalous choledochopancreatico-ductal junction
Biliary atresia or agenesis†
Infantile polycystic disease or congenital hepatic fibrosis
Caroli disease (cystic dilatation of intrahepatic ducts)

Genetic or Chromosomal
Trisomy E
Down syndrome
Donahue syndrome (leprechaunism)

Miscellaneous
Histiocytosis X
Shock or hypoperfusion
Intestinal obstruction
Polysplenia syndrome (with extrahepatic biliary atresia)
Neonatal lupus erythematosus
Dubin-Johnson syndrome
Arthrogryposis, cholestatic pigmentary disease, renal
dysfunction syndrome

Modified from Balistreri WF, Schubert WK. Liver disease in infancy and childhood. *In* Schiff L, Schiff ER (eds). Diseases of the Liver, 7th ed. Philadelphia: JB Lippincott, 1993:1109–1110.
*†*Note:* There may be various types of biliary atresia. The asterisk may represent an idiopathic postnatal obliterative cholangiopathy. The dagger may represent a congenital malformation.

setting has not been established; alternative theories include inhibition of glucuronyl transferase activity and increased enterohepatic circulation of UCB. Kernicterus has not been reported in association with breast-feeding.

No treatment is necessary for physiologic jaundice. If the bilirubin exceeds 20 mg/dl in the breast-fed infant, discontinuing breast-feeding for 24 hours results in a decreased bilirubin level.

If there are any *red flags* (Table 24–4), the hyperbilirubinemia should be investigated further. Any abnormality identified by history or physical examination is a matter of concern. If not already performed, the next step in the evaluation is fractionation of the bilirubin.

UNCONJUGATED HYPERBILIRUBINEMIA

The differential diagnosis of unconjugated hyperbilirubinemia in the neonate and infant is presented in Table 24–2. Unless abnormalities on history and physical examination direct the evaluation more specifically, hematologic evaluation, which may identify causes of increased bilirubin production, should be performed. This includes a complete blood count (CBC) with examination of the smear, a reticulocyte count, a direct Coombs test, blood typing (maternal and infant), and, in conjugated hyperbilirubinemia, possibly a PT and partial thromboplastin time (PTT).

Polycythemia

Neonatal polycythemia, defined as a central hematocrit greater than 65% by venipuncture, is caused by maternal diabetes, maternal-fetal or twin-twin transfusion, intrauterine hypoxemia, endocrine disorders, and delayed cord clamping (see Table 24–2). Polycythemia, by definition of its increased red cell mass, features increased bilirubin production.

Hemolytic Disorders

Reticulocytosis and an increased nucleated red blood cell count, with either a low or normal hematocrit, suggest hemolysis. This can be due to isoimmunization; erythrocyte membrane, hemoglobin, or enzyme defects; or sepsis with disseminated intravascular coagulation (DIC).

Isoimmune Hemolytic Disease. In this group of disorders, maternal antibodies (IgG) to the infant's erythrocytes cross the placenta, resulting in red blood cell destruction. The use of anti-D gamma globulin (Rho-GAM) following delivery in women who are Rh-negative has reduced the incidence of Rh sensitization and erythroblastosis fetalis. If a woman has been sensitized, the fetus can be monitored with serial amniocenteses. If necessary, intrauterine transfusion (via the umbilical vein or less often the intra-abdominal route) can then be performed to prevent the sequelae of severe hemolysis, which include fetal and neonatal anemia, edema, hepatosplenomegaly, and circulatory collapse or a stillborn infant with hydrops fetalis. If the problem has not been recognized prenatally, the infant with Rh incompatibility will present with pallor, hepatosplenomegaly, and rapidly developing jaundice.

The diagnosis is confirmed by demonstrating that the infant is Rh-positive, that the direct Coombs test is positive, and that maternal antibody is coating the infant's red blood cells. These tests will be modified with *in utero* transfusions. Depending on the degree

Table 24–4. **Red Flags in the Evaluation of the Infant with Jaundice**

Onset
  <24 hr of age

Course
  Increases by >5 mg/dl/day
  Persists beyond 14 days of age

Prenatal History
  Maternal infection
  Maternal diabetes mellitus
  Maternal drug use
  Polyhydramnios
  Intrauterine growth retardation

Delivery
  Prematurity
  Perinatal asphyxia
  Small for gestational age

Feeding
  Delayed enteral feeding
  Vomiting
  Poor feeding
  Associated with change in formula

Stools
  Acholic
  Delayed passage of meconium

Family History
  Jaundice
  Anemia
  Liver disease
  Splenectomy
  Cholecystectomy

Physical Examination
  Ill-appearing
  Pallor
  Petechiae
  Chromosomal stigmata
  Abnormal facies
  Microcephaly
  Cataracts
  Chorioretinitis
  Nystagmus
  Optic nerve hypoplasia
  Posterior embryotoxon
  Heart murmur
  Hepatosplenomegaly (or isolated
    hepatomegaly or splenomegaly)
  Ascites
  Acholic stools
  Microphallus
  Hematoma or ecchymoses

Bilirubin
  Total
    >13 mg/dl formula-fed
    >14–15 mg/dl breast-fed
  Conjugated
    >20% of total or >2 mg/dl

of hemolysis, postnatal phototherapy and/or exchange transfusion may be required.

ABO incompatibility causes a less severe form of isoimmune hemolytic disease with a less rapid development of jaundice. It is more common in infants with blood type A or B who are born to mothers with blood type O. Hemolysis develops in only 50% of sensitized infants; of these infants, 50% will have a bilirubin level greater than 10 mg/dl. In addition to showing anemia, reticulocytosis, and spherocytes on the smear, the direct Coombs test will be weakly positive with a positive indirect Coombs test. Although other minor blood group antibodies can also cause hemolysis, this is a rare phenomenon.

Erythrocyte Membrane Defects. Red blood cell membrane defects are relatively uncommon causes of unconjugated hyperbilirubinemia. There is often a family history of hemolysis, transfusions, cholecystectomy for bilirubin stones, or splenectomy. Hemolysis results from fragility of the red blood cell membrane. When the defect is present in infancy, there is anemia, jaundice, and splenomegaly and the smear is often characteristic (e.g., spherocytosis or elliptocytosis). Spherocytes are also seen with ABO incompatability. Membrane defects are all Coombs-negative.

Erythrocyte Enzyme Defects (see Chapter 49). Glucose-6-phosphate dehydrogenase (G6PD) deficiency is common. It is seen more frequently in those with a Mediterranean or Far Eastern ancestry who have complete absence of the enzyme. In these individuals, hemolysis can occur without a precipitant. In blacks, the disease is less severe, and hemolysis is rare without exposure to a drug or toxin or infection that causes an oxidant stress. G6PD deficiency can present as neonatal jaundice on day 2 or 3 of life, alternatively, it may not present until later in childhood if jaundice is associated with an acute hemolytic crisis. The diagnosis is confirmed by documenting deficiency of the enzyme in red blood cells.

Numerous deficiencies of enzymes in the glycolytic pathway have been identified. Pyruvate kinase deficiency is the most common of these rare disorders. Most disorders are thought to have an autosomal recessive mode of transmission and have been identified in only a small number of individuals. They all result in hemolysis. The time of presentation depends on the degree of hemolysis.

Other Considerations

If the hematocrit is normal and there is no evidence of hemolysis or a consumptive process, other explanations for unconjugated hyperbilirubinemia should be sought. Blood and urine cultures rarely identify infectious etiologic agents if the patient is otherwise clinically normal. Obstruction of the gastrointestinal tract should be evident on clinical grounds when vomiting, abdominal distention, and delayed passage of meconium are present. Obstruction should be confirmed with plain abdominal roentgenograms and contrast studies. Clinical examination should also identify cephalohematoma, ecchymoses, congestive heart failure, hypoxia, and acidosis. Thyroxine (T_4) and thyroid-stimulating hormone (TSH) levels should be obtained or checked from the state neonatal screening program to look for evidence of hypothyroidism or hypopituitarism.

Drugs, either maternal or neonatal, and toxins should be identified by careful record review. Examples include oxytocin, excess vitamin K in premature infants, some antibiotics, and phenol disinfectants used in nurseries.

Familial Disorders

Final consideration should be given to one of the familial disorders of bilirubin uptake, storage, and metabolism.

Gilbert syndrome. Gilbert syndrome is a benign condition that occurs in up to 5% of the population. It is thought to have autosomal dominant transmission with variable penetrance. A familial incidence is reported in 15% to 40% of cases. Postulated causes include partial UDPGT deficiency (<50% of normal) or a defect in hepatocyte bilirubin uptake. Affected individuals are generally asymptomatic and may not present with jaundice until the second or third decade of life. Mild jaundice with a bilirubin up to 7 mg/dl can occur transiently with fatigue, exercise, fasting, febrile illness, and alcohol ingestion. Except for showing an increased indirect bilirubin level, all laboratory studies are normal. The diagnosis can be confirmed by documenting a twofold to threefold rise in unconjugated bilirubin during a 24-hour fast.

Crigler-Najjar Syndrome. Crigler-Najjar (type I) syndrome is an autosomal recessive condition that is characterized by marked hyperbilirubinemia (20 to 40 mg/dl) in the neonatal period in an otherwise healthy infant. Kernicterus is universal, and affected individuals usually die with severe neurologic problems. Because UDPGT is completely absent, there is no conjugated bilirubin in the bile or serum and the bile is colorless. There is no decrease in serum UCB levels during phenobarbital administration. The only therapies are exchange transfusion, intensive phototherapy, and liver transplantation.

Arias Syndrome. Known as Crigler-Najjar (type II) syndrome, Arias syndrome is thought to be an autosomal dominant condition with incomplete penetrance. The onset is usually at birth, although it can be in late childhood. There is less than 5% of the normal UDPGT activity. Bile contains bilirubin monoglucuronides. Bilirubin levels, generally 9 to 17 mg/dl, respond to phenobarbital administration with a decrease to near normal. There is no neurologic disease.

Lucey-Driscoll Syndrome. Lucey-Driscoll syndrome is a transient familial neonatal hyperbilirubinemia that appears in the first few days of life and resolves by 2 to 3 weeks of age. However, the bilirubin level can rise to greater than 60 mg/dl in untreated infants, resulting in severe neurotoxicity. This results from inhibition of UDPGT by a substance that has been found in both maternal and infant serum. The condition is treated with exchange transfusion.

Therapy

Treatment of unconjugated hyperbilirubinemia depends on the degree of elevation of bilirubin. Considerable controversy exists over what level is toxic and, therefore, when treatment should be initiated. Because it is lipid-soluble, unconjugated bilirubin can diffuse into the central nervous system, resulting in neurologic toxicity. Most agree that kernicterus does not occur below a bilirubin level of 20 to 25 mg/dl in the healthy, full-term infant without evidence of hemolysis. Kernicterus may occur at lower bilirubin levels in the premature or sick neonate.

Treatment options include phototherapy and exchange transfusion. Phototherapy produces a reduction of bilirubin by 1 to 2 mg/dl in 3 to 12 hours by causing the photoisomerization and photodegradation of unconjugated bilirubin to more water-soluble forms that are more readily excreted in bile and urine respectively. Potential complications include retinal damage, diarrhea, and dehydration. Phototherapy is begun at levels below that for exchange transfusion (~5 mg/dl less) or during preparations for an exchange transfusion.

Exchange transfusion with blood cross-matched against the

mother is indicated for severe anemia and/or hyperbilirubinemia. This decision must be based not only on the hematocrit and bilirubin but also, as importantly, on the infant's age and clinical condition. In term or near-term infants (>2000 g in weight) with evidence of hemolysis, exchange transfusion is indicated if the serum unconjugated bilirubin level is higher than 20 mg/dl or if the bilirubin level does not rapidly respond to phototherapy. Signs of kernicterus (i.e., a high-pitched cry, gaze paralysis, fever, lethargy, and opisthotonic posture) warrant exchange transfusion, no matter what the bilirubin level is.

NEONATAL CONJUGATED HYPERBILIRUBINEMIA

Potential causes of conjugated hyperbilirubinemia in the neonate and infant are extensive (see Table 24–3). It is important to first evaluate the infant for treatable problems (Table 24–5) and institute specific therapy that prevents significant morbidity and may be lifesaving. Figure 24–2 outlines a diagnostic approach when the clinical presentation has not suggested a likely diagnosis.

Common to all of these conditions is the potential for hypoprothrombinemia; therefore, a PT should be obtained. If the PT is prolonged, the infant should be treated with intravenous vitamin K to avoid spontaneous hemorrhage, particularly intracranial. Depending on the degree of hepatocellular damage, vitamin K may not correct the PT.

Hypoglycemia is another danger that is associated with diseases that cause severe hepatic dysfunction as well as with hypopituitarism. The infant may be relatively asymptomatic despite significant hypoglycemia. A serum glucose level can be obtained prior to feeding. If hypoglycemia is present, the infant should receive frequent feedings, continuous feedings, or intravenous dextrose infusions.

Treatable Infections

Bacterial Infection. An infant may rarely be clinically well-appearing with jaundice as the only sign of bacterial infection. Blood and urine specimens for culture should be obtained in infants with unexplained conjugated hyperbilirubinemia. Infection is less likely to be missed in the symptomatic infant who presents with poor feeding, lethargy, vomiting, temperature instability, apnea, and bradycardia or shock. *Escherichia coli* is the most common organism identified in either sepsis or urinary tract infection (often with bacteremia) when jaundice is present. The hyperbilirubinemia may be due to endotoxin-mediated canalicular dysfunction. Less often, other gram-negative bacilli, *Listeria, Staphylococcus,* or *Streptococcus* may be identified as the causative agent. Although sepsis

Table 24–5. Things Not to Miss in the Infant with Conjugated Hyperbilirubinemia

Heart disease	Endocrine disorders
Toxins	Hypopituitarism
Hypoprothrombinemia	Hypothyroidism
Hypoglycemia	Metabolic disorders
Infections	Galactosemia
Sepsis	Tyrosinemia
✱Urinary tract infection	Bile acid abnormalities
Syphilis	Extrahepatic biliary atresia
Toxoplasmosis	Cystic fibrosis
Hepatitis	

Table 24–6. Relative Frequency of the Various Clinical Forms of Neonatal Cholestasis*

Clinical Form	Cumulative (%)	Estimated Frequency (per 10,000 Live Births)
Idiopathic neonatal hepatitis	35–40	1.25
Extrahepatic biliary atresia	25–30	0.70
α_1-Antitrypsin deficiency	7–10	0.25
Intrahepatic cholestasis (with or without bile duct paucity)	5–6	0.14
Bacterial sepsis	2	<0.1
Cytomegalovirus hepatitis	3–5	<0.1
Rubella or herpes simplex hepatitis	1	<0.1
Endocrine disorders (hypothyroidism, panhypopituitarism)	1	<0.1
Galactosemia	1	<0.1

From Balistreri WF, Schubert WK. Liver disease in infancy and childhood. *In* Schiff L, Schiff ER (eds). Diseases of the Liver, 7th ed. Philadelphia: JB Lippincott, 1993:1111.

*Based on more than 500 cases.

accounts for only 2% of the cases of neonatal cholestasis (Table 24–6), it is easily diagnosed and treated.

Syphilis. Syphilis (congenital) is relatively common. With severe infection, the infant will have fever, a diffuse macular-papular rash, hepatosplenomegaly, edema, anemia, and periostitis in addition to jaundice. Nontreponemal serologic tests (Veneral Disease Research Laboratory [VDRL]) may be routinely performed on cord blood. If positive, the diagnosis should be confirmed on serum from the infant. Confirmation requires a positive specific test for syphilis such as the IgM or IgG FTA (fluorescent trepomenal antibody). Treatment is with intravenous penicillin for 10 to 14 days.

Toxoplasmosis. If toxoplasmosis is suspected on clinical grounds, IgM titers should be obtained or the placenta should be examined histologically. Most infected infants will be asymptomatic. Infants with severe congenital infection may have hydrocephaly or microcephaly, intracranial calcifications, chorioretinitis, aseptic meningitis, jaundice, purpura, and hepatomegaly. Postnatal treatment consists of pyrimethamine and sulfadiazine; folinic acid is added to prevent folate deficiency.

Treatable Metabolic Disorders

There are several useful screening modalities: urine-reducing substances (galactosemia), serum and urine amino acids, urine organic acids, quantitative serum bile acids, qualitative analysis of urinary bile acids by fast atom bombardment–mass spectrometry (FAB-MS), the T_4 level, and the TSH level. These can be obtained at the same time as bacterial cultures or checked as part of some state neonatal screening programs (e.g., galactosemia and thyroid).

Galactosemia. Although rare, galactosemia is a life-threatening disorder that can easily be detected. It is an autosomal recessive disorder with deficiency of galactose-1-phosphate uridyl transferase, which is required for conversion of galactose to glucose. As a result, galactose-1-phosphate accumulates; this compound is thought to be hepatoxic. Once lactose (glucose-galactose) is introduced in the infant's diet, vomiting, diarrhea, jaundice, hepatomegaly, and cataracts develop. Affected infants often present with *E. coli* sepsis in the first weeks of life.

Laboratory evaluation may demonstrate elevations of transaminase levels, a prolonged PT, hemolytic anemia, and aminoaciduria. The urine is positive for reducing substances (galactose) if the infant is receiving a lactose-containing formula or breast milk. The diagnosis can be confirmed by documenting deficiency of the enzyme in erythrocytes or leukocytes. Transfusions may cause false-negative results. Treatment consists of eliminating galactose from the diet.

Tyrosinemia and Inborn Errors of Bile Acid Metabolism. Also rare, but readily identifiable, are tyrosinemia and inborn errors of bile acid metabolism. Tyrosinemia is diagnosed by serum and urine amino acids and urine organic acid levels. Treatment involves dietary restriction of phenylalanine, methionine, and tyrosine and, ultimately, liver transplantation. Drug manipulation of tyrosine metabolizing enzymes is a promising therapy under investigational trials. Disorders of bile acid metabolism can be detected by FAB-MS analysis of urine. Treatment consists of oral bile acid therapy.

Hypothyroidism and Hypopituitarism. Jaundice can be a manifestation of both hypothyroidism and hypopituitarism. Hypopituitarism may present with hypoglycemia, microphallus, and signs of hypothyroidism in addition to jaundice. Wandering nystagmus is present when hypopituitarism is associated with septo-optic dysplasia. Treatment of the underlying endocrinopathy leads to resolution of the liver disease.

Other Identifiable Causes of Cholestasis

The next step in the evaluation includes a search for a group of diseases that, while not specifically treatable, can be readily diagnosed.

Alpha₁-Antitrypsin Deficiency. An alpha$_1$-antitrypsin phenotype can detect alpha$_1$-antitrypsin deficiency, which is responsible for 7% to 10% of the cases of neonatal cholestasis. Alpha$_1$-antitrypsin is a protease inhibitor (Pi) that is synthesized in the liver and inactivates trypsin and neutrophil elastase. The normal Pi phenotype, MM, is found in 80% to 90% of the population. There are numerous allelic variants. Lung disease in older patients, is associated with MZ, MS, and SZ phenotypes. Liver disease is associated with the ZZ phenotype and sporadically with other variants. The exact mechanism of liver injury is unclear, and there is variability in expression so that liver disease does not develop in all individuals with the ZZ phenotype. There is also great variability in presentation. Commonly, the disorder presents in early infancy with prolonged conjugated hyperbilirubinemia, failure to thrive, acholic stools, hepatomegaly, and possibly ascites. It may not present until later childhood or even adulthood. Presentations in the older individual include jaundice, ascites, portal hypertension with varices, chronic hepatitis, cryptogenic cirrhosis, or, rarely, hepatocellular carcinoma.

The diagnosis is suggested by serum phenotyping (ZZ) and confirmed on liver biopsy, which demonstrates distinctive periodic acid–Schiff positive and diastase-resistant, glycoprotein-rich inclusions in hepatocytes.

Treatment is supportive. Some individuals do very well with minimal liver dysfunction. Others have progressive liver disease, requiring transplantation. The progression may be rapid or slow.

Cystic Fibrosis. As many as 33% of patients with cystic fibrosis may present with neonatal conjugated hyperbilirubinemia. The incidence is increased in infants with meconium ileus. The diagnosis can be confirmed with a sweat chloride test or by detecting the abnormal gene. Although the cholestasis will resolve, the infant with cystic fibrosis will often have additional hepatobiliary problems later in childhood. These problems may include focal biliary cirrhosis, multilobular cirrhosis, fatty liver, obstruction of the common duct secondary to pancreatic duct sludge or pancreatic fibrosis, cholelithiasis, sclerosing cholangitis, and, rarely, cholangiocarcinoma.

Congenital Viral Infections. Although a number of viral infections have been associated with neonatal cholestasis, routine TORCH (toxoplasmosis, other, rubella, cytomegalovirus, herpes) titers are not indicated. Selected serologic or viral studies should be performed only if there is a high index of suspicion on the basis of the history or physical examination.

Cytomegalovirus Infection. CMV infection is common, but 90% of infants are asymptomatic. The severely affected infant with vertical transmission of CMV can present within the first 24 hours of life with intrauterine growth retardation, conjugated jaundice, hemolytic anemia, thrombocytopenic purpura, and hepatosplenomegaly. Often a low-birth-weight infant presents with microcephaly, periventricular calcifications, and chorioretinitis. The diagnosis can be made by obtaining urine specimens for culture.

There is no effective therapy for the central nervous system involvement. Ganciclovir is an experimental but unproven therapy. The liver disease will resolve, but neurologic sequelae are common. Postnatal acquisition from CMV-positive blood transfusion may produce a sepsis syndrome and hepatitis.

Herpes Simplex. Herpes simplex causes a severe neonatal infection that usually presents at 1 to 2 weeks of age with lethargy, poor feeding, a vesicular rash (60% to 70%), jaundice, hepatomegaly, hepatic failure, temperature instability, encephalitis and DIC. The diagnosis is made by a Tzanck stain of cutaneous scrapings from lesions that demonstrates multinucleated giant cells with intranuclear inclusions and by viral culture of vesicles or cerebrospinal fluid. Polymerase chain reaction (PCR) can also detect herpes simplex DNA in cerebrospinal fluid. Treatment is with intravenous acyclovir. Infants with disseminated infection have a mortality rate of 15% to 35%.

Rubella. Jaundice is present in only 15% to 20% of cases of congenital rubella. Other manifestations include low birth weight, cataracts, heart disease (patent ductus arteriosus), hepatosplenomegaly, and thrombocytopenic purpura. The diagnosis is made by viral isolation.

There is no proven therapy. The liver disease usually resolves completely; the infant is left with other organ sequelae, (such as deafness and microcephaly).

Hepatitis B. Hepatitis B infection presents with jaundice in fewer than 5% of perinatal infections. Perinatal transmission is high when mothers are chronic carriers or when they acquire acute infection in the last trimester. Most infants are asymptomatic, but there is a high incidence of subsequent chronic infection. Once a person is

[handwritten top margin: 2 Common Causes of Conjd Bili— ① EHBA ② Idiopathic Neonatal Hepatitis } ~70% of all cases.]

infected, there is no treatment. <u>Perinatal infection can be prevented with hepatitis B immune globulin and vaccination.</u> It is important to identify mothers who are hepatitis B surface antigen–positive; identification requires universal screening.

Anatomic Abnormalities and Idiopathic Obstructive Cholangiopathies

[handwritten: ✳]

This group includes the two most common causes of neonatal cholestasis—extrahepatic biliary atresia and idiopathic neonatal hepatitis, which together account for 60% to 70% of cases. Ultrasonography, hepatobiliary scintigraphy, duodenal aspiration, and liver biopsy aid in the diagnosis.

Biliary Atresia. In biliary atresia all or part of the extrahepatic biliary tree is obliterated. This condition is thought to be the result of a progressive inflammatory process. Infants are less often icteric from birth and more often develop jaundice at 2 to 6 weeks of age. <u>Infants are usually full term and initially are well-appearing except for jaundice, dark urine, and acholic stools. The family history is negative.</u> There appear to be two forms of biliary atresia:

[handwritten left margin: MAY BE A JAUNDICE FREE INTERVAL]

1. Fewer than 33% have a "fetal form," which has an early onset with no jaundice-free period. There are often associated defects, including cardiac defects, polysplenia, malrotation, and situs inversus. At surgery, no bile duct remnants are found in the hepatic hilum. Cirrhosis develops early.

2. In the "perinatal form," there is a jaundice-free interval following the normal physiologic jaundice and there are no associated anomalies. Remnants of bile ducts are identified in the porta hepatis. Cirrhosis has a later onset.

[handwritten left margin: BIG FIRM LIVER]

<u>At the time of presentation, infants with biliary atresia have an enlarged, firm liver.</u> Pruritus, splenomegaly, ascites, and digital clubbing often develop.

Diagnostic work-up includes exclusion of other identifiable causes of neonatal cholestasis. The work-up should be performed expeditiously, as it is important to identify biliary atresia early because successful surgical establishment of drainage is correlated with age at surgery. The operative success decreases beyond 2 months of age. An <u>ultrasound</u> study helps to exclude other treatable anatomic abnormalities, such as a choledochal cyst. The gallbladder is not found in infants with biliary atresia. Some centers utilize <u>hepatobiliary scintigraphy,</u> which demonstrates uptake of tracer but no excretion into the duodenum if biliary atresia is present. <u>Duodenal aspiration can be performed; there are no bilirubin or bile salts in the aspirate.</u> A liver biopsy is needed regardless of the results of the last two studies, so they are sometimes omitted. Characteristic findings on biopsy are portal and perilobular edema and fibrosis, bile duct proliferation, and bile duct plugs.

The diagnosis is confirmed by intraoperative cholangiogram at the time of surgery. The surgical procedure is that initially described by Kasai and is a *hepatoportoenterostomy.* The porta hepatis is transected, and a loop of intestine is brought up to drain the bile ducts. In a small percentage (5% to 15%), a discrete distal lesion can be used for bile drainage and the surgery is curative. In the remainder, surgery is palliative, allowing time before liver transplantation is needed. If surgery is performed before the infant is 2 months old, there is a 65% to 90% success rate in terms of obtaining some bile flow. This decreases to less than 20% after 3 months of age. The primary postoperative complication is bacterial cholangitis.

Neonatal Hepatitis. Neonatal hepatitis must be differentiated from biliary atresia. The infant with neonatal hepatitis is often premature or small for gestational age. Acholic stools are uncommon. In 15% to 20% of cases, there is a familial incidence. <u>The prothrombin time may be unresponsive to vitamin K.</u>

Neonatal hepatitis is a descriptive term rather than a specific disease entity. The diagnosis is made by exclusion of other causes of cholestasis. <u>Hepatobiliary scintigraphy demonstrates delayed uptake, but there is usually excretion into the duodenum.</u> Biopsy findings include panlobular disarray indicative of <u>severe hepatocellular disease, inflammatory infiltrate in the portal areas, focal hepatocellular necrosis, multinucleated giant cells, and increased extramedullary hematopoiesis.</u>

<u>Treatment is supportive.</u> The outcome is variable and is better for infants with sporadic *(nonfamilial)* cases, approximately 60% of whom recover, 10% have chronic liver disease, and 30% die without liver transplantation. The percentages for recovery and death are reversed in *familial* cases.

[handwritten: Alagille – facies, liver, heart, vertebrae, eye (post⁺ embryotoxon) Renal, AFTT. AD variable penetrance]

Intrahepatic Paucity of Bile Ducts. This condition is defined as the absence or marked reduction in the number of interlobular bile ducts. Jaundice may have its onset in the neonatal period or may not appear until later in childhood. There is a *syndromic* form known as <u>arteriohepatic dysplasia, or *Alagille syndrome*.</u> This is characterized by unusual facies (a <u>triangular face with broad forehead, widely spaced and deep-set eyes, a long nose, and a pointed mandible</u>), vertebral arch defects (butterfly vertebrae, hemivertebrae, decreased interpedicular distance), <u>posterior embryotoxon</u> (ocular), <u>cardiac anomalies (peripheral pulmonic stenosis or tetralogy of Fallot),</u> in addition to <u>cholestasis</u> secondary to paucity of ducts. Renal anomalies and growth retardation are also often present. This appears to be a progressive phenomenon and may not be readily recognizable in neonates. By age 4 to 6 months, pruritus develops and can be severe. <u>Xanthomas appear</u> in association with a markedly elevated cholesterol level. Alagille syndrome is thought to have an <u>autosomal dominant transmission</u> with variable penetrance. Often other family members are recognized as being affected when an infant presents.

The diagnosis is confirmed by liver biopsy. Symptoms often improve over time, and long-term survival is good.

There is a *nonsyndromic* form with cholestasis caused by bile duct paucity but not the other features. The prognosis for this form is less favorable.

Choledochal Cysts. Manifestations include <u>conjugated hyperbilirubinemia with jaundice, vomiting, acholic stools, and hepatomegaly in the neonate.</u> Alternatively, choledochal cysts can present with jaundice, abdominal pain, and a right upper quadrant mass in the older child. There are five types of cystic dilatations of the extrahepatic or intrahepatic bile ducts.

The diagnosis is made by <u>ultrasound</u> studies and confirmed by an <u>intraoperative cholangiogram.</u>

Treatment involves <u>surgical excision.</u> Cholangitis may occur <u>postoperatively.</u> If the cyst is not fully excised, carcinoma can develop in the residual cyst tissue.

[handwritten: RISK OF Ca in residual cyst]

Treatment of Cholestasis

[handwritten: MCT and Vit Supps ADEK]

Some interventions are essential for all infants with cholestasis, no matter what the cause. In these infants, there is malabsorption of fats and fat-soluble vitamins as a result of a decreased concentration of bile salts in the intestinal lumen. Infants should be given a formula containing <u>medium-chain triglycerides,</u> which are digested and absorbed without bile salts. Even with the use of special formulas, infants will have some degree of malabsorption and will require extra calories for growth. Some infants require supplemental nocturnal nasogastric feedings for adequate nutrition. They should be given supplemental vitamins A, D, E, and K to prevent visual problems, rickets, neuropathy, and coagulopathy, respectively. A water-soluble vitamin E preparation, d-α-tocopheryl-polyethylene glycol-1000 succinate (TPGS), forms micelles without bile salts and is therefore readily absorbed. Mixing vitamins A and D with TPGS promotes their absorption.

Ascites can be managed with sodium restriction and diuretics. Pruritus is often severe and is not readily treatable. Several medications have been tried, including ursodeoxycholic acid, antihistamines, cholestyramine, phenobarbital, and rifampin. Ursodeoxycholic acid is beneficial in some infants with cholestasis and helps to improve bile excretion, thus reducing serum bile acid levels. Biliary diversion has been effective in some cases.

JAUNDICE IN THE CHILD AND ADOLESCENT

History

The symptom complex is frequently characteristic of a specific class of disease causing jaundice. The individual with hepatocellular disease generally feels ill. For example, fatigue, anorexia, myalgias, nausea, vomiting, and fever are often seen in those with viral hepatitis or autoimmune hepatitis. Acute biliary obstruction is signaled by right upper quandrant pain, vomiting, fever, and acholic stools in addition to jaundice. Neurologic and psychiatric symptoms may be part of the presentation of *Wilson disease.* Autoimmune hepatitis is often accompanied by manifestations of other autoimmune disorders.

The child's age at the onset of symptoms may be helpful. For example, Wilson disease commonly presents in the preadolescent and adolescent, with only very few cases reported in 3- to 4-year olds.

A careful history should be taken regarding past and present use of prescription, over-the-counter (e.g., acetaminophen), and street drugs. Many medications have been associated with hepatobiliary damage, others with hemolysis. Drug abuse is a risk factor for viral hepatitis and human immunodeficiency virus (HIV). Other risk factors for viral hepatitis include homosexual activity, tattooing, and a history of blood transfusions or dialysis. Alcohol use should be asked about, particularly in the adolescent.

Exposure to viral hepatitis, either by travel to an endemic area or during an outbreak, should be pursued. There is a high transmission rate in day care centers.

The patient's past medical history should be reviewed because some chronic illnesses are associated with specific hepatobiliary complications. These include acquired immunodeficiency syndrome (AIDS), cystic fibrosis, heart disease, hemolytic disorders, hemoglobinopathies, and inflammatory bowel disease.

A family history of inheritable disorders, such as Wilson disease and Alagille syndrome, is always helpful. Less specific but still useful clues are other family members with a history of jaundice, anemia, cholecystectomy, or splenectomy.

Physical Examination

Some patients present with previously unidentified chronic liver disease. Evidence of this on physical examination includes spider angiomas, palmar erythema, dilated abdominal veins, cutaneous excoriation as evidence of pruritus, xanthomas, clubbing of digits, ascites, and splenomegaly with a small liver. Splenomegaly is also a characteristic finding in hemolytic disorders and in some oncologic disorders (see Chapter 23). A large, tender liver is suggestive

of acute viral hepatitis or congestive heart failure. A small liver may be found in patients with severe hepatitis or cirrhosis. A tender gallbladder is indicative of choledocholithiasis. Abnormal neurologic findings, including tremor, fine motor incoordination, clumsy gait, and choreiform movements, suggest Wilson disease. An ophthalmologic examination should be included to look for Kayser-Fleischer rings of Wilson disease or posterior embryotoxon of Alagille syndrome.

Differential Diagnosis

A specific diagnosis may seem highly likely, based on the clinical presentation. In such a case, laboratory evaluation should first be directed at confirming the suspected diagnosis. If no clear diagnosis is readily apparent, the evaluation should proceed as outlined in Figure 24–3. Just as with the infant, an initial step in the diagnosis of jaundice in the older child should be fractionation of the bilirubin to discriminate unconjugated from conjugated hyperbilirubinemia.

UNCONJUGATED HYPERBILIRUBINEMIA

Most causes of unconjugated hyperbilirubinemia in the child and adolescent are secondary to hemolysis, resulting in increased bilirubin production (Table 24–7) (see Chapter 49). A CBC with evaluation of the smear, reticulocyte count, and Coombs test can differentiate hemolytic from non-hemolytic disorders.

Erythrocyte membrane (spherocytosis) and enzyme defects (py-

Table 24–7. Differential Diagnosis of Unconjugated Hyperbilirubinemia in Childhood and Adolescence

Increased Bilirubin Production
Autoimmune hemolytic anemia
   Idiopathic
   Secondary
       Infection (viral, mycoplasma)
       Diseases with autoantibody production
       Immunodeficiency
       Malignancy
Drug-induced hemolytic anemia
Paroxysmal nocturnal hemoglobinuria
Erythrocyte membrane defects
   Hereditary spherocytosis
   Hereditary elliptocytosis
Erythrocyte enzyme defects
   Glucose-6-phosphate dehydrogenase
   Pyruvate kinase
   Hexokinase
   Other
Sepsis with disseminated intravascular coagulation
Reabsorption of hematoma
Transfusion reaction

Decreased Uptake, Storage, or Metabolism
Congestive heart failure
Sepsis
Acidosis
Gilbert syndrome
Arias syndrome → Crigler Najjar type II
Prolonged fasting
Drugs
Portacaval shunt

ruvate kinase, G6PD) may not be apparent until childhood or adolescence. Autoimmune hemolytic anemia is characterized by pallor, abdominal pain, fever, and dark urine in addition to jaundice. Laboratory studies document anemia and reticulocytosis. The direct Coombs test will be positive. This hemolytic anemia can be associated with infection, immunodeficiency, malignancy, or other autoimmune disorders, such as systemic lupus erythematosus, rheumatoid arthritis, thyroid disorders, and chronic autoimmune hepatitis. Most of the time autoimmune hemolytic anemia is idiopathic.

Most of the non-hemolytic causes of unconjugated hyperbilirubinemia will have been identified during the initial assessment. Congestive heart failure and infection should be suspected from physical examination. The child or adolescent with infection severe enough to cause jaundice has other signs of sepsis. If no other explanation is found, Gilbert syndrome or Arias (Crigler-Najjar type II) syndrome should be considered.

CONJUGATED HYPERBILIRUBINEMIA

In the child with conjugated hyperbilirubinemia, the PT and the albumin, glucose, transaminase, and alkaline phosphatase levels should be measured. Albumin and PT determinations provide evidence of hepatocyte synthetic function. Hypoglycemia is another marker of severity of hepatocellular damage. This is important in considering how quickly the evaluation should proceed or how closely the patient should be monitored. For example, the child who has a classic presentation for hepatitis A but also a prolonged PT or hypoglycemia may be in that small group who develop fulminant hepatic failure; these children should be admitted to the hospital and observed very closely. An attempt should be made to correct the PT to differentiate hepatocellular from cholestatic disease. Hypoglycemia should be corrected with frequent meals or intravenous dextrose.

Obstruction

The relative elevation of transaminase and alkaline phosphatase levels in the context of the clinical picture will determine the likelihood of an obstructive etiology. While obstructions occur less commonly in children than in adults, it is important not to miss correctable causes of obstruction that, if left untreated, can cause hepatocellular damage. These patients usually have markedly elevated alkaline phosphatase and minimally elevated transaminase levels. They should be evaluated promptly with ultrasound and possibly ERCP or PTC. The possible causes of obstruction are listed in Table 24–8.

Gallstones. Gallstones are particularly common in children with hemolytic disorders, such as sickle cell disease, thalassemia, erythrocyte membrane defects, erythrocyte enzyme defects, and autoimmune hemolytic anemia. The mean age of presentation is 12 years. Gallstones are also associated with anatomic abnormalities of the biliary tract, cystic fibrosis, ileal dysfunction, obesity, parenteral nutrition, sepsis, prematurity, and adolescent pregnancy. Stones may be found incidentally on abdominal x-ray or ultrasound studies in asymptomatic individuals. Alternatively, gallstones may present with nausea, vomiting, right upper quadrant or nonspecific abdominal pain, and jaundice. Ultrasonography is a very sensitive diagnostic test. Treatment for symptomatic patients is cholecystectomy. ERCP can be used to remove common bile duct stones.

Primary Sclerosing Cholangitis. Primary sclerosing cholangitis

is characterized by dilatation and stenosis of the intrahepatic or extrahepatic bile ducts with surrounding fibrosis resulting from an inflammatory process. It can present from early childhood through adulthood. In adults, it is frequently associated with inflammatory bowel disease, especially ulcerative colitis. It may precede the onset of inflammatory bowel disease by many years. It has also been found in association with histiocytosis X and immunodeficiency states. It can occur in the absence of any underlying condition. The onset may be insidious. Symptoms include diarrhea, abdominal pain, fever, and jaundice.

Diagnostic evaluation includes ultrasound studies, which may show dilated ducts, and cholangiography, ERCP, or PTC, which will demonstrate the characteristic beading of bile ducts. The disorder can progress to cirrhosis with ultimate liver failure. Cholangiocarcinoma has occurred in 10% to 15% of adults. There is no documented efficacy of any therapy except transplantation.

Other Causes. If an obstructive process has been excluded or is less likely, based on a combination of the clinical picture and transaminase levels that are more elevated than the alkaline phosphate levels, the evaluation should focus on infectious, metabolic, toxic, and autoimmune causes.

Infection

Infections are the most common cause of jaundice in the child and adolescent. To diagnose acute hepatitis, the following studies should be obtained: hepatitis A IgM, hepatitis B surface antigen (HBsAg), hepatitis B core IgM (antiHBc), and hepatitis C antibody (anti-HCV). If HBsAg is positive, it may be useful to obtain hepatitis D antibodies as well. Epstein-Barr virus titers may also be useful.

Hepatitis A. Hepatitis A (HAV) infection is usually asymptomatic in children younger than 5 years of age. However, in almost 66% of those between 5 and 17 years of age, a symptomatic illness with

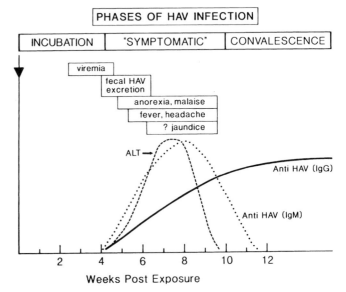

Figure 24–4. Typical course of hepatitis A infection. HAV = hepatitis A virus; ALT = alanine aminotransferase; Ig = immunoglobulin. (Modified from Balistreri WF: Viral hepatitis. Pediatr Clin North Am 35:637, 1988.)

jaundice will develop. Two to 7 days before the onset of jaundice, there is a flu-like illness with symptoms that can include malaise, headache, myalgias, anorexia, vomiting, diarrhea, right upper quandrant pain, and fever. Some children present with cough and coryza. The urine becomes dark, and jaundice and pale or acholic stools develop. Transaminase levels are 10 to 100 times normal.

The diagnosis is confirmed by HAV IgM. Children generally recover within 2 weeks. Occasionally, fulminant hepatitis develops from HAV infection; however, there is no carrier state or chronic hepatitis.

HAV is an enterovirus of the picornavirus group. Transmission is by the fecal-oral route, which may include contaminated water and food, especially shellfish. The greatest fecal excretion is prior to the onset of jaundice when the disease has not yet been recognized (Fig. 24–4). Transmission rates are high in day care centers and institutions for the mentally retarded. The incubation period is 15 to 49 days. Infection can be prevented in 85% to 90% of cases by giving intramuscular immunoglobulin to contacts within 2 weeks of exposure.

Hepatitis B. Hepatitis B (HBV) infection has a more insidious onset than HAV infection but produces the same symptoms. In addition, there may be evidence of arthritis, polyarteritis, urticaria, and nephritis from circulating immune complexes.

There are a number of serologic markers of HBV infection. HBsAg is the first antigenic marker to appear; it disappears after 1 to 3 months if HBV resolves (Fig. 24–5). Hepatitis B surface antibody (anti-HBs) documents recovery and immunity. In patients whose infections resolve, there is a window of 2 to 6 weeks between the disappearance of HBsAg and the appearance of anti-HBs. During this window, anti-HBc may be the only evidence of infection with HBV. Hepatitis B e antigen (HBeAg) correlates with viral replication and thus is a marker of the degree of infectivity. HBV deoxyribonucleic acid (DNA) is a measure of viral replication. The diagnosis of acute infection is made with HBsAg and anti-HBc.

In 1% to 2% of children with HBV, fulminant hepatic failure develops. The severity of hepatic failure for this and other causes and the need for emergent liver transplantation are presented in Table 24–9. Possible additional causes of hepatic failure are listed in Table 24–10. Grading of hepatic encephalopathy is noted in Table 24–11.

Chronic infection, defined as the persistence of HBsAg for at least 6 months, occurs in 90% of neonates, 25% to 50% of children under 5 years of age, and 5% to 10% of adults. HBV is a DNA

Table 24–8. Differential Diagnosis of Conjugated Hyperbilirubinemia in Childhood and Adolescence

Obstructive	**Drug or Toxin** *Continued*
Gallstones	Drugs*
Primary sclerosing cholangitis	Hormones (estrogens, androgens)
Choledochal cyst	Antibiotics (erythromycin, tetracycline)
Bile duct stenosis	Anticonvulsants (valproate, phenytoin)
Anomalies of the choledochopancreaticoduodenal junction	Acetaminophen
Pancreatitis	Salicylate
Caroli disease	Halothane
Congenital hepatic fibrosis	Isoniazid
Tumor	Antineoplastics
Hepatic	Pemoline
Biliary	Toxins
Pancreatic	*Amanita phalloides* (mushroom)
Duodenal	Carbon tetrachloride
	Phosphorus
Infection	Total parenteral nutrition
Hepatitis A	Alcohol
Hepatitis B	
Hepatitis C	**Autoimmune Hepatitis**
Hepatitis D	
Hepatitis E	**Intrahepatic Cholestasis**
Hepatitis GB	Alagille syndrome
Epstein-Barr virus	Familial benign recurrent cholestasis
Cytomegalovirus	Byler syndrome
Human herpesvirus 6	
Herpes simplex virus	**Miscellaneous**
Varicella zoster virus	Dubin-Johnson syndrome
Leptospirosis	Rotor syndrome
Sepsis/shock	Cardiovascular
Liver abscess	Ischemia
	Congestive heart failure
Metabolic Disorders	Cardiomyopathy
Wilson disease	Oncologic
Cystic fibrosis	Leukemia
Cholesterol ester storage disease	Lymphoma
	Graft-versus-host disease
Drug or Toxin	Veno-occlusive disease
Drugs*	Sickle cell disease with intrahepatic sickling
Chlorpromazine	Heat stroke

*Many other drugs have been implicated in the etiology of conjugated hyperbilirubinemia; these are the most commonly cited.

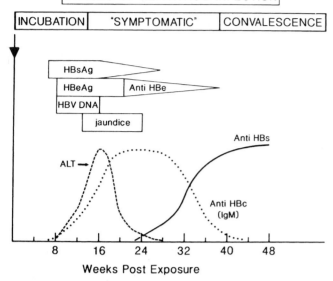

Figure 24–5. Typical course of acute hepatitis B infection. HBV = hepatitis B virus; ALT = alanine aminotransferase; Ig = immunoglobulin; HBc = hepatitis B core (antigen); HBs = hepatitis B surface; HBsAg = hepatitis B surface (antigen); HBe = hepatitis e (antigen). (From Balistreri WF: Viral hepatitis. Pediatr Clin North Am 35:637, 1988.)

virus that is transmitted through blood products, shared needles, and sexual contact; vertically during childbirth; and from occupational exposure. Risk of vertical infection in the infant is greatest in the presence of high maternal HBsAg titer and maternal HBeAg positivity. Infection is prevented by administration of hepatitis B immunoglobulin (HBIG) within 12 hours of birth and a series of three hepatitis B vaccinations.

Hepatitis C. Acute hepatitis C (HCV) infection is often mild and

may be subclinical. Jaundice is unusual but can be seen in severe HCV infection, which resembles HAV and HBV infections clinically. HCV is a rare cause of fulminant hepatic failure. Chronic active hepatitis occurs in 35% to 50% of cases, with cirrhosis in 20% to 25%. It is currently diagnosed by anti-HCV antibodies, as there is no commercially available test for HCV antigen. The utility of anti-HCV is limited by the fact that seroconversion may not occur for up to a year after the onset of symptoms. Therefore, if HCV infection is suspected, the anti-HCV serology studies should be repeated. Transmission may be parenteral or rarely vertical.

Hepatitis D. Hepatitis D (HDV) infection can occur only in the presence of HBV as either a coinfection or superinfection. Its route

Table 24–9. Severity of Hepatic Failure and Criteria for Predicting Death and the Need for Liver Transplantation at King's College Hospital, London*

Causes of Acute Liver Failure	Criteria
Acetaminophen poisoning	pH <7.3 (irrespective of grade of encephalopathy) *or* Prothrombin time >100 sec and serum creatinine >3.4 mg/dl (300 μmol/liter) in patients with grade III or IV encephalopathy
All other causes	Prothrombin time >100 sec (irrespective of grade of encephalopathy) *or* Any 3 of the following variables (irrespective of grade of encephalopathy): age <10 yr or >40 yr; liver failure caused by non-A, non-B hepatitis, halothane-induced hepatitis, or idiosyncratic drug reactions; duration of jaundice before onset of encephalopathy >7 days; prothrombin time >50 sec; serum bilirubin >17.5 mg/dl (300 μmol/liter)

From O'Grady JG, Alexander GJM, Hayllar KM, et al. Early indicators of prognosis in fulminant hepatic failure. Gastroenterology 1989;97:4439–4435.

*Transplantation was considered if the likelihood of survival without it was less than 20%.

Table 24–10. Etiologic Considerations for Hepatic Failure

Early perinatal	Hepatitis B
Herpesvirus	Hepatitis C
Hepatitis B virus	Hepatitis E (especially if
Echoviruses	pregnant)
Adenoviruses	Hepatitis non A, non B
Neonatal	Drugs
hemochromatosis	Acetaminophen
	Isoniazid
Late perinatal	Sodium valproate
Tyrosinemia	Methyldopa
Fructose intolerance	Tetracycline
Galactosemia	Halothane
Epstein-Barr virus	Chemical toxins
Zellweger syndrome	Carbon tetrachloride
Inborn errors of bile acid	Phosphorus
metabolism	*Amanita phalloides*
Alpha$_1$-antitrypsin	Miscellaneous
deficiency	Ischemia/hypotension
Familial hemophagocytic	Wilson disease
syndrome	Leukemia/lymphoma
	α_1-Antitrypsin deficiency
Childhood and young	
adulthood	
Viral infections	
Hepatitis A	

Modified from Russell GJ, Fitzgerald JF, Clark JH. Fulminant hepatic failure. J Pediatr 1987;111:313–319

Table 24–11. Stages of Hepatic Encephalopathy

	Stage 1	Stage 2	Stage 3	Stage 4
Clinical symptoms	Normal level of consciousness with periods of lethargy and euphoria; reversal of day-night sleep pattern	Increased drowsiness, inappropriate behavior, disorientation, agitation with wide swings in affect and mood	Stuporous, sleeping most of time, although arousable; marked confusion; incoherent speech	Comatose; may not respond to noxious stimuli
Signs	Asterixis may be present; patient may have trouble drawing line figures	Asterixis; fetor hepaticus	Asterixis; hyperreflexia and extensor reflexes elicited; rigidity	Reflexes disappear; asterixis cannot be elicited; flaccid limbs
Electroencephalogram	Normal	Abnormal with generalized slowing	Markedly abnormal	Markedly abnormal

From Russell GJ, Fitzgerald JF, Clark JH. Fulminant hepatic failure. J Pediatr 1987;111:313–319.

of transmission is parenteral. As with HBV, it can become chronic. The diagnosis is confirmed by HDV antibody.

Hepatitis E. Hepatitis E (HEV) infection is a recently recognized hepatitis that is similar to HAV in its presentation and mode of transmission. It is a self-limited illness with no chronic state. As with HAV, however, fulminant hepatitis may rarely occur. There is no commercially available serologic test for HEV.

Epstein-Barr Virus. Epstein-Barr viral (EBV) infection can mimic HAV, HBV, or HCV infection. Often there is an exudative pharyngitis and lymphadenopathy. Fatal hepatic necrosis can occur. This is rare but is of particular concern in the immunocompromised host. The diagnosis is confirmed by elevation of EBV IgM titers.

Other Viruses. Other viruses, including herpes simplex, human herpes virus 6 and CMV, can also cause hepatitis, particularly in the immunosuppressed patient.

Wilson Disease

Wilson disease, an inborn error of copper metabolism, can present in a variety of ways (see Chapter 22). The liver involvement may include an acute hepatitis, fulminant hepatic failure, chronic active hepatitis, or cirrhosis. Neurologic symptoms, such as dysarthria, clumsiness, and tremor, may be present in addition or can be the only manifestations. As a result of defective metabolism, copper cannot be excreted and it accumulates in the liver, which causes hepatic necrosis. Copper is then released into the circulation and is ultimately deposited in the central nervous system, kidneys, and cornea. In the kidney, the result is tubular dysfunction; in the cornea, the result is Kayser-Fleischer rings. Wilson disease is an inherited disorder with autosomal recessive transmission that usually presents in the preadolescent or adolescent.

The diagnosis is supported by documenting a low serum ceruloplasmin level, high urinary copper excretion, and increased hepatic copper on liver biopsy. Effective treatment is provided by administration of D-penicillamine, which chelates copper, and by dietary restriction of copper, unless the patient presents in fulminant hepatic failure. In this case, a liver transplant is the only therapy.

Drugs and Toxins

Numerous drugs and toxins associated with hepatic injury (see Table 24–8) should always be considered in the evaluation of

jaundice. The reaction can be idiosyncratic or dose-related. In the latter case, this may be associated with either accidental or purposeful overdose. The presentation can be that of acute hepatitis, fulminant hepatic failure, or cholestatic disease, depending on the drug.

Autoimmune Hepatitis

In children, autoimmune hepatitis often presents acutely with malaise, anorexia, nausea, vomiting, and jaundice; it can also present with evidence of chronic liver disease (see Chapter 22). There may be associated autoimmune problems, such as arthritis, thyroiditis, vasculitis, nephritis, hemolytic anemia, or diabetes mellitus. Autoimmune hepatitis may be associated with inflammatory bowel disease. Laboratory studies demonstrate elevated transaminase levels, mild hyperbilirubinemia, and hypergammaglobulinemia. Children are often found to have anti-LKM (liver-kidney-microsomal) antibodies and a positive antinuclear antibody (ANA).

Liver biopsy is required for diagnosis. Characteristic findings are an inflammatory infiltrate expanding the portal area and moderate to severe piecemeal necrosis. Treatment consists of steroids; occasionally, azathioprine is also required.

REFERENCES

General

Sherlock S, Dooley J. Diseases of the Liver and Biliary System, 9th ed. Oxford, England: Blackwell Scientific Publications, 1993.

Diagnostic Strategies

Frank BB. Clinical evaluation of jaundice: A guideline of the patient care committee of the American Gastroenterological Association. JAMA 1989;262:3031.

Rutledge JC, Ou C-N. Bilirubin and the laboratory: Advances in the 1980's, considerations for the 1990's. Pediatr Clin North Am 1989;36:189.

St. Louis PJ. Biochemical studies: Liver and intestine. *In* Walker WA, Durie PR, Hamilton JR, et al (eds). Pediatric Gastrointestinal Disease: Pathophysiology, Diagnosis, Management. Philadelphia: BC Decker, 1991.

Neonatal Jaundice

Balistreri WF. Neonatal cholestasis. J Pediatr 1985;106:171.

Balistreri WF, Schubert WK. Liver disease in infancy and childhood. *In* Schiff L, Schiff ER (eds). Diseases of the Liver, 7th ed. Philadelphia: JB Lippincott, 1993.

Gourley GR. Jaundice. *In* Wyllie R, Hyams JS (eds). Pediatric Gastrointestinal Disease: Pathophysiology, Diagnosis, Management. Philadelphia: WB Saunders, 1993.

Heubi JE, Daugherty CG. Neonatal cholestasis: An approach for the practicing pediatrician. Curr Probl Pediatr 1990;20:235.

Rosenthal P, Sinatra F. Jaundice in infancy. Pediatr Rev 1989;11:79.

Alagille Syndrome

Alagille D, Estrada A, Hadchouel M, et al. Syndromic paucity of interlobular bile ducts (Alagille syndrome or arteriohepatic dysplasia): Review of 80 cases. J Pediatr 1987;110:195.

Alagille D, Odievre M, Gautier M, et al. Hepatic ductular hypoplasia associated with characteristic facies, vertebral malformations, retarded physical, mental, and sexual development, and cardiac murmur. J Pediatr 1975;86:63.

Riely CA. Familial intrahepatic cholestatic syndromes. Semin Liver Dis 1987;7:119.

Alpha₁-Antitrypsin Deficiency

Balistreri WF. Liver disease associated with α_1-antitrypsin deficiency. *In* Balistreri WF, Stocker JT (eds). Pediatric Hepatology. Bristol, Pa: Hemisphere Publishing, 1990.

Odievre M, Martin J-P, Hadchouel M, et al. Alpha₁-antitrypsin deficiency and liver disease in children: Phenotypes, manifestations, and prognosis. Pediatrics 1976;57:226.

Sveger T. The natural history of liver disease in α_1-antitrypsin deficient children. Acta Pediatr Scand 1988;77:847.

Bile Acid Abnormalities

Balistreri WF. Fetal and neonatal bile acid synthesis and metabolism—clinical implications. J Inherit Metab Dis 1991;14:459.

Setchell KDR, Street JM. Inborn errors of bile acid synthesis. Semin Liver Dis 1987;7:85.

Biliary Atresia

Kasai M, Kimura S, Asakura Y, et al. Surgical treatment of biliary atresia. J Pediatr Surg 1968;3:665.

Ryckman FC, Noseworthy J. Neonatal cholestatic conditions requiring surgical reconstruction. Semin Liver Dis 1987;7:134.

Crigler-Najjar and Arias Syndromes

Arias IM, Gartner LM, Cohen M, et al. Chronic nonhemolytic unconjugated hyperbilirubinemia with glucuronyl transferase deficiency. Am J Med 1969;47:395.

Crigler JF, Najjar VA. Congenital familial nonhemolytic jaundice with kernicterus. Pediatrics 1952;10:169.

Sinaasappel M, Jansen PLM. The differential diagnosis of Crigler-Najjar disease, types 1 and 2, by bile pigment analysis. Gastroenterology 1991;100:783.

Erythrocyte Enzyme Defects

Luzzato L. G6PD deficiency and hemolytic anemia. *In* Nathan DG, Oski FA (eds). Hematology of Infancy and Childhood, 4th ed. Philadelphia: WB Saunders, 1993.

Gilbert Syndrome

Bosma P, Chowdhury J, Bakker C, et al. The genetic basis of reduced expression of bilirubin UDP-glucuronosyltransferase I in Gilbert's syndrome. N Engl J Med 1995;333:1171–1175.

Powell LW, Hemingway E, Billing BH, et al. Idiopathic unconjugated hyperbilirubinemia (Gilbert's syndrome): A study of 42 families. N Engl J Med 1967;277:1108.

Lucey-Driscoll Syndrome

Arias IM, Wolfson S, Lucey JF, et al. Transient familial neonatal hyperbilirubinemia. J Clin Invest 1965;44:1442.

Lucey JF, Arias IM, McKay RJ. Transient familial neonatal hyperbilirubinemia. Am J Dis Child 1960;100:787.

Physiologic and Breast Milk Jaundice

Kivlahan C, James EJP. The natural history of neonatal jaundice. Pediatrics 1984;74:364.

Lascari AD. ''Early'' breast-feeding jaundice: clinical significance. J Pediatr 1986;108:156.

Maisels MJ, Gifford K. Normal serum bilirubin levels in the newborn and the effect of breast feeding. Pediatrics 1986;78:837.

Jaundice in Older Children and Adolescents

Balistreri WF, Schubert WK. Liver disease in infancy and childhood. *In* Schiff L, Schiff ER (eds). Diseases of the Liver, 7th ed. Philadelphia: JB Lippincott, 1993.

Sokol RJ. Fulminant hepatic failure. *In* Balistreri WF, Stocker JT (eds). Pediatric Hepatology. Bristol, Pa: Hemisphere Publishing, 1990.

Autoimmune Hemolytic Anemia

Schreiber AD, Gill FM, Manno CS. Autoimmune hemolytic anemia. *In* Nathan DG, Oski FA (eds). Hematology of Infancy and Childhood, 4th ed. Philadelphia: WB Saunders, 1993.

Autoimmune Hepatitis

Homberg J-C, Abuaf N, Bernard O, et al. Chronic active hepatitis associated with anti–liver/kidney/microsome antibody type 1: A second type of ''autoimmune hepatitis.'' Hepatology 1987;7:1333.

Johnson PJ, McFarlane IG, Eddleston ALWF. The natural course and heterogeneity of autoimmune-type chronic active hepatitis. Semin Liver Dis 1991;11:187.

Maggiore G, Bernard O, Homberg J-C, et al. Liver disease associated with anti-liver-kidney microsome antibody in children. J Pediatr 1986;108:399.

Drugs

Lee W. Drug-induced hepatotoxicity. N Engl J Med 1995;333:1118.

Zimmerman HJ, Mullick FG. Drug-induced hepatic disease. *In* Balistreri WF, Stocker JT (eds). Pediatric Hepatology. Bristol, Pa: Hemisphere Publishing, 1990.

Gallstones

Reif S, Sloven DG, Lebenthal E. Gallstones in children: Characterization by age, etiology, and outcome. Am J Dis Child 1991;145:105.

Hepatitis

Balistreri WF. Viral hepatitis. Pediatr Clin North Am 1988;35:637.
Hoofnagle JH, DiBisceglie AM. Serologic diagnosis of acute and chronic hepatitis. Semin Liver Dis 1991;11:73.
Krugman S. Viral hepatitis: A, B, C, D, and E—infection. Pediatr Rev 1992;13:203.
Krugman S. Viral hepatitis: A, B, C, D, and E—prevention. Pediatr Rev 1992;13:245.
Nowicki MJ, Balistreri WF. Hepatitis A to E: building up the alphabet. Contemp Pediatr 1992;9:118.
Nowicki MJ, Balistreri WF. The C's, D's, and E's of viral hepatitis. Contemp Pediatr 1992;9:23.

Primary Sclerosing Cholangitis

El-Shabrawi M, Wilkinson ML, Portmann B, et al. Primary sclerosing cholangitis in childhood. Gastroenterology 1987;92:1226.
Sisto A, Feldman P, Garel L, et al. Primary sclerosing cholangitis: Study of 5 cases and review of the literature. Pediatrics 1987;80:918.

Wilson Disease

Saito T. Presenting symptoms and natural history of Wilson disease. Eur J Pediatr 1987;146:261.

25 Constipation

Gloria Ana Berenson   Robert Wyllie

It is estimated that approximately 3% of pediatric patients have constipation or fecal soiling and that 10% to 25% of patients of pediatric gastroenterologists experience difficulties with defecation. The number of children from birth to 9 years of age brought to a physician's attention for constipation has increased from approximately 850 per 100,000 visits to 1700 per 100,000 visits in the past three decades. Much of this increase occurred in 0- to 2-year-old patients, with both sexes being equally represented.

The diagnosis of constipation requires careful history taking and interpretation because the history is often obtained from the parents, reflects their observations of the child's stooling behavior, and may be influenced by their perception of what is normal. Constipation may be defined in terms of frequency of bowel movements, consistency, straining activity in passing a stool, or pain associated with the passage of stool. Given the variable range of normal stooling patterns in children, it is very difficult to assign a numeric value to normal bowel frequency. Bottle-fed infants may have four or five stools per day in the first weeks of life; stool frequency gradually decreases to one to two per day by 1 year of age. Breast-fed infants usually pass softer and more frequent stools in the first few months but also show a gradual diminution in stool frequency to one to two bowel movements per day by 1 year of age. Of children aged 1 to 4 years, 85% have one or two bowel movements per day and 96% fall within the range of three bowel movements per day to one bowel movement, every other day. Constipation may also be defined as the difficult passage of hard stools.

The daily bowel habits of children are extremely susceptible to any change in routine or environment. Infants frequently experience at least transient constipation as a result of changes in their diet, such as formula changes or the addition of solid foods. Constipation is often secondary to inadequate intake of dietary fiber, fluid, or both. Young children in the United States have a diet that is poor in fiber content and high in refined sugars. Infrequently, infectious enteritis may present with constipation. An infectious illness, including a diarrheal illness, may also be the initial event that causes constipation. A diaper dermatitis or an anal fissure may cause painful defecation, leading to fecal retention (hoarding), constipation, and if persistent, dilation of the rectal vault, with loss of normal sensation and overflow encopresis.

Patients with chronic constipation have been found to have physiologic abnormalities that can be demonstrated by anorectal manometric evaluation. The most consistent abnormality is a blunted rectal sensation, rendering the patient unable to feel the bolus of stool in the rectum. Other findings include incomplete relaxation of the internal anal sphincter and paradoxical contraction of the external sphincter during attempted defecation. A significant proportion of chronically constipated patients show contraction rather than relaxation of the external anal sphincter during attempted defecation. Patients who have paradoxical anal contraction are less likely to respond to routine medical therapy and have high rates of recurrence of constipation after routine treatment regimens are terminated. These abnormalities may slowly diminish with medical therapy, but they do not resolve, placing these patients at increased risk for recurrent problems, especially if treatment for constipation is withdrawn.

Many children develop constipation at one time in their lives; in most children, it is transient. If problems with defecation persist, an individualized plan of management is successful in most patients.

PHYSIOLOGY OF NORMAL DEFECATION

Normal defecation patterns and behavior depend on a host of factors, including:

1. The abdominal musculature and the diaphragm allow intra-abdominal pressure to build during the Valsalva maneuver.
2. Innervation of the smooth muscle in the colonic wall results in peristalsis necessary to propel the fecal mass to the anorectum.
3. The normal rectum is distensible and can act as a reservoir for the bolus of stool until it can be expelled.
4. The internal anal sphincter is under autonomic control, main-

Table 25–1. Causes of Constipation Presenting in the Neonatal Period

Meconium plug (rule out cystic fibrosis)
Meconium ileus (rule out cystic fibrosis)
Hirschsprung disease
Anatomic anomalies
    Anteriorly displaced anus
    Ectopic anus
    Anal stenosis
    Imperforate anus
Hypothyroidism
Hypercalcemia
Spina bifida
Neuronal intestinal dysplasia types A and B

taining the anal canal closed at rest and maintaining continence. Arrival of a bolus of stool in the anorectum causes the internal anal sphincter to reflexively relax, thus allowing the stool to be expelled.

5. The external anal sphincter and the levator ani muscles work in concert. Voluntary contraction of these muscles causes the anus to close and be lifted, thus decreasing the rectoanal angle and delaying defecation. Relaxation of these muscles allows the rectoanal angle to increase or straighten, facilitating the passage of stool into the anal canal.

6. Transitional epithelium in the anorectal area enables the awareness of the urge to defecate and allows discrimination between the sensations caused by solid, liquid, and gas.

Anomalies in any of these structures can result in significant difficulties of defecation. Several studies have been conducted to measure the colonic transit time in normal and constipated children. Mean colonic transit times have been found to increase with age from approximately 8.5 hours at 1 to 3 months of age to 26 hours at 3 to 13 years of age. Ninety percent of children have total colonic transit times of within 33 hours. Children who show delayed transit have fecal retention in the distal colon, suggesting that the problem is that of expulsion of stool from the distal rectum, or voluntary retention of the stool. Delayed transit in the small bowel or other parts of the colon is rare in children.

DATA COLLECTION AND ASSESSMENT

History

Obtaining a thorough and accurate history is of paramount importance in the evaluation of a child with constipation because much of the initial evaluation and management decision making is based on the presenting history. The differential diagnosis of constipation is different in the various age ranges and the ages at the onset of symptoms (Figs. 25–1 and 25–2). Constipation in the newborn or very young infant or a history of constipation since infancy suggests a diagnosis of Hirschsprung disease (Tables 25–1 and 25–2). The severity and duration of the constipation should be noted, with the frequency, the pattern, and the volume of bowel movements as well as any associated signs and symptoms, such as

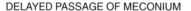

DELAYED PASSAGE OF MECONIUM

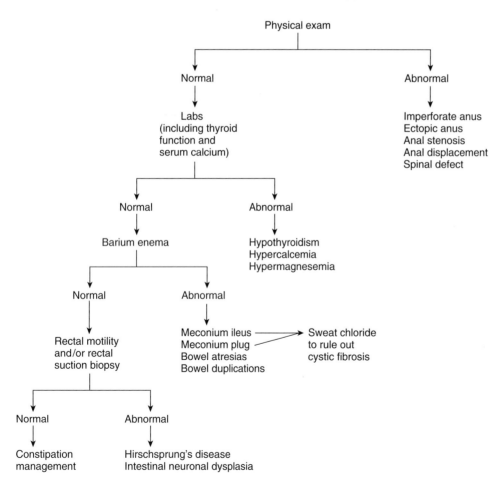

Figure 25–1. Algorithmic approach to the differential diagnosis of delayed passage of meconium.

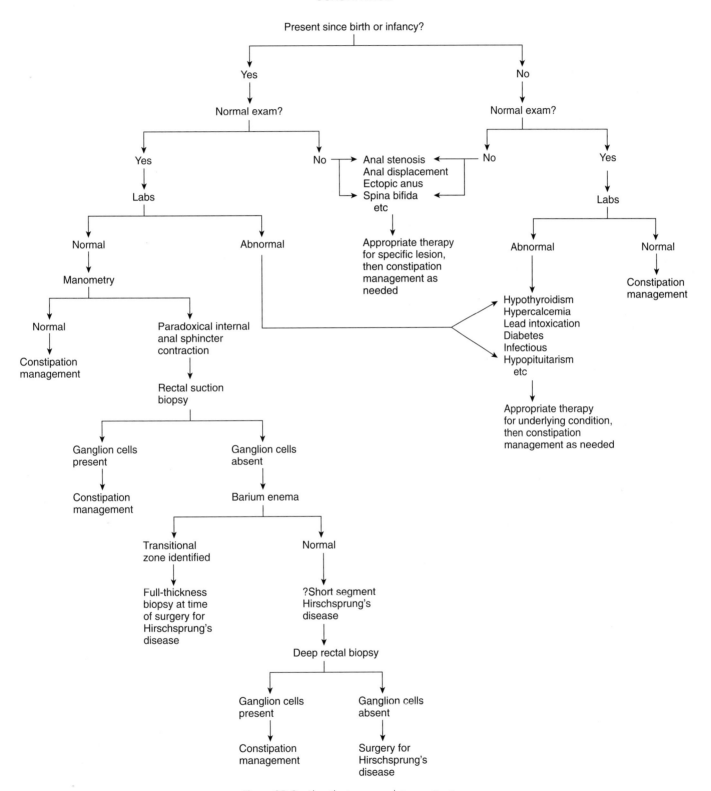

Figure 25–2. Algorithmic approach to constipation.

abdominal pain, intermittent diarrhea alternating with the constipation, blood in the stool, soiling, and changes in appetite or activity level (Table 25–3).

Abdominal pain is a common complaint in constipated patients and when present is often mild, nonspecific, and periumbilical. Older children may describe discomfort in the lower abdomen and a history of relief of pain after a stool is passed. Appetite is often diminished. A diary recording the passage of stools, the timing of meals, and the onset of abdominal pain over a period of several days to a few weeks can aid in the diagnosis of constipation and monitoring of therapy. The past medical history and the family history are important because constipation can be associated with many other illnesses and conditions (Table 27–3).

The child's behavior during defecation should be noted. A history of straining as an index of difficulty in stooling can be misinterpreted by parents, who often view a child's efforts to withhold stool as efforts to pass a bowel movement. Parents often describe a toddler who hides in a corner, with stiffened straight legs, or who may lean into the wall or hold onto a table while "straining." The likely events leading up to this situation are simple to describe to the parents. The young child, having become constipated for many reasons, passes a painful stool. Passage of a large painful stool may be associated with a fissure. If a fissure is present, a small amount of blood is usually passed with the stool. The child associates the passage of stools with pain and will try to prevent further painful episodes by withholding fecal matter. This behavior results in the formation of even larger, harder stools, which are painful to pass, thus establishing a link between pain and defecation that perpetuates the cycle.

Physical Examination

Typically, the child who presents with the chief complaint of constipation (not caused by Hirschsprung disease) is healthy, with normal growth and development. Abnormal growth patterns should alert the physician to the possibility of underlying organic pathology. Abdominal examination is usually benign. Stool may be palpable in the sigmoid and descending colon through the abdominal wall. Occasionally, a large, firm fecal mass extends from the symphysis pubis to the umbilicus, raising concerns of an abdominal malignancy. The abdomen is not tender to palpation; there may be some mild tenderness in the left lower quadrant on palpation of a segment of bowel that is full of stool.

The spine and sacral area should be examined closely—a tuft of hair or a dimple, or a palpable defect in this area should prompt an evaluation to rule out spina bifida occulta or a tethered cord. The perianal area should be examined for evidence of fissures, which suggests the passage of large, hard stools. The examination is facilitated if an assistant gently spreads the patient's buttocks apart while the examiner illuminates the area. Soiling in the underwear may indicate fecal impaction with overflow encopresis. Location of the anus relative to the other perineal structures should be determined to rule out anatomic or structural anomalies, such as anterior displacement of the rectum, as the cause of the constipation. The presence of a normal anal wink, as elicited by gentle stroking of the perianal skin with a sharp object, such as a wooden tongue blade or the corner of a small package of lubricant, gives evidence of intact sacral innervation.

Digital examination can identify such anomalies as anal stenosis.

Table 25–2. Distinguishing Features of Hirschsprung Disease and Functional (Acquired) Constipation

	Functional Constipation	Hirschsprung Disease*
History		
Gender	Males	Males
Onset of constipation	After 2 yr of age	At birth
Prevalence	1%–3% of males	1:5000–1:15000
Encopresis	Common	Very rare
Forced bowel training	Usual	None
Stool size	Very large	Small, ribbon-like
Enterocolitis	None	Possible
Abdominal pain	Common	Rare except with obstruction, toxic megacolon, or enterocolitis
Failure to thrive	Uncommon	Common
Examination		
Abdominal distention	Variable	Common
Poor growth	Rare	Common
Anal tone	Patulous	Tight
Rectal examination	Stool in ampulla	Ampulla empty
Malnutrition	Absent	Possible
Laboratory		
Barium enema	Massive amounts of stool, no transition zone	Transition zone, delayed evacuation (>24 hr)
Rectal biopsy	Normal	No ganglion cells; ↑ acetylcholinesterase staining
Anorectal manometry	Distention of the rectum causes relaxation of the internal sphincter	No sphincter relaxation

Adapted from Behrman RE (ed). Nelson Textbook of Pediatrics. 15th ed. Philadelphia: WB Saunders, 1996:1071.
*Note that ultrashort-segment Hirschsprung disease may have clinical features of functional (acquired) megacolon (e.g., constipation).

Table 25–3. Causes of Constipation in Infants and Children

Functional
  Faulty diet (poor fiber intake, excessive cow's milk, inadequate nutrition)
  Inadequate fluid intake
  Symptoms of irritable bowel syndrome
  Situational
  Depression
  Familial-constitutional

Anatomic
  Anterior anal displacement
  Ectopic anus
  Anal stenosis
  Malrotation
  Colonic anomalies (rectocele, duplications)
  Stricture (postsurgical, sequelae of inflammatory disorders)
  Painful anorectal lesions (fissures, dermatitis, abscess)
  Abnormal abdominal musculature (prune belly, gastroschisis)
  Intestinal neoplasm, extraintestinal pelvic mass (teratoma)

Endocrine
  Hypothyroidism
  Panhypopituitarism
  Diabetes mellitus

Metabolic
  Hypercalcemia
  Metal intoxication (lead, arsenic, mercury)
  Dehydration
  Cystic fibrosis—meconium ileus equivalent
  Hypokalemia
  Acute intermittent porphyria
  Blue diaper syndrome
  Hereditary coproporphyria

Infectious
  Typhoid

Abnormal Innervation
  Aganglionosis
    Congenital: Hirschsprung disease
    Acquired: Chagas
  Neural dysgenesis (pseudo-obstruction syndromes)
  Hyperganglionosis

Spinal Cord Lesions
  Spina bifida and spina bifida occulta
  Tethered cord
  Spinal cord tumors
  Traumatic lesions

Neurologic
  Infant botulism
  Myotonic dystrophy
  Cerebral palsy

Psychologic Illness
  Anorexia nervosa
  Depression

Drugs
  Anticonvulsants
  Antacids (aluminum and calcium)
  Iron
  Barium
  Opiates (codeine, diphenoxylate–atropine sulfate [Lomotil], loperamide [Imodium])
  Antidepressants
  Anticholinergics
  Phenothiazines
  Vincristine
  Calcium channel blockers
  Bismuth
  Clonidine
  Antihistamines
  Diuretics

Other
  Collagen vascular disease (SLE, mixed connective tissue disease, scleroderma)
  Amyloidosis
  Rubinstein-Taybi syndrome
  Williams syndrome (hypercalcemia)

Abbreviation: SLE = systemic lupus erythematosus.

A dilated rectal vault with a large fecal mass is usually seen in chronic constipation. In most patients with Hirschsprung disease, retained fecal material is not encountered within the first few centimeters of the anal canal.

Laboratory Evaluation

Routine laboratory evaluation is usually not helpful in the evaluation of constipation. Analysis is indicated if a metabolic abnormality is suspected on the basis of the history or physical examination. Endocrinologic disturbances, such as hypothyroidism, can be associated with constipation. Stool studies may be obtained to rule out infectious agents, if the patient's history indicates that infection may be present.

A rectal motility evaluation is often helpful in the diagnosis and management of chronic constipation. Anorectal manometry can be used to evaluate the integrity of the muscles and the innervation of the defecatory mechanism. The determination of sensory threshold can give clues to the projected length of therapy. Patients who cannot detect a balloon filled with 120 ml of air usually have encopresis. Hirschsprung disease is ruled out if a reflex relaxation of the internal anal sphincter is present in the face of rectal distention. Manometry and electromyography document the presence of paradoxical contraction of the external anal sphincter on attempted defecation. Anorectal manometry can also be used as a therapeutic modality in biofeedback therapy in patients with constipation and encopresis and in patients with paradoxical external anal sphincter contraction.

Imaging

Plain films of the abdomen are rarely necessary, but if they are obtained, they may demonstrate stool in the large bowel. This information may occasionally be useful in the case of a child with complaints of diarrhea who suffers from fecal impaction and overflow of liquid stools. If Hirschsprung disease is to be evaluated by radiologic studies, the examination of choice is the "unprepped" barium enema. A 24-hour lateral film must be obtained to look for a short segment of Hirschsprung disease in the rectum. In some older children, defecography may provide useful information on the dynamics of defecation and may allow measurement of the rectoanal angle at rest and during straining.

DIFFERENTIAL DIAGNOSIS
(see Tables 25–2 and 25–3)

Anatomic Lesions

HIRSCHSPRUNG DISEASE

Congenital aganglionic megacolon, or Hirschsprung disease, is a common cause of neonatal intestinal obstruction. It occurs in approximately 1:5000 to 1:15,000 live births, with a male-to-female ratio of about 4:1. The disease is rare in premature births, may be familial, and is associated with trisomy 21, Waardenburg syndrome, multiple endocrine neoplasia 2A (MEN-2A) syndrome, and piebaldism. The absence of ganglion cells in both the Meissner (submucosal) plexus and the Auerbach (myenteric) plexus results in an inability of the involved segment of bowel to relax in response to distention from the presence of stool. In the newborn, passage of meconium is often delayed beyond the usual 24 or 48 hours after birth. Most such conditions are diagnosed during infancy; 50% are diagnosed in the first months of life, 75% by 3 months, and 80% by the first year. Diagnosis may be delayed into childhood, and rarely into adolescence or even adulthood in some patients with short segments of disease. These patients complain of constipation, usually starting in infancy.

The lesion begins at the internal anal sphincter and extends continuously into the rectum or the rectosigmoid in 75% to 80% of cases. In 10% of cases, there is total colonic aganglionosis; in another 10%, there is variable involvement of the small intestine in addition to total colonic disease. The most common presentation in the neonate is delayed passage of meconium, followed by lower intestinal obstruction (distention, bile-stained emesis), obstipation, failure to thrive, or rarely intestinal perforation. Meconium plug syndrome may also be present. In addition, if stool is passed immediately after a rectal examination is performed in an obstipated (no stools) or constipated patient, Hirschsprung disease should be suspected.

Anorectal manometry is a valuable diagnostic procedure. Normal internal anal sphincter relaxation with transient rectal distention rules out Hirschsprung disease. Paradoxical contraction of the internal anal sphincter suggests an absence of ganglion cells and is most common in Hirschsprung disease. Absent relaxation has been noted in premature infants, in neonates with infection or sepsis, and in one baby with thyroid aplasia; normal function is seen after appropriate therapy. The sensitivity and specificity of this test vary somewhat among the different age groups (children versus infants versus neonates). This test has a sensitivity that ranges from 0.79 to 0.90, a specificity ranging from 0.97 to 1.00, and a positive predictive value of 0.94 to 1.00.

A plain abdominal film may occasionally reveal distention of the normally innervated bowel proximal to the affected segment. The most useful radiographic test is the unprepped barium enema, which usually demonstrates a small-caliber rectum with a transition in the rectosigmoid to the dilated, obstructed, normal proximal colon. A delayed lateral radiograph 24 hours after the barium enema aids in identifying a transition zone in the sigmoid colon.

A definitive diagnosis of Hirschsprung disease requires histologic confirmation of the absence of ganglion cells; such confirmation may be accomplished by a simple submucosal suction biopsy, which may be performed in the physician's office. Suction biopsy excludes the diagnosis if ganglion cells are present. However, there

may be a 10% false-negative rate. A full-thickness rectal biopsy procedure is reserved for infants with bowel obstruction and for older children with abnormal rectal motilities and suction biopsies in which ganglion cells have not been identified. In patients with undiagnosed Hirschsprung disease acute toxic megacolon or an infectious enterocolitis may develop (*Staphylococcus aureus, Clostridium difficile*). Therapy for these complications includes correcting electrolyte abnormalities (hypokalemia), broad-spectrum parenteral antibiotics, bowel rest, and if needed, emergency colectomy. Treatment for Hirschsprung disease is surgical resection of the affected segment of bowel and various strategies for an ileal or colonic rectal pull-through procedure. *Red flags* to suspect Hirschsprung disease are noted in Table 25–2. Diseases which may mimic Hirschsprung disease and require biopsy diagnosis include other abnormalities of intestinal innervation such as pseudo-obstruction (neural dysgenesis) and hyperganglionosis.

ANTERIOR ANAL DISPLACEMENT

The position of the anus may be described in terms of the anogenital index, that is, the ratio of the distance from the posterior aspect of the vagina or scrotum to the anus, divided by the full distance to the tip of the coccyx. In individuals with a normally placed anus, this value is greater than 0.34 in females and greater than 0.45 in males. There are two forms of displacement of the anus. In the *anterior ectopic* anus, the anal canal and the internal anal sphincter as a unit are displaced anteriorly in the perineum and are separated from the external anal sphincter, which remains posterior in its usual position. On physical examination, it may be possible to elicit an external sphincter anal wink in the usual location, posterior to the opening of the anal canal. Rectal examination often reveals a sharp posterior angulation in the anal canal. In the *anteriorly located* anus, the entire normal anal unit is located in the anterior perineum (Fig. 25–3). Both of these entities are found more commonly in females. Symptoms of constipation often begin in the newborn period and are related to the difficulty in expelling stool through a canal that is angled anteriorly (Fig. 25–3). Where the displacement is severe enough to cause symptoms, it may require surgical correction to relocate the anus and relieve the obstruction.

ANAL STENOSIS

The diagnosis of anal stenosis may be delayed beyond the newborn period, especially if the degree of stenosis is not severe. Any portion of the anal canal or the entire canal may be involved. The diagnosis can be made by digital examination or by endoscophy. Constipation is caused by fecal retention secondary to outlet obstruction. Treatment is by dilation or anorectal myectomy.

IMPERFORATE ANUS

Imperforate anus is usually diagnosed in the nursery. Passage of meconium is delayed or is noted to take place through an abnormal location as a result of the presence of a fistula (rectovaginal, rectovesicular, or rectoperineal). Treatment is surgical; the actual procedure depends on the level and the extent of the defect.

SPINA BIFIDA AND SPINA BIFIDA OCCULTA

Defecation disturbances, most frequently constipation, are common in patients with spina bifida and spina bifida occulta, espe-

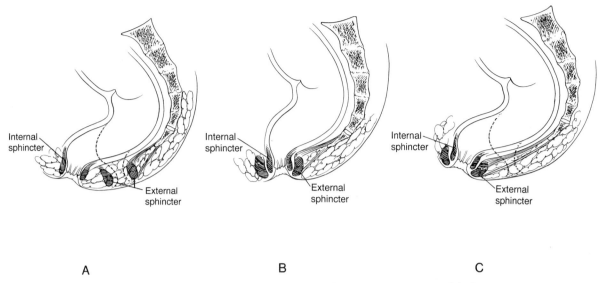

Figure 25–3. *A,* Anterior ectopic anus. *B,* Normal anal anatomy. *C,* Anterior anal displacement.

cially if the defect involves the lumbosacral spine. The spinal and nerve root injury results in poor functioning of the terminal bowel. Voluntary external sphincter control and rectoanal sensation are most often diminished or absent, and the degree of difficulty with defecation is related to the degree and the extent of the injury.

Anticipatory management and education are very important in these patients. Most patients can achieve an acceptable level of continence when they are given a bowel regimen that is individualized to their needs. Dietary fiber, stool softeners, suppositories, and enema continence catheters are treatment options. Biofeedback and pudendal nerve stimulation have been reported to be successful in some patients. In most patients, a combination of treatment modalities allows social continence to be achieved and dramatically improves the patients' quality of life. Treatment of patients with spinal or nerve injury or dysfunction from other causes is similar.

Metabolic Diseases

The appropriate laboratory tests should be performed to rule out the various metabolic and endocrinologic conditions that may present with constipation (see Table 25–3). The most important of these conditions is hypothyroidism. In routine neonatal screening, hypothyroidism presenting solely with constipation is rarely seen. It should be suspected in any infant presenting with constipation and a history of prolonged neonatal jaundice.

Neurologic Diseases

The neurologically impaired child often has constipation for many reasons, including poor intestinal motility, lack of dietary fiber, and poor awareness of rectal vault distension with stool retention. Any illness affecting the spinal cord or sacral nerves, degenerative muscle diseases, cerebral palsy, and demyelinating diseases can result in constipation.

Pharmacologic Side Effects

A complete list of any drugs being taken by the patient should be obtained because many classes of drugs can cause constipation (see Table 25–3).

ENCOPRESIS

Idiopathic constipation is much more common than Hirschsprung disease. Longstanding constipation leads to encopresis, the deposition of stools in the undergarments or other unorthodox locations that persists or occurs beyond the age of formal bowel training. This definition is flexible in that the age by which a child should be toilet trained for feces varies in different cultures. In some cultures, delayed bowel training up to the age of 6 years is normal. It is generally accepted in the United States that healthy children should be bowel trained by the age of 4 years.

Encopresis is thought to be the end result of chronic withholding of stool. As the fecal mass accumulates, it causes rectal distention, increases rectal compliance, and eventually results in blunted or absent sensitivity of the rectum to the presence of liquid stool passing around a firm fecal mass. Children with encopresis usually pass small stools and do not completely empty the rectum. Periodically, they pass huge stools, which may plug the toilet. It is important to specifically question the patient or parents regarding these massive stools because this information is frequently not volunteered in the history.

Encopresis has been incorrectly considered a symptom or manifestation of psychiatric illness. It was thought that the patient retained stools either consciously or subconsciously as a way to rebel, please, or anger caretakers. Although encopresis may be seen in association with emotional and behavioral problems, it is usually the result of painful defecation followed by a pattern of stool withholding, leading to chronic constipation, overflow encopresis, and possibly poor relations with peers as a result of fecal soiling. In the few patients in whom encopresis is truly a manifestation of psychiatric disease, there is often no stool retention and the prognosis for fecal continence with therapy is poor.

Idiopathic constipation with or without constipation may compress the bladder by a dilated rectum, thus causing stasis and urinary tract infections.

MANAGEMENT

The treatment of chronic constipation must be individualized (Table 25–4). Medical therapy is usually protracted, lasting from several weeks to months. The cooperation and compliance of the

Table 25–4. Management of Constipation and Encopresis

Initial Evaluation

  Appropriate studies to rule out underlying disease

  Rectal manometry if clinically indicated

  Education

Initial Bowel Evacuation (1–4 days)

  Mineral oil in large doses (15 ml per year of age or 5 ml/kg of body weight) initially to complete evacuation.

  In severe cases, one or more enemas may be needed to empty the bowel.

  May also give a balanced electrolyte colonic lavage solution orally or via nasogastric tube, if needed.

Maintenance

  Mineral oil titrated to effect (very soft stool without excessive leakage of oil), starting at 5 ml/kg of body weight (not indicated in patients at risk for aspiration or in infants <6 months of age).

  Alternatively, may use lactulose in cases in which mineral oil is contraindicated or not tolerated. Doses must be tailored to individual patient. Some guidelines for initial doses:

  <10 kg (to 1 year): 1 teaspoonful p.o. b.i.d.

  10–20 kg: 1 tablespoonful p.o. b.i.d.

  >20 kg: 2 tablespoonful p.o. b.i.d.

  Recommend increased fiber and fluid intake.

  Toilet training: sitting on toilet for 5–10 minutes b.i.d. after meals.

  Gradual reduction of lubricant over several weeks to months once symptoms have resolved.

Abbreviations: b.i.d. = twice a day; p.o. = orally.

patient and the family are of paramount importance. Providing the family with information on the physiology of constipation and encopresis is essential to ensure compliance. Frequent office visits are needed initially, with the initial follow-up either by telephone or in the physician's office 1 to 2 weeks after therapy is initiated. Once therapy is well under way, follow-up can be performed at longer intervals.

An assessment must be made of the degree of constipation present. Adequate bowel cleansing must be accomplished before bowel softeners are given because they increase the frequency of encopresis in the child with fecal impaction. Some patients object to enemas, and many do not require one. However, a patient who has fecal impaction may require an enema in the physician's office and at home before treatment is initiated. The administration of a balanced electrolyte colonic lavage solution either orally or by gavage may be necessary in selected patients with severe impaction.

Once the bowel is deemed to have been emptied, the patient is started on sufficient doses of mineral oil or lactulose. Both of these agents have proved to be effective. Mineral oil is more palatable if it is served very cold, and it can be mixed with any food or liquid to aid in administration. It should not be used if the patient is at increased risk of vomiting or aspiration. Lactulose is a non-absorbable sugar that is usually well tolerated. Both agents have been found to be safe for use in the treatment of constipation. No nutritional deficiencies have been reported with the use of mineral oil over a 6-month course of therapy. Nonetheless, some practitioners supplement the patient's diet with vitamins.

The child should attempt defecation twice daily, sitting on the toilet with proper foot support for approximately 5 to 10 minutes shortly after meals (breakfast and dinner) to try to take advantage of the gastrocolic reflex. The goal of therapy is for the child to pass one soft stool at least every day. The stools should be soft enough to not cause pain. Eventually, the patient loses the fear of

pain with the passage of stool. Regular evacuation of the rectum allows the rectum to return to normal caliber, with improved compliance and sensory threshold. The addition of dietary fiber as a maintenance measure helps to maintain regular stooling habits and may help to prevent acute recurrences. The efficacy of bulking agents depends on an adequate fluid intake. Manipulation of the diet to increase fiber content is difficult in children, especially in toddlers.

Children who have paradoxical external anal contraction during attempted defecation can greatly benefit from biofeedback therapy. The child must be old enough to understand directions and to cooperate with the exercises. As few as two or three 1-hour sessions can be curative. Additional booster sessions are occasionally needed.

REFERENCES

Bautista Casasnovas A, Varela Cives R, Villanueva Jeremias A, et al. Measurement of colonic transit time in children. J Pediatr Gastroenterol Nutr 1991;13:42–45.

Benninga MA, Buller HA, Taminiau JAJM. Biofeedback training in chronic constipation. Arch Dis Child 1993;68:126–129.

Christophersen ER. Toileting problems in children. Pediatr Ann 1991;20:240–244.

Johanson JF, Sonnenberg A, Koch TR, et al. Association of constipation with neurologic diseases. Dig Dis Sci 1992;37:179–186.

Kot TV, Pettit-Young NA. Lactulose in the management of constipation: A current review. Ann Pharmacother 1992;26:1277–1282.

Lemoh JN, Brooke OG. Frequency and weight of normal stools in infancy. Arch Dis Child 1979;54:719–720.

Liptak GS, Revell GM. Management of bowel dysfunction in children with spinal cord disease or injury by means of the enema continence catheter. J Pediatr 1992;120:190–194.

Sonnenberg A, Koch TR. Physician visits in the United States for constipation: 1958–1986. Dig Dis Sci 1989;34:606–611.

Weaver LT, Ewing G, Taylor LC. The bowel habit of milk-fed infants. J Pediatr Gastroenterol Nutr 1988;7:568–571.

Weaver LT, Steiner H. The bowel habit of young children. Arch Dis Child 1984;59:649–652.

Yoshioka K, Keighley MRB. Anorectal myectomy for outlet obstruction. Br J Surg 1987;74:373–376.

Yoshioka K, Keighley MRB. Randomized trial comparing anorectal myectomy and controlled anal dilatation for outlet obstruction. Br J Surg 1987;74:1125–1129.

Younoszai MK. Stooling problems in patients with myelomeningocele. South Med J 1992;85:718–724.

Hirschsprung Disease

Crocker NL, Messmer JM. Adult Hirschsprung's disease. Clin Radiol 1991;44:257–259.

Low P, Quak S, Prabhakaran K, et al. Accuracy of anorectal manometry in the diagnosis of Hirschsprung's disease. J Pediatr Gastroenterol Nutr 1989;9:342–346.

Luukkonen P, Heikkinen M, Huikuri K, et al. Adult Hirschsprung's disease: Clinical features and functional outcome after surgery. Dis Colon Rectum 1990;33:65–69.

Nagasaki A, Sumitomo K, Shono T, et al. Diagnosis of Hirschsprung's disease by anorectal manometry. Prog Pediatr Surg 1989;24:40–48.

Powell RW. Hirschsprung's disease in adolescents: Misadventures in diagnosis and management. Am Surg 1989;55:212–218.

Rescorla FJ, Morrison AM, Engles D, et al. Hirschsprung's disease: Evaluation of mortality and long-term function in 260 cases. Arch Surg 1992;127:934–942.

Ryan ET, Ecker JL, Christakis NA, et al. Hirschsprung's disease: Associated abnormalities and demography. J Pediatr Surg 1992;27:76–81.

Encopresis

Clayden GS. Management of chronic constipation. Arch Dis Child 1992;67:340–342.

Dahl J, Lindquist BL, Tysk C, et al. Behavioral medicine treatment in chronic constipation with paradoxical anal sphincter contraction. Dis Colon Rectum 1991;34:769–776.

Di Lorenzo C, Flores AF, Reddey SN, et al. Use of colonic manometry to differentiate causes of intractable constipation in children. J Pediatr 1992;120:690–695.

Gleghorn EE, Heyman MB, Rudolph CD. No-enema therapy for idiopathic constipation and encopresis. Clin Pediatr 1991;30:669–672.

Hatch TF. Encopresis and constipation in children. Pediatr Clin North Am 1988;35:257–280.

Keren S, Wagner Y, Heldenberg D, et al. Studies of manometric abnormalities of the rectoanal region during defecation in constipated and soiling children: Modification through biofeedback therapy. Am J Gastroenterol 1988;83:827–831.

Levine MD. The school child with encopresis. Pediatr Rev 1981;2:285–290.

Loening-Baucke VA. Factors determining outcome in children with chronic constipation and faecal soiling. Gut 1989;30:999–1006.

Loening-Baucke VA. Factors responsible for persistence of childhood constipation. J Pediatr Gastroenterol Nutr 1987;6:915–922.

Loening-Baucke V. Persistence of chronic constipation in children after biofeedback treatment. Dig Dis Sci 1991;36:153–160.

Loening-Baucke V, Cruikshank B, Savage C. Defecation dynamics and behavior profiles in encopretic children. Pediatrics 1987;80:672–679.

McClung HJ, Boyne LJ, Linsheid T, et al. Is combination therapy for encopresis nutritionally safe? Pediatrics 1993;91:591–594.

Rappaport LA, Levine MD. The prevention of constipation and encopresis: A developmental model and approach. Pediatr Clin North Am 1986;33:859–869.

Shafik A, Abdel-Moneim K. Fecoflowmetry: A new parameter assessing rectal function in normal and constipated subjects. Dis Colon Rectum 1993;36:35–42.

Swanwick T. Encopresis in children: A cyclical model of constipation and faecal retention. Br J Gen Pract 1991;41:514–516.

Wexner SD, Cheape JD, Jorge JMN, et al. Prospective assessment of biofeedback for the treatment of paradoxical puborectalis contraction. Dis Colon Rectum 1992;35:145–150.

26 Abdominal Masses

Lotta Anveden-Hertzberg   Michael W. L. Gauderer

The discovery of an abdominal mass or abdominal swelling in a child is of great concern to parents and physicians. Most masses are not observed until late in their development. Often, the parents note changes in the abdominal contour of the child or accidently discover a mass while bathing or dressing the child. Abdominal masses may arise from hollow or solid intra-abdominal or retroperitoneal viscera, or they may arise from the abdominal wall (Figs. 26–1 and 26–2). The mass may be life threatening, as in the case of a highly malignant neoplasm; it may have been present since birth and gradually evolved, as in a child with a mesenteric cyst; or it may be caused by something less foreboding such as habit constipation. A child with an abdominal mass usually requires hospitalization and a prompt, accurate, and cost-effective work-up.

DIAGNOSTIC STRATEGIES

Clinical History

The clinical history of the patient helps to identify the most likely tumor category (Table 26–1). The nature of the mass is also related to the age and gender of the child (Table 26–2). The duration and character of the symptoms should be noted. It is important to know if the child has general systemic symptoms such as fatigue, fever, or weight loss. Additionally, gastrointestinal, urogenital, or pulmonary symptoms as well as any complaints of chronic or acute pain should be identified. Abdominal trauma (hematoma of liver-spleen, pancreatic pseudocyst) or exposure to infectious disease may lead to the formation of a cyst, lymphadenopathy, or an abscess. Systemic disease, genetic abnormalities, or anomalies such as aniridia (Wilms tumor) or hemihypertrophy (neuroblastoma, Wilms tumor) are associated with some intra-abdominal tumors. A family history is also pertinent, as is a sexual history, particularly in adolescent girls.

Physical Examination

Special attention should be paid to the general condition of the child and to signs of possible metastatic disease (Tables 26–3 and 26–4). The patient's blood pressure must be determined and may be elevated in patients with Wilms tumor, neuroblastoma, or pheochromocytoma. Any enlarged lymph nodes and their location should be noted, the skin inspected, and the lungs and heart auscultated. In addition, a neurologic examination may reveal signs of nervous system involvement.

To successfully perform abdominal palpation in a child, the physician must approach the patient with the greatest care, gentleness, and respect. It is important that the child cooperate and be able to relax. The abdomen should be examined systematically. With the patient placed in the supine position, the shape of the abdomen should be inspected and any visible masses or the presence of ascites observed. The position of the umbilicus and the presence of any hernias should be assessed. The mass should be located (right or left upper quadrant; right or left lower quadrant) and its size, shape, texture, motility, tenderness, and relation to the midline noted. Any peritoneal irritation must be observed. If there is any suspicion of obstipation or urinary retention, the patient should be re-examined after voiding or defecating (see Table 26–3).

Approximately half of abdominal masses in children are caused by enlargement of the liver (see Chapter 22) or spleen (see Chapter

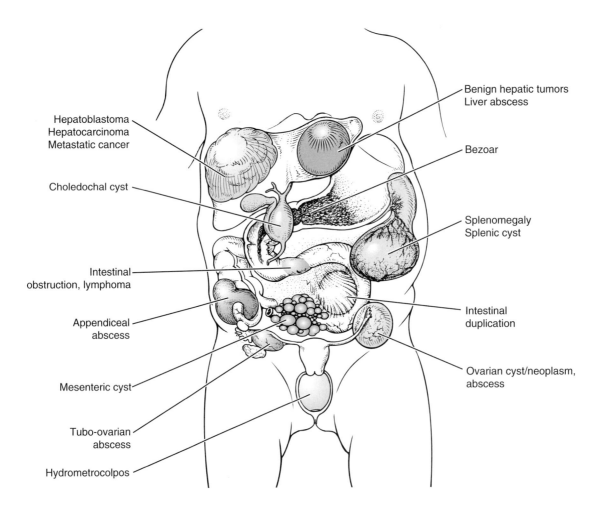

Figure 26–1. Location of select intra-abdominal tumors and masses.

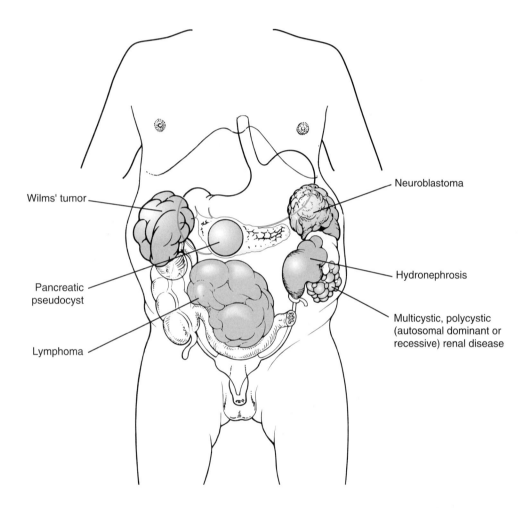

Figure 26–2. Location of select retroperitoneal tumors and masses.

Table 26–1. Stepwise Evaluation of a Mass

1. Clinical history
   Age and gender? General symptoms? Pain? Gastrointestinal symptoms? Urogenital symptoms? Pulmonary symptoms? Family history? Sexual history?

2. Physical examination
   General condition? Lymph nodes? Associated physical findings?

3. Abdominal palpation to locate tumor
   Which quadrant of the abdomen? Which organ most likely affected?

4. Character of tumor
   Soft or hard? Mobile or nonmobile? Crosses midline? Moves with respiration? Tender?

5. Ultrasonography
   Location? Solid or cystic?

6. Depending on the clinical suspicion, evaluation can be continued with one or more of the following:
   a. *Laboratory studies:* hematology, urinalysis, tumor markers (alpha-fetoprotein)
   b. *Imaging studies:* plain radiography of lungs and abdomen, contrast radiography of the gastrointestinal tract, computed tomography, magnetic resonance imaging, pyelography, angiography, scintigraphy

Table 26–2. Age-Related Etiology of Abdominal Masses

Age	Benign	Malignant
Neonate (0–1 mo)	Intestinal duplication Mesenteric/omental cyst Congenital hydronephrosis Cystic kidney diseases Neurogenic bladder Ovarian cyst Renal vein thrombosis Choledochal cyst Mesoblastic nephroma Meconium ileus Hematoma (adrenal, hepatic, splenic)	Neuroblastoma
Infant (0–1 yr)	Intestinal duplication Mesenteric/omental cyst Ovarian cyst Mesoblastic nephroma Liver hamartoma Hepatic cavernous hemangioma Liver hemangioendothelioma Teratoma Intussusception Hepatosplenomegaly Choledochal cyst Megacolon	Neuroblastoma Hepatoblastoma Wilms tumor (rare) Teratoma
Child (2–10 yr)	Mesenteric/omental cyst Choledochal cyst Abscess of the appendix	Neuroblastoma Hepatoblastoma Wilms tumor Leukemia Lymphoma
Adolescent (11–16 yr)	Bezoar Hematocolpos Hydrometrocolpos Pregnancy Inflammatory bowel disease Retroperitoneal hematoma (hemophilia)	Neuroblastoma Hepatocarcinoma Ovarian neoplasm Lymphoma

23), or both. The liver is normally palpated in the right upper quadrant and epigastrium, 1 to 2 cm below the costal margin. It has a sharp edge, is usually nontender, and moves with respiration. The spleen is located in the left upper quadrant and is nonpalpable in most healthy children. It has a rounded edge, moves with respiration, and is more superficial than a renal mass. Next to enlargement of the liver and spleen, lateral flank masses are the most numerous. Renal masses, located in either flank, usually extend downward and do not move with respiration. They rarely cross the midline.

Lower abdominal masses may be caused by constipation or urinary retention. A perforated appendix with resulting abscess formation can cause a right lower quadrant mass. Ovarian or uterine tumors occasionally develop into huge abdominal masses. A rectal examination is necessary in every case of suspected abdominal disease, and examination of the external genitalia is indicated in females with a lower abdominal mass to exclude imperforate hymen.

Laboratory and Imaging Studies

The aim of the laboratory and imaging studies is to obtain the most accurate diagnosis with as few investigations as possible.

Laboratory data, including complete blood count, serum electrolytes, serum amylase, urinalysis, and special tumor markers such as serum alpha-fetoprotein and human chorionic gonadotropin (hepatoma, teratoma), should be obtained. Liver and kidney function tests should be obtained when appropriate.

Plain abdominal radiographs may reveal tumor calcifications, organomegaly, or any displacement of intra-abdominal organs, such as the intestines. Contrast studies can help identify such displacement or diagnose masses within the gastrointestinal tract (Fig. 26–3). Ultrasonography is an excellent screening imaging modality. It is noninvasive, not painful, and can give detailed information on the location and nature of the tumor and adjacent structures (Figs. 26–4). Intravenous pyelography demonstrates obstruction of the

urinary tract or impaired renal function. Angiography can be of great help in identifying displacement or compression of blood vessels as well as the characteristic blood supply of potentially highly vascular neoplasms (Fig. 26–5). This modality provides invaluable information about the tumor, its location and ease of resection, as well as the diagnosis of metastatic disease. However, since angiography is invasive, it should be used very selectively, as in the planning of resection of complex tumors. The most widely used imaging techniques are computed tomography (CT), with or without contrast, and magnetic resonance imaging (MRI) (Fig. 26–6).

NEUROBLASTOMA

Neuroblastoma is the most common abdominal malignancy in childhood. It is of embryonic origin, arising from primitive sympathetic system cells derived from the neural crest. The malignant growth may develop wherever sympathetic tissue is found, but 75% of the tumors are abdominal, and 65% of these originate in

Table 26–3. Location and Nature of Abdominal Masses

Organ	Congenital	Benign	Malignant	Acquired
Liver and biliary tract	Hemangioma Choledochal cyst	Hemangioendothelioma Hamartoma	Hepatoblastoma, lymphoma, leukemia Hepatocarcinoma Sarcoma	Abscess, hematoma Parasitic disease, hydrops of gallbladder
Spleen		Cyst		Splenomegaly (e.g., mononucleosis) Cyst Hematoma
Kidney	Hydronephrosis Cystic disease Duplication		Wilms tumor	Hematoma
Adrenal glands	Neuroblastoma		Neuroblastoma	Hematoma
Stomach	Duplication Teratoma	Leiomyoma Inflammatory pseudotumor	Leiomyosarcoma Adenocarcinoma	Bezoar
Intestines	Duplication Megacolon	Lymphangioma Hemangioma	Carcinoma Lymphoma	Appendiceal abscess, intussusception Obstipation
Mesentery		Mesenteric/omental cyst		Inflammatory bowel disease Parasitic disease, tuberculosis
Pancreas		Cyst	Carcinoma	Pseudocyst
Uterus	Hydrometrocolpos secondary to imperforate hymen	Myoma	Rhabdomyosarcoma	Pregnancy
Ovaries	Cyst Teratoma	Cyst Cystic teratoma Cystic adenoma Granulosa cell tumor	Yolk sac tumor Embryonal carcinoma Dysgerminoma Choriocarcinoma	Tubo-ovarian abscess
Bladder	Urachal cyst Urethral valve	Inflammatory pseudotumor	Rhabdomyosarcoma	Urinary retention
Retroperitoneum	Presacral teratoma Anterior myelomeningocele	Ganglioneuroma	Neuroblastoma	Psoas abscess Aortic aneurysm Hematoma (hemophilia)
Abdominal wall	Hernia	Hemangioma	Rhabdomyosarcoma Hematoma	Rectus sheet hematoma Abscess

the adrenal glands. Neuroblastoma is an unusual tumor in that its behavior is not always predictable: well-advanced lesions may regress spontaneously or mature into benign tumors, while others with a similar histology rapidly progress in spite of intensive multimodal therapy. This tumor has unique biochemical (catecholamines) and immune properties that can aid in the diagnosis but that also produce adverse symptoms and a variable response to the tumor.

The incidence of neuroblastoma is approximately 1 in 10,000 children and is more common in boys than in girls (1.2:1). The tumor primarily affects children younger than 8 years of age, and more than 50% occur in infants younger than 2 years of age.

Neuroblastoma usually presents with an abdominal mass or abdominal discomfort. Catecholamine production by the tumor can occasionally result in flushing, sweating, and irritability, while vasoactive intestinal polypeptides, also produced by the tumor, may rarely cause watery, explosive secretory diarrhea. A variety of neurologic symptoms (opsoclonus-myoclonus) may also be seen, as well as weight loss and anorexia. Many patients have metastases at diagnosis, mainly to regional and distant lymph nodes, bone marrow and bone cortex, liver, and occasionally lungs. Symptoms related to metastases include bone pain and anemia.

Neuroblastoma presents as a solid, often fixed and painful mass crossing the midline. Its position does not change with respiration.

The purpose of the diagnostic studies is to find the exact location and size of the tumor and to determine regional invasion, metastatic disease, and histology. A plain radiograph shows finely stippled tumor calcifications in 50% of cases and also reveals displacement of bowel gas. Ultrasonography distinguishes a solid mass from a cystic mass and determines its position in relation to the kidney. CT further demonstrates calcifications of the tumor and determines the exact position in relation to other intra-abdominal and retroperi-

Table 26–4. Red Flags

1. Lower abdominal mass in girls
   Pregnancy? Imperforate hymen? Torsion of ovarian tumor? Tubo-ovarian abscess? Appendiceal abscess?
2. Nonmobile mass
   Malignancy?
3. Skeletal pain or pathologic fracture
   Metastases (neuroblastoma)? Lymphoma?
4. Sudden increase in size of clothing
   Abdominal mass—malignancy? Ascites?
5. Left-sided varicocele
   Wilms tumor?
6. Systemic signs of weight loss, fever, night sweats, anorexia, petechiae, anemia
   Malignancy? Granulomatous disease? (tuberculosis, inflammatory bowel disease)

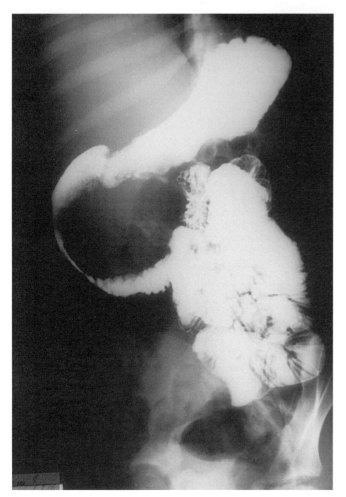

Figure 26–3. A contrast study of the upper gastrointestinal tract shows anterior displacement of the stomach and duodenum by a pancreatic pseudocyst.

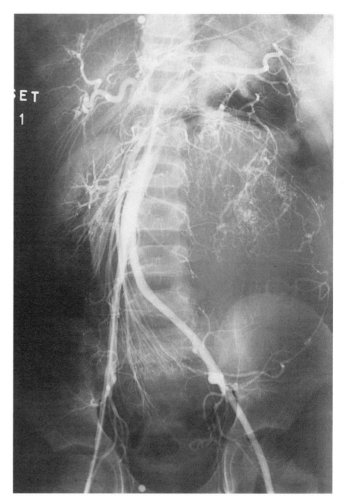

Figure 26–5. Contrast injected into the renal artery disclosing characteristic pathologic vessels of a large left-sided Wilms tumor. This technique has been largely replaced by CT and MRI.

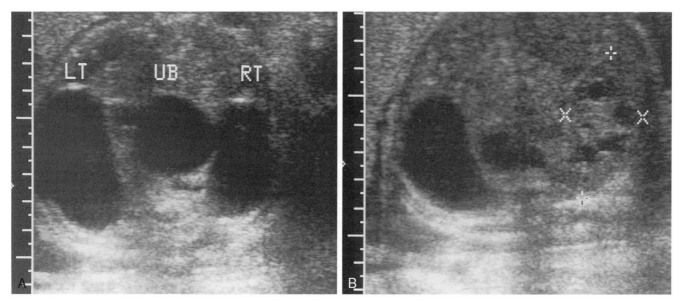

Figure 26–4. Fetal ultrasonography showing bilateral hydronephrosis. *A,* The urinary bladder is seen between the two dilated renal pelvises. *B,* The renal cortex is seen on the right side in the same fetus.

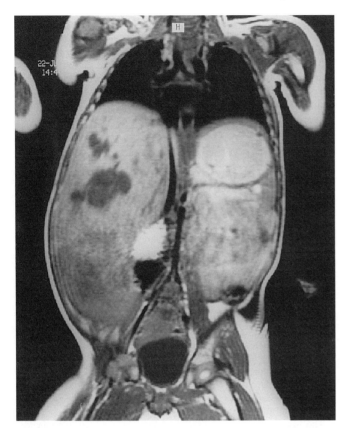

Figure 26–6. MRI scan showing a liver hamartoma in a 13-month-old boy. Note the excellent visualization of the blood vessels. The child presented with abdominal distention, poor appetite, and decreased activity. The liver was nontender and was palpated 15 cm below the costal margin. Operative resection was successful.

toneal organs. It also reveals any intraspinal or intracranial (if a cervical primary) extension of the tumor or its metastases. MRI demonstrates bone marrow metastases with great accuracy. Plain radiographs or isotope bone scans can be used to detect bony cortical lesions. In 90% of patients, the tumor excretes high levels of catecholamines and their metabolites. A 24-hour urine collection to determine levels of homovanillic acid, vanillylmandelic acid, adrenaline, noradrenaline, DOPA, and metanephrine aids in the assessment of the patient.

Surgical resection is the primary treatment of localized neuroblastoma. Adjuvant chemotherapy and radiotherapy are added to the therapy, depending on the stage of the disease and the age of the patient. If the tumor is considered unresectable, a diagnostic open biopsy or a needle biopsy is performed. Bone marrow may also demonstrate classic small round cells forming rosettes. To control the disease, the child may be given chemotherapy and radiotherapy prior to attempted resection. In some, high-dose chemotherapy is followed by bone marrow transplantation.

Staging is based on the regional extension of the tumor, the level of metastatic disease, and the degree of resectability. The outcome of the patient is determined by the age and stage. Children younger than 1 year, especially neonates, have the best prognosis; about 75% of these patients survive. However, for children older than 2 to 3 years, the outlook is guarded.

RENAL MASSES

The most common causes of a renal mass are congenital hydronephrosis (often bilateral), multicystic-dysplastic kidney (often uni-

lateral), and Wilms tumor (nephroblastoma). Ultrasonography immediately reveals whether the mass is solid or cystic, thus directing further investigation. An ectopic or horseshoe midline kidney can also be affected by renal disease, in which case the renal mass is palpated in an unexpected location.

Cystic Abnormalities of the Kidney

A unilateral multicystic-dysplastic kidney usually presents as a flank mass in the newborn. Ultrasonography and intravenous pyelography demonstrate a cystic kidney with absent renal parenchyma and no function. The contralateral kidney should be carefully evaluated for cysts or other abnormalities. Treatment usually consists of surgical excision, since it is believed that a dysplastic kidney increases the child's risk for hypertension, urinary tract infection, tumor, or pain. Alternatively, select patients with small lesions may be managed nonoperatively with long-term follow-up.

In the more serious case of autosomal recessive infantile polycystic disease, both kidneys are affected and there is a family history of the disease. The kidneys are filled with thousands of small cysts derived from the collecting tubules. The clinical presentation varies, depending on the degree of renal failure. Unfortunately, almost 50% of patients experience severe renal insufficiency before the age of 15 years. The neonatal form is fatal without renal transplantation. Abdominal ultrasonography discloses the cystic nature of the condition, while pyelography may show very poor function. Besides supportive treatment (dialysis), the only therapeutic option available at this time is renal transplantation.

Congenital Hydronephrosis

Hydronephrosis secondary to a ureteropelvic stricture may result in a flank mass discovered in the neonatal period or in later childhood. The obstruction can also be caused by an aberrant renal artery or adhesions kinking the ureter. Hydronephrosis is found mainly in young children. It is more common in males and on the left side. The most common presenting symptom in infants is an abdominal mass or urinary tract infection. In older children, distention of the renal pelvis may cause intermittment pain; hematuria can be seen as a result of minor abdominal trauma.

The diagnosis is confirmed with ultrasonography and occasionally intravenous pyelography. Diuretic renal scintigraphy demonstrates the degree of obstruction, and a voiding cystourethrogram excludes ureterovesical reflux and posterior urethral valves (in males). Treatment consists of pyeloplasty with resection of the obstruction and, if necessary, parts of the distended renal pelvis.

With fetal ultrasonography, hydronephrosis can be detected antenatally (see Fig. 26–4). The management of asymptomatic neonates remains controversial, since it has been demonstrated that unilateral neonatal hydronephrosis may improve without operative intervention.

Wilms Tumor (Nephroblastoma)

Wilms tumor is an embryonal renal neoplasm, one of the most common childhood abdominal malignancies. The estimated incidence is close to 1 in 15,000 live births, with a male-to-female ratio of 0.9:1. The mean age at diagnosis is 3.5 years, and at least 90% of the patients present before the age of 8 years. Approximately 5% of children with Wilms tumor have bilateral disease; the mean age in bilateral cases is 2.5 years. Associated conditions include aniridia, hemihypertrophy, genitourinary anomalies, and Beckwith-Wiedemann syndrome.

The etiology of Wilms tumor remains unclear, but evidence of a genetic component is emerging. A subset of patients have other types of renal malignant tumors (no longer classified as Wilms tumor), such as rhabdoid tumors and sarcoma.

Most children present with an asymptomatic abdominal mass discovered accidentally by the parents or a physician during routine examination. Microscopic hematuria is present in about 30%. Rarely, occlusion of the left renal vein may obstruct the left spermatic vein and thus cause left-sided varicocele. Other, less common symptoms or signs include anemia, polycythemia, weight loss, hypertension, or frank hematuria following rupture of the tumor secondary to minor abdominal trauma.

Diagnostic imaging techniques include one or more of the following: plain radiography, ultrasonography, CT or MRI and, less often, intravenous pyelography. Assessment is made of the location, size, and resectability of the tumor; of the presence of local tumor invasion; and of infiltration of the renal vein and inferior vena cava. Metastatic or bilateral disease must be ruled out. Lung metastases from venous infiltration may be present, while bone metastases are rare; this distinguishes Wilms tumor from neuroblastoma.

Treatment includes a transabdominal nephrectomy with early ligation of the renal vein to avoid tumor mobilization. Postoperatively, the team consisting of oncologists, surgeons, pathologists, and radiotherapists decides on further treatment. Chemotherapy and radiotherapy are added, depending on the stage and histology of the tumor. For very large or complex tumors, preoperative chemotherapy has been employed in select patients. In some cases of bilateral disease, partial resections with nephron-sparing surgery is employed. For children with excessive loss of functional renal parenchyma, transplantation is an option. Late effects of treatment with radiation and chemotherapy include second primary malignancies such as leukemia or soft tissue sarcomas, as well as infertility.

Tumor staging is based on radiographic evaluation (metastatic disease) and interpretive findings (tumor size, extrarenal extension of the tumor, tumor spillage, local lymph nodes). The stage determines the prognosis and treatment of the disease. Survival depends on the prognostic factors, the success of treatment, the histology of the tumor, and the age of the patient. Younger patients have a better prognosis. Most children have either stage I or II disease (regional extension of the tumor but complete surgical removal), and most cases of Wilms tumor have favorable histology. Overall, survival currently approaches 90%.

LIVER TUMORS

Hepatomegaly (diffuse enlargement of the liver) or a hepatic mass may be due to infectious diseases (hepatitis, abscess, cyst), as well as benign or malignant lesions. Primary liver tumors are uncommon in children, but about 66% are malignant. Hepatoblastomas predominate, followed by hepatocellular carcinoma, mesenchymoma, and, rarely, sarcoma.

Infectious diseases such as hepatitis may cause hepatomegaly. Hepatic abscesses are due to pathogens such as *Staphylococcus aureus,* anaerobic bacteria, or *Escherichia coli.* Certain conditions, such as chronic granulomatous disease or appendicitis, may predispose the child to this complication. Amebic infection of the liver caused by *Entamoeba histolytica* and parasite infestation with *Echinococcus* may also lead to abscess formation in warm, tropical climates. Abscesses are treated with appropriate antibiotics and surgical or percutaneous drainage.

Benign tumors can be of either mesenchymal or epithelial origin. Mesenchymal tumors include disorders such as hamartomas, cavernous hemangiomas, and infantile hemangioendotheliomas in young children. These conditions present as asymptomatic abdominal masses. Hemangiomas, particularly diffuse ones, may be difficult to resect and should be managed nonoperatively unless complications develop. Hamartomas, which usually present in the first year of life, should be resected. Epithelial lesions include focal nodular hyperplasia, hepatic adenoma, and nonparasitic solitary or multiple cysts.

Hepatoblastoma

Hepatoblastoma is usually found in children younger than 5 years of age; more than half of the cases are diagnosed during the first 2 years of life. It is twice as common in boys. The most common presentation is a child with a palpable abdominal mass, occasionally associated with anemia, nausea, vomiting, weight loss, or abdominal pain. An unusual presentation is precocious puberty resulting from tumor secretion of human chorionic gonadotropin. Elevated levels of serum alpha-fetoprotein are seen in about 90%, and this feature is helpful in the post-therapy monitoring of disease activity.

As in any other liver tumor, initial radiographic evaluation should include plain abdominal radiography to detect calcifications and the mass effect, and ultrasonography to determine the origin, size, and echogenicity of the tumor. Additionally, an abdominal CT or MRI scan can be obtained to define the exact localization and extent of the tumor (Fig. 26–7). Angiography may occasionally be useful to determine resectability. Chest radiography or CT is used to determine the presence of pulmonary metastases.

The tumor is usually solitary and predominantly located in the right hepatic lobe. If deemed resectable after radiographic evaluation (no portal vein or extrahepatic invasion, limited to one lobe) and without metastases, complete surgical removal in combination with chemotherapy is the primary treatment (Fig. 26–8). A significant number of tumors are not resectable at diagnosis. These are treated with preoperative chemotherapy to possibly convert the tumor to a resectable one. Irradiation is an additional but less desirable option.

The prognosis of patients with hepatoblastoma depends on the histology of the tumor and the resectability. Approximately 80%

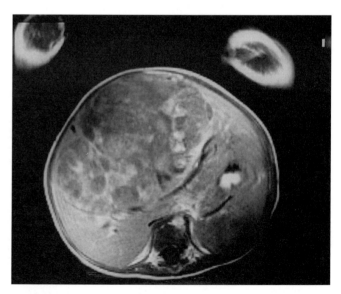

Figure 26–7. Hepatoblastoma examined by CT in an 8-month-old girl. The child presented with hepatomegaly, increased abdominal girth, weight loss, and lethargy. The voluminous tumor occupies a large part of the upper abdominal cavity (see also Fig. 26–8).

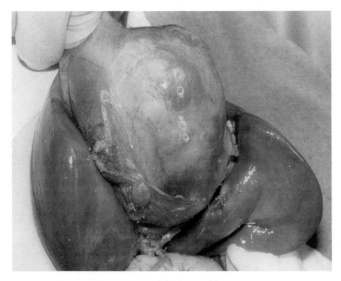

Figure 26–8. Operative picture of the hepatoblastoma seen in Figure 26–7 following biopsy and chemotherapy. Resection was undertaken successfully.

of patients with completely resected tumors survive, whereas those with incompletely resected lesions have a poor prognosis.

Hepatocarcinoma

Hepatocarcinoma, the adult type of liver tumor, usually occurs in an already diseased liver, such as found following hepatitis B or C virus infection, tyrosinemia, galactosemia, biliary atresia, or cirrhosis. It is rare in younger children and has a peak incidence between the ages of 10 and 15 years. The tumor presents as a painful abdominal mass; in more than 65% of patients it is not resectable. The diagnostic evaluation, staging, and treatment of hepatocarcinoma are similar to those of hepatoblastoma.

CONGENITAL DILATATION OF THE BILE DUCTS

Any congenital cystic dilatation of the bile ducts is commonly called choledochal cyst. There are several anatomic varieties of this condition, and the cause remains unknown. The classic choledochal cyst is seen when the common bile duct is grossly dilated. However, the size varies, and the child may remain asymptomatic for many years. About 20% of patients present with the *classic triad* of jaundice, pain, and a right upper quadrant abdominal mass. The jaundice is of the obstructive type with associated pruritus, dark urine, and acholic stool.

Ultrasonography reveals the location, size, and nature of the cyst (Fig. 26–9). If there is any doubt about its origin, a technetium excretion scan can be used to outline the biliary tract and help differentiate it from other lesions such as duodenal duplication. Treatment consists of resection of the cyst and drainage of the hepatic duct into an intestinal segment (Fig. 26–10).

INTESTINAL AND PANCREATIC MASSES

Bezoar

Emotionally disturbed or mentally retarded children occasionally eat their own hair or other undigestible material. Ninety percent of these patients are female, usually in their teens. A trichobezoar (hair) or a phytobezoar (vegetable matter) forms in the stomach and causes partial gastric outlet obstruction. Gastric bezoars may extend into the small intestine. If hair manages to pass the stomach, it collects in the duodenum and causes biliary tract obstruction; if it collects in the ileum, it may lead to intestinal obstruction.

The clinical picture is characterized by poor appetite, vague abdominal discomfort, and intolerance to solid foods. Physical examination reveals a movable mass in the epigastrium. The diagnosis is confirmed with upper gastrointestinal contrast radiography, and the bezoar is removed operatively if it is large.

Duplications

Duplications of the gastrointestinal tract occur anywhere from the esophagus to the anus and are either cystic or tubular. The

Figure 26–9. Ultrasonography of a choledochal cyst in a 3-year-old girl. The patient presented with a 2-year history of intermittent abdominal pain and jaundice and a tender mass.

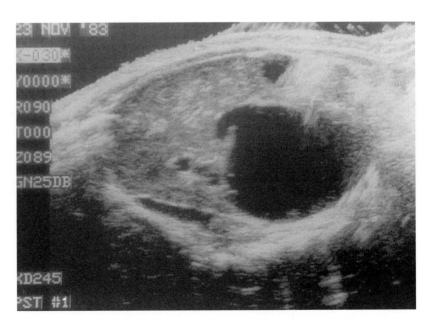

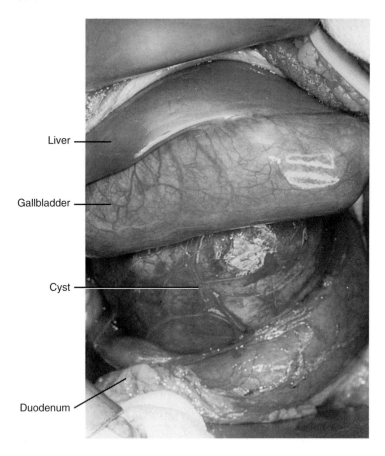

Liver

Gallbladder

Cyst

Duodenum

Figure 26–10. Operative photograph of the choledochal cyst seen in Figure 26–9. The cyst is located between the gallbladder and the duodenum, displacing both.

more common cystic duplications are lined with endothelium and are enclosed in a muscular wall common with the adjacent intestinal segment. Tubular duplications are located on the mesenteric side of the bowel and are either blind or in communication with the bowel. The lining is usually that of the adjacent intestine but may be heterotopic, such as gastric mucosa in a small bowel duplication.

Most duplications are diagnosed during the first years of childhood. The manifestations depend on the size and location of the malformation. Many intra-abdominal duplications present as an asymptomatic palpable mass but may also cause pain, intestinal obstruction, or even volvulus. Ultrasonography differentiates the cystic nature of duplications from solid tumors and also demonstrates the intimate association between the duplication and the bowel wall. Treatment consists of resection of the duplication alone or, more commonly, along with the part of the gut from which the duplication arose, depending on the anatomic location and amount of shared wall and blood supply (Fig. 26–11).

Neoplasms of the Gastrointestinal Tract

Neoplasms of the gastrointestinal tract of infants and children are rare. The symptoms are often nonspecific, and diagnosis tends to be delayed. A gastric teratoma may appear as an epigastric mass, while gastric leiomyosarcomas or leiomyomas present with bleeding.

Non-Hodgkin's lymphoma is the most common malignant tumor of the small intestine and may act as a leading point for an intussusception. Other malignant tumors of the small intestine include leiomyosarcoma, angiosarcoma, and carcinoid tumor. These conditions also occur in the large intestine. Carcinoid tumors are

most commonly found in the appendix, where they can cause obstruction and lead to appendicitis. The colon is the most common site for the rare adenocarcinoma of the gastrointestinal tract in children.

Benign neoplasms of the small and large intestine include hemangiomas, lymphangiomas, leiomyomas, and polyps.

All malignant neoplasms and most benign neoplasms should be resected.

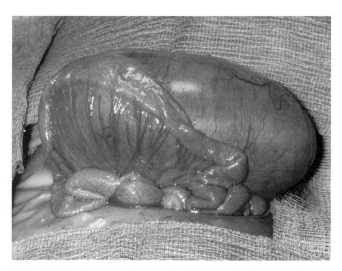

Figure 26–11. Operative photograph of the typical appearance of an intestinal duplication.

Mesenteric and Omental Cysts

Cysts located in the omentum or mesentery are benign, unilocular, or multilocular and contain clear serous fluid. They arise from a developmental abnormality of the lymphatic system resulting in lymphatic obstruction. Most of these cysts are diagnosed during the first 5 years of life. They may be asymptomatic for a long period or present with a distended abdomen, abdominal mass, intestinal obstruction, volvulus, or abdominal pain. The abdomen is usually nontender with a mobile mass. Unlike in ascites, when a child with an abdominal cyst is in the supine position, the flanks do not bulge.

A plain abdominal radiograph shows intestinal gas displaced forward in the case of a mesenteric cyst and backward in the case of an omental cyst. Small amounts of calcification may be seen in the wall of the cyst. Ultrasonography or CT further elucidates the nature, size, and location of the cyst (Fig. 26–12). An ovarian, pancreatic, or choledochal cyst or an intestinal duplication may be difficult to differentiate from a mesenteric or omental cyst. Treatment consists of surgical removal. Often, bowel has to be removed together with a mesenteric cyst because of its intimacy with enteric vessels.

Pancreatic Pseudocyst and Neoplasms

Pancreatic tumors are rare in children and infants and are either cystic or solid, benign or malignant. Functional neoplasms arise from the islet cells, and the clinical presentation is not of an abdominal mass but rather is characterized by the effects of the endocrine substances secreted by the tumor (hypoglycemia caused by insulinoma). Tumors arising from the acinar or ductal parts of the pancreas are nonfunctional and usually present as an abdominal mass. They may be benign (cystadenoma) or malignant (adenocarcinoma). Metastases are common.

Diagnosis is made by ultrasonography and CT and, in cases of suspected endocrine tumors, by measurements of active hormones. Both benign and malignant tumors should be surgically resected. The outlook for pediatric patients with pancreatic neoplasms may be better than in adults.

A pancreatic pseudocyst lacks epithelial lining and is the result of pancreatitis or pancreatic blunt trauma. Often, there is a symptom-free interval of several weeks or months between the trauma

and the appearance of symptoms. Typical signs and symptoms are nausea, abdominal pain, and an epigastric mass. Ultrasonography and an upper gastrointestinal contrast radiography locate the cyst and identify any displacement of the bowel (see Fig. 26–3). The cysts usually undergo spontaneous resolution; however, if this is not the case, they should be drained externally percutaneously or internally to the gastrointestinal tract (see also Chapter 18).

OVARIAN TUMORS

Ovarian tumors in children are uncommon, with an incidence of about 25 in 100,000 children's hospital admissions. They must be considered in any female with lower abdominal pain, an abdominal mass, or precocious puberty. They present at any age from birth to adulthood but occur slightly more frequently in children older than 8 years of age. The risk of malignancy seems to increase with age. Cystic tumors are more common than solid tumors, and the majority of masses are benign. An ovarian lesion may also be the presenting manifestation of other metastatic diseases, such as neuroblastoma or rhabdomyosarcoma. Malignant gonadal tumors (dysgerminoma, gonadoblastoma) are common in females with gonadal dysgenesis (see Chapter 33) and males with cryptorchism. A lower abdominal mass in a female can be due to pregnancy or to imperforate hymen, which leads to hydrocolpos or hydrometrocolpos.

Diagnosis is made by ultrasonography, which provides information on the size, consistency, location, and wall characteristics of the tumor. Abdominal radiography reveals calcifications, and intravenous pyelography identifies ureteral obstruction or displacement. CT can locate local or distant metastases. Since endocrinopathies are present in 5% to 10% of children with ovarian tumors, elevated levels of tumor markers, such as alpha-fetoprotein or human chorionic gonadotropin, should be investigated.

A simple cyst may appear in a neonate as a mobile abdominal mass or may even be detected incidentally by ultrasonography. Small cysts can be followed with ultrasonography and should spontaneously disappear. Larger cysts should be excised, since they can undergo torsion (Fig. 26–13). The symptoms of ovarian torsion in an older child simulate appendicitis or ectopic pregnancy.

All other tumors of the ovaries should be excised, whether benign (cystic teratoma, cystic adenoma, granulosa cell tumor) or malignant (endodermal sinus tumor, yolk sac tumor, embryonal carcinoma, malignant teratoma, adenocarcinoma, dysgerminoma, choriocarcinoma). Great care should be taken to spare as much of the adnexa as possible to preserve future fertility. Depending on the histologic appearance and stage, most malignant lesions should be treated postoperatively with chemotherapy. Survival depends on the nature of the lesion; however, with the exception of highly malignant tumors such as endodermal sinus tumors and embryonal carcinoma, the prognosis is good.

SUMMARY AND RED FLAGS

Although the discovery of an abdominal mass in a child is of great concern, there is good reason for the physician to reassure the parents. The prognosis of most congenital masses is excellent, and with modern diagnostic techniques and advanced, multimodal therapy the prognosis for malignant tumors continues to improve. Red flags suggestive of malignancy are listed in Table 26–4.

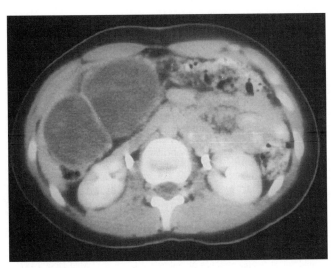

Figure 26–12. CT scan of the abdomen in an 11-year-old boy disclosing a mesenteric cyst in the transverse mesocolon.

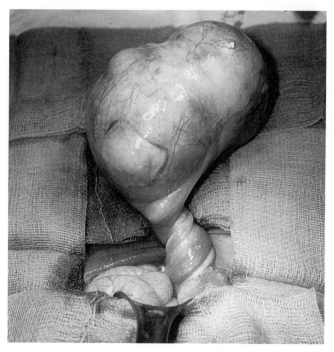

Figure 26–13. Torsion of an ovarian teratoma in a 5-year-old girl. The child presented with acute abdominal pain and a movable mass. A preoperative radiograph showed calcified material in the mass.

REFERENCES

Neuroblastoma

Brodeur GM, Pritchard J, Berthold, et al. Revisions of the international criteria for neuroblastoma diagnosis, staging, and response to treatment. J Clin Oncol 1993;11:1466.

Evans AE, D'Angio GJ, Randolph J. A proposed staging for children with neuroblastoma. Children's Cancer Study Group A. Cancer 1971;27:374.

Grosfeld JL. Neuroblastoma. In Welch KJ, Randolph JG, Ravitch MM, et al (eds). Pediatric Surgery, 4th ed. Chicago: Year Book Medical Publishers, 1986.

Ho PTC, Estroff JA, Kozakewich H, et al. Prenatal detection of neuroblastoma: A ten-year experience from the Dana-Farber Cancer Institute and Children's Hospital. Pediatrics 1993;92:358.

Ng YY, Kingston JE. The role of radiology in the staging of neuroblastoma. Clin Radiol 1993;47:226.

Renal Masses

Atiyeh B, Husmann D, Baum M. Contralateral renal abnormalities in multicystic-dysplastic kidney disease. J Pediatr 1992;121:65.

Koff SA, Campbell K. Nonoperative management of unilateral neonatal hydronephrosis. J Urol 1992;148:525.

Lippert MC. Renal cystic disease. In Gillenwater JY, Grayhack JT, Howards SS, et al (eds). Adult and Pediatric Urology, 2nd ed. St. Louis: Mosby Year Book, 1991.

Wacksman J, Phipps L. Report of multicystic kidney registry: Preliminary findings. J Urol 1993;150:1870.

Wilms Tumor

Caty GC, Shamberger RC. Abdominal tumors in infancy and childhood. Pediatr Clin North Am 1993;40:1253.

Cosentino C, Raffensperger JG, Luck SR, et al. A 25-year experience with renal tumors of childhood. J Pediatr Surg 1993;28:1350.

D'Angio GJ, Breslow N, Beckwith JB, et al. Treatment of Wilms tumor. Results of the Third National Wilms Tumor Study. Cancer 1989;64:349.

Dykes EH, Marwaha C, Dicks-Mireaux C, et al. Risks and benefits of percutaneous biopsy and primary chemotherapy in advanced Wilms tumour. J Pediatr Surg 1991;26:610.

Greenberg M, Burnweit C, Filler R. Preoperative chemotherapy for children with Wilms tumor. J Pediatr Surg 1991;26:949.

Othersen BM. Wilms tumor. In Welch KJ, Randolph JG, Ravitch MM, et al (eds). Pediatric Surgery, 4th ed. Chicago: Year Book Medical Publishers, 1986.

Pais E, Pirson Y, Squifflet JP, et al. Kidney transplantation in patients with Wilms tumor. Transplantation 1992;53:782.

Liver Tumors

Gururangan S, O'Meara A, Macmahon C, et al. Primary hepatic tumours in children: A 26-year review. J Surg Oncol 1992;50:30.

Randolph JG, Guzetta PC. Tumors of the liver. In Welch KJ, Randolph JG, Ravitch MM, et al (eds). Pediatric Surgery, 4th ed. Chicago: Year Book Medical Publishers, 1986.

Touloukian RJ. Nonmalignant liver tumors and hepatic infections. In Welch KJ, Randolph JG, Ravitch MM, et al (eds). Pediatric Surgery, 4th ed. Chicago: Year Book Medical Publishers, 1986.

Weinberg AG, Finegold MJ. Primary hepatic tumors of childhood. Hum Pathol 1983;14:512.

Congenital Dilatation of the Bile Ducts

Kim SH. Choledochal cyst: Survey by the surgical section of the American Academy of Pediatrics. J Pediatr Surg 1981;16:3.

O'Neill JA, Templeton JM, Schnaufer L, et al. Recent experience with choledochal cyst. Ann Surg 1987;205:533.

Intestinal and Pancreatic Masses

Swenson O. Foreign bodies in the gastrointestinal tract. In Raffensperger JG (ed). Swenson's Pediatric Surgery, 5th ed. Norwalk, Conn: Appleton & Lange, 1990.

Duplications

Bower RJ, Sieber WK, Kiesewetter WB. Alimentary tract duplications in children. Ann Surg 1978;188:669.

Holcomb GW, Gheissari A, O'Neill JA, et al. Surgical management of alimentary tract duplications. Ann Surg 1989;209:167.

Ildstad ST, Tollerud DJ, Weiss RG, et al. Duplications of the alimentary tract. Ann Surg 1988;208:184.

Neoplasms of the Gastrointestinal Tract

Berry CL, Keeling JW. Gastrointestinal lymphoma in childhood. J Clin Pathol 1970;23:459.

Dehner LP. Gastrointestinal tract. In Pediatric Surgical Pathology, 2nd ed. Baltimore: Williams & Wilkins, 1987.

Hermann R, Panahon AM, Barcos MP, et al. Gastrointestinal involvement in non-Hodgkin's lymphoma. Cancer 1980;46:215.

Mesenteric and Omental Cysts

Blumhagen JD, Wood BJ, Rosenbaum DM. Sonographic evaluation of abdominal lymphangiomas in children. J Ultrasound Med 1987;6:487.

Kosir MA, Sonnino RE, Gauderer MWL. Pediatric abdominal lymphangiomas: A plea for early recognition. J Pediatr Surg 1991;26:1309.

Takiff H, Calabria R, Vin L, et al. Mesenteric cysts and intra-abdominal cystic lymphangiomas. Arch Surg 1985;120:1266.

Pancreatic Pseudocyst and Neoplasms

Grosfeld JL, Vane DW, Rescorla FJ, et al. Pancreatic tumors in childhood: Analysis of 13 cases. J Pediatr Surg 1990;25:1057.
Jaksic T, Yaman M, Thorner P, et al. A 20-year review of pediatric pancreatic tumors. J Pediatr Surg 1992;27:1315.

Ovarian Tumors

Brown MF, Hebra A, McGeehin K, et al. Ovarian masses in children: A review of 91 cases of malignant and benign masses. J Pediatr Surg 1993;28:930.
Gribbon M, Ein SH, Mancer K. Pediatric malignant ovarian tumors: A 43-year review. J Pediatr Surg 1992;27:480.
Ikeda K, Suita S, Nakano H. Management of ovarian cyst detected antenatally. J Pediatr Surg 1988;23:432.
Young RH, Kozakewich HPW, Scully RE. Metastatic ovarian tumors in children: A report of 14 cases and review of the literature. Int J Gynecol Pathol 1993;12:8.

Genitourinary Disorders

27 Dysuria

Candice E. Johnson

Dysuria is a symptom of urethral irritation that is usually associated with urinary frequency. Children with severe dysuria may demonstrate refusal to voluntarily void. Dysuria in younger children may cause incontinence of urine, whereas adults and older children may have urgency to urinate. The main cause of dysuria in children is bacterial infection of the urethra, bladder, and kidneys. Viruses play a minor role in causing dysuria, and chlamydia urethritis is rare in young children and suggests possible sexual abuse. Causes of mechanical irritation are uncommon. The cause in young adults and adolescent women is entirely different; dysuria represents urinary tract infection (UTI) in only 50%. The other 50% have vaginitis or urethritis caused by sexually transmitted pathogens, including *Chlamydia* species.

Dysuria (and the associated UTI) is an important symptom in children because it may be the first indication of an anatomic lesion, such as obstruction of the urinary tract or vesicoureteral reflux (VUR). Recurrent or persistent UTI in such children can cause kidney damage, leading to end-stage renal disease. Even simple UTIs not accompanied by obstruction or reflux can recur so often that the parents perceive the child as chronically ill. Much attention has been directed at the localization of the site of urinary infection to the upper or lower tract (pyelonephritis versus cystitis) in the hope that the site would determine the long-term prognosis.

Pyelonephritis refers to upper UTIs, as defined by the presence of fever, or flank pain, or both. No other markers of inflammation (elevated C-reactive protein, erythrocyte sedimentation rate, or leukocyte count) are superior to these clinical symptoms in children. Not all cases of pyelonephritis produce fever in adults, but it is generally believed that afebrile pyelonephritis is rare in children. Renal scans are helpful adjunctive tests to localize the infection to the kidney or kidneys.

Cystitis is defined as an afebrile infection without flank pain or tenderness, but including dysuria, or frequency, or both. *Urethritis* is dysuria accompanied by pyuria, but without evidence of significant bacteriuria or bacteria cultured from the urine. *Asymptomatic bacteriuria* is colonization of the bladder (often chronically) with bacteria in amounts exceeding 10^5/ml and by definition is not accompanied by dysuria, urinary frequency or urgency, or daytime enuresis. *Vesicoureteral reflux* is the retrograde flow of urine from the bladder toward the kidney (Fig. 27–1). It is graded I through V, based on the appearance of the calyces and ureter on a voiding cystogram. This is the most common and serious predisposing factor for pyelonephritis identified in children with UTIs.

HISTORY

Neonates

A history that is suggestive of urinary infection in the neonate is the same as that for suspected sepsis. A mother whose vaginal culture is positive for group B streptococci or who presents with fever, prolonged rupture of the amniotic membranes (>18 to 24 hours), uterine tenderness, or preterm labor is at increased risk for having a premature baby with pyelonephritis as part of the neonatal sepsis syndrome. It is also suspected that maternal urinary infection at or near term may increase the risk for neonatal pyelonephritis. The siblings of children with known VUR also have a significant risk of reflux, with or without infection, and they should be screened with a radionuclide cystogram within 4 weeks of birth.

Infants

Infants cannot report dysuria; all infants normally have frequent urination. A UTI should be suspected in any male under 6 months

GRADES OF REFLUX

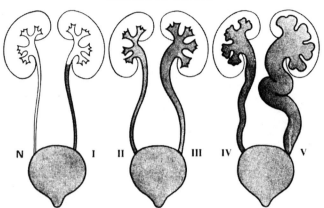

N   I   II   III   IV   V

Figure 27-1. Classifications of grades of vesicoureteral reflux adopted by the International Reflux Study Committee. Grade I, reflux into ureter only. Grade II, reflux into ureter, pelvis, and calyces. There is no dilation, and calyceal fornices are normal. Grade III, mild to moderate dilation and/or tortuosity of the ureter and moderate dilation of the renal pelvis but little or no blunting of the fornices. Grade IV, moderate dilation and/or tortuosity of the ureter and moderate dilation of the renal pelvis and calyces. Grade V, gross dilation and tortuosity of the ureter and gross dilation of the renal pelvis and calyces. Papillary impressions are no longer visible in most of the calyces. There is complete obliteration of the sharp angle of the fornices, but maintenance of papillary impressions in major calyces. N = normal. (From Hellerstein S. Urinary Tract Infections in Children. Chicago: Year Book Medical Publishers, 1982.)

of age with unexplained fever, especially if he is uncircumcised. All infant girls with unexplained fever should have a urinalysis and a catheterized specimen obtained if pyuria is present.

Toddlers

In toddlers, a UTI should be suspected in those with a delayed onset of daytime toilet mastery. However, because of the large variability in daytime dryness (15 months to 4 years), this symptom is unreliable. Nocturnal enuresis is rarely a sign of UTI, but urine cultures should probably be obtained in children not dry at night by 5 years of age. A more significant symptom in toddlers is the acute onset of daytime enuresis after a period of continence. Boys who present with a history of dribbling rather than a strong urine stream should be suspected of having posterior urethral valves; a standard voiding cystourethrogram must be obtained. Girls who present with episodes of squatting or curtsying to stop urination may have a UTI. This behavior arises from uncontrolled bladder contractions against a closed bladder sphincter. Some terms for this are bladder dyssynergia, unstable bladder, uninhibited bladder, and persistence of the infantile bladder. Because many of these children develop VUR and infection, it is important to ask about the voiding pattern in dysuric children.

Uncircumcised males, patients with neurogenic bladders (spina bifida), or patients with renal anomalies (cysts, obstructed hydronephrosis, double collecting systems, ectopic ureter, horseshoe kidney, VUR) are at increased risk for UTI.

Older Children and Adolescents

Because older children are better historians, it is often worthwhile to ask about any urine color change, which suggests the presence of hematuria. A history of anal pruritus is suggestive of pinworms, which may also irritate the urethral area. The child should be questioned about the frequency, character, and size of his or her bowel movements. Bulky stools associated with constipation may predispose the child to a UTI; stool softeners, such as mineral oil or fiber, may be indicated (see Chapter 25).

In the adolescent, a detailed sexual history is mandatory, focusing on cystitis from sexual intercourse or vaginitis. Herpes simplex, *Trichomonas*, *Chlamydia*, and gonorrhea all cause urethritis. The most likely time for this to appear is within 1 month of a new sexual partner. Because the use of a diaphragm for contraception is associated with an increased risk of UTI, adolescents experiencing recurrent UTIs should be offered an alternative method. Similarly, female adolescents should be questioned about voiding before or after intercourse because studies have shown a reduction of UTI with post-intercourse urination.

Finally, young males should be asked about self-injection of bath water or foreign bodies into the urethra. Although this behavior sounds unusual and painful, it is more common than is appreciated (~30% of school-aged boys with a UTI). About 60% of these boys have gross hematuria; there is an increased risk for *Staphylococcus saprophyticus* rather than *Escherichia coli*, to be the infecting agent.

PHYSICAL EXAMINATION

Although infection is the leading cause of dysuria in children, other, less common, causes should be considered. Physical examination of the genitalia and periurethral area may be helpful in finding external perineal irritation or vaginitis; there are no specific physical findings in urinary infection or bladder tumors. The urinalysis replaces the physical examination as the central diagnostic element. Abdominal palpation for a kidney mass should be performed, as should percussion over the costovertebral angle for renal tenderness. A blood pressure measurement should also be obtained at diagnosis and yearly in children with recurrent urinary infections.

In 30% to 40% of patients with pyelonephritis, fever, chills, tachycardia, and occasionally hypotension are present. Such patients have "uro-sepsis" and demonstrate the systemic inflammatory response syndrome that is typical of bacteremic sepsis or septic shock.

Pelvic examination to exclude vaginitis is essential in all sexually active adolescent females when pyuria is absent or when vaginal discharge is reported. Conversely, adolescents with dysuria and pyuria may be assumed to have urinary infection if the urinalysis is free of contaminating squamous epithelial cells. The presence of more than rare epithelial cells suggests contamination of the urine with vaginal white cells and bacteria. The pelvic examination should include cervical cultures for *Neisseria gonorrhoeae* and *Chlamydia* because both organisms can cause urethritis. *Trichomonas* species and clue cells should be checked with a saline preparation, and any lesions suggestive of herpes simplex should be cultured (see Chapter 31).

A cause for dysuria may be found in 90% of young adult women. About 10% may have vaginitis, whereas about 50% have greater than 10^5 bacteria/ml in a midstream urine sample. The remaining 40% of women with fewer than 10^5 bacteria/ml were once considered to have "urethral syndrome" and were believed not to have true bacteriuria. However, by direct bladder sampling, half have positive bacterial cultures of the usual pathogens. One third of the women with urethral syndrome had positive *Chlamydia* cultures from the bladder. Virtually all these women had pyuria, leaving 10% of the original cohort as having no cause for dysuria. This last group probably had mechanical or chemical irritation of the urethra, either from sexual intercourse or bath soaps.

Males with dysuria may also have penile pain or dysuria as a result of phimosis, paraphimosis, balanitis, urethral trauma, epididymitis, or meatal stenosis. *Phimosis* is a scarring or narrowing of the preputial opening and manifests as failure to retract the foreskin (the foreskin is normally difficult to retract in neonates, but by 3 years of age, it is easily retracted). *Paraphimosis*, an emergent disease, is an incarceration of the prepuce behind the glans. Edema, pain, and swelling are present. *Balanitis* is an infection of the prepuce (streptococcus, candida, mixed flora, trichomonas) which may be recurrent and warrants circumcision.

URINALYSIS AND URINE CULTURE

A properly obtained urine specimen for urinalysis and culture is critical for accurate treatment. Numerous studies have shown that over 50% of all positive cultures obtained from a "bagged" specimen are skin contaminants. In the non–toilet-trained toddler, urine may be obtained by a bag only if treatment is not planned that day, and a confirmatory culture may be done the next day. The confirmatory culture may be either a suprapubic aspiration or a catheterized urine specimen. Because aspiration requires a full bladder and infants void every 1 to 2 hours, it is often impractical to wait. Catheterization is more efficient, but it does carry approximately a 1% risk of introducing infection into the bladder.

In the toilet-trained child, a clean-void urine is an adequate specimen. There are several exceptions to this rule. Uncircumcised males have a contamination rate of 5% to 9%, depending on whether or not soap cleansing was used. Therefore, if treatment is needed urgently in such boys, two urine samples should be cultured or catheterization should be performed. Adolescent females may also fail to cleanse adequately, as may obese younger girls. The urine sample should be examined for squamous epithelial cells and should be discarded if more than rare cells are present.

Urinalysis should be performed both microscopically and by the dipstick method to detect the presence of nitrites, hematuria, and leukocyte esterase (Fig. 27–2). Decisions on treatment are usually based on the urinalysis results, not urine culture results, which require 18 to 24 hours of incubation. Fortunately, the sensitivity and specificity of the combination of the presence of leukocyte esterase and nitrite are very high in older children (Table 27–1). The accuracy of these tests in young infants and neonates is much lower. In these patients, presumptive therapy is often begun for presumed sepsis before confirmation of urine, blood, or other cultures.

The usual method of microscopic examination of the centrifuged urine sediment is often unreliable. In the preferred method in adults, a hemacytometer is used to count leukocytes, and a count of greater than 10 cells/mm^3 is correlated with true infection. In children, two studies have examined the use of the hemacytometer; one found 50 cells/mm^3 to correlate well with greater than 10^5 bacteria per milliliter (the colony count definition for UTI in adult females) (Table 27–1). The other study used the centrifuged sediment method and obtained an 80% sensitivity and a 84% specificity for UTI in children (Table 27–1). When this method is combined with an examination for bacteria, the sensitivity increases to 99%. The sensitivity of combining the centrifuged sediment with the hemacytometer method is increased to 84.5%, compared with 65.6% for a standard urinalysis. Specificity remained over 99% for both methods.

Therefore, in the evaluation of older children, a dipstick test for the presence of nitrites and leukocyte esterase should be performed, as should a microscopic examination using a hemacytometer. The presence of leukocytes and bacteria (Table 27–2) even with a negative nitrite test result, suggests a diagnosis of a UTI. The presence of only leukocytes indicates a diagnosis of either vaginitis or *Chlamydia, Mycoplasma hominis,* or *Ureaplasma urealyticum* urethritis if the patient is an adolescent. Alternately, *sterile pyuria* may suggest prior treatment with antibiotics, low-grade bacterial infection, renal abscess, viral cystitis, appendicitis, inflammatory bowel disease, Kawasaki disease, Stevens-Johnson syndrome, tuberculosis, analgesic nephropathy, sarcoidosis, interstitial nephritis, heavy metal toxicity, acute tubular necrosis, Reiter syndrome, renal transplant rejection, nephrotoxic drugs, or nephrolithiasis. The presence of only bacteria with or without a positive nitrite test result may still indicate a UTI because the sensitivity of leukocytes on urinalysis is only 80% to 85%. Neonates and infants may have a UTI in the absence of pyuria or other laboratory evidence other than a positive urine culture. The gold standard for a UTI in a child remains the quantitative urine culture.

The gold standard for a UTI is a positive culture, by the criteria of 10^5 bacteria/ml; nonetheless, 10% of cases have at least 10^4, and 10% have fewer than 10^4 (Table 27–3). Lower colony counts may be indicative of infection in males, in diluted urine, in specimens from suprapubic or catheterized samples, or for various pathogens (for *S. saprophyticus*, colony counts may be as low as 10^2/ml). About 33% of adult women have true cystitis with colony counts of less than 10^5 bacteria/ml; therefore some investigators have suggested a criterion of 10^2 bacteria/ml for dysuric adult women. In children, the use of colony counts as low as 10^2 bacteria/ml will

Table 27-1. Urinalysis Methods in Children

Method	Sensitivity (%)	Specificity (%)	Positive Predictive Value (%)	Negative Predictive Value (%)
Dipstick*				
Leukocyte esterase	79	73	34	95
Nitrite	37	100	100	90
Leukocyte and/or nitrite	83	72	34	96
Microscopy of sediment*				
Leukocytes	80	84	47	96
Bacteria (any)	99	71	37	100
Leukocyte and/or bacteria	99	65	33	100
Unspun urine in counting chamber†				
>5 motile bacteria/mm^3	96	89	75	99
>5 WBC/mm^3	64	92	70	88

*Adapted from Lohr JA, Portilla MG, Geuder TG, et al. Making a presumptive diagnosis of urinary tract infection by using a urinalysis performed in an on-site laboratory. J Pediatr 1993;122:22–25.

†Adapted from Corman LI, Horbison RW. Simplified urinary microscopy to detect significant bacteriuria. Pediatrics 1982;70:133–135.

Abbreviation: WBC = white blood cell.

Dipstick Testing   Store strips at proper humidity and temperature
Test fresh urine (bilirubin and urobilinogen are light - and heat-sensitive)
Mix urine thoroughly (red blood cells will settle to bottom)
Compare reagent strips carefully, under good lighting
Read strip at proper time

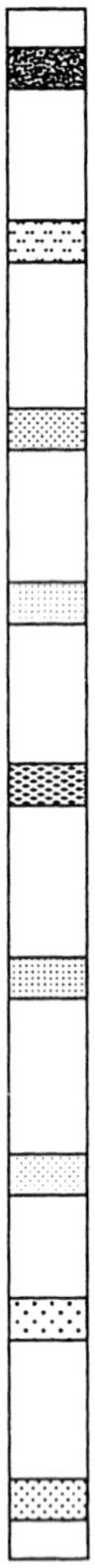

Finding	Normal Result	Method	Source of Error
Leukocytes	Negative (60–120 seconds)	Leukocyte esterase enzyme assay	Possible false-negatives with phenazopyridine HCl (Pyridium), vitamin C, nitrofurantoin
Nitrite	Negative (30 seconds)	Use first morning specimen since reaction may take 4 hours	Bacteriuria will cause positive results; vitamin C, acid pH may cause false-negative results
pH	5 to 7 (immediate)	Methyl red and bromthymol blue indicators for pH 5–9	Bacteriuria increases pH by converting urea to ammonia
Protein	Negative (30–60 seconds)	More sensitive to albumin than globulin; can detect as little as 60 mg/liter of protein	False-positives may be due to very alkaline urine, radiographic dyes
Glucose	Negative (60 seconds)	Glucose oxidase is specific for glucose	False-negatives occasionally seen resulting from tetracycline, aspirin, L-dopa, and vitamin C
Ketones	Negative (60 seconds)	Sodium nitroprusside forms violet dye with acetone, acetoacetate (not beta hydroxybutyrate)	False-positives may be seen with L-dopa, methyldopa (Aldomet), captopril, phenylketones
Urobilinogen	Negative (10–30 seconds)		Many possible false-positives and false-negatives
Bilirubin	Negative (30–60 seconds)		Vitamin C, nitrates may cause false-negatives; rifampin, chlorpromazine may cause false-positives
Blood	Negative (60 seconds)	Red blood cells cause stippling; free hemoglobin, or myoglobin causes diffuse pigment change	Nonspecificity of diffuse pigment change for hemoglobin, myoglobin, and others

Figure 27–2. Dipstick testing. Strips are stored at proper humidity and temperature. Fresh urine is tested (bilirubin and urobilinogen are light-sensitive and heat-sensitive). The urine is mixed thoroughly (red blood cells will settle to bottom). Reagent strips are compared carefully, under good lighting. The strip is read at the proper time. (From Reilly BM. Practical Strategies in Outpatient Medicine, 2nd ed. Philadelphia: WB Saunders, 1991:983.)

Table 27-2. Criteria for Interpretation of Bacteria Visualized During Urine Microscopy

Method	Methodology	Criteria for Significance*	Sensitivity, %	Specificity, %
1. Examination of *unstained, uncentrifuged* urine	1 drop of urine from Pasteur pipette, cover-glassed slide, ×40 objective, low-intensity light, high technical skill	Any/HPF	61–88	65–94
2. Examination of *unstained, centrifuged* urine	10 ml of urine, centrifuge at 2500–3000 rpm for 5 min, 1 drop of sediment from cover-glassed slide, ×40 objective, trained observers	Any/HPF ≥1/HPF >10/HPF	91 93–97 82	84 ≤88 >95
3. Examination of *stained, uncentrifuged* urine	1–2 drops of urine from Pasteur pipette, Gram's stain, observe ≥5 fields, ×100 objective, trained observers	Any/OIF ≥1/OIF ≥2/OIF ≥5/OIF	93 87 94 83	79 89 98 99
4. Examination of *stained, centrifuged* urine	10 ml of urine, centrifuge at 2500–3000 rpm for 5 min, 1–2 drops of sediment from Pasteur pipette, Gram's stain, ×100 objective	Any/OIF ≥1/OIF >5/OIF	97 98 87	66 89 96

From Jenkins RD, Fenn JP, Matsen JM, et al: Review of urine microscopy for bacteriuria. JAMA 1985;255:1596–1660. Copyright 1985, American Medical Association.
*Number of bacteria seen per oil-immersion field correlated with urine culture results ≥10⁵ CFU/ml.
Abbreviations: CFU = colony-forming units; HPF = high-power field; OIF = oil-immersion field.

result in overdiagnosis, which is a problem, since it may lead to unnecessary radiologic evaluation of the urinary tract. Table 27–3 shows that 90% of children with positive suprapubic tap results had at least 10^4 bacteria/ml; therefore, this seems a reasonable criterion for defining infection on clean-void urines. Symptomatic children with less than 10^4 bacteria/ml need a second specimen before treatment. Table 27–4 summarizes the recommended colony counts to define UTI in children. *Escherichia coli* is the dominant pathogen causing UTI in all ages; less common pathogens include *Klebsiella* species, *Proteus* species, *S. saprophyticus*, and enterococcus.

Mixed urine cultures do not always signify a contaminated specimen. Mixed coliform infections are noted in adult women (19% of all positive cultures) who were catheterized to avoid contamination. Mixed infections are also seen in children but require a catheterized specimen to confirm.

Table 27–5 offers clues found in the urinalysis that point to the correct diagnosis. Although microscopic hematuria is common in all UTIs, gross hematuria is more common with cystitis, glomerulonephritis, and renal calculi (see Chapter 29). The presence of red

Table 27-3. Suprapubic Tap Results Compared with Colony Counts on Simultaneous Clean-Void Urines in 272 Symptomatic Children

	Colony Count/ml		
	≤10³	≥10⁴	≥10⁵
Positive tap	20(10%)	18(9%)	161(81%)
Negative tap	55(75%)	9(12%)	9(12%)

From Pylkkanen J, Vilska J, Koskimies O. Diagnostic value of symptoms and clean-voided urine specimen in childhood urinary tract infection. Acta Paediatr Scand 1979;68:341.

Table 27-4. Criteria for Urinary Infection in Children

Suprapubic aspiration	Any growth significant
Catheterization*	10³ bacteria/ml
Clean-void urine (CVU) in symptomatic patient	≥10⁴ bacteria/ml
CVU in asymptomatic patient	>10⁵ bacteria/ml in 2 samples

*The exception is the uncircumcised neonate with a non-retractile foreskin. If colony count is <10⁵ bacteria/ml, a suprapubic aspiration should be performed.

blood cell casts suggests glomerulonephritis, whereas the presence of white cell casts suggests pyelonephritis. The combination of heavy proteinuria and a UTI should suggest infection in a child with reflux nephropathy or a urologic anomaly, such as polycystic kidney disease. Urate crystals may move as a result of brownian motion and resemble motile rods, but they dissolve with gentle heating of the test tube or slide. Finally, breast-fed neonates often produce salmon-colored patches in the urine that are caused by urate crystals filtered on the diaper.

LOCALIZATION METHODS

Tests that differentiate pyelonephritis from cystitis are of importance in the research on UTI and are also clinically useful. If an accurate localization test were available in children, it might select the appropriate children for short-course therapy (for cystitis). Localization to the kidney might identify children who are likely to have radiologic abnormalities, such as VUR. Many available methods are either highly invasive or still in the development stage. The test felt to be the most accurate in adults, the bladder washout test,

Table 27–5. Clues on Urinalysis That Point to the Correct Diagnosis for Dysuria

1. *Gross hematuria* suggests:
   a. Passage of clots from glomerulonephritis, especially Berger disease (IgA nephropathy)
   b. Cystitis
   c. Renal calculi
   d. Trauma
   e. Tumor (rare)
2. *White blood cell casts* suggest pyelonephritis but are rarely seen in children. *Red cell casts* suggest acute glomerulonephritis.
3. *Proteinuria* on yellow urine (little blood present) suggests glomerular damage. Reflux nephropathy and polycystic kidney disease can produce a UTI and proteinuria.
4. *Urate crystals* resemble bacteria but may be dissolved by heating the slide or test tube.
5. *Alkaline pH* in the presence of pyuria suggests a urease-producing bacterium, such as *Proteus*.
6. *Salmon-colored urine* in neonates is urate crystals, not blood. It is not a sign of UTI, but rather of concentrated urine.

Abbreviation: UTI = urinary tract infection.

is not universally accepted as reliable in children. Bladder washout relies on the sterilization of the bladder by topically instilled neomycin, followed by collection by Foley catheter of timed urine aliquots that are assumed to derive from the kidney. Nonetheless, in one study by Hellerstein et al in children with stringently defined clinical pyelonephritis, bladder washout identified only eight of 14

children. Pyelonephritis in children is thought to be more likely if three or more of the following are present: (1) fever greater than 39°C, (2) elevated serum C-reactive protein level, (3) elevated erythrocyte sedimentation rate, and (4) decreased renal concentrating ability measured by a 1-deamino-(8-D-arginine)-vasopressin test. Nonetheless, the positive and negative predictive value of these individual criteria as predictors of a treatable radiologic abnormality are poor (Fig. 27–3). Neither the four individual laboratory tests nor age of the child is any better a positive predictor of abnormalities than the simple presence of fever.

Other localization methods in children include antibody-coated bacteria (ACB) and serum C-reactive protein tests. The ACB method appears to be reliable in adult women but not in children (33% false-negative and 37% false-positive results). C-reactive protein elevation also gives poor results, with many false-negative results.

In adult women, it has been suggested that the failure of a single dose of antibiotic to cure a urinary tract infection may in itself be a localization test. Women who do not respond to single-dose therapy have a higher rate of radiologic anomalies. The predictive value of single-dose failure for predicting urinary tract anomalies in children yields a sensitivity of 60% and a specificity of 58%, which makes it a poor screening test in children.

An important and promising method for localization in children is the ⁹⁹ᵐTc-dimercaptosuccinic acid (DMSA) scan. Approximately 55% to 66% of febrile inpatient children with UTIs have localized renal defects on DMSA scanning performed within 72 hours of admission. This study localizes the infection to the kidney, but the 40% of children with normal results do not necessarily not have pyelonephritis. Nor has this method been used in a series of afebrile outpatients with UTIs. It appears that the subsequent development of permanent renal scars occurs only in areas of nonperfusion on

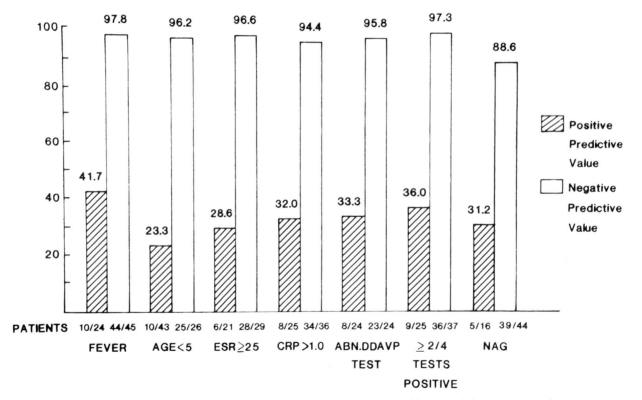

Figure 27–3. Predictive values of a positive or negative test result for a treatable urologic problem on radiologic evaluation after a urinary tract infection in children 2 weeks to 13 years old. The actual number of patients is shown at the bottom of each bar graph. ABN = abnormal. CRP = C-reactive protein; DDAVP = 1-deamino-(8-D-arginine)-vasopressin; ESR = erythrocyte sedimentation rate; NAG = N-acetyl glucosaminidase. (Reproduced with permission from Johnson CE, Shurin P, Marchant C, et al. Identification of children requiring radiologic evaluation for urinary infection. Pediatr Infect Dis J 1985;4:656–663.)

the initial scan; therefore, DMSA scanning may be a clinically useful method of predicting which children are at risk for scarring.

Ultrasonography or computed tomography (CT) demonstrates an enlarged kidney (nephromegaly) in patients with pyelonephritis. In addition, focal renal cellulitis or focal pyelonephritis may produce the sonographic appearance of a decreased density termed a nephronia. Finally, and most uncommonly, these visualizing methods may detect a renal or perinephric abscess. In addition, ultrasonography may detect anomalies of the kidney and ureters; unfortunately, it does not help in the diagnosis of VUR.

Determination of bacteria P-piliation may be a useful localization method; *E. coli* that are P-pili positive cause over 70% of all episodes of pyelonephritis, but only 20% to 30% of cystitis. These pili are surface structures of *E. coli* that adhere to uroepithelium and allow ascent from the bladder to the kidney. They are the main virulence factor of *E. coli* and often occur in combination with hemolysin and O-capsular antigen. They are also believed to cause a higher failure rate for short-course therapy. Few hospital laboratories are now able to perform P-pili testing, but simple commercial kits are available for research studies and future applications.

DIFFERENTIAL DIAGNOSIS

Once the history taking and physical examination of the child are completed, a list of probable diagnoses should be developed. This list determines what laboratory tests or radiologic studies are needed and cost effective. Table 27–6 outlines the causes of dysuria, regardless of patient age.

Tumors of the kidney or ureters can cause dysuria only by passive bleeding that produces clots. Rarely, glomerulonephritis can also produce painful blood clots. Hemorrhagic cystitis, whether caused by chemotherapy or by adenoviral infection, is severely painful. Tumors of the bladder are quite rare in children but can produce urinary retention or dysuria. Fibromas, rhabdomyosarcomas, and hemangiomas may occur. Congenital urethral polyps occur in young boys and may prolapse. In prepubertal girls, the urethra may prolapse and bleed. Labial adhesions are a common problem of unknown cause that may produce either dysuria or a true UTI.

Mechanical irritation of the male urethra may result from water injection, foreign body insertion, renal calculi, or masturbation. In the uncircumcised male, balanitis or penile ulcers may cause dysuria. In infants, recurrent diaper dermatitis may lead to a urethral stricture that requires surgery. Urethral stenosis is no longer believed to cause UTIs in girls or women, despite the fact that thousands of unfortunate women underwent urethral dilatations in the past.

The *frequency-dysuria syndrome* in females is common and may often be a low-colony-count UTI. However, it may also be due to chemical irritants, such as bubble bath, bath soap, douche, or local perfumes. Pinworms play an unknown role in this syndrome, but they should be evaluated by a tape-preparation if anal pruritus is present. Labial adhesions are common in toddlers and may cause dysuria or a true UTI. Urethral prolapse is quite rare but may resemble vaginal trauma when it presents with bleeding.

Sexual abuse frequently causes dysuria, but less often causes a UTI. Although 10% of victims of abuse ranging from 1 to 16 years of age had dysuria or urinary frequency in one study, only two (0.5%) had pyuria and a UTI. However, urine cultures for *Chlamydia* organisms were not performed in this study. It would seem reasonable to obtain urine specimens for culture for *Chlamydia* species in any abused child with pyuria, as well as the standard vaginal and rectal cultures.

Vaginitis can cause dysuria in girls and women. In prepubertal girls in whom a UTI is ruled out, a careful examination of the introitus for discharge or foreign body should be made. Cultures

Table 27–6. Differential Diagnosis of Dysuria

Urinary Tract Infections*
  Urethritis
  Cystitis
  Pyelonephritis
  Adenoviral hemorrhagic cystitis
  Schistosomiasis

Vaginitis*
  Candida albicans
  Trichomonas vaginalis
  Nonspecific vaginitis with clue cells
  Group A streptococci
  Proteus species, *Escherichia coli,* and other enteric pathogens
  Sexual abuse: gonorrhea, chlamydia, and herpes simplex
  Foreign body in vagina
  Herpes simplex

Tumor-Related Dysuria
  Passage of blood clots from kidney tumors (Wilms)
  Chemotherapy-related hemorrhagic cystitis (cyclophosphamide)
  Rhabdomyosarcoma of bladder
  Urethral polyps or diverticula
  Fibromas of the bladder
  Hemangiomas

Mechanical Irritation of the Urethra
  Males
    Water injection or foreign body insertion
    Hypercalciuria or frank calculi
    Balanitis or penile ulcers
    Urethral stricture
    Posterior urethral valves
    Masturbation
  Females
    Hypercalciuria
    Bubble bath or detergent
    Pinworms
    Labial adhesions
    Urethral prolapse
    Sexual abuse

Other
  Appendicitis
  Inflammatory bowel disease

*Common.

for enteric pathogens, group A streptococci, gonorrhea, *Chlamydia* species, and *Candida* species should be obtained if a discharge is seen. A digital rectal examination may palpate foreign bodies in the vagina, but it is often necessary to perform an examination under anesthesia if a foreign body is suspected but is not felt or seen.

Most instances of dysuria are caused by ascending bacterial infection of the urinary tract. About 80% of infections are caused by *E. coli*, 10% by *Klebsiella* or *Proteus* species, and 5% by *S. saprophyticus.* These infections originate in the fecal reservoir and spread to the introitus and urethra and finally into the bladder.

Table 27–7 is a stepwise evaluation scheme for children who are dysuric but have fewer than 10^4 bacteria/ml on a clean-void urine culture. First, a complete history taking and physical examination should be performed. If vaginitis is present, appropriate specimens for culture should be obtained. If anal pruritus is present, a pinworm tape slide should be sent home with the patient for early morning testing. If no vaginitis or anal excoriation is present, one of two strategies is possible: a first morning urine or a catheterized urine specimen can be obtained. The decision of which strategy is

Table 27–7. Stepwise Evaluation Strategy for Children
with Urinary Frequency and/or Dysuria and $<10^4$
Pathogens/ml

1. Check for bubble bath or harsh detergent use in the bath water.
2. Ask about masturbation or foreign body insertion introduction into the penile urethra.
3. If vaginitis is present, obtain cultures for gonorrhea, *Candida, Chlamydia,* and bacteria (group A streptococci, *Escherichia coli*).
4. Examine for pinworms with a tape slide.
5. Obtain a second urine for culture.
   a. First A.M. urine
   b. Catheterized urine sample. ($>10^3$ pathogens/ml indicate urinary tract infection.)
6. Obtain an 8-hour urine specimen for calcium:creatinine ratio.
7. Treat for 3 days with an antibiotic for presumed urethritis.

Table 27–8. Differential Diagnosis of Dysuria and Pyuria
by Age of Child

Neonate
　Sepsis with secondary bacteriuria or candiduria—common especially in preterm infants
　Pyelonephritis secondary to obstructive lesion—rare

Infant
　Asymptomatic bacteriuria (ABU—2% males, 0.5% females)
　Cystitis—rare, except in uncircumcised males
　Pyelonephritis—common
　Sexual abuse—rare

Preschool- and School-Aged Child
　ABU—females only, ~ 1%
　Cystitis—common
　Pyelonephritis—uncommon after age 5 yr
　Vaginitis secondary to *Candida albicans,* group A streptococci, and fecal coliforms—common
　Bubble bath urethritis—common

Adolescent
　Vaginitis secondary to sexually transmitted pathogens—common
　Mechanical irritation from intercourse or masturbation—common
　Cystitis—common
　Pyelonephritis—rare
　ABU—1% of females
　Renal calculi or hypercalciuria—rare
　Appendicitis—rare
　Inflammatory bowel disease—rare

Abbreviation: ABU = asymptomatic bacteriuria.

used should be based on the severity of the symptoms. Commonly, symptoms are mild and self-limited and do not require catheterization. Finally, an 8 to 12 hour urine sample for calcium-to-creatinine ratio should be ordered (a ratio >0.4 is diagnostic of hypercalciuria) to evaluate for renal stones. Most children with hypercalciuria are younger than 8 years; only 50% have hematuria. If no diagnosis is reached after these steps, the severity and duration of dysuria should guide the clinician. Referral to a urologist for cystoscopy may be necessary to diagnose the extremely rare occurrence of a bladder tumor in a child.

DIFFERENTIAL DIAGNOSIS BASED ON AGE
(Table 27–8)

Neonates

　Urinary tract infection in the first month of life has a significantly different epidemiology than that occurring in later infancy and childhood. Boys predominate over girls at a 5:1 ratio; about 5% of these male infants have obstructive uropathy (Fig. 27–4). It was once thought that these infections were all hematogenous, but the high incidences of VUR and obstructive uropathy suggest that many of these infections are ascending. In addition, the rate of UTI in the first year of life is eleven times higher for uncircumcised males than for circumcised males, suggesting that infection originates in the prepuce. Furthermore, the rate of UTI is lower in the first 72 hours than after 72 hours of life. In the first 72 hours, 90% of the urinary infections were accompanied by bacteremia, suggesting the presence of disseminated sepsis. Thereafter, the rate of accompanying bacteremia is 10% to 20%.

　In one prospective screening study of 1762 infants admitted to a neonatal intensive care nursery, 2.4% of patients were bacteriuric, of whom 1.9% were symptomatic and 0.5% were asymptomatic. Of 43 urinary tract infections, only six were associated with bacteremia. Radiologic anomalies were found in 44% of the symptomatic neonates, including three children with hydronephrosis. In another study, hydronephrosis due to obstructive lesions was seen in about 5%, and severe (grade IV of V) VUR was seen in about 19% of neonates with symptomatic UTI. Hence, over 20% of neonates with a urinary tract infection will potentially require urologic surgery.

　When uncircumcised male infants are evaluated for sepsis, a suprapubic aspiration yields a much lower contamination rate than does a catheter specimen. The bladder is a more superficial abdominal organ until the end of infancy and is readily accessible with a 1½-inch-long, 22-gauge needle, inserted perpendicular to the

abdominal wall, 1 to 2 cm above the symphysis pubis in the midline. Negative pressure is applied while the needle is advanced slowly until urine is obtained. No anesthetic or sterile gloves are necessary, but the infant should be cleansed with an antiseptic

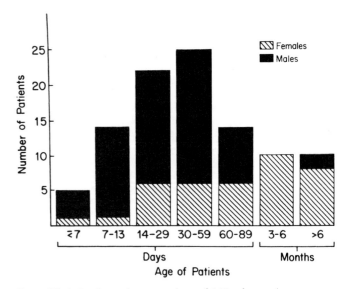

Figure 27–4. Distribution by age and sex of 100 infants with urinary tract infections. (From Ginsburg CM, McCracken GH Jr. Urinary tract infections in young infants. Pediatrics 1982;69:409–412.)

solution and should not have voided for 1 hour before the procedure is performed, to ensure a filled bladder.

Obstructive uropathy can also cause neonatal UTI and sepsis. Many affected neonates are diagnosed based on the results of prenatal ultrasonography, so that antibiotic prophylaxis or immediate surgical correction can prevent sepsis and renal injury. Any neonate with bilateral hydronephrosis should undergo voiding cystourethrography before discharge to rule out posterior urethral valves or bladder neck obstruction. If VUR is found, antibiotic prophylaxis may be begun. Neonates with the more common diagnoses of ureteropelvic junction obstruction and multicystic dysplastic kidney do not usually need prophylaxis; urologic consultation should be obtained.

Infants (< 12 months)

All discussions of UTI in infants must begin with the fact that approximately 0.9% of infant girls and 2.5% of infant boys may have *asymptomatic bacteriuria*. An additional 1.2% of both boys and girls may develop symptomatic UTI before the age of 12 months. UTI is one of the most common bacterial causes of fever without a focus in children under 2 years of age. Nonetheless, the high background rate of asymptomatic bacteriuria may explain why many studies in febrile infants show apparent UTI with no pyuria. These infants may have another (viral) source of fever and coincident asymptomatic bacteriuria. Because no laboratory test can distinguish asymptomatic bacteriuria from pyelonephritis in a febrile infant, all such infants must be treated as if they are infected and should subsequently be radiologically evaluated. Conversely, asymptomatic infants should not be treated if asymptomatic bacteriuria is found, because of the excellent prognosis for spontaneous clearing of colonization.

Several prospective American studies of febrile infants have shown the rate of greater than 10^4 bacteria/ml to be about 5%. Until infants are 3 months of age, males predominate. After 3 months of age, UTIs were uncommon in male infants in one study of predominantly uncircumcised male infants (see Fig. 27–4). Nonetheless, in other studies, some male infants with UTIs present as late as 1 year of age. Bacteremia is less common in patients with UTIs outside the neonatal period (rates range from 6% to 31% in various studies), but fever is seen in most patients. Because pyuria is seen in only about 50% of all infants with UTIs, it is important for a catheterized or suprapubic urine specimen to be obtained from all infants in whom the source of fever cannot be identified. It is impossible to confirm a suspicious urine culture obtained with a urine bag after antibiotic therapy has begun. Therefore, all febrile infants younger than 12 months (and possibly those <24 months) of age require a urinalysis and culture if no other definite source of fever is found.

Should circumcision be recommended in all newborn males? Males who are uncircumcised have a 10-fold increased risk of UTI in infancy. At present, clinicians should leave the decision for circumcision up to the family, unless there is a family history of VUR, in which case circumcision seems prudent.

Preschool- and School-Aged Children

The preschool child (aged 1 to 5 years) poses new problems. This is the age at which toilet training occurs, which may cause dysfunctional voiding patterns, such as urine retention and contractions against a closed sphincter. In males, such problems may not be identified, because the length of the male urethra and meatal position are protective against ascending infection. Girls readily become infected, and bladder edema may then intensify the voiding

problems. Children with daytime incontinence after 4 years of age need a urine culture and possibly cystography. Attempting to void with the sphincter closed generates high intravesicular pressures and may cause VUR, even in the absence of congenital reflux. Urodynamic studies are extremely difficult to perform in toddlers; most investigators recommend a 6-month trial of therapy before cystometric tests are attempted. Anticholinergic therapy and antibiotic prophylaxis are useful for children who have recurrent infections, urgency, and frequency.

In young children, the incidence of asymptomatic bacteriuria is approximately 1% in girls and zero percent in boys. Symptomatic infection is also very rare in boys; hence, when it occurs, a complete radiologic evaluation for anomalies or reflux must be performed.

Sexual abuse is more common in young children than in infants but usually presents with vaginitis, vaginal or rectal bleeding, or abdominal pain (see Chapter 37). Dysuria is not a common single presenting symptom.

Adolescents

In adolescent males, lack of circumcision increases the risk of UTI about threefold, compared with those who are circumcised. Because the risk of UTI is so low in boys of this age group, this is a poor argument in favor of late circumcision. It is useful to obtain a urine culture as well as cultures for *Chlamydia* species and *N. gonorrhoeae* in all dysuric adolescent males. Careful examination of the scrotum for signs of epididymitis is indicated (see Chapter 30).

In adolescent females, cystitis and urethritis are more common in those who are sexually active, especially those using barrier contraception. Both diaphragm, and spermicide and foam, and condom users have a much higher rate of bacteriuria than do those taking birth control pills. Pyelonephritis occurs in nonsexually active adolescents only rarely and should suggest the possibility of (1) neglected UTI symptoms for days to weeks or (2) VUR.

Pitfalls in the diagnosis of UTI are noted in Table 27–9.

ASYMPTOMATIC BACTERIURIA

A decade or two ago, it was commonly recommended to screen all preschool girls for asymptomatic bacteriuria by an annual urine culture. It was widely believed that asymptomatic bacteriuria could lead to silent renal damage and ultimate renal failure. The completion of several long-term prospective studies of school-aged girls with asymptomatic bacteriuria has put such fears to rest. The incidence of asymptomatic bacteriuria is about 1.5%. About 33% of girls with ABU have VUR, and as many as 10% to 25% may have renal scarring. However, the long-term prognosis is excellent, even in patients with ongoing bacteriuria. Treatment with short courses of antibiotics may lead to more episodes of pyelonephritis than did no treatment. No girl with renal scarring will show a decrease in glomerular filtration rate, despite prolonged (median of 3.1 years) bacteriuria. It is strongly recommended that no prophylaxis be administered; treatment is indicated for all symptomatic episodes.

For these reasons, it is best not to screen for asymptomatic bacteriuria. When the condition is found incidentally, the family should be counseled regarding its favorable outcome. Radiologic studies are not indicated unless a symptomatic UTI subsequently develops. The doctor may wish to repeat a urine culture in 3 to 6 months because most cases of asymptomatic bacteriuria clear spontaneously, and the family can be reassured.

Knowledge of asymptomatic bacteriuria may be beneficial when

Table 27–9. Common Pitfalls in the Correct Diagnosis of Dysuria

Neonates

   Assume that significant bacteriuria in a bagged urine specimen is a true UTI, and treat before a confirmatory culture is obtained.

   Fail to obtain a urine culture in a neonate over 3 days of age and miss obstructive uropathy with a secondary infection.

Toddlers and School-Aged Children

   Trusting a urine culture from a bagged urine specimen.

   Accept a laboratory report of "no significant growth" on urine, without knowing that the laboratory reports only $>5 \times 10^4$ CFU/ml as "significant."

   Fail to label a urine as "catheterized specimen," so that the laboratory can plate 0.1 ml as well as 0.01 ml.

   Fail to obtain a cystogram after the first infection, trusting to see reflux on sonogram or intravenous pyelogram.

Adolescents

   Fail to ask about sexual history suggestive of vaginitis, such as a new sexual partner and condom or other birth control device use.

   Treat pyuria as a UTI in a sample contaminated with vaginal leukocytes.

Abbreviations: CFU = colony-forming unit; UTI = urinary tract infection.

an affected young woman becomes pregnant. During pregnancy, asymptomatic bacteriuria increases the risk of pyelonephritis, preterm labor, and the possibility of sepsis in the infant.

TREATMENT

Goals of Therapy

In a child with dysuria, the primary goal is to accurately diagnose the cause of the dysuria rather than to relieve the symptoms, which are often mild. If the child is treated with antibiotics prematurely, that is before definitively cultured proof of infection is obtained, the child may be committed to unnecessary radiologic studies. A similar principle applies to adolescent girls, in whom antibiotic therapy begun for a UTI may mask or only partially treat vaginitis. Only in the febrile child with suspected pyelonephritis should there be urgency to treat before establishing a diagnosis.

Treatment of Cystitis

Once the diagnoses of vaginitis, tumors, renal calculi, and other less common causes of dysuria have been excluded, the diagnostic decision tree in Figure 27–5 applies. In afebrile older children without flank pain, cultures may be obtained, and the condition may be left untreated if pyuria is absent. Those with pyuria or bacteriuria may undergo treatment if the severity of symptoms warrants this. The choice of antimicrobial agent depends only on the cost and the spectrum of resistance in the area of country. In many areas, *E. coli* resistance rates to sulfa drugs and amoxicillin may exceed 50%, making these agents an unwise empiric choice.

Quinolones are widely used in adults, but effects on animal cartilage plates make their use unwise in children under 18 years of age. All other oral agents have cure rates exceeding 80% when they are given for at least 7 days. Nonetheless, administration of amoxicillin or trimethoprim-sulfamethoxazole is considered the treatment of choice for outpatient therapy of UTI in patients with uncomplicated infections.

Once the culture specimen is positive, the next decision is the length of therapy. Although short-course (1- to 3-day) therapy is widely used with success in adult women, it cannot be recommended in most children. Because the recurrence rate after a short course of therapy is higher than that after longer-course therapy, children with undiagnosed VUR may have a second episode of pyelonephritis before radiologic evaluation. However, in some children, short-course therapy is appropriate in children with recurrent UTIs who have completed a normal radiologic evaluation. Short-course therapy enhances compliance and avoids selection of resistant organisms. If short-course therapy is chosen, the drug of choice is trimethoprim-sulfamethoxazole, given for 3 days.

Symptomatic treatment of cystitis in children usually includes oral analgesics and sitz baths of 20 minutes several times daily. Pyridium is not available in oral form for children, but tablets may be given to adolescents for local anesthesia of the urethra.

Treatment of Pyelonephritis

Children with fever, chills, flank pain, or systemic toxicity are assumed to have pyelonephritis. Most, but not all, children with pyelonephritis require inpatient therapy. Infants under 1 to 2 years of age require intravenous antibiotic therapy until bacteremia has been excluded at 48 to 72 hours. In older children, the presence of emesis or anorexia may make compliance with oral therapy difficult. This is especially true in adolescents, who generally should be admitted if they are febrile. Compliance is also a reason for admitting children because pyelonephritis generally requires 10 to 14 days of therapy. Because the dysuria and fever usually resolve in 2 to 3 days, many adolescents discontinue therapy. If outpatient management is selected, a repeat evaluation 24 hours later is mandatory to assess compliance and severity of illness. A second visit on day 4 of treatment should show that the child is afebrile; a repeat urine culture should also be obtained.

Pyelonephritis in the neonate is treated similarly to sepsis. The cultures should include urine, blood, and cerebrospinal fluid. If an antigen test for group B streptococci is desired, the urine should be obtained by suprapubic aspiration or catheter; latex bags have been shown to be contaminated with skin flora, yielding false-positive results. The choice of antibiotics varies with the epidemiologic patterns in each hospital but usually includes ampicillin (100 mg/kg/day for neonates under 7 days of age or 150 mg/kg/day for neonates over 7 days) and an aminoglycoside. Both drugs may be given either intravenously or intramuscularly. The drugs are given for 10 days, unless meningitis is present (in which case the dose of ampicillin is increased and cefotaxime is added) (see Chapter 53). All neonates older than 72 hours who have pyelonephritis should undergo renal sonography to exclude congenital hydronephrosis. Ultrasonography performed in the first 72 hours of life may yield false-negative results because of decreased glomerular filtration rates after birth. At discharge, the neonate should not be given trimethoprim-sulfamethoxazole prophylaxis, because of the possible displacement of bilirubin from albumin by some sulfonamide drugs. The timing of the cystography is controversial, but it should probably be performed before the neonate is discharged, to avoid the need for prophylactic antibiotics.

Treatment of pyelonephritis in older children may be guided by the results of Gram stain of the urine. If cocci are seen, intravenous

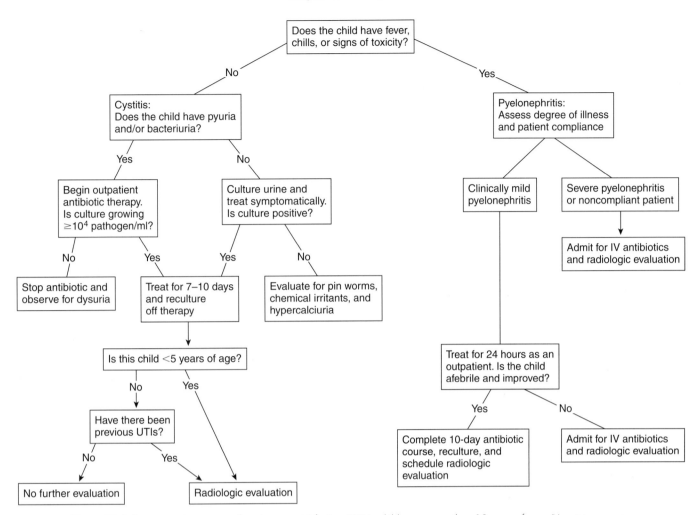

Figure 27–5. Diagnostic decision tree for urinary tract infection (UTI) in children younger than 13 years of age. IV = intravenous.

ampicillin may be given to eliminate enterococci. If bacilli alone are seen, intravenous gentamicin or kanamycin therapy is added to ampicillin therapy. Cefotaxime or a related cephalosporin is also indicated and is often used as single-drug intravenous therapy for presumed gram-negative rod UTI. Ceftazidime, or ticarcillin or piperacillin, and an aminoglycoside are indicated for the rare occurrence of *Pseudomonas* UTI (oncology patient or child with myelodysplasia).

The child should be treated on an inpatient basis until he or she is afebrile for 1 day, the urine shows no motile rods, and the urine culture sensitivities are known. This interval allows selection of an oral agent to complete a 10- to 14-day course. The radiologic evaluation may be obtained on the day of discharge. This schedule increases compliance and eliminates the need for prophylaxis until the studies are obtained. For children who are still febrile on day 3 of treatment, ultrasonography rules out a perirenal abscess or obstructive uropathy.

Follow-Up Monitoring After a Urinary Tract Infection

In all children with a UTI, a urine culture should be obtained 3 to 4 days after therapy, to detect early relapse. This is especially critical for those given short-course therapy. If a child relapses, a second course of therapy, of a full 10-day length, should be given. Early relapse may be a sign of VUR or congenital obstruction; radiologic evaluation is mandatory.

If the post-therapy culture is negative, no further cultures are needed unless the child is awaiting a cystogram. If so, a culture and urinalysis should be performed 1 or 2 days before the cystogram is obtained to avoid performing the study during acute infection. It is no longer believed necessary to obtain specimens for culture monthly for 3 to 6 months in asymptomatic children, because asymptomatic bacteriuria need not be treated.

If a child has had three or more afebrile UTIs in a year, or more than one febrile UTI, oral antimicrobial prophylaxis at bedtime for 6 months is a cost-effective method of preventing a new UTI. In sexually active adolescents, an alternative method is to recommend one tablet of trimethoprim-sulfamethoxazole after each episode of sexual intercourse. Drugs appropriate for prophylaxis are shown in Table 27–10. It is not appropriate to use amoxicillin or cephalosporins for prophylaxis, because they alter bowel flora and may select resistant organisms. Low doses of the three drugs listed in Table 27–10 are concentrated in urine and vaginal secretions and reduce the relapse rate to fewer than 0.1 infections/patient/year. The use of trimethoprim-sulfamethoxazole for several years in children with VUR is highly effective in preventing UTI and allowing resolution of VUR without surgery.

Table 27–10. Prophylactic Antibiotics for Childhood Urinary Infections

	Dose	Timing	Side-Effects	Monthly Cost of Adult Dose
Trimethoprim-sulfamethoxazole (TMP-SMX)	2 mg/kg of TMP component (up to 40 mg) (½ tablet)	Bedtime	Skin rash, Stevens-Johnson (rare)	$2.00
Nitrofurantoin	1–2 mg/kg/day up to 50 mg	Bedtime	GI intolerance, pulmonary fibrosis (rare)	$4.00
Trimethoprim	2 mg/kg up to 40 mg (only tablet form is available)	Bedtime	Few	$9.00

Abbreviation: GI = gastrointestinal.

RADIOLOGIC EVALUATION OF URINARY TRACT INFECTIONS

Vesicoureteral Reflux and Reflux Nephropathy

Radiologic studies normally follow the diagnosis of a UTI rather than precede it, as in most diseases. Figure 27–6 demonstrates renal atrophy and scarring that occur when VUR with recurring infection affect a kidney. The goal of radiologic evaluation is to identify VUR and early scarring to prevent progressive disease.

In a survey of 241 patients who were over 18 years of age and who had UTI and VUR as children, 201 had been medically treated and the rest had been surgically treated because of the severity of VUR. In the surgical group, one patient who had renal failure and three who required a renal transplant died. In the rest of the patients, the outcome was very good: only 8% had hypertension, 4% had an elevated plasma creatinine level, and 6% have had at least one febrile UTI since diagnosis. Seventy-five percent of all ureters no longer show VUR in the medically managed group. None of 198 kidneys that were restudied had developed a new scar. Renal growth was impaired in only four of the 198 kidneys, and these four had shown severe scarring and high-grade VUR at first presentation. There was a direct relationship between severe renal scarring and uncooperative parents or children, suggesting that late presentation or noncompliance with antibiotic therapy may have led to the initial scarring.

This study included only children with VUR, but several other studies have conclusively shown that only about 50% of children developing scars have VUR. Late (>7 days) or inappropriate antibiotic therapy is a risk factor for renal scarring. Acquired renal scars noted on intravenous pyelography were found in only 37 of 4000 children; 32 of the 37 were aged 6 years or younger (Fig. 27–7). Children under 6 years of age who receive delayed or inappropriate treatment for pyelonephritis may develop renal scarring, regardless of whether they have VUR.

Many studies show a poorer prognosis if UTIs continue in children with VUR. Many patients (especially if they are noncompliant) develop progressive scarring, and others develop new scars. Children with high-grade but *sterile* VUR usually show no new scars. Long-term studies have shown that as many as 30% of patients with renal scars as children may develop end-stage disease and require nephrectomy and/or transplantation, or chronic dialysis. Others have lower glomerular filtration rates and higher diastolic blood pressures than those in control patients. These data emphasize the need to carefully identify children with VUR after the first UTI and the need to either operate (for reflux or obstruction) or use medical prophylaxis to prevent recurrent UTI in these children.

Another risk factor for renal scarring may be various virulence factors of *E. coli*. Quite unexpectedly, scarring is more common after infection due to a non–P-piliated (low-virulence) organism. One explanation for this observation is that the P-piliated strains infect only the renal pelvis and invoke a host response before they can invade the parenchyma. Non-piliated strains usually enter the kidney if reflux is present and may cause a slower, more insidious illness without immediate fever. The scarring may even result from the patient's host defense mechanisms, such as the release of interleukin-6 (IL-6) and other cytokines.

Ultrasonography Versus Intravenous Pyelography

Renal ultrasound studies are the least invasive method for studying the kidney, and the most acceptable to parents and children. Ultrasonography excellently evaluates the gross anatomy of the kidney and the collecting system for obstruction; its resolution for parenchymal scarring is limited. It does not show acute density changes of pyelonephritis as well as DMSA scanning, computed tomography, or gallium scanning does. Its two advantages over DMSA scanning are that it shows the collecting system well and it demonstrates a nonfunctional pole of a duplex kidney. Intravenous pyelography, once the gold standard for renal scarring, is now used less often than DMSA scanning. It surpasses renal sonography in the detection of renal scars, and it demonstrates the size and path of the ureter.

DMSA Scans

DMSA scans are quite effective in the evaluation of UTIs. DMSA is a radioisotope bound by the renal tubular cells after intravenous injection, which is probably as much as 100% specific and 87% sensitive for pyelonephritis. DMSA scanning involves placing an intravenous catheter and waiting for 90 to 120 minutes before images can be obtained. DMSA is imaged either by pinhole imaging, which rarely needs sedation, or by single-photon emission computed tomography (SPECT), which usually necessitates sedation in toddlers and infants. Radiation doses to the kidneys are significant, being about 10 times that used during intravenous pyelography. Gonadal radiation doses are similar to those used during intravenous pyelography. The renal collecting system is not seen well on DMSA scanning, so renal sonography must accompany the DMSA scanning to rule out or define obstruction.

Advocates of DMSA scanning believe that a scan obtained during acute illness localizes the infection to the kidney and therefore has clinical value. There are no large series of children with afebrile UTIs who have been studied by DMSA scanning. The focal areas of decreased density (photopenic) that are seen within

Right   **Left**

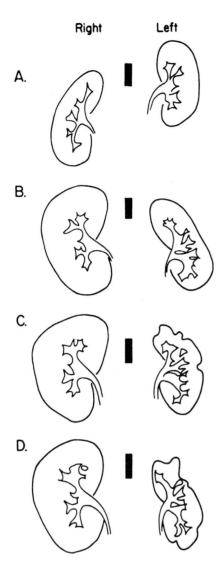

Figure 27–6. Serial tracings of excretory urograms after diagnosis of left-sided vesicoureteral reflux. *A*, 23 months after diagnosis. *B*, 31 months. *C*, 41 months. *D*, 52 months. *Solid bars* indicate the height of first lumbar vertebral body. (From Shindo S, Bernstein J, Arant BS. Evolution of renal segmental atrophy [Ask-Upmark kidney] in children with VUR: Radiographic and morphologic studies. J Pediatr 1983;102:847–854.)

72 hours of the diagnosis of pyelonephritis may resolve in 4 to 6 months. The defects heal slowly in infants and rapidly in adolescents; any defects present after 6 months are permanent scars. Some radiologists suggest that two DMSA scans be obtained in each child with a febrile UTI, one within 72 hours and a follow-up study in 4 to 6 months on all that show abnormalities. In children who have two scans, no new defects appear in kidneys that were normal on the first scan; 30% to 60% of defects resolve. It is unclear what difference in practical management would result from an initially abnormal study. All children with a febrile UTI should undergo 10 days of therapy, as well as post-therapy culture and careful follow-up. Prophylaxis is not currently recommended after a single episode of pyelonephritis. Therefore, the results of DMSA scanning performed during acute illness do not alter clinical management unless old scars are demonstrated. A single study at 4 to 6 months after diagnosis demonstrates all permanent scars and assists in the decision about surgical versus medical management of VUR.

DMSA is not universally available; glycoheptonate scans are a reasonable substitute. ^{99m}Tc glucoheptonate also reveals dynamic excretory data in addition to imaging the cortex.

Voiding Cystography

Renal ultrasonography, intravenous pyelography, and DMSA scanning may all miss significant degrees of VUR. Reflux is graded I through V (see Fig. 27–1) by standard contrast cystograms. Only grades IV and V are usually seen on upper tract studies; ballooning of the pelvocalyceal system requires a full bladder to contract to void. Because the standard cystogram requires placement of a Foley catheter, many doctors and parents are reluctant to obtain this study after only one UTI. Several studies have reported that despite appropriate recommendations, this study is seldom carried out until two or more UTIs occur or the child is hospitalized. In Europe, only infants and children with abnormal sonographic results usually undergo a cystogram.

To increase parental acceptance, *indirect radionuclide cystography* was developed. Here isotope is injected intravenously, and images are made after the child's bladder is filled. Unfortunately, this method may miss 61% of grade II VURs and even 12% of grade IV VURs.

Direct radionuclide cystography is 100% sensitive for VUR. This method requires urinary catheterization, but no sedation is usually needed. The radiation to the gonads is less than that used with standard cystography, and the sensitivity for lower grades of VUR may surpass that of the standard study. It is difficult with this study to grade reflux except into low grade (II and III) and high grade (IV and V). The main drawback of direct radionuclide cystography is the poor resolution of the penile urethra, which makes the study contraindicated in boys when posterior urethral valves may be present. Most clinicians prefer to use standard cystography for the first study after a UTI, even in girls, to allow accurate grading of VUR and to detect ureteroceles, ectopic ureters, and ureteral diverticulae.

To avoid the problems associated with catheter placement, several approaches may be used. First, midazolam (Versed) sedation has been used in toddlers with excellent results. Second, a Child Life worker may use a doll (to practice catheterization) and a book of pictures of the procedure to prepare the child older than 3 years of age. The presence of a parent during the procedure is also reassuring to most children.

Finally, the clinician must remember the siblings of children with VUR. As many as 33% of siblings also have VUR; about 33% have scars seen on DMSA scans, despite lacking a history of known UTI. All siblings younger than 13 years of age should undergo isotopic cystography and DMSA scanning if VUR is found. Alternately, DMSA scanning may be performed, and if no scarring is present in children over 5 years of age, careful follow-up is recommended.

Recommendations for Radiologic Evaluation

Unfortunately, no worldwide consensus exists about the need for a voiding cystogram in children or the role of the DMSA scan. In Europe, it has been traditional to evaluate children over 1 year of age by intravenous pyelography or sonography and proceed to cystography only if the results of the initial study are abnormal. With the development of the DMSA scan, several centers are now recommending this scan as the initial study in children over 1 or 2 years of age. In the United States, most pediatric centers begin evaluation of all children under 5 years with both a sonogram and a cystogram. DMSA scanning or less often intravenous pyelogra-

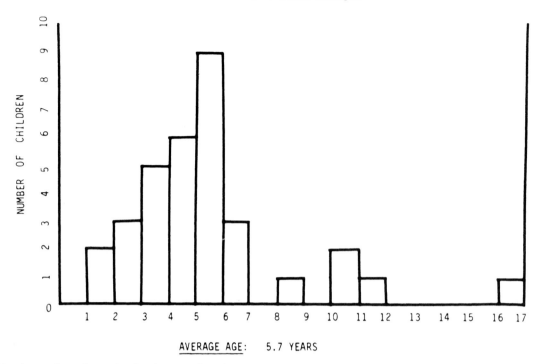

Figure 27–7. Distribution of age (by year) at first detection of renal scarring on intravenous pyelogram. (From Winter AL, Hardy B, Alton G, et al. Acquired renal scars in children. J Urol 1983;129:1190–1193.)

phy is then performed on children with either VUR or suspected renal scarring; the scanning is usually delayed until 4 to 6 months after infection.

Some investigators suggest that all febrile children with a UTI have DMSA scanning, cystography, and ultrasonography within 3 weeks of infection. If scarring is present, a repeat DMSA scan is recommended 4 to 6 months later. For children who are afebrile, cystography is recommended as the initial study. Patients with VUR should have DMSA scanning, while those without VUR need only ultrasonography to exclude obstruction. This approach has several problems. First, many parents refuse to have their child undergo three initial radiologic studies after a single UTI, plus a possible fourth study several months later. Second, radiation to the kidney from two DMSA scans must be balanced against any benefit derived from localizing the infection immediately. Third, the cost of these three studies is $768, compared with $414 if only ultrasonography and cystography are performed. The treatment of children with scarring is presently the same as that of children without scarring; both require antibiotic prophylaxis only if VUR is present. Therefore, it seems logical to reserve the immediate DMSA scan until its utility is demonstrated and to follow the algorithm presented in Figure 27–8. Renal sonography detects obstruction and allows referral to a urologist for appropriate diuretic renography (Table 27–11). The voiding cystogram shows reflux; if the VUR is grade IV or V, a urologic referral is recommended. Children with grade II or III VUR should be placed on bedtime antibiotic prophylaxis and scheduled monthly for urine culture. In 4 to 6 months after infection, a radiologist should be consulted as to the best study to detect scarring.

For children who have VUR and minimal or no scarring, the pediatrician should repeat both studies in 1 to 2 years after infection (using radionuclide cystography to reduce radiation). The decision on when to repeat the radiologic evaluation should be based on the parental acceptance of daily antibiotic therapy, as well as on the severity of VUR and age of the child. The overall mean time to spontaneous resolution of grade I, II, and III VUR is about 2 years.

Grades IV and V tend not to resolve. However, in infants under 1 year of age, severe VUR may disappear in less than 1 year; therefore, these infants require a 1-year follow-up study. All subsequent cystograms should be direct radionuclide studies because the radiation exposure to the gonads is markedly lower in these studies compared with that in a standard contrast cystogram.

There may also be a role for diagnostic restraint in evaluating childhood UTI. Unfortunately, attempts to find a simple blood or urine test to identify children at high risk for radiologic abnormalities such as VUR have been unsuccessful. Approximately 40% of UTIs in children under the age of 5 years are associated with grade II or higher VUR, but the rate declines to 5% after 5 years of age (Fig. 27–9). It is reasonable to defer radiologic studies in *afebrile*

Table 27–11. Red Flags and Indications for Referral to a Pediatric Urologist After a Urinary Tract Infection

1. Grade IV or V VUR
2. Marked bilateral renal scarring on IVP or a DMSA scan taken >4 months after UTI
3. Obstructive lesions
   a. Ureteropelvic junction obstruction
   b. Ureterocele
   c. Ureteral diverticulum
   d. Megaureter
   e. Posterior urethral valves
   f. Neurogenic bladder or markedly trabeculated bladder
4. Noncompliance with antibiotic therapy
5. Failure of kidney growth on yearly sonograms
6. Elevated serum creatinine concentration
7. Hypertension

Abbreviations: DMSA = dimercaptosuccinic acid; IVP = intravenous pyelography; UTI = urinary tract infection; VUR = vesicoureteral reflux.

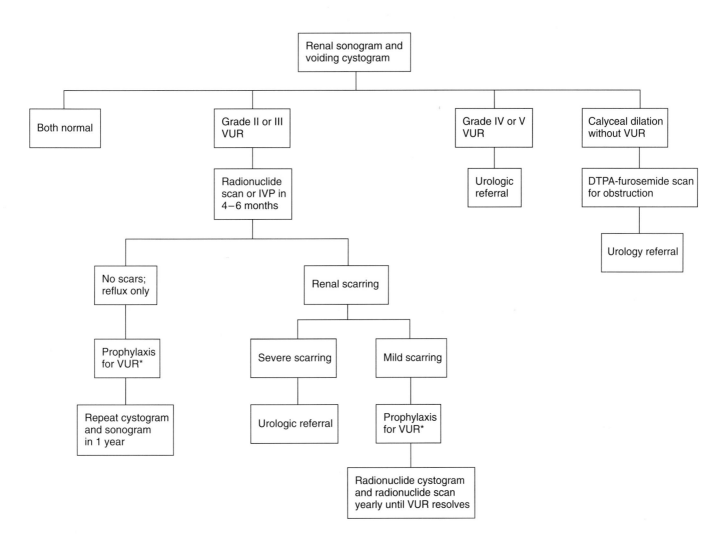

*Trimethoprim-sulfamethoxazole (1–2 mg/kg/day at bedtime)

Figure 27–8. Algorithm for radiologic evaluation of a child with a urinary tract infection. VUR = vesicoureteral reflux; IVP = intravenous pyelography; DTPA = pentetic acid.

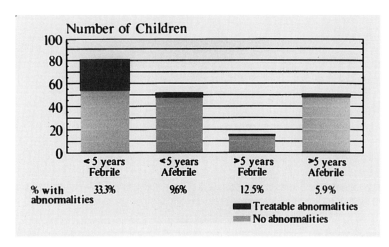

Figure 27–9. Incidence of treatable urologic problems found by radiologic evaluation 4 to 6 weeks after urinary tract infection in children 2 weeks to 13 years old, classified by age at evaluation and presence of fever of at least 38°C rectally or 37°C orally. (Data from Johnson CE at MetroHealth Medical Center, Cleveland, Ohio.)

girls older than 5 years until the second or third UTI. Boys of any age with a UTI require radiologic evaluation. Febrile infections in children older than 5 years are uncommon and are best evaluated immediately, even in adolescents. Renal scarring rarely occurs after 5 years of age in the absence of existing scars, so DMSA scanning or intravenous pyelography may be an adequate evaluation for afebrile girls over the age of 6 years. This approach spares many older girls the need for a cystogram, and allows the clinician to focus efforts on high-risk younger children.

High-risk, "red flag" situations are noted in Table 27–11 and often require referral to a urologist.

REFERENCES

History and Physical Examination

Labbe J. Self-induced urinary tract infection in school-age boys. Pediatrics 1990;86:703–706.

Klevan J, DeJong A. Urinary tract symptoms and urinary tract infection following sexual abuse. Am J Dis Child 1990;144:242–244.

Stamm WE, Counts GW, Running KR, et al. Diagnosis of coliform infection in acutely dysuric women. N Engl J Med 1982;307:463–468.

Urinalysis

Corman LI, Horbison RW. Simplified urinary microscopy to detect significant bacteriuria. Pediatrics 1982;70:133–135.

Hoberman A, Wald ER, Penchansky L, et al. Enhanced urinalysis as a screening test for UTI. Pediatrics 1993;91:1196–1199.

Lohr JA, Portilla MG, Geuder TG, et al. Making a presumptive diagnosis of urinary tract infection by using a urinalysis performed in an on-site laboratory. J Pediatr 1993;122:22–26.

Pylkkanen J, Vilska J, Koskimies O. Diagnostic value of symptoms and clean-voided urine specimen in childhood urinary tract infection. Acta Paediatr Scand 1979;68:341–344.

Saez-Llorens X, Umana MA, Odio CM, et al. Bacterial contamination rates for non-clean-catch and clean-catch midstream urine collections in uncircumcised boys. J Pediatr 1989;114:93–96.

Localization

Avner ED, Inglefinger JR, Herrin JJ, et al. Single-dose amoxicillin therapy of uncomplicated pediatric urinary tract infections. J Pediatr 1983;102:623–627.

Hellerstein S, Duggan E, Weichert E, et al. Localization of the site of

urinary tract infections with the bladder washout test. Pediatrics 1981;98:201–206.

Hellerstein S, Duggan E, Weichert E, et al. Serum C-reactive protein and the site of urinary tract infections. J Pediatr 1982;100:21–25.

Johnson CE, Shurin PA, Marchant CD, et al. Identification of children requiring radiologic evaluation for urinary infection. Pediatr Infect Dis J 1985;4:656–663.

Johnson CE, Vacca CV, Fattler D, et al. Urinary N-acetyl-β-glucosaminidase and the selection of children for radiologic evaluation after urinary tract infection. Pediatrics 1990;86:211–216.

Differential Diagnosis

Alon V, Warady BA, Hellerstein S. Hypercalciuria in the frequency-dysuria syndrome of childhood. J Pediatr 1990;116:103–105.

Klevan JL, DeJong AR. Urinary tract symptoms and urinary tract infection following sexual abuse. Am J Dis Child 1990;144:242–244.

Epidemiology

Ginsburg C, McCracken G. Urinary tract infections in young infants. Pediatrics 1982;69:409–412.

Siegel SR, Siegel B, Sokoloff BZ, et al. Urinary infection in infants and preschool children—five-year follow-up. Am J Dis Child 1980;134:369–372.

Spach DH, Stapleton AE, Stamm WE. Lack of circumcision increases the risk of UTI in young men. JAMA 1992;267:679–681.

Steele BT, DeMaria J. A new perspective on the natural history of vesicoureteral reflux. Pediatrics 1992;90:30–32.

Strom BL, Collins M, West S, et al. Sexual activity, contraceptive use, and other risk factors for symptomatic and asymptomatic bacteriuria. Ann Intern Med 1987;107:816–823.

Visser VE, Hall RT. Urine culture in the evaluation of suspected neonatal sepsis. J Pediatr 1979;94:635–638.

Wettergren B, Jodal U, Jonasson G. Epidemiology of bacteriuria during the first year of life. Acta Paediatr Scand 1985;74:925–933.

Winberg J, Bollgren I, Gothefors L, et al. The prepuce: A mistake of nature? Lancet 1989;1:598–599.

Asymptomatic Bacteriuria

Davison JM, Sprott MS, Selkon JB. The effect of covert bacteriuria in schoolgirls on renal function at 18 years and during pregnancy. Lancet 1984;1:651–655.

Hanson S, Jodal U, Noren L, et al. Untreated bacteriuria in asymptomatic girls with renal scarring. Pediatrics 1989;84:964–968.

Treatment

Rubin RH, Shapiro ED, Andriole VT, et al. Evaluation of new anti-infective drugs for the treatment of urinary tract infection. Clin Infect Dis 1992;15:S216–S227.

Short-Course Therapy

Johnson CE, Maslow JN, Fattlar DC, et al. The role of bacterial adhesins in the outcome of childhood urinary infection. Am J Dis Child 1995;147:1090–1096.

Moffatt M, Embree J, Grimm P, et al. Short-course antibiotic therapy for urinary tract infections in children. Am J Dis Child 1988;142:57–62.

Norrby SR. Short-term treatment of uncomplicated lower UTI in women. Rev Infect Dis 1990;12:458–467.

Pyelonephritis

Hellerstein S. Urinary Tract Infections in Children. Chicago: Year Book Medical Publishers, 1982.

Prophylaxis

Smellie JM, Katz G, Gruneberg RN. Controlled trial of prophylactic treatment in childhood urinary tract infection. Lancet 1978;2:175–178.

Radiology

Renal Scars

Holland NH, Jackson EC, Kazee M, et al. Relation of urinary tract infection and vesicoureteral reflux to scars: Follow-up of thirty-eight patients. J Pediatr 1990;116:S65–S71.

Jacobson SH, Eklof O, Eriksson CG, et al. Development of hypertension and uraemia after pyelonephritis in childhood: 27 year follow-up. Br Med J 1989;299:703–706.

Smellie JM. Reflections on 30 years of treating children with urinary tract infections. J Urol 1991;146:665–668.

Vesicoureteral Reflux

Belman AB, Skoog SJ. Nonsurgical approach to the management of vesicoureteral reflux in children. Pediatr Infect Dis J 1989;8:556–559.

Renal Ultrasonography

Johnson CE, DeBaz BP, Shurin PA, et al. Renal ultrasound evaluation of urinary tract infections in children. Pediatrics 1986;78:871–878.

Radionuclide Scanning

Jakobsson B, Nolstedt L, Svensson L, et al. 99mTechnetium-dimercaptosuccinic acid scan in the diagnosis of acute pyelonephritis in children: Relation to clinical and radiological findings. Pediatr Nephrol 1992;6:328–334.

Rushton HG, Majd M, Jantausch B, et al. Renal scarring following reflux and nonreflux pyelonephritis in children: Evaluation with 99mTechnetium-dimercaptosuccinic acid scintigraphy. J Urol 1992;147:1327–1332.

Sreenarasimhaiah V, Alon U. Uroradiologic evaluation of children with urinary tract infection: Are both ultrasonography and renal cortical scintigraphy necessary? J Pediatr 1995;127:373–377.

Cystography

Eggli DF, Tulchinsky M. Scintigraphic evaluation of pediatric urinary tract infection. Semin Nucl Med 1993;23:199–218.

Majd M, Kass EJ, Belman AB. Radionuclide cystography in children: Comparison of direct (retrograde) and indirect (intravenous) techniques. Ann Radiol 1985;28:322–328.

Radiologic Evaluation Recommendations

Andrich MP, Majd M. Diagnostic imaging in the evaluation of the first urinary tract infection in infants and young children. Pediatrics 1992;90:436–441.

Gleeson FV, Gordon I. Imaging in urinary infection. Arch Dis Child 1991;66:1282–1283.

Johnson CE, Shurin PA, Marchant CD, et al. Identification of children requiring radiologic evaluation for urinary infection. Pediatr Infect Dis 1985;4:656–663.

Rickwood AMK, Carty HM, McKendrick T, et al. Current imaging of childhood urinary infections: Prospective survey. Br Med J 1992;304:663–665.

28 Proteinuria

STARTED 29/3

Robert J. Cunningham III

An approach to the pediatric patient with proteinuria requires a consideration of age, sex, the presence of edema, the presence of hypertension, and a measure of renal function. In many cases, the diagnostic work-up is brief, and it is unusual for a pediatric patient to require a renal biopsy as part of the initial evaluation. Proteinuria may be an inconsequential finding or a manifestation of a more serious disease (Table 28–1). Because many patients with proteinuria often present with edema with or without other nonrenal symptoms, the physician should be familiar with the differential diagnosis of other edematous conditions (Table 28–2).

The definition of significant proteinuria is noted in Table 28–3.

Nephrotic syndrome is a constellation of manifestations and includes proteinuria (Table 28–3), hypoalbuminemia, edema (with or without ascites), and hyperlipidemia (lipiduria). Hyperlipidemia results from the liver's attempt to enhance its production of proteins (including albumin and lipoproteins) to correct the hypoalbuminemia secondary to the large renal losses of albumin and, at times, other larger proteins. Nephrotic syndrome may be a result of many primary etiologic factors, with varying renal pathology and long-term consequences. Most cases of nephrotic syndrome in children are due to *minimal change nephrotic syndrome*, defined as normal histology of the kidney by light microscopy and immune stains.

Table 28–1. Classification of Proteinuria

Nonpathologic Proteinuria
Postural (orthostatic)
Febrile
Exercise

Pathologic Proteinuria
Tubular
Hereditary
Cystinosis
Wilson disease
Lowe syndrome
Proximal renal tubular acidosis
Galactosemia
Acquired
Analgesic abuse
Vitamin D intoxication
Hypokalemia
Antibiotics
Interstitial nephritis
Acute tubular necrosis
Sarcoidosis
Cystic diseases
Homograft rejection
Penicillamine
Heavy metal poisoning (mercury, gold, lead, bismuth, cadmium, chromium, copper)
Glomerular
Persistent asymptomatic
Nephrotic syndrome
Idiopathic nephrotic syndrome
Minimal change
Mesangial proliferation
Focal sclerosis
Glomerulonephritis
Tumors
Drugs
Congenital

From Behrman RE (ed): Nelson Textbook of Pediatrics, 14th ed. Philadelphia: WB Saunders, 1992:1340.

NEPHROTIC SYNDROME IN YOUNG CHILDREN

Minimal Change Disease

Preschool-aged children constitute the most common age group for the presentation of minimal change nephrotic syndrome. Patients often present with asymptomatic edema, which may manifest as swollen or puffy eyes on awakening in the morning from sleep; increasing abdominal girth (increased waist or belt size) from ascites; pedal or leg edema, which causes difficulty in putting on regular-sized shoes; especially after being upright during the daytime, or swelling in other sites, such as the scrotum, penis, vulva, and scalp. Tense edema or ascites may be painful, but it is usually not a primary concern to the patient because it develops gradually and is thus not always painful or tender.

The initial evaluation of a patient with proteinuria is presented in Table 28–4. Indications for a referral to a pediatric nephrologist are described in Table 28–5. If there is obvious edema with proteinuria, the diagnostic evaluation noted in Table 28–4 advances directly to the second phase and, if needed, to the third phase. A biopsy may or may not be indicated, and it is usually avoided until the response to therapy is noted to be poor (Table 28–6).

ETIOLOGY

The evaluation requires that one consider the causes of nephrotic syndrome in early childhood (Table 28–7). These data have been derived from the International Study of Kidney Disease in Children (ISKDC); three diseases constitute 92% of all cases of nephrotic syndrome in childhood:

- Minimal change disease (the most common)
- Focal segmental sclerosis (also called focal glomerular sclerosis), seen in 6.9%
- Membranoproliferative glomerulonephritis (7.5%)

These data were gathered from more than 700 patients with nephrotic syndrome who were older than 1 year of age but younger than age 17. The features of these three common disorders producing nephrotic syndrome are noted in Table 28–8, and they are compared with a common cause of nephrosis in young adults. Nephrotic syndrome in membranous disease may be primary or secondary to other diseases or drugs such as gold, mercury, bismuth, silver, D-penicillamine, trimethadione, probenecid, and captopril.

Systemic diseases also cause childhood nephrotic syndrome but account for 10% of cases. The three foremost considerations are:

Table 28–2. Conditions Leading to Generalized Edema

Diseases of the Kidney
Acute glomerulonephritis
Nephrotic syndrome
Acute renal failure
Chronic renal failure

Heart Failure
Numerous conditions of the heart, pericardium, or lungs leading to low-output congestive heart failure
Noncardiovascular diseases leading to high-output heart failure (e.g., anemia, thyrotoxicosis, beriberi, sepsis)

Diseases of the Liver
Arteriovenous fistulas*
Cirrhosis
Malnutrition (protein)
Obstruction to the great veins
Inferior vena cava
Superior vena cava
Portal vein

Endocrine Disorders
Hypothyroidism
Mineralocorticoid excess

Iatrogenic Causes
Drug administration
Estrogens; oral contraceptives
Antihypertensive agents

Miscellaneous
Hydrops fetalis—immune/nonimmune
Extreme prematurity < 1000 g
Protein-losing enteropathy
Vitamin E deficiency in preterm neonates
Chronic hypokalemia
Chronic anemia (especially myelofibrosis)
Nutritional edema (especially on re-feeding)
Capillary leak syndrome–systemic inflammatory response syndrome

Modified from Baliga R, Lewy JE. Pathogenesis and treatment of edema. Pediatr Clin North Am 1987;34:639–649.
*Usually associated with high-output heart failure.

Table 28–3. Definition of Significant Proteinuria

I. **Qualitative**
   1. 1+ (30 mg/dl) on dipstick examination of 2 out of 3 random urine specimens collected one week apart if urine specific gravity ≤ 1.015
   or
   2. 2+ (100 mg/dl) on similarly collected urine specimens if urine specific gravity ≥ 1.015

II. **Semiquantitative**
   1. Urine protein-to-creatinine ratio (mg/dl:mg/dl) of ≥0.2 on an early morning urine specimen

III, **Quantitative**
   1. *Normal:* ≤4 mg/m²/hour in a timed 12- to 24-hour urine collection
   2. *Abnormal:* 4–40 mg/m²/hour* in a timed 12- to 24-hour urine collection
   3. *Nephrotic range:* ≥40 mg/m²/hour* in a timed 12- to 24-hour urine collection

Modified from Norman ME. An office approach to hematuria and proteinuria. Pediatr Clin North Am 1987;34:545–561.
Example: For a 1 m² child (age 8 years; 60 pounds), abnormal is from 100 to 1000 mg; nephrotic range is greater than 1000 mg.

- Systemic lupus erythematosus
- Anaphylactoid purpura (Henoch-Schönlein purpura)
- Hemolytic-uremic syndrome

These diseases present with other manifestations in addition to the proteinuria and must be considered in any child who presents with systemic illness with significant proteinuria as part of symptom complex.

Minimal change nephrotic syndrome is slightly more common in males than females; the hallmark of this disease is total clearing of the proteinuria with a 1-month course of daily oral prednisone therapy. A common misconception is that neither hematuria nor hypertension is present in children with minimal change disease. As demonstrated in Table 28–8, both hematuria and hypertension may be present in up to 20% of children who were ultimately shown to have minimal change disease. The blood urea nitrogen (BUN) or serum creatinine level may also be elevated in up to 30% of the cases, although an elevation of creatinine beyond 1 to 1.5 mg/dl is rarely seen. Serum complement studies, specifically C3, are invariably normal. Older age, hematuria, hypertension, and

Table 28–4. Work-up of a Child with Proteinuria

I. **Pediatrician's Work-up: Phase I**
   1. Early morning urinalysis to include examination of the sediment
   2. Ambulatory and recumbent urinalyses for dipstick protein

II. **Pediatrician's Work-up Phase II**
   1. Blood electrolytes, BUN, creatinine, serum proteins, cholesterol
   2. ASLO titer, C₃ complement, ANA
   3. Timed 12-hour urine collections, recumbent and ambulatory
   4. Renal ultrasound, IVP, voiding cystourethrogram

III. **Pediatric Nephrologist's Work-up: Phase III**
   1. Renal biopsy
   2. Management of established renal disease

Modified from Norman ME. An office approach to hematuria and proteinuria. Pediatr Clin North Am 1987;34:545–562.
Abbreviations: ANA = antinuclear antibody; ASLO = antistreptolysin O; BUN = blood urea nitrogen; IVP = intravenous pyelogram.

Table 28–5. When to Refer the Child with Proteinuria

Persistent nonorthostatic proteinuria
A family history of glomerulonephritis, chronic renal failure, or kidney transplantation
Systemic complaints such as fever, arthritis or arthralgias, and skin rash
Hypertension, edema, cutaneous vasculitis, or purpura
Coexistent hematuria with or without cellular casts in the spun sediment
An elevated blood urea nitrogen (BUN) and creatinine or unexplained electrolyte abnormalities
Increased parental anxiety

Modified from Norman ME. An office approach to hematuria and proteinuria. Pediatr Clin North Am 1987;34:545–561.

azotemia may occur with minimal change nephrotic syndrome, but the combination of these variables suggests that another etiologic factor may be present.

DIAGNOSIS

Studies that would help confirm that a patient with nephrotic syndrome has minimal change disease include:

- A urinalysis
- A serum C3 level
- A serum cholesterol determination
- A serum albumin level
- BUN
- A serum creatinine level

The urinalysis would be expected to show 3+ to 4+ protein, which correlates to a urine concentration of 300 to 2000 mg/dl. The urine may also test positive for hemoglobin. Microscopic examination of the urine sediment often shows oval fat bodies and/or refractile granular casts, which are seen when there is significant lipiduria. Red blood cells might also be present, but it would be unusual to see red blood cell casts in this clinical situation. Their presence would suggest a diagnosis of post-streptococcal glomerulonephritis or other causes of nephritis (see Chapter 29).

The C3 complement level would be normal in minimal change disease and would be depressed in post-streptococcal glomerulonephritis and some other causes of nephritis (see Chapter 29). If the urine does not demonstrate red blood cells nor test positive for hemoglobin, postinfectious glomerulonephritis is unlikely and C3 determinations are unnecessary.

Table 28–6. When to Consider Renal Biopsy in a Child with Proteinuria

Strong family history of chronic nephritis or unexplained renal failure
Unexplained failure to thrive
Coexistent hypertension and nephrotic syndrome, or evidence of a systemic inflammatory process
Coexistent significant hematuria (≥10 erythrocytes/hpf) with or without erythrocyte casts in the spun sediment
Nephrotic range proteinuria with poor response to prednisone
Renal glomerular insufficiency
Biochemical evidence of renal tubular dysfunction (e.g., renal tubular acidosis, Fanconi syndrome)

Modified from Norman ME. An office approach to hematuria and proteinuria. Pediatr Clin North Am 1987;34:545–561.

Table 28-7. Distribution of Unselected Patients with Nephrotic Syndrome

Histology	No. of Patients (%)	
Minimal change disease	398	(76)
Focal segmental sclerosis	44	(8.6)
Membranoproliferative glomerulonephritis (MPGN)	39	(7.5)
Mesangial proliferation	12	(2.3)
Proliferative glomerulonephritis	12	(2.3)
Membranous nephropathy	8	(1.5)
Chronic glomerulonephritis	3	(0.6)
Unclassified	4	(0.8)
TOTAL	520	100

Adapted from a report of the International Study of Kidney Disease in Children.

The serum cholesterol values are elevated in minimal change nephrotic syndrome and are usually greater than 250 mg/dl. Cholesterol levels in the range of 500 to 600 mg/dl may be common in minimal change nephrotic syndrome, but serum albumin concentrations are invariably less than 2.5 and often less than 2.0 g/dl. Studies that are not of help include complete blood counts and a 24-hour urinary protein determination. A 24-hour urine collection for protein would be redundant, given the obvious clinical edema, the increased serum cholesterol level, and the low serum albumin level. Therapy can be instituted given the information of nephrotic syndrome criteria, and one need not wait for a 24-hour urine collection. Likewise, at this point and given these clinical parameters, a renal biopsy is not indicated because most patients (>90%) with minimal change disease respond to prednisone—a response that may also be considered diagnostic.

TREATMENT

With a presumptive diagnosis of minimal change nephrotic syndrome, it is recommended that patients be placed on a therapeutic course of prednisone, 2 mg/kg per day for 4 weeks, followed by a dose of 1.5 mg/kg given every other morning for another 4 weeks. In most patients, there is total resolution of proteinuria within 21 days of initiating therapy. Patients who do not respond to prednisone therapy should be considered candidates for a renal biopsy (see Table 28–6). There are no data to suggest that more prednisone therapy will increase the response rate. A longer duration of prednisone treatment increases the side effects without concomitant benefit. Therefore, if there is no response, prednisone should be discontinued after the 2-month course and a renal biopsy performed to guide further therapy.

Table 28-8. Summary of Primary Renal Diseases That Present As Idiopathic Nephrotic Syndrome

	Minimal Change Nephrotic Syndrome (MCNS)	Focal Segmental Sclerosis	Membranous Nephropathy	Membranoproliferative Glomerulonephritis (MPGN)	
				Type I	Type II
Frequency*					
Children	75%	10%	<5%	10%	10%
Adults	15%	15%	50%	10%	10%
Clinical Manifestations					
Age (yr)	2–6, some adults	2–10, some adults	40–50	5–15	5–15
Sex	2:1 male	1.3:1 male	2:1 male	Male-female	Male-female
Nephrotic syndrome	100%	90%	80%	60%	60%
Asymptomatic proteinuria	0	10%	20%	40%	40%
Hematuria	10%–20%	60%–80%	60%	80%	80%
Hypertension	10%	20% early	Infrequent	35%	35%
Rate of progression to renal failure	Does not progress	10 years	50% in 10–20 yr	10–20 yr	5–15 yr
Associated conditions	Allergy? Hodgkin's disease, usually none	None	Renal vein thrombosis, cancer, SLE, hepatitis B	None	Partial lipodystrophy
Laboratory Findings	Manifestations of nephrotic syndrome ↑ BUN in 15%–30%	Manifestations of nephrotic sydnrome ↑ BUN in 20%–40%	Manifestations of nephrotic syndrome	Low C1, C4, C3–C9	Normal C1, C4, low C3–C9
Immunogenetics	HLA-B8, B12 (3.5)†	Not established	HLA-DRW3 (12–32)†	Not established	C3 nephritic factor Not established
Renal Pathology					
Light microscopy	Normal	Focal sclerotic lesions	Thickened GBM, spikes	Thickened GBM, proliferation, lobulation	
Immunofluorescence	Negative	IgM, C3 in lesions	Fine granular IgG, C3	Granular IgG, C3	C3 only
Electron microscopy	Foot process fusion	Foot process fusion	Subepithelial deposits	Mesangial and subendothelial deposits	Dense deposits
Response to Steroids	90%	15%–20%	May be slow progression	Not established	Not established

Modified from Couser WG. Glomerular disorders. *In* Wyngaarden JB, Smith LH, Bennett JC (eds). Cecil Textbook of Medicine, 19th ed. Philadelphia: WB Saunders, 1992:560.
*Approximate frequency as a cause of idiopathic nephrotic syndrome. About 10% of adult nephrotic syndrome is due to various diseases that usually present with acute glomerulonephritis.
†Relative risk.
Abbreviations: BUN = blood urea nitrogen; C = complement; GBM = glomerular basement membrane; HLA = human leukocyte antigen; Ig = immunoglobulin; SLE = systemic lupus erythematosus; hepatitis B = hepatitis B virus; ↑ = elevated.

Most patients with nephrotic syndrome respond with total clearing of proteinuria within 10 to 21 days. Total clearing of proteinuria in response to prednisone is an excellent prognostic sign. Very few patients progress to renal failure, although many patients who initially respond to prednisone therapy with total clearing of proteinuria may have relapses and require intermittent prednisone therapy for many years thereafter. Approximately 18% of patients treated with prednisone for minimal change nephrotic syndrome respond to therapy and never relapse.

Patients with recurrent nephrotic syndrome are subgrouped by the ISKDC into *frequent* and *infrequent* relapsers. An infrequent relapser is a patient with fewer than two relapses in any 6-month period; a frequent relapser is a patient with two or more relapses within 6 months. In the treatment of relapses, prednisone should be initiated at a dose of 2 mg/kg/day and continued until the urine tests are negative for protein for 4 consecutive days. Alternate-day prednisone is then given at a dose of 1.5 mg/kg in the morning for another 2 weeks and then discontinued altogether. Relapses are frequent during the influenza virus seasons; any minor upper respiratory infection may trigger a relapse of nephrotic syndrome. Patients who suffer infrequent relapses may be treated safely with prednisone alone. Assuming three relapses a year and clearing of proteinuria in 10 to 12 days after beginning prednisone therapy, a patient would receive approximately 45 days of daily prednisone in a 1-year interval. In addition, the patient would receive 8 weeks of prednisone administered on an alternate-morning schedule. Most patients have few long-term side effects when given this amount of prednisone in this fashion.

The greater problem is the development of frequently relapsing nephrotic syndrome. These patients respond with total clearing of proteinuria after daily prednisone therapy but relapse more frequently than four times a year and may require constant daily prednisone therapy to maintain a remission. Because daily prednisone has significant untoward side effects (growth failure, Cushing facies, osteoporosis, cataracts, infection, hypertension, and glucose intolerance), other therapies need to be considered.

Four strategies are employed in the treatment of patients with frequently relapsing but steroid-responsive minimal change nephrotic syndrome:

- Alternate-day prednisone
- Cyclophosphamide (Cytoxan)
- Chlorambucil
- Cyclosporine

Prednisone

Occasionally, it is possible to maintain the patient in remission on a low dose of alternate-day prednisone therapy. This is well tolerated with minimal toxicity and is the first method employed in an attempt to maintain the patient in remission and avoid the long-term side effects of daily steroids. In many cases, however, patients relapse while receiving alternate-day prednisone therapy, and other therapies need to be considered.

Cyclophosphamide and Chlorambucil

Two immunosuppressive agents used in the treatment of frequently relapsing nephrotic syndrome are Cytoxan and chlorambucil. These drugs are given on a daily basis for approximately 8 weeks. Following the use of either agent, patients have a 70% chance of long-term remission (2½ to 3 years in duration). During this time, patients require no prednisone therapy. Unfortunately, after this time, relapses often recur, and further courses of prednisone therapy are required.

Toxicities of the two drugs differ; the choice of agent is determined by the toxicity profile. Both are equally efficacious in generating long-term remission, and the relapse rate following a 2- to 3-year interval is similar.

Cyclophosphamide. Cytoxan's major toxicities include:

- Hair loss
- Hemorrhagic cystitis
- Leukopenia
- Sterility (particularly in males)
- A possible predisposition to future neoplasia

Hair Loss. Hair loss is the side effect that most often disturbs the patient. It is short-lived, and hair growth returns to normal.

Cystitis. Hemorrhagic cystitis is more dangerous and can be difficult to control. It is not the drug itself but rather a metabolite produced by the liver that is directly toxic to bladder epithelial cells. The resulting irritation may rarely necessitate surgical intervention to control the bleeding. Considering the risk of hemorrhagic cystitis, it is recommended that patients increase their fluid intake by an additional 500 to 1000 ml of fluid each day. This medication should be given in the morning. If a patient forgets to take a morning dose, the medication should not be taken in the evening. The rationale is that following ingestion, the drug is metabolized by the liver and excreted by the kidney. A dose given in the evening may cause the metabolites to remain in contact with the bladder epithelium overnight, which may increase the risk of mucosal bleeding.

Leukopenia. Leukopenia is unusual at the recommended doses; nonetheless, white blood cell counts need to be checked every 2 weeks while patients are receiving the drug.

Sterility. Sterility can be a side effect of Cytoxan therapy. Postpubertal men taking the drug at 2 mg/kg/day have very low sperm counts. Studies of long-term toxicity of Cytoxan therapy have shown that 5 years after completion of the therapeutic course, 20% of men still demonstrate abnormally low sperm counts. Ten years after completion of therapy, 10% still have abnormally low sperm counts, but this percentage approaches that of the normal male population who have not received any chemotherapy. The question as to the effect of Cytoxan therapy on the prepubertal testes has not been studied thoroughly; however, Cytoxan has been used for the treatment of nephrotic syndrome since 1960, and there are multiple reports of patients who have normal fertility and who have fathered children many years after a Cytoxan course. Although this remains a concern that must be discussed with parents, it appears to be more of a theoretical risk than a documented one.

Risk of Neoplasia. The question of neoplasia must be discussed with parents because it has been shown that low-dose Cytoxan therapy given to experimental animals increases the incidence of neoplasia. However, cancer has not been reported in any patient treated with a course of Cytoxan therapy for nephrotic syndrome.

Chlorambucil. The efficacy of chlorambucil parallels that of Cytoxan, but the toxicities differ. There is no evidence that chlorambucil causes hair loss, but leukopenia remains a prominent problem. The white blood cell counts need to be checked every 2 weeks while patients are taking the drug, and the drug should be discontinued if the absolute neutrophil count falls below 1000/mm³. Hemorrhagic cystitis does not occur with chlorambucil. The risk of sterility appears to be similar to that of Cytoxan, although studies have not been as detailed and the follow-up for patients treated with chlorambucil has not been as long as for those treated with Cytoxan.

The one major concern has been reports of lymphoma following chlorambucil treatment of nephrotic syndrome in childhood. Most of the children were treated in France, and the doses of chlorambucil were higher than those given today. Patients who developed lymphoma had received a total dose of chlorambucil of greater than 14 mg/kg. Current guidelines would keep the total chlorambucil dose between 8 and 10 mg/kg. Cancer has not been reported when this drug is given in accordance with these recommendations.

Cyclosporine

A fourth approach to the treatment of frequently relapsing nephrotic syndrome is the use of cyclosporine. Cyclosporine is an immunosuppressive agent developed to prevent solid organ transplant rejection, but it is clear that patients with nephrotic syndrome who respond to prednisone therapy also respond to cyclosporine. For the patient who has frequent relapses of nephrotic syndrome and who has significant steroid toxicity, cyclosporine offers another choice of therapy. Patients require treatment with 5 to 7 mg/kg/day given in divided doses on a 12-hour schedule.

The toxicity of cyclosporine differs from that of prednisone; many children tolerate cyclosporine therapy for years with minimal toxicity. The major side effects of cyclosporine are nephrotoxicity, hypertension, hirsutism, and tremor, which is bothersome both to patients and families. Therefore, the blood pressure and renal function (creatinine, BUN) need to be monitored.

COMPLICATIONS

Even in patients with the frequently relapsing variant of minimal change disease, the incidence of renal failure is only 1%. The reported mortality rate remains higher, at approximately 5%.

Infection

The major cause of death is overwhelming infection, usually secondary to spontaneous bacterial peritonitis, which develops in as many as 10% of patients with nephrotic syndrome at some point in the course of illness. The highest frequency appears when patients are edematous with significant ascites. Peritoneal fluid interferes with macrophage function, whereas ascitic fluid may dilute local complement or immunoglobulin levels altering host defense mechanisms in the peritoneum.

The most common pathogen is *Streptococcus pneumoniae*. *Escherichia coli* and *Staphylococcus aureus* are other etiologic agents that may cause spontaneous peritonitis in patients with minimal change disease. Prior to 1940, the mortality of nephrotic syndrome was approximately 60%. With the use of antibiotics, mortality dropped rapidly to 10% to 15% because penicillin offered an effective treatment for peritonitis. Infections remain the major cause of mortality, and any child with nephrotic syndrome in relapse with evidence of ascites needs to be evaluated quickly if either abdominal pain or fever develops. A blood specimen and paracentesis (Gram stain, culture, neutrophil count, glucose and protein level) should be obtained and the patient started on intravenous cefotaxime (ceftriaxone) and an aminoglycoside without further delay.

Thrombosis

A second serious complication of nephrotic syndrome is spontaneous thrombosis, pulmonary embolus, or both. The blood of patients with nephrotic syndrome is hypercoagulable, and there is an increased incidence of thrombotic phenomenon in these children. Children have lost parts of their lower limbs because of arterial thrombosis, and a number of deaths in children with nephrotic syndrome have resulted from pulmonary emboli. The renal vein is another possible site. Use of streptokinase or urokinase has allowed for more effective treatment of thrombotic complications.

Focal Segmental Sclerosis

DIAGNOSIS

Inspection of the clinical criteria outlined in Table 28–8 does not always allow one to differentiate minimal change disease from focal segmental sclerosis before completion of a course of prednisone therapy. Inability to clear proteinuria completely during prednisone therapy may be the first indication of focal segmental sclerosis. Patients who respond to prednisone initially with clearing of proteinuria but who do not respond to a subsequent course of steroids should also be considered to have focal segmental sclerosis. This figure represents about 7% of those patients who have an initial response to prednisone therapy. A patient who does not respond to prednisone with total clearing of proteinuria should undergo renal biopsy. Focal segmental sclerosis may be primary or secondary to reflux nephropathy, sickle cell nephropathy, reduced renal mass (single kidney), opiate or analgesic abuse, chronic bacteremia (endocarditis), renal transplant rejection, or nephropathy resulting from human immunodeficiency virus (HIV) infection.

TREATMENT

Treatment of focal segmental sclerosis has usually been uniformly poor. Patients have severe and unremitting proteinuria despite treatment with prednisone, chlorambucil, or cyclophosphamide. None of these agents is warranted for treatment of a child once the diagnosis of focal segmental sclerosis is established. The long-term outcome for these patients has been poor; 33% are in renal failure approximately 10 years following diagnosis, and nearly 100% are in renal failure 20 years following diagnosis.

Patients with focal segmental sclerosis present two difficult problems. First, renal function may be maintained reasonably well for years, but massive proteinuria persists. Hence, patients are often edematous for months or years, and stigmata of protein malnutrition may also develop as a result of large protein losses. Symptomatic therapy with a low-sodium diet and judicious use of diuretics is sometimes effective. Dietary manipulation of protein intake is ineffective, even though increasing dietary protein intake is accompanied by a concomitant increase in urinary protein excretion. There is no evidence that protein restriction modifies either serum proteins or prevents progression to renal insufficiency.

The second problem occurs when affected patients progress to end-stage renal failure. Recurrence of the disease in transplanted kidneys occurs 25% to 30% of the time. Therefore, many patients undergo a long period of dialysis prior to receiving a kidney transplant in an effort to diminish the frequency of recurrent disease.

It is now evident that some patients respond to cyclosporine with total clearing of their proteinuria. Early reports indicate that there may be no progression to renal insufficiency. Nonetheless, data are sparse, and it is unknown what percentage of patients with focal segmental sclerosis will respond to cyclosporine; however, a preliminary analysis suggests that between 25% and 60% will respond initially. The new long-term outcome is unknown.

MEMBRANOPROLIFERATIVE GLOMERULONEPHRITIS

Major diagnostic considerations in patients with hypertension, hematuria, older age, and mild to moderate edema should be membranoproliferative glomerulonephritis (MPGN) and systemic lupus erythematosus (SLE) (see Table 28–8). Both diseases are more common in girls and are seen as the girls reach adolescence. There may be proteinuria or nephrotic syndrome accompanying hematuria. In both diseases, cholesterol levels may be normal or minimally elevated in the presence of proteinuria and hypoproteinemia; serum C3 is often reduced. The major laboratory feature that points to SLE is the presence of anti-DNA antibodies (particularly anti–double-stranded DNA). In addition, MPGN is a renal disease without multisystem involvement whereas SLE affects other organ systems (skin, joints, mucous membranes, bone marrow, serous surfaces, heart, lung, and brain).

It is important to identify the patient with possible MPGN because daily prednisone therapy is contraindicated for these individuals; in a number of cases, malignant hypertension has developed following its use. Therefore, if MPGN is suspected, a renal biopsy is indicated before therapy is initiated.

The older patient is a more likely candidate for renal biopsy. Although 80% of the patients with minimal change disease are younger than age 6, MPGN and focal segmental sclerosis increase in frequency with aging. An analysis of ISKDC data shows that at age 6 years, only 6% of the renal biopsies show lesions other than minimal change disease. At age 10 years, the probability of other lesions increases to 28%.

The treatment of MPGN includes low-dose, alternate-day prednisone, the antiplatelet agents dipyridamole (Persantine) and aspirin, and angiotensin-converting enzyme (ACE) inhibitors, which may reduce glomerular hyperfiltration and thus improve proteinuria. Few studies have confirmed the efficacy of any therapy. Few patients progress to renal failure within 5 years, but a large percentage progress slowly and renal insufficiency develops over 10 to 20 years.

NEPHROTIC SYNDROME IN INFANTS

The single group of children for whom the traditional discussion of nephrotic syndrome does not apply is that of infants younger than age 1 year. Nephrotic syndrome that presents very early in life is a much more serious entity, and the prognosis is guarded. In general, the outlook is poorest in younger infants (<6 months of age) and improves as the age at presentation approaches 1 year. Minimal change disease is rarely seen in infants younger than 6 months of age. It begins to appear in infants who present at 6 to 8 months. By 1 year, it is the most common cause of nephrotic syndrome.

The conditions that result in nephrotic syndrome in infants differ markedly from those seen in older children. Secondary causes are more prominent and need to be considered particularly in the newborn or very young infant (Table 28–9).

Table 28–9. Causes of Nephrotic Syndrome in Infants Younger Than 1 Year of Age

I. **Secondary Causes**
  A. Infections
    1. Syphilis
    2. Cytomegalovirus
    3. Toxoplasmosis
    4. Rubella
    5. Hepatitis B
    6. Human immunodeficiency virus
    7. Malaria
  B. Drug reactions
  C. Toxins
    1. Mercury
  D. Systemic lupus erythematosus
  E. Syndromes with associated renal disease
    1. Nail patella syndrome
    2. Lowe syndrome
    3. Nephropathy associated with congenital brain malformation
    4. Drash syndrome-Wilms tumor
    5. Hemolytic uremic syndrome
    6. Renal vein thrombosis

II. **Primary Causes**
  A. Congenital nephrotic syndrome
    1. Finnish type
    2. Non-Finnish type
  B. Diffuse mesangial sclerosis
    1. Minimal change disease
    2. Focal segmental sclerosis
    3. Membranous nephropathy

Adapted from Mauch TJ, Vernier RL, Burk BA, et al. Nephrotic syndrome in the first year of life. *In* Holiday MA, Barratt TM, Avner ED, et al (eds). Pediatric Nephrology. Baltimore: Williams & Wilkins, 1994:791.

It is particularly important to test for syphilis because early institution of penicillin therapy may lead to resolution of the renal disease and may mitigate the involvement of other organ symptoms as well. Congenital toxoplasmosis is also treatable with combination of steroids and pyrimethamine–sulfadiazine–folinic acid. Other congenital infections offer less opportunity for treatment to influence outcome; extrarenal manifestations of these infections are much more serious than the kidney disease.

Primary renal disease causing nephrotic syndrome in early infancy is most often due to either congenital nephrotic syndrome or to diffuse mesangial sclerosis. In both diseases, prognosis for survival is poor unless aggressive supportive therapy and kidney transplantation are undertaken.

Congenital Nephrotic Syndrome

Congenital nephrotic syndrome is divided into the Finnish type and the non-Finnish type. The genetic inheritance of the Finnish type is autosomal recessive, with an estimated incidence of 1 to 2/10,000 births in Finland. In the United States, these patients tend to cluster in areas with populations of Finnish ancestry (e.g., Minnesota). A number of familial cases have been reported in Europe and North America where there is no history of Finnish ancestry. The genetics of these ''sporadic'' cases have not been defined.

Infants with Finnish-type congenital nephrotic syndrome are often premature, with a low birth weight, placentomegaly, increased amniotic fluid alpha-fetoprotein levels, and hypogammaglobulinemia (decreased IgG). There is a male-to-female ratio of 1:1.

The clinical course of both types of congenital nephrotic syndrome is similar, and the outlook is poor. In more than 50% of the patients, proteinuria develops and there is evidence of ascites and edema within the first 2 weeks of life. Patients do not respond to steroid or cytotoxic therapy. Complications are the rule, and frequent bacterial infections occur in more than 85%. Most children die of infectious complications before age 2 years.

Advances in care with a more aggressive approach to these patients has improved survival. Because of the massive proteinuria, patients fail to thrive; they require nasogastric feeding with a high-calorie, high-protein formula. Nephrectomy and peritoneal dialysis are often necessary to control protein losses and allow for adequate growth and control of uremia so that the infant can reach a size and nutritional state sufficient for renal transplantation.

Diffuse Mesangial Sclerosis

Diffuse mesangial sclerosis is the other diagnostic entity seen in infants. This disease is similar to congenital nephrotic syndrome, but it often appears in later infancy and results in less severe protein losses. Patients are often full term and of normal birth weight. The amnionic fluid alpha-fetoprotein is normal, and onset of edema (1 week to 33 months) is later compared with the Finnish type (birth to 3 months). The patients have hypertension, hematuria, and renal insufficiency at presentation. When diffuse mesangial sclerosis is seen in association with a female phenotype, chromosome typing is recommended to look for patients with Drash syndrome (XY gonadal dysgenesis, nephropathy, and Wilms tumor). When this syndrome is present, bilateral nephrectomy and gonadectomy are recommended because the potential for malignancy is very high.

Treatment, as in patients with congenital nephrotic syndrome, consists of renal transplantation. This is curative; neither disease recurs in transplanted kidneys. The major problem is to help these infants achieve the growth and good nutrition necessary for a successful renal transplant.

ASYMPTOMATIC PROTEINURIA DISORDERS

Many patients have proteinuria, but there is no edema, the blood pressure is normal, and serum protein levels are normal. The extent of the work-up must be tailored to the seriousness of the problem (see Tables 28–1, 28–3, and 28–4). Whether or not an evaluation should be performed depends on whether the proteinuria is both persistent and non-orthostatic. The proteinuria that appears in two of four urinalyses is not significant, and the patient would be labeled as having transient proteinuria. Multiple studies have shown that there is no renal pathology in patients who occasionally have proteinuria but at other times have a urine free of protein.

The more common situation is a teenager who demonstrates orthostatic proteinuria. Some patients have protein in their urine when they are standing or sitting but have no protein in their urine when they are recumbent. The simplest way of evaluating the presence of protein is to obtain a first morning urine specimen and compare it with specimens obtained later in the day. The first morning urine specimen is often free of protein, and subsequent urinalysis during the day demonstrates increasing levels of protein. Numerous studies show that individuals who have proteinuria in the upright position only do not have serious pathology. There is no increased incidence of renal disease or hypertension in later life. It is critical to determine that the proteinuria is both persistent and orthostatic before any further evaluation is pursued. Protein should be present in three consecutive urinalyses before one initiates an evaluation for isolated proteinuria. The first step in evaluation is to check for orthostatic proteinuria; a protocol is described in Figure 28–1 and Table 28–10. The five urine samples are collected in separate containers, and qualitative analysis can then be done. Typically observed in patients with orthostatic proteinuria is a pattern of positive samples at 9 P.M. and 12 A.M. The urine excreted at midnight was probably filtered at the glomerular level prior to urination at 9 P.M. If the specimen is again positive for protein only when the patient is standing, no further evaluation is necessary.

For a patient with persistent proteinuria that is non-orthostatic, further evaluation depends on the child's age. An overview of the approach to such a patient is outlined in Figure 28–1.

For the child younger than 7 or 8 years of age who has persistent proteinuria, with normal total protein and serum albumin levels, normal complement, and no other signs of renal disease, there are two options.

One option is to observe the patient carefully with repeated urinalyses every 3 to 6 months and to counsel the parents with regard to swelling and/or ascites, which may develop in association with influenza or an upper respiratory infection. If there is evidence of overt nephrotic syndrome with edema, a decrease in serum albumen and increased serum cholesterol, a trial of daily prednisone therapy is indicated. It is good practice to give patients who have persistent proteinuria—but no evidence of edema or nephrotic syndrome—the pneumococcal vaccine because the major morbid complication of nephrotic syndrome that does develop is pneumococcal peritonitis.

The other option involves instituting prednisone therapy to document that proteinuria has disappeared; this confirms the suspicion that the patient has steroid-responsive nephrotic syndrome.

The rationale for withholding prednisone unless symptoms develop is that the natural history of minimal change disease is to remit; this may occur with or without prednisone administration. If the patient has a more serious lesion, symptoms will develop, at which time evaluation and therapy may be undertaken.

In a patient older than age 8 or 9 years, once the presence of persistent and non-orthostatic proteinuria is established, the next step is to quantify the amount of protein in a 24-hour specimen. If urinary protein excretion is greater than 8 mg/kg/day, a renal

---

Table 28–10. **Test for Orthostatic Proteinuria**

1. Have patient void before bedtime 9:00–10:00 P.M. and save specimen in a labeled container. Dipstick urine for protein, and record result.
2. Patient should then go to bed and lie *flat*. At midnight, patient should void into a container (while in bed and remaining flat). Again, put the urine specimen in a container and label it. Dipstick for protein, and record result.
3. Patient should void again at 5:00–6:00 A.M. (remaining in bed and flat). Again, place specimen in labeled container. Dipstick for protein, and record result.
4. Repeat procedure at 7:00–7:30 A.M. (patient still in bed, still lying flat). Record protein result, and place urine in a labeled container.
5. Patient may then rise. Obtain another urine specimen at 9:00–9:30 A.M. The specimen may be obtained in the standing or sitting position. Place the specimen in a labeled container. Urine should be tested for protein and the result recorded. Patients should bring urine sample with them to the next clinic visit (all five specimens in separate containers).

Note: It is difficult and seemingly silly to have to urinate while lying flat in bed. This is, however, a very important part of the test.

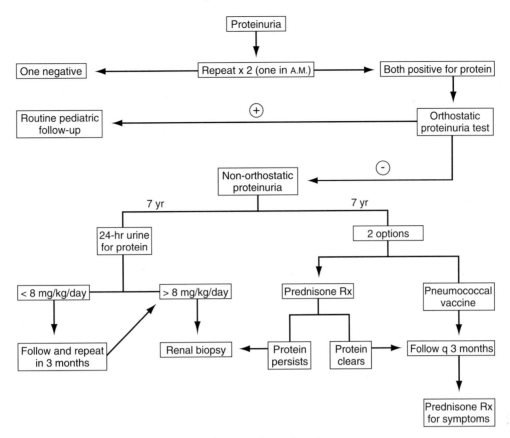

Figure 28–1. Protocol for the evaluation for orthostatic proteinuria.

biopsy is indicated. The choice of 8 mg/kg/day of proteinuria is arbitrary; the ISKDC definition of proteinuria is 8 mg/m²/hour and nephrotic syndrome is defined as 40 mg/m²/hour. Hence, for an average 8-year-old patient who is 30 kg and 1 m², by these definitions proteinuria is a level of 96 mg/day and nephrotic syndrome is a level of 960 mg/day. Renal biopsy is recommended at a level of 240 mg/day of proteinuria. This avoids a biopsy for the patient with minimal proteinuria but does not require full-blown nephrotic syndrome to develop before initiating a definitive work-up. Given the fact that the patient has isolated proteinuria, MPGN or SLE is an unlikely possibility. However, the incidence of focal segmental sclerosis in adolescents is much higher than in the younger child. With the possibility of treatment with cyclosporine and/or angiotensin-converting enzyme inhibitors preventing future renal failure, aggressive evaluation is warranted to identify patients who might benefit from these therapies.

SUMMARY AND RED FLAGS

Asymptomatic proteinuria may be associated with fever, postural mechanisms, and glomerular or tubular dysfunction. Significant proteinuria with edema suggests the nephrotic syndrome, which in most children suggests minimal change nephrotic syndrome. An age less than 1 year or more than 10 years plus hematuria, azotemia, and hypertension are red flags that suggest a cause of nephrosis other than the more benign minimal change disease. Additional red flags include a poor response to prednisone therapy and signs of multiple organ system involvement by a primary systemic disease, such as SLE. Fever and abdominal pain in a patient with nephrotic syndrome should suggest spontaneous primary peritonitis.

REFERENCES

A report of the International Study of Kidney Disease in Children. Nephrotic syndrome in children: Prediction of histopathology from clinical and laboratory characteristics at time of diagnosis. Kidney Int 1978;13:159.

A report of the International Study of Kidney Disease in Children. The primary nephrotic syndrome in children: Identifying of patient with minimal change nephrotic syndrome from initial response to prednisone. J Pediatr 1981;98:561.

A report of the Southwest Pediatric Nephrology Study Groups. Focal segmental glomerulosclerosis in children with idiopathic nephrotic syndrome. Kidney Int 1985;27:442.

Antero M, Brova C, Amend W, et al. Recurrent focal glomerulosclerosis: Natural history and response to therapy. Am J Med 1992;92:375.

Ford DM, Briscoe DM, Shanleg PF, et al. Childhood membranoproliferative glomerulonephritis type I: Limited steroid therapy. Kidney Int 1992;41:1606.

Gorensek MJ, Lebel MH, Nelson JD. Peritonitis in children with nephrotic syndrome. Pediatrics 1988;81:849.

Ingulli E, Tejani A. Incidence, treatment, and outcome of recurrent focal segmental glomerulosclerosis postransplantation in 42 allografts in children—a single-center experience. Transplantation 1991;51:401.

Mauch TJ, Vernier RL, Burk BA, et al. Nephrotic syndrome in the first year of life. *In* Holliday MA, Barratt TM, Avner ED, et al (eds). Pediatric Nephrology. Baltimore: Williams & Wilkins, 1994:788.

Rytand DA, Spreiter S. Prognosis in postural (orthostatic) proteinuria. N Engl J Med 1981;305:618.

Senggutuvan P, Cameron JS, Hartley RB, et al. Recurrence of focal segmental glomerulosclerosis in transplanted kidneys: A analysis of incidence and risk factors in 59 allografts. Pediatr Nephrol 1990;4:21.

Trompeter RS, Lloyd BW, Hicko J, et al. Long-term outcome for children with minimal change nephrotic syndrome. Lancet 1985;1:368.

Vehaskari VM, Rapola J. Isolated proteinuria: Analysis of a school-age population. J Pediatr 1982;101:661.

West CD, McAdams AJ, McConville JM, et al. Hypocomplementemic and normocomplementemic persistent (chronic) glomerulonephritis: Clinical and pathologic characteristics. J Pediatr 1965;67:1089.

Yashikawa N, Kitagawa K, Ohta K, et al. Asymptomatic constant isolated proteinuria in children. J Pediatr 1991;119:375.

Yoshikawa N, Ito H, Akamatsu R, et al. Focal segmental glomerulosclerosis with and without nephrotic syndrome in children. J Pediatr 1986;109:65–70.

29 Hematuria

Ben H. Brouhard

Hematuria is a common urinary complaint in childhood. The presence of blood in the urine by itself rarely indicates a serious or an immediate life-threatening illness. Because of this, screening for asymptomatic hematuria, or the aggressive evaluation of hematuria in general, may be overly de-emphasized. Conversely, the anxiety provoked by blood in the child's urine may cause physicians to perform extensive and costly evaluations.

INITIAL APPROACH TO HEMATURIA

Some general guidelines can be listed for all cases of hematuria, regardless of whether it is gross or microscopic, symptomatic, or asymptomatic. Historically, it is important to inquire about the results of previous urinalyses and the presence or absence of any abnormalities of the urine that might have been present (proteinuria, leukocyturia). Such determinations may help to pinpoint the time of onset of the hematuria. For children with gross hematuria, the number of episodes, how long they last, and the circumstances surrounding the episodes may provide clues to the diagnosis. It is also important to inquire about the presence or absence of hypertension as well as the family history regarding renal abnormalities, hematuria, deafness, renal failure, transplantation, and hypertension.

The physical examination may be unrevealing in patients with renal disease. The initial evaluation must include the urinalysis: "the physical examination of the kidneys." The color of the urine should be noted. A reagent strip may reveal the presence of proteinuria and may also suggest the presence of blood and leukocytes. The heme-positive reagent strip must be confirmed by microscopic examination for the presence of red blood cells. Other elements to be particularly noted by microscopic examination are white blood cells, casts, and crystals (see Fig. 27–2).

Hematuria is categorized as (1) gross hematuria (blood in the urine visible to the naked eye) and (2) microscopic hematuria (red blood cells found only by microscopic examination of the urine). It is also useful to separate gross hematuria into the categories of symptomatic and asymptomatic. Another useful point is to consider whether the blood is originating from the kidney or the lower urinary tract. These four broad categories can be used as points of differentiation, and they provide a framework for the evaluation and the differential diagnosis. There may be overlap in the signs and symptoms of upper versus lower tract bleeding. For example, acute postinfectious nephritis can have manifestations of asymp-tomatic microscopic hematuria with or without proteinuria; it can also present with gross hematuria with nephrotic syndrome range proteinuria (see Chapter 28).

Regardless of whether the blood is gross or microscopic, it must be determined that red blood cells are present in the urine. Certainly, red or brown urine does not always indicate gross hematuria. Table 29–1 indicates causes of colored urine that may be mistaken for gross hematuria. Pink stains in the diapers of infants can often be mistaken for blood; these stains represent urate crystals, which disappear from the urine when acid is added.

Even the reagent strip may not accurately reflect the presence of red blood cells in the urine. The reagent strip, which is impregnated with orthotolidine-peroxide and enhanced with 6-methoxyquino-

Table 29–1. Conditions Other Than Gross Hematuria That Cause Colored Urine

Pink, Red, Coke-Colored, Burgundy	
Disease-associated; multiple causes	
Gross hematuria	Myoglobinuria
Hemoglobinuria	Porphyrinuria
Associated with drug/food ingestion	
Aminopyrine	Nitrofurantoin
Anthrocyanin	Phenazopyridine
Azo dyes	Phenolphthalein
Beets	Pyridium
Blackberries	Red food color
Chloroquine	Rifampin
Deferoxamine mesylate	Rhodamine B
Ibuprofen	Sulfasalazine
Methyldopa	Urates
Dark Brown, Black	
Disease-associated	
Alkaptonuria	Methemoglobinemia
Homogentisic aciduria	Tyrosinosis
Melanin	
Associated with food/drug ingestion	
Alanine	Resorcinol
Cascara	Thymol

From Travis LB, Brouhard BH, Kalia A. An approach to the child with hematuria. *In* Cornfeld D, Silverman B (eds). Dialogues in Pediatric Management. East Norwalk, Conn: Appleton-Century-Crofts, 1985.

lone, turns blue in the presence of hemoglobin or myoglobin (Table 29–2; see also Fig. 27–2). False-negative results for hemoglobin are unusual but have been reported in the presence of high concentrations of ascorbic acid. False-positive results are also unusual but can occasionally occur in urine infected with bacteria that produces bacterial peroxidase. With a positive reagent strip result, it is important to determine whether there are red blood cells in the urine or whether this result may represent free hemoglobin or myoglobin, indicating another disease process and not necessarily disease of the urinary tract. Hemoglobinuria occurs in the setting of brisk hemolysis (often caused by glucose-6-phosphate dehydrogenase deficiency or autoimmune hemolysis), and may be associated with pallor, tachycardia, dyspnea, and reduced exercise tolerance (see Chapter 49). Myoglobinuria frequently follows rhabdomyolysis secondary to viral myositis (influenza, enterovirus) in the setting of tender muscles and weakness. Rhabdomyolysis may also occur in patients with inborn errors of metabolism affecting the muscle and is often noted in these patients after exercise. Both hemoglobin and myoglobin may produce renal tubular injury and thus produce elevated serum blood urea nitrogen and creatinine levels, giving the false impression of primary renal disease. Forced diuresis is indicated in hemoglobinuria and myoglobinuria.

When red blood cells are present, a positive reagent strip result correlates with approximately more than two to five red blood cells per high-power field (hpf) on a fresh centrifuged urine. A result of greater than five red blood cells/hpf in a centrifuged urine is abnormal. Quantitatively, the normal red blood cell excretion has been determined to range from 30,362 to 163,200 per 24 hours, with an upper limit of 240,000 per 24 hours. Although precise values differ, repeated urinalyses yielding greater than five blood cells/hpf and a positive reagent strip result document the presence of abnormal hematuria.

UPPER VERSUS LOWER TRACT BLEEDING

Once the presence of red blood cells is documented, the differential diagnosis is simplified if the abnormality can be categorized

Table 29–2. Hemoglobinuria Without Hematuria

Disease States
Hemolytic anemias—all types
Hemolytic-uremic syndrome
Septicemia
Paroxysmal nocturnal hemoglobinuria

Drugs/Chemicals
Aspidium
Betanaphthol
Carolic acid
Carbon monoxide
Chloroform
Fava beans
Mushrooms
Naphthalene
Pamaquine
Phenylhydrazine
Potassium chlorate
Quinine
Snake venom (and occasionally spider venom)
Sulfonamide

Miscellaneous
Cardiopulmonary bypass
Drowning (freshwater)
Mismatched blood transfusions

From Travis B, Brouhard BH, Kalia A. An approach to the child with hematuria. *In* Cornfeld D, Silverman B (eds). Dialogues in Pediatric Management. East Norwalk, Conn: Appleton-Century-Crofts, 1985.

into upper or lower tract bleeding. The color of the urine should be noted, with brown, smokey, or tea-colored urine indicating blood coming from the upper urinary tract as a result of the acid urine's changing the hemoglobin to hematin, producing a brown color. It is also important to determine whether protein is in the urine samples. The presence of protein may localize the origin of the blood to the glomerulus. Grossly bloody urine coming from the lower urinary tract rarely contains significant amounts of protein. If the blood is bright red, the blood is more likely to be originating from the lower urinary tract. Blood noted at the beginning or end of the stream also indicates lower tract bleeding, whereas blood throughout the stream may suggest the upper tract as the source of the hematuria. The presence of clots points to the lower urinary tract as the source of the blood. When the child presents with isolated microscopic hematuria, a determination of the source of the blood may not be possible.

Another method used to localize the bleeding is determination of the red blood cell morphology. Dysmorphic cells indicate disruption of cell membrane integrity after passing through the glomerular basement membrane, whereas isomorphic cells indicate an origin below the glomerulus. These studies are performed with a phase-contrast microscope. The distinction between dysmorphic and isomorphic red cells has a great deal of overlap; it has been proposed that for a diagnosis of upper tract bleeding, at least 75% of the cells should be dysmorphic, whereas for a diagnosis of lower tract hematuria, no more then 17% should be dysmorphic. Other methods that have been proposed include measurement of mean corpuscular volume of the urinary red cells or use of the red blood cell distribution width, which would be abnormally high in upper tract bleeding.

GROSS HEMATURIA

Symptomatic Hematuria

In the patient with the chief complaint of gross hematuria, it is useful to consider whether the patient is symptomatic or asymptomatic. Symptoms can be divided into two groups: those that originate from the kidney itself and those that are associated with systemic illnesses that affect the kidney secondarily (Table 29–3).

Symptoms arising from the kidney that are associated with gross hematuria are those of stone disease (hypercalciuria with or without an overt stone) and those of urinary tract infection. *Nephrolithiasis* can occur at any age and may cause the symptoms of renal colic, manifested as intense, episodic flank pain often radiating to the groin. In young infants, such pain may be manifested as generalized irritability or abdominal pain. The episode of hematuria, which has been reported in 28% of patients with nephrolithiasis, may begin abruptly without a previous history of hematuria. The physical examination may be unrevealing; the urinalysis may contain crystals, in addition to red blood cells. Family history may also suggest the diagnosis because up to 70% of children with hypercalciuria have a family history of stone disease. The past medical history of furosemide administration to premature neonates, especially those with bronchopulmonary dysplasia, may suggest nephrocalcinosis with gross hematuria. Findings of nephrocalcinosis and nephrolithiasis have been reported when the dose of furosemide of 2 mg/kg/day was given for at least 2 weeks. If stone disease is suspected, a radiographic procedure, such as intravenous pyelography or renal and bladder ultrasonography, should be performed. Ultrasonography is more sensitive (84%) than kidney, ureter, and bladder (KUB) radiography (54%) in detecting calculi. If the presence of a calculi is confirmed, a 24-hour urine collection for calcium, urate, citrate, oxalate, cysteine, and creatinine should be obtained. Patients with nephrolithiasis may have decreased excretion of citrate, thus pro-

Table 29–3. Differential Diagnosis of Symptomatic and Asymptomatic Hematuria

Confirm the presence of red blood cells

Symptomatic
  Renal symptoms
  Urinary tract infections
  Nephrolithiasis
  Urethrorrhagia
  Systemic symptoms
  Henoch-Schönlein purpura
  Tuberous sclerosis

Asymptomatic
  Cystic disease
  Obstruction
  Vascular
  Arteriovenous malformation
  Thrombosis
  Trauma
  Tumor
  Hemoglobinopathies
  Coagulopathies
  Exercise-induced
  Benign familial hematuria (thin
    basement membrane)
  Glomerulonephritis
  Acute, postinfectious
  IgA nephropathy
  Henoch-Schönlein purpura

moting the crystallization of calcium salts. The determination of creatinine excretion is important to ensure that an adequate collection has been obtained (10 to 15 mg/kg/24 hours). Furthermore, hypercalciuria (defined as urinary calcium levels of 4 mg/kg/day) without an overt stone can manifest as gross hematuria with abdominal or flank pain. Indeed, 2.0% to 9.1% of normal children have been reported to have hypercalciuria, and 1.8% have hyperuricosuria. Hypercalciuria can be idiopathic or secondary to another disease, such as renal tubular acidosis (Table 29–4). Hypercalciuria is a frequent cause of hematuria and may represent a risk of future nephrolithiasis. Therapy depends on the cause of the hypercalciuria or the type of stone present.

Urinary tract infection is a common cause of symptomatic, gross hematuria (see Chapter 27). In this circumstance, the infection is usually confined to the bladder; the blood is bright red rather than brown and may contain clots. As many as 25% of children presenting with gross hematuria have a documented symptomatic urinary tract infection; an additional 35% will have a suspected but unproven infection. The urine culture is the *sine qua non* for a diagnosis of urinary tract infection. Symptoms and gross hematuria do not constitute evidence for a diagnosis of urinary tract infection.

Symptoms of *urethritis* with gross hematuria in males suggest *urethrorrhagia*. The symptoms are those of urethritis, but cultures are negative. The most common complaint is blood-stained underwear. The symptoms tend to occur at intervals several months apart and may persist for up to 10 years. Cystoscopy does not show a treatable lesion and may be contraindicated because of the possibility of producing a stricture. Low-dose, long-term antibiotic treatment may help in some cases. The condition appears to be benign and self-limited; reassurance is the treatment of choice.

Gross hematuria with systemic symptoms may be indicative of a generalized process in which the kidney is involved. The triad of abdominal pain, joint pain, and lower extremity purpuric rash with gross hematuria (with or without proteinuria) suggests *anaphylactoid purpura*, also known as *Henoch-Schönlein purpura* (HSP).

HSP affects children between the ages of 3 and 10 years, and males are more often affected than females. In 60% of cases, an upper respiratory tract infection precedes the onset of the disease by 1 to 3 weeks. There is a seasonal variation, with a peak around November to January in the northern hemisphere. The rash is an acute symmetric erythematous maculopapular rash that characteristically starts around the malleoli but extends to the dorsal surface of the legs, the buttocks, and the ulnar side of the arms. These lesions may eventually coalesce into large patches or ecchymoses (palpable purpura) and may persist for up to 2 weeks. Joint pain is present in about 60% to 75% of children with HSP.

The arthralgia or periarticular swelling of HSP affects the knees and ankles most commonly. Abdominal pain, occurring in about 50% of cases, consists of severe colicky abdominal pain with melena or bloody diarrhea; rarely, intussusception may develop. Eighty percent of children have renal involvement, as is revealed by careful inspection of the urine. However, the nephritis, which clinically manifests in only 20% to 30% of patients, occurs after or with the purpura, and rarely precedes it. Between 50% to 70% of children have hematuria with mild or moderate proteinuria. It is not known how many children with HSP have gross hematuria. Usually, the other symptoms cause the child to visit the physician. No pathognomonic laboratory test exists for HSP; 50% of children have elevated serum immunoglobulin A (IgA) concentrations. No specific therapy exists, and 5% to 10% of children go on to have renal failure. These children tend to be more severely affected, with gross hematuria and nephrotic range proteinuria, and show severe lesions on renal biopsy in addition to IgA deposits in the glomerulus.

The presence of epilepsy, developmental delay, and skin manifestations, with an autosomal dominant inheritance pattern suggests *tuberous sclerosis* (see Chapter 58). Hematuria in such patients suggests a diagnosis of renal cysts and/or angiomyolipomas that have bled. The former are uncommon, but latter occur in 50% to 80% of patients with tuberous sclerosis complex. These tumors are

Table 29–4. Causes of Hypercalciuria

  I. *Physiologic Stimuli to Calcium Excretion*
     Sodium excretion
     Acidosis
     Hypophosphatemia

 II. *Increased Filtered Load*
     Hypercalcemia (hyperparathyroidism, dietary, vitamin D
       excess)
     Excess calcium administration

III. *Impaired Renal Tubular Reabsorption of Calcium*
     Loop diuretics
     Selective tubular defects
     Bartter syndrome
     Hereditary hypophosphatemic rickets with hypercalciuria
     Syndrome of hypercalciuria, normocalcemia, growth
       retardation, polyuria, and proteinuria
     Renal tubular acidosis
     Fanconi syndrome

 IV. *Idiopathic Hypercalciuria*
     Absorptive
     Renal leak

  V. *Hypercalciuria of Unknown Cause*
     Medullary sponge kidney
     Diabetes mellitus
     Syndrome associated with total parenteral nutrition

From Milliner DS, Stickler GB. Hypercalcemia, hypercalciuria and renal disease. *In* Edelmann CM (ed). Pediatric Kidney Disease, 2nd ed. Boston: Little, Brown & Co, 1992;1661–1687.

histologically benign and consist of smooth muscle, adipose tissue, and vascular elements. Symptomatic renal tumors are more common in adults. Hematuria, retroperitoneal hemorrhage, and abdominal or flank pain may be present. Ultrasonography suggests the diagnosis, and histology is diagnostic.

Asymptomatic Hematuria

Gross hematuria is often asymptomatic. The presence of brown or smoky urine or significant proteinuria indicates upper tract bleeding, whereas bright red urine or blood denotes lower tract bleeding.

POSTINFECTIOUS NEPHRITIS

Gross hematuria appearing 4 days to 3 weeks after a febrile illness suggests a diagnosis of acute *postinfectious nephritis*. Acute postinfectious glomerulonephritis is the most common cause of acute nephritis. The classic findings are those of hematuria, oliguria, edema, and hypertension. Microscopic hematuria is present in virtually all cases; gross hematuria is present in about 30%. The urine is characteristically described as smoky and coke-colored to tea-colored. The gross hematuria usually disappears in 3 to 5 days, proteinuria disappears in several weeks, and microscopic hematuria resolves in months to 1 year. Group A streptococcal infection is the most well-defined cause of acute nephritis, occurring in 80% of patients with postinfectious nephritis; however, other causes have also been documented, ranging from other bacteria to viruses. The usual age of involvement is school age, and the streptococci usually come from cutaneous infection (impetigo) in the southern states and the pharynx in more northern states.

It is important to document the time of appearance of the hematuria from the infection. It should be between 4 days and 3 weeks; a shorter period of time may suggest IgA nephropathy or exacerbation of a preexisting nephritis. Laboratory confirmation consists of identifying the streptococcal cause and noting the decrease in serum C3 concentration and variable decreases in C4. Determinations of serum creatinine concentration should also be performed because a rapidly progressive decline in renal function can occur. This situation should also suggest additional diseases (the *differential diagnosis* is noted in Tables 29–5 and 29–6).

Differential Diagnosis. Important diseases presenting as an acute proliferative glomerulonephritis include the postinfection nephritis, systemic infections, IgA nephropathy, and HSP. Infectious agents producing post-infectious nephritis other than group A streptococcus have included *Streptococcus viridans, Streptococcus pneumoniae, Staphylococcus aureus, Staphylococcus epidermidis, Corynebacterium* species, *Mycoplasma* species, meningococcus, leptospira, varicella, rubella, cytomegalovirus, Epstein-Barr virus, toxoplasmosis, *Trichinella* species, and *Rickettsia* species. Less common causes of childhood-onset acute proliferative glomerulonephritis include membranoproliferative glomerulonephritis, systemic lupus erythematosus (SLE), familial nephritis, endocarditis, and shunt nephritis; uncommon causes include Wegener granulomatosis and polyarteritis nodosa.

Glomerulonephritis may also be classified by its histologic appearance. In *crescrentic glomerulonephritis,* there is a proliferation in Bowman capsule. This disorder is usually a problem of adolescents who have hypertension, anemia, hypocomplementemia, hematuria (gross in 50% to 80%), proteinuria, and edema. Primary renal diseases include anti–glomerular basement membrane disease, immune complex disease, IgA nephropathy, and membranous and

Table 29–5. Classification of Rapidly Progressive (Crescentic) Glomerulonephritis

Type of RPGN	Frequency
Anti-GBM Antibody–Mediated RPGN	20%
Goodpasture's syndrome	
Idiopathic anti-GBM nephritis	
Membranous nephropathy with crescents	
RPGN-Associated with Granular Immune Deposits	40%
Postinfectious	
Poststreptococcal glomerulonephritis	
Bacterial endocarditis	
''Shunt'' nephritis	
Visceral abscesses, other nonstreptococcal infections	
Noninfectious	
Systemic lupus erythematosus	
Henoch-Schönlein purpura	
Mixed cryoglobulinemia	
Solid tumors	
Primary Renal Disease	
Membranoproliferative glomerulonephritis	
IgA nephropathy	
Idiopathic ''immune complex'' nephritis	
RPGN Without Glomerular Immune Deposits	40%
Vasculitis	
Polyarteritis	
Hypersensitivity vasculitis	
Wegener's granulomatosis	
Idiopathic RPGN	

Modified from Couser WG. Glomerular disorders. *In* Wyngaarden JB, Smith LH, Bennett JC (eds). Cecil Textbook of Medicine, 19th ed. Vol 1. Philadelphia: WB Saunders, 1992:552.

Abbreviations: GBM = glomerular basement membrane; IgA = immunoglobulin A; RPGN = rapidly progressive glomerulonephritis.

membranoproliferative glomerulonephritides. Systemic illnesses producing crescentic glomerulonephritis include postinfectious disease, shunt nephritis (infected ventriculoatrial shunts for hydrocephalus), endocarditis, SLE, HSP, polyarteritis, cryoglobulinemia, and Wegener granulomatosus.

Membranoproliferative glomerulonephritis is categorized into three types:

- Type I manifests as nephritis-nephrosis, hypocomplementemia, subendothelial glomerular deposits, mesangial proliferation, and deposition of immunoglobulins and complement; it is rarely asymptomatic.
- Type II is similar to type I except the deposits are in the lamina densa, the basement membrane demonstrates dense deposits, the mesangial cell proliferation is milder, and only C3 is deposited.
- Type III differs in that asymptomatic hematuria or proteinuria may be present at first, nephritis-nephrosis is unusual at presentation, and deposition of C3 and C5 with few immunoglobulins occurs within the glomerular basement membrane.

Membranoproliferative glomerulonephritis may be secondary to immune complex disease (SLE, HSP, hereditary complement deficiencies, other collagen vascular diseases), infections (bacteremia, human immunodeficiency virus), malignancy (lymphoma), chronic liver disease (hepatitis, cirrhosis, α_1-antitrypsin deficiency), or other lesions (hemolytic-uremic syndrome, sickle cell anemia, partial lipodystrophy, renal graft rejection).

Membranous glomerulopathy involves the glomerular basement

Table 29–6. Summary of Primary Renal Diseases That Present As Acute Glomerulonephritis

Diseases	Poststreptococcal Glomerulonephritis (PSGN)	IgA Nephropathy	Goodpasture's Syndrome	Idiopathic Rapidly Progressive Glomerulonephritis (RPGN)
Clinical manifestations				
Age and sex	All ages, mean 7 yr, 2:1 male	15–35 yr, 2:1 male	15–30 yr, 6:1 male	Mean 58 yr, 2:1 male
Acute nephritic syndrome	90%	50%	90%	90%
Asymptomatic hematuria	Occasionally	50%	Rare	Rare
Nephrotic syndrome	10%–20%	Rare	Rare	10%–20%
Hypertension	70%	30%–50%	Rare	25%
Acute renal failure	50% (transient)	Very rare	50%	60%
Other	Latent period of 1–3 weeks	Follows viral syndromes	Pulmonary hemorrhage; iron-deficiency anemia	None
Laboratory findings	↑ ASO titers (70%) Positive streptozyme (95%) ↓ C3–C9 Normal C1, C4	↑ Serum IgA (50%) IgA in dermal capillaries	Positive anti-GBM antibody	Positive ANCA
Immunogenetics	HLA-B12, D "EN" (9)*	HLA-Bw 35, DR4 (4)*	HLA-DR2 (16)*	None established
Renal pathology				
Light microscopy	Diffuse proliferation	Focal proliferation	Focal → diffuse proliferation with crescents	Crescentic GN
Immunofluorescence	Granular IgG, C3	Diffuse mesangial IgA	Linear IgG, C3	No immune deposits
Electron microscopy	Subepithelial humps	Mesangial deposits	No deposits	No deposits
Prognosis	95% resolve spontaneously 5% RPGN or slowly progressive	Slow progression in 25%–50%	75% stabilize or improve if treated early	75% stabilize or improve if treated early
Treatment	Supportive	None established	Plasma exchange, steroids, cyclophosphamide	Steroid pulse therapy

Modified from Couser WG. Glomerular disorders. *In* Wyngaarden JB, Smith LH, Bennett JC (eds). Cecil Textbook of Medicine, 19th ed. Vol 1. Philadelphia: WB Saunders, 1992:552.
*Relative risk.
Abbreviations: ANCA = antineutrophil cytoplasm antibody; GBM = glomerular basement membrane; GN = glomerulonephritis; Ig = immunoglobulin.

membrane in stages with increasing severity of deposits from scant discrete subepithelial (stage I) to larger, confluent, diffuse, electiondense subepithelial deposits (stage II), to large deposits in an irregularly thickened glomerular basement membrane surrounded by projection spikes of the glomerular basement membrane (stage III), to a thickened glomerular basement membrane with intramembranous deposits and an electron-lucent pattern (stage IV). Membranous glomerulopathy may be idiopathic (primary) or associated with infectious (hepatitis B, congenital syphilis, malaria, filariasis), immune-mediated (SLE, Crohn disease, pemphigus, enteropathy), drug intake (penicillamine), malignancy (neuroblastoma, Wilms tumor, gonadoblastoma), or other diseases (renal transplant graft, Fanconi syndrome, sickle cell anemia, antiglomerular basement membrane–antialveolar basement membrane antibodies, thrombocytopenia with microangiopathic anemia, α_1-antitrypsin deficiency). This disorder rarely manifests with macroscopic hematuria; microscopic hematuria is present in 70%. Renal failure and hypocomplementemia are rare, whereas nephrotic syndrome occurs in 70% (see Chapter 28).

Treatment. Therapy for postinfectious nephritis is symptomatic, with particular attention paid to the hypertension that may be present; the acute morbidity results from hypertensive encephalopathy, congestive heart failure, hypertension, and rarely renal failure. The prognosis of postinfectious nephritis is excellent. The early mortality is 0.5% to 0.8%. The long-term outlook is for complete recovery in 95% of patients. Recurrence due to streptococcal disease has been documented in fewer than 5% of cases. Early treatment of streptococcal disease does not prevent postinfectious nephritis or recurrences (see Chapter 6). However, recurrent hematuria and proteinuria can occur in patients who have a nonspecific upper respiratory febrile illness within 6 weeks of the original episode.

IgA NEPHROPATHY

IgA nephropathy is a common cause of nephropathy that also presents with gross hematuria. The presentation varies from gross hematuria (30%), nephrotic syndrome (6%), acute nephritis (10%), malignant hypertension (8%) to chronic renal failure (6%) and acute renal failure (6%). Although IgA nephropathy is usually asymptomatic, loin pain has been reported in some patients. There is a male predominance, with a peak incidence in late childhood and early adult life. Gross hematuria appears within 48 hours of an upper respiratory tract infection. Between episodes, the urine may be free of blood or may show microscopic hematuria. No pathognomonic laboratory tests exist for IgA nephropathy; however, the serum IgA concentration may be increased during episodes of gross hematuria. The diagnosis can be made with certainty only with renal biopsy when mesangial deposits of IgA are noted, usually in association with the presence of C3 and IgG (see Fig. 29–1). No specific therapy exists for IgA nephropathy; alternate-day steroid therapy may be useful for patients with nephrotic-range proteinuria. The prognosis is not as benign as previously suggested. Thirty percent of adults and 10% of children progress to end-stage renal disease. Recurrence after renal transplantation has been documented.

OTHER CAUSES OF ASYMPTOMATIC HEMATURIA

Asymptomatic gross hematuria occurring after exercise is known as *stress hematuria*. It is characterized by gross hematuria immediately or a few hours after exercise. The episodes are usually of short duration and painless. The blood may be bright red or a darker color. Proteinuria does not occur. No laboratory or radiographic abnormalities exist. An extensive investigation is not warranted. With a decrease in exercise, the hematuria disappears.

Two, less common, familial syndromes can produce asymptomatic gross hematuria: *progressive familial nephritis (Alport syndrome)* and *polycystic kidney disease*. A family history of renal disease, deafness, hematuria, or renal failure suggests a diagnosis of progressive familial nephritis. The first symptoms of hematuria may occur early in life, especially in males. Approximately 72% of children are symptomatic before 6 years of age, and hematuria is the most common sign. The only definitive method of diagnosis is renal biopsy, which shows the characteristic electron microscopic appearance of attenuation, disruption, and lamellation of the glomerular basement membrane. Although no specific therapy exists, genetic counseling is needed. The mode of transmission is unclear; however, the disease is thought to be transmitted by X-linked dominant inheritance.

Some patients with a more common form of familial hematuria demonstrate persistent microscopic and recurrent gross hematuria without deterioration of renal function. This has been called *benign familial hematuria*. Evidence of disease can also be obtained when urinalyses are performed on family members. An autosomal pattern of inheritance has been proposed. Renal biopsy demonstrates normal light and immunofluorescent microscopy with electron micrographs showing attenuation and disruption of the glomerular basement membrane (thin basement membrane disease).

Autosomal dominant polycystic kidney disease, the causative gene for which is located on the short arm of chromosome 16, has been documented in children and infants as early as birth. Gross hematuria may be the first manifestation of this disorder and occurs in 50% of patients; minimal trauma produces hematuria as a result of stretching of the vessels surrounding the cyst. Although the usual presenting manifestations of the disease (hematuria, hypertension, abdominal mass, and uremia in adults) are rarely seen in children, onset in childhood does occur. Adults tend to demonstrate symptoms not seen in children, which include acute and chronic pain (60%), urinary tract infection, and nephrolithiasis (20%). With the use of ultrasonography, it may be more common to detect the disease when the children are asymptomatic. The cysts are bilateral and may involve other organs, the liver most commonly. There are no specific laboratory findings and no specific therapy except genetic counseling.

The mechanism of hematuria in cystic disease may be generalizable to other conditions that produce dilatation of the upper urinary tract. *Hydronephrosis* due to ureteropelvic junction obstruction or vesicoureteral reflux may also result in hematuria when the dilated areas are subjected to even minimal trauma. Occasionally, an isolated cyst could be the cause of the bleeding.

Coagulation abnormalities and *hemoglobinopathies* are rarely found in patients with gross hematuria. Sickle cell disease and sickle cell trait are hemoglobinopathies that cause asymptomatic gross hematuria (see Chapter 49). A combination of low oxygen tension, reduced blood flow, low pH, and high osmolality in the medulla induces sickling and sludging of erythrocytes, resulting in areas of infarction and hemorrhage. The bleeding commonly comes from the left kidney, for unknown reasons. Conventional therapy consists of hydration and rest; recent evidence suggests intravenous desmopressin therapy may also be useful.

Renal tumors are a rare cause of gross hematuria in children. Wilms tumor, the most common pediatric renal malignancy, usually presents as a flank mass found by the parent or physician incidentally (see Chapter 26). Adenocarcinoma is rarely found in children but has been reported in older children and may present as gross hematuria. The diagnosis is suspected radiographically through ultrasonography or computed tomography and is confirmed at the time of surgery.

Bladder tumors are a rare cause of asymptomatic gross hematuria. These can be detected with ultrasonography of the bladder.

Gross hematuria in the neonate (Table 29–7) can originate from thrombotic events associated with an umbilical artery catheter, trauma, hypercoagulable states, or disseminated intravascular coagulation and may be renal venous or arterial thrombosis. Thrombosis can be caused by catastrophic events at the time of delivery, causing trauma or hypotension and decreased perfusion to the kidney. The incidence of renal venous thrombosis ranges from 0.26% to 0.70% of autopsies, with infants younger than 1 year of age accounting for up to 90%. A male predominance (2:1) has been reported. Infants of diabetic mothers are more prone to renal venous thrombosis, possibly as a result of polycythemia, dehydration, trauma, or a hypercoagulable state. Along with hematuria, the physical examination may demonstrate a palpable enlarged kidney on the affected side.

Another group of children that are susceptible to thrombotic events with gross hematuria are children with nephrotic syndrome (associated with a hypercoagulable state). The diagnosis of renal vein thrombosis can be suspected from the patient's history and can be confirmed with a Doppler flow study or an isotope scan. A spectrum of therapies has been advocated, ranging from watchful waiting with careful attention to hemodynamic status, hydration, electrolyte abnormalities, reduction of blood pressure, anticoagula-

Table 29–7. Causes of Hematuria in Neonates and Children

Common	Rare
Neonates	
Thrombosis (renal vein or artery)	Mesoblastic nephroma
Nephrolithiasis (including hypercalciuria)	Factitious
Obstruction	
Reflux	
Cystic disease	
Syphilis (congenital)	
Children	
Glomerulonephritis	Wilms tumor
Postinfectious nephritis	Arteriovenous malformations
Immunoglobulin A nephropathy	Factitious
Henoch-Schönlein purpura	
Systemic lupus erythematosus	
Familial nephritis (Alport syndrome)	
Nephrolithiasis (including hypercalciuria)	
Cystic disease, reflux	
Interstitial nephritis	

tion, and treatment of the underlying abnormality to thrombolytic agents. Nephrectomy, which had been advocated in the past, has been abandoned with the expectation of recovery of renal function without surgery. Follow-up studies have reported that 60% to 80% of patients demonstrate renal atrophy, with 8% to 12% of the total patients developing hypertension.

Bleeding from *arteriovenous malformations* of the kidney can present as asymptomatic gross hematuria. The blood may be bright red as a result of the rapid transit of the blood and urine down the ureter. The blood can be localized to one kidney with cystoscopy; angiography is indicated when the bleeding is so severe that surgery for the malformation would be considered. Hemangiomas of the bladder can also be detected with the use of cystoscopy.

Gross hematuria can also occur from direct injury to the bladder epithelium from *cyclophosphamide*. This problem results from prolonged contact with the toxic metabolites of this drug. Therapy includes increased hydration to ensure adequate urine flow and the use of mesna. The latter drug coats the bladder to prevent contact of the metabolites with the bladder mucosa.

Often the child presents with gross hematuria without history or physical findings that suggest a cause. Laboratory data should then be obtained, including determinations of serum creatinine concentration, complement (low in postinfectious glomerulonephritis, SLE, serum sickness, endocarditis, membranoproliferative glomerulonephritis, hypocomplementemic vasculitis) levels, and urinary calcium to creatinine ratio. The initial radiographic study should be ultrasonography of the entire urinary tract. If all of these results are normal, then cystoscopy should be considered to localize the bleeding to the urethra, bladder, or one or both ureters. If these results are normal or suggest that only one kidney is the source of the bleeding, renal angiography should be considered to detect an arteriovenous malformation. Renal biopsy is seldom indicated for gross hematuria with no other signs or symptoms.

MICROSCOPIC HEMATURIA

Without Proteinuria

In one study, school screening data demonstrated a high prevalence of isolated, often intermittent, asymptomatic microscopic hematuria. The rate varied by sex, age, and definition of hematuria. More girls had microscopic hematuria than boys and fewer children had three of three consecutive positive urines than two of three positive for blood. Half of the children screened had no blood in the urine after the initial positive results of urinalysis. When yearly urinalyses were performed, the disappearance rate of hematuria was 30%. If children have greater than 20 red blood cells/hpf of spun urine, the prevalence of asymptomatic hematuria is much lower than in children with fewer red blood cells/hpf; the likelihood that hematuria persists is higher in the former group. It is imperative that the urinalysis be repeated over the course of 2 to 3 months in patients with isolated asymptomatic microscopic hematuria. Isolated asymptomatic hematuria follows a benign course if the number of red blood cells are few and there is no proteinuria and no hypertension.

If isolated asymptomatic hematuria persists after two to three examinations over 2 to 3 months, then further evaluation is indicated (Table 29–8). The evaluation is similar to that for patients with asymptomatic gross hematuria because those same disease entities can produce microscopic hematuria as well as gross hematuria. It is important to document whether there have been episodes of gross hematuria with persistent microscopic hematuria between episodes, as well as whether there has been a viral or streptococcal illness in the previous several days. Screening of siblings of patients with classic post-streptococcal glomerulonephritis demon-

Table 29–8. Differential Diagnosis of Hematuria with Proteinuria

Proteinuria	No Proteinuria
<40 mg/m²/hr	
Glomerulonephritis	Hypercalciuria
Acute postinfectious	Glomerulonephritis
IgA nephropathy	Acute postinfectious nephritis
Henoch-Schönlein purpura and	IgA nephropathy
other vasculitides	Benign familial hematuria
Hereditary nephritis (Alport)	Factitious
Systemic lupus erythematosus	Juvenile rheumatoid arthritis
Interstitial nephritis	Loin pain/hematuria
	Exercise
	Other vasculitides
	Coagulopathies
	Hemoglobinopathies
≥40 mg/m²/hr; Nephrotic Syndrome	
Minimal lesion	
Focal segmental	
glomerulosclerosis	
Membranoproliferative	
Membranous	

Remember: first confirm the presence of red blood cells.
Abbreviation: IgA = immunoglobulin A.

strated that 30% can have asymptomatic disease. The diagnosis of post-infectious nephritis should be considered even if the usual symptoms are not present.

Other causes of asymptomatic gross hematuria can also present as asymptomatic microscopic hematuria, including HSP, IgA nephropathy, cystic disease, obstructive uropathy, Alport syndrome, benign familial hematuria, and hypercalciuria (see Tables 29–5 to 29–7).

Microscopic hematuria may also be present in children with juvenile rheumatoid arthritis. Juvenile rheumatoid arthritis is the most common type of childhood arthritis and has three types: systemic, polyarthritic, and oligoarthritic (see Chapter 45). The cause is unknown. Renal lesions reported in juvenile rheumatoid arthritis include amyloidosis, glomerulonephritis, necrotizing arteritis, nephritis, urolithiasis, and papillary necrosis. Abnormal urinalysis results can be found in up to 25% of children with polyarticular juvenile rheumatoid arthritis. Hematuria occurs in 8% to 25%; hematuria may also be related to gold therapy or to hypercalciuria.

Loin-pain hematuria syndrome consists of microscopic hematuria (with or without proteinuria) with incapacitating pain. The pain is of such severity that it often leads to narcotic dependency. Nephrectomy with or without autotransplantation is the only treatment. This is an uncommon idiopathic disorder and is a diagnosis of exclusion.

If no cause can be ascertained from the history of the present illness, family history, or physical examination (including urinalyses), the laboratory evaluation should focus on two areas: renal function and renal anatomy. Thus, serum creatinine concentration should be determined as a measure of renal function, and serum complement concentrations could be obtained to document any decreases that would suggest postinfectious nephritis or asymptomatic SLE. A spot urine sample for determination of calcium to creatinine ratio should be performed as a screening test for hypercalciuria. The normal value is less than 0.2.

If all results are normal but the hematuria persists, one may consider factitious hematuria, which is a form of *Münchausen syndrome by proxy* (see Chapter 37). This diagnosis can be confirmed by comparing the red blood cell antigens in the urine to those of the patient. If they are different, factitious hematuria is confirmed.

Renal ultrasonography should be also be performed to define the presence of hydronephrosis, cysts, or tumor (although rare, the latter is a concern to parents). If all results are normal but hematuria persists, renal biopsy may be considered. This test provides a morphologic diagnosis. However, therapy is unlikely to be found for asymptomatic isolated hematuria; most nephrologists would propose close observation with semiannual or annual re-evaluations. If the number of red blood cells increases, the character of the hematuria changes (microscopic to gross), proteinuria appears, hypertension emerges, or serum creatinine concentration increases, then biopsy would be indicated.

Neither cystoscopy nor renal angiography is indicated for children with asymptomatic isolated microscopic hematuria.

With Proteinuria

When the child has blood and protein in the urine, it is important to document the amount of protein. Proteinuria can be determined qualitatively with a dipstick or with sulfosalicylic acid. If the proteinuria is persistent at or above 1+, then quantitation should be undertaken. Proteinuria is defined as a protein level of 4 mg/m²/hour, with nephrotic-range proteinuria being greater than 40 mg/m²/hour. Proteinuria suggests upper tract bleeding. Causes of upper tract bleeding include IgA nephropathy, HSP, and postinfectious nephritis (see Tables 29–5, 29–6, and 29–8 and Chapter 28).

DIFFERENTIAL DIAGNOSIS

Systemic Lupus Erythematosus. A butterfly rash, fever, mouth ulcers, and joint pain suggests a diagnosis of SLE. Cutaneous lesions (butterfly rash, discoid, vasculitis, alopecia, photosensitivity, Raynaud phenomenon) occur in most patients with SLE. Fever occurs in 60% to 70%, weight loss in 30% to 40%, and arthritis (morning stiffness) in 40% to 80% of children. Renal manifestations of SLE occur in over 50% of children. These manifestations range from hematuria (microscopic with some proteinuria), to hypertension, nephrotic syndrome, rapidly progressive glomerulonephritis (see Table 29–5), and acute renal failure. Various glomerular lesions have been associated with SLE, including those of minimal or mesangial disease, focal proliferative nephritis, diffuse proliferative nephritis, and membranous nephritis. Laboratory confirmation rests with the finding of antibodies to DNA, usually with a decrease in serum complement concentration.

The mainstay of therapy of SLE is corticosteroids. Other agents that have been used as adjuncts to this therapy are azathioprine, cyclophosphamide, and nitrogen mustard. The prognosis depends on the renal lesions, the normalization of the complement and a decrease in the antibody titer to DNA. Diffuse proliferative glomerulonephritis is the most severe renal lesion and can lead to end-stage renal failure. Treatment for SLE nephritis includes the usual therapy for SLE, including pulse steroids and renal transplantation.

Previously discussed disease states, such as IgA nephropathy, HSP, and post-infectious nephritis, can also present with hematuria and proteinuria.

Tubulointerstitial Nephritis (TIN). TIN is the term applied to a heterogeneous group of diseases that primarily affect the tubules and interstitial structure of the kidney. Acute TIN is characterized by an abrupt clinical onset with infiltration of the renal interstitium by inflammatory cells. Acute TIN may be an entity unto itself or a part of another process, such as SLE. Tubulointerstitial nephritis has been commonly associated with the use of antibiotics, especially penicillins (methicillin, penicillin) and cephalosporins. Antibiotic-associated TIN is associated with high-dose, long-term antibiotic therapy. The clinical picture is characterized by fever, rash, and eosinophilia, with pyuria, eosinophiluria, hematuria, proteinuria, and nonoliguric renal failure. Hematuria is present in more than 90% of patients with TIN, but casts are rarely seen. With discontinuation of the drug, the presumed hypersensitivity reaction rapidly remits, and renal function returns toward baseline. Other drugs commonly associated with TIN include sulphonamides, rifampin, and tetracyclines. Nonsteroidal agents can produce renal disease both from inhibition of prostaglandin synthesis and by the development of TIN. Diuretics, such as furosemide and the thiazides, have also been incriminated, as have cis-platinum, methyllomustine (CCNU), and lithium. Heavy metals, such as cadmium and lead, can also result in interstitial nephritis. Urate, oxalate, and hypercalcemia also produce interstitial disease.

Miscellaneous Disease. Other systemic diseases that have renal manifestations with hematuria (usually microscopic) and proteinuria are the *systemic vasculitides*. These diseases have characteristic systemic signs and symptoms. Seventy percent to 80% of patients with polyarteritis nodosa demonstrate renal involvement. Other diseases in this category include Wegener granulomatosis, allergic granulomatosis (Churg-Strauss syndrome), Takayasu arteritis, and giant cell arteritis. Patient history and physical examination should help to define the cause of hematuria in these syndromes.

Systemic infections can also affect the kidneys and produce hematuria. *Bacterial endocarditis* can be associated with hematuria and proteinuria; the hematuria may be gross or microscopic. *Shunt nephritis* (ventricular-atrial for hydronephrosis) also characteristically produces hematuria and proteinuria. The renal manifestations of syphilis in infants can manifest as microscopic hematuria.

Nephrotic Syndrome (see Chapter 28). If the proteinuria is of such degree to produce nephrotic syndrome, two categories should be initially considered: secondary and primary. *Secondary* causes of nephrotic syndrome with hematuria as a component can usually be determined by history, physical examination and laboratory evaluation. Such conditions, including HSP, SLE, and occasionally postinfectious nephritis, can present with nephrotic-range proteinuria, as can IgA nephropathy (see Table 29–8).

If the proteinuria is in the nephrotic range (>40 mg/m²/24 hours), then the diagnostic possibilities are those of the idiopathic primary nephrotic syndrome, which have gross or microscopic hematuria (see Table 29–8). The most common cause of primary nephrotic syndrome is minimal lesion syndrome. The pathogenesis of idiopathic nephrotic syndrome and its prognosis are discussed in Chapter 28. It has been estimated that 20% of children with this lesion have microscopic hematuria, and 2% have gross hematuria. Other diagnoses to be considered for a child with nephrotic syndrome and hematuria must include *focal segmental sclerosis,* which has a 50% frequency of hematuria. Because the prognoses of these two histologic lesions with nephrotic syndrome are quite different, the presence of hematuria in the patient with nephrotic syndrome, who responds poorly to therapy, may lead to a renal biopsy. Biopsy is also considered if there is associated hypertension, azotemia, hypocomplementemia, and more often if there is a poor response to steroid therapy (see Chapter 28).

The classic disease causing nephrotic syndrome with gross hematuria, or microscopic hematuria, or both, is that of membranoproliferative glomerulonephritis. The children are usually teenagers; affected patients under 6 years of age are very unusual. Edema, gross hematuria, and hypertension are the predominant symptoms at the time of diagnosis. Laboratory features include an elevated serum creatinine concentration and depressed serum complement concentrations (C3). Treatment is controversial, but alternate low-dose prednisone has been reported to offer some long-term benefit.

Membranous nephropathy is a rare cause of nephrotic syndrome in children. It usually presents with edema and nephrotic syndrome. Microscopic hematuria has been found rarely. Biopsy is the only way to diagnose the disease.

SUMMARY AND RED FLAGS

Blood in the urine can be very concerning to the child, the parents, and the physician. Blood can originate from any place along the urinary tract. Parents are always concerned that hematuria is a manifestation of tumor; this should be addressed initially with reassurance that hematuria as the initial manifestation of a urinary tract tumor is very rare. The history of present illness and the family history as well as associated signs or symptoms can usually direct the appropriate evaluation. If no diagnosis is readily apparent, depending on whether the hematuria is gross or microscopic, further studies may be indicated. Invasive studies, such as cystoscopy, angiography, and renal biopsy, are rarely indicated.

Red flags include absence of red blood cells in the urine (hemoglobinuria-hemolysis, myoglobinuria-rhabdomyolysis), hypertension, azotemia, palpable masses, nephrotic-range proteinuria, hypocomplementemia, and secondary diseases, such as SLE, vasculitis, malignancy, and infections.

REFERENCES

Edelmann CM. Pediatric Kidney Disease, 2nd ed. Boston: Little, Brown & Co, 1992.

Kalalis PP, King LR, Belman AB. Clinical Pediatric Urology, 3rd ed. Philadelphia: WB Saunders, 1992.

Norman ME. An office approach to hematuria and proteinuria. Pediatr Clin North Am 1987;34:545.

Stapleton FB. Isolated hematuria in children. Kidney 1984,17:24.

Travis LB, Brouhard BH, Kalia A. An approach to the child with hematuria and proteinuria. *In* Cornfeld D, Silverman B (eds). Dialogues in Pediatric Management. East Norwalk, Conn: Appleton-Century-Crofts, 1985.

Localization

Oner Q, Ahmed TM, Gesbas N, et al. Identification of the source of hematuria by automated measurement of mean corpuscular volume of urinary red cells. Pediatr Nephrol 1991;5:54.

Pollack C, Pei-Ling L, Gyory AZ, et al. Dysmorphism of urinary red blood cells—value in diagnosis. Kidney Int 1989;36:1045.

Symptomatic Gross Hematuria

DeSanto NG, DiIoria B, Caparsso G, et al. Population based data on urinary excretion of calcium, magnesium, oxalate, phosphate and uric acid in children from Cimilile (southern Italy). Pediatr Nephrol 1992;6:149.

Fivush B. Irritability and dysuria in infants with idiopathic hypercalciuria. Pediatr Nephrol 1990;4:262.

Gearhart JP, Herzberg GZ, Jeffs RA. Childhood urolithiasis: Experiences and advances. Pediatrics 1991;87:445.

Hufnagle KG, Khan SN, Pean D, et al. Renal calcifications: A complication of long-term furosemide therapy in premature infants. Pediatrics 1987;70:360.

Ingelfinger JR, Davis AE, Grupe WE. Frequency and etiology of gross hematuria in a general pediatric setting. Pediatrics 1977;59:557.

Karlowica MG, Katz ME, Adelman RD, et al. Nephrocalcinosis in very low birthweight neonates: Family history of kidney stones and ethnicity as independent risk factors. J Pediatr 1993;122:635.

Perrone HC, Ajzen H, Toporvsec J, et al. Metabolic disturbance as a cause of recurrent hematuria in children. Kidney Int 1991;39:707.

Perrone HS, do Santos DR, Santos MV, et al. Urolithiasis in childhood: Metabolic evaluation. Pediatr Nephrol 1992;6:54.

Sargent JD, Strokel TA, Kresel J, et al. Normal values for random urinary calcium to creatinine ratios in infancy. J Pediatr 1993;123:393.

Southwest Pediatric Nephrology Study Group. Idiopathic hypercalciuria: Association with isolated hematuria and risk for urolithiasis. Kidney Int 190;37:807.

Asymptomatic Gross Hematuria

Abarbanel J, Benet AE, Lask D, et al. Sport hematuria. J Urol 1990;143:887.

Baldree LA, Ault BH, Chesney CM, et al. Intravenous desmopressin acetate in children with sickle trait and persistent macroscopic hematuria. Pediatrics 1977;86:238.

Bernstein J. Renal cystic disease in the tuberous sclerosis complex. Pediatr Nephrol 1993;7:490.

Blumenthal SS, Gritsche C, Lemami J. Establishing the diagnosis of benign familial hematuria: The importance of examining the urine sediment of family members. JAMA 1988;259:2263.

Couser WG. Pathogenesis of glomerulonephritis. Kidney Int 1993;44:S-19.

Gabow PA. Autosomal dominant polycystic kidney disease. N Engl J Med 1993;329:332.

Lew ER, Ross JR, Chon JH. Hematuria and sickle cell disorder. South Med J 1977;70:432.

Meadow SR, Scott DG. Berger disease: Henoch-Schönlein syndrome without the rash. J Pediatr 1985;106:27.

Molteni KH, George J, Messwesmith R, et al. Intrathrombic urokinase reverses neonatal renal artery thrombosis. Pediatr Nephrol 1993;7:413.

Saulsbury FT. Corticosteroid therapy does not prevent nephritis in Henoch-Schönlein purpura. Pediatr Nephrol 1993;7:69.

Microscopic Hematuria

Hisano S, Kwano M, Hotae K, et al. Asymptomatic isolated microhematuria: Natural history of 136 children. Pediatr Nephrol 1991;5:578.

Mrakami M, Yamamoto H, Ueda Y, et al. Urinary screening of elementary and junior high-school children over a 13-year period in Tokyo. Pediatr Nephrol 1991;5:50.

Turi S, Visy M, Visy A, et al. Long-term follow-up of patients with persistent/recurrent, isolated hematuria: A Hungarian multicentre study. Pediatr Nephrol 1989;3:235.

Vehaskari VM. Asymptomatic hematuria—a cause for concern? Pediatr Nephrol 1987;3:240.

Hematuria with Proteinuria

Cameron JS. Tubular and interstitial factors in the progression of glomerulonephritis. Pediatr Nephrol 1992;6:292.

Jones CL, Eddy AA. Tubulointerstitial nephritis. Pediatr Nephrol 1992;6:572.

MeLean RH. Complement and glomerulonephritis—an update. Pediatr Nephrol 1993;7:226.

Roberti I, Reisman L, Churg J. Vasculitis in childhood. Pediatr Nephrol 1993;7:479.

Rottem M, Fauci AS, Hallahan CW, et al. Wegener granulomatosis in children and adolescents: Clinical presentation and outcome. J Pediatr 1993;122:26.

30 Acute and Chronic Scrotal Swelling

Mark A. Wainstein   Jack S. Elder

While some of the causes of acute and chronic scrotal swelling require immediate surgical correction, others are benign and require no further treatment. The differential diagnosis is extensive (Tables 30–1 and 30–2). Optimal treatment requires an expeditious diagnosis that results from a clear understanding of the problem. Failure to make the correct diagnosis or to initiate appropriate therapy, or both, can result in loss of the testis. Consequently, if there is any ambiguity regarding the diagnosis, a pediatric urologist should be consulted.

SCROTAL AND INGUINAL ANATOMY

Inguinal Region

All abdominal muscles and their aponeuroses contribute to the inguinal ligament and canal. The inguinal canal runs obliquely between the external and the internal inguinal rings. The anterior wall of the canal is formed by the external oblique aponeurosis; the floor by the inguinal ligament; the roof by arching fibers of the internal oblique and transversus abdominis muscles; and the posterior wall by the conjoined tendon, formed by the internal oblique and transversus abdominis muscles. The oblique direction of the inguinal canal allows for the posterior and anterior walls to coapt with increases in intra-abdominal pressure.

Testis Descent

The testes develop in the lumbar region of the abdominal cavity between the peritoneum and the transversalis fascia at approximately 7 weeks of intrauterine life. By the eighth week of gestation, the gubernaculum extends from the caudal end of the epididymis through the inguinal canal to insert on the internal wall of the scrotum. The processus vaginalis, a finger-like outpouching of the peritoneum, tracts adjacent to the gubernaculum to form the inguinal canal. As the processus vaginalis descends into the scrotum, it carries extensions of the abdominal wall layers.

The testis normally descends through the inguinal canal into the scrotum before birth. As the testis and the spermatic cord descend through the inguinal canal, they are covered by the three concentric layers of the anterior abdominal fascia (Fig. 30–1). When the testis reaches the scrotum, the processus vaginalis is patent, leaving a connection between the scrotum and the peritoneal cavity. Normally, the processus vaginalis obliterates, leaving a residual tunica vaginalis surrounding the testis. Usually, 1 to 2 cc of clear fluid is in the tunica vaginalis.

Scrotum

The scrotum is partitioned into two separate compartments, each containing a testis, epididymis, and distal spermatic cord. It comprises multiple layers that are continuous with the superficial layers of the anterior abdominal wall. The external location of the scrotum results in the temperature of the testes being 2° to 3° below core body temperature, which allows for normal spermatogenesis.

Testis

The testes are the reproductive organs of the male and are suspended in the tunica vaginalis of the scrotum by the spermatic cords. The epididymis is attached to the testis posteriorly and consists of the caput (upper pole), corpus (body), and cauda (tail) (Fig. 30–2). The cauda epididymis is attached to the vas deferens, which can be palpated as a small rubbery structure in the spermatic cord. The epididymis is responsible for sperm maturation and storage. Each testis relies on three arteries for its blood supply: the testicular artery and the cremasteric and deferential arteries. Each enters the scrotum through the spermatic cord. The testicle receives both sympathetic and parasympathetic innervation. These autonomic nerves carry impulses that produce symptoms of deep visceral pain and associated nausea with testicular stimulation.

Table 30–2. Differential Diagnosis of Scrotal Swelling in Newborns

Hydrocele	Scrotal hematoma
Inguinal hernia (reducible)	Testicular tumor
Inguinal hernia (incarcerated)*	Meconium peritonitis
Testicular torsion*	Epididymitis*

*May be associated with scrotal inflammation.

Table 30–1. Differential Diagnosis of Scrotal Masses in Boys and Adolescents

Painful	Painless
Testicular torsion	Hydrocele
Torsion of testicular appendage	Inguinal hernia (reducible)*
Epididymo-orchitis	Varicocele*
Trauma: testicular rupture, hematocele	Spermatocele
	Testicular tumor*
Inguinal hernia (incarcerated or strangulated)	Paratesticular tumor*
	Idiopathic scrotal edema
Mumps orchitis	Henoch-Schönlein purpura*

*Occasionally associated with discomfort.

433

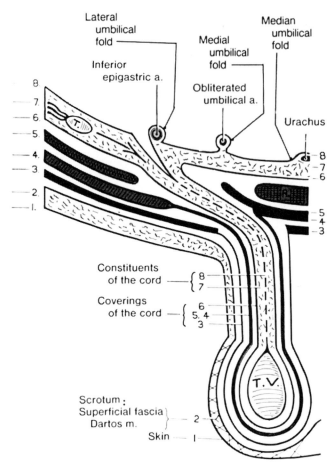

Figure 30–1. Diagram illustrating the inguinal canal and the origin of the layers of the spermatic cord. The drawing demonstrates the eight layers of the abdominal wall, the scrotal wall, and the spermatic cord. The external spermatic fascia is derived from the external oblique aponeurosis; the cremaster muscle and cremasteric fascia are derived from the external oblique and its fascia; and the internal spermatic fascia is derived from the transversalis fascia. T = testis; R = rectus abdominis; TV = tunica vaginalis. (Reproduced with permission from Moore KL. Clinically Oriented Anatomy, 2nd ed. Baltimore: Williams & Wilkins, 1985.)

DIAGNOSTIC STRATEGIES

History

A detailed history is critical in evaluating a boy with acute or chronic scrotal swelling. If there is painful testicular or scrotal swelling, knowing the following characteristics is helpful:

1. *Onset of pain.* Was it associated with trauma or exercise, or did it awaken the patient? Testicular torsion and torsion of a testicular appendage often occur following exercise or minor genital injury. These conditions may also awaken the patient from sleep.

2. *Duration of pain.* Number of hours or days since onset of symptoms.

3. *Evolution of pain.* Sudden versus gradual onset. Testicular torsion tends to occur abruptly, whereas torsion of a testicular appendage and epididymitis typically have an insidious onset.

4. *Associated/radiation of pain.* Is there associated inguinal discomfort, or does the pain radiate from the flank? Inguinal discomfort suggests inguinal pathology such as a hernia. If there is radiation of pain from the flank, renal or ureteral pathology, such as an

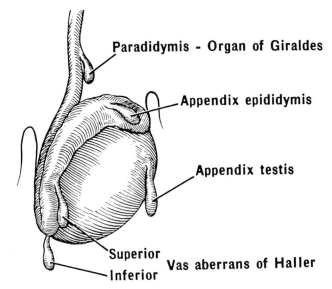

Figure 30–2. Lateral view of the testis showing posterior location of epididymis and testicular appendages. The appendix testis is present in almost all boys, the appendix epididymis is present in approximately 50% of boys, and the other appendages are rarely present. (Reproduced with permission from Kelalis PP, King LR, Belman AB [eds]. Clinical Pediatric Urology, 2nd ed. Philadelphia: WB Saunders, 1985.)

obstructing ureteral calculus, should be considered in the differential diagnosis. Pain with or without swelling of the scrotum includes a large differential diagnosis (Table 30–3).

Although sometimes nonspecific, associated manifestations are also important:

Table 30–3. Etiology of Acute Scrotal Pain

Common
Testicular torsion
Torsion of testicular appendage
Epididymitis (gonorrhea, chlamydial infection in sexually active adolescents)*
Orchitis (mumps, varicella, coxsackievirus, dengue)*
Trauma*
Pain referred to scrotum (nephrolithiasis, ureteropelvic junction obstruction, appendicitis, spinal cord tumor, immunoglobulin A [IgA] nephropathy)

Less Common
Granulomatous orchitis*
Abscess
Infarction
Malignancy (primary testicular neoplasm—e.g., seminoma, embryonal cell—usually painless mass)
Leukemia (primary or relapse—usually painless swelling)*

Uncommon
Drug-induced epididymitis (amiodarone)*
Behçet disease
Sarcoidosis
Polyarteritis nodosa*
Epididymitis (tuberculosis, brucellosis, actinomycosis, leprosy, salmonella, fungal, parasitic, *Nocardia*)
Orchitis (rickettsia, *Nocardia,* toxoplasmosis, cytomegalovirus)
Testicular pyocele
Fournier gangrene*

*Bilateral involvement possible.

1. *General systemic.* Fever, chills, or rigors may suggest an infectious etiology.

2. *Abdominal signs/symptoms.* Nausea, vomiting, or referred abdominal and inguinal pain suggest testicular torsion or epididymitis.

3. *Urologic signs/symptoms.* Dysuria, urinary frequency, hematuria, or penile discharge suggest a urinary tract infection, urethritis, or epididymitis in a sexually active male.

In addition, a thorough medical history is imperative. Significant questions include:

1. History of urinary tract infections, sexually transmitted diseases, or renal calculi.

2. History of any surgical procedures on the groin, scrotum, or abdomen.

3. History of any previous episodes of testicular pain—previous intermittent severe pain in the same testis may be secondary to intermittent torsion of the testis.

Physical Examination

Examination of the scrotal contents should be routine in any male presenting with abdominal, inguinal, or scrotal pain. Inspection, palpation, and transillumination of any mass are integral parts of a thorough physical examination.

Pubertal Development. Has the patient undergone puberty? Testicular torsion is much less common than torsion of the appendix testis in a prepubertal child (Fig. 30–3). Conversely, in an adolescent, testicular torsion and epididymitis (if sexually active) are most common.

Scars in the Inguinal Region. Scars imply previous surgery for hernia, hydrocele, undescended testis, or varicocele.

Scrotal Skin Changes and Fixation. Erythema suggests an underlying inflammatory process but is nonspecific. Fixation of skin over the testis is suggestive of testicular necrosis.

Testis Position Within the Scrotum. An inflamed testis positioned high in the scrotum is suggestive of testicular torsion. Palpation provides information regarding intrascrotal structures. The testis should be evaluated for size and consistency (soft, firm, or hard) and compared to the contralateral side. Accurate localization of pain and swelling of the testis or epididymis, or both, is important. The consistency, size, and relationship to the testis of a paratesticular mass should be noted, along with its reducibility. Any scrotal soft tissue swelling should be evaluated by transillumination. The absence of a cremasteric reflex makes testicular torsion more likely. This reflex is stimulated by gently scratching the medial thigh ipsilateral to the testis; cremasteric muscle contraction causes the scrotum to retract.

Laboratory Data

Basic laboratory data for evaluation of acute and chronic swelling of the testis include urinalysis, urine culture, tests for chlamydia and gonorrhea if sexually active, and complete blood count (see Chapters 27 and 31).

Imaging Studies

Traditionally, prompt surgical exploration was advocated for young males presenting with acute scrotal pain to rule out testicular torsion, which can result in testicular loss within 6 to 8 hours. However, only 29% of boys presenting with acute scrotal pain or swelling, or both, may require immediate surgical intervention. Subjecting all young males to scrotal exploration would result in a large number of unnecessary scrotal explorations. Careful history and physical examination in conjunction with selective imaging studies should result in appropriate recommendations for surgery.

The conditions requiring immediate surgical treatment include testicular torsion, incarcerated inguinal hernia, testicular rupture secondary to trauma, and testicular tumor. While the diagnosis of incarcerated hernia is straightforward, testicular torsion can easily be confused with several conditions that can be managed nonoperatively. The two diagnostic studies most frequently utilized are the radionuclide scrotal (testicular flow) scan and color Doppler

Figure 30–3. Age distribution of testicular torsion, torsion of testicular appendage, and epididymitis. (Reproduced with permission from Hemalatha V, Rickwood AMK. The diagnosis and management of acute scrotal conditions in boys. Br J Urol 1981; 53:455.)

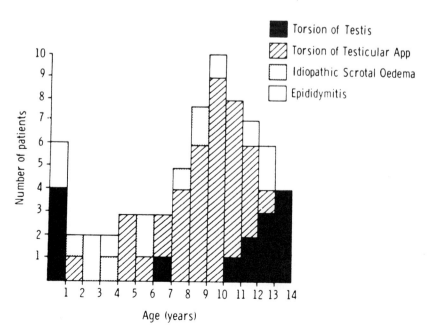

ultrasound. Unfortunately, neither is 100% accurate. Therefore, obtaining either of these studies to determine whether a patient has testicular torsion is appropriate in specific situations:

1. When the clinician is relatively certain that the child does not have torsion and desires confirmation.

2. If the scrotal pain and swelling have been present for more than 48 hours, in which case the likelihood of testicular salvage with testicular torsion is low.

TESTICULAR FLOW SCAN

The ^{99m}Tc-pertechnetate testicular flow scan is accepted for distinguishing between inflammatory and ischemic conditions of the testis. Following intravenous injection of the radionuclide, both flow studies and static images of the testes are obtained. Testicular torsion appears as a "cold spot" of radionuclide deficiency secondary to diminished blood flow. In contrast, inflammatory conditions, such as epididymitis or torsion of the appendix testis, produce normal or increased uptake of ^{99m}Tc. If the testicle has been torsed for greater than 48 hours, often there is a hyperemic rim of tissue surrounding a cold spot, referred to as the "vascular rim."

Accuracy rates of scrotal scintigraphy may be as high as 90% to 95%. Unfortunately, this test is not available at all hospitals. A false-positive scan (incorrectly interpreted as reduced flow—i.e., torsion) can result from a hernia, hydrocele, or spermatocele, which may falsely decrease the radionuclide counts in the region of the testis. A false-negative scan (torsion is present but scan is read as normal) usually occurs in boys with prolonged torsion, in which hyperemia of the scrotal wall is misinterpreted as flow to the testis. Furthermore, if the degree of testicular torsion is "mild" (only 360 degrees), the scan may suggest normal flow, as compared to the obvious reduced flow to the testis if it has undergone more severe torsion (540 to 720 degrees), as is most common. Consequently, nuclear scan results must be correlated with clinical findings.

Another disadvantage of nuclear scanning is the time factor.

Although many institutions can rapidly arrange this study during daytime hours, considerable time delays may be encountered in arranging scans at night or on weekends.

ULTRASONOGRAPHY

Color Doppler ultrasound as well as conventional ultrasound studies can contribute to the diagnosis of scrotal swelling. The Doppler scan, like the nuclear scan, allows assessment of blood flow to the testicle and provides an excellent image of the testis that is easier to interpret than the testicular flow scan. The test is quick, easy to perform, and noninvasive. Published accuracy rates of this modality are 90% to 95%, which compares favorably with scrotal scintigraphy. The study is extremely user-dependent. Furthermore, in the prepubertal age group, the test is much less reliable, as blood flow even to the normal testis can be difficult to demonstrate.

In boys with a suspected testicular tumor or testicular rupture secondary to trauma, a scrotal sonogram should be obtained. If a tumor is present (usually the mass is hypoechoic) sonography can demonstrate that the mass arises from the testis. There are a few benign testicular tumors that are localized and can be excised, sparing the remainder of the testis. In boys with blunt scrotal trauma, an ultrasound scan is sensitive in delineating whether the capsule of the testis, the tunica albuginea, is intact. Furthermore, sonography is helpful in demonstrating the extent of hematoma.

DIFFERENTIAL DIAGNOSIS (Table 30–4)

Testicular Torsion

Testicular torsion is a surgical emergency due to the risk of gonadal loss. The likelihood of testis survival depends on the duration and severity of torsion. Consequently, testicular survival depends on accurate diagnosis and expedient management.

Table 30–4. Differentiation of Acute Painful Scrotal Swelling in Childhood

	Spermatic Cord Torsion	Epididymo-orchitis	Torsion of Testicular Appendage
Age	Perinatal, 10–18 yr, any age possible	Adolescence, but any age possible	2–12 yr
Symptoms and signs	Abrupt onset; may have had previous similar episodes	Gradual onset	Gradual onset
Pain	Localized to the testis and may radiate to groin and lower abdomen	Localization to epididymis; may involve entire testis after 24 hr	Localization to upper pole of testis; may involve entire testis after 24 hr
Fever	Rare	Common	Rare
Vomiting	Common	Rare	Rare
Dysuria	Rare	Common	Rare
Physical examination	Testis may be high riding, swollen, exquisitely tender; scrotal erythema may be present; cremasteric reflex is absent	Testis and epididymis are firm, tender, swollen; scrotal erythema may be present; cremasteric reflex present	Testis is normal or enlarged; firm mass may be seen or felt at upper pole, distinct from epididymis; scrotal erythema may be present; cremasteric reflex present
Pyuria, urinary infection	Rare	Common	Rare
Blood flow (color Doppler; isotope scrotal scan)	Diminished or absent	Increased	Normal or increased

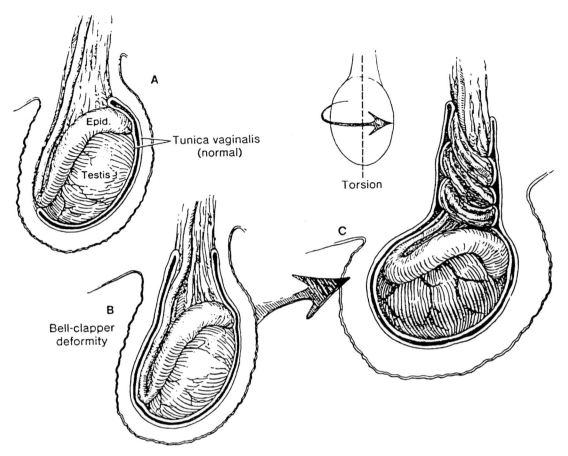

Figure 30–4. *A to C, Mechanism of testicular torsion associated with the bell-clapper deformity. (Reproduced with permission from Fleisher GR, Ludwig S. In* Textbook of Pediatric Emergency Medicine, *3rd ed. Baltimore: Williams & Wilkins, 1993.)*

The incidence of spermatic cord torsion is 1 in 4000 in males younger than 25 years of age. Although testicular torsion can occur at any age, 66% of cases occur between 12 and 18 years of age. In testicular torsion, the testis and spermatic cord rotate or twist on a vertical axis, resulting in obstruction of venous drainage and secondary edema of the spermatic cord with progressive arterial compromise and subsequent infarction (Fig. 30–4). In most cases, there is a predisposing anatomic abnormality that increases the likelihood that the testis can rotate on the spermatic cord. The ''bell-clapper'' abnormality refers to a horizontally positioned testis resulting from a redundant tunica vaginalis or from an abnormal insertion of the epididymis to the testis (Fig. 30–5).

With torsion, patients typically experience the sudden onset of severe testicular pain and swelling. It can occur following minor trauma or exercise or may awaken the patient from sleep. Although the pain is usually localized to the affected hemiscrotum, there can be referred pain to the ipsilateral groin or abdomen. Associated symptoms may include nausea and vomiting. Thirty percent to 50% of patients describe previous episodes of severe scrotal pain that resolved spontaneously. Patients usually have no irritative voiding symptoms.

On examination, the scrotum is erythematous and edematous and the testis is enlarged and extremely tender. The relationship between the testis and the epididymis depends on the degree of testicular torsion; often the epididymis is posterior, as in the normal male. If the individual has been experiencing pain for more than 24 hours, there may be too much inflammation to palpate the epididymis. The testis may be high in the scrotum. Urinalysis should be negative.

Radionuclide testicular flow scan or color Doppler ultrasonography usually demonstrates reduced blood flow. In most cases, how-

ever, the diagnosis of testicular torsion can be made by history and physical examination. If torsion is the likely diagnosis, scrotal exploration should proceed immediately because irreversible histologic damage to the seminiferous tubules occurs within 4 to 6 hours and damage to Leydig cell function occurs within 8 to 12 hours. Significant delay in therapy can result from excessive time spent obtaining adjunctive diagnostic studies. Since no radiologic test is 100% accurate, these studies should be reserved for cases when the clinical impression is against torsion.

If the duration of symptoms is less than 4 to 6 hours, manual detorsion should be attempted. After administration of intravenous morphine (0.1 mg/kg body weight), manual detorsion can be attempted by lifting the scrotum and rotating the testis on its vascular pedicle. Usually, torsion occurs in a medial direction; therefore, the testis should be rotated outward toward the thigh. Successful detorsion is indicated by both relief of pain and a lower testicular position within the scrotum. Although successful manual detorsion may avoid emergent surgery, prompt surgical fixation must be performed because of the risk of recurrence.

Surgical management consists of exploration, detorsion, and evaluation of testicular viability. An infarcted testicle is removed. If the testis is viable, it is fixed to the scrotal wall with nonabsorbable suture, termed *scrotal orchiopexy*. Fixation of the contralateral testis is also necessary because there is a significant risk of contralateral torsion. If detected and treated within 4 hours of the onset of symptoms, the salvage rate approaches 100%; within 12 hours, it falls to 20%; and after 24 hours, infarction is the rule.

Testicular torsion can also occur in the fetus and neonate. In these cases, torsion results from incomplete attachment of the gubernaculum to the scrotal wall and is ''extravaginal.'' When torsion occurs *in utero,* often the infant is born with a large, firm

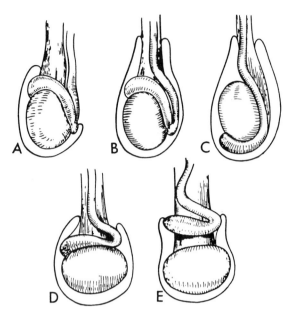

Figure 30–5. Anomalies of suspension associated with intravaginal testicular torsion. *A*, Normal. *B*, Envelopment by the tunica vaginalis. *C*, Inversion of the epididymis. *D, E,* Horizontal lie. Bell-clapper deformity in *B* through *E.* (Reproduced with permission from Kelalis PP, King LR, Belman AB [eds]. Clinical Pediatric Urology, 2nd ed. Philadelphia: WB Saunders, 1985.)

testis that is nontender. Usually the ipsilateral hemiscrotum is ecchymotic. In these cases, the testis always is nonviable because torsion was a remote event. Extravaginal testicular torsion may occur until 30 days beyond term—in these cases, the infant becomes irritable, the testis enlarges, and the scrotum becomes erythematous.

Scrotal imaging studies are unreliable in distinguishing testicular torsion from scrotal hematoma and testicular tumor. Although testicular salvage in neonates with *in utero* torsion is highly unlikely, urgent exploration is recommended to confirm the diagnosis and to perform a contralateral scrotal orchiopexy to protect the solitary testis. If there is a possibility that torsion occurred after birth, there is a slight chance of saving the testis and immediate exploration is warranted.

Torsion of Testicular Appendage

The appendix testis is a vestigial embryonic remnant of the müllerian (mesonephric) ductal system that is attached to the upper pole of the testis. When these appendages are long and pedunculated, they have a tendency to twist at their base, resulting in ischemia and eventual infarction. This entity is most common in boys between 2 and 12 years of age and is rare in adolescents. Torsion of the appendix testis results in progressive inflammation and swelling of the epididymis and testis.

The onset of testicular pain and swelling is usually gradual. Constitutional symptoms are usually less severe than with testicular torsion, but referred pain to the lower abdomen, nausea, and vomiting can occur. The physical examination shows an erythematous and edematous scrotum with underlying testicular enlargement. Palpation of the testis should reveal a 3- to 5-mm tender, indurated mass on the upper pole. In some cases, the torsed appendage may be visible through the scrotal skin, termed the blue dot sign. Later in its clinical course, differentiation from testis torsion becomes increasingly difficult because there is associated reactive orchitis. A clinical diagnosis of torsion of the appendix testis should not be made unless the appendage is palpated or visualized.

The natural history of torsion of the appendix testis is for the inflammation to resolve gradually following infarction of the appendage. Generally, the process is complete within 10 days from the onset of symptoms. Nonoperative treatment is recommended, including bed rest and analgesia with nonsteroidal anti-inflammatory medication for 5 days. The child should be re-examined within 48 hours.

If the likely diagnosis is torsion of the appendix testis but the clinician desires confirmation, color Doppler sonography or a testicular flow scan may be ordered. Either of these studies should demonstrate hyperemia to the testis. On the other hand, if there is any ambiguity regarding the diagnosis, emergency scrotal exploration should be performed to be certain that the child does not have testicular torsion.

Epididymo-orchitis

Epididymitis refers to an inflammatory process that involves the epididymis and usually results from a urethral infection that passes in a retrograde manner through the vas deferens to the epididymis (Fig. 30–6). It is most common in adolescent males and rare in the prepubertal age group. Unless there is a preexisting abnormality of the lower genitourinary tract (neuropathic bladder, urethral stricture), in most postpubertal males epididymitis results from a sexually transmitted disease (see Chapter 31). Organisms responsible include *Chlamydia, Mycoplasma,* and *Neisseria gonorrhoeae.* In prepubertal boys, in contrast, epididymitis is most frequently secondary to a structural abnormality of the lower genitourinary tract, including ectopic ureter, ectopic vas deferens, rectourethral fistula associated with imperforate anus, and urethral stricture. If diagnosed and treated early, the testicle is not involved. In many cases, however, the inflammatory process also involves the testis and is termed epididymo-orchitis. If the infection is bacterial (e.g., *Escherichia coli* or other gram-negative uropathogens) and is not treated for 1 to 2 weeks, testicular infarction can occur.

Adolescent males with epididymitis are usually sexually active. They typically experience testicular pain and swelling that is insidious in onset. Some males also have symptoms of urinary tract infection, including dysuria, urgency, frequency, as well as urethral discharge. Some report transient inguinal pain secondary to in-

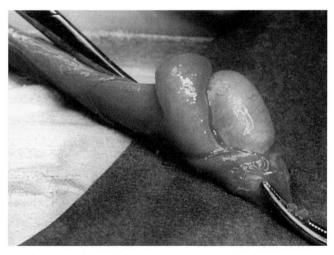

Figure 30–6. A 6-year-old boy with epididymitis. Note the reactive orchitis as well as significant enlargement of the epididymis.

flammation of the spermatic cord prior to the onset of testicular symptoms. On physical examination, fever is common, as is scrotal erythema. The epididymis is tender, enlarged, indurated, and posterior to the testis. Often the testis is also enlarged and tender. A reactive hydrocele may be present and obscures the testicular examination. If there is fixation of skin over the testis, the testis may be nonviable.

The most important laboratory study is the urinalysis, which often shows pyuria or bacteriuria, or both (see Chapter 27). A urine specimen should also be obtained for culture. Not all prepubertal boys with epididymitis have an abnormal urinalysis; rarely, boys with testicular torsion may have evidence of infection. If there is a urethral discharge, a specimen of urethral fluid should be obtained for Gram stain and culture. If the diagnosis is not definitive or if testicular infarction is suspected, a testicular flow scan or color Doppler ultrasound scan may be helpful by showing blood flow to the testis. Sonography also may show evidence of an abscess.

If the urinalysis shows evidence of infection, treatment should include empiric broad-spectrum antibiotics (for *N. gonorrhoeae* and *Chlamydia*, ceftriaxone and doxycyline, respectively) until the culture results are available. Supportive measures include an ice pack, scrotal support, nonsteroidal anti-inflammatory medication for analgesia, and bed rest for 48 hours. If the patient is an adolescent and the urinalysis does not show an obvious urinary tract infection (see Chapter 27), treatment of other genital bacteria should be initiated with doxycycline for 10 to 14 days. If there is evidence of gonorrhea, ceftriaxone therapy should be administered. Finally, in a prepubertal male with epididymitis and no evidence of infection on urinalysis, empiric treatment with a broad-spectrum antibiotic (ampicillin, gentamicin, or cefotaxime) is recommended. All patients should be re-examined periodically until the inflammatory process resolves completely. Approximately 15% of individuals with a testis tumor are initially treated for epididymitis.

Surgical management is reserved primarily for cases in which there is ambiguity regarding the diagnosis and testicular torsion is suspected or if there is a suspected abscess.

Orchitis as an isolated infection is uncommon in boys. Most often, it results from extension of an epididymal inflammatory process. Mumps orchitis occurs most frequently in postpubertal males. The onset of orchitis usually occurs 4 to 6 days after the manifestations of parotitis. As many as 33% of patients with orchitis experience testicular atrophy.

Treatment of orchitis includes broad-spectrum antibiotics until the urine culture result is available. If the primary infection is obviously viral, symptomatic therapy is all that is needed (NSAIDS, scrotal support, ice pack).

Trauma and Hematocele

Blunt scrotal trauma can result in a spectrum of injuries ranging from testicular contusion to rupture of the testis (Fig. 30–7). Testicular injuries usually result from a fall, kick, or direct blow from a blunt object. A detailed history of the nature of the injury aids in recognizing the likelihood of serious testicular injury. With disruption of the tunica albuginea (capsule) of the testis, there is such significant painful scrotal swelling that the testis cannot be palpated. Often there is associated erythema or ecchymosis of the scrotal wall. In most cases of suspected testicular injury, scrotal ultrasonography is performed to assess the integrity of the testis.

In many boys with testicular torsion or torsion of the appendix testis, inexplicably there is a history of recent mild scrotal trauma. Although there is no evidence that these disorders can result from blunt trauma, these diagnoses should be considered if there is not an obvious testicular injury but the scrotal examination is abnormal.

Treatment of scrotal trauma is determined by the extent of the injury. Boys with a small, nonexpanding hematocele and a normal testis are managed nonoperatively with bed rest, scrotal support, and ice. In contrast, a ruptured testis associated with a large hematocele requires urgent surgical exploration and repair.

Varicocele

A varicocele is an abnormal dilation of the veins of the pampiniform plexus in the scrotum. Approximately 5% of adolescent males and 15% of adult men have a varicocele; 15% of these men are infertile. Varicocele is the most common surgically correctable cause of infertility in men. The etiology of infertility is thought to result from the effect of elevated temperature on the testis. Varicoceles are rare in boys younger than 10 years of age. The increased

Figure 30–7. *A,* An 8-year-old boy kicked in the scrotum while doing karate with his brother. Note right scrotal swelling. An ultrasound study showed scrotal hematoma and ruptured testis. *B,* Scrotal exploration shows a nonviable testis. Orchiectomy was performed.

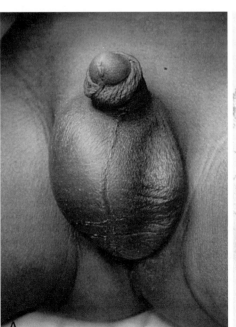
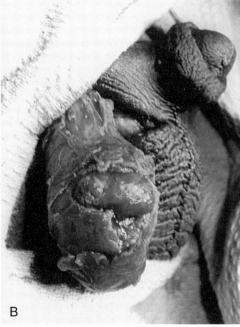

prevalence in adolescents is secondary to the increased testicular blood flow that occurs with puberty. More than 95% involve the left testis, which is secondary to multiple factors, including the long length of the left internal spermatic vein compared with that of the right and the absence of a venous valve at the insertion of the left internal spermatic vein into the renal vein.

A varicocele presents as a painless, paratesticular mass often described as a ''bag of worms.'' Occasionally, patients describe a chronic dull ache in or adjacent to the testis. Physical examination of the patient in both the supine and the upright positions, with and without the Valsalva maneuver, facilitates the diagnosis. Typically, the varicocele is decompressed when the patient is supine and prominent when standing. Measurement of the volume of both testicles is important to document differences in the size of the testis. Approximately 33% of affected boys have an associated volume loss of the left testis. If a varicocele is detected in a boy younger than 10 years old or on the right side (both *red flags*), an abdominal ultrasound is indicated to ascertain whether an abdominal mass is present.

Histologic studies have demonstrated pathologic testicular changes in some adolescents and men with varicoceles, including degeneration of germinal centers, interstitial fibrosis, and impaired spermatogenesis. The goal in treatment of a varicocele is preservation and restoration of spermatogenesis. Because the majority of testicular volume is composed of seminiferous tubules, if the left testis is significantly smaller than the right, one may presume that the varicocele has affected testicular growth. Typically, following varicocelectomy in an adolescent, the testis shows catch-up growth and ultimately is similar in size to the contralateral testicle.

Indications for varicocelectomy in boys and adolescents include:

1. Significant disparity in testicular size.
2. Pain.
3. Diseased or absent contralateral testis.

Surgical repair should also be considered for large varicoceles. Varicocelectomy is accomplished by ligating the dilated veins of the pampiniform plexus through a low inguinal incision or by ligating and dividing the internal spermatic vein through a high transverse inguinal incision or by a laparoscopic approach. All of these techniques may be performed on an ambulatory basis.

Inguinal Hernia

Hernias and hydroceles result from incomplete obliteration of the processus vaginalis. Indirect inguinal hernias result from a patent processus vaginalis that allows a loop of bowel, omentum, or other abdominal organ to pass through the internal inguinal ring. Patients usually present with nontender groin or scrotal swelling, or both, that reduces with minimal pressure (Fig. 30–8). A hernia that cannot be reduced is called an *incarcerated hernia*. A *strangulated hernia*, meaning the vascular supply of the herniated bowel is compromised, is a surgical emergency. Physical signs of incarceration include inguinal or scrotal erythema, pain, signs of bowel obstruction, and inability to reduce the hernia. Infants with an incarcerated hernia have a 10% incidence of ipsilateral testicular infarction secondary to increased pressure on the spermatic cord.

If an incarcerated hernia is suspected, the child is admitted and sedated and manual reduction of the hernia is attempted. Most hernias can be reduced successfully and should be repaired within a short period of time. Children with an easily reducible hernia should also undergo herniorrhaphy within a reasonable time period to reduce the possibility of incarceration or strangulation. Neonates or small infants with an incarcerated hernia may present with painful scrotal swelling without an inguinal mass, but this presentation is unusual in older children.

Surgical correction involves dissection and high ligation of the

hernia sac through a small inguinal incision. This is usually performed as an ambulatory surgical procedure unless the infant is younger than 2 months old or has an associated medical condition (cardiorespiratory compromise) requiring observation.

Hydrocele

A hydrocele is an accumulation of fluid within the tunica vaginalis. Approximately 1% to 2% of male neonates have a hydrocele. In most of these cases, which are noncommunicating hydroceles, the fluid disappears by 1 year of age. Communicating hydroceles, defined by a patent processus vaginalis (Fig. 30–8), tend to persist. Typically, these boys have progressive scrotal swelling over the course of the day that decreases by morning as the hydrocele fluid returns to the abdomen during sleep. In infants that are not walking, the hydrocele usually does not change in size. In an older boy, a noncommunicating hydrocele can result from an inflammatory condition within the scrotum (testicular torsion, torsion of the appendix testis, epididymitis, testis tumor). Communicating hydroceles and hernias differ by the anatomy and contents of the processus vaginalis. In communicating hydroceles, the diameter of the processus vaginalis is much smaller relative to a hernia, allowing only fluid to pass into the scrotum.

On examination, hydroceles are smooth and nontender and can be associated with thickening of the cord structures. Bright transillumination of the scrotum confirms the fluid-filled nature of the mass. If compression of the fluid-filled mass reduces the size of the hydrocele, the presence of an inguinal hernia is the likely diagnosis. Because hydroceles can be associated with testicular neoplasms, the testis should be palpated to document that it is normal. If the diagnosis is uncertain regarding the mass, scrotal ultrasonography is advised.

Treatment depends on several factors. Most hydroceles resolve by 12 months of age following reabsorption of the hydrocele fluid. If the hydrocele is large and tense, however, early surgical correction is recommended for two reasons: (1) it is often impossible to verify that the child does not have a hernia and (2) large hydroceles rarely disappear spontaneously. Hydroceles persisting beyond 12 to 18 months are usually communicating and thus rarely regress; consequently, these hydroceles should be surgically repaired. If left untreated, most eventually progress to an inguinal hernia. Parents should be advised to watch for more severe inguinal or scrotal swelling, or both, which indicates that a hernia has developed.

Surgical repair of hydroceles is essentially identical to a herniorrhaphy. Through an inguinal incision, the spermatic cord is identified, the hydrocele fluid is drained, and a high ligation of the processus vaginalis is performed.

Testicular Tumors

Although testicular and paratesticular tumors are uncommon, they can occur at any age, even in the newborn. In adult men, 98% of testis tumors are malignant. In children, however, only 66% are malignant and are germ cell in origin. Most present as a painless, hard, testicular or paratesticular mass that does not transilluminate. Ten percent to 15% are associated with a hydrocele. Scrotal ultrasonography should be performed to confirm the finding of a testicular mass and may help to delineate the type of testicular tumor. In addition, serum tumor markers—alpha-fetoprotein and human chorionic gonadotropin (hCG)—should be drawn prior to surgical intervention.

Definitive therapy includes surgical exploration through an inguinal incision. Radical orchiectomy involves ligation of the spermatic cord followed by removal of the testis and spermatic cord. If the

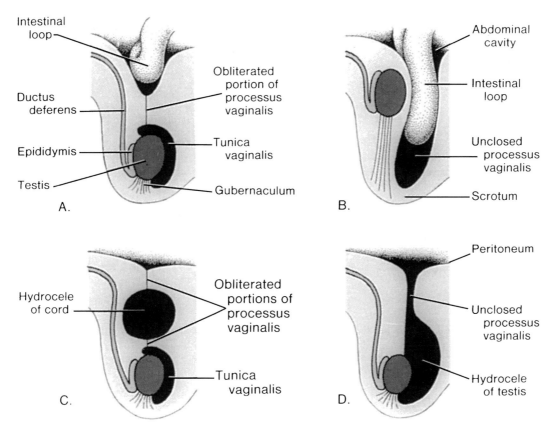

Figure 30–8. Diagrams of sagittal sections of the inguinal region. *A,* Incomplete indirect inguinal hernia resulting from persistence of the proximal processus vaginalis. *B,* Indirect inguinal hernia into the scrotum resulting from persistence of the entire processus vaginalis. Note the presence of an undescended testicle, which is a commonly associated malformation. *C,* Hydrocele of the cord derived from an unobliterated portion of the processus vaginalis. *D,* Communicating hydrocele resulting from peritoneal fluid passing through a patent processus vaginalis. (Reproduced with permission from Moore KL. The Developing Human: Clinically Oriented Embryology, 5th ed. Philadelphia: WB Saunders, 1993:299.)

ultrasound study or surgical exploration suggests the presence of a benign tumor, such as a teratoma or epidermoid cyst, with a significant amount of normal testicular parenchyma, excision of the mass only (''testis-sparing surgery'') may be performed. If the tumor is malignant, a metastatic work-up, including abdominal and chest computed tomography scan, is obtained to evaluate the most common sites of metastatic disease: the retroperitoneum and lung.

Meconium Peritonitis

Antenatal peritonitis may result from intestinal perforation. Although the intestinal perforation may heal, the intra-abdominal meconium may track down the patent processus vaginalis into the scrotum, resulting in the formation of an inflammatory mass. This condition can present as bilateral neonatal hydroceles, which eventually regress into firm, nodular masses involving either or both testicles. Scrotal sonography demonstrates multiple areas of echogenic foci suggestive of calcification. In addition, a plain film of the scrotum shows calcification.

Scrotal Wall Swelling

HENOCH-SCHÖNLEIN PURPURA

Henoch-Schönlein purpura is a systemic vasculitis of unknown etiology that involves the skin, gastrointestinal tract, joints, and

kidney. Most affected patients are younger than 7 years of age. Genitourinary manifestations may include renal parenchymal involvement, ureteritis, renal pelvic bleeding, and acute swelling of the scrotum and spermatic cord. Scrotal wall and testicular involvement has been reported in up to 33% of affected patients.

Typically, a maculopapular purpuric (palpable purpura) rash begins in the lower extremities and buttock region. Later the rash may spread to the scrotum. In some cases, however, the initial manifestation is a scrotal rash. Testicular involvement is indicated by mild to moderate swelling and tenderness of the testes. Differentiation from testicular torsion can be made if the characteristic rash and associated symptoms develop before the acute enlargement of the scrotum. Because these two conditions have been reported to coexist in the same patient, if there is any uncertainty regarding the diagnosis, color Doppler ultrasonography or scrotal scintigraphy should be performed.

ACUTE IDIOPATHIC SCROTAL WALL EDEMA

Acute idiopathic scrotal wall edema is an uncommon entity that accounts for 2% to 5% of acute scrotal swelling. The average patient age is between 4 and 7 years. Patients typically present with the sudden onset of unilateral or bilateral scrotal wall edema associated with mild tenderness. The overlying skin is erythematous, and the edema may extend anteriorly onto the abdominal wall or posteriorly into the perineum. The testicles are easily palpable, normal in size, and nontender. The etiology of this syndrome is unknown, but allergic causes have been implicated.

Therapy consists of bed rest and parental reassurance. Although treatment with antibiotics, antihistamines, and corticosteroids has been proposed, most children improve within 48 to 72 hours regardless of therapy.

IDIOPATHIC FAT NECROSIS

Idiopathic fat necrosis causes acute painful swelling of the scrotum secondary to necrosis of intrascrotal fat. Examination of the underlying testis may be obscured from inflammation within the scrotal wall. The cause of this problem is unknown but may be related to trauma with physical activity. Sonography may help to differentiate this entity from an intrascrotal process.

Treatment is supportive if the diagnosis is made nonoperatively.

FOURNIER GANGRENE

Fournier gangrene of the scrotum usually involves adults but occasionally afflicts infants and children. It occurs primarily in children with severe diaper rash, insect bites, following circumcision, or perianal skin abscess. Other predisposing factors include diabetes mellitus, trauma, instrumentation, urethral stricture, and inguinal or perineal surgery. Symptoms of this life-threatening infection include acute scrotal swelling with tenderness, erythema, and systemic manifestations of fever, chills, and septicemia. The most common organisms identified include *Staphylococcus aureus, Streptococcus, Bacteroides fragilis, E. coli,* and *Clostridium welchii.*

Treatment involves emergency debridement under anesthesia, copious irrigation, and broad-spectrum parenteral antibiotics. Despite aggressive treatment, mortality rates approach 50%.

Red Flags

The most important and common lesions not to miss are noted in Table 30–4; both historical and physical red flags are noted.

REFERENCES

Diagnosic Strategies

Burks DD, Markay BJ, Burkhard TK, et al. Suspected testicular torsion and ischemia: Evaluation with color Doppler sonography. Radiology 1990;175:815.

Eshghi M, Silver L, Smith AD. Technetium 99m scan in acute scrotal lesions. Urology 1987;30:586.

Gilchrist BF, Lobe TE. The acute groin in pediatrics. Clin Pediatr 1992;31:488–496.

Golimbu M, Florio FE, Al-Askari S, et al. Value of scrotal scanning. Urology 1985;25:92.

Kass EJ, Stone KT, Cacciarelli AA, et al. Do all children with an acute scrotum require exploration? J Urol 1993;150:667.

Testicular Torsion

Barada JH, Weingarten JL, Cromie WJ. Testicular salvage and age-related delay in the presentation of testicular torsion. J Urol 1989;142:746.

Jones DJ. Recurrent subacute torsion: Prospective study of effects on testicular morphology and function. J Urol 1991;145:297.

Krarup T. The testes after torsion. Br J Urol 1978;50:43.

Ransler CW, Allen TD. Torsion of the spermatic cord. Urol Clin North Am 1982;9:245.

Skoglund RW, McRoberts JW, Radge H. Torsion of the testis: A review of the literature and an analysis of 70 new cases. J Urol 1970;104:604.

Williamson RCN. Torsion of the testis and allied conditions. Br J Surg 1976;63:465.

Epididymo-orchitis

Beard CM, Benson RC, Kelalis PP, et al. The incidence and outcome of mumps orchitis in Rochester, Minnesota 1935 to 1974. Mayo Clin Proc 1977;52:3.

Siegel A, Snyder H, Duckett JW. Epididymitis in infants and boys: Underlying urogenital anomalies and efficacy of imaging modalities. J Urol 1987;138:1100.

Inguinal Hernia

Puri P, Guiney EJ, O'Donnell B. Inguinal hernia in infants: The fate of the testis following incarceration. J Pediatr Surg 1984;19:44.

Stoker DL, Spiegelhalter DJ, Singh R, et al. Laparoscopic versus open inguinal hernia repair: Randomised prospective trial. Lancet 1994;343:1243.

Other Diagnoses

Adeyokunnu EL. Fournier's syndrome in infants. Clin Pediatr 1983;22:101.

Chaviano AH. Fournier's gangrene in children. Infect Urol 1989;2:137.

Clark WR, Kramer SA. Henoch-Schönlein purpura and the acute scrotum. J Pediatr Surg 1986;21:991.

Kaplan GW. Acute idiopathic scrotal edema. J Pediatr Surg 1977;12:647.

Kogan SJ. Acute and chronic scrotal swellings. *In* Gillenwater JY, Grayhack JT, Howards SS, et al (eds). Adult and Pediatric Urology, 2nd ed. St. Louis: Mosby–Year Book, 1991.

Levy DA, Kay R, Elder JS. Neonatal testis tumors: A review of the prepubertal testis registry. J Urol 1994;151:715.

Loh HS, Jalan OM. Testicular torsion in Henoch-Schönlein syndrome. Br Med J 1974;2:96.

Nemoy NJ, Rosin S, Kaplan L. Scrotal panniculitis in the prepubertal male patient. J Urol 1977;118:492.

Ross J, Kay R, Elder J. Testis sparing surgery for pediatric epidermoid cysts of the testis. J Urol 1993;149:353.

Rushton HG, Belman AB, Sesterhenn I, et al. Testicular sparing surgery for prepubertal teratoma of the testis. J Urol 1990;144:726.

Sawczuk IS, Hensle TW. Varicoceles in children. *In* Resnick MI, Kursh ED (eds). Current Therapy in Genitourinary Surgery, 2nd ed. St. Louis: Mosby–Year Book, 1992.

Skoglund RW, McRoberts JW, Radge H. Torsion of testicular appendages: Presentation of 43 new cases and a collective review. J Urol 1970;104:598.

31 Sexually Transmitted Diseases

Trina M. Anglin

Teenagers currently represent the age group at highest risk for acquisition and transmission of sexually transmitted diseases (STDs). National survey data of high school students demonstrated that 54% have engaged in sexual intercourse, with 39% having had a sexual encounter within the previous 3 months. Adolescents are likely to have multiple sexual partners over relatively short periods of time, to choose partners unwisely, to not recognize the symptoms of STDs, and to use condoms inconsistently. Adolescents who abuse alcohol and drugs and those who are runaways, prostitutes, or delinquents are at especially high risk for acquiring STDs; male teenagers who have sex with other males are at high risk.

HISTORY

The adolescent who seeks medical attention for treatment of a sexually transmitted disease may complain of vague symptoms and attempt to avoid discussing the real problem. Health professionals should always elicit a sexual history from adolescent patients and should gently question the individual for specific information. One should be suspicious of the adolescent patient who just "comes in for a check-up"; the visit may be a call for help.

The general history should be obtained from the patient and a parent or guardian if one accompanies the adolescent patient. If the parent wants time alone with the physician, this visit should be scheduled prior to the physical examination. Generally, the examiner should not spend time alone with a parent after the adolescent patient has shared personal information with the health provider.

Tables 31–1 and 31–2 list a number of issues that must be discussed with the patient who is sexually active. It is critical that the history be thorough and that inquiries be made in a nonjudgmental and nonthreatening manner. Questioning adoles-

Table 31–1. Approach to Clinical Evaluation of Sexually Transmitted Diseases (STDs): Sexual History

Chronology of sexual activity
Date of most recent sexual encounter
Duration of relationship with current partner
Fidelity of self and partner
Numbers of lifetime partners (especially in previous year)
Condom usage (overall consistency, with last and previous encounters)
Contraceptive usage
Vaginal intercourse
Oral intercourse
Anal intercourse
Dyspareunia
Gender of partners
Involuntary sexual encounters (abuse, rape)
Communication and confidentiality

Table 31–2. Approach to Clinical Evaluation of Sexually Transmitted Diseases: Symptoms and General Health

Symptoms (Duration, Intensity, Course)
Urinary (dysuria, urgency, frequency, hematuria)
Vaginal discharge (quantity, color, odor, consistency, pruritus, burning)
Urethral discharge (character, quantity, when it occurs)
Anorectal discharge (character, quantity, when it occurs; bowel movements)
Local pain (character, location: mucosal, abdominal, testicular, inguinal, anal)

Self-Treatment
Over-the-counter medication
Douching
Antibiotic usage

Reproductive Health History
Previous diagnosis and treatment of sexually transmitted diseases
Previous similar symptoms
History of pregnancies or impregnation

Menstruation
Last menstrual period (date, duration, quantity, associated pain or cramping, comparison to usual menses)
Spotting or intermenstrual bleeding

Review of Systems
Skin (rash, pruritus, lesions)
Joints (pain, swelling, redness)
Bowel changes (diarrhea, bleeding)
Constitutional (fever, weight loss, night sweats, malaise, cough, depression)

General Health
Medical problems
Medication usage
Travel

Substance Abuse
Alcohol and illicit drug usage (self and partner)
Needle injection (self and partner)

Partner(s)
Symptoms
STD history
Source(s) of health care

cents about their knowledge of STDs is important, since they might not understand exactly which behaviors could put them at risk for infections. Since some patients infected with STDs may be asymptomatic, gaining insight into sexual activity and orientation is most important. A previous history of an STD places the patient at higher risk for STDs in the future.

Table 31-3. Diagnostic Characteristics of Genital Lesions

Syndrome	Appearance	Number of Lesions	Pain	Adenopathy	Epidemiology in the United States
Herpes	Vesicles and superficial ulcers on erythematous base (1–2 mm)	Multiple	Yes	Bilateral; inguinal; firm; movable; tender	Frequent
Syphilis	Papule and superficial or deep ulcer (5–15 mm)	Single	No	Bilateral; inguinal; firm; movable; nontender	Frequent
Lymphogranuloma venereum	Ulcer resolves quickly (2–10 mm)	Single	Yes	Unilateral; inguinal; fluctuant; may suppurate; tender	Rare
Human papilloma-virus	Anogenital exophytic warts; may resemble cauliflowers or be papular with projections	Single or multiple	No	None	Common
Lice or nits	Tiny (1 mm or less) insects or eggs adherent to hair shaft; excoriations	Multiple	No, but pruritic	None	Common
Chancroid	Deep, purulent ulcers (2–20 mm)	Multiple	Yes	Unilateral; inguinal; fluctuant; may suppurate; tender	Rare

While both children and adolescents may present because they have been sexually abused, the examiner should ask about victimization and abuse in all cases. If the patient has been abused, it is useful to obtain a history of the encounter. If the patient has been a victim of assault, a description of the assault should be obtained and the sites of attempted or successful penetration should be noted. If possible, the offender should be identified. The time interval between the assault and evaluation is important.

Clinical symptoms that should specifically be noted include vaginal or rectal discharge, odor, pruritus, or pain; sore throat; local bleeding; dysuria, urgency or frequency; abdominal pain; warts; and abnormal menstrual bleeding. Activities since the time of assault that must be documented are bathing, douching, urinating, defecating, tooth brushing, or gargling; such activities may interfere with specimen collection. If any antimicrobial drug has been taken, the dosage and frequency should be noted. A history of any known STD, voluntary sexual relationships, or previous sexual assault and relevant medical treatment should be discussed with the patient.

Whether or not a patient has been abused, symptomatic individuals often seek medical attention for an STD. Females commonly present with a vaginal discharge, genital lesions, abdominal pain, dysuria and menstrual spotting. Males may complain of dysuria, genital lesions, testicular pain, urethral discharge or scrotal swelling. A variety of skin rashes may be noted with STDs and may be the reason for seeking medical attention. Constitutional symptoms include fever, malaise, lymphadenopathy and less often arthritis. If the patient has any constitutional symptoms, one should inquire about weight loss, appetite, sleep patterns, energy level, headaches, and weakness.

Patients who present with systemic disease may be more likely to have an infection with the human immunodeficiency virus (HIV), syphilis, herpes simplex virus (HSV), or Reiter syndrome (reactive arthritis).

Male patients who seek medical attention for a urethral discharge or urethritis are likely to have been infected with *Neisseria gonorrhoeae* or *Chlamydia trachomatis*. Both male and female patients who describe genital lesions may have ulcers, vesicles, papules or warts (Table 31–3).

Vaginal discharge in female adolescents is a nonspecific symp-

tom but should lead to the consideration of bacterial vaginosis, trichomonas, or gonorrhea. The character of the discharge, presence of pruritus, and types of home treatments already used are clues that often lead the clinician to a diagnosis. Unfortunately, many adolescents with infections present with few symptoms and they may never seek medical attention for an STD.

PHYSICAL EXAMINATION

A complete physical examination is required whenever an STD is considered in the differential diagnosis. Table 31–4 presents a brief listing of findings that must be sought. If a skin rash is noted, secondary syphilis, Reiter syndrome, or disseminated gonococcal infection must be considered. Secondary syphilis, primary genital herpes simplex virus, or primary HIV infection might also be in the differential diagnosis when a patient complains of headache, stiff neck, and malaise; findings of nuchal rigidity suggest an aseptic meningitis. Gonococcus may rarely cause bacterial meningitis. Generalized adenopathy, weight loss, and skin rash can indicate HIV infection or secondary syphilis. However, because constitutional symptoms are present in a large number of patients with primary herpes simplex virus genital infections, a careful search must be made for vesicles on an erythematous base. The presence of arthritis should alert the clinician to the possibility of Reiter

Table 31-4. Physical Examination

Vital signs
Skin (rash, excoriations, location of lesions, especially palms, soles, face, trunk, extremities)
Oropharynx (inflammation, lesions, exudates, enanthem)
Nodes
Abdominal tenderness, hepatosplenomegaly
Back (costovertebral angle tenderness)
Joints (tenderness, erythema, swelling, warmth)

syndrome or disseminated gonococcal infection. Women with severe abdominal tenderness might have PID with or without a tubo-ovarian abscess; ectopic pregnancy, mesenteric adenitis, Fitz-Hugh Curtis syndrome, ruptured ovarian cyst, adnexal torsion, and appendicitis must also be carefully considered.

Tables 31–5 and 31–6 review the necessary physical examination procedures that should be followed for the male and female adolescent. Table 31–3 should assist the clinician in distinguishing genital lesions associated with some of the more common infectious agents. Table 31–7 offers some clues for approaching the physical examination in the prepubertal girl who presents with vaginal irritation or discharge.

If the clinician suspects that a prepubertal child has been sexually abused, a careful general examination is performed. Anatomic abnormalities (trauma, lacerations, erythema, scarring) of the external genitalia and the anorectal area should be documented; colposcopic magnification and photography are standard (see Chapter 37).

LABORATORY TESTING

Adolescents who present with one STD are at high risk for having another STD. For example, syphilis and HIV testing should

Table 31–5. **Examination of the Female Adolescent**

External Genitalia
Pubic hair sexual maturation rating
Lice and nits
Mucosal estrogenization
Erythema
Edema
Skin and mucosal lesions (erythema, ulcers, warts, fissures, excoriation)
Bartholin and Skene (periurethral) glands
Urethra
Discharge at introitus
Trauma

Speculum Examination (see Chapter 32)
Vagina (erythema, lesions, quantity/color/consistency/odor of vaginal pool)
Cervix (conformation, bleeding, erythema, friability, character of mucus, lesions, colpitis muscularis)

Bimanual
Degree of patient relaxation
Uterus (size, position, mobility, tenderness, consistency)
Adnexae (tenderness, enlargement, mass)
Cervical motion tenderness

Rectum
Lesions of perianal skin or anal verge
Grip
Ampulla (mass, tenderness, feces)
Stool character and Hematest
Rectoabdominal
Rectovaginal

Vaginal Pool Laboratory Testing
pH
Potassium hydroxide odor test and mount (buds, pseudohyphae)
Normal saline mount (% clue cells, % parabasal cells, white and red blood cells per high-power field, trichomonads, yeast buds/pseudohyphae, lactobacilli, or other bacterial morphotypes, sperm/motility)
Gram stain

Cervical Laboratory Testing
Gram stain (white blood cells)

Table 31–6. **Examination of the Male Adolescent**

External Genitalia
Sexual maturation ratings (pubic hair and genitalia)
Lice and nits
Skin lesions (mons, penis and foreskin, scrotum, inguinal region, medial thighs; ulcers, warts, papules, erythema, nodules, excoriation)
Urethral meatus (erythema, lesions, tenderness)
Urethral discharge (quantity, color, consistency)
Scrotum/testes (tenderness, mass, edema)

Rectum
Lesions of perianal skin or anal verge
Grip
Ampulla (mass, tenderness, feces)
Stool character and Hematest
Rectoabdominal

be considered when the diagnosis is gonorrhea. However, information from a carefully obtained patient history correlated with physical findings should suggest the appropriate laboratory evaluations.

Pregnancy testing is indicated when a female adolescent presents with symptoms of an STD. The test results may influence the treatment plan.

HIV Testing

Table 31–8 lists the circumstances in which HIV testing should be considered for children and adolescents (see also Chapter 55).

Localized Symptoms

GENITAL ULCERS

Vesicles atop an erythematous base are most often a result of herpes simplex. Fluid from these vesicles may be sent for herpes culture or for a direct fluorescent antibody (DFA) test. Material from the ''ulcer'' or ''chancre'' associated with syphilis can be examined via dark field for the presence of treponemes (a difficult test), or the material can be air-dried on a slide and a DFA test for *Treponema pallidum* can be performed (highly sensitive and specific).

GENITAL WARTS

The diagnosis of genital warts (human papillomavirus) is usually straightforward. Condylomata lata (secondary syphilis) should also be considered. Since human papillomavirus has been associated with malignant transformation, a Papanicolaou smear is indicated for sexually active female adolescents on a regular basis. Cervical warts, atypical lesions, and those not responding to local treatment require a biopsy.

URETHRAL DISCHARGE IN THE MALE ADOLESCENT

In the symptomatic male patient, both gonorrhea and chlamydia specimens can be obtained for culture by inserting a Dacron or

Table 31–7. Approach to the Physical Examination in Prepubertal Girls with Vaginal Irritation or Discharge

General Physical Examination
  Skin for evidence of viral exanthem, atopic or seborrheic dermatitis, and other lesions
  Evidence of acute respiratory, pharyngeal, or gastrointestinal illness
  Chronic disease
  Inspection of underpants for discharge

Visualization of External Genitalia and Perianal Area
  Supine, lithotomy, or modified lithotomy position (includes labial separation and traction):
    Inflammation and lesions of skin and vulva mucosa
    Evidence of poor toilet hygiene
    Signs of excoriation
    Presence of discharge at introitus
    Presence of pinworms *(Enterobius vermicularis)*
    Degree of estrogenization
    Hymenal configuration
    Evidence of recent or earlier trauma
    Ectopic urethra
    Congenital anomalies
    Evidence of scabies

Visualization of Vagina and Cervix
  Knee-chest position with traction on buttocks and use of otoscope as light source

Vaginal Specimen Collection
  Saline moistened cotton/dacron-tipped nasopharyngeal or urethral swabs or ''catheter within a catheter'' technique to aspirate specimen
  Normal saline preparation for microscopic examination
  Potassium hydroxide preparation
  Cultures for *N. gonorrhoeae, C. trachomatis, Candida,* group A streptococci, anaerobes, and gram-negative enteric bacteria
  Request that laboratory identify and quantify *all* predominant isolates
  Tape test (non-frosted cellophane tape) for pinworms (best performed by parent before child arises in the morning; specimen of tape then applied to microscope slide and brought to laboratory)

Rectoabdominal Examination
  Lithotomy or modified lithotomy position
    Tenderness
    Expression of vaginal discharge
    Palpation of mass or firm foreign body through rectovaginal wall

cotton-tipped thin wired swab into the urethra and gently swirling this for 5 seconds. The first 10 cc of urine can be cultured for *N. gonorrhoeae;* a Gram stain of the urethral discharge revealing gram-negative diplococci within or near leukocytes may also diagnose gonorrhea. If the urethritis is recurrent, specimens for *N. gonorrhoeae, Ureaplasma urealyticum,* herpes simplex virus, *Staphylococcus saprophyticus,* and other bacteria should be obtained. A Gram stain and a normal saline mount to detect *T. vaginalis* should also be performed. Rarely, human papillomavirus causes a urethral infection; cytologic evaluation might be necessary to make this unusual diagnosis.

VAGINAL DISCHARGE

Table 31–9 summarizes the vaginal pool findings in a number of clinical conditions. Vaginal ''clue cells'' (Fig. 31–1) are commonly found in patients with bacterial vaginosis. In general, bacterial culture of vaginal fluid in adolescents is not helpful.

In adolescent females who present with vaginal pruritus, frothy yellow-green (but not purulent) vaginal discharge, a diagnostic test for trichomonads should be performed (Fig. 31–2). A normal saline preparation of vaginal fluid may yield neutrophils and motile trichomonads, and the vaginal pH should be 4.5 or greater and the KOH odor test should be positive.

The female with a mucopurulent vaginal discharge (or a male with a urethral discharge) may have gonorrhea or a chlamydial infection. In females, the ectocervix should be wiped clean of mucus and vaginal secretions. The specimen for *N. gonorrhoeae* should be obtained first by gently swirling a Dacron or cotton-tipped swab in the endocervical canal for 5 seconds. This should be inoculated onto selective media (Thayer-Martin, Martin-Lewis, or New York City) and repeated on the opposite side of the plate after another endocervical specimen is obtained. The culture plate must be placed in a high carbon dioxide environment (e.g., a candle jar or carbon dioxide tablet) and immediately sent to the laboratory. After this is done, the procedure can be repeated but the swab should be placed in a chlamydial transport medium and sent to the laboratory as quickly as possible.

If the discharge resembles cottage cheese and is associated with pruritus or labial erythema, a KOH preparation of the vaginal pool

Table 31–8. Guidelines for Human Immunodeficiency Virus (HIV) Antibody Testing in Adolescents

To Decrease Transmission in Patients Who Are:
  Individuals who consider themselves at risk for HIV infection
  Patients who acquire a sexually transmitted disease
  Intravenous or subcutaneous injecting drug users
  Individuals who report having had multiple sexual partners
  Prostitutes or adolescents who practice ''sex for survival'' or for drugs
  Homeless or runaway adolescents (or who have been in the past)
  Incarcerated adolescents
  Individuals who received a blood transfusion prior to 1985
  Adolescents planning marriage who live in communities with an HIV seroprevalence ≥ 1.0%
  Blood, organ, and semen donors
  Adolescents admitted to hospitals that have a high HIV prevalence (≥1%)
  Male adolescents who have had sexual contact with other males
  Female adolescents who have had sexual contact with bisexual males, hemophiliacs, or other males who are at high risk

To Diagnose in Patients Who Present With:
  Generalized lymphadenopathy
  Unexpected dementia or encephalopathy
  Chronic, unexplained fever, diarrhea, or candidiasis (other than recurrent vulvovaginal candidiasis)
  Unexplained weight loss or wasting syndrome
  Tuberculosis
  Kaposi sarcoma
  Primary lymphoma of the brain
  Generalized herpes virus infection or ulcer persistent for more than 1 month
  Recurrent pneumonia
  Invasive cervical cancer
  Syphilis unresponsive to therapy

Adapted from Centers for Disease Control. Public Health Service guidelines for counseling and antibody testing to prevent HIV infection and AIDS. MMWR 1987; 36:509.

Table 31–9. Vaginal Pool Findings in Common Clinical Conditions

Diagnosis*	Macroscopic Appearance†	Odor	Vaginal pH‡	Normal Saline Mount§	Potassium Hydroxide Mount
Normal	Flocculent, cream-colored	None	≤ 4.5	Normal squames, few PMNs, lactobacilli#	Negative
Candidiasis	Curdy, cream-colored	None	≤ 4.5	Normal squames, few to moderate PMNs, pseudohyphae/buds/mycelia**	Pseudohyphae/buds/mycelia
Trichomoniasis	Bubbly, yellow-green	None to malodorous	≥ 5.0	Many PMNs, motile trichomonads††	Negative
Bacterial vaginosis	Homogeneous, watery, gray	None to fishy‖	> 4.5	Few PMNs, clue cells (≥20% of squames), no or few lactobacilli, preponderance of other bacterial morphotypes	Negative
Cervicitis	Normal to purulent, may be blood-tinged	None to malodorous	Variable	Few to many PMNs	Negative

Adapted from Holmes KK. *In* Holmes KK, Mårdh PA, Sparling PF, Wiesner PJ (eds). Sexually Transmitted Diseases, 2nd ed. New York: McGraw-Hill, 1990:542.

*It is not uncommon for a patient to have more than one infectious diagnosis. For example, trichomoniasis and bacterial vaginosis frequently coexist, and trichomoniasis and a sexually transmitted cervicitis also frequently co-exist. Gonococcal cervicitis is frequently highly inflammatory; the degree of inflammation in chlamydial cervicitis is very variable. Purulent cervical discharge becomes part of the vaginal pool.

†These descriptions are ''classic.'' A ''normal'' macroscopic appearance can be misleading.

‡An elevated vaginal pH is quite sensitive to the presence of an infectious condition, but is nonspecific. *Candida* species prefer an acidic environment. Although a vaginal pH as high as 4.5 is considered normal, it is not uncommon to find motile trichomonads, to meet the other diagnostic clinical criteria for bacterial vaginosis, or to diagnose a sexually transmitted cervicitis (frequently chlamydial) at this pH. Contamination of the vaginal fluid by douching, semen, and cervical secretions can each elevate the pH of the vaginal fluid. pH cannot be determined in the presence of blood.

§Although <5 PMNs per high power field is frequently considered normal, quantification is imprecise because there are no standards for specimen dilution.

‖Fishy amine odor noted or accentuated on addition of 1 drop of 10% potassium hydroxide (KOH).

#A squamous epithelial cell can be diagnosed as a clue cell only if it is in a monolayer and is not folded. To be considered clinically significant, at least 20% (some authorities state 10%) of squames should be clue cells. In bacterial vaginosis, small pleomorphic bacteria and small curved rods are easily visualized at 400× magnification of a normal saline mount. Lactobacilli are uncommon in this condition.

**Pseudohyphae can sometimes be appreciated on the normal saline preparation, but other cellular elements can easily obscure them.

††Flagellar beating or activity should be observed to diagnose trichomoniasis. Trichomonads become less active once cooled below body temperature.

Abbreviation: PMN = polymorphonuclear leukocytes.

should be performed and pseudohyphae should be sought. If the KOH preparation is negative but candidiasis is highly suspected, the vaginal pool should be cultured for *Candida* (Fig. 31–3).

Sexual Abuse

The prevalence of STDs among prepubertal children who are victims of sexual abuse has ranged from 2% to 13%, and the prevalence in adolescent patients is much higher. Children who have evidence of anogenital trauma or a history of oral-genital, genital-genital, anal-genital, or oral-anal contact should be screened for gonorrhea, syphilis, and *Chlamydia*. If no trauma is noted and the child can give an accurate account of the event, screening can be undertaken on a more selective basis. If the perpetrator is known to be at risk for an STD, if the prevalence of STDs in the community is high, if the child is a poor historian, or if the child has symptoms of an STD, appropriate testing should be done. In contrast, the adolescent should always be screened for gonorrhea, syphilis, chlamydial infection, and possibly HIV.

When testing is indicated, the most sensitive and specific tests should be used because the results have profound medicolegal consequences. Patients are evaluated at the time of presentation, 2 weeks after the assault and again at 12 weeks after the assault (Table 31–10).

Diagnosis of the following in prepubertal children requires clini-

cians to report the case as suspected abuse; gonorrhea, syphilis, *Chlamydia*, condylomata acuminata, *Trichomonas*, HSV-1 (unless autoinoculation), and HSV-2. Presumptive treatment of asymptomatic prepubertal children is not recommended.

In contrast, adolescent patients who are sexually assaulted should be evaluated and treated empirically. Therapy includes ceftriaxone, 125 mg IM for 1 dose; doxycycline, 100 mg p.o. b.i.d. for 7 days (or azithromycin, 1 g p.o. for 1 dose); and metronidazole, 2 g p.o. × 1 dose (females only). This regimen does not treat syphilis. HBIG (hepatitis B immune globulin) and the first dose of hepatitis vaccine should be given within 2 weeks of the assault if the patient is unimmunized.

HIV Infection. Children should be screened for HIV in the following circumstances:

- If the perpetrator is known to be HIV-positive or engages in high-risk behavior
- If the child has another STD
- If the child was abused by multiple perpetrators
- If the child lives in an environment with a high HIV prevalence or in which illicit substance use or prostitution may be occurring
- If the parents insist that HIV testing be done

Serum can also be frozen at the time of presentation; this can be

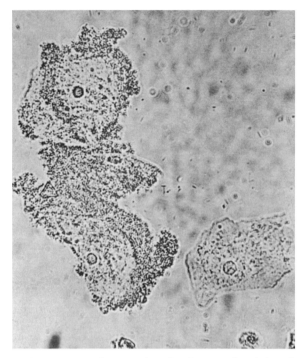

Figure 31–1. Bacteria clinging to the sides of a vaginal epithelia cell ("clue cell") is significant in bacterial vaginosis. (Reproduced by courtesy of Dr. Herman L. Gardner.) (From Huffman JW. Genitourinary infections. *In* Feigin RD, Cherry JD [eds]. Textbook of Pediatric Infectious Diseases, 2nd ed. Philadelphia: WB Saunders, 1992:570.)

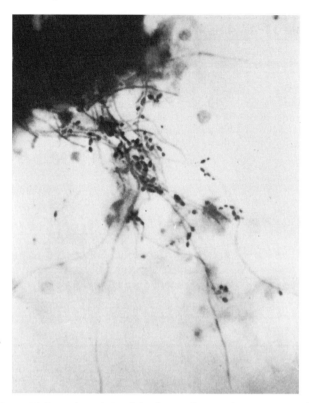

Figure 31–3. Hyphae of *Candida albicans* discovered on wet smear of vaginal discharge. (From Huffman JW. Genitourinary infections. *In* Feigin RD, Cherry JD [eds]. Textbook of Pediatric Infectious Diseases, 2nd ed. Philadelphia: WB Saunders, 1992:564.)

used for future analysis if needed. Follow-up samples should also be obtained 12 weeks and 6 months after the assault.

Syphilis. A standard syphilis test (STS) or Venereal Disease Re-

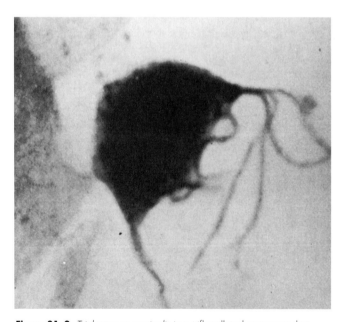

Figure 31–2. *Trichomonas vaginalis* is a triflagellated protozoan that, when motile, is easily identified in wet smears of the vaginal discharge. (From Huffman JW. Genitourinary infections. *In* Feigin RD, Cherry JD [eds]. Textbook of Pediatric Infectious Diseases. Philadelphia: WB Saunders, 1992:568.)

search Laboratory (VDRL) test may be done 12 weeks after the assault. Although nontreponemal tests are always reactive in secondary syphilis, they are nonreactive in 23% to 33% of patients with primary disease. A false-negative result (the prozone phenomenon) can occur if the serum has an extremely high antitreponemal antibody titer. False-positive tests can be a result of *Mycoplasma* and pneumococcal pneumonias, scarlet fever, viral hepatitis, varicella, infectious mononucleosis, IV drug use, pregnancy, or tuberculosis.

The fluorescent treponemal-antibody absorption test (FTA-ABS) is more reliable but remains positive for life. However, false-positive results may occur in Lyme disease and systemic lupus erythematosus (SLE). HIV infection may be associated with unusual serodiagnostic results.

Anogenital Condylomata. In prepubertal children, these are frequently, but not universally, associated with abuse. The long incubation period (2 to 3 months), possible perinatal transmission (up to 20 months of age), and possible autoinoculation or casual spread of cutaneous warts to the anogenital region add to the uncertainty. HPV typing may be of some value.

Systemic Disease

The STDs most often associated with systemic symptoms include HIV, syphilis, Reiter syndrome, herpes simplex, disseminated gonococcemia, and PID (with or without tubo-ovarian abscess).

The adolescent female who presents with acute lower abdominal pain may have appendicitis, an ectopic pregnancy, ovarian cysts (ruptured) or torsion, mesenteric adenitis, pyelonephritis, PID, or a

Table 31-10. Laboratory Evaluation of Children and Adolescents Who Have Been Sexually Abused or Assaulted

Initial Evaluation*
    Normal saline mount of vaginal pool for WBCs, RBCs, trichomonads, clue cells, bacterial morphotypes, and
        sperm
    KOH mount for pseudohyphae/mycelia and blastophores/chlamydospores
    Vaginal pH and KOH odor test†
    Gram stain of any anorectal secretions
    Cultures for *Neisseria gonorrhoeae* and *Chlamydia trachomatis* from all sites of attempted penetration
    Cultures and/or dark field microscopy for lesions resembling syphilis
    Serum samples for syphilis and HIV serology or to preserve for testing later

Follow-up Evaluation 2 Weeks After Assault*
    Repeat examination (cultures are not necessary if patient was treated prophylactically and is asymptomatic
        and vaginal pool is normal or, in the case of a male, no urethral discharge or symptoms are noted)
    Evaluation of vaginal pool as above

Follow-up Evaluation 12 Weeks After Assault*
    STS (VDRL)
    HIV antibody test (if results are positive, test initial serum now)

*Evaluations are based on the premise that the patient sustained an acute assault within several days of the initial evaluation. The protocol should be varied based on the timing of the assault.
    †Fishy amine odor noted or accentuated on addition of 1 drop of 10% KOH.
    Abbreviations: HIV = human immunodeficiency virus; KOH = potassium hydroxide; RBC = red blood cell; STS = serologic test for syphilis; VDRL = Venereal Disease Research Laboratory; WBC = white blood cell.

tubo-ovarian abscess. Although a complete blood count (CBC) with differential is often requested, the results are rarely diagnostic unless hemorrhage has caused anemia. The erythrocyte sedimentation rate (ESR) cannot distinguish most of these entities from one another, but it may be elevated in appendicitis, PID, and tubo-ovarian abscess. In some cases, a pelvic ultrasound study or, less often, compression computed tomography (CT) scans (for appendicitis) may be needed to exclude an ovarian process or ectopic pregnancy (see Chapter 18). A urinary tract infection might be revealed by a urinalysis and culture (see Chapter 27). A pregnancy test should be performed to exclude ectopic pregnancy and to help determine which antibiotics can be used. If PID is suspected, cervical specimens for *N. gonorrhoeae* and *C. trachomatis* should be obtained for culture.

If arthritis, mucocutaneous lesions, lower genital tract inflammation, and conjunctivitis are noted, Reiter syndrome should be suspected. Unfortunately, no laboratory tests are specifically indicative of this disorder. Disseminated gonoccemia may cause fever, rash, arthralgias, and arthritis.

DIAGNOSTIC AND THERAPEUTIC CONSIDERATIONS

Bacterial Vulvovaginitis

Nonsexually transmitted vulvovaginitis in female infants and children is common. In prepubertal girls, the vulvar mucosa is thin and susceptible to inflammation from chemicals and mechanical irritation. Because the labia are not well developed, the vulvar mucosa is not anatomically shielded and is thus vulnerable to irritation. In addition, a girl's hymenal configuration may predispose to vaginitis: a high, small opening may interfere with vaginal drainage, whereas a wide, gaping hymen (e.g., "posterior rim" configuration or following episodes of sexual abuse) permits easy contamination of the vagina by urine and feces.

The most common cause of vulvovaginitis in young girls is a mixed, nonspecific bacterial infection secondary to contamination by urine and feces (in 70% of cases). The usual responsible bacteria are considered to be normal flora: diphtheroids, alpha-hemolytic

streptococci, lactobacilli, and *Escherichia coli*. Other organisms include non-hemolytic streptococci, groups B and D streptococci, beta-hemolytic group A streptococci, *Staphylococcus aureus* and *Staphylococcus epidermidis*, *Klebsiella*, *Pseudomonas*, *Proteus*, and *G. vaginalis*. Anaerobes, *Candida*, *Mycoplasma hominis*, and *U. urealyticum* have also been found. Overgrowth of even normal flora can cause symptomatic vulvovaginitis.

Bloody vaginal discharge in young girls may be caused by *Shigella* or group A streptococcal infections, a foreign body, neoplasm (such as rhabdomyosarcoma), or trauma. Retained toilet paper is a common foreign body. It can usually be flushed out of the vagina with normal saline.

Several vulvar skin disorders can be confused with vulvovaginitis. Lichen sclerosus manifests as white patches on the glabrous skin that are thinned and atrophic and are easily traumatized with resultant bullae (which may be blood-filled) in the vulvar region. Seborrheic dermatitis may present with inflammation and secondary infection of the intertriginous areas; the face and scalp may be involved as well. Labial or vulvar agglutination may be noted and can be secondary to previous vulvovaginitis of unestrogenized epithelia.

Other etiologic factors in premenarchal vulvovaginitis include infection (fungi, pinworms, scabies), irritation (soap, shampoo, detergent), systemic illness (Stevens-Johnson syndrome), and trauma (abuse, play, tight clothing).

Finally, some young girls with emotional or behavioral problems (occasionally caused by sexual abuse) may complain of vulvar symptoms in the absence of any findings on examination. The treatment of vulvovaginitis in prepubertal girls is summarized in Tables 31–11 and 31–12.

Bacterial vaginosis is one of the most common causes of vaginal discharge in adolescents. It is thought to result from the replacement of the normal vaginal flora with organisms such as *G. vaginalis*, *Mycoplasma hominis*, *Mobiluncus* spp., *Bacteroides* spp., and other anaerobes. Bacterial vaginosis may be asymptomatic in almost 50% of females diagnosed with this disorder. Usual symptoms include vaginal odor (49%) and vaginal discharge (50%).

The two strongest clinical signs of bacterial vaginosis are release of a fish odor when vaginal fluid is mixed with a drop of a 10% KOH solution (43%) and presence of clue cells on high power (×400) microscopic examination of a normal saline mount of vaginal fluid (78%). Other signs are a homogeneous white dis-

Table 31–11. Treatment of Nonspecific Vulvovaginitis in Young Girls

Toilet Hygiene
  Wipe in an anterior-to-posterior direction with supervision
  Diaper wipes are useful
  Urinate with knees spread apart

Clothing
  Choose white, cotton underpants
  Wear loose-fitting clothing

Bathing
  Take sitz baths in clear water up to four times a day
  Wash gently with unperfumed soap
  Do not use bubble bath and/or wash hair in bath
  Rinse perineum with clear water, dry gently with towel
  Use a hand-held hair dryer on cool setting to complete drying
  Protect vulvar skin with a bland ointment

Management of Inflammation and Pruritus
  Hydrocortisone cream, 1% applied topically t.i.d.
  Hydroxyzine, 0.5 mg/kg/dose p.o. q.i.d.
       or
  Diphenhydramine, 1 mg/kg/dose p.o. q.i.d.

Antimicrobial Treatment
  See Table 31–12

charge (69%) adherent to the vaginal walls, and a vaginal fluid pH greater than 4.5 (97%). If a patient is found to have clue cells, a positive fish odor test, and a pH higher than 4.5, the chances are virtually 100% that bacterial vaginosis is present. If this is the case, Gram staining is not necessary unless recurrent infections are noted and the organisms need to be characterized (see Table 31–9).

The Centers for Disease Control and Prevention (CDC) recommends that only symptomatic patients be treated (Table 31–13). However, some adolescents may be unaware of their symptoms, leading some authorities to treat all patients with bacterial vaginosis. Partners need not be treated unless the infections are recurrent.

Candidal Vulvovaginitis

Candida is a common microbe that can be isolated from the vagina in 10% to 55% of asymptomatic, healthy women of reproductive age. It is probably a commensal organism that becomes an invasive pathogen under certain circumstances. Increased rates of infection are noted in pregnant females, especially during the third trimester; in oral contraceptive users (the high-dose estrogen pill); in patients with poorly controlled diabetes mellitus; in patients with high-calorie, high-carbohydrate, high-fiber diets; and in patients who are taking corticosteroids or broad-spectrum antibiotics. Most vaginal yeast infections (85% to 90%) are caused by *Candida albicans*. Other candidal species and *Torulopsis glabrata* infections are increasing in frequency.

Acute pruritus and vaginal discharge are the main complaints of symptomatic patients. The discharge may be watery or thick and sometimes resembles cottage cheese. The discharge is odorless. At times, the patient may state that vulvar burning, vaginal soreness, external dysuria, or dyspareunia is present. On examination, the labia can be edematous and erythematous; pustulopapular lesions may exist peripherally. The vaginal mucosa may be erythematous, but the cervix is normal.

If candidiasis is clinically suspected and a normal saline and a KOH preparation of the vaginal discharge do not reveal pseudohy-

phae, mycelia, or blastophores, a specimen for culture may be obtained. Only symptomatic patients should be treated (Table 31–14). Intravaginal prescribed formulations include butoconazole (2% cream for 3 days), clotrimazole (500 mg tablet for 1 dose), miconazole (200-mg suppository for 3 days), ticonazole (6.5% ointment, 5 g × 1) or various formulations of terconazole (see Table 31–14).

Chlamydial Infection

C. trachomatis is the most common sexually transmitted bacterial pathogen in United States adolescents. It causes up to 50% of

Table 31–12. Oral Treatment of Non–Sexually Transmitted Causes of Vulvovaginitis in Prepubertal Females

Group A beta streptococci
  Clindamycin, 8–12 mg/kg/day ÷ t.i.d. or q.i.d. for 10 days
       or
  Penicillin VK, 125–250 mg q.i.d. for 10 days
       or
  Erythromycin, 50 mg/kg/day ÷ t.i.d or q.i.d. for 10 days
       or
  Cephalexin, 25–50 mg/kg/day ÷ t.i.d. or q.i.d. for 10 days

Streptococcus pneumoniae
  Penicillin VK
       or
  Erythromycin
       or
  Cephalexin (see above)

Staphylococcus aureus
  Dicloxacillin, 25 mg/kg/day ÷ q.i.d. for 7–10 days
       or
  Amoxicillin + clavulanate, 40 mg/kg/day (based on amoxicillin) ÷ t.i.d. for 7–10 days
       or
  Cefpodoxime proxetil, 10 mg/kg/day ÷ b.i.d. for 7–10 days
       or
  Cephalexin (see above)
       or
  Clindamycin (see above)
  Cefuroxime, 30 mg/kg/day ÷ b.i.d. for 7–10 days
       or
  Clarithromycin, 15 mg/kg/day ÷ b.i.d. for 7–10 days

Haemophilus influenzae
  Erythromycin ethylsuccinate/sulfisoxazole, 50 mg/kg/day (based on erythromycin) ÷ t.i.d. for 10 days
       or
  Trimethoprim/sulfamethoxazole, 8 mg/kg/day (based on trimethoprim) ÷ b.i.d. for 10 days
       or
  Amoxicillin/clavulanate (see above)
       or
  Clarithromycin (see above)
       or
  Cefixime, 8 mg/kg/day ÷ b.i.d. for 10 days

Shigella
  Trimethoprim/sulfamethoxazole (see above)

Candida
  Fluconazole, 3 mg/kg/day in a single dose for 3–5 days

Enterobius vermicularis
  Mebendazole, 100 mg as a single dose for patient and all household members, then repeated in 2 weeks

Table 31–13. **Treatment of Bacterial Vaginosis**

Nonpregnant Patients
  Metronidazole, 500 mg p.o. b.i.d. × 7 days
or
  2 g p.o. for 1 dose (less effective)
or
  Clindamycin, 300 mg p.o. b.i.d. for 7 days
or
  Clindamycin cream (2%) 5 g (one applicator full) intravaginally
    at bedtime for 7 nights
or
  Metronidazole gel (0.75%) 5 g (one applicator full)
    intravaginally b.i.d. for 5 days

Pregnant Patients (First Trimester)
  Clindamycin cream (2%) 5 g (one applicator full) intravaginally
    at bedtime for 7 nights

Pregnant Patients (Second and Third Trimesters)
  Same recommendations as for nonpregnant patients, but vaginal
    cream or gel is preferred to systemic therapy

Adapted from Centers for Disease Control and Prevention: 1993 Sexually transmitted diseases treatment guidelines. MMWR 1993; 42(RR-14):69.

the cases of nongonococcal urethritis in males. The incubation period is usually 7 to 14 days but may be as long as 35 days. Symptoms in male adolescents may be absent but may include dysuria and urethral discharge. Although these symptoms may eventually resolve, epididymitis and Reiter syndrome may occur later in untreated males.

Female adolescents infected with *C. trachomatis* are frequently asymptomatic. However, because this organism can cause both a urethritis and endocervicitis, some patients may complain of a vaginal discharge, dysuria, or urinary urgency. Some patients have endometritis and present with metrorrhagia or menorrhagia. Salpingitis occurs in some female patients and may result in infertility and ectopic pregnancy. Pelvic examination reveals a mucopurulent discharge from the cervical os, with associated inflammatory changes and friability, in some patients. Perihepatitis may occur (Fitz-Hugh–Curtis syndrome).

For patients suspected of having chlamydial infections and those with suspected gonorrhea, chlamydial specimens should be obtained from the urethra in males and the endocervix in females. In

Table 31–14. **Treatment of Vaginal Candidiasis**

Initial or Infrequent Episodes
  Miconazole or clotrimazole intravaginally for 7 days
or
  Terconazole (Candida tropicalis or Torulopsis glabrata)
    intravaginally for 7 days
or
  Fluconazole, 150 mg p.o. for 1 day

Recurrent Episodes (Three or More per Year)
  Culture organism and treat as above
followed by
  Clotrimazole, 500 mg vaginal tablet intravaginally weekly for
    6 months
or
  Fluconazole, 100 mg p.o. daily for up to 6 months

Adapted from Centers for Disease Control and Prevention: 1993 Sexually transmitted diseases treatment guidelines. MMWR 1993; 42(RR-14):50.
*Terconazole dosing varies: 0.4% cream–5 g for 7 days or 0.8% cream 5 g for 3 days or 80-mg suppository for 3 days.

addition, sexually active males and females should be screened annually.

Infected patients should be treated (Table 31–15), but routine test-of-cure is not universally recommended. However, clinicians should consider more frequent screening of adolescents who have been previously infected.

Gonococcal Infections

Gonorrhea is a disease that must be reported to public health departments; epidemiologic information is therefore readily available. Adolescent females have the highest rate of infection in the United States. Overall, adolescents account for 24% to 30% of all cases of gonorrhea in the United States. In general, gonorrhea in American appears to be a disease of poor urban minority groups with limited access to health care.

N. gonorrhoeae causes a variety of infections. Uncomplicated urogenital infections include urethritis in both male and female adolescents and endocervicitis in females. The incubation period usually ranges from 1 to 14 days. Because the symptoms are nonspecific, gonorrheal infections cannot easily be distinguished from other STDs.

Males usually experience dysuria and a urethral discharge that is initially mucoid. More than 95% of males experience a discharge but are infective prior to the development of symptoms. They eventually become asymptomatic but still remain infective. On physical examination, inflammation of the urethral meatus, variable penile edema, and a urethral discharge can be noted.

Adolescent females frequently have a vaginal discharge and dysuria. Some may experience abnormal uterine bleeding as the organisms ascend to the endometrium. Physical examination may reveal a urethral exudate or a discharge from periurethral glands, the Bartholin duct, and the cervix.

Rectal infections may exist in individuals who practice receptive anal intercourse. Symptoms are variable and may include anal pruritus, a painless mucopurulent rectal discharge, mucus-coated stools, or minimal rectal bleeding. In male patients who have overt proctitis, rectal pain, tenesmus, and secondary constipation may be noted. Physical examination findings may include a perianal discharge and inflammation. In contrast, most female patients with rectal gonorrhea are asymptomatic, as their infections often represent local contamination by a cervicovaginal exudate.

Gonococcal pharyngeal infections are relatively common in the presence of urogenital infection. Although *N. gonorrhoeae* can cause acute pharyngitis and tonsillitis, pharyngeal infections are

Table 31–15. **Antimicrobial Treatment of Uncomplicated** *Chlamydia trachomatis* **Infections**

Recommended Regimens
  Doxycycline, 100 mg p.o. b.i.d. for 7 days (not in pregnancy)
or
  Azithromycin, 1 g p.o. in a single dose

Alternative Regimens
  Ofloxacin, 300 mg p.o. b.i.d. for 7 days (must be > 17 years
    old and not pregnant)
or
  Erythromycin base, 500 mg p.o. q.i.d. for 7 days (recommend
    during pregnancy)
or
  Erythromycin ethylsuccinate, 800 mg p.o. q.i.d. for 7 days

Adapted from Centers for Disease Control and Prevention: 1993 Sexually transmitted diseases treatment guidelines. MMWR 1993; 42(RR-14):50.

largely asymptomatic. Spontaneous resolution in untreated individuals usually occurs within 12 weeks.

Local complications of mucosal urogenital gonococcal infections include epididymitis or proctitis in males. Unilateral scrotal pain or inguinal pain may be noted. In female patients, PID, perihepatitis (Fitz-Hugh–Curtis syndrome) and Bartholin gland abscess formation may occur.

Disseminated gonococcal infection can occur in 0.5% to 3% of patients. Untreated mucosal gonococcal infections can result in a bacteremia and disseminate. This results in acute arthritis (30% to 40%), tenosynovitis (80%), and/or dermatitis (50% to 75%). The skin lesions are usually located on the distal extremities and are usually fewer than 30 (maximum 100) in number. Classically, the lesions are described as tender, necrotic, hemorrhagic pustules on an erythematous base. However, lesions may be in varying stages and may not resemble the classic lesions.

Tenosynovitis and arthralgias occur early, but actual arthritis occurs later. Arthritides are noted in the wrist, metacarpophalangeal, ankle, and knee joints. In general, no more than three joints are involved in any one patient. Fever and elevated white blood cell count are present in 50% to 70% of the patients; a mild chemical hepatitis can also be noted. Individuals with complement deficiency are at a greater risk for recurrent disseminated infections.

In male adolescents, the diagnosis may be made from a urethral culture (or Gram stain) or by sending the first 10 cc of a voided urine for culture. In females, sending two endocervical specimens is the most sensitive technique for accurate diagnosis.

Infected individuals should be treated according to CDC recommendations (Table 31–16). The sexual partner should also be referred for treatment. Patients must receive co-treatment for *C. trachomatis* and should be tested for syphilis. It is thought, but not confirmed, that treatment with ceftriaxone and doxycycline (or erythromycin) may also cure incubating syphilis. If there is a suspicion that the sexual partner will not be treated or if the patient has had frequent infections, more frequent screening should be performed. Hospitalization is required for patients with disseminated disease.

Genital Herpes Simplex Virus Infections

Genital herpes simplex virus infection is the most common cause of genital ulceration in the United States. It has an acute presentation and a recurrent course. HSV is more common in females than males, and approximately 10% of adolescents who have been seen in a family planning clinic had serologic evidence of HSV-2 infection. Most HSV strains isolated from the human genitalia are HSV-2, and most strains isolated from labial, facial, and ocular lesions are HSV-1.

Only 20% to 40% of newly infected individuals report symptoms (asymptomatic primary infection). In general, previous oral-labial HSV-1 infection protects against HSV-2 infection. The initial symptomatic HSV-2 infection usually is painful and more severe than subsequent ones.

The clinical course of primary HSV infection can be divided into three phases.

- In the first phase, vesicles and pustules form within 2 to 12 days of sexual contact (see Table 31–3). They continue to spread over the genital area for a few days before coalescing into large areas of ulceration. Vaginal discharge and dysuria are prominent complaints.
- During the second phase, ulceration occurs and may last for 10 days or more. During this time, systemic constitutional symptoms may occur. These may include fever, headache, backache, malaise, and myalgias; 40% of males and 70% of females are affected. Females usually experience more severe local and systemic disease than males do.
- In the third phase, usually around day 12, local lesions start to heal. Scarring is uncommon. Tender, nonsuppurative inguinal adenopathy develops in the second and third weeks and persists beyond the healing of the mucocutaneous lesions.

HSV-1 and HSV-2 infections from oral-genital contact can result in complaints of a sore throat, which can manifest as an exudative pharyngitis with or without ulceration (see Chapter 6). Tender cervical adenopathy, fever, malaise, headache, and myalgia may be present as well. These symptoms may be similar to streptococcal pharyngitis or Epstein-Barr viral infections.

Symptomatic proctitis from anogenital contact can occur. Symptoms include rectal pain, bloody discharge, urinary retention, local dysesthesia, and impotence. In some patients, fever and other constitutional symptoms are noted.

The most serious complication of primary genital herpes virus in pregnancy is disseminated disease of the newborn. In the adult patient, central nervous system involvement is a potentially serious complication. Meningeal symptoms occur in 36% of women and 13% of men during the initial period of the illness, but hospitalization for aseptic meningitis is rarely needed. Rarely, sacral radiculopathy (urinary retention, obstipation, and sacral anesthesia) or transverse myelitis may occur.

A fairly frequent complication of primary genital herpes infection is the development of nongenital lesions; they are thought to be caused by autoinoculation of virus. This occurs more commonly in women. Disseminated cutaneous and visceral herpetic infection is unusual in immunocompetent individuals, but atopic dermatitis and pregnancy may predispose to dissemination. Hepatitis, pneumonia, thrombocytopenia, and a monoarticular arthritis may occur. HSV can also cause PID by direct extension into the upper genital tract. During the second week of primary HSV infection, vaginal candidiasis develops in about 14% of women.

Recurrent genital herpes is caused by viral reactivation following an asymptomatic period. Within the first year following a primary genital HSV infection, approximately 90% of individuals with HSV-2 and 60% with HSV-1 experience a recurrence. In contrast to the primary infection, the lesions of recurrent infections are usually unilateral (80% to 95%) and involve a much smaller area. The number of lesions is small (five in women and eight in men). Most patients experience pain for 4 to 6 days. Some patients may experience dysuria or tender adenopathy. The mean time to heal is 10 days (maximum 29), and the mean duration of viral shedding

---

Table 31–16. Treatment of Uncomplicated Gonococcal Mucosal Infections in Adolescents

Recommended Regimens
Ceftriaxone, 125 mg IM in a single dose
or
Cefixime, 400 mg p.o. in a single dose
or
Ciprofloxacin, 500 mg p.o. as a single dose (not during pregnancy or nursing or for patients under the age of 18 years)
or
Ofloxacin, 400 mg p.o. as a single dose (see warning for Cipro)
plus
Antimicrobial treatment against *Chlamydia trachomatis* (see Table 31–15)

Alternative Regimen
Spectinomycin, 2 g IM as a single dose (not effective for pharyngeal infection)
plus
Antimicrobial treatment against *C. trachomatis* (see Table 31–15)

Adapted from Centers for Disease Control and Prevention: 1993 Sexually transmitted diseases treatment guidelines. MMWR 1993; 42(RR-14):56.

is 4 days (maximum 20). Asymptomatic shedding may be intermittent and may be responsible for spread of HSV.

Two noninfectious causes of genital ulcers can be confused with HSV infection. Individuals with inflammatory bowel disease have intestinal symptoms, deeper ulcers, and a longer duration of ulcerative lesions. Behçet syndrome may also present with lesions of other mucous membranes as well as central nervous system manifestations. If the clinical diagnosis is not definitive, viral culture of the lesions is recommended (see also Table 31–3 for the differential diagnosis).

HSV is a manageable but not curable chronic disease. Practical therapeutic and management goals include hastening the rate of healing and resolution of symptoms, limiting the frequency and severity of complications, preventing and limiting subsequent clinical recurrences, and decreasing the transmission of HSV infection.

Acyclovir is currently the only recommended treatment for HSV infections in immunocompetent individuals. Acyclovir has demonstrated efficacy in shortening the clinical course and decreasing the frequency of complications in genital infections (primary more significantly than recurrent). Acyclovir also suppresses recurrent episodes; however, it does not eradicate latent virus. Even when given in the acute or primary course of disease, it does not ameliorate the subsequent risk, frequency, or severity of recurrence. Acyclovir does not eliminate viral shedding or the potential for HSV transmission.

Treatment of HSV is summarized in Table 31–17. Acyclovir is not currently recommended for use during pregnancy. Local comfort measures during genital infections may include application with a cotton ball of a diluted Burrows solution and application of topical lidocaine for dysuria.

Patients should be reminded to abstain from sexual activity while lesions are present or during a prodromal period. Condom usage should be encouraged at all times. Information about the risks of neonatal infection must be shared with both male and female adolescents. Female patients should be instructed to inform their obstetric health care provider of the history of HSV infection.

HIV Infection

The biology, natural history, clinical presentation, and management of HIV infection are discussed in Chapter 55. Indications for HIV testing are listed in Table 31–8.

Human Papillomavirus Anogenital Infections

Human papillomavirus (HPV) infections of the anogenital region are considered the most prevalent viral STD. It is thought that 10% to 20% of sexually active individuals are infected with HPV. Most HPV infections are transient; 75% of sexually active individuals may be infected at some point but either never demonstrate clinical evidence of the disease or suppress or lose the infection.

HPV infection can be classified into four categories of disease: latent, acuminate, subclinical, and neoplastic. *Latent infection* is probably the most common type, but patients manifest no symptoms. *Acuminate infection* is the historically classical form and consists of anogenital exophytic condylomas or warts. The warts may be papular or may have finger-like projections. Lesions can coalesce and resemble cauliflowers. In dry areas, such as the penile shaft, lesions may present as keratotic plaques.

In males, HPV can infect the penis, urethra, scrotum, perianal, anal, and rectal areas. In females, the vulvar skin and mucosa, vagina, cervix, perianal area, anus, and rectum can be infected. In general, HPV is a multifocal disease. In women, vestibular and

Table 31–17. Therapy for Genital Herpes Simplex Virus Infections

Initial Clinical Episode
  Acyclovir, 200 mg p.o. 5 times a day for 7–10 days (dose should be doubled in proctitis or in patients who are immunocompromised and have localized disease)
  Acyclovir, 5–10 mg/kg IV q 8 hr for 5–7 days or resolution (for disseminated or systemic disease in patients ill enough to be hospitalized)

Recurrent Episodes*
  Acyclovir 200 mg p.o. 5 times a day for 5 days
            or
  400 mg p.o. 3 times a day for 5 days
            or
  800 mg p.o. 2 times a day for 5 days

Daily Suppressive Therapy†
  Acyclovir, 400 mg p.o. 2 times a day
            or
  200 mg p.o. 3–5 times a day

Adapted from Centers for Disease Control and Prevention. 1993 Sexually transmitted disease treatment guidelines. MMWR 1993;42(RR-14):22.

*Episodic treatment is recommended for patients who have fewer than six episodes per year but who have prolonged or severe recurrences or who have a recognized prodrome preceding lesion development.

†Recommended for patients who have six or more episodes a year or who have human immunodeficiency virus (HIV) infection.

vulvar lesions can cause local burning and pruritus; vaginal lesions can be associated with discharge, pruritus, and postcoital bleeding. Men also experience local pruritus and bleeding of lesions with trauma. Urethral lesions can cause discharge or hematuria.

Subclinical disease is invisible to the eye but is apparent under colposcopic magnification following a 5-minute application of 3% acetic acid. *Neoplastic transformation* of HPV lesions is the most important clinical manifestation of the infection. It is considered a leading cause of cervical carcinoma.

Clinical diagnosis of exophytic condylomas caused by HPV is usually straightforward. However, it is important to distinguish them from the lesions of secondary syphilis (condylomata lata). Condylomata lata are more rounded, and serologic tests for syphilis are strongly positive. A screening STS (VDRL) should be done in a patient who presents with anogenital warts.

The lesions of *molluscum contagiosum* are smooth, firm, dome-shaped, and umbilicated. Rarely, nongenital HPV types can cause warts in the genital region. Although frank neoplasia of the vulva, penis, and anus is extremely rare among adolescents, any atypical lesion or a lesion that responds poorly to treatment should be sampled for biopsy. Routine Papanicolaou (Pap) smears in sexually active women are the most important reason for a decrease in the mortality from cervical cancer. Adolescent girls with an abnormal cervical cytologic or Pap smear should be referred immediately to an experienced gynecologist.

Treatment of HPV infection can range from local therapy for small, exophytic lesions on the external genitalia to ablative therapy in the cervical region. In general, primary care providers should limit therapy to those patients with small lesions on the external genitalia. More extensive lesions; warts in the vaginal, cervical, urethral meatal or anal regions; and complex problems should be referred to more experienced clinicians. Cryotherapy with liquid nitrogen can be applied with a cotton-tipped swab or cryoprobe. A cryoprobe should not be used in the vagina. If a swab is used, apply the liquid nitrogen until the lesion and an area of 10 mm beyond its margins are white. This should be done weekly up to six times. Recurrences are noted in 20% to 40%.

Alternatively, a 0.5% solution of podophyllotoxin (Podofilox) can be used for self-treatment of genital warts that the patient can visualize and easily reach. The solution should be applied twice daily for 3 days, followed by 4 days of no treatment. This cycle can be repeated no more than four times. No more than 0.25 ml of podophyllin should be used per application, and the total area should be less than 10 cm². This therapy is contraindicated during pregnancy. Recurrences are noted in 30% to 60%.

Podophyllin, 10% to 25% in compound tincture of benzoin, can be applied by a health care provider weekly up to six times for an area no larger than 10 cm². The patient should wash the area and remove the chemical within 4 hours. Recurrences are noted in 20% to 60%.

Finally, trichloracetic acid (TCA) (80% to 90%) can be applied by a health care worker directly to the condylomas using a cotton-tipped swab. The adjacent area can be protected by powdering with sodium bicarbonate. This treatment can be repeated weekly up to six times. Recurrences are 36%.

Syphilis

Teenagers account for 10% to 12% of reported cases of syphilis. The rates are highest among black adolescents; syphilis is more common in the southern United States than any other region. The disease is most readily transmitted during sexual contact by organisms living in open lesions of the genital and anal mucosa. Organisms can be transmitted by oral contact. Following inoculation of *T. pallidum,* the incubation period averages 21 days, with a range of 10 to 90 days.

Primary syphilis begins with a papule that progresses to an ulcer over 1 to 3 weeks. More than one lesion can be present. The typical ulcer (chancre) can range in size from 2 to 20 mm, and unless it is secondarily infected, it has a clean base with rounded borders that feel rubbery to palpation. The ulcer is usually painless but can be tender to palpation. The ulcer heals gradually within a few weeks. Almost 50% of patients have bilateral, usually non-tender, nonsuppurative regional lymphadenopathy that can persist for months.

Secondary syphilis represents disseminated infection and develops 6 to 24 weeks following inoculation. Multiple organ systems can be involved, including the skin, lymphatics, gastrointestinal tract, bones, kidneys, eyes, and central nervous system. Most patients have symptoms of fever, malaise, anorexia, weight loss, pharyngitis, laryngitis, arthralgia, and lymphadenopathy. Epitrochlear nodes are suggestive of syphilis. Most patients have a skin rash that manifests as macular, maculopapular, papular, papulosquamous, or, rarely, pustular lesions. Vesicles are not present. The lesions occur on the trunk at first and may be pruritic. Different types of lesions can occur simultaneously. Two thirds of patients have lesions on their palms and soles. Occasional patients may have a temporary patchy alopecia or loss of eyebrows. These closed skin lesions are relatively noninfectious but may persist for months. If a squamous component of the rash is present, it may resemble pityriasis rosea, psoriasis, or lichen planus.

Other types of mucocutaneous lesions are highly infective because they contain large numbers of spirochetes. The plaques of condylomata lata occur in warm, moist intertriginous locations, such as the vulva, scrotum, anal verge, inner thighs, and axillary folds. Mucous patches may occur in the mouth, pharynx, vulva, vagina, cervix, glans penis, and anal canal.

Asymptomatic involvement of the central nervous system can occur in 8% to 40% of patients; cerebrospinal fluid (CSF) demonstrates elevated protein levels and lymphocyte counts. Symptoms of aseptic meningitis develop in only 1% to 2% of patients. Anterior uveitis is rare. Other rare manifestations of secondary syphilis include glomerulonephritis, nephrotic syndrome, hepatitis, arthritis, and periostitis.

Untreated syphilis enters a *latent stage* following resolution of the symptoms and signs of secondary syphilis. During this time, 25% of patients have evidence of an infectious relapse; most of such cases occur within the first year following infection. Tertiary syphilis develops years to decades later.

The diagnosis is made by identifying the organism from exudates or by serologic tests (see Laboratory Testing earlier).

The treatment of primary and secondary syphilis is best achieved with parenteral penicillin G. In primary syphilis, individuals who are HIV-negative and not pregnant may receive a single dose of 2.4 million units of benzathine penicillin G as a single intramuscular injection. If the duration of the disease is not known, this dose is repeated twice more in weekly intervals (7.2 million units total). Single-dose ceftriaxone is not effective.

For nonpregnant, penicillin-allergic patients, doxycycline, 100 mg twice a day for 14 days, may be given. Patients with early syphilis may experience the Jarisch-Herxheimer reaction within the first 24 hours following treatment. This reaction includes acute fever, headache, and myalgias. Sexual partners are treated presumptively for syphilis. Follow-up is necessary for all patients so they can be evaluated clinically and serologically; a fourfold decrease in nontreponemal test titer (VDRL) should occur. HIV testing should also be performed.

Trichomoniasis

Trichomonas vaginalis is a sexually transmitted, unicellular, flagellated, anaerobic protozoan that exists as an extracellular parasite in the human lower genitourinary tract (see Fig. 31–2). It is considered to be the most prevalent nonviral STD in the world. Women appear to be more susceptible and have more acute manifestations. The incubation period ranges from 3 to 28 days. As many as 56% of women have no symptoms, but vaginal discharge, abnormal vaginal odor, vulvar pruritus, dyspareunia, dysuria, and lower abdominal discomfort are the usual findings in women. In males who are symptomatic, urethral discharge has been noted. Vaginal pool findings are summarized in Table 31–9.

All patients with trichomoniasis should be treated. Other STDs should be tested for. The treatment regimen of choice is metronidazole, 2 g orally as a single dose. Partners should also be treated. However, if the male is symptomatic, single-dose regimens fail to cure 40%. The alternative regimen is metronidazole, 500 mg orally twice a day for 7 days. This regimen has a cure rate of 95% in both men and women. If patients are refractory to this regimen, metronidazole, 2 g daily for 3 to 5 days, should be given.

During the first trimester of pregnancy metronidazole is contraindicated. To alleviate symptoms, clotrimazole as 100-mg vaginal suppositories can be used at night for 2 weeks. During the second and third trimesters, a single oral dose of metronidazole may be used.

COMPLICATIONS OF SEXUALLY TRANSMITTED DISEASES

Female Adolescents

PELVIC INFLAMMATORY DISEASE

Pelvic inflammatory disease is a clinical diagnosis that is defined as an infection ascending from the lower female genital tract through the endometrium to the level of the fallopian tubes. It may involve contiguous structures including the ovaries, pelvic peritoneum, and pelvic cavity. It includes endometritis, salpingitis, tubo-ovarian abscess, and pelvic peritonitis. It has a broad clinical spectrum that includes the following presentations: acute, silent, atypical, a residual or chronic syndrome, and postpartum or post-abortal. Unless such a diagnostic procedure as laparoscopy, endometrial biopsy, or ultrasonography is performed, it is difficult to enhance clinical specificity.

PID is common; in 1988, 3% of all female teenagers living in the United States have self-reported a history of PID. PID is important because serious late sequelae can occur in at least 25% of females. Short-term complications include perihepatitis (Fitz-Hugh–Curtis) syndrome, an infection of the liver capsule occurring in 5% to 20% of women) and tubo-ovarian abscess, which affects 7% to 16% of females with PID. Long-term consequences from tubal scarring and occlusion include infertility and ectopic pregnancy. Following PID, a woman's risk of ectopic pregnancy increases sixfold to 10-fold. A third long-term problem after PID is chronic pelvic pain, which affects 12% of women after a single episode.

In 60% to 75% of young women with PID, *C. trachomatis* or *N. gonorrhoeae* is the responsible organism. In addition, a wide variety of anaerobic (*Bacteroides, Peptococcus, Peptostreptococcus*) and facultative aerobic bacteria (*G. vaginalis, Streptococcus* sp., *E. coli, Haemophilus influenzae,* coagulase-negative staphylococci) have been isolated from the fallopian tubes of females with PID. Other bacterial agents have included *M. hominis* and *U. urealyticum.*

Most patients with PID become symptomatic within the first 7 days of a new menstrual cycle. The diagnostic criteria and differential diagnosis of PID are presented in Tables 31–18 and 31–19.

When the diagnosis is suspected, the following laboratory studies should be sent: CBC with differential, ESR or C-reactive protein, urinalysis, and urine culture, cultures for *N. gonorrhoeae* and *C. trachomatis,* a cervical Gram stain, and an STS.

A sensitive pregnancy test should be performed routinely in patients with suspected PID. This will exclude the diagnosis of ectopic pregnancy and guide antibiotic treatment. For patients who are pregnant, inpatient treatment with intravenous antibiotics is recommended by the CDC.

Endometrial biopsy and laparoscopy are usually reserved for when the diagnosis of PID is not completely clear. Endometrial biopsy in minimally invasive, but results take 2 to 3 days. Laparoscopy, the gold standard, is reserved for patients in whom the diagnosis cannot otherwise be made or for patients who are not responding to treatment.

Ultrasonography has an established role in diagnosing a tubo-ovarian abscess in patients with PID. Although routine use is

Table 31–19. Differential Diagnosis of Pelvic Inflammatory Disease

Acute Pain
  Appendicitis
  Ectopic pregnancy
  Adnexal torsion
  Ruptured ovarian cyst
  Pyelonephritis—cystitis
  Psoas—pelvic abscess
  Mesenteric adenitis

Chronic or Recurrent Pain
  Endometriosis
  Pelvic adhesions
  Ovarian cyst
  Chronic intestinal disease (e.g., inflammatory bowel disease)

not recommended, endocervical ultrasonography can help detect uncomplicated PID while pelvic ultrasonography may identify tubo-ovarian abscesses that had not been clinically suspected.

The treatment of PID is summarized in Table 31–20. The CDC suggests hospitalization when the diagnosis is uncertain and problems requiring emergent operative intervention are possible (appendicitis, ectopic pregnancy), when pelvic abscess is suspected, and when the patient is pregnant, has an HIV infection, has a risk of poor compliance, or is severely ill. If nausea and vomiting preclude the use of oral agents, hospitalization is required.

In general, all adolescent patients should be hospitalized for treatment of PID. In addition, if clinical follow-up cannot be ensured, the patient should be admitted for treatment. After treatment is completed, follow-up should occur in 72 hours for those treated as an outpatient and 2 weeks following diagnosis for all patients.

TUBO-OVARIAN ABSCESS

Tubo-ovarian abscess formation is a common complication of PID. The prevalence of tubo-ovarian abscesses during or after PID is 3% to 34%. Although tubo-ovarian abscesses are classically considered to represent the end stage of an upper genital tract sexually transmitted infective process, only 46% of cases are associated with a history of PID. The organisms commonly associated with tubo-ovarian abscesses include *E. coli, Bacteroides fragilis,* other *Bacteroides* species, aerobic streptococci, *Peptococcus,* and *Peptostreptococcus.* In contrast to PID, gonorrheal infection is only rarely reported and there are no reports of *Chlamydia* specimens cultured from tubo-ovarian abscesses.

The symptoms of tubo-ovarian abscesses are similar to those of PID. More than 90% of patients have lower abdominal pain, 60% have fever, and at least 66% have leukocytosis. Patients may appear acutely ill or feel only slightly unwell.

The diagnosis is made by demonstrating an inflammatory adnexal mass. Because examination may be difficult, a pelvic ultrasonography is a useful tool (93% sensitive, 99% specific). Pelvic CT scanning may be helpful if the ultrasound study is not diagnostic.

Patients with tubo-ovarian abscesses can usually be treated medically (75%) and do not require surgical intervention. Abscesses larger than 10 cm in diameter usually necessitate surgical treatment.

Antibiotic regimens recommended by the CDC are similar to the inpatient therapies for PID (Table 31–20). Many clinicians add metronidazole to cefoxitin and doxycycline. However, the minimum duration of parenteral therapy is 7 days. A successful initial clinical response to antimicrobial medical management of a tubo-ovarian abscess is defined as decreased pain, diminished abscess size, defervescence, and a decreased white blood cell count. If a

Table 31–18. Formulating a Diagnosis of Pelvic Inflammatory Disease

Minimal Triad of Physical Examination Findings
  Lower abdominal tenderness
  Adnexal tenderness
  Cervical motion tenderness

*Additional Routine Diagnostic Criteria**
  Oral temperature >38.3°C
  Abnormal cervical or vaginal discharge
  Elevated C-reactive protein or erythrocyte sedimentation rate
  Cervical infection with *Neisseria gonorrhoeae* or *Chlamydia trachomatis*

Elaborate Diagnostic Criteria
  Endometrial biopsy showing endometritis
  Tubo-ovarian abscess on ultrasonography
  Laparoscopic visual confirmation of salpingeal inflammatory changes

*Each additional criterion enhances the specificity of the diagnosis.

Table 31–20. Antimicrobial Treatment of Pelvic Inflammatory Disease*

Inpatient Treatment
(Treat for at least 48 hours after substantial clinical improvement before switching to oral antibiotics)

Regimen A
Either Cefoxitin, 2 g IV q6 hr
                    or
            Cefotetan, 2 g IV q12 hr
                    plus
    Doxycycline, 100 mg IV or p.o. q12 hr, then p.o. b.i.d. for 14 days total

Regimen B
    Gentamicin, 2 mg/kg IV once, then 1.5 mg/kg/dose q8 hr
                    plus
    Clindamycin, 900 mg IV q 8 hr, then 450 mg p.o. q.i.d. for 14 days total

Outpatient Treatment

Regimen A
Either Cefoxitin, 2 g IM
                    plus
        Probenecid, 1 g orally
                    or
    Ceftriaxone, 250 mg IM
                    plus
    Doxycycline, 100 mg p.o. b.i.d. for 14 days

Regimen B
    Ofloxacin, 400 mg p.o. b.i.d. for 14 days
                    plus
Either Clindamycin, 450 mg p.o. q.i.d. for 14 days
                    or
    Metronidazole, 500 mg p.o. b.i.d. for 14 days

*Recommended by the Centers for Disease Control and Prevention, 1993. Metronidazole should not be used in the first trimester of pregnancy; ofloxacin and doxycycline should not be used during pregnancy. Ofloxacin is not recommended for use in patients younger than 18 years of age.

patient does not respond to medical management within 48 to 72 hours, surgical intervention is indicated. If the tubo-ovarian abscess ruptures, immediate operative intervention is mandatory.

Male Adolescents

EPIDIDYMITIS

Epididymitis is an unusual complication of sexually transmitted urethritis. Ascent of *N. gonorrhoeae* or *C. trachomatis* to the epididymis occurs in fewer than 1% of patients. Sexually transmitted epididymitis presents with an abrupt onset of unilateral testicular pain and edema (see Chapter 30).

Treatment must begin at the time of presentation. The recommended regimen consists of ceftriaxone, 250 mg intramuscularly as a single dose followed by doxycycline, 100 mg orally twice a day for 10 days. Teenagers older than 17 years of age may be treated with ofloxacin, 300 mg orally twice a day for 10 days. Bed rest, scrotal elevation, and nonsteroidal anti-inflammatory agents afford symptomatic relief.

Patients should be re-evaluated in 3 days. If significant clinical improvement has not occurred, hospitalization and referral to a urologist may be indicated. Patients who have persistent tenderness and swelling following treatment should be evaluated for tuberculosis, fungal epididymitis, or a neoplasm.

SEXUALLY ACQUIRED REACTIVE ARTHRITIS (REITER SYNDROME)

The risk of an aseptic, reactive arthritis following a bacterial sexually transmitted urethritis is estimated to be 1% to 3%. Among adolescents and adults hospitalized with acute, nontraumatic arthritis, 11% to 13% were given the diagnosis of Reiter syndrome, 33% to 52% had a disseminated gonococcal infection, and 7% to 13% had a non–sexually transmitted septic arthritis. The etiology is poorly understood. Individuals with HLA-B27 haplotype are overrepresented in patients with Reiter syndrome. At least 50% of patients affected have evidence of active *C. trachomatis* infection, whereas 10% have gonorrhea. Gastrointestinal infections with *Shigella, Salmonella, Yersinia,* and *Campylobacter* can also be associated with the development of Reiter syndrome.

The four clinical elements of Reiter syndrome include acute arthritis, lower genital tract infection, conjunctivitis, and mucocutaneous lesions. Not all manifestations may be present initially but may develop over time. Symptoms usually begin within 4 weeks of a sexually transmitted urethritis or gastrointestinal infection. In 80% of cases, the arthritis is polyarticular and may involve more than four joints. Tendon insertion sites, such as the Achilles tendon and plantar fascia (25%), are commonly involved. The arthritis typically starts in the distal weight-bearing joints, including the knees, ankles, and metatarsophalangeal joints. Over the following 2 to 3 weeks, more joints are affected. Almost 50% of the patients have low back pain; sacroiliitis is found radiographically in 5% to 10% of patients. A fusiform dactylitis of a toe or finger (''sausage'' appearance) occurs in 17% of patients.

Ocular manifestations develop in almost half of the patients. Conjunctivitis is most common. Anterior uveitis may occur in 12% of patients. A variety of subtle, painless mucocutaneous lesions can be present initially or may develop over time. Circinate balanitis can be noted in up to 40% of males; it may assume a serpiginous appearance in uncircumcised males or may develop into hyperkeratotic papules in circumcised males. In almost 30% of patients, asymptomatic shallow ulcers of the oropharyngeal mucosa develop. Some skin and nail lesions may even resemble psoriasis.

Patients with Reiter syndrome are frequently systemically ill with malaise, fever, anorexia, and weight loss. In addition, they may have nonspecific electrocardiographic abnormalities as well as atrioventricular conduction disturbances (a prolonged PR interval). Serious but quite rare complications include pericarditis, myocarditis, complete heart block, acute aortitis, peripheral neuropathy, meningoencephalitis, pleuritis, pneumonitis, thrombophlebitis, and amyloidosis.

The clinical course is variable. Approximately two thirds of patients achieve clinical resolution of an initial episode in 3 to 5 months. However, 15% to 30% of patients may have persistence of symptoms for more than a year. More than 50% of patients will experience at least one recurrence of symptoms over several years. About 16% of patients may develop destructive joint disease or spondylitis; crippling foot deformities develop in 5% to 10% of patients.

Reiter syndrome is a clinical diagnosis, and no specific laboratory tests are helpful. Treatment consists of ensuring that the infectious process is cured with antibiotics; anti-inflammatory agents are used to treat the other symptoms.

URETHRITIS: PERSISTENT OR RECURRENT

If the patient has complied with antibiotic treatment for *N. gonorrhoeae* and *C. trachomatis,* recurrent or persistent urethritis

Table 31–21. Red Flags and Things Not to Miss

Diagnosis of More Than One Sexually Transmitted Disease in the Same Patient
If patient is diagnosed with syphilis, gonorrhea or human immunodeficiency virus
If patient reports engaging in unprotected sex with multiple partners
If patient is immunocompromised
If patient has a history of sexually transmitted diseases in the past

Abdominal Pain in a Female Adolescent
Pelvic inflammatory disease
Tubo-ovarian abscess
Ectopic pregnancy
Appendicitis
Ovarian cyst

Fever, Rash, Malaise, Arthalgia
Disseminated gonococcemia
Reiter syndrome
HIV

Pregnancy
Treatment of Partners
Asymptomatic Cervicitis or Urethritis

is unusual. If this does occur, the patient may have engaged in unprotected sexual contact or his partners may not have received appropriate evaluation and treatment. Urethritis is present if at least 5 polymorphonuclear leukocytes per $1000\times$ oil-immersion field are noted. *U. urealyticum, T. vaginalis, S. saprophyticus,* herpes simplex virus, or human papillomavirus infection may be present. Although unusual in adolescents, an infected prostate could continue to serve as a source of recurrent or persistent urethritis.

Microscopy should be performed on the urethral specimen, and cultures for *N. gonorrhoeae* and *C. trachomatis,* should be requested. A normal saline mount should be performed to search for *T. vaginalis.* Alternatively, examining the centrifuged sediment from the first 10 cc of a freshly voided urine sample may reveal the organism.

If poor compliance or re-infection is diagnosed, the patient should be treated with the original regimen. If the patient has not completed the course of doxycycline or erythromycin, a single dose of azithromycin in addition to single-dose treatment of *N. gonorrhoeae* should be considered. Trichomoniasis should be treated with metronidazole. If the patient has been truly compliant and reports sexual abstinence, he should receive a 14-day course of erythromycin if he had been previously treated with doxycycline. If the patient had received erythromycin, 14 days of doxycycline are then in order. It is not known how effectively azithromycin cures urethritis caused by *U. urealyticum.*

RED FLAGS

Red flags are presented in Table 31–21.

REFERENCES

Gonococcal Infections

Hook EW, Handshield H. Gonococcal infections in the adult. *In* Holmes KK, Mårdh PA, Parling PF, et al (eds). Sexually Transmitted Diseases, 2nd ed. New York: McGraw-Hill Information Services, 1990:149–165.

Judson FN. Gonorrhea. Med Clin North Am 1990;74:1353–1366.
Webster LA, Berman SM, Greenspan JR. Surveillance for gonorrhea and primary and secondary syphilis among adolescents, United States: 1981–91. CDC Surveillance Summaries, August 13, 1993. MMWR 1993; 42(No. SS-3):1–11.

Herpes Simplex Virus

Centers for Disease Control and Prevention. 1993 sexually transmitted diseases treatment guidelines. MMWR 1993;42(No. RR-14):22–26.
Mertz GJ. Epidemiology of genital herpes infections. Infect Dis Clin North Am 1993;7:825–839.

Human Immunodeficiency Virus (HIV)

American College of Physicians and Infectious Diseases Society of America. Human immunodeficiency virus (HIV) infection. Ann Intern Med 1994;120:310–319.
Boyer CB, Kegeles SM. AIDS risk and prevention among adolescents. Soc Sci Med 1991;33:11–23.

Pelvic Inflammatory Disease

Centers for Disease Control. Pelvic inflammatory disease: Guidelines for prevention and management. MMWR 1991;40(No. RR-5)1–25.
McCormack WM. Pelvic inflammatory disease. N Engl J Med 1994; 330:115–119.
Weström LV, Berger GS. Consequences of pelvic inflammatory disease. *In* Berger GS, Weström LV (eds). Pelvic Inflammatory Disease. New York: Raven Press, Ltd., 1992:79.

STDs and Vaginal Infections in Adolescents and Children Who Have Been Sexually Assaulted

Adams JA, Harper K, Knudson S. A proposed system for the classification of anogenital findings in children with suspected sexual abuse. Adolesc Pediatr Gynecol 1992;5:73–75.
American Academy of Pediatrics, Committee on Abuse and Neglect. Guidelines for the evaluation of sexual abuse in children. Pediatrics 1991; 87:254–260.
Bays J, Chadwick D. Medical diagnosis of the sexually abused child. Child Abuse Neglect 1993;17:91–110.
Estreich S, Forster GE, Robinson A. Sexually transmitted diseases in rape victims. Genitourin Med 1990;66:433–438.
Finkel MA, DeJong AR: Medical findings in child sexual abuse. *In* Reece RM (ed). Child Abuse: Medical Diagnosis and Management. Philadelphia: Lea & Febiger, 1994.
Glaser JB, Hammerschlag MR, McCormack WM. Sexually transmitted diseases in victims of sexual assault. N Engl J Med 1986;315:625–629.

Syphilis

Chiu MJ, Radolph JD. Syphilis. *In* Hoeprich PD, Jordan MC, Ronald AR (eds). Infectious Diseases (5th ed). Philadelphia: JB Lippincott, 1994;694–714.
Hook EW III, Marra CM. Acquired syphilis in adults. N Engl J Med 1992;326:1060–1069.

Vulvovaginal Infections in Young Girls and Adolescents

Chacko MR, Woods CR. Gynecologic infections in childhood and adolescence. *In* Feigin RD, Cherry JD (eds). Textbook of Pediatric Infectious Diseases, 3rd ed. Vol 1. Philadelphia: WB Saunders, 1992:507–517.

Eschenbach DA, Hillier S, Critchlow C, et al. Diagnosis and clinical manifestations of bacterial vaginosis. Am J Obstet Gynecol 1988; 158:819–828.

Heine P, McGregor JA. *Trichomonas vaginalis*: A reemerging pathogen. Clin Obstet Gynecol 1993;36:137–144.

Horowitz BJ, Giaquinta D, Ito S. Evolving pathogens in vulvovaginal candidiasis: Implications for patient care. J Clin Pharmacol 1992;32:248–255.

Krieger JH, Jenny C, Verdon M, et al. Clinical manifestations of trichomoniasis in men. Ann Intern Med 1993;118:844–849.

32 Menstrual Problems and Vaginal Bleeding

Marjorie Greenfield

Abnormal vaginal bleeding (Table 32–1) is a common problem reported by adolescents. The severity can range from a minor inconvenience to a medical emergency. Ninety-five percent of abnormal bleeding in adolescents is dysfunctional uterine bleeding (DUB). The term "dysfunctional" denotes abnormal bleeding without discernible pelvic pathology; such bleeding is usually caused by a hormonal abnormality. The history, physical examination, and possibly a few blood tests should rule out most other causes of bleeding and allow appropriate management of DUB.

THE OVULATORY MENSTRUAL CYCLE

Hypothalamus

Gonadotropin-releasing hormone (GnRH), a decapeptide secreted in pulses from the hypothalamus, is transported down a portal system to the pituitary. Under normal circumstances, the pulsatile secretion of GnRH from the hypothalamus allows secretion of follicle-stimulating hormone (FSH) and luteinizing hormone (LH) but has only a permissive effect and is not involved in regulation of their blood levels. Factors that interfere with hypothalamic function can reduce production of FSH and LH.

Pituitary

Pituitary gland production of FSH and LH responds to negative feedback of circulating estrogen. There is also a positive feedback mechanism that causes increasing LH when estrogen levels rise

sharply midcycle, producing the "LH surge" (Fig. 32–1). In adolescents, the positive feedback mechanism and LH surge are the last parts of the system to mature.

Ovary

FOLLICULAR PHASE

The ovary controls the menstrual cycle. When estrogen and progesterone levels decline and a menstrual period begins, the pituitary, released from negative feedback inhibition, begins to secrete FSH, stimulating the development of new ovarian follicles. As the dominant follicle emerges, it produces great amounts of estrogen. This rapid rise in estrogen leads to the LH surge; the LH surge triggers ovulation. Estrogen levels do not rise to the level that triggers positive feedback until the follicle is ready for ovulation; the follicle itself controls the timing of ovulation.

LUTEAL PHASE

After ovulation, the follicle becomes a corpus luteum, a factory for progesterone synthesis. After 14 days, if conception has not occurred, the corpus luteum ceases its function, estrogen and progesterone levels decline, and menstruation begins as a result of withdrawal of hormonal support to the endometrial lining. If pregnancy were to occur, chorionic gonadotropin (hCG) from the conceptus would stimulate the corpus luteum to continue producing progesterone.

Endometrium

HISTOLOGIC CHANGES THROUGH THE CYCLE

The characteristic sequence of hormonal changes during the menstrual cycle leads to a synchronous response of the endometrium. Estrogen, in the first half of the cycle, causes the *proliferative phase*, characterized by endometrial growth and thickening.

Table 32–1. Normal and Abnormal Menses

Normal cycle (adolescent): bleeding every 21–40 days for 2–8 days
Normal cycle (adult, ovulatory): bleeding every 21–35 days for 3–7 days
Menorrhagia: prolonged or excessive regular periods
Menometrorrhagia: heavy, irregular periods
Oligomenorrhea: infrequent periods
Intermenstrual bleeding: bleeding between regular menstrual periods
Dysfunctional uterine bleeding: abnormal uterine bleeding not due to local uterine pathology; cause usually hormonal

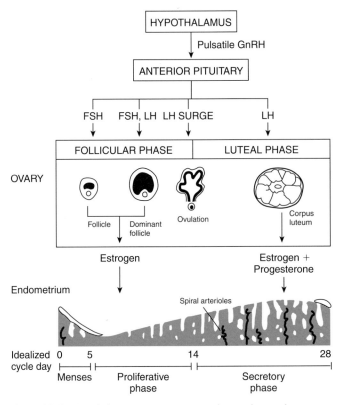

Figure 32–1. Hypothalamic-pituitary-ovarian endometrial axis: changes over time. FSH = follicle-stimulating hormone; GnRH = gonadotropin-releasing hormone; LH = luteinizing hormone. (Adapted from Nesse R. Managing abnormal vaginal bleeding. Postgrad Med 1991; 89:207.)

Progesterone, in the second half of the cycle, causes the *secretory phase*—differentiation of an already estrogenized endometrium, readying it for implantation of a conceptus.

NORMAL CONTROL OF MENSTRUAL BLEEDING

Menstruation occurs when a sequence of hormonally determined events in the endometrium leads to an organized sloughing of the endometrial surface. As estrogen and progesterone levels decline, the spiral arterioles spasm in rhythmic waves and the surface of the endometrium becomes ischemic. As the surface weakens, it loses its integrity, allowing menstrual blood to escape. Thrombin and platelet plugs limit blood loss (see Chapter 51). The superficial endometrium collapses and is shed. Menstrual flow stops as a result of synchronized vasoconstriction, tissue collapse, vascular stasis (clotting of blood in exposed vessels), and estrogen-induced "healing." The self-limited character of menstrual bleeding thus depends on adequate clotting mechanisms and normal ovulatory hormonal events. This becomes important in the attempt to understand causes of abnormal menstrual bleeding.

UTERINE BLEEDING IN THE ADOLESCENT

Normal Adolescent Cycles

Normal adolescent menstrual cycles are not necessarily the same as normal ovulatory adult cycles (see Table 32–1). Among 99 girls

aged 13 to 16 who were evaluated by serial serum progesterone levels, only 33% of cycles in females who were menstruating for less than 1½ yr were ovulatory. Even 5 years from menarche, only 80% of the cycles were ovulatory. This anovulatory state is believed to be due to immaturity of the hypothalamic-pituitary-ovarian (HPO) axis, since the positive feedback mechanism for the LH surge is not yet functional. Anovulatory cycles are, therefore, the norm for young adolescents.

The normal cycle in a teenager is light to moderate bleeding lasting 2 to 8 days every 21 to 40 days. The best explanation for the cyclicity of bleeding in normal but anovulatory adolescents is that although the positive feedback mechanism of ovulation is not developed, there is negative feedback of estrogen on pituitary FSH. As estrogen levels rise, FSH decreases, causing the ovarian follicles to stop producing estrogen. The withdrawal of hormonal support causes the endometrium to slough, an "estrogen withdrawal bleed." As the inhibition of the pituitary is released, FSH increases and the ovarian production of estrogen resumes. This allows for regular "menses" in the anovulatory adolescent. The bleeding is not quite as controlled and consistent as the cycles of estrogen-progesterone withdrawal bleeding in an ovulatory female, but the decline in estrogen levels is effective at decreasing the thickness of the uterine lining enough so that bleeding is not excessive. This pattern, interspersed with occasional ovulatory cycles, appears to control bleeding adequately in most teenagers.

Abnormal Adolescent Menstrual Cycles: Dysfunctional Uterine Bleeding

Problems develop when the negative feedback does not occur and estrogen levels stay constant. Because hormone levels do not decline to allow a withdrawal bleed, a normal cyclic menstrual pattern is not seen. Constant levels of circulating estrogen stimulate the uterine lining to become abnormally thick and unstable. As dyssynchronous breakdown in the endometrial structure occurs, bleeding can be heavy and unpredictable, lasting days to months and leading to hemodynamic instability and anemia. This classic description of severe dysfunctional bleeding may or may not be superimposed on a pattern of oligomenorrhea or amenorrhea.

Developing a Differential Diagnosis

Dysfunctional bleeding presenting as heavy irregular menses is the most common type of abnormal vaginal bleeding in teenagers. Other patterns of bleeding suggest other diagnoses (Table 32–2). Normal menses followed by intermenstrual bleeding may indicate a structural process, such as endometrial polyps or cervicitis, in which the bleeding is not controlled by the hormonal environment. Normal menses with bleeding after intercourse can be from a vaginal or cervical lesion. Dark, possibly foul-smelling blood following the normal menstrual period suggests an obstructed uterine horn or hemivagina with slow leaking of sequestered blood through a fistulous tract. A detailed menstrual history can give clues toward the diagnosis.

In addition to the menstrual history, a sexual history, medical history, review of systems, pelvic examination with a Papanicolaou (Pap) smear and urine pregnancy test are necessary to identify the site and etiology of bleeding (Figs. 32–2 to 32–5). Additional testing is determined by the emerging differential diagnosis (Table 32–3).

Text continued on page 465

Table 32–2. Differential Diagnosis of Abnormal Vaginal Bleeding in Adolescents

	Bleeding Pattern			Evaluation	Treatment
	MR	MMR	IB	**Suggestive Finding:** *Diagnostic Finding*	
Source: Uterus				*Common Causes*	
Anovulation	+	+		No extrauterine source of bleeding seen on examination *Responds appropriately to treatment*	See Table 32–5
Coagulopathy	+			More commonly found in cases of severe bleeding especially if onset at menarche. Family hx, ROS suggestive of clotting disorder; ecchymoses, petechiae seen on exam *Abnormal PT, PTT, platelet count or bleeding time*	Treat coagulopathy; oral contraceptives may help with menorrhagia; complete menstrual suppression sometimes required. See also Chapter 51.
Complication of pregnancy		+		History of late period; pregnancy symptoms (nausea, breast tenderness) *Positive urine or blood pregnanacy test*	See Figure 32–6
Source: Vagina				*Uncommon Causes*	
Injury			+	History *Visible laceration*	Surgical or topical hemostasis, suture or allow to heal by secondary intention
Foreign body (e.g., retained tampon or contraceptive sponge)			+	History, foul discharge *Visible foreign body*	Removal
Cancer			+	Lesion seen, ± abnormal cytology *Biopsy*	Referral to specialist; therapy chosen by type and stage of tumor
Source: Cervix				*Less Common Causes*	
Neoplasia Dysplasia/carcinoma			+	Bleeding point on cervix; abnormal cytology *Colposcopy with directed biopsies*	LEEP, laser, cryotherapy or cone biopsy
Cervical polyp			+	*Polyp seen*	Grasp with clamp or ring forceps and twirl off polyp in office; send specimen to pathologist
Hemangioma			+	Lesion seen	Conservative versus excision or ablation
Infection (cervicitis) (see Chapter 31)					
Herpes			+	Cervical vesicles ± ulceration, ± pelvic pain, tenderness; Pap smear sometimes shows multinucleated giant cells *Culture positive for herpes*	Consider oral acyclovir, if early in primary infection, 200 mg 5× per day × 10 days
HPV			+	Flat or raised warts seen on cervix *Pap smear + colposcopy necessary to differentiate from dysplasia*	Laser, LEEP, cryotherapy, trichloroacetic acid or 5-fluorouracil cream after Pap smear and colposcopy
Chlamydia	±		+	Mucopurulent cervicitis; bleeding may be endocervical *Culture, ELISA, IFA, or DNA probe positive*	Tetracycline, 500 mg p.o. q.i.d., or doxycycline, 100 mg p.o. b.i.d. for 7 days (see current CDC guidelines); partner must be treated
Gonorrhea	±		+	Cervicitis, yellow discharge *Culture, ELISA, or DNA probe—positive*	Ceftriaxone, 250 mg IM, plus empiric treatment for *Chlamydia* (see current CDC guidelines); partner must be treated
Trichomonas			+	Friable inflamed cervix; yellow-green vaginal discharge, pH 7–8 *Saline prep: motile flagellates*	Metronidazole, 2 g p.o. × 1 for patient and sexual partner

Table 32–2. **Differential Diagnosis of Abnormal Vaginal Bleeding in Adolescents** *Continued*

	Bleeding Pattern			Evaluation	Treatment
	MR	*MMR*	*IB*	**Suggestive Finding:** *Diagnostic Finding*	**Treatment**
Source: Uterus				*Less Common Causes*	
Neoplasia Fibroid	±		±	± Enlarged uterus on examination; palpable fibroids *Abnormal findings on ultrasound, and/or hysteroscopy*	PGSI sometimes helpful for menorrhagia; myomectomy via hysteroscope, laparoscope, or laparotomy may be needed
Endometrial polyps			+	History of spotting superimposed on normal menstrual cycle *Hysteroscopy and/or D&C*	D&C
Malignant uterine tumor		±	±	Abnormal Pap smear, enlarged uterus, tissue at cervical os. *Biopsy*	Surgery determined by stage
Ovarian tumor producing estrogen (bleeding is uterine)		+		Adnexal mass on examination or ultrasound *Surgical diagnosis and staging*	Surgery
Foreign body IUD	+		+	No other cause of bleeding (patient ovulatory, not pregnant, no PID) *IUD in uterus; responds to therapy*	PGSI sometimes useful for menorrhagia; removal if PID coexists or if necessary to control bleeding
Infection PID	+		+	Tender uterus and adnexae; purulent cervical discharge ± ↑ WBC or ESR or fever *Clinical diagnosis, tests often positive for gonorrhea, chlamydia*	CDC guidelines (see Chapter 31)
Postpartum or postabortal endometritis ± retained products of conception		+		± ↑ WBC, ESR, fever *Recent pregnancy; tender uterus*	D&C if retained tissue seen on sonogram; broad-spectrum antibiotics, methergine
Congenital partially obstructed hemivagina or uterine horn			+	Foul, dark blood after menses *Abnormal pelvic examination and/or pelvic ultrasound*	Refer for surgical treatment

Abbreviations: CDC = Centers for Disease Control and Prevention; D&C = dilation and curettage; DNA = deoxyribonucleic acid; ELISA = enzyme-linked immunosorbent assay; ESR = erythrocyte sedimentation rate; IB = intermenstrual bleeding; IFA = immune fluorescent antibody; IUD = intrauterine device; LEEP = loop electroexcisional procedure; MR = menorrhagia; MMR = menometrorrhagia; Pap = Papanicolaou; PID = pelvic inflammatory disease; PGSI = prostaglandin synthetase inhibitor (nonsteroidal anti-inflammatory agent); PT = prothrombin time; PTT = partial thromboplastin time; WBC = white blood cell.

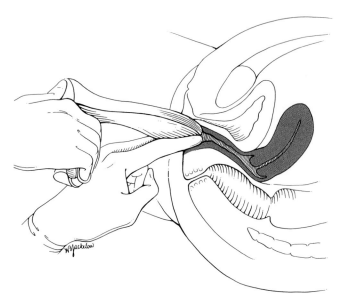

Figure 32–2. Cross-section of the speculum examination. The Huffman vaginal speculum is essential for examining adolescents. With blades 1.5 cm wide and 11 cm long, it is narrow enough to be tolerated by a virginal adolescent and also deep enough to reach the cervix. With one hand (usually the dominant hand), the examiner separates the labia minora and visualizes the introitis. The speculum is then inserted at an oblique angle. (From Swartz MH. Textbook of Physical Diagnosis: History and Examination. Philadelphia: WB Saunders, 1989:400.)

Figure 32–3. Cross-section illustrating the position of the speculum during inspection of the cervix with the speculum. The examiner fully inserts the speculum before opening the blades. *Top,* The angle of insertion is about 45 degrees to the examining table. As the blades are opened, the speculum is carefully maneuvered so that the cervix is fully seen. *Bottom,* The thumb lever is then locked in place. (From Swartz MH. Textbook of Physical Diagnosis: History and Examination. Philadelphia: WB Saunders, 1989:401.)

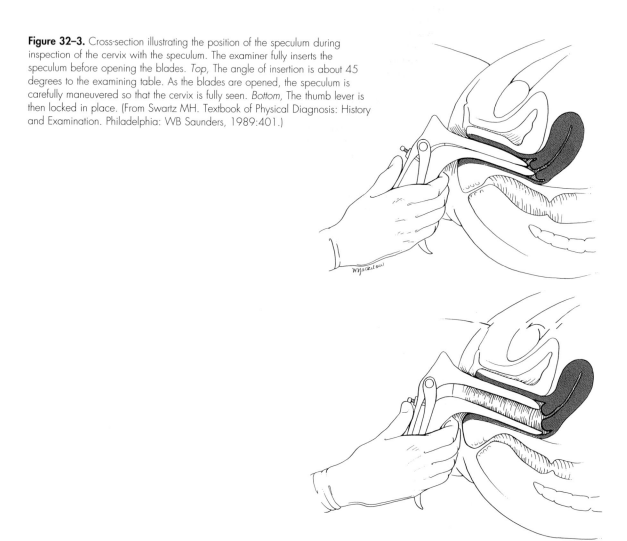

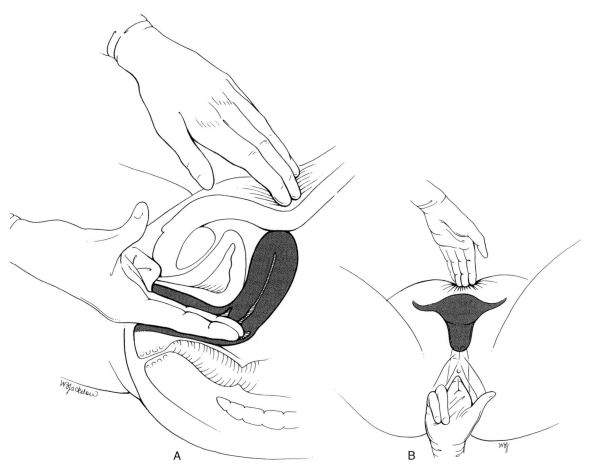

Figure 32–4. The bimanual examination. Palpation of the uterus is performed with one or two fingers of the examiner's dominant hand inside the vagina, with the other hand on the lower abdomen. As the uterus is trapped between the examining hands, pressure with the abdominal hand causes the cervix to move against the inside finger(s), giving the examiner an appreciation of the uterine size, shape, configuration, mobility, and tenderness. An empty bladder facilitates the examination. By pressing the vaginal examining finger(s) into the lateral fornix anteriorly, superiorly and laterally and pressing on the abdomen such that the vaginal and abdominal fingers try to appose, the examiner can palpate the adnexal structures as they move between the examining hands. This gives an appreciation of adnexal size, shape, mobility, and tenderness. A rectoabdominal examination may also be used to assess the uterus or adnexa if a vaginal examination is not tolerated. *A*, Cross-section through the pelvic organs. *B*, Position of the uterus between the examining hands. (From Swartz MH. Textbook of Physical Diagnosis: History and Examination. Philadelphia: WB Saunders, 1989:405.)

Figure 32–5. Obtaining smear for the Pap test. Notice that the longer end of the wooden spatula is placed in the cervical os. (From Swartz MH. Textbook of Physical Diagnosis: History and Examination. Philadelphia: WB Saunders, 1989:403.)

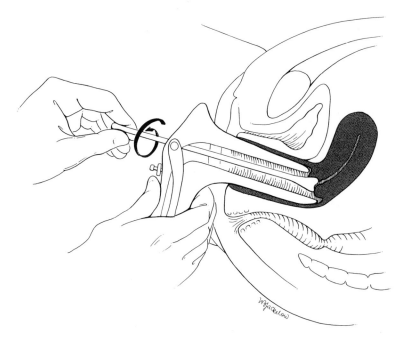

Table 32–3. Diagnostic Approach to Abnormal Uterine Bleeding in Adolescence

Evaluation Method	Comments	When Needed
History		
Menstrual	Last menstrual period, pattern of cycles, recent change, molimina (i.e., premenstrual symptoms) dysmenorrhea	Always
Medical	Pelvic pain, fever, vaginal discharge, coagulopathy, endocrine problems, major illness	Always
Sexual	History of sexual intercourse (including most recent date), birth control used, history of abnormal Pap smear or sexually transmitted infection	Always
Social	Stress, eating disorder, exercise, drugs, alcohol abuse, domestic violence	Always
Medications	Anticoagulants, hormones, drugs with endocrine or coagulation effects	Always
Family history	Clotting disorders, endocrinopathies	Always
Physical Examination		
General	Weight	Always
	Body habitus, hirsutism, Tanner stage	
	Stigmata of endocrine or coagulation disorders	
	Signs of trauma	
Pelvic	To assess source of bleeding and possible cause	Always
External genitalia, vagina, cervix	Cervix and vaginal walls can usually be visualized with a narrow Huffman speculum, even in a young virginal adolescent	
Uterus, adnexa	By rectoabdominal examination if bimanual examination not tolerated	
Rectovaginal or rectoabdominal		
Tests		
Pregnancy test	If urine test results are negative and suspicion is high, check serum hCG	Always, if sexual contact is a possibility
Hemoglobin or hematocrit	With or without retic count, iron studies, ferritin	If bleeding is heavy or objective quantification is desired*
Clotting studies	Platelet count, PT, PTT, bleeding time	In menorrhagia at first period, severe bleeding, family history or personal history of coagulopathy, or failure to respond to treatment
Blood type and screen	Treat Rh-negative teenagers who miscarry with RhoGAM	If pregnant or hemodynamically compromised
Gonorrhea and chlamydial probes	Specimen can be obtained during examination; discarded if results rule out suspicion of infection	If any chance of sexually transmitted infection
Pelvic ultrasound		If bimanual examination results are abnormal or if there is suspicion of congenital anomaly
Hysteroscopy/endometrial sampling		If bleeding is superimposed on normal ovulatory cycles *and* no extrauterine bleeding site is apparent; or if bleeding does not respond to hormonal therapy and coagulation studies and pregnancy test are negative
Heme in urine, heme in stool		If bleeding site is not apparent

*Patient's assessment of menstrual blood loss is notoriously inaccurate. Even pad counts can vary tremendously between women with similar blood loss, although six to eight pads or tampons per day is considered the upper limit of normal. Hematologic parameters can be objective measures of severity of bleeding.

Abbreviations: hCG = human chorionic gonadotropin; PT = prothrombin time; PTT = partial thromboplastin time.

Common Causes of Abnormal Uterine Bleeding

ANOVULATION

The chronic anovulation associated with heavy irregular bleeding poses a problem. In contrast to the cyclical changes in estrogen levels seen with "normal" anovulatory cycles in teens, problematic bleeding is a result of chronic anovulation associated with a steady state of estrogen, FSH, and LH. Constant levels of estrogen provide constant stimulation of endometrial growth and can lead to hemorrhage, anemia, infertility, and endometrial cancer. Only 50% of patients will revert to regular cycles by 4 years after presentation.

COAGULOPATHY

In one study of 56 nonpregnant adolescent girls *admitted* to the hospital for menorrhagia, 19% had coagulopathies. As the severity of the menorrhagia increased, coagulation problems were more likely to be diagnosed. Severe anemia, requirement for transfusion, and hemorrhage at first menses each conferred an even greater chance of finding coagulopathy.

Idiopathic thrombocytopenia purpura, von Willebrand disease, and less often thrombocytopenia caused by systemic disease, such as leukemia, can present with menorrhagia (see Chapter 51). Screening for coagulopathy with a platelet count, prothrombin time (PT), partial thromboplastin time (PTT), and bleeding time is usually adequate. Bleeding time, although inconvenient to obtain, identifies patients with platelet function abnormalities, including some with von Willebrand disease, who have a normal PT and PTT and normal platelet counts.

BLEEDING AND HORMONAL CONTRACEPTIVES

Abnormal bleeding during the first few months of low-dose oral contraceptive (OC) use is common and can be managed with reassurance if pregnancy is not suspected. Bleeding usually normalizes within three to four cycles. Prolonged use of combination estrogen-progesterone oral contraceptives, progestin-only oral contraceptives ("mini-pill"), and injectable or implantable progestin contraceptives may lead to decidualization and atrophy of the endometrium. This thin uterine lining may bleed unpredictably. Endometrial atrophy is best treated with supplemental estrogen, which thickens and stabilizes the uterine lining. Conjugated equine estrogens (e.g., Premarin), 2.5 mg, or ethinyl estradiol, 20 mg taken daily with the oral contraceptive for 7 days, should regulate bleeding for many cycles afterward, but they may need to be taken again months later if the problem recurs. If estrogen supplementation is not successful, other causes of bleeding should be considered.

ILLNESS AND MEDICATION

Medications and illnesses that cause abnormal uterine bleeding do so by their effects on coagulation or on the hormonal milieu (Table 32–4).

Chronic illnesses such as diabetes, cystic fibrosis, and sickle cell anemia can lead to anovulation. Such diseases have the short-term and long-term risks of unopposed estrogen exposure. If the patient's medical condition cannot be improved, cyclic progestins or oral

Table 32–4. Medications That Can Cause Abnormal Uterine Bleeding

Hormonal Effects
  Estrogens: oral estrogens, estrogen patch
  Progestins: oral progestins, progestin-only "mini-pill," injectable or implantable progestin
  Estrogen/progestin: combination oral contraceptives
  Androgens: anabolic steroids, danazol
  Prolactin: many drugs raise prolactin levels, including estrogens, phenothiazines tricyclic antidepressants, benzodiazepines, metaclopromide, and other drugs that deplete dopamine levels or block dopamine receptors

Anticoagulant Effects
  Warfarin, heparin
  Aspirin, other prostaglandin synthetase inhibitors
  Chemotherapeutic agents that result in thrombocytopenia

contraceptives should be considered if there are not contraindications (Table 32–5).

PREGNANCY COMPLICATIONS

Pregnancy can present with abnormal bleeding that may or may not be preceded by an episode of amenorrhea. Particularly abnormal pregnancies, such as ectopic pregnancies or those about to end in miscarriage, may present with abnormal bleeding without a "missed period." The urinary human chorionic gonadotropin (hCG) pregnancy tests used commonly today are positive in 98% of patients with ectopic pregnancies. Highly dilute urine may yield false-negative results. A negative serum hCG level essentially rules out the possibility that abnormal bleeding is caused by a complication of pregnancy (Fig. 32–6).

Table 32–5. Management of Dysfunctional Bleeding

Mild (Hg ≥ 11 mg/dl)
  Reassurance
  Menstrual calendar
  Iron supplementation
  Periodic re-evaluation—2–3 months

Moderate (Hg 9–11 mg/dl)
  Actively bleeding: hormonal hemostasis—oral estrogen protocol,* then as below
  Not actively bleeding: iron supplementation, regulate cycles with cyclic progestins† or oral contraceptives‡ for 3–6 months, then re-evaluate

Severe (Hg ≤ 8 mg/dl or hemodynamically unstable)
  Not actively bleeding: transfusion if necessary, then as for moderate DUB
  Actively bleeding: transfusion/fluid replacement, hormonal hemostasis IV. or oral estrogen protocol, D&C if unable to stop bleeding with IV estrogen, then same as moderate DUB

*See Table 32–7.
†Medroxyprogesterone acetate (Provera) 10 mg/day for 12 days each month.
‡Any 30- to 35-μg estrogen pill.
Abbreviations: D&C = dilation and curettage; DUB = dysfunctional uterine bleeding; Hg = hemoglobin; IV = intravenous.

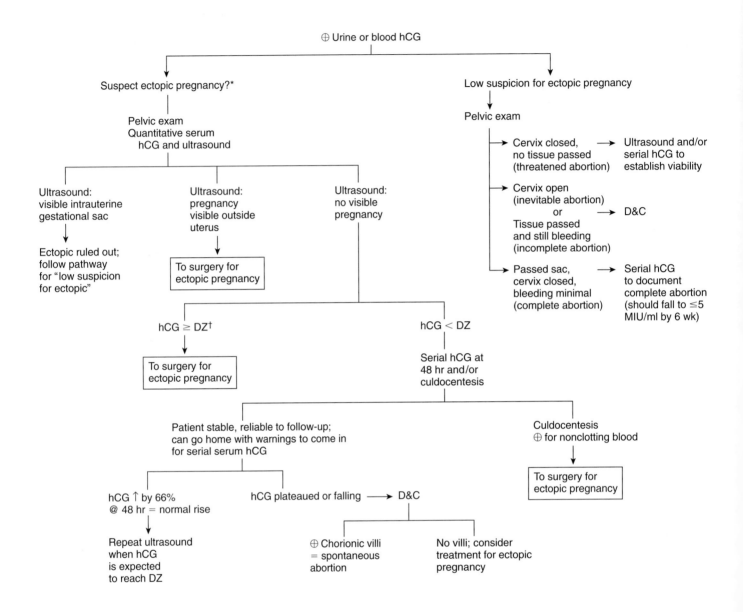

*Patient with pelvic/abdominal pain or risk factors (prior ectopic, prior tubal surgery, prior pelvic inflammatory disease, prior gonorrhea or chlamydial infection, chronic pelvic pain). If ruptured tubal pregnancy suspected (e.g., hemodynamic instability with pelvic pain), may take patient to surgery with only positive pregnancy test or positive culdocentesis.

†DZ (discriminatory zone) is the hCG value at which a normal pregnancy would be expected to be visible on ultrasound. Vaginal probe scanning, which visualizes a pregnancy a few days earlier than abdominal scan, has a lower DZ. Each institution should assess its own DZ based on ultrasound technology and the type of hCG test used. According to the 2nd International Reference Preparation, the DZ for vaginal probe ultrasound is usually ≤ 1500 MIU/ml; DZ for abdominal sonogram it is about 6000 MIU/ml.

Figure 32–6. Evaluation of abnormal bleeding in pregnancy. DZ = discriminatory zone; D & C = dilation and curettage; hCG = human chorionic gonadotropin.

MANAGEMENT OF ABNORMAL BLEEDING
(see Table 32–5)

Acute Management

Treatment and evaluation of severe abnormal bleeding are usually begun simultaneously. The first step is to rule out pregnancy. The urine test can be used to triage the patient; a negative blood hCG level effectively rules out pregnancy. Hemodynamic stability is assessed. Replacement of blood and fluids is used as needed; it is helpful to complete relevant blood work (complete blood count, PT, PTT, bleeding time) before a blood transfusion is started. If the acute bleeding is due to a coagulopathy, it is best controlled by addressing the underlying problem (see Chapter 51). Most patients with bleeding severe enough to require hospitalization are anovulatory. Both estrogens and progestins have been used to stop acute anovulatory bleeding; few studies are available to compare their effectiveness (Table 32–6).

Prevention of Recurrence and Long-Term Follow-Up

Once the initial bleeding is controlled, or if the patient with moderate/severe bleeding is not actively bleeding at presentation, therapeutic goals include prophylaxis against recurrence, prevention of the long-term sequelae of unopposed estrogen stimulation to the endometrium, and treatment of anemia. Although the underlying cause of chronic anovulation may not be found, a basic work-up should be done (see amenorrhea next).

To prevent recurrence of bleeding, cyclic progestins or oral contraceptives are used for 3 to 6 months. This decreases the thickness of the uterine lining and allows for orderly estrogen-progestin withdrawal bleeds. Because the uterine lining is usually quite thick at the onset of treatment, the first progestin withdrawal period may be quite severe but should not last longer than 1 week. This should be explained to the patient so that the heaviness of the next period is not viewed as failure of treatment. As the endometrial height diminishes with each succeeding menstrual period, bleeding should become lighter.

For the teenager who does not need contraception, after 3 to 6 months it is acceptable to discontinue treatment and observe the patient for development of ovulatory cycles. Of the females who have severe dysfunctional bleeding, 50% will have long-term problems with chronic anovulation and its associated risks of recurrent hemorrhage and uterine cancer. Therefore, a few months after treatment is stopped, the clinician should review the patient's menstrual calendar and document ovulation. Prospective documentation of premenstrual symptoms (breast tenderness) or a luteal phase serum progesterone level or a basal body temperature chart is adequate for documenting ovulation (Table 32–7). If the patient remains anovulatory, cyclic progestin or oral contraceptive treatment should be reinstituted to prevent recurrent abnormal bleeding and to diminish the long-term risk of endometrial carcinoma.

In the adolescent who needs contraception, it is best to continue oral contraceptives. There is no evidence that even long-term oral contraceptive use has any effect on the menstrual cycle within 1 year of discontinuance. Females who are anovulatory before using oral contraceptives, however, may well continue to be anovulatory after the pills are stopped.

Failure of anovulatory bleeding to respond to hormonal treatment is an indication to re-evaluate the cause.

AMENORRHEA

Amenorrhea or absence of menstrual periods is a symptom, not a diagnosis. Causes can be grouped into two categories: (1) end-organ or outflow tract anomalies and (2) inadequate hormonal stimulation to the endometrium.

Primary amenorrhea is defined as no menstrual period by age 16

Table 32–6. Medications to Stop Acute Anovulatory Bleeding

Medication	Dose	Comments
Estrogens		Usually causes nausea
IV conjugated equine estrogens (Premarin)*	25 mg IV q 4 hr Maximum 4 doses	One published study only; study showed effectiveness at stopping acute bleeding from many causes
Conjugated equine estrogens (Premarin)*	2.5 mg p.o. q 6 hr for 5 days	
Combination Estrogens/Progestins		May cause nausea, progestin side effects (see below)
High-dose oral contraceptive pills	50 μg estrogen pill q.i.d. for 5–7 days	Outpatient method that provides estrogen and progestin
Progestins		
Medroxyprogesterone acetate (Provera)	10–20 mg p.o. qd bid × 12 days	No comparison studies versus estrogen or oral contraceptives; theoretically less effective if bleeding has been prolonged and endometrial basalis layer is exposed because progestins only "organize" an already estrogenized proliferative endometrium; side effects of progestins are similar to normal premenstrual symptoms: breast tenderness, depression, bloating, water retention
Norethindrone acetate (Norlutate, Aygestin)	5–10 mg p.o. b.i.d. for 12 days	
Megesterol	40–120 mg/day	

*Must be immediately followed by 12–21 days of progestin dominant therapy. Usually oral contraceptives, although medroxyprogesterone acetate, 10 mg, can be used.

Table 32–7. Differentiating Ovulatory from Anovulatory Menstrual Cycles

	Ovulatory	Anovulatory
Menses	There is regularity of interval, flow, and duration, usually 28 ± 7 days lasting 3–7 days	Variable flow, duration, and interval
Dysmenorrhea	Possibly cramps with bleeding†	No cramps or cramps only with passing clot
Molimina* (premenstrual cramps)	Possibly breast tenderness,† fluid retention, abdominal bloating, mood disturbance	None
Mittelschmerz	Possibly midcycle unilateral pelvic pain	None
Basal body temperature (BBT)	Biphasic basal body temperature, taken each day, usually before rising in A.M.	Monophasic basal body temperature
Serum progesterone	High serum progesterone 1–12 days before menses (5 ng/ml)	Serum progesterone ≤1 ng/ml 1–12 days before bleeding

*Best documented prospectively and/or correlated with BBT.
†Presence of these signs in a reliable historian strongly suggests ovulatory cycles.

years or no menses in the absence of signs of puberty by age 13 years. Secondary amenorrhea denotes 3 to 6 months without menstrual bleeding in a previously menstruating female. The evaluation is driven by patient needs and concerns, not necessarily by definitions. A 16-year-old with 8 weeks of amenorrhea may need a pregnancy test. A 10-year-old with stigmata of Turner syndrome need not wait until age 13 for a diagnosis.

Certain processes can only cause primary amenorrhea, such as imperforate hymen or müllerian agenesis (absent uterus). Other processes can cause amenorrhea at any time, depending on when the disease process occurs. For example, if anorexia nervosa develops before menarche, it can cause primary amenorrhea with or without pubertal delay. If it develops later, it may cause secondary amenorrhea.

Congenital anatomic conditions that cause only primary amenorrhea will be suspected by the initial history and physical. Once these few specific diagnoses are ruled out, primary and secondary amenorrhea are evaluated similarly.

Overview of Processes That Lead to Amenorrhea

Causes of amenorrhea may be divided into compartments: end-organ and outflow tract, and then three compartments that lead to inadequate hormonal stimulation to the endometrium: the ovary, the pituitary, and the hypothalamus. The history, physical examination, and a few simple tests can usually identify which compartment has led to the problem. In teenagers, end-organ and outflow tract conditions are most likely congenital, presenting as primary amenorrhea with normal secondary sexual development. Once these are ruled out, the general evaluation for amenorrhea can begin.

Congenital Causes of Primary Amenorrhea in Adolescents with Normal Secondary Sexual Development
(Table 32–8)

OBSTRUCTION TO MENSTRUAL OUTFLOW

Congenital conditions, such as imperforate hymen, transverse vaginal septum, and (rarely) cervical anomalies, can obstruct menstrual outflow. The diagnosis is suspected when cyclic pain and abnormal anatomy are found. A mass (hematocolpos and/or hematometria) may be palpable.

INABILITY OF THE ENDOMETRIUM TO RESPOND TO HORMONAL STIMULATION

Absence of the uterus or, rarely, absence or severe scarring of the endometrium can cause amenorrhea. The most common diagnosis in this category is *müllerian agenesis* with absence of the uterus and proximal vagina. A less common cause is *androgen insensitivity syndrome* (see Chapter 33).

Müllerian Agenesis

Müllerian agenesis, also known as *Mayer-Rokitansky-Küster-Hauser* syndrome, is associated with urinary tract and skeletal anomalies. These females have normal gonadal function and completely normal secondary sexual development. Cyclic abdominal pain, if present, is *Mittelschmerz* (ovulation pain). The vagina is usually a dimple or small in-pouching for which a procedure is needed later in life to allow sexual intercourse. These individuals cannot become pregnant, but with assisted reproductive technology they can provide eggs that can be fertilized with the male partner's sperm and gestated in a surrogate.

Androgen Insensitivity Syndrome

Androgen insensitivity syndrome (AI), formerly known as *testicular feminization*, occurs in phenotypic females who are chromosomally XY and lack androgen receptors. In complete AI, the external genitalia appear female and the vagina is very shallow. The müllerian and wolffian duct systems are absent. At puberty, breasts develop as a result of gonadal estrogens. Axillary and pubic hair are absent. Malignant transformation of intra-abdominal testes can occur, usually after age 25 years. Currently, gonadectomy is recommended after puberty to allow smooth secondary sexual development and prevent the majority of tumors.

Explaining the Diagnosis

The diagnosis of müllerian agenesis or androgen insensitivity can be psychologically traumatic. Just as she is forming her identity

Table 32-8. Congenital Anatomic Causes of Primary Amenorrhea with Normal Breast Development‡

Diagnosis	Müllerian Agenesis	Androgen Insensitivity (AI)	Transverse Vaginal Septum	Imperforate Hymen
Patients with primary amenorrhea*	1:4000 females 15%	1%	3%	1%
Patients with primary amenorrhea and apparent obstruction or absence of vagina*	75%	5%	15%	5%
Chromosomes†	46,XX	46,XY	46,XX	46,XX
Gonads	Ovaries	Testes	Ovaries	Ovaries
Serum testosterone†	Normal female	Normal male (high)	Normal female	Normal female
Vagina	Absent or shallow	Absent or shallow	Obstructed by septum which may be thick or thin, high or low	Obstructed by thin membrane, which may look blue from hematocolpos
Axillary/pubic hair	+	Unless AI is incomplete	+	+
Cyclic pain	±	−	+	+
Uterus	Absent	Absent	Present	Present
Mass	−	−	+ Can present with acute urinary retention as hematocolpos mass obstructs urethra	+ Can present with acute urinary retention
Introitus bulges with Valsalva maneuver	−	−	−	+
Associated anomalies	Urinary tract and skeletal	Inguinal hernias; gonadal malignancy in adulthood	15%; major urinary tract abnormalities	Possibly some increase in urinary tract abnormalities
Treatment	Vaginal dilation or surgical neovagina	Gonadectomy after age 16–18 Vaginal dilation or surgical neovagina	Surgical approach depends on extent and location of septum; may be extensive; should be done as soon as possible	Excision of hymen as soon as possible; diagnostic needle aspiration contraindicated because of risk of infection
Fertility	Advanced reproductive technology required; *in vitro* fertilization, surrogate with uterus to gestate pregnancy	Not fertile	Variable, low septa better prognosis than high septa	Usually fertile

*Data from Reindollar RH.
†Sometimes useful in differentiating Müllerian agenesis from androgen insensitivity.
‡Cervix not visible on pelvic examination. Short vagina; may be absent or obstructed.

as a woman, she discovers she is ''not normal'' and cannot achieve the milestone of menarche. At the same time, she learns of impediments to reproduction and to sexual intercourse. Explanation to the patient that her vagina did not form completely and needs a procedure to help deepen it can give her words for her condition which she can use when she chooses to tell others about it. A multidisciplinary approach with counseling and, if possible, group support or contact with an older female who has been through treatment can be helpful.

Causes of Amenorrhea in Adolescents with Normal Anatomy

Inadequate hormonal stimulation to the endometrium is the most common cause of both secondary amenorrhea and of pubertal delay. There are three general situations that fall under this heading:

- Chronic anovulation
- Hypogonadotropic hypoestrogenism
- Ovarian failure (hypergonadotropic hypoestrogenism)

ANOVULATION

In females with chronic anovulation, the ovary makes estrogen but ovulation does not occur. Since there is no ovulation, there is no cyclic elevation of progestins and there is no progestin withdrawal bleeding. Obesity, stress, hypothyroidism, and hyperprolactinemia can all lead to chronic anovulation. Nonetheless, a cause is usually not found.

Polycystic ovarian syndrome (PCO) is an end result of chronic anovulation. Patients with PCO may have cystic ovaries, hirsutism, obesity, and amenorrhea or dysfunctional bleeding. Insulin resistance (hyperglycemia, frank diabetes) and acanthosis nigricans are sometimes observed. PCO is best considered part of a spectrum of presentations of chronic anovulation. Patients with PCO should be treated as anovulatory. If hirsutism is present, it is evaluated with attention to ruling out the rare case of late-onset congenital adrenal hyperplasia, Cushing syndrome, and tumor of the ovary or adrenal (Fig. 32–7) (see p. 472).

HYPOGONADISM

Ovarian Failure

In patients with hypergonadotropic hypogonadism, FSH and LH levels are in the menopausal range because the ovaries do not make estrogen, which would otherwise provide negative feedback. This ovarian failure may be due to gonadal dysgenesis or the ovaries may appear normal. *Gonadal dysgenesis* is associated with Turner syndrome and other X chromosome deletions and mosaics (see Chapter 33). Some females with Turner syndrome are chromosomally XY/XO mosaic and require gonadectomy at the time of diagnosis to prevent malignant transformation of the gonad. Because of this risk, karyotype must be obtained on all adolescents with unexplained ovarian failure to evaluate for the presence of Y chromosomal material. Other less common causes of ovarian failure include autoimmune oophoritis, galactosemia, and exposure to cytotoxic chemotherapy or radiation therapy. Some ovarian failure is idiopathic.

Hypothalamic Amenorrhea

Another low-estrogen condition is hypogonadotropic hypogonadism. The pituitary, hypothalamus, or both are not appropriately cycling to allow stimulation of the ovary to produce estrogen. FSH and LH levels in these cases are low or normal. This is the situation found in exercise-induced amenorrhea, in anorexia nervosa, and also sometimes in association with hypothyroidism or hyperprolactinemia. Intracranial tumors, such as craniopharyngioma and prolactinoma, can also lead to this condition.

SPECIAL CONSIDERATIONS: AMENORRHEA RELATED TO HORMONAL CONTRACEPTIVES

Amenorrhea that occurs while a person is taking birth control pills or long-acting implantable or injectable progestins is caused by the progestin-dominant hormonal environment provided to the endometrium and by suppression of ovulation. As long as pregnancy has been ruled out, further work-up is generally not necessary. The endometrium in these cases is decidualized and atrophic. Short-term additional estrogen for females taking combination birth control pills usually leads to resumption of menses. Conditions such as eating disorders and stress do not play a role in creating amenorrhea in a female receiving hormone therapy because the hormonal environment is already provided to the endometrium.

Menstrual cycles are expected to revert to normal by 6 months after discontinuance of oral contraceptive pills and by 12 months after the last medroxyprogesterone (Depo-Provera) injection. Beyond that point, evaluation for amenorrhea is indicated.

Evaluation of the Amenorrheic Adolescent

The evaluation for amenorrhea (Table 32–9) is rarely an emergency. An organized history and physical examination with cau-

---

Table 32–9. General Work-up for Amenorrhea in Females with Normal Anatomy and Some Secondary Sexual Development

Visit 1

From History and Physical Examination

1. Some secondary sexual development (for pubertal delay, see Chapter 61)
2. Patent vagina
3. Cervix seen or palpated
4. Uterus palpated or visualized by ultrasonography

Suspect Inadequate Hormonal Stimulation to Endometrium

1. Assess estrogen status, prolactin, and thyroid function
   a. Serum PRL, thyroid-stimulating hormone (TSH)
   b. Serum follicle-stimulating hormone (FSH) if hypoestrogenic state is suspected
   c. For assessment of estrogen status, perform progestin challenge

Schedule Next Visit in 3–4 Weeks

Visit 2

Review Results of PRL and TSH

1. ↑ PRL (or any galactorrhea) requires evaluation for pituitary adenoma. Most cost-effective is coned-down x-ray of the sella turcica. If this is abnormal or if PRL ≥100 ng/mL, CT or MRI is needed to check for pituitary tumor. Many medications can lead to elevation of PRL (see Table 32–4). Any elevation of PRL can lead to ovulatory dysfunction
2. ↑ TSH requires assessment of free T_4. If hypothyroid, thyroid hormone replacement may completely resolve ovulatory dysfunction
3. Even if PRL or TSH levels are abnormal, continue work-up to identify where the patient falls in the spectrum of ovulatory dysfunction (see Fig. 32–7)

Review of Response to Progestin Challenge

1. Was there menstruation-like bleeding?
2. Follow flowsheet to identify hormonal state of the patient (see Fig. 32–7).
3. Remainder of care plan depends on the hormonal state (normal versus low estrogen) and on the compartment that has caused the problem

Abbreviations: CT = computed tomography; MRI = magnetic resonance imaging; PRL = prolactin.

---

tious use of auxiliary tests can usually identify the general category in which the patient fits. Within that category, serious medical conditions can be ruled out before treatment is initiated. Even when there is an obvious predisposing factor, such as intense competitive exercise, the protocol should be followed to allow precise identification of the current hormone state and to rule out serious coinciding conditions.

HISTORY

The patient history should cover general health, including any immediate problems at the time of her birth, major illness, chronic illness, and exposure to chemotherapy or pelvic or central nervous system (CNS) radiation therapy. Pubertal milestones are identified. Eating habits, emotional stress, exercise, sexual activity, birth control method, use of drugs and medications, and any change in weight must be addressed. Review of systems can identify sex hormonal abnormalities, including hirsutism, hot flashes, presence of cyclic abdominal pain, and/or premenstrual symptoms. Is there a breast discharge suggestive of a prolactinoma? Are there symptoms of any other hormonal syndrome, such as hypothyroidism? (See Chapter 50.) Are there any symptoms that might suggest an intracranial tumor, such as significant headaches and visual disturbance?

THE PHYSICAL EXAMINATION

General appearance, pulse, and blood pressure should be noted. Vital signs may be depressed in anorexia nervosa and other starvation states. Weight and height should be plotted on a growth chart. Secondary sexual characteristics may be undeveloped (delayed puberty), normal, or abnormal (hirsutism). Tanner staging (see Chapter 61), observation for evidence of hirsutism or virilization, nipple expression to check for galactorrhea, and palpation of the thyroid are performed. The abdomen should be examined to identify a pelvic mass, which may indicate hematocolpos or pregnancy.

On pelvic examination, external genitalia should be observed for estrogen effect. Are the tissues pink, moist and full, or red, thin and atrophic? Is the vagina patent? Vaginal smear, processed like a Pap smear, can be assessed by the cytologist for estrogen status. Is the cervix visible or at least palpable?

On bimanual examination, if the uterus is palpable, is it normal in size or prepubertal? Are the ovaries palpable? If the digital examination and speculum examination are not tolerated, the vagina can be probed with a swab to determine its length.

On rectovaginal or rectoabdominal examination, are there any masses consistent with hematometria or hematocolpos? If there is evidence of an obstructed or absent vagina, a rectoabdominal examination can be done to check for a mass and identify the uterus if present. Ultrasonography is helpful in corroborating the physical examination.

In females without pubertal development, estrogen levels are low. Visualization of the cervix in these cases is not as important as it is in the pubertal adolescent with delayed menarche because abnormal anatomy is rarely found. The cause of the delay is almost always hypothalamic, pituitary, or ovarian. In the postpubertal girl, if the physical examination demonstrates normal female external genitalia and a patent vagina with visualization or palpation of the cervix, the work-up can then progress to the general evaluation for amenorrhea. The cause is usually in the HPO axis.

Evaluation of the HPO Axis

LABORATORY STUDIES AND THE PROGESTIN CHALLENGE (see Fig. 32–7)

After the history and physical, the examiner should assess for hypothyroidism and prolactinoma with serum thyroid-stimulating hormone (TSH) and prolactin. At the same time, an assessment of the estrogen status of the patient is performed. Because single blood estrogen levels are unreliable, physiologic testing is done by progestin challenge. Progestins cause bleeding only if the endometrium is in a proliferative state from prior estrogen exposure. The progestin challenge test is positive if menstruation-like bleeding occurs within 2 weeks of treatment with 5 days of 10 mg of oral medroxyprogesterone acetate (MPA) or one dose of 150 mg of intramuscular progesterone in oil.*

PROGESTIN CHALLENGE RESULTS

If bleeding occurs after the progestin challenge, there is a functional uterus and outflow tract. The amount of bleeding is roughly proportional to the amount and duration of prior estrogen exposure. If bleeding is similar to a menstrual period, the patient falls into the category of chronic anovulation with an estrogenized endometrium.

Failure of the progestin challenge to lead to menstruation-like bleeding indicates a low-estrogen state or the inability of the uterus to demonstrate bleeding. If there is a question that the patient may have been pregnant for a few days at the time of the progestin challenge, the pregnancy test should be repeated 2 weeks later. If the pelvic findings are entirely normal and the patient has no historical risk factors for Asherman syndrome,† she falls into the category of hypogonadism (hypoestrogenic amenorrhea.) If there is any question of the ability of the uterus to bleed, progestin withdrawal should be repeated after priming the endometrium with estrogen.

THINGS NOT TO MISS

The examiner must never forget that the most common cause of amenorrhea in the general population is pregnancy. One needs to obtain a private history, engender the patient's confidence, and provide confidentiality if requested. When the diagnosis is in doubt, a pregnancy test should be conducted even if the patient does not admit to sexual activity. Commercially available urine pregnancy tests turn positive around the time of the first missed period. Rarely, patients with abnormal pregnancies (ectopic and those about to abort) have hCG levels too low to detect in the urine. A blood hCG level is diagnostic.

Treatment of Amenorrhea

END-ORGAN AND OUTFLOW TRACT ANOMALIES

In all cases of outflow obstruction, it is important to allow menstrual blood to escape, as failure to do so can lead to severe endometriosis and scarring of the reproductive organs. The procedure may be as simple as hymenotomy, or it may involve complicated vaginal and cervical reconstruction. All efforts should be made to preserve reproductive function.

If the uterus is absent, as in müllerian agenesis and androgen insensitivity syndrome, treatment is aimed at creating adequate vaginal depth for satisfactory sexual intercourse once that is desired. These procedures are best held off until the patient is mature and motivated, since they bring with them the demand that she take responsibility for ongoing dilation of her vagina. The presence of a Y chromosome, as in androgen insensitivity, requires surgical gonadectomy. Estrogen replacement therapy is then necessary.

HORMONAL CAUSES OF AMENORRHEA

If the underlying cause is identified, such as hypothyroidism, obesity, or an eating disorder, treatment should be aimed at the

---

*Progesterone in oil is safe to give if the pregnancy test is negative, but not if unprotected sexual intercourse has occurred within the past 2 weeks, allowing for a chance of very early pregnancy. MPA has been associated with some birth defects and should be avoided during pregnancy.

---

†Asherman syndrome or intrauterine scarring is caused by prior dilation and curettage and/or severe uterine infection. The scarred endometrium does not respond to hormones and menses are not observed. This is extremely rare in teenagers.

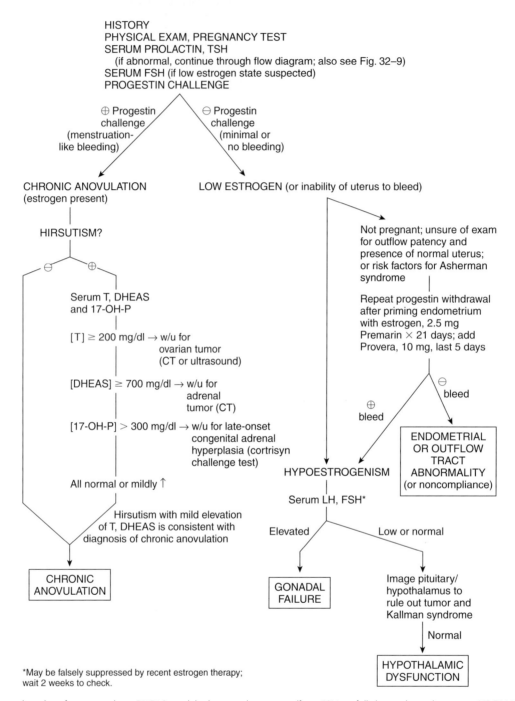

Figure 32–7. General work-up for amenorrhea. DHEAS = dehydroepiandosterone sulfate; FSH = follicle-stimulating hormone; 17-OH-P = 17-hydroxyprogesterone; LH = luteinizing hormone; T = testosterone; TSH = thyroid-stimulating hormone.

specific problem. However, often a specific cause is not found or not easily treated.

Regardless of cause, hormonal replacement is indicated to improve self-image and to prevent the sequelae of untreated sex hormone abnormalities (Table 32–10). In general, hypoestrogenic states require estrogen-progestin hormone replacement therapy or oral contraceptives to complete pubertal development and to prevent osteoporosis, vaginal atrophy, and atherosclerotic heart disease. Patients with chronic anovulation require cyclic progestins at least every few months to bring about withdrawal bleeding. This prevents dysfunctional bleeding, endometrial hyperplasia, and cancer. An alternative is oral contraceptives, which have the added

Table 32-10. Hormone Replacement Options for Amenorrheic Conditions*

	Hormone Replacement	Benefits	Risks
Chronic anovulation (estrogen present)	Medroxyprogesterone acetate, 10 mg p.o./day 12 days/ month every 1–3 months	Diminish risk of sudden menorrhagia and of endometrial hyperplasia/ cancer later in life; create predictable normal menses	Some premenstrual symptoms may occur while the patient is taking progestin; does not provide contraception or address cause of amenorrhea; does not suppress androgens to treat hirsutism
	Low-dose oral contraceptive pills (20–35 μg estrogen)	Same as above; provides contraception; improves hirsutism by suppressing ovarian androgens	Does not address cause of amenorrhea. Some parents object to their daughters taking oral contraceptives: side effects can include nausea, headache, and breakthrough bleeding
Hypogonadism (low-estrogen state)†	Oral medroxyprogesterone acetate, 10 mg/day from days 1–12 of the month (by calendar) plus oral conjugated estrogens 0.625 mg/day	Prevents osteoporosis, heart disease, and atrophic vaginal changes; eliminates hot flashes if present	Does not address cause of amenorrhea; does not provide contraception (if ovulation is possible, given the diagnosis); premenstrual symptoms may occur while the patient is taking progestins; some adolescents prefer oral contraceptives to "medications."
	Low-dose oral contraceptive pills (20–35 μg of estrogen)	Same as above; provides contraception in case of spontaneous ovulation (if that is a possibility); adolescents prefer taking oral contraceptives to taking "medications"	See risks of oral contraceptives above

*These options may need modification based on the individual's response.
†See Chapter 61 for treatment of pubertal delay.

benefit of suppressing ovarian androgens and providing contraception. The length of time to continue therapy depends on whether spontaneous cycles can be expected to resume.

DYSMENORRHEA

Dysmenorrhea is defined as crampy lower abdominal or low back pain temporally associated with menstruation. It is a common problem that causes much suffering and interferes in some cases with school attendance. Sixty percent of 12- to 17-year-old females report some dysmenorrhea; 14% frequently miss school.

Dysmenorrhea is categorized into the very common *primary* dysmenorrhea, associated with no clinically detectable pelvic pathology, and the much less common *secondary* dysmenorrhea, caused by an underlying pelvic abnormality. Primary dysmenorrhea usually begins with the onset of menstrual flow and lasts from hours to a few days. The cramping may be associated with nausea, vomiting, diarrhea, and/or headache. Primary dysmenorrhea begins when the cycles become ovulatory, usually by the third postmenstrual year.

Mechanism of Primary Dysmenorrhea

Primary dysmenorrhea by definition has no clinically discernible pelvic pathology. The pain is due to uterine contractions caused by

prostaglandins originating in the premenstrual secretory endometrium. Women with dysmenorrhea have greater resting uterine tone during menses and more severe contractions than do asymptomatic controls. Treatment with prostaglandin synthetase inhibitors (PGSIs) diminishes these objective findings as well as the sensation of cramps. Release of prostaglandins probably accounts for the other symptoms, such as nausea and diarrhea, often seen with primary dysmenorrhea.

Because it is progesterone from the postovulatory corpus luteum that induces the change from a proliferative to a secretory endometrium, it is only in ovulatory cycles that primary dysmenorrhea occurs. Of note, anovulatory bleeding may cause cramping as a clot passes through the cervix, but as a rule it is not associated with pain.

Secondary Dysmenorrhea

A small percentage of adolescents with menstrual pain have underlying pathology. Table 32–11 presents the differential diagnosis of menstrual pain.

Evaluation of Dysmenorrhea

HISTORY

Routine inquiry allows female patients otherwise disabled from their pain to get treatment. It is important to assess the timing of

Table 32–11. Differential Diagnosis of Dysmenorrhea

	Description of Pain	Occurrence of Dysmenorrhea in Anovulation Cycles	Diagnosis	Treatment
Primary	Crampy lower abdominal/ low back pain ± radiation to upper thighs ± nausea, vomiting, diarrhea, headache; begins at time of menstrual flow; lasts 1–3 days	No	Normal abdominal and pelvic exam; internal pelvic exam can be reserved for sexually active girls and older teenagers	PGSIs and/or oral contraceptives; see Table 32–12
Secondary				
Congenital outflow obstruction (e.g., rudimentary uterine horn, obstructed hemivagina)	Pain begins at menarche and occurs with bleeding	Yes	Pelvic exam with or without ultrasound, with or without laparoscopy; found in 8% of adolescents who underwent laparoscopy for pain	Surgical relief of obstruction
Endometriosis	Increasingly severe dysmenorrhea ± chronic pelvic pain exacerbated during menses	No	Found in 16% to 50% of adolescents who underwent laparoscopy for pelvic pain; pelvic exam may be normal or there may be tenderness of the uterosacral ligaments/*cul-de-sac* and/or ovarian masses; although congenital obstruction of menstrual outflow increases chance of endometriosis, most teenagers with endometriosis have normal anatomy; diagnosis is by laparoscopy	Surgical and/or hormonal therapy
Atypical Secondary Dysmenorrhea				
Pelvic inflammatory disease	Pain during or immediately after menses	Yes	Pelvic exam: tender uterus and adnexae, ± cervicitis, with or without ↑ WBC, with or without ↑ ESR, with or without fever	Follow CDC recommendations (see Chapter 31)
Pregnancy complication	Pain and bleeding may coincide and may be interpreted by the patient as a painful menstrual period	N/A	UCG, or serum hCG	See Figure 32–6

Abbreviations: CDC = Centers for Disease Control and Prevention; ESR = erythrocyte sedimentation rate; hCG = human chorionic gonadotropin; PGSI = prostaglandin synthetase inhibitor; UCG = urinary chorionic gonadotropin; WBC = white blood cell.

pain, the degree of disruption of daily routines, the associated symptoms, the use of and response to over-the-counter medications, and the sexual history. The history helps to differentiate primary from secondary dysmenorrhea. Dysmenorrhea associated with one specific menstrual period in a sexually active adolescent suggests a pregnancy complication or pelvic inflammatory disease (PID). Menstrual pain beginning at menarche or at any other time during which the cycles are believed to be anovulatory suggests outflow tract obstruction because anovulatory bleeding does not cause primary dysmenorrhea. Endometriosis may be difficult to diagnose because its presentation may be similar to that of primary dysmenorrhea. However, endometriosis that is diagnosed in the adolescent is often associated with intermittent non-menstrually related pelvic pain that worsens before and during menses.

EXAMINATION AND TESTING

In the evaluation of dysmenorrhea, an internal pelvic examination can be reserved for sexually active females, older adolescents, and females with atypical presentations. If necessary, a rectoabdominal examination or ultrasound study can diagnose a pelvic mass and may be better tolerated in young virginal adolescents.

If the pain is associated with one particular period, pregnancy and PID should be ruled out. PID is a clinical diagnosis based on history, vital signs, abdominal and pelvic examination, and white blood cell count (see Chapter 31).

The goals of identifying endometriosis in an adolescent with dysmenorrhea include treatment of pain and, if possible, prevention of progression of the disease. If endometriosis is suspected, the benefits of laparoscopy to make the diagnosis should be weighed against the risks.

Treatment of Dysmenorrhea (Table 32–12)

The PGSI group of drugs work by decreasing production of prostaglandins in the endometrium. About 80% of women with primary dysmenorrhea obtain relief of pain and gastrointestinal symptoms with most PGSIs.

Oral contraceptives are successful in diminishing primary dysmenorrhea by inducing atrophy of the endometrium; the result is decreased production of prostaglandins. Because this effect may not be seen initially, PGSIs should be offered concurrently for the first few treatment cycles. Low-dose oral contraceptives, if not contraindicated, are the treatment of choice for dysmenorrhea in sexually active adolescents requiring contraception.

Acupuncture, transcutaneous electrical nerve stimulation (TENS), and calcium antagonists have also shown some promise in treating primary dysmenorrhea.

SUMMARY AND THINGS NOT TO BE MISSED

The examiner should not miss the opportunity to treat the adolescent with primary dysmenorrhea who is suffering in silence.

One should not mistake acute pelvic pain with vaginal bleeding for dysmenorrhea but should consider pregnancy and PID in the differential diagnosis of sudden onset of "menstrual" pain.

The practitioner should consider endometriosis and/or congenital anomaly with partial menstrual outflow obstruction in cases of severe dysmenorrhea with abnormal pelvic findings, poor response to the usual therapies, and/or generalization of pelvic pain beyond the time of the menstrual flow.

VAGINAL BLEEDING IN THE PREPUBERTAL CHILD

Vaginal bleeding is abnormal below age 9 or in the absence of secondary sexual characteristics. Although childhood vaginal bleeding is uncommon, it can be caused by serious problems such as vaginal malignancy, sexual abuse, and intracranial tumors. The source of bleeding in a young girl can be the lower genital tract or the uterus.

Etiology

In a child without signs of puberty, a vulvovaginal source of bleeding is most likely. Common causes within this category include vaginal foreign body, infectious vulvovaginitis, urethral prolapse, vulvar injury, and lichen sclerosis. There are also some common vulvovaginal diagnoses that only rarely present with bleeding. In condyloma acuminatum and vulvar herpes, mild vulvar trauma or secondary infection can lead to bleeding. Scratching can result in bleeding excoriations during a pinworm infestation.

Uncommon lower genital tract conditions, including vaginal or cervical malignancy, vaginal polyps, and hemangiomas of the vagina, vulva, or cervix, can present with vaginal bleeding. Although malignancy is rare, it is found in 12% to 21% of the patients in published series of cases of early childhood vaginal bleeding and must not be missed.

Except for a small amount of endometrial bleeding as the newborn withdraws from relatively high fetal levels of estrogen, *uterine bleeding* is always pathologic in childhood. Possible causes include:

● Precocious puberty
● Isolated premature menarche
● Autonomous estrogen secretion from either an ovarian or adrenal tumor
● Exposure to exogenous estrogen

VULVOVAGINAL SOURCES OF BLEEDING
(Table 32–13, Fig. 32–8)

Vaginal Foreign Body

Vaginal bleeding is more predictive of vaginal foreign body than vaginal discharge. Indeed, the chief complaint of vaginal bleeding without discharge may yield a 50% rate of vaginal foreign body. In contrast, if the bleeding is associated with vaginal discharge, there may be only an 18% chance of finding a foreign body. Usually the foreign body consists of a small wad of what appears to be toilet paper or other fibrous material. This is not palpable on rectoabdominal examination or visible on a sonogram or radiograph. Other items, such as small toys, pen tops, and safety pins, have been reported. The child usually does not recall or does not admit to placing the foreign object in the vagina.

The question remains: How, then, did the foreign material get into the vagina? Hymenal tissue in girls is exquisitely and uncomfortably sensitive to touch, and normal masturbation in girls is thought to involve clitoral and labial manipulation, with fewer than 1% engaging in vaginal or anal penetration. Among girls referred

---

Table 32–12. Treatment of Primary Dysmenorrhea

	Medication	Regimen	Comments
Prostaglandin synthetase inhibitors* (PGSIs)	Ibuprofen, 200 mg	2 tablets p.o. q4–6hr	Over-the-counter
	Mefenamic acid, 250 mg	2 tablets to start, then 1 p.o. q6hr	Suggested in some studies as most effective drug
	Naproxen sodium, 275 mg	2 tablets to start, then 1 p.o. q6hr	
	Naproxen sodium, 550 mg	1 tablet p.o. q12hr	12-hr regimen appealing to patients
Oral contraceptives	Any low-dose pill (≤35 μg estrogen)	21-day active pills; 7-day placebo	Particularly useful if birth control method is needed; may take a few cycles to reach maximum effectiveness

*Aspirin has not been shown to be better than placebo in the treatment of primary dysmenorrhea. PGSI treatment is effective if started at the onset of cramping and bleeding, and it does not need to be started earlier.

Table 32–13. Etiology of Lower Genital Tract Bleeding in Girls

	Diagnostic Features	Management
	Common Causes	
Vaginal foreign body	Vaginal bleeding with or without discharge; usually a wad of toilet paper or other fibers; case reports of small toys, pen tops, safety pins; may be seen on unaided visual examination especially in the knee-chest position; vaginoscopy* is gold standard to make diagnosis and to rule out additional masses in vagina	Removal of foreign body usually resolves bleeding/discharge; persistent or recurrent bleeding is suggestive of additional foreign material; possibility of sexual abuse should be considered
Infectious vulvovaginitis	Vaginal discharge usually reported; may follow URI (group A streptococci) or diarrheal episode (*Shigella*); vulva may look reddened from primary infection or from irritating secretions; wet preparation shows white blood cells; vaginal culture may grow specific organism	If no response to local hygiene measures and specific antibiotics, consider EUA or vaginoscopy to look for another cause (i.e., foreign body); if vulvitis is severe, consider short course of estrogen cream to thicken tissue and promote healing
Urethral prolapse	Careful examination demonstrates red edematous or necrotic mass encircling urethral meatus; vagina can be identified posterior to mass; sometimes occurs after hard Valsalva maneuver; age range: 5–9 yr	Sitz baths with or without estrogen cream or oral or topical antibiotics; usually effective within 2 weeks; urethral catheter if patient cannot void; resection or cautery of mass with anesthesia if local care fails or if patient is symptomatic or tissue is necrotic
Lichen sclerosus	Vulvar ecchymoses and abrasions may be seen with minimal trauma; characteristic white parchment-like thin skin, often in hourglass symmetric pattern around introitus/anus; biopsy is diagnostic but unnecessary when lesion is characteristic; some cases improve at puberty	Recommended good hygiene, prevention of trauma (e.g., loose clothes, padded bicycle seat); no treatment needed in asymptomatic patients; topical corticosteroids can diminish irritation
Trauma	Evaluate for possibility of abuse to determine whether it is safe for patient to be discharged home Straddle injury: evaluate extent of lacerations/stability of hematoma Penetrating injury: evaluate extent of injuries and perform EUA; perform laparotomy if wound extends to vaginal apex; evaluate bladder and rectum if laceration extends there or if urine or stool test is positive for blood	EUA needed when injuries are more than minor; small vulvar hematoma: pressure, ice pack, rest, and evaluation of size stability; large or expanding hematoma: incision or evacuation of clots and ligation of visible vessels or pack; repair lacerations; careful evaluation for abuse or neglect necessary
Malignancy Sarcoma botryoides (embryonal rhabdomyosarcoma of vagina or cervix) or endodermal sinus tumor of vagina	Grape-like mass protruding from vagina; peak age 2 yr; (90% <5 yr); biopsy is diagnostic, but tumor is below epithelium (can be missed); full staging required	Initial treatment is chemotherapy followed by surgery or radiation; exenteration no longer standard first line care
Adenocarcinoma of vaginal or cervix	Vaginoscopy with biopsy; staging required; expect incidence in children to diminish because most adenocarcinomas of the vagina occurred in girls exposed to DES *in utero* and DES off the market for more than 20 years	Radical surgery

Table 32-13. Etiology of Lower Genital Tract Bleeding in Girls *Continued*

	Diagnostic Features	Management
	Uncommon Causes	
Human papillomavirus	Lesions can be single or multiple, 1 mm to large cauliflower-like masses, flesh-toned or pink or white; abrasion or secondary infection with ulceration can lead to vulvar bleeding	Evaluate for sexual abuse especially if diagnosed after age 2 years. Small vulvar condylomata office podophyllin or TCA. Large or resistant to treatment: laser ablation under general anesthesia. Recurrence rate: 25% Cervical/vaginal lesions: laser in OR under general anesthesia. Colposcopy with biopsy if indicated
Genital herpes	Vesicles or ulcers on vulva usually 1–2 mm; can be secondarily infected; culture usually, but not always, for herpes simplex virus	Evaluate for sexual abuse Local care with sitz baths Pain control with acetaminophen or narcotics; primary infection: symptoms can be shortened with oral acyclovir
Pinworms *(Enterobius vermicularis)*	Transparent tape (Scotch tape) test shows eggs; flashlight examination at night can show worms at vagina or anus	Mebendazole; evaluate family members, classmates, and playmates; clean and trim patient's fingernails
Hemangiomas of lower genital tract	Urethral, vulvar, vaginal, and cervical hemangiomas have been reported; appear purple or dark-red and soft; blanching occurs with pressure; overlying epithelium is usually intact, but bleeding occurs when trauma leads to ulceration; biopsy, if done, should be in hospital with blood replacement available	If no reports of malignant degeneration, treatment can be withheld if no symptoms; many spontaneous regressions; successful reported treatments include surgical excision, laser ablation, topical estrogen, and systemic corticosteroids
Vaginal polyps	Visible at vaginoscopy	Excision is diagnostic and therapeutic

*Vaginoscopy. With the availability of fiberoptics, visualization of the full length of the vagina can be performed with only a 3- to 5-mm-diameter instrument. A hysteroscope or cystoscope with saline as the distending medium is ideal. In a cooperative child, fiberoptic vaginoscopy can be accomplished in the office. A bivalve speculum, such as a nasal speculum, can be substituted, if necessary, during examination of prepubertal children under anesthesia.

Abbreviations: DES = diethylstilbestrol; EUA = examination under anesthesia; TCA = trichloroacetic acid; URI = upper respiratory infection.

from a general outpatient pediatric practice to a child gynecology clinic who were subsequently found to have vaginal foreign bodies, most met criteria for confirmed sexual abuse. In light of these data, the approach to evaluation of the girl with a vaginal foreign body needs to include an in-depth assessment for the possibility of sexual molestation (see Chapter 37). A screening interview of the child alone with a trained professional and cultures for sexually transmitted infections are indicated.

Infectious Vulvovaginitis

Vulvovaginitis most commonly presents with discharge or irritation, but vaginal bleeding is sometimes reported. Although most vulvovaginitis is from irritants or mixed bacteria, the most common types of vaginal infection associated with bleeding are group A streptococci, *Shigella*, and on occasion gonococci. Diagnosis is made by visualization of vaginal discharge and a positive culture for a specific pathogen. The treatment for bacterial vulvovaginitis includes either culture-driven or broad-spectrum antibiotic therapy and local hygiene measures, including sitz baths, wiping from front to back after defecation, and appropriate hand washing.

Urethral Prolapse

Urethral prolapse is an eversion of the urethral mucous membrane through the meatus. Careful examination reveals red, friable, and sometimes necrotic tissue at the urethra, which is sometimes mistaken for cervical prolapse or vaginal tumor. Many approaches to treatment have been reported. Local care with sitz baths is often all that is needed. Estrogen cream or broad-spectrum antibiotics have sometimes been used. Surgical resection of the mucosa can be reserved for cases in which initial treatment fails or if bleeding or necrosis is severe.

Trauma

Vulvovaginal trauma in girls is usually caused by straddle injury. Other reported mechanisms of injury include vaginal penetration and tearing resulting from sudden forced stretching of the perineum from leg abduction. Evaluation of the child with vulvovaginal trauma requires a detailed history of how the injury occurred, with attention to the consistency and plausibility of the story. The hymen will be lacerated only if the injury involved penetration into the vagina. A suspicion of sexual abuse requires a report to the proper authorities and evaluation of the ongoing safety of the child (see Chapter 37).

A vulvar laceration that is bleeding but that can be completely visualized is treated with cold packs, pressure, and suturing if necessary. Vulvar hematomas are common and usually self-limited as tissue pressure controls continued expansion. A surgical approach with evacuation of the hematoma and ligation of bleeding vessels can be reserved for situations in which the hematoma is very large or continues to expand. If the bleeding points cannot be isolated, the hematoma cavity can be packed for 24 hours.

Examination with the patient under anesthesia is required to assess for hymenal or vaginal trauma if the apex of the laceration cannot be seen. Hymenal laceration implies that the injury has

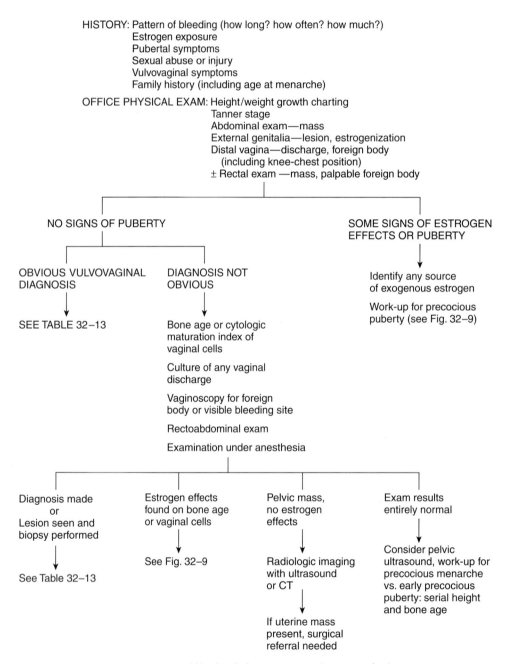

Figure 32–8. Vaginal bleeding below age 9 or without signs of puberty.

penetrated the vagina. Because the vaginal wall is very thin, penetrating vaginal injuries often extend into adjacent structures. If the laceration extends to the vaginal apex, laparotomy is necessary to exclude extension into the peritoneal cavity. Laparoscopy may be inadequate to identify bowel injury or retroperitoneal bleeding. If hematuria is found, a cystourethrogram is recommended to evaluate the bladder and urethra. Urethral obstruction from a hematoma may require suprapubic catheter placement. Homegoing care after initial treatment of vulvar injury includes ice packs for 6 hours, followed by warm sitz baths two to three times a day to promote comfort and help prevent secondary infection.

Malignancy

Vaginal or cervical sarcoma botryoides (embryonal rhabdomyosarcoma) and endodermal sinus tumor can both present as a grape-like mass that is seen at the introitus. The diagnosis of these malignancies is made by biopsy. Because these tumors grow below the epithelium of the vagina, superficial biopsy may not be diagnostic.

Vaginal adenocarcinoma is rare and should become even more rare as the cohort of females exposed to diethylstilbestrol (DES) *in utero* continues to age. DES was taken off the market in 1972, and the youngest people exposed *in utero* are now in their 20s. Vaginal adenocarcinoma is occasionally seen in females who were not DES-exposed.

Lichen Sclerosis

Lichen sclerosis is a hypotrophic dermatologic condition often found in the vulvar area. It appears as a thinning of the skin to a parchment-like appearance. The classic pattern is of an hourglass surrounding the introitus and anus. As a result of the thinness of the epidermis, minor trauma can lead to significant bruising and bleeding. Lichen sclerosis has been misdiagnosed as fungal infection, hemangiomas, sexual abuse, and severe vulvar trauma. The diagnosis is usually clinical, based on the characteristic appearance, but biopsy can be used to confirm if necessary.

UTERINE SOURCES OF VAGINAL BLEEDING

If the external examination and vaginoscopy do not demonstrate a vulvovaginal source of bleeding, uterine bleeding should be suspected. Other indications that the source may be uterine include secondary sexual development, abdominal tumor, or risk factors for precocious puberty, such as previous cranial irradiation or stigmata of McCune-Albright syndrome.

Except for the occasional neonatal estrogen withdrawal bleeding, all uterine bleeding in children is pathologic, usually indicating an estrogenic hormonal effect on the endometrium. Serious underlying conditions, including brain tumor and malignant ovarian tumor, may yield no signs or symptoms other than vaginal bleeding at presentation. Causes of uterine bleeding in children are categorized below (Fig. 32–9) (see Chapter 61).

Precocious Menarche

Cyclic menses with no other secondary sexual characteristics has been termed precocious menarche. The cause is not known, but it is considered a rare form of incomplete precocious puberty. In these children, there is a low increase in serum estrogen levels that does not lead to short stature. Gonadotropin levels are prepubertal. After other sources of vaginal bleeding with examination using anesthesia and vaginoscopy are ruled out, growth rate and/or bone age can be followed over months to ensure that menstruation was not an early sign of precocious puberty. In precocious menarche, normal adult height and fertility are achieved.

Complete Precocious Puberty

Complete precocious puberty denotes that more than one manifestation of puberty has occurred. Growth acceleration and breast development may precede uterine bleeding, but the sequence of pubertal events may be disordered, with uterine bleeding as the initial finding. Adrenarche may or may not occur. The menstrual bleeding may be anovulatory or ovulatory. Causes of complete precocious puberty (see Chapter 61) are as follows:
1. Central or gonadotropin-dependent precocious puberty
2. Peripheral or gonadotropin independent pseudoprecocious puberty
   a. Exogenous estrogen
   b. Estrogen secretory tumors of the ovary or adrenal
   c. Apparent autonomous function of the ovary (McCune-Albright syndrome, follicular cysts of the ovary)
3. Gonadotropin and gonadotropin-like molecules not due to maturation of the HPO axis
4. Mixed peripheral and central precocious puberty.

Other Causes of Uterine Bleeding in Children

Uterine malignancy is extremely rare in premenarchal children. Findings include no secondary sexual characteristics and irregular unregulated bleeding with its source in the uterus. A preliminary diagnosis will be made by abdominal or rectal examination, examination using anesthesia with hysteroscopy, or ultrasonography. Full staging and treatment are carried out according to oncology protocol.

Evaluation (see Figs. 32–8 and 32–9)

HISTORY

The history seeks to differentiate vulvovaginal from uterine causes of bleeding. The pattern of bleeding (''how long, how often, how much''), previous vulvovaginal symptoms or trauma, and any possibility of sexual abuse must be addressed. Estrogen manifestations, including growth spurt, known estrogen exposure, and family history of precocious puberty, should be sought.

PHYSICAL EXAMINATION

The general physical examination includes height, weight, Tanner staging, and abdominal examination. External genitalia should be visualized in the frog-leg position, which can be done with the patient semisitting on an examination table, in stirrups, or in the parent's lap. Vulvar lesions are noted. Is there evidence of estrogen effect? Is there vaginal discharge of fluid, pus or blood? The knee-chest position may allow better visualization of vaginal walls. Specimens for culture, if indicated by signs of vaginitis, can be

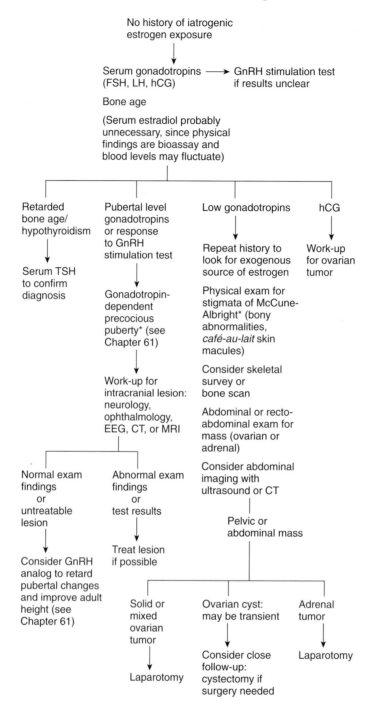

*Follicular cysts are often found with true precocious puberty and with McCune-Albright syndrome. Surgical treatment is not effective at ameliorating pubertal development.

Figure 32–9. Uterine bleeding in a child with estrogen effects or other pubertal findings. CT = computed tomography; EEG = electroencephalography; FSH = follicle-stimulating hormone; GnRH = gonadotropin-releasing hormone; hCG = human chorionic gonadotropin; LH = luteinizing hormone; MRI = magnetic resonance imaging; Tc = technetium; TSH = thyroid-stimulating hormone.

obtained by small Calgiswab, nonbacteriostatic saline lavage with an eyedropper or by the catheter-within-a-catheter technique. Cotton swabs are abrasive as they pass through the hymen, and they should not be used. The rectoabdominal examination can assess for a pelvic mass. Further examination and testing are determined by findings.

The genital examination can be frightening for children. Time

spent developing rapport, engendering the child's trust and assuring the child (truthfully) that she can stop the examination at any time pays off when the examination is completed. The examiner should give as much control as possible, such as letting the child choose who will be in the room and decide whether she wants to climb up to the table or be lifted by her parent. Sometimes an adequate result can be obtained with the girl herself separating the labia and keeping the examiner's hands off. Physicians need to reinforce for her that when it comes to her private parts, "no means no," even in the doctor's office. If the patient is not able to allow an office examination, she can be examined under anesthesia, if necessary.

SUMMARY AND THINGS NOT TO MISS

In the list of causes of vulvovaginal causes of bleeding, the most concerning possibilities include malignancy and sexual abuse. Both diagnoses require a high index of suspicion and may demand persistence on the part of the evaluator.

When bleeding is uterine, it is the underlying cause of the endometrial stimulation that is most important. If the cause cannot be eliminated, attention must be turned to ameliorating peripheral effects of early sex steroid exposure.

REFERENCES

Normal and Abnormal Menstrual Bleeding in the Adolescent

Ataya K, Moghissi K. Chemotherapy-induced premature ovarian failure: Mechanisms and prevention. Steroids 1989;54:607.

Bayer SR, DeCherney AH. Clinical manifestations and treatment of dysfunctional uterine bleeding. JAMA 1993;269:1823.

Christiaens GCML, Sixma JJ, Haspels AA. Morphology of haemostasis in menstrual endometrium. Br J Obstet Gynecol 1980;87:425.

Claessens EA, Cowell CA. Acute adolescent menorrhagia. Am J Obstet Gynecol 1981;139:277.

Livio M, Mannucci PM, Vigano G, et al. Conjugated estrogens for the management of bleeding associated with renal failure. N Engl J Med 1986;315:731.

Romero R, Kadar N, Copel JA, et al. The effect of different human chorionic gonadotropin assay sensitivity on screening for ectopic pregnancy. Am J Obstet Gynecol 1985;153:72.

Amenorrhea

Aiman J, Smentek C. Premature ovarian failure. Obstet Gynecol 1985;66:9.

Buss JG, Lee RA. McIndoe procedure for vaginal agenesis: Results and complications. Mayo Clin Proc 1989;64:758.

Byrne J, Fears TR, Gail MH, et al. Early menopause in long-term survivors of cancer during adolescence. Am J Obstet Gynecol 1992;166:788.

Coney PJ. Effect of vaginal agenesis on the adolescent: Prognosis for normal sexual and psychological adjustment. Adolesc Pediatr Gynecol 1992;5:8.

Corenblum B, Rowe T, Taylor PJ. High-dose, short-term glucocorticoids for the treatment of infertility resulting from premature ovarian failure. Fertil Steril 1993;59:988.

Neinstein LS, Castle G. Congenital absence of the vagina. Am J Dis Child 1983;137:669.

Reindollar RH, Byrd JR, McDonough PG. Delayed sexual development: A study of 252 patients. Am J Obstet Gynecol 1981;140:371.

Rock JA, Zacur HA, Dlugi AM, et al. Pregnancy success following surgical correction of imperforate hymen and complete transverse vaginal septum. Obstet Gynecol 1982;59:448.

Russell JB, Mitchell D, Musey PI, et al. The relationship of exercise to

anovulatory cycles in female athletes: Hormonal and physical characteristics. Obstet Gynecol 1984;63:452.

Dysmenorrhea

Andersch B, Milsom I. An epidemiologic study of young women with dysmenorrhea. Am J Obstet Gynecol 1992;144:655.

Bullock JL, Massey FM, Gambrell RD. Symptomatic endometriosis in teenagers: A reappraisal. Obstet Gynecol 1974;43:896.

Dawood MY, Ramos J. Transcutaneous electrical nerve stimulation (TENS) for the treatment of primary dysmenorrhea: A randomized crossover comparison with placebo TENS and ibuprofen. Obstet Gynecol 1990;75:656.

Hauksson A, Ekstrom P, Juchnicka E, et al. The influence of a combined oral contraceptive on uterine activity and reactivity to agonists in primary dysmenorrhea. Acta Obstet Gynecol Scand 1989;68:31.

Helms JM. Acupuncture for the management of primary dysmenorrhea. Obstet Gynec 1987;69:51.

Owen PR. Current developments: Prostaglandin synthetase inhibitors in the treatment of primary dysmenorrhea. Am J Obstet Gynecol 1984;148:96.

Smith RP. Pressure-velocity analysis of uterine muscle during spontaneous dysmenorrheic contractions in vivo. Am J Obstet Gynecol 1989;160:1400.

Strickland DM, Hauth JC, Strickland KM. Original studies: Laparoscopy for chronic pelvic pain in adolescent women. Adolesc Pediatr Gynecol 1988;1:31.

Teperi J, Rimpela M. Menstrual pain, health and behaviour in girls. Soc Sci Med 1989;29:163.

Ulmsten U. Calcium blockade as a rapid pharmacological test to evaluate primary dysmenorrhea. Gynecol Obstet Invest 1985;20:78.

Vaginal Bleeding in the Prepubertal Child

Blanco-Garcia M, Evain-Brion D, Roger M, et al. Isolated menses in prepubertal girls. Pediatr 1985;76:43.

Cook CL, Sanfilippo JS, Verdi GD, et al. Capillary hemangioma of the vagina and urethra in a child: Response to short-term steroid therapy. Obstet Gynecol 1989;73:883.

Dewhurst J. Lichen sclerosus of the vulva in childhood. Pediatr Adolesc Gynecol 1983;1:149.

Eberlein WR, Bongiovanni AM, Jones IT, et al. Ovarian tumors and cysts associated with sexual precocity. Pediatrics 1960;57:484.

Friedrich WN, Grambsch P, Broughton D, et al. Normative sexual behavior in children. Pediatrics 1991;88:456.

Heller ME, Dewhurst J, Grant DB. Premature menarche without other evidence of precocious puberty. Arch Dis Child 1979;54:472.

Herman-Giddens ME. Vaginal foreign bodies and child sexual abuse. Arch Pediatr Adolesc Med 1994;148:195.

Hill NCW, Oppenheimer LW, Morton KE. The aetiology of vaginal bleeding in children: A 20-year review. Br J Obstet Gynecol 1989;96:467.

Jenny C, Kirby P, Fuquay D. Genital lichen sclerosus mistaken for child sexual abuse. Pediatrics 1981;83:597.

Lyon AJ, DeBruyn R, Grant DB. Transient sexual precocity and ovarian cysts. Arch Dis Child 1985;60:819.

Muram D. Vaginal bleeding in childhood and adolescence. Obstet Gynecol Clin North Am 1990;17:389.

Paradise JE, Willis ED. Probability of vaginal foreign body in girls with genital complaints. Am J Dis Child 1985;139:472.

Richardson DA, Hajj SN, Herbst AL. Medical treatment of urethral prolapse in children. Obstet Gynecol 1982;59:69.

Sanfilippo JS, Wakim NG. Bleeding and vulvovaginitis in the pediatric age group. Clin Obstet Gynecol 1987;30:653.

West R, Davies A, Fenton T. Accidental vulval injuries in childhood. Br Med J 1989;298:1002.

Young RH, Dickersin GR, Scully RE. Juvenile granulosa cell tumor of the ovary. Am J Surg Pathol 1984;8:575.

33 Ambiguous Genitalia

Daniel M. Hoffman   Jack S. Elder

The infant with ambiguous genitalia presents a challenge in diagnosis and management for the physician and parent. Questions of diagnosis and management have profound and lifelong implications for the patient and family. Advances in genetics, endocrinology, and surgical techniques have allowed earlier diagnosis as well as treatment.

EMBRYOLOGY

All embryos possess indifferent internal and external genital structures that will feminize unless they are acted on by a masculinizing influence. Sexual characteristics emerge from common bipotential precursors, and errors are possible at each stage of development. Normal sexual differentiation is the result of a series of well-regulated steps (Figs. 33–1 to 33–3). Initially, the indifferent gonad forms on the genital ridges at 3 to 5 weeks' gestation. Chromosomal information dictates whether this gonad will differentiate into a testis or an ovary. The *SRY* (sex-determining gene Y) gene, which codes for the *testis-determining factor*, is located on the short arm of the Y chromosome (Fig. 33–3). This gene may code for a DNA-binding protein that affects transcription of the testis-determining protein. This gene may sequentially affect autosomal

genes to induce Sertoli cell development in the bipotential primordial gonad. The testis-determining factor causes the primordial germ cells to become organized into testicular cords starting in the sixth week of gestation. By the ninth week, Leydig cells are formed and testosterone production begins.

An ovary will not form without two X chromosomes. Both X chromosomes appear to be active in the germ cell and oocyte from the onset of meiosis to ovulation. In the formation of an ovary, the primitive cords break up into cell clusters that give rise to the ovarian medulla, and in the seventh week of gestation, the surface epithelium gives rise to cortical cords, which eventually develop into follicular cells in the fourth month of gestation. In XX females, the medullary cords regress.

The fetal gonads dictate the development of the genital ducts (Fig. 33–1). At the seventh week of gestation, the fetus has indifferent mesonephric (wolffian) and paramesonephric (müllerian) ducts. These structures complete their development during the third fetal month. In the male, under the influence of local testosterone secreted by the Leydig cells of the fetal testes, the wolffian duct becomes the epididymis, the vas deferens, the seminal vesicle, and the ejaculatory duct (see Fig. 33–1). The testosterone diffuses into the target cells and binds to a cytoplasmic receptor. This receptor-testosterone complex stimulates the differentiation of the wolffian duct structures. The Sertoli cells in the fetal testes secrete müllerian

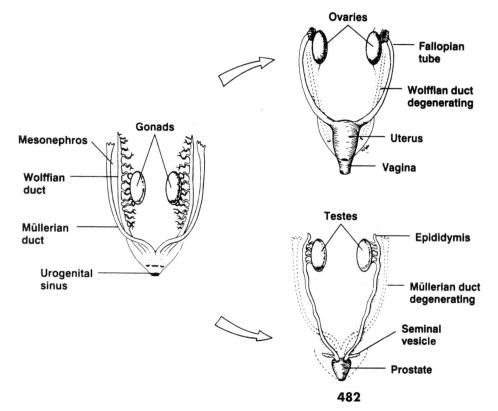

Figure 33–1. Development of the internal genitalia from the indifferent stage. (From Rubenstein SC, Mandell J. The diagnostic approach to the newborn with ambiguous genitalia. Contemp Urol 1994; 6:13–26, copyright Medical Economics.)

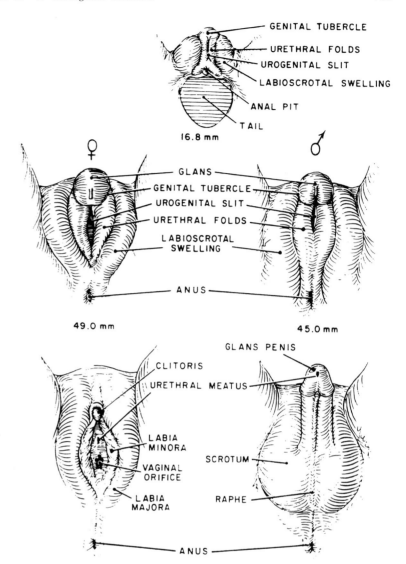

Figure 33–2. Differentiation of male and female external genitalia from indifferent primordia. (From Grumbach MM, Conte FA. Disorders of sex determination. *In* Wilson JD, Foster DW [eds]. Williams Textbook of Endocrinology, Philadelphia: WB Saunders, 1992:853.)

inhibiting substance (MIS), also termed *antimüllerian hormone*. The remnants of the müllerian duct in the male are the appendix testis (a short stalk-like structure on the upper pole of the testis) and the prostatic utricle (a tiny diverticulum in the prostatic urethra).

In the female, the absence of MIS production allows the müllerian ducts to develop into the fallopian tubes, the uterus, and the upper third of the vagina (Fig. 33–1). In the absence of testosterone, the vestigial wolffian duct structures remain as Gartner's duct and the epoophoron and paroophoron.

The external genitalia develop via a common pathway from the cloacal folds starting in the third week of gestation, modifying into the urogenital sinus, the genital tubercle, the urethral folds, and the genital (labioscrotal) swellings (Fig. 33–2). Dihydrotestosterone (DHT) is the active hormone that stimulates the development of the male external genitalia. Testosterone is converted into DHT by the 5α-reductase enzyme, which is present in cells in the urogenital sinus. Intracellular DHT binds to the androgen receptor, causing the genital tubercle and the urethral plate to elongate into the phallus. By the third month of gestation, the urethral folds fuse in the midline to form the urethra and the genital swellings fuse to form the scrotum.

Female external genitalia differentiate in the absence of DHT. The genital tubercle forms the clitoris, the genital swellings become the labia majora, and the urethral folds become the labia minora (Fig. 33–2). The vagina is formed from the urogenital sinus.

By the 15th week of gestation, differentiation of the external genitalia is complete. The male genitalia continue to enlarge throughout the second and third trimesters.

CHROMOSOMAL, PHENOTYPIC, AND GONADAL SEX

Sexual differentiation is a well-regulated sequence of events. Developmentally, chromosomal sex determines gonadal sex, which then determines phenotypic sex. Intersex disorders may be classified according to the stage of the developmental sequence that becomes disrupted, for example, (1) perturbations of chromosomal information, such as Klinefelter syndrome; (2) disorders of gonadal architecture or content, such as true hermaphroditism; and (3) phenotypic anomalies, such as congenital adrenal hyperplasia (CAH).

A simpler organizational scheme for intersex disorders is based on the histology of the gonads (Table 33–1). The five possible classifications are:

- Female pseudohermaphroditism
- Male pseudohermaphroditism
- True hermaphroditism

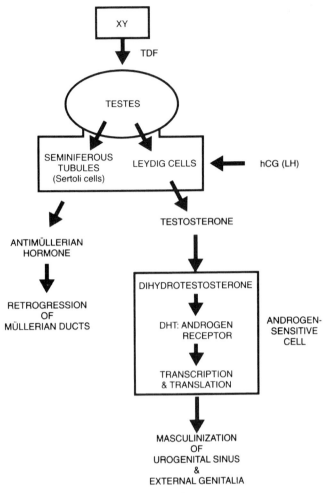

Figure 33-3. A diagrammatic scheme of male sex determination and differentiation. DHT = dihydrotestosterone; hCG = human chorionic gonadotropin; LH = luteinizing hormone; TDF = testis determining factor. (From Wilson JD, Foster DW [eds]. Williams Textbook of Endocrinology, 8th ed. Philadelphia: WB Saunders, 1990:918.)

- Mixed gonadal dysgenesis
- Gonadal dysgenesis.

Because evaluation of a patient with ambiguous genitalia is one of the more delicate tasks undertaken by a physician, a principal advantage of a classification based on the gonads is its relative objectivity.

EVALUATION (Fig. 33–4)

The child with ambiguous genitalia should be examined by a team consisting of a geneticist (dysmorphologist), pediatric endocrinologist, and pediatric urologist. Decisions regarding the evaluation, gender assignment, and long-term management need to be made jointly based on the diagnosis and the future potential for successful sexual function.

History and Physical Examination

A thorough history taking and physical examination must be performed, with full attention given to the history of the pregnancy,

the family history, and the pedigree. Identically afflicted relatives should be identified, but more subtle signs must not be missed. Sudden infant death, infertility, amenorrhea, hirsutism, and variant forms of sexual development in any relative should be investigated. The mother should be questioned about any medication, especially hormones, taken during pregnancy.

On physical examination, the genitalia should be meticulously examined and documented; one important finding is a gonad located in the scrotum or the labioscrotal fold. Any phenotypic male with bilateral impalpable testes or subcoronal hypospadias and cryptorchidism should undergo full evaluation. Rectal examination may disclose a cervix. Other potential findings include hyperpigmentation of the areola and labioscrotal folds (CAH), palpation of the uterus as a thickened structure, hypertension, signs of dehydration and failure to thrive, and associated congenital anomalies.

Diagnostic Studies

Laboratory analysis provides an important tool for the evaluation and treatment of these conditions. An initial study is a karyotype determination. Testing of multiple tissues (blood lymphocytes, skin fibroblasts) may be necessary if chromosomal mosaicism is suspected. Evaluation for Barr bodies in a buccal smear may be inaccurate in the newborn and is generally not obtained.

If the gonads are impalpable, the serum 17-hydroxyprogesterone level should be measured (Fig. 33–5). Serial serum electrolyte levels should also be determined because the most common cause of intersex disorder, CAH (21-hydroxylase deficiency), may cause life-threatening salt wasting (hyponatremia, hyperkalemia, acidosis). Steroid profiles, such as testosterone, androstenedione, adrenocorticotropic hormone (ACTH), plasma renin, and 11-deoxycortisol determinations, may on occasion be necessary.

Voiding cystourethrography and retrograde genitography determine whether the uterus, cervix, and vagina are present. Abdominopelvic ultrasonography should be performed to study the pelvic organs for the presence of a uterus, the inguinal area for the presence of gonads (testes or ovotestes), and for the size and presence of the kidneys and adrenal glands. If the bladder is empty during the study, it should be filled by means of a small feeding tube to allow visualization of the pelvic structures. Inability to discern the cervix or vagina by radiography does not exclude their

Table 33–1. Classification of Intersex Disorders

Disorder	Gonads	Karyotype
Female pseudohermaphroditism	Ovaries only	46,XX
Male pseudohermaphroditism	Testicles only	46,XY
True hermaphroditism	Ovarian and testicular tissue Ovary and testis Ovotestis and testis Ovotestis and ovary Two ovotestes	46,XX, 46,XY and mosaics
Mixed gonadal dysgenesis	Testis and streak gonad	45,XO/46,XY with mosaicism
Pure gonadal dysgenesis	Streak gonads only	46,XX or 46,XY or 45,XO

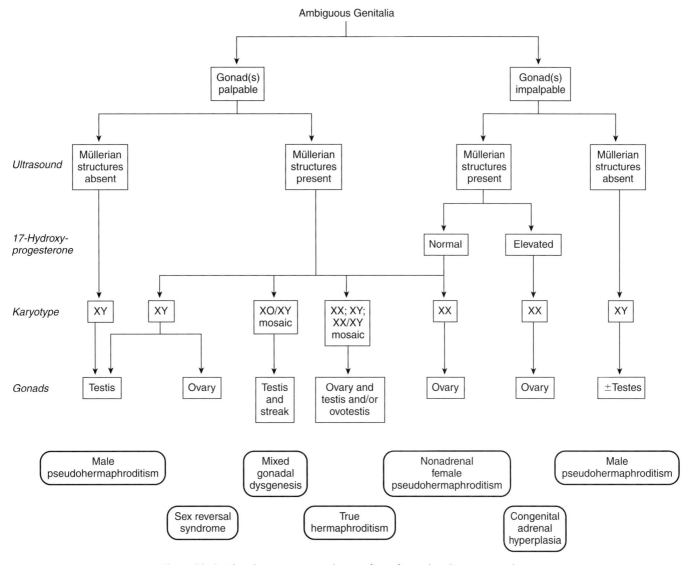

Figure 33–4. Algorithm portraying evaluation of an infant with ambiguous genitalia.

existence. Endoscopy, cystourethroscopy, and vaginoscopy allow more complete examination of the genitalia, and if these tests are performed with contrast under fluoroscopic control, the anatomy may be defined more accurately.

Exploratory laparotomy and gonadal biopsy are used to confirm the gonadal histology and morphology of the wolffian and müllerian duct structures to aid in the assignment of sex. At the time of exploration, high-risk gonadal tissue may be removed if necessary. Laparotomy and biopsy are indicated if the results will affect the sex of rearing or if there is a risk of gonadal malignancy in the future. Regardless of the gonadal sex, if the phallus is too small, the sex of rearing should be female. In the child with a uterus and a well-developed phallus, the sex of rearing may be significantly influenced by the results of gonadal biopsy.

FEMALE PSEUDOHERMAPHRODITISM

Female pseudohermaphroditism occurs in a subject with a 46,XX karyotype who is partially virilized; it is the most common intersex disorder. The ovaries and müllerian derivatives are normally developed, and sexual ambiguity is limited to the external genitalia.

Because patients with this disorder have normal internal structures, they are potentially fertile. The timing of intrauterine exposure to androgen determines the severity of the masculinization. If the differentiating external genitalia are exposed to androgens, there may be complete labioscrotal fusion and possibly a phallic urethra. In contrast, androgen exposure primarily during the second and third trimesters causes only clitoral hypertrophy.

The most common cause of genital ambiguity in the newborn is CAH, the frequency of which is estimated to be 1 in 14,000 births in whites. In the female, CAH results from a deficiency in the activity of one of three enzymes required for cortisol biosynthesis (Table 33–2; see also Fig. 33–5).

Cholesterol is the building block for adrenal hormone synthesis. Through a series of enzymatic reactions, cholesterol is converted to cortisol, aldosterone, and sex hormones (see Fig. 33–5). CAH is caused by a deficiency of an enzyme in this pathway, resulting in decreased synthesis of the desired hormone and an elevated ACTH level, secondary to reduced cortisol feedback on the fetal hypothalamic-pituitary-adrenal axis. The elevated ACTH level causes an overproduction of the precursors of cortisol proximal to the enzyme deficiency, which are then transformed to various androgens, including dehydroepiandrosterone, androstenedione, and androstenediol.

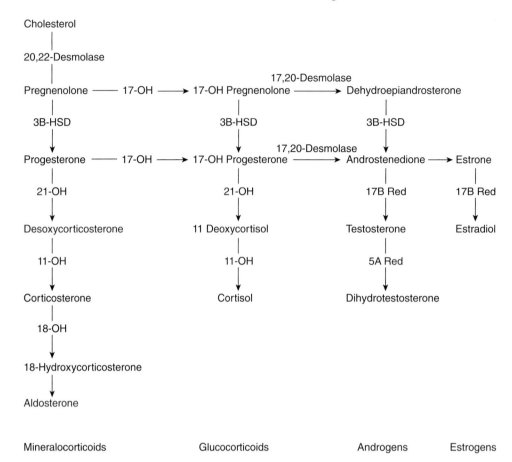

Figure 33–5. Scheme of adrenal steroid biosynthesis. 11-OH = 11 β-hydroxylase; 17-OH = 17 α-hydroxylase; 18-OH = 18-hydroxylase; 21-OH = 21-hydroxylase; 3B-HSD = 3 β-hydroxysteroid dehydroxgenase; 17B Red = 17 β-reductase; 5A Red = 5 α-reductase.

Congenital adrenal hyperplasia is inherited as an autosomal recessive trait with a locus near the HLA locus on chromosome 6. Girls and boys are affected with equal frequency. However, genital ambiguity occurs primarily in girls. The condition in boys is not discovered at birth unless the boys experience a salt-losing crisis, are identified through prenatal screening performed because of the birth of an affected sibling, or have one of the less common enzyme defects. Precocious puberty develops in untreated males with CAH.

Congenital adrenal hyperplasia is the only intersex disorder that can be life-threatening if untreated. More than 90% of the cases are a result of a deficiency of the enzyme 21-hydroxylase, whereas deficiency of the 11β-hydroxylase enzyme accounts for another 5% of cases. Less common are deficiencies of the enzymes 3β-hydroxysteroid dehydrogenase, 17α-hydroxylase, and desmolase.

A 21-hydroxylase deficiency may be mild or severe. The severe, or salt-wasting, type of 21-hydroxylase deficiency is a life-threatening disease. In this form of the disorder, there is impaired secretion of cortisol and aldosterone, resulting in anorexia, vomiting, hyponatremia, hyperkalemia, acidosis, dehydration, and circulatory collapse. This usually occurs after the fifth day of life. Virilization of the external genitalia is variable; the more masculine the phenotype, the more severe the enzymatic defect. Other causes of *adrenal insufficiency* with or without intersex signs in infancy and childhood are noted in Table 33–3; manifestations are noted in Table 33–4.

The second most common cause of CAH, 11β-hydroxylase deficiency, results in decreased production of cortisol and corticosterone and increased production of desoxycorticosterone, a steroid with a salt-retaining effect. This gene is on chromosome 8 and is not linked to HLA. There is marked heterogeneity in the clinical and hormonal manifestations of this defect. Typically, females present with ambiguous genitalia at birth and may become hypertensive either in infancy or later in childhood. Male infants appear

Table 33–2. Causes of Virilization in the Female

Condition	Additional Features
P-450 C_{21} deficiency (21-hydroxylase)	Salt loss in some
3β-Hydroxysteroid dehydrogenase deficiency	Salt loss
P-450 C_{11} deficiency (11β-hydroxylase)	Salt retention/hypertension
Androgenic drug exposure (e.g., progestins)	Exposure by 12th wk of gestation
Mixed gonadal dysgenesis*	Karyotype = 45,X/46,XY
True hermaphrodite	Testicular and ovarian tissue present
Maternal virilizing adrenal or ovarian tumor	Rare, positive history
Idiopathic	Unknown cause

Adapted from Styne DM. Endocrine disorders: *In* Behrman RE, Kliegman RM (eds). Nelson Essentials of Pediatrics, 2nd ed. Philadelphia: WB Saunders, 1994:636.
*Or mosaic Turner syndrome.

Table 33–3. Causes of Adrenal Insufficiency in Infancy and Childhood

Congenital adrenal hypoplasia
　Secondary to ACTH deficiency
　Autosomal recessive
　X-linked

Adrenal hemorrhage

Congenital adrenal hyperplasia
　P-450$_{scc}$ (Cholesterol side chain cleavage) deficiency
　3β-Hydroxysteroid dehydrogenase deficiency
　P-450 C$_{21}$ (21-hydroxylase) steroid dehydrogenase deficiency
　P-450 C$_{11}$ (11β-hydroxylase) deficiency
　P-450 C$_{17}$ (17-hydroxylase) deficiency

Isolated deficiency of aldosterone synthesis
　P-450$_{c11}$ (18-hydroxylase) deficiency
　P-450$_{c11}$ (18-hydroxysteroid dehydrogenase) deficiency

Pseudohypoaldosteronism—end-organ unresponsiveness to aldosterone

Congenital adrenal unresponsiveness to ACTH

Addison disease
　Autoimmune
　Infections of the adrenal gland
　　Tuberculosis
　　Histoplasmosis
　　Meningococcosis
　Infiltration of the adrenal gland
　　Sarcoidosis
　　Hemochromatosis
　　Amyloidosis
　　Metastatic cancer
　Adrenoleukodystrophy

Drugs (suppress adrenal steroidogenesis)
　Withdrawal of steroid therapy given for more than 7–10 days
　Metyrapone
　Ketoconazole

From Styne DM. Endocrine disorders. *In* Behrman RE, Kliegman RM (eds). Nelson Essentials of Pediatrics, 2nd ed. Philadelphia: WB Saunders, 1994:639.
Abbreviation: ACTH = adrenocorticotropic hormone.

Table 33–4. Clinical Manifestations of Adrenal Insufficiency

Cortisol deficiency
　Hypoglycemia
　Inability to withstand stress
　Vasomotor collapse
　Hyperpigmentation (primary adrenal insufficiency with ACTH excess)
　Apneic spells
　Hypoglycemic seizure
　Muscle weakness, fatigue

Aldosterone deficiency
　Vomiting
　Hyponatremia
　Urinary sodium wasting
　Salt craving
　Hyperkalemia
　Acidosis
　Failure to thrive
　Volume depletion
　Hypotension
　Dehydration
　Shock
　Diarrhea
　Muscle weakness

Androgen excess or deficiency (caused by enzyme defect)
　Ambiguous genitalia

From Styne DM. Endocrine disorders. *In* Behrman RE, Kliegman RM (eds). Nelson Essentials of Pediatrics, 2nd ed. Philadelphia: WB Saunders, 1994:639.
Abbreviation: ACTH = adrenocorticotropic hormone.

normal at birth, but hypertension and precocious puberty develop. There is no salt-wasting component to the classic form of this syndrome, but gene mutations can rarely result in a salt-wasting form of the condition.

Other enzyme deficiencies that lead to CAH include deficiencies of 3β-OL dehydrogenase, 17α-hydroxylase, and desmolase. However, these conditions do not cause female pseudohermaphroditism; females with these conditions are not virilized.

Evaluation (Table 33–5)

Patients with CAH and ambiguous genitalia are genetic females with normal ovaries. The karyotype is 46,XX. Because there is no production of testosterone or MIS by the male gonads, the wolffian structures are absent, and the development of the fallopian tubes, the uterus, and the upper vagina is normal. Only the development of the external genitalia is affected in females. Examination of girls with the 21-hydroxylase or 11-hydroxylase enzyme deficiency reveals variable degrees of virilization. With the mildest forms, there is simply clitoral hypertrophy and a normally positioned vagina; in the most severe forms, there is complete labioscrotal

fusion, a long phallus with a urethral opening at its tip, and a high insertion of the vagina on the urethra (Figs. 33–6 and 33–7). The gonads are impalpable because the ovaries do not descend into the inguinal canal or labia unless an inguinal hernia is present. The more severe the virilizing effect, the more severe the enzyme deficit. Any phenotypic male neonate with impalpable testes should be evaluated for CAH.

In the full-term newborn with a 21-hydroxylase deficiency, serum levels of 17-hydroxyprogesterone are typically elevated, ranging from 3000 to 40,000 ng/dl (normal, 100 to 200 ng/dl); in those

Table 33–5. Diagnostic Tests for Suspected Congenital Adrenal Hyperplasia

Test	Finding
Blood	
Karyotype	46,XX
17-Hydroxyprogesterone	Elevated
Testosterone	Elevated
11-Deoxycortisol	Elevated (with 11β-hydroxylase deficiency)
Androstenedione	Elevated
Serial electrolytes	↓ Na, ↑ K
Radiology	
Ultrasonography (pelvis, inguinal canal, adrenal glands)	
Genitogram	

Abbreviations: Na = sodium; K = potassium.

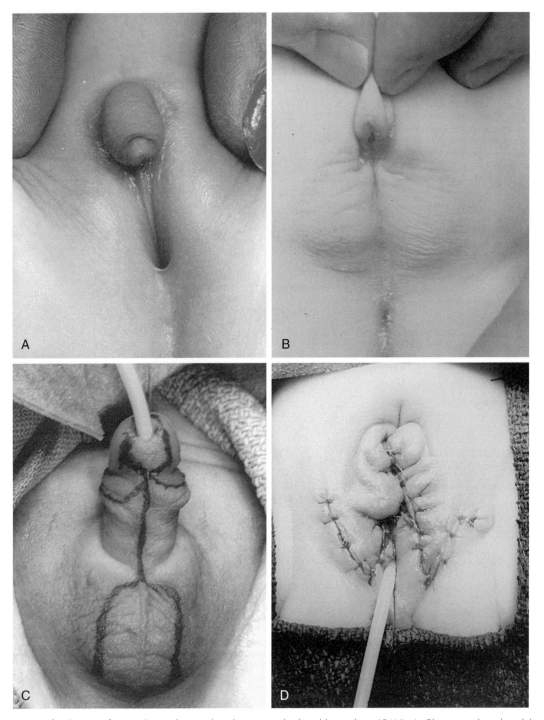

Figure 33–6. Spectrum of virilization of external genitalia in girls with congenital adrenal hyperplasia (CAH). *A,* Clitoromegaly without labioscrotal fusion. *B,* Mild clitoromegaly with labioscrotal fusion. *C,* Severe virilization in a girl with CAH. *D,* Same patient as in *C* after feminizing genitoplasty.

with mild forms, the level is at the upper limit of normal. In premature infants, 17-hydroxyprogesterone levels may be normally elevated (false positive). Measurement of urinary 17-ketosteroid and pregnanetriol level is not usually performed. Salt-losing patients often have hyponatremia and hyperkalemia on a regular or low-salt diet. In newborns, with the 11-hydroxylase deficiency, plasma 11-deoxycortisol and 11-deoxycorticosterone levels are elevated. Radiologic evaluation includes a pelvic ultrasound study to try to identify a uterus and ovaries, an inguinal ultrasound study to try to identify gonads (testes, if present, indicate that the patient does not have CAH), and an adrenal ultrasound study, because

50% of neonates with CAH have adrenal glands that are enlarged or at the upper limit of normal in size.

Treatment

Initial management is directed at correcting or preventing hypoglycemia, hyponatremia, hyperkalemia, hypovolemia, and shock. In addition to saline infusion and correction of electrolyte abnormalities, hydrocortisone therapy is started. When the child is stabi-

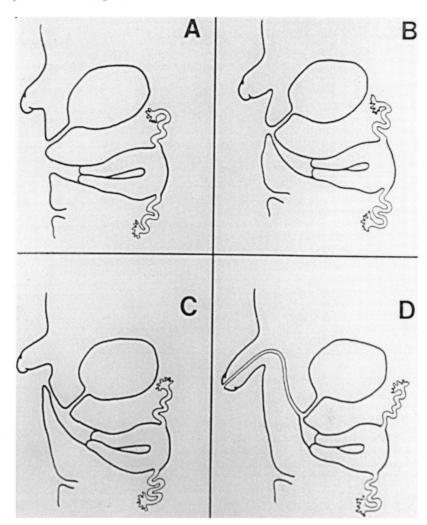

Figure 33–7. Spectrum of external virilization in congenital adrenal hyperplasia. *A*, Clitoromegaly. *B* and *C*, Progressive labioscrotal fusion. *D*, Complete virilization with penile urethra. (From Griffin JE, Wilson JD: Disorders of sexual differentiation. *In* Walsh PC, Retik AB, Stamey TA, Vaughan ED Jr [eds]. Campbell's Urology, 6th ed. Philadelphia: WB Saunders, 1992:1509.)

lized and receiving appropriate doses of glucocorticoids and mineralocorticoids, surgical management is considered. The procedure, termed *feminizing genitoplasty*, involves (1) clitoroplasty, in which the erectile tissue of the clitoris is removed, preserving normal clitoral sensation, and (2) vaginoplasty, in which the lower vagina is exteriorized (Fig. 33–6*D*).

Prenatal Screening

The 21-hydroxylase deficiency is an autosomal recessive condition; consequently, there is a 25% risk that a sibling of an affected child will have CAH. The gene for CAH is closely associated with the HLA class I and HLA class II genes. DNA probes for these genes can be used to define the sequences associated with CAH. If genetic material can be obtained from the embryo or fetus (chorionic villus biopsy at 10 weeks' gestation) of an affected sibling before the external genitalia have completely developed, treatment may be given to prevent virilization of the genitalia. If dexamethasone is administered to the mother at 10 weeks of gestation, it will cross the placenta and suppress the overproduction of cortisol precursors. Amniotic fluid can also be assayed for 17-hydroxyprogesterone as a complementary study. The earlier the initiation of dexamethasone therapy, the less likely that significant virilization will occur in the fetus with CAH.

MALE PSEUDOHERMAPHRODITISM

Male pseudohermaphroditism refers to a chromosomal male (46,XY) with normal testes who undergoes incomplete virilization (Table 33–6). The abnormality includes a spectrum of conditions, including:

1. Failure of target tissue response to testosterone or dihydrosterone.
2. Failure of conversion of testosterone to dihydrosterone.
3. A defect in testicular differentiation.
4. A disorder in testosterone synthesis.
5. A defect in production of müllerian inhibiting substance (MIS).

Although some of these conditions do not result in obvious ambiguous genitalia, in all cases sexual differentiation is abnormal.

Androgen Resistance

Testicular feminization (complete androgen resistance) is an X-linked disorder of patients with a 46,XY karyotype who have an abnormality of the androgen receptor, either qualitatively abnormal or at undetectably low levels. During embryonic development, differentiation of the wolffian ducts and virilization of the external genitalia are inhibited and secretion of MIS causes regression of

Table 33–6. Causes of Inadequate Masculinization in the Male

Condition	Additional Features
Testicular feminization syndrome (complete)*	Female external genitalia, absence of müllerian structures
Testicular feminization syndrome (partial)*	As above with ambiguous external genitalia
Partial androgen insensitivity syndromes	Family history frequently positive
5α-Reductase deficiency	Autosomal recessive, virilization at puberty
Vanishing testis syndrome	Unknown or vascular event; may be >12 weeks' gestation
P-450$_{scc}$ deficiency	Salt loss
3β-Hydroxysteroid dehydrogenase deficiency	Salt loss
P-450$_{c17}$ deficiency	Salt retention/hypertension
17,20-Desmolase deficiency	Adrenal function normal
17β-Hydroxysteroid oxidoreductase deficiency	Adrenal function normal
Dysgenetic testes	Possible abnormal karyotype
Leydig cell hypoplasia	Rare

Adapted from Styne DM. Endocrine disorders. *In* Behrman RE, Kliegman RM (eds). Nelson Essentials of Pediatrics, 2nd ed. Philadelphia: WB Saunders, 1994:636.
*Or androgen insensitivity.

the müllerian ducts. Consequently, affected individuals have bilateral testes; female external genitalia with a short, blind-ending vagina; and wolffian-derived internal duct structures. At puberty, breasts develop but the patients do not menstruate or develop any pubic or axillary hair.

Diagnosis occurs at puberty after evaluation for amenorrhea. Androgen resistance results in increased luteinizing hormone (LH) secretion, which causes elevated levels of testosterone as well as estradiol. The elevated level of estradiol is responsible for breast development. The diagnosis of testicular feminization may be suspected before puberty as a result of detection of inguinal or labial gonads (testes) in a phenotypic female. After puberty, the patient has primary amenorrhea. Markedly elevated serum LH and testosterone levels and a 46,XY karyotype establish the diagnosis. The assignment of female sexual identity should be reinforced.

Treatment includes bilateral orchiectomy because there is a significant risk of gonadal cancer with age. Estrogen replacement then becomes necessary. Because of the underdeveloped müllerian structures, patients are candidates for vaginoplasty, which is usually performed with a segment of large or small bowel.

A spectrum of incomplete androgen resistance syndromes, which are X-linked, has been identified. Müllerian development does not occur, and wolffian duct derivatives usually are hypoplastic. In these syndromes (Reifenstein, Lubs, Gilbert-Dreyfus), development of the external genitalia is variable and ranges from genital ambiguity to severe hypospadias with chordee. The testes are small and are often undescended. Biopsy of the testes reveals azoospermia. At puberty, there is usually poor virilization, absent or sparse axillary and pubic hair, and gynecomastia. Serum LH, testosterone, and estradiol levels are elevated. Gender assignment of these patients depends on their phenotype. Phenotypic males with severe hypospadias and chordee can undergo satisfactory urethral reconstruction and resemble normal males.

5α-Reductase Deficiency

External genital development in the male is stimulated by the 5α-reduced product of testosterone, DHT (see Fig. 33–3). In males

with a 5α-reductase deficiency, there is a small phallus or ambiguous genitalia with perineoscrotal hypospadias, a bifid scrotum, and inguinal or scrotal/labial testes. Because the testes produce MIS, there is a blind vaginal pouch that opens into the urogenital sinus or urethra. However, the wolffian duct derivatives are present. In untreated patients, at puberty the female phenotype transforms into a masculine phenotype with penile/phallic enlargement, scrotal rugation and pigmentation, enlargement and descent of the testes into the labioscrotal folds, and deepening of the voice.

The diagnosis is suggested by a high testosterone-to-DHT ratio, either under basal conditions or after stimulation with human chorionic gonadotropin (hCG). Genitography shows wolffian duct structures. Early diagnosis of 5α-reductase deficiency is important to allow appropriate gender identification.

In many cases, DHT therapy results in significant phallic enlargement and hypospadias repair can then be performed, which results in a satisfactory male appearance. If the genitalia are clearly female, however, bilateral orchiectomy and estrogen replacement are indicated.

Abnormal Testicular Differentiation

If testicular differentiation is abnormal, often genital development may be abnormal.

In the *vanishing testis syndrome*, the testes form but involute during gestation. If testicular regression occurs before 8 weeks' gestation, the embryo has no testosterone or MIS and female external genitalia and müllerian development results. Testicular regression also may occur late in gestation, usually from testicular torsion. In this instance, the individual has a normal phallus but bilateral impalpable testes and absent müllerian derivatives. In these patients, the karyotype is 46,XY. Usually, the baseline gonadotropin levels are high, and the testosterone level is low. After a series of hCG injections, the serum testosterone level should rise dramatically in normal males with functioning testes but is unchanged with the vanishing testis syndrome.

Although the diagnosis of anorchia can be made by endocrine methods, confirmation with laparoscopy is recommended. Management includes treatment with exogenous testosterone at puberty. Patients with this disorder are sterile.

Disorder of Testosterone Synthesis

Five enzymes are involved in the biosynthesis of testosterone:

- 20,22-Desmolase
- 3 β-Hydroxysteroid dehydrogenase
- 17α-Hydroxylase
- 17,20-Desmolase
- 17-Ketosteroid reductase

The first three enzymes also are involved in the production of corticosteroids; thus, a deficiency of one of these enzymes also causes CAH (see Fig. 33–5).

A defect in *desmolase activity* causes severe adrenal and gonadal insufficiency. Because testosterone is not produced, affected males usually have female external genitalia with a blind vaginal pouch, undeveloped wolffian duct derivatives, and no müllerian structures. Sonography demonstrates large, lipid-laden adrenal glands. Death from adrenal insufficiency may occur in infancy. The diagnosis is made by demonstration of low levels of all steroids in urine and plasma and an absent adrenal response to ACTH.

A defect in *3β-hydroxysteroid dehydrogenase* results in reduced testosterone production but increased dehydroepiandrosterone production, allowing some virilization of males; the typical appearance is severe hypospadias with chordee. In its complete form, deficiencies of aldosterone, cortisol, estradiol, and testosterone occur. The usual presentation is adrenal crisis with severe salt loss, although milder forms have been described. The diagnosis is made by detection of the precursors of aldosterone and cortisol, pregnenolone, 17-hydroxypregnenolone, and dehydroepiandrosterone (DHEA). Treatment is similar to that of other patients with CAH.

A defect in the *17α-hydroxylase enzyme* results in impaired synthesis of 17α-hydroxypregnenolone and 17α-hydroxyprogesterone, causing impaired cortisol and sex steroid synthesis. Affected individuals may experience hypertension, hypokalemia, and alkalosis. Because of impaired testosterone synthesis, the external genitalia in males show minimal or no virilization. The diagnosis is suspected in 46,XY males with ambiguous or female genitalia, hypokalemic alkalosis, and hypertension. The diagnosis of 17α-hydroxylase deficiency is confirmed by demonstration of high levels of corticosterone, deoxycorticosterone, progesterone, and pregnenolone, as well as low levels of aldosterone and renin.

A defect in *17,20-desmolase activity* or *17β-hydroxysteroid dehydrogenase* activity causes reduced testosterone secretion and thus ambiguous genitalia in subjects with the 46,XY karyotype. They have virilization of the wolffian duct derivatives and absent müllerian structures. Inguinal or intra-abdominal testes are common. An unusual feature of 17β-hydroxysteroid dehydrogenase deficiency in males is that at puberty significant virilization can occur, often in association with gynecomastia. Affected patients have elevated levels of androstenedione and estrone and low levels of testosterone and estradiol.

In most patients with the 46,XY karyotype with a disorder in testosterone synthesis, the genitalia are female in appearance or ambiguous. If the sex of rearing is decided to be male, early hypospadias repair and orchiopexy are recommended. If a female gender is assigned, however, gonadectomy and clitoroplasty should be performed and vaginoplasty may be necessary at puberty.

Persistent Müllerian Duct Syndrome

Also termed *hernia uteri inguinale*, persistent müllerian duct syndrome is an X-linked condition that results from a defect in the production of MIS, an abnormality in the secretion of MIS, or a lack of response by the müllerian duct to MIS. This form of male pseudohermaphroditism does not cause ambiguous genitalia. The typical presentation is an infant or child with an inguinal hernia and cryptorchidism in whom routine exploration discloses müllerian structures (fallopian tube and uterus) as well as an epididymis and vas. In many cases, transverse testicular ectopia is present.

Treatment includes removal of the müllerian structures; care must be taken not to injure the wolffian duct derivatives.

MIXED GONADAL DYSGENESIS

Mixed gonadal dysgenesis is the second most common cause of ambiguous genitalia in newborns. Most patients have chromosomal mosaicism with a 45,XO/46,XY karyotype. Nearly all have incomplete virilization (Fig. 33–8). Patients reared as females typically have genital ambiguity with phallic enlargement, a urogenital sinus, and varying degrees of labioscrotal fusion. Internal genitalia include a unilateral streak gonad; persistent müllerian duct structures (fallopian tube, uterus, and vagina) ipsilateral to the streak; a contralateral testis, which may or may not be undescended; and frequently a fallopian tube on the side of the testis. Individuals reared as females usually have an intra-abdominal testis, whereas in those with a more masculine phenotype the testis is usually inguinal or scrotal. Approximately 33% of patients have somatic

stigmata of *Turner syndrome* with a shield chest, webbed neck, cubitus valgus, multiple pigmented nevi, and short stature. Approximately 60% are reared as females because of the diminutive phallus, which is usually hypospadiac.

Histologically, the streak gonad is composed of fibrous connective tissue resembling ovarian stroma. The testis lacks germinal elements but at puberty has abundant Leydig and Sertoli cells. Thus, at puberty most patients with a retained testis undergo virilization and the serum testosterone level is in the normal adult range. It is thought that the incomplete virilization at birth represents delayed development of the testis in utero.

Management depends on several factors. First, the testis lacks germinal elements. Second, most patients have significant hypospadias, with a uterus and vagina. Individuals with a male gender assignment must undergo reconstructive surgery, but usually the appearance of the penis can be relatively normal if the corporal bodies of the penis are sufficiently long. Third, gonadal tumors develop in 25% of patients and include seminoma, gonadoblastoma, dysgerminoma, and embryonal cell carcinoma. Tumors may develop in either the testis or the streak gonad. If a tumor develops in an intra-abdominal testis, ipsilateral müllerian structures are always present. Tumors may develop in a scrotal streak gonad but not a scrotal testis. If a tumor is present in a streak gonad, it is also present in the contralateral intra-abdominal testis. Approximately 50% of patients will be less than 148 cm in height. For these reasons, most infants with mixed gonadal dysgenesis are reared as females. If gender assignment is female, early exploratory laparotomy and prophylactic gonadectomy are advisable.

GONADAL DYSGENESIS (Turner Syndrome)

Although patients with gonadal dysgenesis do not have ambiguous genitalia, the condition represents an important disorder of sexual differentiation. The karyotype is 45,XO, and this abnormality affects 1 in 10,000 newborn females. Typical features include short stature, sexual infantilism at puberty, and distinctive somatic abnormalities. At birth, loose skin folds on the neck are apparent, as is lymphedema of the extremities. Later, characteristic facial features become apparent, including prominent low-set ears, epicanthal folds, ptosis, low posterior hair line, and micrognathia. There is a shield chest and often a webbed neck. Associated anomalies may include renal abnormalities, coarctation of the aorta, cubitus valgus, puffy hands and feet, and short fourth metacarpals. Treatment includes estrogen replacement at puberty. All patients are sterile.

PURE GONADAL DYSGENESIS

Individuals with pure gonadal dysgenesis have normal female external genitalia, but the internal structures are similar to those in patients with Turner syndrome (bilateral streak gonads, müllerian duct development, and sexual infantilism). The patients are normal or tall in height and have few congenital anomalies and either a 46,XX or 46,XY karyotype. Those with the 46,XY form often have clitoromegaly. Gonadal tumors may arise in patients with a 46,XY karyotype, and prophylactic gonadectomy is recommended for these individuals. Patients may present with amenorrhea. Virilization indicates the presence of a tumor of one of the streak gonads.

TRUE HERMAPHRODITISM

True hermaphroditism is the least common of the intersex disorders. In a person with this condition, the gonads contain both

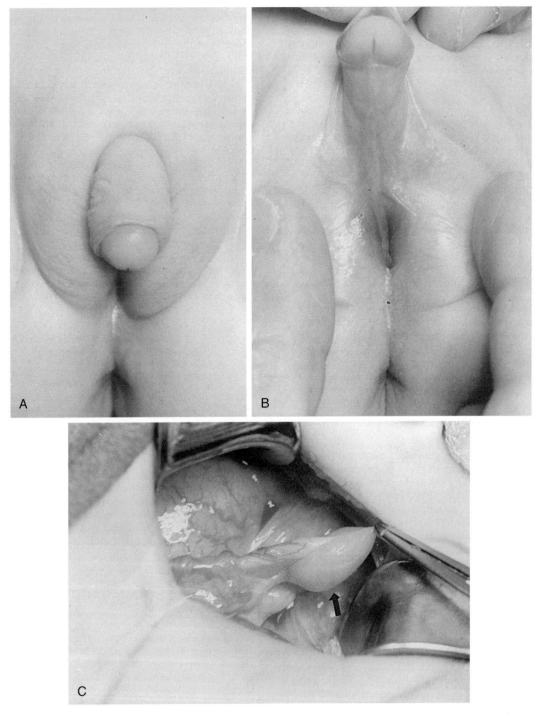

Figure 33–8. Patient with mixed gonadal dysgenesis. *A* and *B,* External genitalia shows normal-sized phallus and hypospadiac urethra. *C,* Laparotomy shows streak gonad *(arrow).*

ovarian and testicular tissue. The patients may have an ovotestis on one side and an ovary or testis on the other (unilateral), bilateral ovotestes (bilateral), or a testis on one side and an ovary on the other (lateral). The most common finding is an ovary on the left side and a testis on the right. Nearly all patients have a urogenital sinus and most have a uterus. The ductal system usually follows from the ipsilateral gonad: a fallopian tube on the side of the ovary and an epididymis on the side of the testicle. If an ovotestis is present, the adjacent ducts may be wolffian, müllerian, or both. If an ovotestis is present, it may be anywhere along the course of normal testicular descent, and often it is associated with an inguinal hernia. The appearance of the external genitalia is variable. Nearly all have incomplete virilization; that is, they have hypospadias.

At puberty, 80% of patients develop gynecomastia and 50% menstruate. Individuals reared as males may show cyclic hematuria. Ovulation is more common than spermatogenesis, but both are uncommon.

Sixty percent of the patients have a 46,XX karyotype, but the *SRY* gene has been detected in many. Twenty percent have a 46,XY karyotype; the remainder demonstrate mosaicism or chimerism. Gonadal neoplasms have been reported in patients with an XY cell line. Because most have a masculine phenotype, approximately 70% have been reared as males.

The primary consideration in these patients is gender assignment. If the phallus is diminutive, the infant should be reared as a female, irrespective of the internal genitalia. If there is both a phallus and vagina, the sex of rearing should be based on the findings at exploratory laparotomy. If a testis is identified that can be placed in the scrotum, the infant should be raised as a male. If there are normal müllerian structures on one side that are associated with an ovary, strong consideration should be given to rearing the infant as a female. After gender assignment, the contradictory gonadal tissue and internal ducts should be excised.

GENDER ASSIGNMENT AND MANAGEMENT

When a baby is born, the parents, the family, and their friends immediately want to know the baby's weight and its sex. If the neonate has ambiguous genitalia, the possible confusion among the medical team regarding gender assignment can have a profound effect on how the baby is viewed and treated by his or her family. Gender assignment in these patients is an emergency.

The initial discussion with the parents should include the fact that the genitalia of the child are incompletely formed and that more extensive testing must be performed before gender assignment. Until a definite sex has been assigned, the newborn should be referred to as "the baby," rather than "he," "she," or "it." The infant should never be alluded to as "half-boy and half-girl." For inquisitive family and friends, the parents may simply state that the baby is quite ill and will need to be hospitalized for several days; most of the time, no further questions regarding the baby's sex will follow. It sometimes takes several days to identify the cause of the ambiguous genitalia; only after the cause is determined can the gender assignment be made. In the unlikely event that an older child is found to have an intersex condition, the assigned gender should not be changed except in very unusual circumstances.

The important factors in gender assignment are (1) the likelihood of having a cosmetically acceptable male or female genital appearance after reconstructive surgery that will allow satisfactory sexual function, (2) the potential for fertility, (3) the potential for sex steroid production, and (4) the likelihood of gonadal tumor formation.

When a neonate with ambiguous genitalia is assigned a male gender, current surgical techniques allow a remarkably normal genital appearance as long as the phallus is satisfactory in size. If the penis is diminutive, it may be necessary to give two or three monthly injections of testosterone enanthate to determine whether there is significant phallic growth potential. Nearly all of these infants have hypospadias, often with chordee (ventral penile curvature). If there is significant chordee, the stretched penile length may be difficult to assess accurately and tends to be underestimated. In the absence of chordee, the stretched penile length is determined with a ruler pressed into the suprapubic fat pad above the symphysis pubis. The measurement includes the tip of the glans to the base (excluding redundant foreskin). The width is measured at midshaft during stretching. A micropenis has a stretched length or width below −2.5 standard deviations of the mean for age. At 40 weeks' gestation, this measurement is approximately 27 to 30 mm for length and 9 to 10 mm for diameter. Clitoral enlargement is present if the clitoris exceeds 6 mm in a term neonate. Gonadal (testis) size is considered small if the longest diameter is less than 0.8 cm. If a male gender assignment is made, the reconstructive procedure can be performed at 6 to 12 months of age, usually with one procedure.

If the patient is assigned a female gender, reconstructive surgery, termed *feminizing genitoplasty*, should be performed as soon as is feasible from a medical standpoint. This procedure involves both a clitoroplasty and a vaginoplasty. If only clitoromegaly is present, only a reduction clitoroplasty is necessary. Reconstructive surgical techniques have allowed this procedure to be performed in a way that allows an excellent cosmetic appearance and satisfactory sexual function. In this procedure, the corporal bodies of the clitoris are removed, and the glans (tip of the phallus) and the neurovascular bundle, which provides sensation, are preserved. In patients with mixed gonadal dysgenesis or true hermaphroditism, reduction clitoroplasty may be performed shortly after laparotomy and gonadal biopsy. In infants with congenital hyperplasia, genitoplasty needs to be deferred until the baby is stable from a medical standpoint. If the vagina opens onto a urogenital sinus, a vaginoplasty must be performed in conjunction with reduction clitoroplasty. In patients born without a vagina, usually bowel vaginoplasty is deferred until puberty.

In a female infant with CAH, the sex of rearing should always be female. With feminizing clitoroplasty, the cosmetic and functional anatomic result should be quite satisfactory. With proper hormonal regulation, these individuals can bear children and the likelihood of tumor formation is no different than that in other women.

In a patient with male pseudohermaphroditism secondary to complete androgen resistance, a female gender assignment is most appropriate. The testes have a 6% to 30% risk of undergoing malignant degeneration in adulthood and therefore should be removed. Timing of gonadectomy is controversial, however, as some investigators recommend the procedure during childhood whereas others advocate waiting until after puberty to allow feminization because of augmented estradiol secretion. If the testes are to be removed after puberty, the caregiver must be careful in explaining to the patient the reason for the procedure and should not refer to the gonads as testicles. After gonadectomy, estrogen support must be initiated.

Individuals with an incomplete form of androgen resistance have a variable phenotypic appearance. The müllerian structures are absent, and the wolffian structures are generally hypoplastic. In some cases, significant virilization occurs at puberty. In general, a male gender assignment should be made only if there is an excellent response with significant phallic growth following parenteral administration of testosterone.

In males with a 5α-reductase deficiency, pseudovaginal perineoscrotal hypospadias is apparent. These boys have normal testes and wolffian duct derivatives, but external virilization is absent. Although some of these males may be assigned a female gender, at puberty marked virilization occurs with penile enlargement, testicular descent, scrotal rugation, and deepening of the voice. Consequently, these patients are good candidates for a male gender assignment if they have an adequate response to parenteral androgens.

In 46,XY males with a disorder in testosterone synthesis, the genital appearance is variable, from female to hypospadiac male. However, the tissue response to testosterone stimulation should be normal. Some of these patients, such as those with a 17β-dehydrogenase defect, eventually restore their capacity for testosterone synthesis and show significant virilization at puberty. All have bilateral testes, which may be intra-abdominal, inguinal, or labioscrotal. In these patients, the enzyme defect should be identified and androgen stimulation initiated to determine whether there is sufficient penile growth response to allow a male gender assignment.

Males with persistent müllerian duct syndrome have a normal penis and wolffian duct derivatives but internally have a fallopian tube or tubes and a uterus. The likelihood of gonadal malignancy is low. These patients are reared as males, but the likelihood of fertility is reduced. Complete excision of the müllerian duct derivatives often results in injury to the vas deferens and is often unnecessary.

In neonates with mixed gonadal dysgenesis, the phenotypic appearance is variable, from predominantly masculine to predominantly feminine. After puberty, the testis contains no spermatogonia. Consequently, the patient is sterile, irrespective of sex assignment. Furthermore, in 25% of cases, a gonadal tumor develops, either in the streak or in the testis. If the patient has a female phenotype, a female gender assignment should be made. However, those with a normal-sized phallus and a scrotal testis can be reared as a male. In such patients, the streak gonad should be promptly removed. If a child with mixed gonadal dysgenesis is reared as a male, the short stature may be treated with growth hormone.

Patients with pure gonadal dysgenesis have bilateral streak gonads and a female phenotype without ambiguous genitalia. Because the risk of tumor development in the streak is 30%, prophylactic gonadectomy is necessary.

Patients with true hermaphroditism have a variable karyotype and phenotype. Gender assignment in these patients can be a difficult decision. In general, ovarian tissue functions better than testicular tissue. For example, the ovary produces estrogen in a cyclic pattern that allows breast development and, in some cases, menses and ovulation. In fact, pregnancy in true hermaphrodites has been reported. On the other hand, spermatogenesis in testicular tissue is uncommon, and testosterone production is often inadequate. Furthermore, testes have a 2% to 3% likelihood of undergoing malignant degeneration. Nevertheless, approximately 70% of affected patients are assigned a male gender. The most important criterion is the phallic size. If the penis is small, one way to test it is to measure the serum testosterone level and reassess stretched penile length after hCG stimulation because a poor response to hCG predicts poor penile growth and masculinization at puberty. After a decision regarding assignment of gender, all discordant gonadal tissue must be removed. In addition, if a female gender assignment is made, feminizing genitoplasty should be performed before hospital discharge.

RED FLAGS

Danger signs include manifestations of adrenal insufficiency, in addition to a male phenotype without palpable testis in the scrotum, hyperpigmentation (increased ACTH production), and hypertension. Although normal at birth, male patients with CAH experience an adrenal crisis once circulating placental-maternal steroid hormones are catabolized and excreted. This phenomenon often occurs between the third and the tenth days of life. The initial diagnosis of the male with salt-losing CAH may be sepsis, pyloric stenosis, meningitis, or other more common neonatal conditions.

REFERENCES

Aaronson IA. True hermaphroditism: Review of forty-one cases with observations on testicular histology and function. Br J Urol 1985;57:775–779.

Allen TD. Disorders of sex differentiation. Urology 1976;7(Suppl):1S–32S.

Amice V, Amice J, Bercovici JP, et al. Gonadal tumor and H-Y antigen in 46,XY pure gonadal dysgenesis. Cancer 1986;57:1313–1317.

Blyth B, Churchill BM, Houle AM, et al. Intersex. *In* Gillenwater JY, Grayhack JT, Howards SS, et al (eds). Adult and Pediatric Urology, 2nd ed. St. Louis: Mosby–Year Book, 1991:2141–2172.

Brosman SA. Mixed gonadal dysgenesis. J Urol 1979;121:344–347.

Bryan PJ, Caldamone AA, Morrison SC, et al. Ultrasound findings in the adrenogenital syndrome (congenital adrenal hyperplasia). J Ultrasound Med 1988;7:675–679.

Elder JS, Duckett JW. Perinatal urology. *In* Gillenwater JY, Grayhack JT, Howards SS, et al (eds). Adult and Pediatric Urology, 2nd ed. St. Louis: Mosby–Year Book, 1991:1711–1810.

George FW, Wilson JD. Embryology of the genital tract. *In* Walsh PC, Retik AB, Stamey TA, et al (eds). Campbell's Urology, 6th ed. Philadelphia: WB Saunders, 1992:1496–1508.

Glassberg KI. Gender assignment in newborn male pseudohermaphrodites. Urol Clin North Am 1980;7:409–421.

Griffin JE, Wilson JD. Disorders of sexual differentiation. *In* Walsh PC, Retik AB, Stamey TA, et al (eds). Campbell's Urology, 6th ed. Philadelphia: WB Saunders, 1992:1509–1542.

Grumbach MM, Conte FA. Disorders of sex differentiation. *In* Wilson JD, Foster DW (eds). Williams Textbook of Endocrinology, 8th ed. Philadelphia: WB Saunders, 1992.

Hughes IA. Management of congenital adrenal hyperplasia. Arch Dis Child 1988;63:1399–1404.

Izquierdo G, Glassberg KI. Gender assignment and gender identity in patients with ambiguous genitalia. Urology 1993;42:232–242.

Martinez-Mora J, Isnard R, Castellvi A, et al. Neovagina in vaginal agenesis: Surgical methods and long-term results. J Pediatr Surg 1992;27:10–14.

Matsumoto T, Kondoh T, Kamei T, et al. Prenatal DNA analysis in four embryos/fetuses at risk of 21-hydroxylase deficiency. Eur J Pediatr 1988;148:228–232.

Mulaikal RM, Migeon CJ, Rock JA. Fertility rates in female patients with congenital adrenal hyperplasia due to 21-hydroxylase deficiency. N Engl J Med 1987;316:178–182.

Nihoul-Fekete C, Lortat-Jacob S, Cachin O, et al. Preservation of gonadal function in true hermaphroditism. J Pediatr Surg 1984;19:50–55.

Savage MO, Lowe DG. Gonadal neoplasia and abnormal sexual differentiation. Clin Endocrinol (Oxf) 1990;32:519–533.

Shapiro E, Santiago JV, Crane JP. Prenatal fetal adrenal suppression following in utero diagnosis of congenital adrenal hyperplasia. J Urol 1989;142:663–666.

Sheldon CA, Gilbert AA, Lewis AG. Vaginal reconstruction: Critical technical principles. J Urol 1994;152:190–195.

Snyder HM, Retik AB, Bauer SB, et al. Feminizing genitoplasty: A synthesis. J Urol 1983;129:1024–1026.

Walsh PC. The differential diagnosis of ambiguous genitalia in the newborn. Urol Clin North Am 1978;5:213–221.

Walsh PC, Migeon CJ. The phenotypic expression of selective disorders of male sexual differentiation. J Urol 1978;119:627–629.

Wilson JD, Harrod MJ, Goldstein JL, et al. Familial incomplete male pseudohermaphroditism, type 1. N Engl J Med 1974;290:1097–1103.

White PC, New MI, Dupont B. Congenital adrenal hyperplasia. Part 1. N Engl J Med 1987;316:1519–1524.

White PC, New MI, Dupont B. Congenital adrenal hyperplasia. Part 2. N Engl J Med 1987;316:1580–1586.

34 Mental Retardation and Developmental Disability

Gregory S. Liptak

DEFINITIONS

Mental retardation is defined as limitations in intelligence and adaptive skills that begin in childhood. The formal definition of mental retardation has been based on the intelligence quotient (IQ) derived from formal testing. Unfortunately, although the IQ score is an average of many abilities, it has been viewed as a single entity. The ability of children to adapt to their environment has been added to the definition. In 1992, the American Association on Mental Retardation (AAMR) defined mental retardation as an IQ less than 70 or 75, with onset before age 18 years and limitations in two or more of the adaptive skills shown in Table 34–1. Although adaptive skills and strengths are more difficult to quantify, the hope is that this information will improve the diagnosis and prevent ''labeling.''

In the past, retarded children have been grouped into categories, including moron, imbecile, and idiot; mild, moderate, severe, and profound; and educable, trainable, and untrainable. Rather than using these classifications, the AAMR recommends that once a child has been diagnosed as being mentally retarded, the strengths and weaknesses in four domains should be described. These domains are intellectual functioning and adaptive skills, psychologic and emotional considerations, physical health and etiologic consid-erations, and environmental considerations. For example, a child could be described as ''a 4-year-old mentally retarded child who has good social skills but needs supports in self-direction and safety.''

The term *developmental disabilities* is used to describe a broader array of conditions, including mental retardation. Developmental disabilities may be isolated, as in the child with vision impairment, or may be multiple, as in the child with delays in fine motor, gross motor, and social functioning.

EPIDEMIOLOGY

Developmental disabilities are common; about 5.5% of patients encountered in a general practice may have cognitive and language disorders, while 4.0% may have motor abnormalities. These disa-bilities and their prevalence rates per 1000 children include (1) mental retardation (10.3), (2) cerebral palsy (2.0), (3) hearing impairment (1.0), and (4) visual impairment. Table 34–2 lists the prevalence of select conditions associated with developmental de-lay. Overall, chromosomal disorders (24%), syndromes (12%), perinatal-postnatal injury (2.6%), intrauterine infection (7%), in-born errors of metabolism (5%), and undetermined factors (18%) account for many causes of severe mental retardation.

Delayed development is not uniformly distributed among all children but is more frequent in certain populations, such as those from low socioeconomic status, including the homeless. The preva-lence of specific conditions that cause developmental delay varies with gender, age (especially since many conditions such as chromo-somal anomalies are associated with high mortality rates and are less frequent after infancy), and location. For example, 5% of the individuals in a town in Northern Quebec carry the gene for hereditary tyrosinemia. The distribution of etiologic factors in chil-dren with mental retardation also differs with the degree of delay. Chromosomal disorders, such as trisomy 21 (Down syndrome), are more common in moderately and severely retarded individuals, whereas environmental deprivation is more common in those with mild retardation. The percentage of children having retardation with an unknown etiology is also greater in the milder group. Additional methods have helped identify the etiology of adolescents with severe retardation and can determine a diagnosis in about 81% of those previously undiagnosed. These new diagnoses include fragile X syndrome, Rett syndrome, and Angelman syndrome.

DIAGNOSIS

Although pursuing a single etiology for delayed development in a child is important to provide insight into prognosis, recurrence

---

Table 34–1. Definition of Mental Retardation

A. Assumptions
  1. Assessments performed on the child are sensitive to differences in culture, language, communication, and behavior.
  2. The demands and constraints of the child's environment (home, neighborhood, school) must be considered.
  3. Even children with limitations have strengths that should be considered.
B. Criteria
  1. Intelligence quotient (IQ) equal to or below 70–75, *plus*
  2. Limitations exist in two or more of the following adaptive skills:
    a. Communication
    b. Self-care
    c. Home living
    d. Social skills
    e. Community use
    f. Self-direction
    g. Health and safety
    h. Functional academics
    i. Leisure
    j. Work
  3. Limitations manifest before age 18 yr.

Table 34-2. Prevalence of Select Conditions Associated with Developmental Delay

Condition	Prevalence per 100,000	Comments
Cerebral palsy	250–270	Represents many etiologies
Significant hearing loss	150	In neonatal period
Down syndrome	98–125	Prevalence at birth
Fragile X syndrome	117	
Meningomyelocele	60–100	Prevalence at birth
Klinefelter syndrome	100	15% have intelligence quotient (IQ) <80
Fetal alcohol syndrome	60–800	
Congenital HIV infection	5–50	Increasing incidence
Blindness	41–88	At 10 yr of age
Infantile hydrocephalus	64	Prevalence at birth
Neurofibromatosis	33	5% have mental retardation
Trisomy 18	30	Prevalence at birth
Trisomy 13	20	Prevalence at birth
Turner syndrome	20	
Prader-Willi syndrome	13–20	In childhood
Galactosemia	14	In infancy
Phenylketonuria	6–12	
Anophthalmia	6	
Rett syndrome	4–5	In girls 2 to 18 yr of age
Histidinemia	3	At birth
Acrocephalosyndactylia (Apert syndrome)	1–2	

risk, therapies, counseling, and linkage with a supportive group, it is not sufficient. Identification of the child's functional abilities, strengths and weaknesses, overall physical health, and environmental factors such as support is critical to optimizing the child's health, development, and functioning. In addition, developmental disability does not have an apparent etiology in many children, or there may be multiple possible causal factors or multiple disabilities. For example, as many as 23% of children with developmental disabilities may have two disabilities, while 6% may have three or more. Even if a specific diagnosis cannot be made, early identification of developmental delay can lead to a program of early intervention or remediation that will improve the child's ultimate functioning.

Identification

Identifying a child who is at increased risk for developmental delay requires a process of selection (screening). The screening process may be minimal, as with the child who has obvious multiple congenital anomalies or when parents tell you that their child's development is delayed; or the screening may require a more formal test, as in the general screening of children who have no apparent risk factors. Once a child is identified as being at increased risk, a comprehensive evaluation needs to be performed to make a diagnosis, evaluate functioning, and develop a plan of care.

The greater the number of biologic risk factors, the greater the likelihood that the child will develop abnormally. For prenatal and perinatal risk factors, a combination of three or more factors predicted later developmental delay; in one study 11% of mothers had three or more risk factors but accounted for 43% of the "disabled" children.

- *Biologic risks* include prematurity, intracranial hemorrhage, intrauterine growth retardation, hypoxic-ischemic encephalopathy, brain anomalies on computed tomography (CT), symptomatic hypoglycemia, severe hyperbilirubinemia, micro- or macrocephaly, congenital infections, acquired infection (men-

ingitis), seizures, maternal drug use, exposure to toxins (lead), severe acute or chronic neonatal lung disease, or congenital malformations.
- *Sociocultural risks* have a profound effect on development and interact with biologic risk factors.

Sociocultural risks include poverty, a lack of prenatal care or health insurance, teenage or single-parent status, maternal mental illness, a history of child abuse or neglect or family violence, poor parenting skills, homelessness, divorce, or disordered attachment (bonding).

Perinatal and other biologic risk factors that can lead to intellectual impairment do not always have the same magnitude of neurodevelopmental consequences for middle-class or upper-class children as they do for poor children.

Except in children with catastrophic circumstances, child-rearing conditions that support and enrich early development may compensate for biologic deficits. Sociocultural conditions such as small family size, higher level of parental education, and fewer changes in residence have a more powerful effect than many biologic risks and seem to be important predictors of developmental functioning beyond infancy.

Screening for Specific Abnormalities

Defects in vision, hearing, and language can have devastating effects on development; early intervention to ameliorate these problems can improve developmental outcomes. All children should be screened on a regular basis for these conditions.

VISUAL DEFECTS

Children at high risk for development of defects in vision (see Chapter 44) include those with strabismus (especially after 4 months of age), hydrocephalus, congenital infection, asphyxia, congenital anomaly of the central nervous system, prematurity with exposure to oxygen, and family history of childhood onset of visual impairment. All neonates should routinely have an evaluation of their fundi for the presence of a red reflex, which can be obscured by cataract or tumor, as well as inspection of the globe, which may be affected by congenital glaucoma. Infants with nystagmus who do not follow visually by 3 months of age, who have dissociation between visual behavior and motor behavior, or whose parents express concern about their vision should have formal ophthalmologic evaluation.

Preschool children should have periodic evaluations of extraocular movements to rule out strabismus and amblyopia using visual inspection of the child's eyes, the Hirschberg light test, and the cover-uncover test. As early in the child's development as possible, specific tests of monocular and binocular vision such as Allen cards (3 to 5 years), the Snellen chart (>5 years), or the Titmus tester (>4 years) should be performed. If physicians fail to adhere to established recommendations for vision screening, the diagnosis of amblyopia may not be made until the child is older than 5 years of age and vision loss cannot be prevented.

LOSS OF HEARING

Screening for hearing should begin in the neonatal period for high-risk newborns by using brainstem auditory evoked potentials. Criteria for classifying a child at high risk include prematurity or low birth weight (usually <1500 g), or both, hereditary hearing loss, use of potentially ototoxic drugs such as aminoglycoside antibiotics and furosemide, craniofacial anomaly (cleft palate), congenital infection, meningitis, hyperbilirubinemia requiring an exchange transfusion, severe neonatal asphyxia, head trauma, persistent fetal circulation, and parental suspicion that the child does not hear. Newborns born weighing 1500 g or less or with gestations of 32 weeks or less, or both, may have an incidence of hearing loss of 15% (14% conductive or unspecified and 1% sensorineural). At 5 years of age, 2% of these high-risk neonates may have severe problems with communication.

For older children, parents should be asked about their child's auditory acuity. Parental concern has a sensitivity of approximately 44%. If parents express concern about their child's ability to hear, the child has recurrent episodes of otitis media, mastoiditis, or one of the perinatal risk factors, a formal audiometric screening is performed. The value of routine screening of all preschool children using audiometry has been questioned.

Table 34–3 lists the latest acceptable age ("limit ages") for the appearance of abilities that may indicate a disorder of hearing. Deaf infants may smile, coo, and babble; however, their vocalizations usually cease after 8 months of age.

Table 34–3. Latest Acceptable Age for Skills Related to Hearing*

Age (mo)†	Activity
3	Not startling to loud sounds
6	Not smiling to voice; not vocalizing
9	Does not localize speech or other sounds
12	Not babbling multiple sounds and syllables
18	No words
24	<50% of speech understandable

Adapted from the Arizona Speech, Language, Hearing Association.
*A child who does not demonstrate the activity by the stated age should have formal audiometry performed.
†Corrected for gestational age.

SPEECH AND LANGUAGE DISORDERS

Disorders of speech and language development are common in childhood, with a prevalence in preschool children of 3% to 20%, and are correlated with subsequent learning problems. The most common cause of delayed language development is global mental retardation. Although the optimal age at which to intervene for a child with abnormal language development is uncertain, the general consensus is that delayed diagnosis decreases the likelihood of successful treatment. A number of screening tests, such as the Language Development Survey (sensitivity 0.87, specificity 0.86 when compared to the Bayley Mental Developmental Index), the Clinical Linguistic and Auditory Milestone Scale (CLAMS) (sensitivity 0.66, specificity 0.79), and the Early Language Milestone Scale (sensitivity 0.87, specificity 0.70 when compared to the Sequenced Inventory of Communication Development), are available; none is completely practical for use in an office setting. A very brief sentence-repetition screening test has a sensitivity of 0.76, specificity of 0.92, positive predictive value of 0.54, and negative predictive value of 0.97 when compared to a standard battery of tests.

OTHER CONDITIONS

For approximately 30 years, mass-population newborn screening for inborn errors of metabolism, which can have profound effects on development, have been performed. New York State screens newborns for phenylketonuria, galactosemia, maple syrup urine disease, homocystinuria, biotinidase deficiency, and hypothyroidism. Screening tests for histidinemia and adenosine deaminase deficiency were removed several years ago because of extremely low yields. Although most of these conditions are extremely rare, early treatment can lead to improved developmental outcomes.

Prenatal screening of alpha-fetoprotein using maternal serum and, if indicated, amniotic fluid obtained during amniocentesis has become widespread. Low levels have been associated with Down syndrome, while elevated levels have been associated with open neural tube defects and other anomalies, such as gastroschisis. Prenatal screening for other specific conditions, such as Tay-Sachs disease, is being performed in high-risk populations.

General Screening

Most pediatricians do not routinely use formal developmental screening tests. When they do screen, the most commonly used test is the Denver Developmental Screening Test (DDST). Some issues have been raised about the soundness of using this test as a screening device. For example, its sensitivity may be only 0.20 when compared with outcomes such as teacher reports, IQ tests, and placement in special education classes. The DDST may fail to identify a high proportion of children who are developmentally at risk because it has very few speech and language items, does not consider attention, and does not consider environmental factors such as educational achievement of the parents, environmental stimulation, and social support. The insensitivity of the DDST is a problem because many physicians use it as the sole basis for referring children for early intervention or special education programs.

It has been recommended that the DDST be used as a "growth curve" to monitor development on a regular basis. Whether this is more advantageous than using the traditional method of history taking, observation, and physical assessment is uncertain. Other checklists that are more comprehensive, such as the Hawaii Early

Learning Profile (for children from birth to 3 years), are available for developmental surveillance.

The DDST has been revised and is called the Denver II. It has low specificity (0.43) when scored the conventional way and low sensitivity (0.56) when scored an alternative way. Many recommend using another screening test, such as the Battelle or the Minnesota inventories.

Screening tests have been utilized by physical and occupational therapists to evaluate neuromotor functioning in infants and preschool children. However, the positive predictive value for longterm functioning for most of these evaluations is modest when used during infancy. Screening tests to predict learning problems in school, such as the Pediatric Examination of Education Readiness (PEER), which takes approximately 30 minutes to administer, and the Einstein, which requires 7 to 10 minutes, have been developed. Both require additional evaluation before they can be recommended for general use. No screening test should be used in isolation from other clinical and social data.

Another strategy for screening children for high risk of developmental delay is to develop an inventory of items that leads to an index of risk. A list of commonly used items is shown in Table 34–4. Although these indices have been shown to have good concurrent sensitivity and specificity, they may not always predict future function because they do not consider environmental and other factors such as attention.

Table 34–4. Items Used to Identify Neonates at Increased Risk for Developmental Delay

Item	Comment
Apgar scores	<3 at 5 min or <5 at 10 min, especially important in term infants
Abnormal EEG	
Neonatal seizures	Hypoglycemia, hypoxic, intracranial hemorrhage, or infection are high risk
Intracranial hemorrhage	Grade III or higher
Hydrocephalus	Especially with other anomalies, thin cortical mantle, or parenchymal lesions
Central nervous system anomalies	Seen on CT scan or ultrasound
Prematurity	<32 wk
Small for gestational age	<3rd percentile (intrauterine growth retardation)
Dysmorphic features	Three or more minor or one or more major
Chromosomal anomaly	Trisomies, fragile X, XO
Ventilation required	Longer than 2 wk
Small head circumference	<3rd percentile
Meningitis	Bacterial (group B streptococci, *Escherichia coli*) Viral (herpes simplex)
Hypoglycemia	Symptomatic
Congenital infection	Cytomegalovirus, toxoplasmosis, syphilis, rubella, herpes simplex, varicella-zoster, HIV
Hyperbilirubinemia	Requiring exchange transfusions
Associated medical problems	Such as retinopathy of prematurity, heart disease, bronchopulmonary dysplasia, necrotizing enterocolitis

Abbreviations: CT = computed tomography; HIV = human immunodeficiency virus.

Table 34–5. Latest Acceptable Age for Skills Related to Motor Functioning

Milestone	Age (mo)*
Roll prone to supine	4.5
Roll supine to prone	6.0
Sit with arms supported	6.75
Sit without support	8.0
Creep	8.5
Come to sitting	9.5
Crawl	9.75
Pull to standing	10.25
Cruise	11.0
Walk independently	14.75

Adapted from Allen MC, Alexander GR. Motor milestones of very preterm infants at risk for cerebral palsy. Dev Med Child Neurol 1992;34:226–232.
*Corrected for gestational age.

An isolated factor such as low birth weight does not predict school failure or low IQ in a simple linear fashion. States in the United States have adopted some of these items to identify children who would benefit from early intervention programs based on Public Law 99-457. A review of the criteria adopted by most states found that these criteria have poor predictive values (0.25 to 0.35) and poor specificities (0.12 to 0.40).

Inventories of risk can be coupled with other screening assessments of the child, the child's environment, or both. Table 34–5 gives the limit ages of motor milestones. In infants who are premature *and* have delays in the achievement of these milestones, cerebral palsy is more likely to occur. The sensitivities and specificities of these items range from 0.70 to 0.94. Similar criteria, based on motor skills, for screening children who have specific conditions, such as spina bifida, have been developed, although most have not had extensive psychometric evaluation. Any risk inventory should be joined with evaluations of the environment, such as the Home Observation for Measurement of the Environment (HOME).

The most commonly used method of general screening is to rely on parental report of the developmental status of the child, which may have a sensitivity of 80%, specificity of 94%, positive predictive value of 76%, and negative predictive value of 95%. In a similar population, parental concerns regarding speech and language problems may have a sensitivity of 83%, specificity of 72%, positive predictive value of 72%, and negative predictive value of 83%.

Formal assessment of a child's development by a parent is available through instruments such as the Infant/Child Monitoring Questionnaire. These questionnaires, which cover children from birth to 48 months of age, can be administered prior to the pediatric visit and reviewed with the family during the visit. Although parental history is important, it should not be the only criteria used to assess children with potential developmental delay but should be followed up with detailed evaluation. A lack of parental concern about a child's development is no guarantee that the development is normal.

Comprehensive Assessment

HISTORY

Once a child is identified as being at risk for developmental delay, a comprehensive evaluation should be obtained by a primary care physician. Further evaluations by specialty physicians, therapists (physical, occupational, speech), psychologists, nurses, nutritionists, social workers, and others may be indicated. Table 34–6

Table 34–6. Information to Be Sought During the History Taking of a Child with Suspected Developmental Disabilities

Item	Possible Significance
Parental Concerns	Parents are quite accurate in identifying developmental problems in their children
Current Levels of Developmental Functioning	Should be used to monitor child's progress
Temperament	May interact with disability or may be confused with developmental delay
Prenatal History	
Alcohol ingestion	Fetal alcohol syndrome; an index of care-taking risk
Illegal drug, toxin, medication exposure	Developmental toxin (e.g., phenytoin); may be an index of care-taking risk
Radiation exposure	Damage to central nervous system (CNS)
Nutrition	Inadequate fetal nutrition
Prenatal care	Index of social situation
Injuries, hyperthermia	Damage to CNS
Smoking	Possible CNS damage
Human immunodeficiency virus (HIV) exposure	Congenital HIV infection
Maternal phenylketonuria (PKU)	Maternal PKU effect
Maternal illness	Toxoplasmosis, rubella, cytomegalovirus, herpesvirus infections
Perinatal History	
Gestational age, birth weight	Biologic risk from prematurity and small for gestational age
Labor and delivery	Hypoxia or index of abnormal prenatal development
Apgar scores	Hypoxia, cardiovascular impairment
Specific perinatal adverse events—see Table 34–4	Increased risk for CNS damage
Neonatal History	
Illness—seizures, respiratory distress, hyperbilirubinemia, metabolic disorder; see also Table 34–4	Increased risk for CNS damage
Malformations	May represent syndrome associated with developmental delay
Family History	
Consanguinity	Autosomal recessive condition more likely
Mental functioning	Increased hereditary and environmental risks
Illnesses (e.g., metabolic disease)	Hereditary illness associated with developmental delay
Family member died young or unexpectedly	May suggest inborn error of metabolism or storage disease
Family member requires special education	Hereditary causes of developmental delay
Social History	
Resources available (e.g., financial, social support)	Necessary to maximize child's potential
Educational level of parents	Family may need help to provide stimulation
Mental health problems	May exacerbate child's conditions
High-risk behaviors (illicit drugs, sex)	Increased risk for HIV infection; index of care-taking risk
Other stressors (e.g., marital discord)	May exacerbate child's conditions or compromise care
Other History	
Gender of child	Important for X-linked conditions
Developmental milestones	Index of developmental delay; regression may indicate progressive condition
Head injury	Even moderate trauma may be associated with developmental delay or learning disabilities
Serious infections (e.g., meningitis)	May be associated with developmental delay
Toxic exposure (e.g., lead)	May be associated with developmental delay
Physical growth	May indicate malnutrition; obesity, short stature associated with some conditions
Recurrent otitis media	Associated with hearing loss and abnormal speech development
Visual and auditory functioning	Sensitive index of impairments in vision and hearing
Nutrition	Malnutrition during infancy may lead to delayed development
Chronic conditions like renal disease or anemia	May be associated with delayed development

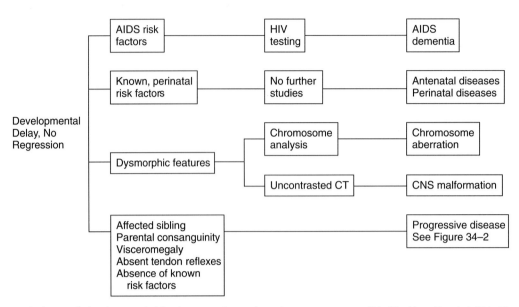

Figure 34–1. Evaluation of infants with developmental delay but no evidence of psychomotor regression. (Modified from Fenichel GM. Clinical Pediatric Neurology: A Signs and Symptoms Approach, 2nd ed. Philadelphia: WB Saunders, 1993:118.)

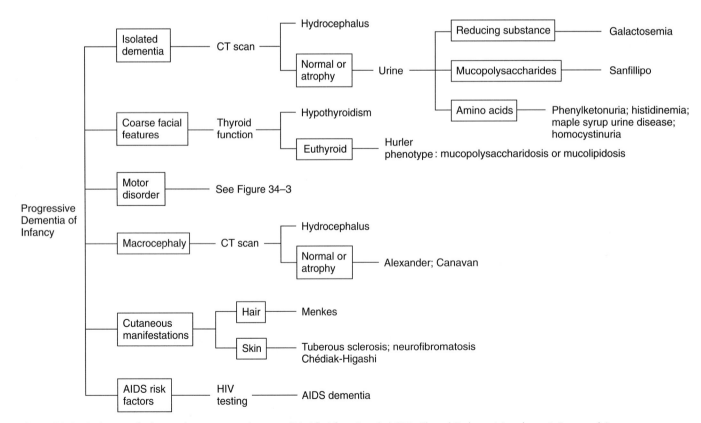

Figure 34–2. Evaluation of infants with progressive dementia. (Modified from Fenichel GM. Clinical Pediatric Neurology: A Signs and Symptoms Approach, 2nd ed. Philadelphia: WB Saunders, 1993:121.)

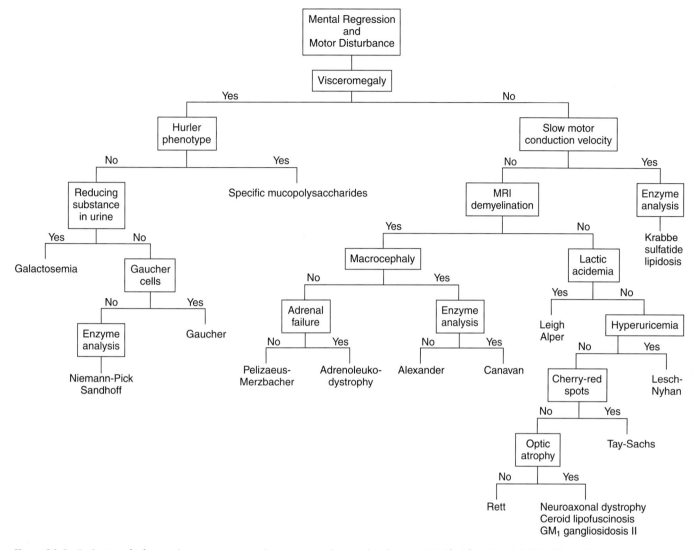

Figure 34–3. Evaluation of infants with progressive mental regression and motor disturbances. (Modified from Fenichel GM. Clinical Pediatric Neurology: A Signs and Symptoms Approach, 2nd ed. Philadelphia: WB Saunders, 1993:131.)

outlines some of the information that should be sought whenever obtaining a history of a child suspected of having developmental delay.

An assessment of the child's current level of functioning and previous developmental milestones should be obtained for all areas of development, including cognitive, fine motor, gross motor, speech and language, and socialization.

Delays isolated to a single, specific area such as expressive language are more likely to be transient than are generalized delays. Because the guidelines of the DDST end at school age, many physicians are unaware of milestones that children achieve after 5 years of age. Guidelines are available, and school records can be used to help evaluate cognitive and social functioning.

If the child's development has deteriorated (regressed) so that the child no longer functions as well as before, a *progressive encephalopathy* is likely. *Progressive* disorders are often a result of metabolic causes, whereas *static* encephalopathies are usually due to structural abnormalities or are the result of a previous trauma (including hypoxia). Table 34–7 lists some extrinsic causes of neurologic deterioration, and Table 34–8 lists some intrinsic causes. More than 300 neurodegenerative disorders have been described; additional classifications based on progression and age are noted in Tables 34–9 and 34–10 and in Figures 34–1 to 34–4.

Neurodegenerative disorders are often categorized as involving white matter, gray matter, basal ganglia, or the entire central nervous system. White matter diseases (adrenoleukodystrophy) affect long tracts and present with loss of motor skills, spasticity, areflexia (if peripheral nerve involvement), or ataxia, while gray matter diseases (gangliosidosis type II) present with seizures and abnormalities of cognition, vision, and hearing. Many disorders classified as "white matter" or "gray matter" present with a mixed picture of signs and symptoms. Diseases that primarily involve the basal ganglia, such as Huntington disease, present with mental deterioration, behavioral changes, rigidity, ataxia, dysarthria, and incoordination. As these diseases progress, neurologic signs and symptoms become less specific.

The history should include prenatal, perinatal, and neonatal events as well as serious acute illnesses, recurrent illnesses, and trauma. Details regarding nutrition and exposure to toxins should be sought. A detailed pedigree of the family should be acquired, outlining the previous two generations to identify any familial conditions similar to the patient's problem and to identify consanguinity.

An evaluation of the home, including family composition, resources, stresses, and social supports, should be sought. Information regarding a typical day from the time the child awakens to the time the child sleeps can provide insights into the child's routine activities, nutritional status, and parent-child interactions (whether the

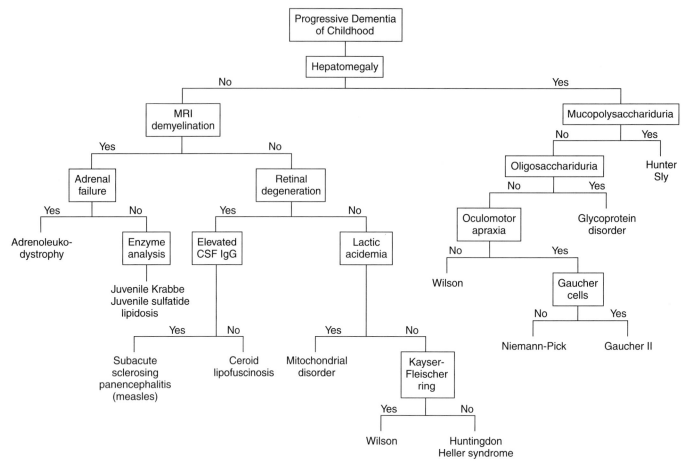

Figure 34–4. Evaluation of children with progressive dementia. (Modified from Fenichel GM. Clinical Pediatric Neurology: A Signs and Symptoms Approach, 2nd ed. Philadelphia: WB Saunders, 1993:138.)

parent spends time playing with the child or participates in stimulating activities). Because a child's temperament can affect the manifestations of developmental delay or even be mistaken for developmental delay or a psychiatric condition (the slow-to-warm-up child who is labeled retarded or depressed by the kindergarten teacher), a temperamental profile should be obtained.

Table 34–7. Select "Extrinsic" Conditions Associated with Developmental Regression

Neoplasms and their therapy
  Leukemia
  Tumors
  Histiocytosis
Increased intracranial pressure
  Hydrocephalus, including ventricular shunt malfunctions
  Subdural hematoma or effusion
  Tumors
Infections
  Encephalitis, including human immunodeficiency virus (HIV) infection
  Meningitis
Endocrine
  Hypothyroidism
  Adrenocortical insufficiency
Other
  Collagen-vascular disease (e.g., systemic lupus erythematosus)

In addition to developing a rapport with the family, the act of taking the history can provide insights into the child's developmental status. While the interview is occurring, the child's interactions with the environment (light, sound) and with people should be observed. The child's general neurologic functioning can also be assessed; level of alertness, facial symmetry, extraocular movements, use and symmetry of extremities, locomotion, and posture should be noticed. Parental interactions with the child should also be noted.

PHYSICAL EXAMINATION

Any child suspected of having developmental delay should have a complete physical examination, which may reveal a recognizable pattern of malformation. Tables 34–11 and 34–12 outline areas that provide clues to the diagnosis. In addition to a qualitative evaluation to obtain a comprehensive view of the child and to determine if the child is ill, precise quantitative measurements include:

- Weight, length (or height), and head circumference
- Facial features, such as inner canthal distance, palpebral fissure length, and ear length
- Hand and foot measurements as well as dermatoglyphics
- Measurement of male genitalia (penile length and testicular volume)

If a child has an unusual appearance, biologic family members should be examined either directly or using photographs to deter-

Table 34–8. Select "Intrinsic" Conditions Associated with Developmental Regression

Age at Onset (yr)	Condition	Comments
< 2—with hepatomegaly (see Chapter 22)	Fructose intolerance	Vomiting, hypoglycemia, poor feeding, failure to thrive (when given fructose)
	Galactosemia	Lethargy, hypotonia, icterus, cataract, hypoglycemia (when given lactose)
	Glycogenosis (glycogen storage disease) types I–IV	Hypoglycemia, cardiomegaly (II)
	Mucopolysaccharidosis types I and II	Coarse facies, stiff joints
	Niemann-Pick disease, infantile type	Gray matter disease, failure to thrive
	Tay-Sachs disease	Seizures, cherry-red macula, edema, coarse facies
	Zellweger (cerebro-hepato-renal) syndrome	Hypotonia, high forehead, flat facies
	Gaucher disease type II	Extensor posturing, irritability
< 2—without hepatomegaly	Krabbe disease	Irritability, extensor posturing, optic atrophy and blindness
	Rett syndrome	Girls with deceleration of head growth, loss of hand skills, hand wringing, impaired language skills, gait apraxia
	Maple syrup urine disease	Poor feeding, tremors, myoclonus, opisthotonos
	Phenylketonuria	Light pigmentation, eczema, seizures
	Menkes kinky hair disease	Hypertonia, irritability, seizures, abnormal hair
	Subacute necrotizing encephalopathy of Leigh	White matter disease
	Cerebro-oculo-facio-skeletal syndrome (of Pena and Shokeir)	Reduced white matter, failure to thrive
	Canavan disease	White matter disease
	Pelizaeus-Merzbacher disease	White matter disease
2–5	Niemann-Pick disease types III and IV	Hepatosplenomegaly, gait difficulty
	Wilson disease	Liver disease, Kayser-Fleischer ring, deterioration of cognition is late
	Gangliosidosis type II	Gray matter disease
	Ceroid lipofuscinosis	Gray matter disease
	Mitochondrial encephalopathies (e.g., myoclonic epilepsy, ragged-red fibers [MERRF])	Gray matter diseases
	Ataxia-telangiectasia	Basal ganglia disease
	Huntington disease (chorea)	Basal ganglia disease
	Hallervorden-Spatz syndrome	Basal ganglia disease
	Metachromatic leukodystrophy	White matter disease
	Adrenoleukodystrophy	White matter disease, behavior problems, falling school performance, quadriparesis
	Subacute sclerosing panencephalitis	Diffuse encephalopathy, myoclonus, may occur years after measles
5–15	Adrenoleukodystrophy	See above for adrenoleukodystrophy
	Multiple sclerosis	White matter disease
	Neuronal ceroid lipofuscinosis, juvenile and adult (Spielmeyer-Vogt and Kufs disease)	Gray matter diseases
	Schilder disease	White matter disease, focal neurologic symptoms
	Refsum disease	Peripheral neuropathy, ataxia, retinitis pigmentosa
	Sialidosis II, juvenile form	Cherry-red macula, myoclonus, ataxia, coarse facies

Table 34–9. Progressive Encephalopathy: Onset Before Age 2 Years

Acquired Immunodeficiency Syndrome Encephalopathy

Aminoacidurias
1. Homocystinuria
2. Maple syrup urine disease
   a. Intermediate form
   b. Thiamine-responsive form
3. Phenylketonuria

Hypothyroidism

Lysosomal Enzyme Disorders
1. Glycoprotein degradation disorders
   a. Mannosidosis type I
   b. Fucosidosis types I and II
   c. Sialidosis type II (infantile form)
2. Mucolipidoses
   a. Type II (I-cell)
   b. Type IV
3. Mucopolysaccharidoses
   a. Type I (Hurler)
   b. Type II (Sanfilippo)
4. Sphingolipidoses
   a. Gaucher disease type II (glucosylceramide lipidosis)
   b. GM_1 gangliosidosis types I and II
   c. GM_2 gangliosidosis (Tay-Sachs, Sandhoff)
   d. Globoid cell leukodystrophy (Krabbe)
   e. Metachromatic leukodystrophy (sulfatide lipidoses)
   f. Multiple sulfatase deficiency
   g. Niemann-Pick type A (sphingomyelin lipidosis)

Mitochondrial Disorders
1. Mitochondrial myopathy, encephalopathy, lactic acidosis, stroke
2. Progressive infantile poliodystrophy (Alper)
3. Subacute necrotizing encephalomyelopathy (Leigh)
4. Trichopoliodystrophy (Menkes)

Neurocutaneous Syndromes
1. Chédiak-Higashi syndrome
2. Neurofibromatosis
3. Tuberous sclerosis

Other Genetic Disorders of Gray Matter
1. Infantile ceroid lipofuscinosis (Santavuori)
2. Infantile neuroaxonal dystrophy
3. Lesch-Nyhan disease
4. Rett syndrome

Other Genetic Disorders of White Matter
1. Alexander disease
2. Galactosemia: transferase deficiency
3. Neonatal adrenoleukodystrophy
4. Pelizaeus-Merzbacher disease
5. Spongy degeneration of infancy (Canavan–Van Bogaert)

Progressive Hydrocephalus

From Fenichel GM. Clinical Pediatric Neurology: A Signs and Symptoms Approach, 2nd ed. Philadelphia: WB Saunders, 1993:116.

mine any resemblance. If the child does not resemble anyone in the family, a new genetic mutation or autosomal recessive condition may be responsible. Examination of the skin of family members may be helpful in conditions such as tuberous sclerosis and neurofibromatosis.

Although the presence of multiple minor physical anomalies has been associated with developmental delay (see Table 34–12), most children with minor anomalies develop normally; predicting that a child will have developmental delay on the basis of these findings alone may lead to a self-fulfilling prophecy whereby an otherwise normal child's development ecomes delayed.

A conscientious neurologic evaluation should be performed. In addition to general mentation and cerebellar signs, a careful motor examination, including evaluation of muscle tone, deep tendon reflexes, and strength, is indicated. Children who are "cute," who have normal motor milestones, or who appear alert may have significant developmental delay.

LABORATORY STUDIES

Routine Blood and Urine Tests

Most children who present with possible developmental delay do not require routine laboratory studies, such as white blood cell counts or electrolyte levels. If a child demonstrates failure to thrive (Chapter 17), developmental regression, or vomiting (see Chapter 20) and lethargy, metabolic screening should be performed (Table 34–13).

The first step is to make certain that the child had a normal neonatal metabolic screening evaluation. Once this has been en-

sured, a metabolic screen of urine can be performed using a group of colorimetric tests (ferric chloride, dinitrophenylhydrazine, reducing substances, nitroprusside, and cetyltrimethylammonium bromide/Berry spot). This battery can be used to screen for phenylketonuria, galactosemia and fructosemia, organic aciduria, amino aciduria, homocystinuria, and mucopolysaccharidosis. In addition, the combination of blood gases, blood lactate, blood ammonia, blood glucose, and urine ketones can help identify children to be evaluated for maple syrup urine disease, organic aciduria, lactic acidosis, urea cycle disorders, and nonketotic hyperglycinemia.

Once suspicions have been narrowed to a group of conditions (on the basis of clinical presentation, laboratory screening tests, and neuroimaging), specific evaluations (such as microscopy or biochemical analyses) of blood, urine, and tissue samples can be undertaken.

Chromosome Analysis

Chromosome-DNA diagnostic techniques, such as karyotyping, banding, hybridization, specific gene identification, and restriction fragment length polymorphism, have allowed precise diagnoses such as the pairing of Prader-Willi and Angelman syndromes (both contiguous gene syndromes) with specific chromosomal anomalies. Other contiguous gene syndromes include Miller-Dieker, Langer-Giedion, aniridia–Wilms tumor, DiGeorge, Alagille, Beckwith-Wiedemann, Palister-Killian, Smith-Magenis, and Wolf-Hirschhorn. Table 34–14 lists some common chromosomal defects that are associated with developmental delay.

All children who have severe developmental delay with multiple congenital abnormalities should have chromosome analyses performed. If the analyses were performed more than 5 years

Table 34–10. Progressive Encephalopathy: Onset After Age 2 Years

Infectious Diseases
1. Subacute sclerosing panencephalitis
2. HIV infection

Lysosomal Enzymes Disorders
1. Glycoprotein degradation disorders
   a. Aspartylglycosaminuria
   b. Mannosidosis type II
2. Mucopolysaccharidoses types II and VII
3. Sphingolipidoses
   a. Gaucher disease type III (glucosylceramide lipidosis)
   b. GM_2 gangliosidosis (juvenile Tay-Sachs)
   c. Globoid cell leukodystrophy (late-onset Krabbe)
   d. Metachromatic leukodystrophy (late-onset sulfatide lipidoses)
   e. Niemann-Pick type C (sphingomyelin lipidosis)

Other Genetic Disorders of Gray Matter
1. Ceroid lipofuscinosis
   a. Late infantile (Bielschowsky-Jansky)
   b. Juvenile
2. Heller syndrome
3. Huntington disease
4. Mitochondrial disorders
   a. Late-onset poliodystrophy
   b. Myoclonic epilepsy and ragged-red fibers (MERRF)
5. Xeroderma pigmentosum

Other Genetic Disorders of White Matter
1. Adrenoleukodystrophy
2. Alexander disease
3. Cerebrotendinous xanthomatosis

Modified from Fenichel GM. Clinical Pediatric Neurology: A Signs and Symptoms Approach, 2nd ed. Philadelphia: WB Saunders, 1993:117.
Abbreviation: HIV = human immunodeficiency virus.

previously, they should be repeated using currently available techniques. For children with developmental delay and hypopigmentation not pathognomonic for a specific condition (e.g., neurofibromatosis), chromosome analysis of cells from peripheral blood should be performed. If these results are normal, a skin biopsy should be performed for analysis of skin fibroblasts, since these may be abnormal while lymphocytes appear normal.

Controversy exists regarding the routine chromosome screening for fragile X syndrome of all children with mental retardation who do not have features suggesting other chromosomal aberrations (e.g., Prader-Willi syndrome). Proponents argue that the knowledge potentially gained regarding prognosis and familial issues outweighs the cost. Others have argued that children should be screened and that only those at high risk should have chromosome analysis. Table 34–15 presents one screening method; a score of 5 or greater leads to a sensitivity of 0.88 and specificity of 0.98 when compared to chromosome analysis. Once fragile X syndrome is identified in a family, molecular studies may be substituted for cytogenetic techniques for subsequent testing.

Whenever a clinician screens a child for a chromosomal anomaly, the physician should provide clinical information to the laboratory performing the chromosome studies, including the child's differential diagnosis, so that the technicians can choose the proper techniques.

Neuroimaging

Ultrasonography. An ultrasound study of the head performed prenatally or during infancy until the anterior fontanelle closes can provide a general anatomic picture of the brain, including a view of the posterior fossa. This technique is insensitive to lesions involving the subdural space, such as subdural hematoma, and depends on the skill of the interpreter more than other imaging studies. It does not expose the child to radiation, nor is sedation required in most instances. Its primary uses include identifying and monitoring intraventricular hemorrhage and hydrocephalus, functions especially useful in the preterm infant.

CT Scans. CT provides greater detail than ultrasonography, including details of bony structures and the subdural space. It can be used with contrast material to further delineate structures, such as tumors, or to differentiate white from gray matter. However, CT exposes the child to irradiation and most young children require sedation.

Magnetic Resonance Imaging (MRI). MRI provides the greatest detail of the nonbony aspects of the central nervous system. It cannot be used in individuals who have ferromagnetic implants or foreign bodies. The scanning time is longer than for CT scanning, and most young children require sedation. The contrast material usually used, gadolinium, is generally safer than the contrast agents used for CT scanning. MRI is superior to CT scanning in the evaluation of lesions of the posterior fossa. MRI can also be used for imaging the spinal cord without the need for lumbar puncture.

Indications for Various Imaging Modalities. Many studies have identified abnormalities of the brains of children with developmental delay on MRI scans that were not evident on CT. These abnormalities include delayed myelination, focal lesions, and hypoplastic white matter. In approximately 33% of children with developmental delay, the MRI scan tends to be abnormal. The result is more likely to show abnormalities if the child has microcephaly or associated neurologic findings, such as seizures; the scan is less likely to be positive if the child has no associated symptoms or is autistic. In most cases, the findings seen on MRI examination are nonspecific and do not help make a definite diagnosis. The MRI scan may help clarify the timing of a lesion. For example, if a child who has cerebral palsy following a difficult labor and delivery at term is found to have periventricular leukomalacia in the first weeks of life, an abnormality that usually occurs prior to 38 weeks' gestation, it is likely that a prenatal event rather than the difficult labor and delivery led to the cerebral palsy.

Although the MRI scan is invaluable in identifying neuroanatomic changes in disorders of development, it generally does not provide a definite diagnosis. Some clinicians believe that identifying a physical factor responsible for developmental delay is reassuring for parents; it is not clear that this justifies the expense of MRI as well as the risk of sedation in most children with developmental delay. Therefore, MRI should be reserved for a limited number of conditions, including:

- Children who have had developmental regression in which the scan can differentiate white from gray matter involvement, can guide subsequent specific metabolic studies, and can identify extrinsic causes of regression, such as leukemia and human immunodeficiency virus (HIV) infection
- Children who have intractable seizures for whom surgical intervention may be of help
- Children thought to have intracranial tumors or masses, including neurofibromatosis, Sturge-Weber syndrome, and tuberous sclerosis
- Children who have evidence of brainstem dysfunction, such as Möbius syndrome or Arnold-Chiari malformation

CT scanning should be performed if intracranial calcifications

Table 34–11. Information to Be Sought During the Physical Examination of a Child with Suspected Developmental Disabilities

Item	Possible Significance
General Appearance	May indicate significant delay in development or obvious syndrome
Stature	
Short stature	Williams syndrome, malnutrition, Turner syndrome; many children with severe retardation have short stature
Obesity	Prader-Willi syndrome
Large stature	Sotos syndrome
Head	
Macrocephaly	Alexander syndrome, Sotos syndrome, gangliosidosis, hydrocephalus, mucopolysaccharidosis, subdural effusion
Microcephaly	Virtually any condition that can retard brain growth (e.g., malnutrition, Angelman syndrome, de Lange syndrome, fetal alcohol effects)
Face	
Coarse, triangular, round, or flat face; hypo- or hypertelorism, slanted or short palpebral fissure; unusual nose, maxilla, and mandible	Specific measurements may provide clues to inherited, metabolic, or other diseases like fetal alcohol syndrome, *cri du chat* (5p- syndrome), or Williams syndrome
Eyes	
Prominent	Crouzon syndrome, Seckel syndrome, fragile X
Cataract	Galactosemia, Lowe syndrome, prenatal rubella, hypothyroidism
Cherry-red spot in macula	Gangliosidosis (GM_1), metachromatic leukodystrophy, mucolipidosis, Tay Sachs disease, Niemann-Pick disease, Farber lipogranulomatosis, sialidosis III
Chorioretinitis	Congenital infection with cytomegalovirus, toxoplasmosis, or rubella
Corneal cloudiness	Mucopolysaccharidosis I and II, Lowe syndrome, congenital syphilis
Ears	
Pinnae, low set or malformed	Trisomies such as 18, Rubinstein-Taybi syndrome, Down syndrome, CHARGE association, cerebro-oculo-facial-skeletal syndrome, fetal phenytoin effects
Hearing	Loss of acuity in mucopolysaccharidosis; hyperacusis in many encephalopathies
Heart	
Structural anomaly or hypertrophy	CHARGE association, CATCH-22, velo-cardio-facial syndrome, glycogenesis II, fetal alcohol effects, mucopolysaccharidosis I; chromosomal anomalies like Down syndrome; maternal PKU; chronic cyanosis may impair cognitive development
Liver	
Hepatomegaly	Fructose intolerance, galactosemia glycogenosis types I–IV, mucopolysaccharidosis I and II, Niemann-Pick disease, Tay-Sachs disease, Zellweger syndrome, Gaucher disease, ceroid lipofuscinosis, gangliosidosis
Genitalia	
Macro-orchidism	Fragile X syndrome
Hypogenitalism	Prader-Willi syndrome, Klinefelter syndrome, CHARGE association
Extremities	
Hands, feet, dermatoglyphics, and creases	May indicate specific entity like Rubinstein-Taybi syndrome or be associated with chromosomal anomaly
Joint contractures	Sign of muscle imbalance around joints—e.g., with meningomyelocele, cerebral palsy, arthrogryposis, muscular dystrophy; also occurs with cartilaginous problems such as mucopolysaccharidosis
Skin	
Café au lait spots	Neurofibromatosis, tuberous sclerosis, Bloom syndrome
"Eczema"	Phenylketonuria, histiocytosis
Hemangiomas and telangiectasia	Sturge-Weber syndrome, Bloom syndrome, ataxia-telangiectasia
Hypopigmented macules, streaks, adenoma sebaceum	Tuberous sclerosis, hypomelanosis of Ito
Hair	
Hirsutism	De Lange syndrome, mucopolysaccharidosis, fetal phenytoin effects, cerebro-oculo-facial-skeletal syndrome, trisomy 18
Neurologic	
Asymmetry of strength and tone	Focal lesion, cerebral palsy
Hypotonia	Prader-Willi syndrome, Down syndrome, Angelman syndrome, gangliosidosis, early cerebral palsy
Hypertonia	Neurodegenerative conditions involving white matter, cerebral palsy, trisomy 18
Ataxia	Ataxia-telangiectasia, metachromatic leukodystrophy, Angelman syndrome

Abbreviations: CHARGE = *C*oloboma *h*eart defects, *a*tresia choanae, *r*etarded growth, *g*enital anomalies, *e*ar anomalies (deafness); CATCH-22 = *C*ardiac defects, *a*bnormal face, *t*hymic hypoplasia, *c*left palate, *h*ypocalcemia–defects on chromosome No. 22; PKU = phenylketonuria.

Table 34–12. **Examples of Minor Anomalies and Associated Syndromes*†**

Head	Flat occiput: Down syndrome, Zellweger syndrome Prominent occiput: trisomy 18 Delayed closure of sutures: hypothyroidism, hydrocephalus Craniosynostosis: Crouzon syndrome, Pfeiffer syndrome Delayed fontanelle closure: hypothyroidism, Down syndrome, hydrocephalus	Teeth	Anodontia: ectodermal dysplasia Notched incisors: congenital syphilis Late dental eruption: Hunter syndrome Wide-spaced teeth: de Lange syndrome, Angelman syndrome
Face	Midface hypoplasia: fetal alcohol syndrome, Down syndrome Triangular facies: Russell-Silver syndrome, Turner syndrome Coarse facies: mucopolysaccharidoses, Sotos syndrome Prominent nose and chin: fragile X syndrome Flat facies: Apert syndrome, Stickler syndrome Round facies: Prader-Willi syndrome	Hair	Hirsutism: Hurler syndrome Low hairline: Klippel-Feil sequence, Turner syndrome Sparse hair: Menkes, argininosuccinicacidemia Abnormal hair whorls/posterior whorl: Down syndrome Abnormal eyebrow patterning: Waardenburg syndrome
		Neck	Webbed neck/low posterior hair line: Turner syndrome
		Chest	Shield-shaped chest: Turner syndrome
Eyes	Hypertelorism: fetal hydantoin syndrome, Waardenburg syndrome Hypotelorism: holoprosencephaly sequence, maternal phenylketonuria effect Inner canthal folds/Brushfield spots: Down syndrome Slanted palpebral fissures: trisomies Prominent eyes: Apert syndrome, Beckwith-Wiedemann syndrome Lisch nodules: neurofibromatosis Blue sclera, osteogenesis imperfecta, Turner syndrome	Genitalia	Macro-orchidism: fragile X syndrome Hypogonadism: Prader-Willi syndrome
		Extremities	Short limbs: achondroplasia, rhizomelic chondrodysplasia Small hands: Prader-Willi syndrome Clinodactyly: trisomies including Down syndrome Polydactyly: trisomy 13 Broad thumb: Rubinstein-Taybi syndrome Syndactyly: de Lange syndrome Transverse palmar crease: Down syndrome Joint laxity: Down syndrome, fragile X syndrome Phocomelia: de Lange syndrome
Ears	Large pinnae/simple helices: fragile X syndrome Malformed pinnae/atretic canal: Treacher Collins syndrome, CHARGE association Low-set ears: Treacher Collins syndrome, trisomies	Spine	Sacral dimple/hairy patch: spina bifida
Nose	Anteverted nares/synophrys: de Lange syndrome Broad nasal bridge: fetal drug effects, fragile X syndrome Low nasal bridge: achondroplasia, Down syndrome Prominent nose: Coffin-Lowry syndrome, Smith-Lemli-Opitz syndrome	Skin	Hypopigmented macules/adenoma sebaceum: tuberous sclerosis *Café au lait* spots and neurofibromas: neurofibromatosis Linear depigmented nevi: hypomelanosis of Ito Facial port-wine hemangioma: Sturge-Weber syndrome Nail hypoplasia or dysplasia: fetal alcohol syndrome, trisomies
Mouth	Long filtrum/thin vermilion border: fetal alcohol effects Cleft lip and palate: isolated or part of syndrome Micrognathia: Robin sequence, trisomies Macroglossia: hypothyroidism, Beckwith-Wiedemann syndrome		

Modified from Levy SE, Hyman SL. Pediatric assessment of the child with developmental delay. Pediatr Clin North Am 1993;40:465–477.
*Increased incidence of minor anomalies have been reported in cerebral palsy, mental retardation, learning disabilities, and autism.
†The presence of three or more minor anomalies places a child at greater risk to have a major anomaly and the diagnosis of a specific syndrome.
Abbreviation: CHARGE = *C*oloboma, *h*eart defects, *a*tresia choanae, *r*etarded growth, *g*enital anomalies, *e*ar anomalies (deafness).

Table 34–13. **Clinical Features Suggestive of Inherited Neurometabolic Disorders**

Encephalopathy	Systemic features
Mental retardation	Urinary odor
Developmental regression	Intrauterine growth
Cerebral palsy	retardation
Spastic diplegia	Failure to thrive
Spastic quadriplegia	Poor suck
Depressed sensorium	Vomiting repeatedly
Lethargy	Weak cry
Irritability	Cardiomyopathy
Stupor	Hepatomegaly
Coma	Fatty liver
Dementia	Fibrosis/cirrhosis
Hypotonia	Hepatosplenomegaly
Seizures	Renal tubular acidosis
Myoclonus	Susceptibility to infections
Infantile spasms	Bone marrow depression
Extrapyramidal symptoms	(neutropenia,
Dystonia	thrombocytopenia,
Opisthotonos	pancytopenia)
Choreoathetosis	Seborrhea
Cerebellar symptoms	Alopecia
Ataxia	Abnormal hair
Microcephaly	Pili torti
Macrocephaly	Trichorrhexis nodosa
Speech problems	
Eye-related problems	
Abnormal movements	
Apraxia	
Cherry-red spot	
Nystagmus	
Optic atrophy	
Tapetoretinal degeneration	

Modified from Chaves-Carballo E. Detection of inherited neurometabolic disorders: A practical clinical approach. Pediatr Clin North Am 1992;39:801–820.

are suspected, as with prenatal infections (toxoplasmosis, cytomegalovirus); if abnormalities of the skull or subdural space are in question; and to identify major malformations, such as holoprosencephaly. CT scanning can be substituted for MRI in children who present with seizures or focal neurologic findings if MRI is not available or if the results of the CT scan can be obtained in a more timely fashion.

Ultrasonography can be used to diagnose and monitor intracranial hemorrhage and hydrocephalus and as a screening test for congenital anomalies of the brain.

Plain skull roentgenograms are helpful in the diagnosis of craniosynostosis and other craniofacial anomalies, such as Apert syndrome.

OTHER TESTS

Other tests can be helpful for identifying specific diagnoses or categories of diseases. For example, analysis of cerebrospinal fluid for elevated protein levels may help in the diagnosis of a disease affecting white matter. Peripheral nerve conduction tests and electromyography may help to confirm that the condition is associated with a peripheral neuropathy. Diminished deep tendon reflexes and prolonged nerve conduction times are noted in Krabbe disease, Refsum disease, metachromatic leukodystrophy, and infantile neuroaxonal dystrophy (see Chapter 39). Skin and muscle biopsies may identify conditions in which abnormal material is stored in

cells, such as neuronal ceroid lipofuscinosis. Brainstem auditory evoked response is useful as an evaluation of hearing in infants and can also be used to evaluate brainstem functioning. Visual evoked response can be useful in determining the integrity of the visual pathways in children who may have problems with vision; however, it cannot determine visual acuity.

FORMAL NEURODEVELOPMENTAL ASSESSMENTS

Standardized evaluations of development are usually indicated in the comprehensive evaluation of a child with developmental delays. These include tests of general intelligence like the Stanford-Binet test, tests of language such as the Peabody Picture Vocabulary Test, tests of fine motor skills like the Bruininks-Oseretsky Test of Motor Integration, and tests of social adaptation like the Vineland Adaptive Behaviour Scales. Tests of educational achievement such as reading comprehension can be useful to identify the child's functional status. Other tests, such as the Halstead-Reitan Neuropsychological Battery and the Bender Visual Motor Gestalt test, can provide information on the child's sensory motor abilities (such as visual spatial integration).

The selection of the test battery should be related to the child's condition. The testing should provide a profile of the child's strengths and weaknesses and not just a series of scores. These results can also serve as a baseline for subsequent monitoring of the child's progress. The tests, which should be administered by trained people, should be adapted for alternate sensory and response modes. For example, the Leiter International Performance Scale has been constructed for use in hearing-impaired children. After the functional assessment has been completed, the child's progress should be monitored in a systematic fashion.

Diagnostic Strategy

Figure 34–5 illustrates a strategy that can be employed to identify and assess individuals with developmental delay. All children should routinely be screened for vision, hearing, and language. Children with abnormal findings should be referred for definitive evaluation. Using developmental surveillance techniques such as evaluation of the family and home environment (obtained as part of a routine history or by using the HOME), a checklist of milestones (such as the Hawaii Early Learning Profile), risk inventories (see Table 34–4), and parental assessments of a child's development (either informally as part of a routine history or formally using a questionnaire such as the Infant/Child Monitoring Questionnaire), the clinician can identify children who are at increased risk for delayed development. This decision should not be made exclusively on the basis of a screening instrument like the DDST.

Children identified at increased risk should have a comprehensive history, physical examination, and evaluation of the environment. If the child has developmental regression, the steps outlined in Figure 34–5 should be followed to determine a specific diagnosis. If the child does not have a terminal condition, formal neurodevelopmental testing should be performed to identify the child's functional profile in order to tailor his or her intervention to maximize development. Continuous monitoring of the child's development should follow the diagnosis.

Children with delayed development *without regression* can be divided into four groups:

1. Children with microcephaly, macrocephaly, multiple physical anomalies, and pigmentary changes should have MRI scan and chromosome analysis. (Those with pigmentary changes should have

Table 34-14. Select Chromosomal Abnormalities in Which Developmental Delay Is a Major Feature

Condition	Incidence	Comments
Trisomy 21	1/700	Down syndrome
Fragile X syndrome	1/800	Macro-orchidism, hyperactivity, autistic-like behavior
47XXY (Klinefelter syndrome)	1/1000	Small testes, problems in language skills
47XXX	1/1000	Girls with learning and language problems; may have 48XXXX
45XO (Turner syndrome)	1/2000	Girls with short stature, broad neck, gonadal dysgenesis; visuospatial deficits common
Prader-Willi syndrome (abnormality of contiguous genes on chromosome 15; inherited from deletions of paternal chromosomes—monoparental disomy)	1/5000	Hypotonia in infancy, obesity, short stature, mild retardation
Angelman syndrome (chromosome anomaly similar to that in Prader-Willi syndrome; inherited from maternal deletion in chromosome 15—monoparental disomy)	?	Ataxia, prognathism, absence of speech, severe retardation, inappropriate laughter
Trisomy 18	1/8000	Multiple congenital anomalies, severe developmental delay
Trisomy 13	1/20,000	Multiple congenital anomalies, severe developmental delay
5p- (*cri du chat* syndrome)	1/100,000	High-pitched cry, small stature, speech and language delays
4p- (Wolf-Hirschhorn syndrome)	1/100,000	Midline deficiencies, profound retardation, seizures
11p- (Wilms tumor, aniridia)	1/100,000	Ambiguous genitalia, aniridia, cataracts
17p- (Miller-Dieker syndrome)	1/100,000	Lissencephaly, microcephaly, seizures, cryptorchidism

Table 34-15. Scoring System for Screening Individuals for Fragile X Syndrome

Category	Score	Criteria
Family history	2	Retarded sibling, maternal uncle, aunt, nephew, niece, first cousin
	1	Any other affected relative
	0	No family history of retardation
Personality	2	Shyness, lack of eye contact followed by friendliness, verbosity, and echolalia
	1	Some of the above characteristics
	0	No characteristic
Ears	2	Large and protruding
	1	Large, not protruding
	0	Other
Face	2	Long jaw, high and wide forehead
	1	Only one finding
	0	No findings
Body habitus	2	Slim, tall, rounded shoulders, hyperextensible fingers, lack of body hair, *or* obese with female fat distribution, striae, soft skin, lack of body hair (for males)
	2	Slim *or* obese (for females)
	1	Only some features
	0	No features

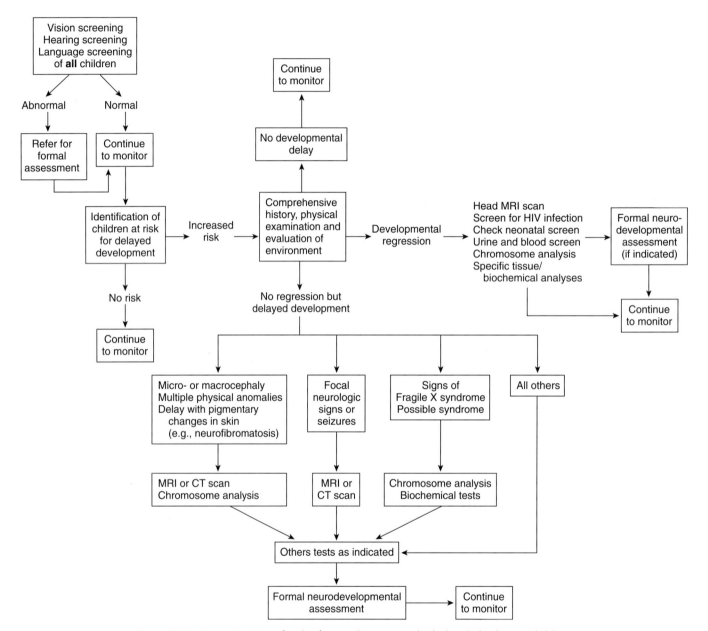

Figure 34–5. Diagnostic strategy for identifying and assessing individuals with developmental delay.

fibroblast sample for chromosome analysis if the lymphocyte sample is negative.)

2. Children who seem to fit a specific syndrome or who have evidence of fragile X syndrome should have chromosome analyses or specific biochemical tests, or both, in order to identify the etiology of the developmental delay.

3. Children with focal neurologic signs or focal or repeated seizures should have an MRI scan, although it is reasonable to forgo this in some instances.

4. All other children with delayed development, as well as those in the previous three groups, should be referred for formal neurodevelopmental assessments.

Because many conditions can cause developmental delay (e.g., more than 600 syndromes have been associated with mental retardation), identifying those in which treatment may dramatically improve the course becomes essential. Table 34–16 lists some "treatable" conditions that cause developmental delay. Although these conditions account for only a small proportion of children with delayed development, early recognition is critical. Enzyme replacement therapy and transplantation of liver, bone marrow, and fetal tissue may offer treatment for several more conditions in the future.

In addition to the primary condition leading to developmental delay, many children experience behavioral or psychologic problems; this is often referred to as "dual diagnoses." Psychiatric illnesses common to children with mild or moderate retardation include adjustment disorders, organic brain disease, affective disorders, and attention deficit with hyperactivity (see Chapter 36). Children with severe delay may experience stereotypic or self-destructive behaviors. Clinicians evaluating these children must be aware that these psychiatric conditions can interfere with functioning as much as the primary condition.

Specific Conditions

HIV INFECTION (see Chapter 55)

One of the conditions to consider in the child who has developmental regression before the age of 2 years is infection with human immunodeficiency virus. Approximately 20% of children infected with HIV prenatally or in the immediate perinatal period have signs and symptoms in the first year of life. The developmental regression or failure to progress (developmental plateau) is usually accompanied by other signs and symptoms, including failure to thrive, diarrhea, hepatosplenomegaly, lymphadenopathy, thrush, parotitis, and recurrent infections, including otitis media and pneumococcal (bacteremia, pneumonia) and prolonged viral infections.

All children with developmental regression in the first 2 years of life should be screened for HIV, especially because current treatment can prolong life, prevent opportunistic infection, and improve developmental functioning. CT and MRI scans of these children usually show cerebral atrophy with abnormalities of white matter; calcifications of the basal ganglia may be present as well. Children with early symptoms have a worse prognosis for survival than those who present later.

A second group of children (80%) with congenital HIV infection present later with a slower, less fulminant course; every year another 8% of children in this group have full-blown acquired immunodeficiency syndrome (AIDS). These children may present with delays in speech and cognition as well as with hyperactivity and difficulties with attention without any other signs or symptoms of HIV infection. Clinicians in areas where HIV infection is frequent screen children with nonspecific developmental delay for HIV infection. Interestingly, treatment with anti-HIV agents such as zidovudine (AZT) has improved the IQ scores and cognitive functioning of infected children who had IQs in the normal range, as well as those with IQs in the 50s. It is estimated that 1500 to 2000 new cases of HIV infection occur annually in neonates in the United States.

Table 34–16. Conditions Associated with Developmental Delay in Which Early Treatment May Significantly Improve the Course of the Disease

Condition	Treatment
Galactosemia	Lactose-free diet
Fructosemia	Fructose-free diet
Hypoglycemia from any cause	Prevent hypoglycemia and/or provide glucose
Lead intoxication	Separate child from source of lead; chelation therapy (?)
Hypothyroidism	Thyroid replacement
Phenylketonuria	Phenylalanine-free diet
Maternal phenylketonuria	Phenylalanine-free diet during pregnancy
Maple syrup urine disease	Diet restricted in branch chain amino acids + dialysis or exchange transfusion
Recurrent otitis media	Antibiotic prophylaxis, pressure-equalizing tubes (?)
Malnutrition	Adequate nutrition
Increased intracranial pressure (e.g., hydrocephalus, neoplasm)	Shunt ventricles or cystic structure
Congenital HIV infection	Prenatal treatment with AZT (zidovudine)
Congenital toxoplasmosis	Prenatal treatment with spiramycin, pyrimethamine and sulfonamide
Dopa-responsive dystonia	Responds to levodopa; may be misdiagnosed as cerebral palsy
Metachromatic leukodystrophy	Bone marrow transplantation
Niemann-Pick disease	Bone marrow transplantation, liver transplantation, implanted amniotic epithelial cells
Adrenoleukodystrophy	Bone marrow transplantation
Mucopolysaccharidosis type I	Bone marrow transplantation
Glycogen storage disease type IV	Liver transplantation
Menkes disease	Parenteral copper histidinate
Lesch-Nyhan syndrome	Allopurinol + bone marrow transplantation (?)
Krabbe disease	Bone marrow transplantation (?)

CEREBRAL PALSY

The term cerebral palsy (CP) refers to a group of conditions characterized by abnormalities of movement and posture following nonprogressive lesions of the immature brain. Cerebral palsy is not a single disorder or pathologic entity but is a heterogeneous collection of conditions. Table 34–17 shows a classification scheme for CP as well as occurrence rates of mental retardation and seizures in children with the various forms.

Cerebral palsy may be the result of prenatal factors such as congenital infections or malformations, perinatal factors like hypoxia or intraventricular hemorrhage, or postnatal factors like central

Table 34–17. Classification of Cerebral Palsy (CP) and Association with Mental Retardation and Seizures

Type	% of All CP	IQ <50 (%)	Seizures (%)
Spastic diplegia	32	33	31
Spastic quadriplegia	24	64	56
Spastic hemiplegia	29	39	67
Dyskinetic	10	30	27
Ataxic	4	1	1

nervous system infection, trauma, or hypoxia such as occurs with near-drowning. CP is more common in preterm births and infants who are small for gestational age (SGA). The incidence of CP per 1000 births by birth weight is 90 for infants weighing less than 1500 g; 23 for SGA infants weighing between 1500 and 2000 g; and 7 for average-for-gestational-age infants weighing between 1500 and 2000 g.

Previously, it was believed that a difficult labor and delivery was a leading cause of CP. Although there are instances when asphyxia related to obstetric conditions such as cephalopelvic disproportion leads to CP, prenatal, often undetected events are more likely causes of CP. Abnormalities of the central nervous system, such as cysts or ischemia, cause CP *and* may also lead to difficult labors and deliveries. Using MRI scans to ''date'' the lesions may help clarify the etiology of the CP in select cases.

Although the lesion in CP is static, the clinical picture of the child may change with maturation. For instance, the child who has a neonatal insult may be hypotonic for the first 6 months of life and then develop spasticity. Dyskinesia (dystonia and athetosis) and ataxia may not develop until the child is 18 months old. Earlier signs that should raise suspicion of CP include difficulty feeding due to abnormal oromotor patterns (tongue thrusting, tonic bite, oral hypersensitivity), irritability, and delayed milestones, including head control. Exaggerated or persistent infantile reflexes such as the asymmetric tonic neck response, hyperreflexia, and asymmetry may occur. The presence of delayed milestones, primitive or exaggerated reflexes, abnormal posture, spasticity, and abnormal neurologic examination should suggest the diagnosis of CP. Repeated examination is necessary to exclude a degenerative condition; persistent subclinical seizures or adverse reaction to anticonvulsants may worsen the clinical condition of children with CP. In addition to seizures and mental retardation, children with CP have an increased occurrence of visual problems, including strabismus, hearing loss, and growth failure. In older children with dyskinetic CP, symptomatic cervical spine degeneration may develop.

If a child with a diagnosis of dyskinetic CP has symptoms that worsen significantly as the day progresses, *dopa-responsive dystonia* should be suspected. This rare but treatable form of dystonia may begin with toe-walking and difficulties with gait and responds dramatically to the administration of levodopa. There is usually no history of preexisting condition that would be consistent with CP. Other unusual inborn errors of metabolism, such as *arginase deficiency* and *glutaric aciduria*, may mimic CP. These conditions cause progressive deterioration, whereas CP does not.

FRAGILE X SYNDROME

The diagnosis of fragile X syndrome is difficult to make clinically, especially in young children. Physical features are neither constant nor specific and are less noticeable in those younger than 3 years of age. Table 34–15 lists some of the associated features.

Others include macro-orchidism in postpubertal males, macrocephaly, flattened nasal bridge, and prominent epicanthal folds. Cognitive abilities vary from learning disabilities to severe impairment, and seizures have been reported in about 20% of these individuals.

Fragile X syndrome is the most common genetic cause of mental retardation and is due to an inheritable unstable DNA in the FMR-1 gene of the X chromosome. A genetic sequence (C-C-G) is duplicated more than 200 times in affected individuals. Males and females with this unstable sequence who have fewer than 200 copies are usually mildly affected or normal (are carriers). When transmitted by a female, this unstable sequence increases in size. Therefore, male carriers who are clinically normal produce female carriers who are also clinically normal. Clinically normal female carriers likely produce males (the 50% that inherit the abnormal X chromosome) who are abnormal. The greater the number of these abnormal sequences in the female, the greater the likelihood that she will have developmental delay and will have abnormal sons.

Controversy exists regarding whether testing for the fragile X site should occur in all retarded children or should be limited to those who have some clinical features of the syndrome. Children with fragile X syndrome often have autistic features, and 5% of boys with a diagnosis of autism have fragile X syndrome. Yet 5% of severely retarded, nonautistic boys also have the fragile X gene. Therefore, it is unlikely that this disorder *per se* is a major cause of autism.

AUTISM

Developmental disorders of cerebral function are often revealed as disorders of language. The differential diagnosis of poor language development in the preschool child includes hearing impairment, mental retardation (of any etiology), expressive dysphasia, and autism. The same child may have features of more than one of these conditions. The diagnosis of autism is based on a constellation of clinical features and does not imply a single etiology. The *Diagnostic and Statistical Manual of Mental Disorders, Fourth Edition (DSM-IV)* requires three criteria on which to base the diagnosis:

1. Impaired reciprocal social interactions.
2. Abnormal verbal and nonverbal communication (eye-to-eye contact).
3. Diminished repertoire of activities and interests, with onset during infancy or childhood.

Children with features of autism who do not meet all the criteria may be designated to have pervasive developmental disorder, not otherwise specified.

Although certain diagnoses have been associated with autism (untreated phenylketonuria, hypomelanosis of Ito), most cases of autism have no known etiology. Abnormalities of the cerebellum and limbic system have been hypothesized but not proven.

Autism has a prevalence of about 50 in 100,000 and is more common in boys. During infancy, autistic children avoid eye contact, do not play with their parents or siblings, act deaf or visually impaired, and do not ''cuddle.'' They have delayed language skills and may have echolalia. They tend to be irritable, require routines in their daily lives, and often have stereotypic behaviors. Visual impairment, deafness, child abuse and neglect, and severe language disorders must be considered in children who present with autistic features. Generally, the degree of aloofness (impaired social relatedness like solitary activities and poor social signals) in children with autism is much more severe than in children with the other disorders.

STORAGE DISEASES

Inborn errors of metabolism and storage diseases may present as an acute encephalopathy (coma, emesis), often a result of organic acidemias or hyperammonemia, or as a chronic progressive encephalopathy (cardiomyopathy, spasticity, hyperreflexia, liver dysfunction), often due to mitochondrial disorders or storage diseases (see Table 34–13).

- *Sphingolipidoses* (Tay-Sachs disease, Niemann-Pick disease, GM_1 gangliosidosis) often demonstrate a cherry-red retinal spot, organomegaly, and mental retardation.
- *Glycoprotein degradation disorders* (e.g., mannosidosis, fucosidosis) may variably manifest coarse facies, mental retardation, hepatosplenomegaly, and vacuolated lymphocytes.
- *Mucopolysaccharidoses* (e.g., the Hurler, Hunter, and Sanfilippo syndromes) may variably demonstrate coarse facies, mental retardation, hepatosplenomegaly, dysostosis multiplex, and corneal clouding.
- *Neuronal ceroid lipofuscinosis* may manifest mental retardation, vision loss, ataxia, and myoclonic seizures.
- *Peroxisomal disorders* (Zellweger syndrome, X-linked adrenoleukodystrophy, Refsum syndrome) variably demonstrate mental retardation with encephalopathy, seizures, blindness, dysmorphic features, and deafness.

CONGENITAL INFECTIONS

Bacteria, parasites, or viruses acquired prior to, during, or after birth may cause central nervous system infection and injury. The diagnosis is based on the clinical manifestations (Table 34–18) and culture or serologic evidence of infection (Table 34–19).

POSTNATAL INFECTIONS

Central nervous system infection during infancy or childhood may cause encephalitis or meningoencephalitis with resultant mental retardation. Bacterial (*Haemophilus influenzae* type b, pneumococcus, *Mycobacterium tuberculosis*; meningococcus) and viral (herpes simplex type 1 or 2, eastern or western equine encephalitis virus, St. Louis encephalitis virus, HIV; rarely, mumps, enteroviruses, or California encephalitis virus) etiologies are common in infancy and early childhood and variably have neurodevelopmental sequelae. Secondary problems due to the infection, such as hearing or visual loss, must also be considered. Late sequelae of prior viral infection such as measles or rubella panencephalitis may appear 10 to 20 years after the initial central nervous system disease and manifest as dementia, poor school performance, and progressive encephalopathy.

Diagnostic Hazards

One of the risks in identifying children as developmentally delayed (or at risk of developmental delay) is that it can alter the perceptions of the child's family, making the child "vulnerable." This might lead to constraints on the child's experiences and diminished expectations of performance. Parents who view the world in a categorical fashion ("if my child is labeled 'at-risk' or 'delayed' or 'retarded,' he will always be that way") may have difficulty abandoning a label once it is applied. For example, if a child is born with a single risk factor, such as prematurity, and if the child has some difficulty during infancy, such as colic or slow weight gain, the parents may stop placing any demands on the child and treat the child as if he or she were retarded. The child, especially if he or she has a passive temperament, may respond to the environment by withdrawing and may indeed have delays in motor and other milestones. Identifying unusual physical characteristics (minor anomalies) may have the same negative effects.

Balanced against the risk of labeling is the need for parents to know their child's condition and to be responsible for informed decisions regarding care. Thus, as soon as the child's condition is fairly certain, this information should be shared with the family in a sensitive fashion with an explanation of the margin of uncertainty. Positive as well as negative information about the child should be transmitted, and an effort should be made to identify the child's and parents' accomplishments during subsequent visits so that the visits are not viewed as entirely "fault finding."

When parents are informed that their child is not normal, they grieve for the "lost" normal child. This process of grieving involves stages that include denial, sadness, anger, and guilt. One parent may be experiencing persistent anger while another is still sad or depressed. This difference in stages may make communication between them exceedingly difficult. Grieving may occur at times other than the initial diagnosis—for example, on the first day of kindergarten for a child with Down syndrome.

These feelings may be expressed in nonfunctional ways, such as denial that leads to unending shopping for professionals who will "cure" the child, or anger that is expressed at the clinician, thereby thwarting a trusting relationship. However, many believe that these emotions are essential steps that allow the parents to release the old dreams and secure new ones. The goal of the therapeutic clinician is not to prevent parents from expressing these feelings or hurrying them through the stages but to accept the parents where they are and to help them understand the normalcy of the stages.

TREATMENT

The treatment of a child with developmental delay or mental retardation includes:

1. Health maintenance.
2. Treatment of the underlying condition (if possible).
3. Treatment of associated conditions (such as hyperactivity or drooling).
4. Relief of symptoms.
5. Anticipatory guidance to prevent secondary conditions.
6. Environmental support.

The overriding goal of these objectives is *to optimize the functional status of the child.*

Health maintenance should be the same as that provided for all children, including immunizations (except pertussis in undiagnosed progressive neurologic disorders), regular monitoring for physical growth and development, and screening for conditions like anemia, tuberculosis, and lead poisoning. For instance, specific growth charts are available for some conditions, including Down syndrome, Prader-Willi syndrome, and fragile X syndrome. Nutritional recommendations are available for children with cerebral palsy.

Except for a few conditions, some of which are listed in Table 34–16, very few conditions that lead to developmental delay can be "cured." Because many of these conditions are rare, medications that may be effective in their treatment could receive the support provided "orphan drugs" under the Orphan Drugs Act.

Treatment of associated conditions depends on knowledge of the condition and the child, which argues for continuity of care. For example, the child with dual diagnoses who has a behavioral or psychiatric problem may benefit from counseling, support, or psychopharmacologic medications. These medications can be used to reduce arousal symptoms and to improve affect, perceptual

Table 34–18. Distinguishing Features of Perinatal Congenital Infections (TORCH)

Agent	Maternal Epidemiology	Neonatal Features
Toxoplasma gondii	Heterophil-negative mononucleosis Exposure to cats or raw meat or immunosuppression High-risk exposure at 10–24 weeks' gestation	Hydrocephalus, abnormal spinal fluid, intracranial calcifications, chorioretinitis, jaundice, hepatosplenomegaly, fever, MR if symptomatic Many infants asymptomatic at birth *Treatment:* pyrimethamine plus sulfadiazine
Rubella virus	Unimmunized seronegative mother; fever ± rash Detectable defects with infection: 　by 8 wk, 85% 　9–12 wk, 50% 　13–20 wk, 16% Virus may be present in infant throat for 1 yr *Prevention:* vaccine	Intrauterine growth retardation, microcephaly, microphthalmia, cataracts, glaucoma, "salt-and-pepper" chorioretinitis, hepatosplenomegaly, jaundice, PDA, deafness, blueberry muffin rash, anemia, thrombocytopenia, leukopenia, metaphyseal lucencies, B- and T-cell deficiency, MR if symptomatic Infant may be asymptomatic at birth
Cytomegalovirus (CMV)	STD: primary genital infection may be asymptomatic Heterophil-negative mononucleosis; infant may have viruria for 1–6 yr	Sepsis, intrauterine growth retardation, chorioretinitis, microcephaly, periventricular calcifications, blueberry muffin rash, anemia, thrombocytopenia, neutropenia, hepatosplenomegaly, jaundice, deafness, pneumonia Many asymptomatic at birth, MR if symptomatic *Prevention:* CMV-negative blood products
Herpes simplex type 2 virus	STD: primary genital infection may be asymptomatic; intrauterine infection rare, acquisition at time of birth more common	*Intrauterine infection:* chorioretinitis, skin lesions, microcephaly, MR *Postnatal:* encephalitis, localized or disseminated disease, skin vesicles, keratoconjunctivitis, MR if CNS *Treatment:* acyclovir
Varicella-zoster virus	Intrauterine infection with chickenpox during first trimester Infant develops severe neonatal varicella with maternal illness 5 days prior to or 2 days after delivery	Microphthalmia, cataracts, chorioretinitis, cutaneous and bony aplasia/hypoplasia/atrophy, cutaneous scars, MR Zoster as in older child *Prevention of neonatal condition:* VZIG *Treatment of ill neonate:* acyclovir
Treponema pallidum (syphilis)	STD Maternal primary asymptomatic: painless "hidden" chancre Penicillin, not erythromycin, *prevents* fetal infection	Presentation *at birth* as nonimmune hydrops, prematurity, anemia, neutropenia, thrombocytopenia, pneumonia, hepatosplenomegaly *Late neonatal* as snuffles (rhinitis), rash, hepatosplenomegaly, condylomata lata, metaphysitis, cerebrospinal fluid pleocytosis, keratitis, periosteal new bone, lymphocytosis, hepatitis, MR possible *Late onset*—teeth, eye, bone, skin, CNS, ear *Treatment:* penicillin
Parvovirus B-19	Etiology of fifth disease; fever, rash, arthralgia in adults	Nonimmune hydrops, fetal anemia *Treatment: in utero* transfusion
Human immunodeficiency virus (HIV)	AIDS: most mothers are asymptomatic and HIV-positive; high-risk history: prostitute, drug abuse, married to bisexual, or hemophiliac	AIDS symptoms develop between 3 and 6 mo of age in 25%–40%; failure to thrive, recurrent infection, hepatosplenomegaly, neurologic abnormalities, MR *Management:* intravenous immunoglobulin, trimethoprim-sulfamethoxazole, AZT
Hepatitis B virus	Vertical transmission common; may result in cirrhosis, hepatocellular carcinoma	Acute neonatal hepatitis; many become asymptomatic carriers *Prevention:* HBIG, vaccine
Borrelia burgdorferi	Lyme disease, erythema chronicum migrans, meningitis, arthritis, carditis *Maternal treatment:* penicillin, ceftriaxone	Prematurity, rash, cortical blindness, fetal death?
Neisseria gonorrhoeae	STD, infant acquires at birth *Treatment:* cefotaxime, ceftriaxone	Gonococcal ophthalmia, sepsis, meningitis *Prevention:* silver nitrate, erythromycin eye drops *Treatment:* intravenous ceftriaxone
Chlamydia trachomatis	STD, infant acquires at birth *Treatment:* oral erythromycin	Conjunctivitis, pneumonia *Prevention:* erythromycin eye drops *Treatment:* oral erythromycin
Mycobacterium tuberculosis	Positive PPD skin test, recent converter, positive chest roentgenogram, positive family member *Treatment:* INH and rifampin ± ethambutol	Congenital rare septic pneumonia; acquired primary pulmonary TB; MR if CNS; asymptomatic, follow PPD *Prevention:* INH, BCG, separation *Treatment:* INH, rifampin, pyrazinamide
Trypanosoma cruzi (Chagas disease)	Central South American native, immigrant, travel Chronic disease in mother	Failure to thrive, heart failure, achalasia *Treatment:* nifurtimox

Modified from Kliegman RM. Fetal and neonatal medicine. *In* Behrman RE, Kliegman RM (eds). Nelson Essentials of Pediatrics, 2nd ed. Philadelphia: WB Saunders, 1994.
Abbreviations: AIDS = acquired immunodeficiency syndrome; AZT = zidovudine; BCG = bacillus Calmette-Guérin; CNS = central nervous system; HBIG = hepatitis B immune globulin; INH = isoniazid; MR = mental retardation; PDA = patent ductus arteriosus; PPD = purified protein derivative; STD = sexually transmitted disease; TB = tuberculosis; VZIG = varicella-zoster immune globulin.

Table 34-19. Microbiologic Diagnosis of
Congenital Infections

Serologic
 Syphilis: nontreponemal (VDRL) or treponemal (FTA-
  ABS)
 Toxoplasmosis: ELISA, Sabin-Feldman dye test
 Rubella: latex agglutination, enzyme immunoassay
 Cytomegalovirus: ELISA
 Herpes simplex viruses: several methods
 Varicella-zoster virus: fluorescent antimembrane antibody
 Lyme disease: ELISA
 Human parvovirus B19: ELISA or RIA
 Arboviruses: antibody capture ELISA (blood or CSF)

Serologic studies should include:
 An acute sample from the infant for agent-specific IgM
  and IgG
 A convalescent sample from the infant for agent-specific
  antibodies
 A maternal sample for agent-specific IgG

Virologic
 Cytomegalovirus: urine, saliva, blood leukocytes;
  occasionally, CSF
 Rubella virus: urine, nasopharyngeal secretions
 Herpes simplex viruses: skin lesions, throat, rectum, CSF
 Varicella-zoster virus: skin lesions
 Enteroviruses: CSF, throat, stool
 Arboviruses: blood, CSF

When the agent is unknown, samples should include urine,
 throat washing, CSF, blood, rectal swab, and fluid from
 skin vesicles, if present.

From Bale JF, Murph JR. Congenital infections and the nervous system. Pediatr Clin North Am 1992;39:669–690.

Abbreviations: VDRL = Venereal Disease Research Laboratory; FTA-ABS = fluorescent treponemal antibody absorption; ELISA = enzyme-linked immunosorbent assay; RIA = radioimmunoassay; CSF = cerebrospinal fluid; IgM = immunoglobulin M.

functioning, cognitive processing, communication, and behavior. Table 34–20 lists some psychopharmacologic medications that may be helpful in the care of children with dual diagnoses. Attention must be paid to the medication and condition. For example, valproic acid is more likely to cause hepatotoxicity in certain conditions, including GM₂ gangliosidosis, spinocerebellar degeneration, Friedreich ataxia, Lafora body disease, Alper disease, and myoclonic epilepsy with ragged-red fibers. Parents and capable children should be informed of the medication prescribed, including its side effects. Some written guidelines for parents and youth are available for psychopharmacologic medications.

Effective relief of symptoms also depends on knowledge of the child and the condition. For example, many children with cerebral palsy have drooling and spasticity. Drooling has been controlled by the use of a scopolamine patch or by surgery. Spasticity has been treated with the injection of botulinum toxin, intrathecal or oral baclofen, and dorsal root rhizotomy.

Anticipatory guidance involves the same categories used in all children, such as safety and nutrition, but may need to be modified because of the unique features of the child's condition. Prevention of secondary conditions requires specific anticipatory guidance. For example, in a child with cerebral palsy, the following conditions listed by category require prevention:

- *General health*—aspiration pneumonia, obesity, malnutrition, falls, decubiti ulcers
- *Neuromuscular*—deformities (contractures) of the foot, knee, hip, and spine

- *Communication*—poor expressive communication
- *Psychosocial*—depression, low self-esteem
- *Quality of life*—employment opportunities, recreation

Although many different conditions can cause developmental delay, children with this problem and their families share many common characteristics, including chronicity of the condition (with no cure in most instances), inability to participate in peer activities, loss of the "ideal" child, increased expense, lost opportunities (such as the parent who cannot return to work because he or she must care for the child at home), need for personal care (because the child cannot be left alone or with a sitter), confusing systems of health care, insurance coverage, and governmental agencies and rules, and social isolation.

Environmental support may be needed and may take the form of family therapy, financial counseling, referral to a disease-oriented volunteer support group, or enrollment in a school or preschool program or a "Big Brothers/Big Sisters" program. Although families should ideally be able to determine their children's needs and procure services, they may need assistance to do so. Care coordination (or case management) is one way of providing environmental support. This consists of:

- Determining the needs of the child and family
- Planning comprehensive care
- Facilitating and coordinating services
- Monitoring to ensure that the families have received the services they need
- Empowering families to become increasingly independent in the care of their child

Although treatment plans differ for different conditions, a mnemonic—MD'S DD BASICS—may help one to remember issues related to the care of children with developmental disabilities. Table 34–21 gives the mnemonic, areas to check, and possible consultations that may be helpful. Specific checklists that can be used to monitor the care of children with specific problems are also available. For instance, Table 34–22 lists areas to monitor in a child with Down syndrome.

Because conventional medical care cannot cure many conditions associated with developmental delay, many alternative therapies have arisen. A number of them, such as patterning to learn motor skills, ingestion of megadoses of vitamins, and the indiscriminate injection of fetal tissue, have largely been disproved. Two more therapies are facilitated communication and auditory training. In

Table 34-20. Select Psychopharmacologic Agents That May Be Useful in the Treatment of Children with Developmental Disabilities

Medication	Possible Indications
Carbamazepine	Mania, bipolar disorder, impulsivity, aggression, seizures, trigeminal neuralgia
Clomipramine	Obsessive-compulsion, depression
Clonazepam	Mania, bipolar disorder, seizure
Clonidine	Manic episodes, attention-deficit hyperactivity disorder, aggression
Fenfluramine	Prader-Willi syndrome (to suppress appetite and control aggression)
Fluoxetine	Obsessive-compulsion, depression
Methylphenidate, dextroamphetamine, pemoline	Attention-deficit hyperactivity disorder
Propranolol	Aggression, impulsivity
Valproic acid	Bipolar disorder, especially rapidly cycling

Table 34–21. Items to Monitor Using the Mnemonic "MD'S DD BASICS" and Potential Consultations to Consider When Providing Primary Care to Children with Developmental Disabilities

MD'S DD BASICS	Things to Check	Potential Consultant(s)
Motor	Ambulation, seating, position, spine	Orthopedist, physiatrist, PT, OT
Diet	Weight, fat stores, diet, feeding problems	Nutritionist/dietitian, speech pathologist, OT
Seizures	Seizure record, drug levels and side effects	Neurologist
Dermatology	Skin breakdown	Nursing, plastic surgeon
Dentistry	Teeth, gums	Dentist
Behavior	Aggression, self-injury, sleep, pica, interfering behavior	Psychologist, psychiatrist
Advocacy	Finances, family support, program aid	Social worker
Sensory	Vision, hearing	Ophthalmologist, audiologist
Infections	Immunizations, environment, lungs, urine	Infection-control nurse
Constipation	Stools, gastroesophageal reflux	Gastroenterologist
Sexuality	Menses, sexual activity, masturbation, contraception, prevention of sexually transmitted diseases	Gynecologist, habilitation program

Adapted from Sulkes S. MD's DD BASICS: Identifying common problems and preventing secondary disabilities. Pediatr Ann 24:245–254, 1995.

Table 34–22. Medical Checklist for the Primary Care Physician Evaluating a Child with Down Syndrome

Age	Condition	Monitoring
Birth to 2 mo	Etiology, recurrence risk	Chromosome analysis and genetic counseling
	Hypothyroidism	TSH, T_3 and T_4
	Congenital heart defect	Pediatric cardiology evaluation, including echocardiography
	Family stress	Referral to Down Syndrome Association
2–12 mo	Refractive errors, cataracts	Pediatric ophthalmologic evaluation
	Hearing loss; recurrent otitis media	Auditory brainstem evoked response
	Delayed development	Formal developmental evaluations
1–12 yr	Delayed development	Enrollment in Early Intervention program
	Hypothyroidism	Annual TSH
	Hearing loss	Auditory testing: annually between 1 and 3 yr and every 2 yr between 3 and 13 yr
	Refractive error	Ophthalmologic exam every 2 yr
	Atlantoaxial instability	Cervical spine roentgenograms at 2 and 12 yr
	Routine care	Dental examination at 2 yr then every 6 mo (remember prophylaxis for subacute bacterial endocarditis, if indicated)
12–18 yr	Hypothyroidism	TSH annually
	Decreased hearing	Auditory testing every 2 yr
	Refractive error	Ophthalmologic examination every 2 yr
	Mitral valve prolapse	Echocardiogram

Abbreviations: TSH = thyroid-stimulating hormone; T_3 = triiodothyronine; T_4 = thyroxine.

facilitated communication, an individual who is familiar with a child who has difficulty communicating (a child with autism) assists the child in some way, such as holding the hands or wrists while the child uses a communication device such as a communication board or keyboard to express ideas. There is evidence that the resulting messages depend more on the facilitator than on the child. The theory behind auditory training is that in certain delayed children, hypersensitivities develop to particular frequencies of sound (e.g., 3000 Hz). Treatment consists of desensitizing individuals to these frequencies by first eliminating those frequencies and then gradually reintroducing them to music played on earphones. Although short-term changes have been observed, there is no convincing evidence yet that this treatment provides any long-term benefit on functioning. Because hope for a cure is difficult for families of a developmentally delayed child to abandon, and because traditional medicine is often ineffective in helping children with delayed development, the clinician should keep an open mind when discussing alternative therapies with families.

REFERENCES

Adesman AR. Is the Denver II developmental test worthwhile? Pediatrics 1992;90:1009–1011.

Ad Hoc Committee on Terminology and Classification. Mental Retardation: Definition, Classification and Systems of Support. Washington, DC: American Association on Mental Retardation, 1992.

Albright AL. Neurosurgical treatment of spasticity: Selective posterior rhizotomy and intrathecal baclofen. Stereotact Funct Neurosurg 1992;58:3–13.

Allen MC, Alexander GR. Motor milestones of very preterm infants at risk for cerebral palsy. Dev Med Child Neurol 1992;34:226–232.

Augustsson I, Nilson C, Engstrand I. The preventive value of audiometric screening of preschool and young school-children. Int J Pediatr Otorhinolaryngol 1990;20:51–62.

Bradley RH, Caldwell BM, Brisby J, et al. The HOME inventory: A new scale for families of pre- and early adolescent children with disabilities. Res Dev Disabil 1992;13:313–333.

Butler M, Meaney F. Standards for selected anthropometric measurements in Prader-Willi syndrome. Pediatrics 1991;88:853–860.

Butler M, Brunschwig A, Miller L, et al. Standards for anthropomorphic measurements in males with fragile X syndrome. Pediatrics 1992;34:481–487.

Capute AJ, Shapiro BK, Wachtel RC, et al. The clinical linguistic and auditory milestone scale (CLAMS): Identification of cognitive defects in motor-delayed children. Am J Dis Child 1986;140:694–698.

Carey JC. Health supervision and anticipatory guidance for children with genetic disorders (including specific recommendations for trisomy 21, trisomy 18 and neurofibromatosis I). Pediatr Clin North Am 1992;39:25–53.

Chamberlin RW. Developmental assessment and early intervention programs for young children: Lessons learned from longitudinal research. Pediatr Rev 1987;8:237–247.

Chaves-Carballo E. Detection of inherited neurometabolic disorders: A practical clinical approach. Pediatr Neurol 1992;39:801–820.

Coplan J, Gleason JR. Quantifying language development from birth to 3 years using the early language milestone scale. Pediatrics 1990;86:963–971.

Einarsson-Backes LM, Stewart KB. Infant neuromotor assessments: A review and preview of selected instruments. Am J Occup Ther 1992;46:224–232.

Escalona SK. Babies at double hazard: Early development of infants at biologic and social risk. Pediatrics 1982;70:670–676.

Frankenburg WK, Dodds J, Archer P, et al. The Denver II: A major revision and restandardization of the Denver developmental screening test. Pediatrics 1992;89:91–97.

Gabrielli O, Salvolini O, Coppa GV, et al. Magnetic resonance imaging in the malformative syndromes with mental retardation. Pediatr Radiol 1990;21:16–19.

Glascoe FP. Can clinical judgment detect children with speech-language problems? Pediatrics 1991;87:317–322.

Glascoe FP, Altemeier WA, MacLean WE. The importance of parents' concerns about their child's development. Am J Dis Child 1989;143:955–958.

Glascoe FP, Byrne KE, Ashford LG, et al. Accuracy of the Denver II in developmental screening. Pediatrics 1992;89:1221–1225.

Harbord MG, Finn JP, Hall-Craggs MA, et al. Myelination patterns on magnetic resonance of children with developmental delay. Dev Med Child Neurol 1990;32:295–303.

Harris SR. Early diagnosis of spastic diplegia, spastic hemiplegia, and quadriplegia. Am J Dis Child 1989;143:1356–1365.

Holm VA, Cassidy SB, Butler MG, et al. Prader-Willi syndrome: Consensus diagnostic criteria. Pediatrics 1993;91:398–402.

Holst K, Andersen E, Philip J, et al. Antenatal and perinatal conditions correlated to handicap among 4-year-old children. Am J Perinatol 1989;6:258–267.

Horwitz SM, Leaf PJ, Leventhal JM, et al. Identification and management of psychosocial and developmental problems in community-based, primary care pediatric practices. Pediatrics 1992;89:480–485.

Iivanainen M, Kaakkola S. Dopa-responsive dystonia of childhood. Dev Med Child Neurol 1993;35:362–367.

Kilmon CA, Barber N, Chapman K. Instruments for the screening of speech/language development in children. J Pediatr Health Care 1991;5:61–70.

Kirby RS, Swanson ME, Kelleher KJ, et al. Identifying at-risk children for early intervention services: Lessons from the Infant Health and Development Program. J Pediatr 1993;122:680–686.

Kjos BO, Umansky R, Barkovich AJ. Brain MR imaging in children with developmental retardation of unknown cause: Results in 76 cases. Am J Neuroradiol 1990;11:1035–1040.

Kopparthi R, McDermott C, Sheftel D, et al. The Minnesota Child Development Inventory: Validity and reliability for assessing development in infancy. J Dev Behav Pediatr 1991;12:217–222.

Laing S, Partington M, Robinson H, et al. Clinical screening score for fragile X (Martin Bell) syndrome. Am J Med Genet 1991;38:256–259.

Lovell RW, Reiss AL. Psychiatric disorders in developmental disabilities. Pediatr Clin North Am 1993;40:579–592.

Najman JM, Bor W, Morrison J, et al. Child developmental delay and socio-economic disadvantage in Australia: A longitudinal study. Soc Sci Med 1992;34:829–835.

Palmer DJ, Garner PW, Lifschitz MH, et al. An exploratory study of the structure and validity of pediatric examination of education readiness (PEER) factors. J Dev Behav Pediatr 1990;11:317–321.

Ramey CT, Ramey SL. Effective early intervention. Ment Retard 1992;30:337–345.

Rapin I. Hearing disorders. Pediatr Rev 1993;14:43–49.

Rescorla L. The language development survey: A screening tool for delayed language in toddlers. J Speech Hear Disord 1989;54:587–599.

Schaefer GB, Bodensteiner JB. Evaluation of the child with idiopathic mental retardation. Pediatr Neurol 1992;39:929–943.

Scheiner AP, Sexton ME. Prediction of developmental outcome using a perinatal risk inventory. Pediatrics 1991;88:1135–1143.

Shonkoff JP, Hauser-Cram P, Krauss MW, ct al. Development of infants with disabilities and their families. Monogr Soc Res Child Dev 1992;6:1–153.

Snow BJ, Tsui JK, Bhatt MH, et al. Treatment of spasticity with botulinum toxin: A double-blind study. Ann Neurol 1990;28:512–515.

Sturner RA, Kunze L, Funk SG, et al. Elicited imitation: Its effectiveness for speech and language screening. Dev Med Child Neurol 1993;35:715–726.

Sugimoto T, Yasuhara A, Nishida N, et al. MRI of the head in the evaluation of microcephaly. Neuropediatrics 1993;24:4–7.

Veen S, Sassen ML, Schreuder AM, et al. Hearing loss in very preterm and very low birthweight infants at the age of 5 years in a nationwide cohort. Int J Pediatr Otorhinolaryngol 1993;26:11–28.

Wasserman RC, Croft CA, Brotherton SE. Preschool vision screening in pediatric practice: A study from the Pediatric Research in Office Settings (PROS) Network, American Academy of Pediatrics. Pediatrics 1992;89:834–838.

Watkin PM, Baldwin M, Laoide S. Parental suspicion and identification of hearing impairment. Arch Dis Child 1990;65:846–850.

Wellesley D, Hockey A, Stanley F. The aetiology of intellectual disability in Western Australia: A community-based study. Dev Med Child Neurol 1991;33:963–973.

Yeargin-Allsopp M, Murphy CC, Oakley GP, et al. A multiple-source method for studying the prevalence of developmental disabilities in children: The Metropolitan Atlanta Developmental Disabilities Study. Pediatrics 1992;89:624–630.

35 The Irritable Infant

Emory M. Petrack

An irritable infant presents a challenge to the parents and physician. Although all infants are irritable at times, an irritable infant is defined as a patient younger than 1 year of age whom the caregiver deems to cry excessively or to be excessively fussy or cranky. This definition encompasses the many categories of infant irritability (Tables 35–1 and 35–2). Most infants with excessive crying or irritability do not have significant underlying pathology. However, there are serious entities that must not be missed during this initial evaluation (Table 35–3), and the clinician faces the challenge to identify these diseases or processes.

DIAGNOSTIC APPROACH

The approach to the crying infant is directed toward a thorough history and physical examination, coupled with the judicial use of laboratory and roentgenographic studies. Patients without prior medical problems (e.g., sickle cell anemia) who cry for more than 2 hours and whose parents believe that this episode is longer than any previous episode represent approximately 0.2% of emergency department visits. The final diagnoses of these irritable infants stress the importance of a thorough and comprehensive evaluation. The history provides important information in directing the evaluation in approximately 20% of cases. The final diagnosis is evident from the initial physical examination in 41%, from initial laboratory or roentgenographic studies in 20% (Table 35–4), and from subsequent follow-up evaluations in 39%.

In 61% of these infants, the crying may be due to a serious underlying cause, defined as a condition with the potential to cause harm if it is not promptly treated.

In 75% of these seriously ill infants, the diagnosis can be made or accurately suspected by the end of the physical examination. Many seriously ill infants with no physical findings may continue to cry excessively after their evaluation. Most infants without serious conditions stop crying excessively after the evaluation. Abnormal physical findings or persistent crying beyond the initial assessment may be predictive of serious illness, with a sensitivity of 100% (95% confidence interval [CI]:90% to 100%), a specificity of 77% (95% CI:54% to 91%), and a positive predictive value of 87% (95% CI:72% to 95%).

As with any potentially ill patient, initial attention is given to the evaluation and stabilization of the airway, breathing, and circulation (Fig. 35–1). Once this is accomplished, the next step is to perform a careful history and physical examination. Every component of the physical examination has the potential to uncover physical findings that may direct the clinician to a specific diagnosis (Table 35–5). Every part of the body should be carefully examined after covering garments are removed. This initial evaluation should be performed with the intent of specifically looking for serious diagnoses (Table 35–3). The evaluation should include a fluorescein examination of the eye to detect a corneal abrasion and retinoscopy to detect retinal hemorrhages from abuse.

The second branch point of this decision tree (see Fig. 35–1) occurs in patients with normal findings on physical examination. This point is based on the consolability of the patient during the evaluation. In patients with normal examination results, very few consolable patients have a serious condition, whereas about 60% of inconsolable patients have a serious illness. Because of the low incidence of serious illnesses in the consolable infant, the clinician should consider nonurgent causes of the crying (Table 35–6). However, the clinician must monitor these patients closely (at 24-hour

Table 35–1. Differential Diagnosis of the Irritable Infant

Central Nervous System
  Encephalitis
  Hydrocephalus
  Intracranial hemorrhage
  Meningitis
  Pseudotumor cerebri
  Tumor

Eyes
  Corneal abrasion
  Foreign body
  Glaucoma

Ears
  Otitis media
  Foreign body

Nose
  Foreign body

Mouth
  Foreign body
  Herpangina
  Herpes stomatitis
  Teething

Respiratory System
  Bronchiolitis
  Foreign body aspiration
  Pneumonia
  Reactive airways
  Upper airway obstruction

Cardiovascular System
  Anomalous coronary artery
  Congestive heart failure
  Supraventricular tachycardia

Gastrointestinal System
  Anal fissure
  Appendicitis
  Constipation
  Feeding problems
  Gastroenteritis
  Gastroesophageal reflux

  Incarcerated inguinal hernia
  Intussusception
  Malrotation
  Volvulus

Genitourinary Tract System
  Testicular torsion
  Tourniquet syndrome of the penis
  Urinary tract infection

Musculoskeletal System
  Cellulitis
  Diskitis
  Fractures
  Osteomyelitis
  Septic arthritis
  Soft tissue injury
  Tourniquet syndrome of the digit

Skin
  Dermatitis
  Insect bites
  Physical abuse

Miscellaneous
  Colic
  Drug ingestion
  Electrolyte disorder
  Fever
  Hypoglycemia
  Hypoxia
  Inborn error of metabolism
  Lactose intolerance
  Neonatal drug withdrawal (from maternal use)
  Parenting difficulties
  Sepsis
  Sickle cell anemia (crisis)
  Vaccine reaction
  Viral syndrome

Table 35–2. Acute and Subacute Causes of Infant Irritability

Acute (<48–72 hours)	Subacute (>3–4 Days)
Infectious	Colic*
Encephalitis	Feeding problems*
Herpangina	Fever
Herpes stomatitis	Parenting difficulties
Meningitis	Dermatitis
Osteomyelitis	Teething
Otitis media	Abdominal pain
Sepsis	Constipation
Urinary tract infection	Gastroenteritis
Viral syndrome	Gastroesophageal reflux
Surgical	Anal fissure*
Appendicitis	Infectious
Hernia*	Diskitis
Intussusception	Encephalitis
Testicular torsion	Herpangina
Volvulus	Herpes stomatitis
	Meningitis
	Osteomyelitis
Cardiovascular	Otitis media
Congestive heart failure	Sepsis
Supraventricular tachycardia	Urinary tract infection
	Viral syndrome
Trauma	Trauma
Minor	Minor
Intracranial hemorrhage	Insect or spider bites
Insect or spider bites, bee sting	
Other	Other
Dermatitis	Drugs
Fever	Foreign body in ear, nose,
Vaccine reaction	eye, oropharynx
Drugs	Toxin exposure
Corneal abrasion	Lactose intolerance
Anal fissure*	Inborn error of
Hair tourniquet	metabolism
Electrolyte disturbances*	Congenital lesions*
Hypoglycemia*	Heart disease
Physical abuse	Glaucoma
Foreign body in ear, nose, eye,	Hydrocephalus
oropharynx	Central nervous system
Sickle cell anemia crisis	abnormality
Hypoxia	
Teething	
Abdominal pain	
Constipation	
Gastroenteritis	
Gastroesophageal reflux	
Colic*	

*Most commonly seen in infants younger than 3 months of age.

intervals or sooner if necessary) for the development of a serious condition.

Because of the high incidence (61%) of serious illness in the persistently inconsolable infant, laboratory studies are needed to assist in the diagnostic process. Any infant who remains inconsolable is best observed in the hospital until a diagnosis can be established. Some ancillary tests that should be considered in this evaluation are:

- A complete blood count and erythrocyte sedimentation rate or a C-reactive protein determination (infection or inflammation)

Table 35–3. Diagnoses Not to Be Missed

> Acute surgical abdomen
> Anomalous coronary artery
> Congestive heart failure
> Corneal abrasion
> Electrolyte disturbance
> Foreign body
> Incarcerated hernia
> Intussusception
> Physical abuse
> Serious infectious illness
> Supraventricular tachycardia
> Testicular torsion
> Tourniquet syndromes

- Analysis of cerebrospinal fluid (meningitis or encephalitis)
- Hemoglobin electrophoresis (sickle cell disease)
- Serum pH and electrolyte levels (electrolyte abnormalities, metabolic diseases)
- Urinalysis and culture (pyelonephritis)
- Stool guaiac (intussusception, gastroenteritis, cow's milk allergy)

Other possible tests include a skeletal survey or bone scan (trauma, abuse), a head computed tomographic (CT) scan (intracranial hemorrhage or hydrocephalus), and amino and organic acid studies (metabolic abnormality).

Despite the complex differential diagnosis of the crying infant, the most likely diagnosis in infants younger than 4 months of age is either normal infant with above-average crying or infantile colic. For infants without colic, the information that the physical examination is normal (coupled with assurances about conditions that have been ruled out) may reduce parental stress. Other issues concerning feeding (overfeeding or underfeeding), teething, and parental stress related to infant care are all important to explore. Caregivers should be questioned about the options for increased support from family or friends during this stressful period. Most

Table 35–4. Contribution of Ancillary Studies to the Diagnosis in Infants with Acute Excessive Crying

Diagnostic Study	No. of Patients in Whom Study Proved Useful (n = 11)	Final Diagnosis (n)
Skeletal radiography	2	Tibial fracture (1) Clavicular fracture (1)
Lumbar puncture/ cerebrospinal fluid analysis	2	Pseudotumor cerebri (1)* Encephalitis (1)
Electrocardiography	2	SVT
CT of the head	2	Pseudotumor cerebri (1)* Subdural hematoma (1)
Barium enema	1	Intussusception
Esophagraphy	1	GE reflux/esophagitis
Amino and organic acid studies	1	Glutaric aciduria
Urinalysis	1	Urinary tract infection

Adapted from Poole S: The infant with acute, unexplained, excessive crying. Pediatrics 1991;88:450–455. Reproduced with permission.
*One patient, with pseudotumor cerebri, required lumbar puncture and head CT to establish the diagnosis.
Abbreviations: CT = computed tomography; GE = gastroesophageal; SVT = supraventricular tachycardia.

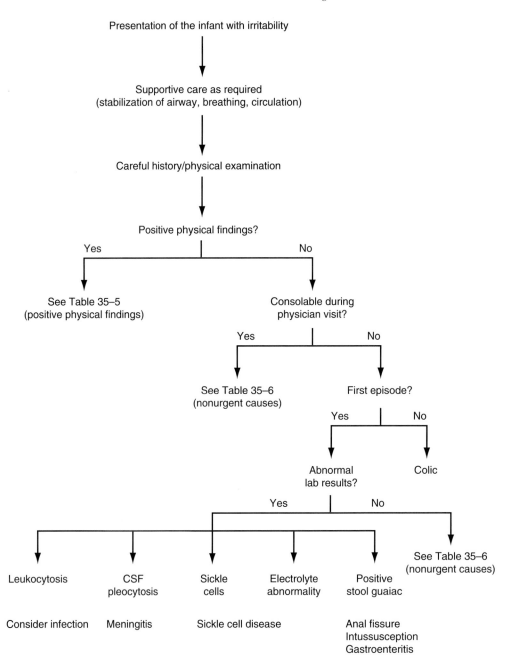

Figure 35–1. Approach to the irritable infant. CSF = cerebrospinal fluid.

importantly, because a definitive diagnosis has not been established, infants in this group should receive follow-up within 24 hours, or sooner if indicated, to ensure that a more serious illness was not missed.

SPECIFIC DIAGNOSES

Infantile Colic (Excessive Crying, Paroxysmal Fussing, Persistent Crying)

Infantile colic is a controversial topic, and there is still marked disagreement regarding its etiology and management. There is a lack of a uniform definition for infantile colic, an inability to incorporate double-blind strategies to assess some of the interven-

tions for it, and an overreliance on maternal recall for documenting length of crying. Furthermore, colic is a relatively self-limited condition that usually lasts less than 3 months. Because of these facts, there may not be enough time to adequately assess the success of a particular therapy. Nonetheless, infantile colic is a common problem that occurs in 20% to 30% of young infants.

DEFINITION

Colic refers to unexplained paroxysms of irritability, fussing, or crying in an infant. Episodes occur more than three times per week, last longer than 3 hours per day, and usually have been present for 3 weeks by the time of presentation to the physician. Paroxysms generally occur in the evenings and usually start between 3 and 21

Table 35–5. Positive Findings on Physical Examination

Physical Finding	Possible Diagnoses	Specific Tests to Consider
Skin	Dermatitis (eczema) Abuse DTP reaction Abrasion, cellulitis Insect bite Viral exanthem	Skeletal survey

Fever with
  Inflamed eardrum
  Increased urination
  Bone tenderness, erythema
	Otitis media
	Urinary tract infection
	Osteomyelitis, arthritis
		UA, urine/blood culture
		CBC, ESR, blood culture, bone scan, arthrocentesis

Tachycardia	Supraventricular tachycardia Congestive heart failure Dehydration Trauma Blood loss, anemia	Electrocardiography CXR Electrolyte level Hematocrit value, UA, CT Hematocrit value
Tachypnea	Hypoxia Respiratory illness Salicylate ingestion Acidosis	Pulse oximetry, ABG, CXR Pulse oximetry, ABG, CXR ABG, salicylate level ABG
Ears	Otitis media Foreign body	
Eyes	Corneal abrasion Foreign body Fundi (hemorrhage, papilledema)	Fluorescein stain Fluorescein stain CT
Nose	Foreign body	
Mouth	Herpangina Stomatitis Teething	

Respiratory findings
  Wheezing
  Rales
	Asthma, bronchiolitis, foreign body
	Pneumonia, CHF
		Pulse oximetry, ABG, CXR
		Pulse oximetry, ABG, CXR

Abdominal findings	Reflux esophagitis Volvulus Intussusception Appendicitis Testicular torsion Gastroenteritis Hernia Anal fissure	pH probe, barium swallow Upper barium study Barium enema Abdominal x-ray, ultrasound studies Nuclear scan, Doppler scan
Genitourinary findings	Testicular torsion Sexual abuse Hair tourniquet	Nuclear scan, Doppler scan
Extremity findings	Trauma Hair tourniquet Osteomyelitis-arthritis	x-ray study x-ray study, bone scan, arthrocentesis
Neurologic findings	Meningitis Pseudotumor cerebri Cerebral palsy	LP Head CT, LP

Abbreviations: DTP = diphtheria, tetanus, pertussis vaccine; CT = computed tomography; UA = urinalysis; LP = lumbar puncture; CHF = congestive heart failure; ABG = arterial blood gas; CXR = chest x-ray study; ESR = erythrocyte sedimentation rate; CBC = complete blood count.

Table 35–6. Nonurgent Causes of Infant Irritability

Colic
Constipation
Feeding problems
Parenting difficulties
Teething
Vaccine reaction
Viral syndrome

days of age and subside by 3 to 4 months of age. In an infant with colic, no underlying disease is responsible for the crying. Crying and fussing are normal parts of early infant development. Normal crying gradually increases from birth until 2 months of age, when the child may cry for a total of 2.5 hours per day. The distinction between normal crying in infancy and colic is not clear. Colic may simply represent a point further along on a continuum of infant behavior.

ETIOLOGY

The etiology of colic is unclear. Colic may not represent a single entity but, rather, may be a common end point for various processes. Some of the proposed theories for the causes of colic are dietary antigens (milk proteins), abnormal peristalsis, excessive gas production, and infant temperament.

Some of the dietary antigens that have been implemented as a possible cause for colic are cow's milk whey or casein and soy protein. Even the maternal consumption of cow's milk has been associated with colic in purely breast-fed infants. However, this is not a consistent finding. Parental consoling of the infant may be more effective than formula changes in crying infants. Counseling (for consoling) consists of instructing parents to maintain diaries and to acknowledge possible needs of the infant that are expressed by crying. Parents can respond by feeding, holding, giving a pacifier, stimulating, or putting the infant to bed. Although crying time may decrease with the elimination of soy or cow's milk protein, the decrease in crying time may be greater with parental consoling. In addition, re-exposure of a diet-treated group to soy or cow's milk antigen may not result in an increase in crying time. Despite the conflicting evidence, dietary protein may play some role in a subset of crying infants. Unfortunately, no specific laboratory test exists for diagnosing dietary protein allergy in relation to infantile colic. The only way to study this phenomenon is through the elimination of, and re-challenge with, the specific antigens.

Another theory of the etiology of colic implicates the role of abnormal peristalsis or excessive intestinal gas. Colicky infants often exhibit intermittent episodes of crying that appear to be associated with pain. The infant seems to achieve relief after the passage of flatus. It is difficult to know whether these episodes of colic are a result of excess gas or whether the excess gas is a result of significant periods of crying with aerophagia. If there is excessive gas, watery diarrhea, and cramps, it is possible that lactose malabsorption is present. A lactose feeding with a hydrogen breath test will confirms this diagnosis. Infants with lactose malabsorption should respond to a non–lactose-containing formula (soy-based, Nutramigen).

The role of abnormal peristalsis and infant crying is suggested by the reduction of infant crying with dicyclomine hydrochloride, which is an anticholinergic agent. Because of the severe side effects of this drug, which include hypersensitivity reactions and apnea, dicyclomine hydrochloride is no longer approved for use in infants under 6 months of age. Drugs that have been shown to have no effect in treating colic are simethicone, dimethicone, phenobarbital,

and alcohol. In addition, several reports have been published of infants presenting with cyanosis and apnea who were treated for colic with the following medications: dimenhydrinate (Dramamine) plus phenobarbital, hyoscyamine sulfate, atropine sulfate, and scopolamine hydrobromide (Donnatal). The clinician must be aware that parental distress from prolonged, unexplained infant crying can lead to the use of inappropriate and even dangerous remedies.

Another theory relates to infant temperament. Some infants have an increased sensitivity to surrounding stimuli, leading to excessive crying. Parental anxiety concerning the crying infant may interact with the infant's native temperament to create an environment that exacerbates the problem. Some aspect of this infant-maternal relationship is frequently associated with a significant number of children with the diagnosis of colic (Fig. 35–2).

CLINICAL FEATURES

The most prominent feature of the infant with colic is significant crying or irritability. It is important to carefully characterize the nature of the crying, including the duration, intensity, and time of day when it occurs. The crying is intense and often inconsolable. Episodes typically occur in the late afternoon or evening. The parent is often quite distressed about the inability to soothe the infant. At times of the day when the infant is not exhibiting this behavior, the activity level, amount of feeding, and general appearance are normal. In addition, there is no suggestion of any other pathophysiologic process (history of fever, cyanosis, trauma).

In infantile colic, both the physical examination and laboratory results are normal. Even though the clinician may suspect infantile colic by the history alone, it is extremely important to proceed through the differential diagnosis of the irritable infant (see Tables 35–1 and 35–2). One must perform a thorough physical examination to rule out other diagnoses (see Fig. 35–1, Table 35–5). If the infant remains inconsolable during the evaluation, the clinician needs to perform a series of laboratory investigations to rule out other conditions (see Fig. 35–1, Table 35–4). If the infant has normal physical findings, is consolable, and has a history consistent with infantile colic, laboratory tests are usually not required.

TREATMENT

Before a management plan is chosen, other serious illnesses must be ruled out; infantile colic may be multifactorial. The initial presentation of colic can be confused with other, more significant, disease processes requiring immediate intervention. It is therefore critical that the practitioner exercise caution in making the diagnosis of colic, especially if irritability is present for only a few hours.

The following approach to the infant with colic is recommended:

1. The level of distress and anxiety that the crying is causing the parents should be recognized and acknowledged with empathy. Severe colic can be associated with an intense level of frustration and anger for the entire family. It is not acceptable to acknowledge colic simply as a developmental phenomenon that the infant will soon outgrow.

2. The parents should be reassured that based on a thorough history and physical examination, no specific problem exists regarding the infant's physical or emotional health. The clinician should acknowledge that the infant appears to be crying more than the average infant and that such crying can be quite stressful for the family.

3. Although still controversial, changing the infant's formula will probably not have a significant impact on most cases of colic. In addition, although some clinicians switch from lactose-based to

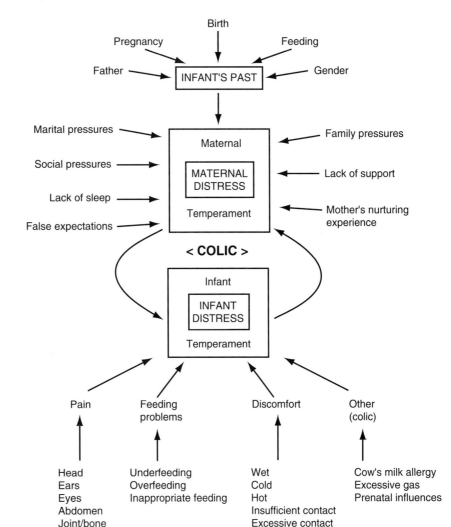

Figure 35–2. Interaction of stresses acting on mother and crying infant. (Adapted from Hewson P, Oberklaid F, Menahem S. Infant colic, distress, and crying. Clin Pediatr 1987;26:74.)

soy-based formulas, soy protein may be as antigenic as cow's milk protein and can cause symptoms of colic. If an allergic cause is suspected, a formula change to a hydrolyzed casein formula (Nutramigen) may be considered. Any improvement, although welcome, may simply reflect a placebo effect. A change in formula for colic may not be without undesirable behavioral consequences, including development of parental anxiety concerning the possibility of an intrinsic abnormality in their infant. Appropriate counseling should help to allay this fear.

4. Although increased carrying of young infants may reduce normal crying time, such a reduction has not been shown to occur in infants with colic. Parents might try to respond to excessive crying by feeding, holding, giving the baby a pacifier, or putting the infant to bed. It has also been suggested that perhaps some background noise or vibration, as occurs during an automobile ride (in an appropriate infant restraint seat), might be useful. The possibility of overstimulation as a cause of colic should also be entertained. If the infant remains inconsolable after 20 to 30 minutes of active intervention, it is probably worthwhile attempting to decrease stimulation by attempting to put the infant to bed in a quiet environment.

5. The use of various medications to reduce colic remains controversial. These medications also have potential serious and life-threatening side effects. No specific drug therapy can be recommended for the treatment of colic.

6. The clinician should give encouragement to the parents that altering the way they handle the crying and interact with the infant during colicky periods should reduce the amount of crying. While not minimizing the impact of colic on the family, the clinician should explain to the family the natural history and usually short course of colic. The primary caregiver should be encouraged to seek support and periodic relief from the infant's care from a family member or a trusted friend.

7. For excessively anxious parents, close follow-up is important. This element is especially critical if the clinician has any doubt concerning the establishment of the correct diagnosis.

Tourniquet Syndromes

In tourniquet syndromes, a filamentous material, such as hair or a thread from clothing, wraps around an appendage, causing ischemia. Some of the reported appendages that can be affected by this syndrome are the fingers, the toes, the penis, and even the uvula. Almost 2% of infants with prolong crying may have a tourniquet syndrome. Hair that is initially moist can tighten on drying after wrapping around an affected appendage. With surrounding edema, the hair may become partially or completely obscured in the skin, which makes the diagnosis difficult to establish. This syndrome should be suspected in any irritable infant who has a well-demarcated line separating normal tissue from a distal, dusky, edematous appendage.

With penile hair strangulation, the distal penis is noted to be swollen, edematous, and sometimes discolored. The hair is often deeply imbedded in a groove that is covered with edematous tissue. Because the hair is often not visible, an erroneous diagnosis of paraphimosis might be made. Failure to recognize penile strangulation can lead to numerous complications, including urethral fistula, gangrene, deformity of the glans, urethral stricture, or loss of part of the penis. Therefore, this diagnosis should be considered in any infant presenting with a swollen penis.

Management of tourniquet syndromes consists of the expeditious removal of the strand. The strand may be dissolved by a hair depilatory agent, removed with tweezers, or cut. Because of the edema obscuring the strand, the only recourse may be to cut the strand through a skin incision perpendicular to the demarcation line. Almost 38% of patients require surgical intervention for penile strangulation. Because of the need to rapidly re-establish tissue perfusion, coupled with the difficulty in removing the strand from edematous tissue, it is important to request surgical consultation as soon as the diagnosis is established.

Teething

Many complaints, ranging from fever to irritability, have been ascribed to teething. Many of the problems for which teething has been held responsible include normal developmental processes and events. For example, teething infants often experience mild fever, drooling, crying, or feeding or sleeping difficulties. Even though teething may be associated with these symptoms, it may not be the cause.

From interviews with parents and pediatricians, the consensus is that teething is associated with irritability. For example, 49 of 64 (77%) pediatricians surveyed believe that teething causes irritability. A longitudinal survey of parental reports of primary tooth eruption supports this notion. Irritability was related to anterior (incisors) and posterior (cuspids and molars) tooth eruption in 69% and 97% of infants, respectively. In addition, of the 19 symptoms accompanying tooth eruption, irritability was the most frequently occurring symptom. Even though tooth eruption may be associated with irritability, teething should be considered as a diagnosis of exclusion in the infant with excessive crying. Just as in the evaluation of the infant with colic, the irritable infant must be evaluated for more serious underlying causes (see Table 35–3).

Management consists of allowing the infant to bite on any appropriate hard object, such as a teething ring, biscuit, pretzel, bagel, or frozen washcloth. Some infants might find rubbing the erupting tooth with the parent's finger to be helpful. Additional relief might be obtained from the use of an analgesic, such as acetaminophen, or the application of a topical anesthetic agent to the site of the erupting tooth. If there is any concern as to the correct diagnosis, close follow-up is mandatory.

Drug Reactions

Although various therapeutic medications and illicit drugs have been said to be responsible for infant irritability, there is little information supporting such an association. In a series of reports, maternal oral decongestants have been associated with infant irritability through their transmission in breast milk. These agents have included dexbrompheniramine, D-isoephedrine, and phenylpropanolamine. Cessation of maternal use led to a rapid improvement in infant behavior. If this effect is caused by maternal transmission, it seems reasonable to suggest that direct treatment of the infant for congestion with these agents may also lead to irritable behavior. Although still controversial, it has been suggested that illicit drugs, including cocaine, opiates, and marijuana, precipitate irritability through breast milk. In the neonate, irritability may also be a symptom of drug withdrawal, resulting from maternal addiction to drugs such as heroin, methadone, amphetamines, or barbiturates during pregnancy. Neonatal drug withdrawal usually occurs in the first week of life but may be delayed 2 to 3 weeks if the mother used methadone. Manifestations include crying, sneezing, emesis, seizures, poor feeding, hiccups, diarrhea, sleeplessness, hyperactivity, and tremors.

Treatment of neonatal drug withdrawal includes replacing the opiate with paregoric or methadone or suppressing symptoms with phenobarbital. Postnatal passive or active exposure to cocaine may also cause acute symptoms. In the evaluation of the irritable neonate, a careful infant and maternal drug history and urine drug toxicology are important to obtain.

Immunization Reactions

Irritability secondary to an immunization is common in infants; most of these reactions follow administration of the diphtheria-tetanus-pertussis (DTP) vaccine. Fretfulness occurs in 70% of infants who receive DTP injections. Although crying usually ceases after the injection, irritability may continue for more than 3 hours in 1% of doses. Some of the irritability associated with the vaccine may be related to the injection rather than the vaccine itself.

Both the pertussis component and the aluminum hydroxide adjuvant of the DTP vaccine may be responsible for reactions. The plain DTP vaccine contains the aluminum hydroxide adjuvant, whereas the absorbed DTP vaccine does not. Irritability or vomiting may occur in 24% of plain DTP doses, compared with only 5% of adsorbed (adjunct and pertussis-removed) DT doses. The onset of reactions usually begins within 8 hours, but 6% of reactions occur more than 24 hours after immunization. The percentages of irritable infants who have received the plain DTP, absorbed DTP, and absorbed DT injection are approximately 44%, 21%, and 15%, respectively. Thus, the injection, the adjuvant, and the pertussis component may all cause irritability.

The irritability associated with the DTP vaccine may be attenuated by acetaminophen. The incidence of fretfulness is reduced approximately 45% with acetaminophen treatment.

SUMMARY AND RED FLAGS

Although at times a simple diagnosis is easily established, the infant with excessive irritability often presents a significant challenge. Establishment of the likely diagnosis combined with exclusion of significant pathophysiology is a prerequisite to the formulation of an appropriate management plan. Through a logical and stepwise approach, the clinician can usually establish the cause and can develop a treatment plan for infant irritability. When the clinician cannot determine the underlying cause of irritability in a particular infant, close follow-up should result in optimal patient care.

Red flags include inconsolability; abnormal level of consciousness or abnormal vital signs; evidence of trauma or anemia (blood loss, sickle cell, leukemia); vomiting; diarrhea; hematochezia and abdominal tenderness or distention; signs of tourniquet syndrome; eye tearing; photophobia or conjunctival irritation; abnormalities of growth, including head circumference; and signs of cardiorespiratory compromise.

REFERENCES

The Irritable Infant

Du J. Colic as the sole symptom of urinary tract infection in infants. Can Med Assoc J 1976;115:334–337.

Harkness M. Corneal abrasion in infancy as a cause of inconsolable crying. Pediatr Emerg Care 1989;5:242–244.

Ludwig S. Shaken baby syndrome: A review of 20 cases. Ann Emerg Med 1984;13:104–107.

Poole S. The infant with acute, unexplained, excessive crying. Pediatrics 1991;88:450–455.

Infantile Colic

Barr R, Kramer M, Pless I, et al. Feeding and temperament as determinants of early infant crying/fussing behavior. Pediatrics 1989;84:514–521.

Barr R, McMullan S, Spiess H, et al. Carrying as colic "therapy": A randomized controlled trial. Pediatrics 1991;87:623–630.

Carey W. The effectiveness of parent counseling in managing colic. Pediatrics 1994;94:37.

Danielsson B, Hwang C. Treatment of infantile colic with surface active substance (simethicone). Acta Paediatr Scand 1985;74:446–450.

Forsyth B, McCarthy P, Leventhal J. Problems of early infancy, formula changes, and mothers' beliefs about their infants. J Pediatr 1985; 106:1012–1017.

Hardoin R, Henslee J, Christenson C. Colic medication and apparent life-threatening events. Clin Pediatr 1991;30:281–285.

Hill D, Menahem S, Hudson I, et al. Charting infant distress: An aid to defining colic. J Pediatr 1992;121:755–758.

Hunziker U, Barr R. Increased carrying reduces infant crying: A randomized controlled trial. Pediatrics 1986;77:641–648.

Illingworth R. Infantile colic revisited. Arch Dis Child 1985;60:981–985.

Lothe L, Lindberg T, Jakobsson I. Cow's milk formula as a cause of infantile colic: A double-blind study. Pediatrics 1982;70:7–10.

Lothe L, Lindberg T. Cow's milk whey protein elicits symptoms of infantile colic in colicky formula-fed infants: A double-blind crossover study. Pediatrics 1989;83:262–266.

Miller A, Barr R. Infantile colic: Is it a gut issue? Pediatr Clin North Am 1991;38:1407–1423.

O'Donovan J, Bradstock A. The failure of conventional drug therapy in the management of infantile colic. Am J Dis Child 1979;133:999–1001.

Parkin P, Schwartz C, Manuel B. Randomized controlled trial of three interventions in the management of persistent crying of infancy. Pediatrics 1993;92:197–201.

Singer J. A fatal case of colic. Pediatr Emerg Care 1992;8:171–172.

St James-Roberts I. Persistent infant crying. Arch Dis Child 1991;66:653–655.

St James-Roberts I. Managing infants who cry persistently. Br Med J 1992;304:997–998.

Taubman B. Parental counseling compared with elimination of cow's milk or soy milk protein for the treatment of infant colic syndrome: A randomized trial. Pediatrics 1988;81:756–761.

Tourniquet Syndromes

Alpert J, Filler R, Glaser H. Strangulation of an appendage by hair wrapping. N Engl J Med 1965;273:866–867.

Curran J. Digital strangulation by hair wrapping. J Pediatr 1966;69:137–138.

Haddad F. Penile strangulation by human hair. Urol Int 1982;37:375–388.

McClure W, Gradinger G. Hair strangulation of the glans penis. Plast Reconstr Surg 1985;76:120–123.

McNeal R, Cruickshank J. Strangulation of the uvula by hair wrapping. Clin Pediatr 1987;26:599–600.

Teething

Honig P. Teething—are today's pediatricians using yesterday's notions? J Pediatr 1975;87:415–417.

Seward M. General disturbances attributed to eruption of the human primary dentition. J Dent Child 1972;39:178–183.

Seward M. Local disturbances attributed to eruption of the human primary dentition. Br Dent J 1971;130:72–77.

Drug Reactions

Chasnoff I, Lewis D, Squires L. Cocaine intoxication in a breast-fed infant. Pediatrics 1987;80:836–838.

Mortimer E. Drug toxicity from breast milk? (Letter.) Pediatrics 1977;60:780–781.

Rogers W. Fussy baby: A new cause. (Letter.) Pediatrics 1979;63:347–348.

Zuckerman B, Bresnahan K. Developmental and behavioral consequences of prenatal drug and alcohol exposure. Pediatr Clin North Am 1991;38:1387–1406.

Vaccine Reactions

Ipp M, Gold R, Greenberg S, et al. Acetaminophen prophylaxis of adverse reactions following vaccination of infants with diphtheria-pertussis-tetanus toxoids-polio vaccine. Pediatr Infect Dis J 1987;6:721–725.

Long S, Deforest A, Smith D, et al. Longitudinal study of adverse reactions following diphtheria-tetanus-pertussis vaccine in infancy. Pediatrics 1990;85:294–302.

Pollock T, Mortimer J, Miller E, et al. Symptoms after primary immunisation with DTP and with DT vaccine. Lancet 1984;2:146–149.

36 Unusual Behaviors

Theodore Reeves Warm   Robert L. Findling

Unusual behaviors in children are common and consist of psychologic conditions that range from variations in normal behavior to life-threatening suicide attempts. Almost 20% of children have a diagnosable psychologic illness that can result in a high degree of stress in the family. These unusual behaviors may be grouped into the following chief complaints: suicide thoughts and attempts, disruptive behaviors, hallucinations, unexplained physical complaints, and delayed development.

HISTORY

The history is the most important tool for identifying the psychologic disorder (Table 36–1). The first step in conducting the history is to ensure the child's safety with regard to either the child hurting himself or herself (suicide attempt) or someone else hurting the child (physical or sexual abuse). After the child's safety is ensured, the history should focus on the stressors that may be precipitating the behavior and on the symptoms that may distinguish which illnesses are causing the behavior.

Besides psychologic illnesses, the clinician should also focus the interview on possible medical causes of these behaviors, including medications side effects, substance abuse, and medical illnesses ranging from encephalopathies to endocrinopathies (e.g., hypothyroidism). Because co-morbidity is common in children with psychologic illnesses, one should consider combinations of illnesses that may cause these symptoms. The clinician should obtain the information from multiple sources, including interviewing the parents and the child separately and interviewing other adults who have spent a significant amount of time with the child (e.g., teacher). Interviewing the child separately provides a better chance of uncovering destructive behaviors (e.g., substance abuse or sexual activity) and of obtaining the child's perspective of the problem. Because of the strong genetic predominance in some of these disorders, a detailed psychiatric family history should be obtained. Often these disorders are undiagnosed; hence, the family history should include both the presence of symptoms and the diagnoses in family members.

Since many of these disorders have symptoms that occur in clusters, a diagnostic manual has been developed that classifies these symptom clusters into individual diagnoses. The *Diagnostic and Statistical Manual of Mental Disorders, Fourth Edition (DSM-IV)* uses descriptive diagnostic criteria that are based on the presence or absence of various symptoms. To use this tool effectively, one needs to know the salient features of these conditions.

SUICIDE THOUGHTS AND ATTEMPTS

Suicide is the third leading cause of death in teenagers. The thought of killing oneself as a solution to a problem is common among grade school and college students. Among grade school students, 9% have thought of suicide, 2% have seriously considered suicide, and 1% have attempted suicide. In college students, there is a fivefold increase in suicide ideation, with 43% thinking of suicide, 15% seriously considering suicide, and 5% attempting suicide. Because of this high prevalence of suicide ideation, the assessment for the risk of suicide is the first part of the evaluation of any child who presents with unusual behaviors. The approach in evaluating suicide ideation is based on whether the child is just thinking of suicide or is making suicide threats or attempts (Fig. 36–1).

Suicide Thoughts

When suicide ideation is present, most parents report that the child has thought of committing suicide. In some cases, however, the office interview may be the first time that the child verbalizes this thought.

Next, the clinician needs to determine the seriousness of these thoughts. To assess risk, the interviewer should focus on the risk factors for completed suicides. These risk factors are male sex, adolescence, conscious plan, available means (medications or firearms), depression, hopelessness, impulsiveness, low frustration level, use of intoxicants, recent death of family member or friend, and previous suicide attempts. Although depression is an important risk factor for suicide, only half of adolescents who attempt suicide have a clinically diagnosable depression. In the nondepressed group, the crucial characteristics for suicide are impulsivity and low frustration tolerance.

Other than for the most frivolous thoughts of suicide, any child or adolescent who is thinking of suicide should be persuaded to discuss this issue with a responsible adult and should be encouraged to seek counseling. If significant risk factors exist for suicide, the patient should be emergently referred to a mental health provider for further evaluation.

Suicide Threats and Attempts

Once the patient's thoughts of suicide have escalated to suicide threats or attempts, the individual's life is in great danger. This is

---

Table 36–1. Essential Elements of Obtaining the Patient History

- Assess suicide potential (ensure safety)
- Interview child alone
- Interview multiple sources
- Obtain family history for symptoms and disorders
- Rule out medical causes, including substance use
- Consider co-morbidities
- Inquire about past mental health referrals

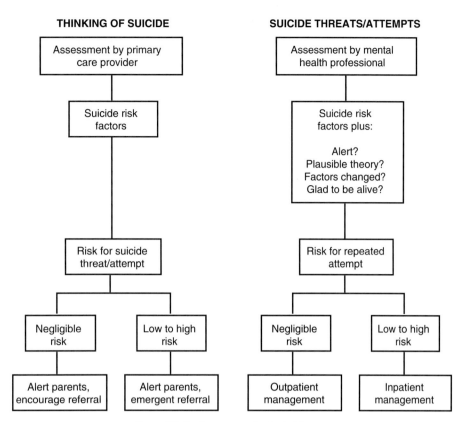

Figure 36–1. Assessment of suicide ideation.

a medical emergency; the patient should be immediately referred to an experienced mental health professional. Because the child's problem-solving abilities and judgment are impaired, someone else must supervise the child's safety. This usually necessitates a psychiatric hospitalization.

Only after suicide risk is accurately assessed can one consider outpatient management. The accuracy of this assessment depends on the patient's cooperating and having a clear consciousness. If the patient is uncooperative, stuporous, or confused, the evaluation results are unreliable, and the patient is assumed to be potentially suicidal. Once the patient is alert, he or she must be able to communicate a plausible theory that led to the suicidal behavior. Without such a theory, the patient has no insight into his or her actions, and hence one cannot predict if the suicide attempt will be repeated. Even with a plausible theory, the crucial factors that led to the act must be changed before one can consider discharging the patient from the hospital.

Finally, the patient must be sincerely glad to be alive. Individuals who have attempted suicide frequently promise that they will not do it again. Because of the high incidence of repeat attempts, these promises are unreliable. The combination of not being remorseful, no plausible theory, and being unable to resolve or change the initiating factors warrants inpatient care.

DISRUPTIVE BEHAVIORS

The disruptive behaviors are the most common chief complaint of unusual behavior presenting to a health care provider's office. These behaviors consist of various diagnoses ranging from Attention-Deficit Hyperactivity Disorder (ADHD) to Schizophrenia. These conditions may be divided into those that are unrelenting and chronic (Fig. 36–2) and those that are episodic and recent in

onset (Figs. 36–3 and 36–4). Disruptive behaviors may be further subdivided into those that may be treated by a primary health care provider and those that should be treated by a mental health specialist.

Chronic Disruptive Behavior

Chronic, disruptive behaviors may be brought to the attention of the health care provider because of an acute crisis (e.g., school failure, destruction of property). In most cases, the consultation is precipitated by changes in the family dynamics that cause the family to be less tolerant of the child's behavior. For example, stress caused by divorce, illness, or work may make a parent more frustrated with the child's behavior and prompt a visit to the child's primary care provider. These chronic behavior disorders consist of ADHD, Oppositional Defiant Disorder (ODD), and Conduct Disorder. Even though these conditions are discussed individually in this chapter, it is common for a child to present with combinations of these disorders (e.g., ADHD plus Conduct Disorder).

TREATMENT BY PRIMARY CARE PHYSICIAN

Attention-Deficit/Hyperactivity Disorder

In the past, ADHD has been called hyperactivity or minimal brain dysfunction. The cardinal features of this condition are hyperactivity (fidgety, on the move), distractibility (short attention span), and impulsiveness (intolerant of delay) (Table 36–2). The preva-

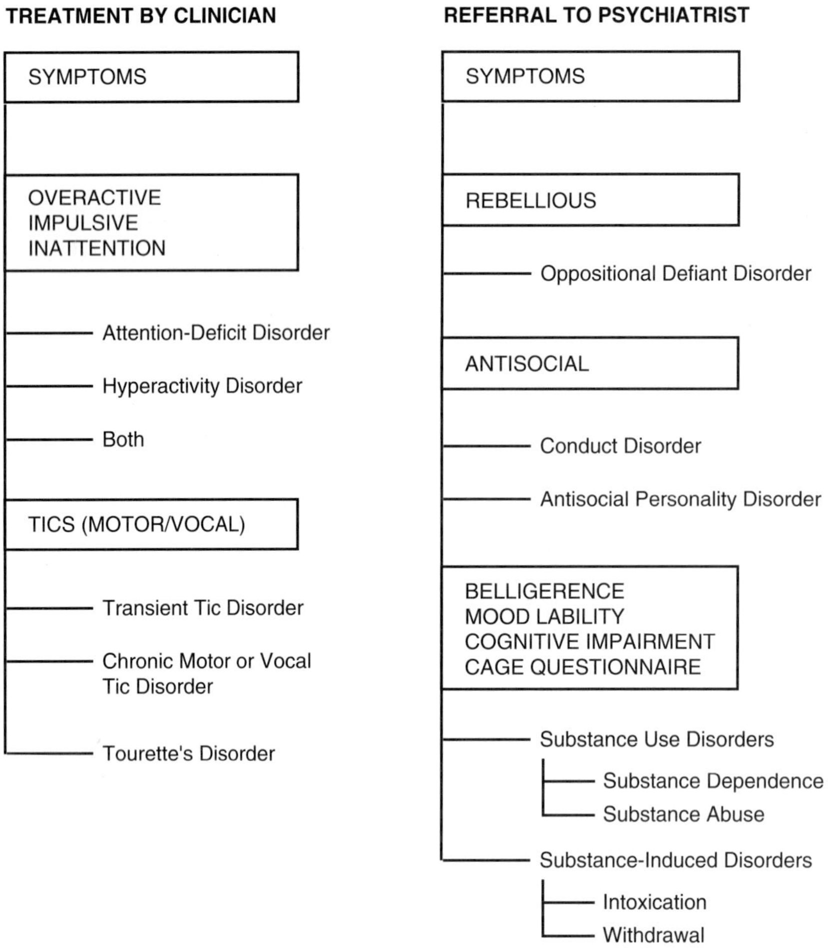

TREATMENT BY CLINICIAN

REFERRAL TO PSYCHIATRIST

SYMPTOMS

OVERACTIVE
IMPULSIVE
INATTENTION

— Attention-Deficit Disorder

— Hyperactivity Disorder

— Both

TICS (MOTOR/VOCAL)

— Transient Tic Disorder

— Chronic Motor or Vocal
Tic Disorder

— Tourette's Disorder

SYMPTOMS

REBELLIOUS

— Oppositional Defiant Disorder

ANTISOCIAL

— Conduct Disorder

— Antisocial Personality Disorder

BELLIGERENCE
MOOD LABILITY
COGNITIVE IMPAIRMENT
CAGE QUESTIONNAIRE

— Substance Use Disorders
     — Substance Dependence
     — Substance Abuse
— Substance-Induced Disorders
     — Intoxication
     — Withdrawal

Figure 36–2. Evaluation of chronic disruptive behaviors. See Table 36–5 for CAGE Questionnaire.

lence of this condition is four to nine times greater in males than in females. The difficulty in diagnosing this disorder is in differentiating age-appropriate hyperactivity/inattentiveness from pathologic behavior. The *DSM-IV* has divided this condition into

---

Table 36–2. Problems in Diagnosis and Treating Attention-Deficit/Hyperactivity Disorder (ADHD)

Problems in Diagnosing ADHD
  No hyperactivity may be present in teenagers; instead, the patient may have only restlessness.
  Differentiating inattention from lack of motivation is difficult.
  Differentiating age-appropriate from pathological behavior (behavioral checklists, teacher's report) is difficult.
  Hyperactive children have normal behavior in quiet, structured settings.
  Sudden onset of hyperactivity is secondary to a stressor and not to ADHD.
  Rule out co-morbidities (learning disabilities, Conduct Disorder, Oppositional Defiant disorder).

Problems in Treating ADHD
  Treatment must be multifactorial and not consist just of stimulants.
  Behavioral modification must have realistic goals, with consistent and frequent rewards.

---

two separate disorders (Attention Deficit with or without Hyperactivity).

To diagnose these conditions, one must note at least six of nine symptoms for inattention or six of nine symptoms for hyperactivity/impulsivity. These symptoms must be present for at least 6 months, be maladaptive, and be inconsistent with child's developmental age.

The nine symptoms of inattention are (1) careless school work, (2) difficulty in sustaining attention, (3) inattentiveness (doesn't listen), (4) failure to finish work, (5) disorganization, (6) avoidance of tasks that require sustained attention, (7) loss of objects necessary for tasks, (8) easy distractibility, and (9) forgetfulness. The nine symptoms of hyperactivity/impulsivity are (1) fidgeting or squirming in one's seat, (2) inappropriately getting out of seat, (3) inappropriately running or climbing on objects, (4) inability to play quietly, (5) often being on the go, (6) talking excessively, (7) stating answers before questions are completed, (8) difficulty in waiting one's turn, and (9) interrupting others.

Some of these symptoms must be present before the child is 7 years of age, they must occur in at least two separate settings (home, school), and they must significantly impair the child's social or academic function.

The chronic hyperactivity of this syndrome may manifest itself in subtle ways. Although hyperactive children move around more than other children, the hyperactivity may be problematic only in certain situations. These circumstances are those in which the child is expected to be sedentary (school, places of worship). In addition, many hyperactive children can sit and be attentive in quiet and relaxed situations, whereas a noisy and active setting (unstructured

TREATMENT BY CLINICIAN   **REFERRAL TO PSYCHIATRIST**

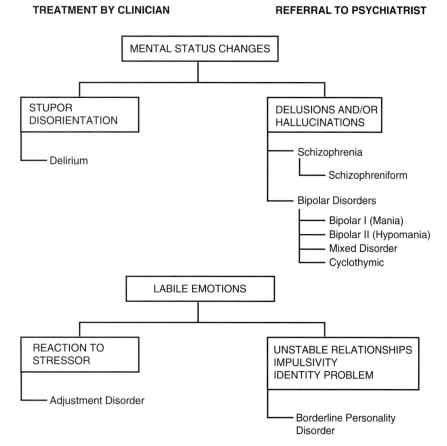

Figure 36–3. Evaluation of episodic disruptive behaviors.

classroom) precipitates the behavior. As children become older, they also become less overtly hyperactive, as is reflected in the *DSM-IV* criteria for hyperactivity, which states that the teenager may only need to feel restless. This restlessness may also significantly contribute to academic underachievement. For example, despite intentions for diligent studying, the restlessness may cause the teenager to feel the need to walk around, which distracts him or her from studies.

The impulsivity component of the hyperactive disorder significantly contributes to the child's morbidity. Just as impulsive children's activities rapidly change, so do their emotions. An impulsive child whose emotions quickly escalate is at risk for potentially aggressive behaviors (hitting, biting). In older children, impulsive aggression is manifested as explosive behavior. Because of their explosive behavior, their inability to wait their turn in a game, and then talking back to teachers, these children have great difficulty with both peer and teacher relations. Impulsivity can also be potentially life-threatening because the child may act before considering the consequences. This may manifest as risk-taking behaviors (sexual activity, substance use) or as actions like running into the street after a ball without checking for oncoming traffic.

Hyperactivity and impulsivity in children are readily apparent to adults; however, the manifestations of inattention and distractibility are not as overtly problematic. Consequently, these symptoms are frequently overlooked. To call attention to this problem, the *DSM-IV* has classified Attention-Deficit Disorder as a separate condition from Hyperactivity. In young children, inattentive behavior consists of shifting from one activity to another and having difficulty finishing tasks. The parents may inappropriately consider these actions to be a problem in behavior or in motivation (''lazy''). In teenagers, inattentive behavior manifests itself as poor school performance.

These individuals may forget to do homework or may need excessively long periods of time to complete assignments because of their inability to focus on their work. Because the assumptions of an inattentive child's character are often inaccurate (lazy, behavior problem), the clinician should consider the diagnosis of Attention-Deficit Disorder (with or without Hyperactivity) in any child who is not achieving his or her potential.

Potential problems in the diagnosis of ADHD are:

- The duration of symptoms
- The definition of abnormal age-specific symptoms
- The absence of symptoms in certain settings

Because ADHD is a chronic disorder, the symptoms should be present for at least 6 months. Acute changes in a child's behavior are usually the result of a recent psychologic stressor and should not be considered a part of ADHD.

The second problem is defining when a symptom is abnormal. Children normally become less active and impulsive as they get older. The classroom teacher is an excellent resource who can determine whether the patient's symptoms are markedly abnormal in contrast to the characteristics of peers. Standardized behavioral checklists (filled out by the parents and teachers) report the degree of patient's abnormal behaviors with regard to an age-specific reference population.

The final problem is the misconception that hyperactive children demonstrate their inattentive, impulsive, and hyperactive behaviors in the examination room. During the structured evaluation, most children with ADHD are attentive and still during a brief outpatient visit. Because of this problem, the clinician should not rely on observations performed in the office but should instead obtain information from multiple sources, including parents, teachers, day

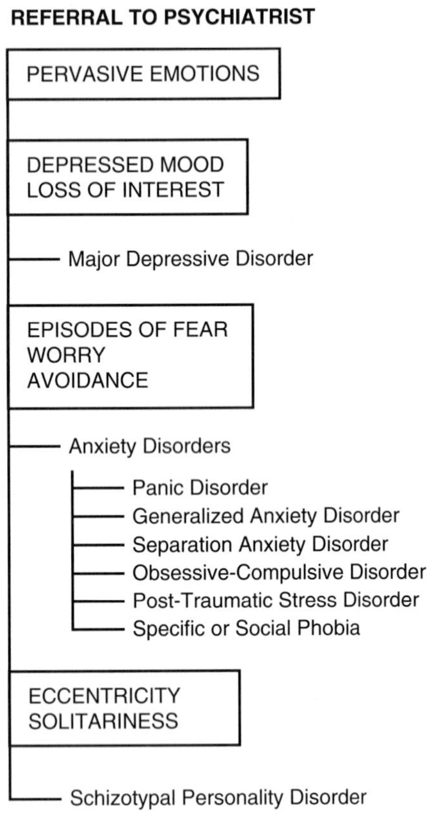

REFERRAL TO PSYCHIATRIST

```
┌─────────────────────────────┐
│  PERVASIVE EMOTIONS          │
└─────────────────────────────┘
  │
┌─────────────────────────────┐
│  DEPRESSED MOOD              │
│  LOSS OF INTEREST            │
└─────────────────────────────┘
  │
  ├──── Major Depressive Disorder
  │
┌─────────────────────────────┐
│  EPISODES OF FEAR            │
│  WORRY                       │
│  AVOIDANCE                   │
└─────────────────────────────┘
  │
  ├──── Anxiety Disorders
  │        ├── Panic Disorder
  │        ├── Generalized Anxiety Disorder
  │        ├── Separation Anxiety Disorder
  │        ├── Obsessive-Compulsive Disorder
  │        ├── Post-Traumatic Stress Disorder
  │        └── Specific or Social Phobia
  │
┌─────────────────────────────┐
│  ECCENTRICITY                │
│  SOLITARINESS                │
└─────────────────────────────┘
  │
  └──── Schizotypal Personality Disorder
```

Figure 36–4. Evaluation of episodic disruptive behaviors with pervasive emotions.

care workers, and even a direct classroom observation by a trained health care professional.

Before settling on a diagnosis of ADHD, the clinician must rule out the various psychiatric and medical causes for these symptoms. Some of the psychiatric illnesses that may resemble this condition or occur with it are learning disorders, oppositional behavior, and other psychiatric illnesses that may better account for the symptoms (pervasive developmental disorders, mood disorders, substance abuse). Because of the high association of learning disorders with ADHD, each evaluation should include an assessment for learning problems. This assessment consists of individual testing by a psychometrician to assess the child's abilities and achievements.

Because of the strong genetic predominance of ADHD, a psychiatric family history should also be obtained. In this family history, the parents may report a feeling of restlessness or a difficulty completing tasks. In the medical evaluation for ADHD, further diagnostic testing should be directed by the results of a thorough history and physical examination. The preschool-aged child should be screened for lead poisoning and iron deficiency, whereas the older child should undergo further diagnostic tests, as directed by the results of history and physical examination, to rule out such conditions as hyperthyroidism, petit mal seizures, hearing loss, and substance abuse.

One of the problems in treating ADHD is that this chronic illness may cause problems throughout the patient's lifetime. Psychotropic medications can reduce some of the outward symptoms of this condition (e.g., hyperactivity); however, the patient can have significant morbidity unless the patient learns how to deal with the learning and behavior problems associated with this condition. Therefore, successful treatment requires a multidisciplinary approach consisting of family education, psychologic counseling, behavior modification, and psychotropic medications.

The first step in treating ADHD is to educate the family with regard to the causes, potential problems, chronicity, and treatment of this condition. Additional important resources are books from the lay press as well as support groups for parents who have children with ADHD. These resources provide parents with a better understanding of their child's problem and its impact on the family unit.

The second step in treating ADHD is to initiate coping skills that can be used to enhance socially appropriate behavior (e.g., task completion, turn-taking in games) at home and in school. These coping skills include establishing a predictable schedule for family activities (bedtime, mealtime routines), distracting the child to another activity when the child's excitement level accelerates, and instituting behavior modification techniques. For behavior modification to be successful, the following elements are essential:

1. Identification of specific behaviors to work on.
2. Selection of tasks small enough to ensure the child some success.
3. An attractive chart for recording success.
4. Reliable rewards with small items or privileges (preferably daily).
5. Small punishments for failure to comply (loss of television or telephone for the evening).
6. Consistent reward and punishment for the corresponding behavior.

Some of the problems in successfully implementing this technique are unrealistic expectations, inconsistency, and delays in rewarding success. In the classroom, the child should be placed in the front to make classroom distractions less apparent to the child.

Many children with ADHD have significant trouble with their self-esteem because of poor school performance, difficulty in peer relations, and intrafamilial discord. To address the child's emotional issues and problems with self-image, the clinician may recommend psychotherapy for the patient.

An important adjunctive therapy for enhancing the success of the psychologic interventions (i.e., education and coping skills) is the administration of psychotropic medications. Parents are often reluctant to agree to administer these medications for behavioral problems. If the clinician explains to the parents that the biologic base for ADHD has become better elucidated (i.e., reduced metabolism in certain areas of the brain), the parents are more receptive to pharmacologic interventions. The psychotropic stimulants commonly used to treat this condition are methylphenidate (Ritalin), magnesium pemoline (Cylert), and dextroamphetamine (Dexedrine). Medications that may be used in combination with the stimulants are the tricyclic antidepressants and clonidine. Other medications that are being evaluated in clinical studies are the serotonin reuptake inhibitors (fluoxetine and sertraline) and the antidepressant bupropion.

If stimulant therapy is initiated, the clinician needs to perform follow-up at regular intervals to assess efficacy (using such parameters as school performance, standardized behavioral checklists) and side effects (e.g., tics, tremors, hypertension, weight loss). Stimulants can cause weight loss by appetite suppression; this effect can be minimized by using the medication only on school days, thus allowing compensatory caloric intake on weekends and holidays.

Because ADHD is associated with long-term dysfunction, children with this disorder are at an increased risk during adulthood for drug abuse, Antisocial Personality Disorder, and vocational underachievement.

Tic Disorders

Because of parental concerns regarding neurologic problems, tic disorders usually first present to the primary care provider. According to *DSM-IV*, tics are motor movements or vocalizations that are sudden, rapid, recurrent, nonrhythmic, involuntary movements. Tics become worse during stress but improve during activities requiring moderate (physical or mental) activity. Muscle spasms differ from tics because they are slower and last longer.

Tics need to be differentiated from medication-induced movement disorders as well as from the abnormal movements associated with various neurologic conditions. These movements are chorea (dancing, random), athetosis (withering, slow finger movements), dystonia (twisting, slow contractions), myoclonus (shock-like jerks), and hemiballismus (violent, unilateral motions). Simple motor tics may consist of eye blinking, neck jerking, or coughing, whereas examples of complex motor tics are repetitive grooming behaviors, deep knee bends, and smelling of objects. Simple vocal tics may be throat clearing or grunting sounds, whereas complex vocal tics may consist of repeating inappropriate words or phrases (coprolalia, repetitive, stereotyped use of obscenities).

According to the *DSM-IV*, conditions that make up the tic disorders are:

- Transient Tic Disorder (motor or vocal tics < 1 year's duration)
- Chronic Motor or Vocal Tic Disorder (motor or vocal tics > 1 year's duration)
- Tourette's Disorder (motor *and* vocal tics > 1 year's duration)

Tourette's Disorder. Tourette's Disorder is a chronic illness consisting of multiple motor and vocal tics of at least one year's duration. The incidence of this condition is 4 to 5/10,000. This illness is inherited as an autosomal dominant condition, with 70% penetrance in female carriers of the gene and 99% penetrance in male carriers. Because of this difference in penetrance, Tourette's Disorder is 1.5 to three times more common in men than in women. The median age for presentation is 7 years, but some cases are reported as early as 2 years. Even though coprolalia is popularly associated with this illness, fewer than 10% of affected patients have this form of complex vocal tics. The *DSM-IV* criteria for Tourette's Disorder are:

1. Multiple motor and vocal tics lasting longer than 1 year with no tic-free intervals longer than 3 months.
2. Age of onset before 18 years.
3. No medical causes (drugs, neurologic diseases) for the tics.

Children with chronic tic disorders frequently have other psychologic conditions, such as ADHD and Obsessive-Compulsive Disorder. In addition, the symptoms of the tics may cause the patient's peers to socially ostracize him or her. Because of the combination of ADHD and obsessive-compulsive behaviors with the tics, these children are not accepted by their peers and frequently frustrate their teachers and family members. This increase in stress can worsen the tics, which can further compound the problem. Because of these issues, the family should receive counseling, which should consist of parental guidance and emotional support for the child.

If the symptoms are not severe, the only necessary therapy may be psychologic support for the child and parental reassurance. If the symptoms become problematic, the patient may need to be treated with low dosages of high-potency antipsychotic drugs, such as haloperidol (Haldol) or pimozide (Orap). Because pimozide can cause the prolongation of the QT interval, an electrocardiogram should be obtained before therapy is initiated and at regular intervals. Because of the controversy that stimulant therapy may enhance the emergence of tics, children with Tourette's Disorder and ADHD may be treated with clonidine for both conditions. In patients with chronic tics and obsessive-compulsive disorders, both conditions may be treated with medications that potentiate serotonin activity (clomipramine, fluoxetine, or sertraline).

TREATMENT BY PSYCHIATRIST

The chronic disruptive behaviors that are difficult to manage and have a high morbidity occur in Oppositional Defiant Disorder, Conduct Disorder, and substance abuse. These conditions are usually referred to a mental health specialist because their treatments are complicated, intensive, and lengthy. The role of the primary care provider is to recognize these conditions and refer the patient to the appropriate mental health specialist. Before initiating a referral, the clinician should inquire about past referrals. Usually, in chronic and severe illnesses, a mental health agency is already involved in the case. These agencies may seem to be unsuccessful partly because of family noncompliance, impatience, and/or dissatisfaction. Hence, the clinician should either reactivate the involved agency or refer the patient to another mental health professional.

Even though all mental health professionals can provide counseling, the following types of professionals offer special services:

- Social workers (knowledge of community resources)
- Psychologist (psychologic testing)
- Chemical dependency unit personnel (detoxification)
- Child and adolescent psychiatrist (coordination of assessment and possible use of psychotropic medications)

All who are not physicians should have the availability of consultation for the appropriate psychotropic medications.

The chronic disruptive disorders often present at times of severe crisis. Unless the child's medical condition warrants (e.g., drug overdose or withdrawal), the pediatric medical department should not be used to resolve conflicts. This is because the patient's behavior may be disruptive to the ward, it may be difficult to discharge the patient to home because it takes time to resolve the conflict, and the family will expect hospitalization for the next crisis. Instead, the family should be counseled that there is no quick solution to this chronic problem. During such a crisis, a temporary respite may be either placement with a relative or the judicious use of a psychiatric residential treatment center.

Oppositional Defiant Disorder

Oppositional Defiant Disorder is a chronic condition in which the patient is stubbornly rebellious to all authority. This behavior is more than just a reaction to a stressful situation or the normal show of independence during early or mid adolescence. These children exhibit a hostile, negativistic, and disobedient behavior for at least 6 months. According to the *DSM-IV*, the patient must exhibit a consistent pattern during a 6-month period of at least four or more of the following behaviors:

1. Frequently loses temper.
2. Often argues with authority figures.
3. Defies rules.
4. Deliberately annoys adults.
5. Blames others for his or her actions.
6. Is easily annoyed by others.
7. Is angry.
8. Is vindictive.

In addition, this diagnosis should not be made if the patient meets the criteria for Conduct Disorder or if the symptoms occur during the course of a mood or psychotic disorder. In mood and psychotic disorders, children exhibit oppositional behavior as a reaction to their illness and hence they should be classified under their mood or psychotic disorder.

The prevalence of ODD ranges from 2% to 16%, depending on the population. In prepubertal children, it occurs more frequently in males; however in adolescents, it occurs equally in both sexes.

Most children present before 8 years of age. Preschool-aged children exhibit increased motor activity and difficulty in being comforted, and they overreact to situations. School-aged children have low self-esteem and a low tolerance to frustration. If the symptoms present before 8 years of age, the patient is at significant risk for developing more severe disruptive behaviors, such as Conduct Disorder or Antisocial Personality Disorder.

Some of the theories on the causes of ODD are learned behavior (secondary gain from defiant behavior), fixation at the negative stage of behavior development (the "terrible twos"), and poor parenting skills. There may also be a genetic component because the disorder commonly occurs in families with mood or psychotic disorders (especially with maternal depression) and with chronic disruptive behaviors (ADHD, ODD).

Children with ODD are at marked risk for other psychological disorders. Because of the association of ADHD with ODD, children with ODD should also be evaluated for ADHD. In addition, these patients are at increased risk for Conduct Disorder, Antisocial Personality Disorder, substance abuse, Major Depressive Disorder, and suicide.

Because of the difficulty in treating ODD, mental health professionals usually manage this condition. Therapy is directed toward treating co-morbid disorders (ADHD, substance abuse, suicide ideation). In addition, various psychotherapeutic modalities (individual, group, family) are employed to improve the child's functioning. The role of the primary care provider is early recognition and referral to a mental health specialist. Success of therapy depends on early intervention before the dysfunctional patterns are firmly established. In addition, the clinician can enhance compliance with psychotherapy by being supportive and by explaining to the family that therapy often takes months and requires family participation.

Conduct Disorder

Children who are not just defiant but are unremorseful for violating the rights of others may be diagnosed as having Conduct Disorder. According to the *DSM-IV*, a child has Conduct Disorder if they have repetitively violated the rights of others and of society. Children with this diagnosis need to have performed three or more of the following, with at least one occurring in the previous 6 months:

1. Aggression to people or animals (intimidation, initiation of fights; use of weapons; cruelty to people; cruelty to animals; rape; confrontational theft, or "mugging").
2. Destruction of property (arson, vandalism).
3. Deceitfulness (nonconfrontational theft, or swindling).
4. Serious violation of rules (curfew violation, running away, truancy before age 13).

For running away to qualify as a symptom, it must occur twice (or once if it was lengthy) and must not be an attempt to escape sexual or physical abuse. Conduct Disorder is subdivided into childhood onset (symptoms occur before 10 years of age) and adolescence onset (symptoms occur after 10 years of age). It is also subdivided by severity of the offense, such as mild (truancy), moderate (vandalism, nonconfrontational theft), and severe (rape, confrontational theft).

The prevalence of conduct disorders ranges from 2% to 9% in females and 6% to 16% in males. Children initially present with lying, initiating of fights, and truancy; as they get older, they progress to more violent acts. In addition, boys are more likely to exhibit acts of violence (fighting and stealing) in contrast to girls, who are more likely to exhibit truancy, runaway behavior, and prostitution. Of concern is that 50% of these children can develop Antisocial Personality Disorder, which is a severe conduct disorder of adulthood that is usually associated with criminal activity. In addition, these children have a high frequency of depression (suicide ideation), personality disorders, anxiety disorders, ADHD, and substance abuse.

Although the cause of Conduct Disorder is unknown, there may be both genetic and psychosocial etiologic factors. The psychosocial risk factors are parental rejection, difficult infant temperament, physical or sexual abuse, early institutional living, and lack of appropriate discipline. A biochemical or genetic cause for this condition has been postulated because of the high prevalence of this condition in families with mood or psychiatric disorders, ADHD, and Conduct Disorder.

Therapy is best managed by a mental health professional because it is complex, lengthy, and difficult. The therapy consists of individual and/or family psychotherapy, judicious use of residential treatment centers, and treatment of co-morbid conditions (substance abuse, ADHD, depression). The behavior in children with conduct disorders can markedly improve if their ADHD is treated with stimulants and their depression is treated with antidepressants. The success of therapy depends on early recognition and intervention before the destructive behaviors are firmly established. The role of the primary care provider is early recognition, referral, and enhancement of compliance with treatment through education and encouragement of family participation.

Antisocial Personality Disorder

Antisocial Personality Disorder consists of chronic, longstanding traits that lead to significant psychosocial dysfunction and distress. This disorder is closely related to Conduct Disorder. According to the *DSM-IV*, three or more of the following symptoms must be present by age 15 and persist beyond 18 years of age:

1. Repeated unlawful acts.
2. Deceitfulness.
3. Impulsivity.
4. Disregard for others.
5. Irresponsibility.
6. Lack of remorse.

This diagnosis should not be made if the symptoms occur as part of schizophrenia or mania.

The personality of patients with Antisocial Personality Disorder consists of superficial charm, lack of empathy, and inflated self-appraisal. Patients with Antisocial Personality Disorder also complain of frequent episodes of tension, inability to tolerate boredom, and depressed mood.

The prevalence in community samples is 3% in males and 1% in females. Based on adoption studies, this disorder is probably caused by both biologic and psychosocial factors. Approximately 50% of patients with conduct disorders progress to Antisocial Personality Disorder. Risk factors for this progression are child abuse or neglect and poor or erratic parenting.

Frequently encountered co-morbid conditions include anxiety disorders, depressive disorders, substance abuse, and ADHD. Patients with Antisocial Personality Disorder are also at increased risk for death by violence (suicide, homicide, accidents) and for neglect or abuse of their own children. The costs of Antisocial Personality Disorder are high with regard to judicial, penal, emotional, financial, and medical costs incurred by either those with this condition or their victims.

Treatment of Antisocial Personality Disorder is very difficult and is often associated with a poor prognosis. Hence, the goal of treatment is prevention of this condition by recognizing its antecedent disorder (Conduct Disorder), which may be amenable to treatment.

Substance Use

The presence of unusual disruptive behaviors can be the result of the intoxication or the withdrawal of a psychoactive agent. Some of these behaviors are belligerence, mood lability, and cognitive impairment. As many as 90% of high school seniors have tried psychoactive drugs (nicotine or ethanol) and almost 60% have tried illicit drugs. In addition, almost 20% of high school seniors drink ethanol to the point of intoxication on a weekly basis. Of the teenagers who drink, more than half of them drink in automobiles. Some of the illicit drugs that teenagers use are tetrahydrocannabinol (THC, found in marijuana), central nervous system (CNS) depressants (benzodiazepine, phenobarbital), hallucinogens (lysergic acid diethylamide [LSD], phencyclidine piperdine [PCP]), opiates (heroin), stimulants (sympathomimetics, amphetamine, cocaine), and inhalants (toluene, freon, nitrous oxide). The *DSM-IV* divides the diagnoses attributable to drugs into substance use (dependence and abuse) and substance-induced disorders (intoxication, withdrawal).

Substance dependence according to the *DSM-IV* consists of three or more symptoms occurring at the same time during a 12-month period:

1. Tolerance (more drug for the same effect).
2. Withdrawal (the drug is needed to suppress symptoms).
3. Drug use that lingers longer than anticipated.
4. Desire or effort to cut down use.
5. Drug-seeking activity.
6. Social or occupational impairment.
7. Continued use despite medical complications (hepatitis with ethanol use).

Substance abuse occurs when any drug use leads to significant adverse consequences, such as repetitive absences from work or school, expulsion from school, driving while impaired, and arrests. The diagnosis of substance abuse does not require tolerance or withdrawal.

The role of the primary care provider is to identify the patients who are using or abusing drugs. This identification can be made by the patient history and the results of the physical examination and urine toxicology testing.

Because of the high prevalence of substance use in teenagers, the clinician should have a high index of suspicion in any patient who presents with psychiatric symptoms, high-risk behaviors (runaway, delinquency), unexplained somatic complaints, and acute changes in behavior or mental status (Tables 36–3 and 36–4). The interview should begin with the parents out of the room and should be conducted in a manner that does not make the patient defensive. The interview may begin with the clinician asking if the patient's friends have ever tried drugs and if the patient has ever partied with them. One series of questions that may assist the clinician in determining if a patient has a substance use disorder is the CAGE questionnaire (Table 36–5). The CAGE questionnaire has a sensitivity of 90% and a specificity of 79% for detecting substance use secondary to ethanol use. This questionnaire may be used for other substances.

To enhance the yield for urine toxicology testing, the clinician should state which drugs are suspected based on the history and physical examination. Some of the physical findings associated with drug (Tables 36–3 and 36–4) use are:

- Red skin (anticholinergic drugs, jimson weed, LSD, THC, alcohol withdrawal)
- Dilated pupils (stimulants, hallucinogens, withdrawal syndromes)
- Pinpoint pupils (opiates)
- Ataxia (CNS depressants)
- Lateral nystagmus (CNS depressants)
- Vertical nystagmus (PCP)

The time period after ingestion in which a drug may be detected in the urine depends on the drug, the amount ingested, and the chronicity of use. The time period after use in which a drug may be detected in urine is:

- Alcohol (12 hours)
- Heroin (24 hours)
- Cocaine (4 to 6 days, as benzoylecgonine)
- Marijuana (single use: 5 days, long-term daily use: 30 days)
- Phenobarbital (33 days)
- PCP (from an overdose: 9 days)

If a clinician identifies a patient as a substance user, the unusual behavior should not be attributed solely to the drug. Instead, the clinician must consider the co-morbid psychiatric conditions associated with drug use, which are ADHD, ODD, Conduct Disorder, Schizophrenia, and mood disorders (suicide ideation). One must also consider the medical conditions associated with drug use, which are human immunodeficiency virus infection, hepatitis B infection, cerebrovascular accidents (resulting from stimulants), violence, accidents, bacterial endocarditis (resulting from intravenous use), asthma (resulting from THC use), and suicide.

If the clinician suspects substance use, the patient should be referred to a mental health specialist because the aftermath of substance use can be catastrophic. The treatment of drug use or abuse consists of detoxification, treatment of co-morbid conditions, and psychologic intervention to help maintain sobriety. Detoxification involves the termination of use of the substance as well as the management of potential withdrawal (opiates, amphetamines, barbiturates, less often, cocaine). The maintenance of sobriety is then attempted by addressing co-existing psychiatric disorders plus implementing psychosocial interventions. These interventions may be through individual, group, or family psychotherapy, which may be delivered through a medical facility or through special community programs (e.g., Alcoholics Anonymous). Although pharmacologic treatment for abuse prevention is sometimes used in adults (such as disulfiram for alcohol abuse), this form of intervention is not often employed with adolescents.

Episodic (Recent) Disruptive Behaviors

Episodic disruptive disorders may either be an acute presentation of an illness in a previously healthy individual or an episodic flare-up of a chronic disorder. These conditions may be subdivided by the patient's mental status (confusion or delusion) and emotional state (labile or pervasive) and the best person to treat the condition (primary care provider or mental health specialist) (see Figs. 36–3 and 36–4).

Mental Status Changes

Delirium

Delirium is characterized by deficits in cognition and in consciousness that occur over a short time period (Table 36–6). According to the *DSM-IV*, the criteria for the diagnosis of delirium are:

1. A disturbance of consciousness with reduced ability to focus or sustain attention.
2. A change in cognition (drowsiness, disorientation) or perceptual disturbances (illusions, hallucinations).
3. An onset over a short period of time.
4. A medical cause for the symptoms.

The symptoms of delirium develop acutely and fluctuate through-

Table 36–3. Immediate Effects, Duration of Action, Toxicity, and Withdrawal Symptoms of Substance Abuse in Adolescents

Substance	Immediate Effects	Duration of Action	Toxicity	Signs and Symptoms of Withdrawal	Treatment of Overdose
Alcohol	Respiratory depression, central nervous system (CNS) depression, ataxia, slurred speech, hypoglycemia	Depends on amount ingested and adolescent's tolerance	Cirrhosis, gastrointestinal hemorrhage, thiamine and folate deficiency, CNS depression, impaired motor performance and mental function, stupor, deep anesthesia, death	Insomnia, restlessness, anxiety, tremulousness, hypertension, tachycardia, diaphoresis; auditory or visual hallucinations or both, seizures, delirium tremens are rare in adolescents	Supportive ventilation if needed
Amphetamine, other stimulants	↑ blood pressure (BP), activity, and alertness; tachycardia; insomnia, anorexia; ↓ fatigue, euphoria; excitation; aggression; hostility	2–8 hr	Agitation; ↑ heart rate, BP, and temperature; hallucinations; paranoia, psychosis; convulsions; death, arrhythmias	Apathy, hallucinations, irritability, excessive sleep, depression, psychosis, suicidal, sudden death	Paranoia with haloperidol; seizures with diazepam
Tobacco	↑ BP and heart rate; ↓ temperature, CNS stimulation, skeletal muscle relaxation	Minutes	CNS stimulation	Restlessness, anxiety, insomnia, agitation, nausea, headache, ↑ appetite, inability to concentrate	None
Cocaine, crack	↑ alertness, exultation, euphoria, insomnia; ↓ appetite; ↑ BP and heart rate, aphrodisiac, local anesthesia	15–30 min	Agitation; ↑ temperature, pulse, and BP; tremors; convulsions, tachyarrhythmias; paranoia, psychosis; myocardial infarction; death	Apathy, long periods of sleep, irritability, depression, suicidal, disorientation	Paranoia with haloperidol; seizures with diazepam; cooling for hyperthermia; nitroprusside, labetalol for hypertension
Inhalants (solvents, gasoline)	Respiratory depression, CNS depression, ataxia, slurred speech, bradycardia	5–30 min	Arrhythmias, hallucinations, seizures, encephalopathy, renal tubular acidosis, peripheral neuropathy, lead poisoning, death	Rare: chills, hallucinations, headache, abdominal pain, muscle cramps, delirium tremens	Organ-specific therapies
LSD, other hallucinogens	Dysphoria; hallucinations; anxiety; paranoia; psychosis; ↑ BP, heart rate, and temperature; dilated pupils; incoordination; ↑ creativity	2–12 hr; can produce exhaustion lasting for days	Long intense "trips"; psychotic reactions not always reversible; flashbacks; suicide attempts; deaths with some drugs	None	Reassurance; haloperidol
Marijuana, hashish	Euphoria, ↓ reaction time, ↓ inhibitions, ↑ appetite	2–4 hr	Dysphoria, acute anxiety attacks, acute psychosis, fatigue, paranoia, lack of motivation	Insomnia, hyperactivity, ↓ appetite	
PCP and PCP analogs	Ataxia, nystagmus, ↑ BP, slurred speech, dysphoria, hallucinations, aggression, paranoia, confusion	Hours to days	Psychosis; convulsions, paranoia; flashbacks; deaths have resulted from suicide, accidents	None	Haloperidol, diazepam
Opioids	Euphoria, ataxia, slurred speech, miosis, stupor	Hours	Respiratory depression, hypothermia, hypotension, pulmonary edema, apnea, coma, death	Increased sympathetic nervous system activity, hunger, antisocial behavior, gooseflesh, diaphoresis, rhinorrhea (flu), yawning; treatment with clonidine	Naloxone; ventilation

Data from Jones RL. Substance abuse. *In* Shearin RB (ed). Handbook of Adolescent Medicine. Kalamazoo, MI, Upjohn Company, 1983, pp 133–152, and Abramewicz M (ed): Treatment of acute drug abuse reactions. Med Lett 29:83, 1987. From Kreipe RE, McAnarney ER. Adolescent medicine. *In* Behrman RE, Kliegman RM (eds). Nelson Essentials of Pediatrics, 2nd ed. Philadelphia: WB Saunders, 1994:244.

Abbreviations: LSD = lysergic acid diethylamide; PCP = phencyclidine.

Table 36–4. Long-Term Effects, Tolerance, Dependence, Adulteration, and Methods of Administration of Substances Adolescents Abuse

Substance	Long-Term Effects	Tolerance	Dependence Psychologic	Dependence Physical	Adulteration or Substitution	Method of Administration
Alcohol	Blackouts; behavioral changes; ↑ accidents; homicide, suicide; gastritis; peptic ulcer; alcoholic hepatitis; fatty liver; pancreatitis	Yes	Yes	Yes	Methanol	Ingested
Amphetamine, other stimulants	Weight loss, insomnia, anxiety, paranoia, hallucinations; skin abscesses and amphetamine psychosis following injections	Yes	High	Yes	More than 90% of speed is adulterated with caffeine, asthma medicatons, PCP, LSD, strychnine, sugars	Ingested, injected
Tobacco	↑ risk of chronic bronchitis, heart disease, and cancer (oral cancer with smokeless tobacco)	Yes	Yes	Yes	No	Smoke inhaled, snuff dipping, chewed
Cocaine, crack	Nasal perforation with snorting, weight loss, insomnia, anxiety, paranoia, hallucinations, soft tissue abscesses with injections	Yes	High	Yes, especially following smoking or injection	Local anesthetics, sugars, PCP	Snorted, smoked, ingested, injected
Inhalants (solvents, gasoline, "white out," etc.)	Liver damage with toluene, trichloroethylene, gasoline; anemia with tetraethyl lead; leukemia with benzene; kidney damage with trichloroethylene	Yes, especially with toluene	Yes	Yes	None	Sniffing rags soaked with the compound, inhaling fumes through the mouth
LSD, other hallucinogens	Flashbacks, pronounced personality changes, ↑ risk of chronic psychosis	Yes, cross-tolerance with mescaline, DMT, and psilocybin	Degree unknown	No	Sold as tablets, in liquids, in microdots in many colors; often adulterated with or substituted for other drugs	Ingested, injected, sniffed
Marijuana, hashish	Great variety involving several body systems; ↓ motivation	Yes	Degree unknown	No	With PCP	Smoke inhaled, ingested
PCP and PCP analogs	Personality disorders, flashbacks, catatonia, neuropsychologic disturbances, increased risk of schizophrenia	Yes	High	Degree unknown	Often added to other drugs or advertised as other drugs	Ingested, injected, smoked
Opioids	↓ motivation, antisocial behavior, crime to support habit, skin abscess, endocarditis, osteomyelitis, nephritis, hepatitis, HIV, amenorrhea	Yes	Yes	Yes	Quinine, sugar	Ingested, injected, subcutaneous (skin-popping), intravenous

Modified from Jones RLK. Substance abuse. *In* Shearin RB (ed). Handbook of Adolescent Medicine. Kalamazoo, MI, Upjohn Company, 1983, pp 133–152. From Kreipe RE, McAnarney ER. Adolescent medicine. *In* Behrman RE, Kliegman RM (eds). Nelson Essentials of Pediatrics, 2nd ed. Philadelphia: WB Saunders, 1994:245.
Abbreviations: DMT = *N,N* = dimethyltryptamine; LSD = lysergic acid diethylamide; PCP = phencyclidine.

Table 36–5. CAGE Questionnaire

C: Have you ever tried to *C*ut down on drinking?
A: Have you ever been *A*nnoyed by criticism of your drinking?
G: Have you ever felt *G*uilty about your drinking?
E: Have you ever had a morning *E*ye opener (a drink to prevent withdrawal symptoms)?

out the course of the illness. Besides altered sensorium, the patient also has reversal of the sleep/wake cycle and may exhibit disruptive behaviors consisting of psychomotor agitation or retardation.

Delirium is caused by global cerebral dysfunction. Hence, any agent that can cause coma can also cause delirium. Some of these causes are represented by the mnemonic AEIOU-TIPS, which stands for: *A*lcohol, *E*ncephalopathy (lead, Reye syndrome, inborn errors of metabolism, encephalitis), *I*nsulin (hypoglycemia or hyperglycemia), *O*piates, *U*remia, *T*rauma, *I*nfection, *P*oisonings, and *S*eizures. Because the aforementioned causes of delirium are potentially life-threatening, an expedient and comprehensive medical evaluation is needed. In addition, if a previously healthy child presents with delirium, the clinician should suspect a pharmacologic ingestion as a cause of these symptoms.

Children with delirium present with perceptual disturbances consisting of misinterpretations (hearing a sound and thinking it is something else), illusions (visual misinterpretations), and hallucinations (seeing something when nothing is actually there). The hallucinations of delirium are different from those of psychoses (Schizophrenia) because they are usually visual and acute in onset, whereas those resulting from psychoses are usually auditory and subacute or chronic (lasting weeks to months). The hallucinations occurring with psychoses may have a delusional component.

The treatment of delirium is directed toward the underlying medical problem. Some patients with delirium may be aggressive and assaultive. A psychiatric consultation may be helpful in differentiating the hallucinations into medical versus psychotic causes and in assisting in the pharmacologic and behavioral or environmental management of the agitated patient. Benzodiazepines, or high-potency antipsychotic agents (haloperidol), or both, may reduce the agitation; however, the dose must be carefully titrated to prevent the side effects of these medications from contributing to the patient's altered sensorium. Because patients with delirium are frightened and confused, their agitated behavior may respond to frequent reassurances, implementation of expected routines, a consistent environment, and frequent reorientation.

If the underlying medical condition for delirium is promptly treated before irreversible CNS damage develops, the patient should make a full recovery. However, if damage has occurred, the patient may develop dementia. *Dementia* is a chronic, irreversible, and possibly progressive disease that includes memory impairment plus one of the following symptoms:

1. Aphasia (inability to name an object).
2. Apraxia (inability to carry out motor activities despite understanding the task and having intact motor abilities).
3. Agnosia (inability to recognize objects).

Table 36–6. Approach and Red Flags for Delirium

1. Symptoms evolve in hours.
2. Level of consciousness waxes and wanes.
3. Urgent medical evaluation (AEIOU-TIPS) required.
4. Review all poisons and medications in the home.
5. Hallucinations are usually visual or tactile.

AEIOU = TIPS = alcohol, encephalopathy, insulin, opiates, uremia, trauma, infection, poisonings, seizures.

4. Problems with executive function (inability to subtract 7 from 100 in a serial manner).

In children, dementia can also present as a loss of developmental milestones or deteriorating school performance.

Schizophrenia

Schizophrenia is a chronic disorder that flares into an active phase of very disruptive behavior (Table 36–7). This disruptive behavior consists of delusions, hallucinations, disorganized speech, and catatonic behavior. According to the *DSM-IV,* the diagnostic criteria for schizophrenia are:

1. Two or more symptoms during a 1-month period of delusions.
2. Hallucinations.
3. Disorganized speech.
4. Catatonic behavior.
5. Negative symptoms, such as a flat affect.
6. Significant social dysfunction.
7. A prodrome (withdrawal, flat affect) of at least 6 months.

In addition, medical causes and mood disorders need to be excluded. The diagnosis of Schizophrenia is further subdivided by the primary symptom complex into the following types: Paranoid, Disorganized, Catatonic, Residual, and Undifferentiated.

During the prodromal phase, the patient may develop increasing negative symptoms, such as social withdrawal, flattening of affect, alogia (speaking in brief sentences), and avolition (lack of desire to do anything). The flat affect may consist of a reduction in body language, lack of eye contact, and emotional unresponsiveness. During this period, the patient may also have unusual beliefs that are not yet up to the magnitude of true delusions or hallucinations. For example, the patient may have magical thinking or may perceive that someone is talking to them but no words are hallucinated. This prodromal state needs to be present for 6 months before the diagnosis of Schizophrenia can be made.

During the acute phase of Schizophrenia, the patient must have at least two symptoms (may be one if it is severely bizarre) for more than 1 month unless the symptoms have been shortened by

Table 36–7. Approach and Red Flags for Psychoses

General
  Strong family history of symptoms or disorders
  Delusions
  Rule out co-morbidities
  Increased suicide risk

Schizophrenia
  Declining function unless treated
  Duration of symptoms > 6 mo
  Symptoms: hallucinations, disorganized speech, flat affect, disorganized/catatonic behavior

Bipolar Disorders*
  Past episodes of mania or hypomania
  Consider in any disruptive behavior that does not respond to treatment

Major Depressive Disorder*
  Can present with behavioral problems and irritability instead of depressed mood
  Do not overattribute to a stressor
  At risk for developing bipolar disorders

*Bipolar and some depressive disorders can also be classified as mood disorders and not psychosis.

treatment. The most common delusions (erroneous beliefs) in this disorder are persecutory (patient is being spied on) followed by referential (events or comments are directed toward the patient). Other less common delusions are somatic (internal organs are replaced by others), religious, and grandiose. The most common hallucinations are auditory, but they may also be from any sensory modality.

For hallucinations to support the diagnosis of Schizophrenia, the patient must have a clear sensorium. The disorganized speech may be incomprehensible (word salad), and the patient may be unable to organize a logical conversation or gives inappropriate answers to questions. The behavior problems consist of inappropriate dress, disheveled appearance, untriggered aggression, and catatonia (decreased response to the environment).

If symptoms have not been present for 6 months, the provisional diagnosis of Schizophreniform Disorder is used. Approximately two thirds of patients with Schizophreniform Disorder have symptoms that last longer than 6 months and hence are reclassified as having Schizophrenia.

The prevalence of Schizophrenia ranges from 0.5% to 1.0%. Even though some cases have been reported in children as young as 5 years of age, most cases of Schizophrenia present between the late teens and early 30s.

Results of monozygotic twin studies support both an environmental and a biologic cause for Schizophrenia. Children with a first-degree, biologic relative with Schizophrenia have a 10-fold increase in Schizophrenia over the general population. Some of the differences noted in the brains of schizophrenic patients are abnormal glucose utilization in the prefrontal cortex, decreased hippocampal and temporal lobe size, enlarged ventricular system, and prominent cortical sulci.

The differential diagnosis of Schizophrenia consists of the same medical causes of delirium and dementia plus the mood disorders and pervasive developmental disorders. In addition, chronic amphetamine or cocaine use or a PCP ingestion may produce symptoms similar to those found in Schizophrenia.

The prognosis of Schizophrenia is poor, with significant morbidity and mortality (suicide, especially early in the illness). This chronic disorder is associated with exacerbations and remissions. Even with optimal therapy, patients with Schizophrenia have significant social deficits, poor initiative, and abnormal thought processes.

The treatment of Schizophrenia consists of the use of antipsychotic agents (haloperidol, thioridazine, trifluoperazine), psychotherapy, and educational interventions. Because of interpersonal difficulties, the patient often benefits from socialization groups plus individual and/or group therapy. The families of patients with Schizophrenia also need emotional support and guidance by either family therapy or multifamily group therapy to deal with this potentially devastating illness. Because of the abnormalities in the thinking process as well as in the neuropsychologic testing, patients often need an individual educational program to meet their special academic needs. Because this disease is difficult to treat, the therapy is best managed by a psychiatrist. The primary care provider may assist in the management by conducting the medical evaluation and by educating the family. Often, families believe the misconception that Schizophrenia is a multiple-personality disorder.

Bipolar Disorders

Bipolar Disorder, formerly called Manic Depressive Disorder, is a mood disorder. The other mood disorder is Major Depressive Disorder. Bipolar Disorder presents acutely, with severe problems in thinking and behavior that lead to significant impairment in functioning (see Table 36–7). Disturbances in thinking associated with mania include racing thoughts (rapidly changes topics), dis-

tractibility, and delusions of grandeur. Problematic behaviors during a manic episode include recklessness (excessive participation in sports, buying sprees), agitation, decreased sleep, and excessive talkativeness.

The bipolar disorders are divided into the following categories:

- Bipolar I Disorder (episodes of mania with or without depression)
- Bipolar II Disorder (major depression with only hypomanic episodes
- Mixed Bipolar Disorder (daily occurrence of both mania and depression
- Cyclothymic Disorder

Cyclothymic Disorder is a chronic, cyclic illness of hypomania and depressive symptoms (no major depressions). Approximately 50% of patients with Cyclothymic Disorder develop Bipolar I or II disorder.

According to the *DSM-IV*, a manic episode consists of abnormally elevated (euphoric), expansive, or irritable mood for at least 1 week unless treated. This mood disturbance should be associated with at least three (four if patient is irritable) of the following symptoms:

1. Grandiosity.
2. Decreased desire for sleep.
3. Talkativeness.
4. Racing thoughts.
5. Distractibility.
6. Excessive goal-directed activity (or psychomotor agitation).
7. Reckless pursuit of pleasure.

Hypomanic episodes consist of the same symptoms except that the symptoms need to be present for a shorter time (4 days), are not associated with any psychotic activity (delusions or hallucinations), and are not severe enough to cause major social or academic dysfunction. About 10% of patients with hypomania progress to mania.

The differential diagnosis of bipolar disorders includes the medical conditions that cause coma or delirium; hence, a detailed medical history and physical examination are warranted. Some specific medical conditions whose presenting symptoms resemble bipolar disease are thyroid disorders (hypothyroidism or hyperthyroidism), cocaine intoxication, antidepressant (amitriptyline) overdose, and substance withdrawal. To evaluate a child with a possible mood disorder, the clinician should obtain a detailed family history because of the high prevalence of these disorders in parents of children with bipolar disorders. Because the parents are often undiagnosed, the questions should be directed toward the presence of the *symptoms* for bipolar disorders (depression and mania or hypomania) in the parents.

Some of the psychiatric disorders that frequently occur with bipolar disorders are eating disorders, ADHD, panic disorders, social phobias, adjustment disorders, and substance-related conditions. These same conditions may present with symptoms that imitate bipolar disorders (e.g., distractibility of ADHD instead of mania). The clinician must decide whether the symptoms are caused by a bipolar disorder or by some other psychiatric disorder. For example, ADHD can be differentiated from mania because the hyperactive behavior of ADHD is more likely to present in childhood and progress to restlessness in the teenager, whereas teenagers with mania present acutely with excessive activity. Because patients with bipolar disorders can also present with hallucinations and delusions, Schizophrenia must be ruled out because of the differences in treatment and prognosis. Likewise, patients initially diagnosed as having Schizophrenia have been found after years of follow-up to have bipolar disorders.

The lifetime prevalence of bipolar I disorders is 0.4% to 1.6%, and that of bipolar II disorders is 0.5%. Approximately 15% of adolescents with recurrent major depression develop bipolar illnesses. A two- to 15-fold increase of bipolar disorders in children of affected parents supports a biologic or genetic cause for this condition. Manic patients have biologic abnormalities in neuroendocrine function (increased cortisol production, absence of dexamethasone nonsuppression) and in the neurotransmitter systems (norepinephrine, serotonin, γ-aminobutyric acid).

Even though bipolar disorders can develop in childhood, most cases first present when the patient is in his or her mid-20s. The natural history of bipolar disorders is a chronic illness with episodes of mania, hypomania, and major depression; 15% of cases have four or more episodes per year. Risk factors for initiation of a manic episode are disruption of the normal sleep cycle (crossing multiple time zones), postpartum period (often have psychoses), and recent major depressions. About 70% of manic or hypomanic episodes are associated with a recent major depression. With therapy, most patients recover fully between episodes; however, 30% of cases of bipolar I and 15% of bipolar II disorders have persistent interpersonal and occupational disorders. Ten percent to 15% of patients with bipolar disorders commit suicide.

Because of the complexity of the therapy coupled with the severe morbidity and mortality of this disorder, bipolar disorders are managed by psychiatrists. Treatment consists of medications and psychotherapy. The most commonly used medication to stabilize mood is lithium carbonate. Other medications used to treat bipolar diseases are carbamazepine, valproic acid, benzodiazepines, and antipsychotic agents. Various forms of psychotherapy (individual, group, and family) are often employed in conjunction with a close liaison with schools to promote scholastic success as well as to maximize intrapsychic, interpersonal, and intrafamilial well-being.

The role of the primary care provider in the management of bipolar disorders is early detection. Children and adolescents may go undiagnosed for years, during which significant dysfunction and suicide may occur. Guidelines that may lead to early diagnosis are:

1. Know and recognize the symptoms for mania and hypomania.
2. Remember that depressed patients often have bipolar disorders.
3. Obtain a careful family history to look for the diagnosis or the symptoms of mood disorders.
4. Consider bipolar illnesses in patients with any disruptive disorder that does not respond to treatment.
5. Assess for drug and/or alcohol use.

Once the primary care provider suspects bipolar disorders, the patient should be referred to a psychiatrist. Because of the manic symptoms (elation, delusions of grandeur) that accompany this disorder, these patients vigorously argue and refuse referral. Stopping the endless arguing often takes several key family members to insist resolutely on the referral.

Labile Emotions

Adjustment Disorder

Adjustment Disorder is used to identify an excessive or maladaptive response to stress. A recognizable stressor is needed to make this diagnosis. Some of the stressors in children and adolescents are:

- Separations
- Painful injuries
- Illness
- Treatment of the illness (hospitalization, surgery)
- Divorce
- Change of residency
- Academic failure
- Conflict with peers

The *DSM-IV* criteria for adjustment disorder are:

1. The symptoms develop within 3 months of the occurrence of the stressor.
2. Significant impairment (social, academic) results.
3. The symptoms do not meet criteria for mood or anxiety disorder.
4. The symptoms do not represent bereavement.
5. The symptoms abate 6 months after termination of the stressor.

This disorder is further subdivided into the patient's symptoms, such as depressed mood, anxiety, and/or conduct disorder.

The prevalence of adjustment disorder ranges from 5% to 20%. Besides the morbidity secondary to the social and/or academic impairment, these patients are at increased risk for suicide. If the stressor is an illness or treatment, the morbidity of the medical condition may increase secondary to noncompliance or failure to seek further medical care. The differential diagnosis of Adjustment Disorder is mood or anxiety disorder, exacerbation of a personality disorder, or Post-Traumatic Stress Disorder. Once the diagnosis of adjustment disorder is made, the primary care provider may intervene with advice, insight, reassurance, and, if necessary, a referral to a mental health professional for short-term counseling.

Borderline Personality Disorder

Borderline Personality Disorder is a chronic personality disorder characterized by intense mood lability, impulsivity, and identity disturbances. Patients with this disorder also have unstable and intense interpersonal relationships. According to the *DSM-IV*, the diagnosis of this condition requires five or more of the following symptoms:

1. Frantic efforts to avoid abandonment.
2. Intense interpersonal relationships alternating between extreme idealization and devaluation.
3. Unstable self-image.
4. Impulsivity.
5. Recurrent suicide attempts.
6. Marked mood reactivity (intense, short periods of anxiety or dysphoria).
7. Feelings of emptiness.
8. Difficulty in controlling anger.
9. Stress-related paranoia.

The prevalence in the general population of Borderline Personality Disorder is 2%, with 75% occurring in females. Risk factors for this illness include abuse, neglect, and early parental loss. A fivefold increase in children with affected parents coupled with the social risk factors suggests both a genetic and a psychosocial cause of this illness.

This chronic disorder usually presents during adolescence or early adulthood as a fulminant crisis around an unstable and intense relationship. These crises often involve a suicide attempt because of the severe impulsivity and mood lability that are characteristic of the disorder. Approximately 10% of the patients successfully commit suicide. The morbidity is compounded by the physical sequelae from these multiple attempts (scarring, mutilation, brain anoxia). Between episodes, the patient appears very reasonable. In addition to their suicide attempts, these individuals commonly quit school, relationships, or work just before reaching a goal, even when success (e.g., graduation, marriage, or promotion) is imminent. Other co-morbid conditions associated with Borderline Personality Disorder are mood disorders, substance use, eating disorders (especially bulimia), ADHD, and Post-Traumatic Stress Disorder. The suicide attempts, the failed opportunities, and the co-morbidities all add to the morbidity of this condition.

Borderline Personality Disorder is difficult to treat. Even though the patients are very reasonable and appealing between the crises, the primary care provider should resist the temptation to treat these patients. The clinician should instead refer the patient to a mental health specialist because of the severe mortality and morbidity of this chronic, recurrent disorder. The patient's intense labile mood may often frustrate and enrage his or her parents. The primary care provider can assist the family during these crises by education and support.

Treatment consists of psychotherapy and the occasional use of psychotropic agents. The course of treatment is often lengthy, with frequent exacerbations and remissions.

Pervasive Emotions

Major Depressive Disorder

Because of the risk of suicide and significant social or academic discord, depression is a serious condition. Even though a child may be pervasively sad, he or she may also present with behavior problems and irritability (see Table 36–7). According to the *DSM-IV*, Major Depressive Disorder consists of at least a 2-week period of a depressive mood (irritability in some children) or loss of interest in pleasurable activities that results in significant impairment. During this period, the patient must have at least five of the following symptoms:

1. Depressed mood (irritability in some children).
2. Loss of appetite or overeating (children not following expected growth curve).
3. Sleep disorders.
4. Fatigue.
5. Feeling of worthlessness or guilt (may be delusional).
6. Poor concentration.
7. Suicide ideation.

These symptoms should not be secondary to bereavement, medical conditions, substance abuse, or bipolar disorders. Patients may also present with somatic complaints, or psychosis, or both. The psychotic symptoms are hallucinations and delusions of guilt, medical illnesses, or punishment.

The occurrence of major depressive disorders in adolescence from a community screened population is 4% to 5%. There is also a threefold increase of major depression in children whose parents have the disorder. Other evidence suggesting a biologic component to the illness are abnormalities on polysomnograms (increased frequency and duration of rapid eye movements in early sleep), electroencephalograms, and abnormal levels of neurotransmitters (dopamine, norepinephrine, serotonin, and γ-aminobutyric acid).

The differential diagnosis of Major Depression encompasses various medical disorders, including neurologic (causes of coma or delirium), endocrine (hypothyroid, hyperparathyroid), side effects from medications (H_2 blockers) and substance abuse or use. As part of the medical evaluation, the patient should be screened for thyroid or parathyroid disorders and for substance abuse. In addition, numerous psychologic conditions may mimic or present along with major depression. In children, these conditions are ODD, Conduct Disorder, ADHD, and anxiety disorders. In adolescents, these illnesses are ODD, Conduct Disorder, ADHD, anxiety disorders, eating disorders, and substance abuse or use.

Major depressive disorders can present at any age; however, the average age of presentation is the mid-20s. Children usually present with social withdrawal and irritability, whereas teenagers present with psychomotor retardation, delusions (guilt, worthlessness), and excessive sleep. Approximately 10% to 15% of children with major depression eventually develop bipolar disorders. Fifty percent of children with major depression have multiple episodes. The episodes of major depression are frequently associated with significant stressors. For example, up to 25% of patients with certain chronic medical conditions (cancer, diabetes) develop Major Depressive Disorder during the course of their medical illness. Besides the social and academic dysfunction caused by the major depression and its associated co-morbid conditions (ADHD, behavior disorders), 15% of patients successfully commit suicide.

The difficulty in diagnosing major depression is that the gravity of the depressive mood is often not apparent to the parents and the clinician. Unlike bipolar disease, these patients do not present with disruptive behaviors. Instead, they present with irritability or meanness. The parents and/or clinician may attribute this behavior to normal adolescence ("just going through a phase"), and hence the appropriate referrals may not be made. These children do not appear sad and deny having any problems. The clinician should have a high index of suspicion of major depression in any child who presents with meanness and irritability. Guidelines for evaluating such a patient are:

1. Assess suicide ideation and ensure safety.
2. Interview multiple sources (coaches, teachers) to determine the child's function and symptoms when the child denies having a problem.
3. Obtain a thorough family history for symptoms and diagnoses of mood disorders.
4. Rule out bipolar disorders (mania and hypomania).
5. Investigate primary or co-morbid conditions (e.g., substance abuse).
6. Consider but do not overattribute the role of stressors to the symptoms.

Emotional reaction to stressors are a normal part of life. The clinician must decide if the reaction to the stressor is normal, an adjustment disorder, or a major depression. Because the treatments for these disorders are different, it is important to recognize the symptoms of major depression and to determine to what degree they are present within the chronologic perspective of an acute stressor.

Treatment of a major depression is usually conducted by a psychiatrist and consists of psychotherapy and psychopharmacologic interventions. The efficacy of antidepressant therapy in children has not been documented. This lack of information may be partly the result of problems in study design and not medication unresponsiveness. When major depression causes significant impairment in function, a trial of antidepressants should be considered because it may reduce the symptoms. Besides medications, psychotherapy (individual, group, and family) is beneficial in treating depressed children. Because major depression often interferes with academic performance, a close liaison with the school system is important to develop an individual education program for enhancing the child's school performance.

The role of the primary care provider is early recognition and referral to reduce the morbidity and mortality of this disease. Because children with major depression often do not present with problematic behavior, the family is reluctant to seek psychiatric care. The primary care provider is a trusted advisor who can encourage a referral to a mental health provider.

Anxiety Disorders

Anxiety Disorders are one of the most prevalent type of psychologic conditions in children and adolescents. These disorders have intense episodes of distress, which consist of fear, worry, avoidance, or terror. The anxiety disorders are:

• Panic Disorder

- Specific Phobia
- Social Phobia
- Obsessive-Compulsive Disorder
- Post-Traumatic Stress Disorder
- Acute Stress Disorder
- Generalized Anxiety Disorder

Some of the medical conditions that present with anxiety symptoms and hence must be ruled out are metabolic disorders (hypoglycemia), endocrine disorders (thyroid or parathyroid), neurologic diseases, ingestion of stimulants (caffeine, psychostimulants), drug withdrawal, and catecholamine-producing tumors (pheochromocytoma, neuroblastoma).

Panic Disorder. According to the *DSM-IV*, panic disorders consist of recurrent unexpected panic attacks, during which one of the attacks is followed by a concern of having additional attacks, worry about the implications of the attack (loss of control), or a significant change in behavior (social avoidance). A panic attack consists of at least four of the following symptoms:

1. Palpitations (tachycardia).
2. Sweating.
3. Shaking.
4. Shortness of breath.
5. Sensation of choking.
6. Chest pain.
7. Nausea.
8. Dizziness.
9. Detachment.
10. Paresthesia.
11. Chills.
12. Fear of dying.
13. Fear of going crazy.

These symptoms may result in hyperventilation syndrome, which causes respiratory alkalosis, tetany, paresthesia, dizziness, or fainting. Panic attacks occur suddenly, peak within 10 minutes, and may occur with agoraphobia. Agoraphobia is an intense anxiety about having a panic attack in a place from which one cannot escape or in which help may not be available. Because of this anxiety, the individual either avoids the situations (being outside the home alone) or endures the situation with marked distress.

The 1-year prevalence rate of panic disorders ranges from 1.5 to 3.5%. Almost 50% of individuals with Panic Disorder also have agoraphobia. The age of onset is bimodal, with the largest peak occurring in adolescence and a smaller one in the mid-thirties.

Patients with panic disorders have a high degree of co-morbidities. Fifty percent to 65% of patients may have Major Depressive Disorder and hence are at risk for suicide. Patients with Panic Disorder are also at great risk for substance abuse because they often seek out pharmacologic agents (THC, alcohol, benzodiazepines) to reduce their symptoms. There is a relatively high frequency of other anxiety disorders such as Social Phobia (15% to 30%), Obsessive-Compulsive Disorders (8% to 10%), and Generalized Anxiety Disorders (25%), occurring with panic disorders. The physical complaints of this disease often cause patients to miss work or school and seek medical care, which adds to the financial cost of the disorder.

The role of the primary care provider is to rule out the medical causes of these symptoms and recognize this anxiety disorder. The patient should be referred to a child psychiatrist for treatment because of the complexities in treatment that result from the high frequency of co-morbidities. Treatment consists of a combination of psychotherapy and medications (tricyclic antidepressants, benzodiazepines).

Generalized Anxiety Disorder. In this condition, the child displays excessive worries and concerns over many issues. According to the *DSM-IV*, the diagnostic criteria for a general anxiety disorder are:

1. Anxiety and worry about various issues for more than 6 months.
2. Difficulty in controlling the worry.
3. Significant dysfunction.

In addition, children should have one (adults should have three or more) of the following symptoms: fatigue, irritability, sleep disturbances, poor concentration, and muscle tension. Patients may also have symptoms of depression (suicide ideation) or somatic complaints (abdominal pain, headaches).

The lifetime prevalence of Generalized Anxiety Disorder is 5%, with most cases developing during childhood and adolescence. The clinical course of this disorder is chronic and fluctuating and worsens with stress. It is also associated with mood disorders, other anxiety disorders, and substance abuse.

Once the condition is recognized by the primary care provider and is referred to a psychiatrist, the treatment consists of reducing stress in the environment, psychotherapy, and medications. The psychotherapy focuses on helping the child obtain a sense of control over this emotional state. As an adjunct to psychotherapy, some children may benefit from the use of anxiolytic medications.

Separation Anxiety Disorder. In this childhood condition, there is excessive anxiety that is developmentally inappropriate at the separation from home or a loved one. According to the *DSM-IV*, the symptoms are present for more than 4 weeks, occur before the age of 18 years, and consist of at least three of the following:

1. Distress with separation (home, loved one).
2. Worry about losing loved ones.
3. Worry about an event (kidnapping) causing separation.
4. Refusal to go to school.
5. Reluctance to be alone.
6. Refusal to fall asleep alone.
7. Repeated nightmares of separation.
8. Somatic complaints.

These symptoms may worsen when the child anticipates a separation.

The prevalence of Separation Anxiety Disorder is 4%, with the onset usually during early childhood. These patients are often demanding and intrusive, which leads to family conflict. Major depressive disorders and Panic Disorder with Agoraphobia are common co-morbidities.

For simple and uncomplicated cases, the primary care provider may institute simple behavioral techniques, such as initiation of brief separations so that the child may see that separation will not lead to catastrophic consequences. For more complex and severe cases (family strife or co-morbidity present), the patient should be referred to a psychiatrist. The treatment includes behavioral and supportive psychotherapy. In addition, some children may benefit from the prudent adjunctive use of anxiolytics (tricyclic antidepressants or benzodiazepines).

Obsessive-Compulsive Disorder. This disorder consists of recurrent behaviors over which the patient has little control. According to the *DSM-IV*, obsessions are recurrent thoughts that are inappropriate and cause marked anxiety. Some common obsessions are:

- Contamination (acquiring an illness from someone or something)
- Doubts (turning off the stove)
- Order (distress with asymmetry)

- Aggression
- Sexual acts

Compulsions are repetitive and excessive acts designed to reduce anxiety (hand washing, checking the stove).

The obsessive-compulsive behaviors must be time-consuming (take > 1 hour per day) or must significantly interfere with one's function. The lifetime prevalence in a community-based sample for Obsessive-Compulsive Disorder is 2.5%. The etiology of this condition is unknown; however, there is a higher predominance in children whose parents have either Tourette's syndrome or Obsessive-Compulsive Disorder.

The presentation usually occurs earlier in males (6 to 15 years of age) than in females (20 to 29 years of age). Children may present with anxiety, stress, poor concentration, or declining school performance. The differential diagnosis includes anxiety disorders, major depression, hypochondriasis, tic disorders, and Obsessive-Compulsive Personality Disorder. In this personality disorder, the patient may have the preoccupation but not the actual obsessions or compulsions.

The co-morbidity associated with Obsessive-Compulsive Disorder includes major depression, anxiety disorders, eating disorders, and Tourette's Disorder. In addition, the obsessions and compulsions may lead to social avoidance, frequent visits to the doctor, and substance abuse. In this chronic disorder, 80% of patients have waxing and waning symptoms with exacerbations secondary to stress, 15% have a progressive deterioration in function, and 5% have occasional episodes with minimal symptoms.

The treatment is directed by a psychiatrist and consists of psychotherapy and psychotropic medications. The psychotherapy is designed to provide patients with a sense of control over their thoughts and behaviors. Medications that potentiate serotonin activity (clomipramine, fluoxetine) may be successful in alleviating the symptoms. Even with therapy, patients have varying degrees of residual function.

Post-Traumatic Stress Disorder. In this condition, the patient has a severe reaction to an extremely threatening stressor. According to the *DSM-IV*, the characteristics of this syndrome may be summarized by the mnemonic T-R-A-U-M-A, which stands for *T*raumatic event, *R*e-experience, *Au*tonomic, symptoms of greater than 1 *M*onth's duration, and *A*voidance. The traumatic event must be very severe (life-threatening) and cause fear and horror in the victim. This event is then re-experienced as thoughts, dreams, or flashbacks (which occur when waking). The patient also experiences intense distress (psychologic and/or physiologic) when exposed to a situation that resembles the traumatic event. The autonomic symptoms consist of sleep disturbances, irritability, poor concentration, or hyperventilation. The avoidance consists of either avoiding circumstances associated with the event (thought, people, places) or withdrawal from relationships (detachment, diminished interest, inability to love). Children's symptoms are similar to those of adults, except that their dreams are more specific nightmares, their fear is manifested in disorganized or agitated behavior, and their re-enactment may consist of repetitive play (airplane crash re-enacted as throwing a toy plane against the wall). In addition, children frequently complain of somatic complaints (e.g., headaches).

The lifetime prevalence of Post-Traumatic Stress Disorder in a community ranges from 1% to 14%; however, it is three to four times greater in those exposed to extreme stress (disaster victims). Patients with this condition have an increased risk for panic disorders, Social Phobia, substance abuse, Obsessive-Compulsive Disorder, Somatization Disorder, and major depressive disorders.

The differential diagnosis includes adjustment disorders, panic disorders, obsessive-compulsive disorders, and psychoses (flashbacks versus hallucinations). In adjustment disorders, the stressor may be anything, whereas in Post-Traumatic Stress Disorder, it must be extreme. In Acute Stress Disorder, the symptoms can simulate Post-Traumatic Stress Disorder except that the symptoms occur soon after an event (<4 weeks) and rapidly resolve (<4 weeks). In Post-Traumatic Stress Disorder, the intrusive thoughts center around the stressor, whereas in Obsessive-Compulsive Disorder, they are unrelated.

Patients with Post-Traumatic Stress Disorder are usually treated by a mental health professional. Treatment generally consists of psychotherapy. In adults, psychotropic medications improve the Post-Traumatic Stress Disorder–related symptoms; however, there has been little research on the use of this therapy in children. Nevertheless, many psychiatrists would consider a medication trial in children who are not responding to psychotherapy.

Specific and Social Phobias. Fears are common throughout childhood; however, phobias are internal fears that cause severe anxiety and distress. According to the *DSM-IV*, diagnostic criteria of a specific phobia are:

1. An intense fear from a particular stimulus.
2. The presence or the thoughts of a stimulus cause anxiety.
3. Stimuli are avoided or endured with great distress.
4. Symptoms lead to significant dysfunction.

Some of the specific phobias are:

- Animals
- Environmental (e.g., heights)
- Blood or injection
- Situational (e.g., enclosed places)

Social phobias are similar to specific phobias except that the stimulus is either social or performance related. The lifetime prevalences of specific and social phobias from a community-based sample are 10% to 11% and 3% to 13%, respectively. The onset of specific phobias is bimodal, with the peaks occurring in childhood and in the mid-twenties, whereas social phobias begin in adolescence. Boys are more likely to have social phobias, and girls are more likely to have specific phobias. In both conditions, the anxiety in children is manifested as clinging, crying, tantrums, and freezing (not moving). In social phobias, the children refuse to participate in group play, stay close to familiar adults, and appear excessively timid in unfamiliar social functions.

Social phobias tend to be chronic, with fluctuations precipitated by stressors. Co-morbid conditions associated with social phobias are other anxiety disorders (Panic Disorder with Agoraphobia), mood disorders, and substance abuse. The co-morbid conditions associated with specific phobias are other anxiety disorders. In both conditions, the phobias can place significant limitations (academic, work, social life) on one's function in society.

Uncomplicated phobias may be managed by primary care providers, using behavioral therapy; however, problematic cases should be referred to a psychiatrist. The primary treatment of phobias is psychotherapy that addresses both the thinking and the behavior associated with the disorder. If significant dysfunction remains, pharmacotherapy with anxiolytics has been reported to be effective in phobic children.

Personality Disorders

Personality disorders consist of chronic, longstanding traits that lead to psychosocial dysfunction and distress. Even though the personality disorders can present with labile erratic emotions (Borderline Personality Disorder, Antisocial Personality Disorder) and anxiety (Obsessive-Compulsive Personality Disorder), Schizotypal Personality Disorder can present with pervasive and eccentric behavior.

Schizotypal Personality Disorder. This personality disorder consists of a longstanding pattern of marked difficulty in forming close relationships coupled with eccentric behaviors. This condition occurs in about 3% of the population. Children present with solitariness, poor peer relations, social anxiety, and peculiar thoughts. These children appear odd and are often teased by their peers. The patients seek treatment for the acute onset of anxiety or depression. Some of these patients may respond to a stressor with a transient psychoses.

According to the *DSM-IV*, this diagnosis can be made if the patient has five or more of the following symptoms:

1. Ideas but not delusions of reference (events occur because of them).
2. Superstitions.
3. Illusions.
4. Odd thinking.
5. Suspiciousness.
6. Rigid affect.
7. Peculiar behavior and/or appearance.
8. Lack of close friends.
9. Excessive social anxiety.

The etiology of this condition is unknown; however, there is a familial tendency for it. The differential diagnosis includes schizophrenia, mood disorders, and pervasive developmental disorders (Asperger Syndrome, Autistic Disorder). Therapy is best directed by psychiatrists and includes psychotherapy (to deal with the acute problem as well as the underlying personality disorder) and psychotropic agents to treat acute manifestations of anxiety, depression, or psychosis.

HALLUCINATIONS

The presence of hallucinations is of extreme concern to parents because it conjures up the image of an uncontrollable, mentally disturbed person. To the primary care provider, hallucinations are a warning that a serious medical or psychologic condition may be present (Fig. 36–5). Because of these concerns, hallucinations require a prompt and urgent evaluation. The first step in the evaluation is to assess the patient's mental status. If the abnormal mental status consists of confusion, one should consider the medical causes of delirium. If delusions are present, Schizophrenia and Mood Disorder must be ruled out. Most hallucinations from delirium are visual, whereas those from psychoses are auditory. Fortunately, most children who present with hallucinations have a normal mental status.

Hallucinations in normal children occur in as many as 5% of children. Even though these hallucinations can be of any sensory modality, they are mostly auditory. The hallucinations may be perceived as chatter or as a voice that chastises the child. Hallucinating children may also have symptoms of anxiety or depression secondary to a recognizable stressor. Most hallucinations in children with a normal mental status can be managed by the primary care provider through reassurance to the parents. In the more extreme cases, a consultation with a child psychiatrist may be necessary to rule out other conditions (acute phobic hallucinations). The contexts in which children with a normal mental status may hallucinate include beliefs (fantasy, cultural), grief, sleep, acute phobic hallucinations, and fever.

Fantasy

The concept of hallucination is based on the assumption that a person can differentiate the real from the imaginary. Children under 3 years of age confuse reality with imagination. By 4 years of age, children understand the concept of "pretend," and by 7 years of age, they understand imagination but act as though it is still real (e.g., imaginary companion). By 10 years of age, some children may consistently and intentionally fail to distinguish reality from imagination. Such children are involved in more fantasy than their classmates and may use it as entertainment or comfort. Occasionally, they may get carried away by their fantasies and become quite fearful. Most of these children proceed to healthy psychologic adjustment; however, the extremes may be an early manifestation of Schizotypal Personality Disorder.

Culture

The hallucinations may be supported by cultural, religious, and parental beliefs. For example, seeing religious visions or hearing voices from God during excitable, fundamentalist religious services are accepted and even encouraged by the participants. Even more common are parental beliefs in supernatural spirits and ghosts. This becomes problematic when adults accept the child's report of a

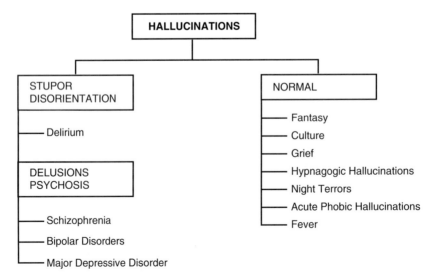

Figure 36–5. Evaluation of hallucinations.

supernatural experience as reality. This acceptance frightens both the child and the adult.

Treatment of these hallucinations consists of recognizing the context (religious service) in which they occurred and reassuring the family that the child is normal. In addition, the child's reality testing would be helped and his or her fearfulness reduced if the family can reassure the child that the hallucination is just imagination and that there is nothing to fear. A problem arises when the family believes in supernatural events. To reduce confrontation, the clinician should first acknowledge that supernatural beliefs are common, determine the extent of the adult's belief in the supernatural, and assess the parent's level of certainty that a supernatural event caused the child's experience. If the parent expresses some uncertainty, acknowledgment of that uncertainty would help the child. If the parents are adamant in their beliefs, they will not be able to reassure their frightened child. In place of the parents, one may need to rely on a trusted family member who is less certain. If asked, the clinician may explain that doctors are scientists who seek explanations that are not supernatural. This approach may avoid a detrimental confrontation between the parents and the health care provider and help the parents decide to reassure their child.

Grief

Hallucinations following the death of a loved person are easily recognized because they are usually visual and occur in the context of grief. These hallucinations can also be auditory, in which the deceased's voice is speaking to the child. The family's reaction and interpretation of these hallucinations are highly dependent on their cultural and religious beliefs. Some families may perceive these events as a supernatural or a religious experience. Even though these hallucinations may be frightening to young children, most find them a reassuring reunion and hence do not present as a problem to the clinician. If these experiences cause a problem, the treatment consists of reassurance from a parent or a recognized religious leader from the family's place of worship.

Hypnagogic Hallucination

Dream-like hallucinations can occur as one falls asleep (hypnagogic) or as one is awakening (hypnopompic). These hallucinations can also occur as part of Post-Traumatic Stress Disorder (flashback) or Narcolepsy (periods of irresistible sleep, cataplexy, and hypnopompic or hypnagogic hallucinations). When these hallucinations occur independently of these syndromes, treatment consists of only reassurance.

Night Terrors

Night terrors are frequently mistaken as hallucinations. This condition is one of the parasomnias, along with sleepwalking and sleep talking. According to the *DSM-IV*, night terrors (Sleep Terror Disorder) consists of episodes in which the child appears to arouse during the night and cries inconsolably. During these episodes, there is intense fear and autonomic arousal (tachycardia, sweating). On arousal, the child has no memory of the event. Episodes of night terrors last from 10 to 20 minutes, during which the child may speak but does not make sense. Even though the child appears to be dreaming during these episodes, night terrors occur during stage 4 deep sleep and not during rapid eye movement sleep.

The prevalence of night terrors ranges from 1% to 6%. It usually begins during early childhood and resolves spontaneously during adolescence. The occurrence of night terrors is inconsistently associated with stressors. Seizure disorders, especially of the temporal and frontal lobes, can produce fear and complex behavior patterns resembling night terrors. Hence, a seizure disorder should be ruled out in patients with persistent and significant symptoms.

Treatment for night terrors consists of education and reassurance. If the night terrors occur in unusually long clusters, a brief course of low-dose benzodiazepine therapy or a tricyclic antidepressant administered at bedtime may interrupt the clusters.

Acute Phobic Hallucinations

Acute phobic hallucination occurs in preschool-aged children and consists of episodes of hallucinations coupled with panic. These hallucinations last from 10 to 60 minutes and occur mostly at night. A child may become very frightened during an episode. For example, the child may state that bugs are crawling over him or her. The child may frantically try to brush them off or run away. Because of the acute change in mental status, this condition must be differentiated from the medical and psychotic causes of hallucinations (delirium).

The actual cause of acute phobic hallucinations is unknown. The symptoms usually last 1 to 3 days and diminish over 1 to 2 weeks. If the condition does not quickly abate, it responds well to low dosages of benzodiazepines.

Fever

During acute illness, preschool-aged children may hallucinate during times of high fevers. These hallucinations are temporary and are not associated with future mental disorders. Management of fever-induced hallucinations consists of ruling out the medical causes of delirium and reassuring the family.

UNEXPLAINED PHYSICAL COMPLAINTS

At times, parents may present to the primary care provider with ''unexplained physical complaints'' on behalf of the child. These complaints may be inconsistent with the results of the physical examination or laboratory tests (severe abdominal pain in a smiling child) and may fail to respond to any medical therapy, or the symptoms may be changed if they are not producing the appropriate response. These unexplained complaints may be caused by overprotectiveness, excessive worry, underlying psychologic conditions, or manipulation. Clinicians can easily become angry when they suspect that they are being manipulated (Table 36–8).

These unexplained physical complaints may be the manner in which a patient copes with a stressor. The patient may not be aware of the stressor, nor may the patient realize that these symptoms emanate from his or her effort to cope with the problem. The clinician should empathize with the patient and begin the conversation with the phrase ''It must be hard for you to . . . (worry or not get satisfactory explanations).'' The clinician should then state the conditions that the child does not have (with serious diseases ruled out) and state that the symptoms are real. The health care provider should address the issue that stress can cause or make symptoms worse and should recommend that the possibility of stress be evaluated while the clinician continues to monitor the patient for other medical illness.

The various conditions that contribute to unexplained physical

Table 36–8. Essential Elements of the Management of Unexplained Physical Complaints

Avoid feeling manipulated or angry
Avoid the following behavior:
   Ordering more tests to prove the child is healthy
   Tricking the patient with a placebo
   Stating that the symptoms do not exist
Proper management consists of
   Addressing parents'/child's worries
   Conducting an appropriate medical evaluation
   Stating what medical conditions are ruled out
   Introducing stress as a possible cause of the symptoms
   Exploring stress while monitoring for other medical illnesses

complaints are organized based on whether the parent or the child is the complainer (Fig. 36–6).

Parent Complaints

Vulnerable Child Syndrome

Vulnerability begins when an apparently healthy child suddenly develops a life-threatening illness. Even though the child may recover completely from the illness, the parents fear that the condition will recur. After a life-threatening illness, parents universally and appropriately rethink the illness to determine whether any warnings were overlooked. After appraising the oversight and/or the absence of warnings, the family usually returns to normal activity except for some increased wariness.

Some parents are so traumatized by this life-threatening event that they live in constant dread of it recurring. They may also manifest some of the features of Post-Traumatic Stress Disorder. These parents are fearfully attentive to every nuance of change in the child and frequently contact the primary care provider prematurely. The child may incorporate this fear and be reluctant to separate from the parent, which delays the development of independence and self-confidence. Because the parents live every day as if it is the child's last, they are reluctant to discipline the child. Consequently, the child does not learn self-control and consideration of others, which can lead to significant personality dysfunction.

During the course of a life-threatening illness, the primary care provider should anticipate the development of the vulnerable child syndrome, warn the parents of this syndrome, and reassure the family that the life-threatening illness will not recur. If the syndrome has already developed, some parents may benefit by realizing that their fears are based on the past and with reassurance can let down their guard.

Hypochondriasis by Proxy

Parents may worry excessively about the child's health because of a preceding life-threatening event (vulnerable child) or mistrust of the medical profession (missed diagnosis in a family member), or as an expression of their own fear of having a serious condition themselves (hypochondriasis by proxy). These parents do not make up the child's symptoms but instead have an exaggerated worry about symptoms. For example, they may seek medical care when

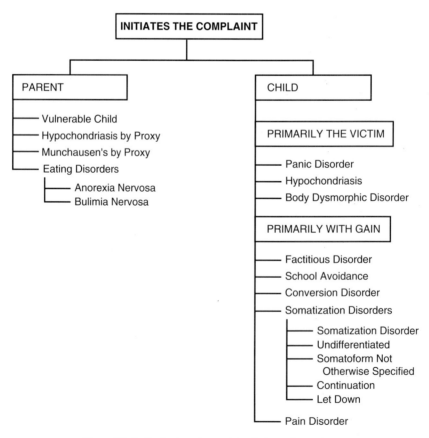

Figure 36–6. Evaluation of unexplained physical complaints.

their child's temperature is only 99.1°F because they fear that their child may have a serious bacterial infection. The evaluation of a parent's excessive concern over the child's health may be further subdivided into specific concerns versus general medical worries.

The specific medical concerns for the child's health are those caused by a prior life-threatening event or by a misfortunate experience with the medical profession. Reassurance after an appropriate and thorough medical evaluation may reduce parental anxiety and worry. In addition, if the parent reveals the past incident that led to distrust of the reassurances of doctors, the clinician may be able to reduce the parent's worry through open discussion on the differences between the past and current events.

If the parent reports that he or she worries about everything, the clinician should determine if this is a recent development or a long-term characteristic. Parents with acute onset of general medical worries about their children may have an anxiety or a depressive disorder. These parents may suffer from a recent stressor and have associated bursts of anxiety (Panic Disorder), fear of being in public (Social Phobia), repetitive preoccupations (Obsessive-Compulsive Disorder), or a sad feeling coupled with fatigue (mood disorder). Because these conditions cause enormous distress in the parent, they merit a referral to a psychiatrist.

Parents with long-term, generalized, and excessive concern of a child's health may have hypochondriasis. Hypochondriasis, according to the *DSM-IV*, is a preoccupation with fears of having a serious disease based on the patient's misinterpretation of the patient's symptoms. In addition these fears are chronic (>6 months in duration) and persist despite an appropriate medical evaluation. The prevalence of hypochondriasis in a general medical practice ranges from 4% to 9%. The onset can occur at any age but usually begins in early adulthood. This condition may cause the deterioration of parent-doctor relationship as a result of frustrations and anger. In addition, it compounds the morbidity by excessive and inappropriate medical testing (which can cause complications from procedures and financial burdens). Even though hypochondriasis is characterized as a chronic condition that waxes and wanes, complete remission can occur. Factors that are favorable to a remission are acute onset, associated medical conditions, lack of secondary gain, and absence of personality disorders.

A simple reassurance does not address the chronic fear or worry expressed by parents with hypochondriasis. The reassurance instead may cause the deterioration of parent-doctor relationship. This deterioration may lead to the referral (by parent or clinician) of the child to a subspecialist for further medical evaluation. Instead of a simple reassurance, the treatment consists of empathy, education of the parents, reassurance about the child's medical health, and referral of the parents to the appropriate mental health professional.

Factitious Disorders (Munchausen Syndrome by Proxy)

According to *DSM-IV*, Factitious Disorder is defined as a condition in which the patient either feigns or produces symptoms and physical findings to fulfill an underlying need to assume the sick role. In addition, there is also no external reward for these symptoms, in contrast to malingering, in which the symptoms result in either economic gain or in avoidance of responsibilities. In Munchausen syndrome by proxy (see Chapter 37), a caregiver feigns or produces the symptoms in a child and then seeks medical care.

The perpetrator in Munchausen syndrome by proxy is usually the mother. The offender may also have had a past history of Factitious Disorder that is quiescent as long as the symptoms can be inflicted on someone else. The victim can be of any age but is usually a toddler. When the victim is an older child, he or she may collaborate with the offender. Usually, the offender focuses on one

victim at a time; however, all siblings in the home are potentially at risk for neglect, abuse, and factitious illness.

The most commonly induced or feigned symptoms in children are:

1. Bleeding (stool or urine contaminated with parent's blood).
2. Diarrhea (laxative induced).
3. Vomiting (emetic use).
4. Fever (injection of bacteria).
5. CNS depression (medication induced).
6. Seizures (hypoxia secondary to smothering or hypoglycemia from insulin injection).
7. Apnea (smothering).
8. Rashes (contact dermatitis).

Potential warning signs for this condition are:

1. Unexplained and prolonged illnesses.
2. Incongruous symptoms and signs.
3. Ineffective medical treatments.
4. Prior episodes of sudden infant death syndrome.
5. Widespread allergies.

In addition, the offending parent may not seem worried about the child's medical condition. Some parents may form an unusually pathologically close relationship with the medical staff; however, there are many exceptions, in which the parent is instead neglectful, disruptive, and argumentative.

Besides the morbidity of the induced symptoms, the mortality rate of this syndrome is as high as 9%. When a clinician suspects Munchausen syndrome by proxy, the first step is to ensure the child's safety, which usually means admission to a medical ward (Table 36–9). The next step is to develop a definitive investigative plan with a multidisciplinary team consisting of mental health professionals, physicians, social services, child abuse specialists, and the legal system to design a system for collecting evidence. This plan may include:

1. Typing the blood in the specimen and comparing it with the child's blood.
2. Toxicology studies of stool (laxatives), vomitus (emetics), or urine (substance use).
3. Species-specific insulin levels (pork/beef) for unexplained hypoglycemia.
4. Surveillance by a hidden video camera (with legal guidance).

Events occurring only in the presence of the offender is circumstantial evidence and by itself will probably not lead to conviction in a court of law. In addition, referring the parent to a mental health provider is unfruitful and rarely results in any evidence being obtained.

Once the evidence is collected, the team should confront the perpetrator in a non-accusatory manner. The offender may confess; however, usually the person denies his or her involvement, becomes angry, and threatens to take the child out of the hospital. During

---

Table 36–9. Essential Elements of the Management of Munchausen's Syndrome by Proxy

1. Maintain high index of suspicion
2. Ensure child's safety
3. Assemble multidisciplinary team
4. Collect evidence before confronting parent with the suspected diagnosis
5. Parental personality is a poor predictor
6. Realize that confrontation rarely results in a confession
7. Present evidence to legal system to determine
   a. Necessity of removal of child from home
   b. Institution of a close monitoring system

this time period, the parent is also at great risk for depression and suicide. Successful psychotherapy for parents with Munchausen syndrome by proxy is rare and cannot guarantee the child's safety. Instead, the multidisciplinary team in conjunction with the legal system needs to decide whether to remove the child from the parents' custody or institute a close surveillance program.

Eating Disorders

Eating disorders (Table 36–10) are included under the heading of parent complaints because it is the concerned parent who initiates the visit to the health care provider and not the adolescent. The eating disorders are Anorexia Nervosa (weight loss with or without induced purging) and Bulimia Nervosa (stable weight, binge eating, and induced purging). These disorders present to the clinician as unexplained physical complaints, such as protracted diarrhea, persistent vomiting, weight loss, and/or amenorrhea. Adolescents who deliberately induce these symptoms to control caloric intake are more concerned about the shape of their body. These patients go to great lengths to hide their intent and symptoms because they know that their parents would object to their actions. Some of the ways of hiding these disorders are wearing baggy clothes to conceal their body, even in hot weather; excessive and vigorous exercise to get into shape for sports or ballet; selection of healthy food because of low-fat or low-calorie content; complaints of allergies ruining the taste and smell of food; and secret purging (induced vomiting and/or diarrhea). Because of this concealment, the detection of these potentially lethal conditions is a diagnostic challenge for the clinician.

Anorexia Nervosa. According to the *DSM-IV*, Anorexia Nervosa is defined as:

1. Refusal to maintain body weight at 85% of what is appropriate for the patient's age or height.
2. Intense fear of gaining weight.
3. Distorted perception regarding one's size.
4. In postpubertal females, an absence of three consecutive menstrual cycles.

The prevalence of Anorexia Nervosa ranges from 0.5% to 1%, with almost 90% of cases occurring in females. Even though this condition is associated with higher socioeconomic status, it can occur in all races and socioeconomic backgrounds. The etiology of anorexia nervosa is unknown; however, it is associated with such factors as psychologic (recent stressor), cultural (industrialized nations with abundance of food), environmental, and biogenetic (twin or family history studies) influences.

Besides the weight loss, patients with Anorexia Nervosa may develop symptoms of depression or withdraw socially secondary to the physiology of semi-starvation. Actual loss of appetite is rare in these patients; instead, they may develop obsessive-compulsive behavior regarding food (e.g., they may collect recipes or hoard food). These patients may also have inflexible thinking or feel the need to control their environment.

Anorexia Nervosa may affect every organ system. The presenting symptoms and signs of Anorexia Nervosa are secondary to malnutrition and purging. The symptoms of malnutrition are fatigue, depression, and amenorrhea. The physical findings of malnutrition are:

- Bradycardia
- Hypothermia
- Hypotension
- Emaciation
- Hair loss
- Yellow skin (hypercarotenemia)
- Lanugo (fine body hair)

Table 36–10. Comparative Characteristics of Anorexia Nervosa and Bulimia Nervosa

Characteristics	Anorexia Nervosa	Bulimia Nervosa
Intense preoccupation with food	Yes	Yes
Weight loss	Severe	Fluctuates
Female	90%–95%	90%–95%
Family history	+ for anorexia nervosa	+ for depression
Methods of weight control	Severe food restrictions, emesis, exercise	Restriction and binges with self-induced vomiting and diuretic and/or laxative purging
Guilt/shame	None	Yes
Denial	Yes	None
Personality	Withdrawn/asexual	Outgoing/heterosexual
Onset (age)	Bimodal (13–14 yr and 17–18 yr)	17–25 yr
Endocrinopathy/metabolism	Amenorrhea, increased growth hormone, osteoporosis, hypercarotenemia, hypothermia	Menstrual irregularities, hypokalemia
Cardiovascular complications	Bradycardia, hypotension, arrhythmias	Ipecac toxicity
Gastrointestinal	Constipation, elevated hepatic enzymes	Gastric dilation and rupture, Mallory-Weiss syndrome, esophagitis, parotid enlargement, dental enamel erosion
Psychiatric	Depression, suicide, obsessional fears	Impulsive behaviors, alcohol-drug addictions, depression, suicide

From Tershakovec AM, Stallings VA. Pediatric nutrition and nutritional disorders. *In* Behrman RE, Kliegman RM (eds). Nelson Essentials of Pediatrics, 2nd ed. Philadelphia: WB Saunders, 1994;66.

If the patient controls caloric intake by vomiting, he or she may present with hypertrophic salivary glands (secondary to gastric irritation), dental erosions (secondary to gastric irritation), and abrasions and/or calluses on the dorsum of the hand (secondary to manual induction of vomiting). The metabolic abnormalities related to starvation and purging consist of:

- Leukopenia
- Anemia
- Hyperamylasemia (resulting from parotid gland irritation from gastric acid)
- Metabolic alkalosis (resulting from vomiting)
- Metabolic acidosis (resulting from laxative abuse)
- Decreased triiodothyronine level
- Hypoproteinemia
- Hypomagnesemia
- Hypocalcemia
- Hypozincemia
- Electrolyte abnormalities (resulting from diuretic abuse, dehydration)

These patients also have regression of the hypothalamic-pituitary-gonadal axis, which results in low serum estrogen levels in females (causing amenorrhea) and low testosterone levels in males.

In evaluating a teenager with unexplained weight loss, one must rule out the medical causes of cachexia (malignancy, inflammatory bowel disease, chronic infections like acquired immunodeficiency syndrome). Questions supporting a diagnosis of Anorexia Nervosa are a dietary history, perception of body shape, and rationalization of behavior (weight loss for ballet).

Once the medical causes for weight loss have been ruled out, one needs to consider the psychologic differential diagnosis for Anorexia Nervosa and its associated co-morbidities. These conditions are Major Depressive Disorder, substance abuse (stimulants), Obsessive-Compulsive Disorder (multiple obsessions besides food), Social Phobia, Body Dysmorphic Disorder, and Bulimia Nervosa. If the depression does not resolve with the correction of the malnutrition, one should also consider the diagnosis of Major Depressive Disorder. In addition, patients who try to control their caloric intake with pharmacologic agents are more likely to exhibit impulsive behavior (sexuality) and substance abuse (stimulants).

Anorexia Nervosa is associated with both life-threatening psychologic (Major Depressive Disorder, suicide) and medical conditions (electrolyte abnormalities, starvation). The lifelong mortality rate secondary to Anorexia Nervosa in patients who require hospitalization is 10%. Some of the possible medical complications of Anorexia Nervosa are osteoporosis (resulting from hypocalcemia with low serum estrogen levels), cardiomyopathy (resulting from ipecac abuse), anemia, sepsis (resulting from malnutrition-induced immunodeficiencies), arrhythmias (resulting from electrolyte abnormalities, prolonged QT_c), and superior mesenteric artery syndrome. The superior mesenteric artery syndrome can occur in any emaciated patient and consists of the artery compressing the stomach. This compression causes intermittent gastric outlet obstruction and results in postprandial vomiting or signs of mesenteric ischemia (e.g., pain).

The treatment of Anorexia Nervosa requires a multidisciplinary approach using the primary care provider (addresses the medical complications), the nutritionist (develops a refeeding plan), and the psychiatrist (treats the underlying syndrome and its co-morbidities). Inpatient management may be necessary, depending on the degree of cachexia coupled with the adolescent's psychologic status (e.g., whether or not suicide ideation is present). The decision about where to admit the patient (medical versus psychiatric unit) is based on the medical stability of the patient and the patient's willingness to cooperate with the nutritionally sound refeeding program. For the medically stable but uncooperative patient, the patient should be admitted to the psychiatric unit, where the focus is on intense behavioral therapy.

The nutritionist can assist in the management by developing a nutritionally sound diet that ensures a safe rate of weight gain. Too rapid a refeeding may result in hepatic steatosis and diarrhea from malabsorption.

The role of the mental health professional is to treat the underlying condition as well as the co-morbidities. The treatment consists of behavior therapy to ensure compliance with the refeeding program as well as various forms of psychotherapies (individual, group, or family). The co-morbidities that also may need to be addressed are depression (suicide ideation), anxiety disorder (Obsessive-Compulsive Disorder, Social Phobia), Body Dysmorphic Disorder, and substance use. Psychopharmacology is unsuccessful in Anorexia Nervosa unless the intent is to treat a co-morbidity (e.g., depression). For most patients, Anorexia Nervosa is a chronic condition requiring long-term psychosocial support and medical monitoring.

Bulimia Nervosa. This condition consists of binge eating with inappropriate means for maintaining weight (purging). The diagnostic criteria for Bulimia Nervosa according to the *DSM-IV* are:

1. Lack of control in eating an excessive amount of food during a set period of time.
2. Inappropriate methods for controlling weight gain (purging).
3. Binge eating or inappropriate methods for controlling weight gain occurring at least twice a week for 3 months.
4. Distorted perception in body shape.
5. Not meeting criteria for Anorexia Nervosa (weight not below 85% for age).

Bulimia Nervosa is twice as common as Anorexia Nervosa and has a later onset (late adolescence). Like Anorexia Nervosa, it is more common in females (90%) and can occur in any socioeconomic background. Almost 90% of patients control their weight gain by purging. Other methods for controlling weight are excessive exercise and fasting before binge eating. In addition, dancers and wrestlers may engage in these behaviors to compete at the lowest possible weight.

Co-morbid psychologic conditions are common in bulimia and include:

- Mood disorders (major depression, especially in those who purge)
- Personality disorders
- Substance use

Approximately 30% of patients who use medications to control weight also have substance use disorders (alcohol, stimulants).

The co-morbid medical conditions of Bulimia Nervosa are associated with vomiting or medication abuse. These conditions are:

- Esophagitis
- Gastritis
- Cardiomyopathy (from ipecac abuse)
- Hypokalemia (from diuretic abuse)
- Kidney stones (from diuretic abuse)
- Metabolic alkalosis (from vomiting)
- Metabolic acidosis (from laxative abuse)
- Increased amylase levels (from salivary gland irritation)

Approximately 30% of teenaged patients with diabetes mellitus may have Bulimia Nervosa. These patients may control their weight gain by reducing their intake of insulin, resulting in the excretion of more glucose in their urine.

The patient's concealment of symptoms coupled with the lack of cachexia makes Bulimia Nervosa difficult to detect. Some patients may present to the clinician because of a parent's detection of binge eating and purging. Physical findings that suggest recurrent vomiting are dental erosion, parotid hypertrophy, callous abrasions on the dorsum of the hand (Russell's sign), and pharyngeal irritation.

In contrast to Anorexia Nervosa, significant medical complications rarely occur in Bulimia Nervosa. Unless serious medical conditions or suicide ideation occur, most patients with Bulimia Nervosa can be treated in an outpatient setting. Treatment is orchestrated by a mental health professional and is directed toward both the underlying condition and the co-morbidities. Patients often respond to individual or group therapy. For other patients, antidepressant medications (e.g., desipramine, fluoxetine) may ameliorate some of the symptoms. For some patients, treatment may be very successful, with remission that persists for years. Unfortunately, for others, Bulimia Nervosa is a disorder of exacerbations, remissions, and chronic residual dysfunction that requires long-term management by a mental health professional.

Child Complaints

One way in which the body responds to a psychologic stressor is through medical symptoms. Evidence that supports a stressor as a cause of the symptom is the potential gain from the symptom and the temporal relationship of the stressor and the symptom. For example, a child may develop chronic fatigue symptoms on the anniversary of his or her mother's death, or a patient's persistent abdominal pain from prior flair-ups of Crohn's disease may prevent the patient from returning to school, despite medical evidence that the disease is in remission. These symptoms seem real to the child and cause a great deal of distress. Some of the extreme presentations of these concerns or complaints are the anxiety disorders (Panic Disorder, Social Phobia, Separation Anxiety Disorder) and the somatoform disorders (Hypochondriasis, Somatization Disorder, Conversion Disorder, Body Dysmorphic Disorder, and Pain Disorder).

The child's complaints may be further subdivided by whether the child primarily suffers (is the victim) or gains (consciously or unconsciously) from the symptoms. Some patients in the victimized group may still receive secondary gain (more attention from parents). In addition, patients with conditions that usually result in secondary gain may obtain relatively little gain compared with the suffering caused by the symptoms. Nevertheless, these disorders can be subdivided based on whether the condition as a whole leads to suffering or to gain (see Fig. 36–6).

To address the psychologic causes for the symptoms, the primary care provider must first rule out the possibility of any medical condition as a cause of the symptoms. Because the psychologic problem lies with the child and not the parents, the child needs to be reassured of his or her health. In addition, the underlying psychologic problem needs to be recognized and treated.

PRIMARILY THE VICTIM

Panic Disorder and Hypochondriasis

Panic Disorder and Hypochondriasis can present with medical symptoms. In Panic Disorder, the patient has recurrent and unexpected panic attacks that are not necessarily preceded by a recognizable stressor. The attacks are characterized by an autonomic discharge, resulting in flushing, sweating, palpitations, chest pain, hyperventilation, dizziness, paresthesias, and an imminent fear of dying. In Hypochondriasis, the child either fears that he or she has a serious illness or focuses on minor discomforts with a worry that he or she may have a life-threatening illness. In addition, these patients may appear sad, irritable, and fatigued, reflecting an underlying anxiety or depressive condition. Treatment centers on an appropriate medical evaluation to reassure the patient, coupled with a referral to a mental health professional to deal with the underlying psychologic condition.

Body Dysmorphic Disorder

Almost all children and teenagers have some concern regarding their physical appearance that leads to some stress. These concerns may be focused on their complexion, their developing bodies (puberty), or the shape of their facial features. According to the *DSM-IV*, patients have Body Dysmorphic Disorder when they are preoccupied with excessive concerns regarding their body's appearance; this preoccupation leads to significant social and academic dysfunction. Their dysfunction may consist of spending hours in front of a mirror worrying about their appearance. Their concern about their appearance may lead to significant public avoidance. In addition, they often seek medical treatment for their perceived disfigurement. Unfortunately, even a result that is cosmetically acceptable to someone else does not alleviate the patient's worry. Because of these concerns, the patient is at significant risk for major depressive disorders and suicide.

The differential diagnosis of Body Dysmorphic Disorder includes eating disorders (preoccupation with weight or body shape), Delusional Disorder (worries persist despite medical assurances), Social Phobia, Major Depressive Disorder, and Obsessive-Compulsive Disorder (multiple obsessions besides body image). Because of the risk of major depression and suicide, these patients should be referred to a psychiatrist for treatment.

PRIMARILY WITH GAIN

Factitious Disorder

Factitious Disorder consists of patients' inducing symptoms or signs in themselves to assume the sick role. There is no financial gain as might be found with malingering. The onset of this disorder usually occurs in early adulthood; however, it can also occur in childhood. Patients are at risk for substance use disorders (using agents to induce symptoms) as well as for complications from associated diagnostic work-ups and unnecessary surgeries. When these individuals are older, they may induce symptoms in their own children (Munchausen syndrome by proxy). On confrontation, they may either change their symptoms or try to seek medical care from someone else. Treatment for this chronic disorder is psychotherapy conducted by a mental health professional.

School Avoidance

School avoidance occurs when a child uses medical symptoms to avoid school unnecessarily. If these symptoms become severe enough (duration > 4 weeks, associated worries of separation, significant dysfunction), they may be an early manifestation of Separation Anxiety Disorder (see Disruptive Behaviors). The symptoms of school avoidance may involve any organ system but are usually abdominal pain, or headaches, or both. These pains are worse in the morning (especially on Mondays). In more severe cases, the symptoms may develop on Sunday evenings. Anxiety about attending school and the pattern of gain are quickly apparent to the primary care provider.

The cause of the anxiety may be a conflict with the teacher or classmates. In adolescents, the anxiety may be due to a recurrent stressor, such as an embarrassing situation (gym class) or conflict with peers. Some factors that may contribute to the development of this disorder are fear of losing one's parents, reduction of fear when the patient stays at home, parental sharing of the worry of loss, recent family tragedy, and an increasing understanding of death (i.e., that it is universal, permanent, and unpredictable). Patients with school avoidance may also have an anxiety disorder (Social Phobia) or Major Depressive Disorder.

Treatment of simple school avoidance consists of correction of school-based fears (e.g., teacher or peers) by parental intervention with the school, reassurance, education of the parents regarding their inadvertent reinforcement of separation anxiety, and immediate return to school. The longer the absence, the harder it is for the child to return. To get the child back to school, the parent may have to either accompany the child to the classroom or institute a stepwise return to the classroom (beginning in the principal's office, then to the library, and finally to the classroom). The child should be referred to a psychiatrist if there is an underlying psychologic disorder (anxiety or depressive disorder) or if the child does not return to school within 1 week, if a grade school child; or within a few days, if a junior high school student. If there is a significant anxiety or depressive component, the psychiatrist may prescribe a temporary course of benzodiazepines or tricyclic antidepressants.

Conversion Disorders

According to the *DSM-IV*, the diagnostic criteria for conversion disorders are:

1. Symptoms associated with voluntary motor or sensory function (not factitious symptoms or pain symptoms).
2. Symptoms preceded by a recent stressor.
3. Symptoms unexplained by a medical evaluation.
4. Symptoms causing significant distress or prompting medical evaluation.

In children under 10 years of age, the presenting symptoms are either gait disturbances or pseudoseizures. Older individuals may present with such symptoms as paralysis of a limb, paresthesias, blindness, or aphonia. These symptoms are relatively easy to identify because they do not follow an anatomic nerve distribution nor do the actions fit the symptoms (blind person never bumping into anything). Pseudoseizures are more difficult to document and may require continuously videotaped EEG telemetry for extended periods of time. The patient may react to the symptoms either with indifference (*la belle indifférence*) or in a dramatic fashion.

The prevalence of conversion disorder is 1 to 30/10,000 patients. The onset is usually in late adolescence to early adulthood. A typical episode is acute, follows a recent stressor, and is of relatively short duration (<4 weeks). Theoretically, the symptoms solve a psychologic conflict (blindness prevents seeing something bad). Some common childhood stressors associated with conversion disorders are grief and incest.

Approximately 25% of the patients have a relapse within a year. Factors that are associated with a favorable prognosis are acute onset; identifiable stressor at time of onset; above-average intelligence; and symptoms of paralysis, aphonia, or blindness. Also associated with conversion disorders are Major Depressive Disorder and personality disorders (Antisocial Personality Disorder).

Management of conversion disorders is usually conducted by a mental health provider. Treatment consists of empathy, a face-saving explanation for the symptoms, explanation of the relationship of stressors to symptoms, reduction of stressors, reassurance that the symptoms will remit, introduction of techniques to reduce stress (relaxation imagery), and a stepwise rehabilitation program with physical therapy. Because of the co-morbidity associated with

this disease, patients need to be monitored for depressive symptoms and suicide ideation. In some cases, patients benefit from dynamic psychotherapy; however, most adolescents with conversion disorders do not engage in reflection on what stressors might be causing their symptoms and hence do not respond well to psychotherapy.

Somatization Disorder

According to the *DSM-IV*, Somatization Disorder (Briquet's syndrome) consists of a preoccupation of multiple physical complaints consisting of at least four pain symptoms, two gastrointestinal symptoms, one neurologic symptom, and one sexual symptom (impotency, menorrhagia). In addition, these multiple symptoms must have occurred over years, must not be produced factitiously or by a medical condition, must have begun before the age of 30 years, and must have caused significant dysfunction. Two milder presentations of somatization disorder, which are more commonly seen in children, are Undifferentiated Somatoform Disorder (one symptom, > 6 months' duration) and Somatoform Disorder Not Otherwise Specified (one symptom, < 6 months' duration).

The prevalence of Somatization Disorder is 0.2% to 2% in females and 0.2% in males. Associated co-morbidities are Major Depressive Disorder, Panic Disorder, substance abuse, and personality disorders (Borderline Personality Disorder and Antisocial Personality Disorder). This is a chronic condition that rarely remits. The psychologic differential diagnosis includes mood disorders (major depression), Schizophrenia with somatic delusions, panic disorders (symptoms occur only during an attack), Generalized Anxiety Disorder, and Factitious Disorder.

Recognition is the major problem in the management of this condition. These patients are often referred to multiple medical subspecialists to reassure the patient. If the underlying psychologic problem is not addressed, reassurance is rarely successful. If reassurance is unsuccessful, patients may become despondent and suicidal. Proper management consists of an appropriate medical evaluation to rule out medical causes for the symptoms, recognition of this psychologic disorder, and prompt referral to a mental health specialist.

Pain Disorder

Pain Disorder is a somatoform disorder in which the patient has significant pain that leads to medical attention. According to the *DSM-IV*, this pain is related to stress and causes significant dysfunction. In addition, it must neither be self-inflicted nor due to any medical condition. The symptoms may occur with or without a previous (but resolved) medical condition.

The actual prevalence of Pain Disorder is unknown; however, it appears to be quite common. The co-morbid conditions associated with pain disorders are substance abuse (to alleviate symptoms), mood disorders (usually with chronic pain), and anxiety disorders (usually with acute pain).

Two methods by which this syndrome may present are the "continuation" syndrome and the "let-down" syndrome. In the continuation syndrome, the symptoms from the medical disease persist in the mind even after the biologic abnormalities have completely resolved. The let-down syndrome occurs in highly successful and hard-working students who are under a lot of stress. These symptoms provide them with a legitimate excuse to escape the rigorous demands imposed by themselves or others. The patient's recognition of the conflict over ambition is important in the resolution of this condition.

Treatment of Pain Disorder consists of an appropriate medical evaluation and prompt referral to a mental health professional. The psychologic treatment is similar to that for Conversion Disorder. In addition, the psychiatrist monitors the patient for the development of co-morbidities.

DELAYED DEVELOPMENT

Delayed development (see Chapter 34) is a broad category of illnesses that can cause specific or general delay. These delays may first be noted by parents (the patient is not developing as fast as siblings), teachers (the patient has academic difficulties), or the primary care provider during a health maintenance examination (developmental screening test). The causes of mental retardation encompass many conditions (see Chapter 34). In over half the cases of mental retardation, a medical condition has caused the development delay. These medical conditions include:

- Heredity (5%)
- Alterations of embryonic development (30%)
- Perinatal or prenatal insults (10%)
- General medical illness of childhood (5%)

Another 15% to 20% of cases are caused by either deprivation or severe mental disorders (pervasive developmental disorders).

The specific delays may be secondary to such conditions as:

- A medical insult (cerebral palsy)
- Learning disorders (reading, mathematics, written expression disorders)
- Developmental Coordination Disorder
- Communication disorders (expressive and/or receptive)
- Psychologic disorders (Selective Mutism)

This part of the chapter concentrates on the psychologic causes of general and specific delay (Fig. 36–7).

Psychologic Causes of General Delay

Pervasive Developmental Disorders

Pervasive developmental disorders cause severe impairment in social development, language development, and/or imaginative play. In addition, these disorders are often associated with severe to profound mental retardation (intelligence quotient [IQ] < 50). The pervasive developmental disorders are

- Autistic Disorder
- Rett Disorder
- Childhood Disintegrative Disorder
- Asperger Disorder

The diagnosis of Pervasive Developmental Disorder Not Otherwise Specified may be used if the patient does not fill the diagnostic criteria for the aforementioned disorders.

Autistic Disorder. According to the *DSM-IV*, the diagnosis of autism is made if the patient has six or more symptoms in the following category: social interaction (at least two symptoms), communication (at least one symptom), and repetitive, stereotypic behavior (at least one symptom). In addition, the symptoms need to occur before the patient is 3 years of age. The problems with social interactions are sparsity of nonverbal communication (body gestures), failure to develop peer relationships, lack of sharing or showing things to others, and lack of emotional reciprocity. In early infancy, parents may notice that these infants do not cuddle well. Affected infants fail to respond to voice to the point that the parent worries that the child is deaf. The language impairments are a delay or a lack of any verbal communication, difficulties in sustaining a conversation, echolalia or nonsensical words, and lack of imaginative play.

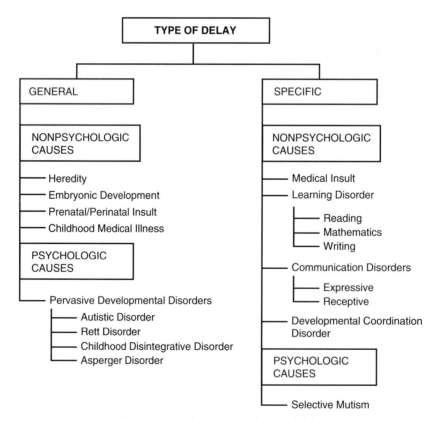

Figure 36–7. Evaluation of developmental delay.

The degree of language impairment is one of the best predictors of prognosis. The stereotypic and repetitious behavior of these children includes intense preoccupation with an interest (mimicking an actor), inflexible adherence to routines (behavioral outbursts when the routines are not adhered to), repetitive motor movements (rocking), and preoccupation with parts of an object.

The prevalence of autistic disorder is 2 to 5/10,000, with over 75% of cases occurring in males. This disorder is probably biologically based because of the neurochemical and neuroanatomic abnormalities occurring in it, coupled with the increased risk of the disorder among siblings in affected families. Some of the medical conditions associated with autistic disorder are encephalitis, phenylketonuria, birth anoxia, and fragile X syndrome.

Children with autistic disorder may be hyperactive, impulsive, and aggressive and may engage in self-injurious activities. These children may also have unusual reactions to stimulation, such as an oversensitivity to touch or a high pain threshold. As these children become older, they may show some willingness to passively engage in social encounters. Older children may also have extraordinary long-term memory (e.g., for songs, baseball statistics) but use the information inappropriately. The co-morbidities of autistic disorder are significant: 25% of affected patients have seizures, and 75% have severe to profound mental retardation (IQ < 50). As adults, about 30% may have some degree of independent living. Because of the severity of the symptoms, depression is common in the patients who have some insight into their condition.

The differential diagnosis of Autistic Disorder includes the other pervasive developmental disorders, communication disorders, Schizophrenia, and mental retardation. Patients with just mental retardation do not have the impairment in social interaction nor the repetitive behaviors associated with Autistic Disorder.

The cornerstone of treatment is to foster the patient's ability to communicate, to develop the patient's social skills, and to facilitate learning. These interventions are usually performed in special education settings. Pharmacologic interventions (haloperidol) are sometimes used to address problematic behaviors.

Rett Disorder

Infants with Rett disorder are normal until 5 months of age. Between 5 and 48 months of age, the toddler experiences decelerated growth of the head circumference, loss of purposeful hand movements (hand wringing), poor gait or truncal movements, loss of social engagement, and severely impaired language development with psychomotor retardation. This condition is extremely rare and has been reported only in females. The loss of skills is persistent and progressive, leading to severe and profound mental retardation. As the patients approach adolescence, there may be some improvement in social interests and developmental milestones. Seizure disorders frequently complicate this disorder.

Childhood Disintegrative Disorder

In this condition, the child is normal until at least 2 years of age. Between 2 and 10 years of age, the patient loses at least two of the following skills: language, social skills, motor skills, bowel or bladder control, and the ability to play. The child also has problems in two of the following areas: social interaction, communications, or repetitive behavior. Autistic Disorder differs from Childhood Disintegrative Disorder in that it occurs earlier (usually in infancy) and causes significant problems in all three areas. Childhood Disintegrative Disorder is a very rare condition.

The etiology is unknown; however, occasionally, a disorder causing developmental regression (metachromatic leukodystrophy) may be associated with it. After the loss of skills, this condition plateaus, from which there may be a slight improvement. Childhood Disintegrative Disorder is also complicated by severe mental retardation and an increased frequency of seizure disorders.

Asperger Disorder

The diagnostic features of Asperger disorder consist of severe impairment in social interactions coupled with restrictive, repetitive behaviors. According to the *DSM-IV*, the diagnostic criteria for Asperger syndrome consist of at least two impairments of social interactions (poor nonverbal communication, failure to develop peer relationships, lack of sharing, lack of emotional reciprocity) coupled with one or more repetitive, stereotypic patterns of behavior (repetitious motor movements, preoccupation with parts, inflexible adherence to rituals, intense preoccupation with a topic). Asperger Disorder differs from Autistic Disorder in that there are no impairments in cognitive function, including language. In addition, patients with Asperger Disorder are curious about the environment and develop appropriate self-help and adaptive (other than social) behavior.

The prevalence of Asperger syndrome is unknown. Preschool-aged children may have motor delay and clumsiness. As the patient gets older, difficulties with social interactions and empathy arise. The duration of this disorder is probably lifelong.

Psychologic Causes of Specific Delay

Selective Mutism

The patient with selective mutism has a persistent failure to speak in certain situations (for instance, the classroom), even though the individual can speak in other situations (at home). These symptoms must last for at least 1 month (but must not include the first month of school). In addition, the symptoms should not be caused by embarrassment from a speech problem (stuttering) or unfamiliarity with a language. Affected children are excessively shy and withdrawn and fear social embarrassment, whereas at home they may be oppositional or controlling.

The differential diagnosis includes communication disorders (not restricted to certain situations), pervasive developmental disorders (absence of language is in all settings), and Social Phobia. Patients with Social Phobia may present with Selective Mutism. Various psychologic interventions have been tried with varying levels of success; however, this condition usually remits spontaneously after several months.

REFERENCES

General References

American Psychiatric Association. Diagnostic and Statistical Manual of Mental Disorders, Fourth Edition. Washington, DC: American Psychiatric Association, 1994.

Canning EH, Hanser SB, Shade KA, et al. Mental disorders in chronically ill children: Parent-child discrepancy and physician identification. Pediatrics 1992;90:692–696.

Lavigne JV, Binns HJ, Christoffel KX, et al. Behavioral and emotional problems among preschool children in pediatric primary care: Prevalence and pediatrician's recognition. Pediatrics 1993;91:649–655.

Whitaker A, Johnson J, Shaffer D, et al. Uncommon troubles in young people: Prevalence estimates of selected psychiatric disorders in a non referred adolescent population. Arch Gen Psychiatry 1990;47:487–496.

Suicide

De Wilde EJ, Kienhorst I, Diekster R, et al. The specificity of psychological characteristics of adolescent suicide attempters. J Am Acad Child Adolesc Psychiatry 1993;32:51–59.

Hergenroeder AC, Kastner L, Farrow J, et al. The pediatrician's role in adolescent suicide. Pediatr Ann 1986;15:787–798.

Pfeffer CR, Klerman G, Hurt S, et al. Suicidal children grow up: Rates and psychological risks of suicide attempts during follow-up. J Am Acad Child Adolesc Psychiatry 1993;32:106–113.

Rudd DM. The prevalence of suicidal ideation among college students. Suicide Life Threat Behav 1989;19:173–183.

Shaffer D, Prudence F. The epidemiology of suicide in children and young adolescents. J Am Acad Child Adolesc Psychiatry 1981;20:545–565.

Chronic Disruptive Behaviors

American Academy of Child and Adolescent Psychiatry. Practice parameters for the assessment and treatment of attention deficit hyperactivity disorder. Washington, D.C.: American Academy of Child and Adolescent Psychiatry, 1991.

American Academy of Pediatrics, Committee on Substance Abuse. Role of the pediatrician in prevention and management of substance abuse. Pediatrics 1993;91:1010–1013.

Biederman J, Newcorn J, Sprich S. Comorbidity of attention deficit hyperactivity disorder with conduct, depressive, anxiety, and other disorders. Am J Psychiatry 1991;148:564–577.

Egan J. Oppositional defiant disorder. *In* Wiener JM (ed). Textbook of Child and Adolescent Psychiatry. Washington, D.C.: American Psychiatric Press, 1991:276–278.

Garfinkel BD, Amrami KK. Assessment and differential diagnosis of attention deficit hyperactivity disorder. Child Adolesc Psychiatr Clin North Am 1992;1:311–324.

Kazdin AE, Bass D, Siegel T, et al. Cognitive-behavioral therapy and relationship therapy in the treatment of children referred for antisocial behavior. J Consult Clin Psychol 1989;57:522–535.

Kelly PC, Cohen ML, Walker WO. Self-esteem in children medically managed for attention deficit disorder. Pediatrics 1989;83:211–217.

Leckman JF, Hardin MT, Riddle MA, et al. Clonidine treatment of Gilles de la Tourette's syndrome. Arch Gen Psychiatry 1991;48:324–328.

Malmquist CP. Conduct disorder: Conceptual and diagnostic issues. *In* Wiener JM (ed). Textbook of Child and Adolescent Psychiatry. Washington, DC: American Psychiatric Press, 1991:279–287.

Mannuzza S, Klein RG, Bessler A, et al. Adult outcome of hyperactive boys: Educational achievement, occupational rank, and psychiatric status. Arch Gen Psychiatry 1993;50:565–576.

Mayfield D, Mcleod G, Hall P. The Cage Questionnaire: Validation of a new alcoholism screening instrument. Am J Psychiatry 1974;131:1121–1123.

Reeves JC, Werry JS, Elkind GS, Zmetkin A. Attention deficit, conduct, oppositional, and anxiety disorders in children: II. Clinical characteristics. J Am Acad Child Adolesc Psychiatry 1987;26:144–155.

Shapiro E, Shapiro A, Fulop G, et al. Controlled study of haloperidol, pimozide and placebo for the treatment of Gilles de la Tourette's syndrome. Arch Gen Psychiatry 1989;46:722–730.

Smith HE, Margolis RD. Adolescent inpatient and outpatient chemical dependence treatment: An overview. Psychiatric Ann 1991;21:105–108.

Stokes A, Bawden HN, Camfield PR, et al. Peer problems in Tourette's disorder. Pediatrics 1991;87:936–942.

Episodic Disruptive Behaviors

Bernstein GA, Borchardt CM. Anxiety disorders of childhood and adolescence: A critical review. J Am Acad Child Adolesc Psychiatry 1991;30:519–532.

Bowen RC, Offord DR, Boyle MH. The prevalence of overanxious disorder and separation anxiety disorder: Results for the Ontario Child Health Study. J Am Acad Child Adolesc Psychiatry 1990;29:753–758.

Charney DS, Deutch AY, Krystal JH, et al. Psychobiologic mechanisms of post traumatic stress disorder. Arch Gen Psychiatry 1993;50:294–305.

Famularo R, Fenton T, Kinscherff R. Child maltreatment and the development of post traumatic stress disorder. Am J Dis Child 1993;147:755–760.

Flament MF, Koby E, Rapoport JL, et al. Childhood obsessive compulsive disorder: A prospective follow-up study. J Child Psychol Psychiatry 1990;31:363–380.

Fristad MA, Weller EB, Weller RA. Bipolar disorder in children and adolescents. Child Adolesc Psychiatr Clin North Am 1992;15:13–29.

Jenson PS, Ryan ND, Prien R. Psychopharmacology of child and adolescent major depression: Present status and future directions. J Child Adolesc Psychopharmacol 1992;2:31–45.

Kutcher SP, Reiter S, Gardner DM, et al. The pharmacotherapy of anxiety disorders in children and adolescents. Psychiatr Clin North Am 1992;15:41–67.

Larson EW, Richelson E. Organic causes of mania. Mayo Clin Proc 1988;63:906–912.

Ludolph PS, Westen D, Misle B, et al. The borderline diagnosis in adolescents: Symptoms and developmental history. Am J Psychiatry 1990;147:470–476.

McClellan JM, Werry JS. Schizophrenia. Psychiatr Clin North Am 1992;15:131–148.

Moreau D, Weissman MM. Panic disorder in children and adolescents: A review. Am J Psychiatry 1992;149:1306–1314.

Petti TA, Vela RM. Borderline disorders of childhood: An overview. J Am Acad Child Adolesc Psychiatry 1990;29:327–337.

Rauch SL, Jenike MA. Neurobiological models of obsessive-compulsive disorder. Psychosomatics 1993;34:20–32.

Stevenson J, Meares R. An outcome study of psychotherapy for patients with borderline personality disorder. Am J Psychiatry 1992;149:358–362.

Weissman MM, Klerman GL, Markowitz JS, et al. Suicidal ideation and suicide attempts in panic disorder and attacks. N Engl J Med 1989;3121:1209–1214.

Weller EB, Weller RA. Mood disorders. *In* Lewis M (ed). Child and Adolescent Psychiatry: A Comprehensive Textbook. Baltimore: Williams & Wilkins, 1991:646–664.

Hallucinations

Kotsopoulos S, Kanigsberg J, Côté A, et al. Hallucinatory experiences in non-psychotic children. J Am Acad Child Adolesc Psychiatry 1987;26:375–380.

Nagera H. The imaginary companion. Psychoanal Study Child 1969;24:165–196.

Schreier HA, Libow JA. Acute phobic hallucinations in very young children. J Am Acad Child Adolesc Psychiatry 1986;25:574–578.

Unexplained Physical Complaints

Agras WS, Rossiter EM, Arnow B, et al. Pharmacologic and cognitive behavioral treatment for bulimia nervosa: A controlled comparison. Am J Psychiatry 1992;149:82–87.

American Psychiatric Association. Practice guidelines for eating disorders. Am J Psychiatry 1993;150:207–228.

Benjamin PY. Psychological problems following recovery from acute life-threatening illness. Am J Orthopsychiatry 1978;48:284–290.

Eminson DM, Postlewaite RJ. Factitious illness: Recognition and management. Arch Dis Child 1992;67:1510–1516.

Fluoxetine Bulimia Nervosa Collaborative Study Group. Fluoxetine in the treatment of bulimia nervosa: A multicenter, placebo controlled, double-blind trial. Arch Gen Psychiatry 1992;43:139–147.

Herzog DB, Keller MB, Sacks NR, et al. Psychiatric co-morbidity in treatment-seeking anorexics and bulimics. J Am Acad Child Adolesc Psychiatry 1992;31:810–818.

Lehmkuhl G, Blahz B, Lehmkuhl U, et al. Conversion disorder (DSM-III-R 300-1), symptomatology and course in childhood and adolescence. Eur Arch Psychiatry Neurol Sci 1989;238:155–160.

Levy JC. Vulnerable children: Parents' perspectives and the use of medical care. Pediatrics 1980;65:956–963.

Maisami M, Freeman JM. Conversion reaction in children as body language: A combined child psychology/neurology team approach to the management of functional neurological disorder in children. Pediatrics 1987;80:46–52.

Meadows R. Management of Munchausen's syndrome by proxy. Arch Dis Child 1985;60:385–393.

Rosenberg D. Web of deceit: A literature review of Munchausen's syndrome by proxy. Child Abuse Negl 1987;2:547–563.

Sharp CW, Freeman CPL. The medical complications of anorexia nervosa. Br J Psychiatry 1993;162:452–462.

Turgay A. Treatment outcome for children and adolescents with conversion disorder. Can J Psychiatry 1990;35:585–587.

Wachsmuth JR, Garfinkel PE. The treatment of anorexia nervosa in young adolescents. Child Adolesc Psychiatr Clin North Am 1993;2:145–160.

Delayed Development

Cook EH, Rowlett R, Jaselskis C, et al. Fluoxetine treatment of children and adolescents with autistic disorder and mental retardation. J Am Acad Child Adolesc Psychiatry 1992;31:739–745.

Ghaziuddin M, Tsai LY, Ghaziuddin N. Brief report: A comparison of the diagnostic criteria for Asperger syndrome. J Autism Dev Disord 1992;22:643–649.

Gillberg C. Outcome in autism and autistic-like conditions. J Am Acad Child Adolesc Psychiatry 1991;30:375–382.

Van Acker R. Rett syndrome: A review of current knowledge. J Autism Dev Disord 1992;22:381–406.

Volkmar FR. Childhood disintegrative disorder: Issues for DSM-IV. J Autism Dev Disord 1992;22:625–642.

Volkmar FR, Nelson DS. Seizure disorder in autism. J Am Acad Child Adolesc Psychiatry 1990;29:127–129.

37 Child Abuse

Robert M. Reece

DEFINITIONS

Local statutes define for local jurisdictions what should legally be considered child abuse. Public Law 93–247, the Child Abuse Prevention and Treatment Act of 1974, defines *child abuse* as "the physical or mental injury, sexual abuse, negligent treatment, or maltreatment of a child under the age of eighteen by a person who is responsible for the child's welfare under circumstances which indicate the child's health or welfare is harmed or threatened thereby."

Kempe (1978) succinctly defines *child physical abuse* as "nonaccidental physical injuries as a result of acts or omissions on the part of the child's parents or guardians." Child-care lapses in environmental control, repetitive accidental poisonings, and failure to provide food, shelter, clothing, medical care, emotional support, or education should all be included as manifestations of maltreatment.

Definitions of *child sexual abuse* depend on the context because there are legal, psychosocial, medical, and cultural situations within which one can define it. Definitions are often omitted from descriptions of child sexual abuse, with the manifestations of the abuse serving to illustrate the phenomenon, thereby avoiding the task of drawing a line between abuse and other events. It is often left to observers, who must claim that they "know it when they see it." But there are definitions, and several are presented here to allow some delineation of this epidemic.

The National Center on Child Abuse and Neglect of the U.S. Department of Health and Human Services defines child sexual abuse as "contacts or interactions between a child and an adult for the sexual stimulation of the perpetrator or another person or sexual contacts or interactions between a child and a significantly older child who has power or control over the child."

The definition of child sexual abuse proposed by Kempe is "the involvement of children and adolescents in sexual activities they do not understand, to which they cannot give informed consent or that violate social taboos."

Legal definitions describe "sexual activity" as being divided into two categories: (1) sexual conduct, or intercourse, and (2) sexual contact, or the touching of the erogenous zones of another person for the purpose of sexually arousing or gratifying either person. Local jurisdictions then define levels of severity attached to the sexual activities described, taking into account the act itself, the age of the victim, and his or her capacity to object or defend against the act.

SEXUAL ABUSE

Incidence

National incidence studies of child sexual abuse suggest a rate of 2.5 cases per 1000 children. Approximately 1% of all children in the United States experience sexual abuse each year. Incidence and prevalence studies are inherently faulty and represent only educated guesses as to the true incidence or prevalence of abuse based on incomplete recognition, reporting, investigation, and substantiation.

Diagnostic Strategies

A child who has been sexually abused may come to the attention of a physician by having told someone of the abuse or by exhibiting—singly or in combination—behavioral or physical signs and symptoms.

Historical information may be derived from:

1. *Witnessed events.* The observation of sexual activity by an adult with a child may be seen by another child or adult. The details of this witnessing need to be clear as to time, what was seen, and the positive identification of the individuals involved.

2. *Admission by the perpetrator.*

3. *Disclosure by the victimized child.* This disclosure can be proximate in time to the event or events (or at a remote time from the event or events) and can be disclosed to an adult caretaker, a trusted friend, or an authority figure (police, child protection worker, teacher, physician, therapist, or other health care provider).

4. *Previous medical encounters.* In some cases, previous medical examinations will have been performed, and this information can provide important data.

MEDICAL HISTORY

A complete medical history, including the prenatal history, obstetric and perinatal events, childhood illnesses and hospitalizations, surgical procedures, and other contact with medical professionals, should be detailed. A careful review of systems may reveal symptoms referable to the present complaint. This exercise helps to avoid the pitfalls of misattribution of medical conditions to sexual abuse, and it also demonstrates good medical diagnostic work if the case comes to trial, where the strength of the legal case may rest on the medical evidence.

FAMILY AND SOCIAL HISTORY

It is the province of the examining physician to gather pertinent family and social history. This should include a description of the social and economic milieu. The marital status of the caretaking parent, the identity of the other members of the household, as well as the status of adult partners and friends who are occasional members of the household should be learned to understand the ecology of the allegation. Inquiries into a history of abuse in the childhood of the adult caretaker or current domestic violence should be made. Is there exposure to high risks of violence, drugs or alcohol, nutritional problems, or diseases? Are there psychiatric disorders apparent in the caretaker or in those with him or her at the time of the visit? Is there a history of emotional disorder in the caretaker or the child? Has there been previous involvement with law enforcement or social service agencies?

The occurrence of allegations of sexual abuse within the context of divorce or custody disputes has brought this situation to the forefront in the public mind. Examination of peer-reviewed literature indicates a very low incidence of sexual abuse in all divorce and custody cases (2%), with a higher incidence of proven "malicious" false allegations (5% to 14%). Nonetheless, all allegations of sexual abuse must be taken seriously and warrant thorough investigations. The emotional landscape of divorce is such that there may also be an increased incidence of all types of abuse perpetrated against the children trapped in these struggles.

BEHAVIORAL SIGNS AND SYMPTOMS

Nonspecific signs and symptoms can occur in a child reacting to a wide range of stresses and conflicts (enuresis, encopresis, disturbed sleep or eating patterns, changes in school performance, mood swings, irritability, temper outbursts). These can be present in sexually abused children but are not specific. Specific symptoms or signs of sexual abuse are the byproduct of inappropriate sexual exposure and are associated with sexual function in some way. Thus, unexpected knowledge in young children about sexual matters, unusual curiosity about sexual or excretory functions, asking others to engage in sexual acts, acting out sexually with toys or other children, or abnormal masturbatory activities are examples of specific symptoms suggestive of sexual abuse.

PHYSICAL SIGNS AND SYMPTOMS

There are also specific and nonspecific physical manifestations and important legitimate reasons for certain presenting complaints that must be taken into account when evaluating a child for possible sexual abuse. A child may have an innocent injury to private parts through play (straddle injury, penetrating injury); have dysuria, abdominal pain, proctitis, vaginitis, or vulvitis from nonsexually acquired infections (streptococcal cellulitis, intravaginal foreign body); or the child may have a nonsexual dermatologic problem (lichen sclerosus et atrophicus, severe contact dermatitis secondary to poor hygiene, seborrheic dermatitis). The 4-year-old child with a foul-smelling vaginal discharge not caused by a foreign body, or vaginal bleeding, or who demonstrates decreased anal tone with accompanying fecal soiling, however, has physical signs that suggest sexual abuse until careful evaluation proves otherwise.

THE MEDICAL INTERVIEW

Because of the nature of the information involved, the diagnostic task of the medical interview in a possible sexual abuse case may intimidate otherwise comfortable pediatricians. One must derive information from the child about what may be confusing, painful, and frightening to him or her and that may be perceived by the child in a completely different way than by adults. The objectives of the interview are to determine:

- the elements of the abuse
- who was involved
- when and how often it occurred
- where it occurred

The initial goal is to make the child comfortable and unafraid. The child and the adult bringing the child for the session should be informed of what will happen during the visit. It is often helpful to address the universal fear of children by assuring them that they are not going to have "shots" or any painful procedure during the course of the examination. The caregiver should be told that the examination does not involve the type of gynecologic examination used for adult women and that nothing is to be inserted into the child's vagina. The child can be reassured that the trusted adult with whom they came can be present during the examination. The caregiver should be interviewed separately from the child, and the interview with the child should be conducted after rapport has been established with him or her.

The first step in interviewing the child is to explain in simple terms that you are a "kid's doctor" and that at first you just want to get to know him or her. This can be done by "making friends" with the child in the form of "getting to know you" questions about his or her friends, pets, neighborhood, school, or interest in sports, television, music, or hobbies. This process can be enhanced by allowing the child to select a beverage or a treat prior to the beginning of the interview. In some clinics, younger children are presented with a choice of small stuffed animals to take home with them, and the animal is used for demonstration of the elements of the examination. The stuffed animal can be used to familiarize the child with the colposcope, allowing the child to look at the toy through the colposcope and then to take a picture of the animal with the flash attachment. This engages the child with the instrument and serves to demystify the process.

The interview must not involve leading questions, must be open-ended, and must use various forms of projective techniques for eliciting information. Projective techniques can include drawing, playing with toys in the room, and using doll houses and dolls (anatomically detailed or not). The interviewer should be supportive, unrushed, and friendly, and the interview should be conducted in a child-friendly environment. If more than one session is required, the same interviewer should ideally conduct the several sessions.

Eliciting information should start with general questions and proceed to more specific ones. Using an approach suggesting ignorance or puzzlement on the part of the examiner instills self-confidence in the child, and it allows the examiner to ask clarifying questions in the form of "I don't really understand what you said about . . ." or "I'm not real sure about one thing that you told me." Establishing the routines in the child's family environment can be a transition from the general discussion about the world outside of the home to the one within the home. It also allows a subtle transition to the more private areas of the child's life:

Where do you sleep?
Who puts you to bed?
Who helps you with your bath?

Once rapport has been established, greater focus can be brought to the issues of possible sexual abuse. The child may be asked if he or she knows the reason for this visit and if he or she could help make you understand what might have happened. This can be augmented by a discussion of "good touch, bad touch" or by asking the child to identify body parts on a picture. The language used by the interviewer influences the success of eliciting accurate information. Developmentally sensitive language should be employed that includes short, single-clause questions; the active voice; the clear use of names over pronouns; single negatives; short, understandable words; simple verbs; and direct statements. The child should be praised for the effort in the interview but not for the content. The use of phrases such as "some children have told me that . . ." or in some other way indicating that this discussion does not necessarily relate to them but to the outside universe is of use by giving the topic at hand an impersonal, abstract cast.

These techniques may elicit the exposition of the events in graphic and lengthy detail or may cause shutdown. The posing of the questions that turn from nonthreatening to threatening requires a sense of timing that experienced interviewers acquire and use intuitively. Most children, if comfortable, will disclose a clear and credible description of their experience.

The Credibility of Children's Histories of Sexual Abuse

From medical, psychosocial, and legal perspectives, it is necessary to evaluate the credibility of a child's recounting of what happened to him or her if sexual abuse is a consideration. Because children are often eager to please and desirous of providing the "right" answer, it is important that the examiner use clearly worded questions that encourage children to provide answers that will be viewed nonjudgmentally. Correct answers or scenarios should not be suggested by the interviewer because children may be influenced and are prone to suggestibility.

The issue of *lying* in childhood has been studied and may be classified. Reasons for lying include to avoid being punished; to get something one could not get otherwise; to protect friends from trouble; to protect oneself from harm; to win the admiration or interest of others; to avoid embarrassment; to maintain privacy; and to demonstrate one's power over an authority. Children do not lie to get into trouble, and the disclosure of sexual abuse, especially since the perpetrator has often intimidated or threatened the child not to tell about "their secret," puts the child at distinct risk. Consequently, when a child discloses sexual abuse to someone who has gained his or her trust, it usually represents the child's desire to escape from further harm and should be accepted as a truthful representation of the events described.

The issue of children's competency in testifying to the events around a sexual abuse allegation becomes a legal question; those doing the medical evaluation have the responsibility to gather information in the most objective manner using the best techniques available and to deliver this information clearly and without bias at the time of legal proceedings.

THE PHYSICAL EXAMINATION

Usually, permission for the performance of a sexual abuse evaluation should be obtained from the legal guardian. If the legal guardian is suspected of being the perpetrator, shielding the perpetrator, or—for some other reason—obstructing the evaluation of the child, some legal consultants believe the authority to perform necessary evaluations is covered under the child abuse reporting statutes. It is advisable in questionable cases to obtain legal advice before proceeding.

The site of the examination and the time of the alleged event or events determine to some extent the approach to the physical examination. If the alleged sexual abuse is thought to have occurred within the last 72 hours and to have involved contact with the perpetrator's genitalia, the collection of forensic evidence is required as an adjunct to the examination (see Chapter 31). If more than 72 hours have elapsed since the alleged contact, and the child is being seen in an emergency setting or where the examiners are inexperienced in conducting such evaluations, the patient should be examined with attention given to treatable acute injury (bleeding, tissue damage needing surgical care) or to signs or symptoms of infection needing culture analysis and treatment. If these are not present and the child is otherwise healthy and is in no danger of being re-exposed to the perpetrator, the child can be scheduled to be examined by professionals familiar with sexual abuse evaluations to avoid needless duplication of interviewing and examinations.

The goals of the physical examination are as follows:

1. "*Primum non nocere*—First, do no harm."
2. Diagnosis and treatment, where necessary, of injured tissue.
3. Diagnosis and treatment of sexually transmitted diseases.
4. Diagnosis and decisions regarding pregnancies in childbearing-age patients.
5. Thorough examination and documentation of medical forensic evidence where indicated.
6. Decisions about disposition and further diagnosis or therapy.
7. Documentation of the findings with a consideration of both medical and legal aspects.

Reiteration of the elements of the physical examination to the caregiver and to the child should be made after the medical interview. This explanation can be made to the child in the presence of the caregiver so that reassurances can be made to the caregiver and interpretation by the caregiver to the child can enhance the compliance of the child. If photocolposcopy is to be done, it should be explained to both the child and the caregiver that the pictures taken are identified only by numbers and that no one will be able to recognize who is in the pictures. Stressing the absence of painful procedures during the examination can be repeated, and the child should be assured that he or she has control over the procedure. Children should be told that the examiner is going to listen to their heart and lungs, look at their eyes, nose, and ears, check to see whether they have any lumps in their tummies, look at their "knees, toes, and bottom" to "make sure they are OK." One can

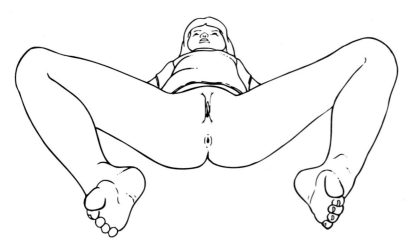

Figure 37–1. Supine frog-leg position for genital examination. (From Giardino AP, Finkel MA, Giardino ER, et al. A Practical Guide to the Evaluation of Sexual Abuse in the Prepubertal Child. Newbury Park, Calif: Sage Publications, 1992:69.)

also state that "if anytime during the examination you want me to stop, just tell me and I'll stop and we'll talk about what I'm doing."

It is also important to tell children that this examination should be done only by a doctor or nurse when their mother (or other trusted caregiver) is present and that no one else is allowed to do this kind of examination. The child should be allowed to ask questions about the examination before it is begun and anytime during the examination. Offering to let the child listen to his or her heart with the stethoscope is also helpful in establishing trust. Enlisting the child's cooperation with any equipment is often useful. If a colposcope is to be used, allowing children to look through the lens and to photograph a toy gains their interest in the instrument. Some colposcopes have been equipped with a long cable so that the child can actually trip the shutter when photographs are to be taken, and this focuses the child's attention on this activity.

A general physical examination should then proceed, with note of any medical findings both of relevance to the sexual abuse issue and to general medical conditions as well. During the examination, the child can be told of what the examiner has seen or heard and what will be done next. Carrying on a conversation with children about subjects of interest to them builds rapport and makes the next phase of the examination easier.

Under no circumstances should the child be forced to undergo any part of the examination. If the child is unable to cooperate after several attempts, consideration can be given to rescheduling the examination. If two attempts at a successful examination have failed, an examination under anesthesia may be scheduled.

Equipment

The conduct of a successful anogenital examination is dependent on the availability of necessary equipment. Although the colposcope is increasingly used in these evaluations and has been successful in augmenting our knowledge about normal and abnormal anogenital findings, its use is not mandatory. It is necessary, however, to have adequate examination tables, optimal lighting, some form of magnification (hand lens or otoscope), and a child-friendly environment for the examination. It is also desirable to be able to provide the child with toys or distracting objects. In addition, the requisite laboratory materials for the collection, transport, culturing, and confirmation of specimens involved in diagnosing sexually transmitted diseases; a microscope and wet mount materials; and experienced medical assistants with knowledge of the need to preserve the chain of evidence are the *sine qua non* of the process. When the need for forensic evidence is present, the availability of a Sex Crimes Kit and the knowledge about the collection and

delivery of such materials, maintaining the legal chain of evidence, must be at hand.

Positions for Examination

Most specialists in sexual abuse employ the supine frog-leg and knee-chest positions, either alone or in combination. The frog-leg position is arguably the most comfortable for the prepubertal child and the most frequently employed (Fig. 37–1). The child can assume this position on a flat table surface with or without stirrups. As the age of the child approaches adolescence, the use of stirrups makes the examination more acceptable because the adductor muscles of the thigh may be less pliant. The knee-chest position is somewhat less natural and comfortable; it is less stable when trying to focus for colposcopic photography (Fig. 37–2). However, some investigators maintain that without employing both positions, the posterior rim of the hymen may be incompletely evaluated.

In both the frog-leg and the knee-chest positions, separation and traction of the labia are necessary to visualize the introitus and the edges of the hymenal membrane. This is usually accomplished by simple lateral movement by the thumbs of the examiner (Fig. 37–3). Traction is carried out by holding the labia majora with the thumbs and forefingers of each hand and drawing these structures toward the examiner and downward (Fig. 37–4). Various movements during this traction enable the floor of the perineum to open,

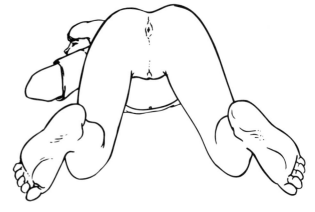

Figure 37–2. Knee-chest position for genital examination of the prepubertal child to supplement the supine frog-leg position. (From Giardino AP, Finkel MA, Giardino ER, et al. A Practical Guide to the Evaluation of Sexual Abuse in the Prepubertal Child. Newbury Park, Calif: Sage Publications, 1992:71.)

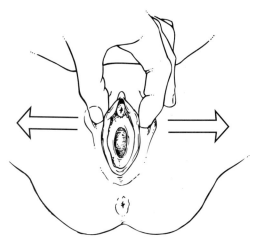

Figure 37–3. Examination of female external genitalia. (From Giardino AP, Finkel MA, Giardino ER, et al. A Practical Guide to the Evaluation of Sexual Abuse in the Prepubertal Child. Newbury Park, Calif: Sage Publications, 1992:73.)

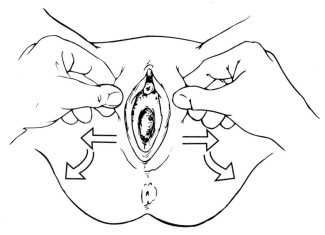

Figure 37–4. Examination of female external genitalia. (From Giardino AP, Finkel MA, Giardino ER, et al. A Practical Guide to the Evaluation of Sexual Abuse in the Prepubertal Child. Newbury Park, Calif: Sage Publications, 1992:72.)

allowing good visualization. Examination of the anus can be done with the child in these same positions or in the left lateral decubitus position (Fig. 37–5).

The appearance of the normal anatomy of the prepubertal female is shown in Figure 37–6. An example of penetrating sexual abuse is noted in Figure 37–7.

TYPES OF SEXUAL ABUSE

Sexual abuse occurs by way of a variety of sexual contacts. Fondling usually produces no physical findings, but when it progresses to digital contact and ultimately penetration, the resulting trauma can range from erythema to abrasion or laceration of the vaginal walls, depending on the amount of force, the penetrating object (finger, penis, instrument), and the degree of penetration involved. Chronic digital abuse can be manifested by changes in the hymenal contour, healed transections, or the attentuations of the hymenal membrane until it is barely visible. When acute penile contact occurs, it can produce erythema, edema, bruising of the vulvar and perivestibular tissue, hymenal distortion, transections, vaginal edema, erythema, or abrasions. In long-standing cases, the vaginal orifice may take on a distinctly dilated character (see Fig. 37–7).

Oral-genital contact by the perpetrator can cause petechiae, edema, bruising, and abrasions, but in most instances no residual trauma is seen.

Anal findings are even more nonspecific owing to the natural distensibility of the anal sphincter. Findings of bruising, laxity of the anal sphincter, and immediate dilation of the anus during the examination, especially in the absence of stool in the rectum, are of concern. Major forced trauma to the anus and perianal structures produces more significant injuries; findings of this magnitude are rare. The perpetrators of child sexual abuse generally intend not to produce discernible injuries, since they want continuing access to their victims.

Classification of Anogenital Findings in Children with Suspected Abuse

The determination of normal and abnormal in the examination of the sexually abused prepubertal female has been difficult. Most children with documented sexual abuse do not have any specific anogenital findings. Only 20% to 25% of known sexually abused children have specific anogenital medical evidence. One classification of medical findings in child sexual abuse examinations includes (Table 37–1):

Class 1: Normal. Variations in the appearance of the hymen, perihymenal tissues, and perianal tissues documented in more than 10% of the subjects in studies of nonabused children.

Class 2: Nonspecific. Findings that may be the result of sexual abuse but may also be due to other nonabusive causes.

Class 3: Suspicious. Findings that are rarely seen in nonabused

Figure 37–5. Hand placement for separation of the buttocks to view external anal tissues with the child in the left lateral decubitus position. (From Giardino AP, Finkel MA, Giardino ER, et al. A Practical Guide to the Evaluation of Sexual Abuse in the Prepubertal Child. Newbury Park, Calif: Sage Publications, 1992:74.)

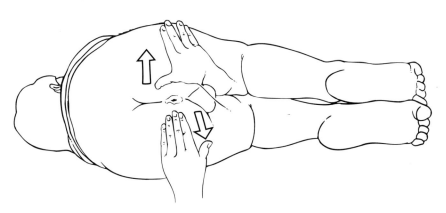

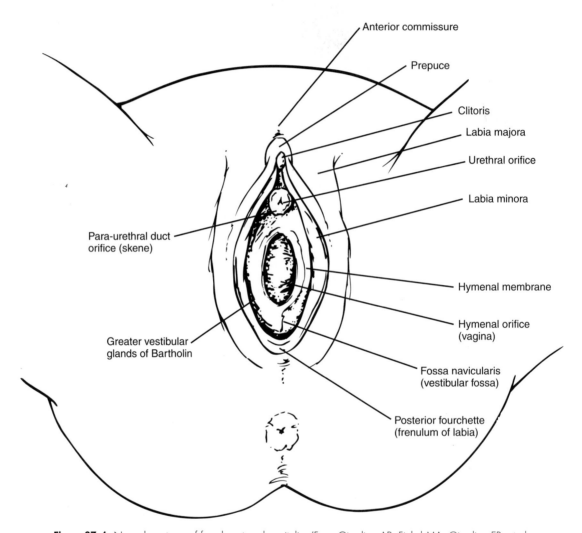

Anterior commissure

Prepuce

Clitoris

Labia majora

Urethral orifice

Labia minora

Para-urethral duct
orifice (skene)

Hymenal membrane

Hymenal orifice
(vagina)

Greater vestibular
glands of Bartholin

Fossa navicularis
(vestibular fossa)

Posterior fourchette
(frenulum of labia)

Figure 37–6. Normal anatomy of female external genitalia. (From Giardino AP, Finkel MA, Giardino ER, et al. A Practical Guide to the Evaluation of Sexual Abuse in the Prepubertal Child. Newbury Park, Calif: Sage Publications, 1992:32.)

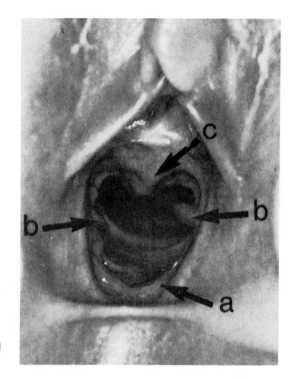

Figure 37–7. A 7-year-old child sexually molested by father and uncle. Labial traction method. Narrow hymenal rim *(arrow a)* with exposed ridges *(arrow b)* at the 3- and 9-o'clock positions. Anterior column *(arrow c)*. Enlarged hymenal orifice. Colposcopic photographs (magnification × 10). (From McCann J. Use of the colposcope in childhood sexual abuse examinations. Pediatr Clin North Am 1990;37:863–881.)

Table 37–1. Proposed Classification of Anogenital Findings in Children

Normal (Class 1)
Periurethral (or vestibular) bands
Longitudinal intravaginal ridges
Hymenal tags
Posterior (inferior) hymenal rim measuring at least
   1-mm wide
Estrogen changes (uniformly thickened, redundant hymen)
Hymenal clefts in the anterior (superior) half of the hymenal
   rim: on or above the 3 to 9 o'clock line, patient supine
Hymenal bumps or mounds
Diastasis ani (smooth area) at 6 or 12 o'clock position in the
   perianal area
Anal tag/thickened fold in midline
Increased perianal pigmentation

Nonspecific (Class 2)
Erythema of vestibule or perianal tissues
Increased vascularity of vestibule or hymen
Labial adhesions
Vaginal discharge
Lesions of condyloma acuminata in a child less than
   2 yr old
Anal fissures
Flattened anal folds
Anal dilation with stool present
Venous congestion of perianal tissues

Suspicious for Abuse (Class 3)
Enlarged hymenal opening (>2 standard deviations above mean
   for age and position)
Immediate venous congestion of perianal tissues with edema
   and/or distorted anal folds
Anal dilation of at least 20 mm with stool not visible in rectal
   vault
Posterior hymenal rim less than 1 mm in all views
Condyloma acuminata in a child older than 2 yr of age
Acute abrasions or lacerations in the vestibule or on the labia
   (not involving the hymen)

Suggestive of Abuse/Penetration (Class 4)
Combination of two or more suspicious anal findings or two or
   more suspicious genital findings
Scar of fresh laceration of the posterior fourchette
Perianal scar

Clear Evidence of Penetrating Injury (Class 5)
Areas in the posterior (inferior) half of the hymenal rim with an
   absence of hymenal tissue, confirmed in knee-chest position
Obvious hymenal transections
Perianal lacerations extending beyond (deep to) the external
   anal sphincter
Recent hymenal-vaginal lacerations
Lacerations through the hymen and posterior fourchette or
   perineum

children and have been noted in children with documented abuse but have not been clearly proven to occur only as a result of abuse.

Class 4: Suggestive of abuse or penetration. Findings, or a combination of findings, that can be reasonably explained only by postulating that sexual abuse or penetrating injury has occurred. This type of finding mandates a report to a law enforcement and child protective service, even if the child is unable to give a clear history of molestation, assuming there is no clear and consistent history of accidental penetrating injury.

Class 5: Clear evidence of penetrating injury. Findings that can have no explanation other than penetrating trauma to the hymen or perianal tissues.

The assessment and likelihood of abuse are noted in Table 37–2.

LABORATORY EVIDENCE

Prepubertal children with sexually transmitted diseases (STDs) are considered the victims of sexual abuse (see Chapter 31). The

---

Table 37–2. Overall Assessment of the Likelihood of Sexual Abuse

Class 1—No Evidence of Sexual Abuse
1:1 Normal examination, no history, no behavioral changes, no witnessed abuse
1:2 Nonspecific findings with another known etiology, and no history or behavioral changes
1:3 Child considered at risk for sexual abuse but gives no history and has nonspecific behavioral changes
1:4 Physical findings of injury consistent with accidental trauma with history given

Class 2—Possible Abuse
2:1 Class 1, 2, or 3 findings in combination with significant behavioral changes, especially sexualized behaviors, but child unable to give history of abuse
2:2 Presence of condyloma or herpes simplex type 1 (genital) in the absence of a history of abuse, with otherwise normal examination
2:3 Child has made a statement but no detailed or consistent history
2:4 Class 3 findings with no disclosure of abuse

Class 3—Probable Abuse
3:1 Child gives a clear, consistent, detailed description of molestation, with or without other findings present
3:2 Class 4 or 5 findings in a child, with or without a history of abuse, in the absence of any convincing history of accidental penetrating injury
3:3 Culture-proven infection with *Chlamydia trachomatis* (child >2 yr of age) in a prepubertal child; also culture-proven herpes simplex type 2 infection in a child, or documented *Trichomonas* infection

Class 4—Definite Evidence of Abuse or Sexual Contact
4:1 The finding of sperm or seminal fluid in or on a child's body
4:2 A witnessed episode of sexual molestation; this also applies to cases in which pornographic photographs or videotapes are acquired as evidence
4:3 Nonaccidental, blunt penetrating injury to the vaginal or anal orifice
4:4 Positive, confirmed cultures for *Neisseria gonorrhoeae* in a prepubertal child, or serologic confirmation of acquired syphilis
4:5 Pregnancy

---

most common STDs acquired through sexual abuse are gonorrhea, chlamydial infection, and syphilis (Table 37–3). Other STDs associated with sexual abuse are herpes simplex, condyloma acuminatum, trichomoniasis, human immunodeficiency virus (HIV) infection, and pediculosis pubis.

The Centers for Disease Control and Prevention (CDC) recommended in 1989 that the following be obtained for sexually abused children:

- Oral, anal, and genital culture specimens for gonorrhea and chlamydia
- A Gram stain of any genital or anal secretions
- A wet preparation for *Trichomonas*
- Culture of lesions consistent with herpes simplex
- Serologic testing for syphilis and HIV, with repeated serologic testing in 12 weeks

When there is history of oral-genital, oral-anal, genital-anal, or genital-genital contact, culture specimens should be obtained from these sites.

Although histories from children, especially the young, cannot supply adequate information as to the type of contact, older children are often able to give quite accurate histories as to the events of sexual contact. More selective testing can be based on the epidemiology of diseases in a given locale. Recent studies have shown a very low recovery of gonorrhea and chlamydia from asymptomatic children. The safest course of action is to adhere to strict guidelines, but clinical judgment based on the circumstances of each individual case should be applied.

For specific therapy of STDs, see Chapter 31.

Collection of Forensic Materials

Five conditions should be adhered to prior to the collection of specimens:

1. Specific details of collection labeling and packaging of specimens should be determined with the processing laboratory.
2. A specimen collection protocol should be used to ensure that all appropriate specimens are collected.
3. Collection kits should be standardized.
4. The procedures for collecting specimens should be explained in advance to the child and his or her caretaker.
5. Proper consent should be obtained before performing the collection.

If forensic evidence is to be gathered, it should be done within 72 hours of the event, since material is rarely recoverable after that time (Table 37–4). The handling of collected specimens should be documented to maintain a chain of evidence to prevent challenges about confusing specimens from different patients.

Differential Diagnosis

The correct diagnosis of sexual abuse in children can lead to intervention that is sometimes life saving. In many cases, the recognition of abuse provides the opportunity for the child to enter a new, protected, and nourishing life. The long-term outcome for some adults in whom the diagnosis was not made in childhood is a life of mistrust and maladjustment. We do not know the outcome in children in whom a misdiagnosis of child sexual abuse set in motion a process that was, in the very least, disruptive and, in the worst case, tragic. It behooves the diagnostician to be aware of the possible reasons for mistaking physical findings for child abuse when the cause is from another source (Table 37–5).

Table 37–3. Incubation, Diagnosis, and Implications of Sexually Transmitted Diseases (STDs) in Prepubertal Children

STDs	Incubation	Diagnosis	Relationship to Sexual Abuse
Gonococcal infection	2–7 days	Culture confirmed by two or more confirmatory tests	Certain*
Syphilis	10–90 days	RPR or VDRL test confirmed by FTA-ABS or MHA-TP test	Certain*
Chlamydial infection	Variable	Culture only: rapid techniques lack adequate specificity	Probable*
Human papillomavirus infection	1–9 mo (? 20 mo)	Inspection, application of acetic acid, or biopsy and viral typing	Probable*
Trichomoniasis	4–20 days	Wet mount of discharge, culture more sensitive	Probable*
Herpes simplex, virus type 2 infection	2–14 days	Culture with viral typing	Probable*
Herpes simplex, virus type 1 infection	2–14 days	Culture with viral typing	Possible
Bacterial vaginosis	7–14 days?	"Clue cells" on wet mount and positive "whiff" test	Uncertain
Genital mycoplasma infection	2–3 wk?	Culture	Uncertain
HIV infection	6 wk to 18 mo	ELISA confirmed by Western blot	Uncertain

From Finkel MA, De Jong AR. Medical findings in child sexual abuse. *In* Reece RM (ed). Child Abuse: Medical Diagnosis and Management. Malvern, Pa: Lea & Febiger, 1994:185–248.
*Except when perinatal transmission is documented.
Abbreviations: RPR = rapid plasma reagin; VDRL = Venereal Disease Research Laboratory; FTA-ABS = fluorescent treponemal antibody absorption; MHA-TP = microhemagglutination–*Treponema pallidum*; HIV = human immunodeficiency virus; ELISA = enzyme-linked immunosorbent assay.

Diagnostic Formulation

Few cases of alleged sexual abuse follow a smooth course from the chief complaint to a firm and unassailable diagnosis. Individuals who provide clear and convincing disclosure information, exhibit behavioral signs and symptoms known to be induced by sexual abuse, and demonstrate definitive anatomic changes secondary to the trauma of sexual abuse may not have their cases supported by the protective and judicial system. Children who provide disclosure information that is borderline or equivocal may be the victims of abuse. It is incumbent on the evaluators to be able to gather meaningful information and to analyze and synthesize it so that a balanced, accurate, and holistic appraisal of the case is accomplished.

The three critical components of diagnosis of child sexual abuse are:

1. The disclosure information.
2. The physical and behavioral signs and symptoms.
3. The positive results of the medical examination.

Foremost in importance are the quality and credibility of the child's description of the events and the techniques used in evincing the information. A disclosure statement is theoretically possible in all cases if child sexual abuse has occurred in a verbal child. This is the best and most reliable evidence. The specificity of a sexualized origin for signs and symptoms determines the value of this category of information. Physical and behavioral symptoms are variably present and can be challenging if it is possible to cast doubt about their origin. The finding of definitive diagnostic anatomic changes is of great value but occurs in a low proportion of cases (15% to 30%). Positive culture or serology results in STDs have value in direct proportion to the STD involved, the detection method used, and the specificity of the STD in sexual abuse.

Reporting Child Abuse

Uniform statutes exist in all 50 states mandating that physicians report to the child protective services bureau in their local jurisdiction all cases in which a "reasonable" suspicion exists that child abuse has occurred. Absolute certainty is not required, and it is recognized that more information needs to be developed by the child protection agency to decide whether a case is founded. Immunity from suit for reporting exists in these laws, and unless it can be proven that malicious intent was present, the reporter who reports in good faith is immune from legal action by caretakers. There are both civil and criminal penalties for failing to report when suspicion exists. Consultation is usually readily available from child protection agencies by telephone on a 24-hour basis if doubt about the need to report exists.

Problems of diagnosis are noted in Table 37–6, and indications for consultation are noted in Table 37–7.

PHYSICAL ABUSE

Two separate domains exist in cases of physical injury in which child abuse could be the pathogenesis. The first domain—a strictly medical one—requires a traditional medical or surgical approach and diagnosis followed by a management strategy. The second domain requires a decision as to whether the observed phenomenon is due to inflicted injury, a medical disease process, or an accidental injury. Standard medical and surgical approaches are the central concerns in the first domain, with optimal management required to obtain the best short-term outcome. Within the second domain lies the challenge of securing the best comprehensive outcome for the child and family. This requires the skills and wisdom of the interdisciplinary team both at the hospital and the community levels.

Table 37–4. Collecting Forensic Specimens in Sexual Abuse Cases

1. Obtain 2–3 swabbed specimens from each area of body assaulted (for sperm, acid phosphatase, P 30, MHS-5 antigen, blood group antigen determinations). The number of swabs required depends on local laboratory. Most laboratories request air-dried specimens, which require drying for 60 min before they can be packaged.

2. Mouth: Swab under tongue and buccal pouch next to upper and lower molars. These areas are locations where seminal fluid is most likely to be persistent.

3. Vagina: Use dry or moistened swab or 2 ml saline wash. Remember that overdilution of secretions may produce false-negative results of tests for acid phosphatase. Secretions may also be collected with a pipette or eyedropper.

4. Rectum: Insert swab at least ½ to 1 inch beyond anus.

5. Specimens should be taken from any other suspicious site on the body. Saline or sterile water–moistened swabs may be used to lift any stains suspected to be dried seminal fluid or blood. An alternate method is to scrape off the dried stains with the back of a scalpel blade into a clean envelope or tube.

6. Make saline wet mount of specimens from all assaulted orifices and examine immediately for presence of motile and nonmotile sperm.

7. Some forensic laboratories request a dry smear of each secretion sample using clean glass microscope slides; others prefer to prepare their own slides from swab specimens.

8. Collect saliva specimen to determine the victim's antigen secretion status. Saliva may be collected using 3–4 sterile swabs or a 2 × 2 gauze pad that the victim placed in the mouth.

9. Obtain a venous blood sample from the victim for antigen secretor status. This sample from the victim will be used in the analysis of the identity of the perpetrator.

10. Save torn or bloody clothes or any clothing when semen staining is suspected, using Wood's lamp. Semen may fluoresce with a blue or green color under the ultraviolet light of the Wood's lamp, although fluorescence under UV light is nonspecific. Various skin infections, congenital or acquired skin pigmentary changes, and chemicals including systemic and topical medications, cosmetics, soaps, and industrial chemicals may fluoresce under UV light.

11. If the victim was wearing a tampon, pad, or diaper during the assault or if a fresh tampon, pad, or diaper was used after the abuse, save this for analysis; seminal fluid products may be found on these items. Plastic bags should be used only on dry specimens and only if directed so by the laboratory. Sealed plastic may promote the growth of *Candida* and other organisms that might destroy some of the evidence.

12. Save any foreign material found on removal of clothing. Fiber analysis or trace analysis may provide evidence that links the specimens to the perpetrator or the location of the abuse.

13. Collect samples of combed pubic hair or scalp hair and fingernail scrapings. These procedures are often considered optional. Pubic hair, scalp hair, or skin fragments from scratching may be used to help identify the perpetrator. Control samples of the victim's body or scalp hair are collected for comparison. Usually, it is recommended that the hairs be plucked rather than cut, although the additional trauma of plucking 10 to 20 hairs from a child may not be warranted unless foreign hair material is found on the child's body. Some protocols recommend considering cutting hairs or collecting plucked hairs at a later time if needed.

14. Specimens should also be taken to screen for sexually transmitted diseases. The recommended procedures are detailed in the text. Swabs should *not* be air dried because air drying kills the organisms and causes the cultures for these diseases to be falsely negative. Specimens for culture should be sent quickly to a microbiology laboratory for processing and not be included with the materials to be processed in the forensic laboratory.

From Finkel MA, De Jong AR. Medical findings in child sexual abuse. *In* Reece RM (ed). Child Abuse: Medical Diagnosis and Management. Malvern, Pa: Lea & Febiger, 1994.

Incidence and Prevalence

In 1992, it was estimated that 2,936,000 children were reported to public social service agencies for abuse or neglect, or both. This represents a 132% increase over the last decade. Approximately 1261 children died from child abuse during that year. In 1990, 27% of the reports were for physical abuse, 45% for neglect, 15% for sexual abuse, 9% for emotional maltreatment, and 4% for other forms of maltreatment.

Neglect occurs when a caretaker responsible for a child either deliberately or by extraordinary inattentiveness permits a child to suffer or fails to provide one or more of the conditions generally deemed essential for developing a person's physical, intellectual, or emotional capacities, or both. A child is *physically neglected* when his or her needs for food, shelter, or clothing are omitted; *emotionally neglected* when he or she is denied nurturing qualities necessary for sound personality development; *medically neglected* when usual and locally accepted minimum levels of preventive, diagnostic, or therapeutic medical services are not provided by parents or guardians; and *educationally neglected* when a caretaker fails to ensure education as provided by state law.

Accident or Abuse?

An accident is defined as an event that occurs incidentally, casually, or by chance. It is presumed that such an event was at least consciously unintentional and that if such circumstances were under conscious control, an attempt would have been made to avert the anticipated event. An intentional event or action is one that occurs voluntarily and assumes conscious—or perhaps even unconscious—control, reflecting an underlying conflict or impulse.

In possible child abuse cases, there is a continuum from what appears to be a volitional act to what appears to be a chance event. The distinction must be made, taking into account the setting of the event (social context, location of encounter), the biases of the observer and the reporter, the type of injury (likelihood of observed

Table 37–5. Conditions Confused with Child Sexual Abuse

Dermatologic Conditions	Injuries	Infections
Erythema and excoriations	Straddle injuries	Vaginitis with organisms not
Diaper rash	Violent abduction of the legs	sexually transmitted
Poor hygiene	Motor vehicle accidents	Group A beta-hemolytic
Candida	Self-destructive behavior in retarded children	streptococcus
Pinworms	Female circumcision	*Shigella*
Allergy/irritants		Pinworms
Bruises	**Anal Conditions**	Nonpathologic *Neisseria* species
Hematologic disorders	Severe or chronic constipation and megacolon	*Haemophilus*
Mongolian spots	Postmortem anal dilation	Varicella
Hypersensitivity vasculitis	Neurogenic patulous anus (myotonic dystrophy)	Molluscum
Purpura fulminans	Fistula	Perinatally acquired
Coining and other folk practices	Inflammatory bowel disease	*Chlamydia*
Phytodermatitis	Pinworms	Syphilis
Other	Lichen sclerosus	Herpes simplex virus (HSV)
Lichen sclerosus	Hemolytic-uremic syndrome	Human papillomavirus (HPV)
Seborrheic, atopic, and contact dermatitis	Rectal polyps or tumor	infection
Lichen planus	Eversion of the anal canal/rectal prolapse	Autoinoculation
Lichen simplex chronicus		HSV type 1
Psoriasis	**Urethral Conditions**	HPV (warts)
	Prolapse	Infection with cyclic/idiopathic
Congenital Conditions	Caruncle	neutropenia
Midline pits, fusion defects, shiny areas	Hemangioma	Non–sexually transmitted disease
Prominent median raphe	Polyps	causes of genital ulcers
Midline tags	Papilloma	
Linea vestibularis	Cyst	
Distasis recti (depressed fan-shaped areas)	Condyloma	
Genital hemangiomas	Sarcoma botryoides	
	Prolapsed bladder or ureterocele	

From Bays JA. Conditions mistaken for child sexual abuse. *In* Reece RM (ed). Child Abuse: Medical Diagnosis and Management. Malvern, Pa: Lea & Febiger, 1994:386–404.

injury or injuries being due to an accidental mechanism), and the future risk to the child, if it is at all predictable.

The approach, however, both to the medical or surgical diagnosis and to the determination of the etiology of the observed condition is a traditional medical one: accurate and comprehensive historical investigation, thorough physical examination, and discerning selection of laboratory and imaging modalities to establish the extent and complexity of the disease state and how it came to be.

Table 37–6. Pitfalls in the Diagnostic Process—Twelve Costly Errors

1. A desire not to make the diagnosis.
2. Failure to assemble past information on medical conditions and medical encounters.
3. Too great a reliance on the information developed by others.
4. Transference-countertransference with custodial parent (formation of alliances or development of hostilities).
5. Overinterpretation or underinterpretation of signs and symptoms.
6. Overinterpretation or underinterpretation of physical findings.
7. Failure to know about conditions mistaken for sexual abuse.
8. Faulty laboratory techniques resulting in either false-positive or false-negative reports.
9. Use of techniques easily challenged in court.
10. Impatience about arriving at a diagnostic conclusion.
11. Failure to understand normative data with regard to psychosexual development.
12. Failure to prepare adequately for court appearances.

Several questions help to distinguish accidental from inflicted injury:

1. What is the age of the patient? Developmental stages of childhood determine what kinds of injuries are likely to be seen. The motor skills of the child determine what the child could have done to incur injury. What can they do at a particular stage of development? What are they likely to be doing? What are the normal behaviors of a child at particular ages? Is the child "hyperactive" either in the eyes of his or her caretakers or in actual fact? Is the child a "daredevil"? Is the child obstreperous, combative, or possessive of a "high annoyance potential" and therefore more likely to be disciplined harshly?

2. Is the history plausible? Could this injury have been sustained in the manner described?

3. Does the history change with changing information supplied to the caretaker? Adjustments in the account of the injury may be made by caretakers to fit the evolving information, indicating that the history is being tailored to fit the new information.

4. Does the history change when related in subsequent accounts by other family members?

Table 37–7. When to Seek Consultation

1. If one is not prepared to work in an interdisciplinary group.
2. If one is not prepared to see the case through from initial encounter through the investigation and ultimate legal resolution.
3. If one's knowledge base about any of the components of the evaluation is too narrow.
4. If there are areas of uncertainty about the diagnosis.

5. Are there nonfamilial eyewitnesses to the injury?

6. Was the injury unwitnessed by the caretaker? The lack of information as to how a serious injury has occurred should raise the index of suspicion for an abusive origin.

7. Is the demeanor of the caretakers defensive, belligerent, hostile, or passive and not in keeping with the seriousness of the patient's condition?

8. Is the social situation in which the injury occurred a high-risk environment? The presence of community or intrafamilial violence, substance abuse, chaotic living arrangements, poverty, social isolation, transient lifestyles, mental health aberrations, or discord among family members should serve as *red flags*.

9. Can the described mechanism of injury account for the observed injury? The concept of the discrepant history is a central one in distinguishing between accidental and inflicted injury. Often the injury is explained by claiming that it was caused by a fall. A large literature has emerged that discounts falls from short distances as being responsible for serious injuries, but short falls—down steps, off beds, couches, or tables, and in baby walkers—are often erroneously cited as the mechanisms of injury for serious injuries in actual abuse cases. The role of torsion must be considered in fractured bones, and it should be remembered that for a torsion injury to exist, one end of a long bone must be fixed and tremendous torsional force must be applied to the long axis of the bone to cause such injuries. The issue of how much force is required to produce injuries must be addressed and a conclusion reached on the basis of information derived from the literature on actual trauma victims.

10. What else might produce the clinical picture?

Head Injuries

More fatalities and long-term morbidity are due to abusive head injury than to any other form of maltreatment. The types of abusive head injuries range from asymptomatic tissue swelling, to mild to moderate bruising, to skull fracture, to intracranial bleeding and diffuse axonal shearing injury and brain swelling resulting in stupor, coma, and death. When a child younger than 3 years of age comes for medical care with a serious head injury without a readily apparent major trauma history (motor vehicle accident, fall from heights over 10 feet), the chances of this being an inflicted injury are quite high.

DATA COLLECTION

While a seriously head-injured child is being evaluated and treated medically, it is crucial for a detailed, analytic—but not challenging or accusatory—history to be obtained from the caretakers. The person collecting the history should ideally be someone with experience in child abuse cases who does not have immediate responsibility for the medical treatment required by the child.

It is the rule that abusing parents will tell a misleading story about how the ''accident'' happened and are sometimes quite inventive in describing the event. Gentle probing, with inquiries and request for clarification about questionable portions of the history by repeating the inquiry but in the form of a different question, will often elicudate the mechanism of injury and show discrepancies in the history.

The history of the pregnancy, labor and delivery, and neonatal course as well as a history of family diseases is important, with particular attention to bleeding and clotting disorders, neurologic diseases, metabolic and bone disease, or other genetic conditions of the family. This comprehensive evaluation will save returning to the caretakers for missing data as the case progresses. The

medical history of the child, including previous injuries and serious illnesses or hospitalizations, along with a review of systems, should be obtained. Exploration of the social milieu with attention to the living arrangements and the relationships of household members should be done.

PHYSICAL EXAMINATION

The physical examination of the child with a head injury involves the risk of ignoring less urgently compromised organ systems (see Chapter 41). Bleeding visceral organs are the most glaring and potentially disastrous omissions, but overlooking cutaneous injuries can deprive the diagnostician of important clinical data because of the fleeting nature of these injuries. Likewise, inspection of the oral cavity for intraoral lesions is important, as is a search for scalp lesions hidden under the hair. The neck should be carefully inspected for signs of injury (strangulation, hand- or finger-inflicted bruising). The presence of bruises on the back or thighs or in the perineum should also be noted. *Photodocumentation* of such injuries is highly desirable.

The examination of the fundi is of utmost importance. This should ideally be carried out by pupillary dilation and indirect opththalmoscopic inspection, but in lieu of that capability, by direct ophthalmoscopy. Although retinal hemorrhages are the most common finding in child abuse, other lesions may also be seen. These include retinal detachment, optic nerve injury, and cupping of the optic nerve secondary to raised intracranial pressure. Although retinal hemorrhages are not pathognomonic for inflicted head trauma, they are present in a high percentage of abuse cases, are not present in most accidental head trauma cases, and are seldom seen in children who have undergone cardiopulmonary resuscitation.

LABORATORY STUDIES

Children with head trauma severe enough to be admitted to the hospital should also have laboratory studies to support diagnoses of associated trauma in other organ systems, to anticipate hematologic and biochemical alterations sometimes attendant to head trauma, and to document and monitor their neurologic status. These studies are listed in Table 37–8.

Table 37–8. Laboratory Studies in Physical Abuse

Complete blood count with morphology; serial hematocrit levels
Serum electrolytes, blood urea nitrogen, creatinine, serum and urine osmolality
Urinalysis
Liver function studies (aspartate aminotransferase, alanine aminotransferase, bilirubin, alkaline phosphatase)
Serum and urinary amylase
Creatine phosphokinase
Cultures of blood, urine, cerebrospinal fluid (if safe to perform lumbar puncture)
Prothrombin time, partial thromboplastin time, platelet count
Stool for blood
Arterial blood gases

IMAGING STUDIES

In most instances of moderate to severe head injury, the first imaging modality should be computed tomography (CT) scanning without contrast, since it is readily available in most hospitals and can be performed safely with life-support systems operating during

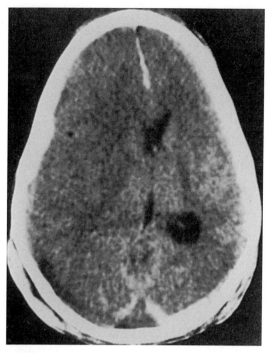

Figure 37–9. A 3-month-old abused infant. Unenhanced CT image reveals generalized right-sided decrease in brain density owing to diffuse cerebral edema. The right lateral ventricle is effaced, and there is a shift of midline structures to the left. Posterior as well as anterior subdural interhemispheric hemorrhage is also present. (From Merten DF, Carpenter BLM. Radiologic imaging of inflicted injury in the child abuse syndrome. Pediatr Clin North Am 1990;37:815–839.)

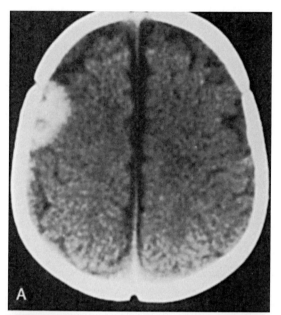

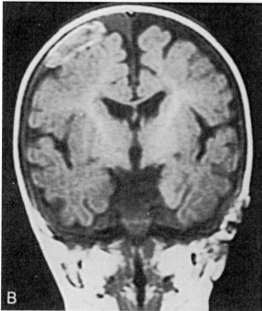

Figure 37–8. A 6-month-old infant with seizures. A, Axial unenhanced CT image reveals a focal acute high-density hematoma over the right cerebral convexity. There is generalized enlargement of the extracerebral spaces, reflecting either chronic subdural hematoma or brain atrophy. B, Coronal T1-weighted MRI scan shows the acute right convexity subdural hematoma as a high-signal-intensity mass. A lower-signal-intensity subacute subdural hematoma surrounds the acute lesion. There is also generalized brain atrophy with increased extracerebral space; the normal cerebrospinal fluid over the left cerebral convexity is of lower signal intensity than the subacute hematoma over the right convexity. (From Merten DF, Carpenter BLM. Radiologic imaging of inflicted injury in the child abuse syndrome. Pediatr Clin North Am 1990;37:815–839.)

the procedure (Figs. 37–8 and 37–9). Bone windows should be employed along with the standard scan. Plain radiographs of the skull usually show existing skull fractures better than CT but are of no value in demonstrating the more important evidence of intracranial bleeding or parenchymal brain injury. Magnetic resonance imaging (MRI) is ordinarily used as a confirmatory test rather than an initial one owing to the longer scan times and need for life support, but MRI gives superior detail in showing parenchymal changes and smaller subdural hematomas (see Fig. 37–8).

CT scans of the abdominal viscera are valuable when liver function studies show elevation of the transaminases or there is reason to believe hepatic damage is present, or both. Likewise, if splenic or renal laceration is suspected, CT will delineate these injuries.

Skeletal radiologic surveys are recommended in serious head trauma, since the diagnosis of abuse may be made or supported if unsuspected or occult traumatic injuries are found in other parts of the appendicular skeleton. Such accompanying skeletal fractures are seen in about 50% of the cases of abusive head injury. Posterior rib fractures are characteristic and are present in some cases of shaken infants. They can be demonstrated with bone scan scintigraphy for new-onset fractures or with follow-up thoracic films in 10 to 14 days to see callus formation at the fracture site (Fig. 37–10).

The types of injuries in serious abusive head injury include skull fractures, subdural or subarachnoid bleeding (see Fig. 37–8), cerebral edema (see Fig. 37–9), diffuse axonal shearing injuries, parenchymal tears and contusions, and injuries to the cervical spinal cord. The *shaken baby syndrome (shaken-impact syndrome)* occurs in infants, usually under 1 year of age but is described in children as old as 2 years of age, and consists of violent shaking or shaking plus impact. Shaking and impact by throwing the child against a surface with the resultant deceleration are the responsible

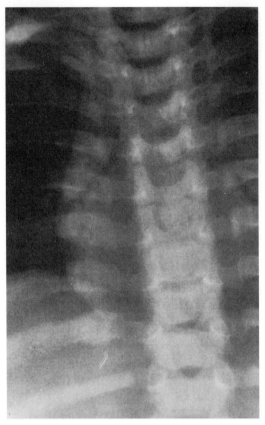

Figure 37–10. A 7-month-old infant with an "accidental" skull fracture. Chest radiograph reveals multiple healing fractures of the right sixth through ninth ribs adjacent to the costovertebral junctions. (From Merten DF, Carpenter BLM. Radiologic imaging of inflicted injury in the child abuse syndrome. Pediatr Clin North Am 1990;37:815–839.)

forces producing the subdural hematoma, diffuse axonal shearing, and consequent cerebral edema leading to raised intracranial pressure. Whether shaking alone or shaking plus impact is required to cause the damage is debated. The clinical picture is one of neurologic devastation, resulting in death in 27% and long-term neurologic morbidity in the majority (57% to 65%) of the survivors.

Abdominal and Thoracic Injuries

Abdominal and thoracic injuries, which constitute the second most common cause of fatality in child abuse, account for between 6% and 8% of all physical abuse. Most of these are abdominal injuries. Reported fatality rates are between 40% and 50% of cases.

The following features distinguish abusive abdominal injuries from accidental abdominal injuries:

1. Abusive injuries are more common in younger children (median age 2.6 years versus 7.8 years in accidental cases).

2. Vague histories account for the abusive injuries; 70% of the injuries in the accidental group are due to motor vehicle accidents and 20% to falls from great heights.

3. Delayed medical care is sought for abusive injuries, in contrast to the accidental group, in which there is prompt care.

4. Abusive injuries occur to hollow viscera most often, whereas a solid organ is more often injured in the accidental group.

5. The mortality rate in the abused group is 53%, but it is 21% in accidental cases.

There is a hierarchy of injury to the abdominal organs, with hollow viscera being the most common; 90% of these are in the duodenum or jejunum. The remainder are in the terminal ileum. The second most common organ for abusive injury is the liver, particularly the more midline portion, and the third most common is the pancreas.

CLINICAL MANIFESTATIONS

The manifestations of abdominal injury can be quite striking, with distention, exquisite tenderness, vomiting, shock, or unconsciousness. Most children with abdominal injuries, either inflicted or accidental, have no obvious abdominal wall cutaneous injuries. Some children have only minimal signs and symptoms; often there are injuries to other parts of the body, making attention to the abdomen less of a priority. Rapid deteriorization can occur if blood loss is not identified and treated.

LABORATORY STUDIES

The pertinent laboratory studies are listed in Table 37–8.

IMAGING STUDIES

The initial imaging study to diagnose abdominal or thoracic injury is the plain radiograph. Two frontal views of the abdomen, one supine and one erect, are recommended. If the child is too ill for an erect view to be obtained, a horizontal-beam cross-table lateral view can be used. This technique usually identifies obstruction, perforation (pneumoperitoneum), hemoperitoneum, or ascites. If there is obstruction, contrast media can be used to localize the lesion. Barium is the preferred contrast medium unless perforation is suspected, in which case a water-soluble contrast medium should be used. A frontal view of the chest is recommended for possible thoracic injuries, including rib fractures. A skeletal survey should also be obtained at the earliest possible opportunity, especially in severely injured children, since future opportunities may not occur and important forensic evidence may be lost. Contrast studies of the genitourinary tract are rarely indicated since the advent of CT scanning, but a voiding cystourethrogram may be needed if lower urinary tract rupture needs delineation.

The CT scan is the most useful imaging technique for evaluation of solid organ injuries. Contrast studies are better for showing hollow organ lesions; the contrast CT scan may demonstrate extravasation or a leak of contrast material, which is usually an indication for surgical exploration. Most intramural hematomas without perforation do not require intervention but resolve with supportive care unless there are bleeding complications. Abdominal ultrasonography also helps identify solid organ trauma and hematoma formation (liver, spleen, pancreas, renal).

Clues to thoracic and abdominal trauma are noted in Table 37–9.

Skeletal Injuries

The actual incidence of skeletal injuries in child abuse is unknown, although an estimate of fractures in abused children younger than 1 year of age is as high as 70%. Nearly 50% of these fractures are clinically unsuspected, and almost 50% involve more than one bone. It is axiomatic that the vast majority (80%) of abuse

Table 37–9. Types of Thoracic and Abdominal Injuries

Organ	Injury	Signs/Symptoms/Diagnostic Findings
Hypopharynx	Traumatic perforation	Feeding difficulty, drooling, palatal abrasion, sloughing lesion pharynx
Esophagus		Coughing, blood-tinged sputum Interstitial emphysema, emesis, mediastinitis, rib fractures on x-ray study
Stomach	Traumatic perforation	Shock and collapse Distended abdomen Free peritoneal air on plain x-ray study
Duodenum	Blunt abdominal trauma	High intestinal obstruction Gastric dilatation Vomiting
Jejunum, ileum	Blunt trauma	Possible peritonitis secondary to perforation Obstruction
Colon, rectum	Blunt trauma Anal penetration	Lower abdominal pain Pain, constipation
Genitourinary tract	Sexual abuse Sadistic abuse	Bruising, abrasions, tears of external genitalia Rupture of bladder
Liver	Blunt trauma	Abdominal distention Shock, collapse Elevated aspartate aminotransferase, alanine aminotransferase, bilirubin Computed tomography (CT) or ultrasound evidence of injury
Spleen	Blunt trauma	Peritoneal irritation, left shoulder pain Blood loss, shock Associated rib fractures CT or ultrasound evidence of injury
Pancreas	Deep epigastric blunt trauma	Abdominal distention, tenderness Elevated amylase CT or ultrasound evidence of injury

fractures are seen in children younger than 18 months and that only 2% of fractures in this age group are of accidental origin.

The importance of the skeletal survey, especially in children with head and visceral injuries, cannot be overstated in suspected child abuse in children younger than the age of 2 years because of the high likelihood of discovery of unsuspected fractures.

The differential diagnosis of skeletal trauma is noted in Table 37–10.

TYPES OF FRACTURES

Extremity Fractures. These are the most common abusive fractures; certain types of extremity fractures are more specific for abuse. The metaphyseal fracture of the long bones has long been identified as the most specific for inflicted injury and is considered pathognomonic for abuse (Fig. 37–11). This so-called "corner fracture," "bucket-handle fracture," "metaphyseal flag," or "metaphyseal fragmentation fracture" is a planar fracture through the primary spongiosa region of the end of the long bones, producing a disc-like fragment at this site. The fractured portion of the bone, depending on the projection of the x-ray beam, appears as a fragment (corner fracture) or a semilunar loop (bucket-handle fracture). The torsional forces required to produce these lesions are those associated with the shaken baby syndrome or the application of rotational vectors to the long bones.

The most common long bone fracture in child abuse involves the diaphysis, occurring four times more frequently than metaphyseal fractures. The femur, humerus, and tibia are the long bones most often affected by transverse or oblique/spiral fractures. There are no specific types or locations for abusive fractures, emphasizing the need for careful history taking, attention to the age of the child, and use of the skeletal survey for children under 2 years of age.

Toddler fractures—accidental oblique fractures of the tibia in the child 9 months to 3 years old—can occur without the knowledge of caretakers and produce symptoms of limp, disinclination to bear weight on the affected leg, or pain on standing. Fractures resulting from abuse may also involve the forearms and, rarely, the clavicle. Fractures of the hands and feet, scapulae, and pelvis are unusual in child abuse.

Rib Fractures. Often unsuspected clinically and discovered by skeletal surveys, rib fractures nevertheless constitute 25% of fractures seen in abuse (see Fig. 37–10). Most of these are posterior fractures, occurring near the costovertebral articulation owing to the levering action of the costovertebral transverse process articulating surface. The second most common location is in the midaxillary line. The fracture line in posterior fractures is usually on the anterior (visceral) surface of the rib, while the fracture line in the midaxillary fracture is on the outer surface of the rib. Because these fractures are produced by compressions of the thorax while the child is being held during shaking or forcefully picked up in anger by a caretaker, they are often multiple and bilateral. Overlying bruises of the thoracic wall may be observed but are often absent. Unless the fractures have been present long enough to produce callus, they may not be discernible on plain radiography; in these cases, bone scintigraphy is most useful.

Vertebral Body Fractures. These fractures are being diagnosed

Table 37-10. Differential Diagnosis of Skeletal Trauma

Obstetric trauma	Neuromuscular disease
Prematurity	Congenital insensitivity to
Nutritional-metabolic	pain
defects	Cerebral
Scurvy	palsy–myelodysplasia
Rickets	Skeletal dysplasia
Secondary	Osteogenesis imperfecta
hyperparathyroidism	Infantile cortical hyperostosis
(renal	(Caffey disease)
osteodystrophy)	Neoplasm and associated
Menkes syndrome	diseases
Mucolipidosis II (I-cell	Leukemia
disease)	Metastatic neuroblastoma
Toxicity	Histiocytosis X
Methotrexate	Innocent trauma
osteodystrophy	Toddler's fracture
Prostaglandin therapy	Normal variant
Hypervitaminosis A	Physiologic periosteal new
Infection	bone
Congenital syphilis	
Osteomyelitis	

Adapted from Brill PW, Winchester P. Differential diagnosis of child abuse. *In* Kleinman PK: Diagnostic Imaging of Child Abuse. Baltimore: Williams & Wilkins, 1987:221; and Radkowski MA. The battered child syndrome: Pitfalls in radiological diagnosis. Pediatr Ann 1983;12:894.

more frequently and may be more common than once thought. They are anterior vertebral body compression fractures and are thought to be caused from hyperflexion during shaking or other violent handling.

Skull Fractures. Skull fractures are classified as *simple* and *complex*. Simple fractures are linear and do not cross suture lines; complex fractures are multiple, crossing suture lines, displaced, comminuted, diastatic, or depressed. Complex fractures do not result from trivial trauma, and although they can be the result of accidental trauma, such trauma nearly always has a consistent history. Complex skull fractures alleged to have been acquired by falls from short heights or in unwitnessed falls are highly suspicious for abuse.

IMAGING TECHNIQUES

The skeletal survey is the preferred diagnostic technique for suspected child abuse. Although radionuclide scintigraphy has cer-

Table 37-11. Elements of the Skeletal Survey

Skull: Frontal and lateral (lateral to include the cervical spine)
Spine: Frontal and lateral thoracolumbar spine (lateral to include the sternum)
Chest: Frontal (for rib and spinal detail)
Extremities:
  Upper: Frontal (to include shoulder and hands*)
  Lower: Frontal (to include lower lumbar spine, pelvis, and feet†)

From Merten DF, Cooperman D, Thompson G. Skeletal manifestations of child abuse. *In* Reece RM (ed). Child Abuse: Medical Diagnosis and Management. Malvern, Pa: Lea & Febiger, 1994:23–54.
*Separate views of the hands and feet in larger infants and children.
†At least two views of each fracture should be obtained.

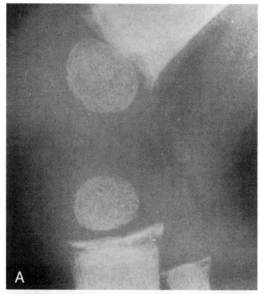
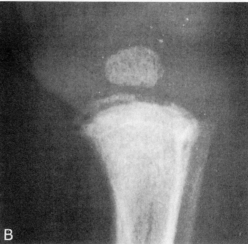

Figure 37-11. Metaphyseal fracture. *A*, Lateral view of the knee in a 5-month-old infant reveals a complete metaphyseal fracture of the tibia and an incomplete fracture of the fibula. There are corner fractures of the femur. *B*, Bucket-handle fracture of the tibia in a 3-month-old infant. (From Merten DF, Carpenter BLM. Radiologic imaging of inflicted injury in the child abuse syndrome. Pediatr Clin North Am 1990;37:815–839.)

tain useful applications (acute subtle fractures, rib fractures), it is not without inherent technical shortcoming and is dependent on the level of competence of the radiologist interpreting it. Table 37–11 details the views recommended for the skeletal survey.

DATING OF FRACTURES

Physicians are often asked to pinpoint the time of injury in child abuse cases. The ability to narrow the time frame is limited, but there are some precepts of value (Table 37–12).

Cutaneous Injuries

The most common manifestations of child abuse are cutaneous injuries. The types of lesions include bruises, abrasions, lacerations,

Table 37–12. Dating Fractures

Category	Early (Days)	Peak (Days)	Late (Days)
1. Resolution of soft tissues	2–5	4–10	10–21
2. Periosteal new bone	4–10	10–14	14–21
3. Loss of fracture line definition	10–14	14–21	
4. Soft callus	10–14	14–21	
5. Hard callus	14–21	21–42	42–90
6. Remodeling	3 months	1 yr	2 yr to epiphyseal closure

From O'Connor JF, Cohen J. Dating fractures. *In* Kleinman PK (ed). Diagnostic Imaging in Child Abuse. Baltimore: Williams & Wilkins, 1987.

Table 37–13. Location of Cutaneous Injuries

Inflicted	Accidental
Upper arms	Shins
Trunk	Hips (iliac crest)
Upper anterior legs	Lower arms
Side of face	Prominences of spine
Ears and neck	Forehead
Genitalia	Under chin

Adapted from Pascoe JM, et al. Patterns of skin injury in non-accidental and accidental injury. Reproduced by permission of Pediatrics 1979;64:245.

petechiae, ecchymoses, and burns (Figs. 37–12 and 37–13). The important characteristics of skin lesions when trying to distinguish inflicted injuries from accidental ones are the location (Table 37–13), pattern, presence of multiple lesions of different ages, and failure of new lesions to appear during hospitalization or removal of the child from the caretaker.

The inflicting instrument may be discerned from the shape of the skin lesion (Fig. 37–14). The typical lesion left by a looped electric cord used for whipping may appear elliptic; a belt, buckle, or wire coat hanger leaves a bruise conforming to its shape; the human hand may leave parallel linear stress petechiae, representing the spaces between the fingers, or scalloping lesions conforming to the metacarpal-phalangeal junction; adult human bites leave characteristic lesions, which can be measured and compared with the dentition of the alleged perpetrator; gags leave downturned lesions at the corners of the mouth; lesions around the neck suggest ligatures applied in that location; ligatures applied to wrists and ankles to restrain the child leave rope burns or pressure lines to those structures; bruises of the upper arms or in the rib cage suggest encirclement bruises resulting from hard pressure applied during shaking or violent handling.

Dating of bruises is imperfect owing to the variability of skin color, healing characteristics, and varying age groups of the children involved in abuse. However, it is of value to make an estimate based on the coloration of healing bruises. Recent bruises (up to 48 hours old) are usually reddish purple; 2- to 3-day-old bruises take on a brownish-purple hue; 4- to 7-day-old bruises are brownish green; and yellow bruises are usually more than 10 days old.

Photodocumentation of bruises with color photography, with clear identification of the patient and the date the photograph is taken, can be of great value if legal proceedings occur.

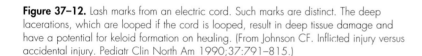

Figure 37–12. Lash marks from an electric cord. Such marks are distinct. The deep lacerations, which are looped if the cord is looped, result in deep tissue damage and have a potential for keloid formation on healing. (From Johnson CF. Inflicted injury versus accidental injury. Pediatr Clin North Am 1990;37:791–815.)

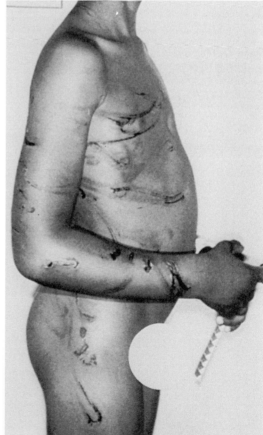

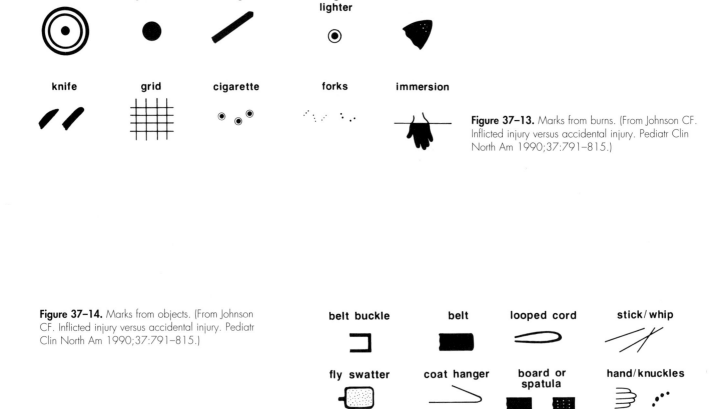

hot plate   light bulb   curling iron   car cigarette lighter   steam iron

knife   grid   cigarette   forks   immersion

Figure 37–13. Marks from burns. (From Johnson CF. Inflicted injury versus accidental injury. Pediatr Clin North Am 1990;37:791–815.)

Figure 37–14. Marks from objects. (From Johnson CF. Inflicted injury versus accidental injury. Pediatr Clin North Am 1990;37:791–815.)

belt buckle   belt   looped cord   stick/whip

fly swatter   coat hanger   board or spatula   hand/knuckles

bite   sauce pan   paddles   hair brush   spoon

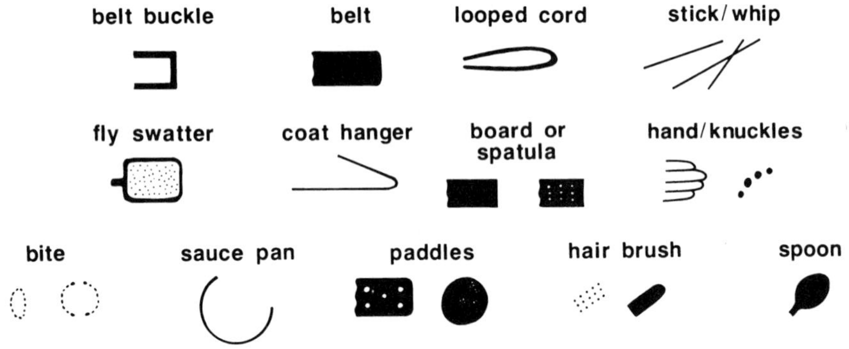

Table 37-14. Inflicted Versus Accidental Burns

	Inflicted	Accidental
History	Burns attributed to sibling Unrelated adult seeks medical care Differing accounts of injury Treatment delay >24 hr Prior "accidents" No parental concern Lesion incompatible with history	Compatible with observed injury
Location	Buttocks, perineum, genitalia Ankles, wrists Palms, soles	Front of body Random and injury-specific
Pattern	Sharply demarcated edges Stocking-glove distribution Full thickness Symmetric Burns older than history indicates Burn neglected, infected Numerous lesions of varying ages Pattern of burn consistent with instrument Large area of uniform, dry contact burn	Associated irregular splash burns Partial thickness Asymmetric One traumatic event

Burns

Between 12% and 30% of burns in children are nonaccidental, and burns represent approximately 10% of all abuse cases; 87% of inflicted burns are scald burns, and 13% are flame injuries. The peak age of burn victims is 13 to 24 months. The classic lesion is the immersion burn involving the buttocks and ankles, sustained when a child is held in extremely hot water and producing either a doughnut lesion of the buttocks, sparing the portion of the buttocks resting against the relatively cooler porcelain of the tub, and showing sharp demarcation lines on the upper margins of the hot water–skin interface. This lesion, plus the stocking-glove immersion burns, are easy diagnoses, since they are so obviously due to restraint of the child. Likewise, burns of the palms and soles are diagnostic for inflicted injury unless the caretaker has an unusually convincing history of a mechanism of injury. Table 37–14 summarizes the distinguishing characteristics of inflicted versus accidental burns.

Nonaccidental burns also seem to carry a higher correlation with social pathology than other forms of child abuse. Most inflicted burn cases either are known to the state's protective service agencies or have been previously admitted to the hospital with a variety of diagnoses, including failure to thrive, poisoning, lead intoxication, fractures, head injuries, and previous burns.

Poisoning

Although reports of intentional poisoning of children are small in number, the true incidence is difficult to determine. Repetitive accidental poisoning in childhood may have no relationship to home safety but is intimately associated with parental psychopathology and disturbed family relationships. The clinical indicators of abuse by poisoning are noted in Table 37–15.

Poisoning may include household agents (salt, pepper, talc, water, caustic agents, air freshener, laxatives), drugs of misuse (cocaine, alcohol-ethanol or isopropyl, opiates, barbiturates, LSD, PCP, marijuana), prescription drugs (barbiturates, anticonvulsants, insulin, imipramine, opiates, phenothiazines), or others (arsenic, ipecac, acetaminophen, aspirin, mineral oil, epsom salt, ethylene glycol) (see Chapter 41).

Munchausen Syndrome by Proxy

Munchausen syndrome by proxy (MSBP) is a bizarre form of child abuse whereby the child is the victim of a form of mental illness of the mother, the psychodynamics of which are poorly understood. The condition is defined as a circumstance in which:

1. Illness is simulated or produced by a parent (almost invariably the mother) or someone who is *in loco parentis*.
2. The child comes for medical assessment and care, usually persistently, often resulting in multiple medical procedures.
3. Knowledge about the etiology of the child's illness is denied by the perpetrator.

Table 37-15. Clinical Indicators of Abuse by Poisoning

Age
  <1 year or between 5 and 10 yr

History
  Nonexistent, discrepant, or changing
  Does not fit child's development
  Previous poisoning in this child
  Previous poisoning in siblings
  Does not fit circumstances or scene
  Third party, often a sibling, is blamed
  Delay in seeking medical care

Toxin
  Multiple toxins
  Substances of abuse
  Bizarre substances

Presentation
  Unexplained seizures
  Life-threatening events
  Apparent sudden infant death syndrome
  Death without obvious cause
  Chronic unexplained symptoms that resolve when the
    child is protected
  Other evidence of abuse or neglect

From Bays JA. Clinical indicators of abuse by poisoning. Personal communication.

Table 37-16. **Munchausen Syndrome by Proxy (MSBP): Methods of Fabrication and Corresponding Diagnostic Strategies**

Presentation	Method of Simulation and/or Production	Method of Diagnosis
Bleeding	1. Warfarin poisoning	1. Toxicology screen
	2. Phenophthalein poisoning	2. Diapers positive
	3. Exogenous blood applied	3. Blood group typing (major and minor) ^{51}Cr labeling of erythrocytes
	4. Exsanguination of child	4. Single blind study Mother caught in the act
	5. Addition of other substances (paint, cocoa, dyes)	5. Testing; washing
Seizures	1. Lying	1. Other MSBP features/retrospective
	2. Poisoning Phenothiazines Hydrocarbons Salt Imipramine	2. Analysis of blood, urine, IV fluid, milk
	3. Suffocation/carotid sinus pressure	3. Witnessed Forensic photos of pressure points
Central nervous system depression	1. Drugs Lomotil Insulin Chloral hydrate Barbiturates Aspirin Diphenhydramine Tricyclic antidepressants Acetaminophen Hydrocarbons	1. Assays of blood, gastric contents, urine IV fluid; analysis of insulin type
	2. Suffocation	2. See apnea and seizures
Apnea	1. Manual suffocation	1. Patient with pinch marks on nose Video camera (hidden) Mother caught Diagnosis of exclusion
	2. Poisoning Imipramine Hydrocarbon	2. Toxicology (gastric/blood) Chromatography of IV fluid
	3. Lying	3. Diagnostic process of elimination
Diarrhea	1. Phenophthalein/other laxative poisoning	1. Stool-diaper positive
	2. Salt poisoning	2. Assay of formula/gastric content
Vomiting	1. Emetic poisoning	1. Assay for drug
	2. Lying	2. Admit to hospital
Fever	1. Falsifying temperature	1. Careful charting, rechecking, urine temperature
	2. Falsifying chart	2. Careful charting, rechecking Duplicating temperature chart in nursing station, urine temperature
Rash	1. Drug poisoning	1. Assay
	2. Scratching	2. Diagnosis of exclusion
	3. Caustics applied/painting skin	3. Assay/wash off

Modified from Rosenberg PA. Munchausen syndrome by proxy. *In* Reece RM (ed). Child Abuse: Medical Diagnosis and Management. Malvern, Pa: Lea & Febiger, 1994:266–279.

4. Acute symptoms and signs in the child abate when the child is separated from the perpetrator (see Chapter 36).

The goal of the diagnostic process is to gather evidence that the illness is simulated or faked (Table 37–16). The strategy of this process is to gather the team of caregivers in the hospital setting and discuss the evolving information on a regular basis. It is wise to alert the child protection agency, law enforcement, and prosecuting attorney's office that such a case is being investigated and sometimes to involve them at the outset of the investigation. A child psychiatrist and child psychologist should be added to the team, and the hospital legal counsel, if not a member of the child protection team, should also attend the meetings.

Covert video surveillance is sometimes employed in these cases and should be done with the full understanding of the ward team, the hospital administration, and the legal department. There are arguments about the use of covert video surveillance, but those who favor its use argue that the goal of the hospital should be to render a diagnosis and to protect children; there are sometimes no other options than to collect data in this fashion.

Extremely careful notes in the chart (or alternate record) are essential because the details are the most important ingredients in the formulation of the diagnosis. When the case comes to court, it is essential that all involved with the proceeding are prepared to present their information and are sure of their facts. The ultimate outcome of the child's well-being rests on this. Seldom does an opportunity to diagnose MSBP on a subsequent admission occur.

The long-term outcome is poorly researched, often because of the disappearance of the families and the short history of the condition.

REFERENCES

General

American Academy of Pediatrics. The child as witness, report of the Committee on Psychosocial Aspects of Child and Family Health. Pediatrics 1992;89:513.

Reece RM. Child Abuse: Medical Diagnosis and Management. Malvern, Pa: Lea & Febiger, 1994.

Saywitz KJ. Developmental considerations for forensic interviewing. Interviewer 1990;3:15.

Sexual Abuse

Adams JA. Classification of anogenital injuries: An evolving process. APSAC Advisor 1993;6:11–13.

Bays JA. Conditions mistaken for child sexual abuse. *In* Reece RM (ed). Child Abuse: Medical Diagnosis and Management. Malvern, Pa: Lea & Febiger, 1994:386–404.

Ekman MAM. Kids' testimony in court: The sexual abuse crisis. *In* Edman P (ed). Why Kids Lie. New York: Scribner's, 1989.

Finkel MA, DeJong AR. Medical findings in child sexual abuse. *In* Reece RM (ed). Child Abuse: Medical Diagnosis and Management. Malvern, Pa: Lea & Febiger, 1994:185–248.

Giardino AP, Finkel MA, Giardino ER, et al. A Practical Guide to the Evaluation of Sexual Abuse in the Prepubertal Child. Sage Publications, 1992.

Heger A, Emans SJ. Evaluation of the Sexually Abused Child. New York: Oxford University Press, 1992.

Jones D, McGraw M. Reliable and fictitious accounts of sexual abuse to children. J Interpersonal Violence 1987;2:27–45.

Physical Abuse

Duhaime AC, Alario A, Lewander W, et al. Head injury in very young children: Mechanisms, injury types and ophthalmologic findings in 100 hospitalized patients younger than 2 years of age. Pediatrics 1992;90:179.

Duhaime AC, Gennarelli T, Thibault L, et al. The shaken baby syndrome: A clinical, pathological and biomechanical study. J Neurosurg 1987;66:409.

Hight DW, Bakalar H, Lloyd J. Inflicted burns in children. JAMA 1979;242:517.

Kempe CH. Sexual abuse, another hidden epidemic. Pediatrics 1978;62:382.

Kleinman PK. Diagnostic Imaging of Child Abuse. Baltimore: Williams & Wilkins, 1987.

Kleinman PK, Marks S, Blackbourne B. The metaphyseal lesion in abused infants: A radiologic and histopathologic study. Am J Roentgenol 1986;146:895.

Ledbetter DJ, Hatch E, Feldman K, et al. Diagnostic and surgical implications of child abuse. Arch Surg 1988;123:1101.

Merten DF, Radkowski M, Leonidas J. The abused child: A radiological reappraisal. Radiology 1983;146:377.

O'Connor JF, Cohen J. Dating fractures. *In* Kleinman PK (ed). Diagnostic Imaging of Child Abuse. Baltimore: Williams & Wilkins, 1987.

Pascoe JM, Hildebrant M, Tarrier A, et al. Patterns of skin injury in non-accidental and accidental injury. Pediatrics 1979;64:245.

Reece RM, Grodin M. Recognition of non-accidental injuries. Pediatr Clin North Am 1985;32:41–60.

Worlock T, Stower M, Barbor P. Patterns of fractures in accidental and non-accidental injury in children. A comparative study. Br Med J 1986;293:100.

Neurosensory Disorders

Started 30/3/97

38 Headaches in Childhood

Bruce H. Cohen

Headaches are a common reason why children make a special visit to their doctor's office or an emergency department. The term headache refers to a nonspecific symptom that consists of any pain or discomfort in the skull, face, facial structures, and pharynx. The pain from headaches affects the quality of life and is an important cause of lost time from school. A classification of headaches is noted in Table 38–1. A headache may also be the initial presenting symptom of a serious medical condition (Tables 38–2, 38–3 and 38–4).

PATHOPHYSIOLOGY

Because no pain receptors exist in the brain, a headache is a result of referred pain from other parts of the head and neck. Intracranial structures that mediate pain include the dura, large arteries, and venous structures (venous sinuses). Extracranial structures that may cause pain include the periosteum, pharynx, orbit, sinus, middle ear, teeth, and muscles of the neck, face, and head. The cranial structures are innervated by the fifth, ninth, and tenth cranial nerves. The structures of the posterior scalp and neck are innervated by the upper cervical spinal cord roots. Pain results from traction or inflammation of vessels or dura, dilatation of vessels, or sustained contraction of the scalp or neck muscles. Diseases of the extracranial structures (sinusitis) can also cause headaches by referred pain.

DIAGNOSTIC APPROACH

History

An accurate patient history guides the physician toward the diagnosis. For example, because the description of aura and pain from classic migraine headaches is so typical, the physician can be confident of the diagnosis if the results of the examination is normal (Table 38–5). Older children usually provide accurate details; parents need to assist younger children in providing the patient history.

The patient history should begin with a general medical history, which includes information about current illnesses, chronic medical problems, and past and current medications (Table 38–6). The next step is to define the headache pattern (pain profile; Tables 38–7 and 38–8). In most cases, a single phenotypic headache is present. If the patient has more than one type of headache, the physician must obtain a specific history for each type (Table 38–9). Patients should be questioned as to the onset, the frequency, and the dura-

tion of the pain, as well as any changing patterns of headache frequency. The severity of pain may be constant or may escalate through the duration of the headache. Special note should be made if the pain awakens the patient from sleep, or if the headache is present when the patient wakes up in the morning, which may indicate increased intracranial pressure (ICP). Once the headache pattern has been defined, the physician should have a precise sense of the temporal pattern of the headaches.

The patient should be asked to localize the pain (Figs. 38–1 to 38–3). If the pain is unilateral, a note should be made if the pain is always on one side or either side at different times (Table 38–10). The patient may be able to characterize the quality of the pain and to report if the pain is sharp or dull, and constant or throbbing.

It is important to determine the intensity of the discomfort; however, the clinician must be careful in determining how the intensity is ascertained. Pain is a subjective symptom with a significant emotional component that may be subject to the influences of age, culture, duration, and previous encounters with physicians. In addition, the intensity of the headache does not necessarily correlate with the seriousness of the disease. For example, a patient may unintentionally exaggerate the pain for attention. Likewise, the clinician should never dismiss the patient who has a mild chronic headache as not having a serious medical problem. Headaches caused by brain tumors may initially be mild but persistent, whereas pain caused by muscle contraction headaches can be quite severe.

A common method for ranking the severity of pain is the "1 to 10 scale," in which the patient ranks the pain using an integer between 1 (mildest) and 10 (worst). This scale is most helpful for assessing chronic headaches or for trying to determine the efficacy of treatment. In older patients, descriptive phrases, such as mild, moderate, severe, and excruciating, may suffice. In children who may have difficulty verbalizing the pain, the nine-face interval scale or the linear analog scale is more reliable (Fig. 38–4).

The family history and the events that surround the onset of the headache may also assist in the diagnosis. Family history is important to obtain because of the genetic component in some headaches, such as migraines and aneurysms. The patient should recall events around the onset of headaches, such as trauma, intake of particular foods or food additives (Table 38–11), physical activities (exertional headache), or presence of an aura (migraine). The clinician should note any symptoms that suggest neurologic dysfunction, such as hemiparesis, visual loss, diplopia, scotomas, vertigo, and hemisensory phenomena. Response to medication can be helpful information, and the physician should ask about both over-the-counter medication and prescription medication, including medication that has not been prescribed for the patient. In patients with recurring headaches, a headache diary helps with the diagnosis and with the assessment of the efficacy of a particular therapy (see Table 38–9).

Table 38-1. 1988 International Headache Society Classification

Migraine without aura
  1. At least five attacks fulfilling 2 to 4
  2. Attacks last 2 to 72 hours
  3. At least two of the following:
    Unilateral
    Pulsating
    Moderate to severe intensity
    Aggravated by routine physical activity
  4. During headache at least one of the following:
    Nausea or vomiting
    Photophobia and phonophobia

Migraine with aura
  1. At least two attacks fulfilling 2
  2. At least three or more of the following:
    One or more reversible symptoms indicating focal
      cerebral cortical or brainstem dysfunction
    At least one aura symptom develops gradually
      over 4 or more minutes, or two or more
      symptoms occur in succession
    No aura lasts more than 60 minutes
    Headache follows aura with a free interval of <1
      hour

  3. Typical auras include
    Homonymous visual disturbance
    Unilateral paresthesias
    Unilateral weakness
    Aphasia or other speech difficulty
Episodic tension
  1. At least 10 episodes fulfilling 2 to 4
  2. Headache lasting 30 minutes to 7 days
  3. Two or more of the following:
    Pressing/tightening quality
    Mild to moderate intensity
    Bilateral
    Not aggravated by routine activity
  4. Both of the following:
    No nausea or vomiting
    Phonophobia or photophobia is absent
Chronic tension type
  1. Average headache frequency >15 days/month for >6 months
      fulfilling 3 and 4 listed above for episodic tension
Headache associated with trauma
Headache associated with disorder of sinuses or other facial or cranial
  structures

Headache Classification Committee of the International Headache Society: Proposed classification and diagnostic criteria for headache disorders, cranial neuralgias, and facial pain. Cephalalgia 1988;8:9–96 (Suppl 7).

Table 38-2. Differential Diagnosis of Headache

 1. Vascular headache of migraine type
    a. Classic migraine
    b. Common migraine
    c. Cluster headache
    d. Hemiplegic and ophthalmoplegic migraine
    e. ''Lower half'' headache

 2. Muscle-contraction (tension) headache

 3. Combined headache: vascular and muscle-contraction

 4. Headache of nasal vasomotor reaction

 5. Headache of delusional, conversion or hypochondriacal states

 6. Nonmigrainous vascular headaches
    a. Systemic infections
    b. Miscellaneous: hypoxic states, carbon monoxide poisoning,
       chemical vasodilator effects (e.g., nitrates), caffeine
       withdrawal, cerebral ischemia, postconcussion or
       postconvulsive states, ''hangovers,'' hypoglycemia,
       hypercapnia, hypertensive states, pheochromocytoma

 7. Traction headache
    a. Primary or metastatic tumors: meninges, brain, or
       vasculature
    b. Hematomas: epidural, subdural, parenchymal
    c. Abscesses: epidural, subdural, parenchymal
    d. Post–lumbar puncture headache
    e. Pseudotumor cerebri

 8. Headache due to overt cranial inflammation
    a. Intracranial: meningitis, subarachnoid hemorrhage,
       iatrogenic (postoperative, postpneumoencephalogram, etc),
       arteritis, phlebitis
    b. Extracranial: vasculitis, cellulitis
 9. Ocular headache
    Increased intraocular pressure, ocular muscle contraction,
    trauma, tumor, inflammation
10. Aural headache
    Trauma, inflammation, infection, tumor of the ear
11. Nasal/sinus headache
    Allergic, infectious, inflammatory, traumatic, tumor of the
    nose and/or paranasal sinuses
12. Dental headache
    Infection, trauma, tumor, inflammation, iatrogenic
    Temporomandibular joint syndrome
13. Cranial/neck headache
    Disorders of cervical spine, cervical nerve roots, scalp/
    neck muscles, tendons, ligaments
14. Cranial neuritides
    Traction, trauma, inflammation, infection, tumor
15. Cranial neuralgia
    Trigeminal
    Glossopharyngeal

Chronic post-traumatic headache is often multifactorial, usually
  related to 1b, 2, and/or 13 above.

Adapted from the Ad Hoc Committee on Classification of Headache, National Institute of Neurological Diseases and Blindness, JAMA 1962;179:717–719.

Table 38–3. Systemic Infection in Which Headache May Be a Prominent Symptom

Common Illness	Uncommon Illness	Uncommon, but Most Serious
Viremia	Typhoid fever	Meningitis (bacterial, viral)
Influenza	Tularemia	Brain abscess
Pharyngitis	Toxoplasmosis	Retropharyngeal abscess
Otitis media	Cytomegalovirus infection	Cervical osteomyelitis
Sinusitis	Mumps	Suppurative intracranial thrombophlebitis
Mononucleosis	Measles	Subdural empyema
Pneumonococcal pneumonia	Poliomyelitis	Encephalitis
Mycoplasma pneumonia	Psittacosis	Septicemia
	Dengue	Endocarditis
	Trichinosis	Rocky Mountain spotted fever
	Q fever	Malaria
	Legionnaires disease	
	Leptospirosis	
	Typhus	

Adapted from Reilly BM. Practical Stategies in Outpatient Medicine, 2nd ed. Philadelphia: WB Saunders, 1991:90.

Physical Examination

Many patients lack physical signs (see Table 38–8). Some serious diseases present early in their course with a normal physical examination. When the results of the neurologic examination are abnormal (see Table 38–7), a structural brain lesion is possible and a neuroimaging study is warranted. Besides the neurological examination, in which particular attention should be paid to signs of papilledema, focality, increased ICP, or abnormal visual field defects, abnormalities found on the ophthalmologic (Table 38–12) and general physical examination (blood pressure, occult head and neck infection, generalized-systemic diseases) may suggest pathology of other cranial structures that will lead the clinician toward a diagnosis.

Sudden Severe Headache

A sudden and severe headache is alarming and usually prompts a doctor's visit. The approach to the patient with an acute, severe headache is different from that to the patient with recurrent headaches. A diagnostic approach for a sudden and severe headache is outlined in Figure 38–5. The physician must note that every patient with migraines (and other non–life-threatening headaches) has a first severe headache. This headache may even be associated with an abnormal neurologic state, fever, or other worrisome features.

Table 38–4. Headache: Systemic and Metabolic Causes

Common	Uncommon
Hyperthyroidism	Carbon monoxide poisoning
Hypothyroidism	Toxic hemoglobinopathies
Anemia	Pheochromocytoma
Polycythemia	Parathyroid disease
Hypoxemia	Cushing disease
Hypercarbia	Addison disease
Hypoglycemia	Vitamin A intoxication
Hypertension	Lead poisoning
Uremia	Cranial neoplasm
Hyponatremia	Chronic leukemia-lymphoma

Adapted from Reilly BM. Practical Stategies in Outpatient Medicine, 2nd ed. Philadelphia: WB Saunders, 1991:111.

Magnetic resonance imaging (MRI) (Table 38–13) and laboratory tests may be indicated in the evaluation of an acute, severe headache (Fig. 38–5). Additional indications for neuroimaging (MRI or CT) include an abnormal neurologic examination, reduced visual acuity, poor growth, neuroendocrine manifestations (galactorrhea, secondary amenorrhea), behavioral changes, seizures, increased headache frequency, and increased pain with awakening, coughing, straining, or position changes.

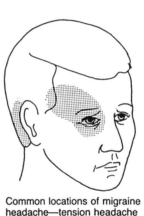

Common locations of migraine headache—tension headache may also be unilateral

Common locations of tension headache—migraine may occur in the same location

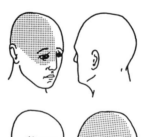

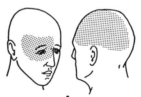

A

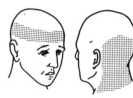

"Hatband" distribution

Occipital distribution

B

Figure 38–1. Common location of migraine *(A)* and tension *(B)* headaches. (From Reilly BM. Practical Strategies in Outpatient Medicine, 2nd ed. Philadelphia: WB Saunders, 1991.)

Table 38–5. **Clinical Features of Most Common Chronic Headache Syndrome**

	Classic Migraine	Common Migraine	Muscle Contraction
Prodrome	Visual or neurologic	None (or vague)	None
Quality	Throbbing, pulsatile	Throbbing	Tight, squeezing
			Sometimes throbbing
Location	Unilateral	Usually unilateral	Usually bilateral
Associated symptoms	Nausea, vomiting, photophobia	Usually nausea; anorexia	Depression
Usual duration	Several hours	Several hours	Highly variable
Usual frequency	Several per year	1–2 per month	Daily or several per week
Patient's typical response	Hibernates in dark room	"Sick"	Rarely interrupts usual activities
	Tries to sleep	Can't work	"I can live with it"
	Frightened by prodrome		

Modified from Reilly BM. Practical Strategies in Outpatient Medicine, 2nd ed. Philadelphia: WB Saunders, 1991:101.

SPECIFIC HEADACHE DISORDERS

Muscle Contraction Headaches

Most children and adolescents experience an occasional muscle contraction headache, usually in response to stress, exhaustion, or hunger (see Table 38–5 and Fig. 38–1). Frequent muscle contraction headaches occur in about 15% of older children. Younger children may also have muscle contraction headaches; however, muscle contraction headaches do not cause persistent headaches in this age group. These headaches can be annoying, painful, and disabling. In addition, a muscle contraction headache may often accompany other headache disorders or be the end result of a migraine.

Table 38–6. **Headache History**

General Medical History
Presence of other acute medical problems or symptoms
Chronic medical problems
Current medication
Previous medication used for headaches
Previous long-term medication
Intake of caffeine, vitamin A, alcohol, cocaine

Pattern
When did the headaches begin?
Frequency and change in frequency
Duration of headaches
Pattern to the time of day
Presence of headaches on weekends, weekdays
Are headaches preceded by a warning?

Description of Pain
Location
Quality
Intensity
Effects of position

Associated Factors
Trauma
Are headaches associated with other activity?
Does any medication make the headache better?
Do the following occur before, during, or immediately after the headache: visual disturbance, vertigo, weakness, nausea, vomiting, changes in sensorium?

Family History
Migraines
Aneurysm

CLINICAL FEATURES

These headaches have a typical pattern and are usually chronic and non-progressing. Patients awaken feeling well, with the pain beginning gradually and escalating throughout the day. The pain is constant, squeezing, and located in a band extending from the front of the head, across the temples, and toward the occiput or neck (see Fig. 38–1). Nausea and photophobia may accompany these headaches but are not a constant feature. In patients with longstanding pain, the headaches can assume characteristics of migraines.

Chronic muscle contraction headaches are defined as headaches occurring at least 15 days a month for at least 6 months. Often, the child or adolescent has daily headaches. A detailed psychosocial history is important because it may uncover the cause for the headache. For example, adjustment disorders and depression may be either the primary cause or a secondary reaction to chronic pain. Sleep disturbances, school absences, and chronic analgesic use are common in this group. A negative psychosocial history can also occur in patients with chronic muscle contraction headaches. In some highly motivated and successful children, the headaches may be a reaction to the stress associated with achievement. In this instance, school attendance is usually perfect and the patient continues to achieve in all realms.

Patients with muscle contraction headaches have normal neuro-

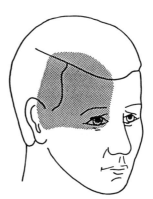 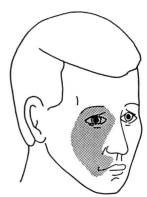

Ocular disease?
Frontal sinusitis?
Temporomandibular syndrome?
Temporal arteritis?
Tension headache?
Migraine?
Cluster?

Ocular disease?
Maxillary sinusitis?
Dental infection?
Allergic/vasomotor rhinitis?
Nasopharyngeal tumor?
Trigeminal neuralgia?
Migraine?
Cluster?

Figure 38–2. Periorbital headache. (From Reilly BM. Practical Strategies in Outpatient Medicine, 2nd ed. Philadelphia: WB Saunders, 1991.)

Table 38–7. Headache Disorders Associated with Neurologic Signs

Headache Disorder	Pain Profile	Neurologic Sign
Classic migraine	AI	Visual disturbance
Complicated migraine	AI	Hemiparesis, aphasia, paresthesia, alteration in sensorium
Basilar artery migraine	AI	Ataxia, visual disturbance, vertigo, tinnitus, paresthesia
Acute confusional migraine	AI	Alteration in sensorium, stupor, agitation, fugue state
Ophthalmoplegic migraine	AI	Paresis of eye movement, dilated pupil, ptosis
Vasculitis	CN, AI	Seizure, changes in sensorium
Brain neoplasm or mass	CP	Papilledema, focal deficit
Hydrocephalus	CP, AI	Papilledema, bilateral sixth nerve palsies, increased motor tone, impaired upward gaze and Parinaud syndrome
Pseudotumor cerebri	CP	Papilledema, constricted visual fields, enlarged blind spot
Subarachnoid hemorrhage, ruptured aneurysm	AS	Changes in sensorium, focal neurologic signs
Subdural or epidural hemorrhage	CP	Focal neurologic signs, papilledema, changes in sensorium
Sagittal sinus thrombosis	AS	Papilledema, focal neurologic deficits, changes in sensorium, seizures
Meningitis; encephalitis	AS	Papilledema, focal neurologic deficits, changes in sensorium, seizures
Optic neuritis	AS	Papillitis, decreased visual acuity, afferent pupillary defect

Abbreviations: AI = acute intermittent; AS = acute, singular (occurs only with the causative condition); CP = chronic progressive; CN = chronic non-progressive.

logic and physical findings except for tenderness along the affected muscles. These muscles often feel tight, and palpation can trigger the pain. There are no available laboratory tests to diagnose these headaches.

TREATMENT

Patients usually do not seek the advice of a physician for the occasional muscle contraction headache because rest and over-the-counter analgesics (acetaminophen or ibuprofen) usually alleviate the pain. In contrast, patients with chronic, frequent headaches may require a multidisciplinary approach to their management. For

Table 38–8. Headache Disorders with No Neurologic Signs

Headache Disorder	Pain Profile
Muscle contraction	CN, AI
Common migraine	AI, CN
Cluster	AI
Hypertension, uncomplicated	AI, CN
Fever	AS
Ice cream headache	AS
Anoxia	AS
Caffeine withdrawal	AS, AI
Coital headache	AS, AI
Early hydrocephalus or brain mass	CP
Cough headache, uncomplicated	AI
Meningitis, uncomplicated	AS
Sinusitis, dental or pharyngeal abscess	AI
Temporomandibular joint syndrome	CN
Postconcussive syndrome	CN
Conversion disorder	CN

Abbreviations: AI = acute intermittent; AS = acute, singular (occurs only with the causative condition); CP = chronic progressive; CN = chronic non-progressive.

example, some may benefit from physical therapy through the use of progressive range-of-motion exercises aimed at strengthening the neck muscles. Other patients may benefit from the assistance of a psychologist. Besides addressing underlying adjustment disorders, the psychologist can assist by teaching the patient stress management (relaxation techniques, biofeedback). It is important for the patient to realize that certain types of stress are normal. In addition, the patient needs to know that stress is not going to be eliminated and that he or she must learn to cope. To reduce stress, the daily schedule should be regulated, with a focus on exercise, proper diet, and sleep. Because caffeine, nicotine, and alcohol may contribute to the headaches, the patient should avoid using these drugs. If the headaches are affecting the activities of normal childhood and adolescence, individual therapy, family therapy, or both are warranted.

Over-the-counter analgesics are the most appropriate treatments for the occasional severe headache. Aspirin is contraindicated in children and teens because of the risk of Reye syndrome (see Chapter 41). Other medications for treating patients with chronic headaches exist; however, the clinician must be careful to ensure that these medications are used properly and are not abused. In addition, treating only the symptom and not the cause (stress) may actually prolong the patient's condition and expose the patient to the potential side effects of the medications. Benzodiazepines, narcotics, and barbiturates should be avoided because of their

Table 38–9. The Headache Diary for Recurring Headaches*

Date
Time of onset
Time of resolution
Maximum level of pain (mild, moderate, or severe, *or* 1–10)
Associated phenomena:
  Sleep
  Food
  Position, Valsalva
  Other

*If more than one type of headache exists, the types should be defined and labeled, and separate data recorded for each type.

Table 38–10. Differential Diagnosis of Commonly Confused Chronic Unilateral Headache Syndromes

	Common Migraine	Cluster	Trigeminal Neuralgia	TMJ Syndrome	Tension*
Prodrome	None	None	None	None	None
Quality	Throbbing	Ache, severe	Sharp, ''electric'' jabs	Dull ache	Dull ache
Location	Hemicranial Periorbital	Periorbital	Cheek, jaw, lower lip	Preauricular, jaw spreading to temple, eye, and neck	Temple, occiput and neck
Associated symptoms	Nausea	Tearing; rhinorrhea	None	Limited jaw motion or ''clicking''	Depression; muscle tightness
Usual duration	3–8 hours	½–2 hours	10–60 seconds, repetitively over 1–3 hrs	Several hours, or constant	Hours–days, constant
Usual frequency	1–2 per month	1–4 per day, during cluster‡	Daily† but episodic	Daily†	Daily†
Patient's typical response	''Sick'' Quiet	Pace the floor, agitated	Avoid trigger points	Depression Teeth grinding	Depression

Modified from Reilly BM. Practical Strategies in Outpatient Medicine, 2nd ed. Philadelphia: WB Saunders, 1991:102.
*Tension headache is usually bilateral but may be confused with these syndromes when unilateral.
†Frequency of these syndromes is highly variable, but daily occurrence is common.
‡A typical cluster will last several weeks.

addiction potential, although these agents can be used rationally and successfully in the responsible patient who has infrequent and severe muscle contraction headaches. Ergot alkaloids should also be avoided because of their addictive properties and the high incidence of side effects in children. The calcium channel blockers and beta blockers are helpful only if there is a significant migrainous component to the headache.

Some patients may benefit from prophylactic therapy. In these patients, a single, daily standard dose of ibuprofen, naproxen, or amitriptyline may prevent headaches. Amitriptyline given at dosages far below what is effective in the treatment of depression can have an excellent effect in preventing muscle contraction headaches. Because amitriptyline can cause sleepiness, it is usually given as a single bedtime dose, with a dose ranging from 25 to 75 mg (adolescent age dose).

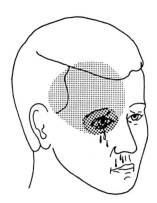

Periorbital or frontotemporal location is usual

Tears and nasal stuffiness, often unilateral, accompany the headache

Duration is usually brief (1 hour)

Figure 38–3. Cluster headache. (From Reilly BM. Practical Strategies in Outpatient Medicine, 2nd ed. Philadelphia: WB Saunders, 1991.)

Vascular Headaches

MIGRAINE HEADACHES

Types of Migraines

Common and Classic Migraines. Migraine headaches are the most common vascular type of headache (see Fig. 38–1 and Tables 38–1, 38–5, and 38–10). By 15 years of age, at least 5% of children have had a migraine headache. Migraine and migraine variants also occur in early childhood but at an unknown prevalence. The general description of this headache type makes the diagnosis usually straightforward. A family history of migraines and a past history of motion (car) sickness are common in patients with migraines.

With a few exceptions, childhood migraines are very similar to those in adults. During childhood, migraines affect more boys than girls, which is contrary to the adult experience. In children, the headaches are less frequent, shorter in duration, and respond better to treatment. Vomiting and abdominal pain are also more common in children than in adults.

The pattern of migraines is highly variable. Migraines may be sporadic; however, they can also occur at almost any interval. Without prophylactic treatment, most patients have between one and four migraines a month. There is often no temporal pattern, although in some patients the headaches may cluster around a certain event. In postpubertal women, migraines may cluster around particular phases of the menstrual cycle. Unless the migraines tend

Table 38-11. Possible Dietary Precipitants of Migraine

Ripened cheeses (cheddar, Emmentaler, Stilton, Brie, Camembert, brick, blue, Swiss, Gouda, Roquefort, mozzarella, Parmesan, provolone, Romano)	Fermented sausage and aged, canned, cured, or processed meats (bologna, salami, pepperoni, summer sausage, hot dogs), bacon
Pickled herring	Canned soups with monosodium glutamate
Chocolate	Pizza
Anything fermented, pickled, or marinated	Hot fresh yeast breads, coffee cake, doughnuts, sourdough bread
Olives, pickles	Chicken livers
Sour cream, yogurt, buttermilk, chocolate milk	Brewer's yeast, meat tenderizers, seasoned salt
Sauerkraut, onions	Citrus foods
Sunflower seeds	Tea, coffee, cola
Nuts, peanut butter	Banana
Beans, except string beans	Foods containing large amounts of monosodium glutamate (Chinese foods)
Avocados, figs, raisins, papaya, passion fruit, red plums	
Alcoholic beverages	Corn
	Egg

Data from Diamond S, et al. Modern Medicine, July 1986, pp 76–86; and Mansfield LE: Postgrad Med 1988;83:46. Reprinted from Reilly BM. Practical Strategies in Outpatient Medicine, 2nd ed. Philadelphia: WB Saunders, 1991:116.

to cluster, patients rarely have pure migraines more than twice a week. Mild or moderate headaches often occur between the more severe migraine attacks.

The migraine is composed of two vascular phases: vasoconstriction and vasodilatation. In the *classic migraine*, the headache is preceded by an aura, which is caused by vasoconstriction and diminished blood flow to the affected region of the brain. The aura associated with the classic migraine is visual and may consist of blurred vision, scotomas, flashing lights, zigzag lines, and hemi-

anopsia. Sensory auras are less common than visual auras and consist of numbness or tingling, which may be followed by weakness. Transient hemiparesis (hemiplegic migraine), aphasia, and alteration of consciousness (confusional migraine) are rare auras. With *common migraines*, there is no specific aura; however, the patient may feel fatigued or ill immediately before the headache.

The vasodilation phase usually causes the pain. The onset of the pain is gradual and develops over minutes to an hour. Some patients, however, have a sudden onset of severe pain. Less severe migraines consist of a dull, constant pain. As the severity increases, the pain becomes throbbing. The headache is often unilateral but may be bilateral. The pain may be frontal or facial, instead of the more typical temporal location. As the headache proceeds, the pain can generalize to the entire cranium. In children with basilar artery migraines, the pain is occipital. Intense nausea and vomiting often accompany migraines. Skin pallor is also a common finding. Because most patients are sensitive to motion, light, and noise during a migraine attack, they search for a dark and quiet place to sleep. The patient usually awakens within 2 to 12 hours feeling fatigued but otherwise well.

Certain factors are known to trigger migraine attacks in susceptible patients. Patients need to be questioned regarding the temporal association of their migraines with these factors because eliminating the precipitant may prevent some or all of the migraines. The most common identified precipitants to migraines are specific foods and food additives, such as chocolate, hard cheeses, tomatoes, onions, yeast, and beans (see Table 38–11). Because caffeine withdrawal can precipitate a migraine attack, all caffeinated beverages should be avoided. Some of the food additives that may trigger a migraine are sulfites, nitrites, and monosodium glutamate (MSG). MSG is found in Chinese-style foods, canned and dehydrated soups, proprietary spices (seasoned salts), and many packaged foods. Because food additives are commonly used in the food industry, susceptible patients are advised to read all labels. Aside from foods, other precipitants include menstruation, hunger, estrogen (oral contraceptives), lack of sleep, stress, heat, and exertion.

Some patients with migraines are extremely sensitive to exertion, especially on hot days. Their headaches may be precipitated by strenuous activities, such as summer practice sessions for varsity

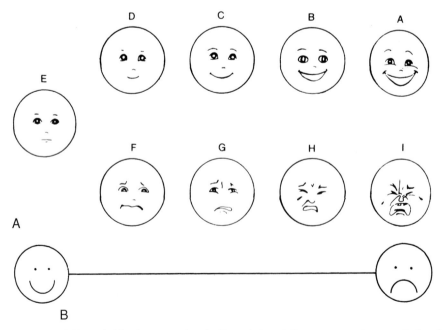

Figure 38–4. Assessing pain in young children. *A,* Nine-face interval scale. Faces A through D represent varying magnitudes of positive affect; faces F through I represent varying magnitudes of negative affect. *B,* Linear analog scale; the child places an X on the line to identify the relative severity of headache. (Adapted from Beyer JE, Wells N. The assessment of pain in children. Pediatr Clin North Am 1989;36:846.)

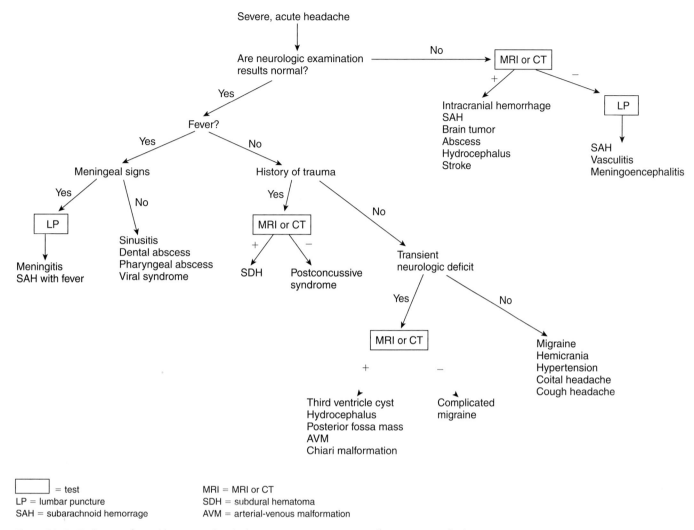

Figure 38–5. Evaluation of a sudden, severe headache. AVM = arteriovenous malformation; LP = lumbar puncture; MRI = magnetic resonance imaging; CT = computed tomography; SAH = subarachnoid hemorrhage; SDH = subdural hematoma. *Boxes* indicate tests.

sports or a marching band. The headaches may be prevented by proper dress and prophylactic indomethacin therapy.

Complicated Migraine. Patients with a complicated migraine have neurologic deficits that persist during and after the headache. These deficits include hemisensory symptoms, hemiparesis, aphasia, visual loss, and alteration in consciousness. In most cases, the neurologic deficit precedes the headache. These symptoms usually last about as long as the headache but can last for days. Permanent neurologic deficits are rare but can occur if the vasoconstriction is severe and causes infarction.

Complicated migraines begin in childhood and evolve into the more typical migraine pattern as the patient gets older. In some children with this disorder, their attacks are precipitated by mild head trauma, such as striking the head against a wall or using the head to hit a soccer ball.

Basilar Artery Migraine. The basilar artery is more prone to involvement in childhood migraines, which leads to brainstem or occipital lobe dysfunction. The headache is usually occipital and may be extremely intense. Neurologic abnormalities include ataxia, nausea, and vomiting. In some patients, the headache may be a minor component of the syndrome. Visual changes can also occur

and can include vivid visual images. Vertigo, tinnitus, and paresthesia are less common symptoms that accompany a basilar artery migraine.

Acute Confusional Migraine. This disorder begins after 5 years of age and usually converts into typical migraines as the patient gets older. The onset of acute confusional migraine begins with an alteration in consciousness, which can include varying degrees of lethargy, agitation, and stupor. A fugue-like state has also been described with these migraines. Attacks last a few hours, with the child eventually falling asleep. The child awakens without memory of the incident.

Ophthalmoplegic Migraine. Cranial nerve palsies, usually of the third cranial nerve, may accompany this type of a migraine. Physical findings usually include pupillary dilatation and ptosis. Other cranial nerves involved during these headaches are cranial nerve IV (causing loss of downward and medial eye movement) and cranial nerve VI (causing loss of lateral eye movement). The ophthalmoplegia may persist for a few weeks after the headache. In younger children, a headache may not be associated with this disorder. An MRI study is warranted because ophthalmoplegia,

Table 38-12. **Conditions That May Cause New Headache and Eye Signs**

Diagnosis	Distinguishing Features
Headaches with Visual Loss	
Headache with Monocular Visual Loss	
Optic neuropathies	
Nonarteritic optic neuropathy	Sudden visual loss; funduscopy may be normal
Optic neuritis	Usually decreased pupillary light reflex, disc blurring with hyperemia of the fundus sometimes with painful extraocular movements
Infiltrative neuropathies	Progressive, *more gradual* visual loss—pituitary tumors, intracranial aneurysms, increased intracranial pressure common cause
Ophthalmic transient ischemic attack (amaurosis fugax)	Typically brief (3–5 min), sudden visual loss, hypercoaguable states, sickle cell anemia, cocaine ingestion, carotid bruit possible
Ophthalmic migraine	More gradual onset of visual loss than amaurosis fugax, lasts longer (25–30 min), and often followed by typical headache
Iritis (uveitis)	Conjunctival injection, miosis, photophobia
Meningovascular syphilis	May mimic temporal arteritis; positive VDRL in CSF (and pleocytosis)
Acute glaucoma	Sick, nausea and vomiting, tender on hard globe, pupil dilated, cornea "steamy," "red eye"
Panophthalmitis	Bacterial, rarely spirochetal or fungal
Headache with Binocular Visual Loss	
Iritis (bilateral)	Gradual visual loss, abnormal eye examination
Basilar migraine	Usually young female with other vertebrobasilar neurologic symptoms—ataxia, vertigo, weakness, loss of consciousness
Vertebrobasilar transient ischemia	Hypercoagulable state, sickle cell anemia, other vertebrobasilar symptoms—vertigo, dysarthria, leg weakness
Chiasmal tumor	Often *bitemporal hemianopia,* enlarged sella turcica on tomograms of skull
Increased intracranial pressure: benign intracranial hypertension	Fluctuating headache, papilledema
Episodic hypoglycemia	*Transient* episode in which visual symptoms may (occasionally) predominate, often followed by headache
Presyncope (usually cardiac)	Transient episode sometimes followed by headache
Headache with Homonymous Hemianopia	
Classic migraine	Typical history
Posterior cerebral transient ischemia	Trauma, Arnold-Chiari crisis, sickle cell, hypercoagulable states, with other neurologic symptoms
Occipital lobe disease (neoplasm, hemorrhage)	Visual loss and headache occasionally may be only manifestation
Headache with Ophthalmoplegia	
Intracranial aneurysm (especially posterior communicating artery)	Third cranial nerve paresis, *pupil dilated*
Diabetic neuritis	Third cranial nerve paresis, *pupil normal*; eye usually very painful
Ophthalmoplegic migraine	Typical history—usually third cranial nerve
Temporal arteritis	Mild *ptosis* occasionally observed without other visual symptoms
Basilar meningitis	Usually chronic symptoms with abnormal spinal fluid
Cavernous sinus disease or parasellar disease	Paresis of third through sixth cranial nerves
Brain tumor or other causes of hydrocephalus	Bilateral sixth cranial nerve paresis–often a "false localizing" sign
Exophthalmos of any cause	Proptosis
Syphilis	CSF VDRL
Nasopharyngeal carcinoma	Usually when cancer advanced and involving base of skull
Multiple sclerosis	Episodic neurologic deficits of different types, occurring widely spaced over time; optic atrophy sometimes a clue
Idiopathic (Tolosa-Hunt syndrome)	Probably granulomatous, may be responsive to corticosteroid therapy
Headaches with Pupillary Asymmetry	
Headache with Unilateral Dilated Pupil	
Transtentorial herniation due to mass effect	Decreased mental status with usually obvious neurologic compromise
Intracranial aneurysm	Other cranial nerve findings (third)
Optic neuritis	
Acute glaucoma	

Table 38–12. **Conditions That May Cause New Headache and Eye Signs** *Continued*

Diagnosis	Distinguishing Features
Headaches and Unilateral Constricted Pupil (and/or Horner's Syndrome)	
Cluster headache	Typical history
	Ptosis, miosis *during* headache
Mediastinal neoplasm with intracranial metastases or superior vena cava obstruction	Chest x-ray diagnostic
	Unilateral ptosis, miosis, anhydrosis
Raeder's paratrigeminal neuralgia	Steroid-responsive
Spontaneous carotid artery dissection	Pulsatile tinnitus, ocular bruit, head and neck pain

Adapted from Reilly BM. Practical Strategies in Outpatient Medicine, 2nd ed. Philadelphia: WB Saunders, 1991:96.
Abbreviations: VDRL = Venereal Disease Research Laboratory; CSF = cerebrospinal fluid.

even if transient, is associated with serious conditions, such as aneurysms and tumors.

Amaurosis fugax (ophthalmic transient ischemia) manifests as monocular visual loss lasting minutes; in childhood, it is often due to migraines.

Migraine Status. Most migraines last 6 to 12 hours; however, some patients are susceptible to prolonged headaches. A prolonged headache may last for days and is usually associated with protracted vomiting and dehydration. Diagnosis is based on a propensity for previous prolonged migraine attacks.

Treatment of Migraines

Treatment can help most patients with migraine headaches. If precipitating factors can be identified, they should be avoided. If medication is necessary, the physician and patient must decide whether the goal is to prevent the migraines (prophylactic management) or to stop or lessen the headache once it starts (abortive management). The choice of treatment depends on the age of the patient and the frequency of the headaches. The adverse effects of the medication need to be balanced against its efficacy.

Abortive Management. Abortive management is effective in older children and adolescents who can identify the stereotypic aura and can self-administer the medication. This management strategy is difficult because the patient needs to carry the medication at all times. If abortive therapy is used, the medication should be taken at the first symptom, whether it be the aura or the headache. Occasionally, a patient may find adequate relief with a simple over-the-counter analgesic. Prescription medications that may abort the migraine attack contain isometheptene mucate (Midrin) or butalbital (Fiorinal). These formulations also include analgesics, such as aspirin, acetaminophen, and codeine. Caffeine is another common component in these preparations, which augments the analgesic effects. Ergot derivatives are useful agents in adults. Their use in children is not recommended because of the high incidence of adverse reactions. An antiemetic may be needed with an analgesic used to treat a severe migraine. If possible, patients should rest and try to fall asleep. Sleep relieves symptoms, and many patients awaken free of pain.

Sumatriptan, a serotonin agonist, is effective in aborting the migraine attack in most patients. This medication is self-administered orally or by subcutaneous injection. Relief occurs in minutes after the injection. The adult dose is 6 mg. Even though the drug has not been approved for use in children by the Federal Drug

Administration, a dose of 3 mg has been used safely and effectively in children older than 10 years. Because sumatriptan can precipitate spasms of coronary arteries, it should not be used in children with cardiac disease.

The physician must be aware that drug-dependent states can develop, even with non-narcotic medications. Therefore, medication use needs to be monitored carefully. If a patient is using analgesics more than 1 day a week, abortive management should be considered to be unsuccessful and should be abandoned.

Prophylactic Management. For children with frequent migraines (every 1 to 2 weeks), daily medication is a more appropriate choice (Table 38–14). The most commonly used prophylactic medications are beta blockers, amitriptyline, and cyproheptadine. The goal is to prevent as many headaches as possible at a dose that has tolerable side effects. Medication should be started at a low dose to minimize sedation and other adverse effects. The dose should be increased every 1 to 2 weeks if the headaches are not controlled. If side effects develop that cannot be tolerated, the medication should be tapered and another begun in its place.

In the younger patient, cyproheptadine (an antihistamine with serotonin antagonist properties) should be the first choice because it is very well tolerated. The major side effects are excessive appetite and weight gain; this drug may not be acceptable to teenagers. Dose escalation is usually in 2-mg increments every 1 to 2 weeks.

The beta blockers (e.g., propranolol) are second-line medications and are generally well tolerated. The major dose-limiting effects include fatigue, weight gain, and cardiovascular beta blockade. Because of these effects, this medication can interfere with the lifestyle of active teenagers and athletes. This group of medications is an excellent choice if the headaches are controlled at a dose below that which causes beta blockade. Dose escalation is usually in weekly increments of 10 to 20 mg. Long-acting (sustained-release) preparations are available once the headaches are controlled.

Amitriptyline, a tricyclic antidepressant with serotonin antagonist properties, is usually a good choice for teenagers with migraines. In addition to controlling migraines, amitriptyline is also effective for those with mixed migraine–tension headache disorders. Because of the sedative properties of amitriptyline, a single daily bedtime dose is usually administered. The starting dose is 10 mg at bedtime, with dose escalation of 10 mg every 1 to 2 weeks until adequate control is achieved. Dose-limiting side effects include dry mouth, weight gain, fatigue, and constipation. Most older patients cannot tolerate more than 75 mg a day. A pretreatment electrocardiogram should be obtained because tricyclics prolong the Q-T interval. This medication should not be prescribed if a prolonged Q-T

Table 38–13. Neuroimaging Studies

When to Order a Neuroimaging Study
 The "thunderclap headache" or "worst headache of my life."
 The first severe headache.
 Abnormal neurologic findings.
 Chronic or progressive headaches.
 Unilateral headaches that never alternate sides.
 Headache associated, even briefly, with alteration of sensorium.
 Presence of papilledema.
 Meningeal signs without fever.

Advantages of Magnetic Resonance Imaging (MRI)
 Most vascular malformations are detected.
 Accurate detection of tumors in temporal lobes and posterior fossa, and small tumors that obstruct CSF flow (quadrigeminal plate and third ventricular).
 Paranasal sinuses usually included in the examination without special request.
 More sensitive for detecting transependymal CSF in cases of borderline hydrocephalus.
 Diagnostic for Chiari malformations.
 Magnetic resonance angiography can detect many aneurysms.
 Magnetic resonance venography can detect cortical vein and dural sinus thrombosis.

Advantages of Computed Tomography (CT)
 Less expensive and easier access than MRI.
 If imaging only for sinusitis, a simple sinus CT costs the same as sinus roentgenography.
 Shorter imaging time, important in evaluating ill patients.
 May be used in patients with pacemakers, metal implants (surgical clips), and cosmetic tattoos (MRI may turn off pacemakers, dislodge the clips, while tattoos distort the image).

Abbreviation: CSF = cerebrospinal fluid.

interval is found because it may precipitate severe, ventricular arrhythmias (torsades de pointes) that are refractory to treatment.

NON-MIGRAINE, VASCULAR HEADACHES

Cluster headaches rarely occur before adolescence (see Fig. 38–3) and are more common in men than in women. Episodes of pain are intermittent, with long periods of remission, hence the name "cluster." Cluster pain is localized to the eyes and temples but can spread to other parts of the head. The pain begins suddenly and rapidly increases to an excruciating level. Most cluster headaches last 30 minutes to 2 hours. The headaches occur in bouts lasting from 4 to 8 weeks, with 1 or 2 bouts occurring a year. During these periods, alcohol should be avoided because it can precipitate a headache. Lacrimation, rhinorrhea, sweating, and nasal stuffiness usually accompany the headache. These headaches usually occur at a particular time of day, with most occurring at night.

The management of cluster headaches is directed at both the prophylaxis of headaches during clusters and the treatment of acute headache. The acute headache can be treated with the inhalation of ergotamine and intranasal lidocaine. Prophylactic agents include calcium channel blockers, lithium, and prednisone.

VASCULITIS HEADACHES

Vasculitis, which is caused by collagen vascular disease, is an important cause of headaches in adults, although in children vascu-

litis rarely presents as headaches. Instead, the headaches may be part of the constellation of symptoms associated with this illness. Because of the increased risk of systemic hypertension in patients with vasculitis, it is important to include a blood pressure measurement as part of the complete history and physical examination. When systemic lupus erythematous and mixed connective tissue disorders affect the central nervous system, children often have seizures and mental status changes. These changes can occur with or without headaches.

HYPERTENSION-RELATED HEADACHES

Systemic hypertension, both acute and chronic, may be associated with headaches. The pain is probably caused by alterations in the regulation of cerebral blood flow. Acute hypertension typically occurs in a child with post-streptococcal glomerulonephritis, renal failure or collagen vascular disease. Although hypertension is an uncommon cause of headaches in children, the diagnosis of hypertension is straightforward and treatment of the hypertension alleviates the headaches. Many patients with hypertension have no headaches.

Headaches can be part of malignant hypertension syndrome, in which case retinal exudates and microscopic hematuria are usually present. Severe hypertension can also cause an intracerebral hemorrhage. Use of cocaine causes headaches through various mechanisms, including hypertension, vasoconstriction, hypersensitivity vasculitis, and subarachnoid hemorrhage.

FEVER-RELATED HEADACHES

Headaches are common in febrile patients, regardless of the source of the fever (see Table 38–3). The pain is usually bifrontal and bitemporal but may also involve the occiput and neck. The pain may be throbbing and may increase with neck flexion. Any abnormalities seen during the neurologic examination (nuchal rigidity, altered mental status) suggest that factors other than fever may be the source of the headache and must be evaluated.

ICE CREAM HEADACHES

This common headache affects about 33% of children and 90% of patients with migraines. This disorder occurs more in the summer. Within 30 seconds of quickly ingesting a cold drink or ice cream, a severe, boring pain develops deep inside the head. The pain lasts for only several seconds to a minute. Once this condition is recognized, no further evaluation or treatment is necessary.

CHRONIC PAROXYSMAL HEMICRANIA

Chronic paroxysmal hemicrania consists of frequent and intense unilateral headaches (see Table 38–10). This disorder is much more common in women than in men. Although it usually begins in adulthood, chronic paroxysmal hemicrania can affect older children and adolescents. The average headache lasts about 10 minutes (range, a few minutes to 45 minutes). Patients can have as many as 10 to 20 attacks a day, and the pain can awaken the patient from sleep. Sudden head movement can also precipitate an attack.

This headache responds dramatically to indomethacin therapy. Relief of symptoms occurs within a few days of beginning the medication. Other nonsteroidal anti-inflammatory drugs (NSAIDs)

Table 38–14. Medication for Migraine Prophylaxis

Medication	Formulation	Starting Dose	Dose Increments	Maximum Dose*	Dose-Limiting Side Effects
Cyproheptadine	Tablets: 4 mg Syrup: 2 mg/5 ml	2 mg	2 mg	0.2–0.4 mg/kg/ day or 4 mg q.i.d.	Weight gain, sedation
Propranolol†	Tablets: 10, 20, 40, 60, 80, 90 mg Long-acting capsules: 60, 80, 120, 160 mg	10–20 mg	10–20 mg	4 mg/kg/day or 240 mg/day	Sedation, weight gain, hypotension, constipation, heart block Should not be used in persons with asthma, IDDM
Amitriptyline	Tablets: 10, 25, 50, 75 mg	10 mg	10 mg	75 mg/day or 2 mg/kg/day	Sedation, weight gain, dry mouth, constipation, urinary retention
Verapamil	Tablets: 80 mg	80 mg	80 mg	80 mg t.i.d.	Sedation, constipation, hypotension

*Maximum effective dose for migraine. Dosages higher will probably not be helpful.
†Propranolol will mask signs of hypoglycemia.
Abbreviations: IDDM = insulin-dependent diabetes mellitus; q.i.d. = four times daily; t.i.d. = three times daily.

are of no benefit. Because the symptoms of chronic paroxysmal hemicrania are similar to those of vascular malformations of the brain, a neuroimaging study should be performed to rule out these malformations before the diagnosis of chronic paroxysmal hemicrania is made.

ANOXIA AND CARBON MONOXIDE HEADACHES

Anoxia, hypoxia, and carbon monoxide poisoning may produce headaches through dilatation of cerebral arteries, which in turn causes an increase in cerebral blood flow. In children with illnesses that predispose one to hypoxia (chronic lung disease, obstructed sleep apnea), treatment should be directed at alleviating the source of the hypoxia. High altitudes can also lead to an acute hypoxic state, in which case symptoms can be treated with altitude descent, acetazolamide, and dexamethasone.

Low-level carbon monoxide poisoning should be suspected in any child with chronic headaches. The diagnosis is difficult to confirm with an arterial hemoglobin carbon monoxide level because the half-life of HgbCO in room air is only 4 hours. Hence, the level may be normal in only a few hours after exposure. One way of diagnosing and treating this condition is removal of the cause of the exposure. Some sources of carbon monoxide exposure are heavy urban traffic in which one is a car passenger, methylene dichloride paint strippers, kerosene space heaters, a gasoline engine running in an attached garage, cigarette smoking, and faulty home furnaces. In severe carbon monoxide poisoning, the patient is treated with 100% oxygen (carboxyhemoglobin half-life, 50 minutes) or hyperbaric oxygen (2 to 3 atm; carboxyhemoglobin half-life, 30 minutes) until the HgbCO level is less than 15% and both the metabolic acidosis and mental status changes have resolved.

CAFFEINE WITHDRAWAL HEADACHES

The threshold for withdrawal for each person is variable, but when caffeine is ingested in sufficient quantities for prolonged

periods of time, sudden withdrawal can lead to vascular headaches. In the most common scenario, consumption occurs on weekdays, and because of schedule differences, the caffeinated beverage is not consumed on the weekend. This syndrome is easily diagnosed by history or by use of a headache diary. Treatment is removal of all sources of caffeine from the diet, such as tea, coffee, caffeinated soft drinks, "pep" pills, and diet pills.

COITAL HEADACHES

The coital or orgasmic headache is associated with orgasm. The basis of this headache is thought to be vascular. This disorder occurs more frequently in men and has been reported in adolescence. It is not related to the level of sexual arousal, the degree of physical activity, or the type of sexual act. Orgasmic headaches usually occur immediately before or during orgasm. Propranolol and indomethacin are successful in preventing this headache.

Traction Headaches

One of the greatest concerns in the evaluation of a child with headaches is whether or not the headache is caused by increased ICP. Increased ICP causes headaches by generating traction on the dura and vessels at the base of the brain. Some processes (brain tumors, pseudotumor cerebri) result in constant headaches because of continuous increased ICP. Other conditions (colloid cyst of the third ventricle) may cause intermittent headaches through transient increases in ICP.

PERSISTENTLY INCREASED INTRACRANIAL PRESSURE

Neoplasms and Hydrocephalus

In children with headaches, a concern about a brain tumor is probably the key reason patients request, and doctors order, an imaging study. The mechanism of brain tumors that cause headaches may be either due to increased ICP or to direct traction on the dural or vascular structures. Headaches due to hydrocephalus can develop rapidly, whereas traction from tumor growth causes a slow and progressive headache. However, at the time of presentation, most patients with headaches due to tumors or hydrocephalus have chronic and progressive headaches, in which the frequency and severity of pain escalate over time. Tumors may produce hydrocephalus by obstructing CSF flow.

With or without a brain tumor, hydrocephalus usually causes a generalized headache. Slowly developing hydrocephalus initially causes mild pain, whereas rapidly developing hydrocephalus causes severe pain. Most patients with hydrocephalus have morning headaches that lessen after arising. Some patients do not follow this pattern and have constant pain.

When the headache is solely a result of tumor without accompanying hydrocephalus, the location of the headache may or may not be related to the tumor site. Patients with posterior fossa tumors usually have occipital pain, but if hydrocephalus is also present, the pain may be generalized. It is important to note that many patients with brain tumors have no particular pattern to their headaches. Initially, their pain may be mild, and over-the-counter analgesics provide adequate pain relief. If the pain pattern is typical, the severity and frequency of pain increase slowly.

The examination often reveals abnormal findings, including papilledema and neurologic deficits. Common focal neurologic findings include eye movement abnormalities, facial weakness, swallowing difficulties, hemiparesis, and ataxia. Non-lateralizing signs include increased motor tone and bilateral sixth nerve palsies. Increased motor tone may not be a constant finding and may appear as transient shivering. Tenderness or rigidity of the neck is a sign for increased ICP. Macrocephaly is present in young children with unfused cranial sutures and in those with long-standing hydrocephalus. Other signs of hydrocephalus are a bulging fontanelle and widened cranial sutures. The head growth chart is especially important in evaluating children with hydrocephalus. Head growth is abnormal if the plot of sequential head circumferences crosses percentile lines. Papilledema is usually absent in children with an open fontenele and may also be absent in children with posterior fossa tumors (with or without hydrocephalus).

The *Parinaud syndrome* is the triad of upward-gaze paresis, poor pupillary reaction to light, and retraction nystagmus on convergence. This constellation of physical findings is seen in patients with hydrocephalus or tumors in the pineal region. The presence of Parinaud syndrome always warrants neuroimaging.

Increased ICP that is caused by hydrocephalus and/or brain tumors should be suspected in any child with chronic progressive headaches, abnormal neurologic examination results, nuchal rigidity, or abnormal head growth. Patients with these signs and symptoms should have a neuroimaging study (see Table 38–13).

Non-neoplastic Masses

Non-neoplastic masses, such as hemorrhage, cysts, and abscesses, can also cause headaches. Intracranial hemorrhage should be suspected in any child with a concussion causing amnesia or loss of consciousness or with a head injury resulting in abnormal neurologic examination results (e.g., altered mental status, focal findings). Most intracranial hemorrhages are detected by the initial neuroimaging study performed immediately after the injury; however, some subdural and fewer epidural hematomas may take weeks to develop after the trauma.

Cysts are classified as arachnoid, epidermoid, and dermoid. Slow-growing cysts often have headache patterns similar to those of neoplasms. Epidermoid and dermoid cysts can have sinus tracts that communicate with the skin. If these cysts become infected, their clinical presentation resembles a brain abscess.

A brain abscess should be considered in any child with a right-to-left cardiac shunt, chronic mucosal surface infections (sinus, otitis, dental), and a recent onset of persistent, chronic headaches. Patients with a brain abscess may present with progressive neurologic dysfunction and may deteriorate quickly.

Aneurysmal Rupture

Arterial aneurysms may be congenital (berry) or due to an infectious process (mycotic). Rupture of an arterial aneurysm is rare in children. The rupture produces an excruciating headache, known as a *thunderclap headache*. Patients state that this is "the worst headache of my life." The pain is acute in onset and associated with nuchal rigidity, emesis, and changes in sensorium. The neurologic examination may be non-focal. Computed tomography (CT) reveals blood in the cisterns and meninges in 85% of cases. If the CT shows no pathology, a lumbar puncture is necessary in all patients thought to have a ruptured aneurysm. The spinal fluid in a ruptured aneurysm is bloody, or xanthochromic, or both. In half of the cases, patients report having headaches before having the headache associated with the rupture. These earlier headaches may be due to leakage of blood from the aneurysm. If one suspects a leaking or ruptured aneurysm, rapid neurologic and neurosurgical care is mandatory. Arteriovenous malformations may produce similar manifestations.

Pseudotumor Cerebri

Even though pseudotumor cerebri is also known as benign intracranial hypertension, it is associated with significant morbidity. The headache in pseudotumor cerebri can be intermittent or constant and may resemble a migraine. Papilledema is usually present at the time of presentation. In severe cases, the retinal blind spot may enlarge and the visual fields may become constricted. This syndrome is more common in older children and adolescents, females, and obese individuals.

Pseudotumor cerebri may be either idiopathic or secondary to a variety of medical conditions (Table 38–15). Because papilledema is a common finding in this syndrome, a neuroimaging study must be performed before the lumbar puncture to rule out other causes of papilledema (tumor, hydrocephalus) (see Table 38–13). The opening pressure from the lumbar puncture in pseudotumor cerebri is elevated (range, 240 mm H_2O to 600 mm H_2O). The results of the physical examination (except papilledema and visual field changes), neuroimaging studies, and cerebrospinal fluid (CSF) studies are usually normal.

In the evaluation of a patient with pseudotumor cerebri, a detailed history and physical examination is needed to rule out the many secondary causes of this syndrome (Table 38–15). One such secondary cause of increased ICP is obstruction of the draining venous sinuses by infection or dehydration. For example, infection of the middle ear and mastoid can spread to involve the sigmoid sinus, causing partial or complete obstruction of venous drainage. This process is also known as *otitic hydrocephalus* and leads to a pseudotumor cerebri syndrome.

The goal of treatment is to lower ICP and alleviate the headaches. Lumbar puncture is a fast, reliable, but temporary method for achieving both goals. Most patients require multiple lumbar punctures before their symptoms resolve. If the visual fields are affected, the treatment must be aggressive, with serial lumbar punctures, until the fields return to normal. If symptoms persist despite serial lumbar punctures, a lumbar-to-peritoneal drain or

Table 38–15. Conditions Associated with Pseudotumor Cerebri

Intracranial venous drainage obstruction
   Mastoiditis and lateral (sigmoid) sinus obstruction
   Extracerebral mass lesions
   Congenital atresia or stenosis of venous sinuses
   Head trauma
   Cryofibrinogenemia
   Polycythemia vera
   Paranasal sinus and pharyngeal infections

Cervical or thoracic venous drainage obstruction
   Intrathoracic mass lesions and postoperative obstruction of
     venous return

Endocrine dysfunction
   Pregnancy
   Menarche
   Marked menstrual irregularities
   Oral contraceptives
   Obesity
   Withdrawal of corticosteroid therapy
   Addison disease
   Hypoparathyroidism
   "Catch-up" growth after deprivation, treatment of cystic
     fibrosis, correction of heart anomaly
   Initiation of thyroxine treatment for hypothyroidism
   Adrenal hyperplasia
   Adrenal adenoma

Hematologic disorders
   Acute iron-deficiency anemia
   Pernicious anemia
   Thrombocytopenia
   Wiskott-Aldrich snydrome

Vitamin metabolism
   Chronic hypervitaminosis A
   Acute hypervitaminosis A
   Hypovitaminosis A
   Cystic fibrosis and hypovitaminosis A
   Vitamin D–deficiency rickets

Drug reaction
   Tetracycline
   Perhexiline maleate
   Nalidixic acid
   Sulfamethoxazole
   L-Asparaginase
   Indomethacin
   Penicillin

Prophylactic antisera

Miscellaneous
   Galactosemia
   Galactokinase deficiency
   Lyme disease
   Sydenham's chorea
   Sarcoidosis
   Roseola
   Hypophosphatasia
   Paget disease
   Maple syrup urine disease
   Turner syndrome

Adapted from Burg FD, Ingelfinger JR, Wald ER (eds). Gellis and Kagan's Current Pediatric Therapy, 14th ed. Philadelphia: WB Saunders, 1993:67.

optic sheath decompression may be necessary to provide long-term drainage for the spinal fluid. In obese patients, weight loss may also be helpful. Corticosteroids provide quick relief from the headache and associated visual impairment. Because steroids can cause rapid weight gain, their use should be avoided if at all possible.

TRANSIENT INCREASED INTRACRANIAL PRESSURE

Cough headaches are intermittent headaches caused by transient increases in ICP that result from activities that elevate intrathoracic pressure (exertion, coughing, bending). The pain is maximum and severe at the onset of the activity and then resolves in seconds. Patients are usually asymptomatic between events. Cough headaches are much shorter than are exercise-induced vascular headaches, which may be caused by both benign and life-threatening conditions. Structural causes of cough headache include brain tumors and Chiari malformations. The results of the physical examination are usually normal, even when structural lesions cause this syndrome. To rule out these structural lesions, patients with cough headaches should undergo MRI.

Colloid cyst of the third ventricle is another life-threatening condition that causes cough headaches. With changes in position, this cyst functions as a ball-valve and intermittently impedes the flow of cerebrospinal fluid (CSF). This obstruction causes transient increases in ICP. Sometimes, the patient may be asymptomatic during these episodes of increased ICP. At other times, the patient may experience severe intermittent headaches, increased muscle tone (posturing) that resembles shivering, coma, and death. The ICP returns to normal when position is changed, or when the increased CSF pressure overcomes the obstruction. Physical findings are normal between events.

The diagnosis is made by neuroimaging studies (MRI). Treatment consists of CSF diversion or removal of the cyst.

DECREASED INTRACRANIAL PRESSURE

Abnormally low ICP causes headaches by the same mechanism as that of increased ICP: traction on the dura and vessels at the base of the brain. The most common cause of a headache from decreased ICP is the lumbar puncture. This headache can occur after any lumbar puncture but is more commonly associated with older children, use of larger-bore spinal needles, and multiple attempts at obtaining CSF. Patients describe a severe headache within seconds after assuming an upright position. The headache disappears soon after lying down.

Treatment consists of bed rest until the leak seals. A blood patch is used when bed rest fails to seal the leak. This procedure consists of injecting the patient's own blood into the epidural space, thus "patching" the dural leak. Other causes of low-pressure headaches include CSF leaks from fractures or tumors at the base of the skull.

Headaches Caused by Inflammation

Any inflammatory process involving the head or neck can cause headaches. The pain may be from direct inflammation of the brain and dura (meningitis) or it may be referred from extracranial inflammation (sinusitis, dental abscesses) (Table 38–16).

INTRACRANIAL INFLAMMATION

With meningitis and meningoencephalitis, the headache is acute in onset and generalized. Fever, nuchal rigidity, alteration in sensorium, and abnormal neurologic findings usually accompany an inflammatory process of the meninges.

EXTRACRANIAL INFLAMMATION

The headache associated with sinusitis can be acute or chronic. The headache is frontal or ocular when the frontal or maxillary sinuses are involved. When the ethmoid or sphenoid sinuses are infected, the headache can be frontal or occipital. Some of the symptoms and signs associated with sinusitis are purulent rhinorrhea, halitosis, cough (worse at night), tenderness to palpation over the sinuses or teeth, and fever. In addition, these patients may have a past medical history of allergic rhinitis or previous sinusitis. If a radiographic study is needed to confirm the diagnosis, a sinus CT is preferred over routine sinus roentgenograms because CT is more sensitive in diagnosing sinusitis and costs the same.

The headaches from dental abscesses may be aching or knifelike. Dental abscesses can be a complication of dental caries, tooth extractions, and root canal procedures. The examination results may be normal, or the examination may reveal gingival swelling, redness, or pain.

Inflammation of the eye and orbit usually causes localized pain

(Table 38–16). The signs and symptoms of periorbital cellulitis are periorbital redness and tenderness, whereas in orbital cellulitis, the patient may have chemosis, proptosis, ophthalmoplegia, and visual loss. A corneal abrasion should always be suspected in the irritable infant and in the patient with excruciating eye pain. Diagnosis is made by fluorescein examination of the cornea (see Chapter 44).

Optic neuritis (inflammation of the optic nerve) often causes ipsilateral retro-orbital pain. Optic neuritis may occur as a single entity, or it can be part of the presentation of multiple sclerosis. This disorder is rare in children but common in adolescents. The ophthalmologic examination shows papillitis (resembling papilledema), afferent pupillary defect, and decreased visual acuity. Often, the findings may be normal except for decreased visual acuity. A neuroimaging study should be performed because of the ocular findings and to rule out multiple sclerosis. Optic neuritis is treated with intravenous corticosteroids.

Miscellaneous Causes of Headaches

TEMPOROMANDIBULAR JOINT SYNDROME

Malocclusion of the temporomandibular joint (TMJ) can cause chronic headaches. The pain is localized to the side of the affected joint. Some patients report constant pain, whereas others have pain only with jaw movement. An identifying ''click'' occurs when the patient opens the mouth. Not every person with a click has TMJ syndrome, and not everyone with TMJ syndrome has headaches. Gum chewing may exacerbate the pain associated with TMJ syndrome. In patients without TMJ syndrome, gum chewing may cause headaches through overuse of the temporalis muscles. Patients with

---

Table 38–16. Chronic Facial Pain: Differential Diagnosis

Orbital Pain	Nasal/Cheek Pain	Dental/Jaw Pain
Ocular disease	Sinusitis	Toothache
Migraine	Facial cellulitis	TMJ syndrome
Cluster	Neoplasm (nasopharynx, sinus)	Sinusitis
Sinusitis	Vasomotor rhinitis	Neoplasm
Orbital cellulitis	Allergic rhinitis	Trigeminal neuralgia
Tolosa-Hunt syndrome	Trigeminal neuralgia	Parotid disease
Intracranial aneurysm	Midline granuloma	Atypical odontalgia
Cavernous sinus disease	Wegener granulomatosis	Postherpetic neuralgia
Giant cell arteritis	TMJ syndrome	
Neoplasm	Dental disease	
Graves disease	Postherpetic neuralgia	
Neoplasm, frontal lobe	Atypical odontalgia	
Trigeminal neuralgia	Cluster	
Postherpetic neuralgia	**Poorly Localized/Vague**	
Ear/Periauricular Pain	Sinus disease	
Chronic external otitis	TMJ syndrome	
Relapsing polychondritis	Depression	
Cholesteatoma	Conversion reaction	
TMJ syndrome	Neoplasm	
Migraine	Muscle contraction	
Carotidynia		
Glossopharyngeal neuralgia		
Thyroiditis		
Muscle contraction		
Carotid aneurysm		
Cervical spine disease		
Neoplasm		

Adapted from Reilly BM. Practical Strategies in Outpatient Medicine, 2nd ed. Philadelphia: WB Saunders, 1991:106.
Abbreviation: TMJ = temporomandibular joint.

symptomatic TMJ syndrome often find relief with the use of a bite plate worn during sleep.

POSTCONCUSSIVE SYNDROME

Chronic headaches can occur as part of the postconcussive or post-traumatic syndrome. The headache is generally constant and may have qualities of both chronic muscle contraction and migraine headaches. For example, some patients may have nausea, vomiting, and visual auras. Other features of this syndrome are fatigue, dizziness, vertigo, poor memory, decreased reaction times, and inability to concentrate. The neurologic findings are usually normal. Symptoms begin soon after the head injury (within 1 to 7 days) and can persist for years. About 70% of patients recover within a year, but 15% are still symptomatic after 3 years. The pathophysiology of this syndrome is unknown.

Even though postconcussive syndrome is more common in those with a past history of psychological or psychosomatic illness, it is a true phenomenon. A neuroimaging study may be necessary to rule out the presence of a chronic subdural hematoma, which is rare. Patient education is the most important element of treatment. Some patients may also benefit from psychotherapy. NSAIDs, amitriptyline, and propranolol may be helpful, but narcotics should be avoided because of their addictive potential in the treatment of chronic headaches.

OCCIPITAL NEURALGIA

The greater occipital nerve is a continuation of the C2 nerve root, which innervates the posterior scalp. Irritation or inflammation of this nerve can produce occipital pain that may be intermittent or persistent. The pain is described as ranging from ''pins and needles'' to lancinating. On physical examination, affected patients have decreased sensation and tenderness to palpation over the posterior scalp. Whiplash injury, atlantoaxial subluxation, and arthritis are associated with this syndrome. Some patients respond to carbamazepine, NSAIDs, and physical therapy. In severe cases, repeated nerve blocks with steroids and a local anesthetic provide relief.

CONVERSION DISORDER

Headaches associated with conversion disorders are very difficult to diagnosis and treat accurately. The frequency and severity of these headaches increase without lasting relief from any pharmacologic or physical therapy. Some patients appear as if they are in pain, whereas others look perfectly normal despite claiming to be in considerable pain. Secondary muscle contraction pain can occur, which further complicates the diagnosis. The neurologic findings in conversion disorders are normal. As patient and family anxiety grows, the physician's anxiety also increases, resulting in the ordering of many blood tests and neuroimaging studies.

The two problems in treating conversion disorder headaches are (1) to convince the family that there is no physical cause for these headaches and (2) to uncover the origin of the conversion disorder. The physician with a pre-established rapport with the family is clearly at an advantage in convincing the family that no physical cause exists for the headaches. The origins of a conversion disorder are difficult to uncover and require the finesse of an experienced therapist. Psychologic intervention is mandatory, not only to identify the source of the problem but also to offer appropriate consoling.

SUMMARY AND RED FLAGS

Headaches are a common cause of morbidity in children. Although muscle contraction and migraine headaches are the most common causes of headaches in children, the clinician must rule out life-threatening conditions in the evaluation of each patient with a headache. A thorough history and physical examination are the best diagnostic tools aiding the clinician in determining which patients have a serious and life-threatening cause for their headaches. The red flags from this evaluation are thunderclap headache, cough headache, the first severe headache, chronic or progressive headaches, persistently unilateral headaches, any abnormal neurologic findings, meningeal signs, papilledema, and alterations of sensorium. Patients with these *red flags* need an emergent and complete evaluation that includes neuroimaging studies (see Table 38–13).

REFERENCES

Appleton R, Farrell K, Buncic JR, et al. Amaurosis fugax in teenagers. Am J Dis Child 1988;142:331–333.

Bartleson JD, Swanson JW, Whisnant JP. A migrainous syndrome with cerebrospinal fluid pleocytosis. Neurology 1981;31:1257–1262.

Batemen DN. Sumatriptan. Lancet 1993;341:221–224.

Blau JN. Behaviour during a cluster headache. Lancet 1993;342:723–725.

Blau JN. Classical migraine: Symptoms between visual aura and headache onset. Lancet 1992;340:355–356.

Blau JN. Migraine: Theories of pathogenesis. Lancet 1992;339:1202–1207.

Diamond S. Headache. Med Clin North Am 1991;75(3).

Diamond S, Dalessio DJ. The Practicing Physician's Approach to Headache, 4th ed. Baltimore: Williams & Wilkins, 1986.

Editorial. Migraine related stroke in childhood. Lancet 1991;337:825–826.

Gautier J-C. Amaurosis fugax. N Engl J Med 1993;329:426–428.

Goadsby PJ, Zagami AS, Donnan GA, et al. Oral sumatriptan in acute migraine. Lancet 1991;338:782–783.

Hockaday JM. Management of migraine. Arch Dis Child 1990;65:1174–1176.

Hockaday JM. Migraine in Childhood. London: Butterworths, 1988.

Igarashi M, May WN, Golden GS, et al. Pharmacologic treatment of childhood migraine. J Pediatr 1992;120:653–657.

Jain N, Rosner F. Idiopathic intracranial hypertension: Report of seven cases. Am J Med 1992;93:391–395.

Lance JW. Treatment of migraine. Lancet 1992;339:1207–1209.

Lessell S. Pediatric pseudotumor cerebri (idiopathic intracranial hypertension). Sur Ophthalmol 1992;37:155–166.

Mathew NT. Headache. Neurol Clin North Am 1990;8(4):781–992.

Raskin NH. Headache, 2nd ed. New York: Churchill Livingstone, 1988.

Rooke ED. Benign exertional headache. Med Clin North Am 1968;52:801–808.

Shinnar S. An approach to the child with headaches. Int Pediatr 1991;6:140–148.

Smith M. Comprehensive evaluation and treatment of recurrent pediatric headache. Pediatr Ann 1995;24:452–457.

Stewart WF, Lipton RB, Celentano DD, et al. Prevalence of migraine headache in the United States. JAMA 1992;267:64–69.

Welch KMA. Drug therapy of migraine. N Engl J Med 1993;329:1476–1483.

39 Hypotonia and Weakness

Warren Cohen

IDENTIFICATION OF MUSCLE WEAKNESS AND HYPOTONIA

Hypotonia (abnormally diminished muscle tone) may be acute or chronic, progressive or static, isolated or part of a complex clinical situation; it affects children of all ages (Table 39–1). It may or may not be associated with weakness (Tables 39–2 to 39–5). The evaluation of children with hypotonia can be simplified by a thoughtful, analytic approach to the differential clues that are useful in identifying an underlying cause (Tables 39–6 and 39–7); (Figs. 39–1 to 39–3).

Hypotonia is usually defined functionally as diminished resistance to movement observed by the examiner as a limb is passively moved through a range of motion about a joint. The assessment of muscle tone can be made by several observations in addition to passive movement of the joints, including:

- Evaluation of spontaneous posture
- Extent of mobility of joints
- Response to flapping of distal extremities
- Response to postural changes

The method of evaluating muscle tone and strength depends on the age of the patient.

Muscle tone is the observable phenomenon of sustained muscle contraction that is continuous even while the child is resting. Tone arises as the result of sustained contraction of resting muscles in response to the stimulation of stretch receptors that are located within muscle. The steady, sustained stretch of muscles produced by gravity is the stimulus that results in normal resting postural tone. Hypertonia is defined as abnormally increased muscle tone. Hypotonia (decreased muscle tone) may be associated with weakness and hyperextensibility (increased mobility of joints). The descriptive but imprecise term *floppy infant* is often used to refer to an infant with hypotonia.

The maintenance of normal muscle tone requires the integrity of the entire central and peripheral nervous systems, from the cerebral cortex, cortical white matter pathways, basal ganglia, cerebellum, brainstem, spinal cord, peripheral nerve, neuromuscular junction, and muscle (Table 39–6). Diseases that affect the function of the nervous system at any level may result in abnormal muscle tone (see Tables 39–6 and 39–7). Many infants with hypotonia have disorders of the brain. Most older children and adolescents with hypotonia have a disorder of the motor unit (anterior horn cell, peripheral nerve, neuromuscular junction, and muscle) (Fig. 39–4).

THE HYPOTONIC INFANT

Clinical Evaluation

In an infant, historical information must include a complete obstetric history as well as accurate data about perinatal events, diet, toxic exposure, and family diseases.

MUSCLE STRENGTH

Muscle strength cannot be measured directly in infants, as in older children (Table 39–8), but numerous clinical clues allow the careful observer to identify muscle weakness. The most important of these is the spontaneous posture. The weak infant has diminished or no spontaneous movement, often in striking contrast to the usual vigorous and plentiful movements of the normally active infant with normal strength (Fig. 39–5). The lower extremities are abducted and the lateral surfaces of the thighs lie against the examination table while the upper extremities lie extended alongside the body or flexed in a flaccid position beside the head. With marked weakness, there are no movements that overcome the pull of gravity. The immobility of the weak infant results in flattening of the occipital bone, with a flattened appearance of the posterior skull often associated with hair loss in the occipital region. When placed in a sitting posture, the infant droops forward, the shoulders droop, the head falls forward, and the arms hang limply.

PASSIVE TONE

Passive tone can be assessed by evaluating the passive resistance to movement of the limbs through a range of motion at the joints. Evaluation of the shoulders, elbows, wrists, hips, knees, and ankles is especially helpful. The examiner will sense a "looseness" of the limbs as the limbs are passively moved.

Additionally, grasping the midportion of the infant's limb and passively flapping the extremity allow the examiner to evaluate the degree of limpness of the distal extremity. In the hypotonic infant, the hands and feet wave limply; in the normal infant, the ankle and wrist are maintained fairly rigidly in line with the rest of the extremity.

Even in normal infants, there is a wide variation of muscle tone. Passive muscle tone varies during the course of the day and is particularly diminished following feeding and following activity prior to sleep. There is profound hypotonia in all infants during sleep. Tone can also be affected by the position of the head. The child whose head is turned to one side may be manifesting an asymmetric tonic neck response, with increased extensor tone on the side of the body to which the head is turned and increased flexor tone on the contralateral side. This asymmetry of tone may be elicited even in the child who does not exhibit the typical "fencer's" posture of the asymmetric tonic neck response. Therefore, examination of the infant should always be conducted while the head is in the midline; the same is true for eliciting muscle stretch reflexes. Striking hypotonia can also be associated with heart failure, sepsis, or acidosis; tone in infants may be modified by the baby's general health.

JOINT EXTENSIBILITY

The extent to which the joints may be extensible provides an indirect clue to the presence of hypotonia. Examination of the

Text continued on page 595

Table 39–1. Causes of Hypotonia and Weakness in Infancy and Childhood

Common

Systemic	Connective Tissue	Cerebral	Spinal Cord	Anterior Horn Cell	Peripheral Nerve	Neuromuscular Junction	Muscle
Sepsis Heart failure Acidosis Failure-to-thrive Hypoxia Renal failure Hypoglycemia Down syndrome Prader-Willi syndrome Noonan syndrome Fragile X syndrome	Stickler syndrome Marfan syndrome Achondroplasia	Hypoxic-ischemic brain injury Brain malformation Intrauterine infection Postnatal brain injury	Myelodysplasia Spinal cord tumor Epidural abscess Transverse myelitis Trauma (transection or compression)	Spinal muscular atrophies	Postinfectious polyneuropathy (Guillain-Barré syndrome) Toxic neuropathies Isoniazid Vincristine Nitrofurantoin Zidovudine	Botulism Infantile myasthenia Transient neonatal myasthenia	Duchenne muscular dystrophy Becker muscular dystrophy Myotonic dystrophy Inflammatory muscle disease (dermatomyositis-myositis)

Uncommon

Systemic	Connective Tissue	Cerebral	Spinal Cord	Anterior Horn Cell	Peripheral Nerve	Neuromuscular Junction	Muscle
Amino acid disorders Organic acid disorders Urea cycle disorders Scurvy Rickets Sotos syndrome Angelman syndrome Rett syndrome Smith-Lemli-Opitz syndrome	Ehlers-Danlos syndrome Osteogenesis imperfecta Velocardiofacial syndrome	Progressive encephalopathies Mitochondrial disease	Neonatal spinal cord transection Hypoxic-ischemic myelopathy Arteriovenous malformation	Möbius syndrome	Chronic inflammatory demyelinating polyneuropathy Hereditary motor and sensory neuropathy (Charcot-Marie-Tooth disease) Déjérine-Sottas disease Familial dysautonomia	Toxic organophosphate poisoning Postneuromuscular blocking agents (vecuronium)	

Rare

Systemic	Connective Tissue	Cerebral	Spinal Cord	Anterior Horn Cell	Peripheral Nerve	Neuromuscular Junction	Muscle
Lowe syndrome Zellweger syndrome Neonatal adrenal leukodystrophy Mucolipidosis IV Tay-Sachs disease Gangliosidosis Mannosidosis		Miller-Dieker syndrome Walker-Warburg syndrome		Poliomyelitis Incontinentia pigmentii Fazio-Londe disease Infantile neuroaxonal dystrophy GM_2 gangliosidosis Anterior spinal artery occlusion Arthrogryposis	Refsum disease Giant axonal neuropathy Metachromatic leukodystrophy Krabbe disease		Other muscular dystrophies Congenital myopathies Metabolic myopathies Mitochondrial myopathies Arthrogryposis

591

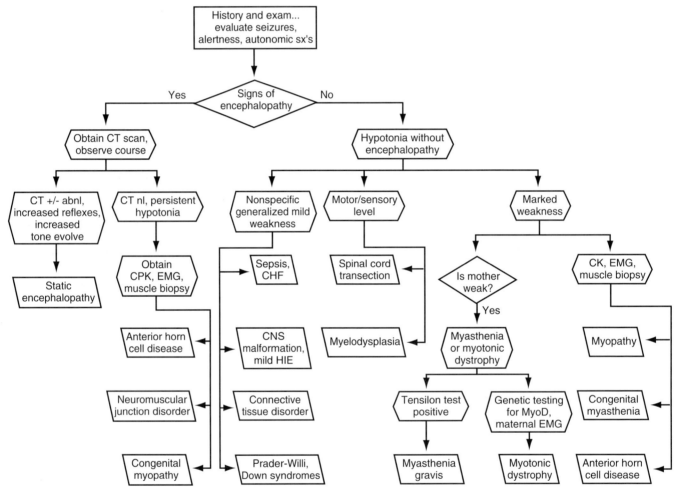

Figure 39–1. Approach to the floppy newborn. SX = signs; CT = computed tomography; EMG = electromyography; CPK (CK) = creatine phosphokinase; nl = normal; abnl = abnormal; CNS = central nervous system; CHF = congestive heart failure; HIE = hypoxic-ischemic encephalopathy; MyoD = myotonic dystrophy.

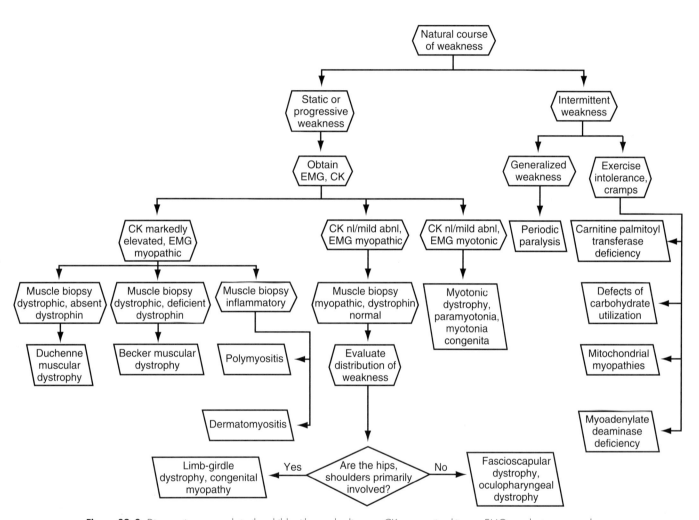

Figure 39–2. Diagnostic approach to the child with muscle disease. CK = creatine kinase; EMG = electromyography.

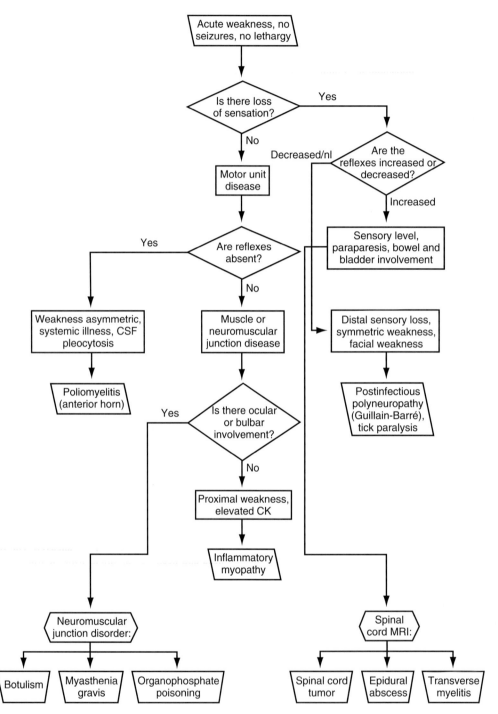

Figure 39–3. Diagnostic approach to the child with acute weakness. CSF = cerebrospinal fluid; CK = creatine phosphokinase; MRI = magnetic resonance imaging.

Table 39–2. Nonparalytic Conditions: Hypotonia Without Significant Weakness

1. Disorders of the central nervous system
   a. Nonspecific mental deficiency
   b. Birth trauma, intracranial haemorrhage, intrapartum asphyxia and hypoxia
   c. Hypotonic cerebral palsy
   d. Metabolic disorders: lipidoses (leucodystrophies); mucopolysaccharidoses; aminoacidurias; Leigh's syndrome
   e. Chromosomal abnormalities
      Down's syndrome
2. Connective tissue disorders
   Congenital laxity of ligaments
   Ehlers-Danlos and Marfan syndromes
   Osteogenesis imperfecta; arachnodactyly
3. Prader-Willi syndrome
4. Metabolic; nutritional; endocrine
   Organic acidaemias; hypercalcaemia; rickets; coeliac disease; hypothyroidism; renal tubular acidosis

Modified from Dubowitz V: Muscle Disorders in Childhood, 2nd ed. London: WB Saunders Co Ltd, 1995:459.

extent of mobility at the elbows, wrists, hips, and knees is especially helpful. The hypotonic infant may assume unusual postures in the presence of joint hyperextensibility. The "scarf sign" is a particularly useful sign of hyperextensibility in the newborn and young infant. With the infant in a semireclining position, the infant's hand is pulled across the chest toward the opposite shoulder and the position of the elbow is noted on completion of the maneuver. The presence of joint hyperextensibility is confirmed if the elbow passes the midline; this is suggestive of hypotonia.

depends on gestational age

POSTURAL REFLEXES

Three postural reflexes are particularly helpful in evaluating muscle tone in the infant.

Traction Response. The traction response is the most useful and

Table 39–3. Acute Generalized Weakness

Infectious Disorders
1. Acute infectious myositis
2. Acute inflammatory polyradiculoneuropathy (Guillain-Barré syndrome)
3. Enterovirus infections

Metabolic Disorders
1. Acute intermittent porphyria
2. Hereditary tyrosinemia

Neuromuscular Blockade
1. Botulism
2. Tick paralysis

Periodic Paralysis
1. Familial hyperkalemic
2. Familial hypokalemic
3. Familial normokalemic

Modified from Fenichel GM: Clinical Pediatric Neurology: A Signs and Symptoms Approach. Philadelphia: WB Saunders, 1993:187.

Table 39–4. Progressive Proximal Weakness

Spinal Cord Disorders
Juvenile Spinal Muscular Atrophies
1. Autosomal recessive
2. Autosomal dominant
3. GM_2 gangliosidosis (hexosaminidase A deficiency)

Myasthenic Syndromes
1. Familial limb-girdle
2. Myasthenia gravis
3. Slow channel syndrome

Myopathies
1. Muscular dystrophies
   a. Duchenne and Becker dystrophies
   b. Facioscapulohumeral syndrome
   c. Limb-girdle dystrophy
2. Inflammatory myopathies
   a. Dermatomyositis
   b. Polymyositis
   c. Inclusion body myositis
3. Metabolic myopathies
   a. Acid maltase deficiency
   b. Carnitine deficiency
   c. Debrancher enzyme deficiency
   d. Lipid storage myopathies
   e. Mitochondrial myopathies
   f. Myophosphorylase deficiency
4. Endocrine myopathies
   a. Adrenal cortex
   b. Parathyroid
   c. Thyroid

Modified from Fenichel GM: Clinical Pediatric Neurology: A Signs and Symptoms Approach. Philadelphia: WB Saunders, 1993:171.

most sensitive of these reflexes. With the infant lying supine, the infant's hand is grasped and the infant is pulled up to a sitting position (Fig. 39–6). Once the sitting posture is attained, the head is held erect in the midline. During the maneuver, the examiner notes the infant's attempt to counter the traction by flexion of the arms.

In an infant under 3 months of age, the plantar grasp should also be evident. Additionally, there should be flexion at the elbow, knee, and ankle in response to the maneuver. The degree to which the head and neck pull up along with the trunk depends on the child's age (Fig. 39–6).

In premature infants less than 33 weeks of gestation, there is no traction response. From 33 weeks to term, the infant has head lag but responds to the traction maneuver by flexing the neck flexors in an attempt to lift the head. The term infant exhibits a traction response with minimal head lag, and when the sitting posture is attained, the head may be held erect momentarily and then fall forward.

By age 3 months, there should be no head lag and the head should be aligned with the plane of the back as the child is pulled to sitting. The absence of flexion of the limbs in response to the examiner's pull and the presence of head lag inappropriate for age suggests hypotonia.

Axillary Suspension. The response to axillary suspension allows assessment of generalized and shoulder girdle tone. The infant is held under the arms and lifted; the infant is suspended from the axillae without the thorax being grasped. In infants with normal tone and strength, the shoulder girdle muscles exert enough strength to allow the infant to be suspended from the axillae without slip-

Table 39–5. Progressive Distal Weakness

Spinal Cord Disorders

Motor Neuron Diseases
1. Juvenile amyotrophic lateral sclerosis
2. Spinal muscular atrophies
   a. Genetic forms
   b. Nonfamilial Asian

Neuropathies

1. Hereditary motor sensory neuropathies (HMSN)
   a. HMSN I: Charcot-Marie-Tooth
   b. HMSN II: neuronal Charcot-Marie-Tooth
   c. HMSN III: Déjérine-Sottas
   d. HMSN IV: Refsum
2. Other genetic neuropathies
   a. Familial amyloid neuropathy
   b. Giant axonal neuropathy
   c. Pyruvate dehydrogenase deficiency
   d. Sulfatide lipidoses: metachromatic leukodystrophy
   e. Other leukodystrophies
3. Neuropathies with systemic diseases
   a. Drug-induced
   b. Systemic vasculitis
   c. Toxins
   d. Uremia
4. Idiopathic neuropathy
   a. Chronic axonal neuropathy
   b. Chronic demyelinating neuropathy

Myopathies

1. Hereditary distal myopathies
2. Myotonic dystrophy

Scapulo(humeral) Peroneal Syndrome

1. Bethlem myopathy
2. Emery-Dreifuss syndrome
3. Scapulohumeral syndrome with dementia
4. Scapuloperoneal neuronopathy

Modified from Fenichel GM. Clinical Pediatric Neurology: A Signs and Symptoms Approach, 2nd ed. Philadelphia: WB Saunders, 1993:181.

ping through the examiner's grasp. Additionally, the infant's head is held midline and the legs are held with some flexion at the hips, knees, and ankles. The hypotonic infant will droop with legs extended and head falling forward, and the absence of resistance of the muscles of the shoulder girdle allows the infant to slip through the grasp of the examiner as the baby's arms fling upward.

Ventral Suspension. The response to ventral suspension allows assessment of tone of the trunk, neck, and extremities (Fig. 39–6). The examiner holds the infant, who is lying prone. The infant is supported only by the examiner's hand on the abdomen. A normal infant will hold the head erect and the back straight and will hold the extremities with some flexion at the elbows, hips, knees, and ankles. A full-term neonate makes intermittent attempts to hold the head straight, maintains the back straight, and can flex the limbs. The hypotonic infant droops in the examiner's palm, as if in the shape of an inverted U, with the head and legs dangling limply.

Diagnostic Approach

A careful perinatal history is obtained to identify possible features suggestive of perinatal hypoxic-ischemic brain injury. The infant who has a neurologic dysfunction attributable to perinatal asphyxia should have demonstrated evidence of an acute encephalopathy during the neonatal period (disturbance of consciousness, poor feeding, seizures, autonomic dysfunction).

A computed tomography (CT) or magnetic resonance imaging (MRI) study of the head is helpful to identify evidence of brain malformation, intrauterine infection, hypoxic brain injury, intracranial hemorrhage, or hydrocephalus. If the history suggests seizures, an electroencephalogram (EEG) should be obtained.

An ophthalmologic evaluation should be requested to detect evidence of ocular malformation (cataracts, microphthalmia, optic hypoplasia), evidence of intrauterine infection (chorioretinitis), or retinal/macular abnormality (retinitis pigmentosa, cherry-red spot) (see Chapter 44).

In some cases, requesting a hearing evaluation or brainstem auditory evoked response may be appropriate. A lumbar puncture is necessary only if acute or chronic (intrauterine) meningitis is suspected.

Figure 39–1 summarizes the approach to the floppy newborn. After a careful history and physical examination, it should be determined whether or not the infant is exhibiting signs of encephalopathy. If so, a CT scan of the head is obtained to determine the presence of any anatomic abnormalities. If the scan does not reveal an anatomic abnormality and if the neonate exhibits increased reflexes and tone over time, a diagnosis of *static encephalopathy* can be made. If hypotonia persists, anterior horn cell disease, congenital myopathy, or neuromuscular junction disease should be considered (see Table 39–1, Table 39–6, and Fig. 39–4).

If the baby is not encephalopathic, the practitioner should determine whether a systemic disease is present (*Prader-Willi syndrome* or *Down syndrome*). Is there a motor-sensory level consistent with myelodysplasia or spinal cord injury?

If the baby is markedly weak, is the mother also weak, or does she display myotonia? If so, transplacental-derived transient neonatal myasthenia gravis or myotonic dystrophy, respectively, is a possibility (Table 39–9). If not, myopathy, congenital myasthenia, infant botulism (Table 39–10), or anterior horn cell disease must be considered (see Tables 39–4 and 39–5).

COMMON DISORDERS

Hypoxic-Ischemic Encephalopathy

Hypoxic-ischemic encephalopathy is a general term that describes a child with sustained hypoxic and ischemic injury (most commonly in the neonatal period) resulting in varying degrees of mental and motor developmental impairment. The typical child with severe hypoxic-ischemic encephalopathy is markedly hypotonic during the newborn period and demonstrates other manifestations of encephalopathy (seizures, poor suck, poor feeding, impaired alertness). Over the course of weeks to several months, signs of hyperreflexia and hypertonia begin to evolve, generally in a rostral-caudal progression. In some infants, hypotonia persists and is the prominent motor sign. The term *hypotonic cerebral palsy* is often used to describe this group. In most of the infants, however, signs of spasticity or dyskinetic movements develop and these children make up the more common spastic cerebral palsy and dyskinetic cerebral palsy groups.

The diagnosis is established by a nonprogressive but often evolving clinical course, with supportive evidence provided by the perinatal history and by CT or MRI findings. Important intervention issues include physical therapy, referral for early services, special education, nutritional counseling, prevention of contractures, adaptive seating, and adaptive equipment.

Table 39–6. Distinguishing Features in Motor Weakness

	Upper Motor Unit		Lower Motor Unit			
	Brain	*Spinal Cord*	*Anterior Horn Cell*	*Peripheral Nerve*	*Neuromuscular Junction*	*Muscle*
Deep tendon reflexes	Normal to ↑	↓ Acutely; ↑	↓ To absent	↓ To absent (lost early)	Normal	Normal to ↓ (lost late)
Strength	Normal	↓	↓	↓	↓	↓
Tone	↑ (Spasticity)	↓ Acutely; ↑	↓ (Flaccid)	↓	↓	↓
Level of consciousness	↓	Normal	Normal	Normal	Normal	Normal
Fasciculations	Absent	Absent	Present	Rare	Absent	Absent
Primitive reflexes, including Babinski	Present	±	Absent	Absent	Absent	Absent
Atrophy	Less prominent	Less prominent	Present	Present	Absent	Present; pseudohypertrophy
Sensation	Normal	Absent below lesion	Normal	±	Normal	Normal
Location	Generalized; may be hemiplegic	Below lesion	Symmetric for SMA; asymmetric for poliomyelitis	Symmetric for GBS; asymmetric for mononeuritis; usually distal	Symmetric	Symmetric; usually proximal
Creatine phosphokinase	Normal	Normal	Normal	May be elevated	Normal	↑

Abbreviations: SMA = Spinal muscular atrophy; GBS = Guillain-Barré syndrome.

Table 39–7. Common Causes of Hypotonia and Weakness

	Hypoxic Ischemic Encephalopathy	Brain Malformation	Spinal Cord Transection	Transverse Myelitis	Spinal Cord Tumor	Spinal Muscular Atrophy	Polio-myelitis	Guillain-Barré	Myasthenia Gravis	Botulism	Myopathy
Dysmorphism, malformation		√									
Seizures, MR, lethargy	√	√									
Motor/sensory level			√	√	√						
Hypotonia	√	√	√	√	√	√	√	√	√	√	√
Hypertonia	√	√	√	√	√						
Reflexes increased	√	√	√	√	√						
Reflexes decreased	√	√	√	√	√	√	√	√		√	Decreased or normal
Proximal weakness						√					√
Distal weakness								√			
Abnormal CT/MRI	√	√	√	√	√						
Abnormal NCV								√			
Abnormal EMG	√	√	√	√	√	√	√	√	√	√	√
Acute onset weakness	Initially		√	√	√		√	√	√	√	√ Inflammatory, metabolic myopathies
Chronic progressive weakness						√	√		√		√

Abbreviations: CT = computed tomography; MRI = magnetic resonance imaging; MR = mental retardation; SMA = spinal muscular atrophy; NCV = nerve conduction velocity; EMG = electromyography.

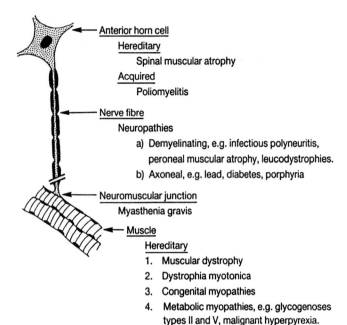

Anterior horn cell
   Hereditary
      Spinal muscular atrophy
   Acquired
      Poliomyelitis

Nerve fibre
   Neuropathies
      a) Demyelinating, e.g. infectious polyneuritis,
          peroneal muscular atrophy, leucodystrophies.
      b) Axoneal, e.g. lead, diabetes, porphyria

Neuromuscular junction
   Myasthenia gravis

Muscle
   Hereditary
    1. Muscular dystrophy
    2. Dystrophia myotonica
    3. Congenital myopathies
    4. Metabolic myopathies, e.g. glycogenoses
       types II and V, malignant hyperpyrexia.

   Acquired
    1. Dermatomyositis/polymyositis
    2. Endocrine myopathies, e.g. thyrotoxic
    3. Iatrogenic, e.g. steroid myopathy

Figure 39–4. Disorders of the lower motor neurone: anatomical approach. (From Dubowitz V. Muscle Disorders in Childhood, 2nd ed. London: WB Saunders Co Ltd, 1995:2.)

Brain Malformations

Brain malformation can arise as a result of a chromosomal disorder, as a component of a multiple malformation syndrome, or as an isolated abnormality of brain morphogenesis. When associated with chromosomal disorder or multiple malformation syndromes, the other associated features are the primary clues to diagnosis. In isolated brain malformation, the primary features are microcephaly (in most) and cognitive and motor developmental impairment. The MRI scan can detect abnormalities of development of the hemispheric structures (agenesis of the corpus callosum, holoprosencephaly), abnormalities of cortical cellular migration (lissencephaly, pachygyria), and cerebral heterotopias as well as brainstem and cerebellar malformations.

UNCOMMON DISORDERS

Progressive Encephalopathies of Infancy

Progressive encephalopathies of infancy account for a small number of children with persistent hypotonia (see Chapter 34).

Table 39–8. Grading Muscle Strength

0: No contraction
1: Minimal contraction only
2: Moves in horizontal plane but not against gravity
3: Moves against gravity but not against resistance
4: Moves against gravity and minimal resistance
5: Moves against gravity and full resistance

Table 39–9. Clinical Features of Congenital Myotonic Dystrophy

Clinical Feature	% of Cases Exhibiting Feature
Reduced fetal movements	68
Polyhydramnios	80
Premature birth (<36 wk)	52
Facial diplegia	100
Feeding difficulties	92
Hypotonia	100
Atrophy	100
Hyporeflexia or areflexia	87
Respiratory distress	88
Arthrogryposis	82
Edema	54
Elevated right hemidiaphragm	49
Transmission via mother	100
Neonatal mortality	41
Infant death in sibs	28
Mental retardation in survivors	100

From Volpe JJ. Neurology of the Newborn, 3rd ed. Philadelphia: WB Saunders, 1995:635.

These disorders are recognizable by a progressive deterioration of neurologic function and by diagnostically specific clues. The infant with a progressive encephalopathy develops normally for a period of time, then plateaus in developmental progress, followed by regression, with loss of previously acquired skills (see Chapter 34). Hypotonia is a feature of many of these disorders, at least at some point during the course of the illness (Tay-Sachs disease), and some disorders feature hypotonia as the result of associated polyneuropathy (Krabbe and metachromatic leukodystrophies). Progressive disorders that may be associated with hypotonia include neonatal adrenoleukodystrophy, mannosidosis, fucosidosis, Gaucher disease types 2 and 3, GM_1 gangliosidosis, infantile neuroaxonal dystrophy, infantile Refsum disease, Krabbe leukodystrophy, metachromatic leukodystrophy, mucolipidosis type IV, and Tay-Sachs disease. The diagnosis of these disorders is based on recognition of clinically suggestive clues and specialized biochemical and molecular genetic testing. If such a disorder is suspected, the infant should be referred to appropriate genetic and neurologic specialists for evaluation.

Table 39–10. Infantile Botulism versus "Congenital Myasthenia"

	Infantile Botulism	"Congenital Myasthenia"
Generalized hypotonia and weakness	+	+/−
Facial weakness, ptosis	+	+
Pupillary abnormality	+	−
Constipation	+	−
Response to anticholinesterase	−	+
Electromyography	Incremental response	Decremental response

Modified from Volpe JJ. Neurology of the Newborn, 3rd ed. Philadelphia: WB Saunders, 1995:628.

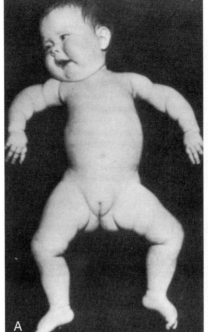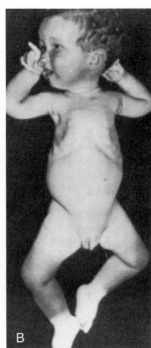

Figure 39–5. Werdnig-Hoffmann disease: characteristic postures. Six-week-old *(A)* and 1-year-old *(B)* infants with severe weakness and hypotonia from birth. Note the frog-leg posture of the lower limbs and internal rotation ("jughandle") *(A)* or external rotation *(B)* at shoulders. Intercostal recession is especially evident in *B*, and facial expressions are normal (From Volpe JJ. Neurology of the Newborn, 3rd ed. Philadelphia: WB Saunders, 1995:609.)

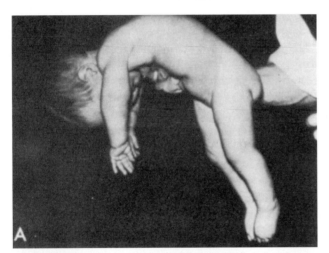
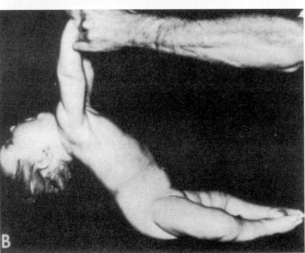

Figure 39–6. Werdnig-Hoffmann disease: clinical manifestations of weakness of limb and axial musculature in a 6-week-old infant with severe weakness and hypotonia from birth. Note the marked weakness of the limbs and trunk on ventral suspension *(A)* and of the neck *(B)* on pull to sit. (From Volpe JJ. Neurology of the Newborn, 3rd ed. Philadelphia: WB Saunders, 1995:609.)

Mitochondrial Diseases

Mitochondrial diseases often affect both the brain and muscle and clinically manifest hypotonia, probably as a combination of both cerebral dysfunction and myopathy (Tables 39–11 and 39–12). The diagnosis is based on recognition of clinical symptoms, presence of lactic acidosis, presence of ragged red fibers on muscle histologic examination, and mitochondrial abnormalities identifiable on a muscle electron microscopic examination. The diagnosis of many mitochondrial diseases is possible by specific mitochondrial DNA testing. Other inborn errors of metabolism may produce hypotonia by central mechanisms (organic acidurias, hyperammonemia) or by interfering with muscle metabolism (Table 39–13).

Brain Malformation Syndromes

Some specific brain malformation syndromes are associated with a striking degree of hypotonia.

Miller-Dieker Syndrome. A cortical malformation, lissencephaly, produces severe developmental impairment and hypotonia early in life, and hypertonia develops later. There is a somewhat characteristic recognizable facies, and many infants have a demonstrable deletion of the short arm of chromosome 17.

Walker-Warburg Syndrome. The combination of brain malformation (polymicrogyria, cerebellar malformation) and an associated congenital muscular dystrophy produces marked hypotonia in infancy.

Table 39–11. Clinical Features of Mitochondrial Disease

Nervous System

1. Ataxia
2. Central apnea
3. Deafness
4. Dementia
5. Hypotonia
6. Mental retardation
7. Neuropathy
8. Ophthalmoplegia
9. Optic atrophy
10. Retinitis pigmentosa

Heart

1. Cardiomyopathy
2. Conduction defects

Kidney

1. Aminoaciduria
2. Hyperphosphaturia

Skeletal Muscle

1. Exercise intolerance
2. Myopathy

From Fenichel GM. Clinical Pediatric Neurology: A Signs and Symptoms Approach, 2nd ed. Philadelphia: WB Saunders, 1993:205.

Table 39–12. Mitochondrial Disorders

Complex I (NADH—Coenzyme Q Reductase)

1. Congenital lactic acidosis, hypotonia, seizures, and apnea
2. Exercise intolerance and myalgia
3. Kearns-Sayre syndrome
4. Metabolic encephalopathy, lactic acidosis, and stroke (MELAS)
5. Progressive infantile poliodystrophy
6. Subacute necrotizing encephalomyelopathy

Complex II (Succinate—Coenzyme Q Reductase)

1. Encephalomyopathy (?)

Complex III (Coenzyme QH₂—Cytochrome *c* Reductase)

1. Cardiomyopathy
2. Kearns-Sayre syndrome
3. Myopathy and exercise intolerance with or without progressive external ophthalmoplegia

Complex IV (Cytochrome *c* Oxidase)

1. Fatal neonatal hypotonia
2. Menkes syndrome
3. Myoclonus epilepsy and ragged-red fibers (MERRF)
4. Progressive infantile poliodystrophy
5. Subacute necrotizing encephalomyelopathy
6. Transitory neonatal hypotonia

Complex V (Adenosine Triphosphate Synthase)

1. Congenital myopathy
2. Neuropathy, retinopathy, ataxia, and dementia
3. Retinitis pigmentosa, ataxia, neuropathy, and dementia

Modified from Fenichel GM. Clinical Pediatric Neurology: A Signs and Symptoms Approach, 2nd ed. Philadelphia: WB Saunders, 1993:206.

THE HYPOTONIC OLDER CHILD

Clinical Evaluation

POSTURE AND STRENGTH

Observation of the child's spontaneous posture may suggest the presence of weakness. Muscle strength can be observed as the child is asked to perform functional tasks, including pulling to sit spontaneously from a prone position, arising to stand from a sitting or lying position (Gower sign) (Fig. 39–7), standing on one leg independently, hopping, walking, running, and climbing stairs. The wheelbarrow maneuver can be used to functionally assess strength in the upper extremities. In the child above age 5 or 6 years, manual muscle testing can be performed if the child is cooperative (see Table 39–8). The examiner evaluates each muscle group independently, comparing the child's muscle strength in resistance to the examiner's. The child with muscle weakness will have difficulty performing motor tasks and may exhibit unusual postures (lordosis) or might manifest the Gower maneuver (see Fig. 39–7) or toewalking and on manual muscle testing may be easily overcome by the examiner's strength.

PASSIVE TONE

Passive muscle tone is more consistent during the waking hours in the child than in the infant. The major joints should be moved

Table 39-13. Glycogenoses That Affect Muscle

Type	Enzyme Deficiency	Eponymous or Other Names	Subunit; Isozyme	Gene Location	Clinical Features	Other Tissues/ Systems Affected
II	α-1,4-Glucosidase (acid maltase)	Pompe's disease	—	17(q23–q25)	(a) Severe form: generalized resembles infantile spinal muscular atrophy (b) Mild form: resembles limb girdle dystrophy	Heart, nervous system, leucocytes, liver, kidneys ? Heart
III	Amylo-1,6-glucosidase ("debranching enzyme")	Limit dextrinosis Forbes' disease Cori's disease	—	NK	Infantile hypotonia Mild weakness	Hepatic Hypoglycaemia Ketosis Leucocytes Cardiac
IV	α-1,4-Glucan: α1,4-glucan 6-glycosyl transferase ("branching enzyme"; amylo (1,4→1,6) transglucosidase)	Amylopectinosis	—	NK	Usually no muscle symptoms In some wasting or weakness	Hepatomegaly Cirrhosis Liver failure Cardiac
V	Muscle phosphorylase	McArdle's disease	M	11q13	Exercise intolerance Muscle cramps Fatigue Myoglobinuria	None
VII	Phosphofructokinase	Tarui's disease	M	1(cen–q32)	Exercise intolerance Muscle cramps Fatigue Myoglobinuria	Haemolytic anaemia
VIII	Phosphorylase *b* kinase		α β	Xq12–q13 16q12–q13	Exercise intolerance Muscle stiffness Weakness	Liver Cardiac
IX	Phosphoglycerate kinase		A	X(q13)	Exercise intolerance Muscle cramps Fatigue Myoglobinuria	Haemolytic anaemia Central nervous system
X	Phosphoglycerate kinase		M	7	Exercise intolerance Muscle cramps Fatigue Myoglobinuria	
XI	Lactate dehydrogenase		M	11	Exercise intolerance Muscle cramps Fatigue Myoglobinuria	

Modified from Dubowitz V. Muscle Disorders in Childhood, 2nd ed. London: WB Saunders Co Ltd, 1995:178.
Abbreviation: NK = Not known.

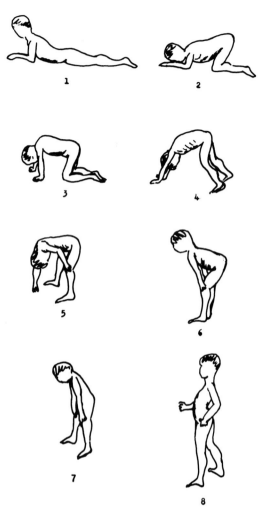

Figure 39–7. The Gowers maneuver showing sequence of postures used in getting up from the ground. *1,* Lying prone. *2, 3,* Getting on to hands and knees. *4,* Legs and arms extended and legs brought as close as possible to arms. *5,* Hand placed on knee. *6,* Both hands on knees, knees extended. *7,* Hands moving alternately up thighs "climbing up himself." *8,* Erect posture. (From Dubowitz V. Muscle Disorders in Childhood, 2nd ed. London: WB Saunders Co Ltd, 1995:42.)

through a range of motion and the extent of resistance noted. Flapping the distal extremities provides a useful clue to passive tone. Lifting the lower extremity briskly at the knee while the patient lies supine is a useful test of muscle tone. In the normal child, the foot briefly drags along the examination table, then lifts with the leg. In the hypertonic child, the leg remains extended stiffly at the knee. In the hypotonic child, the lower leg hangs limply and the foot drags along the examination table as the knee is raised.

JOINT EXTENSIBILITY

The hypotonic child demonstrates hyperextensibility of joints, especially at the elbows, wrists, knees, and ankles. Examination of the small muscles of the fingers may also be helpful.

Diagnostic Approach

The diagnosis of a particular neurologic disorder depends on the location of the lesion (i.e., which part of the nervous system is impaired or abnormal), the patient's age, and whether or not the condition is progressive or static. Tables 39–1 and 39–6 summarize the features of common causes of hypotonia; Figure 39–2 outlines an algorithm for determining the etiology of muscle weakness in a child (see also Tables 39–2 to 39–5).

Anatomic Localization

The initial approach is to identify the location of dysfunction along the axis of the nervous system. Disorders of the cerebral cortex commonly cause hypotonia in infants and children, a phenomenon that is much less common than in adult neurologic disease. In children, more than one component of the nervous system may be affected, and the net result is neurologic dysfunction resulting in hypotonia. Some progressive neurologic disorders affect both the brain and peripheral nerves (metachromatic leukodystrophy, a lipid storage disorder, and some mitochondrial disorders). Other progressive disorders may affect both brain and muscle (Walker-Warburg syndrome, neonatal myotonic dystrophy, and some mitochondrial disorders).

Sometimes disturbance of function at one site conveys a predilection for injury to another site in the nervous system. Children with congenital muscle weakness (congenital myopathy) are likely to have severe respiratory impairment at birth that results in secondary anoxic injury to the brain. Because hypotonia is nonspecific with regard to localizing the site of nervous system dysfunction, the evaluation of the child with hypotonia must begin with a search for other clues that might identify the location of the abnormality in the central or peripheral nervous system.

Is the Problem a Systemic Disorder?

Systemic disorders (see Table 39–1) are a common cause of generalized hypotonia in infants and even in toddlers and children. Hypotonia is commonly seen in association with sepsis and other infections, heart failure, failure to thrive, hypercalcemia, renal failure, hypothyroidism, acidosis, hypoxia, hyperammonemia, hypoglycemia, rickets, scurvy, amino and organic acid disorders, severe malnutrition, and other chronic disorders. This observation warrants a careful search for a systemic or metabolic abnormality in children with hypotonia, particularly (but not exclusively) when the onset of hypotonia is acute (Table 39–3 and Fig. 39–3). Most of these disorders cause hypotonia by causing a disturbance of cerebral cortex function.

Frequently overlooked causes of hypotonia are those that are not traditionally considered to be neurologic disorders. Connective tissue disorders often produce a clinical picture similar to neurologic causes of hypotonia in infancy and early childhood, with associated delay of developmental milestones (velocardiofacial syndrome, achondroplasia, Marfan syndrome, Ehlers-Danlos syndrome). Several congenital disorders regularly feature hypotonia as a result of a combination of abnormalities of neurologic, muscle, and connective tissue function, including Soto syndrome, Prader-Willi syndrome, Angelman syndrome, Noonan syndrome, Rett syndrome and Smith-Lemli-Opitz syndrome. (These are described later.)

DIAGNOSTIC CONSIDERATIONS

Any child with hypotonia and weakness should be evaluated for clues suggestive of a systemic disorder. Laboratory evaluation, such as electrolytes, tests of renal function, thyroid function tests, and acid-base balance, should be considered for common metabolic disorders. Laboratory evaluation should also be considered for uncommon metabolic disorders in infants and children with chronic hypotonia, especially those with other neurologic findings and those with recurrent bouts of lethargy, pronounced hypotonia, vomiting, or acidosis. Appropriate metabolic screening tests include plasma and urine amino acid quantification, urine organic acid quantification, blood ammonia, blood lactate, and pyruvate.

Cytogenic studies should be done for any hypotonic child who additionally demonstrates microcephaly, growth retardation, congenital malformations, dysmorphism, global developmental delay, or features of specific disorders (Down or Prader-Willi syndrome.)

Connective tissue disorders should be considered, especially if joint hyperextensibility and hypotonia are disproportionate to the extent of weakness and in the absence of other neurologic abnormalities or microcephaly. The diagnosis of these disorders is generally based on clinical criteria, but increasingly molecular genetic testing is becoming available (see Table 39–2).

If unusual neurologic or dysmorphic features are present, specific disorders, such as Rett syndrome, Angelman syndrome, Prader-Willi syndrome, Noonan syndrome, Soto syndrome, must be considered. Fragile X mental retardation is also often associated with mild hypotonia.

COMMON DISORDERS

Down Syndrome

The child with Down syndrome generally has stereotypic and recognizable features, including microcephaly, up-slanted palpebral fissures, epicanthal folds, a flat nasal bridge, a protuberant tongue, excess posterior nuchal skin, and simian palmar creases. Hypotonia and associated weakness are an almost constant finding in the infant. As the child with Down syndrome grows, generally the muscle strength improves but the hypotonia persists.

The diagnosis is established by chromosome analysis. Important intervention issues include genetic counseling, referral for early intervention therapeutic services, special education, and monitoring for medical complications, including hypothyroidism, hearing loss, and atlantoaxial dislocation.

Prader-Willi Syndrome

Prader-Willi syndrome presents in the newborn period or early infancy with marked hypotonia and with virtually no other identifiable symptoms. As the child grows, the phenotypic features become more apparent, including microbrachycephaly, almond-shaped palpebrae, short stature, and small hands and feet. At age 3 to 6 years, the child has a disorder of appetite that results in ravenous food-seeking behaviors, impaired satiety, and eventual marked obesity. Weakness associated with the disorder is most prominent in the neonate and infant and gradually improves while the hypotonia persists.

The molecular diagnosis can be obtained by chromosome analysis in many of the children and by a fluorescence *in situ* hybridization (FISH) study or by a study for uniparental disomy in the remainder. Because the clinical findings are nonspecific during the early months, such testing should be performed in any neonate or infant with hypotonia of unknown etiology. Important intervention issues include genetic counseling, referral for early services, special education, nutritional counseling, behavior management, and monitoring for medical complications of the disorder, including glucose intolerance and complications of morbid obesity.

UNCOMMON DISORDERS

Metabolic Disorders

Metabolic disorders that are associated with hypotonia include the following (see Tables 39–1 and 39–11 to 39–13):

- Amino acid and organic acid disorders
- Lowe syndrome
- Peroxisomal disorders (infantile Refsum, infantile adrenoleukodystrophy, Zellweger syndrome)
- Acyl coenzyme A (CoA) dehydrogenase deficiencies
- Storage disorders (mannosidosis, Krabbe disease, sialuria, mucolipidosis IV, Tay-Sachs disease)

Neurologic Disorders

Neurologic disorders associated with hypotonia are often recognizable by unusual neurologic features, including:

- Angelman syndrome (awkward gait, inappropriate laughter, seizures)
- Rett syndrome (autism, loss of hand use, characteristic wringing hand movements)

Congenital Malformation Syndromes

Congenital malformation syndromes are recognizable by their characteristic features and include:

- Soto syndrome (macrocephaly, macrosomia, down-slanted palpebrae, mild ventriculomegaly)
- Noonan syndrome (short stature, down-slanted palpebrae, ear abnormalities, congenital heart disease, wide-spaced nipples and shield chest, pectus deformities)
- Lowe syndrome (cataracts, aminoaciduria, hypotonia)

Connective Tissue Disorders

Connective tissue disorders associated with hypotonia, and particularly with joint hyperextensibility, can also generally be recognized by their associated symptoms, including:

- Stickler syndrome (micrognathia, Pierre-Robin cleft palate)
- Velocardiofacial syndrome (congenital heart disease, cleft palate)
- Achondroplasia (disproportionate short stature)
- Ehlers-Danlos syndrome (skin bruising and scarring, skin hyperelasticity)
- Marfan syndrome (tall stature, long, thin arms and fingers, ectopic lens, blue sclera, aortic dissection, mitral valve prolapse)
- Osteogenesis imperfecta (bone fractures)

Is the Problem in the Cerebrum or Cerebellum?

Several clues suggest that hypotonia is due to abnormality of cerebral function. The presence of associated symptoms attributable to dysfunction of the cerebral cortex is the most useful, including:

- Acute impairment of consciousness
- Acute or chronic impairment of cognitive abilities (mental status examination or poor school grades, respectively)
- Seizures

Delayed language and social development are typical of chronic problems. The presence of microcephaly or macrocephaly is also an important clue. The presence of brisk reflexes, clonus, an asymmetric tonic neck response, and the Babinski sign suggests possible cerebral cortical dysfunction (upper motor neuron disorder). The presence of dysmorphism or of congenital malformations suggests the possibility of a cerebral malformation. Congenital ocular malformations (e.g., microphthalmia or optic hypoplasia) are frequently associated with congenital brain malformation.

The presence of signs of hypertonia mixed with signs of hypotonia strongly suggests a cerebral origin of hypotonia. This may seem paradoxical, but it is often overlooked that many children with cerebral causes of hypotonia have signs of hypotonia as well as hypertonia. This may occur as an evolutionary phenomenon in the development of spasticity, as the typical course of cerebral palsy is characterized by hypotonia in infancy with later development of spasticity. In some children with cerebral dysfunction, the coexistence of signs of hypotonia and hypertonia is persistent. Thus, an infant with hypotonia of the neck and trunk musculature who also exhibits scissoring of the lower extremities or persistent fisting of the hands (typical signs of hypertonia) can be presumed to have a cerebral cause of neurologic dysfunction.

Signs of cerebellar dysfunction are often useful diagnostic clues (see Chapter 43). The cerebellum helps to maintain normal muscle tone, and diseases of the cerebellum typically are associated with some degree of hypotonia. Associated features of ataxia, titubation, dysmetria, and impairment of coordination indicate cerebellar disease.

Is the Problem in the Spinal Cord?

Classically, spinal cord dysfunction produces spastic weakness of all four extremities or paraparesis of the lower extremities (Tables 39–14 to 39–16). However, particularly after acute injury to the spinal cord—and in some chronic disorders of the spinal cord—hypotonia may be the prominent motor sign. The typical associated findings of hyperreflexia, clonus, Babinski signs, and sensory loss (with a sensory level) are important clues, as is the disparity between the weakness and sensory impairment of the extremities in contrast to the normal strength and function of the head and neck.

The possibility of spinal cord injury resulting from birth trauma is frequently overlooked as a cause of hypotonia in the newborn. A history of a lengthy, difficult delivery should suggest spinal cord injury, and care should be taken not to falsely attribute motor dysfunction in these infants to anoxic brain injury. *This is a diagnosis that should never be missed,* as neurosurgical intervention is often required. To make matters more confusing, many spinal cord–injured neonates indeed also have anoxic encephalopathy because of the usually traumatic nature of the delivery.

Finally, the extent to which the hypotonia of neonatal hypoxic-ischemic injury is caused by hypoxic injury to the spinal cord has not yet been fully evaluated. Any child with suspected spinal cord injury deserves neuroradiologic evaluation.

If spinal cord injury is suspected in any aged patient:

1. Immobilize the head and neck of any child or newborn in whom spinal cord trauma is suspected.
2. Examine the back for evidence of tenderness, bony displacements, myelodysplasia, midline hairy tuft, dermal sinus, hemangioma, or pigmentary abnormality.
3. Obtain a spine sonogram in infants if spinal abnormality is suspected on the basis of midline cutaneous abnormality of the back.
4. Obtain spine films and an MRI study of the spine when spinal cord dysfunction is evident and when spinal trauma is suspected.
5. Obtain neurosurgical consultation when structural abnormality of the spine is identified or strongly suspected.
6. Administer very-high-dose intravenous methylprednisolone (Solu-Medrol) for all traumatic spine injuries while obtaining neurosurgical intervention. (Solu-Medrol, 30 mg/kg, is given over 45 minutes, followed by 5.4 mg/kg/hour for 23 hours).

COMMON DISORDERS

Meningomyelocele, a congenital malformation of the spine, spinal cord, and overlying meninges, affects 1 in 500 to 1 in 2000 live-born infants, with some degree of geographic variation of incidence. The spinal defect is obvious at birth except in more mild abnormalities that are covered by skin. The degree to which the lower extremities are hypotonic and flaccid depends on the location of the spinal defect. The presence of an Arnold-Chiari malformation and associated hydrocephalus must be evaluated in every patient with a CT scan.

Intervention issues are complex and include early neurosurgical repair, physical therapy, orthopedic management, urologic management, neurosurgical management of hydrocephalus, special education, adaptive seating, and genetic counseling.

UNCOMMON DISORDERS

Spinal Cord Transection

Spinal cord transection in the newborn has been discussed. The practitioner should be particularly concerned regarding difficult deliveries (breech, internal versions, star gazing fetal position).

Spinal Cord Tumor

Spinal cord tumor (primary or metastatic) usually presents with subacute onset of spastic weakness of the extremities but occasionally may present as hypotonia (Table 39–14). Rapid diagnosis with MRI and medical (prednisone, irradiation) or neurosurgical interventions are essential.

Transverse Myelitis

Transverse myelitis is a common cause of acute hypotonia and weakness. As with any spinal cord lesion, the localization is suggested by an identifiable motor-sensory level, impairment of bowel and bladder function, and hyperreflexia and Babinski signs. The diagnosis is made by MRI scan and lumbar puncture findings, with abnormal signal intensity of the cord segment involved on MRI scan and with mild pleocytosis and elevated cerebrospinal fluid protein. Treatment with steroids has been traditional, but its benefit is not entirely well established.

Epidural Spinal Abscesses

Epidural spinal abscesses may present in a similar manner except with more back pain and local tenderness. Drainage and antibiotics are necessary.

Table 39–14. Spinal Cord Syndromes

Site	Mechanism	Manifestation
Complete—upper cord (above T10)	Space-occupying lesion Trauma	Flaccid symmetric weakness, paralysis, loss of sensation below lesion, areflexia (in spinal shock), reflexes return and are ↑ after recovery from spinal shock, distended bladder, positive Babinski, positive Beevor sign*
Conus medullaris (T10–L2)	Space-occupying lesion Trauma	Symmetric weakness—paralysis, ↑ knee deep tendon reflexes, ↓ ankle deep tendon reflexes, saddle perineum sensory loss, no Babinski sign
Cauda equina (below L2)	Space-occupying lesion Tethered cord (?) Trauma	Asymmetric weakness, loss of deep tendon reflexes, sensory deficit, no Babinski sign
Anterior cord	Flexion-rotation force from anterior dislocation or compression fracture of vertebral body ($\pm$ ischemia of anterior spinal artery)	Weakness and reduced pain and temperature sensation
Central cord	Hyperextension injury; tumor, hemorrhage, syringomyelia	Flaccid weakness of arms (lower motor neuron lesion) with strong and spastic lower extremities (upper motor neuron lesion) Sacral sensation with bowel and bladder are partially affected
Posterior cord	Hyperextension (fractures of posterior vertebra)	Significant ataxia (loss of proprioception); strength and pain and temperature sensations may be spared or less affected
Brown-Séquard	Laceration (stabs), lateral space-occupying lesions: hemisection	Strength is affected on the side of the lesion; pain and temperature sensation is affected on the contralateral side

*Beevor sign = superior displacement of umbilicus in paraplegia when attempting to lift shoulders off an examining table.

Is the Problem in the Motor Unit?

The functional unit of the anterior horn cell, peripheral nerve, neuromuscular junction, and muscle fiber make up the motor unit (see Fig. 39–4). Disorders that affect the motor unit present a common clinical picture characterized by preservation of cognitive function and alertness, absence of seizures, characteristically diminished or absent muscle stretch reflexes, and hypotonia (see Tables 39–2 and 39–4 to 39–6). Muscle atrophy is frequently associated with motor unit disorders, but it can also occur in cerebral causes of hypotonia.

It is not always easy to determine at the bedside which component of the motor unit is abnormal (anterior horn cell, peripheral nerve, neuromuscular junction, or muscle), but the following guidelines are useful.

Anterior horn cell disease is suggested by hypotonia, weakness, absent reflexes, and fasciculations (see Figs. 39–5 and 39–6). The presence of fasciculations of muscle usually cannot be appreciated

Table 39–15. Spinal Paraplegia

Congenital Malformations
1. Arachnoid cyst
2. Arteriovenous malformations
3. Atlantoaxial dislocation
4. Caudal regression syndrome
5. Dysraphic states
   a. Chiari malformation
   b. Myelomeningocele
   c. Tethered spinal cord
6. Syrinogomyelia

Familial Spastic Paraplegia
1. Autosomal dominant
2. Autosomal recessive
3. X-linked recessive

Infections—Inflammatory
1. Asthmatic amyotrophy
2. Diskitis
3. Epidural abscess
4. Herpes zoster myelitis
5. Polyradiculoneuropathy
6. Tuberculous osteomyelitis

Neonatal Cord Infarction

Transverse Myelitis
1. Devic disease
2. Encephalomyelitis
3. Idiopathic

Trauma
1. Concussion
2. Epidural hematoma
3. Fracture dislocation
4. Neonatal cord trauma

Tumors
1. Astrocytoma
2. Ependymoma
3. Neuroblastoma
4. Other

Modified from Fenichel GM. Clinical Pediatric Neurology: A Signs and Symptoms Approach, 2nd ed. Philadelphia: WB Saunders, 1993:262.

Table 39–16. Motor Involvement in Spinal Cord Lesions

Affected Cord Segment	Motor Involvement
C1–4	Paralysis of neck, diaphragm, intercostals, and all four extremities
C5	Spastic paralysis of trunk, arms, and legs; partial shoulder control
C6–7	Spastic paralysis of trunk and legs; upper arm control; partial lower arm control
C8	Spastic paralysis of trunk and legs; hand weakness only
T1–10	Spastic paralysis of trunk and legs
T11–12	Spastic paralysis of legs
L1–S1	Flaccid paralysis of legs
S2–5	Flaccid paralysis of lower legs; bowel, bladder, and sexual function affected

From Swartz MH. Textbook of Physical Diagnosis: History and Examination, 2nd ed. Philadelphia: WB Saunders, 1994:496.

Table 39-17. Typical Electrophysiologic Features of Neuropathies and Myopathies

	Nerve Conduction Velocity	F-response	H-reflex	Electromyography
Inflammatory myopathy or dystrophy	Normal	Normal	Normal	Fibrillations; positive sharp waves; small motor units
Metabolic myopathy	Normal	Normal	Normal	Small motor units
Axonal neuropathy	Normal	Normal	Normal	Fibrillations; positive sharp waves; fasciculations; large motor units with distal predominance
Demyelinating neuropathy	Slowed diffusely	Delayed or absent diffusely	Delayed or absent	Normal motor units
Radiculopathy	Normal	Delayed or absent in damaged root	Delayed or absent if S1 is involved	Fibrillations; positive sharp waves; fasciculations; large motor units if chronic
Motoneuron disease	Normal	Normal	Normal	Fibrillations; positive sharp waves; fasciculations; large motor units diffusely

From Wyngaarden JB, Smith LH Jr, Bennett JC (eds). Cecil Textbook of Medicine, 19th ed. Vol 2. WB Saunders, 1988:2038.

in infants because of the presence of subcutaneous fat. Fasciculations might be seen on the tongue, but they must be distinguished from normal quivering movements of the tongue. Muscle enzymes are usually normal or slightly elevated, and nerve conduction studies are usually normal (Table 39–17). The electromyogram (EMG) may demonstrate fibrillations and large motor unit potentials that are reduced in number.

DIAGNOSTIC CONSIDERATIONS

The patient is examined for distribution of weakness, reflexes, and the presence of tongue fasciculations. Creatine kinase levels and an EMG are obtained, and a lumbar puncture is performed when acute poliomyelitis is suspected.

A muscle biopsy is indicated when spinal muscular atrophy is suspected.

COMMON DISORDERS

Anterior Horn Cell Disease

Spinal muscular atrophy represents a group of heterogeneous genetic disorders characterized by degeneration of anterior horn cells in the spinal cord (Table 39–18). *Werdnig-Hoffmann disease* is the prototype for the spinal muscular atrophies and is inherited as an autosomal recessive trait. Manifestations begin early in life and even occasionally in the prenatal period (e.g., decreased fetal

movements, congenital contractures, polyhydramnios due to poor swallowing, poor respiratory effort at birth). Neonates and young infants experience progressive weakness and hypotonia, which result in poor head and body control and a flaccid, motionless, extended posture with alert facies (see Figs. 39–5 and 39–6). Fasciculations may be noted in the tongue, over muscles with little subcutaneous fat, and as a fine tremor of the outstretched fingers.

The diagnosis is confirmed by fibrillation potentials on EMG and a denervation pattern on muscle biopsy. Supportive care is all that can be offered. Patients with delayed onset and of intermediate or less severe disease have a better prognosis than patients with Werdnig-Hoffmann disease (>65% mortality by 2 years of age).

Neuropathies

Neuropathies are characterized by hypotonia, weakness, and diminished or absent reflexes (Tables 39–19 and 39–20; see Fig. 39–3). Neuropathies may be primarily motor or sensory, and the child's symptoms may be either acute or chronic weakness or discomfort caused by paresthesias and dysesthesias. In chronic sensory neuropathies, the child may sustain injuries (e.g., burns or even bone fracture) that are unnoticed. Autonomic symptoms associated with some neuropathies include orthostatic hypotension, gastrointestinal dysmotility, and abnormalities of sweating. Generally, the reflexes in neuropathies are diminished disproportionately to the extent of muscle weakness; that is, the reflexes may be markedly reduced or absent while the muscle strength is only mildly diminished. Nerve conduction studies and EMG demonstrate slowing of nerve conduction velocities and features that suggest either primary axonal involvement (fibrillations, normal or mildly

Table 39-18. Spinal Muscular Atrophy: Clinical Classification

Type	Disease	Onset	Course	Age at Death
1, Severe	Werdnig-Hoffman	Birth to 6 months	Never sit	Usually < 2 years
2, Intermediate	—	< 18 months	Never stand	> 2 years
3, Mild	Kugelberg-Welander	> 18 months	Stand alone	Adult

From Munsat TL. Workshop Report: International SMA [Spinal Muscular Atrophy] Collaboration. Neuromuscular Disord 1991; 1:81. Reprinted in Dubowitz V. Muscle Disorders in Childhood, 2nd ed. London: WB Saunders Co Ltd, 1995:327.

Table 39–19. Mnemonic for Peripheral Neuropathy—"CHANCE-IT"

Collagen Vascular Diseases	Hereditary	Autoimmune	Nutrition	Cancer	Endocrine	Infectious	Toxin or Trauma
Periarteritis nodosa	HMSN	GBS	Vitamin deficiencies	Eaton-Lambert	Diabetes mellitus	Diphtheria	Tick-toxin
	HSAN	Immunizations	(B_1, B_6, B_{12}, E)		Hyperthyroidism	Lyme (cranial)	INH
	HSN				Hypothyroidism	Leprosy	DDC
		Chronic inflammatory			Acromegaly (entrapment)	HIV	DDC
SLE	Metabolic (porphyria)	polyneuropathy				*Campylobacter* (GBS)	Organophosphates
Vasculitis	Refsum disease					Herpes-zoster	Lead
Angiitis	Leukodystrophies (e.g.,					Rabies	Mercury
	Krabbe,						Thallium
Granulomatous (sarcoidosis)	metachromatic)						Arsenic
Wegener granulomatosis	Amyloid (familial)						Vincristine
Henoch-Schönlein purpura							Uremia
	Congenital						Chloramphenicol
	abetalipoproteinemia						Nitrofurantoin
Mononeuritis multiplex							Acrylamide
	Fabry disease						Cyanide
	Tangier disease						N-Hexane
							Buckthorn toxin
							Carbon monoxide
							Entrapment
							Obstetric trauma

Abbreviations: SLE = systemic lupus erythematosus; HMSN = hereditary motor-sensory neuropathy—Charcot-Marie-Tooth syndrome; HSAN = hereditary sensory-autonomic neuropathy—Riley-Day syndrome (dysautonomia); HSN = hereditary sensory neuropathy; INH = isoniazid; DDI = dideoxyinosine; DDC = dideoxycytidine; GBS = Guillain-Barré syndrome.

Table 39–20. Polyneuropathies with Possible Onset in Infancy

Axonal
1. Familial dysautonomia
2. Hereditary motor-sensory neuropathy type II
3. Idiopathic with encephalopathy
4. Infantile neuronal degeneration
5. Subacute necrotizing encephalopathy

Demyelinating
1. Acute inflammatory demyelinating polyneuropathy (Guillain-Barré syndrome)
2. Chronic inflammatory demyelinating polyneuropathy
3. Congenital hypomyelinating neuropathy
4. Globoid cell leukodystrophy
5. Hereditary motor-sensory neuropathy type I
6. Hereditary motor-sensory neuropathy type III
7. Metachromatic leukodystrophy

Modified from Fenichel GM. Clinical Pediatric Neurology: A Signs and Symptoms Approach, 2nd ed. Philadelphia: WB Saunders, 1993:158.

slow nerve conduction velocity) or demyelination (marked slowing of nerve conduction velocity) (see Table 39–17).

Guillain-Barré syndrome is an acute demyelinating polyneuropathy that frequently follows an upper respiratory tract infection or *Campylobacter*-associated diarrhea. There may be paresthesias; nonetheless, the disorder is characterized by ascending motor weakness and areflexia that are usually first manifest by a foot-slapping gait due to weak dorsiflexion muscles of the foot and absent ankle deep tendon reflexes. The weakness is usually symmetric, and it ascends and progresses over various periods of time (usually 1–2 weeks) and may cause serious respiratory compromise by producing weakness of the respiratory muscles (intercostals). Therefore, all patients must be tested for respiratory function (negative inspiratory forces, arterial blood gases). A Miller-Fisher variant also involves ophthalmoplegia and ataxia, whereas autonomic nervous system involvement may produce hypotension or hypertension and bradyarrhythmias or tachyarrhythmias. In addition to an abnormal nerve conduction velocity, the cerebrospinal fluid protein level is usually elevated (no corresponding elevation in cells: cyto-albumin dissociation) within 3 weeks of the illness.

Treatment includes careful monitoring of respiratory status, autonomic dysfunction, and strength. Intravenous immunoglobulin may be of value (it may result in relapse, requiring additional treatment). Plasma exchange has proved to be of great value for severely affected patients, but it is much more invasive than high-dose intravenous immunoglobulin.

Muscle and Neuromuscular Junction Disorders

Neuromuscular junction disorders must be differentiated from *muscle diseases*. Both are characterized by hypotonia, weakness, and normal to diminished reflexes (see Tables 39–5 and 39–6). The degree of muscle weakness is usually more pronounced than the extent of loss of reflexes, just the reverse of the case observed in neuropathies. Disorders of the neuromuscular junction are identifiable by EMG response to repetitive stimulation and by response to edrophonium chloride (Tensilon) intravenously (see Tables 39–10 and 39–17 and Fig. 39–8). In most muscle disorders, weakness is most prominent in the proximal muscles (Fig. 39–7) and the sensory examination is normal. The creatine kinase level is elevated in many but not all muscle disorders. The nerve conduction velocities will be normal, and the EMG will demonstrate

fibrillations and small motor unit potentials. The muscular dystrophies (Table 39–21) and other myopathies (see Table 39–4) are typical of muscle disorders and usually produce progressive proximal muscle weakness (Table 39–4).

Myopathies

Muscular dystrophy, most commonly and typically *Duchenne muscular dystrophy,* is an X-linked recessive trait (1 in 3600 liveborn males). Most neonates and young infants are not obviously symptomatic. Poor head control may be noted, but early motor milestones are achieved on time (sitting, walking). Nonetheless, the walking child may assume a hyperlordotic posture by 1½ to 2 years of age; the Gower sign, demonstrating proximal leg weakness, is often present by age 3 years (see Fig. 39–7). The typical waddling antalgic Trendelenburg gait is often noted by 5 to 6 years of age. Eventually, there is muscle atrophy; the calves may be enlarged (pseudohypertrophy) because of proliferation of fat and collagen with possibly some muscle hypertrophy.

With time, proximal muscle weakness makes ambulation difficult and the patient will require a wheelchair for ambulation. Nonetheless, with progression, respiratory muscle failure eventually develops; pulmonary insufficiency is aggravated by thoracic kyphoscoliosis. Additional complications include myocardiopathy, mental retardation (20% to 30%), contractures, scoliosis, and malignant hyperthermia on exposure to various anesthetic agents.

The diagnosis of Duchenne muscular dystrophy is suspected by the history (including the family history) and physical examination plus an elevated serum creatinine phosphokinase (often 10,000 to 30,000 IU/L). The diagnosis is confirmed by muscle biopsy or genetic testing for mutations in the dystrophin gene. Treatment is supportive and includes exercise, physical therapy, bracing, seating, special education, and emotional support. Most patients succumb by age 20 to 25 years.

Myotonic dystrophy is a common muscle disorder of childhood that is distinct in that it causes primarily a distal distribution of muscle weakness and is associated with myotonia, a phenomenon characterized by persistent muscular contraction with apparent delay in relaxation of muscles. A child with myotonia will have difficulty releasing a ball after gripping it tightly or letting go of a doorknob after grasping it.

In *congenital myotonic dystrophy,* the newborn infant appears with severe generalized hypotonia and weakness, often with swallowing and sucking difficulty, facial diplegia, and congenital joint contractures (talipes equinovarus, arthrogryposis). In *childhood onset myotonic dystrophy* the phenomenon of myotonia is often the first symptom and is usually described by the child as "stiffness," which is often exacerbated by exposure to cold temperatures. Myotonia usually is present by age 10 years, but significant distal muscle weakness is not usually evident until the end of the second decade. This is a slowly progressive disorder with multisystemic involvement, including the development of cataracts, premature male-pattern baldness, facial muscle atrophy resulting in "hatchet face" appearance, cervical kyphosis, cardiac arrhythmias, and testicular atrophy. Useful diagnostic tests include EMG (which reveals a characteristic electrical pattern of myotonia), muscle biopsy, and molecular genetic studies.

Dermatomyositis

See Chapter 45.

Neuromuscular Junction Disorders

Myasthenia gravis is due to the presence of anti-acetylcholine receptor antibodies, which produce neuromuscular blockade at the

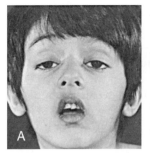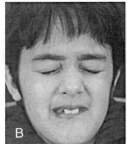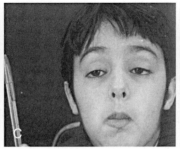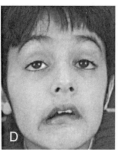

Figure 39–8. Congenital myasthenia. This child was referred at 4 years of age with a history of swallowing difficulty. By 2 years, his walking had not progressed further and he was unable to run or climb stairs. His parents had also noted some ptosis in the first year. On examination he had obvious ptosis, limited ocular movement, associated weakness of facial movement, an expressionless face, open mouth and an inability to close the eyes tightly (A). There was general hypotonia with joint laxity. The child got up from the floor with a Gowers sign and could not stand on one leg or run. A diagnosis of myasthenia was confirmed by demonstrating response decrement to repeated ulnar nerve stimulation. A definite improvement in the ptosis and his ability to get up from the floor was noted after IV edrophonium chloride (Tensilon). He was treated with pyridostigmine and showed a definite improvement, but with time he needed an increased dose and frequency. His performance improved after each dose and tended to wane as the next dose became due. He still had a Gowers sign on rising from the floor, marked ptosis, external ophthalmoplegia, and facial weakness (B–D). The parents are first cousins, so that this is probably a case of autosomal recessive infantile (congenital) myasthenia. (From Dubowitz V. Muscle Disorders in Childhood, 2nd ed. London: WB Saunders Co Ltd, 1995:414.)

level of the neuromuscular junction. Antibodies may be acquired by the transplacental route (transient neonatal myasthenia gravis) in infants born to mothers with this disease. Congenital-infantile myasthenia gravis (a permanent disease) is less common than that acquired in older childhood. In all types, the cranial nerves are most often affected, producing ptosis (Table 39–10; Fig. 39–8) and diplopia, followed by facial weakness and dysphagia. The pupillary light response is intact, although the deep tendon reflexes may be reduced; these reflexes are never completely lost. Generalized motor weakness ensues. The disease is characterized by rapid fatigue of muscles; patients are more symptomatic as the day progresses.

The diagnosis is suspected by the history of fatigability of extraocular muscles and is confirmed by the presence of anti-acetylcholine receptor antibodies and a positive edrophonium test. This short-acting cholinesterase inhibitor acutely elevates the level of acetylcholine in the neuromuscular junction, thus overcoming the receptor blockade. Ptosis, ophthalmoplegia, and fatigability are rapidly corrected (in seconds) but return to baseline levels within 1 to 2 minutes.

Therapy includes long-acting cholinesterase inhibitors (neostigmine, pyridostigmine) and atropine if the former drugs produce untoward muscarinic effects (e.g., increased secretions.) Prednisone is useful because of the autoimmune nature of the disease. Thymectomy in noncongenital or nonfamilial cases or plasmapheresis may also be of value. Hashimoto thyroiditis with resultant hypothyroidism may complicate myasthenia gravis. Neonatal myasthenia gravis is transient, and anticholinesterase therapy is needed for a few days to a few weeks after birth.

Infantile botulism is caused by the germination of *Clostridium*

botulinum organisms in the infant's gastrointestinal tract with local endogenous toxin production. Toxin is absorbed into the circulation and eventually inhibits the release of neuronal acetylcholine in the peripheral nervous system.

Infantile botulism is common between the ages of 2 and 6 months of life; infants are often breast-fed and may have a prior history of constipation. The source of *C. botulinum* includes honey, corn syrup, soil, and dust. Manifestations include lack of fever, poor feeding (poor sucking and swallowing), constipation, a weak cry and smile, hypotonia, ptosis (see Table 39–10), mydriasis, ileus, bladder atony, and hypotonia. Respiratory arrest and inappropriate antidiuretic hormone secretion may ensue. There is a descending paralysis, as symptoms are usually first noted in the cranial nerves.

Food-borne botulism is manifested after ingestion of preformed toxin in poorly canned foods. The child has nausea and vomiting with dilated pupils, diplopia dysphagia, dysarthria, dry mouth, and hypotonia.

The diagnosis of infant botulism is confirmed by recovery of the organism or the toxin from stool, blood, or food. Treatment is supportive, with careful attention to respiratory function and nutrition. No antitoxin or antibiotics are needed. Aminoglycoside antibiotics may exacerbate weakness, as they have neuromuscular blocking effects. In food-borne botulism, antitoxin and penicillin therapy are indicated.

SUMMARY AND RED FLAGS

In the infant, hypotonia is more commonly associated with systemic diseases that indirectly affect the central nervous system.

Table 39–21. Muscular Dystrophies

	Genetic Type	Age at Onset (yr)	Age at Disability (yr)	Pattern of Weakness
Duchenne	X-linked	0–5	10–15	Proximal
Becker	X-linked	5–15	15–25	Proximal
Limb-girdle	Autosomal recessive	10–30	20–40	Proximal
Facioscapulohumeral	Autosomal dominant	10–30	30–50	Proximal arm, face
Myotonic	Autosomal dominant	10–30	30–50	Distal limbs, face
Scapuloperoneal	Autosomal dominant	20–30	30–50	Proximal arm, distal leg
Emery-Dreifuss	X-linked	5–15	25–50	Proximal arm, distal leg

From Fenichel GM. Clinical Pediatric Neurology: A Signs and Symptoms Approach, 2nd ed. Philadelphia: WB Saunders, 1993:174.

However, a variety of disorders are related to the nervous system and require immediate attention. Meningomyelocele is usually discovered in the delivery room. As with an encephalopathic infant, any child with an acute neurologic process deserves thorough investigation. Hypotonia and weakness can arise from dysfunction at many potential sites of the nervous system. An accurate diagnosis requires careful anatomic localization.

Acute weakness, paralysis, or loss of function also warrants immediate attention and follow-up. Ascending motor weakness with absent deep tendon reflexes that develop over a few days suggests Guillain-Barré syndrome and is a medical emergency. In addition, spine pain, a motor and sensory level, bowel and bladder dysfunction, and upper motor neuron signs strongly suggest a lesion in the spinal cord and constitute a medical *and* possibly a surgical emergency.

REFERENCES

Muscle Disorders

Buist NRM, Powell BR. Approaches to the evaluation of muscle diseases. Int Pediatr 1992;7:320–326.

Bushby KMD: Recent advances in understanding muscular dystrophy. Arch Dis Child 1992;67:1310–1312.

Darras B: Molecular genetics of Duchenne and Becker muscular dystrophy. J Pediatr 1990;117:1–15.

Mendell JR, Moxley RT, Griggs RC, et al. Randomized, double-blind six-month trial of prednisone in Duchenne's muscular dystrophy. N Engl J Med 1989;320:1592–1598.

Miller G, Wessel HB. Diagnosis of dystrophinopathies: Review for the clinician. Pediatr Neurol 1993;9:3–9.

Pearse RG, Höweler CJ. Neonatal form of dystrophia myotonica. Arch Dis Child 1979;54:331–338.

Ptacek LJ, Johnson KJ, Griggs RC. Genetics and physiology of the myotonic muscle disorders. N Engl J Med 1993;328:482–488.

Reardon W, Newcombe R, Fenton I, et al. The natural history of congenital dystrophy: Mortality and long-term clinical aspects. Arch Dis Child 1993;68:177–181.

Rutherford MA, Heckmatt JZ, Dubowitz V. Congenital myotonic dystrophy: Respiratory function at birth determines survival. Arch Dis Child 1989;64:191–195.

Smith PEM, Calverley PMA, Edwards RHT, et al. Practical problems in the respiratory care of patients with muscular dystrophy. N Engl J Med 1987;316:1197–1206.

Peripheral Neuropathy

Epstein MA, Sladky JT. The role of plasmapheresis in childhood Guillain-Barré syndrome. Ann Neurol 1990;28:65–69.

Gruenewald R, Ropper AH, Lior H, et al. Serologic evidence of *Campylobacter jejuni/coli* enteritis in patients with Guillain-Barré syndrome. Arch Neurol 1991;48:1080–1082.

Hodson AK. Peripheral neuropathy in childhood: An update in diagnosis and management. Pediatr Ann 1983;12:814–820.

Hund EF, Borel CO, Cornblath DR, et al. Intensive management and treatment of severe Guillain-Barré syndrome. Crit Care Med 1993;21:433–446.

Jansen PW, Perkin RM, Ashwal S. Guillain-Barré syndrome in childhood: Natural course and efficacy of plasmapheresis. Pediatr Neurol 1992;9:16–20.

Lewis DW, Berman PH. Progressive weakness in infancy and childhood. Pediatr Rev 1987;8:200–208.

Lupski JR, Chance PF, Garcia CA. Inherited primary peripheral neuropathies: Molecular genetics and clinical implications of CMT1A and HNPP. JAMA 1993;270:2326–2330.

Moore PM, Cupps TR. Neurological complications of vasculitis. Ann Neurol 1983;14:155–167.

Rantala H, Uhari M, Niemel M. Occurrence, clinical manifestations, and prognosis of Guillain-Barré syndrome. Arch Dis Child 1991;66:706–709.

Ropper AH. The Guillain-Barré syndrome. N Engl J Med 1992;326:1130–1136.

Van Der Meché FGA, Schmitz PIM, Dutch Guillain-Barré Study Group. A randomized trial comparing intravenous immune globulin and plasma exchange in Guillain-Barré syndrome. N Engl J Med 1992;326:1123–1128.

Winer J: Guillain-Barré syndrome revisited. BMJ 1992;304:65–66.

Neuromuscular Junction

Drachman DB. Myasthenia gravis. N Engl J Med 1994;330:1797–1810.

Editorial. Spinal muscular atrophies. Lancet 1990;336:280–282.

Havard CWH, Fonseca V. The natural course of myasthenia gravis. BMJ 1990;1409–1410.

Horslen SP, Clayton PT, Harding BN, Hall NA, Keir G, Winchester B. Olivopontocerebellar atrophy of neonatal onset and disialotransferrin developmental deficiency syndrome. Arch Dis Child 1991;66:1027–1032.

Wessel HB. Spinal muscular atrophy. Pediatr Ann 1989;18:421–427.

40 Paroxysmal Disorders

Andrew Bleasel   Elaine Wyllie

DEFINITIONS

An *epileptic seizure* is a paroxysmal alteration in behavior, motor function, or autonomic function or a combination of these, occurring in association with excessive synchronous neuronal activity in the central nervous system (CNS).

A *convulsion* is a generalized tonic-clonic (grand mal) seizure in which bilateral tonic or tonic-clonic motor involvement of the upper and lower limbs occurs in association with loss of consciousness.

Epilepsy is a disorder in which there are *recurrent* unprovoked epileptic seizures; unprovoked seizures are spontaneous seizures without remediable precipitating stimuli or environments.

Nonepileptic paroxysmal disorders comprise a variety of episodic behavioral and motor phenomena causing people to seek medical advice. These episodes may result from physiologic processes, intercurrent organic illness, or psychiatric illness.

Acute symptomatic seizures are defined as those seizures occurring in association with a transient acute structural or metabolic insult to the CNS.

The term *ictal* refers to the events or phenomena occurring during an epileptic seizure.

The term *interictal* describes behavior or clinical observations in patients between epileptic seizures, most often used in reference to electroencephalogram (EEG) findings.

EPIDEMIOLOGY AND ETIOLOGY OF CHILDHOOD SEIZURES AND EPILEPSY

The incidence of "recurrent afebrile seizures" among children younger than 14 years of age has been estimated to be 45.6 to 83.1 in 100,000. It is highest in younger children, and in those younger than 1 year of age it is 72.7 to 249.6 in 100,000. If "active epilepsy" is defined by the number of patients with epilepsy taking antiepilepsy drugs (AEDs), the *prevalence* of active epilepsy in the community is between 4.3 and 9.3 in 1000. Epilepsy is more common than cerebral palsy but less common than mild and severe mental retardation.

The number of children having at least one afebrile seizure during childhood is high, approximately 1% before the age of 14 years; most seizures occur before age 3. Most children who experience a seizure will not go on to have epilepsy. If one includes febrile seizures, approximately 3.5% of children experience a seizure by the age of 15 years. Of children experiencing seizures, most (>50%) have febrile convulsions; 13% have acute symptomatic seizures other than febrile convulsions; 8% have single, unprovoked seizures of unknown cause; and 25% have chronic epilepsy. The incidence of acute symptomatic seizures is highest in the first year of life (212 in 100,000); the commonest etiologies of these predominantly neonatal seizures are infection and metabolic insults. After age 4 years, head injury becomes the commonest cause of acute symptomatic seizures, closely followed by infection, with other known causes being much less frequent.

Between 69% and 76% of children (neonates to adolescents) with active (chronic) epilepsy have no identifiable etiologic factors for their epilepsy. Population-based studies report the following presumed causes for 24% of children with symptomatic epilepsy: developmental (epilepsy in association with neurologic abnormalities present since birth), 13%; infection, 5%; head trauma, 3%; and miscellaneous causes, 2%. Other identifiable causes include tumors, neuroblast migration disorders, vascular malformations, and cerebral infarction.

HISTORY AND PHYSICAL EXAMINATION

The assessment of children presenting with unexplained episodes of disturbed consciousness or abnormal movements depends almost entirely on the history taking, as there are rarely any abnormal physical signs; few investigations provide conclusive diagnostic results. By their very nature, paroxysmal disorders are not present most of the time. The history often needs to be obtained exclusively from the parents of very young children. Witnesses to the episodes are the most informative sources, and it is imperative that witnesses, if other than the parents, are sought and interviewed. A description of the events from the patient should be obtained whenever possible. Even young children can provide potentially diagnostic symptoms, and parents may sometimes unwittingly mis-

represent symptoms otherwise informative to a physician. It is valuable to have parents and witnesses mimic the behavior or events witnessed; this may clarify the nature of ictal motor activity.

The history and physical examination must also explore possible underlying causes, such as perinatal hypoxia-asphyxia, metabolic or degenerative disease, cerebral tumors, or neurocutaneous disease (most commonly tuberous sclerosis or Sturge-Weber syndrome) (Table 40–1).

SEIZURE CLASSIFICATION

Table 40–2 outlines the International League Against Epilepsy (ILAE) 1981 proposal for a clinical and EEG classification of epileptic seizures.

Partial Seizures

Seizures in which "the first clinical and EEG changes indicate initial activation of a system of neurons limited to part of one cerebral hemisphere" are termed *partial seizures* and are further classified according to whether consciousness is preserved or lost during the seizures.

Simple partial seizures do not involve loss or impairment of consciousness. The clinical symptoms and signs of simple partial seizures reflect the functional anatomy of the region of the brain undergoing the abnormal neuronal discharge at the time they are manifested. In all cortical areas there may be spread of a focal seizure beyond the region of onset, and this may be reflected in a march of motor or sensory symptoms in contralateral body parts if the seizure activity spreads to primary motor or sensory cortex. Certain cortical areas do not produce symptoms when involved by focal seizure activity, and seizures beginning in a so-called silent cerebral area may produce symptoms and signs only on spread to eloquent cortex.

Focal motor seizures produce clonic movements of the limb or limbs contralateral to the primary motor cortex involved with the seizure activity. Other focal motor seizures include version of the head and eyes, vocalization, and speech arrest. Involvement of primary *somatosensory* or *special sensory* cortex produces crude somatosensory experiences such as paresthesia or numbness, often with a dysesthetic quality, and visual, auditory, olfactory, or gustatory phenomena. Symptoms arising from special sensory cortex seizures vary in complexity according to the extent of involvement of the association cortex surrounding the primary special sensory cortex (flashes of uncolored light compared with structured visual hallucinations). Focal seizures involving the limbic system, including certain regions of the frontal and temporal lobes, produce *psychic symptoms,* such as distorted memory experiences, sensations of unreality or detachment, distorted time sense, fearfulness, depression or a sense of well-being, distorted perceptions of surroundings, objects or self, and structured hallucinations.

When consciousness is impaired, the seizure is classified as a *complex partial seizure.* Impairment of consciousness is defined as an alteration in awareness of external stimuli; this may be combined with a loss or impairment of responsiveness to external stimuli. Assessment of consciousness during seizures is often difficult. It is possible to be unresponsive on the basis of an aphasia, an apraxia, paralysis, or even distraction without being unaware or unconscious of one's surroundings. At the same time, it is possible to be responsive to external stimuli but have altered awareness, often demonstrated by complete amnesia for peri-ictal events, implying that memory was not laid down during the seizure because of neuronal dysfunction. It is difficult to distinguish between ictal unresponsiveness caused by neurologic deficit or distraction and

Table 40–1. Selected Neurocutaneous Syndromes

Clinical Syndromes and Findings	Investigations
Sturge-Weber Syndrome	
Facial hemangioma, "port-wine stain" upper face, division of cranial nerve V; bilateral in 30%, absent in 5%, associated truncal and limb hemangiomas in 45%	
Intracranial leptomeningeal angiomatosis	CT scan; calcification, MRI scan with gadolinium
Epilepsy in 70%–90%, usually before 2 yr and before hemiparesis, intractable in 35%	EEG; attenuation of background rhythms, epileptiform discharges
Mental retardation in 50%–60%	
Hemiparesis in 30%, often with hemisensory deficit and hemianopia	
Tuberous Sclerosis	
Diagnostic criteria	
Any one of the following:	
Facial angiofibroma (adenoma sebaceum, nasolabial folds, and nose: become more prominent with age) or periungual fibromas	Physical examination
Cortical tubers, subependymal nodule, giant cell astrocytoma	MRI examination, T_1 and T_2 sequences, with gadolinium
Multiple retinal hamartomas (usually asymptomatic) or multiple renal angiomyolipomas (usually asymptomatic, may manifest as hematuria, hypertension, or renal failure)	Dilated eye examination and renal ultrasound, abdominal CT scan
Or any two of the following:	
Infantile spasms (seizures in 90%, most commonly generalized; infantile spasms and myoclonus)	History and physical, EEG; focal or generalized abnormalities
Hypomelanotic papules (ash leaf spots; in 80%–90%, 1–2 cm oval or leaf-shaped)	Wood's lamp (UV light) examination in darkened room
Single retinal hamartoma	Dilated eye examination
Subependymal or cortical calcification on CT scan	CT scan of the brain
Single renal angiomyolipomas or cysts	Renal ultrasound or abdominal CT scan
Cardiac rhabdomyomas (single or multiple, may obstruct outflow, cause arrhythmias or conduction defects)	Echocardiography, EKG
First-degree relative with tuberous sclerosis (autosomal dominant disorder, 80% of cases represent new mutations)	Must examine parents and do cardiac echo, MRI scans
Also associated:	
Mental retardation in 50%–66%	
Shagreen patches; hamartomatous skin lesion in lumbosacral region in 20%	
Pulmonary involvement, fibrosis	Chest x-ray
Skeletal abnormalities	Hand, feet (cystic), long bone (sclerotic) x-ray changes
Epidermal Nevus Syndrome	
Hamartomatous lesions; subclassified according to most predominant histologic and clinical features (e.g., linear nevus sebaceus, see below)	Careful examination of scalp, skin folds, and conjunctiva, dilated eye examination
Sporadic, affects males and females equally. CNS abnormalities are common with epidermal nevus syndrome, including seizures (25% of patients), mental retardation, and neoplasia. Also skeletal abnormalities, including kyphoscoliosis and hemiatrophy.	Spine and limb x-rays as appropriate
Linear nevus sebaceus; hairless verrucous yellow-orange or hyperpigmented plaques occurring on the face and scalp	
Epilepsy in 76%	
Mental retardation in 60%	
Associated neuroblast migration disorders	MRI scans of the brain
Malignant transformation of the skin lesion	
Other Neurocutaneous Syndromes Associated with Seizures	
Neurofibromatosis; cutaneous lesions include *café au lait* spots, axillary freckling, neural tumors; seizure type includes generalized tonic-clonic, partial complex, and partial simple-motor	MRI scan of the brain — Skin biopsy; ophthalmology examination
Incontinentia pigmenti; involvement includes linear papular-vesicular cutaneous lesions at birth—later pigmentation, ocular and dental anomalies; female-to-male ratio >20:1 (males may die *in utero*); seizure type includes neonatal onset and later generalized tonic-clonic	
Hypomelanosis of Ito (incontinentia pigmenti achromians)	

Table 40–2. The International League Against Epilepsy Classification of Epileptic Seizures

Partial Seizures

Simple partial seizures
With motor signs
With somatosensory or special sensory symptoms
With autonomic symptoms or signs
With psychic symptoms
Complex partial seizures
Simple partial onset followed by impairment of consciousness, with or without automatisms
With impairment of consciousness at the onset, with or without automatisms
Partial seizures, secondarily generalized seizures
Simple partial, complex partial, or simple to complex partial before generalizing; the evolution may be to generalized tonic-clonic, tonic, or clonic seizures

Generalized Seizures

Absence seizures
Simple, complicated, atypical
Myoclonic seizures
Clonic seizures
Tonic-clonic seizures
Tonic seizures
Atonic seizures

Unclassified Epileptic Seizures

unresponsiveness due to altered awareness and loss of consciousness.

An *aura* is ''that portion of a seizure that is experienced before loss of consciousness occurs.'' The aura that precedes a complex partial seizure is itself a simple partial seizure, as noted in patients who experience auras in isolation without progression to impairment of consciousness. An aura may be suspected if the patient notes a change in behavior before seizures, such as indicating an epigastric discomfort or seeking help before altered consciousness develops.

Automatisms are semipurposeful movements that usually occur with impairment of consciousness either during or after an epileptic seizure. They may be a perseveration of an activity in progress at ictal onset or novel semipurposeful movements arising during the seizure. They are most often a mixture of masticatory oral and lingual movements or simple fragmentary limb movements, such as fidgeting with a held object or clothing; they can involve walking or running and vigorous large-amplitude movements of the limbs and trunk. Studies of recorded complex partial seizures in childhood have shown automatisms to be common but to differ somewhat from those noted in adults. In infants, oroalimentary automatisms are more likely than gestural automatisms and must be distinguished from the normal behavior of infants.

Generalized Seizures

Generalized seizures are defined as ''those in which the first clinical changes indicate initial involvement of both hemispheres.'' Motor involvement, if present, is bilateral, as are the initial EEG changes. Consciousness is impaired in most generalized seizures but not in all; for instance, brief myoclonic seizures and some atonic seizures may not be associated with any impairment of consciousness.

Absence seizures (''petit mal'') begin with sudden interruption of activity and staring; they are usually brief and end abruptly without postictal confusion. *Simple absences* consist of only a motionless blank stare. Absence seizures more typically have added motor features and may then be referred to as *complicated absences*. Clonic motor activity may occur, most often involving only the eyelids and facial muscles, but it may be so marked as to be manifested as generalized myoclonic jerks of the trunk and limbs. Changes in muscle tone are common; increased tone is usually maximal in the axial musculature and may be predominantly flexor or extensor, symmetric or asymmetric. Alternatively, there may be a loss of muscle tone associated with the seizure such that the head droops, objects are dropped, or the person slumps; falling is unusual. Automatisms may be seen in 40% to 50% of absence seizures and are more common in absences of long duration. Lip smacking, swallowing, fumbling or searching hand movements, or ambulation can appear during the seizure, or preictal activities may be continued in a slow, automatic fashion. Paroxysmal alterations in autonomic function may also accompany absence seizures, including pupillary dilatation, pallor, flushing, sweating, salivation, piloerection, or a combination of these. *Atypical absences* are described as absence seizures with a less abrupt beginning and end, with more pronounced changes in muscle tone, and of longer duration. Table 40–3 compares the clinical features of absence seizures, complex partial seizures, and episodic daydreaming or staring spells.

Tonic-clonic seizures are perhaps the most dramatic of the epileptic seizures. The tonic phase begins with sudden sustained contraction of facial, axial, and limb muscle groups, and there may be an initial involuntary stridorous cry or a moan secondary to contraction of the diaphragm and chest muscles against a partially closed glottis. The tonic contraction is maintained for seconds to tens of seconds, during which time the child will fall if standing, will be apneic, and may become cyanosed, may bite the tongue, and may pass urine. The clonic phase of the seizure begins when the tonic contraction is repeatedly interrupted by momentary relaxation of the muscular contraction. This gives the appearance of generalized jerking as the contraction resumes after each relaxation. At the end of the clonic phase, the body relaxes and the patient is unconscious with deep respiration. If roused, the patient is confused, may complain of muscle soreness, and will usually wish to sleep. The tonic-clonic sequence and the unconscious postictal state are very important historical points in the differential diagnosis of psychogenic convulsive events and epileptic tonic-clonic seizures.

Myoclonic jerks are ''sudden, brief, shock-like'' contractions of muscles. They may involve the whole body or a portion of the axial musculature such as face and trunk, or they may be limited to the limbs. They can be isolated or repetitive, irregular or rhythmic. Myoclonus may arise from cortical, brainstem, and spinal cord neuronal groups. Some forms of myoclonus of brainstem or spinal origin occurring without other seizure types are not regarded as epileptic myoclonus but thought of as movement disorders.

Generalized clonic seizures may occur without a preceding tonic phase, and the postictal phase is usually shorter than for tonic-clonic seizures.

Generalized tonic seizures begin as in tonic-clonic seizures. The tonic contraction subsides without the intervening relaxation-recontraction clonic phase. The extent of muscle involvement may vary from patient to patient and from seizure to seizure in a single patient. A massive generalized contraction produces facial grimacing, neck and trunk flexion or extension, abduction of the arms, and flexion of the hips. Subtle tonic seizures may produce only facial grimacing and slight neck and trunk flexion. Tonic seizures may be accompanied by pronounced autonomic activity with diaphoresis, flushing, pallor, and tachycardia even when the muscular contraction is slight.

Atonic seizures are characterized by a sudden decrease or loss of postural muscle tone. The extent of muscle involvement, and thus the clinical manifestations, may vary; an atonic seizure may be limited to a sudden head drop with ''slack jaw'' or may result

Table 40–3. Differential Diagnosis of Episodic Unresponsiveness Without Convulsions

Clinical	Absence Seizures	Complex Partial Seizures	Staring, Inattention
Frequency	Multiple daily	Rarely >1–2/day	Daily, situation-dependent (e.g., may occur only at school)
Duration	Often <10 sec, rarely >30 sec	Average duration >60 sec, rarely <10 sec	Seconds to minutes
Aura	Not present	May be present	Not present
Abrupt interruption of child's activity	Yes (e.g., speech arrest mid-sentence, pause while eating, playing, or fighting)	Yes	Activities such as play or eating are not abruptly interrupted, no sudden onset
Eyelid flutter	Common	Uncommon but may be present	No
Myoclonic jerks	Common	Uncommon	Not present
Automatisms	Occur in longer absences, usually mild	Frequent and often prominent	No
Postictal impairment	None	Postictal confusion and malaise are typical, drowsiness may also occur	No
EEG	Generalized 3-Hz spike and wave complexes	Regional epileptic discharges (most often frontal or temporal)	Normal
MRI scan	Normal	Focal structural lesions not uncommon (e.g., tumor)	Normal
First-line medication	Valproate, ethosuximide	Carbamazepine, phenytoin, valproate	—

in a fall due to loss of axial and limb muscle tone. The latter are referred to as "drop attacks," and these unprotected falls often result in facial laceration or head injury.

Some seizures cannot be classified into the above groups, often because they were not witnessed, and the ILAE has created an *unclassified epileptic seizure* group.

Status epilepticus exists when epileptic seizures are prolonged or are frequently repeated without recovery between the seizures. The time most often given for the purposes of definition is 30 minutes or longer. Status epilepticus is most commonly characterized as convulsive or nonconvulsive status epilepticus. Convulsive status epilepticus may involve repetitive or prolonged generalized tonic-clonic, myoclonic, or tonic seizures. Nonconvulsive status epilepticus may involve repeated or continuous absence or complex partial seizures with an altered state of consciousness varying from slightly clouded but ambulant to stuporous, lasting hours or even days. A rare but striking example of partial status epilepticus is *epilepsia partialis continua,* in which brief focal motor seizures involving a part of a limb or the face occur repeatedly, without alteration of consciousness, in the setting of a variety of focal cerebral insults.

CLASSIFICATION OF EPILEPSIES AND EPILEPTIC SYNDROMES

Table 40–4 presents the ILAE classification of epilepsies and epileptic syndromes with two broad divisions: epilepsies with generalized seizures and epilepsies with partial seizures. These two categories are divided into symptomatic, or cryptogenic, epilepsy and idiopathic epilepsy. *Symptomatic epilepsies* have a known etiology, and idiopathic epilepsies have no known cause other than a possible genetic predisposition. *Cryptogenic epilepsy* is thought to be symptomatic but without an identifiable etiology. Most epileptic syndromes are manifested in childhood.

Neonatal Period

The paroxysmal disorders seen in the neonatal period (birth to 8 weeks) are given in Table 40–5.

PAROXYSMAL NONEPILEPTIC DISORDERS

Jitteriness

Jitteriness or tremulousness is a common movement disorder of neonates. It can be confused with seizures, especially if superimposed on normal tonic postural reflexes. Jitteriness characterized by rhythmic alternating movements of all extremities with equal velocity in flexion and extension only occasionally has a clonic appearance. Jitteriness is not accompanied by eye deviation or staring, is stimulus-sensitive, and can usually be stopped by gentle passive flexion of the moving limb.

Although jitteriness is not epileptic, it is still not to be ignored, and a specific cause should be sought. Common associations of jitteriness in the newborn are hypoxic-ischemic encephalopathy, hypoglycemia, hypocalcemia, drug withdrawal, and maternal drug abuse. Jittery neonates may be more likely to have seizures and epileptiform EEG abnormalities than unaffected neonates. However, jitteriness may also appear in otherwise healthy infants. In this case, there are no associated insults or identifiable etiologic factors and the children develop normally. Jitteriness then seems to behave as a benign movement disorder, resolving by 10 to 14 months but often earlier.

Another rare disorder, *familial trembling chin syndrome,* may appear in the neonatal-infancy period and cause concern. This unusual condition may have some relationship to familial essential tremor.

Table 40–4. International League Against Epilepsy Classification of Epilepsies and Epileptic Syndromes

Localization-related (focal, partial) epilepsies
  Idiopathic
    Benign childhood epilepsy with centrotemporal spikes
    Childhood epilepsy with occipital paroxysms
  Symptomatic
    The subclassification within this group is currently determined by the anatomic location suggested by the clinical history, predominant seizure type, interictal and ictal EEG, and imaging studies. Thus, SPS, CPS, or secondarily generalized seizures arising from frontal lobes, parietal, temporal, occipital, multiple lobes, or an unknown focus
  Localization-related but uncertain symptomatic or idiopathic

Generalized epilepsies
  Idiopathic
    Benign neonatal familial convulsions
    Benign neonatal convulsions
    Benign myoclonic epilepsy in infancy
    Childhood absence epilepsy (pyknoepilepsy)
    Juvenile absence epilepsy
    Juvenile myoclonic epilepsy (impulsive petit mal)
    Epilepsy with grand mal seizures on awakening
    Other generalized idiopathic epilepsies occur not conforming exactly to the above syndromes
  Cryptogenic or symptomatic generalized epilepsies
    West syndrome (infantile spasms)
    Lennox-Gastaut syndrome
    Epilepsy with myoclonic astatic seizures
    Epilepsy with myoclonic absences
  Symptomatic
    Nonspecific etiology
      Early myoclonic encephalopathy
    Specific disease states presenting with seizures

Epilepsies and syndromes in which it is undetermined whether they are focal or generalized
  With both generalized and focal seizures
    Neonatal seizures
    Severe myoclonic epilepsy in infancy
    Epilepsy with continuous spike waves during slow-wave sleep
    Acquired epileptic aphasia (Landau-Kleffner syndrome)
  Without unequivocal generalized or focal features
    All cases with GTCS in which the EEG findings do not allow classification as definitely generalized or localization-related (e.g., sleep GTCS)

Special syndromes
  Situation-related seizures
    Febrile convulsions
    Isolated seizures or isolated status epilepticus
    Acute symptomatic seizures (e.g., alcohol withdrawal seizures, eclampsia, uremia)

Abbreviations: CPS = complex partial seizures; GTCS = generalized tonic-clonic seizures; SPS = simple partial seizures.

Benign Neonatal Sleep Myoclonus

Myoclonic jerks may appear during sleep in some healthy, neurologically normal neonates. It has been reported within hours of birth and may disappear over the next few months or persist into childhood. The jerks can be bilateral and synchronous or asymmetric; they may migrate between muscle groups during an episode. They are repetitive but do not disturb sleep. These jerks have been described in all stages of sleep but are most prominent in quiet sleep; they are not confined to sleep onset.

Features distinguishing this phenomenon from epilepsy are lack of associated seizures, presence exclusively during sleep with disappearance on awakening, normal EEGs, and normal psychomotor development.

ACUTE SYMPTOMATIC SEIZURES AND OCCASIONAL SEIZURES

Classification

Most neonatal seizures are acute symptomatic seizures. The number of children who will continue to have seizures beyond the neonatal period is relatively small. Neonatal seizures, defined as paroxysmal alterations in behavior, motor function, or autonomic function, have been classified according to the clinical features of the ictus as subtle, tonic, clonic, and myoclonic. However, not all of these clinical seizure types have ictal EEG patterns. The classification of neonatal seizures reflects the ''variable, poorly organized and often subtle'' clinical expression of epileptic seizures at this age. Typical generalized tonic-clonic or absence seizures are not seen at this age, perhaps because of the limited capacity of the neonatal brain for interhemispheric synchrony.

- *Clinical seizures consistently associated with an EEG seizure pattern.* Clonic seizures with focal or multifocal jerking of the face or extremities fit this category, as do focal tonic seizures with focal tonic posturing of a limb or asymmetric posturing of the axial musculature.
- *Clinical seizures sometimes associated with an EEG seizure pattern.* Myoclonic seizures consist of single or multiple flexor jerks of the upper or lower limbs. An ictal EEG pattern is not always seen in this group, although one may be present in some cases of focal and generalized myoclonus. Focal and generalized myoclonic seizures may often not be associated

Table 40–5. Paroxysmal Disorders of the Neonatal Period

Paroxysmal Nonepileptic Disorders
  Jitteriness
  Benign neonatal sleep myoclonus

Acute Symptomatic Seizures and Occasional Seizures
  Hypoxic-ischemic encephalopathy
  Intraventricular hemorrhage
  Acute metabolic disorders*
  Sepsis-meningitis
  See Table 40–7

Epileptic Syndromes
  Benign idiopathic neonatal convulsions
    Familial
    Nonfamilial
  Symptomatic focal epilepsy
    Brain tumor
    Neuroblast migration disorders
    Inherited metabolic disease; mitochondrial disorders
  Early-onset generalized epileptic syndromes with encephalopathy
    Early myoclonic encephalopathy
    Early infantile encephalopathic epilepsy

*Hypoglycemia, hypocalcemia, hypomagnesemia, hyponatremia, hypernatremia.

with an ictal EEG pattern; fragmentary (multifocal) myoclonus is not always associated with ictal EEG.

- *Clinical seizures not consistently associated with an EEG seizure pattern.* These include motor automatisms characterized by a diversity of signs, including any of the following: wide-eyed staring, rapid blinking, eyelid fluttering, drooling, sucking, repetitive limb movements such as "rowing" or "swimming" with the arms or "pedaling" with the legs, apnea, hyperpnea, and vasomotor skin color changes. This group may be subtle seizures and include tonic eye deviation.

Generalized tonic seizures are manifested as tonic extension of the limbs or flexion of the upper limbs and extension of the lower limbs, sometimes mimicking decerebrate or decorticate posturing. The question has arisen whether abnormal posturing or automatisms without an ictal EEG pattern are epileptic seizures at all or rather brainstem-mediated release phenomena in very ill encephalopathic neonates. Instead of an EEG seizure pattern, infants with subtle seizures typically have suppressed background rhythms. Generalized tonic seizures and focal and multifocal myoclonus are also often not associated with ictal EEG patterns, and when seen in stuporous or comatose children the jerks may not be epileptic.

Some simple clinical observations should guide the assessment of neonates with episodic abnormal behaviors. Epileptic behaviors are typically repetitive and stereotyped but not provoked by stimulation of the child nor increased with increasing intensity of a stimulus. Nonepileptic movements may disappear with repositioning of a limb or the child. Gentle restraint of a limb should be able to suppress or abort nonepileptic motor activity, whereas epileptic movements will still be palpable. Apneas or tachyarrhythmias or bradyarrhythmias suggesting autonomic activation are not typical of nonepileptic phenomena. The association of abnormal eye movements with unusual behavior or limb movements suggests a seizure rather than nonepileptic behavior.

Diagnostic Investigations

EEG monitoring can be useful in the evaluation of suspicious fluctuations in vital signs in neonates who are paralyzed and intubated or comatose or in the neonate with subtle but repetitive episodes of unusual behavior.

Proper treatment must include a thorough search for the cause of the seizures, as many conditions require specific treatment. The possible etiologic factors are numerous and diverse (Tables 40–6 and 40–7). The most common cause is hypoxic-ischemic encephalopathy (60% to 65%); however, it is important to make a positive diagnosis of this historically and to exclude conditions such as local anesthetic toxicity, pyridoxine-dependent seizures, and metabolic encephalopathies that may masquerade as perinatal asphyxia with seizures. The initial routine investigation and more detailed investigations suggested for a neonate with seizures are listed in the beginning of Table 40–7.

Prognosis

The prognosis for normal development following neonatal seizures depends on the cause of the seizures. Approximately 56% of neonates with seizures develop normally, 29% have neurologic sequelae such as mental retardation, motor deficits, and seizures, and 15% die. The likelihood of recurrent seizures is 15% to 20% overall. Generalized myoclonic jerks may be the harbinger of infantile spasms in later months. In relation to the major causes of seizures in the neonatal period, 50% of neonates with hypoxic-ischemic encephalopathy–related seizures develop normally, but

Table 40–6. Etiology of Neonatal Seizures

Age 1–4 Days

Hypoxic-ischemic encephalopathy
Drug withdrawal, maternal drug use of narcotic or barbiturates
Drug toxicity; lignocaine, penicillin
Intraventicular hemorrhage
Acute metabolic disorders
  Hypocalcemia
    Perinatal asphyxia, small for gestational age
    Sepsis
    Maternal diabetes or hyper- or hypoparathyroidism
  Hypoglycemia
    Perinatal insults, prematurity, small for gestational age
    Maternal diabetes
    Sepsis
  Hypomagnesemia
  Hypo- or hypernatremia
    Iatrogenic or inappropriate antidiuretic hormone secretion
Inborn errors of metabolism
  Galactosemia
  Hyperglycinemia
  Urea cycle disorders
Pyridoxine deficiency (must consider at any age)

Age 4–14 Days

Infection
  Bacterial meningitis, viral encephalitis
Metabolic disorders
  Hypocalcemia
    Diet, milk formula
  Hypoglycemia, persistent
    Inherited disorders of metabolism: galactosemia, fructosemia, leucine sensitivity
    Anterior pituitary hypoplasia, pancreatic islet cell tumor
    Beckwith syndrome
Drug withdrawal, maternal drug use of narcotic or barbiturates
Benign neonatal convulsions, familial and nonfamilial
Kernicterus, hyperbilirubinemia

Age 2–8 Weeks

Infection
  Herpes simplex encephalitis, bacterial meningitis
Head injury
  Subdural hematoma, child abuse
Inherited disorders of metabolism
  Aminoacidurias, urea cycle defects, organic acidurias
  Neonatal adrenoleukodystrophy
Neuroblast migration disorders
  Lissencephaly
  Focal cortical dysplasia
Tuberous sclerosis, Sturge-Weber syndrome

fewer than 10% of neonates with seizures and intraventricular hemorrhage develop normally. Neonates with seizures due to CNS infection (congenital-TORCH, acquired bacterial meningitis, herpes simplex virus), hypoglycemia, structural brain malformations, and birth trauma do poorly, while those with seizures due to hypocalcemia (in the absence of asphyxia) usually do well.

The EEG may add prognostic information; children with a normal background are unlikely to have any neurologic deficits, but severe abnormalities of the background rhythms, such as burst-suppression patterns, suppression of background rhythms, and electrocerebral silence, are associated with a 90% chance of a poor outcome, including death. Moderate abnormalities of the EEG in the form of amplitude asymmetries and patterns immature for the

Table 40–7. Selected Inherited Disorders of Metabolism and Neurodegenerative Diseases Associated with Seizures in Neonates and Infants

Disorder	Clinical Features and Laboratory Findings	Investigations
Neonates		
All of these disorders are rare. The clinical features are nonspecific and will usually not distinguish between the inherited disorders of metabolism in neonates; however, they may suggest that a search for these diseases is warranted: Autosomal recessive inheritance, another sibling with a metabolic or degenerative disorder Normal immediately after birth with symptoms and signs developing in the first days to weeks of life Food intolerance; vomiting, diarrhea, not settling after feeds Lethargy, may become stuporous after feeding Hypotonia Seizures; tonic, clonic, subtle neonatal seizures, myoclonus in some disorders Late signs: weight loss, failure to thrive, psychomotor retardation		Initial investigations in neonatal seizures: Urinalysis, ketones, glucose, 2,4-DNPH screen Serum Na^+, K^+, Ca^{++}, Mg^{++}, glucose, blood urea nitrogen, creatinine Serum ammonia, lactate, and pyruvate Liver function tests, complete blood count, arterial blood gases Urine and blood cultures Lumbar puncture and CSF analysis EEG CT or MRI scan may be indicated
Amino acid acidurias Maple syrup urine disease	May detect an unusual maple syrup odor to urine, severe metabolic acidosis and increased anion gap, urine positive for ketones, boiled urine reacts with 2,4-DNPH to give yellow precipitate.	Serum and urine amino acid analysis Elevated serum leucine, isoleucine, and valine

Organic acidurias
  Propionic acid
  Methylmalonic acid
  Isovaleric acid
  Glutaric acid
	Hyperammonemia, metabolic acidosis and increased anion gap, ketosis, low blood urea nitrogen. Secondary elevation of lactate and hypoglycemia may be present, and secondary carnitine deficiency may occur. Note glycine may be elevated in these disorders. Thrombocytopenia, neutropenia, and anemia. Characteristic body odor in some of these disorders.	Serum and urine organic acid analysis
		Serum carnitine

Urea cycle disorders	Hyperammonemia without ketoacidosis or hematologic abnormalities.	Urine orotic acid and serum citrulline
Nonketotic hyperglycinemia D-glycericacidemia	Intractable seizures and severe encephalopathy, often with coma, within the first weeks of life. May have the clinical syndrome of early myoclonic encephalopathy; myoclonic seizures, burst-suppression pattern on EEG, severe psychomotor retardation.	Elevated urine and plasma glycine, normal organic acid pattern and ammonia
Pyridoxine dependency	No specific clinical features, must suspect in all neonatal seizures without alternate etiology and especially those not responding to simple measures.	Therapeutic trial of pyridoxine, must give high dose for a period of weeks

Peroxisomal diseases
  Zellweger syndrome
  Adrenoleukodystrophy
  Refsum disease
	Characteristic facies
	Neonatal form
	Infantile form
		Serum very long chain fatty acid analysis

Infants		
Pyruvate dehydrogenase deficiency	Metabolic acidosis and increased anion gap, lactic acidosis with normal lactate-to-pyruvate ratio (20:1), hyperammonemia may be seen, normoglycemic. Serum, urine, and CSF alanine may be elevated.	Serum lactate and pyruvate Serum, urine, and CSF amino acids
Pyruvate carboxylase deficiency	Lactate-to-pyruvate ratio is normal or elevated. The clinical features are nonspecific; encephalopathy, hypotonia, and seizures. Intermittent hyperventilation may be present. Both these disorders can present later in childhood with developmental delay and episodic symptoms such as ataxia and vomiting.	

Table continued on following page

Table 40–7. Selected Inherited Disorders of Metabolism and Neurodegenerative Diseases Associated with Seizures in Neonates and Infants *Continued*

Disorder	Clinical Features and Laboratory Findings	Investigations
Biotinidase deficiency	Refractory seizures, rash, alopecia. Lactic and organic acidosis.	
Amino acid acidurias		
Phenylketonuria	Onset in infancy with developmental delay and seizures, seizures occur in about 25%, and the infant may have severe epilepsy with West syndrome. A deficiency of phenylalanine hydroxylase causes the accumulation of phenylalanine and phenylacetic acid.	Detection and quantification of urinary and plasma amino acids
Phenylketonuria variant with biopterin deficiency	Hypotonia and seizures develop at or after 6 mo of age, generalized motor seizures, erratic myoclonus and oculogyric seizures.	Detection and quantification of urinary and plasma amino acids Blood sample and skin biopsy
GM₂ gangliosidosis Tay-Sachs disease	Abnormalities appear in the first weeks to months of life with irritability and acoustic startle or myoclonus in the first months, not seizures. There is developmental delay and cherry-red macular spots. Seizures develop in the second year of life; erratic myoclonus, partial seizures, and slowing of background rhythms on EEG.	Hexosaminidase A deficiency detectable in blood lymphocytes and cultured fibroblasts
Sandhoff disease	Similar phenotype to Tay-Sachs disease	Hexosaminidase A and B deficiency detectable in blood lymphocytes and cultured fibroblasts
GM₁ gangliosidosis Pseudo–Hurler disease	Dysmorphic features, developmental delay appears with decreased responsiveness in the first weeks of life, then arrest of development after 3–6 mo of age. Seizures are frequent without specific characteristics. Cherry-red spots at maculae. In the other mucopolysaccharidoses, Hunter, Hurler, and Sanfilippo, seizures are not often a prominent feature.	Skin biopsy β-Galactosidase deficiency found in cultured fibroblasts
Leigh disease (subacute necrotizing encephalopathy)	A clinical syndrome resulting from various enzyme disorders, usually presenting in infancy with regression of motor skills, hypotonia, lethargy, respiratory disorders (typically hyperventilation and apnea), and seizures. Other features are nuclear and supranuclear oculomotor paralysis, brainstem dysfunction, choreoathetosis, cerebellar ataxia, and pyramidal signs.	MRI scan of the brain may show midbrain periaqueductal signal abnormalities Muscle biopsy for oxidative metabolism analysis and mitochondrial DNA studies
Menkes disease	Sex-linked inheritance, long arm X chromosome. Hypotonia, failure to thrive, abnormal temperature regulation, hypothermia or hyperthermia, fragile wiry hair, poor pigmentation, generalized seizures, often have infantile spasms.	Deficiency of serum copper and ceruloplasmin
Krabbe disease	Appears before 3–6 mo of age, rigidity develops in an irritable crying infant. Opisthotonic posturing of the neck and trunk. Generalized motor seizures may occur but must be distinguished from tonic spasms. The children become blind with optic atrophy.	Skin biopsy Galactocerebroside deficiency
Angelman syndrome	Delayed from birth, characteristic facies, ataxia with jerky limb movements, inappropriate laughter (''happy puppet''), seizures in 86% of patients	Chromosome 15 abnormality
Early infantile type of ceroid lipofuscinosis	Massive myoclonus 3–18 mo, hypotonia, ataxia, impaired vision, dementia. Vanishing EEG. No enzymatic defect identified, diagnosis must be made on clinical features and skin biopsy showing ceroid.	Skin biopsy, biopsy
Other rare metabolic disorders with encephalopathy seizures in infancy		
Glutaric aciduria type II, multiple acyl-CoA dehydrogenase deficiency		Dicarboxylic aciduria
Medium-chain acyl-CoA dehydrogenase deficiency		Hypoglycemia, hypoketonuria, increased medium-chain fatty acids
Canavan–van Bogaert disease		Increased urinary *N*-acetylaspartic acid

Abbreviations: CSF = cerebrospinal fluid; DNPH = dinitrophenylhydrazine.

patient's conceptional age are associated with intermediate outcomes and are of less value in isolation of other clinical data.

Treatment

The primary treatment of neonatal seizures is the treatment of the underlying cause. Some neonates also require treatment with an antiepileptic medication. The most commonly used AED in this setting is phenobarbital. At an intravenous loading dose of 18 to 20 mg/kg, phenobarbital should produce a serum level of approximately 18 to 20 mg/L, as the volume of distribution for phenobarbital in neonates is very close to 1 L/kg (Table 40–8). A maintenance dose of 3 to 5 mg/kg keeps serum levels in this range. The serum level can be increased to 40 to 60 mg/L with further loading doses before consideration of a second drug for persistent seizures. Frequent estimations of serum levels are needed, and some free levels should be determined during the course of treatment with high total levels, as protein binding in neonates is lower than in older children and adults.

If a self-limited or correctable short-term insult is the cause, one might load with phenobarbital and give no maintenance therapy, simply observing for recurrent seizures. Another alternative would be to load with phenobarbital and give maintenance doses throughout an illness, or to load and treat for a maximum of 3 months if the time period during which the child is at risk for seizures is uncertain.

In the setting of refractory seizures with adequate serum levels of phenobarbital and no treatable exacerbating factors, phenytoin is most commonly chosen as a second drug, usually added to phenobarbital. An intravenous loading dose of 15 mg/kg can be used, but it must not be infused at rates faster than 1 mg/kg/minute because of the risk of cardiac arrhythmias. The half-life of phenytoin may vary between 6 and 140 hours, with a mean of 30 hours in neonates. The maintenance dose may be difficult to predict; thus, frequent serum levels are indicated. Protein binding is lower than in older children.

Other agents that have been used include diazepam infusions and, less often, paraldehyde or lidocaine infusion (see Table 40–8).

EPILEPTIC SYNDROMES

Benign Idiopathic Neonatal Convulsions, Familial and Nonfamilial

Some neonatal seizures occur in otherwise well neonates without perinatal risk factors or identifiable causes that remit spontaneously and are not followed by developmental delay; these include benign idiopathic neonatal convulsions and benign familial neonatal convulsions.

Benign idiopathic neonatal convulsions are common and may account for 2% to 7% of neonatal seizures. The disorder is sometimes referred to as "fifth-day fits," although the seizures may begin between 1 and 7 days of age. The seizures are typically focal and multifocal clonic seizures that may rarely develop into status epilepticus. The seizures remit within hours or days. Although normal at the onset of seizures, neonates may become drowsy and hypotonic during the seizures and for a few days after they remit. The distinctive interictal EEG pattern is referred to as *theta pointu alternant*: intermittent theta rhythms in the rolandic area, often asynchronous between the hemispheres and associated with sharp waves. This pattern may occur in 60% of neonates with benign idiopathic neonatal convulsions but is not specific for the disorder, being seen after other causes of status epilepticus. Normal interictal EEGs have also been reported. Long-term follow-up data are not yet complete, but the majority of children appear to have normal psychomotor development and no increased risk for the development of epilepsy at an older age. Currently, this diagnosis may be made only after exclusion of other causes of neonatal seizures, and the diagnostic work-up must include a lumbar puncture with examination of the cerebrospinal fluid and a computed tomography (CT) scan to exclude neonatal stroke (see Chapter 42).

Benign familial neonatal convulsions are less common. There is a distinctive family history of transient neonatal seizures showing autosomal dominant inheritance. The onset of seizures is usually between 2 and 4 days after birth, but some outliers may have onset of seizures at 1 and 3 months of age. The neonates are otherwise healthy without risk factors for seizures. The seizures have usually been brief clonic seizures, but some neonates have tonic seizures. This group differs from the nonfamilial cases in that the seizures may persist longer, the interictal EEG is generally nonspecific (*theta pointu alternant* is reported in very few cases), and later seizures occur more frequently, in approximately 11% of infants. Linkage studies have demonstrated genetic markers on the long arm of chromosome 20 in some kindreds.

Symptomatic Focal Epilepsy

Neuroblast Migration Disorders. Disorders of cell migration within the CNS may result in profound anatomic abnormalities and dysfunction or a spectrum of lesser abnormalities, ranging from focal areas of cortical dysgenesis and clinical deficits to subcortical collections of neurons (heterotopia) seen only under the microscope. Migrational abnormalities are rare and are commonly associated with seizures.

Lissencephaly or agyria describes a profound abnormality characterized by a smooth brain without development of the normal gyral pattern and sulci; there are often large heterotopia in the white matter, and neuroimaging studies may reveal the appearance of a "double cortex."

Hemimegencephaly is characterized by gross enlargement of one

Table 40–8. Neonatal Antiepileptic Drugs, Pharmacokinetic Parameters

Antiepileptic Routes of Administration		% Protein-Bound	Volume of Distribution (L/kg)	Loading Dose (mg/kg)	Half-Life (hr)	Maintenance Dose (mg/kg/day)	Therapeutic Range (mg/L)
Phenobarbital	IV, p.r., p.o.	24	0.81–0.97	20	40–400	3–4	10–30
Phenytoin	IV, p.o.	70	0.9	15–20	6.9–140*	18–20	10–20
Diazepam	IV, p.r.	84	1.3–2.6	0.5–1	31–75	3–12	0.3–0.7
Lidocaine	IV	20	2.75	2–3	1–1.5	4	0.5–4

*Great variation, shorter if exposed to enzyme-inducing drugs (e.g., phenobarbital) and within first 2 to 3 weeks of life.
Abbreviations: IV = intravenously; p.o. = orally; p.r. = rectally.

cerebral hemisphere with no normal cortical development within that hemisphere and often recognizable magnetic resonance imaging (MRI) scan abnormalities in the ''normal-sized'' hemisphere. More restricted abnormalities may occur in the form of limited area of gyral enlargement and distortion called *pachygyria.*

Schizencephaly refers to unilateral or bilateral clefts in the cerebral hemispheres, usually with abnormal arrangement (polymicrogyria) of the cortical gray matter lining the clefts.

Porencephaly describes fluid-filled cavities within the brain. Porencephalic cysts communicate with both the subarachnoid space and the ventricular system and are not lined by cortical gray matter but rather by gliotic tissue, as they result from loss of tissue as a consequence of insults during development, typically infarction.

Early-Onset Generalized Epileptic Syndromes with Encephalopathy

Early myoclonic encephalopathy appears in neonates before 2 to 3 months of age, usually within the first 2 weeks of life. Myoclonus appears at the onset but may be fragmentary. Partial motor seizures, massive myoclonus, or infantile spasms may also occur. The EEG does not show hypsarrhythmia but rather a suppression-burst pattern that may later evolve into a hypsarrhythmia pattern. There is a failure or arrest of psychomotor development and a high rate of mortality before 12 months of age. A number of patients have had nonketotic hyperglycemia or congenital malformations of the nervous system. Familial cases with identifiable etiologic factors have also been reported.

Early infantile encephalopathic epilepsy has an onset during the same period. The child experiences only infantile spasms without other seizure types, and the EEG shows a suppression-burst pattern. The prognosis for remission from seizures and for normal development is very poor.

There appear to be neonates in whom the EEG features and clinical course of these two syndromes overlap; these syndromes may evolve into West syndrome.

Infancy

The paroxysmal disorders of infancy (8 weeks to 2 years) are shown in Table 40–9.

PAROXYSMAL NONEPILEPTIC DISORDERS

Infantile Syncope

Cyanotic Infant Syncope (Breath-Holding Spells). Cyanotic infant syncope describes episodes of loss of consciousness followed by tonic stiffening in crying infants upset by minor injury, fright, or frustration. They have also been called breath-holding spells, anoxic seizures, or convulsive syncope, but cyanotic infant syncope may be a better term because the loss of consciousness appears to be the result of transient impairment of cerebral perfusion. The subsequent tonic posturing in the typical attack is not epileptic but is thought to share a brainstem origin with decerebrate or decorticate posturing. In rare cases, typical infant syncope may evolve into a true generalized tonic-clonic seizure or even status epilepticus, presumably triggered by the anoxia.

Cyanotic infant syncope is common, seen in 4.6% of a large cohort of children followed from birth, and can be mistaken for tonic-clonic seizures. A thorough history is usually sufficient to

Table 40–9. Paroxysmal Disorders of Infancy

Paroxysmal Nonepileptic Disorders

More Common

>Infantile syncope
>>Cyanotic breath-holding spells
>>Pallid syncope
>Sleep disorders
>>Jactatio capitis (head banging)

Less Common

>Shivering attacks
>Paroxysmal torticollis
>Extrapyramidal drug reactions, dystonia
>Gastroesophageal reflux with dystonia
>Rumination
>Stereotypic movements, autism, Rett syndrome, deaf and blind children
>Withholding, constipation
>Masturbation
>Spasmus nutans
>Opsoclonus
>Benign paroxysmal vertigo
>Myoclonus
>Nonepileptic; anxiety, excitement, acute metabolic encephalopathy
>Benign myoclonus of early infancy
>Hyperekplexia
>Alternating hemiplegia of childhood

Acute Symptomatic Seizures and Occasional Seizures

More Common

>Febrile convulsions
>Meningitis, encephalitis

Less Common

>Head injury, child abuse
>Poisoning
>Intercurrent medical illness, renal, liver disease, cardiac right-to-left shunt and embolism
>Metabolic disease, rickets

Epileptic Syndromes

More Common

>Symptomatic focal epilepsy

Less Common

>West syndrome
>Early myoclonic encephalopathy
>Early infantile encephalopathic epilepsy
>Neuroblast migration disorders
>Neurocutaneous disorders
>>Tuberous sclerosis
>>Sturge-Weber syndrome
>>Incontinentia pigmenti
>>Epidermal nevus syndrome
>Severe myoclonic epilepsy in infancy

diagnose this condition. The peak incidence is between 6 and 18 months of age, but the phenomenon may occur in neonates or in children as old as 6 years of age. The typical clinical picture is an infant who is frightened or frustrated by an event or surprised by some relatively minor injury and begins to cry vigorously, then becomes apneic and cyanotic before becoming unconscious, stiff, or limp. The crucial diagnostic point is the history of an external event, however minor, precipitating the episode. The striking features that are so easily confused with an epileptic seizure are the tonic posture or the clonic movements that may occur after the child has lost consciousness. The child should regain consciousness rapidly without a prolonged postictal state, although there may be a tendency to sleep. The differential diagnosis is noted in Table 40–10.

Although the attacks appear to be unpleasant for the child, they do not result in late sequelae and do not require intensive investigation, nor do they respond to any form of medical therapy. Treatment with an AED such as carbamazepine, phenytoin, or valproate may decrease the frequency or severity of postsyncopal convulsions in the rare child with epileptic seizures triggered by the anoxic event. It is important to explain the mechanisms underlying the phenomenon and reassure the parent of their benign and self-limited nature.

Pallid Infant Syncope. Pallid infant syncope occurs in response to transient cardiac asystole in those with a hypersensitive cardioinhibitory reflex. This form is less common but more alarming and more likely to lead to presentation to the emergency department or referral. There is minimal crying, perhaps only a gasp, and no obvious apnea before the loss of consciousness. Again there is a precipitating event, the child appears to lose consciousness after minimal injury or fright, collapses limply, and then may have posturing and clonic movements before regaining consciousness. Ocular compression can produce transient cardiac asystole in more than 50% of patients with a clinical diagnosis of pallid infant syncope compared with only 6% of patients with cyanotic infant syncope. The procedure is not in general use and is of uncertain clinical utility.

Pallid infant syncope, if frequent and troublesome or if followed by prolonged generalized tonic-clonic convulsions, can be treated with atropine, which blocks the vagus nerve–mediated asystole. Most children require no medical treatment. The differential diagnosis is noted in Table 40–10.

Sleep Disorders

Also referred to as head banging or rocking, jactatio capitis nocturna consists of rhythmic to-and-fro movements of the head or rocking of the body. It occurs typically at the transition from wakefulness to sleep; early in the evening or after arousal during the night, however, it may be seen from deeper stages of non–rapid eye movement (NREM) sleep and rapid eye movement (REM) sleep. This behavior is quite common, occurring in up to 15% of children; it begins in infancy or early childhood but may persist up to 10 years of age. The child is not awake during the episode and does not remember the events, which can go on for prolonged periods but usually last less than 15 minutes.

Clonazepam at bedtime may be helpful if the episodes are prolonged, threaten to injure the child, or appear to be interfering with normal sleep patterns. In most cases, it is sufficient to ensure that the bed area is padded to prevent injury.

Shivering Attacks

Shivering or shuddering attacks are brief episodes characterized by sudden flexion of the head and trunk associated with a rapid tremulous contraction of the musculature. The appearance is exactly that of a sudden brief shudder experienced normally when exposed to cold. In this condition, however, the shuddering occurs repeatedly. Some infants experience more than 100 brief shudders per day. There may be clustering, with intervals of several weeks free of the episodes. The child may assume a characteristic posture with flexion of head, trunk, and elbows and adduction of elbows and knees.

The attacks have been described in children between the ages of 4 months and 10 years, although most often the onset seems to be

Table 40–10. Differential Diagnosis of Infantile Syncope

Clinical	Infantile Syncope	Pallid Syncope	Tonic-Clonic Seizures	Infantile Spasms
Age range	1–6 yr, peak 6–18 mo	1–6 yr	All ages	4–12 mo
Precipitating factors	Present (e.g., minor trauma, frustration, fright)	Present (e.g., minor trauma, frustration, fright)	Usually none	None
Occurrence in sleep	Never	Never	Common	At transition from awake to sleep and sleep to awake
Sequence of events	Crying → exhale, apnea → cyanosis, loss of consciousness, opisthotonos → relaxation, resumes breathing	Upset, usually not crying → sudden pallor → limp fall with faint → tonic posture or clonic jerks may occur	Sudden loss of consciousness → increased tone followed by synchronous jerking of body and limbs → unconsciousness; duration 1–2 min	Sudden sustained flexion or extension of proximal limbs and trunk; duration 2–20 sec; seizures usually occur multiple times daily
Postictal symptoms	Usually minimal, may be lethargic and irritable	Usually minimal, quick return to normal	Usually marked, unconscious initially, then confused and lethargic	Rapid return to preictal state
Interictal EEG	Normal	Normal	Frequently abnormal with epileptiform discharges but may be normal	Abnormal background and epileptiform discharges
Ictal EEG	Reflects global cerebral hypoxia, diffuse rhythmic slowing → suppression → slowing with return of consciousness	Reflects global cerebral hypoxia, diffuse rhythmic slowing → suppression → slowing with return of consciousness	EEG seizure patterns, postictal diffuse suppression then slowing	High-amplitude slow-wave transient → diffuse suppression
Pathophysiology	Respiratory arrest without asystole	Vagal bradycardia or temporary asystole	Primary CNS event	Primary CNS event, age-related epileptic seizure

in infancy and early childhood. The phenomenon is nonepileptic and benign, eventually disappearing. Some children and their relatives have been reported to have an essential tremor. The shuddering is faster and of lower amplitude than myoclonus and is paroxysmal, not sustained, as occurs with a tremor.

Paroxysmal Torticollis

Torticollis is an abnormal posturing of the head and neck, with the head flexed toward the shoulder and the neck rotated with the chin turned toward the opposite shoulder (see Chapter 53). The posturing is paroxysmal, although variable in duration, lasting minutes or days, and there is no loss of consciousness. Some children have associated pallor, agitation, and vomiting, and the disorder has been suspected to be due to labyrinthine dysfunction similar to benign paroxysmal vertigo of childhood. The disorder is self-limited and remits in early childhood. There appears to be some association with migraine in patients later in life and among their relatives.

There are a variety of causes of torticollis in children (see Chapter 53). In older children, torticollis may occur as a focal dystonia persisting to adulthood. Familial cases have been described, and in some the torticollis may be the earliest manifestation of a more generalized dystonia. Sustained abnormal posturing should prompt appropriate radiologic investigations to exclude inflammatory or neoplastic disorders of the upper cervical spinal cord, posterior fossa, cervical spine, or soft tissues of the neck. Gastroesophageal reflux may very rarely present with dystonic posturing of the neck and upper trunk. Adverse extrapyramidal reactions to phenothiazines and related drugs may produce dystonic posturing of the neck and trunk, usually in association with ocular deviation or nystagmoid eye movements.

Masturbation

Episodes of genital self-stimulation may occur in young children. Infant girls may assume stereotyped posturing with tightening of the thighs or applied pressure to the suprapubic or pubic area, not associated with manual stimulation of the vulva or rhythmic movements. The episodes vary in duration from minutes to hours and are often accompanied by irregular breathing, facial flushing, and diaphoresis. Such behavior has been mistakenly thought to be a result of abdominal pain or seizures.

Spasmus Nutans

Spasmus nutans is a rare disorder of unknown etiology characterized by nystagmoid eye movements, head nodding, and torticollis. Head nodding may develop before the nystagmus and can be horizontal, vertical, or mixed. Both the head movements and the nystagmus may be paroxysmal, allowing confusion with seizures. There is no loss of consciousness during an episode. Small-amplitude rapid eye movements are typical; they tend to be asymmetric between the eyes and may even be monocular. The eye movements vary in prominence with different directions of gaze.

This is a self-limited disorder with onset between 4 and 18 months of age and not persisting beyond 3 years, although nystagmus alone may persist in some children. Investigations should include imaging of the optic nerves and chiasma, as some cases have been associated with local tumors.

Benign Paroxysmal Vertigo

Benign paroxysmal vertigo may be confused with seizures, as attacks develop suddenly, are accompanied by ataxia, and may cause the infant to fall. There is pallor, distress, and assumption of a motionless, often supine, position but no loss of consciousness; older children can recall the event. There may be vomiting; nystagmus should be visible during the episode. Attacks last seconds to minutes and vary in frequency, sometimes occurring daily. Older children can identify symptoms of nausea and vertigo and are less likely to be thought to be experiencing seizures. The children are normal between attacks. Vestibular function testing should be abnormal (see Chapter 43).

Treatment for repeated attacks may include dimenhydrinate (5 mg/kg/24 hours).

Benign Myoclonus of Early Infancy

This uncommon syndrome may resemble the cryptogenic form of infantile spasms at onset, with bilateral myoclonic jerks developing in a previously normal infant. However, this is a benign, probably nonepileptic condition occurring in infants 3 to 8 months of age and disappearing after a period of weeks or months. The pattern of myoclonus may differentiate it from infantile spasms, including predominant involvement of the head, neck, and upper limbs with adversive head movements or tremors without involving the lower limbs.

The EEG is normal and remains normal throughout the illness. Myoclonic movements are not accompanied by an EEG seizure pattern. These abnormal movements may require monitoring to establish the nonepileptic diagnosis. There is no arrest of normal development or regression as is seen in West syndrome. Most important, the myoclonus remits, not persisting beyond 2 years of age, and no other seizure patterns appear following its cessation.

Alternating Hemiplegia of Childhood

Alternating hemiplegia of childhood is an unusual and rare syndrome of episodic hemiplegia, movement disorders, and cognitive and behavioral abnormalities that usually presents in infancy with the following diagnostic criteria:

1. Onset before age 18 months, often before 6 months.
2. Recurrent episodes of fluctuating hemiparesis or hemiplegia affecting both sides of the body and disappearing during sleep.
3. Other paroxysmal phenomena: tonic fits, dystonic posturing, choreoathetosis, nystagmus and other paroxysmal oculomotor disturbances, and autonomic dysfunction, occurring during or between hemiplegic episodes.
4. Progressive cognitive and neurologic deficits.

The pathophysiology remains unknown, although there is a report of an autosomal dominant inheritance pattern with a chromosomal translocation. The differential diagnosis includes paroxysmal choreoathetosis and dystonia syndromes, hemiplegic migraine, transient ischemic attacks associated with cerebral vascular abnormalities such as moyamoya disease or cardiac emboli, mitochondrial disorders, hyperviscosity, sickle cell anemia crises, inherited disorders of metabolism (pyruvate dehydrogenase deficiency and Leigh disease), and epileptic seizures with postictal paralysis (see Chapter 42).

Symptomatic treatment is available with flunarizine, a calcium channel blocker, lessening the duration, severity, and frequency of hemiplegic attacks in some patients.

ACUTE SYMPTOMATIC SEIZURES AND OCCASIONAL SEIZURES

Febrile Convulsions

Febrile convulsions in children are common and are defined as seizures occurring between the ages of 6 months and 5 years in association with a fever in the absence of intracranial infection or other identifiable cause. Patients with a history of previous afebrile seizures are not included. The temperature elevation is variable; physicians would use a temperature of greater than 38° to 38.5°C. The highest incidence of febrile convulsions is between 1 and 2 years of age, and 85% of febrile convulsions occur before the age of 4 years. A number of prospective community-based surveys have shown that the incidence is between 2% and 5%; it is slightly more common in males.

The seizures are usually brief with bilateral clonic or tonic-clonic motor involvement without any postictal paralysis or a prolonged postictal state of confusion or drowsiness. The seizures generally occur well within the first 24 hours of a febrile illness, not necessarily when the fever is highest; they may be the first indication of illness. Complicated or severe febrile convulsions are defined as those lasting longer than 15 minutes, recurring during a single febrile illness, having unilateral or focal features, or followed by postictal paralysis. Seizures occurring late in a febrile illness, especially with an exanthem, should raise suspicions of an encephalitis or meningitis. Abnormal behavior associated with a febrile delirium and even violent shivering may be mistaken for seizure activity, especially if the latter is associated with pallor or perioral cyanosis.

Evaluation. The initial investigation must include a search for the cause of the febrile illness. The commonest causes of fever in children at this age are viral infections of the upper respiratory and gastrointestinal tracts and otitis media. Urinary tract infections and fever following immunization are also common. It is essential that primary CNS infection be ruled out as the cause of both the fever and the seizures, and a lumbar puncture (LP) may occasionally need to be performed. It is suggested that children younger than 12 months of age should routinely have an LP when presenting with a febrile seizure; many would not do an LP in an otherwise healthy child with an uncomplicated febrile seizure over the age of 2 years. An LP must be performed if there is any suspicion of intracranial infection (an ill-looking child who does not recover rapidly with lowering of the fever) and when features of the seizure or postictal state suggest a focal or lateralized seizure (see Chapter 53). In a child with focal seizures, fever, and encephalitis, herpes simplex encephalitis must be suspected.

Electroencephalography and neuroradiologic imaging have no place in the assessment of simple febrile convulsions, but CT or MRI scans and EEG may be part of the work-up if an underlying CNS infection is suspected or a preexisting neurologic deficit has been revealed by the history.

Treatment. Treatment of a child still convulsing on arrival at the hospital should include prompt attention to protection of the airway and circulation. The fever should be lowered by undressing the child and sponging with tepid water and giving acetaminophen per rectum at 10 to 15 mg/kg. If the convulsion does not cease promptly with lowering of the fever, rectal diazepam should be administered at 0.3 to 0.5 mg/kg. Some children may require hospital admission for observation and administration of regular antipyretics. The family should be advised that future fevers above 38°C be treated with regular acetaminophen or ibuprofen, tepid water sponging, and cool oral fluids.

There is no increased mortality from febrile convulsions, and the mental and neurologic development can be expected to be normal following a simple febrile convulsion. However, approximately 30% of febrile convulsions recur in future febrile illness, and the parents should be warned of this. Recurrence is most likely in the first 6 to 12 months after the initial febrile convulsion. Other factors that increase the chance of recurrence are onset at a young age, preexisting neurologic abnormalities, and family history of epilepsy.

Most would advise no treatment for almost all children with febrile convulsions. Rare exceptions include children presenting with prolonged (>15 minutes) seizures and children younger than 12 months old with multiple recurrences, especially if the circumstances are such that the patient will continue to be at risk of contracting febrile illness (in a day care center). In such cases, one option would be intermittent rectal or oral diazepam during febrile illnesses. One regimen involves treatment with 5 mg rectal diazepam every 8 to 12 hours (if younger than 3 years of age) and with 7.5 mg every 8 to 12 hours (if older than 3 years) if the temperature is above 38°C. If this is ineffective or impractical, chronic phenobarbital or valproate could be considered for the rare child with prolonged or very frequent febrile convulsions.

Informing and reassuring parents of the benign nature and usual course of febrile convulsions are very important and may be of greater value than any medication.

Prognosis. There appears to be an increased risk for the development of epilepsy in later life among children suffering febrile convulsions. The risk is as high as 7% in a study with a mean follow-up of 18 years. Risk factors included existence of a prior neurologic abnormality, prolonged convulsions (>30 minutes), focal or lateralized features to the seizure, and repeated convulsions within 24 hours. The incidence of epilepsy rose from 4% in those without risk factors to 49% in those with three risk factors. Risk factors specifically for epilepsy with generalized seizures were greater than three febrile seizures and epilepsy in a first-degree relative, which suggests that febrile convulsions in these individuals may be a manifestation of an increased predisposition to epilepsy. For epilepsy with partial seizures, the risk factors were prolonged convulsions, focal features to the seizure, and repeated seizures within 24 hours, suggesting either a causative role for febrile convulsions in partial epilepsy or a preexisting brain lesion. The number of recurrences of febrile seizures has not been shown to be a risk factor for later epilepsy. There is no evidence that AED treatment of febrile seizures affects the risk for later development of afebrile seizures.

EPILEPTIC SYNDROMES

West Syndrome

West syndrome, or severe encephalopathic epilepsy in infants, is characterized by infantile spasms, the EEG pattern hypsarrhythmia, and developmental delay. It is a severe form of epilepsy, usually with evidence of diffuse cerebral dysfunction and a poor prognosis in most cases. The incidence is about 1 in 4000 to 6000 infants, with onset between 3 and 12 months of age; peak onset is 4 to 8 months.

The spasm is a brief bilateral tonic contraction of muscles of the trunk, neck, and limbs, usually symmetric. The extent of muscle involvement varies from a powerful contraction "jackknifing" the body to minimal contraction of truncal muscles causing only stiffening. The classic spasm, "salaam attack," begins with a jerk-like contraction of trunk and limb musculature, which is maintained for a few seconds. Spasms may involve truncal flexion, extension, or both. Eye movements are commonly associated with the spasm either as deviation or as repetitive nystagmoid jerks. Apnea is common but tachypnea is uncommon. Children may cry or even appear to giggle at the end of the spasm. The seizures occur daily, frequently with hundreds being recorded per 24-hour period, often clustered together. Seizures may increase during the transitions from sleep to wakefulness and wakefulness to sleep.

EEG Features. The EEG pattern hypsarrhythmia is a high-amplitude (>300 μV) chaotic slowing of generalized distribution without interhemispheric synchronization and with multifocal sharp waves throughout. Hypsarrhythmia is more frequent in younger infants and early in the course of the disorder, and it is more common to find some modified variant of it. The commonest ictal EEG pattern is that of a generalized high-voltage slow-wave transient followed by generalized electrodecrement of the EEG.

Differential Diagnosis. Differential diagnosis for the seizures themselves can include intestinal colic, exaggerated startle or Moro reflexes, or normal myoclonic jerks on going into or out of sleep. Two myoclonic syndromes occur in this age group and must be distinguished from infantile spasms: (1) benign myoclonus of early infancy (see preceding neonatal section) and (2) benign myoclonic epilepsy.

Benign myoclonic epilepsy is a rare syndrome described in previously normal infants with onset between 4 months and 3 years. The infant has brief repetitive myoclonic jerks that involve the head and upper limbs and rarely the lower limbs; they occur daily in drowsiness and wakefulness. The ictal EEG shows 3-Hz spike and wave or polyspike activity during the events. The background EEG rhythms interictally are normal, as opposed to the hypsarrhythmic background of West syndrome. There are no other seizure types, and the infant does not have associated behavioral or cognitive disturbances.

The long-term prognosis is favorable for development and remission of seizures following response to treatment with antiepileptic medication. Some patients have had tonic-clonic seizures later in adolescence.

An EEG pattern of suppression-burst activity heralds a poor prognosis, and some groups have proposed that infants with a consistent EEG pattern of this nature and a much earlier onset of seizures may have distinct epileptic syndromes separable from the majority of patients with West syndrome. These related syndromes are discussed in the preceding neonatal section: *early infantile epileptic encephalopathy* and *early myoclonic encephalopathy*. Both present earlier than typical West syndrome, usually in the first weeks of life; the former features tonic seizures like infantile spasms and an EEG pattern of suppression-burst activity, and the latter features erratic fragmentary myoclonus, other partial and generalized seizure types, and suppression-burst pattern on EEG.

Evaluation. Investigation of patients with infantile spasms is directed at determining the cause, if possible, and then classification into cryptogenic and symptomatic groups. The commonest etiologic factor found is perinatal hypoxic-ischemic insult. Other important associations include intrauterine infection, prematurity, intracranial hemorrhage, neuroblast migration disorders, tuberous sclerosis, head injury, CNS infection, and inborn errors of metabolism. Approximately 10% to 15% of patients have no identifiable underlying etiology found on investigation and a history of normal development prior to the onset of their illness; this subset is referred to as *cryptogenic,* or *idiopathic, West syndrome.* The cryptogenic subset of patients is likely to have a much better long-term outcome, with

38% normal or mildly impaired compared with only 5% in the symptomatic patients.

About 50% of infants go on to have other seizure types when spasms cease. The infantile spasms are age-related, and persistence of the epilepsy in most of the patients is associated with loss of the spasms and development of other seizure types, such as tonic seizures, simple partial seizures, and tonic-clonic seizures.

Treatment. Treatment with corticosteroids aborts the spasms in a significant number of infants. Regimens vary, including initial doses of adrenocorticotropic hormone (ACTH; 20 to 30 units/day or 150 units/m²/day) or prednisone (2 mg/kg/day). The spasms should cease and the EEG pattern improve if the child has responded. After 1 to 2 weeks at maximum doses, the corticosteroid is gradually decreased until it is discontinued altogether after 2 to 3 months.

There are a number of important side effects of corticosteroid therapy: hypertension, hyperglycemia, electrolyte imbalance, immune suppression, cataract formation, and transient radiologic evidence of cerebral atrophy. The parents must be warned of these side effects and of the change in body habitus to be expected. Before therapy, baseline serum electrolytes, serum glucose, blood pressure, and EEG should be obtained. During therapy, electrolytes, glucose, and blood pressure must be monitored; the skin creases, mouth, and perineum must be inspected regularly for fungal infection; and any fever or deterioration in the child's condition must be promptly investigated.

Severe Myoclonic Epilepsy in Infancy

Severe myoclonic epilepsy in infancy is a rare cryptogenic generalized epilepsy appearing in the first year of life. The syndrome differs from the myoclonic syndromes already described (early myoclonic encephalopathy and early infantile encephalopathic epilepsy) by its later onset and the EEG findings.

The child may present with febrile or afebrile seizures, usually with normal psychomotor development preceding the onset of seizures, although often with a family history of epilepsy. The seizures are generalized or unilateral clonic seizures; myoclonic seizures appear later, between 8 months and 4 years of age; and partial seizures and atypical absences may occur. The interictal EEG may be normal initially and only later show fast generalized spike and wave epileptiform discharges and focal abnormalities.

The seizures are usually refractory to AEDs, and psychomotor development eventually becomes retarded. Ataxia and signs of pyramidal tract dysfunction may become apparent.

Childhood

The paroxysmal disorders of childhood (2 to 12 years) are given in Table 40–11.

PAROXYSMAL NONEPILEPTIC DISORDERS

Migraine and Migraine Equivalents

Migraine is a common disorder, and some episodes may be confused with seizures because of their paroxysmal nature and association with neurologic deficits or altered consciousness (see Chapter 38).

Table 40–11. Paroxysmal Disorders of Childhood

Paroxysmal Nonepileptic Disorders

More Common

Breath-holding spells
Migraine and migraine equivalents, recurrent abdominal pain,
  cyclic vomiting
Tic
Withholding, constipation
Daydreaming, staring spells
Sleep
  Head banging (jactatio capitis)
  Pavor nocturnus
  Somnambulism, somniloquy

Less Common

Syncope
Spasmodic torticollis
Drug reactions, dystonia
Paroxysmal choreoathetosis
Gastroesophageal reflux
Benign paroxysmal vertigo
Myoclonus, nonepileptic; anxiety, excitement, acute metabolic
  encephalopathy
Hyperekplexia
Masturbation
Stereotypic movements, autism, deaf and blind children
Munchausen syndrome by proxy
Hyperventilation
Psychogenic seizures
Transient global amnesia

Acute Symptomatic Seizures and Occasional Seizures

More Common

Febrile convulsions

Less Common

Brain tumor
Meningitis, encephalitis
Head injury, child abuse
Poisoning
Intercurrent medical illness, renal, liver disease, cardiac
  right-to-left shunt and embolism
Metabolic disease, rickets

Epileptic Syndromes

More Common

Benign partial epilepsies
Symptomatic focal epilepsy
Childhood absence epilepsy

Less Common

Epilepsia partialis continua (Kojewnikow syndrome)
Rasmussen encephalitis
Hemiconvulsion hemiplegia syndrome
Epilepsy with myoclonic absences
Lennox-Gastaut syndrome
Myoclonic astatic epilepsy
Landau-Kleffner syndrome
Epilepsy with continuous spike and wave during slow-wave
  sleep

In *cyclic vomiting,* recurrent attacks of nausea, vomiting, and abdominal pain occur on a daily or weekly basis. There is no clouding of consciousness, although the child may become dehydrated and acidotic, requiring hospitalization. Typically, there are symptom-free intervals lasting weeks to months. Migraine may develop later, or there may be a strong family history of migraine, and there appears to be some overlap with migraine (see Chapter 20).

Tic Disorders

Tics are common. They are sudden, brief, purposeless involuntary movements or utterances that occur repetitively (see Chapter 36). Tics may be thought to be myoclonic seizures, and indeed some tics may have a rapid myoclonic character. Myoclonus cannot be suppressed by the patient and may have an ictal EEG correlate and be associated with other seizure types.

Table 40–12 outlines some of the clinical features of episodic abnormal movements that may appear in children.

Sleep Disorders

Night Terrors and Confusional Arousals. *Night terrors* are a common phenomenon in children and are most frequent in boys aged 5 to 7 years. Up to 15% of children younger than 7 years have experienced some form of these episodes. The attacks are characterized by sudden arousal from sleep, often screaming in terror, then crying with agitation and tachycardia. There may be vigorous and potentially injurious motor activity in older children, such as running or hitting the bed or wall. The striking feature of these episodes is the inconsolable but seemingly awake child. The episodes arise out of slow-wave NREM sleep, usually occurring 1 to 2 hours after bedtime, and are not responses to dream imagery (i.e., not nightmares). Episodes last several minutes. Prior sleep deprivation, febrile illness, emotional stress, and some medications (sedatives/hypnotics, neuroleptics, stimulants, antihistamines) may be precipitants. In contrast to the experience of nightmares, children are amnestic for the events and their distress in night terrors.

Confusional arousals are less dramatic attacks with similar origin from slow-wave sleep and are more typical in the younger child. The child stirs and begins crying and whimpering inconsolably. These arousals may be prolonged in infants, lasting up to 30 to 40 minutes.

In both of these types of episodes, the EEG demonstrates the arousal from NREM sleep and that the patient does not fully awaken; the EEG shows persistent delta slowing or a mix of slow activity and the patient's normal background rhythms.

There is no specific treatment for these events, and parents should be educated about their nature and reassured that they are self-limited. It is generally impossible to ignore these events, and although efforts to calm the child may seem to prolong the attacks, it is probably best if a parent sits with the child if only to prevent injury. Frequent disruptive attacks or those with potentially injurious motor activity may be decreased by short-term treatment with low-dose tricyclic antidepressants or benzodiazepines.

Somnambulism. Somnambulism, or sleepwalking, is common in childhood: approximately 15% of children have walked in their sleep, especially in the 2- to 3-year-old age group, and 2.5% are habitual sleepwalkers, having episodes at least once a month. The age of onset peaks between 4 and 10, and 8 and 15 years. There is a family history of sleepwalking and other parasomnias in 60% to 80% of patients. These episodes of apparent unresponsiveness and "automatisms" could be mistaken for complex partial seizures or a postictal state.

Table 40–12. Abnormal Involuntary Movements

Movement	Characteristics	Associations
Tic	Brief involuntary movements (motor tics) or sounds (phonic or vocal tics) occurring against a background of normal motor activity. Tics may be *simple*: sudden, brief movements such as shrugging a shoulder, blinking, or grimacing, or *complex*: more coordinated movement that might appear purposeful such as hitting or touching. Snorting, sniffing, and throat clearing are examples of simple phonic tics, and short utterances, echolalia, and coprolalia are complex phonic tics.	Idiopathic tic disorders Tourette syndrome
Tremor	Movements due to rhythmically alternating contractions of a muscle group and its antagonists. The movements may involve proximal and axial muscles. Classified as *resting, postural,* or *action* tremors according to the response to these maneuvers.	Physiologic tremor Essential tremor
Chorea	Random, brief limb movements of variable duration; these can be incorporated into voluntary movements by the patient. The term is derived from the word for a "dance."	Lupus Wilson disease Postinfectious state
Athetosis	Slow, writhing movements of the extremities, often the distal extremities. The movements are random. Often involuntary movements of this type have some features of chorea and are termed *choreoathetoid.*	Kernicterus
Dystonia	Sustained muscle cocontraction of agonist and antagonist muscle groups, frequently causing twisting and repetitive movements or abnormal postures. The velocity of the movements varies, usually being sustained at the height of the involuntary contraction for a second or longer. The duration also varies in different syndromes of dystonia; in spasmodic torticollis there may be rhythmic jerks or spasms into the abnormal posture. Subclassified by extent—*focal, segmental, multifocal,* and *generalized*—and by relationship to movement—*action* and *rest.*	Idiopathic (inherited) syndromes Postlesional syndromes
Myoclonus	Rapid, brief muscle jerks with an irregular or occasionally rhythmic quality; can be epileptic or nonepileptic in origin.	Encephalopathies Idiopathic and symptomatic epilepsies
Ballismus	Wild, large-amplitude, irregular limb movements.	Postlesional syndromes
Asterixis	Repetitive movements due to sudden, brief, irregular lapses in posture of an extremity.	Metabolic encephalopathies
Dyskinesia	Sometimes used as a general term to describe abnormal involuntary movements.	

Hyperekplexia

A startle response is normally seen in children and adults in response to sudden, unexpected stimuli. The typical response consists of a facial grimace, eye blink and brief head nod, shoulder elevation, abduction of the arms with elbow flexion, truncal flexion, and knee flexion. Startle is exaggerated with anxiety, fatigue, and sleep deprivation. Hyperekplexia is characterized by an excessive startle response interfering with daily living, usually causing patients to fall stiffly in the posture of the startle response and sustaining injury, with preserved consciousness. A history of infantile stiffness of the trunk and limbs and nocturnal myoclonus is present in many. There appears to be an infantile expression of the disorder, with severe hypertonia occurring with handling; the hypertonia may be so severe as to cause apnea, bradycardia, and even sudden death.

Generalized seizures have been reported in some cases, and mental retardation and delayed motor development appear to be common. The background EEG is usually normal. There may be some improvement with clonazepam or sodium valproate therapy. Linkage analysis has assigned the gene to the long arm of chromosome 5 in one five-generation pedigree. Familial cases with autosomal dominant inheritance patterns have been described as well as apparently sporadic cases.

In some epileptic syndromes, such as the *Lennox-Gastaut syndrome,* generalized seizures may be precipitated by sudden unexpected stimuli. This phenomenon has been termed *startle-induced epileptic seizures,* or *startle epilepsy.* Startle-induced seizures can normally be differentiated from nonepileptic startle responses by the presence of other seizure types and EEG abnormalities.

Self-Stimulatory Behavior

Repetitive purposeless movements may be performed by physically and intellectually handicapped children and by autistic children in settings of low stimulation. Combined with unresponsiveness, these behaviors may be mistaken for automatisms in complex partial seizures in a group at higher than normal risk of epilepsy and of having an abnormal EEG. The important features that distinguish such behavior from epileptic activity are the setting in which it occurs, the variable content and duration of the "attacks," and the failure of the episodes to ever interrupt more stimulating activities. However, it may be very difficult to determine the nature of the episodes by interview, and video and EEG monitoring may be required for diagnosis.

Munchausen Syndrome by Proxy

Munchausen syndrome describes a consistent simulation of illness by a person leading to unnecessary investigations and treatments. When parents pursue such deception and cause their children to be investigated and treated, the situation is referred to as

Munchausen syndrome by proxy. Presentations include neurologic illness, and a history of paroxysmal loss of consciousness or seizures is common. The syndrome is described in children under 6 years of age, and the mother is often the perpetrator. The mother often has some paramedical training (see Chapters 36 and 37).

Seizures refractory to carefully prescribed antiepileptic medication must always prompt a review of the diagnosis, and one must also be careful to consider fabricated presentations of paroxysmal disorders.

ACUTE SYMPTOMATIC SEIZURES AND OCCASIONAL SEIZURES

Febrile convulsions remain one of the most common causes of occasional seizures in early childhood. Head injury is more common in childhood than in infancy, but the list of other potential causes of seizures, including brain tumor, intracranial infection, and poisoning, is very similar.

EPILEPTIC SYNDROMES (Table 40–13)

Benign Partial Epilepsies of Childhood

Partial seizures and focal EEG discharges usually suggest the presence of a localized cerebral lesion. There are a group of idiopathic partial epilepsies beginning in children without abnormalities on neurologic examination or neuroimaging studies and frequently with a family history for epilepsy. The benign partial epilepsies of childhood (BPEC) are characterized by partial seizures and focal epileptiform discharges, both with age-dependent spontaneous recovery, in the absence of anatomic lesions.

Clinically, the seizures begin between 18 months and 12 years of age, most often at 8 to 10 years; there is no neurologic or intellectual deficit or developmental delay. The seizures are brief and stereotyped in an individual, although they vary among patients. The seizures do not have a prolonged postictal deficit, are usually infrequent, and respond well to AED treatment. The focal epileptiform discharges occur with normal background rhythms in sleep and wakefulness. The sharp waves or spikes have a characteristic morphology and are often very frequent, increasing during sleep. Rare generalized epileptiform discharges may occur, but if they are prominent, the diagnosis of BPEC should be questioned.

The most well-defined form of BPEC is *benign epilepsy with centrotemporal spikes and seizures,* often referred to as *benign rolandic epilepsy.* Brief hemifacial motor seizures with anarthria and drooling are typical. Consciousness is typically preserved, although this may not be true with longer seizures. A somatosensory aura involving the tongue, cheek, or gums may precede the hemifacial motor seizure. Many seizures occur at night as tonic-clonic seizures, presumably secondary generalized with unwitnessed partial onset. Onset is between 3 and 13 years, with a peak onset at 9 to 10 years; there is a male-to-female predominance of approximately 3:2.

Management depends on seizure frequency; if the typical EEG discharges have been found in a child without seizures or following a first seizure, there is usually no indication to treat with AEDs. If seizures are infrequent and nocturnal, the option of no treatment should be discussed. AED treatment should be considered for patients experiencing more frequent seizures, troublesome seizures during the day, or seizures associated with any morbidity such as postictal headaches or lethargy. The seizures are usually easily controlled with a variety of AEDs, including carbamazepine, phenytoin, or valproate.

The seizures of BPEC resolve spontaneously before 16 years of age, so all treated patients should have AED withdrawal at least by that time. The EEG may be helpful in deciding when to withdraw treatment, as the discharges are also age-related, tending to become blunter and lower in amplitude before disappearing. One should withdraw treatment in patients older than 14 years who are seizure-free for 1 to 2 years with normal EEGs; one should strongly consider trial of withdrawal in patients 10 to 14 years who are seizure-free with a normal EEG. Younger patients with active EEGs are likely to have recurrence of seizures with AED withdrawal.

Benign partial epilepsy of childhood with occipital paroxysms forms a subset of BPEC. The seizures begin with visual symptoms (amaurosis, phosphenes, visual illusions, hallucinations) consistent with an occipital origin. Hemiclonic seizures or the automatisms of temporal lobe complex seizures often follow, according to whether the seizure spreads to suprasylvian or infrasylvian regions. The EEG shows high-amplitude sharp waves or spike and wave complexes recurring at 1 to 0.5 Hz posteriorly, usually maximal in the occipital regions. The discharges are present when the eyes are closed and should disappear with eye opening.

Symptomatic Focal (Localization-Related) Epilepsy

The most common seizure type in symptomatic focal epilepsy in children is complex partial. Complex partial seizures may arise from temporal, frontal, parietal, or occipital lobes, most often from the temporal lobe. The etiology of focal epilepsy in childhood is diverse and includes birth asphyxia, later anoxic episodes, head injury, neoplasms (usually slowly growing gliomas or rarer embryologic-origin tumors), infection, neuroblast migration disorders, the cerebral lesions of neurocutaneous syndromes, vascular malformations, and cerebral infarction. Mesial temporal sclerosis is the most common finding in temporal lobes resected to treat refractory focal epilepsy in adults. The incidence of mesial temporal sclerosis in childhood non–idiopathic focal epilepsy has not yet been determined. MRI is a crucial diagnostic procedure and can reveal a variety of structural abnormalities.

Symptomatic focal epilepsy commonly evolves as a medically refractory disorder, yet in some patients it can be amenable to surgical resection of the epileptic focus. The investigation of children for epilepsy surgery is a highly specialized process that follows documentation of medical intractability (see "Choice of Antiepileptic Drugs" later). Concordant evidence of a single epileptogenic region within the brain must be found with ictal video and EEG monitoring, both structural (MRI scans) and functional (single photon emission computed tomography [SPECT] and positron emission tomography [PET] scans) neuroimaging and neuropsychologic evaluation. If a focus can be demonstrated, it must be shown that resection of that area of the brain will not cause loss of sensorimotor or cognitive function. As most of the intractable focal epilepsies have temporal foci, the risk of postoperative memory dysfunction must be addressed. In seizures with foci from extratemporal sites, it may be necessary to map cortical sensorimotor and language function by cortical stimulation to determine the limits of a surgical resection.

Childhood Absence Epilepsy

Childhood absence epilepsy is an idiopathic generalized epilepsy beginning in previously normal children between 3 and 12 years of age, with peak incidence at 6 to 7 years of age; girls are more frequently affected. It accounts for only about 8% to 10% of

Table 40–13. Selected Inherited Disorders of Metabolism and Neurodegenerative Diseases Associated with Seizures in Childhood and Adolescence

Disorder	Clinical Features and Laboratory Findings	Investigations
Syndrome of Progressive Myoclonus Epilepsy (PME)		
Multiple specific disorders cause the clinical syndrome of PME:		
Prominent myoclonus: irregular, repetitive, spontaneous, or with action; stimulus-sensitive		
Associated seizure types: usually tonic-clonic but also tonic, absence, and partial		
Progressive neurologic deterioration, with prominent ataxia and other motor signs developing later		
Progressive dementia, varies in degree between the specific disorders		
Most cases are caused by the following five disorders:		
Unverricht-Lundborg syndrome	Onset 8–15 yr, myoclonus and generalized tonic-clonic (GTC) seizures, cerebellar ataxia, slowly progressive but mild cognitive decline. Patients have long survival compared with those with other disorders in this group.	Clinical diagnosis must exclude other causes of PME syndrome
Myoclonus epilepsy and ragged-red fibers (MERRF)	Onset 5–12 yr (range 3–62 yr), myoclonus, GTC seizures, progressive ataxia, dementia. Other features include deafness, optic atrophy, neuropathy, myopathy, pyramidal signs, dysarthria, and nystagmus. There may be clinical overlap with other mitochondrial encephalomyopathies; mitochondrial encephalomyopathy with lactic acidosis and stroke-like episodes (MELAS) and Kearns-Sayre syndrome.	Serum and CSF lactate and pyruvate. Muscle biopsy; light microscopy, electron microscopy (EM), biochemical analysis of oxidative metabolism, and DNA studies.
Lafora body disease	Onset 10–19 yr, generalized clonic, GTC seizures, and partial seizures with visual auras; myoclonus develops later and becomes very disabling; severe dementia. Death within 5.5 yr of disease onset. Lafora bodies, intracellular amyloid inclusions, are found in skin, muscle, neurons, and hepatocytes.	Biopsy of skin must include eccrine sweat glands (i.e., axilla) to exclude Lafora bodies
Neuronal ceroid lipofuscinosis	Onset 2–4 yr, severe epilepsy, myoclonic, GTC, atonic, atypical absence seizures (not tonic vs. Lennox-Gastaut syndrome), progressive severe dementia, ataxia, pyramidal and extrapyramidal signs, visual loss later, usually death in adolescence. Dilated eye examination must be done. EEG; marked photic sensitivity to 1-Hz stimulation, electroretinogram (ERG) and visual evoked potential (VEP) abnormalities.	Skin, conjunctival or rectal mucosal biopsy. Skin biopsy is the most practical and least morbid. Lipopigment accumulation in lysosomes, best seen in eccrine secretory cells. The inclusions have a characteristic morphology on EM that differs between the different subtypes of neuronal ceroid lipofuscinosis.
Late infantile form (Jansky-Bielschowsky disease)		
Juvenile form (Batten-Spielmeyer-Vogt disease)	Onset 4–10 yr, usually presents with decreased visual acuity secondary to retinal degeneration, psychomotor delay, cerebellar and extrapyramidal signs, later onset of seizures; GTC seizures and myoclonus. Progressive severe dementia accompanies the other neurologic signs. Death in early adulthood. ERG and VEP abnormalities.	EEG, ERG, and VEP
Adult onset (Kufs disease)	Onset 11–50 yr, dementia, psychiatric symptoms, cerebellar and extrapyramidal signs are most prominent, seizures often tonic, visual disturbances are less common, fundi normal, EEG; marked photic sensitivity to 1-Hz stimulation.	

Table 40–13. Selected Inherited Disorders of Metabolism and Neurodegenerative Diseases Associated with Seizures in Childhood and Adolescence *Continued*

Disorder	Clinical Features and Laboratory Findings	Investigations
Sialidosis		
Type I	Onset 8–20 yr, decreased visual acuity and macular "cherry-red spot," action- and stimulus-induced myoclonus, cerebellar ataxia, no dementia or decreased survival. May have a peripheral neuropathy.	Urine specimen, blood sample for cultured leukocytes, and skin biopsy to obtain cultured fibroblasts for enzyme analysis
Type II	Onset 10–30 yr, seen in Japanese. Dysmorphic features and PME syndrome. Elevated excretion of urinary sialylated oligosaccharides, enzyme analysis shows deficiency of α-*N*-acetylneuraminidase (type I) additional deficiency of β-galactosidase (type II).	
Less common causes of PME syndrome in this age group:		
Juvenile neuronopathic Gaucher disease	PME, supranuclear palsy and splenomegaly, no dementia. Pancytopenia on CBC, leukocytes show low β-glucocerebrosidase activity.	CBC, leukocytes for enzyme analysis
Dentatorubral-pallidoluysian atrophy	Seen in Japanese, PME is one presentation	Clinical diagnosis in life
Neuroaxonal dystrophy	May appear as PME, also chorea, lower motor neuron signs; axon spheroids in neurons, may see in autonomic nerve endings around eccrine secretory coils.	Peripheral nerve biopsy, skin biopsy
Late onset GM$_2$ gangliosidosis	Acoustic stimulus–sensitive, myoclonus, severe dementia, dystonia, pyramidal signs, may see cherry-red spot at maculae.	Hexosaminidase A activity
Hallervorden-Spatz disease		Clinical diagnosis in life
Action myoclonus–renal failure syndrome	Described in French Canadians, tremor, PME, and later proteinuria and renal failure, no dementia.	Clinical diagnosis, renal function
Other Rare Disorders with Seizures in Childhood and Adolescence		
Juvenile Huntington disease	Onset >3 yr, developmental delay, dystonia, GTC, atypical absence, myoclonic seizures, may have parkinsonian features.	
Alpers syndrome	Progressive neurologic degeneration of childhood. A clinical syndrome; now suspected to be a mitochondrial encephalopathy. Normal at birth, then failure to thrive with developmental delay, myoclonic jerks, seizures, episodes of status epilepticus, hypotonia, visual loss followed by spastic quadraparesis. May have epilepsia partialis continua. The spectrum of clinical features includes deafness, ataxia, chorea, and liver disease.	Muscle biopsy
Rett syndrome	Girls, onset of symptoms 1–2 yr, delay or regression in motor development, loss of language, ataxia, "hand wringing" mannerism. Seizures occur later; myoclonic, partial, and GTC. Episodes of apnea, ataxic breathing, and hyperventilation, pyramidal signs.	Muscle biopsy for mitochondrial enzyme analysis and histology, although etiology unknown
Maple syrup urine disease	Less severe forms may present late, even in adulthood, with episodic symptoms of encephalopathy and ataxia. ? Seizures.	Urine and serum amino acids
Porphyria	Late adolescence, after puberty, 15% of affected patients have seizures during an acute attack of porphyria.	Urinalysis

school-age children with epilepsy. There is a family history of epilepsy in approximately 15% to 25% of patients. The absence seizures are simple or more often complicated with mild automatisms or other motor features. Absences are very frequent, occurring daily, although responding well to therapy. The EEG is normal apart from runs of 3-Hz spike and wave complexes; clinical seizures are associated with discharges lasting more than 2 to 3 seconds. The discharges and often clinical seizures can be produced by hyperventilation. Failure to produce seizures during hyperventilation with good effort is very unusual in untreated patients. Prognosis is generally favorable, with remission in approximately 80% of cases by late adolescence; rarely, absences may persist into adulthood. Generalized tonic-clonic seizures occur in 40% to 50% of patients with childhood absence epilepsy. They typically develop years after the onset of absences, in adolescence or adulthood, and may appear after remission from the absence seizures. Usually, the tonic-clonic seizures are infrequent and medically controlled.

Treatment with ethosuximide or valproate controls absence seizures in most patients. However, ethosuximide offers no protection against tonic-clonic seizures, whereas valproate is also effective against tonic-clonic seizures. Therefore, valproate is the drug of choice if both seizure types are present. If either ethosuximide or valproate proves ineffective after an adequate trial at maximum tolerated doses, a trial of the other should be commenced. Combination ethosuximide and valproate therapy has been effective in controlling absence seizures in some patients not controlled on either drug alone. Clonazepam may also be effective in controlling absence seizures, but it is associated with sedative and behavioral side effects.

Epilepsia Partialis Continua and Rasmussen Encephalitis

Epilepsia partialis continua, or Kojewnikow syndrome, describes continuous partial motor seizures usually manifesting as repetitive clonic jerks of the face, upper limb, lower limb, or larger portion of one half of the body that continue in this localized fashion for hours to days or months. These focal seizures with occasional secondary generalization are caused by circumscribed rolandic or perirolandic cortical processes that include vascular lesions, focal cortical dysplasia, neoplasms, and unidentified focal areas of atrophy.

The focal seizures in this condition are generally impossible to control with AEDs, and assessment toward surgical management of the epilepsy with a limited cortical resection may be necessary. The risk of motor and sensory deficits limits possible resections, and careful mapping of the site of seizure onset and its relationship to functional cortex is required. Mitochondrial encephalomyopathies (MELAS) and an inherited disorder of metabolism (nonketotic hyperglycinemia) have also been reported to cause epilepsia partialis continua.

Rasmussen encephalitis is a clinically defined syndrome of predominantly lateralized cerebral dysfunction, with onset of seizures between 2 and 10 years of age. A variety of seizure types can occur, including focal motor seizures and complex partial seizures with secondary generalization, myoclonus, and epilepsia partialis continua, and they are intractable to management with AEDs. The disorder is characterized by a progressive hemiparesis, language disturbances if the dominant hemisphere is affected, and intellectual decline. Progressive hemispheric atrophy, maximal in the central, temporal, and frontal regions, can be documented with neuroimaging studies. The pathologic specimens show nonspecific changes of microglial nodules, perivascular inflammatory cells, and neuronal loss, suggesting an encephalitis, although no etiologic agent has been identified. Worsening of the neurologic deficits can be expected over time, although the seizures may lessen and even "burn out."

Functional hemispherectomy, done early in the course of the disease before complete hemiparesis, should control seizures, arrest the motor deterioration, and in most cases lead to stabilization or even improvement in language and intellectual function. However, there is a significant morbidity and mortality associated with the surgery, and the child is left with a paretic upper limb.

Lennox-Gastaut Syndrome

The Lennox-Gastaut syndrome is characterized by generalized seizures and epileptiform discharges against the background of delayed mental development and behavioral problems beginning between 1 and 8 years of age. The patients have a mixed seizure disorder with multiple seizure types; the typical seizures are axial tonic seizures, atypical absences, and atonic seizures, although patients may also have tonic-clonic, myoclonic, and complex partial seizures. The seizures are not easily controlled and usually frequent, often several a day. Episodes of status epilepticus are common, and nonconvulsive stupor with continuous spike and wave discharges or a stuporous state with repeated tonic seizures is typical. The waking EEG has abnormally slow background activity, and the EEG correlates of sleep may also be poorly organized. The epileptiform abnormalities consist of slow (<3 Hz) spike and wave discharges, multifocal spikes, or sharp waves and paroxysmal fast activity (>10 Hz) in sleep.

AEDs are always indicated but rarely able to control seizures completely. More often, some reduction in frequency and severity of seizures may be obtained. As in all seizure disorders, monotherapy should be attempted with substitution of another agent if the initial drug proves ineffective. However, because of multiple seizure types, patients commonly need combinations of AEDs. Valproate should be used as a first-line agent for patients with atonic, tonic, and myoclonic seizures and may be helpful with tonic-clonic seizures. Patients with refractory tonic-clonic seizures or partial seizures as well as generalized seizures may benefit from the addition of phenytoin or carbamazepine to valproate. Combinations of AEDs must be monitored carefully for drug toxicity and unwanted interactions. Carbamazepine has been reported to exacerbate atypical absences in some patients. Barbiturates may be effective, although they are often poorly tolerated, and drug-related drowsiness may exacerbate tonic seizures in some patients. Second-line agents include clonazepam. Felbamate has been reported to improve control of the debilitating tonic or atonic "drop attacks" in patients with this syndrome. Felbamate also causes bone marrow suppression and aplastic anemia.

An issue perhaps peculiar to this notoriously refractory seizure disorder is the need to consider what level of seizure activity can be tolerated in a particular patient. For instance, the best control achieved may be infrequent daytime tonic seizures in the setting of daily absences and frequent nocturnal tonic seizures. AED toxicity may be particularly noxious in these patients, leading to increased numbers of falls, worsening behavior, lethargy, and exacerbation of seizures.

A major source of morbidity and an important management issue is repeated injurious falls associated with tonic and atonic seizures. Appropriate restriction in daily activities and the wearing of helmets with face protection are often required. Division of the anterior portion of the corpus callosum has been successful in controlling the falls associated with tonic or atonic seizures, but not all patients benefit, and seizure control is not complete.

Myoclonic Astatic Epilepsy

Although sometimes seen as a variant of the Lennox-Gastaut syndrome, myoclonic astatic epilepsy has been described as a distinct entity. Patients have a mixed seizure disorder with myoclonus, atypical absences, and tonic-clonic seizures but not tonic seizures. The term astatic refers to loss of station or posture with abrupt falling during myoclonic seizures. The peak age of onset is between 2 and 5 years and ranges from 7 months to 6 years. Approximately one third of patients have a family history of epilepsy.

Compared to the interictal EEG in Lennox-Gastaut syndrome, that in myoclonic astatic epilepsy shows faster generalized spike and wave and polyspike and wave epileptiform discharges. The absence of tonic and partial seizures and the EEG findings distinguish this syndrome from Lennox-Gastaut syndrome.

The course is variable, but a large proportion of patients have a favorable one. A certain small group of children with an apparently unfavorable, even catastrophic-looking initial clinical presentation may respond well to valproate therapy and have spontaneous remission of seizures.

Adolescence

The paroxysmal disorders of adolescence (12 to 18 years) are shown in Table 40–14.

PAROXYSMAL NONEPILEPTIFORM DISORDERS

Syncope

Loss of consciousness with falling are the salient features of syncope (see Chapter 43).

Table 40–15 compares the clinical features of syncope and tonic-clonic seizures.

Psychogenic Seizures

Nonepileptic paroxysmal abnormal behaviors (psychogenic seizures) may be a manifestation of psychiatric illness or emotionally based. Psychiatric disease may be mistaken for epilepsy, in particular panic attacks in the setting of an anxiety neurosis.

Panic attacks may begin without the patient being able to identify an external precipitant, and then the sense of dread or fear may be mistaken for a psychic aura. Many of the symptoms experienced result from hyperventilation and tachycardia, including palpitations, paresthesia, formication, lightheadedness, and carpopedal spasm. There may be some apparent disturbance of consciousness. Historically, the sequence of events is important, especially the hyperventilation and attendant symptoms. The patient may be encouraged to hyperventilate in the office to see if symptoms are reproduced; hyperventilation must continue for 3 to 5 minutes with good effort for a negative result to be clinically useful.

Rage attacks may occur and be confused with epileptic seizures; often seen in intellectually impaired patients, they represent intense frustration in the face of an inability to vent the frustration in other ways or to communicate it. Rage attacks may also occur in children with a normal intelligence quotient (IQ) or in athletes taking anabolic steroids.

Psychogenic seizures are common. Among adults, 20% of referrals with refractory seizures are found to be suffering from psychogenic seizures; in children, the number is smaller (4%). Psychogenic seizures may appear as a manifestation of a conversion disorder. Psychogenic seizures or hysterical seizures probably occur

Table 40–14. Paroxysmal Disorders of Adolescence

Paroxysmal Nonepileptic Disorders

More Common

 Syncope
 Migraine
 Psychogenic seizures
  Dissociative states, conversion disorders
  Panic attacks, hyperventilation
  Episodic rage (uncommon)
  Malingering (uncommon)
 Daydreaming
 Sleep
  Nocturnal myoclonus, hypnic jerks
  Narcolepsy
  Somnambulism
  Somniloquy

Less Common

 Paroxysmal choreoathetosis
 Tremor
 Tic
 Drug reactions, dystonia
 Transient global amnesia

Acute Symptomatic Seizures and Occasional Seizures

More Common

 Drug abuse
 Head injury
 Meningitis and encephalitis

Less Common

 Brain tumor
 Intercurrent medical illness, endocrine disorder, systemic
  neoplasia

Epileptic Syndromes

More Common

 Symptomatic localization-related epilepsy
 Juvenile myoclonic epilepsy

Less Common

 Juvenile absence epilepsy
 Epilepsy with generalized tonic-clonic seizures on awakening
 Epilepsia partialis continua (Kojewnikow syndrome)
 Rasmussen encephalitis
 Progressive myoclonic epilepsy (see Table 40–9)

in a dissociative state. Typically, they are characterized by marked motor activity such as pelvic thrusting, arching of the back, thrashing of the limbs, and even self-injury. The episodes may have a gradual onset with buildup of motor activity, and they usually last longer than epileptic seizures (Table 40–16). There is often irregular respiration, gasping, or moaning. These attacks have been described as a "macabre pastiche of intercourse"; there is an association between such behavior and sexual abuse in childhood. Other forms that the psychogenic seizure may take include a gradual slump to a motionless supine position with unresponsiveness and eyes closed, often with some flickering of the eyelids, referred to by some as a "swoon."

Deliberate simulation of an epileptic attack may occur in some patients with epilepsy in an effort to manipulate their environment or circumstances, and in this case the diagnosis may include school refusal.

Evaluation. The interictal EEG is repeatedly normal in patients

Table 40–15. Differential Diagnosis of Syncope

Clinical	Syncope	Tonic-Clonic Seizures
Precipitating factors	Almost always, patient standing, warm environment, fright, pain	Usually none, although sleep deprivation or awakening may be contributory
Prodrome	Lightheaded, dizzy, queasy, vision dims, loss of color, "gray out"; may be averted by putting head down or recumbency	May have an aura
Occurrence in sleep	Never	Common
Evolution	Limp faint → fall → motionless unconsciousness often with pallor, clammy skin, may have tonic phase with generalized stiffening	Sudden loss of consciousness → increased tone, massive truncal flexion or extension followed by synchronous jerking of body and limbs with rubor or cyanosis and sweating → unconscious
Incontinence	Rare	Occasional
Self-injury	Rare	Common
Degree of postictal confusion	Minimal	Marked
Family history	Often positive for syncope	May be positive for seizures
Interictal EEG	Usually normal	Frequently abnormal, epileptiform discharges

with psychogenic seizures. For definitive diagnosis, it may be necessary to record a clinical episode. In patients with frequent events, this may be accomplished with a few days of continuous video and EEG monitoring.

In some cases, spontaneous events may not occur during a reasonable period of video and EEG monitoring. Some centers attempt to induce suspected psychogenic seizures during video and EEG monitoring by suggestion, hyperventilation, photic stimulation, or administration of an intravenous "convulsant drug" (saline) or skin patch containing only alcohol. While injection or

Table 40–16. Differential Diagnosis of Psychogenic Seizures

Clinical	Psychogenic Seizures	Epileptic Seizures
Age at onset	Usually >8–10 yr, predominantly female, 15%–30% male	Any age, no sex predominance
Duration of seizures	May be very prolonged	Usually seconds to minutes
Evolution	May have a very gradual onset and ending	Usually more abrupt onset
Quality of convulsive movements	Thrashing, asynchronous limb movements, often with partial responsiveness	Usually rhythmic and synchronous with loss of consciousness
Stereotypic attacks	Typically variable	Typically stereotyped
Examination during the seizure	May resist examination, combative	Usually unresponsive and amnestic for ictal events
Self-injury	Rare	Common in GTC seizures
Incontinence	Rare	Common in GTC seizures
During sleep	No, may be nocturnal but while awake	Common
Changes in seizure frequency with medication	Rare	Usual
Interictal EEG	Repeatedly normal	Often abnormal
Ictal EEG	No EEG seizure patterns, normal rhythms while unresponsive	EEG seizure patterns
Pitfalls in diagnosis	1. Psychologic factors may not be immediately apparent. 2. Misleading information may be given by parents (Munchausen syndrome by proxy).	1. Asynchronous vigorous automatisms are found in frontal lobe seizures. 2. Bilateral limb movements and posturing without loss of consciousness occur in supplementary motor area (SMA) seizures. 3. EEG seizure patterns may be absent during some seizures—e.g., auras, SMA seizures.

Abbreviation: GTC = generalized tonic-clonic.

patch procedures are clinically useful if typical attacks are precipitated and recorded on video and EEG, there are ethical considerations raised by such a practice. The issue is complicated, and although some physicians and psychiatrists are opposed to induction (trickery) procedures, there may be a role for these techniques in certain children with suspected psychogenic seizures in whom spontaneous attacks could not be recorded.

Serum prolactin or creatinine kinase levels may also be helpful in the differential diagnosis of psychogenic seizures and epilepsy. Serum prolactin elevation can be seen within 30 minutes after a tonic-clonic or temporal or frontal complex partial seizure but not after a psychogenic seizure. The test specimen must be compared with a baseline serum prolactin level collected at the same time of day, not within 24 hours of one of the episodes. Marked elevation of serum creatinine kinase can be seen for 2 to 3 days after a tonic-clonic convulsion but generally not after a psychogenic seizure. However, elevation of creatinine kinase reflects muscle damage, and a vigorous psychogenic episode with injury will also be followed by elevation of creatinine kinase.

Treatment. Treatment of psychogenic seizures must include an identification of underlying psychosocial and psychiatric problems by psychiatric personnel. Presentation of the nonepileptic diagnosis to the patient following monitoring of a typical spell must be positive ("These attacks are not epileptic and will not require chronic medication or further neurologic investigation") and truthful ("We don't know exactly what is causing them, but emotional factors are clearly playing a major role").

The prognosis of psychogenic seizures in the pediatric population is much better than in adults, with 80% of patients seizure-free at 3-year follow-up.

ACUTE SYMPTOMATIC SEIZURES AND OCCASIONAL SEIZURES

The causes of acute symptomatic seizures in adolescence include those described in the preceding neonatal and childhood sections except for febrile convulsions. Head injury as a cause may be more common among adolescents, with participation in contact sports and motor vehicle accidents occurring in the middle to late teen years. Street drug abuse must be considered as a cause of altered mental state or coma; drugs of abuse can be associated with seizures.

EPILEPTIC SYNDROMES

Juvenile Myoclonic Epilepsy

Juvenile myoclonic epilepsy has onset in adolescence, at between 12 and 18 years of age. The hallmark of the disorder is early-morning myoclonus involving axial and upper limb muscles, usually with sparing of facial muscles. Episodes typically occur on awakening. Tonic-clonic seizures occur in the majority of patients and are the reason for seeking medical attention. The history of early-morning myoclonic jerks may not be volunteered and should be asked of all patients presenting with generalized tonic-clonic seizures. The patients may not have identified the myoclonus and instead describe nervousness, shakiness, or clumsiness for the first 1 to 2 hours of a morning. Fatigue, sleep deprivation, physical and mental stress, and alcohol exacerbate the seizures. The tonic-clonic seizures typically begin with a clustering of repeated myoclonic jerks. Absence seizures occur in 15% to 40% of patients. Neuro-

logic examination and IQ are normal. The interictal EEG shows spike and wave complexes at 3.5 to 6 Hz.

The AED is valproate. The seizures are well controlled in 80% to 90% of patients, but lifelong treatment is required, as relapse is common even after prolonged seizure-free intervals. It is estimated that more than 90% of patients relapse following cessation of AEDs within the first 6 to 12 months.

Linkage analysis of patients with this syndrome and of their family members has suggested that the disorder is linked to chromosome 21.

Juvenile Absence Epilepsy

Compared with childhood absence epilepsy, juvenile absence epilepsy has a later onset, at about the time of puberty, and the seizures are less frequent (less than daily). Neurologic examination and IQ are normal. The EEG shows generalized spike and wave discharges, usually at rates faster than 3 Hz. Tonic-clonic seizures may occur, usually on awakening, more frequently than in childhood absence epilepsy.

The treatment is the same as that for childhood absence epilepsy, but the prognosis for complete remission on therapy is less favorable than in childhood.

Epilepsy with Generalized Tonic-Clonic Seizures on Awakening

This idiopathic generalized epilepsy involves generalized tonic-clonic seizures occurring exclusively or more than 90% of the time within 2 hours of awakening or in an early-evening period of relaxation. Sleep deprivation and disruption are often potent precipitants of seizures. The age at onset of the seizures is usually between 10 and 20 years; a family history of epilepsy occurs in approximately 10% to 13% of cases. Myoclonic and absence seizures may also be present, and the distinction between juvenile myoclonic epilepsy and juvenile absence epilepsy is not clear. EEG may show generalized spike and wave complexes or polyspikes.

The AED is valproate, although barbiturates may be very effective. Prognosis for complete control of seizures on therapy is very good: 65% to 79% of patients have remitted with therapy. Avoidance of precipitating factors that disrupt sleep patterns (shift work, alcohol) is important. The relapse rate if AEDs are stopped is high (83%).

DIAGNOSTIC EVALUATION OF A SEIZURE DISORDER

EEG Studies

Following a detailed history and physical examination, the EEG is the next step in the evaluation of the child. An EEG also contributes to the specific diagnosis of patients with epilepsy syndromes. The incidence of EEG epileptiform activity in normal children without a history of seizures is very low (<2%); many positive records show benign focal epileptiform discharges of childhood. The incidence of epileptic seizures in patients with focal spikes is 83%, while for generalized spikes it is probably much lower. In a child with suspected seizures, the finding of focal or generalized epileptiform activity on the EEG supports a diagnosis of epilepsy, while repeatedly negative EEG studies argue against such a diagnosis and should prompt the physician to consider alternative diagnoses and to attempt to record the episodes.

An EEG should include at least 20 to 30 minutes of recording. The recording should include hyperventilation (3 to 5 minutes), photic stimulation, and sleep, all of which potentially activate epileptiform discharges, increasing the diagnostic yield. Hyperventilation produces absence seizures in about 80% of children with childhood absence epilepsy. Intermittent photic stimulation produces generalized epileptic discharges in a number of the generalized epileptic syndromes, including juvenile myoclonic epilepsy, childhood absence epilepsy, symptomatic generalized epilepsy, and juvenile absence epilepsy. Sleep and sleep deprivation also increase the yield of EEG records with interictal epileptiform activity. Awake and asleep recording performed after sleep deprivation probably has the highest yield. Recording of the EEG during light NREM sleep can easily be achieved by administration of sedative agents such as chloral hydrate. If benign focal epilepsy of childhood is suspected, a period of recording in sleep is essential; a negative EEG study performed in wakefulness and sleep argues against the diagnosis. In juvenile myoclonic epilepsy, discharges may appear only in the mornings on awakening in some individuals. It is often impractical to monitor overnight, but it may be possible to use ambulatory EEG monitoring if diurnal EEG with sleep and awakening has been unhelpful and the diagnosis is still in question.

Repeated outpatient EEGs after earlier negative studies may provide positive studies by increasing the total sampling time. In those not responding to treatment, repeated studies may reveal previously unrecorded focal or generalized discharges that would support a modification of AED therapy. Overnight recording in the hospital, if available, provides for prolonged sampling of the interictal EEG in wakefulness and spontaneous sleep. For any patient with refractory seizures or an uncertain diagnosis, the use of video and EEG monitoring is usually helpful in clarifying the diagnosis. Defining the exact seizure type or types may lead to modification of drug treatment or consideration of epilepsy surgery, or a nonepileptic paroxysmal disorder may be discovered.

Neuroimaging Studies

For evaluation of epilepsy, MRI is superior to CT. Any patient with focal epilepsy should have an MRI scan of the brain unless the syndrome is clearly that of benign focal epilepsy of childhood with centrotemporal spikes. MRI should also be performed in the other benign focal epilepsies of childhood, as these syndromes are less clearly defined and may be mimicked by structural lesions.

Structural neuroimaging is becoming increasingly important in the assessment of candidates for surgical resection to control intractable seizures.

Evaluation of the First Seizure

There is no clinical sign or diagnostic investigation that determines with certainty if a child presenting with a first seizure has epilepsy or has had an isolated seizure. The assessment of patients with a first seizure must include a search for etiologic agents and features that may predict the risk of recurrence of seizures. Factors to be considered include the circumstances of the seizure, the health of the child in the days or hours before the seizure, the recent sleep patterns, and the chance of inadvertent or willful ingestion of prescription or street drugs.

A number of prospective studies have addressed the recurrence risk following a first unprovoked seizure, usually defined as a seizure or flurry of seizures within 24 hours in patients older than 1 month with no history of a previous unprovoked seizure. The rate of recurrence from studies that combine adults and children is between 27% and 62%; the variability is related to the time of assessment in each study and the rigor with which patients with a previous unprovoked seizure were excluded. In a pediatric population, the recurrence rate is probably 40% to 50%.

The most important predictor of recurrence appears to be the existence of an underlying neurologic disorder or deficit or a history of a neurologic insult. The existence of mental retardation or cerebral palsy is a common antecedent to epilepsy, as is a history of significant head injury. An EEG with generalized or focal epileptiform discharges or with focal or generalized slowing also predicts recurrence. Partial seizures are more likely to be associated with recurrence, although patients with such seizures are also more likely to have an existing neurologic deficit or an abnormal EEG with epileptiform discharges. The duration of the first seizure or a presentation in status epilepticus does not seem to be associated with a higher incidence of recurrence. A family history of epilepsy, somewhat surprisingly, is not a predictor of recurrence. Earlier age of onset, in particular before the age of 12 months, has been associated with a higher risk of recurrent seizures.

Treatment with AEDs lowers the recurrence rate by about 50%. However, most believe that the majority of patients with a first seizure should not be treated. In adults or adolescents, the issues of driving and employment are paramount and may influence the decision to treat or not to treat a first seizure. In children, there is almost no indication for chronic AED treatment in response to a single seizure, and the implications of a second seizure are less pronounced. If there is a second seizure, the risk of further seizures increases significantly. The decision to begin AED therapy is usually made after a patient has had two or more seizures in a short interval of time (6 to 12 months).

ANTIEPILEPTIC DRUGS

The goal of AED therapy is to use a single AED in adequate dosages to completely control seizures. If seizures recur, the dose of an AED should be gradually increased to achieve the maximum tolerated dose for the patient without causing symptoms of drug toxicity. Therapeutic ranges are derived from population studies looking at the serum levels of patients controlled on an AED and those experiencing side effects. The therapeutic levels should be used as a guide to determine the initial dose used. They should not be interpreted as the ''normal'' levels; the ''therapeutic'' level is that which controls the individual's seizures without causing symptoms of toxicity.

If one agent does not control the seizures after an adequate trial of therapy, another AED should be substituted and tried as monotherapy. An adequate trial of therapy uses the maximum tolerated dose of an AED for a period of time in which several of the patient's seizures (or clusters of seizures) would usually occur or for at least 2 months, whichever is longer. Changes in AED doses and regimens should be performed gradually, and due regard must be given to time taken to reach steady-state serum concentrations on the new regimen (Tables 40–17 and 40–18).

If the child with epilepsy fails to achieve complete control of seizures on an adequate trial of monotherapy with one of the first-line drugs, an alternative first-line drug should be substituted as monotherapy, followed, if unsuccessful, by a trial of monotherapy with one of the more recent AEDs. Drug changes can be made gradually on an outpatient basis; the existing AED can be reduced by 20%, and the new AED commenced at the usual starting dose (see Table 40–17). Each week, the dose of the new AED can be increased with a corresponding reduction in the previous AED until the new drug is at the desired maintenance dose and the previous AED has been ceased. The physician must warn the parents and child that AED toxicity or an increase in the seizure frequency may occur during the change-over period. The parents should be

Table 40–17. Antiepileptic Drugs

Antiepileptic Drug	Indication	Introduction	Maintenance Dose (mg/kg/day)	Side Effects	Monitoring of Serum Levels
First-Line Drugs					
Carbamazepine	Partial seizures and secondarily GTCS	No loading dose	10–30 as t.i.d.	Drowsiness, vertigo, diplopia, hyponatremia (SIADH), dose–dependent neutropenia, rash 4%–10% Rare: serious blood dyscrasia	Yes
Ethosuximide	Absence seizures Trial use in symptomatic generalized epilepsy with falls	Add 33% of maintenance dose every 7 days	10–40 as t.i.d., with meals	Nausea, gastrointestinal discomfort, headache Rare: aplastic anemia	No
Phenytoin	Partial seizures and secondarily GTCS	Loading p.o.	5–10 as b.i.d.	Ataxia, diplopia, gingival hyperplasia, coarsening of facial features Chronic use: cerebellar atrophy Rare: Stevens-Johnson syndrome	Yes
Valproate	Primary GTCS, myoclonus and absence seizures	No loading dose	15–30 as b.i.d. or t.i.d.	Weight gain, hair loss, tremor at high dose Rare: hepatotoxicity, pancreatitis, encephalopathy	Yes
Second-Line Drugs					
Phenobarbital (PB)	Partial seizures and GTCS	6–8 mg/kg p.o. for 2 days, then maintenance dose	3–4 as q.d. or b.i.d.	Drowsiness, behavioral changes; hyperactivity	Yes
Primidone (PRM)	Partial seizures and secondarily GTCS	Begin with PB, increasing over 3 days, then add PRM	5–20 as b.i.d. or t.i.d.	Acute reaction: nausea, vomiting, vertigo Sedation	Yes
Third-Line Drugs					
Acetazolamide	Absence seizures May use as trial in refractory generalized epilepsy	33% of maintenance dose for 1 wk, then gradual increase over weeks	10–20 as b.i.d. or t.i.d.	Altered taste, paresthesia, initial drowsiness, cross-reactivity with sulfonamide allergy Rare: renal calculi precipitation, hepatic coma in liver failure	No
Clonazepam	Infantile spasms Myoclonus, reflex epilepsy Second-line therapy for absence seizures and partial seizures	0.01–0.03 mg/kg/day for 1 wk, then increase by 0.25–0.5 mg/day each week	0.03–0.1 as b.i.d. or t.i.d.	Sedation, drooling, behavioral change: irritable, aggressive, hostile	No
Clorazepate	Adjunct in partial seizures and secondarily GTCS	0.3 mg/kg/day for 1 wk, then increase by 0.4–3 mg/day each week	1.0–3.0 as b.i.d.	Sedation, ataxia, drooling	No
Drugs for Special Circumstances					
Diazepam	Prophylactic rectal use in febrile convulsions Status epilepticus	0.5–0.7 q8h when fever >38.5°C See Table 40–21		Sedation, ataxia, vertigo IV use; respiratory depression and apnea, hypotension	No
Lorazepam	Status epilepticus	0.03–0.22 mg/kg, IV bolus See Table 40–21		IV use; respiratory depression and apnea, hypotension	No

Table continued on following page

Table 40–17. Antiepileptic Drugs *Continued*

Antiepileptic Drug	Indication	Introduction	Maintenance Dose (mg/kg/day)	Side Effects	Monitoring of Serum Levels
		More Recent Drugs			
Clobazam	Second-line therapy for partial seizures Adjunct in Lennox-Gastaut syndrome	Begin at night with 33% of maintenance dose	0.5–1 as b.i.d.	Sedation	No
Felbamate	Partial seizures Adjunct in symptomatic generalized epilepsy	Add 25% of maintenance dose every 4 days	30–45 as t.i.d.	Headache, insomnia, anorexia, nausea and vomiting Rare: aplastic anemia, hepatitis	No
Gabapentin	Adjunct in refractory partial seizures	Add 25% of maintenance dose every 2 days	15–45 as t.i.d. or q.i.d.	Drowsiness, fatigue, ataxia, nonspecific dizziness	Uncertain
Lamotrigine	Adjunct in refractory partial seizures and Lennox-Gastaut syndrome	Begin 25 mg q.d., second weekly increases; 25 mg b.i.d., 50 mg b.i.d., 100 mg b.i.d. If on valproate, begin 25 mg q.o.d.	2.5–15 as t.i.d. or q.i.d.	Marked changes in half-life dependent on concomitant AED use Rash, ataxia, drowsiness, diplopia	May be useful with polytherapy
Nitrazepam	Infantile spasms Myoclonic seizures, reflex epilepsy Adjunct in symptomatic generalized epilepsy	Add 25% of maintenance dose every week	0.25–1 as b.i.d.	Sedation, impaired swallowing, drooling, ataxia	No
Oxcarbazepine	Partial seizures	Add 25% of maintenance dose every week	10–30 as b.i.d. or t.i.d.	Rash less common than with carbamazepine, hyponatremia	Yes
Vigabatrin	Partial seizures Tuberous sclerosis and West or Lennox-Gastaut syndrome	Begin 500 mg q.h.s.: increase by 500 mg/day each week	10–50 as b.i.d. or q.i.d.	Drowsiness, fatigue, gastrointestinal upset, weight gain Depression and psychosis reported in adults	No

Abbreviations: GTCS = generalized tonic-clonic seizures; t.i.d. = three times a day; SIADH = syndrome of inappropriate antidiuretic hormone secretion; p.o. = orally; b.i.d. = twice a day; IV = intravenous ; q.i.d. = four times a day; q.h.s. = every bedtime; q.d. = every day; q.o.d. = every other day.

given a written dose schedule to follow and easy access to medical advice. More rapid medication changes, especially if barbiturates are to be ceased, often require that the patient be admitted to the hospital for observation during the change-over period.

Only about 10% of patients achieve better control with the addition of a second drug to the first, and there is very little evidence that more than two drugs benefit patients. However, there are some exceptions, and in rare instances patients with specific syndromes may benefit from the use of multiple AEDs. Carbamazepine and phenytoin have often been given in combination to patients with poorly controlled epilepsy. This combination can be very effective in some patients. However, it is usually very difficult to achieve adequate serum levels of both drugs because of their hepatic enzyme–inducing properties, and any adverse effects may be additive. As a general rule, the combination is best avoided. The process of monotherapy trials should be efficient, with close follow-up of patients experiencing persistent seizures and regard to the factors listed in Table 40–19 as possible causes of refractory seizures. Failure to respond to two to three AEDs in monotherapy at maximum tolerated doses should prompt a referral for assessment in a specialty epilepsy program with consideration of epilepsy surgery.

It is important to design dose schedules that are realistic. Dosing more often than three times a day results in a high incidence of poor compliance. Parents must be advised to be careful with other prescribed and over-the-counter medications; upper respiratory tract infection remedies containing antihistamines may cause excessive drowsiness in children taking an AED. Many medications may interfere with the AED metabolism; the antibiotic erythromycin may precipitate drug toxicity by decreasing carbamazepine clearance. Table 40–20 sets out the usual indications for monitoring AED serum levels.

Choice of Antiepileptic Drugs

FOCAL EPILEPSIES

Partial Seizures and Secondary Generalized Tonic-Clonic Seizures

Phenytoin (PHT), carbamazepine (CBZ), phenobarbital (PB), and primidone (PRM) are equally effective in controlling partial and secondary generalized tonic-clonic seizures in adults. In the symptomatic focal epilepsies, only approximately 35% to 50% of patients become seizure-free with AED monotherapy, with another 20% to 30% experiencing a greater than 75% reduction in seizure frequency. First-line treatment in this group of seizures has been

Table 40–18. Antiepileptic Drugs, Pharmacokinetic Parameters in Children

Antiepileptic Drug	Half-life (hr)	Therapeutic Range (mg/L)*	Molecular Weight
First-Line Drugs			
Carbamazepine	5–20†	8–12	236.26
Ethosuximide	30–60‡	40–100	141.17
Phenytoin	10–60	10–20	252.26
Valproate	5–15	50–100	144.21
Second-Line Drugs			
Phenobarbital	35–125	15–45	232.23
Primidone	3–20	6–12	218.25
Third-Line Drugs			
Acetazolamide	10–15§	10–14	222
Clonazepam	20–30	20–75	315.5
Clorazepate‖	55–100	NA	408.9
Drugs for Special Circumstances			
Diazepam	6–23	0.3–0.7	284.8
Lorazepam	8–25	NA	321.2
More Recent Drugs			
Clobazam#	10–30	NA**	300.5
Felbamate	14–20	20–80	238.24
Gabapentin	5–9	2.0–3.0	171.24
Lamotrigine	12–48††	2.0–4.0	256.09
Nitrazepam	20–30	0.1–0.2	281.3
Oxcarbazepine‡‡	10–15	8–20	252.28
Vigabatrin§§	5–8	NA**	129.16

*To convert to μmol/L: (1000/mol. wt.) × concentration (mg/L) = concentration (μmol/L).

†Carbamazepine causes autoinduction of hepatic metabolism over first 2 to 6 weeks of therapy, clearance increases, half-life shortens, and serum level can be expected to drop despite compliance with original dose.

‡Ethosuximide half-life is shorter in infants and younger children.

§Acetazolamide is bound to carbonic anhydrase; this complex dissociates very slowly, so the biologic half-life is several days.

‖Clorazepate acts as a pro-drug and is converted to *N*-desmethyldiazepam, the active form of clorazepate; the figures for protein binding, volume of distribution, and half-life are for *N*-desmethyldiazepam. There is no established target level for monitoring.

#*N*-Desmethylclobazam is the major active metabolite, and its much longer half-life (mean 42 hours, range 30 to 100 hours) must be considered.

**There is no established target level for monitoring.

††Used as monotherapy, lamotrigine has a half-life of about 24 hours; with phenobarbital, phenytoin, or carbamazepine (hepatic enzyme inducers), it is reduced to 12 hours; and with valproate (hepatic enzyme inhibition), it is increased to 48 hours.

‡‡Oxcarbazepine (10,11-dihydro-10-oxycarbamazepine) has a half-life of 1 to 2.5 hours. It is converted to an active metabolite, 10,11-dihydro-10-hydroxycarbamazepine; the figures for protein binding, half-life, and serum levels are for the 10-hydroxy compound.

§§The biologic half-life is approximately 5 days as a result of the irreversible inhibition of GABA transaminase by vigabatrin.

with CBZ or PHT. While the barbiturates and also the benzodiazepines have been shown to be effective, the sedative and cognitive side effects prevent them from being drugs of first choice, and they are generally reserved for patients in whom first-line drugs are not effective or tolerated. Valproate (VPA) is also effective against partial seizures in children, although large comparative studies are not available. Other, more recent drugs, including lamotrigine, vigabatrin, and gabapentin (see Table 40–17), have also been shown to have efficacy for the treatment of refractory partial seizures, but their place in the order of management is not yet defined.

IDIOPATHIC GENERALIZED EPILEPSY

Primary Generalized Tonic-Clonic Seizures

It is widely thought that VPA should be the drug of first choice for primary generalized tonic-clonic seizures, especially if they occur in association with absence seizures or myoclonic seizures. PHT, CBZ, and valproate are equally effective in controlling primary generalized tonic-clonic seizures in adults, and between 60% and 70% of patients can become seizure-free. Phenytoin does not control any associated absence seizures, and CBZ may exacerbate absence seizures, although the latter is more likely to occur with atypical absences in the symptomatic generalized epilepsies. PB and PRM are not the drugs of first choice because of potential adverse effects.

Absence Seizures

Ethosuximide and VPA are the two drugs of first choice for these seizures. Monotherapy with valproate controls absence seizures in more than 90% of children with childhood absence epilepsy. Ethosuximide and valproate have been successfully combined in patients with refractory absence seizures. Clonazepam is also effective but has the disadvantages of sedation and development of tolerance with chronic treatment.

Table 40–19. Management of Seizures Refractory to Medical Therapy

Incorrect Diagnosis?

Review seizure type
   Complex partial seizures mistaken for absence seizures, reflex epilepsy with uncontrolled precipitating factors, photosensitivity, reading epilepsy
Repeat EEG with hyperventilation, photic stimulation, and sleep recording
If negative, consider nonepileptic paroxysmal disorders
Continuing seizures: admit for video/EEG monitoring to record the event (may need to withdraw antiepileptic drug [AED])

Inappropriate Medication?

Review anticonvulsant levels
   A second AED may have caused a drop in the serum level of a first-line drug
Review seizure type
   Phenobarbital and carbamazepine may exacerbate atypical absences
   Drowsiness caused by phenobarbital and benzodiazepine may exacerbate tonic seizures in symptomatic generalized epilepsy
   Phenytoin often worsens the function of patients with progressive myoclonus epilepsy syndromes

Noncompliance with Medication or Medical Advice?

Check AED levels, ask patient to record medication doses taken
   Noncompliance with AED therapy
Check sleep habits, drug use, arrange review by social worker, psychiatrist
   Inability to cope with epilepsy and avoidance of precipitating factors; adolescent, low intelligence, dysfunctional home situation
Review all prescribed and over-the-counter medications, urine drug screen for drug abuse
   Exacerbation by other medications or toxins

Intercurrent Illness or Metabolic Complication of Another Medication?

Obtain serum Na^+, K^+, glucose, Ca^{++}, Mg^{++}, and creatinine levels, liver function studies, complete blood count, pregnancy test

Intractable Epilepsies

1. Up to one third of symptomatic focal epilepsy is refractory to current medical therapy.
   After adequate trial of two first-line medications and available new AEDs, refer for epilepsy surgery program assessment
2. Symptomatic generalized epilepsies such as West syndrome and Lennox-Gastaut syndrome are often refractory.
   Need to reassess goals of therapy
   Refer for surgical assessment if recurrent falls due to tonic or atonic seizures in older child
3. Epilepsy with progressive neurologic deterioration—e.g., brain tumor, inherited disorders of metabolism, degenerative neurologic disease, progressive myoclonus epilepsy, phakomatosis, systemic or cerebral vasculitis.
   Review history, family history, and physical examination, repeat neuroimaging studies, repeat EEG studies, see Tables 40–7 and 40–13

Myoclonic Seizures

Specific myoclonic syndromes associated with absence seizures and tonic-clonic seizures, such as juvenile myoclonic epilepsy, are usually treated with valproate, with a very good response against seizures. Approximately 80% of patients with this epilepsy can become seizure-free, although lifelong treatment is required with juvenile myoclonic epilepsy. Clonazepam is also useful in myoclonic syndromes, although sedation occurs and it does not tend to be useful in the long term because of tolerance; there are even some reports of exacerbation of seizures with long-term high-dose clonazepam. Exacerbation of seizures is particularly frequent with this drug when abrupt withdrawal is attempted. Clonazepam must be withdrawn very gradually, and the daily dose is reduced by only 0.25 mg every 3 weeks.

SYMPTOMATIC GENERALIZED EPILEPSIES

Tonic, Atonic, and Atypical Absence Seizures

These seizures may be found in combination with mental retardation in patients with the Lennox-Gastaut syndrome. These patients are often refractory to conventional AED therapy. Drugs useful in the treatment of these seizures include valproate and benzodiazepines such as clonazepam and clobazam. Valproate monotherapy should be introduced first, although complete control of seizures is likely to occur in only 10% to 30% of patients. The maximum tolerated dose should be tried for at least 1 to 2 months before trying another monotherapy. CBZ and PHT are often not effective, and CBZ may exacerbate absence seizures in the Lennox-Gastaut syndrome. PRM and PB often have unacceptable side effects of drowsiness or worsening intellectual handicap at the doses needed to control seizures; sedation may increase the frequency of tonic seizures.

Because of the refractory nature of these seizures, patients often end up on a combination of drugs, and AED toxicity can be a great problem, exacerbating a patient's tendency to fall and injure himself or herself. A benzodiazepine, such as clonazepam or clobazam, in combination with valproate is often chosen in this setting. Felbamate has been shown to be a useful drug as adjunctive treatment of tonic and atonic seizures in the Lennox-Gastaut syndrome but the risk of serious toxicity limits its use.

Status Epilepticus

Convulsive status epilepticus is a medical emergency and requires prompt management to control the seizures and investigations to identify precipitating factors. Studies of adults and children presenting with status epilepticus show that 33% have no history of epilepsy and are presenting for the first time in status, another third have a history of chronic epilepsy, and in another third an acute systemic or neurologic illness or insult has caused status epilepticus. Status epilepticus is more likely to develop in patients with symptomatic localization-related and generalized epilepsies than in those with idiopathic epilepsy; however, one of the most common precipitants of status epilepticus, cessation or disruption of a regular AED, affects both groups. Other important causes of status epilepticus include systemic febrile illnesses, intracranial infections, poisoning, acute metabolic disorders, and head injury.

Table 40–20. Indications for Antiepileptic Drug Serum Level Monitoring

Introduction and stabilization of a new medication
Alteration in seizure pattern or frequency
Change in the dosage of an anticonvulsant
To establish the lowest effective dose
Commencement or withdrawal of other medications that interfere with anticonvulsants
Symptoms of toxicity
To check patient compliance

The goals of the emergency management of status epilepticus are:

1. Maintain normal cardiorespiratory function and cerebral oxygenation.
2. Stop clinical and electrical seizure activity and prevent its recurrence.
3. Identify precipitating factors.
4. Correct any metabolic disturbances and prevent systemic complications such as cardiovascular collapse, cardiac arrhythmia, pneumonia, and renal failure.
5. Further evaluate patients and treat the etiology of the status epilepticus.

Table 40–21 sets out a plan of initial assessment and management of convulsive status epilepticus. The benzodiazepines, lorazepam and diazepam, offer a rapid anticonvulsant action when given intravenously but must be combined with a primary AED. The benzodiazepines are sedating, will depress respiration and the patient's ability to protect his or her airway, and may cause hypotension. Either PHT or PB could be used in conjunction with the benzodiazepines, but PHT is less sedating than PB. If the status epilepticus consists of frequent, repeated generalized seizures with return of consciousness between episodes, immediate attention to PHT or PB loading is more appropriate than bolus doses of benzodiazepines because the latter alters the level of consciousness and complicates the assessment. Paraldehyde (2:1 paraldehyde:vegeta-ble oil, 0.3 ml/kg per dose, repeat doses every 2 to 4 hours) and lidocaine (bolus of 2 to 3 mg/kg, then infusion of 4 to 10 mg/kg/hour, monitor levels) have been used to treat status epilepticus in the past and may find a role in special circumstances today (multiple drug allergy). Valproate can be given rectally as Depakene and may be the appropriate therapy for patients with known idiopathic and symptomatic generalized epilepsies when stable or instead of PHT or PB.

Nonconvulsive status epilepticus may arise when frequent complex partial seizures or absence seizures occur. In both of these settings, discrete seizures may not be identifiable; instead, the child may present with confusion, clouded consciousness, and partial responsiveness or a stuporous state, lasting hours or even days. This clinical picture is more typical of absence status. In complex partial status, probably a less common phenomenon, it is more likely that obvious fluctuations in the level of responsiveness with automatisms occur, suggesting repeated seizures and intervening postictal confusion. This form of status epilepticus is not a medical emergency, cardiorespiratory function is not endangered, and, in practice, treatment is sometimes delayed until a suspected diagnosis is confirmed by EEG recording. However, delay in therapy is not advisable, especially if complex partial status is suspected, in which case treatment should follow that outlined for convulsive status epilepticus.

In absence status, intravenous benzodiazepines are usually effective but should be used in conjunction with oral or rectal VPA, ethosuximide, or clonazepam.

Table 40–21. Management of Convulsive Status Epilepticus

Priority	Examination and Laboratory Investigations	Management
On arrival	Airway patency and respiratory rate, inspect pharynx, chest auscultation BP, pulse, temperature Level of consciousness: response to command, pain Serum Na, K, glucose, creatinine, Ca, and Mg levels, CBC, liver function studies, AED levels Serum and urine toxin screen Arterial blood gases, CXR	Airway protection; suction pharynx, NPO, give supplemental oxygen Rectal antipyretic to lower temperature if >38°C, acetaminophen (10–15 mg/kg) IV access and administer: 25% glucose IV (2–4 ml/kg) *and** lorazepam IV (0.1 mg/kg as bolus) *and* phenytoin (PHT) IV (20 mg/kg at <3 mg/kg/min), with EKG monitor and collection of serum level after loading dose If immediate IV access is not possible, give diazepam (0.3–0.5 mg/kg) rectally and arrange for central line or intraosseous access
After initial treatment	Neck stiffness, fundoscopy, signs of trauma, skin rashes, symmetry of motor function and reflexes	If febrile, urine and blood cultures, viral titers If any suspicion of head injury, obtain urgent CT scan
If seizures continue	Patient's level of consciousness will become depressed with lorazepam and phenobarbital (PB), and an EEG will be required to assess adequacy of therapy	Arrange ICU bed and consider intubation, give further bolus of lorazepam (0.5 mg/kg) and push PHT serum level above 30 mg/L with further loading dose In ICU setting, if seizures continue with PHT levels 30–40 mg/L, add PB (20 mg/kg IV loading over 15–30 min) Continued clinical or electrical seizures may require induction of pentobarbital therapy: elective intubation and ventilation, arterial-line BP monitoring, loading dose of 6 mg/kg followed by IV infusion of 2–5 mg/kg/hr titrated by EEG monitoring to achieve burst-suppression pattern, maintain for 24–48 hr and review
After stabilization or in tandem with escalating therapy	Lumbar puncture (LP); if acute febrile illness without papilledema, focal neurologic signs, do not wait for CT/MRI scan	If LP is delayed and intracranial infection suspected, cover with antibiotic and antiviral therapy

*Give lorazepam if actively convulsing; this may not be required in patients with serial seizures, who can be quickly loaded with phenytoin.
Abbreviations: BP = blood pressure; Na = sodium; K = potassium; Mg = magnesium; CBC = complete blood count; AED = antiepileptic drug; CXR = chest x-ray; NPO = nothing by mouth; IV = intravenous; CT = computed tomography; ICU = intensive care unit; MRI = magnetic resonance imaging.

Stopping Antiepileptic Drugs

Most children (60% to 75% of patients) remain seizure-free following the withdrawal of AEDs after a seizure-free interval on medication for more than 2 years. If relapse occurs, it is generally in the first few months after ceasing medication, and 60% to 80% of the relapses occur before 12 months. Those patients with underlying neurologic disorders and deficits are more likely to relapse. Patients with multiple seizure types also have a higher rate of relapse. A long duration of epilepsy before remission carries a slightly higher risk of relapse. The EEG is a strong predictor in idiopathic epilepsy; if frequent epileptic discharges are recorded in generalized epilepsy, the rate of relapse is higher. The EEG recorded at the time of medication withdrawal is less useful as a predictor of relapse in focal epilepsy.

Most recommend that children who have been seizure-free for 2 years undergo a trial of AED withdrawal; however, in benign partial epilepsy of childhood, consideration must be given to the age-dependent nature of seizure expression. Juvenile myoclonic epilepsy also deserves special consideration because even following a prolonged seizure-free period on medication, the frequency of relapse is very high, and AED therapy must be continued throughout life in order to remain seizure-free.

LIFESTYLE

Parents should be encouraged to let their children lead a normal lifestyle, although some activities are inherently more dangerous for people with epilepsy than for those without. Generally, climbing to significant heights and bathing or swimming alone are not safe for children with active epilepsy. Parents should be instructed to keep a seizure diary for their children and bring it to each clinic visit. In following children with epilepsy and their families, one must stress the importance of avoiding overprotection of the child. Participation in sports and other school activities should be encouraged within the limits of avoiding dangerous activities such as rock climbing and scuba diving, in which even a brief loss of awareness could result in serious injury or death. If seizures are well controlled, minimal restrictions apply: the child should be advised against climbing and against bathing and swimming alone (one should encourage children and parents to continue swimming but always with a supervisor who could assist them). In children with active seizures characterized by loss of consciousness, the physician has to make judgments based on an individual assessment considering the nature of the seizures, their frequency, and the degree of supervision during the activity in question. Driving restrictions vary from state to state; however, it is advisable that a teenager be seizure-free for at least 2 years before applying for a driver's permit. Generally, heavy-impact contact sports such as football are best avoided in children with active epilepsy but are not contraindicated in children in remission.

Parents are best advised about basic first aid for seizure patients. First aid for generalized tonic-clonic seizures involves assisting the child to a supine position lying semiprone (head to side), with any hyperextension or flexion of the neck corrected. The airway is adequately maintained if the patient is semiprone and the head turned toward the ground. No attempt should ever be made to place any object in the patient's mouth during a tonic-clonic seizure: the risk of swallowing or biting the tongue does not exist, while the risk of breaking teeth or causing soft tissue trauma is very high.

In older adolescents, some advice regarding birth control may be necessary, and it is important that the matter be raised as a routine issue rather than provided on request, as many adolescents will be unaware of the interaction of AEDs and oral contraceptives or shy about broaching the subject.

RED FLAGS

Red flags include signs of raised intracranial pressure, focality, and signs suggestive of syndromes. In addition, a positive family history, neurodevelopmental delay, trauma, exposure to drugs, and multiple organ system dysfunction should also be considered as red flags.

REFERENCES

General

Commission on Classification and Terminology of the International League Against Epilepsy. Proposal for revised clinical and electroencephalographic classification of epileptic seizures. Epilepsia 1981;22:489–501.

Commission on Classification and Terminology of the International League Against Epilepsy. Proposal for revised classification of epilepsies and epileptic syndromes. Epilepsia 1989;30:389–399.

Dodson W, Pellock J. Pediatric Epilepsy: Diagnosis and Therapy. New York: Demos, 1993:57–61.

Wyllie E. The Treatment of Epilepsy: Principles and Practice. Philadelphia: Lea & Febiger, 1993.

Neonatal Period

Parker S, Zuckerman B, Bauchner H, et al. Jitteriness in full-term neonates: Prevalence and correlates. Pediatrics 1990;85:17–23.

Resnick T, Moshe S, Perotta L, Chambers H. Benign neonatal sleep myoclonus: Relationship to sleep states. Arch Neurol 1986;43:266–268.

Shuper A, Zalzberg J, Weitz R, et al. Jitteriness beyond the neonatal period: A benign pattern of movement in infancy. J Child Neurol 1991;6:243–245.

Acute Symptomatic Seizures and Occasional Seizures

Mizrahi E, Kellaway P. Characterization and classification of neonatal seizures. Neurology 1987;37:1837–1844.

Painter M. Therapy of neonatal seizures. Cleve Clin J Med 1989;56:S124–131.

Volpe J. Neonatal seizures: Current concepts and revised classification. Pediatrics 1989;84:422–428.

Epileptic Syndromes

Miles D, Holmes G. Benign neonatal seizures. J Clin Neurophysiol 1990;7:369–379.

Plouin P. Benign idiopathic neonatal convulsions (familial and non-familial). *In* Roger J, Bureau M, Dravet C, et al (eds). Epileptic Syndromes in Infancy, Childhood and Adolescence. London: John Libbey, 1992:3–11.

Early-Onset Generalized Epileptic Syndromes with Encephalopathy

Aicardi J, Levy Gomes A. The myoclonic epilepsies of childhood. Cleve Clin J Med 1989;56:S34–39.

Lombroso C. Early myoclonic encephalopathy, early infantile epileptic encephalopathy, and benign and severe infantile myoclonic epilepsies: A critical review and personal contributions. J Clin Neurophysiol 1990;7:380–408.

Infancy

Pallid Infant Syncope

Lombroso C, Lerman P. Breath-holding spells (cyanotic and pallid infantile syncope). Pediatrics 1967;39:563–581.

McWilliam R, Stephenson J. Atropine treatment of reflex anoxic seizures. Arch Dis Child 1984;59:473–485.

Stephenson J. Reflex anoxic seizures (''white breath-holding''): Nonepileptic vagal attacks. Arch Dis Child 1978;53:193–200.

Sleep Disorders

Sallustro C, Atwell F. Body rocking, head banging, and head rolling in normal children. J Pediatr 1978;93:704–708.

Shivering Attacks

Holmes G, Russman B. Shuddering attacks. Am J Dis Child 1986;140:72–73.

Vanasse M, Bedard P, Andermann F. Shuddering attacks in children: An early manifestation of essential tremor. Neurology 1976;26:1027–1030.

Paroxysmal Torticollis

Gilbert G. Familial spasmodic torticollis. Neurology 1977;27:11–13.

Synder C. Paroxysmal torticollis in infancy. Am J Dis Child 1969;117:458–460.

Masturbation

Fleisher D, Morrison A. Masturbation mimicking abdominal pain or seizures in young girls. J Pediatr 1990;116:810–814.

Spasmus Nutans

King R, Nelson L, Wagner R. Spasmus nutans. Arch Ophthalmol 1986;104:32–35.

Benign Paroxysmal Vertigo

Basser L. Benign paroxysmal vertigo of childhood. Brain 1964;87:141–152.

Benign Myoclonus of Early Infancy

Lombroso C, Fejerman N. Benign myoclonus of early infancy. Ann Neurol 1977;1:138–143.

Alternating Hemiplegia of Childhood

Aminian A, Strashun A, Rose A. Alternating hemiplegia of childhood: Studies of regional cerebral blood flow using 99Tc-Hexamethylproylene amine oxime single-photon emission computed tomography. Ann Neurol 1993;33:43–47.

Acute Symptomatic Seizures and Occasional Seizures

Annegers J, Hauser W, Shirts S, et al. Factors prognostic of unprovoked seizures after febrile convulsions. N Engl J Med 1987;316:493–498.

National Institutes of Health. Febrile seizures: Long-term management of children with fever associated seizures. Pediatrics 1980;66:1009–1012.

Nelson K, Ellenberg J. Prognosis in children with febrile seizures. Pediatrics 1978;61:720–727.

Verity C, Butler N, Golding J. Febrile convulsions in a national cohort followed up from birth. I. Prevalence and recurrence in the first five years of life. Br Med J 1985;290:1307–1310.

Verity C, Butler N, Golding J. Febrile convulsions in a national cohort followed up from birth. II. Medical history and intellectual ability at 5 years of age. Br Med J 1985;290:1311–1315.

Epileptic Syndromes

Dravet C, Bureau M, Genton P. Benign myoclonic epilepsy of infancy: Electroclinical symptomatology and differential diagnosis from the other types of generalized epilepsy of infancy. Epilepsy Res Suppl 1992;6:131–135.

Hrachovy R, Frost J. Severe encephalopathic epilepsy in infants: Infantile spasms. *In* Dodson W, Pellock J (eds). Pediatric Epilepsy: Diagnosis and Therapy. New York: Demos, 1991:135–145.

Severe Myoclonic Epilepsy in Infancy

Dravet C, Bureau M, Roger J. Severe myoclonic epilepsy in infants. *In* Dravet C, Bureau M, Dreifuss FE, et al (eds). Epileptic Syndromes in Infancy, Childhood and Adolescence. London: John Libbey, 1985:58–67.

Childhood

Paroxysmal Nonepileptic Disorders

Rothner A. The migraine syndromes in children and adolescents. Pediatr Neurol 1986;2:121–126.

Tic Disorders

Erenberg G, Rothner A. Tourette syndrome: Diagnosis and management. Int Pediatr 1987;2:149–153.

Sleep Disorders

Mahowald M, Ettinger M. Things that go bump in the night: The parasomnias revisited. J Clin Neurophysiol 1990;7:119–143.

Hyperekplexia

Aguglia U, Tinuper P, Gastaut H. Startle-induced epileptic seizures. Epilepsia 1984;25:712–720.

Ryan S, Sherman S, Terry J, et al. Startle disease, or hyperekplexia: Response to clonazepam and assignment of the gene (STHE) to chromosome 5q by linkage analysis. Ann Neurol 1992;31:663–668.

Self-Stimulatory Behavior

Donat J, Wright F. Episodic symptoms mistaken for seizures in the neurologically impaired child. Neurology 1990;40:156–157.

Epileptic Syndromes

Holmes G. Benign focal epilepsies of childhood. Epilepsia 1993;34:S49–61.

Lerman P, Kivity S. The benign partial nonrolandic epilepsies. J Clin Neurophysiol 1991;8:275–287.

Symptomatic Focal (Localization-Related) Epilepsy

Duchowny M. Complex partial seizures of infancy. Arch Neurol 1987;44:911.

Wyllie E, Rothner A, Luders H. Partial seizures in children: Clinical features, medical treatment, and surgical considerations. Pediatr Clin North Am 1989;36:343–364.

Childhood Absence Epilepsy

Holmes G, McKeever M, Adamson M. Absence seizures in children: Clinical and electrographic features. Ann Neurol 1987;21:323–352.
Penry J, Porter R, Dreifuss F. Simultaneous recording of absence seizures with videotape and electroencephalography. A study of 374 seizures in 48 patients. Brain 1975;98:427–440.
Porter R. The absence epilepsies. Epilepsia 1993;34:S42–48.

Epilepsia Partialis Continua and Rasmussen Encephalitis

Bancaud J. Kojewnikow's syndrome (epilepsia partialis continua) in children. *In* Roger J, Bureau M, Dravet C, et al (eds). Epileptic Syndromes in Infancy, Childhood and Adolescence. London: John Libbey, 1992:363–379.
Rasmussen T, Andermann F. Rasmussen's syndrome: Symptomatology of the syndrome of chronic encephalitis and seizures: 35-year experience with 51 cases. *In* Lüders HO (ed). Epilepsy Surgery. New York: Raven Press, 1991:173–182.

Lennox-Gastaut Syndrome

Beaumanoir A. The Lennox-Gastaut syndrome. *In* Dravet C, Bureau M, Dreifuss FE, et al (eds). Epileptic Syndromes in Infancy, Childhood and Adolescence. London: John Libbey, 1985:89–99.

Myoclonic Astatic Epilepsy

Henriksen O. Discussion of myoclonic epilepsies and Lennox-Gastaut syndrome. *In* Dravet C, Bureau M, Dreifuss FE, et al (eds): Epileptic Syndromes in Infancy, Childhood and Adolescence. London: John Libbey, 1985:100–104.

Adolescence

Jeavons P. Non-epileptic attacks in childhood. *In* Rose FC (ed). Research Progress in Epilepsy. London: Pitman, 1983:224–230.
Wyllie E, Friedman D, Lüders H, et al. Outcome of psychogenic seizures in children and adolescents compared with adults. Neurology 1991;41:742–744.

Epileptic Syndromes

Janz D. Juvenile myoclonic epilepsy: Epilepsy with impulsive petit mal. Cleve Clin J Med 1989;56:S23–33.
Wolf P, Goosses R. Relation of photosensitivity to epileptic syndromes. J Neurol Neurosurg Psych 1986;49:1386–1391.

Diagnostic Evaluation of a Seizure Disorder

Drury I. Epileptiform patterns in children. J Clin Neurophysiol 1989;6:1–39.
So N. Recurrence, remission, and relapse of seizures. Cleve Clin J Med 1993;60:439–444.

Antiepileptic Drugs

Bourgeois B. Childhood epilepsy: Pharmacological considerations. Acta Neurol Scand Suppl 1992;140:23–27.
Mattson R, Cramer J, Collins J, et al. Comparison of CBZ, phenobarbital, phenytoin and primidone in partial and secondary generalized tonic-clonic seizures. N Engl J Med 1985;313:145–151.
Mattson R, Cramer J, Collins J, et al. Valproate in the treatment of partial and secondary generalized tonic-clonic seizures in adults: A comparison with CBZ. N Engl J Med 1992;327:765–771.
So N. Recurrence, remission, and relapse of seizures. Cleve Clin J Med 1993;60:439–444.

41 Delirium and Coma

James B. Besunder   John F. Pope

Coma, delirium, or any alteration of consciousness can be considered brain failure and necessitates a rapid, methodical approach to evaluation and treatment. The causes of coma are numerous, diverse, and, in some cases, life-threatening.

DEFINITIONS

Consciousness is the state of awareness of self and environment. Coma is lack of any awareness of self or environment, even in the presence of painful or other external stimulation. Many terms have been used to describe the levels of consciousness between full awareness and coma. Table 41–1 presents a practical approach to defining levels of impaired consciousness. *Delirium* is an abnormal mental state characterized by irritability, agitation, lack of contact with the environment, and confusion. Periods of lucidity may alternate with the delirious state, and the patient is often very frightened by this changing mental status. Patients may proceed rapidly from delirium or lethargy to coma. *Any alteration in the level of consciousness, be it defined as delirium, lethargy, obtundation, stupor, or coma, must be managed as a life-threatening emergency until proven otherwise.*

Terms such as *lethargy, obtundation, stupor,* and *coma* are qualitative descriptions that do not precisely define an individual's level of consciousness. Many rating scales have been developed to objectively evaluate the level of awareness in a patient; this allows different observers to follow the progression of the patient's mental status over time. The scales can be used to direct the level of intervention necessary to treat the patient and may provide prognos-

Table 41–1. States of Altered Consciousness or Unresponsiveness

Coma: A state of unarousable unresponsiveness; even strong exteroceptive stimuli fail to elicit recognizable psychological responses. Unresponsive to pain.

Stupor: Spontaneous unarousability interruptable only by vigorous, direct external stimulation. Responsive only to pain.

Hypersomnia, pathologic drowsiness, obtundation: Terms applied to an increase above the patient's normal sleep/wake ratio, often accompanied during wakefulness by reduced attention and interest in the environment. Responsive to pain and other stimuli.

Delirium: An acute or subacute reduction in awareness, attention, orientation, and perception (''clouding of consciousness''), usually fluctuating and accompanied by abnormal sleep/wake patterns and often psychomotor disturbances.

Syncope: Brief loss of consciousness due to global failure of cerebrovascular perfusion.

Dementia: A sustained or permanent multidimensional or global decline in cognitive functions.

Vegetative state: A sustained, complete loss of cognition, with sleep/wake cycles and other autonomic functions remaining relatively intact. The condition can either follow acute, severe bilateral cerebral damage or develop gradually as the end stage of a progressive dementia

Locked-in state: Preservation of intellectual activity accompanied by severe or total incapacity to express voluntary responses as a result of damage to or dysfunction of descending motor pathways in the brain or peripheral motor nerves Most, but not all, such patients can use vertical eye movements to signal by code.

Adapted from Plum F. Neurology/disturbances of consciousness and arousal. *In* Wyngaarden JB, Smith LH, Bennett JC (eds). Cecil Textbook of Medicine, 19th ed. Philadelphia: WB Saunders, 1992:2049.

tic information. The most widely used grading system is the Glasgow Coma Scale (Table 41–2).

The Glasgow Coma Scale is a 15-point scale that evaluates three areas of central nervous system (CNS) function. A score of 15 indicates full function as assessed by the scale, whereas a score of 3 indicates no function. The first area of assessment is *eye opening,* which evaluates the arousability and alertness of the patient. Spontaneous eye opening indicates intact arousal mechanisms but does not imply awareness. Eye opening in response to speech may be a response to any verbal stimulation; it does not imply a response to a command to open the eyes. Eye opening in response to pain is tested by application of a painful stimulus to the extremities, not to the face. Facial pain may elicit a grimace, preventing opening of the eyes. Patients with facial injuries and periorbital edema may not be capable of opening their eyes, rendering this part of the scale unevaluable.

Verbal responses require a high degree of integration within the CNS. Oriented responses indicate awareness of person, place, and time. Patients should know why they are in the hospital as well as the day, month, and year. Confused speech denotes that the patient can respond to questions and engage in conversation but that the responses are disoriented or inappropriate. Inappropriate words imply that the patient can make intelligible utterances but that speech is used only in an exclamatory or random way, often through shouting and swearing. Nonspecific sounds are moans, groans, and other utterances containing no recognizable words. Lack of verbal response may be due to conditions other than a

depressed level of consciousness. Tracheal intubation, aphasia, and language barriers are examples of situations or conditions that may make the verbal area of the Glasgow Coma Scale unevaluable. In the intubated patient, this area of the scale is often assigned the letter ''T,'' indicating tracheal intubation and the inability to rate verbal responses.

Motor functioning reflects mentation as well as the integrity of the major CNS pathways. A score of 6 is given if the patient follows commands. If the patient does not follow commands, a painful stimulus is applied via pressure to the nail bed of a finger. The response to this stimulus may be flexion, withdrawal, extension, or no response. If the response is withdrawal, another painful stimulus must be applied to the trunk, head, or neck to determine whether there is localization. A localizing response indicates that stimuli at more than one area cause the patient to purposefully move the extremity to remove the irritant. Withdrawal of the upper extremity consists of abduction of the shoulder and flexion of the elbow. Withdrawal is typically a rapid movement. The flexion response, or *decorticate posturing,* is a slow adduction of the shoulder, flexion of the arm, wrist, and fingers along with extension, internal rotation, and vigorous plantar flexion of the lower extremity. The extensor response, or *decerebrate posturing,* involves the adduction and internal rotation of the shoulder and pronation of the forearm.

For purposes of gauging global brain function, the best motor response from any limb is taken as the score. Variation in response from one side of the body to the other is indicative of an asymmetric brain lesion. If the patient has a right hemiparesis, there may be a withdrawal response of the left arm and no response to painful stimulation of the right arm. With an asymmetric brainstem injury, the patient may demonstrate decorticate posturing on one side and decerebrate posturing on the opposite side. In these instances, it is important to describe the patient's response in addition to assigning a score. Spinal cord lesions resulting in paralysis or significant orthopedic injuries to the extremities render the motor portion of the Glasgow Coma Scale unevaluable.

The Glasgow Coma Scale is not intended to take the place of a complete neurologic evaluation (Table 41–3); it is considered as another vital sign in a patient with mental status changes. The scale

Table 41–2. Glasgow Coma Scale

Activity	Best Response	Score
Eye opening	Spontaneous	4
	To speech	3
	To pain	2
	None	1
		1–4
Verbal	Oriented	5
	Confused	4
	Inappropriate words	3
	Nonspecific sounds	2
	None	1
		1–5
Motor	Follows commands	6
	Localizes pain	5
	Withdraws in response to pain	4
	Flexion in response to pain	3
	Extension in response to pain	2
	None	1
		1–6
TOTAL SCORE		3–15

Adapted from Teasdale G, Jennet B. Assessment of coma and impaired consciousness. Lancet 1974;2:81.

Table 41-3. The Neurologic Examination in Coma

1. Guarantee vital functions.
2. Feel the scalp for hematomas (overlying fracture lines); be sure the neck is not fractured; test *gently* for stiff neck.
3. Test language. Test arousability by words, loud sounds, noxious stimuli. If vocalizations occur, check quickly for appropriate phrases, actual words, and presence or absence of aphasia.
4. Do a neuro-ophthalmologic examination.
   Funduscopy (if difficult can be deferred until patient is stabilized)
      Papilledema? (increased intracranial or venous sinus pressure)
      Hemorrhages (subarachnoid hemorrhage; hypertensive encephalopathy; hypoxic-hypercarbic encephalopathy)
   Pupils
      Light reaction. Use bright flashlight and, if necessary, magnifying glass to be certain. Absence means potentially fatally deep sedative poisoning or acute or chronic structural brainstem damage.
      Equality. 15% of normals have mild anisocoria but new or >2 mm dilation means parasympathetic (third nerve) palsy.
   Extraocular movements. Absence acutely means deep drug poisoning, severe brainstem damage, polyneuropathy, or botulism.
      Dysconjugate at rest means an acute third, fourth, or sixth nerve palsy or internuclear ophthalmoplegia. Tonic conjugate deviation toward a paralytic arm and leg means forebrain seizures or a contralateral pontine destructive lesion; away from the paralytic arm and leg means forebrain gaze paralysis.
      Spontaneous eye movements. In coma patients, nystagmus, bobbing, independently moving eyes all mean brainstem damage.
      Oculocephalic (away from direction of head turning) or oculovestibular (toward cold caloric irrigation) responses. Absence of responses means drugs or severe brainstem disease; dysconjugate responses with equal pupils mean internuclear ophthalmoplegia, with unequal pupils mean third nerve disease.
5. Examine the motor systems.
   Strength
      Unilateral weakness or motionlessness of arm and leg means contralateral supraspinal upper motor neuron lesion, most often cerebral; if of arm, leg, and face, contralateral cerebral lesion. Occasionally arm and leg weakness can reflect contralateral brainstem lesion.
      All four extremities weak or motionless implies metabolic disease; less likely is brainstem disease (tone and reflexes increased) or peripheral disease (tone and reflexes decreased).
   Attempt to elicit reflex posturing
      Arm flexed, leg extended—contralateral deep cerebral-thalamic lesion
      Arm and leg extended—thalamic or mesencephalic lesion
      Arms extended and legs flexed or flaccid—pontine lesion
      Legs flexed, arms flaccid—pontomedullary or spinal lesion
      Compare side-to-side reflexes and examine plantar responses.
6. Seek seizure activity or abnormal movements. (1) Generalized? (2) Focal? (3) Multifocal? (4) Myoclonic?
   Control 1 immediately, 2 and 3 deliberately; if 4, treat underlying disease.
   Acute tremor, asterixis, multifocal myoclonus—seek metabolic cause.
7. Inspect breathing
   Regular hyperpnea: metabolic acidosis; pulmonary infarction; congestive failure or alveolar infiltration; sepsis; salicylism; hepatic coma
   Cyclically irregular (Cheyne-Stokes): low cardiac output plus bilateral cerebral or upper brainstem dysfunction
   Irregularly irregular gasping, slow or weak: lower brainstem dysfunction (including hypoglycemia, drug effects), less often peripheral ventilatory paralysis
8. Proceed with laboratory tests and emergency management as described in text.

Adapted from Plum F. Neurology/sustained impairments of consciousness. *In* Wyngaarden JB, Smith LH, Bennett JC (eds). Cecil Textbook of Medicine, 19th ed. Philadelphia: WB Saunders, 1992:2057.

can be used as an objective measure of improvement or worsening of the patient's level of consciousness over time. Interventions are often based on the score. Most patients with traumatic brain injury should undergo endotracheal intubation if their score is 8 or less. Deterioration of a patient's score by 2 or more points indicates a need for quick re-evaluation of the patient and the possible need for interventions such as tracheal intubation and diagnostic studies such as a brain computed tomographic (CT) scan. The score has been used to assign a prognosis to patients with brain injury, particularly with traumatic brain injury; about 36% of children who suffer a traumatic brain injury with scores of 3 to 5 will die, compared with 1.7% of patients with scores of 6 or greater. It may take a mean of 23 days for patients with initial scores of 3 to 5 to become cognizant, versus 4 days in patients with scores of 6 or greater. The eventual outcome of patients is often related to the initial Glasgow Coma Scale score. Patients with an initial score of 3 to 5 do more poorly than those with scores of 6 or greater. Nonetheless, some patients with scores of 3 to 5 do recover independent function.

The Glasgow Coma Scale score has also been used as a prognostic indicator in nontraumatic coma. Children presenting after near-drowning with an initial score of 6 or greater have a good outcome. Patients presenting with a score of 5 or less have a high probability of mortality or profound neurologic sequelae, although a patient with a score of 4 or 5 may survive with minimal impairment. A score of 3 on transfer to an intensive care unit has been associated with nearly 100% poor outcome in near-drowning.

The Glasgow Coma Scale was designed and validated in adult patients, and the normal verbal and motor responses in this scale are not achievable during the first few years of life. Many groups have developed modified coma scales for children. The modifications are based on a child's age-appropriate developmental abilities. The reliability and clinical applicability of any scale are dependent on the interobserver variability of that scale. The greater the variability, the less reliable the scale. The Pediatric Glasgow Coma Scale appears to be a reliable scale for use in children 5 years of age or younger (Table 41-4).

Other scales have been developed to measure the level of con-

Table 41–4. Pediatric Glasgow Coma Scale

Activity	Best Response	Score
Eye opening	Spontaneously	4
	To speech	3
	To pain	2
	None	1
Verbal	Oriented	5
	Words	4
	Vocal sounds	3
	Cries	2
	None	1
Motor	Obeys commands	5
	Localizes pain	4
	Flexion to pain	3
	Extension to pain	2
	None	1

Normal Total Score Based on Age

Birth–6 months	9
7–12 months	11
1–2 years	12
2–5 years	13
> 5 years	14

Adapted from Simpson D, Reilly P. Pediatric Coma Scale. Lancet 1982;2:450.

sciousness in specific disease states, such as poisonings, Reye syndrome, and hepatic failure. Reed classification of coma has been used in the setting of poisoning or intoxication (Table 41–5) and evaluates increasing depths of coma encountered with CNS depressant drugs. The cardiovascular system is included in this classification because toxic ingestions may depress myocardial contractility or cause vasodilation.

A staging system used in Reye syndrome is presented in Table 41–6. The Reye syndrome scale is similar to the Glasgow Coma Scale but has the additional feature of evaluation of brainstem function by observation of pupillary and oculocephalic reflexes. The Glasgow Coma Scale and Reye syndrome staging scale are

Table 41–5. Reed Classification of Coma

Grade 0*	Asleep Can be aroused Will answer questions
Grade 1*	Comatose Withdraws from painful stimuli Intact reflexes
Grade 2*	Comatose Does not withdraw from painful stimuli No respiratory, circulatory depression Intact reflexes
Grade 3†	Comatose Reflexes absent No respiratory, circulatory depression
Grade 4†	Comatose Reflexes absent Respiratory or circulatory problems

Adapted from Ellenhorn MJ, Barceloux DE. Medical Toxicology, Diagnosis and Treatment of Human Poisoning. New York: Elsevier Science, 1988:17.
*Good prognosis.
†Very serious, may need measures to enhance elimination.

Table 41–6. Staging of Reye's Syndrome

Stage I: Lethargy, follows verbal commands, normal posture, purposeful response to pain, brisk pupillary light reflex, and normal oculocephalic reflex.

Stage II: Combative or stuporous, inappropriate verbalizing, normal posture, purposeful or nonpurposeful response to pain, sluggish pupillary reaction, conjugate deviation on doll's eye maneuver.

Stage III: Comatose, decorticate posture, decorticate response to pain, sluggish pupillary reaction, conjugate deviation on doll's eye maneuver.

Stage IV: Comatose, decerebrate posture and decerebrate response to pain, sluggish pupillary reflexes, and inconsistent or absent oculocephalic reflex.

Stage V: Comatose, flaccid, no response to pain, no pupillary response, no oculocephalic reflex.

From Tasker RC, Dean JM, Rogers MC. Reye syndrome and metabolic encephalopathies. *In* Rogers MC (ed). Rogers Textbook of Pediatric Intensive Care, 2nd ed. Baltimore: Williams & Wilkins, 1992:792.

based on the central syndrome of rostral-caudal deterioration. The central syndrome describes the constellation of clinical findings in patients as brainstem function becomes impaired at progressively lower levels by compression from above (Fig. 41–1). Neurologic function in a patient with hepatic encephalopathy is graded using the scoring system in Table 41–7. This scale focuses more on cortical functioning and less on evolution of the central syndrome. Patients with grade IV hepatic encephalopathy have cerebral edema from liver failure and may show signs of the central syndrome. The cerebral edema in Reye syndrome is a direct effect of the disease process, distinct from hepatic failure. This distinction explains the differences in the Reye's and hepatic encephalopathy scales.

DIFFERENTIAL DIAGNOSIS

The differential diagnosis of delirium and coma in the child is extensive. The etiology of coma in children without head injuries commonly includes intracranial infections (meningitis, encephalitis), ischemia, epilepsy, metabolic diseases, child abuse, and cerebral vascular accidents. Approximately 25% of children from a large series of comatose patients have traumatic brain injuries. Table 41–8 presents causes of mental status changes in children. As can be seen, some diagnoses (subdural hematoma, hydrocephalus, cerebral edema) apply to more than one category. The age of the patient can help one differentiate the likely causes of coma, although there is considerable overlap (Table 41–9).

MANAGEMENT APPROACH

The approach to the child with an alteration of consciousness can be divided into four parts: (1) stabilization (2) rapid neurologic assessment (3) reversal of immediately treatable toxic or metabolic causes, and (4) determination of level of CNS function and of the cause of the coma (Fig. 41–2, p. 649).

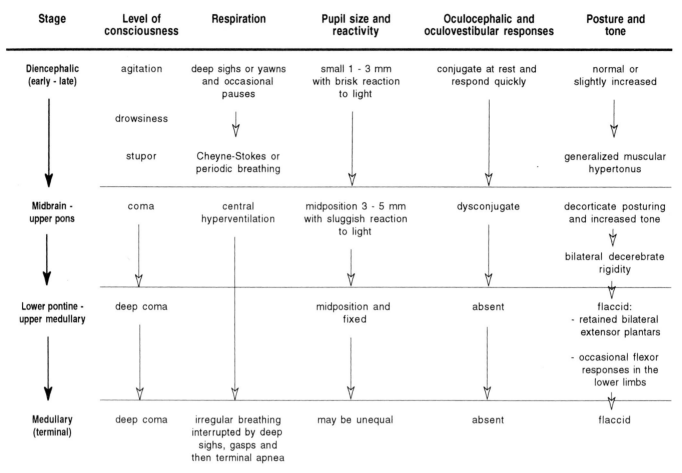

Stage	Level of consciousness	Respiration	Pupil size and reactivity	Oculocephalic and oculovestibular responses	Posture and tone
Diencephalic (early - late)	agitation	deep sighs or yawns and occasional pauses	small 1 - 3 mm with brisk reaction to light	conjugate at rest and respond quickly	normal or slightly increased
	drowsiness				
	stupor	Cheyne-Stokes or periodic breathing			generalized muscular hypertonus
Midbrain - upper pons	coma	central hyperventilation	midposition 3 - 5 mm with sluggish reaction to light	dysconjugate	decorticate posturing and increased tone
					bilateral decerebrate rigidity
Lower pontine - upper medullary	deep coma		midposition and fixed	absent	flaccid: - retained bilateral extensor plantars - occasional flexor responses in the lower limbs
Medullary (terminal)	deep coma	irregular breathing interrupted by deep sighs, gasps and then terminal apnea	may be unequal	absent	flaccid

Figure 41–1. Rostral-caudal deterioration in coma. (From Tasker RC, Dean JM, Rosen MC. Reye syndrome and metabolic encephalopathies. *In* Rogers MC (ed). Textbook of Pediatric Intensive Care, 2nd ed. Baltimore: Williams & Wilkins, 1992:778.)

Stabilization

ABCs

The initial step is a rapid but meticulous evaluation of the patient's *a*irway, *b*reathing, and *c*irculation, including determination of vital signs. Obtunded, stuporous, or comatose patients usually require intubation unless their mental status is improving or can be readily reversed. Intubation may be necessary not only to secure an airway but also to treat hypoventilation, to protect the airway if a gag reflex is not present, and to facilitate hyperventilation therapy in a child with suspected intracranial hypertension. *Manipulation*

Table 41–7. Classification of Hepatic Encephalopathy

Grade 0:   Normal

Grade I: Altered spatial orientation, sleep patterns, and affect

Grade II: Drowsy but arousable, slurred speech, confusion, and asterixis

Grade III: Stuporous but responsive to painful stimuli

Grade IV: Unresponsive, with decorticate or decerebrate posturing possible

From Rogers EL, Perman JA. Gastrointestinal and hepatic failure. *In* Rogers MC (ed). Textbook of Pediatric Intensive Care, 2nd ed. Baltimore: Williams & Wilkins, 1992:1151.

of the neck, particularly extension, should be avoided when an airway is being stabilized or secured unless a cervical spine injury can be ruled out.

Attention is next directed toward an assessment of the circulation; this mandates evaluation of vital signs, presence and volume of peripheral pulses, and adequacy of end-organ perfusion. Blood pressure must be sufficiently high to support perfusion of vital organs. Patients may be in shock with a normal blood pressure and may manifest tachycardia and often tachypnea. In early shock, except for septic shock, peripheral pulses are diminished compared with central pulses. As shock progresses and stroke volume decreases, the pulse pressure narrows and the peripheral pulses become weak or "thready" and finally nonpalpable. Early septic shock or "warm" shock is often characterized by a widened pulse pressure and bounding pulses.

End-organ perfusion is best evaluated in the skin, kidneys, and brain. The skin should be checked for temperature, color, and capillary refill. Cool extremities, pallor, mottling, peripheral cyanosis, and delayed capillary refill of more than 2 seconds indicate poor perfusion. As perfusion worsens, the coolness of the extremities extends proximally. Urine output may not be helpful in the initial evaluation of a patient, but it becomes an important marker to follow during therapy. As renal perfusion improves, urine flow rate increases. The patient's alteration in consciousness may be a consequence of shock. In early stages of shock, the patient is typically lethargic or confused. Lethargy alternating with combativeness is often seen. Infants older than 1 to 2 months of age should normally focus on their parents' faces. Failure to recognize parents is a sign of poor perfusion. Infants may also be irritable

Table 41–8. Etiologic Classification of Altered Mental Status in Children

Infectious	Metabolic/Systemic	Toxic*	Traumatic*	Anatomic	Hypoxic-Ischemic	Epileptic	Vascular	Psychologic
Viral	Hypoglycemia*	Sympathomimetics	Concussion*	Tumor	Cardiac arrest	Postictal state*	Embolism	Conversion disorders*
Aseptic meningitis*	Inborn errors of metabolism*	Anticholinergics	Cerebral contusion	Hydrocephalus	Cardiac arrhythmia	Status epilepticus*	Spontaneous intraparenchymal hemorrhage	Catatonic schizophrenia
Encephalitis*	Hyperammonemia	Phenothiazines	Epidural hematoma	Hydrocephalus with shunt malfunction	Severe shock	Absence status	Subarachnoid hemorrhage	
? Reye syndrome	Hepatic failure	PCP	Subdural hematoma	Subdural hematoma	Near-drowning	Complex partial seizure	Vasculitis	
? Hemorrhagic shock and encephalopathy syndrome	Renal diseases	LSD	Brainstem contusion	Epidural hematoma	Neonatal asphyxia*		Lupus erythematosus	
Postinfectious encephalomyelitis	Uremic encephalopathy	Marijuana	Diffuse axonal shear injury	Brain abscess	Hypoxemic respiratory failure		Hypertensive encephalopathy	
Systemic infection with shock	Hypertensive encephalopathy	Cocaine	Cerebral edema*	Subdural empyema	Carbon monoxide poisoning		Acute confusional migraine*	
Bacterial	Dialysis encephalopathy (dysequilibrium syndrome)	Heavy metals (lead)	Intraparenchymal hemorrhage	Epidural empyema	Cyanide toxicity			
Meningitis*	Hyperosmolar states	Salicylates	Intraventricular hemorrhage (neonate)*	Cerebral edema	Anaphylaxis			
Brain abscess	Hypernatremia	Organophosphates and carbamates	Obstructive hydrocephalus	Intracranial hemorrhage	Asthma			
Epidural empyema	Hyperglycemia–diabetes mellitus*	Antihistamines	Post-traumatic seizure	Cerebrovascular accident				
Subdural empyema	Hypo-osmolar states	Industrial solvents (inhaled)	Fat embolism					
Systemic infection with shock	Hyponatremia*	Alcohols						
Toxic shock syndrome	Rapid decrease in osmolality in hyperosmolar states	Narcotics						
Fungal	Endocrine disorders	Sedative-hypnotics						
Fungal meningitis	Adrenal insufficiency	Barbiturates						
Fungal brain abscess	Hyperthyroidism and hypothyroidism	Carbon monoxide						
Protozoan	Hypoparathyroidism	Tricyclic antidepressants						
Meningitis	Mineral abnormalities	Carbamazepine						
Abscess	Hypercalcemia, hypocalcemia, hypermagnesemia and hypomagnesemia, hypophosphatemia	Cyanide						
Postimmunization encephalopathy	Hypercapnia	Methaqualone						
	Hypoxia*							
	Shock*							
	Vitamin deficiency and dependency states							
	Nicotinic acid							
	Pantothenic acid							
	Pyridoxine							
	Thiamine							
	Vitamin B$_{12}$							
	Intussusception encephalopathy							
	Methemoglobinemia							
	Acidosis							
	Alkalosis							
	Porphyria							
	Reye syndrome							
	? Hemorrhagic shock and encephalopathy syndrome							
	Mitochondrial encephalopathies							

*Common.

Abbreviations: LSD = lysergic acid diethylamide; PCP = phencyclidine piperdine.

Table 41–9. Common Causes of Altered Mental Status Based on Age

Neonate	Infant	Child	Adolescent

Hypoglycemia	Meningitis
	  Bacterial
	  Viral
		Meningitis
		  Bacterial
		  Viral
			Meningitis
			  Bacterial
			  Viral
			  Encephalitis

Birth asphyxia	Trauma
	  Abuse/shaken baby syndrome
		Encephalitis	Intentional ingestion
			  Recreational drug/alcohol use
			  Suicide gesture or attempt
			  Often involves multiple agents

Congenital anomalies of the central nervous system	Asphyxia
	  Apparent life-threatening event
	  Intentional suffocation
		Trauma	Trauma

Systemic infection with shock	Systemic infection with shock	Ingestion	Seizures
Cardiogenic shock	Ingestion	Reye syndrome	Diabetic ketoacidosis
Congenital infection	Inborn errors of metabolism	Systemic infection with shock	Systemic infection with shock
Bacterial meningitis	Hypoglycemia	Seizure	Toxic shock syndrome
Inborn errors of metabolism	Hyponatremia	Near-drowning	Reye syndrome
Hypocalcemia	Hypernatremia	Hypoglycemia	Spontaneous intracranial hemorrhage
Intraventricular hemorrhage	Hypocalcemia	Intussusception encephalopathy	Psychologic
Seizures	Encephalitis	Diabetic ketoacidosis	
Birth trauma	Postimmunization encephalopathy		
	Hemorrhagic shock and encephalopathy syndrome		
	Intussusception encephalopathy		
	Seizures		

and have a weak cry. As shock progresses, changes in level of consciousness become more profound. The child may progress from responding to voice to responding to pain only and may subsequently become unresponsive.

HISTORY

During stabilization, a patient history must be obtained, by another physician or nurse, if available. Pertinent questions should focus on the recent history preceding the change in mental status, the past medical history, and a family history, particularly of seizures or encephalopathy. Did the child sustain any traumatic injuries in the previous few days? Has the child been febrile, or are there other signs or symptoms of infection or systemic disease? A dietary history in infants presenting with a depressed level of consciousness is paramount and may raise suspicion of hypoglycemia (fasting or emesis) or hyponatremia (ingestion of free water). *Exposure to drugs or toxins should be suspected in any patient with a sudden onset of unexplained symptoms (coma, seizures) or a gradual onset of symptoms preceded by a period of confusion or delirium.* A thorough history focusing on patient, environmental, and toxic factors should be elicited.

Rapid Neurologic Assessment

After stabilization, the next phase in management is a rapid neurologic assessment (see Table 41–3), which should take no more than a few minutes. The primary goal is to identify patients with a potentially rapidly progressive intracranial process that may be life-threatening, such as an expanding mass lesion (subdural or epidural hematoma) and to identify patients who are rapidly deteriorating. A secondary objective is to provide prognostic and triage information to other personnel who may be involved with the child in the future. This information permits comparisons of sequential examinations and is important in the patient who receives medications (neuromuscular blockers, CNS depressants) in the emergency department that may obscure subsequent neurologic findings. The rapid assessment includes an evaluation for traumatic injuries, focal neurologic findings, brainstem dysfunction, and clinically significant intracranial hypertension.

TRAUMATIC INJURIES

Traumatic injuries can result in life-threatening illnesses at any age, including newborns. The head and neck should be carefully inspected and the skull palpated for evidence of trauma (Table 41–10). In infants, a bulging fontanelle represents raised intracranial pressure, which may have various causes. In the absence of a febrile illness, trauma, including that caused by shaken baby syndrome (child abuse), should be suspected in any infant with a bulging fontanelle. Retinal hemorrhages are often present on funduscopic examination in children with the shaken baby syndrome (see Chapter 37).

FOCAL NEUROLOGIC FINDINGS

The presence of focal findings is determined by examination of a child's pupils for asymmetry in size or reactivity and examination

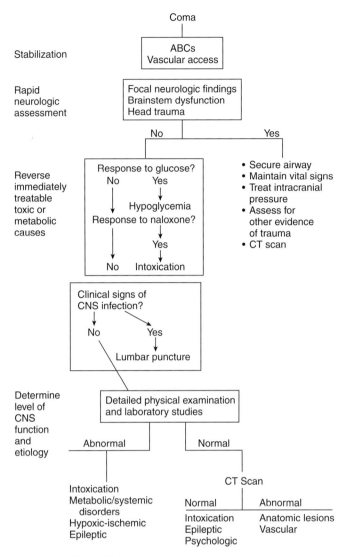

Figure 41-2. Management approach to coma.

Table 41-10. Signs of Head Trauma Possibly Associated with Intracranial Pathology

General	Signs of Basilar Skull Fracture
Lacerations	Hemotympanum
Hematomas	CSF rhinorrhea
Ecchymosis	CSF otorrhea
Swelling	Racoon eyes
Palpable crepitations	Battle sign
Step-off of skull	

Abbreviation: CSF = cerebrospinal fluid.

to upper medullary lesions, whereas medullary lesions result in ataxic or irregular breathing, slow regular breathing, or agonal respirations.

Absent or asymmetric corneal reflexes or abnormal oculocephalic or oculovestibular reflexes also suggest serious brainstem involvement.

INTRACRANIAL HYPERTENSION

Indications of clinically significant intracranial hypertension are usually apparent during an assessment of pupillary responses, vital signs, and motor response (Tables 41–11 and 41–12). A unilaterally fixed and dilated pupil in a patient who is not awake represents uncal herniation precipitated by an increase in intracranial pressure in the supratentorial space. Impending central herniation from increased pressure on the caudal brainstem may be preceded by *Cushing triad* of hypertension, bradycardia, and apnea. All three components are not necessarily present, however. Decerebrate or opisthotonic posturing should also be considered a sign of raised intracranial pressure in an unresponsive patient. A lateral rectus palsy (cranial nerve VI) may also be an early sign of intracranial hypertension. A history of headaches, persistent vomiting, or ataxia may also suggest raised intracranial pressure.

A child with focal neurologic findings or brainstem dysfunction

of the motor system for asymmetric movement of the extremities or face. The motor response is part of the Glasgow Coma Scale.

BRAINSTEM DYSFUNCTION

Brainstem function is evaluated by observing the child's respiratory pattern, assessing corneal reflexes, and testing oculocephalic (doll's eyes) or oculovestibular (cold caloric) reflexes. *The oculocephalic reflex should not be checked unless a cervical spine injury has been ruled out.* Significant brainstem dysfunction is rarely associated with a normal breathing pattern (Fig. 41–3). Cheyne-Stokes respiration is a pattern of breathing observed in the presence of bilateral hemispheric or diencephalic dysfunction. It may also precede transtentorial herniation. Periods of hyperpnea alternate with shorter apneic phases. The hyperpneic periods have a characteristic, smooth, crescendo-decrescendo pattern.

Central neurogenic hyperventilation is encountered with midbrain dysfunction; patients with this problem are tachypneic and hyperpneic. Apneustic breathing is associated with damage in the mid to lower pontine region. This pattern is characterized by a prolonged pause at full inspiration. Clusters of breaths separated by periods of apnea may be observed in patients with low pontine

Table 41-11. Signs of Incipient Downward Herniation

	Central	Uncal
Arousal	Impaired early, before other signs	Impaired late, usually with other signs
Breathing	Sighs, yawns, sometimes Cheyne-Stokes respirations	No early change
Pupils	First small reactive (hypothalamus), then one or both approach midposition	Ipsilateral pupil dilates, followed by somatic third nerve paralysis
Oculocephalic responses	Initially sluggish, later tonic conjugate	Unilateral third nerve paralysis
Motor signs	Early hemiparesis opposite to hemispheric lesion followed late by ipsilateral motor paresis and extensor plantar response	Motor signs late, sometimes ipsilateral to lesion

From Plum F. Neurology/sustained impairments of consciousness. *In* Wyngaarden JB, Smith LH, Bennett JC (eds). Cecil Textbook of Medicine, 19th ed. Philadelphia: WB Saunders, 1992:2050.

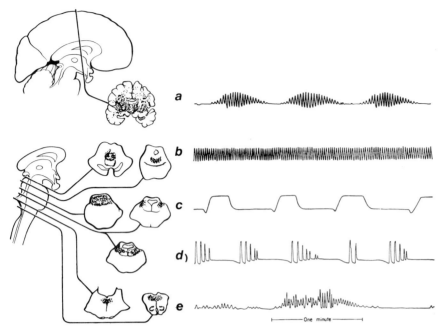

Figure 41–3. Abnormal respiratory patterns associated with pathologic lesions (shaded areas) at various levels of the brain. Tracings by chest-abdomen pneumograph, inspiration reads up. *a,* Cheyne-Stokes respiration. *b,* Central neurogenic hyperventilation. *c,* Apneusis. *d,* Cluster breathing. *e,* Ataxic breathing. (Adapted from Plum F, Posner JB (eds). The Diagnosis of Stupor and Coma, 3rd ed. Philadelphia: FA Davis, 1982:34.)

has a rapidly progressive intracranial lesion until proven otherwise. These children require an emergent head computed tomography (CT) scan and an assessment for other life-threatening injuries if trauma is suspected. Vital signs should be monitored frequently. Intubation is performed before CT scanning if the Glasgow Coma Scale score is 8 or less or if signs of increased intracranial pressure are present. If raised intracranial pressure is suspected, the child should be hyperventilated and given mannitol before CT scanning. Children with altered mental status and a suspected head injury but without focal findings or brainstem dysfunction should also have an emergent CT scan performed. If their score is 8 or less, an airway should be secured before they undergo scanning.

The absence of a history of trauma or physical findings suggestive of a rapidly progressive intracranial process does not preclude a traumatic or an anatomic cause of coma. A child may have a subarachnoid hemorrhage (ruptured aneurysm, arteriovenous malformation) or hydrocephalus without any of the aforementioned signs or symptoms of raised intracranial pressure.

Reversal of Immediately Treatable Toxic or Metabolic Causes

Hypoglycemia and narcotic intoxication are two rapidly reversible causes of coma. Hypoglycemia is a medical emergency that

Table 41–12. Characteristics of Supratentorial Lesions Leading to Coma

---

Initiating symptoms usually cerebral-focal: aphasia; focal seizures; contralateral hemiparesis, sensory change, or neglect; frontal lobe behavioral changes; headache.

Dysfunction moves rostral to caudal: e.g., focal motor → bilateral motor → altered level of arousal.

Abnormal signs usually confined to a single or adjacent anatomic level (not diffuse).

Brain stem functions spared unless herniation develops.

From Plum F. Neurology/sustained impairments of consciousness. *In* Wyngaarden JB, Smith LH, Bennett JC (eds). Cecil Textbook of Medicine, 19th ed. Philadelphia: WB Saunders, 1992:2050.

must be reversed because sustained hypoglycemia may result in permanent neurologic damage (see Chapter 63). When vascular access is achieved, blood can be obtained for laboratory studies, including a blood glucose level determination. However, *once an intravenous catheter has been placed, all unresponsive children should receive 0.5 to 1.0 g/kg (2 to 4 ml/kg) of 25% dextrose unless a diagnosis other than hypoglycemia is apparent.* If the child's mental status improves or there is laboratory confirmation of hypoglycemia, the dextrose bolus should be followed by a continuous infusion of glucose and electrolytes to prevent rebound hypoglycemia. Naloxone (0.01 to 0.1 mg/kg) is also administered to all children who have marked depression of consciousness without an obvious cause, particularly if hypoventilation is observed. Miosis is not a necessary finding because ingestion of multiple agents, including narcotics, may not result in small constricted pupils. Large ingestions of narcotics may require larger single doses of naloxone because of the competitive nature of its antagonistic effect, or they may require multiple doses because its half-life is shorter than that of the narcotic ingested.

Another reversible cause of coma is a benzodiazepine ingestion. Flumazenil, a specific competitive antagonist of benzodiazepines, should not be routinely administered to unresponsive children in the emergency department. There are no compelling data suggesting that flumazenil reverses respiratory depression. Administration of flumazenil to a patient who has ingested multiple agents can precipitate seizures, particularly if the concomitant ingestion can cause seizures (e.g., tricyclic antidepressants).

The next question to be answered is whether there are clinical signs or symptoms of meningitis or encephalitis. Specifically, the child should be assessed for the presence of a bulging fontanelle, nuchal rigidity, and Kernig or Brudzinski signs (see Chapter 53). Prior administration of antibiotics does not affect meningeal irritation. Most (85%) children with meningitis have an alteration in mental status (53% lethargic, 22% stuporous, 10% comatose). Focal neurologic findings or seizures may be seen in children with meningitis.

If meningitis is suspected, a lumbar puncture including measurement of the opening pressure, should be performed unless the procedure is contraindicated (Table 41–13). If a contraindication exists, the child should be stabilized, receive empirical antimicrobial therapy, and undergo head CT scanning. The patient should undergo lumbar puncture as soon as it is no longer contraindicated.

Table 41–13. **Contraindications to Lumbar Puncture**

Clinically important cardiorespiratory compromise in a neonate or young infant

Signs of raised intracranial pressure (pupillary changes, ptosis, hypertension, bradycardia, posturing, cranial nerve VI palsy, retinal changes)

Skin or soft tissue infection overlying area where lumbar puncture to be performed

Focal neurologic findings

Suspected brain abscess (illness duration greater than expected for meningitis; focality)

If a patient presents with sudden nuchal rigidity not preceded by a prodromal illness, a subarachnoid hemorrhage should be suspected and a CT scan performed before the lumbar puncture.

Level of Central Nervous System Function and Etiology

The coma can be initially considered stable if (1) focal neurologic findings are not present, (2) there is no evidence of significant brainstem dysfunction, (3) intracranial pressure is not raised, (4) there is no evidence of head trauma or CNS infection, and (5) the child does not have a rapidly reversible toxic or metabolic cause. A detailed physical examination and laboratory evaluation can then be undertaken to determine the level of CNS function and the cause of the coma.

PHYSICAL EXAMINATION

Coma can be thought of as resulting from hemispheric or brainstem (including reticular activating formation) dysfunction. The dysfunction in either location may be produced by anatomic or nonstructural causes (referred to as metabolic causes in this discussion (see Table 41–8). The origin of coma (hemispheric versus brainstem) and its cause (metabolic versus structural) can be elucidated by evaluation of pupillary size and reactivity, eye movements, respiratory pattern, and motor responses. *Pupillary light reflexes are generally preserved in metabolic encephalopathy, whereas their absence strongly suggests a structural lesion.* The only exception to the latter is drug effect, particularly with potent anticholinergic compounds, such as glutethimide, atropine, or scopolamine, which produce fixed and dialted pupils. Pupillary size and reactivity are normally determined by the balance between sympathetic and parasympathetic stimulation, which result in pupillary dilation and constriction, respectively. A unilaterally dilated and fixed pupil is a sign of uncal herniation with entrapment of the oculomotor nerve. Parasympathetic fibers innervating the eye accompany the oculomotor nerve. Sympathetic fibers originate from at least four hypothalamic nuclei so that diencephalic dysfunction results in small, reactive pupils. Hypothalamic damage often results in ipsilateral miosis associated with a *Horner syndrome* (miosis, ptosis, and anhidrosis).

Anhidrosis, in contrast to that observed with cervical lesions, involves the entire ipsilateral half of the body. This is an important clinical finding in that it may portend imminent transtentorial herniation. Injury to nuclei located in the midbrain disrupts both sympathetic and parasympathetic pathways, resulting in mid-sized, fixed pupils. Damage to the midbrain tectal regions also produces midposition or slightly large, fixed pupils. In contrast to nuclear damage, however, accommodation may be intact, so that pupillary size fluctuates spontaneously. Pontine lesions, principally hemorrhage, interfere with descending sympathetic fibers, causing symmetrically small pupils that may require a magnifying glass to detect a light reflex. Lateral medullary lesions may also produce a Horner syndrome, whereas central herniation results in fixed, dilated pupils. Figure 41–4 summarizes pupillary findings in comatose patients.

Evaluation of eye movements is helpful in differentiating hemispheric from brainstem causes of coma. Frontal regions of the cerebral hemispheres are responsible for voluntary eye movements, the quick phase of nystagmus, and control over brainstem reflexes that determine eye movements. Bilateral hemispheric depression may result in roving eye movements if brainstem function is intact.

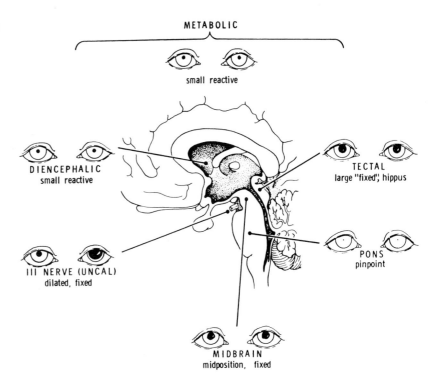

Figure 41–4. Pupils in comatose patients. (Adapted from Plum F, Posner JB (eds). The Diagnosis of Stupor and Coma, 3rd ed. Philadelphia: FA Davis, 1982:46.)

METABOLIC
small reactive

DIENCEPHALIC
small reactive

TECTAL
large "fixed", hippus

III NERVE (UNCAL)
dilated, fixed

PONS
pinpoint

MIDBRAIN
midposition, fixed

Because stimulation of a frontal gaze center causes conjugate deviation of the eyes to the opposite side, tonic lateral deviation of the eyes implies a seizure emanating from the contralateral hemisphere. Eye deviation may also result from an ipsilateral hemispheric injury with unopposed stimulation from the undamaged hemisphere or from a contralateral pontine lesion. The degree of eye deviation is usually more dramatic with hemispheric damage than with brainstem damage.

If the patient's eyes are not moving, then reflex eye movements are tested by the oculocephalic and oculovestibular responses (Fig. 41–5). These maneuvers involve the same major neuronal pathways. Afferent fibers from the labyrinth, cerebellum, and cervical muscles reach the vestibular nuclei (cranial nerve VIII) in the medulla. Fibers from the vestibular nuclei then course to the ipsilateral abducens nuclei (cranial nerve VI). Fibers from the abducens nuclei then decussate in the midpons and ascend in the medial longitudinal fasciculus to reach the contralateral oculomotor nuclei (cranial nerve III). Positive reflexes indicate the absence of cortical input on an intact brainstem.

The *oculocephalic* reflex is elicited by rotating the child's head from side to side and observing the eye movements. If brainstem function is intact, the eyes deviate in a direction opposite to the head movement. Both left and right lateral rotation should be tested. This reflex should then be tested in a vertical plane by rapidly flexing and extending the neck. A positive response is upward gaze when the neck is flexed and downward deviation when the head is extended. *Such maneuvers are contraindicated if cervical spine injury is suspected.*

The *oculovestibular* reflex is tested by instilling ice water into the ear canal. The ear canal must be visualized to ensure that there is no obstruction and that the tympanic membrane is intact. The head is then placed at a 30-degree angle from the horizontal so that the semicircular canal is vertical, and up to 120 ml of ice water is then injected slowly into the external ear canal over a few minutes through an angiocatheter. After a minimum of 5 minutes, the other ear may be tested; this interval allows time for the oculovestibular system to re-equilibrate. A positive response in an awake patient is nystagmus with the slow component toward the

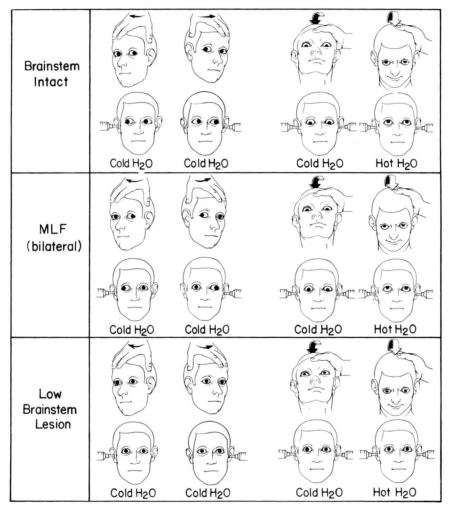

Figure 41–5. Ocular reflexes in unconscious patients. The upper section illustrates the oculocephalic *(above)* and oculovestibular *(below)* reflexes in an unconscious patient whose brainstem ocular pathways are intact. In the middle portion of the drawing, the effects of bilateral medial longitudinal fasciculus lesions on oculocephalic and oculovestibular reflexes are shown. The left portion of the drawing illustrates that oculocephalic and oculovestibular stimulation deviates the appropriate eye laterally and brings the eye, which would normally deviate medially, only to the midline, since the medial longitudinal fasciculus, with its connections between the abducens and oculomotor nuclei, is interrupted. The lower portion of the drawing illustrates the effects of a low brainstem lesion. On the left, neither oculovestibular nor oculocephalic movements cause lateral deviation of the eyes because the pathways are interrupted between the vestibular nucleus and the abducens area. Likewise, in the right portion of the drawing, neither oculovestibular nor oculocephalic stimulation causes vertical deviation of the eyes. (Adapted from Plum F, Posner JB (eds). The Diagnosis of Stupor and Coma, 3rd ed. Philadelphia: FA Davis, 1982:55.)

irrigated ear and the fast component away from the stimulus. With bilateral hemispheric depression, the fast phase of nystagmus dissipates, and the eyes are tonically deviated toward the irrigated ear. Both the oculocephalic and oculovestibular reflexes are absent in patients with low brainstem lesions because neurotransmission between the vestibular and abducens nuclei is interrupted. In those with damage to the medial longitudinal fasciculus, the ipsilateral eye fails to adduct on irrigation of the contralateral ear canal. However, the opposite eye abducts normally. For example, with a lesion in the left medial longitudinal fasciculus, the right eye abducts but the left eye does not adduct in response to irrigating the right ear canal. This reaction is due to disruption of fibers between the abducens and the contralateral oculomotor nuclei (Fig. 41–5).

In addition to assessing ocular motility, the examiner should test corneal reflex and determine the presence or absence of a blink. The absence of a blink in response to a loud noise or bright light implies dysfunction of the pontine reticular formation secondary to either metabolic or structural causes. Unilateral absence of a blink implies a facial nerve lesion. The afferent limb of the corneal reflex is carried by the trigeminal nerve (cranial nerve V). The normal effector response involves both upward deviation of the eye (oculomotor nerve) and closure of the eyelid (facial nerve). A normal reflex suggests that the integrity of pathways between the midbrain and the pons has not been violated.

Examination of the motor system includes observation of body position, spontaneous movements, and response to noxious stimuli (Fig. 41–6). A normal body position usually denotes an intact brainstem, as does spontaneous, nonposturing movements. Hemiparesis or hemiplegia implies a structural lesion in the contralateral hemisphere or subcortical region or an ipsilateral spinal cord injury. The presence of hypertonia or hyperreflexia suggests previous corticospinal tract disease or an acute brainstem injury at the midbrain-pontine level. It can also be observed in patients with severe metabolic derangements, such as hepatic coma, hypoglycemia, anoxia, and uremia. Hypotonia implies bilateral hemispheric dysfunction or a medullary or spinal cord lesion. In patients with severe

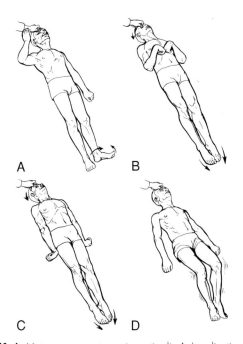

Figure 41–6. Motor responses to noxious stimuli. *A,* Localization of pain as patient attempts to remove stimulus. *B,* Decorticate posturing. *C,* Decerebrate posturing. *D,* Flaccid patient with no response. (Adapted from Plum F, Posner JB (eds). The Diagnosis of Stupor and Coma, 3rd ed. Philadelphia: FA Davis, 1982:66.)

depression of brain function, motor function can be assessed only after the application of a noxious stimulus, such as a sternal rub or increasing subungual pressure to the fingernails or toenails. Ascending sensory pathways to the cerebral hemispheres are intact, and descending motor pathways are functioning to some degree if the response to a noxious stimulus includes verbalization or eye opening or a normal motor response, such as localization of the stimulus, withdrawal of the limb, or movement away from the stimulus.

Decorticate posturing implies hemispheric dysfunction with an intact brainstem (Fig. 41–6). Decerebrate posturing is more ominous (Fig. 41–6). Opisthotonos with clenched teeth is a severe form of decerebration. This response usually suggests brainstem compression or a severe structural injury to the midbrain-pontine region. It can also occur in association with severe metabolic diseases, such as hepatic coma, anoxia, and hypoglycemia. Less commonly, decerebrate posture may represent delayed cortical demyelination after a hypoxic-ischemic injury. Pontomedullary or spinal cord damage is associated with a flaccid response to noxious stimulation.

A patient's breathing pattern is also helpful in localizing the area of CNS dysfunction (see Brainstem Dysfunction). Hyperventilation can be observed not only in midbrain structural lesions but also in toxic-metabolic encephalopathies as a primary response to stimulation of the respiratory center (salicylate, theophylline, hepatic coma) or as a compensatory response to a metabolic acidosis. This pattern is also seen with raised intracranial hypertension, as may occur in a child with meningitis. Hypoventilation with a normal rhythm, particularly if associated with a symmetrically depressed motor examination, usually implies global CNS depression secondary to drug ingestion.

A detailed physical examination should be performed next and may provide further clues to the cause of the coma (Table 41–14). Several laboratory or ancillary studies should be obtained in all patients, whereas ordering of other studies depends on clinical suspicions formulated from the history and physical examination (Table 41–15). Patients with suspected anatomic causes of coma should undergo emergent head CT scanning, whereas those with a suspected CNS infection should undergo a lumbar puncture. Other studies to consider are electrocardiography to rule out conduction abnormalities, seen with many drugs; liver function studies; blood ammonia determination; mineral determinations, such as calcium, magnesium, and phosphorus; and a measured serum osmolality. An *osmolal gap* as well as an anion gap should be calculated. The osmolal gap is the difference between the measured and calculated serum osmolality (normal is <5 to 10 mOsm/kg H_2O). Table 41–16 summarizes the differential diagnoses of an elevated anion or osmolal gap. Toxicology screens may be of value with suspected ingestions; however, the results must be interpreted cautiously. Because toxicology screens are not standardized, a "negative" result does not rule out an undetermined ingestion. Screening for certain agents, such as methanol and ethylene glycol, needs to be requested specifically, whereas tests for other compounds may yield false-negative results.

If physical examination and laboratory studies do not yield a diagnosis, a head CT scan should be obtained to rule out anatomic or vascular causes. If these results are normal, the most likely causes of coma are intoxication, psychologic, or related to seizure. An electroencephalograph is indicated if encephalitis, encephalopathy, or seizure disorder is suspected.

TOXIC ENCEPHALOPATHY

Toxic compounds are common causes of altered consciousness in children. More than 90% of poisonings in young children are accidental and involve a single substance. To make an accurate

Table 41–14. **Physical Examination and Diagnosis of Coma**

System	Sign	Disorder
Skin	Dry	Dehydration, myxedema, adrenal insufficiency, anticholinergic poisoning
	Wet	Syncope
	Pigment	Addison disease
	Nevi	Tuberous sclerosis with seizures
	Petechiae	Bacteremia, subacute bacterial endocarditis, idiopathic thrombocytopenic purpura
	Cyanosis	Hypoxia, congenital heart disease with cerebral embolism, methemoglobinemia
	Erythema	Carbon monoxide, atropine, or mercury intoxication
	Butterfly rash	Lupus erythematosus, tuberous sclerosis
	Desquamation	Vitamin A intoxication, scarlatina
	Nail changes	Splinter hemorrhage—endocarditis
		Mycotic infection and hypoparathyroidism
		Periungual fibroma (tuberous sclerosis)
Breath odor	Fruity	Diabetic ketoacidosis; amyl nitrate, alcohol, isopropyl alcohol poisonings
	Feculent	Hepatic encephalopathy
	Garlic	Selenium toxicity, arsenic poisoning, organophosphate poisoning
	Almonds	Cyanide poisoning
	Wintergreen	Methyl salicylate poisoning
	Ammoniacal	Uremia
	Acrid (pear-like)	Paraldehyde, chloral hydrate poisoning
Scalp	Contusions	Trauma
	Vasodilation	Sagittal sinus thrombosis
Eyes	Chemosis	Cavernous sinus thrombosis
	Periorbital ecchymosis	Blow-out orbital fracture
	Subhyaloid hemorrhage	Subarachnoid hemorrhage
	Vasospasm	Hypertensive encephalopathy
Ears	Hemorrhage	Basilar skull fracture
	Otitis media	Brain abscess, lateral sinus thrombosis
Nose	Cerebrospinal fluid rhinorrhea	Basilar skull fracture
Mouth	Scarred tongue	Seizure disorder
	Pigmentation	Addison disease
	Lead lines	Plumbism (lead intoxication)
Neck	Rigid	Meningitis, pneumonia, subarachnoid hemorrhage, encephalitis
Thyroid	Enlarged	Myxedema, thyrotoxicosis
Heart	Murmur	Subacute endocarditis, brain abscess
Abdomen	Hepatomegaly	Leukemia, hepatic failure, heart failure
Extremities	Fracture	Trauma, fat embolism
	Ecchymosis	Trauma, hemorrhagic diathesis

Adapted from Tait VF, Dean JM, Hanley DF. Evaluation of the comatose child. *In* Rogers MC (ed). Textbook of Pediatric Intensive Care, 2nd ed. Baltimore: Williams & Wilkins, 1992:741.

Table 41-15. Laboratory Evaluation of Metabolic Brain Disease

Test	Reason for Test
Immediate	
Glucose	Hypoglycemia, hyperosmolar coma
Na⁺	Osmolar abnormalities
Ca²⁺	Hypercalcemia or hypocalcemia
BUN	Uremia
Arterial blood pH, PCO₂, PO₂, oxygen saturation	Acidosis, alkalosis, hypoxia, CO or methemoglobin
Lumbar puncture	Infection, hemorrhage, meningeal carcinomatosis
Later	
Liver function tests, ammonia level	Hepatic coma, Reye syndrome, urea cycle defect
Sedative drug levels	Overdose
Blood and CSF culture	Sepsis, encephalitis, meningitis
Full electrolytes, including Mg²⁺	Electrolyte imbalance
Coagulation profile	Intravascular coagulation
EEG	Seizure disorder

Adapted from Plum F. Neurology/sustained impairments of consciousness. *In* Wyngaarden JB, Smith LH, Bennett JC (eds). Cecil Textbook of Medicine, 19th ed. Philadelphia: WB Saunders, 1992:2053.
Abbreviations: BUN = blood urea nitrogen; CSF = cerebrospinal fluid; EEG = electroencephalogram.

Table 41-16. Toxins and Disease States Causing Elevated Anion and/or Osmolal Gaps

Anion Gap	Osmolal Gap
Ethanol	Ethanol
Ethylene glycol	Ethylene glycol
Methanol	Methanol
Toluene	Acetone
Iron	Propylene glycol
Isoniazid	Ethyl ether
Salicylates	Isopropyl alcohol
Paraldehyde	Mannitol
Strychnine	Trichloromethane
Renal failure	Renal failure
Diabetic ketoacidosis	Diabetic ketoacidosis
Lactic acidosis	

diagnosis, the health care provider must have a high index of suspicion of an intoxicated state. Children in certain age groups are statistically at greater risk of being poisoned. Forty-four percent and 59% of all cases of poisonings reported to Poison Control Centers occur in children younger than 3 and 6 years of age, respectively. Intentional ingestions are far more common in adolescents. One's index of suspicion should be heightened not only by the age of the patient but also by the history of the present illness; *a poisoning should be suspected in a previously healthy child who presents with a sudden onset of unexplained symptoms (seizures, mental status changes, vomiting, hematemesis) or a gradual onset of symptoms preceded by a period of confusion or delirium.* A correct diagnosis is usually established by integrating information from the history, physical examination, and ancillary tests and then identifying a *toxidrome,* a symptom complex associated with a given class of ingested drug. The most important aspects of the physical examination to identify a toxidrome are the level of consciousness, the vital signs, and the pupillary examination.

LEVEL OF CONSCIOUSNESS

Table 41-17 lists common agents responsible for different changes in mental status. Toxic exposures may also occur via routes other than the oral route; organophosphates may be absorbed through the skin, whereas other compounds, such as carbon monoxide, are inhaled.

PUPILLARY EXAMINATION

When the pupils are evaluated for size and reactivity, the presence of nystagmus should also be noted (Table 41-18). Most drugs

Table 41-17. Changes in Level of Consciousness Observed with Specific Drug Intoxications

Level of Consciousness			
Coma	*Agitation*	*Confusion and/or Hallucinations*	*Seizures*
Anticholinergics	Sympathomimetics	Anticholinergics	Cocaine
Antihistamines	Methylxanthines	Psychotropics	Amphetamines
Cholinergic agents	Phencyclidine	Lysergic acid diethylamide	Methylxanthines
Sedative-hypnotics	Salicylates	Mescaline	Tricyclic antidepressants
Alcohols	Alcohol	Marijuana	Cholinergic agents
Narcotics		Antihistamines	Neuroleptics
Neuroleptics			Salicylates
Tricyclic antidepressants			Camphor
Phencyclidine			Isoniazid
Salicylates			Phenytoin
Heavy metals			Antihistamines
Hypoxia			
Carbon monoxide			
Cyanide			

Table 41–18. Effect of Drugs on Pupillary Findings

Pupillary Finding		
Dilated	*Constricted*	*Nystagmus*
Sympathomimetics	Narcotics	Barbiturates
Anticholinergics	Phenothiazines	Alcohol
Cocaine	Cholinergic agents	Phenytoin
Tricyclic antidepressants	Benzodiazepines	Carbamazepine
Glutethimide	PCP	PCP
LSD	Clonidine	Glutethimide

Abbreviations: LSD = lysergic acid diethylamide; PCP = phencyclidine piperdine.

cause horizontal nystagmus; however, phenytoin may produce upbeat nystagmus, whereas phencyclidine may cause rotary nystagmus.

TEMPERATURE

Although fever is typically indicative of infection or a metabolic disturbance, such as the hemorrhagic shock and encephalopathy syndrome, many toxic compounds may induce hyperthermia (Table 41–19). The most common causes of fever in intoxicated children include anticholinergic compounds, antihistamines, salicylates, and sympathomimetic agents. Hypothermia may also be a sign of drug exposure (Table 41–20). Sedative-hypnotic agents, including ethanol, are common causes of hypothermia.

HEART RATE AND BLOOD PRESSURE

Bradycardia or tachycardia may result directly from the autonomic effect of a drug or may be a reflex response to a change in

Table 41–19. Compounds and Conditions Inducing Hyperthermia

Muscular Hyperactivity or Rigidity
    Amoxapine
    Amphetamines
    Cocaine
    Ethanol or sedative-hypnotic withdrawal
    Lithium
    LSD
    MAO inhibitors
    Phencyclidine
    Tricyclic antidepressants

Increased Metabolic Rate
    Dinitrophenol
    Pentachlorophenol
    Salicylates
    Thyroid hormone

Impaired Heat Dissipation or Thermoregulation
    Anticholinergic agents
    Antihistamines
    Antipsychotic agents
    Tricyclic antidepressants

Other/Unknown Mechanisms
    Metal fume fever

Adapted from Olson KR, Pentel PR, Kelley MT. Physical assessment and differential diagnosis of the poisoned patient. Med Toxicol 1987;2:40.
Abbreviations: LSD = lysergic acid diethylamide; MAO = monoamine oxidase.

Table 41–20. Compounds and Conditions Inducing Hypothermia

    Ethanol
    Sedative-hypnotic agents (e.g., barbiturates, benzodiazepines)
    Hypoglycemia
    Isopropyl alcohol
    Narcotics
    Phenothiazines
    Tricyclic antidepressants

Adapted from Olson KR, Pentel PR, Kelley MT. Physical assessment and differential diagnosis of the poisoned patient. Med Toxicol 1987;2:41.

blood pressure. Intoxication with a beta blocker, calcium channel blocker, alpha$_2$-adrenergic agonist (clonidine), or a cholinergic agonist (organophosphate) characteristically presents with bradycardia with or without hypertension. In mild clonidine ingestions or in the early stage of a clonidine intoxication, the patient may be hypertensive as a result of the partial alpha$_1$-agonist effect of the drug. Bradycardia may be a reflex response to the precipitation of hypertension by a vasoconstrictor agent, such as an ergotamine or an alpha-adrenergic agonist, such as phenylpropanolamine. On the other hand, beta-adrenergic agonist or anticholinergic agent intoxication usually presents with tachycardia as part of the symptom complex. Intoxication with drugs that possess both alpha- and beta-adrenergic agonist properties may present with both tachycardia and hypertension, whereas several classes of compounds may cause hypotension with a reflex tachycardia. Examples of the latter include direct vasodilators or alpha-adrenergic blockers (hydralazine, phenothiazines, tricyclic antidepressants) and compounds that cause third-space fluid losses (acute iron intoxication). The anticholinergic properties of the phenothiazines and tricyclic antidepressants contribute to the tachycardia seen with these agents. Cholinergic compounds, such as organophosphates and carbamates, may cause tachycardia instead of bradycardia because acetylcholine is the neurotransmitter found at nicotinic receptors in sympathetic chain ganglion.

RESPIRATIONS

Tachypnea or hyperpnea may result from a central effect of a drug (salicylates, methylxanthines) or from a metabolic acidosis (salicylates, alcohols) in addition to structural CNS lesions or

Table 41–21. Skin Manifestations of Intoxication

Manifestation	Toxin/Condition
Bullous lesions	Barbiturates, carbon monoxide, sedative hypnotics, narcotics
Diaphoresis	Cholinergic agents (organophosphates), sympathomimetics, mercury, arsenic, salicylates
Dry skin (and mucous membranes)	Anticholinergics, antihistamines, narcotics
Diffuse erythema	Anticholinergics, carbon monoxide, cyanide, boric acid, mercury
Cyanosis	Hypoxia, methemoglobinemia, ergotamines
Needle tracks	Opiates, phencyclidine, amphetamine

cardiopulmonary compromise. Slow or shallow breathing should always raise the suspicion of drug ingestion, particularly with CNS depressants, such as narcotics and sedative hypnotics. Hypoventilation may also be a presenting symptom of a clonidine overdose as a result of its opiate-like effects. Organophosphate or carbamate intoxications may also present with hypoventilation as a primary symptom as a result of weakness of respiratory muscles.

Odors emanating from the breath or clothing may offer invaluable clues as to the diagnosis. Not only do certain metabolic diseases, such as diabetic ketoacidosis and hepatic failure, produce characteristic breath odors, but so do a number of chemical compounds, including cyanide (bitter almonds); isopropyl alcohol, methanol, salicylate (acetone); methyl salicylate (wintergreen); arsenic, thallium, organophosphates (garlic); turpentine (violets). Inspection of the skin and mucous membranes may also be helpful (Table 41–21).

Although a single sign or symptom may be attributable to many classes of drugs, combinations of symptoms *(toxidrome)* allow one to narrow down the number of possible agents. Sympathomimetic agents, anticholinergics, and tricyclic antidepressants (TCAs) all cause mydriasis and tachycardia. If these symptoms occur in a patient with a prolonged QRS interval on an electrocardiogram, the most likely cause is a tricyclic compound, whereas if the former symptoms occur in a diaphoretic, tremulous patient, a sympathomimetic agent would be suspected. Table 41–22 outlines toxidromes of common classes of compounds ingested by children.

Management of most ingestions includes prevention of further absorption and supportive therapy. The decision to perform gastric decontamination (by inducing emesis, performing gastric lavage, or using activated charcoal) should be individualized. Gastric decontamination should be withheld if a nontoxic substance is ingested, if a nontoxic quantity of a toxic compound is ingested, if absorption is complete, or if a caustic agent is ingested. Under these circumstances, gastric decontamination carries risks but no benefits. Induction of emesis is contraindicated in patients with a depressed mental status or who are at risk for a sudden deterioration of their mental status.

Very few specific antidotes exist for substances that are ingested. If an antidote exists, its use depends on the patient's prognosis if it were not administered. Not all children require treatment with

Table 41–22. Toxidromes of Common Classes of Drugs

Drug Class	Level of Consciousness	Pupils	Vital Signs	Other
Sympathomimetics (amphetamines, cocaine, ephedrine, methylphenidate [Ritalin])	Agitation; psychosis	Dilated	↑ HR; ↑ BP; ↑ T	Tremors, sweating, arrhythmias; seizures
Anticholinergics (antihistamines, scopolamine, atropine, jimson weed, nightshade, phenothiazines, tricyclics)	Confusion; hallucinations	Dilated	↑ HR; ↑ T; ± ↑ BP	Flushed; dry skin and mucous membranes; urinary retention; ↓ bowel sounds
Opiates	Euphoria; coma	Pinpoint	↓ RR; ± ↓ HR; ± ↓ BP	Shallow respirations; dry mucous membranes
Cholinergic syndrome (organophosphates; carbamates, bethanichol, *Amanita* mushrooms)	Coma	Miosis	↓ or ↑ HR; ↓ or ↑ BP	Salivation, lacrimation, urination, defecation; bronchorrhea; muscle twitching before flaccidity; seizures
Sedative-hypnotics (alcohol, barbiturates, benzodiazepines)	Coma	± Miosis	↓ RR—shallow; hypothermia; ↓ BP	Ataxia; nystagmus; slurred speech
Neuroleptics (phenothiazines, butyrophenones)	Coma	Miosis (except thioridazine [Mellaril])	↑ HR; ↓ BP; ↓ T or ↑ T	Dystonic reactions; ataxia; neuroleptic malignant syndrome; prolonged QT
Tricyclic antidepressants	Confusion; agitation; coma	Dilated	↑ HR; ↓ or ↑ BP; ↑ T; ↓ RR	Quinidine-like effect–prolonged QRS or QT interval and ventricular arrhythmias; seizures; anticholinergic effects (see above)
Salicylates	Disorientation; hyperexcitability; coma (severe)	—	↑ T; ↑ RR + depth	Vomiting; tinnitus; metabolic acidosis; hypokalemia
Carbon monoxide	Lethargy; coma	—	—	Headache, nausea, flu-like syndrome, dizziness, blurred vision
Theophylline	Agitation	—	↑ HR; ↓ BP; ± ↑ RR; ± ↑ T	Protracted vomiting; tremors, seizures, arrhythmias
Phencyclidine	Delirium; combativeness; catatonia; coma	Miosis	—	Rotary nystagmus; seizures

Abbreviations: BP = blood pressure; HR = heart rate; RR = respiratory rate; T = temperature.

Table 41–23. Specific Toxins and Their Antidotes

Toxin	Antidote
Acetaminophen	*N*-Acetylcysteine
Anticholinergics	Physostigmine
Arsenic	Dimercaprol
Benzodiazepines	Flumazenil
Beta blockers	Glucagon*
Calcium channel blockers†	Calcium
Carbamate insecticides	Atropine
Carbon monoxide	Oxygen
Cyanide	Amyl nitrite or sodium nitrate + sodium thiosulfate
Digitalis	Digoxin-specific Fab antibody fragments
Ethylene glycol	Ethanol
Heparin	Protamine
Iron	Deferoxamine
Lead	EDTA; dimercaprol; dimercaptosuccinic acid; penicillamine
Mercury	Dimercaprol
Methanol	Ethanol
Narcotics	Naloxone
Nitrites	Methylene blue
Organophosphates	Atropine; pralidoxime
Phenothiazines‡	Diphenhydramine or benztropine
Salicylates	Sodium bicarbonate
Tricyclic antidepressants	Sodium bicarbonate
Warfarin	Vitamin K

*May reverse cardiac toxicity.
†Usually requires saline infusion as well for bradyarrhythmias or conduction abnormalities.
‡Dystonic reactions only.
Abbreviation: EDTA = ethylenediaminetetraacetic acid.

N-acetylcysteine after acetaminophen poisoning. If the patient is asymptomatic and has a serum acetaminophen concentration in a nontoxic range when plotted on the Matthew-Rumack nomogram, *N*-acetylcysteine therapy is not indicated. Table 41–23 presents a partial list of available antidotes. Although not a true antidote, sodium bicarbonate is included as an antidote for salicylate and tricyclic antidepressant ingestions because its use can reduce symptoms by reducing tissue distribution of these compounds.

Some drugs lend themselves to procedures aimed at enhancing drug elimination from the body. These include changing urinary pH (alkalinization to enhance salicylate excretion), using multiple doses of charcoal (theophylline, phenobarbital, carbamazepine), and

Table 41–24. Indications for Extracorporeal Drug Removal*

Patient-Related
   Severe intoxication refractory to medical management (e.g., refractory seizures)
   Impairment of normal excretion routes that may lead to prolonged intoxication

Drug-Related
   Ingestion and probable absorption of a potentially lethal dose determined after gut decontamination
   Documentation of a potentially lethal drug level
   Presence of a significant quantity of a compound that is metabolized to a toxic metabolite (e.g., methanol)

*Patient-related and drug-related criteria for extracorporeal drug removal. Only one criterion needs to be met.

performing extracorporeal drug removal (peritoneal or hemodialysis, charcoal hemoperfusion, exchange transfusion). Either patient-related or drug-related criteria should be met before the institution of extracorporeal drug removal (Table 41–24). When the management approach is not known, a resource such as a poison control center, Poisondex, or a clinical pharmacologist should be consulted.

TRAUMA

Infants with head trauma may have evidence of intracranial hypertension: bulging fontanelle, decerebrate posturing, and tachypnea. The clinical picture in a young infant may be confused with meningitis. *In the absence of a febrile illness, trauma should be suspected and the patient should be treated in accordance with a rapidly progressive intracranial process.*

Serious head injury in infants is most commonly a result of physical abuse (see Chapter 37). Except for uncomplicated skull fractures, 95% of serious intracranial injuries in infants younger than 1 year of age result from child abuse. Approximately 80% of deaths from head injuries in children younger than 2 years of age are due to nonaccidental trauma. The shaken baby syndrome is noted in a child who is usually younger than 6 to 12 months of age (see Chapter 37). The head is relatively large and the neck muscles weak in these infants. The child is typically held by the arms or trunk and is shaken, causing a rapid acceleration and deceleration of the head. This leads to tearing of bridging cerebral veins and development of subdural hematomas. The subdural collections are usually seen bilaterally but may be small over the

Table 41–25. Diagnostic Criteria for Hemorrhagic Shock–Encephalopathy Syndrome

Clinical	Laboratory	Exclusion Criteria
Shock	Falling hemoglobin level (>3 g/dl below admission level)	Known infectious and metabolic disorders
Coma and seizures	Falling platelet count (<150 × 10⁶/L)	Reye syndrome
Bleeding	Prolonged PT and PTT	Toxin-mediated shock syndromes
Diarrhea	Low fibrinogen level	
Oliguria	Elevated fibrin degradation products	
	Elevated blood urea nitrogen concentration	
	Elevated plasma creatinine concentration	
	Elevated aspartate aminotransferase and alanine aminotransferase levels	
	Metabolic acidosis	

Adapted from Levin M, Pincott JR, Hjelm M, et al. Hemorrhagic shock and encephalopathy: Clinical, pathologic, and biochemical features. J Pediatr 1989;144:195.
Abbreviations: PT = prothrombin time; PTT = partial thromboplastin time.

convexities of the brain. A more common CT finding is a subdural collection of blood in the interhemispheric fissure in the parietal and occipital region. Subdural hematomas are invariably the result of trauma in infants. If they result from birth trauma, the infant is symptomatic within 24 to 48 hours of delivery. Therefore, a subdural hematoma in a previously asymptomatic infant is not a "chronic" subdural hematoma from birth trauma.

Approximately 50% of children present without an antecedent history to explain the clinical findings; 10% have a history of a minor fall, 10% have seizures, and 10% present in respiratory arrest. There are often no external signs of trauma, and the only findings on physical examination are retinal hemorrhages and signs of raised intracranial pressure, particularly a bulging fontanelle. Retinal hemorrhages have been seen in 75% to 90% of cases. Some infants may present with less severe injuries and more subtle symptoms, such as poor feeding, lethargy or irritability, and vomiting.

In suspected cases of physical abuse a careful search for other injuries should be undertaken both by physical examination and radiography (see Chapter 37).

HEMORRHAGIC SHOCK–ENCEPHALOPATHY

Hemorrhagic shock–encephalopathy (HSE) is characterized by the sudden onset of encephalopathy, shock, seizures, coagulopathy, bleeding, and hepatic and renal impairment in young children. Table 41–25 outlines diagnostic criteria for HSE, which has been reported in patients from 17 days of age to 15 years. The median age of onset is 5 months, with 87% of cases occurring before 1 year of age. There is no seasonal or geographical variation. The clinical course is usually fulminant with profound disseminated intravascular coagulation and bleeding from all venipuncture sites. The shock state is severe resulting in extreme metabolic acidosis. Renal and hepatic failure develop, and the patients often succumb to cerebral edema with subsequent herniation. The mortality rate is 60% to 70%, and most survivors have a poor neurologic outcome.

The etiology is unknown. A viral etiology has been postulated, but no pathogens have been isolated. The occurrence of high fever in most patients has raised the question of thermal stress as a trigger of this syndrome in susceptible hosts. The high temperatures may also indicate a relationship to myopathic processes, such as malignant hyperthermia or neuroleptic malignant syndrome.

METABOLIC DISORDERS

Inborn errors of metabolism are complex and encompass many conditions. Table 41–26 presents a partial list of inborn errors of metabolism that may present in the neonate with lethargy, seizures, and coma. The clinical manifestations of metabolic disease in the

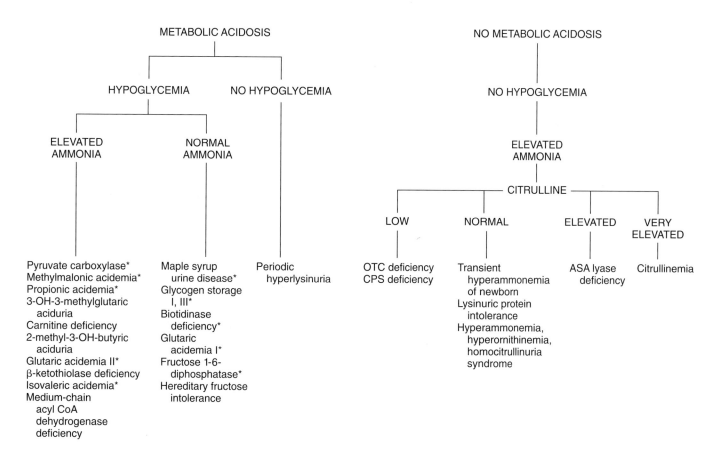

*Ketonuria.

Figure 41–7. An approach to evaluation of metabolic disorders in which symptoms are similar to those of Reye syndrome. In disorders with metabolic acidosis, the most useful diagnostic test is evaluation of organic acids. In the second group, plasma amino acids are most helpful. ASA = argininosuccinic acid; CPS = carbamoyl phosphate synthetase. OTC = ornithine transcarbamoylase. (Adapted from Green CL, Blitzer MG, Shapira E. Inborn errors of metabolism and Reye syndrome: Differential diagnosis. J Pediatr 1988;113:156.)

Table 41–26. Inborn Errors of Metabolism Presenting with Seizures, Lethargy, and Coma in the Neonatal Period

Disorders of Carbohydrate Metabolism	Disorders of Amino Acid Metabolism	Organic Acidemias	Urea Cycle Defects	Lysosomal Storage Disorders	Other
Fructose-1, 6-biphosphatase deficiency	Maple syrup urine disease	Methylmalonicacidemia	Carbamyl phosphate synthetase deficiency	Farber disease	Congenital adrenal hyperplasia
Galactosemia	Hypervalinemia	Propionicacidemia (ketotic hyperglycinemia)	Ornithine transcarbamylase deficiency	Fucosidosis	Hypophosphatasia
Hereditary fructose intolerance	Periodic hyperlysinemia	Isovalericacidemia	Citrullinemia		Menkes kinky hair syndrome
Glycogen storage disease, types I and III	Hyper-β-alaninemia	3-Methylcrotonyl CoA carboxylase deficiency	Argininosuccinicaciduria		Hereditary oroticaciduria
Pyruvate carboxylase deficiency	Nonketotic hyperglycinemia	Multiple carboxylase deficiency			Fatty acyl-CoA dehydrogenase deficiencies
Phosphoenolpyruvate carboxykinase deficiency	Pyroglutamic aciduria	Multiple acyl-CoA dehydrogenase deficiencies			Primary systemic carnitine deficiency
	Hyperornithemia-hyperammonemia-homocitrullinuria (HHH) syndrome	Hydroxymethylglutaryl (HMG)-CoA lyase deficiency			Zellweger syndrome
	Lysinuric protein intolerance	2-Methyl-3-hydroxybutyricacidemia			Neonatal adrenoleukodystrophy
	Methylenetetrahydrofolate reductase deficiency	D-Glycericacidemia			
	Sulfite oxidase deficiency				

Adapted from Burton BK. Inborn errors of metabolism: The clinical diagnosis in early infancy. Pediatrics 1987;79:359.
Abbreviation: CoA = coenzyme A.

Table 41-27. Clinical Manifestations of Inborn Errors of Metabolism in the Neonatal Period

Lethargy
Coma
Seizures
Increased or decreased muscle tone
Poor suck and feeding
Vomiting
Diarrhea
Tachypnea and/or hyperpnea
Respiratory failure
Jaundice
Unusual odors
Cardiomegaly
Hepatomegaly

Table 41-29. Laboratory Evaluation of Suspected Metabolic Disease

Plasma ammonia
Arterial blood gas
Plasma amino acids
Plasma carnitine
Plasma pyruvate and lactate
Urinary amino acids
Urinary organic acids

neonate can be nonspecific (Table 41–27). The infants are often thought to have sepsis and are evaluated and treated for presumptive infection. The presence of a documented infection does not preclude metabolic disease because these infants are prone to infection (galactosemia and *Escherichia coli* sepsis). A family history of a previous infant dying from an unexplained illness or other children in the family with neurologic disorders may provide clues to a metabolic etiology. Laboratory abnormalities that may be seen in metabolic disease are listed in Table 41–28.

Infants with *urea cycle defects* often manifest altered mental status, coma (recurrent), and emesis and cannot metabolize ammonia to urea, leading to accumulation of ammonia in the blood. These disorders are inherited as autosomal recessive traits, except for ornithine transcarbamoylase (OTC) deficiency, which is X-linked. Carbamyl phosphate and ornithine cannot be metabolized to citrulline in the absence of the enzyme OTC. In this defect, carbamyl phosphate is shunted to produce orotic acid, which is detected in the urine, and plasma citrulline levels are low or absent.

The keys to the diagnosis of inborn errors of metabolism in the neonate are a high degree of suspicion, the appropriate screening studies, and if the results are positive, a more detailed laboratory evaluation under the guidance of a specialist in metabolic diseases (Table 41–29).

Metabolic encephalopathy resulting from inborn errors of metabolism (partial, incomplete, stress, or fasting exacerbated) or from renal, hepatic, or toxic causes may also manifest in older children or adolescents. There may or may not be a family history or personal history of recurrent lethargy, emesis, repeated hospitalizations, or personality changes. Encephalopathy in older patients that results from endogenous (ammonia, organic acids, hypoglycemia, urea) or exogenous substances (opiates, barbiturates) may manifest within a wide range of symptoms (Table 41–30). The electroencephalograph may be of value in addition to the screening and specific tests noted in Tables 41–15, 41–28, and Figure 41–7 (see p. 659).

REYE SYNDROME

Reye syndrome is classically seen within 2 weeks after a prodromal viral infection, such as varicella, influenza B, or influenza A. There is a strong association between aspirin use and Reye syndrome, which led to the warning against the use of aspirin in children and adolescents. Reye syndrome can be seen in children of any age and has a peak incidence between ages 5 and 15 years. This syndrome is usually heralded by the abrupt onset of repeated vomiting, followed by combativeness and mental status changes, which can range from delirium to coma. Cerebral edema and increased intracranial pressure can develop. The mortality is high; death is usually secondary to cerebral herniation or myocardial depression from drugs used to treat intracranial hypertension.

Laboratory studies reveal an elevated serum ammonia concentration and elevated hepatic enzyme levels. The serum ammonia level may be initially normal, particularly during stage I (see Table 41–6). The patients may also be hypoglycemic and have a metabolic acidosis. Patients with Reye syndrome have microvesicular fatty metamorphosis of the liver, with swelling and disruption of hepatic mitochondria.

The incidence of Reye syndrome has decreased dramatically in the 1980s and it is now an uncommon diagnosis. Reye syndrome should be thought of as a syndrome and not as a specific disease. A distinct etiologic factor has not been discovered, but the syndrome may represent a response to several different insults in susceptible hosts. Many genetic metabolic diseases may present with a picture similar to that of Reye syndrome. Although inborn errors of metabolism usually present in infancy, some may present later. Findings of hypoglycemia, acidosis, or hyperammonemia in any patient with altered mental status should lead one to consider a metabolic etiology. Figure 41–7 outlines an approach to the patient who presents with mental status changes, vomiting, and a Reye-like illness. Additional causes of hyperammonemia are valproic acid–induced hyperammonemia and the rare syndrome of elevated ammonia seen after high-dose chemotherapy for malignancy.

Table 41-28. Laboratory Evidence of Metabolic Disease

Acidosis,* alkalosis
Hypoglycemia
Hyperammonemia
Elevated liver enzyme levels
Direct hyperbilirubinemia
Urine-reducing substance
Urine ketones

*High anion gap if increased organic acids (ketoacids, lactic acid) are produced. Normal anion gap if associated renal tubular acidosis (type I glycogen storage disease, galactosemia) is present.

Table 41-30. Characteristics of Metabolic Encephalopathy

Confusion, lethargy, delirium often precede or replace coma
Motor signs, if present, usually symmetric
Bilateral asterixis, myoclonus appear
Pupillary reactions usually preserved; tonic calorics often present
Sensory abnormalities usually absent
Hypothermia common
Abnormal signs reflect incomplete brain dysfunction at multiple anatomical levels

From Plum F. Neurology/sustained impairments of consciousness. *In* Wyngaarden JB, Smith LH, Bennet JC (eds). Cecil Textbook of Medicine, 19th ed. Philadelphia: WB Saunders, 1992:2052.

Table 41–31. Criteria for Diagnosis of Brain Death

1. **Nature and duration of coma must be known**
   a. Known structural disease or irreversible systemic metabolic cause
   b. No chance of drug intoxication or hypothermia; no paralyzing or potentially anesthetizing drugs recently given for treatment
   c. Body temperature must be above 34°C
   d. Hypotension excluded
   e. Six-hour observation of no brain function is sufficient in cases of known structural cause when no drug or alcohol is involved in causation or treatment; otherwise, 12 hours plus negative drug screen required (24 hours with anoxic injury). Observation period may be shortened with the use of a confirmatory test (EEG, cerebral perfusion scan)
2. **Absence of cerebral and brain stem function**
   a. No behavioral or reflex response to noxious stimuli above foramen magnum level including absent corneal, gag and cough reflexes
   b. Midposition or fully dilated fixed pupils
   c. No oculovestibular response to 50 ml ice water calories
   d. Apneic off ventilator with oxygenation for 10 minutes with arterial $pCO_2 \geq 60$ mmHg
   e. Systemic circulation may be intact
   f. Purely spinal reflexes may be retained
3. **Supplementary (optional) criteria**
   a. EEG isoelectric for 30 minutes at maximal gain
   b. Brain stem–evoked responses reflect absent function in vital brain stem structures
   c. No cerebral circulation present on angiographic examination or cerebral perfusion scan

Modified from Plum F. Neurology/brain death. *In* Wyngaarden JB, Smith LH, Bennett JC (eds). Cecil Textbook of Medicine, 19th ed. Philadelphia: WB Saunders, 1992:2059.
Abbreviation: EEG = electroencephalogram.

SUMMARY AND RED FLAGS

Delirium and coma are common and potentially serious manifestations of a diverse group of life-threatening but potentially reversible disorders. Common causes vary by age, but toxic ingestion, trauma, seizures (postictal), infections, and metabolic disturbances, including inborn errors of metabolism, must be considered. Red flags include family or personal histories compatible with these disorders, signs of increased intracranial pressure, rapidly progressive rostral-caudal deterioration, and the eventual determination of brain death (Table 41–31).

REFERENCES

Coma Scales

Fenichel GM (ed). Altered states of consciousness. *In* Clinical Pediatric Neurology: A Signs and Symptoms Approach. Philadelphia: WB Saunders, 1988:42.

Lieh-Lai MW, Theodorou AA, Sarnaik AP, et al. Limitations of the Glasgow Coma Scale in predicting outcome in children with traumatic brain injury. J Pediatr 1992;120:195.

Rowley G, Fielding K. Reliability and accuracy of the Glasgow Coma Scale with experienced and inexperienced users. Lancet 1991;337:535.

Simpson D, Reilly P. Pediatric coma scale. Lancet 1982;2:450.

Simpson DA, Cockington RA, Hanieh A, et al. Head injuries in infants and young children: The value of the Pediatric Coma Scale. Childs Nerv Syst 1991;7:183.

Teasdale G, Jennett B. Assessment of coma and impaired consciousness: A practical scale. Lancet 1974;2:81.

Yager JY, Johnston B, Seshia S. Coma scales in pediatric practice. Am J Dis Child 1990;144:1088.

Differential Diagnosis

Huff JS, Montes J. Coma. *In* Reisdorff EJ, Roberts MR (eds). Pediatric Emergency Medicine. Philadelphia: WB Saunders, 1993:1015.

Plum F, Posner JB. The pathologic physiology of signs and symptoms of coma. *In* Plum F, Posner JB. The Diagnosis of Stupor and Coma. Philadelphia: FA Davis, 1982:1.

Seshia SS, Seshia MMK, Sachdeva RK. Coma in childhood. Dev Med Child Neurol 1977;19:614.

Vannucci RC, Wasiewski WW. Diagnosis and management of coma in children. *In* Pellock JM, Myer EC (eds). Neurologic Emergencies in Infancy and Childhood, 2nd ed. Stoneham: Butterworth-Heinemann, 1993:103.

Approach To Coma

Bates D. The management of medical coma. J Neurol Neurosurg Psychiatry 1993;56:589.

Chamberlain JM. Algorithm for pediatric trauma. *In* Eichelberger MR (ed). Pediatric Trauma: Prevention, Acute Care, Rehabilitation. St. Louis: Mosby–Year Book, 1993:145.

Feigen RD. Central nervous system infections, bacterial meningitis beyond the neonatal period. *In* Feigin RD, Cherry JD (eds). Textbook of Pediatric Infectious Diseases, 3rd ed. Philadelphia: WB Saunders, 1992:401.

Geiseler JP, Nelson KE, Levin S, et al. Community-acquired purulent meningitis: A review of 1,316 cases during the antibiotic era, 1954–1976. Rev Infect Dis 1980;2:725.

Malouf R, Brust JCM. Hypoglycemia: Causes, neurological manifestations, and outcome. Ann Neurol 1985;17:421.

Toxicology

Fine JS, Goldfrank LR. Update in medical toxicology. Pediatr Clin North Am 1992;39:1031.

Fleisher GR, Kearney TE, Henretig F, et al. Gastric decontamination in the poisoned patient. Pediatr Emerg Care 1991;7:378.

Goldberg MJ, Spector R, Park GD, et al. An approach to the management of the poisoned patient. Arch Intern Med 1986;146:1381.

Litovitz TL, Holm MA, Clancy C, et al. 1992 annual report of the American Association of Poison Control Centers Toxic Exposure Surveillance System. Am J Emerg Med 1993;11:494.

Nice A, Leikin JB, Maturen A, et al. Toxidrome recognition to improve efficiency of emergency urine drug screens. Ann Emerg Med 1988;17:676.

Olson KR, Pentel PR, Kelley MT. Physical assessment and differential diagnosis of the poisoned patient. Med Toxicol 1987;2:52.

Trauma

Billmire ME, Myers PA. Serious head injury in infants: Accident or abuse. Pediatrics 1985;75:340.

Bruce DA, Zimmerman RA. Shaken impact syndrome. Pediatr Ann 1989;18:482.

Committee on Child Abuse and Neglect. Shaken baby syndrome: Inflicted cerebral trauma. Pediatrics 1993;92:872.

Hemorrhagic Shock–Encephalopathy

Bowham JR, Meeks A, Levin M, et al. Complete recovery from hemorrhagic shock and encephalopathy. J Pediatr 1992;120:440.

Chesney JP, Chesney RW. Hemorrhagic shock and encephalopathy: Reflections about a new devastating disorder that affects normal children. J Pediatr 1989;114:254.

Levin M, Pincott JR, Hjelm M, et al. Hemorrhagic shock and encephalopathy: Clinical, pathologic, and biochemical features. J Pediatr 1989;114:194.

Inborn Errors of Metabolism

Burton BK. Inborn errors of metabolism: The clinical diagnosis in early infancy. Pediatrics 1987;79:359.

Rizzo WB, Kaplowitz PB. Metabolic and endocrine disorders. *In* Pellock

JM, Meyer EC (eds). Neurologic Emergencies in Infancy and Childhood, 2nd ed. Stoneham: Butterworth-Heinemann, 1993:344.

Reye Syndrome

Consensus conference. [NIH] Diagnosis and treatment of Reye's syndrome. JAMA 1981;246:2441.

Greene CL, Blitzer MG, Shapira E. Inborn errors of metabolism and Reye syndrome: Differential diagnosis. J Pediatr 1988;113:156.

Reye RDK, Morgan G, Baral J. Encephalopathy and fatty degeneration of the viscera: A disease entity in childhood. Lancet 1963;2:749.

Tasker RC, Dean JM, Rogers MC. Reye syndrome and metabolic encephalopathies. *In* Rogers MC (ed). Textbook of Pediatric Intensive Care, 2nd ed. Baltimore: Williams & Wilkins, 1992:778.

42 Stroke in Childhood

Michael J. Rivkin

Most cases of acute lateralized body weakness result from abnormalities of the blood supply to a portion of the central nervous system. *Stroke* serves as a term to denote the sudden onset of symptoms attributable to such an interruption of cerebral or spinal perfusion.

Childhood stroke has been reported in all racial and ethnic groups and occurs with an incidence of 2.5 cases per 100,000 population per year. The sequelae are not trivial. In addition to lasting lateralized weakness, learning disabilities, disturbances of language, visual deficits, and seizures may persist.

Brain damage resulting from stroke occurs in one of two general forms:

1. *Ischemia* consists of inadequate brain or spinal cord perfusion with consequent dearth of oxygen or other blood-delivered substances necessary for normal metabolic function.

2. *Hemorrhage* occurs when blood is released into the extravascular cranial space. In this circumstance, focal injury of brain or spinal tissue occurs as a result of pressure exerted by the space-occupying mass of blood.

Ischemic injury of brain occurs as a result of one of three mechanisms:

● Embolism
● Thrombosis or
● Diminished systemic perfusion

Embolic damage to brain occurs when material formed at a site in the vascular system proximal to brain lodges in a blood vessel, thus blocking cerebral perfusion. Emboli originate most commonly from the heart, arising from a thrombus on cardiac chamber walls or from vegetations on valve leaflets. Artery-to-artery emboli are composed of clot or platelet aggregates that originate in vessels proximal to brain but ultimately come to rest and to occlude flow in vessels critical for cerebral perfusion. Systemic vein–to–cerebral artery emboli (paradoxical emboli) are possible in the presence of right-to-left shunts with cyanotic congenital heart disease or a patent foramen ovale.

Thrombosis denotes vascular occlusion due to a localized process within a blood vessel or vessels. Although atherosclerosis underlies most thrombotic processes affecting adults, it is not common in children. Localized luminal clot formation occurs in polycythemia or in a hypercoagulable state. Alternatively, anatomic abnormalities may lead to clot formation or mechanical obstruction as is found in fibromuscular dysplasia, arteritis (vasculitis), or arterial dissection.

If *systemic pressure declines* enough to compromise cerebral perfusion, the central nervous system may sustain injury due to diminished perfusion. Cardiac pump failure (congenital heart disease or its surgical repair) and systemic hypotension due to hypovolemia represent common causes of hypotensive cerebral ischemic injury. With diminished cerebral perfusion, brain injury is more diffuse than the more focal injuries characteristic of thrombotic and embolic cerebral events.

Intracranial *hemorrhage* arises in one of two neuropathologic patterns.

1. *Subarachnoid* hemorrhage occurs when blood flows from the intracranial vascular bed and onto the surface of the brain to mix with cerebrospinal fluid in the subarachnoid space. The most common source of such intracranial bleeding in early childhood is an arteriovenous malformation. Ruptured intracranial aneurysms also cause subarachnoid hemorrhage, especially in older children.

2. *Intracerebral* hemorrhage denotes bleeding into the parenchyma of the brain. Severity and region of deficits consequent to intraparenchymal hemorrhage are determined by the extent and location of bleeding in the brain.

The location or focality of the resultant deficit after a stroke depends on whether the event occurred in cortex, subcortical areas, brainstem, or cerebellum. Although many strokes result in permanent deficits, some cause only temporary ones. *Transient ischemic attacks* (TIAs) are brief episodes of focal, nonconvulsive neurologic deficit attributable to interruption of cerebral perfusion. Similar to stroke, the onset is abrupt. However, the episode must last less than 24 hours; recovery must be complete. Progression of symptoms marks stroke when the underlying process, either ischemia or hemorrhage, widens its central nervous system domain with resultant expansion of symptoms and signs.

Whether short-lived or fixed, deficits are commonly motor. Loss of strength may occur as a lateralized weakness involving one half of the body *(hemiparesis)* or as complete loss of strength *(hemiplegia)*. *Diparesis* or *diplegia* involves weakness of the legs and is found primarily in premature infants who have suffered bilateral hypoxic-ischemic brain injury, in term neonates after intracranial hemorrhage that has led to posthemorrhagic hydrocephalus, and in children suffering spinal cord injury below the neck. Involvement of cerebellum often manifests as gait ataxia or impairment of fine motor coordination. Stroke occurring in brainstem is reflected by cranial nerve dysfunction in the distribution of the vascular event. If sensory or motor long tracts running between brain and spinal cord are involved, dysfunction of these systems may be involved.

Distinction among the three processes underlying stroke—embolism, thrombosis, and hemorrhage—is possible using clinical features (Table 42–1). Thrombotic strokes are often heralded by TIAs. The episode frequently bears a stepwise tempo, and neurologic symptoms may appear haltingly. The cerebrospinal profile is normal. Embolic strokes are infrequently preceded by TIAs. Onset of the episode is abrupt, and neurologic symptoms are manifested immediately. A mild to moderate headache may accompany neurologic symptoms. Lumbar puncture yields normal cerebrospinal fluid. Intracerebral hemorrhage is frequently marked by headache. Severe headache of sudden onset marks subarachnoid hemorrhage, in particular. Prodromal symptoms generally do not occur. However, previous seizures may suggest the existence of an arteriovenous malformation, while previous episodes of headache may be attributable to leaks from intracranial aneurysms. Consciousness is often lost, although it may be regained after a short while. Cerebrospinal fluid is bloody if subarachnoid hemorrhage has occurred or if intraparenchymal bleeding reaches the ventricular system.

The signs of stroke found on physical examination often reflect interruption of the motor pathways extending from cortical upper motor neurons to the spinal cord lower motor neuron, the anterior horn cell. "Upper motor neuron" motor deficits seen in stroke patients may result from events occurring at any of several levels in the central nervous system: cerebral cortex, subcortical white matter, brainstem, or spinal cord. Despite the vast neurologic terrain in which stroke may occur, characteristics common to its occurrence at each of these locations can be found. A group of muscles is always involved. Never are individual muscles affected in isolation. The group of muscles affected may initially be flaccid and powerless, but the paralysis is rarely permanently complete.

Spasticity serves as the chronic functional manifestation of upper motor neuron injury due to stroke. The *antigravity muscles*, con-sisting of arm flexors and leg extensors, are most commonly affected. As a result, arms assume a position of flexion and pronation while legs become extended and adducted. If the involved extremity is rapidly moved so that the affected muscles are quickly stretched, a short interval of free movement occurs until an abrupt catch is encountered, eventually to give way grudgingly to progressively easier passive movement *(clasp-knife rigidity)*. Enhancement of deep tendon reflex response has been attributed to the interruption of descending inhibitory pathways as well as to increased activity of the gamma neuron reflex loop.

Clonus, repetitive muscle contraction in response to tendon percussion or stretch, further reflects the enhanced response of tendon reflexes resulting from upper motor neuron injury in stroke. Reflex elicitation at one point, such as at the bicep, may provoke reflex responses in adjacent muscle groups such as brachioradialis or finger reflexes. Such *spread* of reflex responsiveness is commonly seen in patients whose upper motor neuron pathways have been injured by stroke. Features of upper motor neuron injury are compared with those of lower motor neuron injury in Chapter 39.

The causes of stroke in children differ from those in adults. Stroke in adults is associated largely with hypertension or atherosclerosis and their respective hemorrhagic and ischemic consequences. Stroke in children is more commonly caused by or related to congenital heart disease, infection, metabolic disorders, hematologic diatheses, and collagen-vascular disease (Table 42–2). Nonetheless, despite the most thorough evaluation, etiology escapes detection in 25% to 33% of pediatric patients.

THE SETTINGS OF STROKE IN CHILDREN

The neonatal (Table 42–3) and adolescent age groups each carry risks for stroke not shared equally by the large number of children whose ages lie between 1 and 13 years. The clinical presentations and causes of stroke are best considered with respect to each of three pediatric age groups: neonates, children between 1 and 13 years of age, and adolescents.

Neonates

HYPOXIC-ISCHEMIC ENCEPHALOPATHY

Brain injury consequent to asphyxia, hypoxia, or ischemia is an important cause of neonatal neurologic morbidity. Tissue oxygen deficiency is presumed to underlie the neurologic injury caused by

Table 42–1. Stroke in Children: Characteristics of Stroke by Mechanism

Mechanism	Onset	Pace of Deficit Onset	Location	TIAs	Neck Pain*	Headache	Impaired Consciousness
Embolism	Sudden	Abrupt	Remote site of origin	Rare	None	Common	Seldom found unless infarction is large
Thrombosis	During sleep or in the setting of hypotension	Stepwise	*In situ*	Yes	None	Rare	Unusual
Hemorrhage	Rapid	Abrupt or rapid in progression	In subarachnoid space or in brain parenchyma	None	Yes	Yes	Frequent in subarachnoid hemorrhage and in large parenchymal hemorrhages

*Meningismus.
Abbreviation: TIAs = transient ischemic attacks.

Table 42–2. Causes of Stroke in Children

I. **Cardiac Disease**
  A. Congenital
    1. Aortic stenosis
    2. Mitral stenosis
    3. Ventricular septal defects
    4. Patent ductus arteriosus
    5. Cyanotic congenital heart disease involving right-to-left shunt
  B. Acquired
    1. Endocarditis
    2. Kawasaki disease
    3. Cardiomyopathy
    4. Atrial myxoma
    5. Arrhythmia
    6. Paradoxical emboli through patent foramen ovale
    7. Rheumatic fever
    8. Prosthetic heart valve
II. **Hematologic Abnormalities**
  A. Hemoglobinopathies
    1. Sickle cell (SS) disease
    2. Sickle (SC) disease
  B. Polycythemia
  C. Leukemia/lymphoma
  D. Thrombocytopenia
  E. Thrombocytosis
  F. Disorders of coagulation
    1. Protein C deficiency
    2. Protein S deficiency
    3. Factor V resistance to activated protein C
    4. Antithrombin III deficiency
    5. Lupus anticoagulant
    6. Oral contraceptive pill use
    7. Pregnancy and the postpartum state
    8. Disseminated intravascular coagulation
    9. Paroxysmal nocturnal hemoglobinuria
    10. Inflammatory bowel disease (thrombosis)

III. **Inflammatory Disorders**
  A. Meningitis
    1. Viral
    2. Bacterial
    3. Tuberculosis
  B. Systemic infection
    1. Viremia
    2. Bacteremia
    3. Local head and neck infections
  C. Drug-induced inflammation
    1. Amphetamine
    2. Cocaine
  D. Autoimmune disease
    1. Systemic lupus erythematosus
    2. Juvenile rheumatoid arthritis
    3. Takayasu arteritis
    4. Mixed connective tissue disease
    5. Polyarteritis nodosum
    6. Primary CNS vasculitis
IV. **Metabolic Disease Associated with Stroke**
  A. Homocystinuria
  B. Pseudoxanthoma elasticum
  C. Fabry disease
  D. Sulfite oxidase deficiency
  E. Mitochondrial disorders
    1. MELAS
    2. Leigh syndrome
V. **Intracerebral Vascular Processes**
  A. Ruptured aneurysm
  B. Arteriovenous malformation
  C. Fibromuscular dysplasia
  D. Moyamoya disease
  E. Migraine headache
  F. Postsubarachnoid hemorrhage vasospasm
  G. Hereditary hemorrhagic telangiectasia
  H. Sturge-Weber syndrome
  I. Carotid artery dissection
VI. **Trauma and Other External Causes**
  A. Child abuse
  B. Head trauma/neck trauma
  C. Oral trauma
  D. Placental embolism
  E. ECMO therapy

Abbreviations: ECMO = extracorporeal membrane oxygenation; MELAS = mitochondrial encephalomyopathy, lactic acidosis, and stroke; CNS = central nervous system.

hypoxic-ischemic insults. An oxygen deficit may be incurred by either *hypoxemia* or *ischemia.* Hypoxemia is defined as a diminished oxygen content of blood. Ischemia is characterized by reduced blood perfusion in a particular tissue bed. Commonly, hypoxemia and ischemia occur simultaneously or in sequence. Ischemia is likely to be the more important of these two insults.

Asphyxia denotes an impairment in gas exchange, which results not only in a deficit of oxygen in blood but also in an excess of carbon dioxide and thereby acidosis. Further, sustained asphyxia usually results in hypotension and ischemia, consistent with the likely predominant importance of ischemia as the final common pathway to brain injury. Asphyxia is the most common clinical insult resulting in brain injury during the perinatal period.

Evidence of hypoxic-ischemic injury to the neonatal nervous system is reflected by a constellation of signs noticed early in the postpartum period (hypoxic-ischemic encephalopathy [HIE]). The asphyxiating event or events may occur at any point in the ante-, intra-, or postpartum periods. On the basis of admittedly imprecise historical data, it has been concluded that insults sustained by the fetus during the antepartum period account for approximately 20% of cases of HIE. Maternal cardiac arrest or hemorrhage leading to transplacental and fetal hypotension represents such prenatal insults. Intrapartum events, such as abruptio placentae, uterine rupture, and traumatic delivery, may account for 35% of cases of HIE. In an additional 35% of infants displaying signs of HIE, markers of intrapartum fetal distress and antepartum risk, such as maternal diabetes, intrauterine growth retardation, or maternal infection, are found. Postpartum difficulties, such as cardiovascular compromise, persistent fetal circulation, and recurrent apnea, account for approximately 10% of HIE cases. Postpartum difficulties are found more commonly in premature than in term infants. Therefore, for at least 65% of cases of neonatal HIE, difficulties of the intrapartum period alone do not explain the encephalopathy.

Recognition of neonatal HIE requires careful observation and examination of the newborn in the context of a detailed history of pregnancy, labor, and delivery. Newborns who have sustained hypoxic-ischemic insults severe enough to cause permanent neurologic injury usually demonstrate abnormalities on neurologic exam-

Table 42–3. Causes of Stroke in Neonates

1. Hypoxic-ischemic encephalopathy
2. Cerebral venous thrombosis
3. Congenital coagulopathies, including hypercoagulable states
4. Intracranial hemorrhage
5. Intraventricular hemorrhage
6. Polycythemia
7. Familial porencephaly
8. Organic acidemias
   a. Methylmalonic acidemia
   b. Propionic acidemia
   c. Isovaleric acidemia
9. Unknown presumed emboli (placental, patent ductus arteriosus) of *in utero* onset

ination. Nonetheless, if the hypoxic-ischemic damage has occurred well in advance of parturition, it may be asymptomatic in the neonate.

Mild HIE (stage 1) may be characterized by hyperalertness or by mild depression of the level of consciousness, which may be accompanied by uninhibited Moro and brisk deep tendon reflexes, signs of sympathetic activity (dilated pupils), and a normal or only slightly abnormal electroencephalogram (EEG). Typically, these symptoms last less than 24 hours. Moderate encephalopathy (stage 2) may be marked by obtundation, hypotonia, diminished number of spontaneous movements, and seizures. Infants with severe HIE (stage 3) are ill for greater than 24 hours and are comatose. In addition, they are markedly hypotonic and display bulbar and autonomic dysfunction. The EEG is abnormal and may demonstrate a burst-suppression pattern or seizures, or it may be isoelectric.

Neonates with moderate or severe HIE may show variation in level of consciousness during the first days after birth. Initially, depression of level of alertness may appear to improve after the first 12 to 24 hours of life. However, specific signs of improving alertness such as visual fixation or following are lacking. In addition, other persistent or progressive neurologic deficits, as well as functional deterioration of other extraneural systems, are inconsistent with a true improvement in neurologic state. Coma may persist, supervene, or even progress to brain death by 72 hours of life. If the infant survives through 72 hours without losing all cerebral function, a variable amount of improvement may be observed.

Diffuse hypotonia accompanied by a dearth of movement constitutes the most frequently observed motor deficit found early in the course of neonatal HIE. By the end of the first day, patterns of weakness may emerge that reflect the distribution of cerebral injury from a generalized hypoxic-ischemic insult. Term infants may demonstrate quadriparesis with predominant proximal limb weakness. This pattern of weakness derives from ischemia in the watershed or parasagittal regions of brain, which correspond to the border zones of circulation between the anterior and the middle cerebral arteries and the middle and the posterior cerebral arteries. Premature infants may have weakness primarily in the lower extremities because of perinatal ischemic injury of motor fibers subserving the legs. These fibers lie dorsal and lateral to the external angles of the lateral ventricles. Focal injury consequent to focal ischemia (stroke) may result in focal deficits reflective of the vascular territory in which the injury has occurred. These patterns are relatively subtle. As many as 70% of infants with moderate or severe HIE experience seizures by the end of the first day of life.

Focal and multifocal ischemic brain injury may occur during the perinatal period. Such injury, most often infarction, occurs in a vascular distribution. Prenatal cerebral infarctions have been identified by intrauterine ultrasonography. In one autopsy study of neonates, 32 of 592 (5%) infants had cerebral infarcts. Among neonates surviving only a few hours after birth, several had infarcts with subacute or chronic histologic characteristics, indicating that the ischemic insult occurred before parturition. Focal seizures are the heralding sign of neonatal stroke. While clinical signs corresponding to the area of infarction are expected, they may be absent. Neonatal strokes may follow uneventful deliveries and may occur in otherwise normal infants. Stroke may accompany asphyxia, coagulopathy, polycythemia, and sepsis. A predilection for these ischemic lesions to occur in the territory of the middle cerebral artery, especially the left, has been noted and remains unexplained.

A direct relationship between motor and cognitive deficits at 1 year of age and the severity of acidosis observed at birth in asphyxiated and symptomatic neonates has been described. The extent of these sequelae is dependent not only on the occurrence of asphyxia but also on its duration. The three stages of HIE also correlate with outcome at 1 year of age. Those neonates with mild (stage 1) HIE or those who demonstrate moderate (stage 2) HIE for less than 5 days usually develop normally. Persistence of moderate encephalopathy or appearance of severe (stage 3) HIE is associated with seizures and motor and cognitive delay during follow-up. Children with mild HIE as neonates tend to be free of handicap in motor, cognitive, and school performance. Greater impairment of performance in each of these developmental spheres is found among children who exhibit moderate or severe neonatal HIE.

The likelihood of long-term neurologic sequelae after HIE is increased by the presence of neonatal seizures. Electroencephalography may provide valuable prognostic information after the occurrence of seizure. Interictal background abnormalities, such as a burst-suppression pattern, persistently low voltage, and electrocerebral inactivity, are highly correlated with poor outcome. Conversely, infants with normal EEGs or those revealing only maturational delay have much more favorable prognoses.

Neuroimaging is useful in determination of prognosis. Head ultrasonography has shown that severe periventricular intraparenchymal echodensities followed by evidence of tissue injury (cyst formation) correlate with later motor and cognitive deficits in premature infants. Magnetic resonance imaging (MRI) performed early in the neonatal course of hypoxic-ischemic brain injury provides useful prognostic information. Most infants with MRI evidence of basal ganglia "hemorrhage," periventricular leukomalacia, or multicystic encephalomalacia after asphyxia will ultimately demonstrate neurodevelopmental abnormalities.

IDIOPATHIC CEREBRAL INFARCTION IN THE TERM NEONATE

Focal seizures have been identified as the most common clinical feature indicating the presence of stroke in the full-term nonasphyxiated infant. Even though lateralized findings on neurologic examination may be found, they need not be present as hallmarks of cerebral infarction. Further, diminished movement of extremities on the side of the focal seizure may represent a postictal Todd paralysis rather than paresis from upper motor neuron injury due to cerebral infarction. The recognition of focal seizure as a manifestation of cerebral infarction is important, since this may serve as the only sign of the cerebrovascular event. Initially, other neurologic signs may be absent. However, as the child grows, motor or cognitive impairment may become progressively more apparent during the first 1 to 3 years of life.

The cause of the cerebral infarction frequently escapes detection among neonates who have not been subjected to prenatal asphyxia. Indeed, in 37 of 51 reported cases of neonatal stroke, a cause could not be identified. Causes of neonatal stroke that have been identified include embolic and thrombotic etiologies. Interestingly, a left hemispheric location has been noted to be the most common area involved; the reason for this neuroanatomic predilection has not been discovered. Emboli from placenta may lodge in cerebral vessels and result in stroke. In addition, congenital heart defects involving right-to-left shunts through septal defects or a patent ductus arteriosus serve as settings for embolic stroke in neonates. Coagulopathies due to congenital defects of coagulation (Factor VIII, protein C or S, or antithrombin III deficiency) or to sepsis-induced disseminated intravascular coagulation may underlie neonatal embolic stroke. Fetal head trauma during labor and delivery resulting in endothelial damage to cerebral vessels can lead to thrombosis and resultant focal ischemia of brain. Polycythemia and hypotension can each lead to intravascular stasis and rheologic abnormalities, leading to cerebrovascular thrombosis in neonates. Meningitis and encephalitis cause thrombosis as a result of vascular inflammation, leading to hemostasis and thrombosis.

Evidence of localized dysfunction of brain found on EEG consists of focal, persistent voltage reduction or of marked focal slowing and sharp wave activity. In some instances, EEG evidence of clinically observed seizures may be found. Each of these findings may exist while the EEG remains relatively normal over other regions of brain. The areas of electrical abnormality should correspond to the affected areas of brain revealed by neuroimaging. Cranial computed tomography (CT) demonstrates a low-density region that eventually evolves into atrophy. Visualization of the involved area should not require contrast enhancement. MRI demonstrates low or isointense signal intensity on T1-weighted images and high signal intensity on T2-weighted images as a result of increased water content in the infarcted region of brain.

Treatment is both supportive and symptomatic. Anticonvulsant treatment is given if seizures have occurred (see Chapter 40). Phenobarbital is the preferred drug and is administered as a loading dose of 20 mg/kg. Maintenance therapy of 3 to 5 mg/kg/day is sufficient. Attention should be given to hydration state, acid-base balance, and hematocrit.

Estimation of developmental outcome is difficult. The periods of follow-up reported in neonatal stroke series have been highly variable. While seizures frequently abate, chronic motor deficits often become apparent. MRI evidence of cerebral infarction may be helpful. Most infants with evidence of marked white matter damage, or cystic/multicystic encephalomalacia, have proved to have neurodevelopmental abnormalities on short-term follow-up.

POLYCYTHEMIA

Neonates are much more commonly polycythemic (central venous hematocrit >65%) than are older children. Polycythemia has been estimated to be present in 1.5% of newborns. It is most commonly encountered in neonates who are born at high altitude, who are small for gestational age, infants of diabetic mothers, or recipients in twin-twin transfusion syndrome; it is seen less often in neonatal hyperthyroidism or adrenogenital syndrome. Clinical signs of the elevated hematocrit are present in some but not all affected infants and include plethora, acrocyanosis, impaired renal function, poor feeding, apnea, tachypnea, hypoglycemia, and hyperbilirubinemia (indirect). Neurologic symptoms include jitteriness, irritability, lethargy, seizures, and focal motor deficits.

Most cases of polycythemia are idiopathic or secondary to acquired abnormalities of oxygen delivery (such as maternal smoking). Nonetheless, polycythemias bearing autosomal dominant or recessive inheritance patterns have been described. These familial polycythemias are associated with mutant hemoglobins, creating abnormalities of oxygen delivery.

Polycythemia and its resultant hyperviscosity may contribute to stroke in neonates. Inadequate cerebral perfusion and cerebrovascular thrombosis cause cerebral ischemia. Although most of the systemic complications of polycythemia resolve with adequate treatment, neurologic signs frequently do not. Cerebral infarction

resulting from polycythemia-related ischemia causes deficits that resolve either slowly or not at all. Neurologic sequelae may be present in up to 35% of neonates with symptomatic polycythemia.

If signs of polycythemia are found in a neonate, further evaluation should be undertaken. Venous or arterial hematocrit, rather than capillary hematocrit, should be measured. If family history and physical examination suggest a hereditary polycythemia, hemoglobin electrophoresis should be undertaken. Routine hemoglobin electrophoresis does not elucidate high-oxygen-affinity hemoglobinopathies in all cases. If clinical suspicion is high, the heat instability test for unstable hemoglobins and oxygen dissociation assays can be utilized. Neuroimaging should be used to assess for cerebral infarction.

Treatment of symptomatic patients consists of hematocrit reduction by a partial exchange transfusion until the hematocrit is reduced to 50% to 55%. The equation to calculate the amount of blood removed and the amount of normal saline or albumen infused is

$$\text{volume (ml)} = \frac{(\text{current hematocrit} - 50) \times \text{weight in kilograms} \times 90 \text{ ml}}{\text{current hematocrit}}$$

NEONATAL CEREBRAL VENOUS THROMBOSIS

Thrombosis may occur in cerebral veins that conduct deoxygenated blood from the parenchyma to the dural sinus system. These sinuses—the sagittal, straight, transverse, cavernous, and petrous—then convey the blood to the jugular veins. Occlusion of flow anywhere in these venous conduits leads to ischemia, infarction, and even hemorrhage. Infection, dehydration, polycythemia, congenital heart disease, and protein C deficiency have all been implicated as causes of cerebral venous thrombosis in neonates. However, often no cause is found for this occlusion of the cerebral venous system in neonates. Adjacent areas of brain parenchyma reveal neuropathologic changes typical of infarction.

The only signs may be lethargy and focal seizures. The features of slowly developing focal motor deficits, headache, and cranial nerve dysfunction found in older children and adults with cerebral venous thrombosis is seldom observed.

Neuroimaging reveals the venous stasis best if MR phase imaging, which detects blood flow, or MR venography is performed as well as conventional T1- and T2-weighted images. Treatment of underlying infection, metabolic disorder, or coagulopathy is necessary. However, if the cerebral venous thrombosis appears to be idiopathic, no anticoagulation is necessary. Follow-up has been limited, but neurologic prognosis appears good in the idiopathic cases.

INTRACRANIAL HEMORRHAGE IN THE NEONATE

Intracranial hemorrhage occurs in neonates in one of four different neuroanatomic distributions:

- Subdural (SDH)
- Subarachnoid (SAH)
- Intraparenchymal (IPH)
- Intraventricular (IVH)

While SDH occurs more commonly in the term infant, the other three types of hemorrhage are more common in premature infants.

Subdural Hemorrhage

SDH in neonates usually results from head trauma during birth. Thus, factors of labor and delivery promoting the application of increased force on the fetal head are liable to promote SDH. Cephalopelvic disproportion, rigidity of the bony pelvis, prolonged duration of labor, unusual presentations, or the need for prolonged manipulation or forceps application may each generate increased forces on the fetal head and cause SDH. As a result, shearing forces may create tears in the vein of Galen or tears of superficial cerebral veins. If forces are extreme, tears at the junction of falx and tentorium can generate large subdural blood collections in the relatively small posterior fossa, culminating in compression of the brainstem and cerebellar tonsillar herniation. The incidence of SDH has steadily declined recently as a result of improved obstetric practice.

Clinical features of SDH depend on the location and size of the hemorrhage. Tentorial laceration (Fig. 42–1) can cause stupor or even coma. Pupillary and extraocular movement abnormalities are common. Dystonic postures such as retrocollis or opisthotonos are seen. Finally, abnormalities of respiratory pattern regulation such as apneustic or ataxic respirations are seen and signify imminent respiratory arrest. Less severe SDHs in the posterior fossa evolve more slowly and cause less severe brainstem dysfunction. Subdural collections of blood over the cerebral surfaces due to tears of superficial cerebral veins may be asymptomatic. Minimal manifestation consists of irritability. With time the blood may liquify and draw water into the area by osmotic forces, thus expanding the size of the lesion. If the collection is sufficiently large, seizures occur. Greater pressure may cause oculomotor dysfunction accompanied by pupillary dilation and ablated pupillary light responses.

SDH may escape diagnosis in the first few weeks of life and appear later as a chronic subdural effusion; in this situation, one must suspect child abuse (see Chapter 37). Such an occurrence is marked by a rapidly enlarging head circumference and increased transillumination of the skull. Symptomatic subdural hemorrhage is often treated with subdural taps (through the anterior fontanel) to remove the blood and relieve the pressure.

Subarachnoid Hemorrhage

Blood can occupy the subarachnoid space in one of two ways. First, blood may reach the subarachnoid space after hemorrhage has occurred in the cerebral parenchyma or in the periventricular region. Second, SAH may result from disruption of the superficial leptomeningeal arteries or of the fragile vessels bridging the subarachnoid space; disruption of either vascular structure leads to direct bleeding into the subarachnoid space, so-called primary SAH. Primary SAH commonly occurs after hypoxic-ischemic brain insults and after fetal head trauma.

Clinically, mild SAH is the most common type, occurring as an occult phenomenon with few if any manifestations. Greater amounts of blood collecting over the convexities may result in focal motor deficits and often benign seizures. Large SAH accumulating over the convexities has been associated not only with seizures but with infarction of underlying cerebral cortex. The presence of accompanying infarction is indicated by the occurrence of focal seizures. A history of difficult labor and delivery may be associated with large SAH. Cerebral infarction in the setting of SAH has been observed more commonly in term infants than in premature infants.

When SAH is mild, the neurologic outcome can be good. Even in cases of SAH accompanied by seizure or cerebral infarction, the prognosis is often favorable. Adverse consequences appear to be more dependent on the severity of any underlying intrapartum trauma or hypoxic-ischemic brain injury.

Intraparenchymal and Intraventricular Hemorrhage

IPH of brain occurs in both term and preterm infants. Cerebral hemorrhage in the absence of IVH occurs most commonly in term infants. Hemorrhage into the parenchyma of the cerebral hemispheres can be due to head trauma, vascular malformation, coagulopathy, tumor, or infarction. Vitamin K deficiency should be considered in breast-feeding full-term neonates who present with intracranial hemorrhage. In the absence of recognized coagulation or anatomic abnormalities, cerebral hemispheric IPH has been attributed to hemorrhagic infarction. In premature infants, parenchymal hemorrhage most often occurs in conjunction with severe IVH. Hemorrhage from the friable, unsupported germinal matrix leads to accumulation of intraventricular blood and, often, ventricular distention. These events, in turn, cause impairment of blood flow in the medullary veins located in the periventricular white matter, preventing blood drainage into the greater cerebral venous system. Eventually, the periventricular venous congestion leads to ischemia and a resultant venous infarction.

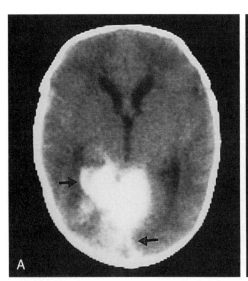
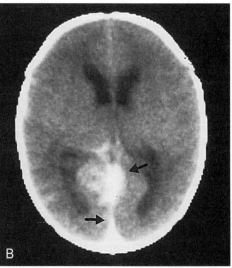

Figure 42–1. *A* and *B*, Generalized tonic seizures, lethargy progressing to coma, and irregular respiratory pattern were observed in a 1-day-old term infant. Cranial CT scan demonstrates a hyperdense region emanating from the falx and tentorium *(arrows)* due to traumatic tear of tentorium resulting in hemorrhage from straight sinus.

Developmental outcome in term infants with IPH depends on the location and extent of the underlying cause. The occurrence of posthemorrhagic hydrocephalus or of moderate to severe asphyxia predicts abnormal outcomes, including motor impairment or cognitive delay. In premature infants, the simultaneous occurrence of IVH with IPH carries high risk for major motor deficits and marked cognitive impairment.

EVALUATION OF STROKE IN INFANTS

Head ultrasonography detects areas of increased echogenicity in the cerebral cortex. In especially severe cases of ischemia, increased echogenicity of injured subcortical structures such as thalamus and basal ganglia can be appreciated. Ischemic cortical injury involving the territory of the middle cerebral artery (frontal and parietal lobe regions surrounding the central sulcus) is better revealed by ultrasonography than are other vascular territories. The principal advantages of cranial ultrasound are its easy portability to the bedside and its lack of radiation exposure to the infant.

CT of the brain is useful, particularly for evaluation of term infants after a suspected cerebral insult. Diffuse injury appears as abnormal generalized attenuation throughout the cerebral parenchyma with loss of the distinction between gray and white matter; this abnormality may represent cerebral edema. Focal and multifocal brain injury is readily detected by cranial CT.

MRI scans obtained within the first 4 days of life in term infants with signs of severe HIE reveal white matter abnormalities and indistinct gray matter–white matter junctions on T2-weighted images. Subsequent images can show chronic changes such as cerebral atrophy, paucity of white matter, delayed myelination, and ventriculomegaly. MRI has proved useful in documenting delay of myelination, a sequel to perinatal ischemic white matter injury not readily discerned with CT. This additional capability has provided a potential explanation for subtle motor deficits found in children who have ischemic brain injury in the perinatal period. As observed in MRI studies of adults, neonatal focal cerebral ischemic injuries may be identified early in their course. MRI also detects neonatal hypoxic-ischemic injuries of basal ganglia not well detected by either head ultrasonography or CT. Moreover, MRI is the procedure of choice in the neonatal period for identification of venous thrombosis.

Laboratory testing for the wide variety of etiologic factors underlying stroke should be conducted. The etiologies include infection, liver dysfunction, coagulopathy, organic and amino acid inborn errors of metabolism, urea cycle disorders, and mitochondrial abnormalities.

Children, Ages 1 to 13 Years

When stroke occurs in children, focal symptoms are reported and corresponding localized deficits are noted on the neurologic examination, which correlate neuroanatomically with the involved region of the central nervous system. In older children able to cooperate, findings elicited are helpful in localizing the site of the cerebrovascular event. Lateralized weakness often signifies injury to the contralateral hemisphere, including the regions governing movement. Such motor impairment accompanied by cranial nerve dysfunction on the side of the head *opposite* to the side of extremity weakness suggests brainstem infarction at a location above the pyramidal decussation. Findings of the sensory examination also may be helpful. Preservation of primary sensory modalities provides assessment of spinothalamic axis (pain and temperature) and posterior column (proprioception) integrity. Loss of pain and temperature sensation on one side of the body, combined with

motor weakness, and proprioceptive deficits on the other, places the cerebrovascular event in the spinal cord. If the same distribution of motor and sensory disturbances occurs but is accompanied by cranial nerve dysfunction, a brainstem site of injury is likely. Finally, impairment of cortically based sensations such as graphesthesia and stereognosis on one side of the body implies a *contralateral* hemispheric cause of the observed cortical sensory deficit.

Analysis of language function in the older child may provide help in localizing the region of the cerebrovascular event. Unilateral lesions of the dominant hemisphere involving frontal lobe immediately anterior to the motor strip supplying the face results in a characteristic speech disturbance. *Broca (nonfluent) aphasia* consists of the patient's inability to utter or to write the words or phrases he or she wishes to express. While the patient knows the thoughts he or she wishes to express, the volitional motor function for written or oral expression cannot be mustered. Infarction in the more posterior superior temporal lobe results in an aphasia of a different type. *Wernicke aphasia* is characterized by marked impairment of auditory comprehension. Comprehension of written matter may be impaired as well. While the patient remains fluent in speech, language is peppered with unintelligible utterances that are meaningless (neologisms) or are similar but incorrect versions of the intended word (paraphasias). The larger the injury to this region, the more severe the impairment of language. Speech in most right-handed people and in 50% of left-handed people is governed by the left hemisphere (so-called left hemispheric dominance). The remaining minority share right hemispheric dominance.

The causes of stroke in 1- to 13-year-old children may be considered in two general groups: (1) ischemic stroke and (2) intracranial hemorrhage. The ischemic category comprises embolic, thrombotic, and hypotensive causes of stroke. The category of intracranial hemorrhage includes both intraparenchymal and subarachnoid hemorrhage.

ISCHEMIC STROKE IN CHILDREN

Congenital Heart Disease

Congenital heart disease remains the most common diagnosable cause of stroke in childhood. Children with cyanotic congenital heart disease (right-to-left shunts or mixing lesions) face the greatest risk (see Chapter 15). An embolic stroke constitutes the most common cerebrovascular event. Cardiac defects involving right-to-left shunts allow emboli originating in peripheral venous circulation to bypass their filtration and removal by the pulmonary vascular bed. Thus, emboli entering the heart via venous return may be shunted to the peripheral arterial circulation, only to lodge in the cerebrovascular tree (Fig. 42–2).

Patent foramen ovale contributes significantly to the occurrence of stroke in children and young adults. Echocardiographic evaluation of young patients who have had stroke reveal patent foramen ovale or evidence of right-to-left shunting in many. Transesophageal echocardiography conducted with Valsalva bubble studies for evidence of direct right-to-left flow serves as the most useful diagnostic test.

Valvular defects can cause stroke. Mitral valve prolapse may contribute to the occurrence of embolic stroke in the young. Small emboli are dislodged from the abnormal valve leaflets. Mitral valve prolapse has been estimated to underlie 20% to 30% of strokes in patients younger than 30 years old. Echocardiography in both two-dimensional and M modes proves most helpful in discerning the cardiac valvular abnormality. Rheumatic valvular disease (mitral, aortic), once a common cause of embolic stroke, has become an infrequent cause of childhood stroke. Infected valves in bacterial endocarditis pose considerable risk for the occurrence of embolic

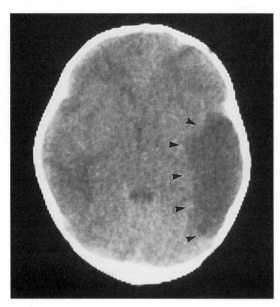

Figure 42–2. Cranial CT scan of a 3-month-old boy with trisomy 21 and tetralogy of Fallot who, following cardiac catheterization, had focal seizures involving the right face and arm. Region of hypodensity in left hemisphere *(arrowheads)* reflects infarction of the left middle cerebral artery territory, most likely due to embolic occlusion of that vessel.

stroke (native, prosthetic, rheumatic, or congenitally abnormal valve). Infective mitral and aortic valvular vegetations may dislodge and travel distally to occlude cerebral arteries. The most common organisms found are streptococci and staphylococci (see Chapter 16). Even after vegetations have been successfully sterilized, they may embolize and cause stroke. Emboli from infected valvular vegetations may embolize, travel to the cerebral vasculature, and seed the adventitia of the cerebral vessel. The resultant infection and inflammation results in weakening of the vessel and development of a *mycotic aneurysm.* Aneurysms may lie dormant for some time before their rupture leads to subarachnoid or intraparenchymal hemorrhage and resultant neurologic signs.

Procoagulopathies

Several disorders of coagulation can lead to embolic or thrombotic stroke. Adverse consequences of antiphospholipid antibodies have been identified in all age groups. Children, adolescents, and young adults experience the cerebrovascular consequences of these antibodies most often. Antiphospholipid antibodies including the lupus anticoagulant (LAC), are polyclonal antibodies found in serum that are able to bind to both neutral and negatively charged phospholipids (see Chapter 51). LAC and anticardiolipin antibodies (aCLs), were first associated with thrombotic or embolic cerebrovascular events in patients with systemic lupus erythematosus (SLE). Subsequently, patients suffering stroke with no evidence of underlying immune-mediated illness other than the LAC or aCL antibody were found. The antibody prolongs the partial thromboplastin time (PTT) *in vitro* but acts as a procoagulant *in vivo.* The presence of these antibodies in a patient who concurrently smokes cigarettes, is positive for antinuclear antibodies, or suffers from hyperlipidemia may impart a higher risk for stroke than if the patient carries the antibody alone. The antibody's presence is indicated by a prolonged PTT and a falsely positive serum Venereal Disease Research Laboratory (VDRL) result. The antibody's presence can be conclusively demonstrated functionally and immuno-

logically. While cerebral infarction and TIAs constitute the most frequently observed neurologic manifestations related to the presence of these antibodies, migraine headache, seizures, and monocular visual disturbances are also associated. Therapy for patients with antiphospholipid antibodies who have suffered stroke has not been fully substantiated by randomized prospective study. Nonetheless, low-dose anticoagulation has been advocated.

Absence of specific serum proteins that act as inhibitors of coagulation may lead to stroke in children. Two of these proteins, *protein S* and *protein C*, have been associated with thrombotic or embolic cerebrovascular disease in the young. Protein C and its cofactor protein S act as anticoagulants and synergistically attenuate coagulation by deactivating the activated forms of Factors V and VIII. Absence of (or resistance to) either of these proteins tips the scale of balanced coagulation toward increased spontaneous clotting and can result in stroke. *Antithrombin III* opposes the action of the activated forms of Factors II, IX, X, XI, and XII through the irreversible formation of inactivating complexes with these factors. Deficiencies of proteins S and C as well as of antithrombin III may cause arterial thrombotic or embolic stroke or venous infarction. While their deficiencies are often congenital, they may be acquired through liver disease or nephrotic syndrome. A screening battery of tests, including prothrombin time (PT), PTT, and specific immunologic and functional testing for the proteins-suspected of being deficient is essential for diagnosis. Treatment with anticoagulation therapy following stroke has been recommended.

Cancer and its treatment may predispose children to cerebrovascular ischemic events. Promyelocytic leukemia and its treatment have been observed to provoke disseminated intravascular coagulation leading to stroke. Lymphoreticular cancers more than solid tumors have been linked to thrombotic and embolic strokes. In addition, dural sinus and cerebral venous thrombosis have been found after therapy with L-asparaginase (Fig. 42–3). TIAs following induction chemotherapy for acute lymphoblastic leukemia have been observed. Finally, cranial radiation therapy may induce an occlusive vasculopathy, leading to focal cerebral ischemia.

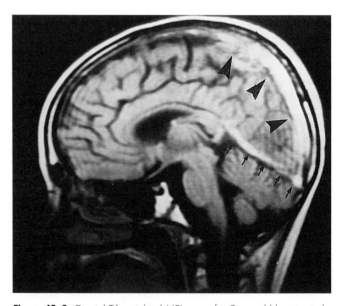

Figure 42–3. Cranial T1-weighted MRI scan of a 9-year-old boy treated with L-asparaginase for acute lymphoblastic leukemia who experienced new headache, seizures, and lethargy. Bright signal in superior sagittal sinus *(arrowheads)* and in straight sinus *(arrows)* denotes L-asparaginase–induced cerebral venous thrombosis.

Table 42–4. Autoimmune Disorders Associated with Central Nervous System Involvement

Disorder	CNS Manifestations
1. Systemic lupus erythematosus	Migraine headache, seizures, stroke, cerebellar dysfunction, transverse myelopathy, aseptic meningitis, psychosis
2. Mixed connective tissue disease	Seizures, stroke, cerebellar dysfunction, trigeminal neuropathy
3. Polyarteritis nodosum	Migraine headache, stroke, subarachnoid hemorrhage, seizures
4. Wegener granulomatosis	Migraine headache, subarachnoid hemorrhage, stroke
5. Takayasu arteritis	Seizure, stroke
6. Henoch-Schönlein purpura	Headache, stroke, seizures, chorea
7. Primary CNS vasculitis	Headache, stroke, seizure

Autoimmune Disorders

Autoimmune disorders may cause neurologic disturbance and cerebrovascular involvement (Table 42–4). Symptoms of abrupt onset with accompanying deficits referable to the central nervous system (CNS) have long been associated with SLE. A CNS vasculitis had been presumed to underlie the CNS manifestations of SLE. However, autopsy study of patients suffering from SLE revealed a virtual absence of cerebrovascular inflammation. Rather, small areas of infarction relate to proliferative changes in cerebral arterioles leading to luminal occlusion. Large areas of infarction are related more likely to LAC-derived thromboembolism or to embolism from the sterile cardiac valve leaflet vegetations associated with SLE (Libman-Sacks endocarditis). Additional causes of CNS illness include thrombocytopenic hemorrhage, steroid-induced pseudotumor or psychosis, and CNS infection.

True cerebral arterial vasculitis may be an isolated disease or seen in association with autoimmune disorders. Neuropathologic evidence of polymorphonuclear leukocyte or monocyte infiltration leading to intimal proliferation and vessel wall necrosis is found. The inflammation affects blood flow and predisposes to thrombosis.

Stroke may occur in the course of *polyarteritis nodosa*. Involvement of the CNS is found in 20% to 40% of such patients.

Wegener granulomatosis, a necrotizing vasculitis of the upper pulmonary system, rarely affects the CNS; stroke is uncommon. When the CNS is affected, extension of sinus or nasal inflammation into the basilar skull frequently has occurred.

Mixed connective tissue disease (MCTD), which clinically overlaps with polymyositis, SLE, and progressive systemic sclerosis, can involve the CNS. Cranial neuropathy, most commonly trigeminal nerve dysfunction, has been the most frequently cited deficit. Stroke manifesting as sudden-onset hemiparesis and aphasia has been reported in children afflicted with MCTD.

Takayasu arteritis, involving the aorta and its principal branches, has been associated with thrombotic stroke. Inflammation-induced luminal constriction leading to thrombosis is thought to cause cerebral ischemia in children. Angiographic improvement of vessels in the carotid tree is observed with immunosuppressive treatment. Necrotizing arteritis with inflammatory infiltrate has been found in both meningeal and cerebral vessels of children suffering from *Henoch-Schönlein purpura*. Both fixed and transient deficits may occur in this disorder.

Treatment with steroids or other immunosuppressive agents proves most helpful in these disorders. Long-term anticoagulation has not been studied.

Inflammation of cerebral vessels may also occur in the course of *bacterial meningitis*. The subarachnoid arteries become immersed in exudate. The vessel wall is affected by the inflammatory process. If allowed to proceed long enough, thrombophlebitis ensues. Vascular occlusion with consequent features of stroke results. Antibiotics combined with steroids early in the course of treatment form the cornerstone of therapy.

Metabolic Disorders Causing Stroke

Homocystinuria, a disorder of homocysteine metabolism, can cause thrombotic stroke in children. Abnormal homocysteine metabolism results from one of three inheritable enzymatic defects. The most striking phenotype results from deficiency of cystathionine synthetase, the enzyme that facilitates the catabolism of homocysteine to cystathionine. Accumulation of not only homocysteine but also methionine results. Children affected by this autosomal recessive disorder (Table 42–5) have marfanoid habitus, global developmental delay, lens dislocation, and thromboembolism. Thromboemboli may travel to cerebrovascular beds, causing stroke. Serum hyperhomocysteinuria injures the vascular endothelium. The denuded vessel wall then becomes a site for thrombosis. The resulting thrombus may remain at its site of origin or it may embolize to a distal locus. Therefore, stroke may have thrombotic or embolic characteristics. Both arterial and venous infarcts may result. Treatment is dietary and aimed at reducing levels of homocysteine in serum. Pyridoxine administration and methionine restriction are effective in 30% to 40% of treated patients.

Sulfite oxidase deficiency, another autosomal recessive disorder, results in the accumulation of serum sulfite. The associated phenotype may result from deficiency of either the enzyme or its associated and essential pterin-containing molybdenum cofactor. Mental retardation, seizures, lens displacement, and acute hemiplegia result. The mechanism of the stroke-like episodes has not been fully elucidated. It is possible that ischemic mechanisms are not involved and that direct metabolic neurotoxicity accounts for the sudden onset of deficits resembling those of stroke. Sulfites, and *S*-sulfo-

Table 42–5. Common Genetic Causes of Stroke

Thrombotic/Embolic Stroke

1. Homocystinuria
2. Fabry disease
3. Sickle cell disease
4. Fibromuscular dysplasia
5. Paroxysmal nocturnal hemoglobinuria
6. Resistance to activated protein C

Hemorrhage

1. Factor VIII deficiency
2. Factor IX deficiency
3. Factor XI deficiency
4. Familial intracranial aneurysms
5. Sickle cell disease
6. Familial cavernous angioma

Unknown Mechanism

1. Familial porencephaly
2. Organic acidemia
3. Mitochondrial disorders

Adapted from Natowicz M, Kelley RT. Mendelian etiologies of stroke. Ann Neurol 1987;22:173.

cysteine accumulates in urine. Dietary attempts to reduce sulfite accumulation have been unsuccessful.

Fabry disease, a lipid storage disease attributable to ceramide trihexosidase deficiency, results in accumulation of the sphingolipid trihexoside in kidney, vascular endothelium, and cornea. Symptoms become apparent in childhood or adolescence. Angiokeratomas and painful paresthesia often constitute the first symptoms. Renal failure follows. However, because of endothelial accumulation of sphingolipid in vessel walls, cerebrovascular occlusion results in stroke. Recurrent stroke is common in this rare X-linked disorder. Supportive care and treatment designed to improve renal function and minimize pain are instituted.

Mitochondrial disorders include in their phenotype recurrent and sometimes catastrophic stroke. The syndrome of MELAS (mitochondrial encephalomyopathy, lactic acidosis, and stroke) presents in childhood and is due to a mutation of mitochondrial DNA. The most common biochemical finding is a deficiency of complex I of the electron transport chain. An elevated serum or cerebrospinal fluid lactate level serves as its chemical signature, and molecular confirmation of the diagnosis can be secured from blood. While some features of MELAS are shared by other mitochondrial syndromes, hemiparesis of abrupt onset is fairly specific for this syndrome. Excruciating headache resembling migraine may precede the stroke-like episodes. Seizures and sensorineural hearing loss are almost always present at some point in the course of the illness. Neuropathologic study of brain from patients with MELAS has shown cystic cavities and necrosis of cortex with relative sparing of white matter.

Other metabolic disorders have been associated with stroke in childhood. Urea cycle defects, especially ornithine transcarbamoylase deficiency presenting in girls, can cause stroke. Deficiency of arginase, another important enzyme of the urea cycle, has been observed in association with hemiparesis and diparesis of subacute onset. Finally, familial lipoprotein disorders, especially those featuring a dearth of high-density lipoprotein or an abundance of triglycerides, have been associated with stroke in children. In most cases, a family history of hyperlipidemia is found.

Moyamoya Disease

Moyamoya disease commonly affects children under the age of 15 years and presents with TIAs or sudden-onset fixed motor deficits. Progressive narrowing and occlusion of the intracranial portion of the internal carotid arteries are characteristic. Endothelial proliferation, fibrosis, and intimal thickening mark the vascular pathology. Resultant proliferation of collateral vessels from the basilar skull circulation creates an intricate latticework of compensatory blood flow. The appearance on angiography is characteristic and consists of a fine vascular network located at the base of the brain. *Moyamoya* means "something hazy like a puff of smoke drifting in the air" (Fig. 42–4).

Children usually present with acute hemiplegia as a result of uncompensated occlusion of the internal carotid artery. Because the anatomic abnormality is often bilateral, the hemiplegia may alternate. Disturbance of fine motor function has been observed. Chorea has been reported in association with moyamoya syndrome. Although the vascular abnormality may be congenital, moyamoya syndrome can occur as a sequel to a primary disorder causing internal carotid artery occlusion. It has been found in children with sickle cell disease, neurofibromatosis, tuberculous meningitis, and fibromuscular dysplasia. Evidence suggesting a hereditary etiology in some cases has been reported in Japan.

Optimal treatment has not been determined. Evidence of inflammation has not been found. Calcium channel blockers have been reported to increase collateral vessel diameter, improve perfusion, and ameliorate neurologic symptoms. Several surgical procedures (extracranial-intracranial or dural-intracranial bypass) designed to re-establish effective perfusion of endangered brain have been performed.

Sickle Cell Disease

Acute hemiplegia may be found in children with sickle cell disease (see Chapter 49). Cerebral infarction occurs in approximately 6% of patients. Most often cerebral infarction occurs in the setting of sickle crisis. Neurologic signs include hemiparesis, aphasia, and visual disturbances. Neuroimaging studies, particularly MRI, reveal that stroke occurs in watershed distributions between two cerebrovascular territories, affecting both the gray and white matter of the cortex. The pathophysiologic mechanisms proposed encompass both large vessel sickling, leading to thrombotic hypoperfusion, as well as diminished flow in small cerebral vessels due to the decreased compliance of sickled erythrocytes. Cerebral vessels reveal endothelial proliferation, disruption of the elastic lamina, and stenosis. Cerebral hyperemia thought to be caused by vasodilation has been suggested as a mechanism contributing to the occurrence of watershed infarctions in sickle cell patients. Recurrences are common. Exchange transfusion diminishes the observed hyperemia and reduces the occurrence of stroke in these patients. Children who have suffered large strokes demonstrate correspondingly multifaceted deficits of cognitive function. Those in whom focal strokes have occurred show more subtle neuropsychologic deficits.

Subarachnoid hemorrhage also occurs among children with sickle cell disease. The frequency of SAH is less than that of infarction, occurring in less than 2%. While ruptured cerebral aneurysm is frequently found in adult sickle cell patients suffering SAH, it is absent in children with sickle cell disease suffering SAH. The clinical findings of SAH differ from those of infarction in sickle cell patients. Severe headache, vomiting, and alteration in mental state mark SAH in children with sickle cell disease. Meningeal signs and focal neurologic deficits may be found on examination. Angiography should be performed on all patients to detect any surgically correctable vascular lesion underlying the hemorrhage. Medical therapy consisting of transfusion therapy has been suggested.

INTRACRANIAL HEMORRHAGE

Coagulopathies

Although some coagulation disturbances may predispose a patient to ischemic stroke (hypercoagulable states), others may promote intracranial bleeding (see Chapter 51). The hemophilias (A and B) are X-linked disorders that may result in intracranial bleeding. Bleeding may occur in either intraparenchymal or subarachnoid locations. Hemophilia A arises from factor VIII deficiency. Males affected by this disorder may experience intracranial bleeding in association with head trauma. Unfortunately, spontaneous intracranial bleeding unassociated with head trauma also occurs. The risk of spontaneous bleeding rises with the severity of factor VIII deficiency.

Hemophilia B derives from a deficiency of factor IX. Intracranial bleeding is seen less frequently in this patient group than in patients with hemophilia A. Hemophilia B is encountered much less frequently than hemophilia A, and this difference may account for the less frequent observation of intracranial bleeding. Clinical symptoms depend on the intracranial location of the hemorrhage. If the bleeding occurs in the subarachnoid space, symptoms of severe headache, nuchal rigidity, and meningismus are found. Mental

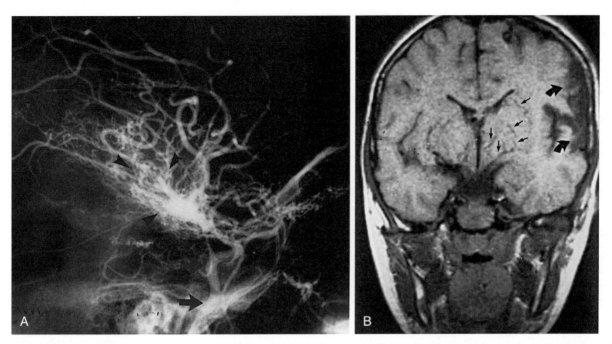

Figure 42–4. Sudden onset of right hemiparesis in a 6-year-old boy. *A,* Cerebral angiogram shows left internal carotid artery *(arrows)* leading to a highly arborized, telangiectatic network of vessels *(arrowheads)* typical of moyamoya disease. The typical middle cerebral artery vascular tree is absent. *B,* Cranial coronal MRI scan of the same patient shows region of low signal in the middle cerebral artery territory and denotes infarction *(curved arrows).* Flow voids in the basal ganglia *(straight arrows)* are radiographic manifestations of the basilar collateral circulation typical of this vascular anomaly.

status is frequently altered. If bleeding occurs within brain parenchyma, focal features, including hemiparesis, may be found.

Thrombocytopenia

Severe thrombocytopenia rarely leads to cerebral hemorrhage, especially if the etiology is idiopathic thrombocytopenic purpura. Thrombocytopenia due to bone marrow failure (drug-induced suppression, aplastic anemia, malignancy) may pose a greater risk. Significant risk of intracranial hemorrhage is thought not to occur until the platelet count is less than 20,000/mm³. Small petechial hemorrhages into white matter are thought to be more common than large parenchymal hemorrhages.

Causes of thrombocytopenia include idiopathic thrombocytopenic purpura, infection, and malignancy (replacement of bone marrow or drug-induced suppression). The features of these underlying causes dominate the clinical picture (see Chapter 51).

Vascular Malformations

Arteriovenous malformation (AVM) of the brain is the most common cause of intracranial hemorrhage in preadolescent children. The malformation represents a developmental anomaly that presents with hemorrhage much more frequently in children than in adults. The AVM consists of dilated vascular channels, some of which reveal the highly muscularized walls of arterioles. Gliotic neural tissue resides in and among the vascular branches of the malformation. More common in males, the most frequent presenting events associated with AVM in children are seizures and hemorrhage. The vast majority of AVMs reside in the cerebral hemispheres, while 10% arise in the posterior fossa.

The clinical features of AVM hemorrhage consist of those found in intraparenchymal hemorrhage. Focal features depend on the area of brain in which the bleeding has occurred. Once hemorrhage has occurred, a higher mortality rate has been observed in children than in adults harboring hemorrhagic AVMs. The risk of hemorrhage from an unruptured AVM is approximately 3% per year.

Initially, treatment of AVMs consisted of anticonvulsant therapy for secondary seizures. Surgery was reserved for those AVMs that bled at presentation. The introduction of MRI has led to better localization of the malformation (Fig. 42–5). In addition, percutaneous selective embolization of portions of or of the entire AVM has permitted the resection of AVMs thought previously to be inoperable. AVMs residing in critical regions of the CNS not amenable to surgery have been treated with stereotactic radiosurgery. Promising results have been obtained. Radiation damage to the CNS has complicated the recovery of approximately 3% of patients receiving this therapy.

Intracranial aneurysms constitute the most common cause of intracranial bleeding in all patients under the age of 20 years and are more frequent in males. Unlike aneurysms in adults, the most common site of aneurysmal bleeding in children is along the intracranial portion of the internal carotid artery. The vertebral and basilar arteries are other common sites of intracranial aneurysm in children. In addition, intracranial aneurysms discovered in children tend to be larger than those found in adults. While most aneurysms constitute vascular developmental anomalies, other causes exist, including mycotic aneurysms associated with bacterial endocarditis (Fig. 42–6). Acquired cerebral artery aneurysms have been reported in children infected with the human immunodeficiency virus. Intracranial aneurysms are found with increased frequency relative to the general pediatric population among patients suffering from polycystic renal disease, those with aortic coarctation, and those with Ehlers-Danlos syndrome. Intracranial aneurysms have been noted to exist in close association with AVMs in some pediatric cases.

All patients should be studied with angiography after aneurysmal bleeding. Patients should be closely observed for development of hydrocephalus and increased intracranial pressure. Aneurysmal bleeding resulting in significant subarachnoid hemorrhage can pre-

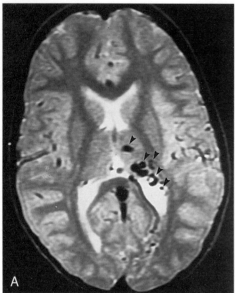 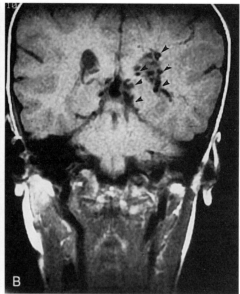

Figure 42–5. Cranial MRI scan of a 6-year-old girl with recurrent headache. *A,* Axial view demonstrates flow voids deep in the left hemisphere near the lateral ventricle *(arrowheads)* consistent with arteriovenous malformation. *B,* Coronal view through parietal lobes also demonstrates numerous flow voids *(arrowheads)* indicative of arteriovenous malformation.

cipitate cerebral vasospasm. Vasospasm, in turn, can cause a secondary cerebral infarction. Vasospasm occurs most commonly 7 to 10 days after the aneurysmal bleeding. Prophylaxis is the most effective treatment for vasospasm. Maintenance of blood pressure through intravascular volume expansion has been shown to reduce the incidence of posthemorrhagic vasospasm. Early enthusiasm for treatment with calcium channel blockers has attenuated.

EVALUATION OF STROKE IN CHILDREN

Neuroimaging provides the foundation of evaluation. Intracranial blood is rapidly seen with CT. The early stages of ischemic stroke, however, are detected with difficulty. MRI provides evidence of ischemia in the early stages of stroke. Magnetic resonance angiography (MRA) has provided reliable information about the blood flow in and the structure of large intracranial vessels. Small intracranial vessels are poorly resolved by MRA, and invasive contrast angiography remains the neuroradiologic procedure of choice for full elucidation of the cerebral vasculature. Laboratory studies helpful in the evaluation of the child who has suffered stroke are determined by the patient's clinical features. Table 42–6 provides a synopsis of the tests most commonly employed.

Adolescents

The causes of adolescent stroke include those discussed for preadolescent children. Determination of stroke mechanism—embolic, thrombotic, or hemorrhagic—remains important. Nonetheless, stroke among adolescents may also be caused by other etiologies not commonly found in neonates or preadolescent children.

FIBROMUSCULAR DYSPLASIA

Fibromuscular dysplasia involves arteries throughout the body. First described in renal arteries, the pathologic features of fibromuscular dysplasia have been found in carotid, vertebral, and intracranial arteries. Fibromuscular dysplasia involves irregularly spaced focal zones of fibrous and muscular hyperplasia of the media, disruption of the elastic lamina, and eventration of the media. The constricted regions of vascular fibrosis alternate with regions of luminal dilation to create the characteristic beaded appearance on angiography. Fibromuscular dysplasia is more common in young females and has been found in adolescents; with carotid involvement, a bruit may be auscultated in the neck. If renal arteries are affected, hypertension may be present. Neurologic symptoms signifying cerebrovascular involvement most commonly consist of TIAs and mild strokes. A thrombotic mechanism is presumed but has never been proven.

No treatment for symptomatic patients is established, although arterial dilation using metal dilators or transluminal angioplasty has been recommended.

SEXUAL ACTIVITY, ORAL CONTRACEPTION, AND THE PUERPERIUM

Sexual intercourse generates marked increases in systemic blood pressure. Sustained hypertension elevates the risk of hypertensive intracranial hemorrhage. The risk for such a hemorrhage is heightened by the existence of an intracranial aneurysm or arteriovenous hemorrhage.

Oral contraceptives have been associated with stroke in young women. In some series, the combination of migraine headache and concurrent oral contraceptive use has been cited as a risk factor for stroke.

Pregnancy and the postpartum state have been considered periods of hypercoagulability. In addition, venous stasis increases. These two factors are believed to promote the occurrence of cerebral venous thrombosis and resultant cerebral venous infarction in pregnant and immediately postpartum females. Frequently, the initial manifestation is headache. Seizures, either focal or generalized, are common. Acute hemiparesis is the most common focal feature on neurologic examination. Papilledema can appear as intracranial pressure rises due to resultant venous outflow obstruction in the head. The appearance of these signs or symptoms in a gravid or postpartum adolescent should raise suspicion about the existence of underlying cerebral venous thrombosis.

Diagnosis is made with cranial neuroimaging; MRI provides the best noninvasive assessment. If seizures occur, anticonvulsant treatment should be initiated. Once the diagnosis is confirmed, anticoagulants should be administered.

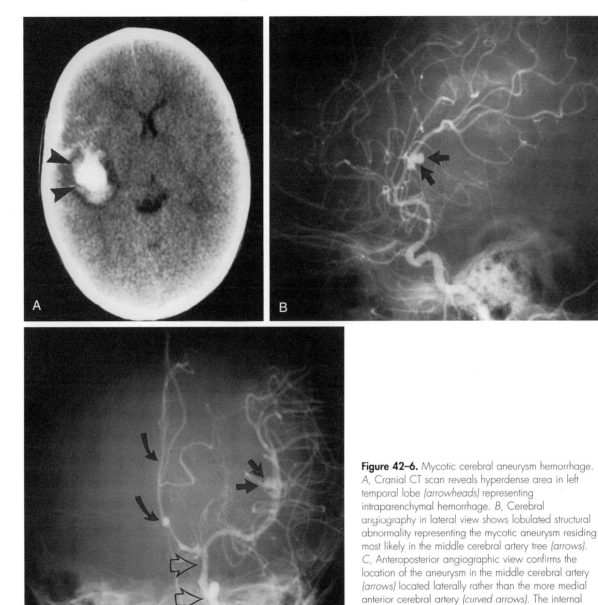

Figure 42–6. Mycotic cerebral aneurysm hemorrhage. *A,* Cranial CT scan reveals hyperdense area in left temporal lobe *(arrowheads)* representing intraparenchymal hemorrhage. *B,* Cerebral angiography in lateral view shows lobulated structural abnormality representing the mycotic aneurysm residing most likely in the middle cerebral artery tree *(arrows).* *C,* Anteroposterior angiographic view confirms the location of the aneurysm in the middle cerebral artery *(arrows)* located laterally rather than the more medial anterior cerebral artery *(curved arrows).* The internal carotid artery *(open arrows)* gives rise to both the anterior and the middle cerebral arteries.

COCAINE USE

Subarachnoid hemorrhage can result from cocaine use. The probability of this occurrence is higher in cocaine users with occult intracranial aneurysms or arteriovenous malformations. Irrespective of the method of cocaine administration, subarachnoid hemorrhage may occur. Cocaine produces tachycardia, hypertension, and vasoconstriction. The resultant sudden rise in systemic blood pressure is thought to precipitate subarachnoid hemorrhage. Ischemic lesions have also been found. Nonetheless, intracranial hemorrhage appears to occur more commonly than ischemic infarction.

Treatment is supportive, with reduction of hypertension, hyperthermia, and tachycardia.

Causes of Stroke Unrelated to Age

PHARYNGEAL INFECTION

Pharyngeal infections have been associated with stroke due to thrombotic occlusion of the carotid arteries in their cervical course.

Stroke in childhood due to carotid occlusion more commonly occurs in the intracranial segment of the carotid artery. Infections of the cervical region such as tonsillitis, pharyngitis, cervical lymphadenitis, and necrotizing fasciitis have been found in children experiencing acute hemiplegia. In these instances, angiography has shown occlusion of the internal carotid artery located in its cervical segment. Neuroimaging has demonstrated ischemic infarction of the cortical region served by the middle cerebral artery, which arises from the carotid circulation. It is speculated that the soft tissue infection leads to an inflammatory arteritis. Vessel wall inflammation and direct pressure on the artery then lead to intravascular thrombosis and occlusion. Neurologic symptoms are noted in a patient with evidence of infection: fever, lethargy, sore throat or neck, difficulty swallowing, or cervical lymphadenopathy.

In these cases, prompt and aggressive antibiotic treatment constitutes the cornerstone of care. In some cases, surgical debridement of the infected area is necessary. Thrombolytic agents have been used to recanalize the occluded carotid artery. However, standardized, controlled trials of such treatment have not been performed.

Table 42–6. Neuroradiologic, Laboratory, and Cardiovascular Assessment of Stroke in Children

I. **Neuroradiologic Assessment**
   A. Rapid detection of intracranial blood
      1. Cranial CT
      2. Cranial MRI also detects extravascular blood but is not as rapidly obtained as cranial CT images
   B. Detection of brain parenchymal changes related to stroke
      1. Cranial MRI
      2. Cranial CT reveals changes later in course than MRI
   C. Detection of abnormal vascular structure
      1. Percutaneous cerebral angiogram provides the most complete and accurate demonstration of extracranial and intracranial vasculature
      2. Cranial MRA
II. **Laboratory Assessment**
   A. Disturbance of RBC, WBC, or platelet number
      1. Hematocrit
      2. Platelet count
      3. WBC count with differential
   B. Disturbance of coagulation
      1. PT, PTT
      2. Antithrombin III level
      3. Protein C level, protein S level; resistance to protein C assay
      4. Lupus anticoagulant detection, anticardiolipin antibody, antiphospholipid antibody
   C. Metabolic disturbances
      1. Serum electrolytes, glucose
      2. Serum amino acids
      3. Urine organic acids
      4. Serum/CSF lacate and pyruvate
      5. Urine toxic screen
   D. Disturbance of hemoglobin
      1. Hemoglobin concentration
      2. Hemoglobin electrophoresis
   E. Inflammatory disturbances
      1. ESR
      2. ANA, RF
      3. CSF studies: glucose, protein cell counts, special stains, cultures
   F. Lipid and lipoprotein disturbances
      1. Serum triglycerides
      2. Serum cholesterol; if high, obtain fasting HDL
III. **Cardiovascular Assessment**
      1. ECG
      2. Standard and transesophageal echocardiogram

Abbreviations: ANA = antinuclear antibodies; CSF = cerebrospinal fluid; CT = computed tomography; ECG = electrocardiogram; ESR = erythrocyte sedimentation rate; HDL = high-density lipoproteins; MRA = magnetic resonance angiography; MRI = magnetic resonance imaging; PT = prothrombin time; PTT = partial thromboplastin time; RBC = red blood cell; WBC = white blood cell; RF = rheumatoid factor.

HEAD AND NECK TRAUMA

Head and neck trauma is an important cause of stroke in children. Neurologic symptoms may be delayed more than 24 hours in their appearance relative to the time of inciting trauma. Stroke due to carotid artery injury has been well documented. Most often, these cerebrovascular events occur after head and neck trauma sustained in motor vehicle accidents, bicycle accidents, fights, or falls. Hemiparesis is a common symptom at presentation if the cause resides in the carotid artery. Carotid angiography reveals internal carotid artery occlusion. The site of occlusion most often exists at the level of the carotid bifurcation. Pathologically, an intimal tear is found with attendant thrombus blocking the arterial lumen. In some cases, arterial dissection is found.

Vertebral artery injury due to trauma may cause stroke in children. Traction injuries of the neck appear to cause vertebral artery injury. The vertebral artery is most vulnerable to traumatic injury at its atlantoaxial portion. The resultant strokes occur in the vertebrobasilar portion of the cerebral circulation. Symptoms are referable to the structures receiving blood from this system—brainstem, cerebellum, occipital, and temporal lobes. Clinical symptoms of vertebrobasilar stroke include difficulty swallowing, ataxia, facial weakness, tinnitus, vertigo, anisocoria, extraocular movement palsies, dysmetria, cortical blindness, and mental status changes. Because both the sensory and the motor long tracts course through the brainstem, symptoms of general sensorimotor impairment may be found. Vertebral artery injury in children has been reported in the setting of athletic endeavor or automobile accidents. The resultant vertebrobasilar strokes are due to thrombosis or to vertebral artery dissection. Anticoagulation with antiplatelet agents has been proposed as therapy.

MIGRAINE HEADACHE

Stroke may occur in the setting of migraine headache. The occurrence of focal motor deficits during a migraine headache denotes *complicated migraine* (see Chapter 38). Acute hemiparesis has been well documented during these episodes and is believed to reflect the involvement of the cerebral circulation derived from the carotid artery. Symptoms such as ataxia, cortical blindness, and cranial nerve dysfunction correlate with vertebrobasilar circulation involvement. Focal symptoms may be fixed or may occur as TIAs.

Initially, an association between migrainous stroke and discharged emboli from mitral valve prolapse was hypothesized, but studies have not supported the association. While oral contraceptives confer hypercoagulability thought to predispose to stroke, the postulated additive risk for stroke with migraine headaches and oral contraceptives has been challenged. Angiographic studies on patients with focal deficits consistent with stroke in the setting of migraine headache reveal vasoconstriction of vessels in either the vertebrobasilar or the carotid circulations. The neuroanatomic position of the constricted vessels correlated with the location of the observed deficits. Ischemia provoked by vasoconstriction during prolonged migraine has been hypothesized as the mechanism of stroke in these patients.

Calcium channel blockers have been used for treatment, but definitive studies of their efficacy are awaited.

SUMMARY AND RED FLAGS

Acute hemiplegia most frequently represents stroke. Critical to the diagnosis of stroke are a history and physical examination that is consistent with the occurrence of stroke. Since stroke occurs most often in children as a consequence of an underlying process, circumspect consideration of the child's condition to determine whether such a predisposing condition exists will help make the diagnosis with much greater accuracy.

Red flags in children with stroke include manifestations of underlying primary processes (e.g., trauma, medications, inborn errors, malignancy, coagulopathy), depressed level of consciousness, a positive family history of early-onset stroke (younger than 30 years of age), signs of increased intracranial pressure (see Chapter 41), a carotid bruit, hypertension, and the presence of prior TIAs.

Not all hemiplegia nor all other focal deficits represent acute cerebrovascular events. Hemiparetic seizures, with their most striking features of acute lateralized weakness and preserved mental state, have been described as a form of partial epilepsy. In addition, seizures can be followed by a postictal (Todd) paralysis that may mimic the motor deficit of stroke. A search for history of previous seizures is essential. A postictal paralysis is short-lived and is unassociated with neuroradiologic characteristics of recent stroke. Preservation of consciousness, a feature not shared by generalized seizures, may help differentiate between epilepsy and cerebrovascular events. The EEG can be helpful in establishing the occurrence of seizure, but the diagnosis remains a clinical one.

Metabolic disturbances may cause focal motor deficits resembling stroke. Hypoglycemia and hyponatremia may each mimic stroke. Similarly, transient hemiparesis unassociated with radiologic changes typical of stroke have been observed in juvenile diabetes mellitus. Survey for the existence of conditions that include these metabolic disturbances is important. Serum electrolyte and glucose levels should be obtained. Similarly, severe anemia causing reduced oxygen delivery to the brain may cause evanescent focal motor deficits; evaluation of an hematocrit is essential in any patient suspected of having suffered stroke.

Alternating hemiplegia of childhood may mimic stroke in children. This disorder appears to be sporadic in its occurrence. Early in its course, oculomotor and extrapyramidal features predominate, but eventually acute episodes of lateralized weakness supervene. The first symptoms of this disorder appear before the age of 18 months. Repeated episodes of lateralized hemiplegia are prominent. However, bilateral hemiplegia may occur. Extrapyramidal symptoms, oculomotor dysfunction, and dysautonomic features may also be present. Symptoms disappear in sleep. Developmental delay or mental retardation is present in all cases. Flunarizine, a calcium channel blocker, has shown some promise as a treatment in its apparent ability to reduce the frequency and duration of hemiplegic attacks. Experience with this drug is limited. Further study of this and other potential therapies are necessary.

Finally, multiple sclerosis may present in childhood with visual or motor disturbances suggesting ischemic stroke; lesions will change in "space and time" and are not often compatible with a neuroanatomic site distal to an arterial supply. MRI reveals demyelination in multiple sclerosis and other demyelinating processes.

REFERENCES

General

Caplan LR. Stroke: A Clinical approach. Stoneham, Mass: Butterworth-Heinemann, 1993:22–53.
Kerr LM, Anderson DM, Thompson JA, et al. Ischemic stroke in the young. J Child Neurol 1993;8:266.
Riela A, Roach S. Etiology of stroke in children. J Child Neurology 1993;8:201–220.
Schoenberg BS, Mellinger JF, Schoenberg DG. Cerebrovascular disease in infants and children: A study of incidence, clinical features, and survival. Neurology 1978;28:763.

The Settings of Stroke in Children

Hypoxic-Ischemic Encephalopathy

Rivkin M, Volpe J. Hypoxic-ischemic brain injury in the newborn. Semin Neurol 1993;13:30.

Idiopathic Cerebral Infarction in the Term Neonate

Butler I. Cerebrovascular disorders of childhood. J Child Neurol 1993;8:197.

Coker S, Beltran R, Myers T, et al. Neonatal stroke: Description of patients and investigation into pathogenesis. Pediatr Neurol 1988;4:219.
Lanska M, Lanska D, Horwitz S, et al. Presentation, clinical course and outcome of childhood stroke. Pediatr Neurol 1991;7:333.
Sran S, Baumann R. Outcome of neonatal stroke. Am J Dis Child 1988;142:1086.

Polycythemia

Barron T, Gusnard D, Zimmerman R, et al. Cerebral venous thrombosis in neonates and children. Pediatr Neurol 1992;8:112.
Black V, Lubchenco L, Koops B, et al. Neonatal hyperviscosity: Randomized study of effect of partial plasma exchange transfusion on long-term outcome. Pediatrics 1985;75:1048.

Neonatal Cerebral Venous Thrombosis

Rivkin M, Anderson M, Kaye E. Neonatal idiopathic cerebral venous thrombosis. 1992;32:51.

Intracranial Hemorrhage in the Neonate

Bergman I, Bauer R, Barmada M, et al. Intracerebral hemorrhage in the full-term infant. Pediatrics 1985;75:488.
Volpe J. Intraventricular hemorrhage in the premature infant—current concepts I, II. Ann Neurol 1989;25:3.

Children Ages 1 to 13 Years

Congenital Heart Disease

Bogousslavsky J, Regli F. Ischemic stroke in adults younger than 30 years of age. Arch Neurol 1987;44:479.
Jones H, Shekert R, Geraci J. Neurologic manifestations of bacterial endocarditis. Ann Intern Med 1969;71:21.
Lechat P, Mas J, Lascault G, et al. Prevalence of patent foramen ovale in patients with stroke. N Engl J Med 1988;318:1148.

Procoagulopathies

Infante-Rivard C, David M, Gauthier R, et al. Lupus anticoagulants, anticardiolipin antibodies and fetal loss. N Engl J Med 1991;325:1063.
Israels S, Seshia S. Childhood stroke associated with protein C or S deficiency. J Pediatr 1987;111:562.
Levine S, Deegan M, Futrell N, et al. Cerebrovascular and neurologic disease associated with antiphospholipid antibodies: 48 cases. Neurology 1990;40:1181.
Pihko H, Tyni T, Virkola K, et al. Transient ischemic cerebral lesions during induction chemotherapy for acute lymphoblastic leukemia. J Pediatr 1993;123:18.

Autoimmune Disorders

Belman A, Leicher C, Moshe S, et al. Neurologic manifestations of Shoenlein-Henoch purpura. Pediatrics 1985;75:687.
Devinsky O, Petito C, Alonso D. Clinical and neuropathological findings in systemic lupus erythematosus: The role of vasculitis, heart emboli and thrombotic thrombocytopenic purpura. Ann Neurol 1988;23:380.
Graf W, Milstein J, Sherry D. Stroke and mixed connective tissue disease. J Child Neurol 1993;8:256.
Kohrman M, Huttenlocher P. Takayasu arteritis: A treatable cause of stroke in infancy. Pediatr Neurol 1986;2:154.
Sigal L. The neurologic presentation of vasculitic and rheumatologic syndromes. Medicine 1987;66:157.

Metabolic Disorders Causing Stroke

Christodoulou J, Qureshi I, McInnes R, et al. Ornithine transcarbamoylase deficiency presenting with stroke like episodes. J Pediatr 1993;122:423.

Glueck C, Daniels S, Bates S, et al. Pediatric victims of unexplained stroke and their families: Familial lipid and lipoprotein abnormalities. Pediatrics 1982;69:308.

Goto Y, Horai S, Matsuoda T, et al. Mitochondrial myopathy, encephalopathy, lactic acidosis, and stroke-like episodes (MELAS): A correlative study of the clinical features and mitochondrial DNA mutation. Neurology 1992;42:545.

Scheuerle A, McVie R, Beaudet A, et al. Arginase deficiency presenting as cerebral palsy. Pediatrics 1993;92:995.

Tulinius M, Holme E, Kristiamsson B, et al. Mitochondrial encephalomyopathies in childhood, I and II. J Pediatr 1991;119:242.

Moyamoya Disease

Karasawa J, Touho H, Ohnishi H, et al. Long-term follow-up after extracranial-intracranial bypass surgery for anterior circulation ischemia in childhood moyamoya disease. J Neurosurg 1992;77:84.

McLean M, Gebarski S, Van der Spek A, et al. Response of moyamoya disease to verapamil. Lancet 1985;1:163.

Rooney C, Kaye E, Scott R, et al. Modified encephaloduro-arteriosynangiosis as surgical treatment of childhood moyamoya disease: Report of 5 cases. J Child Neurol 1991;6:24.

Sickle Cell Disease

Craft S, Schatz J, Glauser T, et al. Neuropsychologic effects of stroke in children with sickle cell anemia. J Pediatr 1993;123:712.

Pavlakis S, Bello J, Prohovnik I, et al. Brain infarction in sickle cell anemia: Magnetic resonance imaging correlates. Ann Neurol 1988;23:125.

Wang W, Kovnar E, Tonkin I, et al. High risk of recurrent stroke after discontinuance of five to twelve years of transfusion therapy in patients with sickle cell disease. J Pediatr 1991;118.

Coagulopathies

Eyster M, Gill F, Blatt P, et al. Central nervous system bleeding in hemophiliacs. Blood 1978;51:1179.

Silverstein A. Intracranial bleeding in hemophilia. Arch Neurol 1960;3:141.

Thrombocytopenia

Woerner S, Abildgaard C, French M. Intracranial hemorrhage in children with idiopathic thrombocytopenic purpura. Pediatrics 1981;67:453.

Vascular Malformations

Broechler J, Thron A. Intracranial arterial aneurysms in children. Neurosurg Rev 1990;13:309.

Brown Y, Wiebers K, Forbes G. Unruptured intracranial aneurysms and arteriovenous malformations: Frequency of intracranial haemorrhage and relationship of lesions. J Neurosurg 1990;73:859.

Ito M, Yishuhara M, Wachi A, et al. Cerebral aneurysms in children. Brain Dev 1992;14:263.

Konsiolka D, Humphreys R, Hoffman H, et al. Arteriovenous malformations of the brain in children: A forty year experience. Can J Neurol Sci 1992;19:40.

Adolescents

Fibromuscular Dysplasia

Corrin L, Sandok B, Houser O. Cerebral ischemic events in patients with carotid artery fibromucular dysplasia. Arch Neurol 1981;38:616.

Smith D, Smith L, Hasso A. Fibromuscular dysplasia of the internal carotid artery treated by operative transluminal balloon angioplasty. Radiology 1985;155:645.

Sexual Activity, Oral Contraception, and the Puerperium

Adams H, Butler M, Biller J, et al. Nonhemorrhagic cerebral infarction in young adults. Arch Neurol 1987;43:713.

Bousser M, Chiras J, Bories J, et al. Cerebral venous thrombosis—a review of 38 cases. Stroke 1985;16:199.

Toffol G, Biller J, Adams H. Nontraumatic intracerebral hemorrhage in young adults. Arch Neurol 1987;44:479.

Cocaine Use and Stroke

Cregler L, Mark H. Medical complications of cocaine abuse. N Engl J Med 1986;315:1495.

Klonoff D, Andrews B, Obana W. Stroke associated with cocaine use. Arch Neurol 1989;46:989.

Causes of Stroke Unrelated to Age

Pharyngeal Infection

Bush J, Givner L, Whitaker S, et al. Necrotizing fasciitis of the parapharyngeal space with carotid artery occlusion and acute hemiplegia. Pediatrics 1984;73:343.

Shillito J. Carotid arteritis: A cause of hemiplegia in childhood. J Neurosurg 1964;21:540.

Tagawa T, Mimaki T, Yabuuchi H, et al. Bilateral occlusions in the cervical portion of the internal carotid arteries in a child. Stroke 1985;16:896.

Head and Neck Trauma

Garg B, Ottinger C, Smith R, et al. Strokes in children due to vertebral artery trauma. Neurology 1993;43:2555.

Hope E, Bodensteiner J, Barnes P. Cerebral infarction related to neck position in an adolescent. Pediatrics 1983;72:335.

Lewis D, Berman P. Vertebral artery dissections and alternating hemiparesis in an adolescent. Pediatrics 1986;78:610.

Migraine Headache

Bogousslavsky J, Regli F, Van Melle G, et al. Migraine stroke. Neurology 1988;38:223.

Caplan L. Migraine and vertebrobasilar ischemia. Neurology 1991;41:55.

Conditions Resembling Stroke

Bourgeois M, Aicardi J, Goutieres F. Alternating hemiplegia of childhood. J Pediatr 1993;122:673.

Casaer P. Flunarizine in alternating hemiplegia in childhood. Neuropediatrics 1987;18:191.

Hanson P, Chodos R. Hemiparetic seizures. Neurology 1978;28:920.

Yarnell P. Todd's paralysis: A cerebrovascular phenomenon. Stroke 1975;6:301.

43 Syncope and Dizziness

David A. Lewis

Dizziness is a nonspecific symptom that generally requires some elaboration by the patient for the physician to know what the patient exactly means. The description of the feeling is critical in distinguishing whether the sensation is due to vertigo, disequilibrium, lightheadedness, or presyncope (Table 43–1). Although the differential diagnoses of these entities overlap, there are conditions that are most specific to each. All of the above are conditions of older children who are capable of articulating the abnormal sensation they feel. Children younger than 6 years of age may present with nausea, vomiting, ataxia, or frank syncope.

Syncope is the transient loss of consciousness and postural tone that results from inadequate cerebral perfusion. Syncope is a common phenomenon in children and adolescents and is usually benign. It is critical to distinguish between syncope associated with exertion or activity versus syncope "at rest" (see below). The history of the event, obtained from the patient or witnesses, will be critical in establishing the differential diagnosis.

Presyncope is the feeling that one is "about to pass out." The patient feels as if he or she is going to lose consciousness but does not. Presyncope may or may not reflect the same pathophysiology as true syncope. The diagnostic approach to presyncope, however, is essentially the same as for syncope.

Dizziness must be considered a change in mental status. It may potentially herald serious underlying central nervous system dysfunction. Dizziness must be better defined to distinguish *vertigo* from *lightheadedness*. The principal distinction is the description of motion; swaying, whirling, or spinning is characteristic of vertigo. Lightheadedness often accompanies hyperventilation and is therefore frequently associated with psychologic distress, including anxiety, depression, and panic attacks. The history surrounding episodes of lightheadedness is vital to formulating the differential diagnosis.

The last of the "dizzy" feelings is *disequilibrium*. Disequilibrium refers to "balance problems" without vertigo. The characteristic historical feature is difficulty ambulating. A fairly rare complaint among children, disequilibrium in the young is most often due to vestibular dysfunction or ataxia.

The common trait among all the "dizzy" feelings is primary or secondary central nervous system dysfunction. Dizziness should be considered an alteration in the patient's level of consciousness and must be taken seriously.

SYNCOPE

Syncope is a common phenomenon among children and adolescents. As many as 15% of children have a syncopal event between the ages of 8 and 18 years. Under age 6 years, syncope is very unusual except in the setting of seizure disorders and primary cardiac dysrhythmias. Syncope in children provokes great anxiety in parents, teachers, and other children. Fainting episodes cause a large number of visits to pediatricians, family physicians, and emergency departments and a surprising number of admissions to community and children's hospitals. The differential diagnosis of syncope is noted in Table 43–2.

The pathophysiology of syncope seems to follow a common pathway with many inciting stimuli. Cerebral perfusion is compromised by a transient decrease in cardiac output as a result of vasomotor changes decreasing venous return, primary dysrhythmia, or impairment of cerebral vascular tone. Adolescents subjected to a head-up tilt table test report blurred vision and constriction of visual fields prior to losing consciousness as well as nausea, pallor, sweating, and dizziness, which are accompanied by hypotension (systolic blood pressure < 60 mmHg), bradycardia (heart rate < 40 beats/minute) with an occasional junctional rhythm and even asystole (Fig. 43–1). Symptoms are relieved by returning to the supine position.

Several situational factors can exacerbate this response, including:

- Warm temperature
- A confined space, such as being in a crowded room

Table 43–1. Syncope and Dizziness

Patient complaint	"My head is spinning." "The room is whirling."	"I feel I might pass out." "I feel faint."	"I feel unsteady." "My balance is off."	"I feel dizzy." "I feel disconnected, drugged."
Diagnosis	Vertigo	Presyncope	Disequilibrium	Lightheadedness
Usual cause	Vestibular disorders	Impaired cerebral perfusion	Sensory and/or central neurologic dysfunction	Anxiety and/or depressive disorders
Key differential diagnoses	Peripheral (labyrinthine-cochlear) vs. Central neurologic disorder	Neurocardiogenic (vagal) vs. Cardiac syncope vs. Neuropsychiatric syncope	Sensory deficit vs. Central neurologic disease	Anxiety/depression vs. Hyperventilation vs. Medication effects

Modified from Reilly BM. Practical Strategies in Outpatient Medicine, 2nd ed. Philadelphia: WB Saunders, 1991:163.

Table 43–2. Syncope and Dizziness: Etiology

Diagnosis	History	Symptoms	Description	Heart Rate/Blood Pressure	Duration	Postsyncope	Recurrence
Neurocardiogenic (Vasodepressor)	At rest	Pallor, nausea, visual changes	Brief ± convulsion	↓/↓	<1 min	Residual pallor, sweaty, hot; recurs if child stands	Common
Other Vagal							
Vasovagal	Needlestick	Pallor, nausea	Brief; convulsions rare	↓/↓	<1 min	Residual pallor; may recur if child stands	Situational
Micturition	Post-voiding	Pallor, nausea	Brief ± convulsion	↓/↓	<1 min		(+)
Cough (deglutition)	Paroxysmal cough	Cough	Abrupt onset	May not change	<5 min	Fatigue or baseline	(+)
Carotid sinus	Tight collar, turned head	Vague, visual changes	Sudden onset, pallor	Usually ↓/↓	<5 min	Fatigue or baseline	(+)
Hypoglycemia	Fasting, insulin use	Gradual hunger, weakness, sweating	Pallor, sweating, loss of consciousness rare	No change or mild tachycardia	Variable	Relieved by eating only	(+)
Neuropsychiatric							
Hyperventilation	Anxiety	SOB, fear, claustrophobia	Agitated, hyperpneic	Mild ↓/↓	<5 min	Fatigue or baseline	(+)
Syncopal migraine	Headache	Aura, migraine, nausea	± pallor	No change	<10 min	Headache, often occipital	(+)
Seizure disorder	Anytime	± aura	Convulsion ± incontinence	No change or mild tachycardia	Any duration	Postictal lethargy + confusion	(+)
Hysterical	Always an "audience" present	Psychologic distress	Gentle, graceful swoon	No change	Any duration	Normal baseline	(+)
Breath-holding (hypoxic)	Agitation or injury	Crying	Cyanosis ± convulsion	↓/↓ Frequent asystole	<10 min	Fatigue, residual pallor	(+)
Cardiac Syncope							
LVOT obstruction	Exercise	± chest pain, SOB	Abrupt during or after exertion, pallor	↑/↓	Any duration	Fatigue, residual pallor, and sweating	(+)
Pulmonary hypertension	Anytime, especially exercise	SOB	Cyanosis and pallor	↑/↓	Any duration	Fatigue, residual cyanosis	(+)
Myocarditis	Post-viral exercise	SOB, chest pain, palpitations	Pallor	↑/↓	Any duration	Fatigue	(+)
Tumor or mass	Recumbent, paroxysmal	SOB ± chest pain	Pallor	↑/↓	Any duration	Baseline	(+)
Coronary artery	Exercise	SOB ± chest pain	Pallor	↑/↓	Any duration	Fatigue, chest pain	(+)
Dysrhythmia	Anytime	Palpitations ± chest pain	Pallor	↑ or ↓/↓	Usually <10 min	Fatigue or baseline	(+)

Abbreviations: LVOT = left ventricular outflow obstruction; SOB = shortness of breath; ± = with or without.

- Anxiety
- Sudden surprise

The response is due to imbalance of parasympathetic and sympathetic tone, which results in peripheral vasodilation, including venodilation but no augmentation of venous return, because there is no accompanying increase in large skeletal muscle activity to augment systemic venous return and maintain cardiac filling. Subsequent vagal output results in inappropriate bradycardia and further compromises cardiac output. The child faints and becomes supine, which restores systemic venous return to the right heart. At the same time, awakening is accompanied by increased sympathetic

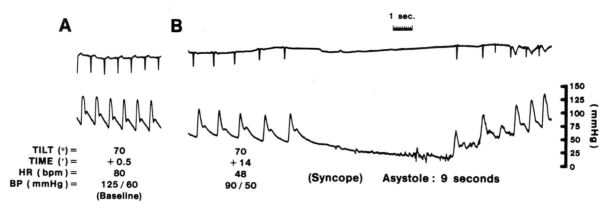

Figure 43–1. *A*, Baseline heart rate (HR), blood pressure (BP), and rhythm 0.5 minutes after tilt to 70 degrees. *B*, Bradycardia and hypotension progressing rapidly to asystole with prompt recovery on returning to the supine position. This is an example of the cardioinhibitory response to orthostatic stress. (From Sra JS, Murthy VS, Jazayeri MR, et al. Use of intravenous esmolol to predict efficacy of oral beta-adrenergic blocker therapy in patients with neurocardiogenic syncope. J Am Coll Cardiol 1992;19:402–408.)

output, which restores the heart rate. The episode tends to be brief but may recur if the patient is "helped up" too quickly. The scenario in which this combination of events might be most dangerous is a hot, closed telephone booth in which a patient cannot become supine and restore cardiac output. The magnitude of this vagal response should not be underestimated. In studies utilizing isoproterenol, despite the powerful β_1-adrenergic stimulation, susceptible patients become profoundly bradycardic and experience junctional rhythm and even asystole.

When one is obtaining the history of a syncopal episode, attention should be paid to the time of day, time of last meal, activities leading up to the event, and associated symptoms (palpitations, racing heart beat, chest pain, headache, shortness of breath, nausea, diaphoresis, visual changes, and hearing changes). Details such as the patient's position when symptoms appeared, duration of the episode, and characterization of the patient's appearance during and immediately following the episode are also important. Almost without exception, the physical examination in children and adolescents will be normal. Therefore, the history becomes the most important piece of information developing the differential diagnosis, evaluation, and management plan.

Neurocardiogenic Syncope

Neurocardiogenic syncope is a type of autonomic dysfunction that is also referred to as *vasodepressor syncope, vasovagal syncope,* and *reflex syncope.* Three mechanisms appear to exist:

1. The first response is primary bradycardia with subsequent hypotension (see Fig. 43–1).
2. A primary vasodepressor response is characterized by hypotension, with the heart rate being relatively preserved.
3. A mixed response features simultaneous hypotension and bradycardia.

The common pathway resulting in central nervous system dysfunction is cerebral hypotension and is also known as the *Bezold-Jarisch reflex* (Fig. 43–2). For most children and adolescents, prodromal warning signs herald the impending episode and can, after the first episode, allow the child enough time to prevent fainting by sitting with the head between the knees or by lying supine.

If the history suggests the diagnosis of neurocardiogenic syncope with a normal physical examination and electrocardiogram (ECG),

treatment may be empirically started. The first line of treatment is the use of salt supplementation (1 g/day orally) with the mineralocorticoid fludrocortisone acetate (Florinef) (0.1 mg/day orally). The average patient will gain about 1 kg of water weight into the circulating volume over 2 to 3 weeks, and the increased volume will allow blood pressure to be maintained even in the face of vasodilation. A repeat tilt test during therapy is sometimes done.

A second therapeutic choice is usually β-adrenergic receptor blockade, typically with atenolol or metoprolol. A second tilt test may be performed. Further therapies include theophylline or pseudoephedrine, and diisopyramide.

An alternative to empiric therapy with repeated tilt testing is the baseline tilt test, followed shortly thereafter with a therapeutic trial of the short-acting beta blocker esmolol and retilting immediately. If esmolol does not prevent a vasodepressor response, the patient is returned to the supine position, esmolol is stopped, and a phenylephrine infusion is begun. The patient is then tilted again. If this does not prevent symptoms during a 30-minute tilt, the patient is returned to the supine position and the phenylephrine infusion is discontinued. One liter of normal saline is then infused over 15 to 20 minutes, and the patient is again tilted to 70 degrees for 30 minutes. Tilt testing can be performed with or without invasive blood pressure monitoring. Outpatient therapy is then chosen according to which therapeutic challenge prevented the development of symptoms during a 30-minute tilt to 70 degrees. This then generally obviates the need for a tilt test during therapy.

There are several causes of autonomic or neurocardiogenic syncope. Excessive vagal tone may be primary or secondary to breath-holding, cough, swallowing (deglutition syncope), micturition or defecation, carotid sinus pressure sensitivity, and orthostasis. Of these, *breath-holding episodes* are among the most common and frightening, representing a frequent mechanism of syncope in children under age 6 years. Typically, the child is startled or agitated, and a period of crying terminates with prolonged expiration, visible cyanosis, and collapse. Not surprisingly, these episodes result in a great deal of parental anxiety. That anxiety is magnified when monitoring illustrates that the episode is accompanied by reflex increase in vagal tone often accompanied by asystole for 15 to 30 seconds. Most children "outgrow" these episodes, which rarely affect future central nervous function, such as cognition. So-called and rare "malignant breath-holding" spells have been treated with placement of permanent cardiac pacemakers with less than convincing results in affecting mortality. There may be some role for preventing the potential cerebral injury associated with profound hypotension during prolonged or repeated episodes of asystole.

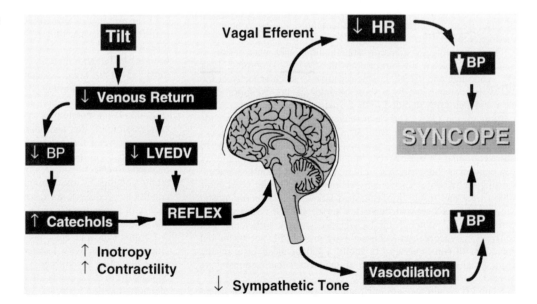

Figure 43–2. Tilt table testing: the Bezold-Jarisch reflex. HR = heart rate; BP = blood pressure; LVEDV = left ventricular end-diastolic volume.

Nonetheless, most patients and families are treated expectantly with reassurance about the benign nature of the usual breath-holding spells.

Reflex vagal bradycardia has been described in association with hair brushing, swallowing, stretching, orthodontic maneuvers, anomalies of the cervical spine, and dental trauma. Many of these may actually be forms of carotid sinus sensitivity. Cough syncope probably is related to prolongation of high intrathoracic pressure that results in decreased venous return and subsequent decreased cardiac output.

The prodromal history is very important in neurocardiogenic or autonomic syncope. Syncope without warning implies a primary cardiac etiology and carries much greater morbidity and potential mortality.

Cardiac Syncope

A variety of cardiac conditions can result in hypotension and syncope. Table 43–2 lists several potential cardiac causes of syncope, both structural and arrhythmogenic. Diseases that produce hypotension (orthostatic, supine) frequently produce syncope or presyncope. Cardiac function and structure are usually normal before the episode; during the predisposing illness, cardiac filling pressures are often reduced because of reduced venous return from hypovolemia or decreased peripheral vascular resistance (peripheral pooling of blood). Dehydration from diarrhea and vomiting, hyperthermia, hyperpyrexia, heat exhaustion, polyuria (diabetes mellitus), or poor intake from anorexia, together with the systemic effects of the primary illness, may produce orthostatic or true hypotension and syncope. Toxins, as in *toxic shock syndrome,* may also contribute to orthostatic or true hypotension. Prolonged bed rest, combined with poor fluid intake during an illness, may also result in syncope or presyncope when the child arises to leave the bed. In most of these situations, intravenous fluid administration (normal saline, lactated Ringer's) is sufficient to restore intravascular volume and venous return to alleviate postural or supine hypotension. Refractory hypotension suggests more serious pathology, such as anaphylaxis, toxic shock syndrome, myocardial disease, or septic shock.

Dysrhythmias are common and are usually the most silent between episodes (see Chapter 12). Supraventricular tachycardia, ventricular tachycardia, and heart block are the most common and may be primary or may result from medications or illicit drugs. Postsurgical and acquired heart block carry a high mortality. One of the more common causes of acquired heart block is Lyme disease. Heart block may necessitate temporary pacing to maintain cardiac output.

Primary cardiac conduction abnormalities that may result in syncope include Wolff-Parkinson-White (WPW) syndrome, long QT syndrome, and catecholamine-sensitive ventricular tachycardia. WPW is characterized by a short PR interval, pre-excitation seen as a widened QRS duration with a "delta wave" on the proximal portion of the QRS. The delta wave represents the presence of accessory electrical tissue from atria to ventricle, with rapid antegrade conduction causing excitation of ventricular tissue prior to atrioventricular (AV) node–His bundle stimulation. If that pathway can conduct in the retrograde fashion, a re-entrant circuit is created, causing tachycardia. This greatly shortens the diastolic ventricular filling time and results in diminished left ventricular end-diastolic volume, with subsequent decreased stroke volume and decreased cardiac output. Although the tachycardia is rarely sufficiently fast to result in syncope, some children have profound hypotension and rapid loss of consciousness. In adults, a similar mechanism results from atrial flutter or fibrillation if the ventricular response rate is fast.

Long QT syndromes are inherited abnormalities in the electrical

recovery (repolarization) of the heart. Prolongation of the repolarization phase results in the risk of simultaneous depolarization, the "R-on-T" phenomenon, which causes disorganized ventricular electrical stimulation characterized by Torsades de pointes coarse ventricular tachycardia, a potentially lethal dysrhythmia. There is usually a family history of sudden death. Some have theorized that long QT syndromes may be responsible for some of the incidence of sudden infant death syndrome as well. Acquired prolongation of the QT interval may also be seen in electrolyte abnormalities (hyperkalemia) and with a variety of medications, including primary antiarrhythmic drugs (procainamide, quinidine, disopyramide, amiodarone), phenothiazines, antibiotics (erythromycin), antihistamines (Hismanal), and tricyclic antidepressants (imipramine, desipramine, Tofranil), which are used commonly in children with attention deficit hyperactivity disorder. For this reason, a toxicology screen may be warranted if there is any question of QT prolongation.

Patients who are status post corrective or palliative surgery for congenital cardiac disease are at risk for some dysrhythmias that might result in syncope. Sinus node disease (in patients undergoing atrial surgery) may result in "tachy-brady" episodes that can be associated with hypotension. Ventricular dysrhythmias are particularly common after repair of tetralogy of Fallot, double-outlet right ventricle, truncus arteriosus, and pulmonary atresia involving right ventriculotomy with subsequent ventricular scar formation.

Uncorrected structural heart disease is a relatively rare cause of a sudden decrease in cardiac output. However, hypertrophic cardiomyopathies, particularly idiopathic hypertrophic subaortic stenosis can result in obstruction of left ventricular outflow with resultant high transmural pressure and secondary cardiac ischemia, which can be fatal. This type of obstruction is exacerbated by high sympathetic tone, which causes increased contractility and is a frequent mechanism of the presentation of syncope associated with exercise in competitive athletics. The presence of an outflow tract murmur in the setting of syncope, especially if there is a positive family history, warrants evaluation with both electrocardiography and echocardiography. Any condition that impedes left ventricular outflow (valvar aortic stenosis, subaortic stenosis), left ventricular inflow or filling (mitral stenosis, pericardial tamponade), or blood flow through the pulmonary vasculature (pulmonary hypertension) may also result in syncope. In almost all cases characteristic physical findings lead the clinician to the diagnosis. Pulmonary hypertension may be associated with cyanosis, as in *Eisenmenger syndrome,* in which case there is cerebral hypoxia due to right-to-left shunting as well as decreased left ventricular output due to poor transpulmonary flow and decreased left ventricular filling (see Chapter 15).

Other rare causes of cardiac syncope are coronary artery abnormalities, intracardiac tumors or masses, and inflammatory cardiac diseases (myocarditis). Masses or tumors, such as myxomas, fibromas, and rhabdomyomas, tend to produce paroxysmal symptoms, which are often associated with position changes, especially in the recumbent position. Coronary artery anomalies are usually not accompanied by signs of ischemia. Rather, the most common (Fig. 43–3) presentation is syncope or sudden cardiac death from compression of the anomalous left main coronary artery as it courses between the pulmonary outflow and the aortic root. This usually occurs in the competitive athlete whose hypertrophied heart responds to catecholamine stimulation during activity and inadvertently compresses the anomalous coronary artery. Inflammatory conditions predispose to dysrhythmias, such as heart block associated with Lyme disease and ventricular tachycardia associated with myocarditis.

Cardiac syncopal episodes can be accompanied by brief tonic-clonic seizure activity known as *Stokes-Adams syndrome.* Originally described in children with heart block, the seizure activity appears 10 to 20 seconds after the onset of asystole and is usually of short duration with no subsequent postictal phase. This may

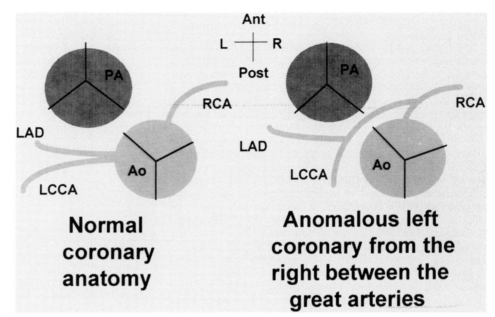

Figure 43–3. Coronary artery anomalies associated with sudden death. Ant = anterior; post = posterior; PA = pulmonary artery; L = left; R = right; Ao = aorta; LAD = left anterior descending coronary artery; LCCA = left circumflex coronary artery. RCA = right coronary artery.

explain why so many children with cardiac syncope frequently see a neurologist.

Neuropsychiatric Syncope

Primary neurologic causes of syncope are much more unusual in otherwise healthy children and adolescents than in adults. Convulsive disorders must be considered if there is a history of an aural prodrome, focal or generalized tonic-clonic activity, and a prolonged postictal phase of lethargy or confusion. Prolonged postevent lethargy is unusual with usual causes of syncope if the vital signs have returned to normal. Seizures are the most likely cause of syncope in the recumbent patient. Absence seizures may lack the aura, motor activity, and postictal confusion and must be distinguished from narcolepsy and temporal lobe seizures, which may have variable motor activity that sometimes appears purposeful but with more gradual loss of consciousness (see Chapter 40).

A premonitory aura may herald vertebrobasilar vascular spasm, which appears to occur in syncope associated with migraines. There may be a history of visual changes on only one side, and there is usually a somewhat longer onset and duration to the loss of consciousness. Hemodynamic status remains stable throughout the episode. The patient frequently complains of headache after regaining consciousness.

Patients with a history of panic attacks or histrionic personalities may become syncopal secondary to hyperventilation. The mechanism is not completely understood but may involve the interaction of cerebral blood flow in response to hypocapnia and respiratory alkalosis. The history of the episode is again critical, and witnesses are especially helpful. The patient frequently relates a feeling of suffocation, smothering, shortness of breath, or chest tightness. In retrospect, the patient may also admit to numbness and tingling of the extremities and visual changes.

Hypoglycemia should always be included as a cause of syncope, but it is exceedingly rare in children and adolescents. Certainly in the patient with insulin-dependent diabetes, hypoglycemia remains an important concern. As the blood glucose level drops, the patient feels weak, hungry, sweaty, agitated, and confused and eventually experiences altered mental status. Onset is gradual, and the patient remains hemodynamically stable (see Chapter 63).

Hysterical syncope is a diagnosis of exclusion. The patient is usually an adolescent and always has episodes in the presence of an audience. The patient is unusually calm in describing the episodes and relates details that may indicate no loss of consciousness. During the episode, there are no associated hemodynamic changes and no pallor, sweating, or respiratory changes. Typically, the patient falls gracefully and gently without injury. The key is to define what secondary gain is obtained by the patient via the syncopal charade.

Evaluation of the Syncopal Child

HISTORY

Most children and adolescents who have a syncopal episode can be evaluated by their pediatrician. The history of the event is the critical information for most patients. A detailed account of what the patient felt immediately prior to losing consciousness, what the patient was doing, what the posture or position was, how the patient looked, how long the episode lasted, and associated signs or symptoms direct the practitioner and the diagnostic work-up. A thorough and detailed family history is necessary to discover risk for sudden death, dysrhythmia, congenital heart disease, seizures, and metabolic disorders. Medication history, including nonprescribed, prescribed, and illicit drugs, as well as any accessible medication of other family members should be gathered.

PHYSICAL EXAMINATION

Any person who suffers a syncopal episode should undergo a thorough physical examination, with special attention to the cardiovascular and neurologic systems. The examination should include obtaining vital signs with the patient supine and after standing for 5 to 10 minutes. Careful auscultation for the presence of an outflow tract murmur radiating to the neck, abnormally loud second heart sound, or the presence of a long decrescendo diastolic murmur at the apex leads to more involved diagnostic testing. In most cases, patients with syncope have normal physical findings.

DIAGNOSTIC TESTS

The history and physical examination guide the practitioner in determining the diagnostic tests. Because the child or adolescent who has had a syncopal episode is often evaluated hours or days after the episode, testing serum glucose and electrolytes may not be of value. All patients presenting with syncope need an ECG. The ECG should be inspected for the rhythm, with special attention to non-sinus rhythms and bradycardia. Measurements of the intervals should be performed manually regardless of any preprogrammed measurements printed on the ECG. Abnormalities of the PR, QRS, or QT/QTc interval imply an underlying conduction abnormality. The P-wave, QRS, and T-wave amplitudes may indicate chamber enlargement or hypertrophy, each of which carries an increased risk for dysrhythmia. In the patient with a history of palpitations associated with syncope, a 24-hour (ECG) Holter monitor with an event recorder monitor may help capture the cardiac rhythm when the patient is symptomatic. If a heart murmur is appreciated, if there is a family history of sudden death or cardiomyopathy, or if the ECG is at all questionable, a cardiology consultation should be obtained and two-dimensional, Doppler, and color flow echocardiography should be performed. If the syncopal event is associated with exercise, a graded treadmill exercise stress test should be performed with full ECG and blood pressure monitoring. Patients with primary dysrhythmias may require cardiac catheterization and electrophysiologic testing with invasive monitoring. Patients with positional syncope with autonomic symptoms should undergo tilt table testing with autonomic function testing utilizing rhythmic breathing, carotid massage, Valsalva maneuver, and diving reflex elicited with ice to the face.

Patients exhibiting prolonged loss of consciousness, seizure activity, and a postictal phase of lethargy or confusion should be referred for neurologic consultation and electroencephalography (EEG). Without this history, the reported positive yield of EEG is less than 1 in 300 studies. Likewise, imaging studies generally have an exceptionally low yield in the absence of abnormality on physical examination.

SUMMARY AND RED FLAGS

The evaluation of the syncopal child or adolescent relies heavily on the ability to perform a thorough, detailed history and physical examination. Hypotension, both supine and orthostatic, is a major red flag. Laboratory tests, except for the ECG, which is mandatory, are generally of limited value unless guided by pertinent positives or negatives in the history and physical examination. The ECG allows screening for red flags (dysrhythmias), such as WPW, heart block, and long QT syndrome as well as hypertrophic cardiomyopathies and myocarditis. The most common identifiable etiologic factor in otherwise healthy children and adolescents is neurocardiogenic or vasodepressor syncope, a usually benign and transient condition.

VERTIGO

The characteristic description of vertigo is the illusion of motion, usually described as spinning or whirling (see Table 43–1). The perception of motion may be internal ("my head or eyes are spinning") or external ("the room is spinning or moving"). The sensation is usually rotatory, but it can be linear ("it feels like the swaying of a boat"). The patient's description is critical although potentially vague; further questioning may lead to the rather discrete differential diagnosis of vertigo.

The presence of associated symptoms may help if the patient's description leaves doubt about the type of dizziness. Nausea and vomiting frequently accompany vertigo, as do auditory changes, such as tinnitus, ear fullness, and unilateral deafness. This is especially important in small children who are unable to articulate the feeling of vertigo. Because middle ear infection can cause peripheral vertigo, some of the many children seen with otitis media and vomiting may in fact have peripheral vertigo and secondary vomiting. If the dizziness usually occurs with abrupt changes in the position of the head, vertigo should be suspected. All vertigo reflects dysfunction of the vestibular-cochlear system.

The vestibular-cochlear apparatus with its associated reflex pathways is very complex. Dysfunction of the vestibular-cochlear apparatus is usually *central* (brainstem and eighth cranial nerve) or *peripheral* (distal or peripheral to the eighth cranial nerve).

Central vestibular disease refers to disorders of the brainstem, especially at the level of the vestibular nuclei or oculomotor nuclei or cerebellum (Table 43–3). Underlying causes of central vestibular dysfunction include:

Table 43–3. Differences Between Peripheral and Central Vestibular Dysfunctions

Symptom/Sign	Peripheral	Central
Severity of vertigo	Marked	Often mild
	Nausea and vomiting common	
Nystagmus	Bilateral	Bilateral or unilateral
	Unidirectional	Bidirectional or unidirectional
	Rotatory/horizontal	May be vertical
	Never vertical	Usually no change with visual fixation
	Fast phase usually opposite to side of lesion	
	Improves with visual fixation	
	Begins within 2–10 sec	Begins immediately
	Fatigues with time	Persistent
	Habituates	Reproducibly repetitive
Direction of environmental spin	Toward fast phase of nystagmus	Variable
Direction of past pointing	Toward slow phase of nystagmus	Variable
Direction of Romberg fall		
Tinnitus/deafness	Often present	Usually absent
Examples	Labyrinthitis	Multiple sclerosis
	Ménière's disease	Vertebrobasilar ischemia (see Table 43–5)
	Positional vertigo (see Table 43–4)	

Modified from Reilly BM. Practical Strategies in Outpatient Medicine, 2nd ed. Philadelphia: WB Saunders, 1991:191.

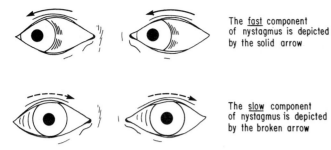

The **fast** component of nystagmus is depicted by the solid arrow

The **slow** component of nystagmus is depicted by the broken arrow

Figure 43–4. (Fast) nystagmus to the right. The appearance of the eyes is that of "frantic," jerky eye movements to the right—the direction of the fast component. (From Reilly BM. *Practical Strategies in Outpatient Medicine*, 2nd ed. Philadelphia: WB Saunders, 1991:192.)

- Acute vascular ischemic or thromboembolic events
- Acute demyelinating diseases
- Pharmacologic vertigo (alcohol, barbiturates, benzodiazepines)
- More indolent causes include tumors of the brainstem or cerebellum and chronic demyelinating diseases.

Peripheral vertigo is generally unilateral and results in stimulation of the autonomic nervous system with resultant intense nausea, vomiting, pallor, and diaphoresis (see Table 43–3). Peripheral vertigo can be caused by the following:

- Middle ear infections
- Paroxysmal positional vertigo
- Labrynthitis
- Vestibular neuronitis
- Ménière disease
- Trauma

Patients suffering from acute ongoing peripheral vertigo appear very ill and very uncomfortable.

Acute ongoing vertigo is always accompanied by nystagmus. The rapidity of onset and the severity determine the severity of the nystagmus. Patients who complain of intermittent vertigo frequently do not have nystagmus between episodes. Figures 43–4 to 43–6 illustrate the appearance of central and peripheral vertigo–related nystagmus. Nystagmus in children with peripheral vestibular dysfunction is usually suppressed by visual fixation. Using an ophthalmoscope, the physician covers and uncovers the contralateral eye, inhibiting and permitting fixation. Peripheral nystagmus is frequently bilateral, unidirectional (slow and fast components in the same direction), and rotatory or horizontal (clockwise or counterclockwise). Therefore, nystagmus that is bidirectional, vertical, or unilateral should be considered central in origin.

Peripheral vestibular dysfunction has characteristic findings that can be elicited on physical examination. Deviation from these findings should imply central dysfunction and should direct the diagnostic work-up to the central nervous system. Central vestibular dysfunction is much less common than peripheral vertigo and has

Figure 43–5. Peripheral nystagmus. *A*, In this case, nystagmus (fast right) affects each eye equally (bilateral), is unidirectional (the direction of fast and slow components stays the same in all gaze directions), and is horizontal and rotatory (i.e., the eyes move in the horizontal plane and in a counterclockwise direction during nystagmus). *B, Horizontal/ rotatory* nystagmus, which occurs on vertical gaze, is *not* vertical nystagmus. *C*, In this instance, nystagmus (fast left) is horizontal/rotatory, unidirectional (fast component is always to the left), and bilateral. (From Reilly BM. *Practical Strategies in Outpatient Medicine*, 2nd ed. Philadelphia: WB Saunders, 1991:192.)

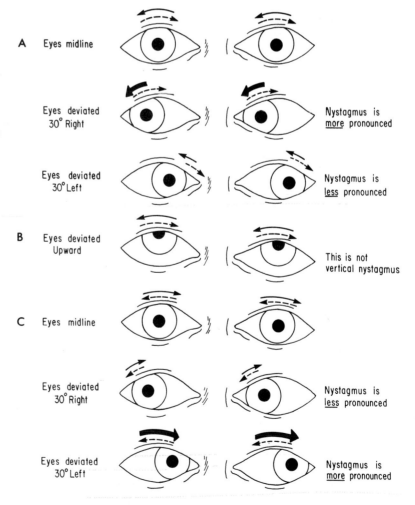

A Eyes midline

Eyes deviated 30° Right — Nystagmus is **more** pronounced

Eyes deviated 30° Left — Nystagmus is **less** pronounced

B Eyes deviated Upward — This is not vertical nystagmus

C Eyes midline

Eyes deviated 30° Right — Nystagmus is **less** pronounced

Eyes deviated 30° Left — Nystagmus is **more** pronounced

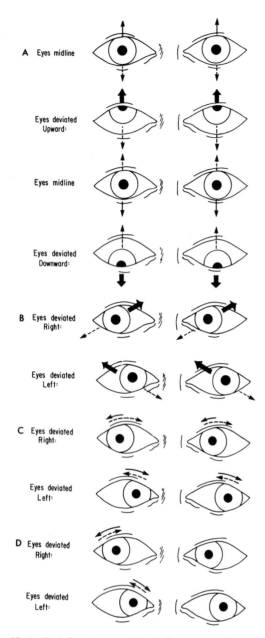

Figure 43–6. Central nystagmus. *A,* Vertical nystagmus. *Upper panel:* The fast (upward) component of vertical nystagmus is more prominent on upward gaze. *Lower panel:* The fast component of vertical nystagmus is "downbeating" and is even more prominent on downward gaze. *B,* Vertical nystagmus may persist on horizontal eye movements as well—this is still vertical nystagmus. *C,* Bidirectional nystagmus. The fast and slow components in this case change direction in different gaze directions. *D,* Unilateral nystagmus. Nystagmus in this instance affects only the right eye (and also changes direction—it is bidirectional as well). (From Reilly BM. Practical Strategies in Outpatient Medicine, 2nd ed. Philadelphia: WB Saunders, 1991:194.)

the patient perceives the environment spinning, and the direction of the nystagmus is important in localizing the lesion. Such patients have an abnormal neurologic examination, and all of the abnormalities are explainable on the basis of vestibular or cochlear dysfunction.

Patients with acute ongoing peripheral vestibular dysfunction frequently cannot walk and often have abnormal Romberg test findings (Fig. 43–8). They may complain of double vision and fine motor discoordination. Associated symptoms, such as dysarthria, dysesthesias, weakness, blindness, true diplopia, or hemiplegia, strongly imply a central mechanism, frequently of vascular origin. These are ominous findings, especially in the child with hemophilia, sickle cell disease, a history of congenital heart disease, or dysrhythmia. Likewise, the simultaneous presence of dysphagia, aphasia, pathologic reflexes, or unilateral cerebellar dysfunction (dysmetria, dysdiadochokinesia) with vestibular dysfunction is of central origin.

To make the diagnosis of acute ongoing peripheral vestibular dysfunction, the following must be demonstrated:

1. Vertigo must be a symptom.
2. Nystagmus must be carefully evaluated and must be of the peripheral type (bilateral, unidirectional, rotatory/horizontal).
3. There can be no neurologic signs or symptoms that cannot be explained by peripheral vestibular dysfunction.

Most patients do not have ongoing vertigo but give an episodic history. Provocational maneuvers of the head, such as the Nylen-Bárány maneuver, are utilized to elicit their symptoms (Fig. 43–9). Table 43–4 demonstrates the various types of peripheral vestibu-

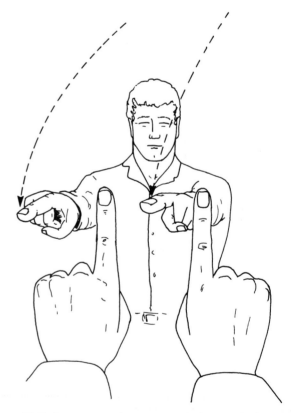

Figure 43–7. Past pointing. The patient is asked to raise the hands over the head and then, with the eyes closed, touch the examiner's fingers. This figure illustrates abnormal past pointing to the right—past pointing often points toward the side of the vestibular lesion. (From Reilly BM. Practical Strategies in Outpatient Medicine, 2nd ed. Philadelphia: WB Saunders, 1991:195.)

a more serious underlying cause and a higher morbidity and mortality.

The patient with peripheral vertigo typically falls toward or past-points (Fig. 43–7) to the side of the lesion. The patient's surroundings appear to spin in the opposite direction, away from the lesion and in the same direction as the fast component of the nystagmus. The relationship of the direction that the patient falls, the direction

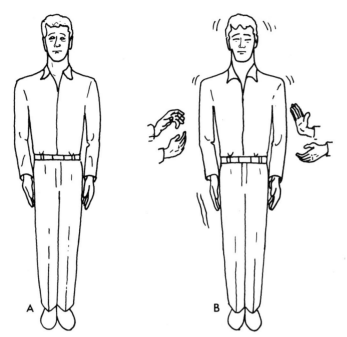

Figure 43–8. The Romberg test. The patient stands upright, feet together, arms at sides. The examiner should stand next to the patient. The test is performed in two stages: with the patient's eyes open and then with the eyes closed. Even a normal person may experience mild subjective disequilibrium and "waver" with his eyes closed. Thus, the Romberg test can sometimes simulate the feeling of disequilibrium. *A,* With his eyes open, the patient can stand unsupported without difficulty. *B,* With his eyes closed, the patient loses his balance. This test result suggests peripheral neuropathy or vestibular dysfunction or both. Cerebellar disease more often results in inability to maintain this posture with the eyes either open or closed. (From Reilly BM. Practical Strategies in Outpatient Medicine, 2nd ed. Philadelphia: WB Saunders, 1991:168.)

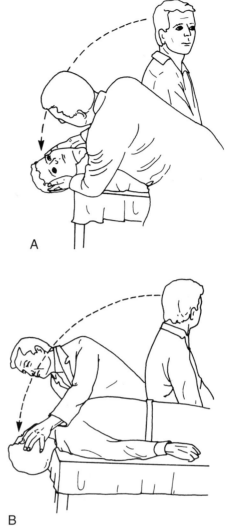

Figure 43–9. *A, B,* Patients are first observed, seated, with the eyes straight ahead. Any spontaneous nystagmus at rest, on horizontal gaze (no more than 30 degrees from the midline), or on vertical gaze is noted and analyzed. Extraocular movements are tested. Patients turn their head 30 to 45 degrees to one side and are then lowered quickly backward to the supine position, such that the head is extended down over the end of the examining table to about a 30-degree subhorizontal angle *(A).* The patient is now lying down, head turned to one side, and inclined backward, one ear facing the floor, with the examiner supporting the patient's head and neck. This position is maintained for 30 seconds. The patient's eyes are observed while in the midline and while they are looking down toward the floor. Induction of nystagmus is often accompanied by the onset of vertigo and a frantic urge to get up (especially when peripheral vestibular disease is the problem). The patient is then brought back to the upright position, the eyes are observed for 30 to 60 seconds (nystagmus may then occur again), and the maneuver is repeated, turning the head now down to the opposite side *(B).* During the Nylen-Bárány maneuver, *positional* nystagmus should be observed for: (1) the direction of slow/fast components; (2) the head position that elicits nystagmus; (3) the latency of onset of nystagmus (the time between assumption of the head position and the onset of nystagmus); (4) the persistence or fatigue of nystagmus (does nystagmus wane as the head position is maintained, or does it continue unabated?); (5) the intensity of vertigo induced; and (6) the presence or absence of habituation (does repeating the test in the vulnerable position cause a lesser or absent nystagmus response—habituation—or not?). (From Reilly BM. Practical Strategies in Outpatient Medicine, 2nd ed. Philadelphia: WB Saunders, 1991:204.)

lopathy. Parainfectious (otitis media, upper respiratory tract) and a post-traumatic etiology are common in children and adolescents. Table 43–5 similarly demonstrates the characteristics of central vertigo; Table 43–3 illustrates differentiating features of positional nystagmus for peripheral versus central vertigo.

To treat persistent peripheral vertigo, the patient is asked to remain still in a dark room with the eyes closed. If symptoms of peripheral vertigo remain distressing to the patient, symptomatic treatment, including sedating (Phenergan) or less sedating (meclizine) antivertiginous agents or transcutaneous scopolamine patches, may be indicated. Specific therapy may be needed for suppurative infections (labrythitis, otitis media, mastoiditis), and central nervous system lesions producing central vertigo.

Paroxysmal positional vertigo is common in adolescents and is characterized by brief (<30 seconds) episodes of disturbing vertigo when the patient turns over in bed, looks up or over the shoulder, or flips the head to move hair away from the face. Between occurrences, there may be anxiety and apprehension about recurrence. The paroxysms can occur at any time of day, but they tend to cluster in the morning. Physical findings, including hearing, cranial nerves, and cerebellar function, are normal. The Nylen-Bárány maneuver (Fig. 43–9) elicits a characteristic response and the patient's symptoms very reliably. Generally a benign, if annoying, condition, positional vertigo has a variable duration. Although it is usually transient, it can recur over a period of years. Most patients learn to avoid the positional maneuvers that provoke their episodes.

Table 43–4. **Peripheral Vestibulopathy**

Syndrome	Usual Presentation	Typical Course	Hearing Loss?	Diagnosis	Treatment
(Benign) paroxysmal positional vertigo	Paroxysmal, brief, purely positional vertigo	Often polyphasic illness with gradual improvement but intermittent brief recurrences for weeks/months. Does not cause ongoing severe vertigo	No	History Nylen-Bárány maneuvers	Wait
Vestibular neuronitis	Acute onset, severe vertigo, sometimes following viral respiratory infection	Severe ongoing vertigo for many hours or a few days. Monophasic illness. Resolves spontaneously. No hearing loss	No	Clinical history. Normal hearing. Peripheral nystagmus. Rapid (hours–days) resolution without recurrence	Wait
Infectious labyrinthitis	Usually mild vertigo accompanying obvious sinusitis, otitis media or serous otitis	Resolves over several days with resolution of otitis/sinusitis. Very rarely: severe purulent labyrinthitis, mastoiditis, meningitis	No, unless conductive loss due to otitis associated	ENT examination: otitis media? serous otitis? sinusitis?	Treat otitis, sinusitis: decongestants
Toxic vestibulopathy	Vertigo and/or hearing loss associated with use of toxic drugs	Usually dose related and reversible after withdrawal or dose reduction of offending drug	Depends on drug, but sensorineural deafness is common with aminoglycosides, aspirin, loop diuretics, platinum; hearing is usually normal with alcohol and quinidine	Peripheral vertigo with or without hearing loss while/after taking vestibulotoxic drugs; most are reversible with discontinuation of drug	Discontinue or adjust dose of drugs
Ménière's disease	Episodic attacks of severe vertigo, usually with associated ear fullness and/or hearing loss	Duration of attack usually several hours; patient well before and after attacks unless hearing loss progresses and persists	Usually sensorineural (90% unilateral) audiometry	Typical history with recurrences	Low-sodium diet. Diuretics. Surgery?
Cervicogenic vestibulopathy	Brief positional vertigo, associated with head and neck movements	Usually recurrent, brief, nondebilitating vertigo in patients with cervical spondylosis or other craniovertebral disease (rheumatoid arthritis, Klippel-Feil deformity)	No (but unrelated presbycusis common in this age group)	Typical history. Nylen-Bárány maneuvers not consistent with benign positional vertigo. Exclude: Vertebrobasilar ischemia. Carotid sinus hypersensitivity	Vestibular exercises
Cholesteatoma	Recurrent, often positional vertigo in patients with a history of chronic otitis, TM perforation, mastoiditis	Indolent progression of symptoms	Conductive	Usually visible (at superior border of tympanic membrane) on otoscope examination of ear	Surgery

Table 43–4. **Peripheral Vestibulopathy** *Continued*

Syndrome	Usual Presentation	Typical Course	Hearing Loss?	Diagnosis	Treatment
Otosclerosis	Progressive hearing loss, sometimes with intermittent vertigo	Indolent progressive hearing loss	Conductive	Family history Audiometry	Surgery
Labyrinthine hemorrhage	Sudden severe vertigo, usually in a patient on systemic anticoagulants (Coumadin)	Gradual resolution over a few days	Variable	Syndrome similar to vestibular neuronitis, but history of anticoagulation is key	Wait Adjust and/or discontinue anticoagulants
Post-traumatic					
Basilar (temporal bone) fracture	Severe vertigo, often with profound hearing loss immediately after head trauma	Gradual (days–weeks) resolution of vertigo; hearing loss, facial nerve injury often permanent	Often: sensorineural	X-ray: fracture Hemotympanum? CSF otorrhea? Facial paresis?	Depends on extent of injury
Postconcussive	Ongoing, often mild/chronic vertigo following concussion, without fracture	Gradual resolution but often delayed for months–years	No	Persistent/chronic symptoms without evidence of other post-traumatic syndromes	Wait
Cupulolithiasis	Classic benign positional vertigo, but following head trauma	See benign positional vertigo (above)	No	Clinical history Nylen-Bárány maneuvers Exclude fistula!	Wait
Perilymphatic fistula	Trauma may be remote or indirect (swimming, diving injuries, for example) Usually, positional vertigo, recurrent; or mild persistent vertigo	Post-traumatic vertigo that does not improve over time	Often: mixed or sensorineural	Clinical history Positive fistula test Valsalva maneuver: symptoms worsen?	Surgery
Whiplash	Positional vertigo, worse with neck extension or turning, following deceleration neck injury	Gradual but slow improvement with resolution of neck symptoms	Usually none	Clinical history Exclude fractures and fistulas	Wait Physical therapy
Ossicular disruption	Hearing loss, acute vertigo, following head/facial trauma	Gradual (days) resolution of vertigo; hearing loss persists	Conductive	Clinical history Audiometry Exclude fistula	Surgery

Modified from Reilly BM: Practical Strategies in Outpatient Medicine, 2nd ed. Philadelphia: WB Saunders, 1991:196–197.
Abbreviations: CSF = cerebrospinal fluid; ENT = ear-nose-throat; TM = tympanic membrane.

Table 43–5. Central Vertigo

Cause	Usual Age at Onset	Clinical Clues	Diagnosis	Treatment
Vertebrobasilar ischemia	Young—migrainous	Known (suspected) vascular disease: hypertensive, diabetic Almost always accompanied by brainstem symptoms and signs: diplopia, dysarthria, dysesthesias, motor weakness	TIA: clinical history Stroke: neurologic examination CT scan may be unreliable MRI more sensitive Angiography?	TIA: aspirin rarely, surgery Stroke: observe; rarely, anticoagulant
Cerebellar hemorrhage	Middle-aged	Hypertensive, anticoagulated, post-traumatic Sudden headache: diplopia, ataxia usually more prominent than vertigo	CT scan	Small hemorrhage: watch for worsening Large hemorrhage: surgical evacuation
Cerebellopontine angle tumors (Most: acoustic neuroma)	Middle-aged Young—neurofibromatosis II	Hearing loss, tinnitus much more prominent than vertigo Mild disequilibrium Early: normal neurologic examination, except sensorineural hearing loss Later: Cranial nerves V and VII abnormal; papilledema?	Audiometry: retrocochlear, sensorineural hearing loss CT scan, MRI Internal auditory canal tomography ENG, ABER	Surgery
Multiple sclerosis	Young (average age 30)	Optic neuritis Internuclear ophthalmoplegia Spastic paraparesis/incontinence Vertigo first isolated symptom in only 10% of cases	Multiplicity of symptoms and signs dissociated in time and space MRI scanning CSF: oligoclonal bands	Steroids Long-term management
Drug toxicity	Any age	Alcohol, sedatives, tranquilizers, opiates, anticonvulsants	Discontinue drug	Discontinue drug
Basilar migraine	Young	Vertigo part of headache syndrome Usually positive family history	Clinical history	See Chap. 38
Vertiginous (temporal lobe) epilepsy	Young	Vertigo as aura to loss of consciousness Very rare	Clinical history Exclude other diagnoses EEG	Anticonvulsants
Cranial neuropathy	Variable	Many types, all uncommon: Herpes zoster—external ear/palate skin lesions and cranial nerve VIII symptoms Postinfectious—following viral syndromes: polyneuritis and/or cerebellitis and/or encephalitis Chronic meningitis—syphilis, tuberculosis, sarcoid, carcinomatous Vasculitis—Cogan's syndrome, Wegener's, temporal arteritis, syphilis Head and neck carcinoma Vascular compression syndromes		

Others: Heredofamilial disorders (Friedreich's, spinocerebellar degeneration, olivopontocerebellar degeneration)
Cerebellar degeneration (alcohol, cancer)
Tumor of brainstem, cerebellum
Syrinx cervical cord
Post-traumatic concussion

Modified from Reilly BM: Practical Strategies in Outpatient Medicine, 2nd ed. Philadelphia: WB Saunders, 1991:200.
Abbreviations: ABER = auditory brainstem evoked response; CT = computed tomography; CSF = cerebrospinal fluid; ENG = electronystagmography; EEG = electroencephalogram; TIA = transient ischemic attack.

Evaluation of the Patient with Vertigo

HISTORY

The history is critical to the diagnosis of the vertiginous patient. A careful, detailed description of the prodrome and the actual symptoms including timing, duration, direction of the spinning, associated symptoms, preceding infections (especially of the upper respiratory tract, such as otitis media or sinusitis), medications, and a history of trauma, including swimming and diving, must be documented. A past history of vertigo or any other neurologic condition is important.

PHYSICAL EXAMINATION

Special attention must be paid to the head, ears, eyes, nose, and throat (HEENT) examination. Good visualization of the tympanic membranes and their mobility is necessary along with testing both air and bony conduction via a tuning fork (Figs. 43–10 and 43–11).

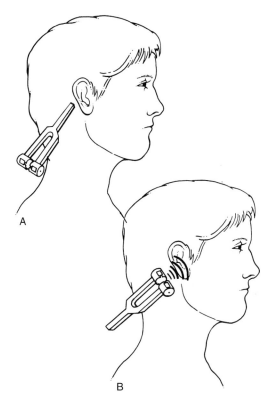

Figure 43–10. The Rinne test. The tuning fork is first placed on the mastoid process *(A)*. When the sound can no longer be heard, the tuning fork is placed in front of the external auditory meatus *(B)*. Normally, air conduction is better than bone conduction. (From Swartz MH. Textbook of Physical Diagnosis: History and Examination. Philadelphia: WB Saunders, 1989:175.)

Visualization of the fundi is important. Palpation and percussion of the paranasal sinuses may be helpful in older children but is rarely useful in patients under 6 to 8 years of age. Testing all the cranial nerves, including the olfactory nerve, should be done in an organized manner.

The neurologic examination must include evaluation of the gait, Romberg test, visual fields, and visual acuity. If nystagmus is not present, the Nylen-Bárány maneuver (see Fig. 43–9) should be performed and the presence or absence of nystagmus noted carefully. In most children and adolescents, the physical examination is normal with only subtle findings when the symptoms are provoked.

DIAGNOSTIC TESTS

The history and physical examination will direct the diagnostic work-up and determine which tests need to be performed. Imaging studies important in the work-up of the vertiginous patient include the computed tomography (CT) scan and magnetic resonance imaging (MRI). Both techniques allow visualization of the inner ear and the labyrinthine apparatus as well as the brainstem and cerebellum. If an infectious etiology is suspected, it may be useful to perform a lumbar puncture as long as an increased intracranial pressure is not suspected. In the setting of trauma, the simple use of the pneumatic otoscope may allow the examiner to perform a "fistula test," reproducing or worsening the patient's symptoms because of an abnormal communication to the labyrinthine system. If hearing loss is a feature, audiometry and evoked response testing should be considered. A summary of diagnostic tests and their outcomes (diagnoses) is noted in Table 43–6.

SUMMARY AND RED FLAGS

Vertigo is characterized by the perception of movement, particularly rotational movement, and can be a most distressing and incapacitating phenomenon. The history and physical examination, especially the HEENT and neurologic examinations, usually lead to the diagnosis, with laboratory tests and imaging studies generally having a confirmatory role. The history and examination should allow the examiner to distinguish between peripheral and central vestibular dysfunction.

In children and adolescents, peripheral vertigo is far more common than central vertigo. However, in certain at-risk populations, such as children with sickle cell disease, hemophilia, congenital heart disease (especially children with right-to-left shunts or mixing lesions), and children receiving warfarin (coumadin), the central causes resulting from hemorrhagic and thromboembolic phenomena must be remembered. Chronicity, persistence, vertical nystagmus, and signs of increased intracranial pressure are red flags. Because the diagnosis of vertigo requires that the patient be able to articulate the perception of movement, it is a difficult diagnosis to make in small children and must be carefully distinguished from other movement impairments, especially disequilibrium.

DISEQUILIBRIUM

When a "dizzy" patient describes feeling unsteady on his or her feet, off balance, or uncoordinated, the patient is describing a disturbance in the body's equilibrium system. The fundamental complaint is difficulty in walking, not from weakness but from a feeling of lack of control.

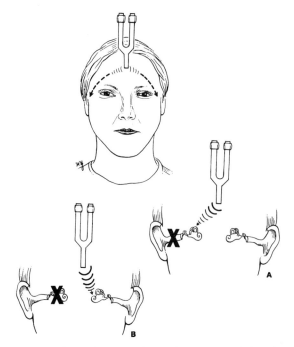

Figure 43–11. The Weber test. When a vibrating tuning fork is placed on the center of the forehead, the sound is heard in the center without lateralization to either side (normal response). *A,* In the presence of a conductive hearing loss, the sound is heard on the side of the conductive loss. *B,* In the presence of the sensorineural loss, the sound is better heard on the opposite (unaffected) side. (From Swartz MH. Textbook of Physical Diagnosis: History and Examination. Philadelphia: WB Saunders, 1989:176.)

Table 43–6. Algorithmic Approach to Diagnosis of Dizziness in Children

Presenting Complaint	Clinical and Laboratory Findings	Likely Diagnosis
Acute onset with hearing loss (all ages)	Fever +, infection +, toxin +, vomiting +	Labyrinthitis
	Fever −, tinnitus +, ear pressure +, vomiting +	Ménière's syndrome
	Head trauma +, barotrauma +, exertion +	Perilymphatic fistula, concussion
	Fever −, head trauma −, infection −	Vascular occlusion
Recurrent paroxysmal vertigo with no hearing loss		
Patient 16 months to 4 or 5 years	Nystagmus +, EEG normal, ENG ±	Benign paroxysmal vertigo
	Torticollis +, GE reflux +, EEG normal, ENG ±	Paroxysmal torticollis
Teen or older patient	Postinfection +, vomiting +, EEG normal, ENG + PPN	Vestibular neuronitis
All ages	Positional vertigo only, vomiting +, EEG normal, ENG + PPN	Paroxysmal positional vertigo
	Headache +, vomiting +, EEG normal, ENG ±	Migraine
Recurrent paroxysmal vertigo with no hearing loss but with loss of consciousness ± (all ages)	Headache +, vomiting +, EEG post. slow, ENG +	Migraine
	Headache −, vomiting −, EEG +, ENG +	Seizures
	Headache −, vomiting −, EEG normal, ENG normal	Hyperventilation
Chronic unremitting vertigo	Neurologic signs +, hearing loss +, cranial nerve deficits +, CT scan of brain +, MR image of brain +	Cerebellopontine angle tumor, cholesteatoma, cerebellar tumor, ependymoma
	Neurologic signs absent, metabolic work-up normal, CT scan brain −, MR image brain −	Panic attacks, conversion reaction, depression
	Neurologic signs absent, metabolic work-up abnormal	Metabolic disorder

From Eviatar L: Dizziness in children. Otolaryngol Clin North Am 1994;27:565.

Abbreviations: + = positive, present; − = negative, absent; ± = positive or negative, present or absent; PPN = paroxysmal positional nystagmus; ENG = electronystagmography; EEG = electroencephalogram; CT = computed tomography; MR = magnetic resonance; GE = gastroesophageal.

Walking is a very complex activity. The constant integration of visual, vestibular, and proprioceptive afferent information regarding the changing spatial orientation is performed using all levels of the central nervous system—the cerebral cortex, cerebellum, brainstem, spinal cord, and peripheral neuromuscular system. These spatial data are then utilized by the efferent system, producing both voluntary and involuntary movements and spatial adjustments (Fig. 43–12). Disturbances in any of these pathways can result in difficulty with locomotion.

Disequilibrium, therefore, may result from any perceptual distortion of spatial orientation. The most common is visual impairment, which any child who has played "pin the tail on the donkey" or "blind man's bluff" can attest. Humans depend a great deal on visual perception to orient in space. Vestibulocochlear dysfunction can also severely impair a person's ability to ambulate. Peripheral neuropathies affecting proprioceptive function impair the ability of the central nervous system to accurately perceive the position of the limbs with respect to one another and to either the ground or the body. Disorders causing diffuse damage to the integrative mechanism or cortical or cerebellar diseases, can impair proprioception as well. Likewise, efferent motor disability produces impairment of locomotion by producing weakness or apraxias (Table 43–7).

The diagnosis of the etiology of disequilibrium, therefore, requires a well-organized, thorough history and physical examination, especially the neurologic examination. A single cause of disequilibrium is sometimes found; however, it is more common for the impairment to result from effects on multiple pathways—afferent, integrative, and efferent.

The history is critical in patients complaining of dizziness or difficulty ambulating. In children this includes a detailed developmental history, because the differential diagnosis varies significantly for children who were walking and then stop and for those

who do not achieve that milestone. In the younger child, it may be very difficult to determine whether refusal or reluctance to walk is related to imbalance, pain, or weakness. Nausea and vomiting are usually associated with vertigo but tend to be rare with disequilibrium. Nausea and vomiting may accompany a viral illness that results in an acute cerebellar ataxia and thus may precede the onset

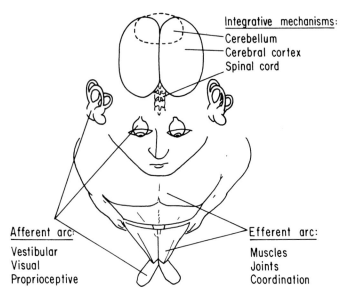

Figure 43–12. The afferent, integrative, and efferent components of the equilibrium system. (From Reilly BM. Practical Strategies in Outpatient Medicine, 2nd ed. Philadelphia: WB Saunders, 1991:166.)

Table 43–7. Disequilibrium

Cause	Clues	Gait/Romberg	Treatment
Most Common			
Multiple sensory deficits	Visual impairment? Hearing/vestibular dysfunction? Neuropathy? Spondylosis/degenerative joint disease? Neuropathy? Weakness?	Timid: slow, short stepped, apprehensive Remarkably improved with sensory assist (cane, companion) Romberg: normal or sensory	Sensory assist Correct/improve any/some of sensory deficits
Hyperventilation/anxiety disorders	Young, healthy, anxious patient with *episodic "spells"* of disequilibrium; or Constant, chronic, elusive disequilibrium with or without obvious medical/psychosocial stress	Usually normal gait Romberg: normal or "Nonphysiologic"	
Vestibular disorders	*Chronic* unilateral vestibulopathy may cause ongoing disequilibrium: Ménière's disease, cholesteatoma, fistula, acoustic neuroma, drug-induced vestibulopathy	Usually normal gait May veer to side of vestibular lesion Romberg: sensory	
Drug-induced	Central nervous system agents: tranquilizers, barbiturates, sedatives, alcohol, H_2 blockers, beta blockers, calcium agents, indomethacin Vestibulotoxic agents: aspirin, loop diuretics, aminoglycosides, quinidine	Timid and/or ataxic gait Romberg: normal or cerebellar Romberg sensory or normal	Discontinue or adjust dose of offending drug
Alcoholic	Heavy alcohol abuse may cause cerebellar and/or sensory degeneration Nystagmus uncommon	Ataxic gait Romberg: cerebellar or sensory	Often some (but incomplete) recovery from neuropathy with alcohol abstinence, vitamin therapy, physical therapy, nutritional therapy Cerebellar dysfunction often permanent, but abstinence, vitamins, nutrition may help
Painful ambulation	Arthritis? Claudication? Pain is limiting factor!	Limping? Waddling? Normal gait? Romberg: usually normal	Find cause
Fear of falling	Normal examination No apraxia or ataxia Rarely, phobic	Timid gait Romberg: Often cerebellar but fluctuates, inorganic	Reassure Rarely, phobic desensitization
Less Common			
Hypothyroidism	Weight gain or poor growth, cold intolerance, hoarseness, fatigue	Usually normal gait Severe: ataxic gait	Thyroid hormone
Hypoglycemia	Episodic; usually postprandial	Romberg: usually normal	Find cause! (drug-induced, postprandial, insulinoma, etc.)
Apraxia	Usually diffuse cortical dysfunction or frontal lobe disease Usually apraxic in execution of other skilled movements (e.g., combing hair, brushing teeth)	Apraxic gait Romberg: normal	Find cause: CNS tumor, subdural hematoma, normal-pressure hydrocephalus, multi-infarct state
Peripheral neuropathy	Diabetes, alcoholism, pernicious anemia Only very severe (proprioceptive) neuropathy causes gait disorder	Sensory gait: footdrop and/or circus clown Romberg: sensory	Find cause: often irreversible
Cerebellar disease (nonalcoholic)	See Table 43–8	Ataxic gait Romberg: cerebellar	Find cause (see Table 43–8)
Spasticity	Multiple sclerosis, spinal cord tumor/trauma Legs: Weak, hyper-reflexic, clonus Often bowel/bladder dysfunction	Spastic, scissors gait Romberg often normal	Find cause: cord lesion, demyelinating disease, myelitis, etc.

Table continued on following page

Table 43–7. **Disequilibrium** *Continued*

Cause	Clues	Gait/Romberg	Treatment
Normal-pressure hydrocephalus	Urinary incontinence Cognitive impairment Gait disturbance	Ataxic/apraxic	CSF shunt
Hemiplegia	Prior cerebrovascular accident Hemiparesis on neurologic examination	Hemiplegic gait Romberg often normal (if able to perform at all)	Find cause
Proximal myopathy	Severe bilateral proximal leg weakness: hip diesase, muscular dystrophy, myositis, etc.	Waddling gait Romberg normal	Find cause
Hysterical	Unpredictable, intermittent or bizarre "Secondary gain"	Gait varies: sometimes normal, timid, limping, apraxic Romberg: Often cerebellar, but fluctuates, inorganic	Exclude organic causes Ongoing medical psychiatric treatment

Modified from Reilly BM. Practical Strategies in Outpatient Medicine, 2nd ed. Philadelphia: WB Saunders, 1991:172–173.
Abbreviations: CNS = central nervous system; CSF = cerebrospinal fluid.

of disequilibrium. If nausea is simultaneous to the disequilibrium, drug or alcohol intoxication must be considered. Morning nausea or vomiting can be seen with increased intracranial pressure, as in hydrocephalus and posterior fossa tumors. Any history of head trauma, especially in the toddler, and any history of congenital heart disease with the potential for paradoxical embolization, including septic emboli resulting in brain abscess, must be taken seriously.

It is important to distinguish acute intermittent ataxia from more chronic or progressive forms (Tables 43–8 to 43–10). Drugs and

Table 43–8. **Cerebellar Ataxia**

"Midline" (Ataxia, Nystagmus)	"Lateralizing" (Ataxia, Limb Incoordination, Dysarthria)
Acute	
Drug/alcohol intoxication-ingestion*	Ischemia/stroke: embolic, vasculitis
Post-traumatic	Hemorrhage: cerebellar, subdural
Cerebellar hemorrhage	Post-traumatic
Migraine	Abscess
Viral cerebellitis (varicella, etc)*	Viral cerebellitis (varicella, etc.)*
Subacute	
Normal-pressure hydrocephalus	Primary neoplasm
Hypothyroidism	Metastatic neoplasm
Demyelinating disease	Demyelinating disease
Remote cancer effect	
Midline cerebellar tumor*	
Chronic	
Heredofamilial	Primary neoplasm
Cervical spondylosis	Arnold-Chiari malformation
Metabolic disease (rare)†	Familial spinocerebellar degeneration
	Metabolic disease†

Adapted from Dreyfus PM, et al: Cerebellar ataxia: Anatomical, physiological, and clinical implications. West J Med 128:499–511, 1978; and from Reilly BM. Practical Strategies in Outpatient Medicine, 2nd ed. Philadelphia, WB Saunders, 1991:168.
*Common.
†Ataxia-telangiectasia, Hartnup disease, Refsum disease, abetalipoproteinemia, etc.

postviral cerebellitis are common causes of acute sudden-onset ataxia. Varicella-associated postinfectious acute cerebellar ataxia usually comes after the infection, but in rare instances it may occur before or during chickenpox. Its nature is benign. Metabolic disorders may cause intermittent symptoms provoked by fever, as in maple syrup urine disease, ataxia-telangiectasia, Hartnup disease, Refsum disease, abetalipoproteinemia, and some enzyme deficiencies. These must be distinguished from hypothyroidism, demyelinating disorders, muscular dystrophies, and neoplasms of the posterior fossa, brainstem, and spinal cord.

Progressive ataxias tend to carry poor prognoses. Age of onset can be used to distinguish some causes, with posterior fossa tumors and neuroblastoma generally occurring within the first decade, Friedreich ataxia and Duchenne muscular dystrophy during the late first to second decades, and multiple sclerosis and diabetic peripheral neuropathy in the second decade.

Observation of the child's gait is an important component of the physical examination. Enough room should be found to allow the child to initiate walking, to proceed in a straight line for 10 to 20 paces, and to turn and return. The normal child, older than 2 to 3 years of age, initiates walking without hesitation and steps smoothly with a consistent stride length and height and a narrow base. The arms should swing freely and rhythmically, alternating with the feet, and there should be little sway in the trunk. When the child stops, there should be no hesitation again and no wavering or compensation. The observer should practice watching children walk to develop a sense for each part of the complex motion.

One of the most common gait abnormalities in children is the *wide-based gait*. Again, careful observation of toddlers at various stages of development will familiarize the observer with the transition from the wide-based, lurching steps of a 12-month old to the smooth, sure, rhythmic stride of children over 2 to 3 years of age. Excessive trunk sway is typical of cerebellar ataxia. Waddling tends to be due to proximal muscle weakness with a forward leaning, stiff appearance. It is important to distinguish an unsteady gait with irregular steps from a limp or a sensory deficit resulting in a high step with a slapping foot plant (see Chapter 46).

In the toddler, passive range of motion as well as active range of motion should be performed to assure the observer that there is no joint or muscle pain. Reflexes, including the Babinski sign, should be carefully performed. Testing the sensory system in the toddler, especially proprioception, vibration, and two-point discrimination, can be a challenge. The Romberg test may also be difficult in younger children.

The Romberg test helps to distinguish between cerebellar disequilibrium and sensory input impairment (see Fig. 43–8). To be

Table 43–9. Congenital Causes of Chronic Ataxia

Disorder	Age of Presentation	Clinical Manifestations	Mechanism of Ataxia, Diagnoses, and Treatment
Cerebellar hypoplasia	Early infancy (occasionally delayed)	Developmental delay, hypotonia, athetosis, chorea, delayed walking, ataxic gait	Absent cerebellar granular cells; CT shows small cerebellum
Vermal aplasia Dandy-Walker malformation	Early infancy	Macrocephaly, enlarged occipital region; ataxia	Hydrocephalus and cystic dilation of the fourth ventricle; treatment is by shunting of hydrocephalus and/or the posterior fossa cyst
Joubert syndrome	Early infancy	Neonatal episodic hyperpnea and apnea; hypotonia, nystagmus	MRI and CT demonstrate agenesis of the superior cerebellar vermis
Arnold-Chiari malformation	Variable	Headache, neck pain, lower cranial nerve dysfunction, nystagmus, ataxia; this variety does not have associated myelomeningocele	MRI and CT demonstrate a caudal fourth ventricle; distortion of the brainstem; treatment is by posterior fossa decompression
Hydrocephalus	Variable	Macrocephaly, vomiting, ataxia	CT and MRI demonstrate enlarged lateral ventricles; in aqueductal stenosis, the third ventricle is particularly large, whereas the fourth ventricle is normal or small

From Behrman RE, Kliegman RM: Nelson Essentials of Pediatrics, 2nd ed. Philadelphia: WB Saunders, 1994:688.
Abbreviations: CT = computed tomography; MRI = magnetic resonance imaging.

reliable, the Romberg test requires some cooperation from the patient. Patients who can hold their position with only a minimal waver with their eyes closed have intact cerebellar and proprioceptive pathways. If the Romberg test is "positive," the observer must distinguish between midline and lateralizing cerebellar disease. Ataxia with nystagmus is characteristic of midline cerebellar disease. Older children can be asked to also perform a heel-to-toe Romberg test. Lateralizing cerebellar diseases usually also manifest dysmetria on finger-to-nose testing or the heel-shin maneuver; they may also show signs of dysdiadochokinesia with impairment of rapid, fine, alternating movements, such as sequential opposition of the thumbs and each fingertip or repetitive pronation supination patting the hands on the knees, palm, and back. To perform these maneuvers, the patient must be old enough to cooperate and follow directions. Table 43–8 briefly demonstrates midline versus lateralizing cerebellar ataxias.

Evaluation of the Patient with Disequilibrium

HISTORY

A detailed developmental history, especially in the younger child, is obtained. The family history should also be complete. The examiner should check for prodromal illnesses, especially viral (varicella) in nature.

Is there any history of trauma?

What is the character of the disability?

Does the child feel unsteady standing, starting to walk, stopping, or turning?

How do the parents characterize the child's gait?

Are there associated symptoms, such as nausea, vomiting, pain, or vertigo?

Does the child take or have access to any medications or alcohol?

Is the disequilibrium intermittent or constant?

Are there any other medical conditions of note?

PHYSICAL EXAMINATION

A thorough general physical examination should precede a very detailed neuromuscular examination. Presence of a goiter, cutaneous lesions of neurofibromatosis, or tuberous sclerosis may point to a diagnosis immediately. The neuromuscular examination should proceed from head to toe in an organized and systematic fashion. Muscle tone, bulk, and symmetry of the face, trunk, and extremities are important. Cranial nerves should be examined, as should the sensory system (dermatome by dermatome). During the motor examination, the physician should isolate muscle groups and joints prior to assessing overall function by observing the gait more than once. The Romberg test should be performed in all patients old enough to cooperate, as should the lateralizing cerebellar tests, such as the finger-to-nose and rapid, alternating movements. Attention to detail in the history and physical examination usually yields a diagnosis.

DIAGNOSTIC TESTS

Other than for drug ingestion, obvious peripheral neuropathies or myopathies, focal extremity infections, or varicella-associated cerebellar ataxia, CT or MRI is the principal diagnostic test for children and adolescents with disequilibrium. Metabolic tests and thyroid function tests will be suggested by either history or physical findings. Especially in younger children, imaging is necessary to rule out the posterior fossa tumors and demyelinating diseases. The lumbar puncture and analysis of the cerebrospinal fluid may also be indicated in cases preceded by a viral or infectious prodrome. When weakness is associated with the disequilibrium, there may be a place for electromyography and nerve conduction studies (see Chapter 39).

SUMMARY AND RED FLAGS

Because disequilibrium involves impairment of ambulation, it is seen only in toddlers and older children. Ataxia, however, can be

Table 43–10. Hereditary Causes of Ataxia

Disorder	Usual Age of Onset	Hereditary Pattern	Clinical Characteristics	Etiology and Treatment
Friedreich ataxia	2–16 yr	Recessive	Ataxia, scoliosis, pes cavus, posterior column sensory loss, areflexia, cardiomyopathy	Supportive
Ataxia-telangiectasia	Early infancy (1–2 yr)	Recessive	Ataxia, oculomotor apraxia, sinopulmonary infections, telangiectasia of conjunctiva and skin	B and T cell dysfunction; cellular immunity is impaired; supportive
Machado-Joseph disease	12–15 yr	Dominant	Cerebellar, pyramidal, extrapyramidal degeneration; anterior horn cell disease; Portuguese ancestry	Supportive
Metachromatic leukodystrophy	1–2 yr	Recessive	Ataxia, peripheral neuropathy, spasticity, optic atrophy, dementia	Supportive
Refsum disease	4–7 yr	Recessive	Ataxia, neuropathy, retinitis pigmentosa, ichthyosis	Phytanic acid hydroxylase deficiency; phytol-free diet
Leigh disease	Infancy to adolescence	Recessive	Ataxia, lactic acidosis, hypotonia, abnormalities of respiration	Some Leigh disorders of pyruvate metabolism; supportive
Wilson disease	Infancy to adulthood	Recessive	Hepatic disease, tremor, dystonic, athetosis, chorea	Ceruloplasmin deficiency; penicillamine
Abetalipoproteinemia	5–15 yr	Recessive	Ataxia, dysmetria, fat malabsorption, acanthocytosis, retinitis pigmentosa, sensory loss	Low-fat diet; vitamin E and A supplementation
Juvenile gangliosidosis	3–5 yr	Recessive GM_1 or GM_2 forms	Ataxia, spasticity, rigidity, dementia	None available
Ramsay Hunt syndrome	7–10 yr	Sporadic	Ataxia, tremor, myoclonus, dementia	Supportive
Marinesco-Sjögren syndrome	Infancy to 5 yr	Recessive	Cataracts, ataxia, growth failure, mental retardation	Supportive
Juvenile sulfate lipidosis (juvenile MLD)	Infancy to 5 yr	Recessive	Dementia, ataxia, spasticity, aryl sulfidase A deficiency	Supportive

Modified from Behrman RE, Kliegman RM: Nelson Essentials of Pediatrics, 2nd ed. Philadelphia: WB Saunders, 1994:689.
Abbreviation: MLD = metachromatic leukodystrophy.

seen in children before they are walking, and it may portend serious pathology, including posterior fossa tumors, leukodystrophies, metabolic disorders, and familiohereditary disorders. The history must be obtained carefully, with attention to developmental milestones, family history, and specifics of prodromal illnesses (chickenpox), associated symptoms, and a description of the gait. The physical examination must also be detailed and methodical, with special emphasis on the neuromuscular examination. Imaging studies of the central nervous system are usually required, especially in the younger child in whom the specter of neoplasms is greatest.

LIGHTHEADEDNESS

Lightheadedness is the most difficult to characterize without using the term "dizzy." The lightheaded patient's description is vague and nonspecific. Terms such as "woozy," "spaced-out," "dreamy," "giddy," or "drugged" are not infrequent. The key for the clinician is to elicit an adequate description from the patient to rule out vertigo, disequilibrium, and presyncope. The differential diagnosis for lightheadedness is then rather short by comparison to the other "dizziness" conditions (Fig. 43–13). Because of this, dizziness simulation tests are useful to distinguish the patient's complaint from atypical descriptions of vertigo, disequilibrium, and presyncope. The distinction between lightheadedness and presyncope is the most difficult to establish.

Besides the Nylen-Bárány maneuver (see Fig. 43–9), dizziness simulation tests include voluntary hyperventilation for 3 minutes, voluntary Valsalva maneuver, caloric testing of the ears, carotid massage, and tilt table testing. These may all be used to distinguish lightheadedness from vertigo, disequilibrium, and presyncope. In the patient who complains of lightheadedness, voluntary hyperventilation usually reproduces his or her symptoms. Voluntary hyper-

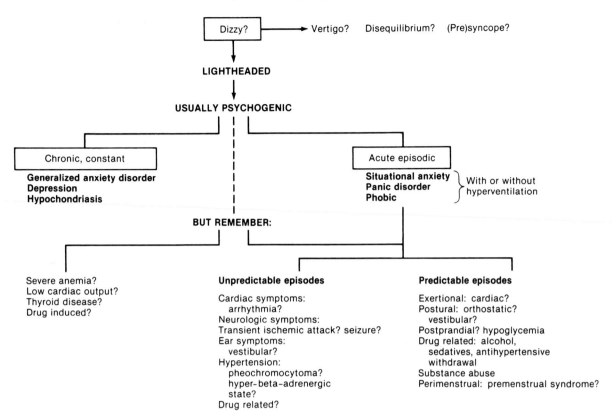

Figure 43–13. Lightheadedness. (From Reilly BM. *Practical Strategies in Outpatient Medicine*, 2nd ed. Philadelphia: WB Saunders, 1991:206.)

ventilation in normal subjects produces a variety of symptoms (Table 43–11). This test is predictive only if the patient's symptoms are precisely reproduced and all other investigations are negative.

Lightheadedness that is episodic frequently follows a pattern related to the underlying psychogenic disorder: phobic disorders, post-traumatic stress syndrome, panic attacks, and anxiety disorders. Such situational anxieties, phobias, or panic attacks may occur with or without hyperventilation. Careful history taking is the key to recognizing the pattern. If the history is that of constant lightheadedness ("always there"), the etiology is almost always psychogenic. This is a somatization generally of anxiety disorder or occasionally depression. The clinician must still remain cautious with predictable episodes, because postural episodes, drug-related episodes, and perimenstrual episodes can follow a pattern and represent physiologic abnormalities that predispose to lightheadedness.

Especially if the episodes of lightheadedness are unpredictable, the clinician is advised to consider a broader differential diagnosis. Severe anemia, low cardiac output, thyroid disease, and some medications may produce occasional lightheadedness. Of greater concern are episodes of lightheadedness associated with other symptoms, especially chest pain, seizures, confusion, and visual or auditory changes. Likewise, exertional lightheadedness must be pursued to definitively rule out a cardiac dysrhythmia.

If hyperventilation reproduces the patient's symptoms, it is not the diagnosis in and of itself. Hyperventilation is a feature of many psychogenic syndromes and may be acute or chronic. Part of the performance of the hyperventilation should be educating the patient to the feelings and to the scenario leading to the hyperventilation reaction. Even rather young children can then be trained to regulate their breathing to avoid the symptoms. However, this does not address the underlying cause of the hyperventilation reaction; that requires patient, nonjudgmental, longer-term counseling and careful categorization of the underlying disorder by the *Diagnostic and*

Statistical Manual of Mental Disorders, Fourth Edition (*DSM-IV*) criteria (see Chapter 36). The clinician should not hesitate to consult a psychiatrist to facilitate this process as well as treatment of the definitive psychogenic disorder.

Evaluation of the Patient with Lightheadedness

HISTORY

The patient is encouraged to describe symptoms without using the word "dizzy." The examiner should listen for descriptions suggesting vertigo, disequilibrium, or presyncope and should establish whether there is any pattern to the occurrence of the feeling of lightheadedness. The child, parents, or siblings are asked about associated symptoms, such as diaphoresis, hyperpnea, pallor or flushing, headache, and chest pain. It is probably best not to pursue psychiatric questioning at the very beginning of a relationship, so as not to give the impression that somatic symptoms are being minimized. However, after the more serious physiologic disorders are ruled out by history, physical, or diagnostic testing, the psychogenic disorders should be pursued.

PHYSICAL EXAMINATION

After a thorough general physical examination, including examination of the fundi, a full, detailed neurologic examination should be performed. In addition to allowing primary cardiac, endocrine, or neurologic disorders to be ruled out, the examination allows the

Table 43–11. Symptoms Associated with Hyperventilation

General	*Neurologic*
Fatigue	Dizziness
Diffuse weakness	Paresthesias (especially distal)
Insomnia	Unsteadiness
Nightmares	Impaired memory and/or
Headache	concentration
''Feel cold''	Slurred speech
Sweats	Blurred vision
Cardiovascular	*Gastrointestinal*
Palpitations	Globus hystericus
Tachycardia	Mouth dryness
Precordial pain	Dysphagia
Raynaud's phenomenon	Bloating
Respiratory	Belching/flatulence
Shortness of breath	Abdominal pain
Chest pain	*Psychic*
Sighing respirations	Tension
Yawning	Anxiety
''Can't get deep breath''	Depression
Paroxysmal nocturnal	Apprehension
dyspnea	
Unexplained cough	
Dry mouth	
Musculoskeletal	
Muscle spasm	
Tremors	
Twitching	
Tetany	

From Reilly BM. Practical Strategies in Outpatient Medicine, 2nd ed. Philadelphia: WB Saunders, 1991:208.

clinician to gain the confidence of the patient and demonstrates the physician's concern about the patient's complaints. Dizziness simulation maneuvers, especially the Nylen-Bárány maneuver and voluntary hyperventilation, should be performed. Along the way, the patient should be given feedback, reassurance, and information about the purpose of various maneuvers in the physical examination.

DIAGNOSTIC TESTS

In general, diagnostic testing is again directed by the history and physical examination. In the setting of lightheadedness, tests are generally done to rule out potentially serious cardiovascular and neurologic conditions. The dizziness simulation tests are very important and should be performed in precisely the same fashion in every patient to maximize their reliability.

SUMMARY AND RED FLAGS

Lightheadedness must be distinguished from vertigo, disequilibrium, and presyncope. Frequently the patient's description of the sensation is vague and uncertain. A pattern of the appearance of the symptoms may suggest an underlying cause. The coexistence of any other symptoms must be carefully sought. Physical findings are generally normal, including the neurologic examination; specific attention is given to cerebellar, vestibular, and sensory function. Voluntary hyperventilation in the supine position frequently

reproduces the patient's lightheadedness. Hyperventilation may be acute or chronic and is a symptom itself, rarely a diagnosis.

Treatment must address the underlying psychogenic cause in order to be successful. Signs of depression as well as suicidal ideation must be determined.

REFERENCES

General

Drachman DA, Hart CW. An approach to the dizzy patient. Neurology 1972;22:323–334.
Eviatar L. Dizziness in children. Otolaryngol Clin North Am 1994;27:557–571.
Samuels MA. The dizzy patient: A clear-headed approach. Clin Exp 1984;19:23–40.

Syncope

Kapoor WN. Diagnostic evaluation of syncope. Am J Med 1991;90:91–106.
Kapoor WN, Smith MA, Miller NL. Upright tilt testing in evaluating syncope: A comprehensive literature review. Am J Med 1994;97:78.
Linzer M. Syncope. Am J Med 1991;90:1–5.
Ruckman RN. Cardiac causes of syncope. Pediatr Rev 1987;9:101–108.
Schatz IJ. Orthostatic hypotension. Arch Intern Med 1984;144:773–777.
Scott WA. Evaluating the child with syncope. Pediatr Ann 1991;20:350–359.
Shalev Y, Gal R, Tchou PJ, et al. Echocardiographic demonstration of decreased left ventricular dimensions and vigorous myocardial contraction during syncope induced by head-up tilt test. J Am Coll Cardiol 1991;18:746–751.
Thilenius OG, Quinones JA, Husanyi TS, Novak J. Tilt test for diagnosis of unexplained syncope in pediatric patients. Pediatrics 1991;87:334–338.

Vertigo

Dunn DW, Snyder H. Benign positional vertigo of childhood. Am J Dis Child 1976;176:1099.
Fisher CM. Vertigo in cerebrovascular disease. Arch Otolaryngol 1967;85:529–534.
Hotson JR. Clinical detection of acute vestibulocerebellar disorders. West J Med 1984;140:910–913.
Katsarkas A, Kirkham TH. Paroxysmal positional vertigo: A study of 255 cases. J Otolaryngol 1978;7:320–330.

Disequilibrium

Dreyfus PM, et al. Cerebellar ataxia: Anatomical, physiological and clinical implications. West J Med 1978;128:499–511.
Kinast M, et al. Cerebellar ataxia, opsoclonus and occult neural crest tumor. Am J Dis Child 1980;134:1057.
Weiner HL, Bresnan MJ, Levitt LP. Pediatric Neurology for the House Officer, 2nd ed. Baltimore: Williams & Wilkins, 1982:60–64.

Lightheadedness

Lum LC. Hyperventilation: The tip and the iceberg. J Psychosom Res 1975;19:375–383.
Magarian GJ. Hyperventilation syndromes: Infrequently recognized common expressions of anxiety and stress. Medicine 1982;61:219–236.
Tiwari S, Bakris GL. Psychogenic vertigo: A review. Postgrad Med 1981;70:69–77.

44 Eye Disorders

Dennis M. Super

Children often present to their primary care provider with common eye problems such as vision impairment, shaking eyes *(nystagmus)*, the red eye, and straying eyes *(strabismus)*. The causes may range from variations of normal to life-threatening illnesses. With a focused and comprehensive evaluation, the primary care provider should be able to diagnose and treat some of these conditions plus know when to refer to the appropriate specialist. A brief review of the anatomy is noted in Figures 44–1 and 44–2 and Table 44–1.

VISUAL IMPAIRMENT

In assessing a vision problem, the clinician must determine whether the underlying disorder is a refractive error, an organic disease affecting the visual system, developmental amblyopia, a psychogenic disorder, or a visual processing disorder (Fig. 44–3 and Tables 44–2 and 44–3).

History

Whenever possible, the history should be obtained from both the parents and the child. Issues to be addressed include:

- The nature of the blurred vision (generalized versus focal)
- The presence of double or "ghost" images
- A decrease in color or night vision
- Bilaterality or unilaterality
- Abnormal visual sensations

The history is often based solely on the observations of family and friends. Observations suggesting a visual impairment are inability to track objects, viewing objects too closely, squinting, roving or wandering eyes (Table 44–4), head tilting, bumping into objects, and reading problems. These historical findings serve as potential *red flags* for detecting severe ocular pathology (Table 44–5).

The clinician should also inquire about past illness as well as the family history (neurocutaneous syndromes, inborn errors of metabolism, and hereditary forms of optic atrophy and cataracts). A past history of birth asphyxia may explain cortical *amaurosis* (blindness) in the infant, whereas a recent viral illness may be the cause of the sudden loss of vision secondary to acute optic neuritis.

Examination

The basic examination must include the following:

- An evaluation of the visual acuity and visual fields

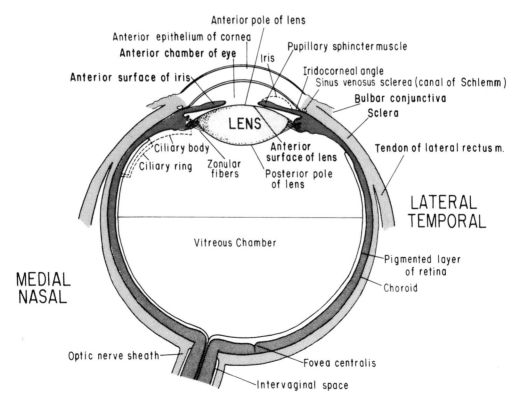

Figure 44–1. Anatomy of the eye, as seen in cross-section. (Modified from Reilly BM. Practical Strategies in Outpatient Medicine, 2nd ed. Philadelphia: WB Saunders, 1991:36.)

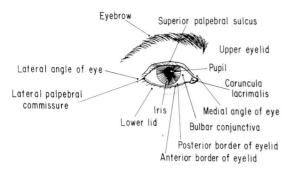

Figure 44–2. Frontal view of the eye. (From Reilly BM. Practical Strategies in Outpatient Medicine, 2nd ed. Philadelphia: WB Saunders, 1991:36.)

- Assessment of the pupils, ocular motility, and alignment
- General inspection of the eye
- Ophthalmoscopic examination of the ocular media and fundi

Examination by an ophthalmologist also includes:

- Biomicroscopy (slit-lamp examination)
- Refraction
- Tonometry (measurement of ocular pressure)

VISUAL ACUITY

For children who can recognize letters, pictures, or both, a variety of charts may be used to assess far vision. These charts consist of:

1. The Snellen acuity test (rows of letters or numbers, with each subsequent row becoming smaller in size).
2. The modified Snellen acuity test (only the letters HOTV are used instead of the entire alphabet).
3. The "illiterate" or *tumbling E test* (instead of letters, the open end of the E faces up, down, right, or left) (Fig. 44–4).
4. The Allen picture test (pictures are used instead of letters).

The test should be conducted in a relaxed and supportive manner.

The test is started with the child 20 feet away from the chart with both eyes open. In young children or those with attention problems, the distance may be reduced to 10 or 15 feet with charts calibrated for the reduced distance. If the child cannot name the letters or pictures, the child may match cards to the corresponding letter (HOTV chart) or to the facing of the E (tumbling E test). After the child reads the chart with both eyes open, the examiner must test each eye individually by covering the opposite eye with an occluder. During this test, the examiner should note whether the child is squinting, posturing as a compensation, peaking around the occluder, memorizing the chart, or obtaining clues from others in the room. The smallest line that the child can accurately read represents the acuity for far vision. The number associated with this line (i.e., 20/200) represents the distance at which a person with normal vision can see that line (200 feet) in contrast to the child being tested (20 feet).

In testing near acuity (reading vision), a Lebensohn chart or a Rosenbaum card is held 14 to 15 inches away from the patient's eye. The results are recorded in the Jaeger or printer's point system. If vision is severely impaired, the child should hold the card as close as desired to read the smallest possible print. This distance is useful for school purposes.

In infants, toddlers, and mentally retarded individuals, behavioral responses are used to assess vision. The examiner notes the child's response to toys or food items (raisins, breakfast cereals, candies) of various sizes and records the size of the item and the greatest distance at which the child regards, follows, or reaches for the object. In addition, noting the child's fixation preference can also provide evidence of visual impairment. For example, if the child objects to the covering of the right eye along with the inability to fixate with the left eye, there may be significant visual impairment of the left eye.

Perception of light and rotating optokinetic targets are qualitative tests to determine whether a child can see; these tests should not be equated with the ability to perceive form or detail (acuity). Signs of light perception include (1) fixation on a stationary, moving, or flashing light source; (2) wincing or aversion to bright light; (3) a change in affect in response to a change in illumination; and (4) "eye popping" (exaggerated eye opening in response to dimming the lights). Optokinetic nystagmus develops in response to fixating on a moving target (e.g., a striped tape or drum). The examiner can also assess a child's visual acuity by using a series of moving targets with smaller gradations between the lines on each target.

Table 44–1. The Extraocular Muscles

Ocular Muscle	Innervation	Functions
Lateral rectus	Abducens (cranial nerve VI)	Abduction—moves eye outward.
Medial rectus	Oculomotor (cranial nerve III)	Adduction—moves eye inward.
Superior rectus	Oculomotor (cranial nerve III)	Elevation: action increases as eye is abducted; becomes nil when eye is adducted.
		Intorsion: action increases as eye is adducted.
		Adduction.
Inferior rectus	Oculomotor (cranial nerve III)	Depression: action increases as eye is abducted; becomes nil when eye is adducted.
		Extorsion: action increases as eye is adducted.
		Adduction.
Inferior oblique	Oculomotor (cranial nerve III)	Extorsion: action increases as eye is abducted.
		Abduction.
		Elevation: action increases as eye is adducted; becomes nil when eye is abducted.
Superior oblique	Trochlear (cranial nerve IV)	Intorsion: action increases as eye is abducted.
		Abduction.
		Depression: action increases as eye is adducted; becomes nil when eye is abducted.

From Harley RD. Pediatric Ophthalmology, 2nd ed. Philadelphia: WB Saunders, 1983:789.

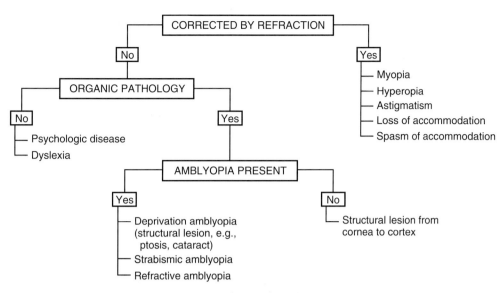

Figure 44–3. Evaluation of visual impairment.

Table 44–2. **Childhood Amaurosis (Blindness): Principal Neurologic Considerations**

Congenital Malformations
  Optic nerve hypoplasia
  Congenital hydrocephalus
  Hydranencephaly
  Porencephaly
  Micrencephaly
  Encephalocele, particularly occipital type

Phakomatoses
  Tuberous sclerosis
  Neurofibromatosis (special association with optic glioma)
  Sturge-Weber syndrome
  von Hippel–Lindau disease

Tumors
  Retinoblastoma
  Optic glioma
  Perioptic meningioma
  Craniopharyngioma
  Cerebral glioma
  Posterior and intraventricular tumors when complicated by
    hydrocephalus

Neurodegenerative Diseases
  Cerebral storage disease
    Gangliosidoses, particularly Tay-Sachs disease (infantile
      amaurotic familial idiocy), Sandhoff variant, generalized
      gangliosidosis
  Other lipidoses and ceroid lipofuscinoses, particularly the
    late-onset amaurotic familial idiocies such as those of
    Jansky-Bielschowsky and of Batten-Mayou-Spielmeyer-
    Vogt
  Mucopolysaccharidoses, particularly Hurler's syndrome and
    Hunter syndrome

Leukodystrophies (dysmyelination disorders), particularly
  metachromatic leukodystrophy and Canavan's disease
Demyelinating sclerosis (myelinoclastic diseases), especially
  Schilder disease and Devic neuromyelitis optica
Special types: Dawson disease, Leigh disease, the Bassen-
  Kornzweig syndrome, Refsum disease
Retinal degenerations: "retinitis pigmentosa" and its variants, and
  Leber congenital type
Optic atrophies: congenital autosomal recessive type, infantile and
  congenital autosomal dominant types, Leber disease, and atrophies
  associated with hereditary ataxias—the types of Behr, of Marie,
  and of Sanger-Brown

Infectious Processes
  Encephalitis, especially in the prenatal infection syndromes due to
    Toxoplasma gondii, cytomegalovirus, rubella virus, *Treponema
    pallidum*
  Meningitis; arachnoiditis
  Optic neuritis
  Chorioretinitis

Hematologic Disorders
  Leukemia with CNS involvement

Vascular and Circulatory Disorders
  Collagen-vascular diseases
  Arteriovenous malformations—intracerebral hemorrhage,
    subarachnoid hemorrhage

Trauma
  Contusion or avulsion of optic nerves or chiasm
  Cerebral contusion or laceration
  Intracerebral, subarachnoid, or subdural hemorrhage

Drugs and Toxins

Modified from Harley RD. Pediatric Ophthalmology, 2nd ed. Philadelphia: WB Saunders, 1983:777.
Abbreviation: CNS = central nervous system.

Table 44–3. Causes of Monocular Visual Loss

Disorder	Timing	Pattern of Loss	Other Clues	Fundus Appearance	Pupil
Refractive error	Gradual*	Varies	Improves with pinhole	Normal	Normal
Cataract	Very gradual	Tunnel?	Opacity visible	Normal	Normal, but red reflex decreased
Corneal disease	Acute or chronic	Murky	Opacity visible or positive fluorescein uptake	Normal	Normal, but red reflex decreased
Iritis	Acute or chronic	Murky	Pain Ciliary flush	Normal	Small Disfigured?
Open-angle glaucoma	Gradual	Varies	Elevated pressures	Normal	Normal
Angle-closure glaucoma	Acute	Varies	Pain Steamy cornea Patient ill	Normal	Dilated Fixed
Central retinal occlusion	Acute	Varies	Painless Abrupt	Pale with cherry-red macula	Normal
Retinal detachment	Acute	Varies	Painless Floaters	Unremarkable or diagnostic	Afferent pupillary defect if extensive
Vitreous hemorrhage	Acute	"Dark"	Cannot see in the eye!	Obscured	Normal, but red reflex decreased
Amaurosis fugax	Acute Transient	5–10 minutes	Carotid or heart disease, migraine	Normal	Normal
Migraine	Acute Transient	5–30 minutes	Headache Prior history Scintillations	Normal	Normal
Optic neuropathy	Gradual or acute	Central scotoma	Toxins? Multiple sclerosis? Pituitary tumor? Virus?	Normal Pale optic disc?	Afferent defect?
Diffuse retinopathy	Gradual	Varies	Genetic? AIDS?	Retinal lesions	Afferent defect?
Papilledema (chronic)	Late	Varies	CNS tumor? Pseudotumor cerebri Hypertensive crisis?	Diagnostic	Normal
Endophthalmitis	Varies	Varies	Corneal infection? Penetrating injury? Systemic infection? Hypopyon?	Varies Often obscured	Varies

Modified from Reilly BM. Practical Strategies in Outpatient Medicine, 2nd ed. Philadelphia: WB Saunders, 1991:60.
*Refractive error may be more acute when caused by diabetes mellitus.
Abbreviations: CNS = central nervous system; AIDS = acquired immunodeficiency syndrome.

The smallest gradation that elicits the nystagmus corresponds to the child's visual acuity.

VISUAL FIELDS

Visual fields can be assessed in young children by either of two methods. With the *confrontation method,* the examiner sits face to face with the patient and moves an object (a finger or toy) from the periphery toward the center of the field until the patient reports seeing the object. Each eye is tested individually. The *attraction technique* uses the element of surprise. The examiner brings an interesting object in from the periphery (testing each quadrant in turn) and notes when the child looks toward the object or reaches for it.

Both techniques are sufficient to detect significant visual field defects, such as *bitemporal hemianopsia* (chiasmal lesion), *homonymous hemianopsia* (cerebral lesion), or constricted vision (retinal degeneration). If a more detailed map of the defect is needed, perimetry and scotometry testing using standard instruments can often be accomplished in school-aged children.

COLOR VISION

By means of standard test plates, color vision can be evaluated in any child capable of naming or tracing simple figures. A change in color vision may be a sign of optic nerve or retinal disease. Congenital color vision defects (*dyschromatopsia*) are common in males, whereas complete congenital absence of color vision (*achromatopsia*) is a rare defect associated with poor acuity, nystagmus, and *photophobia* (abnormal intolerance to light).

PUPIL TESTING

Visual defects can be localized by the reaction of the pupils to near gaze, their direct and consensual response to light, and the

Table 44–4. Causes of Nystagmus and Poor Vision From Birth

I. **Opacities of the Media**
 Bilateral corneal opacities
 Bilateral cataracts
II. **Retinal Disorders**
 A. Ophthalmoscopically visible
  1. Optic nerve
   a. Optic atrophy
   b. Developmental anomalies
    Hypoplasia
    Coloboma
  2. Macular disease
   a. Infections—''coloboma''
   b. Developmental
    Hypoplasia
    Traction
  3. Rare bilateral association
    (e.g., retinal dysplasia, posterior PHPV)
 B. Ophthalmoscopically variable
  1. Achromatopsia (rod monochromatism)
  2. Leber congenital amaurosis
  3. Congenital stationary night blindness X-linked with myopia
III. **Systemic Diseases**
 A. Neurologic disorders (e.g., hydrocephalus)
 B. Metabolic disorders (e.g., Lowe syndrome)
 C. Chromosomal abnormalities (e.g., Down syndrome)
 D. Somatic malfunctions (e.g., De Lange syndrome)
IV. **Disturbances of Higher Centers—Etiology Unknown**
 A. Congenital nystagmus
 B. Spasmus nutans
 C. Latent nystagmus
 D. Occlusion nystagmus

Modified from Nelson LB, Calhoun JH, Harley RD. Pediatric Ophthalmology, 3rd ed. Philadelphia: WB Saunders, 1991:84.
Abbreviation: PHPV = persistent hyperplastic primary vitreous (this is often unilateral).

reaction to reduced light (Fig. 44–5). By noting how the pupil responds to these different tests, one can assess the *afferent conduction system* (response to light), the *parasympathetic efferent pupillomotor system* (near gaze), and the *sympathetic efferent pupillomotor system* (reduced light). In addition, by noting the size and shape of the pupil, one can detect abnormalities of the iris, such as aniridia and synechiae.

Response to Near Gaze

If the pupil does not constrict normally on near gaze, the problem may be a defect in the parasympathetic efferent pupillomotor system, a structural iris defect, or pharmacologic *mydriasis* (pupil dilation). Because the efferent parasympathetic fibers travel with the oculomotor nerve (third cranial nerve), increased intracranial pressure causing early uncal herniation may damage these fibers, resulting in a dilated and unreactive pupil *(Hutchinson pupil)* (see Chapter 41). Since this is potentially a medical emergency, the patient with any neurologic symptoms coupled with a dilated and unreactive pupil must be emergently evaluated and treated. Other causes of a dilated, unreactive pupil are the accidental or purposeful use of mydriatic agents (eyedrops, systemic drugs, or toxins) and the presence of structural iris defects (aniridia, coloboma, sphincter tears, and synechiae).

In some patients, a *tonic pupil* may develop. The tonic pupil is

larger than normal, reacts poorly to light, has a slow and sustained contraction to near gaze, and redilates slowly. The tonic pupil is usually unilateral and may occur after either a viral illness or trauma to the eye or orbit. The pupil typically shows denervation hypersensitivity to dilute parasympathomimetic agents (methacholine 2.5%, pilocarpine 0.125% eyedrops).

Response to Light

If the pupil constricts well on near gaze (i.e., if the efferent parasympathetic system is intact) but does not constrict to light, there is a problem in the anterior or pregeniculate visual pathway, which consists of the retinas to the optic tract.

In unilateral lesions anterior to the chiasm (retina or optic nerve), the patient's pupils constrict normally when light is shined into the eye with normal visual pathways; however, both pupils fail to react when light is shined into the side that has the lesion. The examiner can elicit this finding by having the patient gaze at a distant object (which eliminates the near gaze reflex), by shining the light repetitively from one eye to the other, and by observing the direct and consensual pupillary response to the light in each eye. This pupillary finding may develop even before funduscopic findings occur in diseases of the optic nerve, such as tumors, injury, and neuritis.

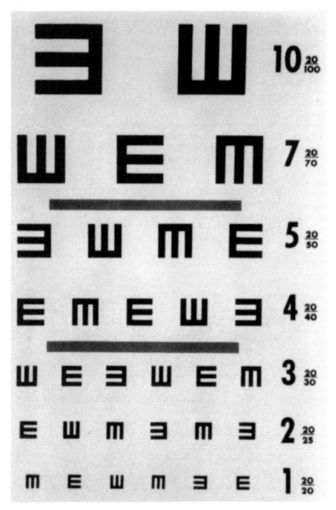

Figure 44–4. Testing visual acuity. Illiterate or tumbling E test. (From Nelson LB, Calhoun JH, Harley RD. Pediatric Ophthalmology, 3rd ed. Philadelphia: WB Saunders, 1991:97.)

Table 44–5. "Red Flags" by History for Visual Impairment

	Possible Pathology
Child's Complaint	
Generalized blurred vision	
Far vision only	Myopia
Near vision only	Hyperopia, disorder of accommodation
Both far and near	Astigmatism or defect of visual pathways
Focal blurred vision (veil, shadow)	
Unilateral	Ipsilateral retinal or optic nerve
Bilateral	Chiasmal, postchiasmal, or bilateral prechiasmal lesion
Ghost /double vision	
With binocular vision	Cranial nerve or extraocular muscle
With monocular vision	Ocular media or macular disease
Changes in special visions	
Poorer color vision	Retinal or optic nerve disease
Poorer night vision	Retinal disease (retinitis pigmentosa)
Visual sensations	
Floaters, spots	Uveitis, retinal detachment, or hemorrhage
Shimmering lines or scotoma	Migraines
Visual hallucinations	Cerebral lesion, psychogenic
Parent's Observations	
Age-appropriate infant does not track	Severe ocular (myopia, cataracts) or systemic (meningitis) pathology
Objects viewed too closely	Decreased visual acuity related to refractive error; ocular or neurologic disorder
Squinting	Decreased visual acuity related to refractive error; ocular or neurologic disorder
Roving or wandering eyes	Nystagmus or strabismus; rule out ocular or neurologic disorder
Head tilting	Compensatory posturing for nystagmus, strabismus, astigmatism, or visual field defect
Bumping into objects	Visual field defect, decreased visual acuity
Reading problems	Visual impairment, visual processing disorder

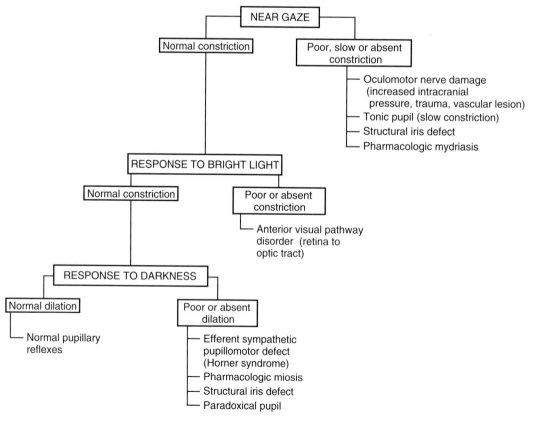

Figure 44–5. Pupillary reflexes in assessment of visual problems.

In patients with retinal disorders (achromatopsia, Leber congenital retinal amaurosis) and optic nerve disorders, the pupils may react *paradoxically* to dim light by constricting instead of dilating. When lights in the room are turned off, the pupils briskly constrict and then slowly redilate. The reason for this paradoxical response is not clear.

Response to Reduced Light

If the pupil reacts to light and near gaze but does not dilate in reduced light, there is either a defect in the sympathetic efferent pupillomotor system, pharmacologic *miosis* (constriction), with eyedrops, systemic drugs, or toxins, or a structural iris defect, particularly synechiae. The sympathetic fibers originate in the hypothalamus *(first-order neurons),* traverse the brainstem, and synapse in the lower cervical and upper thoracic spinal cords. Next, the fibers *(second-order neurons)* exit the spinal cord and synapse in the superior cervical ganglion. Fibers leaving the superior cervical ganglion *(third-order neurons)* then follow the carotid artery to the ophthalmic artery. From there, they join the nasociliary nerve and proceed to innervate (via the long ciliary nerve) the iris dilator muscle. Any lesion along this pathway can cause miosis.

Lesions in the head and neck (from the lateral medulla to the long ciliary nerve) may damage this sympathetic pathway and result in *Horner syndrome.* This syndrome consists of *ptosis* (paralysis of Muller's muscle), miosis, iris heterochromia (especially if the insult occurred in infancy), ipsilateral impairment of facial sweating, and cutaneous vasoconstriction. Horner syndrome may be secondary to birth injury (part of *Klumpke palsy*), thoracic surgery, vertebral anomalies, enterogenous cysts, or tumors of the mediastinum or neck (neuroblastoma).

INSPECTION AND OPHTHALMOSCOPY

The eye itself should be examined methodically, beginning with the inspection of the globe and assessment of clarity of the ocular media and finishing with a detailed funduscopic examination. The globe should be noted for its size, redness, protrusion, and alignment. Corneal opacification can best be detected by bright light tangentially focused on the cornea. Even though slit-lamp examination is the best method for assessing optical clarity, direct ophthalmoscopy is also effective in detecting problems in the ocular media.

Using the refractive power of the ophthalmoscope, the clinician focuses on the cornea (~ +20 diopters), lens (~ +15 diopters), and vitreous (~ +15 to 0 diopters). The examiner notes any opacifications or cloudiness of these structures as well as any dislocation of the lenses. Opacities in the lens and the vitreous appear as dark areas surrounded by the red reflex. With direct ophthalmoscopy, the fundus is then examined; any abnormalities of the optic disc, macula, chorioretinal pattern, and vessels are noted. Since the risk of precipitating acute angle-closure (narrow-angle) glaucoma is minimal in children, the use of short-acting mydriatics (1% tropicamide or 2.5% phenylephrine) may facilitate ophthalmoscopy. Even though these short-acting mydriatics* are relatively safe, systemic absorption may occur, causing adverse reactions (hypertension, bradycardia, or anaphylaxis). Hence, these agents should be used cautiously in premature infants and are contraindicated in any patient being observed for signs of increased intracranial pressure because they may mask signs of an early uncal herniation. The ophthalmologist may obtain a better view of the periphery of the retina through the use of indirect ophthalmoscopy. Some of the ocular pathologic features detected by these abnormalities *(red flags)* in inspection and direct ophthalmoscopy are summarized in Table 44–6.

---

*Time of onset of maximal mydriasis/cycloplegia of tropicamide is 15 to 30 minutes, duration of maximal effect 10 to 20 minutes, and recovery 30 to 240 minutes.

Table 44–6. "Red Flags" by Inspection and Direct Ophthalmoscopy in Evaluating Visual Impairment

Physical Finding	Possible Pathology
Inspection	
Globe	
Small	High hyperopia, persistent hyperplastic primary vitreous, phthisis bulbi (shrinkage related to deteriorating eye disease)
Large	Glaucoma, high myopia
Red eye	Inflammatory disease (infection, uveitis), trauma, tumor, glaucoma
Protrusion	Retrobulbar or orbital infection/tumor, hyperthyroidism
Sunken	Orbital fracture, Horner syndrome, atrophy, microphthalmia
Misalignment	Impairment of extraocular muscles: congenital weakness, muscle entrapment (tumor/trauma), cranial nerve palsy (infection, tumor, stroke, congenital)
Ophthalmoscopy	
Cloudy cornea	Anterior segment dysgenesis (Peter anomaly), glaucoma, trauma, infection, metabolic storage diseases (mucopolysaccharidoses)
Lens	
Cloudy	Cataracts (congenital versus systemic diseases)
Dislocated	Homocystinuria, Marfan syndrome
Cloudy vitreous	Retinoblastoma, detached retina, endophthalmitis, uveitis, hemorrhage
Optic disc	
Pale	Optic atrophy (congenital, trauma, tumor, hydrocephalus, degenerative neurologic disease)
Swollen	Increased intracranial pressure, optic neuritis
Hemorrhage	Optic neuritis, increased intracranial pressure
Retina/choroid	
Abnormal color	Retinitis pigmentosa (spicule pattern), chorioretinitis (atrophy with hyperpigmentation), Tay-Sachs disease (cherry-red macula)
Exudates	Diabetes mellitus, Coats disease, increased intracranial pressure
Hemorrhage	Hypertension, diabetes mellitus, increased intracranial pressure, trauma, blood disorders
Phakomata	Tuberous sclerosis (yellow plaques, nodules), von Hippel–Lindau disease (reddish globular mass), Sturge-Weber syndrome (choroidal hemangioma), neurofibromatosis (yellow plaques)
Blood vessels	
Constricted	Hypertension
Microaneurysm	Diabetes mellitus

REFRACTION

The function of the lens is to bend (focus) parallel light rays onto the curved retina to generate a sharp and bright image on the retina. Refractive errors occur when the lens does not properly focus these light rays onto the retina. The only light rays that do not need to be bent to fall correctly on the retina are those that are perpendicular to the lens.

Physical findings suggestive of a refractive error contributing to the visual loss include (1) a dull red reflex, (2) a diopter other than 0 needed to focus clearly on the retina, and (3) improved visual acuity with the *pinhole test*. In the pinhole test, the child views the eye chart through a small hole in the center of a 3 × 5 inch card. This pinhole (as in squinting) allows only light rays that are perpendicular (central parallel rays) to the lens to fall on the retina. If the decrease in visual acuity is due to refractive error, the child then sees a sharper image through the pinhole.

The ophthalmologist uses both objective techniques, such as retinoscopy, and subjective techniques in order to quantify refractive errors. After the pupils have been dilated with both a mydriatic and a cycloplegic agent, the examiner performs retinoscopy by focusing a beam of light onto the retina through lenses of various power placed in front of the patient's eye. This method is precise and can be done at any age. In the subjective method, the examiner places various lenses in front of the eye and asks the patient to report which lenses provide the clearest image.

Differential Diagnosis

The process of evaluating visual impairment can be simplified by answering the following:

Can the visual problem be corrected by refraction?
Is there a structural or organic defect of the visual pathway?
Has the lesion caused the development of amblyopia?

If the answer to all three questions is "no," the visual problem may be secondary either to a psychologic problem (conversion reaction or factitious disorder) or to a defect in processing graphic symbols (dyslexia) (see Fig. 44–3).

REFRACTIVE ERRORS

Refractive errors include *myopia* (nearsightedness), *hyperopia* (farsightedness), and *astigmatism.* Refractive errors may be similar *(isometropia)* or different *(anisometropia)* between both eyes.

Myopia

In patients with myopia the parallel rays of light in the resting (nonaccommodating) eye are focused in front of the retina. The symptoms of myopia are squinting, viewing an object too closely, and complaining of blurred far vision. Myopia is relatively common during childhood.

The incidence and degree of myopia increase with age, especially during growth spurts, as in adolescence. Because some forms of myopia are hereditary, children of myopic parents should be screened for myopia at an early age. Myopia may be associated with other ocular abnormalities, such as *keratoconus* (central conical protrusion of the cornea), cataracts, *ectopia lentis* (dislocated lens), *spherophakia* (overly spherical lens), *glaucoma,* and medullated (myelinated) nerve fibers. In addition, there is an increased prevalence of myopia in premature infants, especially with retinopathy of prematurity, and in many genetic conditions (Marfan and Stickler syndromes).

Although myopia is usually the simple *(physiologic)* form with a healthy globe, some children have *pathologic* myopia that is associated with thinning of the sclera, choroid, and retina. Pathologic myopia is often associated with some degree of uncorrectable vision impairment. Since myopic patients are at a greater risk for retinal detachment, they should also take appropriate safety precautions, such as wearing polycarbonate spectacles, molded polycarbonate goggles, and appropriate head gear for sports.

If myopia is sufficient to produce visual symptoms, *concave* (minus) lenses in the form of spectacles or contact lenses are prescribed to correct the refractive error (e.g., −3.75 diopters). Prescription changes may be needed every 1 to 2 years (more frequently during growth spurts).

Hyperopia

In patients with hyperopia (farsightedness), the parallel rays of light in the nonaccommodating (nonfocusing) eye are focused behind the retina. The process of accommodation (focusing), which alters the shape of the lens, can compensate for some degrees of hyperopia. Because children have a tremendous range of accommodation, moderately hyperopic children can see clearly without any visual symptoms. Severely hyperopic children may be unable to compensate through accommodation and may complain of blurred near vision and squinting. In addition, the greater accommodative effort may lead to symptoms of "eyestrain," which consist of headaches, fatigue, or eye rubbing. These symptoms may lead to a lack of interest in reading or in prolonged close work (school work). Some children may also cross their eyes (accommodative *esotropia*) secondary to hyperopia coupled with the increased accommodative effort. If hyperopia is severe enough to produce symptoms, *convex* (plus) lenses, usually in the form of glasses, are prescribed to correct the refractive error.

Astigmatism

In the patient with astigmatism, the refractive power differs in various meridians of the eye. In most cases, astigmatism is due to an irregular curvature of the cornea; however, lens abnormalities may also cause astigmatism. Even mild forms of astigmatism may produce blurring of vision (far and near), leading to squinting, fatigue, headaches, and lack of interest in close work. Cylindric or spherocylindric lenses (usually glasses) are used to improve vision and comfort.

Infants and children with corneal distortion secondary to scarring (trauma or infection) or to external compression (ptosis or hemangioma of eyelid) are at an increased risk for astigmatism, anisometropia, and attendant *amblyopia* ("lazy eye"). Early detection, optical correction, and occlusion therapy are essential for optimal binocular vision development.

Anisometropia

In patients with anisometropia, the refractive error of one eye differs significantly from that of the other eye. This difference can lead to amblyopia because the child uses the better eye for definitive vision. Anisometropia may initially be detected by comparison of the red reflex between the two eyes. The affected eye will have the duller red reflex. Early detection and treatment of anisometropia are essential for the development of optimal visual function.

DISORDERS OF ACCOMMODATION

During accommodation, the ciliary muscle contracts; this action releases tension on the suspensory fibers of the lens (zonules). With the relaxation of these fibers, the lens becomes more convex, which bends light (focuses) to a greater degree. A progressive decrease in accommodative ability normally occurs with increasing age (*presbyopia*). Usually symptoms of presbyopia begin in the fourth decade of life, but presbyopia may occur as early as the first decade.

Loss of Accommodation

Any lesion of the parasympathetic fibers of the third cranial nerve (midbrain to eye) may cause the loss of accommodation. Causes may include tumors, trauma, vascular lesions (strokes), degenerative diseases, metabolic disorders (diabetes mellitus, Wilson disease), toxins, inflammatory diseases (acute polyneuritis), and infections (encephalitis, meningitis, herpes zoster, botulism, diphtheria, and syphilis). The most common cause of accommodative paralysis is the use of drugs, especially cycloplegic eyedrops. Since loss of accommodation primarily affects near vision, reading glasses or bifocals can be used as needed to provide clear vision.

Spasm of Accommodation

In patients with spasm of accommodation, the ciliary muscle tone is increased, which results in *pseudomyopia* (blurred distant vision). Because of the increase in ciliary muscle tone, the child may complain of frontal headaches with nausea and vomiting. The symptoms may be accentuated with close work. Accommodative lesions can result from irritative lesions of the midbrain and third cranial nerve, infections (diphtheria), encephalitis, meningitis, intraocular inflammation, medications (morphine, digitalis, sulfonamides), and trauma. Accommodative spasms may also occur with diabetes mellitus, Graves disease, and migraines. Cycloplegic eyedrops and glasses can be used to relieve symptoms.

ORGANIC VISION DISORDERS

Any malformation or disease process of the visual system (from the cornea to the cerebral cortex) may affect vision. A practical clinical approach to this large differential diagnosis is based on the age of presentation (infancy verses childhood), mode of onset (acute versus chronic), and symptoms or physical findings (see Table 44–6).

Congenital and Infantile Vision Defects

Visual impairments that present soon after birth may be secondary either to congenital malformations of the visual system or to perinatal insults (congenital infections, anoxia, birth trauma). Infants with severe visual impairment may have nystagmus, strabismus, or an inability to fixate and follow objects. In addition, the physical findings can range from a cloudy cornea to retinal hemorrhages (Table 44–7). In some diseases, multiple areas of the eye may be involved. For example, neonatal herpes simplex infection can cause keratitis, chorioretinitis, and optic atrophy. Retinopathy of prematurity, congenital cataracts, and glaucoma are common causes of visual impairment in infants.

Retinopathy of Prematurity. A perinatal insult, presumably hyperoxia, disrupts the development of the retinal vascular bed. Normally, beginning at 16 weeks' gestation, retinal angiogenesis begins

to proceed from the optic disc to the periphery, reaching the outer nasal rim by 36 weeks' gestation (ora serrata retinae, or the irregular margin of the pars optica) and the temporal rim by 40 weeks' gestation. Even though hyperoxia is usually associated with retinopathy of prematurity, other perinatal insults, such as hypoxia, acidosis, and hypercarbia, may disrupt the process of angiogenesis and leave a well-demarcated avascular sector in the retina. As cell division resumes, revascularization takes place at this demarcation line, causing a ridge followed by a proliferation of vessels out of the retina and into the vitreous. Traction on the retina from these abnormal vessels may then lead to retinal detachment.

In approximately 90% of the infants with retinopathy of prematurity, the process spontaneously arrests and regresses, resulting in little or no visual disability. In the remaining infants, the disease can progress to severe myopia, retrolental membrane (*leukocoria*, or "white eye"), cataracts, glaucoma, and retinal detachments. The loss of visual acuity can then lead to strabismus, amblyopia, and nystagmus. The end stage is often a painful or degenerated, phthisic (wasting) eye.

Any infant with a birth weight under 2000 g or a gestational age of less than 33 weeks who has required supplemental oxygen therapy should be evaluated for retinopathy of prematurity. A detailed retinal examination should be performed at 4 to 9 weeks of age. The timing of this examination is based on the stability of the infant, the number (and severity) of risk factors for retinopathy of prematurity, and the increased chance of adverse reactions to mydriatic or cycloplegic drops in premature infants.

Besides correcting any visual impairments with surgery (such as cataract removal) and refraction, cryotherapy to the avascular retina may reduce progression of the disease.

Cataracts. A cataract, which occurs when the lens becomes opacified, is one common cause of leukocoria (white pupillary reflex) (Table 44–8; Figs. 44–6 to 44–8). The degree of opacification may disrupt the clear visual axis, which may lead to visual impairment and blindness. Cataracts are the most common cause of blindness in developed countries and account for 15% to 20% of all cases of childhood blindness. In addition, about 1 in 250 newborn infants have some form of lens opacification.

Lens opacifications can represent a clinically insignificant variation of normal development or a severe systemic disease that threatens both the infant's vision and life (Table 44–9). One variation of normal development is the opaque vacuoles that form around the Y sutures of the lens in premature infants. Cataracts of prematurity usually resolve spontaneously in a few weeks, whereas those from remnants of fetal structures (pupillary membrane, hyaloid vessels) are persistent but rarely interfere with vision.

A common cause of childhood cataracts is trauma, which may be accidental (a misplaced forceps during a delivery) or intentional (child abuse). The clinician should suspect abuse if any child presents with an isolated cataract (see Chapter 37). Other causes of cataracts include congenital infections (36%), idiopathic (31%), simple mendelian inheritance (23%), and genetic syndromes or metabolic diseases (10%) (see Table 44–9). Other ocular pathology, including aniridia, subluxation of the lens, coloboma, anterior persistent hyperplastic primary vitreous, and retinopathy of prematurity, may be associated with the development of cataracts and may further reduce the visual acuity.

Treatment. The treatment of cataracts depends on the infant's risk for *sensory deprivational amblyopia* (see Amblyopia). A dense monocular cataract, which carries a high risk for development of amblyopia, should be operated on as soon as possible, no later than 16 weeks of age and preferably in the first 2 weeks of life. Partial bilateral cataracts may be initially managed with nonsurgical therapy. Whenever the cataract significantly interferes with vision,

Table 44–7. Organic Causes of Vision Loss in Infancy

Condition	Physical Finding	Comment
Corneal Disease		
Corneal forceps injury	Cloudy cornea	May lead to astigmatism and amblyopia; associated with intraocular hemorrhage, retinal detachment, or glaucoma
Sclerocornea	Opaque cornea	Scleralization of cornea; familial or sporadic; early keratoplasty possibly needed to provide vision
Anterior microphthalmia	Small cornea	Familial inheritance; associated with congenital cataracts, glaucoma, and/or colobomata
Anterior Chamber Diseases		
Peter anomaly	Corneal opacity with iridocorneal/lenticulocorneal adhesions	Maldevelopment of anterior segment of eye; associated with glaucoma and lens abnormalities
Persistent pupillary membrane	Bands or membranes obscuring pupil	Rupture of vessels in membranes may lead to hyphema; membrane may need to be removed to restore vision
Glaucoma	Tearing, enlarged eye, photophobia, cloudy cornea, pale optic disc	Increased intraocular pressure leading to blindness (optic nerve damage). Causes: anomalies of anterior segment, intraocular hemorrhage, ocular inflammatory disease, intraocular tumors. Treatment: surgery
Iris and Lens Disorders		
Aniridia	Large, irregular, unreactive pupil	Hypoplasia of iris. Type I: dominant; or recessive (ataxia, mental retardation); type II: deletion of chromosome 11, associated with mental retardation, genitourinary anomalies, and Wilms tumor
Cataracts	Lens opacity	Multiple causes, ranging from familial inheritance to drugs
Anterior PHPV	Leukocoria (white pupillary reflex), lens opacity, cloudy cornea, small lens and eye	Persistence of fetal hyaloid vascular system, resulting in fibrovascular plaque on back of lens. As plaque contracts, ciliary process and lens become distorted. Complications: glaucoma, cataract, intraocular hemorrhage, rupture of posterior capsule. Treatment: removal of membrane, lens aspiration. Prognosis: poor visual outcome
Retinal and Optic Nerve Disorders		
Posterior PHPV	Fibroglial veils around disc/macula, vitreous opacities (membrane, vessels)	Persistence of posterior fetal hyaloid vascular system; remnants of vascular system may cause traction detachment of retina
Chorioretinitis	Diffuse or local retinal atrophy demarcated by hyperpigmentation	Inflammation of posterior uveal tract with retinal involvement. Causes: toxoplasmosis, histoplasmosis, herpes simplex, cytomegalic inclusion virus, syphilis, tuberculosis, and toxocariasis. Other complications: glaucoma, detached retina
Retinoblastoma	Leukocoria	Neoplastic tumor with locus on chromosome 13; high incidence of secondary malignancy; poor prognosis with extraorbital metastasis
Retinopathy of prematurity	Leukocoria, cloudy vitreous; retinal white lines and ridges	Insult (hyperoxia) to vascularization of retina; associated with myopia and retinal detachment
Leber congenital retinal amaurosis	Normal findings to degeneration of retina	Failure of both rods and cones in retina; reduced or absent response to electroretinography; autosomal recessive
Achromatopsia	Color unable to be detected	Failure of cone system in retina; autosomal recessive or X-linked; diagnosed with ERG
Congenital stationary night blindness	Disc anomalies, poor night vision	Defect in rod system of retina; autosomal recessive, dominant, or X-linked recessive
Optic nerve hypoplasia	Pale, small optic disc; peripapillary halo of pigmentation	Secondary to failure in differentiation or degeneration of retinal ganglion cell axons. Some causes: septo-optic dysplasia (hypopituitary, midline CNS defects), chromosomal defects (trisomy 13), albinism, fetal drug exposure (phenytoin, ethanol), infant of diabetic mother, CNS defects (hydrocephalus, anencephaly, encephalocele)
Optic nerve aplasia	Absent retinal vessels and optic disc	Maldevelopment of optic nerve; associated with severe eye and CNS anomalies
Morning glory disc anomaly	Enlarged, funnel-shaped disc	Associated with retinal detachments and midline defects (cleft palate, encephalocele, agenesis of corpus callosum)
Coloboma	White, wedge-shaped retinal defect; visual field loss	Malclosure of embryonic fissure that leaves a gap in the retina, hence exposing sclera; defect may extend to lens; associated with many congenital syndromes
Aicardi syndrome	Retinal lacunae, coloboma of optic disc	Occurs mostly in females; associated with agenesis of corpus callosum, seizures, mental retardation, and vertebral anomalies
Albinism	Photophobia; blue-gray to yellow-brown iris; macular hypoplasia	Defect in formation of melanin, resulting in lack of pigment in eyes and sometimes skin; increased risk of skin cancer with hypopigmented skin

Abbreviations: PHPV = persistent hyperplastic primary vitreous; ERG = electroretinogram; CNS = central nervous system.

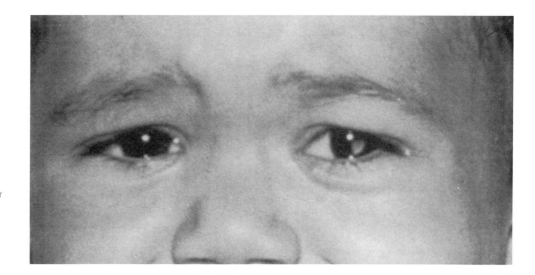

Figure 44–6. Leukocoria, left eye, was first noted by the child's mother when the patient was 18 months old. (From Harley RD. Pediatric Ophthalmology, 2nd ed. Philadelphia: WB Saunders, 1983:1228.)

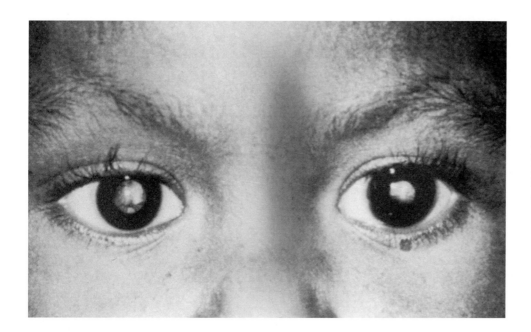

Figure 44–7. Bilateral "cat's eye" reflex (leukocoria) in an infant with bilateral retinoblastoma. (From Harley RD. Pediatric Ophthalmology, 2nd ed. Philadelphia: WB Saunders, 1983:25.)

Figure 44–8. Leukocoria. Cataract, posterior synechia formation, and keratic precipitates in a patient with chronic anterior and posterior uveitis. (From Nelson LB, Calhoun JH, Harley RD. Pediatric Ophthalmology, 3rd ed. Philadelphia: WB Saunders, 1991:273.)

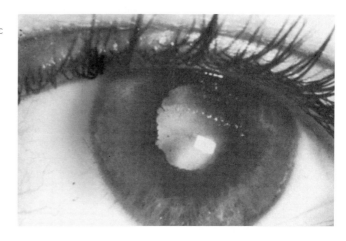

Table 44–8. Differential Diagnosis of Leukocoria (White Pupillary Reflex)

> *Common Causes*
>> Cataracts
>> Cicatricial retinopathy of prematurity
>> Larval granulomatosis (toxocariasis)
>> Persistent hyperplastic primary vitreous
>> Retinal detachment
>> Retinoblastoma
>> Retinoschisis
>
> *Other Causes*
>> Atrophic chorioretinal scars
>> Endophthalmitis
>> Exudative retinopathy (Coats disease)
>> Fundus coloboma
>> Leukemic ophthalmopathy
>> Incontinentia pigmenti
>> Medullated nerve fibers
>> Morning glory disc anomaly
>> Norrie disease
>> Organized vitreous hemorrhage
>> Phakomatoses
>> Retinal gliosis
>> Retinal dysplasia
>> Medulloepithelioma
>> Hemangioma
>> Hamartoma
>> Glioneuroma

the lens should be surgically removed to provide a clear visual axis; the resulting aphakic (absent lens) refractive error should be corrected with glasses, contact lenses, refractive corneal surgery, or lens implants; and any sensory deprivation amblyopia should be treated.

Prognosis. The prognosis varies according to the nature of the cataract, age of onset, duration and extent of preoperative amblyopia, the presence of other ocular abnormalities, and the occurrence of surgical complications. In the first 3 years after surgery, approximately 20% of patients will have postoperative complications, including chronic glaucoma, retinal detachment, and secondary membrane formation. Even with optimal therapy, aphakic patients may end up with reduced peripheral vision and decreased visual acuity.

Glaucoma. Glaucoma occurs when the intraocular pressure builds up in the anterior chamber. The resulting damage to the eye leads to a reduction in vision. The pressure increases when the flow of aqueous humor out of the anterior chamber is impeded through the trabecular meshwork or the canal of Schlemm (see Fig. 44–1).

The incidence of *infantile glaucoma* (before 3 years of age) is approximately 2 in 10,000 (Fig. 44–9). Half of these cases are due to a congenital abnormality of the drainage system, such as a mesodermal membrane covering the drainage system *(primary glaucoma)* (Table 44–10). In the remaining cases, another ocular process impinges on a normal drainage system *(secondary glaucoma)*. The causes of secondary glaucoma are:

- Maldevelopment of the anterior segment of the eye (Peters anomaly, Rieger anomaly)
- Aniridia
- Persistent hyperplastic primary vitreous
- Retinopathy of prematurity
- Tumors (Sturge-Weber syndrome, neurofibromatosis, retinoblastoma)
- Subluxation of the lens (Marfan syndrome, homocystinuria)

- Inflammation (congenital rubella, uveitis)
- Trauma (hyphema)
- Other congenital syndromes (trisomy 21, Pierre Robin anomalad, Rubinstein-Taybi syndrome)

Although *juvenile open-angle glaucoma* may occur in older children, secondary glaucoma is usually the cause of glaucoma in this age group.

The presenting symptoms of children with primary infantile glaucoma, in order of frequency, are tearing (55%), photophobia (41%), corneal haziness (41%) (Table 44–11), and corneal enlargement (32%) (Table 44–12); however, 21% may present without the classical symptoms of infantile glaucoma (tearing, photophobia, and blepharospasm). On physical examination, 92% have either corneal clouding (secondary to corneal edema) or corneal enlargement (diameter > 12 mm) (see Fig. 44–9). Other symptoms and physical findings are blepharospasm (eyelid closure secondary to corneal epithelial breaks, iritis, or glare from corneal edema), optic atrophy, cupping of the optic nerve head, and a decrease in visual acuity or visual fields.

Treatment. The goal of therapy for glaucoma is to control ocular pressure and prevent optic nerve damage. Treatment is primarily surgical and consists of either *goniotomy* (a linear incision through the trabecular meshwork) or *trabeculotomy* (an opening between Schlemm's canal and the anterior chamber). The success rate for both procedures is 70% to 80%. When these treatments fail, the patient may require cyclodestructive procedures (cyclocryotherapy) or even enucleation (for pain control in a blind eye). The patient may also need medical therapy to control intraocular pressure

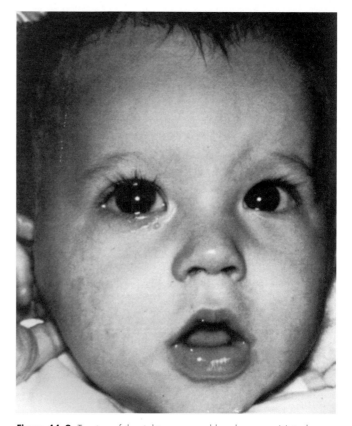

Figure 44–9. Tearing of the right eye caused by glaucoma. Note the increased corneal diameter of the right eye. (From Nelson LB, Calhoun JH, Harley RD. Pediatric Ophthalmology, 3rd ed. Philadelphia: WB Saunders, 1991:260.)

Table 44–9. Differential Diagnosis of Cataracts

Developmental Variants

Prematurity (Y suture vacuoles) with or without retinopathy of prematurity

Genetic Disorders

Simple Mendelian Inheritance

Autosomal dominant (most common)
Autosomal recessive
X-linked

Major Chromosomal Defects

Trisomy disorders (13, 18, 21)
Turner syndrome (45 X)
Deletion syndromes (11p13, 18p, 18q)
Duplication syndromes (3q, 20p, 10q)

Multisystem Genetic Disorders

Alport syndrome (hearing loss, renal disease)
Alström disease (nerve deafness, diabetes mellitus)
Apert syndrome (craniosynostosis, syndactyly)
Cockayne syndrome (premature senility, skin photosensitivity)
Conradi syndrome (chondrodysplasia punctata)
Crouzon syndrome (dysostosis craniofacialis)
Hallermann-Streiff syndrome (microphthalmia, small pinched nose, skin atrophy, and hypotrichosis)
Hypohidrotic ectodermal dysplasia (anomalous dentition, hypohidrosis, hypotrichosis)
Ichthyosis (keratinizing disorder with thick, scaly skin)
Incontinentia pigmenti (dental anomalies, mental retardation, cutaneous lesions)
Lowe syndrome (oculocerebrorenal syndrome: hypotonia, renal disease)
Marfan syndrome
Meckel-Gruber syndrome (renal dysplasia, encephalocele)
Myotonic dystrophy
Nail-patella syndrome (renal dysfunction, dysplastic nails, hypoplastic patella)
Marinesco-Sjögren syndrome (cerebellar ataxia, hypotonia)
Nevoid basal cell carcinoma syndrome (autosomal dominant, basal cell carcinoma erupts in childhood)
Peter anomaly (corneal opacifications with iris-corneal dysgenesis)
Reiger syndrome (iris dysplasia, myotonic dystrophy)
Rothmund-Thomson (poikiloderma: skin atrophy)
Rubinstein-Taybi syndrome (broad great toe, mental retardation)
Smith-Lemli-Opitz syndrome (toe syndactyly, hypospadias, mental retardation)
Sotos syndrome (cerebral gigantism)
Spondyloepiphyseal dysplasia (dwarfism, short trunk)
Werner syndrome (premature aging in 2nd decade of life)

Inborn Errors of Metabolism

Abetalipoproteinemia (absent chylomicrons, retinal degeneration)
Fabry disease (alpha-galactosidase A deficiency)
Galactokinase deficiency
Galactosemia (galactose-1-phosphate uridyl transferase deficiency)
Homocystinemia (subluxation of lens, mental retardation)
Mannosidosis (acid alpha-mannosidase deficiency)
Niemann-Pick (sphingomyelinase deficiency)
Refsum syndrome (phytanic acid alpha-hydrolase deficiency)
Wilson disease (accumulation of copper leads to cirrhosis and neurologic symptoms)

Endocrinopathies

Hypocalcemia (hypoparathyroidism)
Hypoglycemia
Diabetes mellitus

Congenital Infections

Toxoplasmosis
Cytomegalovirus infection
Syphilis
Rubella
Perinatal herpes simplex infection
Measles (rubeola)
Poliomyelitis
Influenza
Varicella-zoster

Ocular Anomalies

Microphthalmia
Coloboma
Aniridia
Mesodermal dysgenesis
Persistent pupillary membrane
Posterior lenticonus
Persistent hyperplastic primary vitreous
Primitive hyaloid vascular system

Miscellaneous Disorders

Atopic dermatitis
Drugs (corticosteroids)
Radiation
Trauma

Idiopathic

---

preoperatively or intraoperatively or when surgery is only partially effective.

Systemic agents used to control pressure are mannitol and carbonic anhydrase inhibitor (acetazolamide); topical agents are more commonly used and include miotics (pilocarpine) and beta-adrenergic blockers (timolol, levobunolol). Besides the control of intraocular pressure, the visual outcome depends on the correction of refractive errors, the treatment of amblyopia, and the presence of other ocular pathology (cataracts, corneal opacities, and retinal disease).

PROGRESSIVE VISION LOSS IN CHILDHOOD

In children with progressive vision loss, the primary considerations in the differential diagnosis are:

● Tumors affecting the visual pathways

● Hydrocephalus
● Progressive retinal disorders
● Optic atrophy or neuropathy

Although corneal opacifications (infections, trauma), cataracts (trauma, corticosteroids), secondary glaucoma, and uveitis (inflammation secondary to trauma, corneal keratitis or ulcer, rheumatoid arthritis) can all cause progressive vision loss, they are usually readily apparent on physical examination. Disease of the retina and optic pathways, however, can be insidious and difficult to diagnose and often requires an extensive diagnostic evaluation and a multisubspecialty approach.

Tumors

Optic Glioma. The most common tumor of the optic pathway in childhood is the optic glioma (*juvenile pilocystic astrocytoma*).

Table 44–10. **Childhood Glaucomas**

I. **Primary Genetically Determined Glaucoma**
  A. Congenital open-angle glaucoma
  B. Juvenile glaucoma
  C. Primary angle-closure glaucoma
  D. Primary glaucomas associated with systemic or ocular abnormalities
    1. Associated with *systemic* abnormalities
      a. Sturge-Weber syndrome
      b. Neurofibromatosis
      c. Pierre Robin anomalad
      d. Oculocerebrorenal syndrome (Lowe syndrome)
      e. Rieger syndrome
      f. Hepatocerebrorenal syndrome
      g. Marfan syndrome
      h. Rubinstein-Taybi syndrome
      i. Infantile glaucoma associated with mental retardation and paralysis
      j. Oculodental-digital syndrome
      k. Syndrome of microcornea, absent frontal sinuses, and open-angle glaucoma
      l. Mucopolysaccharidosis
      m. Trisomy 13
      n. Hurler disease
      o. Cutis marmorata telangiectasia
    2. Associated with *ocular* abnormalities
      a. Aniridia
      b. Congenital ocular melanosis
      c. Sclerocornea
      d. Familial hypoplasia of iris
      e. Anterior chamber cleavage syndrome
      f. Iridotrabecular dysgenesis and ectropion uveae
      g. Posterior polymorphous dystrophy

II. **Secondary Glaucoma**
  A. Traumatic glaucoma
    1. Acute
      a. Angle concussion
      b. Hyphema
    2. Late onset with angle recession
    3. Atriovenous fistula
  B. Intraocular neoplasm
    1. Melanoma
    2. Melanocytoma
    3. Juvenile xanthogranuloma
    4. Retinoblastoma
    5. Leukemia
  C. Uveitis
    1. Open-angle
    2. Angle blockage
      a. Synechial angle-closure
      b. Iris bombé with pupillary block
  D. Lens-induced glaucoma
    1. Subluxation-dislocation and pupillary block
    2. Spherophakia and pupillary block
    3. Phacolytic glaucoma
  E. Glaucoma after surgery for congenital cataract
    1. Lens material blockage of trabecular meshwork
    2. Pupillary block
    3. Chronic open-angle glaucoma
  F. Steroid glaucoma
  G. Glaucoma secondary to rubeosis
    1. Retinoblastoma
    2. Coats disease
    3. Medulloepithelioma
  H. Secondary angle-closure glaucoma
    1. Retinopathy of prematurity
    2. Microphthalmos
    3. Nanophthalmos
    4. Congenital iris-lens membrane
  I. Glaucoma associated with increased venous pressure
    1. Idiopathic
    2. Orbital disease

From Nelson LB, Calhoun JH, Harley RD. Pediatric Ophthalmology, 3rd ed. Philadelphia: WB Saunders, 1991:259.

Gliomas of the visual pathways account for approximately 5% of all primary central nervous system tumors in childhood. This tumor may develop anywhere along the visual pathway, but the most common location is the optic chiasm. Patients present with unilateral vision loss (optic nerve involvement), bitemporal hemianopsia (chiasma involvement), proptosis (exophthalmos), eye deviation, optic disc swelling, and disc pallor. If the glioma involves the chiasm, the child may also present with signs of increased intracranial pressure, pituitary dysfunction, and hypothalamic disorders (e.g., *diencephalic syndrome* consisting of euphoria, hyperalertness, and emaciation). In up to 15% of patients with neurofibromatosis type I, an optic glioma may develop, accounting for almost 25% of all optic gliomas. The natural history often follows a slow, relatively benign course.

The management is controversial because of the difficulty in predicting which tumors will become malignant. Optic gliomas resulting in unsightly proptosis or nearly complete loss of vision in one eye should be resected. In patients with relatively intact vision, the clinician may elect to follow the patient with serial neuroimaging studies every 6 months and visual acuity and visual field determinations every 3 months. If the tumor is progressing in size or if vision is deteriorating, the tumor should be resected. Because resection of an intrachiasm optic glioma results in blindness, a biopsy is performed to confirm the diagnosis, an intraventricular shunt is applied to control secondary hydrocephalus, and any pituitary dysfunction is treated. A subtotal resection may also be done if the tumor is compressing the optic pathways or is causing occlusion of the third ventricle. If the tumor continues to progress, radiotherapy or further subtotal resections are performed. Various chemotherapy programs (actinomycin D and vincristine) may reduce tumor growth and thus delay the need for radiotherapy in younger children.

Craniopharyngioma. Another tumor that commonly affects vision, *craniopharyngioma* accounts for almost 9% of all primary central nervous system tumors in childhood. This tumor originates from the embryonic rests of Rathke's pouch. As the tumor grows, it causes compression of the optic chiasm, the pituitary, and the third ventricle, which results in visual loss (bitemporal hemianopsia), pituitary dysfunction (diabetes insipidus, short stature, hypothyroidism, and so forth), and increased intracranial pressure (papilledema, optic atrophy, and abducent paresis with noncomitant esotropia). Almost 90% of these tumors show calcification on neuroimaging studies.

Treatment involves surgical removal of the tumor and possible

Table 44-11. *STUMPED:* **Differential Diagnosis of Neonatal Corneal Opacities**

Diagnosis	Laterality	Opacity	Ocular Pressure	Other Ocular Abnormalities	Natural History	Inheritance
S—Sclerocornea	Unilateral or bilateral	Vascularized, blends with sclera, clearer centrally	Normal (or elevated)	Cornea plana	Nonprogressive	Sporadic
T—Tears in endothelium and Descemet's membrane						
Birth trauma	Unilateral	Diffuse edema	Normal	Possible hyphema, periorbital ecchymoses	Spontaneous improvement in 1 month	Sporadic
Infantile glaucoma	Bilateral	Diffuse edema	Elevated	Megalocornea, photophobia and tearing, abnormal angle	Progressive unless treated	Autosomal recessive
U—Ulcers						
Herpes simplex keratitis	Unilateral	Diffuse with geographic epithelial defect	Normal	None	Progressive	Sporadic
Congenital rubella	Bilateral	Disciform or diffuse edema, no frank ulceration	Normal or elevated	Microphthalmos, cataract, pigment epithelial mottling	Stable, may clear	Sporadic
Neurotrophic—exposure	Unilateral or bilateral	Central ulcer	Normal	Lid anomalies, congenital sensory neuropathy	Progressive	Sporadic
M—Metabolic (rarely present at birth) (mucopolysaccharidoses IH, IS; mucolipidoses type IV)*	Bilateral	Diffuse haze, denser peripherally	Normal	Few	Progressive	Autosomal dominant
P—Posterior corneal defect	Unilateral or bilateral	Central, diffuse haze or vascularized leukoma	Normal or elevated	Anterior chamber cleavage syndrome	Stable; sometimes early clearing or vascularization	Sporadic, autosomal recessive
E—Endothelial dystrophy						
Congenital hereditary endothelial dystrophy	Bilateral	Diffuse corneal edema, marked corneal thickening	Normal	None	Stable	Autosomal dominant or recessive
Posterior polymorphous dystrophy	Bilateral	Diffuse haze, normal corneal thickness	Normal	Occasional peripheral anterior synechiae	Slowly progressive	Autosomal dominant
Congenital hereditary stromal dystrophy	Bilateral	Flaky, feathery stromal opacities; normal corneal thickness	Normal	None	Stable	Autosomal dominant
D—Dermoid	Unilateral or bilateral	White vascularized mass, hair, lipid arc	Normal	None	Stable	Sporadic

From Nelson LB, Calhoun JH, Harley RD. Pediatric Ophthalmology, 3rd ed. Philadelphia: WB Saunders, 1991:210.
*Mucopolysaccharidosis IH (Hurler syndrome); mucopolysaccharidosis IS (Scheie syndrome).

Table 44-12. **Differential Diagnosis of Enlarged Cornea**

	Simple Megalocornea	Anterior Megalophthalmos	Primary Infantile Glaucoma with Buphthalmos
Inheritance	Autosomal dominant (?)	X-linked recessive (male preponderance)	Sporadic
Time of appearance	Congenital	Congenital	First year of life
Bilaterality	Bilateral Symmetric	Bilateral Symmetric	Unilateral or bilateral Asymmetric
Natural history	Nonprogressive	Nonprogressive	Progressive
Symptoms	None	None	Photophobia, epiphora
Corneal clarity	Clear	Clear or mosaic dystrophy	Diffuse edema, tears in Descemet's membrane
Intraocular pressure	Normal	Elevated in some adults	Elevated
Corneal diameter	13–18 mm	13–18 mm	13–18 mm
Corneal thickness	Normal	Normal	Thick
Keratometry	Normal	Normal. ↑ astigmatism	Flat
Gonioscopy	Normal	Excessive mesenchymal tissue	Excessive mesenchymal tissue
Globe diameter (A scan)	23–26 mm	23–26 mm	27–30 mm
Major ocular complications	None	Lens dislocation, cataract <40 years, secondary glaucoma	Optic disc damage, late corneal edema
Associated systemic disorders	None	Occasionally Marfan and other skeletal abnormalities	None consistent

From Nelson LB, Calhoun JH, Harley RD. Pediatric Ophthalmology, 3rd ed. Philadelphia: WB Saunders, 1991:201.

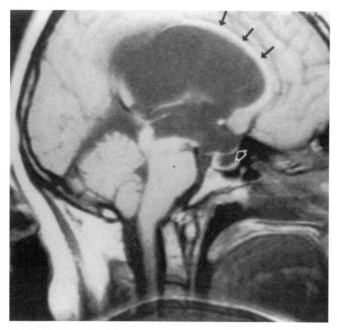

Figure 44–10. Sagittal MRI scan of obstructive hydrocephalus. The lateral ventricles are massively distended, resulting in thinning of the corpus callosum *(black arrows)*. The third ventricle is distended, producing distortion of the optic chiasm *(white arrowhead)*. (From Nelson LB, Calhoun JH, Harley RD. Pediatric Ophthalmology, 3rd ed. Philadelphia: WB Saunders, 1991:475.)

radiotherapy. In up to 88% of the patients, the tumor can be completely resected, resulting in a 10-year disease-free rate exceeding 70%. With subtotal resections, fewer than 50% of the patients survive 10 years. Radiotherapy can reduce recurrence rates and enhance survival; it is used primarily in subtotal resections because of the neurodevelopmental morbidity (cortical atrophy, decreased intelligence, seizures) in young children. Mortality is secondary to recurrence of tumor or complications from the management of hypopituitarism (hypotension, hypoglycemia, and electrolyte abnormalities of adrenal crises and hypernatremia of diabetes insipidus).

Other Tumors. Other suprasellar tumors affecting vision are hypo-

thalamic gliomas, germinoma, and arachnoid cysts. Depending on the location, size of the lesion, and rate of growth, various cerebral tumors (astrocytomas) and vascular lesions may present with visual field deficits, decreased visual acuity, papilledema, and ocular motor signs.

Hydrocephalus

Progressive hydrocephalus affects vision by direct compression on the chiasm or posterior visual pathways (Fig. 44–10). This compression then leads to ischemia and optic nerve atrophy. The hydrocephalus may be secondary to a congenital defect (Arnold-Chiari malformation, aqueductal stenosis), a secondary process obstructing the third ventricle (hemorrhage, tumor), or a ventricular shunt malformation. Other ocular findings of hydrocephalus are papilledema (Fig. 44–11), sixth cranial nerve paresis (esotropia, *diplopia* [double vision], compensatory posturing), nystagmus, and *Parinaud syndrome* (setting-sun sign: downward deviation of the eyes; pressure on the quadrigeminal plate causing vertical gaze palsy, eyelid retraction, pupillary dysfunction).

Retinal Disorders

Degenerative diseases of the retina and macula can be due to either primary diseases of the retina or other ocular pathology or systemic illnesses. Usually these illnesses produce a gradual loss of vision; however, if the process should cause an acute deterioration of the macula, the patient may present with a sudden loss of vision.

Macular Dystrophies

The *macular dystrophies* affecting vision are Stargardt disease (fundus flavimaculatus) and Best vitelliform degeneration. The macula may also be damaged by various metabolic disorders (Tay-Sachs, Sandhoff variant, metachromatic leukodystrophy, Niemann-Pick disease) and by retinal ischemia (occlusion of the central retinal artery), which results in a "cherry-red macula" (Table 44–13).

Stargardt disease is an autosomal recessive disease causing bilateral macular degeneration. Initially, the macula is gray with pigmented spots, followed by depigmentation and chorioretinal atro-

Table 44–13. Conditions in Which a Macular Cherry-Red Spot Occurs

	Frequency of Occurrence of Sign
I. Localized ocular conditions	
Retinal ischemia	
Contusion of globe	
II. Systemic conditions	
Generalized gangliosidosis	<50%
Tay-Sachs disease (G_{M2} type I)	All cases
Sandhoff disease (G_{M2} type II)	Most cases
Metachromatic leukodystrophy (sulfatide lipidosis)	Occasional cases
Niemann-Pick disease (sphingomyelin-cholesterol lipidosis type A)	Most cases
Farber's lipogranulomatosis (ceramide lipidosis)	Uncertain
Cherry-red spot myoclonus syndrome (sialidosis type I)	All cases
Sialidosis type II	All cases
Other Illnesses With Macular Lesions Resembling a Cherry-Red Spot	
Adult Niemann-Pick disease	
Gaucher disease	

Modified from Nelson LB, Calhoun JH, Harley RD. Pediatric Ophthalmology, 3rd ed. Philadelphia: WB Saunders, 1991:460.

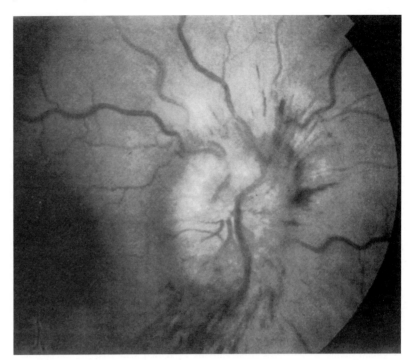

Figure 44–11. Acute papilledema with streak peripapillary hemorrhages, distention of the retinal venous system, and marked optic disc edema. Note the absence of a central cup. (From Nelson LB, Calhoun JH, Harley RD. Pediatric Ophthalmology, 3rd ed. Philadelphia: WB Saunders, 1991:475.)

phy. The illness usually presents by 8 to 14 years of age and often results in a central vision loss up to 20/200.

Best vitelliform degeneration is an autosomal dominant condition that presents at 5 to 15 years of age. Initially, the macula is yellow (yolk-like) and then degenerates into pigmented lesions and chorioretinal atrophy.

Retinal Degeneration. The retinal degenerations caused by a process originating in the retina are Coats disease, retinoschisis, familial exudative vitreoretinopathy, and retinitis pigmentosa.

Coats Disease. *Coats disease* affects primarily boys in the first decade of life. It is an exudative retinopathy caused by leakage of fluid from telangiectasis of retinal vessels. This exudative process can cause leukocoria, retinal detachment, glaucoma, and cataracts. Treatment consists of photocoagulation or cryotherapy.

Retinoschisis. The retina splits into an inner and outer layer, and cystoid macular changes, retinal detachment, and vitreous hemorrhages result. This X-linked condition affects males in early infancy.

Familial Exudative Vitreoretinopathy. In this autosomal dominant condition, aberrant blood vessels and neovascularization of the retina are present. These abnormalities result in vitreoretinal adhesions that cause traction on the retina.

Retinitis Pigmentosa. This progressive retinal degeneration usually begins in late childhood; however, it can also present in infancy (Leber congenital retinal amaurosis). Symptoms include impairment of dark adaptation, leading to night blindness, and progressive loss of peripheral visual fields, leading to central vision loss. The physical findings are arteriolar attenuation, pallor of the optic disc, and rarefaction with clumping of retinal pigment ("bone spicule" pattern). Retinal function, as measured by electroretinog-

raphy (ERG), is reduced or absent even prior to the development of symptoms. This condition may occur as an isolated ocular illness, often inherited as an autosomal recessive, autosomal dominant, or X-linked disorder.

Retinitis pigmentosa may also be associated with the following syndromes and inborn errors of metabolism:

- Usher syndrome (sensorineural hearing loss)
- Kearns-Sayre syndrome (external ophthalmoplegia)
- Lawrence-Moon-Biedl syndrome (obesity)
- Sjögren-Larsson syndrome (ichthyosis)
- Sphingolipidosis
- Lipofuscinosis
- Mucopolysaccharidosis
- Abetalipoproteinemia
- Refsum syndrome (phytanic acid α-hydrolase deficiency)

The retinal findings of cystinosis and congenital rubella syndrome may resemble retinitis pigmentosa, but they rarely affect vision.

Systemic Damage

Retinal damage may also come from systemic illnesses, such as bacterial endocarditis, hypertension, phakomata (hamartomatous disorders), and diabetes mellitus, or from an ocular process causing a retinal detachment.

In bacterial endocarditis, 40% of patients will have retinal damage from emboli causing hemorrhages, hemorrhages with white centers (Roth spots), papilledema, and (rarely) occlusion of the central retinal artery. The initial funduscopic sign of hypertension is narrowing of the arterioles, which then progresses to retinal edema, flame-shaped hemorrhages, "cotton-wool patches," and papilledema.

Impaired vision may also result from retinal tumors of the hamartomatous disorders:

- Choroidal hemangiomas (Sturge-Weber syndrome)
- Hemangioblastoma, a reddish, globular retinal mass in von Hippel–Lindau disease
- Glial hamartoma (raised yellow, multicystic tumor in tuberous sclerosis)
- Benign astrocytic proliferations (whitish-yellow plaques in tuberous sclerosis and neurofibromatosis)

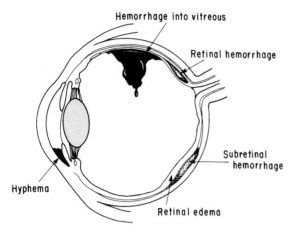

Figure 44–12. Various types of ocular hemorrhage following blunt trauma to the globe. (From Reilly BM. Practical Strategies in Outpatient Medicine, 2nd ed. Philadelphia: WB Saunders, 1991:68.)

Retinal Detachment. A retinal detachment occurs when the neuroretina separates from the pigmented epithelium. In children, this separation is usually associated with traction on the retina (non-rhegmatogenous detachment) from vitreous or retinal scar tissue (retinopathy of prematurity) rather than from an accumulation of fluid between the layers (rhegmatogenous detachment). The accumulation of fluid may be from inflammation, hemorrhage (trauma) (Fig. 44–12), or neoplasm. Other ocular conditions that increase one's susceptibility to retinal detachment are high myopia, ectopia lentis, and aphakia. Symptoms of a detached retina are loss of vision, strabismus, nystagmus, and leukocoria. Prompt surgical intervention may be necessary to salvage vision.

Optic Atrophy

In patients with optic atrophy, the optic nerve axons degenerate, resulting in a gradual loss of vision. The funduscopic signs are a pale optic disc coupled with the enlargement of the optic cup (secondary to the loss of substance to the nerve head). The most common causes of optic atrophy in children are hydrocephalus and intracranial tumors, which cause optic atrophy through ischemic compression of the visual pathways. Optic atrophy may also be associated with longstanding papilledema (pseudotumor cerebri), inborn errors of metabolism (mucopolysaccharidoses, sphingolipidoses, ceroid lipofuscinoses, leukodystrophies, Menkes kinky hair disease), demyelinating scleroses (Schilder disease), congenital infections, congenital syndromes (incontinentia pigmenti, osteopetrosis, Conradi syndrome, Cockayne syndrome), and diabetes mellitus. It may also occur as an autosomal dominant disorder with mild visual loss and a recessive disorder with severe visual loss. Because of this differential diagnosis, optic atrophy in childhood without an obvious cause warrants an extensive investigation.

Acute Vision Loss in Childhood. Acute vision loss in children may be secondary to the following:

- Optic neuritis
- Psychogenic disorders
- A progressive visual loss disorder that now involves the macula
- A vascular insult to the eye or brain (central retinal artery occlusion, migraine, cerebral vascular accident)

In the child with optic neuritis, inflammation and demyelination of the optic nerve lead to acute loss of vision. There may also be pain on movement of the globe. Funduscopic findings can be normal (retrobulbar neuritis) or may reveal exudates and hemorrhages of the optic disc (papillitis) and retina (optic neuroretinitis). The causes of optic neuritis include:

- Viral infections (measles, mumps, varicella, infectious mononucleosis)
- Bacterial meningitis
- Demyelinating sclerosis (Schilder disease, multiple sclerosis, neuromyelitis optica)
- Lymphoma infiltrating the optic nerve
- Toxins (lead)
- Drugs (vincristine, chloramphenicol)

In most cases, there is some improvement in vision within 1 to 4 weeks after onset. High-dose intravenous corticosteroids may reduce inflammation and improve vision.

AMBLYOPIA

Amblyopia (''lazy eye'') is defined as poor visual acuity in one or both eyes despite correction of any refractive error. The incidence of amblyopia is up to 2% in a general pediatric population. This condition occurs when the normal process of visual development is disrupted. In order for visual development to occur, a sharp image needs to be focused on the macula and transmitted to the visual cortex for processing and recognition of the retinal images. This cortical process begins rapidly at birth, with vision reaching its full potential and stability by the time a child is 10 years old. Risk factors for amblyopia are the early onset, duration, and severity of the impaired monocular stimulation. The causes include strabismus (misalignment of the eyes), refractive errors, and deprivation.

Strabismic Amblyopia

Strabismus (see later) is the most common cause of amblyopia. When the eyes are misaligned, each retina perceives different images. The child then effectively uses only one macula at a time for definitive seeing while suppressing the visual image from the other. If the infant alternates fixation by using each eye part of the time for definitive seeing, the risk of amblyopia is relatively low. If the child develops a fixation preference for one eye, the deviating or misaligned eye is at great risk for amblyopia because of the lack of normal use of the misdirected macula. In congenital esotropia (cross-eye, or convergent strabismus), up to half of the infants will develop a fixation preference. Strabismic amblyopia is usually unilateral.

Refractive Amblyopia

The infant or child with uncorrected anisometropia (refractive asymmetry) is at risk for amblyopia in the eye with the higher refractive error secondary to the macular blur and the impaired sensory stimulation. The refractive asymmetry may be secondary to astigmatism, myopia, or hyperopia.

In hyperopia, amblyopia may occur when the refractive difference between the two eyes is greater than 1 diopter. Through the accommodative process, which occurs equally in both eyes, the vision will be clear in the less hyperopic eye but still blurred in the more hyperopic eye. This blurred vision may result in amblyopia in the more hyperopic eye. If the hyperopia is so severe in both eyes to the point that the accommodative process cannot produce a clear vision in any eye (hyperopia > 5 diopters), the child is at risk for bilateral amblyopia. If one eye is myopic, the infant may use the normal or mildly hyperopic eye for fixation during both far and near gaze.

In mild myopia, some infants may use the myopic eye for near gaze and the normal or hyperopic eye for far gaze. If each eye is used at different times in order to generate a clear vision, the risk for amblyopia is reduced. In myopia a difference of greater than 3 diopters between the eyes is potentially amblyogenic.

Deprivation Amblyopia

Sensory deprivation caused by any obstruction that prevents light from reaching the retina may result in amblyopia. The obstructions that block the visual axis may be diseases of the eyelid (severe ptosis, hemangioma) or opacities of the ocular media (corneal scars, cataracts, or hemorrhages). The most critical stage of visual development occurs during the first weeks of life, when the site for central visual acuity (fovea) is recognized by the visual cortex. For this process to take place, an image must be focused on the macula during this period. If this process does not occur, the result is severe amblyopia. The resulting amblyopia is usually more severe from unilateral than bilateral lesions.

Treatment

The patient is provided with a clearly focused retinal image, which ensures proper placement of the image on the retina, and is forced to use the amblyopic eye. For the infant with a congenital cataract, the cataract is removed in a timely fashion to provide a useful visual axis, the resultant refractive error (aphakia) is promptly corrected in order to focus the image on the retina, and occlusion therapy is prescribed for the better eye to force use of the amblyopic eye. In unilateral amblyopia secondary to anisometropia, occlusion therapy is used following optical correction. In bilateral amblyopia secondary to high isometropia, only optical correction is needed.

For the child with strabismic amblyopia, occlusion therapy is usually done prior to surgery to first improve vision and fixation of the deviating eye. This improved vision and fixation enhance the chance of surgical correction to result in binocular vision. If the amblyopia is associated with accommodative esotropia, optical correction is followed by occlusion therapy.

Occlusion therapy involves covering the better eye to force the use of the amblyopic eye. A self-adhesive eye patch is used to ensure total occlusion and to prevent peaking. Pirate-like black patches and opaque occluders attached to glasses are usually ineffective because children can easily remove or peek around them. If the child cannot tolerate the self-adhesive patch because of local skin irritation, occlusion therapy can still be conducted either by using an opaque contact lens or by blurring the vision of the better eye with cycloplegic eyedrops or with a high-power contact lens.

Occlusion therapy must be monitored closely to prevent deprivation amblyopia in the eye that is being covered. As a rule, 1 week of occlusion therapy per year of age is prescribed between follow-up visits. For example, in a 3-year-old, the initial patching is for 3 weeks, followed by an assessment of visual acuity at the end of this period. If more occlusive therapy is needed, another 3-week interval is prescribed and the process is repeated until maximal visual acuity is reached. Once maximal acuity has been reached, part-time maintenance patching may be required up to age 10 years, which is when visual maturity and stability are usually attained. If the child is left with a significant vision defect despite optimal treatment, every effort must be made to protect the better eye through appropriate safety precautions, such as avoidance of contact sports, and the use of impact-resistant (polycarbonate) glasses for routine use and sports goggles for non-contact sports.

The success of therapy depends not only on early treatment but also on compliance. Children resist therapy because of the severity of the visual impairment of the amblyopic eye, the cosmetically unacceptable appearance of the occluder, and the ridicule from their peers.

Prognosis and Prevention

The prognosis varies with (1) the nature of the amblyogenic factors, (2) the age of onset of the insult, (3) the severity of the vision impairment, (4) the age of initiation of treatment, and (5) compliance with treatment. Generally, the earlier the onset, the more profound the effect on visual development and the more urgent the need for intervention. The window of opportunity for successful intervention in an infant with a unilateral congenital cataract may be limited to the first weeks of life, although cataracts that develop later in childhood (after some initial visual development has taken place) have a less damaging effect on visual development and a better prognosis.

PSYCHOGENIC VISION DISORDERS

The clinician must determine whether visual symptoms are of organic or psychogenic origin. Some of the psychologic conditions that may present with visual symptoms are factitious disorders, school avoidance, and conversion disorders (see Chapter 36). The greatest incidence of psychogenic cause of vision loss occurs in older school-aged children (8 to 15 years), with girls being more affected than boys.

Besides complaining of vision loss or blurring, the children with a psychogenic cause of the visual symptoms may also complain of abnormal visual sensations (spots, lines, or patterns, often in color), diplopia, polyopia, and a visual field defect. In addition to visual symptomatology, the spectrum of psychogenic ophthalmic manifestations in these children may also include ocular discomfort ("eyestrain," asthenopia, or painful eye), headaches, exaggerated sensitivity to light, disorders of accommodation and convergence, blinking, and lid tics. Some children may even exhibit self-destructive behavior, such as gouging their eyes or pulling out their eyelashes.

Red Flags

The *red flags* that should alert the clinician to the possibility of a psychogenic vision problem are inconsistency, suggestibility, and the child's affect during the examination.

Inconsistency. If the cause of vision loss is organic, the symptoms will be consistent across a variety of situations. If the vision is so poor as to interfere with school work, it should also interfere with one's performance in sports and in video games.

Suggestibility. Leading the patient to believe that the vision will be clearer as the examiner has the patient look through lenses of negligible power often yields a dramatic improvement in acuity. Similarly, a patient's visual field loss may expand to normal after

Table 44–14. The Red Eye

Condition	Etiology	Signs/Symptoms	Treatment
Bacterial conjunctivitis	*H. influenzae, H. aegyptius, S. pneumoniae, Neisseria gonorrhoeae: S. aureus, Yersinia,* cat-scratch bacillus less common	Mucopurulent unilateral or bilateral discharge, normal vision, photophobia usually absent Conjunctival injection and edema (chemosis); gritty sensation	Topical antibiotics: systemic ceftriaxone for *Gonococcus, H. influenzae*
Viral conjunctivitis	Adenovirus, ECHO virus, coxsackievirus	As above; may be hemorrhagic, unilateral enlarged preauricular lymph nodes	Self-limited
Neonatal conjunctivitis	*Chlamydia trachomatis, Gonococcus,* chemical (silver nitrate), *S. aureus*	Palpebral conjunctival follicle or papillae; as above	Ceftriaxone for *Gonococcus* and erythromycin for *C. trachomatis*
Allergic conjunctivitis	Seasonal pollens or allergen exposure	Itching, incidence of bilateral chemosis (edema) greater than that of erythema, tarsal papillae	Antihistamines, steroids, cromolyn
Keratitis	Herpes simplex, adenovirus, *S. pneumoniae, S. aureus, Pseudomonas, Acanthamoeba,* chemicals	Severe pain, corneal swelling, clouding, limbus erythema, hypopyon, cataracts; contact lens history with amebic infection	Specific antibiotics for bacterial/fungal infections; keratoplasty, acyclovir for herpes
Endophthalmitis	*S. aureus, S. pneumoniae, Candida albicans,* associated surgery or trauma	Acute onset, pain, loss of vision, swelling, chemosis, redness; hypopyon and vitreous haze	Antibiotics
Anterior uveitis (iridocyclitis)	JRA, Reiter syndrome, sarcoidosis, Behçet disease, Kawasaki disease, inflammatory bowel disease	Unilateral/bilateral; erythema, ciliary flush (in circumcorneal area), irregular pupil, iris adhesions; pain, marked photophobia, small pupil, poor vision, no discharge	Topical steroids, plus therapy for primary disease
Posterior uveitis (choroiditis)	Toxoplasmosis, histoplasmosis, *Toxocara canis*	No signs of erythema, decreased vision, no discharge	Specific therapy for pathogen
Episcleritis/scleritis	Idiopathic autoimmune disease (e.g., SLE, Henoch-Schönlein purpura)	Localized pain, intense erythema, unilateral; blood vessels bigger than in conjunctivitis; scleritis may cause globe perforation, no discharge	Episcleritis is self-limiting; topical steroids for fast relief
Foreign body	Occupational exposure	Unilateral, red, gritty feeling; visible or microscopic size	Irrigation, removal; check for ulceration
Blepharitis	*S. aureus, S. epidermidis,* seborrheic, blocked lacrimal duct; rarely molluscum contagiosum, *Phthirus pubis, Pediculus capitis*	Bilateral, irritation, itching, hyperemia, crusting, affecting lid margins	Topical antibiotics, warm compresses
Dacryocystitis	Obstructed lacrimal sac: *S. aureus, H. influenzae, Pneumococcus*	Pain, tenderness, erythema and exudate in area of lacrimal sac (inferomedial to inner canthus); tearing (epiphora); possible orbital cellulitis	Systemic, topical antibiotics; surgical drainage
Dacryoadenitis	*S. aureus, Streptococcus,* CMV, measles, EBV, enteroviruses; trauma, sarcoidosis, leukemia	Pain, tenderness, edema, erythema over gland area (upper temporal lid); fever, leukocytosis	Systemic antibiotics; drainage of orbital abscesses

Table 44–14. The Red Eye *Continued*

Condition	Etiology	Signs/Symptoms	Treatment
Orbital cellulitis (postseptal cellulitis)	Paranasal sinusitis: *H. influenzae, S. aureus, S. pneumoniae, Streptococcus* Trauma: *S. aureus* Fungi: *Aspergillus, Mucor* sp. if immunodeficient	Rhinorrhea, chemosis, vision loss, painful extraocular motion, proptosis, ophthalmoplegia, fever, lid edema, leukocytosis	Systemic antibiotics, drainage of orbital abscesses
Periorbital cellulitis (preseptal cellulitis)	Trauma: *S. aureus, Streptococcus* Bacteremia: *H. influenzae,* pneumococcus, *Streptococcus pyogenes*	Cutaneous erythema, warmth, normal vision, minimal involvement of orbit; fever, leukocytosis, toxic appearance	Systemic antibiotics

Data from Am J Med 1985; 79:545; BMJ 1988; 296:1720; Infect Dis Clin North Am 1988; 2:99; Lancet 1991; 338:1498; Pediatr Ann 1993; 22:353. Modified from Behrman RE, Kliegman RM. Nelson Essentials of Pediatrics, 2nd ed. Philadelphia: WB Saunders, 1994:357–358.

Abbreviations: JRA = juvenile rheumatoid arthritis; SLE – systemic lupus erythematosus; CMV = cytomegalovirus; EBV = Epstein-Barr virus; ECHO = enteric cytopathogenic human orphan.

the examiner suggests to the patient that the pupils will be "opened" following the administration of dilating drops.

Affect and Behavior During Testing. Some children are indifferent despite the purported severity of the disability, whereas others may appear annoyed, resentful, or belligerent. On reading the visual acuity chart, the child may stop abruptly and refuse to cooperate with the examiner. In addition, many youngsters may exhibit exaggerated grimacing, elaborate contortions, and frequent sighs during testing.

Etiology

Whether the symptoms are of conscious or unconscious origin, a precipitating factor often can be identified. The symptoms may be a response to problems at home (illness, divorce, abuse) or in school (peer relationships, school failure, trying to maintain a high level of achievement). Some children willfully feign a vision problem because they want glasses or attention. In each case, it is the physician's responsibility to perform a thorough examination to rule out any organic causes of visual loss, to demonstrate that the patient is capable of normal visual function, and to begin to address the psychogenic nature of the problem.

Evaluation

For an assessment of visual symptoms, the child's response should be physiologically sound. For an assessment of visual acuity, the measurement of acuity should be identical regardless of the chart used (letter E, Snellen, or picture chart), the distance at which the child stands from the chart (adjusted for the shorter distance), and the use of a "zero power" lens despite suggestions from the examiner to the contrary. In a child who is blind in one or both eyes, the affected eye should be unable to fixate on an object (e.g., the patient's image on a tilted mirror), and there should not be any optokinetic nystagmus in response to a moving target in front of the patient.

In the assessment of a constricted visual field, the field constriction of psychogenic origin does not change proportionately when

the test distance or object size is adjusted (the "tubular" field). In addition, the patient may involuntarily glance toward an object suddenly brought into view from the periphery.

Ophthalmologists have additional techniques that may be effective for accurate assessment of visual function:

- High-power lenses to surreptitiously blur the vision of one eye while having the patient read with both eyes open
- Polarizing lenses and vectograph charts
- Red-green goggles and colored charts to demonstrate intact vision in one or both eyes
- Prisms to elicit diplopia or tell-tale refixation movements as the patient views the chart with both eyes open
- The Worth four-dot test to assess whether the patient sees with both eyes or has diplopia

When all else fails, quietly hinting that a few eyedrops might "clear things up" is often sufficient to get a child to read the 20/20 line.

Treatment

The approach to management should be supportive and nonpunitive. The clinician should never embarrass the child, accuse the patient of "faking," show anger, or subject the child to punishment. Glasses or medication that reinforces the concept of organic disease should be avoided. Reassurance and positive suggestion usually are sufficient to ease the child's symptoms. If symptoms persist or recur, the child should be referred to a psychologist or psychiatrist for further evaluation and management.

THE "RED EYE" AND VISION LOSS

Although not always associated directly with vision loss, the red eye is always an important consideration and represents a diverse group of primarily inflammatory processes (Tables 44–14 to 44–16). Vision may be affected if the patient purposefully keeps the lids closed or the inflammation produces sufficient lid edema to force the lids shut. In addition, nonconjunctival inflammation, such as uveitis (see Table 44–16), scleritis, episcleritis, or iritis, may acutely or chronically impair vision.

Table 44-15. Conjunctivitis: Differential Diagnosis

Etiology	Clinical Findings				
	Unilateral or Bilateral	*Discharge*	*Lids*	*Onset/Course*	**Treatment**
Viral* (usually adenovirus)	Bilateral	Thin, mucoid	Follicular	Gradual Upper respiratory tract infection? Preauricular adenopathy	Compresses
Herpes simplex	Unilateral	Thin, mucoid	Follicular	Gradual Keratitis Dendritic ulcer	Idoxuridine
Bacterial	Unilateral or bilateral	Purulent	Papillary, purulent	Gradual	Topical antibiotics
Gonococcal	Unilateral	Purulent	Edema, inflamed	Hyperacute	Systemic antibiotics
Chlamydial	Unilateral or bilateral	Thin, mucoid	Follicular	Indolent Persistent Neonate Sexually active	Oral erythromycin or tetracycline (>10 years of age)
Allergic	Bilateral	Watery	Papillary	Gradual Seasonal	Topical vasoconstrictors Systemic antihistamine Topical steroids
Vernal	Bilateral	Watery	Giant papillary	Adolescents Seasonal	Cromolyn?
Contact lens irritation	Bilateral	Watery	Giant papillary	Lenses	Adjust lens Change solution
Chemical	Unilateral or bilateral	Watery	Variable	Acute	Irrigate Remove irritant

Modified from Reilly BM. Practical Strategies in Outpatient Medicine, 2nd ed. Philadelphia: WB Saunders, 1991:46.
*Undifferentiated viral conjunctivitis, not due to herpesvirus infection.

The differential diagnosis of the red eye is noted in Table 44–14, and the differential diagnosis of conjunctivitis is presented in Table 44–15. An example of the ciliary flush of iritis is noted in Figure 44–13. Patients with iritis, iridocyclitis, or uveitis may require slit-lamp examination to confirm the diagnosis while the examiner looks for signs of more systemic non-ocular manifestations compatible with the differential diagnoses of these disorders (see Table 44–16). Posterior uveitis (choroiditis) usually is not associated with a "red eye."

STRABISMUS

Strabismus (misalignment of the eyes, or "straying eye") is a common ocular problem and is encountered in almost 5% of children. Other terms used for strabismus are "squint," "wall-eye," "cross-eye," and "lazy eye." Strabismus can have significant effects on both vision and cosmesis. Although strabismus is often an isolated ocular problem in an otherwise healthy child, it may also be the presenting sign of a serious underlying disease of the eye or brain, such as tumor, infection, or degenerative disease.

Definitions

Normal alignment of the eyes is referred to as *orthophoria.* Orthophoria occurs when both visual axes consistently intersect on the object of regard; this results in an image that falls simultane-

ously on both maculae. Abnormal alignment and movement of the eyes are described in Table 44–17. Eye deviations may occur singly or in various combinations.

History

The patient history focuses on the clarification of the presenting complaint, the frequency and circumstances eliciting the deviation, the age of onset, associated signs and symptoms, and the general health of the child. Parents often have trouble describing abnormal eye movements. Some of the terms they may use include "lazy eye," "crossing," "turning," "drifting," "rolling," and "unable to focus." In addition, parents may say that their child's eyes cross when they actually deviate outward. The examiner should ask the parent to point to the eye that they think is deviating and indicate the direction in which they think it is turning.

Both the frequency and circumstances in which the abnormal movements occur can help the clinician to determine the cause of the condition. For example, the eye deviation may be frequent or persistent (*heterotropia*) or may occur only under special circumstances, such as fatigue (*heterophoria*). The gaze that is associated with the deviation may also determine the cause of the abnormality. Parents may report the following associations: eye crossing with only near gaze (*esotropia* secondary to hyperopia and accommodation), out-turning only with distant gaze (*exotropia* secondary to myopia), and divergence of the eyes with upward gaze (overreaction of the inferior oblique muscles).

The examiner should inquire about the onset and course of the

Table 44–16. Uveitis in Childhood

Anterior Uveitis
  Juvenile rheumatoid arthritis (pauciarticular)
  Sarcoidosis
  Trauma
  Tuberculosis
  Kawasaki disease
  Ulcerative colitis
  Reiter syndrome
  Spirochetal (syphilis, leptospiral)
  Heterochromic iridocyclitis (Fuchs)
  Viral (herpes simplex, herpes zoster)
  Ankylosing spondylitis
  Stevens-Johnson syndrome
  Idiopathic
  Drugs

Posterior Uveitis (choroiditis—may involve retina)
  Toxoplasmosis
  Parasites (toxocariasis)
  Sarcoidosis
  Tuberculosis
  Viral (rubella, herpes simplex, human
    immunodeficiency virus, cytomegalovirus)
  Subacute sclerosing panencephalitis
  Idiopathic

Anterior and/or Posterior Uveitis
  Sympathetic ophthalmia (trauma to other eye)
  Vogt-Koyanagi-Harada syndrome (uveo-oto-cutaneous
    syndrome: poliosis, vitiligo, deafness, tinnitus,
    uveitis, aseptic meningitis, retinitis)
  Behçet syndrome
  Lyme disease

signs and symptoms to determine whether the strabismus is due to a recognizable syndrome or to a slowly growing brainstem neoplasm. When the strabismus is not caused by an underlying ocular or neurologic disease, the onset and the course of symptoms and signs follow well-established, recognizable patterns. The usual age of onset for infantile esotropia, accommodative esotropia, and cyclic esotropia is approximately 2 to 3 months, 2 to 3 years, and 3 to 4 years, respectively (Fig. 44–14). Strabismus resulting from a congenital disorder of eye movement *(Duane syndrome)* or from the severe vision impairment of a congenital ocular anomaly (congenital cataract) is usually evident early in infancy. When a child presents with acquired strabismus or when the signs do not conform to one of the recognizable patterns of strabismus, the possibility of an underlying ocular or neurologic disease process must be considered. Because the onset of acquired paralytic strabismus can be insidious, a review of old photographs can be helpful in documenting age of onset and course of signs.

The examiner should inquire about associated signs and symptoms. The child with recent-onset strabismus may complain of double vision or may rub, cover, or squint one eye. To avoid diplopia, the child with paralytic strabismus may also exhibit compensatory posturing. The child with a right fourth nerve palsy tends to tilt the head down and toward the left.

Finally, the examiner asks about the child's birth history and general health and development. Early-onset strabismus is more frequent in children with a history of prematurity, perinatal problems, and developmental delay. In children with acquired strabismus, the examiner should probe for signs and symptoms of recent injury, infection, or developmental or neurologic regression.

Since many of the conditions that predispose to strabismus are familial (hyperopia, myopia), it is important to investigate the family history for ocular pathology and eye movement disorders.

Examination

Every child presenting with strabismus needs a comprehensive ophthalmologic examination. This includes a careful evaluation of sensory function (visual acuity, stereoacuity), cycloplegic refraction, inspection of the eye and adnexae, and ophthalmoscopy. A detailed evaluation of ocular motility and binocular alignment (cover tests, corneal light reflex test) (Fig. 44–15) is also mandatory.

OCULAR MOTILITY

The examiner tests the movement of all the extraocular muscles by having the child follow an interesting target, such as a colorful toy, with the head held still. Both eyes are open to test for versions and vergences. If an abnormality is noted, the examiner evaluates the ductions of each eye individually by covering one eye and having the child follow the target in all directions with the open eye. If any abnormality is noted or if the child will not cooperate, the abnormality may be confirmed by reflexive testing *(doll's-eye maneuver)*. Provided there is no neurologic contraindication to rapidly turning the head (cervical neck injury), the examiner elicits the doll's-eye response by rapidly turning the child's head in order to induce deviation of the eye in the opposite direction. If mechanical restriction is impeding ocular motility (orbital wall fracture with ocular muscle entrapment), the ophthalmologist can perform *forced duction testing.* Following proper anesthesia, the examiner grasps the epibulbar tissues with forceps and tests the freedom of movement of the globe in various directions.

BINOCULAR ALIGNMENT

The principal methods for assessing binocular eye alignment are the cover tests and the corneal light reflex test (see Figs. 44–15 and 44–16).

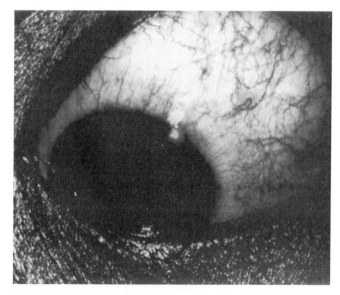

Figure 44–13. Ciliary flush associated with iritis. Note the straight, radially oriented vessels extending out from the iris. (From Reilly BM. *Practical Strategies in Outpatient Medicine,* 2nd ed. Philadelphia: WB Saunders, 1991:41.)

Table 44-17. Description of Eye Alignment and Movement

Normal Ocular Alignment: Orthophoria

Latency
  -phoria: development of abnormality only during certain conditions (fatigue, illness, cover test)
  -trophia: abnormality present during normal conditions; deviation may be constant or intermittent

Direction of Deviation
  Eso-:   inward, horizontal deviation (''crossing'')
  Exo-:   outward, horizontal deviation (''wall-eye'')
  Hyper-:   upward, vertical deviation
  Hypo-:   downward, vertical deviation
  Incyclo-: nasal torsional deviation of the superior pole of the cornea
  Excyclo-: temporal torsional deviation of the superior pole of the cornea

Equality of Deviation
  Concomitant: misalignment is equal in all positions of gaze
  Noncomitant: misalignment varies significantly in different positions of gaze

Neuromuscular Dysfunction
  Paralytic: Misalignment secondary to a cranial nerve palsy, muscle weakness, or mechanical restriction (usually
                   noncomitant)
  Nonparalytic: No underlying neuromuscular dysfunction; usually concomitant but can be noncomitant

Tandem Movements of Both Eyes
  -version: Both eyes move in same direction (conjugate); direction of movement: leve- (left); dextro- (right); supra- (up);
                infra- (down)
  -vergence: Eyes move in opposite directions (disconjugate); convergence (inward movement), divergence (outward movement)

Cover Tests

The *cover-uncover test* and the *alternate cover test* depend on the ability of each eye to fixate on a target; they can be used only when the child's vision and attention are adequate. The target should be of sufficient detail to elicit interest and to control fixation and accommodation. In infants or developmentally impaired children, the target is an attractive object (small toy).

Cover-Uncover Test. The *cover-uncover* test is used to detect heterotropia. With the child fixating on a distant target, the examiner covers one eye while observing the other eye for any movement. Each eye is covered in turn for 2 to 3 seconds. If either eye moves as the other is covered, the patient has *heterotropia*. If neither eye moves, the child may still have *heterophoria*. To determine if the child is orthophoric, the alternate cover test must be performed.

Alternate Cover Test. The patient fixates on the target while each eye is covered in turn for 2 to 3 seconds. The covering is rapidly and repeatedly shifted from eye to eye. This prevents fusion or simultaneous use of the two eyes for the duration of the test. No movement of either eye indicates orthophoria. If either eye moves to refixate on the target, the patient has a heterophoria or a heterotropia. If the cover-uncover test result is normal but the alternate cover test result is abnormal, the child has heterophoria.

The direction of movement identifies the type of *heterophoria* or *heterotropia*. If an eye drifts in nasally and then shifts temporally during fixation, the child has an esodeviation (esotropia, esophoria) (see Table 44-17). The amount of deviation can be measured by using prisms to neutralize the degree of misalignment. The ophthalmologist uses prisms of increasing power held in front of the eye during the cover test until the movement of the deviating eye is eliminated.

Corneal Light Reflex

The corneal light reflex tests (see Figs. 44-15 and 44-16) are performed when the child cannot cooperate with the cover tests. In the *Hirschberg* corneal reflex test, a source of light is directed toward the child's eyes and the position of the light's reflection is assessed. If the reflections are centered in the pupils of both eyes simultaneously, the eyes are ''straight.'' In esodeviation, the light reflections are displaced temporally; in exodeviation, the reflections are displaced nasally. Each 1 mm of displacement of the light reflection indicates approximately 7 degrees of strabismus. The degree of deviation can be measured by introducing prisms of increasing power before one or both eyes to center the reflections of light in the pupils.

In addition to the light reflex test, one must differentiate concomitant (misalignment equal in all gazes) from noncomitant strabismus; the examiner must assess binocular alignment not only in forward gaze using a distant target (primary position) but also in all other positions of gaze (looking right, left, straight up, straight down, and combinations of these—looking up and to the right). To assess the effect of accommodative convergence (near gaze), alignment is also checked with the child focusing on a detailed target (a letter, number, picture, or small toy) at ⅓ meter in front of the eyes.

SENSORY TESTS

Strabismus can interfere with the normal cortical development of visual acuity and stereopsis (three-dimensional vision). Because of the strabismus-induced diplopia, the child suppresses the image from the deviating eye. If the child alternates the fixation preference by using each eye part of the time for definitive seeing, the risk of amblyopia is low. If a fixation preference develops, however, the risk of amblyopia is great in the deviating eye through lack of normal stimulation of the macula. Because of these potential com-

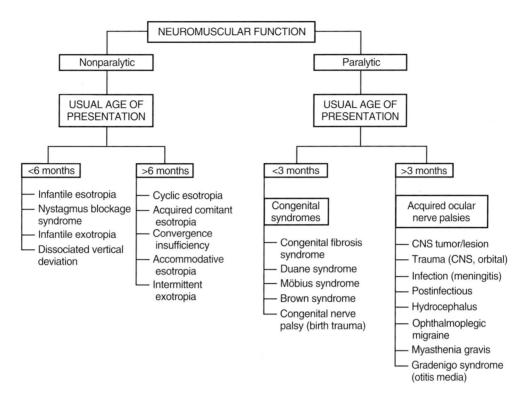

Figure 44–14. Evaluation of strabismus. CNS = central nervous system.

plications of strabismus, visual acuity, fixation patterns, and stereopsis (Titmus Fly Test, random dot stereogram) need to be assessed during the evaluation of abnormal eye movements.

Nonparalytic Strabismus

Most infants and children with strabismus have nonparalytic strabismus; there is no underlying cranial nerve palsy, muscle weakness, or mechanical restriction of eye movement. In most cases, the nonparalytic strabismus is caused by an ill-defined defect in cortical control of eye movement. In some cases, it may be caused by ocular defects, such as cataracts, lesions of the optic nerve, high refractive error, or anisometropia. On the basis of the

history and physical findings, most nonparalytic strabismus can be classified into one of the following clinically distinctive types.

INFANTILE (CONGENITAL) ESOTROPIA SYNDROME

Infantile esotropia consists of all cases of nonparalytic esotropia that present by 6 months of age. Most cases occur in the first 2 to 3 months of life. "Congenital" esotropia refers to only those cases that are truly evident at birth.

Conditions that need to be differentiated from infantile (or congenital) esotropia syndrome are the intermittent transient eye crossing that occurs in normal newborns and *pseudostrabismus.* Approx-

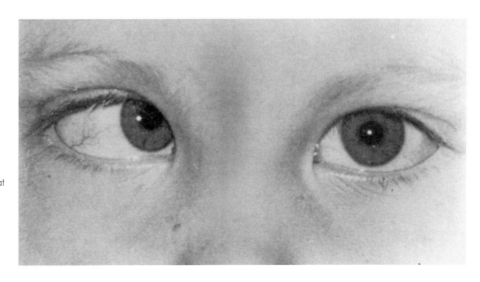

Figure 44–15. Corneal light reflex test reveals an asymmetrically placed reflex that is laterally displaced in the right eye. This indicates an inward deviation of the eye (esotropia). (From Lavrich JB, Nelson LB. Diagnosis and treatment of strabismus disorders. Pediatr Clin North Am 1993;40:739.)

imately 1% of normal neonates have transient esotropia that resolves by 6 months of age; in the infantile esotropia syndrome, the esotropia becomes worse as the infant gets older. In pseudostrabismus, the alignment is normal but the eyes have the appearance of in-turning (an optical illusion) because of the broad flat nasal bridge or prominent epicanthal folds (Fig. 44–16).

The degree of crossing may vary in the first months, but it usually develops into a large degree of esotropia by age 6 months. In some infants, a fixation preference for one eye develops, which predisposes the deviating eye to amblyopia. Fortunately, many infants cross-fixate, which reduces their risk for amblyopia. Infants who cross-fixate may appear to have bilateral sixth nerve palsies (pseudopalsy) because they do not abduct freely on looking to either side. Full abduction can be demonstrated by reflexive testing *(doll's-head maneuver)* or by covering one eye for hours or days to force the use of the other eye.

The usual treatment consists of extraocular muscle surgery. The goal is to straighten the eyes before age 2 years to allow development of the best binocular function. In most cases, surgery consists of the symmetric recession (weakening) of both medial recti. In some cases, resection strengthening of the lateral rectus muscle is performed in conjunction with recession of the medial rectus muscle. The initial operation is usually successful, with only 15% to 30% of patients requiring additional surgery. The family should be prepared for the possibility that postoperative consecutive exotropia may develop, which necessitates a second surgical procedure.

Children with infantile esotropia usually have a normal range of hyperopia and rarely need glasses prior to surgery. In infants with higher degrees of hyperopia, glasses may be needed to keep the eyes straight after surgery. Even though it is unusual, accommodative esotropia can develop in the first 6 months of life. If there is a high degree of hyperopia coupled with variable esotropia, glasses usually are tried preoperatively to treat a possible accommodative esotropia. If amblyopia is present or suspected, occlusion therapy is used as needed either before or after surgery. Other problems that may develop following the onset of infantile esotropia are dissociated vertical deviation, an ''A'' or ''V'' pattern of strabismus (described later), oblique muscle overreaction, and nystagmus.

NYSTAGMUS BLOCKAGE SYNDROME

Nystagmus blockage syndrome is characterized by early-onset esotropia in association with infantile-onset nystagmus. The nystagmus decreases when the fixating eye is adducted and increases when the fixating eye is abducted. When one eye is covered, the child exhibits compensatory posturing, which consists of turning the head toward the open eye. This posturing allows the patient to use the viewing eye in the adducted position, which results in less nystagmus. Various surgical techniques are used to correct the esotropia in infants with nystagmus blockage syndrome.

ACCOMMODATIVE ESOTROPIA

In many children, crossing of the eyes is related to activation of accommodation. Accommodative esotropia commonly occurs in children with moderate to high hyperopia; the degree of esotropia is usually relatively equal on both distant and near gaze. Accommodative esotropia may also occur in children with mild hyperopia or even myopia secondary to a high ratio of accommodative convergence to accommodation (AC:A). In such cases, the degree of esotropia is significantly greater on near gaze than on distant gaze.

Accommodative esotropia usually appears at age 2 to 3 years (range, infancy to 8 years). The crossing may begin intermittently, with gradual progression of severity, or it may develop abruptly. Parents may coincidentally attribute the onset of the esotropia to a recent illness, injury, or behavioral problem. Other symptoms associated with accommodative esotropia are squinting, covering or rubbing the eye, and turning the head to avoid diplopia.

Optical correction for the full amount of the refractive error (by cycloplegic refraction) is the principal treatment. If the accommodative esotropia is associated with mild hyperopia or myopia (high AC:A ratio), bifocal lenses are usually prescribed to control the greater degree of crossing on near gaze than on distant gaze. The bifocal lens should be large and high enough to bisect the pupil. The outcome with optical correction alone is very good, and the need for glasses usually diminishes with age. Most adolescents with proper refractive therapy for accommodative esotropia will have good binocular vision without the need for glasses; however, others may need lifelong refractive correction to maintain normal binocular alignment and optimal visual function.

During the treatment period with glasses, many parents are upset that the eyes cross whenever the spectacles are removed. The examiner should explain that this is expected until the underlying condition resolves and that it does not represent a treatment failure. In addition, children often refuse to wear the glasses, complaining they are ''too strong'' or that they make things look blurry. With time, they will adjust to the therapy.

In most cases, surgery is recommended only for residual crossing that cannot be controlled with glasses. Children with both accommodative and nonaccommodative esotropia require glasses and

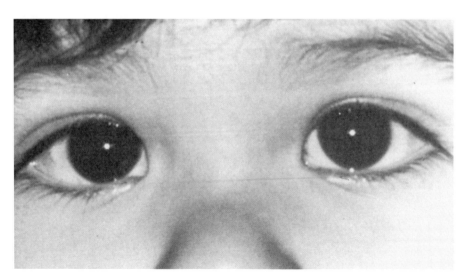

Figure 44–16. A child with pseudoesotropia. Note that the wide nasal bridge and prominent epicanthal folds create the illusion of an esotropia. The corneal light reflexes are centered in each eye; therefore the eyes are straight. (From Lavrich JB, Nelson LB. Diagnosis and treatment of strabismus disorders. Pediatr Clin North Am 1993;40:741.)

surgery. It is also possible that some patients whose accommodative esotropia was well controlled with glasses may eventually deteriorate (decompensated esotropia) and ultimately may require surgery.

Some ophthalmologists use topical miotic (constricting) eye-drops. These agents must be used cautiously because they are long-acting anticholinesterase inhibitors, depleting plasma cholinesterase (which may result in prolonged neuromuscular blockade with succinylcholine), and may cause iris cysts and cataracts.

The goals of therapy are to prevent amblyopia and to promote normal binocular vision. Nevertheless, amblyopia may develop and the child will require a period of occlusion therapy to achieve and maintain optimal visual acuity. Parents must understand that the purpose of occlusion therapy is to improve visual acuity and not to "straighten" the eyes.

CYCLIC ESOTROPIA

Cyclic esotropia is a rare type of strabismus characterized by cyclic episodes of large-angle esotropia alternating with periods of orthophoria, or small-angle esotropia. The onset is usually age 3 to 4 years (range, birth to adulthood). The cycles usually last for 24 to 48 hours, but they can persist for weeks or even years. With time, the esotropia may become constant. The etiology of cyclic esotropia is unknown, but in some cases there is a family history of strabismus.

The response to treatment varies. Glasses usually are tried first and may be effective; in many cases, surgery is curative. The usual procedure is bilateral recession of the medial recti, or unilateral recession of the medial rectus with resection of the lateral rectus of the same eye.

ACQUIRED COMITANT ESOTROPIA

Occasionally, a child will present with acute onset of a large-degree, acquired esotropia. Initially, the esotropia is intermittent, but the deviation soon becomes constant. The esotropia is nonaccommodative and nonparalytic. In some cases, the onset follows a period of occlusion of one eye (occlusion therapy, edematous eyelid, bandage from surgery). When there is no identifiable precipitating factor, the possibility of an underlying disease (tumor, trauma, infection) must be considered in all children who present with acquired, unexplained esotropia. Surgery is required to restore normal alignment.

INFANTILE EXOTROPIA

The early onset of exotropia (before age 6 months) in healthy infants is relatively rare. Infantile exotropia is a large-degree exotropia that begins intermittently and progresses rapidly to a constant deviation. Amblyopia is rare because the infants tend to alternate fixation. Conditions that need to be differentiated from infantile exotropia are the intermittent transient eye crossing of normal newborns and pseudostrabismus. Approximately 0.8% of normal neonates will have transient exotropia that resolves by 6 months of age; in infantile exotropia, the deviation becomes worse as the infant gets older. In pseudoextropia, the alignment is normal but the eyes have the illusion of out-turning because of the appearance of the face.

Treatment consists of correction of any refractive error (myopia, astigmatism, or anisometropia) and early surgical correction to straighten the eyes.

INTERMITTENT EXOTROPIA

Almost 80% of divergent strabismus in children takes the form of intermittent exotropia. The usual age of onset is 2 to 3 years (range, 6 months to 6 years). In many cases, divergent deviation is progressive, evolving through the following stages:

1. Exophoria on far gaze with orthophoria on near gaze.
2. Intermittent exotropia on far gaze with orthophoria or exophoria on near gaze.
3. Exotropia on far gaze with exotropia or intermittent exotropia on near gaze.
4. Exotropia on both far and near gaze.

The deviation is often more apparent with fatigue and illness. The child may also squint or cover one eye, especially in bright sunlight.

Treatment consists of correcting any refractive error and occlusion therapy for associated amblyopia. Surgical correction is performed if the deviation progresses to the point of interfering with the child's ability to maintain an adequate degree of binocular fusion. Surgery may be postponed if the child can maintain normal binocular alignment most of the time and if the child's condition can be monitored carefully. In most cases, bilateral recession of the lateral recti is done. In other cases, recession of the lateral rectus is done in combination with resection of the medial rectus in one or both eyes.

CONVERGENCE INSUFFICIENCY

Convergence insufficiency consists of exodeviation on near gaze or exodeviation greater on near gaze than on distant gaze. There is a subnormal near point of convergence. This convergence insufficiency during near gaze produces the following symptoms of *asthenopia*: fatigue, diplopia, headaches, tearing, and blurred vision.

The most effective therapy for improving fusion and alleviating symptoms is orthoptic treatment, which consists of convergence exercises that can be done at home. The use of base-in prisms also may be helpful. In the rare case in which orthoptic therapy and base-in prisms fail to relieve the symptoms, the medial recti may need to be resected.

"A" AND "V" PATTERNS

Children with horizontal strabismus may exhibit an A or V pattern with upward gaze. In A pattern esotropia, the degree of crossing is greater on upward gaze; in V pattern esotropia, the deviation is greater on downward gaze. The opposite is true for exotropia. For example, the A pattern exotropia produces a greater degree of divergent deviation on downward gaze; in V pattern exotropia, the deviation is greater on upward gaze. Associated with these patterns may be an overreaction of one of the oblique muscles, which produces a vertical "overshoot" of the eyes on gaze to either side. Patients with an A or V pattern strabismus may show compensatory posturing with the chin tilted up in A esotropia or V exotropia and down in V esotropia or A exotropia.

DISSOCIATED VERTICAL DEVIATION

Dissociated vertical deviation (DVD) is characterized by upward deviation of an eye when binocular fusion is interrupted. When this occurs in both eyes, the term *double dissociated vertical deviation* (DDVD) is used. DVD (or DDVD) most commonly occurs in association with infantile esotropia. DVD may also occur in patients with unilateral vision loss (cataracts, corneal scarring) occurring in infancy or early childhood. Both torticollis and manifest latent nystagmus are commonly associated with DVD. The eye deviation rarely causes diplopia; however, it is a cosmetic problem. The treatment is usually surgical.

Paralytic Strabismus

An underlying cranial nerve palsy, muscle weakness, or mechanical restriction of eye movement must be considered in every child presenting with incomitant strabismus, diplopia, or abnormal head posture. Congenital impairment of eye movement may result from birth trauma, perinatal infection, and developmental defects affecting the cranial nerves and extraocular muscles. Acquired palsies should alert the physician to the possibility of tumor, infectious processes, trauma, neuromuscular disease, and neurodegenerative illnesses. Localization of the lesion depends on careful assessment of the ocular motility (see Table 44–1) and alignment, associated signs, such as lid and pupillary abnormalities (see Fig. 44–5), proptosis, vision and fundus changes, and systemic or neurologic manifestations.

THIRD NERVE PALSY

The oculomotor nerve innervates the medial, superior, and inferior rectus muscles; the inferior oblique; the levator palpebrae and the sphincter pupillae and ciliary muscle. The principal signs of third nerve palsy are impairment of adduction, elevation and depression of the eye, ptosis of the upper eyelid, and impaired pupillary constriction and accommodation (see Fig. 44–5). The affected eye tends to deviate downward and outward.

Third nerve palsy may be either congenital or acquired. The most frequent cause of an acquired third nerve palsy in children is trauma, followed by infection (meningitis, orbital cellulitis) and tumor. Rare causes include intracranial aneurysm, ophthalmoplegic migraine (recurrent episodes of third nerve palsy with headache), and myasthenia gravis.

During recovery in some children with third nerve palsy, especially from trauma, aberrant regeneration of nerve fibers to the pupil and eyelid may develop. For example, on attempted inward or downward movement of the eye, the ptotic lid may elevate or retract and the pupil may constrict. Over time, these abnormal signs may become less apparent.

The main principles of treatment (congenital or acquired) are prevention of and therapy for amblyopia. The amblyopia may be secondary to either deprivation (ptosis) or strabismus (exotropia with *hypotropia*). Some children may also require optical correction for the accompanying defect in accommodation. Once the amblyopia has resolved and an adequate time has passed to allow for spontaneous recovery (6 to 12 months), the strabismus and ptosis can be surgically corrected. The strabismus surgery is complicated by all of the extraocular muscles involved and their corresponding force vectors. The ptosis may be corrected by slinging the upper eyelid to the frontalis muscle.

FOURTH NERVE PALSY

The fourth cranial nerve innervates only the superior oblique muscle, which causes *intorsion* (inward rotation) and depression of the eye. A fourth nerve palsy may be unilateral or bilateral and

may result in different symptoms. Most fourth nerve palsies are congenital and bilateral.

A unilateral fourth nerve palsy results in *torticollis* (the head is turned and tilted to the opposite side) and vertical strabismus when the head is straightened. The torticollis is an attempt to maintain fusion by compensating for the excyclotorsion (see Table 44–17) that results from the unopposed inferior oblique muscle. The hypertropia occurs because of the torsional action of the corresponding incycloductor (superior rectus muscle). This hyperdeviation worsens when the head is tilted to the affected side. Hence, a patient with a left fourth nerve palsy will have a right head tilt and a left hypertropia when the head is straightened.

In bilateral fourth nerve palsies, right gaze results in left hypertropia and left gaze produces right hypertropia. The head position is usually normal, because fusion is not possible secondary to bilateral excyclotorsion. Bilateral fourth nerve palsy may produce a V pattern esotropia and excyclotorsion that worsens in downward gaze. Children may adapt a chin-down position (avoiding downward gaze) in order to minimize symptoms from this pattern.

Congenital or early-onset isolated fourth nerve palsy usually becomes apparent when a child develops sufficient head control to demonstrate a head tilt. Underaction of the superior oblique muscle and overreaction of the ipsilateral inferior oblique muscle can usually be detected when the child is old enough to allow an analysis of full eye movement. The most common cause of acquired fourth nerve palsy is closed head trauma followed by postinfectious palsy and posterior fossa tumor.

Ocular torticollis must be considered in any child who presents with head tilt. Patching of one eye may help to differentiate ocular torticollis from a musculoskeletal abnormality; posture improves in patients with ocular torticollis when the affected eye is covered. Even though head tilting maintains fusion and reduces the risk for amblyopia, any associated amblyopia should be treated with occlusion therapy.

The treatment is extraocular muscle surgery. If surgery is unduly delayed, permanent musculoskeletal changes of the head and face may occur.

SIXTH NERVE PALSY

The abducent nerve innervates only the lateral rectus muscle. The sixth nerve palsy results in varying degrees of abduction deficit. Other associated signs are abducting nystagmus, esotropia increasing in gaze toward the affected lateral rectus, esotropia greater on distant gaze than on near gaze, and the face turned toward the affected muscle (which preserves binocular vision).

True congenital sixth nerve palsy is rare and should be distinguished from Duane syndrome, Möbius syndrome, and the pseudoabducent palsy (cross-fixation in babies with infantile esotropia).

Acquired sixth nerve palsy is an ominous sign that requires the immediate evaluation for brain tumors, especially brainstem glioma, and causes of increased intracranial pressure, such as hydrocephalus, head trauma, and meningitis. Other acquired causes of a sixth nerve palsy are vascular malformations, demyelinating diseases, varicella, myasthenia gravis, *Gradenigo syndrome,* and postinfectious sixth nerve palsy.

In *Gradenigo syndrome,* inflammation from otitis media, mastoiditis, or a tumor extends into the petrous bone, meninges, and inferior petrosal sinus. This edema causes entrapment of the sixth nerve against the petrosphenoidal ligament. The trigeminal and the facial nerve may also be involved. Symptoms may consist of facial pain and weakness, diplopia, weakness of the lateral rectus muscle, photophobia, lacrimation, and corneal hypoesthesia (decreased sensitivity to touch).

In benign (postinfectious) sixth nerve palsy, the muscle weakness may be secondary to the neurotropic effect of a virus. This weakness may develop either during the prodrome of a viral exanthem or 1 to 3 weeks after a viral illness. Recovery is usually complete by 12 weeks. Recurrent episodes may also occur. Before a diagnosis of benign sixth nerve palsy is made, the serious causes of acquired sixth nerve palsies must be ruled out.

Management consists of the prevention and treatment of strabismic amblyopia, followed by surgical correction of any residual esotropia. This surgery should be scheduled following the completion of the diagnostic evaluation, the treatment of the underlying cause for the acquired weakness, and the plateauing of any spontaneous recovery.

DUANE SYNDROME

Duane syndrome is a congenital disorder of eye movement caused by anomalous innervation of the horizontal rectus muscles. When the recti contract, the globe is retracted into the orbit. The disorder usually affects the left eye, is unilateral, and occurs more often in females. Duane syndrome usually occurs as an isolated finding without any genetic pattern, but it may also be inherited as an autosomal dominant condition. It may also occur with the following abnormalities and syndromes: hearing impairment, auricular malformation, syndactyly, hemivertibrae, limb malformations, *Goldenhar syndrome* (oculoauriculovertebral dysplasia), and Klippel-Feil anomaly (short neck, vertebral anomalies).

The co-contraction of the rectus muscles results in globe retraction and narrowing of the palpebral fissure during adduction. There may also be an associated esotropia or exotropia. In many cases, adduction also causes an upshoot or downshoot of the affected eye. In order to minimize diplopia (and to preserve binocular vision), often the child exhibits compensatory posturing.

Treatment primarily consists of occlusion therapy for associated amblyopia. In selected cases, surgery may be done in an effort to correct associated strabismus and to improve the head posture.

MÖBIUS SYNDROME

The characteristic features of Möbius syndrome are congenital facial diplegia and defective abduction. The child appears expressionless because of the facial palsies, which are asymmetric. Often the lower face may be spared. The abduction defect may be unilateral or bilateral. The defect is usually complete, and esotropia is common. On EMG, the facial muscles show no activity; the lateral and medial recti may show co-contraction. The *traction (forced duction) test* result is usually abnormal and probably related to fibrotic changes in the extraocular muscles. Weakness of orbicularis muscle may also result in *ectropion* (eversion of the lid margin), *epiphora* (outflow of tears), and exposure keratopathy. *Bell's phenomenon* (upward rolling of the eyes on attempted lid closure) may partially protect the eye from the development of exposure keratopathy.

Patients with Möbius syndrome may also have various musculoskeletal anomalies (e.g., dysgenesis of the limbs, syndactyly, polydactyly, pectoral defects) and neurologic problems (e.g., mental retardation, third nerve palsy [ptosis], corneal anesthesia, hearing impairment, and palatal and lingual palsy). The palatal and lingual palsy may hinder the child's abilities to eat and to protect the airway, which leads to aspiration pneumonitis.

The underlying defect in Möbius syndrome is probably agenesis of cranial nerve nuclei, primarily the sixth and seventh. This condition may be familial, but perinatal insults (trauma, illness, and use of various drugs, particularly thalidomide) have been implicated in some cases.

Treatment for the ocular problems of Möbius syndrome includes

correction of refractive errors, occlusion therapy for any associated amblyopia, and prevention of exposure keratopathy. Even though surgery can be done in an attempt to straighten the eyes, normal ocular function cannot be restored.

BROWN SYNDROME

In the child with Brown syndrome, there is restricted or absent elevation of the eye in the adducted position. This syndrome may be congenital or acquired.

Congenital Brown syndrome is caused by a developmental abnormality of the superior oblique tendon. The tendon abnormality may be a shortening or thickening, or there may be persistent connective tissue trabeculae between the tendon and the trochlea. Approximately 10% of cases are bilateral. This condition may be familial.

Acquired Brown syndrome may follow trauma or surgery of the sinus in the region of the trochlea. It may also occur with inflammatory processes, particularly sinusitis, juvenile rheumatoid arthritis, and occasionally tumor.

Other ocular signs that may occur include an associated downward deviation of the affected eye on adduction, exotropia on upward gaze (V pattern), and a widening of the palpebral fissure on adduction. To maintain binocular vision, the child may raise the chin or turn the head so that the affected eye can be brought into abduction. Parents often first notice the apparent upward overshoot of the normal eye rather than the limited upward movement of the affected eye.

The diagnosis can be confirmed by the traction (forced duction) test.

Treatment for both types consists of occlusion therapy for any associated amblyopia. Although some cases may improve with time, surgery may be helpful for the congenital disorder. Acquired inflammatory Brown syndrome may respond to treatment with corticosteroids.

CONGENITAL FIBROSIS SYNDROME

Congenital fibrosis syndrome (strabismus fixus) is a developmental abnormality of the extraocular muscles and levator palpebrae. The primary features are ptosis and external ophthalmoplegia. The limitation of ocular movement is caused by an increase in fibrotic tissue in the extraocular muscles coupled with anomalous insertions of tissue on the globe. This condition is usually bilateral but occasionally may present in a limited, unilateral form. This syndrome occurs as an isolated finding and occasionally may be familial (autosomal dominant).

Vertical movements of the eyes are affected more than horizontal movements. The eyes usually are fixed in down gaze, resulting in a compensatory chin-up posturing. Other ocular findings are nystagmoid convergence on attempted upward movement, divergence on attempted down gaze, exotropia, ptosis, myopia, and astigmatism. Amblyopia commonly occurs in congenital fibrosis syndrome. The traction (forced duction) test is abnormal.

Treatment consists primarily of occlusion therapy for associated amblyopia coupled with correction of any refractive error. Surgery can be done in an effort to improve the eye position and head posture. Because the protective Bell's phenomenon is absent, correction of the ptosis must be done cautiously because it increases the child's risk for exposure keratopathy.

THE SHAKING EYE

The conditions causing oscillating eye movements range from congenital idiopathic nystagmus to life-threatening neoplasms (Figs. 44–17 and 44–18).

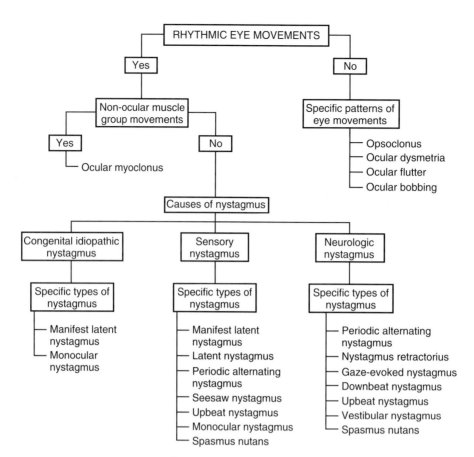

Figure 44-17. Differential diagnosis of oscillating eye movements.

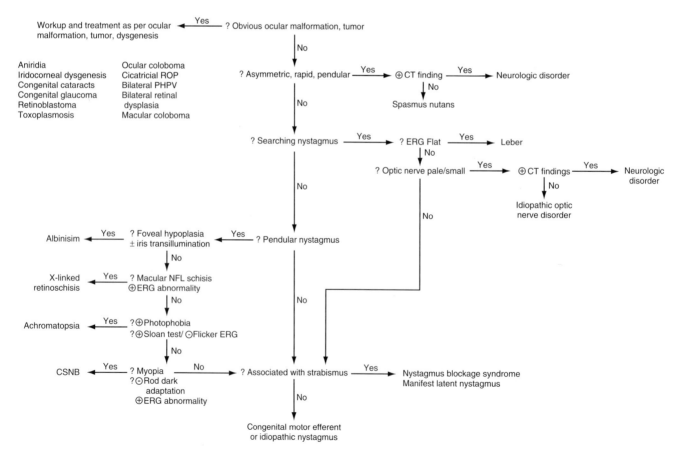

Figure 44-18. Algorithm for the work-up of an infant with nystagmus. $\oplus$ = positive; $\ominus$ = negative; ERG = electroretinogram; ROP = retinopathy of prematurity; PHPV = persistent hyperplastic primary vitreous; NFL = nerve fiber layer; CSNB = congenital stationary night blindness. (From Nelson LB, Calhoun JH, Harley RD. Pediatric Ophthalmology, 3rd ed. Philadelphia: WB Saunders, 1991:493.)

History

The clinician needs to clarify the parents' description, determine the age of onset, and ascertain whether there are any associated symptoms. Parents describe their child's abnormal ocular movements with terms such as "shaking," "shimmying," "jumping," "jiggling," "wobbling," "roving," "darting," or "dancing." Whereas all of these terms suggest the possibility of nystagmus, they could also describe other ocular disorders, such as strabismus or ocular bobbing. The clinician should determine the character, direction, and circumstances that elicit the abnormal eye movements. Abnormal eye movements occurring before 4 months of age are usually of congenital or perinatal origin; those occurring after 4 months are usually related to acquired illnesses (tumors, infection).

Additional signs and symptoms that may assist in the evaluation of oscillating eye movements are visual problems, photophobia, abnormal head movements, tinnitus, and oscillopsia. A history of vision impairment (problems with acuity, color vision, or night vision) suggests an underlying disease of the eye or visual pathways. Photophobia in a child with nystagmus may be a clue to achromatopsia (lack of color vision), albinism, aniridia (lack of iris), cataracts, or glaucoma. A description of abnormal head movements (nodding or bobbing) or abnormal posture (head tilt or face turn) suggests the possibility of congenital idiopathic nystagmus, *spasmus nutans,* and certain brain tumors. A history of vertigo, tinnitus, or hearing loss might pinpoint the cause of nystagmus to a vestibular problem (see Chapter 43). *Oscillopsia* (subjective sensation of movement of the environment) occurs in acquired rather than congenital disorders. All of these symptoms should be ascertained to determine whether the nystagmus is related to congenital, sensory, or neurologic problems.

The examiner should inquire about the child's birth history (any perinatal insults), general health and development, and the possible exposure to any prescription or over-the-counter medications, illicit drugs, or toxins. Since some of the causes of nystagmus are hereditary, a detailed family history should also be obtained.

Physical Examination

The physical examination should delineate the nature of the abnormal eye movements coupled with a detailed and focused ophthalmologic evaluation to rule out any ocular causes for these movements. In delineating the eye movements, the examiner should carefully observe the basic characteristics of the eye movements under a variety of circumstances. A hand-held magnifying glass or the magnification power of an ophthalmoscope can be used to discern fine details. Videotaping and electronystagmography (ENG) may also be used to record and analyze the abnormal eye movements.

DESCRIPTION OF EYE MOVEMENTS

Nystagmus is the repetitive rhythmic oscillations of one or both eyes. It is described on the basis of waveform, direction, amplitude, frequency, and velocity.

The two basic *waveforms* are "pendular" and "jerk." In pendular nystagmus, both phases (to and fro) of the oscillation are equal. In jerk nystagmus, one phase is faster than the other. Jerk nystagmus is described by the direction of the rapid phase. For example, in right jerk nystagmus, each cycle consists of a relatively slow movement toward the left with a more rapid movement toward the right. Pendular and jerk nystagmus can occur in both sensory and neurologic nystagmus.

The *direction* refers to the plane in which the nystagmus occurs. The plane may be horizontal, vertical, rotary (with torsional movement around the anteroposterior axis of the eye), or circumrotary (a wide-ranging combination of vertical and horizontal movements).

Amplitude is the length of eye excursion away from the fixation point. On ENG, it is measured in degrees of an arc; on physical examination, it is described as "large," "medium," or "small."

Frequency is the number of oscillations per second. Clinically, frequency is described as "high" or "low."

Velocity refers to the number of degrees the eyes move per second. Velocity is best measured by ENG. Saccades (reflecting bursts of neuronal activity that originate in brain stem nuclei) have velocities exceeding 500 degrees per second. These bursts of neuronal activity are used in refixating from one target to another. An example of saccades is the rapid-phase movements of jerk nystagmus. Pursuit movements are slower. These movements are initiated by the desire to follow a moving target or to maintain fixation on a target during movement of the head or body.

It should be noted whether the oscillations are symmetric (same waveform, frequency, amplitude, and direction) or asymmetric (dysconjugate, monocular) in both eyes. If the oscillations are intermittent, the situations that affect the movements should be recorded. Some of these are different directions of gaze, change of head position, fixation, intensity of light, sleep, and eyelid closure.

OPHTHALMOLOGIC EXAMINATION

Diseases of the eye that impede visual function are a common cause of nystagmus *(sensory nystagmus).* For example, almost 80% to 90% of children presenting with nystagmus in primary gaze within the first year of life have an underlying vision defect. In addition, oscillating eye movements by themselves can hinder visual acuity. Consequently, the examiner should perform a detailed ophthalmologic examination that concentrates on visual function, evaluation of the pupils, and general inspection of the eye along with careful ophthalmoscopy.

Vision acuity often is subnormal in the presence of abnormal eye movements. The question is whether the abnormal eye movements are due to an underlying vision defect (sensory nystagmus) or whether the vision impairment is secondary to the shaking eyes. This differentiation depends on other ocular findings, such as refractive errors, pupil abnormalities, and funduscopic findings. In some cases, special studies, such as ERG, visual evoked potential (VEP) testing, and neuroimaging (computed tomography [CT] and magnetic resonance imaging [MRI]), are required to resolve this issue.

A complete assessment of visual function should be performed, consisting of:

- Refraction
- Ascertainment of visual fields (a tumor may be affecting the visual pathways)
- Evaluation of color vision (achromatopsia)
- Dark adaptation (congenital stationary night blindness, retinitis pigmentosa)

If the eye movements vary in different positions of gaze, the acuity may vary accordingly. Acuity is usually best in the steadiest position of gaze *(null position).*

If the movements vary with gaze, acuity should be measured in each of these positions.

If the oscillations diminish or "dampen" with convergence, both near and far vision should be measured; near visual acuity may be significantly better than distance visual acuity.

High refractive errors may cause the oscillation of the eyes or may be associated with other illnesses that cause the nystagmus (Leber congenital retinal amaurosis, albinism). If the refractive error is causing the nystagmus, the abnormal movements may resolve with correction of the refractive error.

The pupil should be assessed for both structure and function. Some structural defects of the pupil and iris associated with sensory nystagmus are:

- Albinism (iris transillumination)
- Aniridia
- Coloboma
- Lisch iris nodules (an iris tumor associated with neurofibromatosis)

A subnormal response to light (afferent defect) or a paradoxical pupil response (constriction rather than dilatation in reduced light) would be evidence for an underlying disorder of the retina or optic nerve (see Fig. 44–5).

Ophthalmoscopy may reveal an abnormality of the eye itself (cataracts, hemorrhage) causing sensory nystagmus or a neurologic disease (hydrocephalus resulting in papilledema or optic atrophy) causing neurologic nystagmus. However, a normal funduscopic appearance does not always rule out significant disease. Certain retinal disorders (achromatopsia, congenital stationary night blindness) or early stages of brainstem tumors may produce nystagmus but have normal funduscopy. Electrodiagnostic tests (ERG, VEPs) and neuroimaging (CT, MRI) may be necessary to determine the cause of the nystagmus.

Nystagmus

Oscillating eye movements may be *rhythmic* (nystagmus) or *nonrhythmic*. On the basis of etiology, nystagmus may be classified as (1) congenital idiopathic, (2) sensory, or (3) neurologic. Within these general classifications are a number of special types of nystagmus (e.g., seesaw nystagmus, nystagmus retractorius) (Table 44–18; see Table 44–19 and Fig. 44–17).

CONGENITAL IDIOPATHIC NYSTAGMUS

Congenital idiopathic nystagmus (CIN) affects approximately 1 in 1000 children. This condition is often familial (autosomal dominant, autosomal recessive, or X-linked).

Typically, CIN appears within the first 3 months of life. The nystagmus may be pendular, jerk, or a combination of the two. The pendular nystagmus on forward gaze may convert to jerk nystagmus on lateral gaze. The nystagmus is usually horizontal and remains horizontal on upward and downward gaze. The amplitude is usually greatest soon after onset and diminishes over time. The patient does not experience oscillopsia. The nystagmus disappears in sleep.

The eye oscillations, along with the lack of response to the surroundings, may lead parents to believe that their baby is blind. When acuity can eventually be measured, most children with this condition have vision in the range of 20/60 to 20/200. Usually, near acuity is better than distance acuity. When one eye is occluded or subjected to reduced illumination, the nystagmus often worsens (manifest latent nystagmus). This may adversely affect acuity during monocular testing.

To compensate, the child may either tilt or shake the head. About 30% of patients with CIN have a *null point,* a position of gaze in which the nystagmus decreases and the vision improves. To maintain this position of gaze, patients with a null point often exhibit compensatory posturing. They turn the head or face away from the preferred position of gaze to bring the eyes and the null point toward the midline. Abnormal head shaking may dampen the effect of the nystagmus. The direction and rate of the head shaking often differ from those of the eye movement.

The actual defect in CIN is unknown, but there is evidence supporting a possible defect in the complex mechanism for maintaining steady fixation. Eye movement recordings on ENG in patients with CIN show that the eyes deviate from the target in an accelerating slow-phase movement and return to the fixation point with a fast-phase (jerk) movement. These patients also have abnormalities in response to optokinetic stimulation. Normally, to follow

Table 44–18. Specific Patterns of Nystagmus

Pattern	Description	Associated Conditions
Latent nystagmus	Conjugate jerk nystagmus toward viewing eye	Congenital vision defects, occurs with occlusion of eye
Manifest latent nystagmus	Fast jerk to viewing eye	Strabismus, congenital idiopathic nystagmus
Periodic alternating	Cycles of horizontal or horizontal-rotary that change direction	Caused by both visual and neurologic conditions
Seesaw nystagmus	One eye rises and intorts as other eye falls and extorts	Usually associated with optic chiasm defects
Nystagmus retractorius	Eyes jerk back into orbit or toward each other	Caused by pressure on mesencephalic tegmentum (Parinaud syndrome)
Gaze-evoked nystagmus	Jerk nystagmus in direction of gaze	Caused by medications, brainstem lesion, or labyrinthine dysfunction
Gaze-paretic nystagmus	Eyes jerk back to maintain eccentric gaze	Cerebellar disease
Downbeat nystagmus	Fast phase beating downward	Posterior fossa disease, drugs
Upbeat nystagmus	Fast phase beating upward	Brainstem and cerebellar disease, and some visual conditions
Vestibular nystagmus	Horizontal-torsional or horizontal jerks	Vestibular system dysfunction
Asymmetric or monocular nystagmus	Pendular vertical nystagmus	Disease of retina and visual pathways
Spasmus nutans	Fine, rapid, pendular nystagmus	Torticollis, head nodding; idiopathic or gliomas of visual pathways

a rotating target or to fixate on a target during movement of the head or body, there is a slow pursuit movement of the eyes in the direction of the target, followed by a rapid return or refixation movement. This physiologic response is referred to as *optokinetic nystagmus* ("railroad nystagmus"). In patients with congenital idiopathic nystagmus, there may be reversal of this response, with the fast phase occurring in the direction of the movement of the target. In some patients, the gaze may be abnormal during optokinetic stimulation, with the eye movements being greater or less than the target movements.

The evaluation of a child with CIN begins with a thorough examination to rule out underlying ocular or neurologic disease. Although the clinical picture of CIN is distinctive, electrophysiologic and neuroimaging studies are often necessary to confirm the diagnosis and to rule out the potentially life-threatening causes of nystagmus, such as tumors.

Treatment of congenital idiopathic nystagmus consists of early optical correction of any significant refractive error (including astigmatism), reduction of nystagmus through induced convergence, and normalization of head position with improved utilization of the null point through prisms or surgery. Bilateral *base-out prisms,* sometimes in conjunction with concave (minus) lenses, can be used to induce convergence in an effort to dampen the nystagmus and improve the acuity. Prismatic spectacles are thick and heavy and are not well accepted by patients. In patients with a null point, prismatic spectacles may also be used with the base of the prism over each eye directed away from the null point ("yoke" prisms) to improve head posture. In patients who cannot tolerate prismatic spectacles, eye muscle surgery may shift the null point toward the midline and thus improve the head posture. If the null point is toward the left, the following surgery would be done: recession (weakening) of the left lateral and right medial rectus muscles and resection (strengthening) of the right lateral and left medial rectus muscles.

SENSORY NYSTAGMUS

Sensory nystagmus is caused by a vision deficit due to an abnormality of the eye or visual pathways. Sensory nystagmus is the most common cause of nystagmus in infants and accounts for almost 80% to 90% of cases in which nystagmus occurs in primary gaze.

In infants with bilateral congenital or perinatal vision defects, nystagmus often develops within the first 3 to 4 months of life. The nystagmus may be pendular or jerk, and the direction may be horizontal, vertical, or rotary. Some infants exhibit roving eye movements (multidirectional, large-amplitude, and low-frequency). Similar eye movements may be seen in children who become blind later within the first few years of life. Abnormal eye movements usually are less common in children with cortical vision loss than in those with ocular or anterior visual pathway disease.

Many causes of congenital or early-onset sensory nystagmus will be readily apparent on examination of the eye. Some of these conditions are ocular colobomata and microphthalmia, anterior segment dysgenesis and glaucoma, aniridia, cataracts, optic nerve hypoplasia, albinism, and chorioretinitis. In some conditions, the diagnosis may not be obvious on ophthalmoscopic examination (achromatopsia, congenital stationary night blindness, and Leber congenital retinal amaurosis). Even though associated signs (photophobia, paradoxical pupil, refractive error) may provide clues to their diagnosis, the definitive diagnosis often depends on electrophysiologic studies.

Tumors affecting the visual pathway, such as gliomas of the optic nerves or chiasm and hypothalamus, and craniopharyngiomas, are a major cause of sensory nystagmus in children. The possibility of tumor must always be kept in mind, even when funduscopic findings (papilledema, optic atrophy) are not evident. Neuroimaging is always warranted in infants and children with unexplained vision loss and nystagmus.

NEUROLOGIC NYSTAGMUS

A variety of congenital and acquired disorders of the nervous system may cause nystagmus in infants and children. Examples of conditions that may cause neurologic nystagmus include:

- Infections (meningitis, encephalitis, brain abscess)
- Trauma
- Encephalopathy (hypoxia, toxic)
- Intracranial tumors and vascular lesions
- Hydrocephalus
- Demyelinating neurodegenerative diseases (multiple sclerosis)
- Metabolic disorders (e.g., sphingolipidoses)
- Neurodevelopmental syndromes

In some conditions, there may be a combination of sensory and neurologic problems that is causing the nystagmus.

SPECIAL TYPES OF NYSTAGMUS

Some types of nystagmus are clinically distinctive. Many have important diagnostic implications (see Table 44–18).

Latent and Manifest Nystagmus. *Latent nystagmus* is a conjugate jerk nystagmus that develops when one eye is occluded or subjected to reduced light. This form of nystagmus does not occur under binocular viewing conditions. The initiating slow phase is of decelerating velocity with the fast jerk toward the viewing eye. Latent nystagmus is commonly associated with congenital vision defects, amblyopia, and strabismus.

Manifest latent nystagmus is present when both eyes are open but when only one eye is being used for vision (suppression of the other eye). The initiating slow phase is of a decreasing velocity with the fast jerk toward the viewing eye. Manifest latent nystagmus usually occurs in association with strabismus (especially esotropia, exotropia, and sometimes hypertropia). There may also be coexistent congenital idiopathic nystagmus.

Periodic Alternating Nystagmus. In this form of nystagmus, there are repetitive cycles of horizontal or horizontal rotary nystagmus that periodically change direction. The cycle begins with jerking of the eyes to one side for a few minutes, followed by a quiet interlude of seconds. After the quiescent period, the eyes then beat (jerk) to the other side for a period of minutes. The cycle repeats itself over and over again. During the height of the oscillations, there is oscillopsia and decreased visual acuity. This form of nystagmus may be associated with congenital or acquired illnesses, such as vision defects, albinism, head trauma (cerebral concussion, basal skull fracture), vascular lesions, encephalitis, multiple sclerosis, cerebellar disease, posterior fossa tumors, craniocervical junction lesions, and anti-epileptic drugs.

Seesaw Nystagmus. The seesaw form is a rare variant of dissociated nystagmus characterized by reciprocal vertical movements. As one eye rises and intorts, the other eye falls and extorts. The etiology is unclear. It is usually associated with lesions of the optic chiasm and bitemporal hemianopsia; in children it may be a sign of suprasellar tumors, particularly gliomas or craniopharyngioma.

Seesaw nystagmus has been reported in septo-optic dysplasia, albinism, and head trauma. A congenital form has been reported that is not associated with either ocular or neurologic abnormalities.

Nystagmus Retractorius. Nystagmus retractorius, or *convergence-retraction nystagmus,* is characterized by repetitive jerking of the eyes into the orbit or toward each other. It is usually seen in association with vertical gaze palsy secondary to pressure on the mesencephalic tegmentum (Parinaud syndrome, sylvian aqueduct syndrome). The etiology may be a central nervous system lesion, such as a neoplasm (pineal tumor) or a vascular or inflammatory condition.

Gaze-Evoked Nystagmus. The fast phase is always in the direction of the gaze (right beating on right gaze; up beating on upward gaze). The most common cause is sedative or anticonvulsive medication. Brainstem or labyrinthine dysfunction may also cause this condition.

A subtype of gaze-evoked nystagmus, called *gaze-paretic nystagmus,* indicates difficulty in maintaining eccentric gaze. As the eyes drift from the eccentric position, they then jerk back (corrective saccade) into the proper position. Gaze-paretic nystagmus is seen primarily with cerebellar disease.

Downbeat Nystagmus. Downbeat nystagmus occurs in the primary gaze position with the fast phase beating downward. This form of nystagmus is at maximal intensity when the eyes are deviated laterally and slightly below the horizontal position rather than on extreme downward gaze; it may also be intermittent. Downbeat nystagmus is usually associated with lesions in the posterior fossa near the craniocervical junction. In children, it is usually a sign of Arnold-Chiari malformation. Other causes include spinocerebellar degeneration, hydrocephalus, the toxic effects of certain drugs (anticonvulsants), alcohol, vitamin B_{12} deficiency, and brainstem encephalitis.

Upbeat Nystagmus. Upbeat nystagmus occurs in the primary gaze position with the fast phase beating upward. It is usually associated with masses in the fourth ventricle and lesions of the brainstem and cerebellar vermis. In rare instances, it may occur during drug intoxication, organophosphate poisoning, meningitis, or multiple sclerosis. It may also be seen in children with Leber congenital retinal amaurosis, although in time the upjerking nystagmus may change to the more typical horizontal nystagmus that is associated with vision impairment. Even though the nystagmus in congenital idiopathic nystagmus is usually horizontal, it may occasionally be upbeating.

Vestibular Nystagmus. Vestibular nystagmus (see Chapter 43) is a horizontal-torsional or purely horizontal jerk nystagmus that is due to dysfunction of the vestibular system (end-organ, nerve, or nuclear complex). The intensity of the nystagmus increases on gaze toward the direction of the fast phase and decreases on gaze in the direction of the slow phase. Vertigo is usually associated with the nystagmus. End-organ causes include labyrinthitis, Ménière syndrome, vascular disease, and trauma. Nuclear causes include brainstem lesions (tumors, demyelinating disease).

The COWS (*cold-opposite, warm-same*) mnemonic is helpful in localizing the side of the lesion. In normal subjects, stimulating an ear with cold water produces nystagmus that beats in the opposite (cold-opposite) direction, whereas stimulating an ear with warm water produces nystagmus that beats toward the same (warm-same) side. Destructive lesions (tumors) produce signs mimicking the effects of cold water irrigation; irritative lesions (inflammation) produce signs mimicking the effects of warm water irrigation.

Monocular (Asymmetric) Nystagmus. Children with uniocular vision loss of early onset (cicatricial retinopathy of prematurity, longstanding vitreous hemorrhage, dense amblyopia) may have monocular nystagmus. It is often a pendular vertical nystagmus of small amplitude, with low velocity and low frequency. Asymmetric nystagmus also may be seen with certain visual sensory disorders, such as rod and cone dystrophies. Optic pathway gliomas may present with asymmetric or purely monocular nystagmus that may occur alone or in association with other features of *spasmus nutans.* Rarely is congenital idiopathic nystagmus monocular or asymmetric.

Spasmus Nutans. Spasmus nutans consists of nystagmus, head nodding, and torticollis. These three signs may occur together or in various combinations. The nystagmus is very fine, rapid, and pendular. It is usually bilateral, asymmetric and horizontal, but it may also be vertical. The head nodding tends to be oblique and is usually slower than the nystagmus.

Spasmus nutans is usually a benign, self-limited condition that presents within the first year of life and resolves without sequelae by 3 years of age. Its etiology is unknown. Similar signs may occur in children with brain tumors, particularly gliomas of the anterior visual pathways and hypothalamus. Even when the clinical picture suggests "typical" spasmus nutans, neuroimaging studies would be prudent in children presenting with asymmetric or monocular nystagmus to rule out a central nervous system neoplasm.

Other Abnormal Eye Movements

Not all oscillating eye movements are nystagmus. Some abnormal eye movements are either nonrhythmic or associated with contractions of other muscle groups. These movements are important because they follow clinically distinct patterns that have important diagnostic implications (Table 44–19).

OPSOCLONUS

Opsoclonus is nonrhythmic, chaotic, multidirectional conjugate movements of varying amplitude and rate. The eyes appear to flit around in unpredictable repetitive bursts of activity. The movements often are aggravated by attempted fixation or refixation. Opsoclonus usually persists in sleep and can be detected even when the eyelids are closed.

The onset of opsoclonus usually is sudden, and most cases occur in early childhood. It is associated with hydrocephalus as well as diseases of the cerebellum and brainstem. The most common cause is encephalitis (coxsackievirus B, St. Louis encephalitis, varicella, mumps, and poliomyelitis). There may be associated myoclonus and trunk and limb ataxia. Opsoclonus may be the presenting manifestation of *neuroblastoma.* How this tumor causes opsoclonus is unknown (possible cross-reacting antibody to the tumor and nervous tissue); the abnormal eye movements cease when the tumor is treated.

OCULAR DYSMETRIA

Ocular dysmetria is pathologic hypermetria (overshoot) of the eyes on rapid refixation from one position to another. The over-

Table 44–19. Specific Patterns of Non-nystagmus Eye Movements

Pattern	Description	Associated Conditions
Opsoclonus	Multidirectional conjugate movements of varying rate and amplitude	Hydrocephalus, diseases of brainstem and cerebellum, neuroblastoma
Ocular dysmetria	Overshoot of eyes on rapid fixation	Cerebellar dysfunction
Ocular flutter	Horizontal oscillations with forward gaze and sometimes with blinking	Cerebellar disease, hydrocephalus, or central nervous system neoplasm
Ocular bobbing	Downward jerk from primary gaze, remain for a few seconds, then drift back	Pontine disease
Ocular myoclonus	Rhythmic to-and-fro pendular oscillations of the eyes, with synchronous non-ocular muscle movement	Damage to red nucleus, inferior olivary nucleus, and ipsilateral dentate nucleus

shoot is followed by oscillations of decreasing amplitude until the eyes come to rest and accurate fixation is attained. These abnormal eye movements are best seen on refixation from lateral gaze back to the primary position. Ocular dysmetria indicates cerebellar dysfunction and may occur with tumors, vascular lesions, or degenerative disease.

OCULAR FLUTTER

Ocular flutter consists of intermittent horizontal oscillation of the eyes of only a few seconds in duration. These oscillations occur spontaneously on forward gaze and occasionally on blinking. Flutter represents a disturbance of the pause cells in the pontine paramedian reticular formation. Flutter and opsoclonus represent a continuum of ocular motor instability.

Flutter may occur in patients with acute cerebellar disease or in patients with hydrocephalus. Like opsoclonus, it also may occur as a paraneoplastic phenomenon.

OCULAR BOBBING

In ocular bobbing, the eyes repeatedly jerk downward from the primary position, remain for a few seconds, and then slowly drift back to midposition. The downward jerks may be dysconjugate. Ocular bobbing occurs in gravely ill, stuporous or comatose patients with extensive disease of the pons. In adults, it is associated with pontine infarction or hemorrhage. It has also been reported in association with pontine tumors in childhood.

OCULAR MYOCLONUS

Ocular myoclonus consists of continuous, rhythmic to-and-fro pendular oscillation of the eyes, usually in the vertical plane. The eye movements occur in association with synchronous, rhythmic movement of non-ocular muscles. The non-ocular muscles most frequently involved are those of the soft palate, tongue, face, pharynx, larynx, and diaphragm. Myoclonus usually indicates damage in the triangle formed by the ipsilateral red nucleus, inferior olivary nucleus, and contralateral dentate nucleus of the cerebellum and their interconnecting fiber tracts.

SUMMARY AND RED FLAGS

Ocular manifestations of vision loss, strabismus, and nystagmus may be due to local ocular pathology or to significant neurologic disease. Impaired visual function in one eye due to strabismus, cataracts, or other conditions early in life may produce irreversible amblyopia. *Red flags* are discussed in Tables 44–5 and 44–6 and throughout the chapter.

REFERENCES

Refraction

Gordon RA, Donzis PB. Refractive development of the human eye. Arch Ophthalmol 1985;103:785.
Mäntyjärvi MI. Changes of refraction in schoolchildren. Arch Ophthalmol 1985;103:790.
Sturner RA, Green JA, Funk S, et al. A developmental approach to preschool vision screening. J Pediatr Ophthalmol Strabismus 1981;18:61.
Teller DY, McDonald MA, Preston K, et al. Assessment of visual acuity in infants and children: The acuity card procedure. Dev Med Child Neurol 1986;28:779.

Amblyopia

Flynn JT, Cassady JC. Current trends in amblyopia therapy. Ophthalmology 1978;85:428.
Jastrzebski G, Hoyt CS, Marg E. Stimulus deprivation amblyopia in children: Sensitivity, plasticity, and elasticity (SPE). Arch Ophthalmol 1984;102:1030.
Kushner BJ. Functional amblyopia associated with organic ocular lesions. Am J Ophthalmol 1981;91:39.
Smith KH, Baker DB, Keech RV, et al. Monocular congenital cataracts: Psychological effects of treatment. J Pediatr Ophthalmol Strabismus 1991;28:245.
Tommila V, Tarkkanen A. Incidence of loss of vision in the healthy eye in amblyopia. Br J Ophthalmol 1981;65:575.
Von Noorden GK. A reassessment of infantile esotropia: XLIV Edward Jackson Memorial Lecture. Am J Ophthalmol 1988;105:1.

Organic Vision Disorders

Bardelli AM, Hadjistilianou T. Congenital glaucoma associated with other abnormalities in 150 cases. Glaucoma 1987;9:10.

Barsoum-Homsy M, Chevrette L. Incidence and prognosis of childhood glaucoma: A study of 63 cases. Ophthalmology 1986;93:1323.

Beck RW: The optic neuritis treatment trial. Arch Ophthalmol 1988; 106:1051.

Biglan AW, Brown DR, Reynolds JD, et al. Risk factors associated with retrolental fibroplasia. Ophthalmology 1984;91:1504.

Birch EE, Stager DR. Prevalence of good visual acuity following surgery for congenital unilateral cataract. Arch Ophthalmol 1988;106:40.

Boger WP III, Walton DS. Timolol in uncontrolled childhood glaucomas. Ophthalmology 1981;88:253.

Burns RP, Lourien EW, Cibis AB. Juvenile sex-linked retinoschisis: Clinical and genetic studies. Trans Am Acad Ophthalmol Otolaryngol 1971;75:1011.

Chang M, McLean IW, Merritt JC. Coats' disease: A study of 62 histologically confirmed cases. J Pediatr Ophthalmol Strabismus 1984;21:163.

Cross HE, Jensen AD. Ocular manifestations in the Marfan syndrome and homocystinuria. Am J Ophthalmol 1973;75:405.

CRYO-ROP group: Multicenter trial of cryotherapy for retinopathy of prematurity: Three month outcome. Arch Ophthalmol 1990;108:195.

Flickinger JC, Torres C, Deutsch M. Management of low-grade gliomas of the optic nerve and chiasm. Cancer 1988;61:635.

Francois J. Differential diagnosis of leukocoria in children. Ann Ophthalmol 1978;10:1375.

Frank JW, Kushner BJ, France TD. Paradoxic pupillary phenomenon: A review of patients with pupillary constriction to darkness. Arch Ophthalmol 1988;106:1564.

Gelbart SS, Hoyt CS, Jastrebski G, et al. Long-term visual results in bilateral congenital cataracts. Am J Ophthalmol 1982;93:615.

Hayreh SS. Optic disc edema in raised intracranial pressure: VI. Associated visual disturbances and their pathogenesis. Arch Ophthalmol 1977; 95:1566.

Hing S, Speedwell L, Taylor D. Lens surgery in infancy and childhood. Br J Ophthalmol 1990;74:73.

Hoyt CS. Autosomal dominant optic atrophy: A spectrum of disability. Ophthalmology 1980;87:245.

Juan Verdaguer T. Juvenile retinal detachment. Am J Ophthalmol 1982;93:145.

Kline R, Klein BEK, Moss SE, et al. The Wisconsin epidemiologic study of diabetic retinopathy: II. Prevalence and risk of diabetic retinopathy when age at diagnosis is less than 30 years. Arch Ophthalmol 1984; 102:520.

Kohn BA. The differential diagnosis of cataracts in infancy and childhood. Am J Dis Child 1976;130:184.

Lessell S, Rosman P. Juvenile diabetes mellitus and optic atrophy. Arch Neurol 1977;34:759.

Listernick R, Charrow J, Greenwald MJ, et al. Optic gliomas in children with neurofibromatosis type I. J Pediatr 1989;114:788.

McPherson SD Jr, Berry DP. Goniotomy vs external trabeculotomy for developmental glaucoma. Am J Ophthalmol 1983;95:427.

Nyboer JH, Robertson DM, Gomez MR. Retinal lesions in tuberous sclerosis. Arch Ophthalmol 1976;94:1277.

Packer RJ, Sutton LN, Bilaniuk LT, et al. Treatment of chiasmatic/hypothalamic gliomas of childhood with chemotherapy: An update. Ann Neurol 1988;23:79.

Pike MG, Jan JE, Wong PK. Neurological and developmental findings in children with cataracts. Am J Dis Child 1989;143:706.

Pruett RC, Schepens C. Posterior hyperplastic primary vitreous. Am J Ophthalmol 1970;69:535.

Repka MX, Miller NR. Optic atrophy in children. Am J Ophthalmol 1988;106:191.

Seidman DL, Nelson LB, Calhoun JH, et al. Signs and symptoms in the presentation of primary infantile glaucomas. Pediatrics 1986;77:399.

Shields JA, Augsburger JJ. Current approaches to the diagnosis and management of retinoblastoma. Surv Ophthalmol 1981;25:347.

Topilow HW, Ackerman AL, Wang FM. The treatment of advanced retinopathy of prematurity by cryotherapy and scleral buckling surgery. Ophthalmology 1985;92:379.

Weiss AH, Beck RW. Neuroretinitis in childhood. J Pediatr Ophthalmol Strabismus 1989;26:198.

Strabismus

Archer SM, Sondhi N, Helveston EM. Strabismus in infancy. Ophthalmology 1989;96:133.

Baker JD, Parks MM. Early-onset accommodative esotropia. Am J Ophthalmol 1980;90:11.

Harley RD. Paralytic strabismus in children: Etiologic incidence and management of the third, fourth and sixth nerve palsies. Ophthalmology 1980;87:24.

Harley RD, Rodrigues MM, Crawford JS. Congenital fibrosis of the extraocular muscles. J Pediatr Ophthalmol Strabismus 1978;15:346.

Hiatt RL. Medical management of accommodative esotropia. J Pediatr Ophthalmol Strabismus 1983;20:199.

Ing M. Early surgical alignment for congenital esotropia. Ophthalmology 1983;90:132.

Kalpakian B, Choy AE, Sparkes RS. Duane syndrome associated with features of the cat-eye syndrome and mosaicism for a supernumerary chromosome probably derived from number 22. J Pediatr Ophthalmol Strabismus 1988;25:293.

Katz NNK, Whitmore PV, Beauchamp GR. Brown's syndrome in twins. J Pediatr Ophthalmol Strabismus 1981;18:32.

Kornder LD, Nursey JN, Pratt-Johnson JA, et al. Detection of manifest strabismus in young children: 1. A prospective study. Am J Ophthalmol 1974;77:207.

Kornder LD, Nursey JN, Pratt-Johnson JA, et al. Detection of manifest strabismus in young children: 2. A retrospective study. Am J Ophthalmol 1974;77:211.

Magoon EH. Botulinum toxin chemo-denervation for strabismus in infants and children. J Pediatr Ophthalmol Strabismus 1984;21:110.

Richard JM, Parks M. Intermittent exotropia: Surgical results in different age groups. Ophthalmology 1983;90:1172.

Nystagmus

Antony JH, Ouvrier RA, Wise G. Spasmus nutans: A mistaken identity. Arch Neurol 1980;37:373.

Kushner BJ. Ocular causes of abnormal head postures. Ophthalmology 1979;86:2115.

Miller MT, Ray V, Owens P, et al. Möbius and Möbius-like syndromes (TTV-OFM, OMLH). J Pediatr Ophthalmol Strabismus 1989;26:176.

Scott WE, Kraft SP. Surgical treatment of compensatory head position in congenital nystagmus. J Pediatr Ophthalmol Strabismus 1984;21:85.

Shetty T, Rosman NP. Opsoclonus in hydrocephalus. Arch Ophthalmol 1972;88:585.

Smith JL, Walsh FB. Opsoclonus-ataxic conjugate movements of the eye. Arch Ophthalmol 1960;64:244.

Smith JL, Zieper I, Gay AJ, et al. Nystagmus retractorius. Arch Ophthalmol 1959;62:864.

Orthopedic Disorders

45 Arthritis

Arthur J. Newman

Disorders of joint functions may be due to, result in, or be associated with abnormalities of muscles, tendons, fascia, nerves, blood vessels (as in vasculitis, vaso-occlusion), and skin, as well as the joints (e.g., synovium, cartilage, bone) themselves (Fig. 45–1). Arthralgia and myalgia without demonstrable pathology may also cause symptoms of musculoskeletal malfunction. Many of these illnesses are generally referred to as musculoskeletal diseases, rheumatic diseases, connective tissue diseases, or immune disorders (Table 45–1). All organ systems may be involved, but at some time, arthritis is present in most cases; arthritis may represent a minor annoyance in a major illness (e.g., rheumatic fever, leukemia, or systemic lupus erythematosus [SLE]).

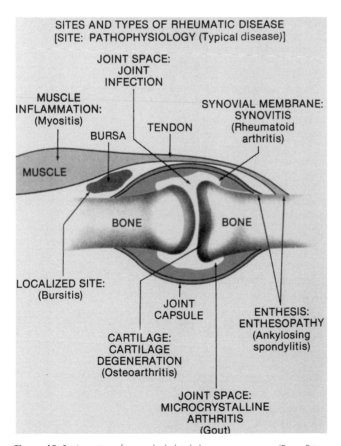

Figure 45–1. Location of musculoskeletal disease processes. (From Fries JF. Approach to the patient with musculoskeletal disease. In Wyngaarden JB, Smith LH, Bennett JC [eds]. Cecil Textbook of Medicine, 19th ed. Philadelphia: WB Saunders, 1992:1488.)

Arthritis can be defined as swelling, tenderness, heat, and limitation of motion of a joint. It may be associated with varying severity of pain, non-use, or misuse. There are more than a hundred illnesses in which arthritis or arthralgia may play a role (Tables 45–1, 45–2, and 45–3). An etiologic explanation is available for bacterial or viral arthritis; only hypotheses exist to explain the pathophysiology of the other types. Diagnostic tests often yield nonspecific findings. The diagnosis of most of these connective tissue diseases is made by obtaining a comprehensive history, performing a thorough physical examination, and obtaining laboratory values to support the more likely possibilities. Occasionally, diagnostic criteria (SLE, Kawasaki disease, rheumatic fever) aid in the diagnosis.

Many rheumatic diseases tend to evolve slowly, and many years may separate a patient's first symptom, perhaps thrombocytopenia, from a disease that can subsequently be identified as SLE. Even when a diagnosis is made, the illness may subsequently involve organs not overtly affected at the time of diagnosis. The changeable aspect of rheumatologic diseases frustrates patients, families, and physicians. There is often a significant delay in diagnosis. Relapses and remissions occur without obvious cause, rendering evaluation of therapy and prognosis difficult. The physician caring for a child with a chronic illness must encourage the family to allow youngsters to develop independently and to accomplish tasks for themselves.

HISTORY

One or two sentences, preferably in the patient's or parent's words, will point out what the family wants remedied. The physician must always keep in mind that "fixing" is what the family wants. A diagnosis is desirable, but only secondary to restoration of function. A diagnosis may not be made with certainty at presentation, but a subsequent visit or visits may permit the physician to resolve this indecision.

The examiner of sports-minded older children or adolescents frequently encounters patients who minimize and even deny complaints and are at odds with the parent's estimation of the severity of their symptoms. Children may be stoic and may be unwilling to face ridicule and ostracism by classmates with whom they need to appear equal. Conversely, a small percentage of children, particularly those who have functional disorders, will exaggerate their symptoms. Despite the absence of positive physical findings or laboratory studies corroborative of their complaints, such children maintain that they have extremely severe pain and that they are disabled. They have often convinced their parents of their infirmity, and the family is unwilling to discard an organic illness in favor of one that is emotionally based.

Young children cannot offer a satisfactory history. The first

Table 45–1. Diagnostic Classification of Juvenile Arthritis and Pediatric Rheumatic Diseases

Connective Tissue Diseases
Juvenile rheumatoid arthritis
Systemic lupus erythematosus
Scleroderma
Dermatomyositis
Necrotizing vasculitis
  Polyarteritis (includes Kawasaki disease)
  Hypersensitivity vasculitis (includes Henoch-Schönlein
    purpura and serum sickness)
  Wegener granulomatosis
  Giant cell arteritis
  Behçet disease
  Miscellaneous
Mixed connective tissue disease and overlap syndromes
Eosinophilic fasciitis
Sjögren syndrome

Seronegative Spondyloarthropathies
Juvenile ankylosing spondylitis
Inflammatory bowel disease
  Crohn disease
  Ulcerative colitis
Psoriatic spondyloarthritis
Reiter syndrome

Degenerative Joint Disease

**Arthritis, Tenosynovitis, and Bursitis Associated with
  Infectious Agents**
Direct
  Bacterial arthritis
    Gram-positive cocci (*Staphylococcus* species and others)
    Gram-negative cocci (gonococcus and others)
    Gram-positive rods
    Mycobacteria
  Viral arthritis (rubella, mumps, parvovirus, Epstein-Barr
    virus)
  Fungal arthritis
  Lyme arthritis
  Toxic synovitis of the hip
  Whipple disease
Indirect (reactive arthritis)
  Bacterial (includes acute rheumatic fever, intestinal bypass,
    postdysenteric *Shigella, Yersinia* species, post-
    meningococcal or *Haemophilus influenzae* immune
    complexes)
  Viral (hepatitis B)

Rheumatic Diseases Associated with Immunodeficiency
Selective IgA deficiency
Agammaglobulinemia and hypogammaglobulinemia
Complement component deficiencies

**Metabolic and Endocrine Diseases Associated with Rheumatic
  States**
Crystal-induced arthritis (gout, pseudogout, chondrocalcinosis)
Biochemical abnormalities
  Amyloidosis (includes familial Mediterranean fever)
  Vitamin C deficiency (scurvy)
  Specific enzyme deficiency states (including Fabry disease,
    Farber disease, alkaptonuria, Lesch-Nyhan syndrome)
  Hyperlipidemias (types II, IV)
  Mucopolysaccharidoses
  Hemoglobinopathies (sickle cell anemia, thalassemia)
  Hemophilia
  Connective tissue disorders (Ehlers-Danlos syndrome,
    Marfan syndrome, pseudoxanthoma elasticum,
    and others)

Endocrine diseases
  Diabetes mellitus
  Acromegaly
  Hyperparathyroidism
  Thyroid disease (hyperthyroidism, hypothyroidism)
Other hereditary or congenital disorders
  Arthrogryposis multiplex congenita
  Hypermobility syndromes
  Myositis ossificans progressiva

Neoplasms
Malignant
  Primary (e.g., synovioma, synoviosarcoma)
  Metastatic (osteosarcoma)
Benign
  Osteoid osteoma
Diffuse
  Leukemia and lymphoma
  Neuroblastoma
  Histiocytosis

Neuropathic Disorders
Charcot joints
Compression neuropathies
Reflex sympathetic dystrophy

**Bone and Cartilage Disorders Associated with Articular
  Manifestations**
Osteoporosis
  Generalized
  Localized (regional)
Osteomalacia
Hypertrophic osteoarthropathy
Avascular necrosis (includes Legg-Calvé-Perthes disease)
Osteochondritis dissecans
Congenital dysplasia of the hip
Slipped capital femoral epiphysis
Costochondritis (includes Tietze syndrome)
Osteolysis and chondrolysis

Nonarticular Rheumatism
Myofascial pain syndromes
  Generalized (fibromyalgia)
  Regional
Low back pain and intervertebral disc disorders
Tendinitis (tenosynovitis) or bursitis
Ganglion cysts
Fasciitis
Ganglion cysts
Chronic ligament and muscle strain
Vasomotor disorders
  Erythromelalgia
  Raynaud phenomenon

Miscellaneous Disorders
Trauma (the result of direct trauma)
Plant-thorn synovitis
Pancreatic disease
Sarcoidosis
Villonodular synovitis
Internal derangement of joints (includes chondromalacia
  patellae, loose bodies)

Arthromyalgia
Growing pains
Psychogenic rheumatism

Table 45–2. Differential Diagnosis of Monarticular Arthritis

Usually Monarticular	Often Polyarticular
Common	
Septic arthritis	Rheumatoid arthritis
Bacterial	Psoriatic arthritis
Tuberculous	Reiter syndrome
Fungal	Chronic articular hemorrhage
Lyme disease	Most JRA and juvenile spondylitis
Avascular necrosis	Erythema nodosum/sarcoidosis
Hemarthrosis	Serum sickness
Coagulopathy	Acute hepatitis B
Warfarin (Coumadin)	Rubella
Trauma/overuse	Henoch-Schönlein purpura
Pauciarticular JRA	Systemic lupus erythematosus
Congenital hip dysplasia	Lyme disease
Osteochondritis dissecans	Parvovirus
Reflex sympathetic dystrophy	Dialysis arthropathy
Hemoglobinopathies	Crystal-induced arthropathies
Stress fracture	Immune complex postbacteremia
Osteomyelitis	(meningococcus, *Haemophilus*
Osteogenic sarcoma	*influenzae*)
Metastatic tumor	
(neuroblastoma, leukemia)	
Synovial	
osteochondromatosis	
Hypermobility	
Rare	
Pigmented villonodular	Undifferentiated connective tissue
synovitis	disease
Plant-thorn synovitis	Relapsing polychondritis
Familial Mediterranean fever	Enteropathic disease
Synovioma	Ulcerative colitis
Synovial metastasis	Regional enteritis
Intermittent hydrarthrosis	Whipple disease
Pancreatic fat necrosis	Chronic sarcoidosis
Gaucher disease	Hyperlipidemias types II and IV
Behçet disease	Still disease
Regional migratory	Pyoderma gangrenosum
osteoporosis	Pulmonary hypertrophic
Sea urchin spine	osteoarthropathy
Amyloidosis (myeloma)	Chrondrocalcinosis-like
Uric acid arthropathy	syndromes due to ochronosis,
	hemochromatosis, Wilson
	disease
	Rheumatic fever
	Paraneoplastic syndromes

Modified from McCune WJ. Monarticular arthritis. *In* Kelley WN, Harris ED, Ruddy S, et al. (eds). Textbook of Rheumatology, 4th ed. Vol 1. Philadelphia: WB Saunders, 1993:369.

Abbreviation: JRA = juvenile rheumatoid arthritis.

problem the examiner faces is the delineation of the parts of the body that are malfunctioning. Failure to ambulate is usually due to an affliction of the lower extremities, but the primary illness may be present in the spine or the abdominal cavity. Referred pain may fool the physician into considering a problem involving the knee, for example, when in fact disease of the hip may be present.

In general, problems involving the locomotor system may be traumatic or nontraumatic. Trauma may be denied but may still be the major etiologic factor, whether accidental or resulting from child abuse (see Chapter 37). History, physical examination, and x-ray evaluation usually disclose the site of injury. Unusual bruis-

ing, tender muscle swellings, and burns may be further clues to trauma and abuse.

The description of the onset of the illness is important. Some children manifest no complaint but one or more swollen joints are seen while the children are being dressed, undressed, or in the bath. Some have gait disturbances or are unwilling to walk (see Chapter 46). The younger the patient with arthritis, the less likely that pain and the more likely that stiffness is a major symptom. Failure to use a limb properly is more likely to occur early in the day, and morning stiffness is almost a *sine qua non* for the diagnosis of juvenile arthritis. Similarly, stiffness may be noted after an afternoon nap, a period of inactivity in the classroom, a car ride, or watching a movie. Children may be suspected of malingering because they function poorly in the morning and well later in the day. Symptoms frequently recur in the evening after activity, and increased activity one day may be followed by greater stiffness the next. Symptoms may be aggravated by inclement weather.

Lower extremity disease is usually recognized first because disorders of ambulation cause visible limp (see Chapter 46). Upper extremity limitations are often silent until marked inability to function occurs. To elicit this information, one must ask specific questions regarding problems performing such tasks as making a fist, removing lids from jars, or opening car doors. When visible swelling has been described, the physician must attempt to identify the following:

1. *Location.* Is the swelling over a joint or does it represent periarticular swelling, bursitis, tendinitis, Osgood-Schlatter disease of the tibial tubercle, or soft tissue swelling? Have finger rings become too tight, or are they difficult to remove?

2. *Color.* Is the swelling skin colored, slightly pink, or fiery red?

Table 45–3. Diseases in Pediatric Age Group That Can Produce Acute or Chronic Arthritis

Rheumatic Diseases	*Heritable Disorders*
Juvenile rheumatoid arthritis	Sickle cell diseases
Systemic lupus	Hemophilia
erythematosus	Mucopolysaccharidosis
Rheumatic fever	Immune deficiency
Juvenile ankylosing	syndromes
spondylitis	
Dermatomyositis	*Neoplastic Diseases*
Scleroderma	Leukemia
Sjögren syndrome	Lymphoma
Polyarteritis	Neuroblastoma
Anaphylactoid purpura	
(Henoch-Schönlein)	*Miscellaneous*
Inflammatory bowel disease	Trauma
Psoriatic arthritis	Legg-Calvé-Perthes
Reiter syndrome	disease
Sarcoidosis	Slipped capital femoral
Kawasaki disease	epiphysis
Serum sickness	Reflex neurovascular
	dystrophy
Infectious Diseases	Discitis
Septic arthritis	Toxic synovitis
Viral arthritis	Hypermobility syndrome
Osteomyelitis	Erythema nodosum
Reactive or postinfectious	Familial Mediterranean
arthritis (postdysentery,	fever
urethritis, *Haemophilus*	
influenzae,	
meningococcal)	
Lyme disease	

Modified from Brewer EJ. Pitfalls in the diagnosis of juvenile rheumatoid arthritis. Pediatr Clin North Am 1986;33:1015–1032.

Very red joints suggest infection, rheumatic fever, or malignancy rather than juvenile arthritis. Black and blue swelling may be due to trauma or purpura.

3. *Temperature.* Joints involved by inflammatory disease are usually warm to the touch.

4. *Duration.* Persistence of involvement of a particular joint for at least 6 weeks is a requirement for the diagnosis of juvenile arthritis, whereas migratory polyarthritis of short duration is suggestive of rheumatic fever, bacteremia, viremia, or malignancy.

Inquiries should be made as to the presence or absence of fever. This is seldom helpful in the diagnosis of juvenile arthritis, with the exception of systemic-onset juvenile arthritis (SOJA). In SOJA, spikes of temperature to 39° to 41°C occur daily or even twice daily, with fever-free periods or even moderate hypothermia interspersed (Fig. 45–2). During the periods of high fever, the child may appear acutely ill and hyperirritable; during fever-free hours, the child is apparently well. Despite the rapid rise and marked elevation in temperature, shaking chills are uncommon, and febrile seizures are rare. Marked temperature elevations are seen in Kawasaki disease as well as in SOJA. When present in association with other rheumatic diseases, high fever usually suggests an infectious complication. Arthritis of immune complex deposition may present 5 to 10 days after therapy for meningococcal or *Haemophilus influenzae* type b bacteremia or meningitis. Arthritis before 5 days of therapy have passed may represent septic arthritis. In both conditions, fever occurs.

It is essential to inquire as to the presence of a rash. *Still's disease* (SOJA) is associated with the presence of an evanescent, occasionally pruritic, macular rash in about 50% of cases (Fig. 45–3). When it is present, it usually occurs at the time of fever peaks. When it is pruritic, it is not unusual to see it linearly at sites where scratching has occurred (Koebner phenomenon). The rash is seen particularly on the face, chest, upper arms, and upper legs. After the acute febrile disease has subsided, the rash may continue to come and go for months.

Other eruptions may be seen in children with arthritis. Palpable purpura, especially over the posterior aspect of legs and buttocks, suggests Henoch-Schönlein purpura. The circular expanding rash of *erythema chronicum migrans* is a valuable clue to the diagnosis of Lyme arthritis (Fig. 45–4). A sun-sensitive malar eruption is often seen in patients with SLE. An erythematous facial rash with discoloration of eyelids, Gottron papules over the knuckles, and a scaly eruption of elbows and knees are defining elements in the diagnosis of dermatomyositis. Similar findings, along with swelling

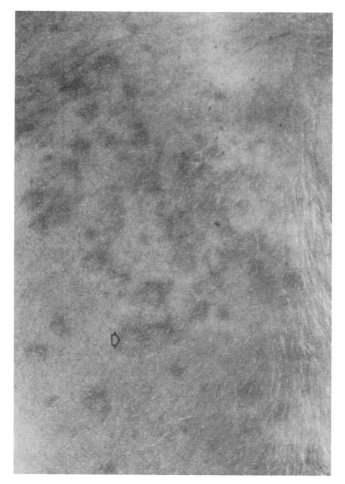

Figure 45–3. Rheumatoid rash. This was a faintly erythematous (salmon-colored), macular rash that was most prominent over the back but involved the extremities and face as well. The individual lesions were transient, appeared in crops, and generally conformed to a linear distribution. Some of the lesions had central clearing (arrow). (From Cassidy JT. Juvenile rheumatoid arthritis. In Kelley WN, Harris ED, Ruddy S, et al. [eds]. Textbook of Rheumatology, 4th ed. Vol 2. Philadelphia: WB Saunders, 1993:1193.)

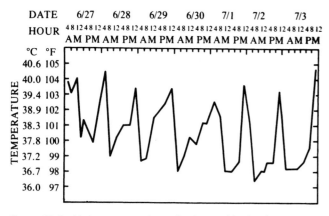

Figure 45–2. High, intermittent fever of a 3-year-old girl with systemic onset of juvenile rheumatoid arthritis. Most of the febrile spikes occurred in the late evening to early morning hours and were accompanied by a rheumatoid rash. (From Cassidy JT. Juvenile rheumatoid arthritis. In Kelley WN, Harris ED, Ruddy S, et al. [eds]. Textbook of Rheumatology, 4th ed. Vol 2. Philadelphia: WB Saunders, 1993:1193.)

of the hands and Raynaud phenomenon, raise the possibility of mixed connective tissue disease. Angioneurotic swellings may be seen with Henoch-Schönlein purpura and SLE. The latter diagnosis may also be suggested by chronic urticaria. Hereditary angioneurotic edema is also a consideration.

Oral, nasal, genital, and perirectal ulcers can be seen in children with arthritis who have inflammatory bowel disease (IBD), or Behçet disease. Mouth ulcers are common in patients with SLE. They are also seen with great regularity in normal preteens and teenagers with dental braces.

Patches of indurated skin, sometimes with a reddish border, may occur in morphea. If the patches are present in a linear pattern, usually unilaterally, the diagnosis of linear scleroderma should be kept in mind.

Petechial rashes in children with arthritis are seen in Henoch-Schönlein purpura, chronic meningococcemia, vasculitic phenomena, particularly SLE, and other vasculitides (Table 45–4) as well as in leukemia and other malignancies.

Skin appendages include hair and nails. Alopecia is seen often in SLE. Pitted nails are seen frequently in psoriatic arthritis, whereas grossly distorted nails are another feature of SLE. Beau's

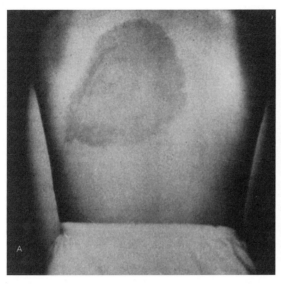 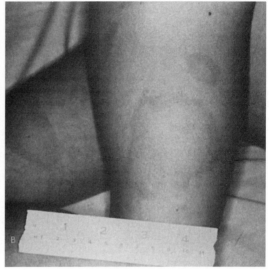

Figure 45–4. Two patients are seen, one with erythema migrans (A), the other with secondary annular lesions (B). The lesions began as red macules that expanded to form large rings. In A, the outer border is an intense red, the middle shows partial clearing, and the center is indurated. In B, the outer rims are red, and centers show nearly complete clearing. (From Steere AC, et al. Erythema chronicum migrans and Lyme arthritis: The enlarging clinical spectrum. Ann Intern Med 1977;86:685.)

lines, a horizontal depression in the nails, are seen after Kawasaki disease.

Chronic erythema nodosum may accompany the arthritis of sarcoidosis, IBD, or Behçet disease. Other lumps include nodules seen and felt under the skin, particularly near the site of tendon insertions, vertebral processes, or the scalp; in the presence of arthritis, these lumps may be rheumatoid nodules or those of rheumatic fever.

Involvement of the skin is one of the six criteria for the diagnosis of Kawasaki disease (see Chapter 50). The rash appears in any form, from the most nondescript to lesions resembling erythema multiforme. Peeling of the skin of the tips of the fingers and of the perineum is expected in the convalescent stage.

A review of systems is particularly important; it is helpful to begin at the top and work down.

Hair loss is frequently seen in patients with SLE. The condition of the scalp is also of interest because psoriasis frequently affects this area.

One should inquire about the presence of recurrent parotid swelling, often misdiagnosed as mumps. This symptom may be associated with dry eyes or dry mouth, as in the sicca syndrome. Parotid swelling is common in Sjögren syndrome, sarcoidosis, and AIDS.

Iritis is seen in two forms, chronic and acute (see Chapter 44). The chronic type may give rise to few if any symptoms until serious loss of vision has occurred. Acute iritis may cause pain, perilimbal erythema, and photophobia and is likely to attract the family's attention. Iritis is often mistaken for conjunctivitis. Because the hallmark of conjunctivitis is eye discharge, its absence should raise the possibility of iritis.

One must inquire about sun sensitivity, which may be manifested by feelings of illness after sun exposure or the development of a rash or even a petechial eruption. Muscle weakness is an important complaint, but confusion regarding this symptom may arise because pain may limit the child's performance and be mistaken for weakness.

Dysphagia may be encountered in children with dermatomyositis or in those with mixed connective tissue disease. Esophagitis can give rise to difficulties in swallowing.

A history of severe chest or abdominal pain may be suggestive of pleural or peritoneal irritation (serositis, e.g., SLE, familial Mediterranean fever); substernal chest pain associated with respiratory distress in a child who prefers to sit upright and lean forward is most suggestive of pericarditis (SLE, rheumatic fever, viral). A history of previous convulsions or psychotic behavior may be elicited in a child with SLE. Dark urine may be reported by patients with hepatic involvement (jaundice), hemolysis, myoglobinuria, or hematuria. The patient and family should be asked about the presence of *Raynaud phenomenon*, typically a three-color progression from white to purple to pink, seen in hands or feet on exposure to cold, cigarette smoke, or even stress.

Urinary tract problems may be encountered in children with Reiter disease. Diarrhea, especially bloody diarrhea accompanied

Table 45–4. **Classification of Necrotizing Vasculitis in Childhood**

Leukocytoclastic (Hypersensitivity or Allergic) Vasculitis
Henoch-Schönlein purpura
Hypersensitivity angiitis and other small vessel disease

Polyarteritis
Infantile
Kawasaki disease
Older children
Cutaneous
Miscellaneous

Associated with Rheumatic Diseases
Systemic lupus erythematosus and mixed connective tissue
Dermatomyositis
Juvenile arthritis
Others

Allergic Granulomatous Angiitis
Churg and Strauss (allergic granulomatosis)
Wegener granulomatosis
Lymphoid granulomatosis

Giant Cell Arteritis
Takayasu disease
Temporal arteritis and adult giant cell arteritis

Modified from Fink CW. Vasculitis. Pediatr Clin North Am 1986;33:1203–1219.

by mucus, may be suggestive of IBD. This symptom may occur before or many years after the development of arthritis.

Information about sexual behavior should be elicited, but these questions may have to be asked with the parent or guardian absent from the room.

Arthritis is a systemic disease, and one is often able to elicit a history of increased fatigability and increased naps in children with disseminated disease. Behavior changes, particularly hyperirritability, are almost always reported in children with Kawasaki disease, diskitis, or SOJA. Absence of this irritability should raise doubts about the diagnosis of these conditions.

Weight loss and anorexia are characteristic of systemic diseases. Marked weight loss and exceptional fatigue and weakness are reported in children with dermatomyositis and SLE as well as in older children with SOJA. Profound muscle weakness with dark urine is suggestive of rhabdomyolysis, which may follow infection or be present in the metabolic myopathies.

Close attention must be paid as well to intellectual, social, and emotional aspects of the child's illness. Cognitive defects are routinely reported in children with SLE. Problems in school or at home may be reflected in musculoskeletal pain and in nonperformance. As an attention-getting device, musculoskeletal pain can be very convincing.

One must inquire whether the child has visited or lived in areas where Lyme disease is endemic (upper Midwest, northeastern United States). A history of exposure to other infectious diseases or the recent acquisition of streptococcal pharyngitis (see Chapter 6), varicella, parvovirus, rubella, or other infectious agents may be of great help. Immunizations, particularly the measles, mumps, rubella vaccine, may be followed by the development of arthritis.

One must obtain a history of previous medications, their dosages, and their possible side effects. Over-the-counter anti-inflammatory drugs are often prescribed, but they may have been prescribed in inadequate doses, or if they were prescribed properly, compliance may not have been satisfactory. Maximal benefit from nonsteroidal drugs may take as long as 6 to 8 weeks. Medications properly prescribed and properly administered may have been discontinued before adequate response could be noted. The properties and side effects of medications should be known or determined. Parents and children may have phobias about certain medications, such as corticosteroids or acetylsalicylic acid, and these must be investigated. Medication-induced serum sickness, SLE, or erythema multiforme may be associated with arthritis.

Questions should be proposed regarding back pain, neck pain, and heel pain. These questions are relevant in patients with arthritis or those with a spondyloarthropathy (Table 45–5). A history of

Table 45–5. The Spondyloarthropathies in Children

	Ankylosing Spondylitis	Reiter Syndrome	Inflammatory Bowel Disease	Reactive Arthritis	Psoriatic Arthritis
Sex	Boys > girls	Boys > girls	No predilection	Boys > girls	Girls > boys
Age at onset	8/yr or older	Occasional in young children, usually over 8 yr	Over age 4 yr	Older children	Over age 2 yr
Joint manifestations	Pauciarticular Lower limb Sacroiliitis Axial arthritis Enthesopathy	Pauciarticular Sacroiliitis Enthesopathy	Pauciarticular Occasional spondylitis	Pauciarticular-transient	Pauciarticular or polyarticular
Extra-articular manifestations	Eye: acute iritis Heart: aortitis	Eye Skin Genitourinary tract Fever	Those of bowel disease: erythema nodosum, growth failure, etc.	Underlying gastroenteritis or urethritis	Psoriatic rash Nail pitting
Laboratory	HLA-B27 Radiographic sacroiliitis	HLA-B27	HLA-B27 in those with spondylitis	Stool culture positive: HLA-B27	None specific
Pathogenesis	Often familial	May follow infectious disease, such as *Shigella*	Arthritis related to bowel disease	Reaction to infection with *Yersinia, Shigella, Salmonella, Chlamydia, Campylobacter* species	Unknown
Diagnosis	Clinical	Clinical	Clinical, demonstration of bowel disease	Demonstration of gastrointestinal or genital infection	Clinical
Natural history	Chronic May cause spinal fusion	Episodic May recur Occasional chronic destructive arthritis	That of underlying bowel disease Peripheral arthritis, benign; spondylitis, chronic	Self-limited arthritis	Arthritis may be chronic
Therapy	NSAIDs Physical therapy	NSAIDs	Bowel disease (see Chapter 19) NSAIDs, physical therapy	That of infection	NSAIDs Remittive agents Physical therapy Skin care

Modified from Behrman RE. Nelson Textbook of Pediatrics, 14th ed. Philadelphia: WB Saunders, 1992:623.
Abbreviation: NSAID = nonsteroidal anti-inflammatory drug.

Table 45–6. **Some Dermatologic Associations of Rheumatic Diseases**

Edema	Angioneurotic edema, serum sickness, reflex sympathetic dystrophy, Kawasaki disease, Raynaud syndrome, scleroderma, mixed connective tissue disease, hereditary angioneurotic edema
Cyanosis	Hypertrophic pulmonary osteoarthropathy
Petechiae and purpura	Rule out *infection* and *leukemia*
Vasculitis	Meningococcemia, lupus, Henoch-Schönlein purpura (more on lower extremities), psychogenic purpura, Wegener granulomatosis
Local loss of hair	Scleroderma, SLE
Nails	Pits—psoriasis Deformed—lupus
Capillary distortions (nail bed)	Dermatomyositis, Raynaud syndrome, scleroderma
Loss of finger pads	Raynaud syndrome, vasculitis
Nodules	Rheumatoid arthritis, rheumatic fever
Erythema nodosum	Streptococcal infection, tuberculosis, sarcoidosis, fungal infections, inflammatory bowel disease
Erythematous rashes	SOJA, erythema chronicum migrans, erythema multiforme, lupus, Kawasaki disease, *infection*
Rash on elbows and knuckles	Dermatomyositis and psoriasis
Calcium deposits	Dermatomyositis
Skin ulceration	Raynaud syndrome, mixed connective tissue disease, lupus, necrotizing vasculitis, Reiter syndrome, Behçet syndrome, inflammatory bowel disease
Pallor (anemia)	Rule out *leukemia, SOJA,* juvenile arthritis, lupus, mixed connective tissue disease

Abbreviations: SLE = systemic lupus erythematosus; SOJA = systemic-onset juvenile arthritis.

migratory polyarthritis involving large joints suggests rheumatic fever, whereas small joint involvement is more suggestive of juvenile arthritis. The duration of arthritic symptoms may also be of help because it is unusual for any single joint in patients with rheumatic fever to be involved for more than 2 to 3 days; it is equally unusual to have joint involvement for more than a total of 3 to 4 weeks.

Results of x-ray studies or bone scans as well as biopsy material are commonly available from previous hospital encounters. In particular, synovium may have been harvested when a child's complaints have suggested an orthopedic disease. Biopsies of the salivary gland, the skin, and rarely the vocal cord may yield important information.

The family history is of great importance not only for the presence of arthritis or SLE but also for the presence of psoriasis or colitis. These illnesses run in families and may precede the development of arthritis (or follow it) by many years. Unusual flexibility or frequent joint dislocations in family members should be identified, because hypermobility and collagen abnormalities are often familial and produce arthritis.

PHYSICAL EXAMINATION

The physical examination is second in importance only to the history and begins at the moment the patient enters the room. A mental note is made of the patient's gait and the presence of

apparent discomfort, fear, and anxiety. During the history taking, the examiner notes whether the child rotates the neck or the whole body in response to a question as well as how the hands are used.

Children should be requested to remove their own clothes without parental help to see whether the fingers are adept at such tasks as untying shoe laces and removing shoes and socks. The child who can externally rotate the hip and flex the knee to remove the shoe may be unwilling to perform the same maneuver during the more formal part of the examination. The patient should be asked to walk or run, to walk on toes and heels, and to hop. The room must be warm and well lit.

The younger child may be unwilling or afraid to climb onto the examining table. Such children may be examined more satisfactorily while they are sitting on the parent's lap. Although this situation is not optimal, it is certainly better than examining a frightened, uncooperative patient on an examining table. Children old enough to cooperate are first asked to walk to the scale, where they can be measured for height and weight. When the child then climbs onto the examining table, the physician should note whether the child pushes up with the palmar or the dorsal side of the hand. The latter is used almost always if arthritis affects the wrist.

After observing the child's face and skin (Table 45–6) for pallor, malar rash, jaundice, eyelid discoloration, petechiae, and swelling of the parotid or other facial area, the physician should begin the formal examination with inspection of the patient's hands.

The dorsal sides of the hands are inspected for knuckle enlargement, sausage digits (Fig. 45–5), rash over knuckles or between knuckles, periungual hemorrhages, cyanosis, or pallor. *The most*

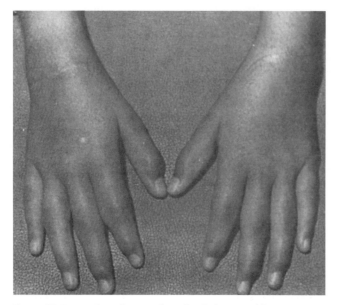

Figure 45–5. Hands and wrists of a girl with rheumatoid factor–negative polyarticular juvenile rheumatoid arthritis. Note the symmetric involvement of the metacarpophalangeal joints, proximal interphalangeal joints, and distal interphalangeal joints. Both wrists are also affected. (From Behrman RE. Nelson Textbook of Pediatrics, 14th ed. Philadelphia: WB Saunders, 1992:613.)

common mistake made in joint examination is failure to examine all the joints, not merely those about which the patient complains. The nails may be deformed, clubbed, or pitted. The palmar surface may be erythematous, with vasculitic lesions. Marked swelling of one or more of the flexor tendons may be noted, and the hand may be kept clawed. There may be atrophy of thenar or hypothenar eminences.

The patient should be asked to extend the fingers and then to make a fist. The older child should be requested to squeeze the smallest sphygmomanometer cuff, inflated to 20 mmHg. The physician records the pressure generated. Children who may be malingering often give only tentative squeezes, but on repeated testing they can be coaxed to exert maximal pressure.

The examiner must then evaluate each finger joint. After feeling gently for synovial thickening, the examiner compresses each joint between the thumb and forefinger while exerting sufficient pressure to whiten the examiner's nail. This should be accomplished both with the joint at rest and in motion. Pain responses should be noted and graded, as should limitations of normal range of motion.

Some children have "wet" arthritis, others "dry" arthritis. In patients with the former condition, the joints are boggy and swollen and on inspection are easily perceived to be enlarged. In others, little is seen on inspection but their joints may be equally tender and limited when properly examined. In some youngsters, synovial cysts form around affected joints and excellent range of motion is maintained. The apparent giving way of the capsule around the joints acts almost like a safety valve and reduces the intra-articular pressure. A *Baker cyst* behind the knee is such a protrusion, but cysts may also be seen around the elbow and other joints. The examiner notes whether the patient's hands deviate medially, which is common in childhood arthritis, or laterally, as seen in adult disease. If the hands are kept in a clawed position, the examiner has to determine whether this is due to involvement of the palmar flexor tendons or to immobility of the joints. Tendinitis may be the equivalent of synovitis for certain children.

Wrists are frequently involved in childhood arthritis, but limitation of motion of these joints frequently escapes the parent's attention unless a definite swelling is visualized on the dorsum of the wrist. Thumb pressure on the dorsum of the wrist, while alternately in flexion and extension, may reveal tenderness and limitation of motion. Involvement of the wrist may also be responsible for poor grip.

The elbow joint can be easily palpated. In addition to flexion and extension, pronation and supination should be evaluated and compared with normal standards. Many young children, particularly girls, may hyperextend the elbows. This is frequently noted when the child is asked to elevate the hands over the head. This hyperextension may call attention to *hypermobility*. The examiner will want to see if other criteria, such as the ability to touch the thumb to the palmar surface of the forearm and to extend the metacarpophalangeal joints to 90 degrees or better, are present. The other criteria include hyperextensibility of the knees and ability to touch the floor without bending the knees while placing the hands flat on the ground.

Examination of the shoulder includes palpation of the acromioclavicular joint. The patient is then asked to extend the arms above the head, This should be done with the arms elevated from the side of the body rather than from the front. In addition to examining the shoulder for mobility, the physician should also test the muscle strength of the proximal upper arm muscles. The child should be requested to keep the arms at shoulder height, with elbows bent, while the examiner exerts pressure to attempt to force the arms down. Even very young children may exert sufficient force to resist this attempt.

The child should be asked to extend and then flex the neck, to place the chin on each shoulder, and finally to place the ear on each shoulder. This exercise gives a good idea of neck mobility. The sternoclavicular joint may then be palpated.

At this point, the patient should be asked to lie down for an examination of the feet. Each toe and metatarsophalangeal joint should be examined individually. The lower legs should be uncovered and examined under a strong light. Petechial and vasculitic lesions may be seen. Both the inner and posterior surfaces of the legs as well as the buttocks should be visualized. Petechiae, bruises, lesions of erythema nodosum, or nodules should be assessed. The examiner should press on the Achilles tendon and on its enthesis attachment to the calcaneus. The examiner should strongly stroke the sole of the foot to look for fasciitis. The ankle joint can be examined by moving the foot in an up-and-down position, whereas the subtalar joint can be examined with side-to-side movement.

Examination of the knee is accomplished with the patient lying down and in a relaxed posture. The synovium of the knee can be easily palpated, particularly on the medial side, especially when the examiner's hands (one from above and one from below the knee) are brought together to squeeze fluid into the synovial space. The skin of the knee should be examined for the presence of a rash similar to that seen over the elbow, which suggests dermatomyositis. The cigarette paper scars of the child with Ehlers-Danlos syndrome are frequently found over the knees and suggest abnormalities in collagen formation. The tibial tubercle should be palpated for evidence of Osgood-Schlatter disease. The knee should be flexed and extended over its full range.

With the patient lying supine and relaxed, patellar mobility should be evaluated. The patellae may be pushed medially or laterally to the point at which the patient feels threatened that subluxation may occur. The examiner should also push the patella in a caudal direction and ask the patient to perform straight leg raising. Contraction of the quadriceps pulls the patella cephalad and causes it to rub against the distal femur. Pain occasioned by this maneuver strongly suggests the *patella-femoral compression syndrome* (also known as *chondromalacia patellae*). The circumference of each thigh should be measured several centimeters above the top of the patella. Atrophy of muscles in this area is often seen with synovial involvement of the knee. Patients with arthritis are expected to have warm joints, and examination using the back of the examiner's hand placed on the joints may corroborate excessive warmth.

The hip joint should be examined for discomfort as well as for limitation of flexion, extension, abduction, and adduction. The examiner can assess limitation of internal and external rotation by rolling the patient's thighs as though the legs were rolling pins and the examiner were attempting to roll a pizza dough.

The child should be asked also to flex one knee while placing the foot on the examining table. The opposite leg should be raised against the examiner's hand to gauge the extent of muscular weakness of the hip flexors.

When the examination of the hip is complete, the patient should be asked to stand and flex forward and backward as well as side to side. An anterior Schober test may be performed by asking the patient to bend over and then measuring the degree of back movement. This is accomplished by making a mark over the lumbar spines in the midline at the dimples of Venus, and measuring 10 cm up and 5 cm down, with the patient in the standing position, and again with forward bending. Less than 6 cm of back movement suggests a stiff back.

With the child in this position, one can examine the back for scoliosis, which may be present because of the abnormal vertebral development. Scoliosis may appear to be present if one leg is longer than the other (see Chapter 47). Leg length is measured by measuring from the anterior-superior iliac spine to the medial malleolus with the patient supine (see Chapter 46). Erroneous measurements may occur if the child cannot extend one or both legs fully. Differences in leg length occur frequently if only one knee is involved in the arthritic process. The involved leg is usually longer.

In addition to the musculoskeletal examination, a full evaluation of other body systems is indicated for each patient. In particular, blood pressure determinations may help to identify children with unsuspected renal disease. Visual problems may be present in the child with iritis, which may have preceded the development of other connective tissue disease symptoms. The presence of nasal or oral ulcers may be helpful in the diagnosis of SLE or Behçet disease. Genital and perirectal ulcers are seen in children with IBD or Behçet disease. Neurologic examination is mandatory in all children, especially those with apparent weakness.

LABORATORY STUDIES

The history and physical examination suggest the correct diagnosis in perhaps 90% of patients in whom a diagnosis can be made. Laboratory tests may serve to confirm or refute these first impressions, and they provide a baseline from which to assess improvement or worsening.

Although few children with juvenile arthritis are severely anemic when the illness commences, moderate anemia (9 to 11 g) frequently develops in those with pauciarticular and polyarticular disease. Children with SOJA may develop profound anemia (5 to 8 g). Severe anemia at presentation should alert the examiner to the possibility of malignancy or SLE. Similarly, most children with juvenile arthritis and SOJA develop and maintain thrombocytosis of 400,000 to more than a million platelets per cubic milliliter. Thrombocytopenia at presentation again suggests malignancy or SLE.

Leukocytosis is the rule in patients with SOJA (and with septic pyogenic arthritis), although a normal white blood cell count may be seen in those with SOJA or septic arthritis. Leukopenia has been reported in SOJA or juvenile arthritis but is excessively rare and should again raise the question of neoplasm or SLE.

Red blood cell morphology in patients with active connective tissue disease usually demonstrates hypochromic microcytic cells. This is the usual finding in what has been called the *anemia of*

chronic disease. In patients in whom spherocytosis is described, the physician should consider the possibility of autoimmune hemolytic anemia and should perform a Coombs test, a reticulocyte count, and an ANA. Positive results on these tests suggest a diagnosis of SLE.

A Westergren sedimentation rate is elevated in 80% of children with juvenile arthritis. Levels greater than 100 mm/hour are seen commonly in those with SOJA. Elevation of the C-reactive protein level is often used as a screening test, and on rare occasions this value may be elevated when the sedimentation rate is normal. The sedimentation rate, C-reactive protein level, and platelet count serve as acute phase reactants. One or more are elevated in 80% of children with active juvenile arthritis. It is disconcerting, however, to see normal levels in some children with polyarticular disease and elevated levels in children with monoarticular arthritis.

A dipstick urine examination may be helpful in children with suspected Henoch-Schönlein purpura or sarcoidosis, and possibly unsuspected SLE, by revealing proteinuria (see Chapter 28) or hematuria (see Chapter 29). A follow-up 24-hour urine sample for total protein level and total calcium excretion may be indicated.

An antinuclear antibody (ANA) determination is positive if it is reported in a dilution of 1:160 or higher. Most physicians accept a positive titer of 1:20 or 1:40 as within normal limits, leaving a titer of 1:80 difficult to interpret. The pattern of ANA staining is of lesser value. The ANA level is elevated in about 35% of children with juvenile arthritis and serves as a reasonable confirmation of a suspected diagnosis. Because the ANA level is elevated in 95% of children with SLE, a negative test result usually precludes that diagnosis. The ANA level is, perhaps, even more useful in pointing to a group of patients with juvenile arthritis who are at risk for chronic iritis. Of the patients destined for this complication, almost 90% have an elevated ANA level. The presence of HLA-DR5 may be even more useful, but it is a research tool.

Rheumatoid factor detected by latex agglutination identifies an immunoglobulin M (IgM) autoantibody directed against human IgG. Although present in only 15% of children with juvenile arthritis (and almost never in those under the age of 7 years), it serves to delineate a group of primarily teenaged females who have a symmetric, rapidly progressive, erosive form of arthritis identical to that seen in adults. This group has a greater tendency to develop subcutaneous nodules and acute iritis than does the larger group of children who are rheumatoid factor negative (seronegative). Tests for rheumatoid factor should be repeated several times. Elevations may be found transiently following various infections (endocarditis, congenital infections, mononucleosis) and may lead to a false diagnosis of juvenile rheumatoid arthritis. The determination of the presence and the quantity of IgA, IgM, and IgG is often helpful. Many children with active rheumatic diseases have markedly elevated levels of IgG (in a polyclonal manner) and variation in the levels of this immunoglobulin that frequently parallel the activity of the disease. Elevation of the serum level of IgA is noted in some patients with Henoch-Schönlein purpura. Some believe that there is an increase in the incidence of connective tissue disease in children who lack serum IgA completely. Such children may also be at risk for transfusion reactions if they have anti-IgA antibodies and receive transfusions with blood containing IgA.

If muscle weakness or dysphagia seems to be significant in the patient's complaint, tests of muscle enzymes should be ordered. Even in the absence of such complaints, these tests should be performed in children with the characteristic rash of dermatomyositis. For this purpose, aldolase, lactic acid dehydrogenase (LDH), serum aspartate transaminase (SGOT), and creatine phosphokinase (CPK) determinations are indicated. Ninety percent of patients with inflammatory myositis have an elevation of one or more of these enzymes. False-positive results may be obtained if the child has recently suffered an injury, or even if the child has undergone difficult venipuncture.

Patients who are thought to be at risk for SLE should be exam-

Table 45–7. Classification of Synovial Effusions*

Gross Examination	Normal	"Noninflammatory"	Inflammatory	Septic
Volume (knee)	<1 ml	Often >1 ml	Often >1 ml	Often >1 ml
Viscosity	High	High	Low	Variable
Color	Colorless to straw	Straw to yellow	Yellow	Variable
Clarity	Transparent	Transparent	Translucent	Opaque
WBCs/mm³†	<200	200–2000	2000–75,000	Often >100,000+
PMN†	<25%	<25%	Often >50%	>85%
Culture	Negative	Negative	Negative	Often positive
Mucin clot	Firm	Firm	Friable	Friable
Glucose	Nearly equal to blood	Nearly equal to blood	<50 mg/dl lower than blood	>50 mg/dl lower than blood

From Schumacher HR. Synovial fluid analysis and synovial biopsy. *In* Kelley WN, Harris ED, Ruddy S, et al. (eds). Textbook of Rheumatology, 4th ed. Vol 1. Philadelphia: WB Saunders, 1993:562.
*See Tables 45–8 and 45–9 for diseases in the noninflammatory and inflammatory groups.
†WBC count and PMN percentage are less if organism is less virulent or partially treated.
Abbreviations: PMN = polymorphonuclear neutrophils; WBC = white blood cell.

ined for the presence of anti–double-stranded DNA, Smith, and ribonucleoprotein antibodies. Complement components C3 and C4 are frequently depressed in children with active SLE. A low-functioning complement CH_{50} may be present in those with active SLE. A false-positive Venereal Disease Research Laboratory (VDRL) result might support the diagnosis of SLE. It might also point to the presence of the anti-phospholipid antibody syndrome. Additional tests for anti-cardiolipin antibodies and lupus anticoagulants are indicated if this syndrome is suspected. The syndrome may exist as a part of SLE, or it may be a syndrome in its own right.

A child with suspected vasculitis and particularly one with dermatomyositis or Kawasaki disease may demonstrate elevated levels of factor VIII–associated antigen (von Willebrand factor). It is thought that this is a sensitive indicator of disease activity in such patients.

If the history elicits, or physical examination demonstrates, swollen parotid glands, the examiner might suspect Sjögren syndrome or sarcoidosis. The diagnosis of Sjögren syndrome would be supported by the findings of positive test results for anti–SS-A or anti–SS-B (known also as anti-Ro or anti-La, respectively). The diagnosis of sarcoidosis might be supported by the findings of elevated serum calcium and angiotensin-converting enzyme (ACE) levels, hyperglobulinemia, noncaseating granulomas on biopsy, or positive findings on gallium scan.

Unexplained subcutaneous swelling (edema, angioedema) of 3 or 4 days' duration in the absence of pruritus demands the performance of a test for C1 esterase inhibitor by both quantitative and functional methods. Low values on this test confirm the diagnosis of hereditary angioneurotic edema.

The rare case of simultaneous respiratory and renal disease justifies testing for P and C-ANCA (anti-neutrophil cytoplasmic antibody), or a test for anti-GBM (glomerular basement membrane) antibody. C-ANCA is usually elevated in Wegener granulomatosis; anti-GBM in Goodpasture syndrome.

Most serum chemistry determinations are within normal limits in children with connective tissue disease except for the rare patient who may present in renal failure with either SLE or Henoch-Schönlein purpura. Children who have SLE occasionally present with jaundice and may have markedly abnormal liver function test results. Of children with SOJA who are treated with aspirin, 50% may also have elevation levels of transaminases.

Patients suspected of having Lyme disease (endemic area, tick bite, erythema chronicum migrans) should be tested for Lyme antibody by the enzyme-linked immunosorbent assay (ELISA) technique, and positive results should be confirmed by Western blot analysis. Tests for antibodies to Epstein-Barr virus, parvovirus, or other viral agents may also be indicated.

JOINT FLUID ASPIRATION

With the exception of pyogenic arthritis caused by streptococcal or gonococcal infections, most children with more than one joint involved are thought to have connective tissue disease.

All patients with suspected septic arthritis or osteomyelitis should undergo joint aspiration (Tables 45–7 to 45–11). Cultures and smears of joint fluid may reveal the presence of bacteria (Table 45–11). Appropriate intravenous antibiotic therapy must be initiated at once (Table 45–12). Surgical drainage may also be indicated. Commonly involved joints are noted in Table 45–13. It is far better to presumptively treat a child with antibiotics for suspected septic

Table 45–8. Relatively Noninflammatory Joint Effusions (Leukocyte Count <2000/mm³)

Osteoarthritis
Traumatic arthritis
Acromegaly
Gaucher disease
Hemochromatosis
Hyperparathyroidism
Ochronosis
Mechanical derangement
Erythema nodosum
Villonodular synovitis
Tumors
Aseptic necrosis
Ehlers-Danlos syndrome
Sickle cell disease
Amyloidosis
Hypertrophic pulmonary osteoarthropathy
Pancreatitis
Osteochondritis dissecans
Wilson disease
Epiphyseal dysplasias
Glucocorticoid withdrawal

Modified from Schumacher HR. Synovial fluid analysis and synovial biopsy. *In* Kelley WN, Harris ED, Ruddy S, et al. (eds). Textbook of Rheumatology, 4th ed. Vol 1. Philadelphia: WB Saunders, 1993:563.

Table 45–9. **Inflammatory Joint Effusions (Leukocyte Count >2000/mm³)**

Rheumatoid arthritis
Psoriatic arthritis
Reiter syndrome
Ulcerative colitis
Regional enteritis
Ankylosing spondylitis
Juvenile rheumatoid arthritis
Rheumatic fever
Collagen-vascular disease
   Systemic lupus erythematosus
   Scleroderma
   Polymyositis
   Polychondritis
   Polyarteritis
Polymyalgia rheumatica
Sjögren syndrome
Wegener granulomatosis
Goodpasture syndrome
Henoch-Schönlein purpura
Familial Mediterranean fever
Whipple disease
Behçet syndrome
Erythema nodosum
Sarcoidosis
Multicentric reticulohistiocytosis
Erythema multiforme (Stevens-Johnson)
Post-*Salmonella,* post-*Shigella,* post-*Yersinia* arthritis
Infectious arthritis
   Parasitic
   Viral (hepatitis, mumps, rubella, parvovirus, human
     immunodeficiency virus, others)
   Fungal
   Mycoplasmal
   Bacterial (staphylococcal or gonococcal infection, tuberculosis,
     others)
   Spirochetal (Lyme disease, syphilis)
Subacute bacterial endocarditis
Crystal-induced arthritis
   Gout
   Pseudogout
   Post–intra-articular steroid injection
   Apatite arthritis
   Oxalosis
Hyperlipoproteinemias
Serum sickness
Hypogammaglobulinemia
Leukemia
Hypersensitivity angiitis

Modified from Schumacher HR. Synovial fluid analysis and synovial biopsy. *In* Kelley WN, Harris ED, Ruddy S, et al. (eds). Textbook of Rheumatology, 4th ed. Vol 1. Philadelphia: WB Saunders, 1993:563.

arthritis and be mistaken than to risk the loss of a joint through delay. Because *H. influenzae* type b and *Staphylococcus aureus* produce septic arthritis (also consider *Salmonella* and *Streptococcus pneumoniae* in patients with sickle cell anemia) in children younger than 4 to 6 years of age, appropriate antibiotics may include ceftriaxone or cefotaxime with nafcillin or methicillin (or vancomycin if methicillin-resistant *S. aureus* or pneumococcus is suspected). Gonococcal septic arthritis often develops in adolescents; therapy includes ceftriaxone or cefotaxime initially, followed by penicillin if the organism is a gonococcus sensitive to penicillin (see Chapter 31).

A diagnostic dilemma arises when a child is first seen with only a single involved joint. If the history and physical examination are typical of those encountered with connective tissue disease, a joint aspiration may not be indicated. Aspiration is performed with appropriate analgesia and sterile precautions; the fluid is submitted for microscopic smear, cell count, culture, and crystal analysis. The white blood cell count in the joint fluid of patients with juvenile arthritis may range from a few thousand cells to over 100,000 cells per cubic milliliter. Thus, interpretation and differentiation from septic arthritis may not be possible using cell count alone.

BIOPSY

Synovial Biopsy

If a patient with monarticular arthritis has a negative ANA and rheumatoid factor, has normal immunoglobulins, and is free of iritis, the question arises as to whether the patient has a connective tissue disease. If no other clues, such as involvement of a second joint, development of iritis, or abnormal blood values, present within 12 months, an orthopedist could perform a synovial biopsy. The results may support the diagnosis of juvenile arthritis or may provide an alternate diagnosis. Biopsy may also be helpful in a patient with suspected sarcoid arthritis because noncaseating granulomas may be seen. Very rarely, the biopsy may disclose a synovial tumor. Foreign body fragments may be phagocytosed by synovial tissue and may not be visible on arthroscopic examination. Therefore, complete synovectomy may be needed both for diagnosis and for therapy.

Skin Biopsy

Skin biopsy may be helpful to confirm a suspected diagnosis of erythema nodosum or vasculitis, although it is not usually necessary. Similarly, skin biopsy and immunofluorescent studies of nonexposed as well as exposed skin may support the diagnosis of SLE. Biopsy of the sural nerve may be indicated in children with suspected vasculitis and may be performed if a nerve conduction of that nerve is abnormal.

Renal Biopsy (see also Chapters 28 and 29)

Renal biopsy is indicated in children with lupus nephritis or Wegener granulomatosus. A patient whose renal biopsy reveals

Table 45–10. **Hemarthroses**

Trauma with or without fractures
Pigmented villonodular synovitis
Tumors
Hemangioma
Hemophilia or other bleeding disorders
Von Willebrand disease
Anticoagulant therapy
Myeloproliferative disease
Thrombocytopenia
Scurvy
Ruptured aneurysm
Arteriovenous fistula
Idiopathic
Intense inflammatory disease

Modified from Schumacher HR. Synovial fluid analysis and synovial biopsy. *In* Kelley WN, Harris ED, Ruddy S, et al. (eds). Textbook of Rheumatology, 4th ed. Vol 1. Philadelphia: WB Saunders, 1993:563.

Table 45–11. Synovial Fluid Examination in the Diagnosis of Bacterial Arthritis

Procedure	Important Technical Aspects	Diagnostic Yield
Culture	Plate immediately or inoculate in blood culture bottles	Nearly 100% positive in nongonococcal bacterial arthritis but only 25–50% positive in gonococcal arthritis
Gram stain smear	Best yield if centrifuge fluid. False-positive gram-positive from precipitated mucin	75% positive with gram-positive cocci, 50% with gram-negative bacilli, less than 25% in gonococcal arthritis
Leukocyte count and differential leukocyte count	Generally greater than 50,000 cells/mm³ and greater than 80% PMNs	Significant overlap with noninfectious arthritis (RA, crystal-induced)
Glucose	Less than 50% of fasting, simultaneous blood sugar	Helpful but often not present and may be seen in RA
Detection of bacterial cell wall antigens	Counterimmuno-electrophoresis or similar immune test	Generally not useful, except in *Haemophilus influenzae* and *Streptococcus pneumoniae* arthritis
Concentration of fatty acids	Lactate dehydrogenase or lactic acid levels are more practical than gas liquid chromatography, which is too cumbersome	Elevated values may be of diagnostic utility in partially treated cases but are nonspecific. Low or normal values are helpful in excluding bacterial arthritis

Modified from Goldenberg DL. Bacterial arthritis. *In* Kelley WN, Harris ED, Ruddy S, et al. (eds). Textbook of Rheumatology, 4th ed, Vol 2. Philadelphia: WB Saunders, 1993:1451.
Abbreviations: PMN = polymorphonuclear neutrophil; RA = rheumatoid arthritis.

diffuse proliferative glomerulonephritis is a candidate for the use of cytotoxic drugs. In addition, valuable information may be obtained as to the possibility of a therapeutic response. A patient whose renal biopsy reveals active disease is more likely to respond than one with chronic changes.

ELECTROMYOGRAPHY AND NERVE CONDUCTION STUDIES

Patients with suspected dermatomyositis can be expected to have a typical pattern of muscle degeneration as shown on an electromyogram (EMG). The technician must select muscles known to be involved rather than selecting muscles at random. If biopsy is contemplated, needle studies should be performed on only one side of the body because disruption of muscle fibers by the needle may confuse the microscopic picture.

Table 45–12. Treatment of Bacterial Arthritis

1. Aspirate any possible infected joint immediately. Remove as much fluid as possible and perform synovial fluid culture, Gram stain, leukocyte count and differential leukocyte count, glucose with simultaneous blood glucose determinations, and crystal analysis.
2. If the fluid is purulent or if organisms are seen on the Gram stain smear, start antibiotics immediately:
   a. Organisms identified on Gram stain. If gram-positive cocci, start nafcillin or (if in hospital with methicillin-resistant *Staphylococcus aureus*) vancomycin. If gram-negative cocci, start ceftriaxone. If gram-negative bacilli, start an aminoglycoside and third-generation cephalosporin.
   b. Negative Gram stain: In children younger than age 2, cover for penicillin-resistant *Haemophilus influenzae*, staphylococci, and gram-negative bacilli. In compromised hosts and intravenous drug users, cover for methicillin-resistant *S. aureus* and gram-negative bacilli.
3. When the specific bacterium is identified, adjust antibiotics if necessary. Administer antibiotics parenterally and in doses used to treat bacteremia.
4. Drain all purulent fluid with closed needle aspiration, arthroscopy, or arthrotomy.
5. Reassess adequacy of treatment clinically and with serial synovial fluid analysis. If inadequate therapeutic response, obtain serum and synovial fluid bactericidal concentrations and evaluate the efficacy of drainage.
6. Treat 4–8 wk for *S. aureus,* 2 wk for gonococcus. Treat intravenously until improvement occurs and then by mouth if organism is isolated and serum levels while on oral antibiotics are equal to those with intravenous therapy.

Modified from Goldenberg DL. Bacterial arthritis. *In* Kelley WN, Harris ED, Ruddy S, et al. (eds). Textbook of Rheumatology, 4th ed. Vol 2. Philadelphia: WB Saunders, 1993:1458.

Nerve conduction studies may be helpful in patients who have SLE with neuropathy or in patients with periarteritis, to indicate the areas of nerve involvement. Abnormal results on conduction studies of the sural nerve may indicate a biopsy site in patients with periarteritis nodosa.

If a patient with suspected dermatomyositis has a characteristic history, typical physical examination, laboratory values showing elevated muscle enzyme levels, and abnormal EMG, many physicians do not recommend a muscle biopsy, believing that the diagnosis of dermatomyositis is on secure ground.

Table 45–13. Affected Joint Distribution in Adults and Children with Nongonococcal Bacterial Arthritis

Joint	Percentage of Cases	
	Adults	*Children*
Knee	55	40
Hip	11	28
Ankle	8	14
Shoulder	8	4
Wrist	7	3
Elbow	6	11
Others	5	3
(More than one joint, usually two)	(12)	(7)

From Goldenberg DL. Bacterial arthritis. *In* Kelley WN, Harris ED, Ruddy S, et al. (eds). Textbook of Rheumatology, 4th ed. Vol. 2. Philadelphia: WB Saunders, 1993:1450.

DIAGNOSTIC IMAGING

In addition to routine laboratory evaluation, diagnostic imaging is often helpful to substantiate a diagnostic possibility and to follow the progress of the patient's illness. Diagnostic imaging refers to techniques that include (1) radiography, (2) computed tomography (CT), (3) ultrasonography, (4) radioisotope imaging such as bone scan or gallium scan, (5) magnetic resonance imaging (MRI), and (6) magnetic resonance angiography (MRA).

Radiography

X-ray examination of affected joints is rarely initially helpful, although soft tissue swellings and displacement of fat pads may signal synovial swelling. *It is imperative that x-ray studies be obtained of both extremities, whether or not only one appears to be involved.* Minimal changes may be significant when one extremity is compared with the normal contralateral extremity. X-ray studies of the knees in the anteroposterior projection should always be ordered with the patient in the standing position. The patient's body weight may be sufficient to make evident the narrowing of the joint space, which can be interpreted as loss of cartilage in the affected joints. Radiographs may reveal alterations in bone density resulting from loss of bony tissue after only a short period of inflammation or immobility. Bony erosions are a later finding.

Radiographs that demonstrate metaphyseal rarefaction are frequently seen in children with leukemia or other neoplasia. Punched-out areas of dactylitis are seen in sickle cell disease. Periosteal elevation is seen in children with arthritis, osteomyelitis, tumor, and hypertrophic pulmonary osteoarthropathy. Tunnel and horizon views of the knee may disclose a fragment of bone loose in the joint space in osteochondritis dissecans. Fragmentation of the tibial tubercle may be seen in adolescents with Osgood-Schlatter disease. Chest films may reveal pleural or pericardial effusions, hilar or paratracheal lymphadenopathy, or lesions suggestive of sarcoidosis or tuberculosis.

Ultrasonography

Ultrasound studies are occasionally helpful in delineating a swollen synovial membrane, particularly in the hip, but are not as sensitive as MRI. Ultrasonography is of great usefulness in examining abdominal contents and in exploring the pericardium for pericarditis. Pericarditis in rheumatologic diseases is usually mild, with minimal fluid accumulation, and thus cannot be ruled out on the basis of the results of physical examination, electrocardiogram, or chest x-ray study (see Chapter 14). Echocardiograms can also demonstrate poor cardiac muscle contractility in patients with myocardial involvement or dilated coronary aneurysms in those with periarteritis nodosa and Kawasaki disease.

Bone Scan

Bone scans may be helpful in identifying the site of inflammatory disease, particularly in patients who are unable to localize discomfort, and in confirming a diagnosis of reflex sympathetic dystrophy (Table 45–14). In contradistinction to adults, who usually show increased uptake of radioactive material, children with reflex sympathetic dystrophy more often have cold extremities with decreased isotope uptake. The radiologist may inadvertently report that one extremity is "hot," when in reality it is the other extremity that is

Table 45–14. Reflex Sympathetic Dystrophy

Age: approx. 9 years
Girls > and usually older than boys
Prolonged dysfunction after an injury
Swelling and tenderness of an extremity (distal, proximal)
Bizarre posturing of a hand or foot
Refusal to move extremity
Causalgia; evidence of autonomic dysfunction (cool, mottled skin; increased sweating)
Radiographs: osteoporosis, soft tissue swelling; positive bone scan
Rx: Gradual guided return to normal activity

From Cassidy JT. Miscellaneous conditions associated with arthritis in children. Pediatr Clin North Am 1986;33:1033–1052.
Abbreviation: Rx = treatment.

"cold". Although bone scans often show increased uptake at the site of septic arthritis or osteomyelitis, there are false-negative results if the scans are obtained too early in the process. Clinicians must therefore follow their instinct and experience when prescribing antibiotic therapy rather than entirely trusting the bone scan results.

The bone scan may be particularly helpful in identifying the site of an osteoid osteoma not visible on routine radiographs (see Chapter 47). It may identify the location of discitis in a child with back pain (see Chapter 47). Subsequent CT or MRI may be required to identify the extent of the lesion. Bone scans may also identify diffuse bone involvement due to neuroblastoma, leukemia, or child abuse.

SPECIFIC DISEASES

Juvenile Arthritis

Juvenile arthritis (JA), juvenile rheumatoid arthritis (JRA), and juvenile chronic arthritis (JCA) are terms often used synonymously to represent a group of illness that have in common (1) the presence of arthritis, (2) the persistence of arthritis for 6 weeks or longer in the same joint or joints, and (3) the onset of items 1 and 2 in a patient younger than 16 years of age. Juvenile arthritis is commonly divided into three main subtypes if it is present for 6 months (Table 45–15).

CLASSIFICATION

Systemic-Onset Juvenile Arthritis

Systemic-onset juvenile arthritis (Still disease, SOJA) is seen primarily in younger patients, with a slight preponderance of males. The patients have very high swinging fevers (see Fig. 45–2). Fifty percent have an evanescent rash present at fever peaks (see Fig. 45–3). They often have extra-articular disease, such as pericarditis or pleural effusion, hepatosplenomegaly, and lymphadenopathy. Laboratory tests usually reveal leukocytosis, thrombocytosis, modest anemia (at presentation), an elevated C-reactive protein level, and an elevated sedimentation rate. In these children, arthritis sometimes develops months or years after the onset of the febrile illness. The differential diagnoses include other causes for obscure fevers, in particular, infections and malignancies (see Chapter 59).

The mainstays of treatment of SOJA include aspirin, 70 to 100 mg/kg/day; naproxen (Naprosyn), 10 to 20 mg/kg/day; and tolmetin

Table 45-15. Classification of Juvenile Rheumatoid Arthritis

Mode of Onset	Percent of all JRA Cases	Incidence Age (yr)	Sex	Clinical Findings	Laboratory Findings	Prognosis
Systemic	30	<10	1.5:1 F:M	Fever, rash; polyarticular arthritis; heart, liver, spleen, and lymph nodes involved; iridocyclitis seen occasionally	Anemia, leukocytosis, ESR elevated; ANA + 10%; RF −	All disease mortality in this group (1%–2% of all JRA patients); 40% evidence of joint destruction
Pauciarticular (<5 joints)	45	<10	6:1 F:M	Lower extremity arthritis	ANA +, ESR elevated 50% HLA-DR5	Continuous—25% Arthritis rarely erosive; 5-year remission 60%
Subtype 1	10	<10	Almost all female	Iritis	ANA + 90%; HLA-DR5, DRW6, DRW8	10% functional blindness 55%—acute iritis 45%—chronic iritis
Subtype 2 (HLA-B27 +)	15	>10	Mostly males	Heel pain, tendinitis, SI joint and lumbar spine arthritis later	HLA-B27 +	Juvenile ankylosing spondylitis later (maybe)
Subtype 3 (arthritis only)	20	<10	Mostly female	No iritis or HLA-B27 +		Best outlook for recovery
Polyarticular (>4 joints)	<25			Acute or insidious onset symmetric arthritis; upper and lower extremities	ESR elevated (50%)	Mortality—0 Duration longer, more crippling 25% remission
Subtype 1 (RF +)	10	>10	Mostly female	Resembles adult RA	RF + HLA-DR4	More crippling
Subtype 2 (RF −)	15				RF −	Less crippling than RF +

Modified from Brewer EJ, Giannini EH, Person DA: Juvenile Rheumatoid Arthritis, 2nd ed. Philadelphia, WB Saunders, 1982:3. Reprinted and modified in Brewer EJ. Pitfalls in the diagnosis of juvenile rheumatoid arthritis. Pediatr Clin N Am 1986;33:1015–1032.

Abbreviations: ANA = antinuclear antibody; ESR = erythrocyte sedimentation rate; HLA = human leukocyte antigen; JRA = juvenile rheumatoid arthritis; RA = rheumatoid arthritis; RF = rheumatoid factor; SI = sacroiliac.

(Tolectin), 20 to 30 mg/kg/day. Prednisone is used primarily in patients with serositis who are particularly toxic and ill.

POLYARTICULAR JUVENILE ARTHRITIS

Polyarticular *seropositive* arthritis (JRA) is usually seen in girls over 9 to 10 years of age, is symmetric, and progresses rapidly to erosive disease.

Polyarticular *seronegative* arthritis is seen in both sexes, with females predominating. It has a variable course and may become inactive in adolescents.

PAUCIARTICULAR JUVENILE ARTHRITIS

Pauciarticular (four or fewer involved joints) arthritis is usually asymmetric; it is common in very young girls. Many children have only knee involvement. If these children are ANA-positive, they are at risk for visual loss secondary to chronic iritis. The iritis may occur at times when the joint disease is quiet. Severe joint involvement, particularly hip involvement, is rarely seen in small children with pauciarticular disease and iritis.

Pauciarticular joint disease in older children may be associated at onset, preceded by, or followed by IBD. Similarly, psoriasis may occur before, during, or after the development of joint disease.

Some patients in this group manifest the SEA syndrome (*s*eronegativity, *e*nthesitis, *a*rthritis), and may progress to classic ankylosing spondylitis. Reiter syndrome is seen less commonly and often follows diarrhea rather than sexually acquired urethritis.

DIAGNOSIS

The differential diagnosis includes rheumatic (Table 45–16), nonrheumatic (Table 45–17), and spondyloarthropathy diseases (see Table 45–5). The diagnosis of Lyme disease must be considered (Table 45–18), especially in patients with a history of residence or travel to a location in which the disease is endemic or in those who have erythema chronicum migrans (see Fig. 45–4). The treatment for Lyme disease is noted in Table 45–19.

TREATMENT

Anti-inflammatory drugs are used in the treatment of juvenile arthritis. To date, only tolmetin and naproxen have been approved for use in children. Concomitant therapy with misoprostol, ranitidine (Zantac), or cimetidine (Tagamet) may prevent gastritis or ulcer formation; methotrexate, 10 mg/m^2/week, has been helpful in alleviating symptoms. Whether methotrexate is capable of arresting the disease process is not yet clear. Long-term adverse effects thus

Table 45–16. Differential Diagnosis: Rheumatic Disease

	Rheumatic Fever	Juvenile Rheumatoid Arthritis	Systemic Lupus Erythematosus	Kawasaki Disease	Dermatomyositis
Sex	No predilection	Dependent on subgroup	Girls > boys	No predilection	Girls 3:2
Age at onset	3 yr or older	1 yr or older	Usually over age 8 yr	4 yr or younger	2 yr or older
Joint manifestations	Transient migratory arthritis—large joints	Pauciarticular or polyarticular Chronic (6 wk or more)	Arthralgia Transient arthritis Chronic arthritis	Pain and swelling of hands and feet Arthritis occasionally	Joint contractures; arthritis occasionally
Extra-articular manifestations	Fever Cardiac disease Chorea Rash, nodules	Dependent on subgroup: Systemic juvenile rheumatoid arthritis: fever, rash, etc. Pauciarticular iridocyclitis	Occasionally multisystem disease, including nephritis	Fever Eye, oral, cutaneous lesions Lymphadenopathy Coronary vasculitis	Rash Muscle weakness, pain Gastrointestinal and respiratory system
Laboratory	Prior streptococcal infection ECHO or ECG evidence of carditis	May have antinuclear antibodies, rheumatoid factor	Antinuclear antibodies Autoantibodies Low complement DNA antibody	Abnormal coronary vessels on ECHO	Abnormal "muscle enzymes," electromyogram, muscle biopsy
Pathogenesis	Post-streptococcal	Unknown	Immune complex disease	Unknown	Unknown
Diagnosis	Clinical (Jones criteria)	Clinical (juvenile rheumatoid arthritis criteria)	Clinical plus laboratory (systemic lupus erythematosus criteria)	Clinical (Kawasaki criteria)	Clinical Rash plus myositis Muscle biopsy
Natural history	Arthritis—transient: carditis may cause permanent damage	Chronic: arthritis may be destructive	Chronic or recurrent, may be fatal	Self-limited (often) Coronary vasculitis May be fatal	Chronic May be fatal
Therapy	Anti-inflammatory, group A streptococci prophylaxis to prevent recurrence	Anti-inflammatory Physical therapy	Anti-inflammatory Corticosteroid Cytotoxic agents	Intravenous globulin Aspirin	Corticosteroid Cytotoxic agents

From Behrman RE (ed). Nelson Textbook of Pediatrics, 14th ed. Philadelphia: WB Saunders, 1992:620.
Abbreviations: ECG = electrocardiogram; ECHO = echocardiography.

far seem to be mild. Rare hepatic fibrosis secondary to methotrexate use has been noted. Subcutaneous or intramuscular methotrexate may be more effective than oral dosing. Folic acid (1 mg/d) is given orally to prevent methotrexate toxicity. Systemic steroids are indicated for life-threatening conditions, such as severe pericarditis or arytenoid–vocal cord arthritis with airway obstruction. Hydroxychloroquine (Plaquenil), in a dose less than or equal to 6 mg/kg/day, is occasionally helpful (eye precautions—red ball color examination every 3 months). Intramuscular gold may be administered in a dose approaching 1 mg/kg/week, with special attention paid to possible renal, bone marrow, and skin toxicity. Oral gold has been of limited usefulness in childhood, as has D-penicillamine. Deflazacort is not available at this time in the United States, but if it is introduced, it may make possible the use of oral steroids in larger than customary doses without causing the growth interruption that is currently inevitable when doses of prednisone of 5 mg or more are given daily.

Intra-articular corticosteroids are useful when one or two joints

are particularly troublesome. After injection, intensive physical and occupational therapy can often overcome contractures due to muscle spasm. The importance of physical medicine, including active range-of-motion exercises, and appropriate splinting cannot be overemphasized.

Arthroplasty provides the opportunity to salvage function in many joints that have been seriously eroded by rheumatic disease activity. Growth should be complete before this modality is used. Asymmetric leg growth may occur in children with unilateral lower limb arthritis. The orthopedist may have to intervene just before puberty to even leg lengths.

Special dental care may be necessary in children whose mandibular growth is abnormally slow and whose jaws may not accept the full complement of 32 adult teeth. A surgical unit offering care to children with arthritis must provide an anesthesiologist capable of giving anesthesia to a child with a small mandible, a limited gape, and limited neck extension.

A team caring for a child with juvenile arthritis must include an

Table 45–17. Diagnosis: Nonrheumatic Conditions

	Septic Arthritis	Lyme Disease	Osteomyelitis	Viral Arthritis	Childhood Malignancy	Structural, Genetic	Growing Pains, Psychogenic
Sex	Any	Any	Any	Girls > boys	Any	Any depending on condition	Growing pains; boys > girls; Psychogenic; girls > boys
Age at onset	<4 yr: *Haemophilus influenzae* Teenage: Gonococcus Any age: *Staphylococcus aureus*	Over age 2 yr	Any	More common in older children and adults	Any	Any	Growing pains, 2–8 yr; Psychogenic, 6 yr or older
Joint manifestations	85% monoarticular joints swollen, hot, painful	Pauciarticular; episodic, recurrent	Sterile joint effusion adjacent to the area of bone infection	Transient arthritis—often polyarticular	Severe bone/joint pain, night pain	Local bone/joint pain or dysfunction	None or bizarre Features of reflex sympathetic dystrophy
Extra-articular manifestations	Fever, signs of sepsis, signs of gonococcal disease	Flu-like illness, erythema migrans, CNS, neurologic, cardiac	Fever, signs of sepsis, bone pain	Those of underlying virus	Those of underlying malignancy; no high fever, rash, or morning stiffness	Those of underlying conditions, dysmorphic features, structural abnormalities	Growing pains—none; psychogenic—bizarre
Laboratory	Cultures: joint fluid, blood, genital	Serologic: antibody to *Borrelia burgdorferi*	Culture: blood, bone: bone scan	Viral culture Serologic: rise in antibody titers	Hematologic abnormalities, abnormal radiograph or scan	Demonstration of abnormal structure or metabolic abnormality	Normal
Pathogenesis	Direct bacteremic synovial infection; occasional immune complex mechanism in gonococcal and meningococcal arthritis	*B. burgdorferi*—synovial and systemic infection	Direct bacteremic infection of bone, sympathetic joint effusion	Direct viral synovial infection, immune complex in some	Direct primary bone tumor or periarticular or bony infiltrate of malignant cells	Idiopathic or genetic	No organic disease
Diagnosis	Demonstration of organisms in joint fluid	Serologic	Demonstration of organisms: blood, bone; bone scan (early), x-ray (late)	Clinical, serologic, or viral culture	Bone marrow tissue biopsy	Recognition of condition or syndrome	Clinical
Natural history	Joint destruction if untreated	Chronic, recurrent; may cause long-term CNS, skin, ocular disease	Bone/joint destruction if untreated	Arthritis transient	Joint manifestations may wax/wane	Chronic	Growing pains benign; psychogenic may become chronic and disabling
Therapy	Specific antibiotic	Specific antibiotic	Specific antibiotic	Symptomatic	That of underlying malignancy	That of underlying conditions	Recognition, reassurance, psychosocial attention

Modified from Behrman RE (ed). Nelson Textbook of Pediatrics, 14th ed. Philadelphia: WB Saunders, 1992:619.
Abbreviation: CNS = central nervous system.

750

Table 45–18. Manifestations of Lyme Disease by Stage*

System†	Early Infection		Late Infection
	Localized Stage 1	*Disseminated Stage 2*	*Persistent Stage 3*
Skin	Erythema migrans	Secondary annular lesions Malar rash Diffuse erythema or urticaria Evanescent lesions Lymphocytoma	Acrodermatitis chronica atrophicans Localized scleroderma-like lesions
Musculoskeletal		Migratory pain in joints, tendons, bursae, muscle, bone Brief arthritis attacks Myositis‡ Osteomyelitis‡ Panniculitis‡	Prolonged arthritis attacks Chronic arthritis Peripheral enthesopathy Periostitis or joint subluxations below acrodermatitis
Neurologic		Meningitis Cranial neuritis, Bell palsy Motor or sensory radiculoneuritis Subtle encephalitis Mononeuritis multiplex Myelitis‡ Chorea‡ Cerebellar ataxia‡	Subtle mental disorders Axonal polyneuropathy Leukoencephalitis Encephalomyelitis Spastic parapareses Ataxic gait Dementia‡
Lymphatic	Regional lymphadenopathy	Regional or generalized lymphadenopathy Splenomegaly	
Heart		AV nodal block Myopericarditis Pancarditis	Cardiomyopathy
Eyes		Conjunctivitis Iritis‡ Choroiditis‡ Retinal hemorrhage or detachment‡ Panophthalmitis‡	Keratitis
Liver		Mild or recurrent hepatitis	
Respiratory		Nonexudative sore throat Nonproductive cough Adult respiratory distress syndrome‡	
Kidney		Microscopic hematuria or proteinuria	
Genitourinary		Orchitis‡	
Constitutional symptoms	Minor	Severe malaise and fatigue	Fatigue

From Steere AC: Lyme disease. N Engl J Med 1989; 321:586. Reproduced by permission of *The New England Journal of Medicine.*
*The staging system provides a guideline for the expected timing of the different manifestations of the illness, but this may vary in an individual case.
†The systems are listed from the most to the least commonly affected.
‡Since the inclusion of these manifestations is based on one or a few cases, they should be considered possible but not proven manifestations of Lyme disease.
Abbreviation: AV = atrioventricular.

ophthalmologist to perform the slit-lamp examinations required by all affected children. It is recommended that children who are ANA-positive have slit-lamp examinations every 3 to 4 months for 7 years; those who are ANA-negative may go 6 months between examinations. After age 7 or 8, children in either group who have not previously been affected by chronic iritis may be examined at yearly intervals. A nutritionist as well as a social worker and a competent psychologist are also necessary for the support of these children.

Systemic Lupus Erythematosus

Systemic lupus erythematosus is a disease of unknown origin with a predilection for females, patients of African-American or Asian-American origin, and multiple family members. Symptoms of SLE may be induced by various drugs, of which the most common are anticonvulsants, such as ethosuximide (Zarontin), or antihypertensive drugs, such as hydralazine. Procainamide, isoniazid, phenytoin, propylthiouracil, and griseofulvin are additional drugs.

DIAGNOSIS

Although any organ system may be involved at any time during the disease, the high frequency of joint involvement brings the rheumatologist into early contact with most patients with SLE

Table 45-19. Treatment Regimens for Lyme Disease

System	Regimen
Early infection* (local or disseminated) Adults	Doxycycline 100 mg orally 2 times/d for 10 to 30 d† *or* Tetracycline 250 mg orally 4 times/d for 10 to 30 d† *or* Amoxicillin 500 mg orally 4 times/d for 10 to 30 d†
Children (age 8 yr or less)	Amoxicillin 250 mg orally 3 times/d *or* 20 mg/kg/d in divided doses for 10 to 30 d† Alternative in case of allergy to penicillin Erythromycin 250 mg orally 3 times/d *or* 30 mg/kg/d in divided doses for 10 to 30 d†‡
Arthritis* (intermittent or chronic)	Doxycycline 100 mg orally 2 times/d for 30 d *or* Amoxicillin and probenecid 500 mg of each orally 4 times/d for 30 d *or* Ceftriaxone‖ 2 g IV once a day for 14 d *or* Penicillin‖ 20 million U IV in 6 divided doses for 14 d
Neurologic abnormalities* (early or late)	Ceftriaxone‖ 2 g IV once a day for 14 to 30 d§ *or* Cefotaxime 2 g IV 3 times a day for 14 to 30 d§ *or* Penicillin G‖ 20 million U IV in 6 divided doses daily for 14 to 30 d§ Alternatives in case of allergy to penicillin or cephalosporin in drugs
(early)	Doxycycline 200 mg orally 2 times/d for 30 d
(early or late)	Vancomycin 1 g b.i.d. for 14 to 30 d‡
Facial palsy alone	Oral regimens may be adequate

Cardiac abnormalities
  First-degree AV block
    (PR interval >0.2 sec)
	Oral regimens, as for early infection

High-degree AV block	Intravenous regimens, as for neurologic abnormalities
Acrodermatitis	Oral regimens for 1 month are usually adequate

Modified from Steere AC. Lyme disease. N Engl J Med 1989;321:586. Reproduced by permission of *The New England Journal of Medicine*.
*Treatment failures have occurred with any of the regimens given. Retreatment may be necessary.
†The duration of therapy is based on clinical response.
‡These antibiotics have not yet been tested systematically for this indication in Lyme disease.
§For early neurologic abnormalities, 2 weeks of therapy is generally adequate. The appropriate duration of therapy is not yet clear for patients with late neurologic abnormalities, and 4 weeks of therapy may be preferable.
‖Pediatric doses of ceftriaxone (100 mg/kg/d) or penicillin (300,000 U/kg/d) are appropriate for young children.
Abbreviations: AV = atrioventricular; IV = intravenously.

(Tables 45–20 and 45–21). Joint disease, although painful, is rarely deforming. In patients with the diagnosis of juvenile arthritis, SLE subsequently develops in almost 10%.

Patients with bleeding phenomena, jaundice, pallor, abdominal pain, dyspnea, edema or anasarca, muscle weakness, skin rash, seizures or psychosis, hair loss, or mouth or nose ulcerations may ultimately prove to have SLE.

Laboratory findings are essential to confirm the diagnosis of SLE. Ninety-five percent of patients have a positive test result for antinuclear antibodies (Table 45–22). Because the test for ANA is highly sensitive, but not specific for the diagnosis of SLE, patients should also have an ANA screen, including tests for anti–double-stranded DNA antibodies. These tests can be performed by the Farr technique or by use of the unicellular organism *Crithidia*. An additional test would be for the Smith (Sm) antigen. Both the Sm and the anti-DNA, while positive in only 35% to 40% of patients with SLE, are highly specific.

Patients whose SLE is active often have low levels of complement components C3 and C4. The CH_{50} level, which is a general measure of complement activity, may be low as well. Complement deficiencies of C1 to C4 (often familial) are seen in patients who may develop SLE or lupus-like syndromes. It may be necessary to test for individual complement components if the CH_{50} level remains low when C3 and C4 levels have returned to normal.

The ANA profile usually includes tests for the presence of ribonucleoprotein (RNP), which produces a speckled pattern on the ANA test. The presence of anti-RNP suggests the patient's diagno-

sis to be mixed connective tissue disease. The clinical characteristics of this illness include the presence of Raynaud phenomenon and hand swelling. A barium swallow often reveals esophageal dysmotility.

Systemic lupus erythematosus may involve any organ system (see Table 45–21). Although only 50% of children have lupus nephritis at the time of diagnosis, 85% will have it within 5 years. Central nervous system SLE, manifested by psychosis and migraine or seizure disorder, is a common problem.

TREATMENT

The mainstay of therapy is prednisone, which is simultaneously the best and worst of drugs. The side effects of prednisone include weight gain and hirsutism, with resulting cushingoid appearance. Loss of bony matrix is seen, which may play a role in the development of aseptic necrosis, especially of the hip. Cataracts may develop. Personality changes, muscle weakness, pancreatitis, and even psychosis may result from corticosteroid therapy.

Sufficient prednisone is used to suppress symptoms, and, it is hoped, correct abnormal laboratory values. An attempt may be made to normalize C3 and C4 determinations while lowering anti-DNA titers. Long-term corticosteroid therapy should be accompanied by the administration of vitamin D and calcium to prevent osteopenia. Steroid-treated patients may develop disseminated vari-

Table 45–20. 1982 Revised Criteria for Diagnosis of Systemic Lupus Erythematosus*

Criterion	Definition
Malar rash	Fixed erythema, flat or raised, over the malar eminences, tending to spare the nasolabial folds
Diskoid rash	Erythematous raised patches with adherent keratotic scaling and follicular plugging; atrophic scarring may occur in older lesions
Photosensitivity	Skin rash as a result of unusual reaction to sunlight (elicited by patient history or physician observation)
Oral ulcers	Oral or nasopharyngeal ulceration, usually painless, observed by a physician
Arthritis	Nonerosive arthritis involving two or more peripheral joints, characterized by tenderness, swelling, or effusion
Serositis	Pleuritis—convincing history of pleuritic pain or rub heard by a physician or evidence of pleural effusion *or* Pericarditis—documented by ECG or rub or evidence of pericardial effusion
Renal disorder	Persistent proteinuria greater than 0.5 g/day or greater than 3+ if quantitation not performed *or* Cellular casts—may be red blood cell, hemoglobin, granular, tubular, or mixed
Neurologic disorder	Seizures—in the absence of offending drugs or known metabolic derangements (e.g., uremia, ketoacidosis, or electrolyte imbalance) *or* Psychosis—in the absence of offending drugs or known metabolic derangements (e.g., uremia, ketoacidosis, or electrolyte imbalance)
Hematologic disorder	Hemolytic anemia—with reticulocytosis *or* Leukopenia—less than 4,000/mm³ total on two or more occasions *or* Lymphopenia—less than 1,500/mm³ on two or more occasions *or* Thrombocytopenia—less than 100,000/mm³
Immunologic disorder	Positive LE cell preparation *or* Anti-DNA antibody to native DNA in abnormal titer *or* Anti-Sm—presence of antibody to Sm nuclear antigen *or* False-positive serologic test result for syphilis known to be positive for at least 6 mo and confirmed by negative *Treponema pallidum* immobilization or fluorescent treponemal antibody absorption test
Antinuclear antibody	An abnormal titer of antinuclear antibody by immunofluorescence or an equivalent assay at any point in time and in the absence of drugs known to be associated with "drug-induced lupus syndrome"

From Tan EM, Cohen AS, Fries JF, et al. The 1982 revised criteria for the classification of systemic lupus erythematosus. Arthritis Rheum 1982;25:1271.

*The proposed classification is based on 11 criteria. For the purpose of identifying patients in clinical studies, a person shall be said to have systemic lupus erythematosus if any four or more of the 11 criteria are present, serially or simultaneously, during any interval of observation.

Abbreviations: ECG = electrocardiogram; DNA = deoxyribonucleic acid; LE = lupus erythematosus; Sm = Smith.

cella or recurrent zoster and are subject to infection with both common and opportunistic infectious agents.

Hydroxychloroquine and cytotoxic drugs, particularly cyclophosphamide (Cytoxan) in oral or parenteral form; methotrexate; and azathioprine (Imuran) are also prescribed. Patients taking hydroxychloroquine should have eye examinations every 3 to 4 months.

Patients with SLE must avoid sun exposure. When participating in outdoor activities, they should use a sunscreen. Birth control for sexually active females may be accomplished with the administration of medroxyprogesterone (Depo-Provera) or the insertion of levonorgestrel (Norplant). Oral estrogen contraceptive agents are thought to be capable of exacerbating SLE.

Dermatomyositis

Dermatomyositis is an illness of uncertain etiology. The symptoms usually come on gradually, and many months may elapse between the onset of symptoms and the diagnosis. In some patients skin manifestations may be prominent without overt muscle involvement; in the majority, however, the motor weakness as well as rash gradually develops. Characteristic skin lesions include a heliotrope colored rash over the eyelids, extending onto the face. Scaly patches over the metacarpophalangeal and proximal interphalangeal joints, Gottron papules, and additional scaly patches may be noted over the elbows and knees. When the rash appears in the absence of marked weakness, it is frequently ignored or misinterpreted as being eczema or a nonspecific dermatitis.

The muscle weakness is usually progressive, and patients are eventually unable to arise from the floor without using their hands. The weakness in this illness is proximal and is identified by testing the muscle power, particularly of the deltoids and hip flexors. In addition, most patients experience great difficulty in keeping their heads off the examining table for 1 minute while they are in the supine position. They also may have difficulty sitting up from a supine position. Nail fold capillary microscopy usually demonstrates capillary distortion, and areas of blood vessel drop out.

Table 45–21. Additional Manifestations of Systemic Lupus Erythematosus

Systemic	*Gastrointestinal*
Fever	Pancreatitis
Malaise	Mesenteric arteritis
Weight loss	Serositis
Fatigue	Hepatomegaly
	Hepatitis (chronic–lupoid)
Musculoskeletal	Splenomegaly
Myositis, myalgia	
Arthralgia	*Renal*
	Nephritis
Cutaneous	Nephrosis
Raynaud phenomenon	Uremia
Alopecia	Hypertension
Urticaria	
Panniculitis	*Reproduction*
Livedo reticularis	Infertility
	Repeat abortions
Neuropsychiatric	Neonatal lupus
Personality disorders	Congenital heart block
Stroke	
Peripheral neuropathy	*Hematologic*
Chorea	Anticoagulants (factors
Transverse myelitis	VIII, IX, XII, others
Migraine headaches	causing hemorrhage)
Mononeuritis multiplex	Antiphospholipid antibodies
	(lupus anticoagulant
Cardiopulmonary	causing thrombosis)
Endocarditis	
Myocarditis	*Treatment-Induced*
Pneumonitis	Steroid toxicity
Pulmonary hemorrhage	Immunosuppression
	Opportunistic infections
Ocular	
Episcleritis	
Sicca syndrome	
Retinal cytoid bodies	

Modified from Kredich DW. Rheumatic diseases of childhood. *In* Behrman RE, Kliegman RM (eds). Nelson Essentials of Pediatrics, 2nd ed. Philadelphia: WB Saunders, 1992:289.

DIAGNOSIS

The evaluation of a patient with suspected dermatomyositis should include a muscle evaluation by a physical or occupational therapist. This examination serves many purposes. It delineates the extent and degree of muscle involvement and serves as a guide for the electromyographer because it indicates which muscles are involved so that electromyography may be performed on affected muscles. It also serves to direct the surgeon, who may be called on to perform a muscle biopsy, to select a muscle involved by the disease. The chances of finding demonstrable pathology are greater when an involved muscle is evaluated. MRI may demonstrate a characteristic appearance to the muscle.

A barium swallow is indicated for all patients with dermatomyositis because dysmotility of the esophagus may result in subsequent aspiration, pneumonia, or even death. Similarly, pulmonary function studies are indicated because breathing may be compromised by involvement of either intercostal muscles or diaphragm.

In addition to routine blood counts and evaluation of muscle enzymes, thyroid function studies should be obtained because hypothyroidism may produce a disease similar to, if not identical to, dermatomyositis. Coxsackievirus studies may indicate elevated titers and has led to the suspicion that this virus may be a causative agent for dermatomyositis.

TREATMENT

Drug therapy for the dermatomyositis consists of the use of prednisone, 1 to 2 mg/kg in divided doses initially, and in single daily morning doses subsequently. Larger doses are used until muscle strength improves, and muscle enzymes study results are normal. The dosage of prednisone should be tapered over several months.

Relapses may occur as the corticosteroid dosage is tapered and require an increase in dosage. If it is not possible to lower the steroid level to a dosage compatible with body growth, alternative therapies should be considered. Methotrexate, in particular, and other cytotoxic agents have been used. Cyclosporine has achieved a degree of popularity, but its toxic effects suggest that its use should be limited to patients refractory to other modalities. Some patients have shown a dramatic and satisfactory response to the use of intravenous immunoglobulin.

Ongoing physical and occupational therapy may be necessary to treat and prevent contractures, which are seen as a result of muscle strength imbalance. Joint disease is often present in patients with dermatomyositis but usually plays a minor role. It can usually be controlled with small doses of anti-inflammatory drugs, if the steroids being administered for the muscle disease are unsuccessful at controlling symptoms.

A later, frequent, and bothersome aspect of dermatomyositis is the development of areas of calcification in skin and muscles. This is thought to be a healing phenomenon in areas where muscles have become necrotic. These deposits of calcium are frequently excreted through the skin and may need to be removed surgically.

The prognosis of dermatomyositis is variable because relapses may occur over many years, but the eventual outcome has improved markedly since the introduction of steroids.

Scleroderma

MORPHEA

In children, scleroderma is usually seen as *morphea* or "linear" scleroderma. Although either of these forms may turn into systemic sclerosis, this phenomenon is rare.

Morphea is the description given to patches of hard skin, which can occur at any place on the body and can be of any size or shape, although the lesions are usually less than 4 cm in diameter. The lesions are nontender but may have a raised reddish or purplish border. Biopsy reveals excessive collagen in the dermis, replacing hair follicles and blood vessels. Morphea is usually asymptomatic but may be unsightly. Therapy for small lesions is not indicated. The lesions may soften at puberty.

LINEAR SCLERODERMA

The same pathologic process described for morphea may be present in linear scleroderma, with sheets or bands of collagen and connective tissue. These occur in a linear distribution, usually unilaterally but occasionally bilaterally, involving upper and lower extremities, and, not uncommonly, the skin of the abdomen, chest, or back. The skin atrophies and shrinks somewhat, causing a scarred appearance. This process, if it occurs on the extremity of a young child, may seriously interfere with growth, resulting in a marked discrepancy in limb length between affected and unaffected sides. Although not painful, movement of the affected limb is progressively limited, and a claw hand or a shrunken foot may be the end result of this illness. When a patch of linear scleroderma

Table 45–22. Autoantibodies Found in Patients with Systemic Lupus Erythematosus and Other Autoimmune Diseases

Specificity	Comments
Nuclear	Present in most but not all patients
Native DNA	Essentially restricted to SLE
Denatured (single-stranded) DNA	May also cross-react with double-stranded DNA; high titers in SLE; lower titers in other diseases
Histones H1, H3-H4	SLE
Histones H2A-H2B	More common in drug-induced SLE
Sm	In 25%–60% of SLE patients, but not found in other diseases
Nuclear ribonucleoprotein	Found in SLE, but highest titers in "mixed connective tissue disease"; multiple small proteins and combined RNA have been discovered
Nucleolar antigens	Scleroderma, SLE, Sjögren syndrome
SS-B (La, Ha)	Sjögren syndrome, SLE
SS-A (Ro)	Sjögren syndrome, SLE
Proliferating cell nuclear antigen	SLE
RANA	Especially in rheumatoid arthritis (Epstein-Barr virus)
DNA-RNA hybrids, double-stranded RNA	SLE
Cytoplasmic	Less information available on these
Ribosomal ribonucleoprotein	SLE
Mitochondria	Primary biliary cirrhosis, SLE
Microsomal antigens	Chronic active hepatitis, malignancies
Lysosomes	SLE
Single-stranded RNA, tRNA	SLE
SS-B and SS-A	Sjögren syndrome, SLE
Cell membrane determinants	Common in SLE
Red cells	May occur without important hemolysis
White cells	Granulocytes, T cells, B cells
Platelets	Common without thrombocytopenia
Lipomodulin	SLE, RA, others (?)
Receptors	Insulin, IL-2, others
MHC class II	Interferes with immune functions
Others	
Mitotic spindle and intracellular supporting proteins	SLE and other rheumatic diseases
Immunoglobulins	JRA, RA, SLE, Sjögren syndrome, others
Clotting factors	SLE and other diseases
Phospholipids (e.g., cardiolipin)	SLE, others or without other disease (idiopathic)
Thyroid antigens	Thryoid diseases, SLE, Sjögren syndrome

Modified from Steinberg AD. Systemic lupus erythematosus. *In* Wyngaarden JB, Smith LH, Bennett JC (eds). Cecil Textbook of Medicine, 19th ed. Philadelphia: WB Saunders, 1992:1524.

Abbreviations: RANA = RA nuclear antigen; RA = rheumatoid arthritis; JRA = juvenile rheumatoid arthritis; IL-2 = interleukin-2; MHC = major histocompatibility complex; SLE = systemic lupus erythematosus; Sm = Smith; RNA = ribonucleic acid; DNA = deoxyribonucleic acid.

occurs over the eyelid and forehead, an indentation may result, known as *coup en sabre* phenomenon.

Although this condition is notoriously resistant to therapy, current recommendations suggest the use of D-penicillamine, with or without accompanying corticosteroids. It is not uncommon around adolescence to see previously very hard and indurated skin soften somewhat, and on rare occasions hair may regrow in the affected skin.

Raynaud phenomenon and dermal capillary abnormalities are not usually seen in linear scleroderma. When they occur, progression to systemic sclerosis is more likely. Joint disease is not a major manifestation of linear scleroderma, although joint limitation may occur if the skin over the joints becomes bound down.

Laboratory studies are frequently unrevealing, although occasional patients may test positive for ANAs. Familial occurrence of scleroderma is rare but does occur.

Reflex Sympathetic Dystrophy (RSD)

Reflex sympathetic dystrophy is a syndrome of unknown origin that is seen infrequently in childhood (see Table 45–14). It is poorly understood and goes under many names, including "reflex neurovascular dystrophy," "causalgia," "shoulder-hand syndrome," and "Sudeck atrophy." The presentation is usually dramatic. After a very minor injury or an injury that is not always acknowledged by the patient, pain, swelling, color, and temperature change of one or more extremities may occur. The hand or foot is kept in an awkward position, and the patient resists movement. The pain may be so intense that the patient is thought perhaps to have sustained a fracture.

On examination, the child is found not to use the affected extremity, which is frequently cooler than, though occasionally warmer than, the opposite extremity. This syndrome usually occurs in teenaged and pre-teenaged girls, although boys may rarely be affected. Laboratory and x-ray studies reveal no abnormalities, but bone scan shows a decreased (or increased) uptake of radioactive material on the affected side.

In children, atrophy rarely occurs, particularly if the patient can be encouraged to use the extremity. Physical therapy is usually successful over a period of time in returning the child to normal function. Relapses may occur. Biofeedback techniques may also be helpful. Only in rare instances is nerve block indicated. Because of the failure of movement of the extremity, these children are frequently suspected of having arthritis, and the correct diagnosis can be made only if the examining physician considers the possibility of reflex sympathetic dystrophy.

Rheumatic Fever

Rheumatic fever is an acute illness of children 4 years of age and older (see Chapters 6 and 16). It occurs in patients who have had previous infections with β-hemolytic streptococci.

Although arthritis is the most common and most dramatic symptom of rheumatic fever, it does not lead to permanent joint damage. Characteristically, the patient displays evidence for migratory polyarthritis and fever. Although excessively painful and tender in the earlier descriptions, the disease manifestation seems to have been modified with time, so that currently most patients complain of only moderate discomfort. The joints may be erythematous. As a rule, only larger joints are affected, and the presence of swollen small joints, such as fingers, should alert the examiner to the probability that the patient has juvenile arthritis, in which streptococcal disease may also be incidentally found. As a rule, in rheumatic fever, each joint is involved for only 3 to 4 days, and the entire period of joint involvement lasts no longer than 6 weeks.

If a febrile illness, a new murmur, migratory polyarthritis, and evidence of recent streptococcal infection are present, rheumatic fever should be suspected.

SUMMARY AND RED FLAGS

The differential diagnosis of arthritis is extensive. A good history and physical examination, especially over time, are helpful in making a diagnosis and initiating therapy in most patients. Potential pitfalls in diagnosis are noted in Table 45–23.

Red flags include manifestations suggestive of septic arthritis (fever, single joint, erythema, extreme tenderness, leukocytosis), malignancy (polyarthritis, night and nonarticular bone pain, absence of high fever, absence of obvious swelling or stiffness, positive radiographic changes, and abnormal complete blood count), Lyme disease, Kawasaki disease, and other treatable disorders. Multiorgan system involvement may be primary (SLE, rheumatic fever) or secondary to therapy and must be considered so as to avoid

---

Table 45–23. **Potential Pitfalls in Diagnosis**

DO'S
1. Examine all joints.
2. Order x-ray studies of both affected and contralateral joints.
3. Ask parents to photograph swelling and rashes.
4. Insist on regular slit-lamp examinations even if arthritis is inactive.
5. Treat suspected septic arthritis or osteomyelitis even if the diagnosis is unsure.
6. Encourage patient independence.

DON'TS
1. Rule out organic disease if laboratory findings are negative.
2. Rule out organic disease if physical findings are normal at the patient's first visit.
3. Be worried about high fevers in children with systemic-onset juvenile arthritis.
4. Expect total compliance with the prescribed regimen.
5. Accept laboratory results at odds with your experience—repeat tests if necessary.
6. Be afraid to say "I don't know."

---

ongoing extra-articular involvement, which may be more life-threatening than the articular process.

REFERENCES

General

Cassidy JT, Petty RE. Textbook of Pediatric Rheumatology, 2nd ed. New York: Churchill Livingstone, 1990.

Jacobs JC. Pediatric Rheumatology for the Practitioner, 2nd ed. New York: Springer Verlag, 1993.

Kelley WN, Harris ED, Ruddy S, et al. Textbook of Rheumatology, 4th ed. Philadelphia: WB Saunders, 1993.

Septic Arthritis

Baker DG, Schumacher HR. Acute monoarthritis. N Engl J Med 1993; 329:1013–1020.

Dubost J-J, Fis I, Denis P, et al. Polyarticular septic arthritis. Medicine 1993;72:296–310.

Epersen E, Frimodt-Moller N, Thamdrup Rosdahl V, et al. Changing pattern of bone and joint infections due to *Staphylococcus aureus:* Study of cases of bacteremia in Denmark, 1959–1988. Rev Infect Dis 1991;13:347–358.

Jackson MA, Burry VF, Olson LC. Pyogenic arthritis associated with adjacent osteomyelitis: Identification of the sequela-prone child. Pediatr Infect Dis J 1992;11:9–13.

Unkila-Kallio L, Kallio MJT, Eskola J, et al. Serum C-reactive protein, erythrocyte sedimentation rate, and white blood cell count in acute hematogenous osteomyelitis of children. Pediatrics 1994;93:59–62.

Systemic Lupus Erythematosus

Cervera R, Khamashta MA, Font J, et al. Systemic lupus erythematosus: Clinical and immunologic patterns of disease expression in a cohort of 1,000 patients. Medicine 1993;72:113–124.

Groen H, Ter Borg EJ, Postma DS. Pulmonary function in systemic lupus erythematosus is related to distinct clinical, serologic, and nailfold capillary patterns. Am J Med 1992;93:619–627.

Mills JA. Systemic lupus erythematosus. N Engl J Med 1994;330:1871–1878.

Molta C, Meyer O, Dosquet C, et al. Childhood-onset systemic lupus erythematosus: Antiphospholipid antibodies in 37 patients and their first-degree relatives. Pediatrics 1993;92:849–853.

Waltuck J, Buyon JP. Autoantibody-associated congenital heart block: Outcome in mothers and children. Ann Intern Med 1994;120:544–551.

Yang L-Y, Chen W-P, Lin C-Y. Lupus nephritis in children: A review of 167 patients. Pediatrics 1994;94:335–340.

Juvenile Rheumatoid Arthritis

Giannini EH, Brewer EJ, Kuzmina N, et al. Methotrexate in resistant juvenile rheumatoid arthritis. N Engl J Med 1992;326:1043–1049.

Hadchouel M, Prieur A-M, Griscelli C. Acute hemorrhagic, hepatic, and neurologic manifestations in juvenile rheumatoid arthritis: Possible relationship to drugs or infection. J Pediatr 1985;106:561–566.

Miller ML. Juvenile rheumatoid arthritis. Curr Probl Pediatr 1994;24:190–198.

Ostrov BE, Goldsmith DP, Athreya BH. Differentiation of systemic juvenile rheumatoid arthritis from acute leukemia near the onset of disease. J Pediatr 1993;122:595–598.

Section on Rheumatology and Section on Ophthalmology. Guidelines for ophthalmologic examinations in children with juvenile rheumatoid arthritis. Pediatrics 1993;92:295–296.

Shaikov AV, Maximov AA, Speransky AI, et al. Repetitive use of pulse therapy with methylprednisolone and cyclophosphamide in addition to oral methotrexate in children with systemic juvenile rheumatoid arthritis: Preliminary results of a long-term study. J Rheumatol 1992;19:612–616.

Woo P. Cytokines in childhood rheumatic diseases. Arch Dis Child 1993;69:547–549.

Other Causes of Arthritis

Arnold JMO, Teasell RW, MacLeod AP, et al. Increased venous alpha-adrenoceptor responsiveness in patients with reflex sympathetic dystrophy. Ann Intern Med 1993;118:619–621.

Bielory L, Gascon P, Lawley TJ, et al. Human serum sickness: A prospective analysis of 35 patients treated with equine anti-thymocyte globulin for bone marrow failure. Medicine 1988;67:40–57.

Calin A. Differentiating the seronegative spondyloarthropathies: How to characterize and manage Reiter's syndrome and reactive arthritis. J Musculoskel Med 1986;3:21–27.

Kunnamo I, Kallio P, Pelkonen P, et al. Serum-sickness-like disease is a common cause of acute arthritis in children. Acta Paediatr Scand 1986;75:964–969.

Larsson L-G, Baum J, Mudholkar GS, et al. Benefits and disadvantages of joint hypermobility among musicians. N Engl J Med 1993;329:1079–1082.

Pinals RS. Polyarthritis and fever. N Engl J Med 1994;330:769–774.

Wilder RT, Berde CB, Wolohan M, et al. Reflex sympathetic dystrophy in children. J Bone Joint Surg 1992;74A:910–919.

46 Gait Disturbances

George H. Thompson

Gait disturbances are common musculoskeletal complaints that produce significant anxiety and concern in parents. Although most gait disturbances are benign and resolve with normal growth and development, others are pathologic in origin and require treatment. It is important that the physician understand the various mechanisms and causes of gait disturbances (Table 46–1), their clinical features, and the appropriate diagnostic procedures and be able to identify treatment options.

GAIT CYCLE

The normal gait cycle is described by foot placement. The gait cycle begins with right heel strike, followed by left toe-off, left heel strike, and right toe-off, and ending with right heel strike. These five events describe one gait cycle and include two phases—stance and swing. The stance phase is the period of time during which one of the two feet is on the ground. The swing phase is a portion of the gait cycle during which a limb is being advanced forward without ground contact.

Measuring the duration of the gait cycle makes possible the calculations of the time required for each of the five phases of gait. During normal gait, the duration of each phase includes weight acceptance, 11%; single limb stance, 39%; weight release, 11%; and swing phase, 39%. Velocity, cadence, step length, stride length, and step width may be calculated from the timed and measured gait cycle.

DEVELOPMENT OF GAIT

Central nervous system maturation is necessary for the development of normal gait and accounts for the normal progression of developmental milestones. The normal milestones for locomotion include independent sitting at 6 months of age, crawling at 9 months, walking without assistance at 12 to 15 months, and running at 18 months. A normal 1-year-old child has a wide-based stance and a rapid cadence with short steps, and the elbows are flexed and reciprocal arm motion is not present. Foot strike occurs without an initial heel strike. A 2-year-old child shows increased velocity and step length and diminished cadence when compared with a 1-year-old child. Most of the adult gait patterns are present in children by 3 years, with changes in velocity, stride, and cadence continuing to 7 years of age. The gait characteristics of a 7-year-old child are similar to those of the adult.

CLINICAL EVALUATION

The evaluation of a child with an abnormal gait begins with a careful history and is followed by a thorough physical examination, with the physician paying special attention to clues identified by the history. Diagnostic studies, such as radiographs and laboratory tests, are ordered when appropriate.

History

The physician should inquire about the pregnancy and delivery, the age at which developmental milestones occurred, the presence of any systemic illnesses, and the family history for any congenital musculoskeletal abnormalities or syndromes. With respect to the gait disturbance, it is important to inquire when it was first observed, whether it is unilateral or bilateral, whether it is associated with any injuries or intercurrent systemic illness, and whether there has been a history of improvement or worsening with time.

Physical Examination

Many of the common gait disturbances can be diagnosed from the patient's clinical history. However, all children presenting with

Table 46-1. Mechanisms of Gait Disturbances

Mechanical
    Trauma, fracture, sprain
    Sports injury, overuse injury
    Child abuse
    Dysplastic lesions
    Short leg

Osseous
    Legg-Calvé-Perthes disease
    Slipped capital epiphysis
    Osteomyelitis
    Discitis
    Osteoid osteoma
    Osgood-Schlatter

Articular
    Developmental hip dysplasia
    Septic arthritis
    Toxic synovitis
    Rheumatic disease (JRA, SLE)
    Hemophilia
    Ankylosis of a joint

Neurologic
    Guillain-Barré syndrome (other peripheral neuropathies)
    Intoxication
    Cerebellar ataxia
    Brain tumor
    Lesion occupying spinal cord space
    Posterior spinal column disorders
    Myopathy
    Hemiplegia
    Sympathetic reflex dystrophy
    Cerebral palsy

Hematologic
    Sickle cell pain crisis
    Leukemia, lymphoma
    Metastatic tumor
    Primary bone tumor
    Histiocytosis

Other
    Soft-tissue infection
    Kawasaki disease
    Conversion reaction
    Gaucher disease
    Phlebitis
    Scurvy
    Rickets
    Peritonitis

Modified from Behrman R, Kliegman R (eds). Nelson Essentials of Pediatrics, 2nd ed. Philadelphia: WB Saunders, 1994:711.
Abbreviations: JRA = juvenile rheumatoid arthritis; SLE = systemic lupus erythematosus.

gait disturbance require very careful evaluation of the musculoskeletal and neurologic systems.

GENERAL MUSCULOSKELETAL EXAMINATION

The musculoskeletal examination begins with the child's ambulating in the examining room or adjacent hallway. The child must be adequately undressed and be observed from a distance while walking so that the trunk and lower extremities can be clearly visualized. The position of the thighs, knees, and lower legs, as well as the feet should be observed during ambulation. Gait observation, plus the clinical history, allows diagnosis of most of the common gait disturbances—torsional variations (in-toeing and out-toeing), toe-walking (equinus gait), and limping.

Limping is categorized into either painful (*antalgic*) or nonpainful (*Trendelenburg gait*), depending on the length of the stance phase. In an antalgic gait, the stance phase is shortened because the child decreases the time spent on the painful extremity. In a Trendelenburg gait, which is indicative of underlying proximal muscle weakness (muscular dystrophy) or hip instability (developmental hip dysplasia), the stance phase is equal between the involved and uninvolved sides, but the child leans over the involved side to shift the center of gravity over the involved extremity for balance. If the disorder is bilateral, it produces a waddling gait.

When the child is walking, the observer records the direction of the long axis of the foot with respect to the direction in which the child is walking. This defines the line of progression and is useful in the evaluation of in-toeing or out-toeing.

After the child's gait has been assessed, a careful musculoskeletal examination of both the upper and lower extremities is performed. Although most of the findings in gait disturbances are confined to the lower extremities, it is important to assess the upper extremities and spine because they may be part of an underlying disease process. The range of motion of all joints should be assessed, and they should be palpated for evidence of tenderness, effusion, synovial thickening, and increased warmth.

Examination of the lower extremities, the most important part of a child with a gait disturbance, should include measurement of leg lengths as well as assessment of the hip, knee, ankle, and subtalar joints. The thighs, lower legs, and feet are inspected for evidence of asymmetry, soft tissue swelling, or injury. Palpation for areas of increased warmth or tenderness is performed. The shape of the foot is assessed for possible intrinsic deformity. Spinal cord evaluation is also performed as subtle neurologic abnormalities may produce a gait disturbance (tethered spinal cord, tumor).

Leg Length Measurements

The most accurate clinical method to measure leg lengths is to have the child stand on a firm, level surface, such as the floor or countertop, with the examiner standing behind the child and placing index fingers over the lateral aspect of each iliac crest. The presence or absence of a pelvic obliquity can be observed. It is then possible to place blocks of various heights beneath the foot on the short side until the pelvis is level. The height of the block indicates the amount of leg length discrepancy. Clinical measurements obtained by use of a tape measure can also be performed but are much less accurate. The most common method is performed by measuring from the anterior superior iliac spine to the distal aspect of the medial malleolus. However, these landmarks are sometimes difficult to palpate accurately, and there can be a considerable margin of error.

Joint Assessment

The range of motion of the hips, knees, ankles, and subtalar joints of both extremities must be assessed. Hip flexion is measured along with any flexion contractures. With the hip in extension, the degrees of abduction, adduction, internal rotation, and external rotation are measured, preferably with a goniometer, and recorded. Hip rotation is most accurately measured with the child in the prone position with the knees flexed. Knee flexion and extension, ankle dorsiflexion, and plantar flexion as well as subtalar motion must be assessed and recorded.

Spinal Evaluation

Spinal mobility should also be assessed because intraspinal abnormalities, such as discitis and tumors, may initially be manifested as a gait disturbance. The child's ability to forward flex and reverse lumbar lordosis is a sign of normal mobility (see Chapter 47). Areas of tenderness and muscle spasm are determined by palpation.

NEUROLOGIC EVALUATION

After the musculoskeletal examination, a careful neurologic evaluation is performed. Many gait disturbances have a neurologic cause or association. This examination should include muscle strength testing, sensory assessment (particularly, specific level of potential sensory deficits), deep tendon reflexes, and pathologic reflexes, such as the Babinski sign (up-going toes—extensor plantar response).

RADIOGRAPHIC ASSESSMENT

The need for radiographic evaluation is based on the differential diagnosis. For many gait disturbances, radiographic assessment is not required. When necessary, plain radiographs of the lower extremities, pelvis, or spine are obtained first, followed by special diagnostic studies, such as scanograms for leg length discrepancy, technetium bone scan for localization of occult lesions or osteomyelitis, and computed tomography (CT) for assessment and localization of specific lesions. Magnetic resonance imaging (MRI) can be very helpful in the diagnosis of occult or soft tissue lesions and intraspinal pathology.

LABORATORY TESTS

Tests such as complete blood count, erythrocyte sedimentation rate, and rheumatoid factor and antinuclear antibody determinations are indicated if an infectious or inflammatory disorder is suspected. Other tests may be indicated for the diagnosis of specific disorders. Electromyography, nerve conduction studies, muscle biopsies, and nerve biopsies are frequently necessary in the diagnosis of myopathic or neuropathic disorders (see Chapter 39). Determinations of creatine phosphokinase, aldolase, and aspartate transaminase levels are important in the evaluation of striated muscle function and should be ordered in all patients suspected of an underlying myopathy.

GAIT DISTURBANCES

The most common categories of gait disturbances of childhood are classified into three groups:

- Torsional variations (in-toeing and out-toeing)
- Toe-walking (equinus gait)
- Limping (antalgic and Trendelenburg gait)

Table 46–2. Common Causes of In-Toeing and Out-Toeing

In-Toeing	Out-Toeing
Medial (internal) femoral torsion	Lateral (external) femoral torsion
Medial (internal) tibial torsion	Lateral (external) tibial torsion
Metatarsus adductus	Calcaneovalgus feet
Talipes equinovarus (clubfoot)	Hypermobile pes planus

Torsional Variations

Torsional variations, in-toeing and out-toeing of the lower extremities, are the most common gait disturbances that cause parents to seek advise from the pediatrician. Most variations do not require treatment because the disorder improves and resolves with normal growth and development; however, they produce anxiety in parents and require that the physician have a clear understanding of the cause and natural history to appropriately reassure the family.

The common causes of in-toeing and out-toeing are listed in Table 46–2. The presence of in-toeing or out-toeing does not imply an abnormality of the foot but, rather, only the direction in which the foot is pointing during ambulation. The causes of torsional variations can occur from proximal (hip) to distal (foot) in the involved extremity. Some causes, such as clubfeet, are obvious, whereas others are subtle.

Normal Developmental Alignment

It is imperative to understand the effects of *in utero* position on the alignment of the lower extremities of infants and young children. In the typical *in utero* position, the hips are flexed, abducted, and externally rotated, and the knees are flexed and the lower legs internally rotated. The feet are in a supinated position against the posterolateral aspect of the opposite thigh. The musculoskeletal examination of an infant characteristically shows 20- to 30-degree hip flexion contractures, 50 to 60 degrees of abduction, 80 to 90 degrees of external rotation in extension, and minimal or no internal rotation. The knees have a 20- to 30-degree flexion contracture, and internal tibial torsion is present. These are normal findings. The increased external rotation of the hip is not due to femoral retroversion but, rather, to a posterior hip capsule contracture, which begins to resolve at the time of independent ambulation.

The combination of external rotation at the hip and internal rotation of the lower leg produces a bowed appearance of the lower extremities in the weight-bearing position. It is not true bowing but rather a torsional combination. After ambulation, this physiologic bowing resolves over a 6- to 12-month period.

Physiologic genu valgum (*knock-knees*) is seen between 3 and 4 years of age. This is true genu valgum and not the result of torsional variations. This condition, too, resolves with growth, and normal adult knee alignment is obtained between 5 and 8 years of age. Assessment of the tibiofemoral angle (clinically and radiographically) in children between birth and 16 years of age reveals a mean varus alignment of 15 degrees in newborns. This figure decreases to approximately 10 degrees by 1 year of age. Neutral alignment occurs between 18 and 20 months of age. The maximum valgus of 12 degrees occurs by 3 to 4 years of age. The results are similar for boys and girls. By 7 years of age, the valgus alignment corrects to that of a normal adult (8 degrees in females, 7 degrees in males). Overall, 95% of developmental physiologic genu varum and genu valgum resolves with growth. This is also true for children with more pronounced physiologic varus (16 to 35 degrees)

	Right	Left
Foot-progression angle (FPA)		
Hip rotation (extension)		
• Internal rotation		
• External rotation		
Thigh-foot angle (TFA)		
Foot shape		

Figure 46–1. Torsional profile for recording the measurements of the foot progression angle, hip rotation in extension, thigh-foot angle, and foot shape. This allows comparison between the right and left sides as well as with subsequent evaluations.

or valgus (15 to 20 degrees), although in some children, the condition may not completely correct until adolescence.

Torsional Profile

The torsional profile aids in the diagnosis and sequential treatment of children with torsional variations (Fig. 46–1).

FOOT PROGRESSION ANGLE

The foot progression angle represents the direction of the long axis of the foot with respect to the direction in which the child is walking (Fig. 46–2). Inward rotation is given a negative value and outward rotation a positive value. A normal foot progression angle in children and adolescence is 10 degrees (range, −3 to 20 degrees). The foot progression angle defines whether the gait is normal or if there is an in-toeing or out-toeing gait. The latter is considered abnormal when the foot progression angle exceeds 20 degrees. The recording of the angle allows a method for comparison during follow-up evaluations because it is virtually impossible to remember the degree of in-toeing or out-toeing from one evaluation to the next.

HIP ROTATION

Hip rotation in extension is assessed with the child in the prone position and the knees together and flexed 90 degrees (Fig. 46–3).

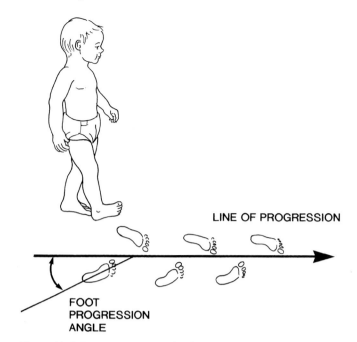

LINE OF PROGRESSION

FOOT PROGRESSION ANGLE

Figure 46–2. Foot progression angle. The long axis of the foot is compared with the direction in which the child is walking. If the foot points outward, the angle is positive. If the foot points inward, the angle is negative.

In this position, the hip is in neutral alignment. As the lower leg is rotated outwardly, internal rotation of the hip is produced, whereas inward rotation produces external rotation. This is due to the anatomic shape of the proximal femur. The femoral neck normally makes a 135-degree angle with the femoral shaft. Typically, there is anterior angulation between the axis representing the femoral neck and the transcondylar axis of the distal femur. This angulation is known as femoral anteversion. Femoral anteversion decreases from approximately 40 degrees at birth to 15 degrees by maturity. A newborn hip typically externally rotates in extension to 80 to 90 degrees and has a limited internal rotation of zero to 10 degrees. Normally, there is approximately 45 degrees of internal and external rotation by 1 year of age. Hip rotation should be symmetric. Asymmetric rotation is often indicative of a hip disorder and necessitates radiographs of the pelvis. The mean hip internal rotation in extension in older male children is 50 degrees (range, 25 to 65 degrees) and for females is 40 degrees (range, 15 to 60 degrees). The degree of hip rotation must be recorded so that it can be compared with that seen in subsequent examinations.

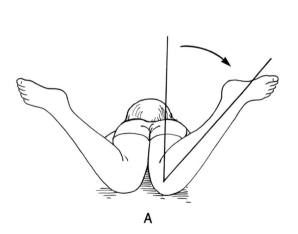
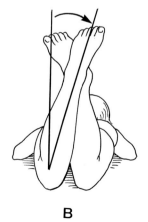

Figure 46–3. Hip rotation in extension. The child is in the prone position, with the knees flexed 90 degrees. The lower leg is vertically oriented. This is considered the neutral position. Outward rotation (A) of the leg produces internal hip rotation, inward rotation (B) produces external hip rotation.

A   B

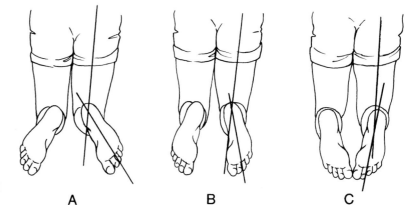

Figure 46–4. Thigh-foot angle. With the child in the prone position and the knees flexed and approximated, the long axis of the foot can be compared with the long axis of the thigh. The long axis of the foot bisects the heel and the third or middle toe. External tibial torsion *(A)* produces excessive outward rotation. Normal alignment *(B)* is characterized by slight external rotation. Internal tibial torsion produces inward rotation *(C)*.

THIGH-FOOT ANGLE

With the child in the prone position and the knees approximated and flexed 90 degrees, the long axis of the foot in the neutral or simulated weight bearing position can be compared with the long axis of the thigh (Fig. 46–4). Inward rotation is given a negative value, whereas outward rotation is given a positive value. Inward rotation is indicative of internal tibial torsion, and outward rotation represents external tibial torsion. This angle must be accurately measured and recorded. The mean thigh-foot angle is 10 degrees (range, −5 to 30 degrees) from middle childhood through adult life. Infants have a mean thigh-foot angle of −5 degrees (range, −35 to 40 degrees) as a consequence of the normal *in utero* position.

FOOT SHAPE

With the child again in the prone position, the shape of the foot is easily assessed (Fig. 46–5). This position is very helpful in the assessment of children with metatarsus adductus or a calcaneovalgus foot. The mobility of the ankle and subtalar joint can also be evaluated with the child in this position.

In-Toed Gait

INTERNAL FEMORAL TORSION

Internal femoral torsion is the most common cause of in-toeing in children 2 years of age or older. It occurs more commonly in females than males (2:1). Most affected children have the common autosomal dominant condition generalized ligamentous laxity. The etiology of femoral torsion is controversial. Some believe that it is congenital, secondary to excessive or persistent infantile femoral anteversion, whereas others believe that it is acquired, secondary to abnormal sitting habits.

Clinical Examination. Clinical features of internal femoral torsion demonstrate that the entire lower leg is inwardly rotated during gait. Characteristically, there will be 80 to 90 degrees of internal rotation of the hip in the prone, extended position (Figs. 46–6A and *B*). External rotation, as a consequence, is limited to zero to 10 degrees. Features of generalized ligamentous laxity are present, including elbow and finger hyperextension, wrist and thumb hyperabduction, knee hyperextension, and hypermobile pes planus. In-

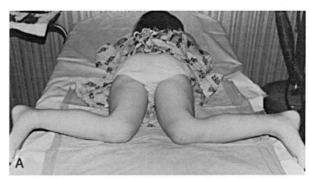
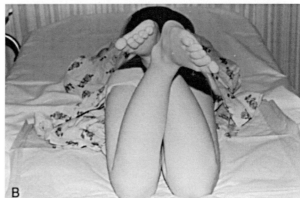

Figure 46–6. *A,* Clinical photograph of a 5-year-old girl demonstrating internal femoral torsion. She has approximately 80 degrees of internal rotation bilaterally. *B,* External rotation is limited to approximately 15 degrees, for a total arc of rotation of 90 to 95 degrees.

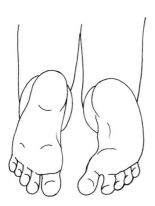

Figure 46–5. Foot shape. In the same position for measurement of the thigh-foot angle, the shape of the foot can also be evaluated. In this illustration, the left foot has normal alignment and the right foot demonstrates metatarsus adductus.

volved children commonly sit in the "television" or "W"-style position. It is felt that this position allows the lower leg to act as a lever, thereby producing the torsional changes in the biologically plastic femora. This condition has also been called excessive femoral anteversion, implying an abnormality of the proximal femur. However, the torsion actually occurs throughout the femoral shaft and results in a change in the normal alignment between the hip and the knee.

Radiographic Evaluation. Radiographic evaluation of internal femoral torsion is not routinely necessary. Results of anteroposterior radiography of the pelvis are normal, but there may be the appearance of a relatively vertical femoral neck angle, or coxa valga. However, if the radiograph is repeated with the legs in 15 degrees of abduction and internal rotation, the femoral neck angle is typically normal.

Treatment. The treatment of internal femoral torsion is predominantly by observation. Correction of abnormal sitting habits usually allows this variation to resolve with normal growth and development. It takes 1 to 3 years for complete correction to occur, depending on the age of the child when the sitting habits are corrected. The correction of sitting habits can be very difficult in preschool-aged children, and improvement frequently does not occur until these children reach school age. The use of nighttime orthoses or daytime twister cables is of no value and may produce a compensatory external tibial torsion. The combination of internal femoral and compensatory external tibial torsion produces a genu valgum deformity. This can eventually result in patellofemoral malalignment, with patella subluxation or dislocation and pain.

Children 10 years of age or older may not have enough remaining musculoskeletal growth for spontaneous correction to occur. After these older children have been followed up for 1 to 3 years without documentation of improvement (torsional profile) or if there is significant cosmetic or functional disability, surgical intervention may be necessary. The procedures advocated include proximal femoral varus derotation osteotomy and simple derotation osteotomy of either the proximal or the distal femur. Sufficient derotation is performed to allow for equal internal and external hip rotation postoperatively.

It was once believed that internal femoral torsion was associated with bunions, back pain, degenerative osteoarthritis of the hip and knee, and decreased athletic ability. This is no longer accepted as true. The only significant long-term problem is abnormal gait and the potential for patellofemoral malalignment.

INTERNAL TIBIAL TORSION

Internal tibial torsion is the most common cause of in-toeing in children under 2 years of age and is secondary to normal *in utero* positioning. This condition is commonly seen during the second year of life and may be associated with metatarsus adductus.

Clinical Examination. The degree of tibial torsion can be measured by the prone thigh-foot angle (torsional profile) (see Fig. 46–4). It can also be measured with the child supine and the knees flexed 90 degrees. The measurements should be recorded on each visit to the physician to document improvement.

Radiographic Evaluation. Radiographic assessment is of no value in the evaluation of internal tibial torsion.

Treatment. Treatment of internal tibial torsion is predominantly conservative. This is a physiologic condition, and spontaneous resolution with normal growth and development can be anticipated. Significant improvement usually does not occur until the child begins to pull to stand and walk independently. Thereafter, it takes 6 to 12 months and occasionally longer for complete correction to occur. If there has been no documented improvement by 2 to 3 years of age, the use of a nighttime orthosis, such as a Denis Browne splint, may be considered. The effectiveness of night splints is controversial because of the lack of prospective studies on this issue. Persistent internal tibial torsion in an older child or adolescent is rare and may require surgical derotation.

METATARSUS ADDUCTUS

Metatarsus adductus is a common problem of infants and young children. It occurs equally in males and females and is bilateral in approximately 50% of cases. Metatarsus adductus has hereditary tendencies and is more common in the firstborn than in later children as a result of increased molding effect from the more rigid primigravida uterus and abdominal wall. This condition is associated with acetabular hip dysplasias, as approximately 10% of children with metatarsus adductus have hip dysplasia.

Clinical Examination. Clinically, the forefoot is adducted and occasionally supinated. The hindfoot and midfoot are normal. The lateral border of the foot is convex, the base of the fifth metatarsal is prominent, and the medial border of the foot is concave. There is usually an increased interval between the first and second toes, with the great toe being held in an inwardly rotated or varus position. The ankle range of motion is normal. Forefoot mobility can vary from flexible to rigid. This parameter is assessed by stabilizing the hindfoot and midfoot in a neutral position and applying pressure over the first metatarsal head with the opposite hand. In the walking child with an uncorrected or partially corrected metatarsus adductus, there will be an in-toed gait, abnormal shoe wear, and possible discomfort from shoe pressure.

Radiographic Evaluation. Radiographs of the foot are not necessary for routine metatarsus adductus because they do not demonstrate forefoot mobility. Anteroposterior and lateral weight-bearing radiographs demonstrate adduction of the metatarsals at the tarsometatarsal joint and an increased intermetatarsal angle between the first and second metatarsals. The midfoot and hindfoot are usually normal. Radiographs should be obtained if there are any clinical abnormalities of the midfoot or hindfoot.

Treatment. Treatment of metatarsus adductus is primarily conservative. The feet may be classified into three types of deformities, depending on forefoot flexibility.

- *Type I.* The feet are flexible and can be placed into an overcorrected or abducted position. Voluntary correction can usually be elicited by stimulating the peroneal musculature by stroking the lateral border of the foot. These feet usually require no treatment and may be observed.
- *Type II.* These feet correct to the neutral position both passively and actively. The feet may benefit from a trial of modified shoes, such as straight or reversed last shoes. Commercially available orthoses may also be used. The shoes or orthoses are worn full time (22 hours per day) and re-evaluated at 4- to 6-week intervals. If the condition has improved, the treatment can be continued. If it has not improved, serial plaster casts may be necessary.

- *Type III.* Type III deformities are rigid and do not correct passively or actively. These feet are treated with serial plaster casts. The forefeet are manipulated before each cast application to stretch the medial soft tissue contractures. Short leg walking casts are applied with the hindfoot held in the neutral position and the forefoot abducted. The casts are changed at 1- to 2-week intervals. Usually, complete correction can be obtained in 4 to 6 weeks, depending on the age of the child and the severity of the deformity. The best results are obtained when the casting is initiated before 8 months of age. Once correction has been achieved, corrective shoes or orthoses may be used for an additional 2 to 3 months to maintain correction. A mild hallux varus may persist for several years after conservative treatment and may be of concern to the parents. This is commonly called the "searching toe" and eventually disappears with growth and development.

Significant metatarsus adductus persisting or presenting after 4 years of age may require surgical correction. Children 4 to 6 years of age with a fixed deformity undergo soft tissue releases. This treatment may consist of a medial release with release of the tendinous portion of the abductor hallucis muscle and capsulotomies of the first metatarsal–medial cuneiform and the medial cuneiform–navicular joint or capsulotomies of all the tarsometatarsal joints. Serial casting is then carried out until forefoot correction has been obtained. This process usually requires 2 to 3 months. Children 6 years of age or older usually do not benefit from soft tissue releases alone and require metatarsal osteotomies to achieve satisfactory correction.

TALIPES EQUINOVARUS (CLUBFOOT)

A clubfoot represents a deformity not only of the foot but of the entire lower leg. It is classified into three groups:

1. The congenital clubfoot is usually an isolated abnormality.
2. The *teratologic* form is associated with a neuromuscular disorder, such as myelodysplasia (spina bifida), arthrogryposis multiplex congenita, or a syndrome complex.
3. Positional clubfoot is a normal foot that has been held in the deformed position *in utero* (oligohydramnios). Usually, a clubfoot is an obvious abnormality.

Out-Toed Gait

EXTERNAL FEMORAL TORSION

External femoral torsion, also known as femoral retroversion, is a very rare disorder unless it is associated with a slipped capital femoral epiphysis (SCFE).

Clinical Examination. External femoral torsion shows limitation of internal rotation and excessive external rotation when the hip is examined in the extended position. Typically, the hip externally rotates 70 to 90 degrees, whereas internal rotation is only zero to 20 degrees. External femoral torsion is usually a bilateral disorder when it occurs idiopathically. If the deformity is unilateral, especially in an obese older child or a young adolescent, the presence of an SCFE must be ruled out.

Radiographic Evaluation. Anteroposterior and Lauenstein (frog) lateral radiographs of the pelvis are necessary in any child or adolescent presenting with external femoral torsion, especially those who are obese, have nontraumatic anterior thigh or knee pain (referred pain), or have unilateral deformity. Approximately 20% of children with an SCFE have simultaneous bilateral involvement. The typical changes of SCFE include widening of the physis and an abnormal relationship between the capital femoral epiphysis and the femoral neck. The femoral neck appears to be slipped inferiorly and posteriorly when, in actuality, the femoral neck is rotating anteriorly and superiorly.

Treatment. The treatment of idiopathic external femoral torsion is usually observation. It is a very rare disorder that usually causes no significant functional impairment. If the femoral retroversion is due to an SCFE, the slip is treated surgically. The most common treatment today is *in situ* pinning with single or multiple cannulated screws.

Occasionally, persistent femoral retroversion after SCFE can produce functional impairment, such as a severe out-toed gait and difficulty in opposing one's knees in the sitting position. The latter can be very disabling to females. Should this occur, a derotation osteotomy (proximal or distal) to restore the normal relationship between the proximal and distal femur is beneficial.

EXTERNAL TIBIAL TORSION

External tibial torsion is a relatively common disorder that is usually associated with a calcaneovalgus foot (Fig. 46–7*A* and *B*). It is secondary to a normal variation in *in utero* positioning. In this condition, the plantar surface of the foot is against the wall of the uterus, forcing it into a hyperdorsiflexed, everted position. This results in the calcaneovalgus foot and because of the externally rotated position, it also produces the external tibial torsion. When the alignment of the lower leg and the foot is combined with the normal increased external rotation of the hip in the newborn, it produces a very out-toed or externally rotated appearance of the lower extremity.

Clinical Examination. External tibial torsion is indicated by an abnormally positive thigh-foot angle (torsional profile) (see Fig.

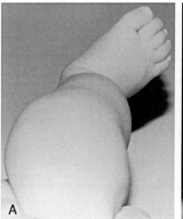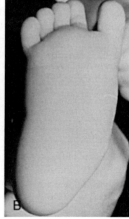

Figure 46–7. *A*, Clinical photograph of a 2-month-old infant girl demonstrating excessive external tibial torsion. This reverse or anterior thigh-foot angle shows approximately 50 degrees of external tibial torsion. *B*, A calcaneovalgus foot with forefoot abduction and increased hindfoot valgus in the same infant. There is also hyperdorsiflexibility of the foot in the ankle.

46–4), at typically 30 to 50 degrees. It is almost always associated with the calcaneovalgus foot.

Radiographic Evaluation. Radiographic assessment for external tibial torsion is not necessary.

Treatment. The treatment of external tibial torsion is observation. This condition follows the same clinical course as internal tibial torsion. Significant improvement does not occur during the first year of life. With the onset of independent ambulation, spontaneous improvement begins to occur and is typically complete by 2 to 3 years of age.

CALCANEOVALGUS FOOT

The calcaneovalgus foot is a relatively common finding in the newborn and is secondary to *in utero* positioning (see Fig. 46–7*B*). This condition is manifested by a hyperdorsiflexed foot with varying degrees of eversion and forefoot abduction. It is usually associated with external tibial torsion. These variations are typically unilateral but occasionally may be bilateral.

Clinical Examination. The infant presents with an out-toed position of the involved extremity. The dorsum of the foot can easily be brought into contact with the anterior aspect of the lower leg, and the forefoot has an abducted appearance. The increased dorsiflexion should not be confused with the neonatal gestational age classification of Dubowitz. There is usually normal or almost normal ankle plantar flexion. External tibial torsion of 30 to 50 degrees is a common associated finding.

Three other conditions must be distinguished from a calcaneovalgus foot: (1) vertical talus, (2) posteromedial bow of the tibia, and (3) neuromuscular abnormalities, such as paralysis of the gastrocnemius muscle. The differentiation is usually made clinically by physical examination of the foot, lower leg, and neurologic systems, and appropriate radiographs.

Radiographic Evaluation. Simulated weight-bearing anteroposterior and lateral radiographs of the foot may be necessary to differentiate between the calcaneovalgus foot and a congenital vertical talus. In a calcaneovalgus foot, the radiographs either are normal or reveal an increase in hindfoot valgus. In the congenital vertical talus, the hindfoot is in equinus while the midfoot and forefoot are dorsally displaced, producing a rocker-bottom appearance. Anteroposterior and lateral radiographs of the tibia and fibula are necessary if there is bowing of the lower leg.

Treatment. In the typical calcaneovalgus foot, no treatment is necessary. The hyperdorsiflexion of the foot resolves during the first 3 to 6 months of life. Occasionally, resistant feet may require passive stretching, taping, or casting into a plantar flexed position. Usually, by the time the child begins to pull to stand and walk independently, the calcaneovalgus foot has resolved. The external tibial torsion, however, persists and follows the same natural history of internal tibial torsion.

HYPERMOBILE PES PLANUS

Hypermobile, flexible, or pronated feet are common sources of concern to parents. In general, children with this deformity are asymptomatic and have no limitation of activities. The family frequently thinks that the child is out-toeing because of the pronation of the midfoot and hindfoot, which may allow the forefoot to become abducted. Flexible flatfeet are also common in neonates and toddlers as a result of the associated laxity in the bone-ligament complexes of the feet and the abundant fat in the area of the medial longitudinal arch. The child usually demonstrates significant improvement by 6 years of age. In the older child, flexible flatfeet are usually secondary to generalized ligamentous laxity, an autosomal dominant condition. Most children and adolescents with flexible flatfeet are asymptomatic.

Clinical Examination. In the non–weight-bearing position in the older child with a flexible flatfoot, the normal medial longitudinal arch is visible, but in the weight-bearing position, the foot becomes pronated with varying degrees of pes planus and hindfoot valgus. Instead of weight-bearing over the lateral column of the foot, the weight is shifted medially, producing pronation. Subtalar motion is examined with the ankle in the neutral position and should be normal or slightly increased. Loss of subtalar motion may indicate a *rigid flatfoot*. Common causes of rigid flatfeet include tendo Achilles contracture, tarsal coalition, and neuromuscular disorders. Rigid flatfeet may also be a familial trait. Evaluation of other joints, especially the elbows, hands, and knees, usually demonstrates generalized ligamentous laxity in patients with flexible flatfeet.

Radiographic Evaluation. Routine radiographs of asymptomatic flexible flatfeet are usually not indicated. Standing, anteroposterior, and lateral weight-bearing radiographs are obtained, if necessary. The most common indication is the presence of pain (Table 46–3 for differential diagnosis). Anteroposterior radiographs reveal an increase in the talocalcaneal angle (>25 degrees) caused by the excessive hindfoot valgus. The lateral view shows distortion of the normal straight line relationship between the long axis of the talus and the first metatarsal and flattening of the normal medial longitudinal arch.

Treatment. Treatment of flexible flatfeet is conservative. Children with this problem do not predictably have symptoms related to their flatfeet; therefore, modified shoes and orthoses do not significantly alter the clinical or radiographic appearance of the feet. The diagnosis of flexible flatfeet is usually not possible until after 6 years of age. Treatment is indicated only for symptoms not attributable to other causes or to abnormal shoe wear. Feet that are symptomatic with vigorous physical activity usually respond readily to the use of commercially available medial longitudinal arch supports. Custom-made supports are usually more expensive and in most cases not more effective than commercially available supports. When the child has excessive heel valgus, pronation, or abnormal shoe wear that is unresponsive to a commercially or custom-made arch support, the use of a UCB (University of California, Berkeley) orthosis may be beneficial. This orthosis holds the hindfoot in the corrected position and restores the medial longitudinal arch.

Equinus Gait (Toe-Walking)

Toe-walking is probably the least common of the three categories of gait disturbances. Toe-walking can be a normal finding in children up to 3 years of age. Persistent toe-walking thereafter or acquired toe-walking at a later age is considered abnormal and

Table 46-3. Differential Diagnosis of Foot Pain

	Age (Yr)	
0–6	*6–12*	*12–20*
Poor-fitting shoes	Poor-fitting shoes	Poor-fitting shoes
Foreign body		Stress fracture
Fracture	Enthesopathy (JRA)	
Osteomyelitis*	Foreign body	Foreign body
		Ingrown toenail
		Bunion
Juvenile rheumatoid arthritis (JRA)	Accessory navicular	Metatarsalgia
	Pes cavus	Pes cavus
		Ganglion
Leukemia	Tarsal coalition	Plantar fasciitis
Drawing of blood	Hypermobile flatfoot	Avascular necrosis of metatarsal (Freiberg infarction) or navicular bone (Köhler disease)
	Trauma (sprains)	Sever disease
		Achilles tendinitis
		Trauma (sprains)
		Plantar warts
Tumor†	Tumor	Tumor†
	Osteomyelitis	

Modified from Behrman R, Kliegman R (eds). Nelson Essentials of Pediatrics, 2nd ed. Philadelphia: WB Saunders, 1994:726.
*Osteomyelitis may be hematogenous or secondary to a puncture wound.
†Soft tissue mass, osteoid osteoma, synovial sarcoma, lipoma, digital fibroma, hemangioma, subungual exostosis, Ewing sarcoma.

requires careful evaluation. The differential diagnosis for persistent or acquired toe-walking includes:

1. Neuromuscular disorders, such as cerebral palsy, Duchenne muscular dystrophy, or spinal cord abnormality resulting from a tethered spinal cord or diastematomyelia.
2. Congenital tendo Achilles contracture.
3. Leg length discrepancy.
4. Habitual toe-walking.

The differentiation of toe-walking can usually be determined from the history and the physical examination. The examiner should establish the time of onset, the amount of time a child spends walking on his or her toes, whether it can be voluntarily corrected, and whether there has been improvement or worsening over time.

NEUROMUSCULAR DISORDERS

The neuromuscular disorder most likely to produce an equinus gait, either unilateral or bilateral, is cerebral palsy. The most common type of cerebral palsy is spastic diplegia, a disorder in which the lower extremities are more involved than the upper extremities. Prematurity is a common risk factor for spastic diplegia. It can be symmetric or asymmetric, with one side being slightly more involved than the other. Spastic diplegia tends to produce a bilateral equinus gait. Spastic hemiplegia, in which only one side is involved, is usually due to birth trauma (asphyxia, *in utero* stroke) or underlying congenital malformation and results in unilateral toe-walking.

Acquired or late-onset toe-walking is usually a result of a developing neuromuscular disorder, such as Duchenne muscular dystrophy. As muscle deterioration progresses and as muscle is replaced by fat and fibrous tissues, equinus and other contractures occur. There is usually a history of progressive clumsiness and frequent episodes of falling. The diagnosis of muscular dystrophy is usually made when the child is between 3 and 5 years of age. The diagnosis is confirmed by markedly elevated creatine phosphokinase levels and by muscle biopsy.

Clinical Examination. The clinical examination of a child with toe-walking secondary to cerebral palsy shows either a tendo Achilles contracture or a spastic equinus gait without contracture and abnormal neurologic findings. These findings include increased muscle tone, spasticity, hyperactive deep tendon reflexes, and pathologic reflexes, such as a positive Babinski sign. Hamstring tightness, in addition to ankle equinus, may be a subtle sign of underlying mild cerebral palsy.

Children with Duchenne muscular dystrophy typically demonstrate pseudohypertrophy of the calves in addition to equinus contracture. They have proximal muscle weakness first, then generalized weakness, and perhaps (depending on the stage of progression) decreased or absent upper extremity and knee deep tendon reflexes. Ankle reflexes are usually preserved.

Radiographic Evaluation. Radiographic evaluation of a child with toe-walking is rarely necessary. CT or MRI of the brain may occasionally be required during the evaluation of a possible neuromuscular disorder.

Other Testing. Dynamic electromyography and gait analysis studies can occasionally be helpful in distinguishing between toe-walking due to mild cerebral palsy and a congenital tendo Achilles contracture. Serum muscle enzyme (creatine phosphokinase, aspartate transaminase, aldolase) levels and muscle biopsies are required for children with suspected Duchenne muscular dystrophy or other myopathies.

Treatment. The treatment of an equinus gait secondary to a neuromuscular disorder depends on an accurate diagnosis. The type of treatment depends on the severity of the involvement. In a spastic equinus gait without contracture, physical therapy and orthoses (daytime, nighttime, or both) may be beneficial. If a contracture has developed, serial casting may be performed in young children, whereas surgical lengthening of the tendo Achilles is usually necessary in the older child.

CONGENITAL TENDO ACHILLES CONTRACTURE

Congenital tendo Achilles contracture is a common cause of an equinus gait in young children, especially in bilateral cases. The foot cannot be dorsiflexed to the neutral or plantigrade position. The birth and developmental history and the neurologic findings are normal. A positive family history for tendo Achilles contracture, male predominance, and learning disabilities are common findings.

Clinical Examination. Examination of the ankle shows a 10- to 15-degree fixed equinus contracture. The assessment of a tendo Achilles contracture should be performed with the hindfoot held in a slightly supinated position to bring the calcaneus beneath the talus. If this position is not used, dorsiflexion of the foot produces hindfoot valgus with the appearance of more dorsiflexion than is actually present. In congenital tendo Achilles contractures, no other musculoskeletal or neurologic abnormalities are present. Muscle strength and deep tendon reflexes are normal; no pathologic reflexes are present.

Radiographic Evaluation. Radiographs are not necessary unless an associated abnormality within the foot is thought to be present. Should this occur, anteroposterior and lateral weight-bearing radiographs of the foot should be obtained.

Treatment. The treatment of congenital tendo Achilles contracture consists of serial casting in the young child. This method has a relatively high success rate, and the risk of recurrence after satisfactory correction is low. In an older child or a younger child who has not responded to serial casting, surgical lengthening of the tendo Achilles is necessary. This procedure can be performed either percutaneously or by an open Z lengthening. This is followed by 4 to 6 weeks of immobilization in a short leg cast. Postoperative orthoses are usually not required.

LEG LENGTH DISCREPANCY

Leg length discrepancy is a common cause for a unilateral equinus gait in the older child and adolescent. Usually, mild discrepancies (1 to 2 cm) can be adequately compensated for during normal gait with minimal, if any, limping or toe-walking. Greater discrepancies may result in toe-walking. This is the child's preferred method of ambulation because the equinus equalizes leg lengths and prevents limping.

The differential diagnosis of a leg length discrepancy is extensive (Table 46–4). A developmentally dislocated hip in the older child may also present as a leg length discrepancy and toe-walking.

Clinical Examination. Examination of a child with a leg length discrepancy shows shortness of the involved extremity; this can be measured by placing blocks of various heights beneath the foot until the pelvis is level. The range of motion of the joints, especially the hips, of the involved extremity must be assessed. The neurologic examination is also important. Children with subtle neurologic disorders, such as cerebral palsy, may also have a very mild leg length inequality that contributes to an equinus gait.

Radiographic Evaluation. Children with a leg length discrepancy require radiographic assessment of the lower extremities. Leg lengths can be measured radiographically by either an orthoroentgenogram or a scanogram. The orthoroentgenogram consists of overlapping exposures centered on the hips, knees, and ankles on a long cassette. The measurements of the lengths of the femur and tibia are made directly from the film. The advantage of this type of radiograph is that it shows associated angular deformities. A scanogram consists of three strip exposures of the hips, knees, and ankles on a standard-sized cassette with a radiographic ruler adjacent to the extremity. This is the most accurate method of assessment, but it does not demonstrate angular deformities. An anteroposterior radiograph of the left hand and wrist for bone age from the Greulich-Pyle atlas is also obtained. This allows a relatively accurate prediction as to when skeletal maturity will occur.

Treatment. The treatment of leg length discrepancy depends on the function of the child and the magnitude of the discrepancy at skeletal maturity. Usually, discrepancies of 2 cm or less at maturity do not require treatment, as these do not produce a functional impairment or limp. The normal mechanisms of gait allow compensation for these mild discrepancies without limping. Discrepancies between 2 and 5 cm are best managed by an appropriately timed epiphysiodesis (surgical closure of an epiphysis), of the distal femoral, or proximal tibial epiphysis, or both, of the long extremity. Discrepancies greater than 5 cm may require lengthening of the femur, tibia, or both, depending on the severity of the shortening and the location.

HABITUAL TOE-WALKING

Habitual toe-walking occurs in a child who is walking on his or her toes voluntarily. Toe-walking occurs relatively commonly in young walkers. Their history and physical examination are entirely normal. This is a diagnosis of exclusion.

Clinical Examination. The findings in the examination of the child with habitual toe-walking are normal. The ankle range of motion is full, and there is no evidence of an underlying neuromuscular disorder.

Radiographic Evaluation. Radiographic evaluation is not indicated in a child with habitual toe-walking.

Treatment. The treatment of habitual toe-walkers is observation. As the child becomes heavier and the central nervous system matures, the toe-walking should resolve. Occasionally, an older child who has habitual toe-walking may benefit by a short course of short leg walking casts. This may disrupt the toe-walking pattern and allow the child to develop a more normal gait. Habitual toe-walking is a very frustrating condition because no true abnormality is present, and the gait disturbance is voluntary. Fortunately, most habitual toe-walking ultimately resolves with growth and development.

Table 46–4. Etiology of Leg Length Discrepancy

Shortening	Lengthening
Congenital	*Congenital*
Hemiatrophy*	Hemihypertrophy*
Skeletal dysplasias	Local vascular malformation
Short femur	
Proximal focal femoral deficiency*	
Fibular, tibial hemimelia	
Developmental dysplasia of the hip*	
Tumor—Developmental	*Tumor—Developmental*
Neurofibromatosis	Neurofibromatosis
Multiple exostosis	Soft tissue hemangioma
Enchondromatosis (Ollier disease)	Arteriovenous malformation
Osteochondromatosis	Hemihypertrophy with Wilms tumor
Fibrous dysplasia (Albright syndrome)	Aneurysm
Punctate epiphyseal dysplasia	
Dysplasia epiphysealis hemimelia (Trevor disease)	
Radiation therapy prior to skeletal maturity (physeal arrest)*	
Resection of benign or malignant neoplasm	
Infection	*Infection—Inflammation*
Osteomyelitis*	Metaphyseal osteomyelitis
Septic arthritis	Rheumatoid arthritis
Tuberculosis	Hemarthrosis (hemophilia)
Trauma	*Trauma*
Physeal injury*	Metaphyseal, diaphyseal fracture
Failed joint replacement	Diaphyseal operations (bone grafts, osteotomy,
Atrophic nonunion	osteosynthesis, periosteal stripping)
Overlapping, malposition of fracture fragments*	
Burns	
Neuromuscular Disease	
Poliomyelitis	
Cerebral palsy*	
Myelomeningocele	
Peripheral neuropathy	
Focal cerebral lesions (hemiplegia)	
Other	
Legg-Calvé-Perthes disease*	
Slipped capital femoral epiphysis	

Adapted from Moseley C. Leg-length discrepancy. Pediatr Clin North Am 1986:33, 1385; and Tachdjian M. Pediatric Orthopedics, 2nd ed. Philadelphia: WB Saunders, 1990. Reprinted and modified from Behrman RE (ed). Nelson Textbook of Pediatrics, 14th ed. Philadelphia: WB Saunders, 1992:1702.
*Common.

Limping

Limping is another common gait disturbance. Limping is divided into antalgic or Trendelenburg gaits, depending on the presence or absence of pain, and the duration of the stance phase between the normal and the abnormal sides. The differential diagnosis of limping is extensive. Most causes involve the lower extremity, but spinal disorders can also produce limping or difficulty walking, especially if there is spinal cord or peripheral nerve involvement. Painful (antalgic) gaits are predominantly due to trauma, infection, neoplasia, and rheumatologic disorders. Trendelenburg gaits are generally caused by congenital, developmental, or neuromuscular disorders. Thus, antalgic gaits are due to acute disorders, whereas Trendelenburg gaits are usually due to chronic disorders. The type of gait, the presence or absence of systemic systems, and the anatomic location of the symptoms can usually be determined by the history and physical examination. Occasionally, this can be difficult, especially in the young child who is a poor historian.

The common causes of limping according to age are listed in Table 46–5.

ANTALGIC GAIT

Congenital Origin

Tarsal Coalition. Tarsal coalition, also called *peroneal spastic flatfoot*, is a common foot disorder that is characterized by a painful, rigid valgus or pronation (flatfoot) deformity of the midfoot and hindfoot in association with peroneal muscle spasm but without true spasticity. This condition represents a congenital fusion or failure of segmentation between two or more tarsal bones. However, any condition that alters the normal motion of the subtalar joint may produce the clinical appearance of a tarsal coalition. Thus, congenital malformation, inflammatory disorders (e.g., juvenile rheumatoid arthritis), infection, neoplasms, and trauma involving the subtalar joint can present with pain, limping, or other symptoms similar to a tarsal coalition.

The most common coalitions occur between the calcaneus and navicular (calcaneonavicular) and the middle or medial facet between the talus and calcaneus (talocalcaneal). Coalitions can be fibrous, cartilaginous, or osseous. The incidence of tarsal coalition

Table 46–5. **Common Causes of Limping According to Age**

Age	Antalgic	Trendelenburg	Leg Length Discrepancy

Toddler (1–3 yr)	Infection
	  Septic arthritis
	    Hip
	    Knee
	  Osteomyelitis
	  Discitis
	Occult trauma
	  Toddler's fracture
	Neoplasia
		Hip dislocation
		Neuromuscular disease
		  Cerebral palsy
			Negative

Child (4–10 yr)	Infection
	  Septic arthritis
	    Hip
	    Knee
	  Osteomyelitis
	  Discitis
	Transient synovitis of the hip
	Legg-Calvé-Perthes disease
	Rheumatologic disorder
	  Juvenile rheumatoid arthritis
	Trauma
	Neoplasia (benign, malignant)
		Hip dislocation
		Neuromuscular disease
		  Cerebral palsy
			Positive

Adolescent (11+ yr)	Slipped capital femoral epiphysis Rheumatologic disorder Juvenile rheumatoid arthritis Trauma Neoplasia (benign, malignant)		Positive

is approximately 1%, and it appears to be inherited as an autosomal dominant trait. Approximately 60% of calcaneonavicular and 50% of talocalcaneal coalitions are bilateral.

Clinical Examination. The onset of symptoms is insidious and usually occurs during late childhood or early adolescence. Although mild limitation of subtalar motion and a valgus or pronated hindfoot may have been present since early childhood, the onset of symptoms varies with the age at which the fibrous or cartilaginous coalition begins to ossify and further decrease motion. The talonavicular coalition ossifies between 3 and 5 years, the calcaneonavicular coalition between 8 and 12 years, and the middle facet talocalcaneal coalition between 12 and 16 years of age. The pain is typically felt laterally in the hindfoot and radiates proximally along the lateral malleolus and distal fibula into the peroneal muscle region. Symptoms are usually aggravated by sports or other vigorous activities and are relieved by rest. The foot is pronated both in the weight-bearing and the non–weight-bearing positions. Subtalar joint motion is diminished or absent, and attempts at motion produce pain.

Radiographic Evaluation. The diagnosis of tarsal coalition is made radiographically. The initial radiographs should include anteroposterior and lateral weight-bearing radiographs of the foot and an oblique radiograph. The latter is necessary in making the diagnosis of a calcaneonavicular coalition. Beaking of the anterior aspect of the talus in the lateral view suggests a talocalcaneal coalition. Axial views of the hindfoot can be useful in the diagnosis of a middle facet talocalcaneal coalition. CT is the diagnostic procedure of choice for this coalition.

Treatment. Treatment of symptomatic tarsal coalition varies ac-

cording to the type of coalition, the age of the patient, the extent of the coalition, and the presence or absence of degenerative osteoarthritis. It can be either nonoperative or operative. Nonoperative treatment consists of cast immobilization, shoe inserts, or orthotics. Operative management usually involves excision of the coalition and interposition of muscle (calcaneonavicular), fat, or tendon (middle facet talocalcaneal) to prevent re-formation of the coalition. Resections are effective in relieving pain, improving subtalar motion, and allowing resumption of normal activities. However, if significant degenerative osteoarthritis is present, a triple arthrodesis may be necessary. Only occasionally does nonoperative treatment yield complete relief of symptoms and restoration of normal function.

Developmental Origin

Legg-Calvé-Perthes Disease. Legg-Calvé-Perthes disease (LCPD) is idiopathic avascular necrosis (osteonecrosis) of the capital femoral epiphysis (CFE) and the associated complications in an immature growing child. This disorder is caused by an interruption of the blood supply to the CFE. It occurs predominantly in males (4 to 5:1) and is bilateral in approximately 20% of affected children. Children with LCPD have delayed skeletal or bone age, disproportionate growth, and mildly short stature. Secondary osteonecrosis is seen in patients with sickle cell anemia.

Clinical Examination. The clinical onset of LCPD typically occurs between 2 and 12 years of age, with a mean age of 7 years. Most children present with a limp and *mild* or intermittent pain in the anterior thigh or knee. This has been referred to as a "painless limp." Pertinent early physical findings include antalgic gait; mus-

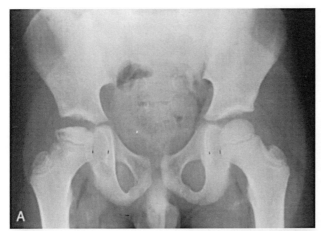
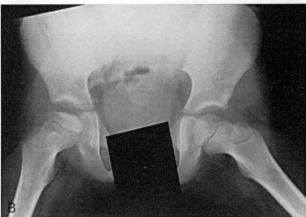

Figure 46–8. *A,* Anteroposterior radiograph of the pelvis demonstrating Legg-Calvé-Perthes disease (LCPD) of the right hip. The capital femoral epiphysis (CFE) is collapsing, and there is mild widening of the medial joint space. The left CFE is normal. *B,* Lauenstein (frog) lateral radiograph of the pelvis demonstrating limited hip abduction caused by LCPD.

cle spasm with mild restriction of hip motion, especially abduction and internal rotation; proximal thigh atrophy; and mild shortness of stature.

Radiographic Evaluation. The diagnosis is typically made from anteroposterior and Lauenstein (frog) lateral radiographs of the pelvis (Figs. 46–8*A* and *B*). The radiographic characteristics can be divided into five distinct stages, depending on the interval from the onset of symptoms: (1) cessation of CFE growth, (2) subchondral fracture, (3) resorption or fragmentation, (4) reossification, and (5) healed, or residual, stage. The symptoms are usually most pronounced during the phase of the subchondral fracture and fragmentation. A child with LCPD has a potential for collapse and extrusion of the femoral head, resulting in a permanent deformity. If plain radiographs do not demonstrate LCPD in suspected cases, technetium bone scanning or MRI is helpful.

Treatment. Legg-Calvé-Perthes is a local, self-healing disorder. Prevention of femoral head deformity and secondary degenerative osteoarthritis in adulthood are the only indications for treatment. The four basic treatment goals are (1) elimination of hip irritability, (2) restoration and maintenance of a good range of hip motion, (3) prevention of capital femoral epiphyseal collapse, extrusion, or subluxation, and (4) attainment of a spherical femoral head at healing. Current treatment methods use a concept of containment.

The femoral head is contained within the acetabulum so that the latter acts as a mold for the reossifying CFE. This task may be accomplished by nonsurgical containment using abduction casts or orthosis or by surgical containment with proximal femoral varus osteotomy, pelvic osteotomy, or both. The long-term results favor operative containment, and satisfactory results occur in approximately 85% of cases.

Slipped Capital Femoral Epiphysis. Slipped capital femoral epiphysis is the most common adolescent hip disorder. It generally occurs in those who are either obese and have delayed skeletal maturation or those who are tall and thin and have had a recent growth spurt. It can also occur as a complication of an underlying endocrine disorder, such as hypothyroidism and pituitary disorders. When a SCFE occurs before puberty, a hormonal abnormality or systemic disorder should be suspected. Studies of the histopathology of SCFE have indicated that mechanical factors are the ultimate cause of slippage. The initial abnormality is most likely secondary to endocrine changes during early adolescence. Obesity produces high shear forces across a weakened and obliquely oriented CFE, resulting in slippage.

Clinical Examination. The physical findings depend on the degree of slippage and the classification. The disorder is classified as either stable or unstable. In an unstable or acute SCFE, the CFE is separated from the femoral neck. This is extremely painful, and the adolescent is unable to stand or bear weight on the involved extremity. In a stable or chronic SCFE, the most common type, the CFE and femoral neck are in continuity and the slippage is occurring slowly by plastic deformation. The adolescent has an antalgic, out-toed gait. The hip range of motion demonstrates a lack of internal rotation and an increase in external rotation. Also, as the hip is flexed, it becomes progressively more externally rotated. Limitation of flexion and abduction in extension may also be present as a result of the deformity of the proximal femur.

Radiographic Evaluation. The diagnosis of SCFE is confirmed radiographically. Anteroposterior and Lauenstein (frog) lateral radiographs of the pelvis must be obtained (Fig. 46–9*A–D*). Both hips should be visualized on each radiograph for simultaneous comparison. The earliest sign of SCFE is widening of the physeal plate without slippage. This is considered a *pre-slip condition.* If slippage occurs, the CFE remains in the acetabulum while the femoral neck rotates anteriorly and superiorly, resulting in a varus, retroverted femoral head and neck. The severity of slippage can be classified radiographically by the degree of displacement of the CFE on the femoral neck.

Treatment. The goals of treatment are to prevent further slippage and minimize complications. This is achieved by performing an epiphysiodesis of the CFE. The technique selected depends on the classification and severity of slippage. The most common method is *in situ* internal fixation with a single or multiple cannulated screw.

Complications include chondrolysis and avascular necrosis of the CFE. These occur in approximately 5% of cases and can be another cause of limping.

Trauma

Sprains, Strains, and Contusions. *Sprains* refer to ligamentous injuries, whereas *strains* are muscle injuries. *Contusions* are the

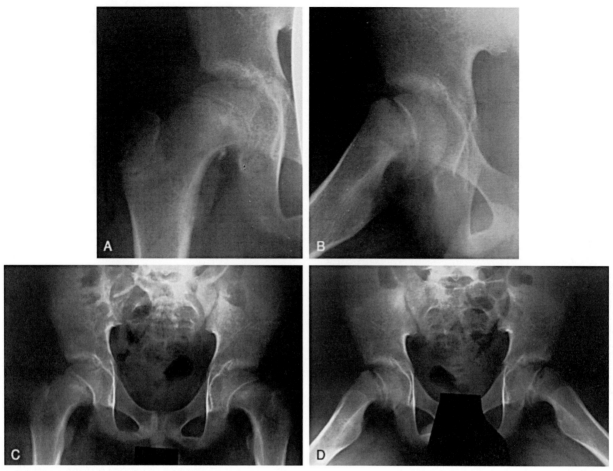

Figure 46–9. *A,* Anteroposterior radiograph of the right hip in a 13-year-old obese boy who had been limping and complaining of anterior thigh and knee pain for approximately 2 months. There is a mild stable or chronic slipped capital femoral epiphysis (SCFE). Klein's line, a line drawn along the superior aspect of the femoral neck, does not bisect the lateral portion of the CFE, thereby indicating slippage. Also, the physis is wide and irregular. *B,* Lauenstein (frog) lateral radiograph clearly demonstrates the slippage of the CFE with respect to the femoral neck. *C,* Anteroposterior radiograph of the pelvis demonstrates an asymptomatic mild stable or chronic left slipped capital femoral epiphysis. It is always important to order radiographs of the pelvis rather than individual views of the right or left hip. *D,* Lauenstein lateral radiograph confirms bilateral slipped capital femoral epiphysis.

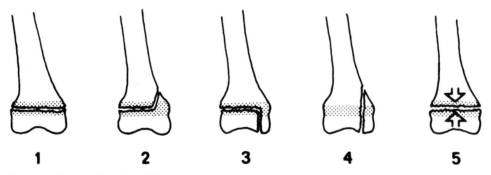

Figure 46–10. Salter-Harris classification of epiphyseal fractures.

1, The epiphysis separates from the metaphysis. The germinal cells remain with the epiphysis, usually uninjured. Healing is rapid and growth is seldom arrested.

2, Similar to type 1, except that a small piece of metaphysis breaks free to remain with the epiphysis. Healing is rapid and growth is usually normal. Types 1 and 2 are the most common.

3, Separation passes a variable distance along the physis, then crosses the epiphysis. Accurate reduction of the intra-articular fracture is necessary to prevent later traumatic arthritis. Open reduction may be needed. Growth disturbances are not usually a problem.

4, The fracture extends from the joint, across the physis, and into the metaphysis. This usually requires open reduction to prevent unilateral growth arrest and traumatic arthritis from malposition.

5, This is a crushing injury that leads to death of the germinal cells of the physis and arrest of growth. This type is rare.

(1–5, From Behrman RE [ed]. Nelson Textbook of Pediatrics, 14th ed. Philadelphia: WB Saunders, 1992:1722.)

result of a direct injury and involve the skin and the subcutaneous tissues as well as underlying muscle.

Sprains are divided into three grades:

- *Grade I*: mild with only slight stretching of the ligament
- *Grade II*: a moderate injury with partial tearing of the ligament but normal stability and
- *Grade III*: a severe injury with ligamentous disruption and instability.

Strains, sprains, and contusions of the lower extremities are among the most common injuries in children and adolescents that produce limping. There is usually a history of trauma, and the location is readily apparent because of soft tissue swelling, ecchymoses, and pain. Most of these injuries occur during athletic activities, but they can also be the result of simple (occult or witnessed) falls or other minor injuries.

Clinical Examination. In sprains, the physical examination typically reveals that the involved ligament is tender to direct palpation. There may be soft tissue swelling as well as ecchymoses. The range of motion of the involved joint is typically decreased because of pain. Occasionally, a mild joint effusion or hemarthrosis may be present.

Strains involve the muscles, and there is usually tenderness to palpation, soft tissue swelling, and pain with joint motion as a result of stretching of the involved muscle. A palpable defect within the muscle is uncommon except in the most severe injuries. These injuries usually limit the excursion of the muscle and its associated joints.

Radiographic Evaluation. In children who sustain sprains, strains, or significant contusions, anteroposterior and lateral radiographs should be obtained of the involved area. A word of caution is necessary regarding sprains. In children, ligaments are usually stronger than the adjacent physes or growth plates. Therefore, a physeal injury may be present and may have the same clinical features as a sprain (Fig. 46–10). This is especially true with lateral ankle injuries. It is more likely that a Salter-Harris type 1 separation of the distal fibular epiphysis has occurred rather than a true ligament injury. This condition should be suspected when there is more tenderness to palpation over the lateral malleolus than over the ligaments. If plain radiographs are normal, stress radiographs may be necessary for the diagnosis to be made. This concept also applies to the knee, and the examiner must always keep this in mind when a knee sprain is thought to be present.

Treatment. Treatment of sprains, strains, and contusions is usually symptomatic unless there is a grade III sprain or a physeal fracture. In the latter, cast immobilization is necessary.

Occult Fractures. Occult fractures of the tibia are a relatively common cause of limping or perhaps refusal to bear weight in very young children. They can also occur in the femur and fibula. These fractures can be the result of very innocuous trauma, such as tripping while walking, stepping on a toy, or falling from a height. Frequently, especially in very young children, the injury may not have been observed, and the child cannot convey to the parents what happened. This can result in a very confusing appearance.

The most common occult fracture in early childhood is the "toddler's fracture" of the tibia. This is an oblique fracture of the distal third of the tibia without an associated fibula fracture. It most commonly occurs in children younger than 4 years of age. Occult tibia fractures can also occur in the metaphyseal regions, usually distally, but only rarely in the diaphysis. Diaphyseal fractures are more commonly the result of child abuse.

Clinical Examination. Physical findings in a child with an occult fracture can be very subtle. There is usually minimal, if any, soft tissue swelling. There is mild tenderness and perhaps increased warmth to palpation over the fracture. Occasionally, the increased warmth may be indicative of osteomyelitis. Stress examination of the involved bone increases discomfort.

Radiographic Evaluation. Anteroposterior and lateral radiographs are obtained in the evaluation for an occult fracture (Figs. 46–11*A*, *B*). Frequently, these reveal no abnormality. The characteristic finding of a toddler's fracture is a faint oblique fracture line crossing the distal one third of the tibia. Occasionally, oblique radiographs may be helpful in revealing the fracture. If plain radiographs are normal, if the child has no systemic symptoms, and if an occult fracture of the tibia is suspected, simple immobilization in a long-leg cast for 1 to 2 weeks followed by another set of radiographs usually reveals the fracture and evidence of healing. If, however, the child has systemic symptoms, such as low-grade fever and osteomyelitis is thought to be present, a technetium bone scan should be obtained. This has been demonstrated to be effective in distinguishing between occult fractures and early osteomyelitis.

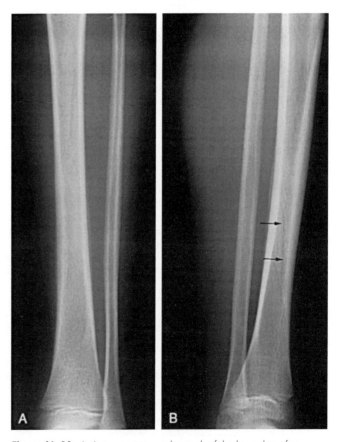

Figure 46–11. *A,* Anteroposterior radiograph of the lower leg of a 2-year-old girl who had been limping on the left lower leg for approximately 1 week. There was no observed trauma. No obvious abnormality is visible in this view. *B,* Lateral radiograph showing a faint oblique fracture line *(arrows).* This is characteristic of the "toddler's fracture." There is already early subperiosteal new bone or callus formation posteriorly.

Treatment. An occult fracture, such as toddler's fracture, is treated with simple cast immobilization. Usually within 1 to 2 weeks, there will be evidence of subperiosteal new bone formation even if a fracture line is not visible. The fractures typically heal satisfactorily within 2 to 4 weeks. A hip spica cast may be necessary for an occult fracture of the proximal femur.

Neoplasia

Neoplastic lesions of the musculoskeletal system in children are common. Fortunately, most are benign. Neoplastic lesions, benign or malignant, that involve bone, cartilage, or soft tissue of the spine, pelvis, and lower extremities can present as a mass, can cause pain, and can produce an antalgic gait. Night pain is a common characteristic of both benign and malignant primary or metastatic tumors. Osseous lesions can usually be diagnosed on plain radiographs, whereas those of cartilage or soft tissue may require MRI or other special imaging studies for diagnosis.

Benign Neoplasms. The most common benign lesions that produce limping include a unicameral (simple) bone cyst and osteoid osteoma (Table 46–6). Other less common benign lesions that can produce pain and limping include eosinophilic granuloma of bone,

Table 46–6. Benign Bone Tumors and Cysts

Disease	Characteristics	Roentgenography	Treatment	Prognosis
Osteochondroma (osteocartilaginous exostosis)	Common; distal metaphysis of femur, proximal humerus, proximal tibia; painless, hard, nontender mass	Bony outgrowth, sessile or pedunculated	Excision, if symptomatic	Excellent; malignant transformation rare
Multiple hereditary exostoses	Osteochondroma of long bones; bone growth disturbances	As above	As above	Recurrences
Osteoid ostoma	Point tenderness; pain relieved by aspirin; femur and tibia; predominantly found in males	Osteosclerosis surrounds small radiolucent nidus, 1 cm	As above	Excellent
Giant osteoid osteoma (osteoblastoma)	As above, but more destructive	Osteolytic component; size greater than 1 cm	As above	Excellent
Enchondroma	Tubular bones of hands and feet; pathologic fractures, swollen bone; Ollier disease if multiple lesions are present	Radiolucent diaphyseal or metaphyseal lesion; may calcify	Excision or curettage	Excellent; malignant transformation rare
Nonossifying fibroma	Silent; rare pathologic fracture; late childhood, adolescence	Incidental roentgenographic finding; thin sclerotic border, radiolucent lesion	None or curettage with fractures	Excellent; heals spontaneously
Eosinophilic granuloma	Age 5–10 yr, skull, jaw, long bones; pathologic fracture; pain	Small, radiolucent without reactive bone; punched out lytic lesion	Biopsy, excision rare; irradiation	Excellent; may heal spontaneously
Brodie abscess	Insidious local pain; limp; suspected as malignancy	Circumscribed metaphyseal osteomyelitis; lytic lesions with sclerotic rim	Biopsy; antibiotics	Excellent
Unicameral bone cyst (simple bone cyst)	Metaphysis of long bone (femur, humerus); pain, pathologic fracture	Cyst in medullary canal, expands cortex; fluid-filled unilocular or multilocular cavity	Curettage; steroid injection into lesion; bone graft	Excellent; some heal spontaneously
Aneurysmal bone cyst	As above; contains blood, fibrous tissue	Expands beyond metaphyseal cartilage	Curettage, bone graft	Excellent

From Thompson GH. Common orthopaedic problems of children. *In* Behrman RE, Kliegman RM (eds). Nelson Essentials of Pediatrics, 2nd ed. Philadelphia: WB Saunders, 1994:744.

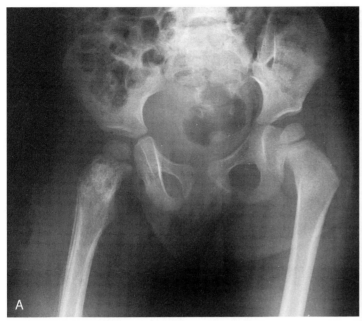

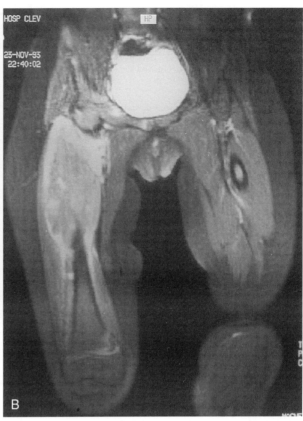

Figure 46–12. *A,* Anteroposterior pelvic radiograph of a 2-year-old girl who had been limping for 4 months. There is an extensive destructive lesion on the right proximal femur. *B,* A large soft-tissue mass is demonstrated in MRI scan. The preoperative diagnosis was Ewing sarcoma, but at biopsy the diagnosis was acute lymphoblastic leukemia.

osteochondroma, and chondroblastoma. The latter typically involves the epiphysis, especially of the proximal humerus.

In unicameral bone cysts, the symptoms are usually due to a nondisplaced pathologic fracture. Occasionally, a displaced fracture may occur. The most common location for a unicameral bone cyst is the proximal humerus, followed by the proximal femur. These can occur in any of the bones of the lower extremities, including the foot.

Osteoid osteomas have a highly vascularized nidus, which incites an intense, painful, inflammatory reaction. This results in sclerosis of the surrounding bone. The pain is typically worse at night and is characteristically relieved by aspirin.

Radiographic Evaluation. Most benign neoplasms are visible on anteroposterior and lateral radiographs of the symptomatic area. Characteristics of benign lesions include well-circumscribed lesions without periosteal new bone formation or soft tissue mass. If a lesion is suspected but not visible on plain radiographs, such as may occur in an osteoid osteoma, a technetium bone scan may be helpful in localizing the lesion. Further evaluation can be achieved with CT or MRI.

Treatment. The diagnosis and treatment of benign neoplasms are usually surgical. Biopsy is usually necessary to obtain a histologic diagnosis. Unicameral bone cysts can be managed by steroid injections or curettage and bone grafting. Osteoid osteomas usually require resection to relieve symptoms. Other benign lesions are usually excised at the time of biopsy.

Malignant Neoplasms. Malignant lesions of the musculoskeletal system are relatively uncommon. Leukemia is the most common childhood malignancy, and frequently is accompanied by musculo-

skeletal complaints (Fig. 46–12*A, B*). Other common malignancies involving the musculoskeletal system include osteogenic sarcoma, Ewing sarcoma, and intraspinal tumors, such as astrocytomas (Table 46–7). The latter tends to produce neurologic symptoms, such as muscle weakness, as the cause of limping. The other lesions may produce a mass, bone weakness, and possible pathologic fractures. Weight loss, fever, and pain are common associated complaints.

Clinical Evaluation. A careful musculoskeletal and neurologic examination is necessary for any child with a suspected neoplasm. In many cases, a mass, either in the involved bone or in adjacent soft tissues, may be palpable. These are typically tender. Increased warmth is also commonly present. These lesions are frequently adjacent to joints and may result in decreased range of motion. Neurologic evaluation may show evidence of muscle weakness or abnormal reflexes, suggesting spinal cord or peripheral nerve involvement.

Radiographic Evaluation. Anteroposterior and lateral radiographs of the involved area will usually reveal the presence of a neoplasm. Characteristics of a malignant osseous lesion include bone destruction, permeative or infiltrative appearance, periosteal new bone formation (Codman triangle), and an associated soft tissue mass (see Table 46–7). Radiographic abnormalities associated with acute leukemia include diffuse osteopenia, metaphyseal bands, periosteal new bone formation, geographic lytic lesions, sclerosis, and permeative distraction. Posteroanterior and lateral standing radiographs of the spine are necessary in the initial evaluation of a suspected spinal lesion. Additional studies, such as technetium bone scanning or MRI, may be helpful in localizing the lesion. CT and angiography may also be necessary in the preoperative assessment of malignancies.

Table 46–7. Comparison of Osteogenic and Ewing Sarcoma

	Osteogenic Sarcoma	Ewing Sarcoma
Age	> 10 yr	< 10 and > 10 yr
Race	Both	White
Sex (M:F)	1.5:1	1.5:1
Cell	Spindle cell, osteoid	Nonosseous, small round cell
Predisposition	Retinoblastoma Radiotherapy Alkylating agents	None
Site	Metaphysis, epiphysis; distal femur > proximal tibia > proximal humerus	Diaphysis, medullary cavity, cortical bone, soft tissue; femur > pelvis > tibia > humerus
Presentation	Local pain	Pain, fever, increased ESR, FUO, weight loss
Roentgenogram	Lytic, sclerotic Sunburst pattern	Mottled, lytic Onion skin pattern
Differential diagnosis	Ewing sarcoma, osteomyelitis	Osteomyelitis, eosinophilic granuloma, lymphoma, neuroblastoma, rhabdomyocarcoma
Metastasis	Lung, bones Skip lesions in the same bone	Lung, bones
Treatment	Surgery, chemotherapy Limb salvage if resectable and the patient is near adult height	Surgery, radiotherapy Chemotherapy
Outcome	50%–60% survival	60% survival without metastasis, 5%–15% with metastasis, primary site dependent
Poor prognosis	Age < 10 yr, large tumor size (> 15 cm), symptoms < 2 months, metastasis	Pelvis, soft tissue tumor, increased LDH, metastasis, increased circulating PMN, decreased circulating lymphocytes

Adapted from Behrman RE (ed). Nelson Textbook of Pediatrics, 14th ed. Philadelphia: WB Saunders, 1992:1312.
Abbreviations: M = male; F = female; ESR = erythrocyte sedimentation rate; FUO = fever of unknown origin; LDH = lactate dehydrogenase; PMN = polymorphonuclear neutrophils.

Treatment. Treatment of malignant lesions is complex. When they occur in the extremities, amputation or limb salvage procedures are usually performed. For intraspinal lesions, excision is required. Occasionally, associated spinal fusions may be necessary to prevent a postoperative spinal deformity. Chemotherapy and radiation are common adjunctive therapies.

Infection

Septic Arthritis/Osteomyelitis. Bone and joint infections are a common cause of limping in toddlers and children. When the infection is confined to the synovium of a joint and the surrounding bone is not involved, the condition is termed *septic arthritis*. If the primary focus of the infection is within bone, even if the joint is secondarily involved, the condition is termed *osteomyelitis*.

Osteomyelitic processes can be acute, subacute, or chronic.

Acute osteomyelitis commonly involves the femoral neck, the distal femoral metaphysis, and the proximal tibial metaphysis, although other areas can also be involved. Acute septic arthritis usually involves the hip, knee, or ankle. Children with these infections may be acutely ill.

Subacute osteomyelitis, which has a very distinct and different presentation, occurs most commonly about the knee (Fig. 46–13A, B). These children are usually afebrile and have night pain. Their hematologic studies are normal. Radiographs show sclerotic metaphyseal lesions that occasionally cross the growth plate into the epiphysis. Culture specimens are positive only occasionally, and they invariably show *Staphylococcus aureus*.

Chronic osteomyelitis is exceedingly uncommon but is associated with open bone injuries following trauma (fractures, penetrating wounds).

Clinical Examination. Young children as well as older children with bone and joint infections may exhibit the clinical signs of bacteremia and infection, including elevated temperature, white blood cell count, erythrocyte sedimentation rate, and C-reactive protein level. Some infants just present with "pseudoparalysis." When the hip joint is involved the child holds the hip in a position of flexion, abduction, and external rotation. This position unwinds the hip capsule and allows it to hold the greatest volume of intracapsular fluid. This initially decreases pressure, but as the pus continues to accumulate, even this position fails to relieve symptoms. A hip joint effusion is usually not palpable, but there may be overlying soft tissue swelling and tenderness to palpation.

Infections about peripheral joints, such as the knee, are more easily diagnosed. There is typically a joint effusion and perhaps soft tissue swelling, erythema, and increased warmth over the metaphysis if osteomyelitis is present. Osteomyelitis typically presents with point tenderness over the involved site; with continued bone destruction and rupture of pus into the periosteum, tenderness becomes more diffuse. Infections can also occur about the ankle and foot. The foot is less common except as a sequela to puncture wounds through a tennis shoe, producing the classic *Pseudomonas aeruginosa* (or *S. aureus*) osteomyelitis-osteochondritis.

Radiographic Evaluation. Plain radiographs are usually not particularly helpful in the early diagnosis (first 7 to 10 days) of osteomyelitis, as they are usually normal, but must be obtained in the assessment of the child. Ten to 14 days of active infection must pass before there is radiographic evidence of bone destruction or periosteal bone elevation. Technetium bone scanning or MRI can be very helpful in establishing an early diagnosis.

If a septic process about the hip is suspected, an ultrasound study may be beneficial in demonstrating an effusion. If this is present, arthrocentesis or hip aspiration is necessary. The fluid is sent for analysis, including a cell count, determinations of protein and glucose levels, and Gram stain as well as cultures and sensitivi-

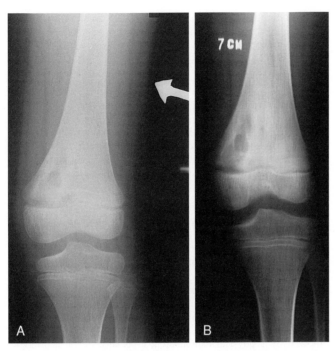

Figure 46–13. *A*, Anteroposterior radiograph of the distal femur in a 12-year-old girl with limping and nighttime knee pain for 6 months. There is a lucent lesion with surrounding sclerosis in the metaphysis. The lesion crosses the epiphysis; this is characteristic of a subacute osteomyelitis. *B*, Anteroposterior tomography clearly demonstrates the lucent nature of the lesion and its surrounding sclerosis.

ties. Infections of peripheral joints, such as the knee, are more readily diagnosed by arthrocentesis.

If an osteomyelitis of a metaphyseal region is suspected, the subperiosteal space and bone may be directly aspirated with a large-bore needle. If pus is not obtained, infection can usually be confirmed by technetium bone scan or MRI.

The material that is obtained from aspiration of the joint or bone should be sampled for culture and sensitivity. Unfortunately, even in an acute infection, these results are not always positive (blood cultures are also not uniformly positive). *S. aureus* is the most common organism that produces osteomyelitis; it is also the most common organism that produces septic arthritis in children 5 to 15 years of age. *Haemophilus influenzae* type b needs to be considered as a cause of septic arthritis in children younger than age 5, but its incidence is declining as a result of immunization. The gonococcus is the most common cause of septic arthritis in sexually active adolescents. Neonatal osteoarticular infection is often due to group B streptococcus or *S. aureus*, rarely to gram-negative organisms or *Candida* species. Patients with sickle cell anemia develop osteomyelitis due to *Salmonella* species or *S. aureus* and septic arthritis due to pneumococcus.

Treatment. Treatment of septic arthritis and osteomyelitis of the hip is always by surgical drainage (see Chapter 45) because the increased intracapsular pressure can tamponade the intracapsular vessels that supply the capital femoral epiphysis, resulting in avascular necrosis. If osteomyelitis involves the femoral neck, a single drill hole into the neck may be required to enhance drainage. Septic arthritis of peripheral joints, such as the knee and ankle, may be aspirated, treated with empiric antibiotics (nafcillin, methicillin, cefotaxime, ceftriaxone), and observed while one is awaiting the results of cultures and sensitivities. The need for surgical drainage is based on the clinical response over a 24- to 48-hour period. If

osteomyelitis is suspected but no pus is present within the metaphysis, this condition can also be treated empirically. In the cellulitic phase of early osteomyelitis before abscess formation, antibiotics alone can be used. When pus (abscess) is present, however, incision and drainage usually result in a more rapid resolution of infection and prevent secondary damage to the adjacent physeal plate.

Treatment of *S. aureus* osteomyelitis takes 4 to 6 weeks; this may be accomplished by an initial regimen of intravenous antibiotics; once signs of improvement occur (decreased erythrocyte sedimentation rate, decreased leukocyte count, decreased pain, negative blood culture, and decreased fever—usually after 10 to 14 days), oral antibiotics may be substituted. The bacteria must be available for minimal inhibitory concentration (MIC) serum determination, the family should be highly compliant, and follow-up should be ensured.

Discitis. See Chapter 47.

Rheumatologic

Hip Monoarticular Synovitis. Transient monoarticular synovitis of the hip is a most common cause of limping in children. It can occur in all age groups, but the mean age of onset is 6 years, with most patients being 3 to 8 years of age. Hip monoarticular synovitis is characterized by acute onset of monoarthritic hip pain, an associated limp, and mild restriction of hip motion, especially abduction and internal rotation. The pain is felt in the groin, anterior thigh, or knee. Any child with nontraumatic anterior thigh or knee pain must be carefully evaluated for hip pathology because these are the sites of referred pain. Septic arthritis and osteomyelitis must be excluded before this diagnosis can be confirmed.

The etiology of this disorder remains uncertain. Suspected causes include (1) active or recent systemic viral syndrome, (2) trauma, and (3) allergic hypersensitivity. Approximately 70% of affected children have a nonspecific viral upper respiratory infection 7 to 14 days before the onset of symptoms.

Clinical Examination. The patient is usually ambulatory, and the hip is not held in the position of flexion, abduction, or external rotation unless a significant effusion has developed. The child walks with an antalgic (painful) gait on the involved side and is usually afebrile. Laboratory findings are usually within normal limits, but occasionally a minimal elevation of the white blood cell count or sedimentation rate may be seen.

Radiographic Evaluation. Anteroposterior and Lauenstein (frog) lateral radiographs of the pelvis are necessary in children with transient monoarticular synovitis to rule out the presence of other lesions. The radiographs in synovitis are normal. Occasionally, ultrasound of the hip may be useful in demonstrating a joint effusion. Technetium bone scans may be necessary in difficult or unusual cases; these results are always normal.

Treatment. The treatment of monoarticular synovitis of the hip is symptomatic. Bed rest and non–weight bearing until these symptoms resolve, followed by limited activities for 1 to 2 weeks thereafter, constitute the treatment of choice. The child should be maintained on limited activities until the symptoms have completely resolved. A rapid return to normal activities may result in exacerbation.

When the diagnosis of monoarticular synovitis is in doubt, a hip

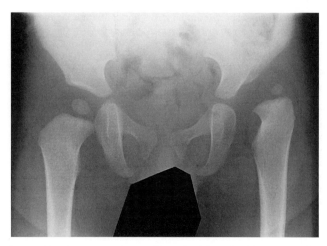

Figure 46–14. Anteroposterior radiograph of the pelvis of an 18-month-old girl demonstrating a developmental dislocation of the left hip. The acetabulum is severely dysplastic, and the femoral head is displaced laterally and superiorly. Shenton's line is markedly disrupted, and there is delayed ossification in the capital femoral epiphysis (CFE) compared with the normal right hip.

arthrocentesis may be necessary. The fluid that is aspirated shows a very low white blood cell count, and the cultures are negative.

TRENDELENBURG GAIT

Developmental Origin

Developmental Dislocation of the Hip. Developmental dislocation of the hip is a very common disorder affecting infants (Fig. 46–14), but its presence after walking age is relatively uncommon. Unfortunately, no matter how careful the initial screening evaluation, a small number of children are seen each year with a late diagnosis of developmental dislocation. When the problem occurs unilaterally, the child walks with a mild Trendelenburg gait or demonstrates toe-walking. With bilateral involvement, the child stands with an increased lumbar lordosis and has a waddling gait. A developmentally dislocated hip is asymptomatic. There is functional impairment resulting from a lack of stability and associated muscle weakness, particularly in the hip abductors (gluteus medius).

Clinical Examination. The most common physical finding in the older child with a developmentally dislocated hip is limited hip abduction on the involved side. There may be a mild hip flexion contracture and apparent shortening of the extremity. The greater trochanter lies above a line between the anterior-superior iliac spine and the ischial tuberosity (Nélaton line). In bilateral dislocations, the physical findings are more symmetric but there is still limitation of hip abduction. Positive Trendelenburg signs are present on the involved side. The normal response to a Trendelenburg test occurs when the patient stands on the uninvolved leg and the abductor muscles are able to maintain balance by elevating the contralateral pelvis. A positive Trendelenburg sign, due to pain or weakness, is demonstrated when the abductor muscles are unable to maintain pelvic balance and the patient compensates by leaning to the affected side.

Radiographic Evaluation. The diagnosis of developmental dislocation of the hip can be made from routine anteroposterior and frog lateral radiographs of the pelvis (see Fig. 46–14). Specialized studies, such as MRI and CT, are usually not necessary at this age. Ultrasound study is not usually necessary in the older child because the capital femoral epiphysis is now ossified.

Treatment. Treatment of developmental dislocation of the hip in the older child is usually surgical. The procedure consists of an open reduction of the hip with a pelvic osteotomy, femoral varus shortening derotation osteotomy, or a combination of both. The procedure selected depends on the age of the child and the severity of the deformity of the acetabulum and proximal femur.

Leg Length Discrepancy. Lower extremity inequality in older children and adolescents has been discussed earlier in this chapter.

Neuromuscular Origin

Cerebral Palsy. Children with a spastic hemiplegia or diplegia may have an associated painless limp caused by muscle spasticity and concomitant weakness of the antagonists. Usually, the diagnosis can be determined by the history of prematurity or birth trauma, followed by a physical examination, especially of the neurologic system. The neurologic examination shows evidence of increased muscle tone, spasticity, hyperactive deep tendon reflexes, and pathologic reflexes, such as Babinski signs.

SUMMARY AND RED FLAGS

Conditions associated with limp must be divided into acute, painful lesions and chronic, painless lesions. Infection and trauma must be considered as emergencies, as should conditions that are limb or articular threatening, such as osteoarthritis of the hip, avascular necrosis, or SCFE. In addition, signs of spinal cord involvement (see Chapter 47) suggest acute processes that warrant immediate attention to prevent permanent paralysis.

Red flags include acute hip pain, fever with limp, neurologic manifestations, point tenderness, the presence of a mass, and signs of weight loss.

REFERENCES

General

Salenius P, Vankka E. The development of the tibiofemoral angle in children. J Bone Joint Surg 1975;57:239–261.

Staheli LT. Lower limb. *In* Staheli LT. Fundamentals of Pediatric Orthopaedics. New York: Raven Press, 1993:4.1–4.25.

Statham L, Murray MP. Early walking patterns of normal children. Clin Orthop 1971;79:8–24.

Sutherland DH, Olshen R, Cooper L, et al. The development of gait. J Bone Joint Surg 1980;62:336–353.

Thompson GH. Pediatric orthopaedics (spine, hips, lower extremities and feet). *In* Marcus RE (ed). Orthopaedics: Problems in Primary Case. Practice Management Information Corporation, 1991:209–300.

Rotational Abnormalities

Femoral/Tibial Torsion

Hubbard DD, Staheli LT, Chew PE, et al. Medial femoral torsion and osteoarthritis. J Pediatr Orthop 1988;8:540–542.

Miller F, Merlo M, Liang Y, et al. Femoral version and neck shaft angle. J Pediatr Orthop 1993;13:382–388.

Ruwe PA, Gage JR, Ozonoff MB, et al. Clinical determination of femoral anteversion: A comparison of established techniques. J Bone Joint Surg 1992;74:820–830.

Stuberg W, Temme J, Kaplan P, et al. Measurement of tibial torsion and thigh-foot angle using goniometry and computed tomography. Clin Orthop 1991;272:208–212.

Svenvingsen S, Terjesen T, Auflein M, et al. Hip rotation and in-toeing gait: A study of normal subjects from four years until adult age. Clin Orthop 1990;251:177–182.

Metatarsus Adductus

Bleck EE. Metatarsus adductus: Classification and relationship to outcomes of treatment. J Pediatr Orthop 1983;3:2–9.

Crawford AH, Gabriel KR. Foot and ankle problems. Orthop Clin North Am 1987;18:649–666.

Farsetti P, Weinstein SL, Ponseti IV. The long-term functional and radiographic outcomes of untreated and non-operatively treated metatarsus adductus. J Bone Joint Surg 1994;76:257–265.

Talipes Equinovarus (Clubfeet)

Bill PL, Versfeld GA. Congenital clubfoot: An electromyographic study. J Pediatr Orthop 1982;2:139–142.

Cowell HR, Wein BK. Current concepts review: Genetic aspects of clubfoot. J Bone Joint Surg 1980;62:1381–1384.

Cummings RJ, Lovell WW. Current concepts review: Operative treatment of congenital idiopathic clubfoot. J Bone Joint Surg 1988;70:1108–1112.

Drvaric DM, Kuivila TE, Roberts JM. Congenital clubfoot: Etiology, pathoanatomy, pathogenesis, and the changing spectrum of early management. Orthop Clin North Am 1989;20:641–647.

Simons GW. Complete subtalar release in clubfeet: I. A preliminary report. J Bone Joint Surg 1985;67:1044–1055.

Thompson GH, Richardson AB, Westin GW. Surgical management of resistant congenital talipes equinovarus deformities. J Bone Joint Surg 1982;64:652–665.

Calcaneovalgus Foot

Meehan P. Other conditions of the foot. *In* Morrissy RT. Lovell and Winter's Pediatric Orthopaedics. Philadelphia: JB Lippincott, 1990:997–998.

Hypermobile Pes Planus

Bordelon FL. Hypermobile flatfoot in children: Comprehension, evaluation and treatment. Clin Orthop 1983;181:7–14.

Staheli LT, Chew DE, Corbet M. The longitudinal arch: A survey of 882 feet in normal children and adults. J Bone Joint Surg 1987;69:426–428.

Wenger DR, Mauldin D, Speck G, et al. Corrective shoes and inserts as treatment for a flexible flatfoot in infants and children. J Bone Joint Surg 1989;71:800–810.

Equinus Gait (Toe-Walking)

Neuromuscular Disorders

Thompson GH, Hoffer MM. Orthopedic surgery in cerebral palsy. J Neurol Rehab 1992;5:97–112.

Congenital Tendo Achilles Contracture

Griffin PP, Wheelhouse WW, Shiavi R, et al. Habitual toe-walkers: A clinical and electromyographic gait analysis. J Bone Joint Surg 1977;59:97–101.

Hicks R, Durinick PT, Gage JR. Differentiation of idiopathic toe-walking and cerebral palsy. J Pediatr Orthop 1988;8:160–163.

Leg Length Discrepancy

Canale ST, Russell TA, Holcomb RL. Percutaneous epiphysiodesis: Experimental study and preliminary clinical results. J Pediatr Orthop 1986;6:150–156.

Green SA. Limb lengthening. Orthop Clin North Am 1991;22:555–734.

Gruelich WW, Pyle SI. Radiographic Atlas of Skeletal Development of the Hand and Wrist, 2nd ed. Stanford, Calif: Stanford University Press, 1959.

Moseley CF. Leg length discrepancy. Orthop Clin North Am 1987;18:529–535.

Paley D. Current techniques of limb lengthening. J Pediatr Orthop 1988;8:73–92.

Shapiro F. Developmental patterns in lower extremity length discrepancies. J Bone Joint Surg 1982;64:639–651.

Timperlake RW, Bowen JR, Guille JT, et al. Prospective evaluation of 53 consecutive percutaneous epiphysiodeses of the distal femur and proximal tibia and fibula. J Pediatr Orthop 1991;11:350–357.

Limping

General

Phillips WA. The child with a limp. Orthop Clin North Am 1987;18:489–501.

Tarsal Coalition

Cowell HR, Elener V. Rigid painful flatfoot secondary to tarsal coalition. Clin Orthop 1983;177:54–60.

Danielsson LG. Talo-calcaneal coalition treated with resection. J Pediatr Orthop 1987;7:513–517.

Leonard MA. The inheritance of tarsal coalition and its relationship to spastic flat foot. J Bone Joint Surg 1974;56:520–526.

Pineda C, Resnick D, Greenway G. Diagnosis of tarsal coalition with computed tomography. Clin Orthop 1986;208:282–288.

Scranton PE Jr. Treatment of symptomatic talocalcaneal coalition. J Bone Joint Surg 1987;69:533–539.

Legg-Calvé-Perthes Disease

Bos CFA, Bloem JL, Bloem RM. Sequential magnetic resonance imaging in Perthes disease. J Bone Joint Surg 1991;73:219–224.

Fulford GE, Lunn PG, MacNichol MF. A prospective study of nonoperative and operative management of Perthes disease. J Pediatr Orthop 1993;13:281–285.

Herring JA, Neustadt JB, Williams JJ, et al. The lateral pillar classification of Legg-Calvé-Perthes disease. J Pediatr Orthop 1992;12:143–150.

Hoffinger SA, Rab GT, Salamon PB. ''Metaphyseal'' cysts in Legg-Calvé-Perthes disease. J Pediatr Orthop 1991;11:301–307.

Martinez AG, Weinstein SL, Dietz FR. The weight-bearing abduction brace for the treatment of Legg-Perthes disease. J Bone Joint Surg 1992;74:12–21.

Mukherjee A, Fabry G. Evaluation of the prognostic indices in Legg-Calvé-Perthes disease: Statistical analysis of the hips. J Pediatr Orthop 1990;10:153–158.

Thompson GH, Salter RB. Legg-Calvé-Perthes disease: Current concepts and controversies. Orthop Clin North Am 1987;18:617–635.

Wenger DR, Ward WT, Herring JA. Current concepts review: Legg-Calvé-Perthes disease. J Bone Joint Surg 1991;73:778–788.

Slipped Capital Femoral Epiphysis

Abraham E, Garst J, Barmada R. Treatment of moderate to severe slipped capital femoral epiphysis with extracapsular base of neck osteotomy. J Pediatr Orthop 1993;13:294–302.

Aronson DD, Carlson WE. Slipped capital femoral epiphysis: A prospective study of fixation with a single screw. J Bone Joint Surg 1992;74:810–819.

Aronson DD, Loder RT. Slipped capital femoral epiphysis in black children. J Pediatr Orthop 1992;12:74–79.

Betz R, Steel HH, Emper WD, et al. Treatment of slipped capital femoral epiphysis: Spica cast immobilization. J Bone Joint Surg 1990;72:587–600.

Carney BT, Weinstein SL, Noble J. Long-term follow-up of slipped capital femoral epiphysis. J Bone Joint Surg 1991;73:677–674.

Krahn TH, Canale ST, Beaty JH, et al. Long-term follow-up of patients with avascular necrosis after treatment of slipped capital femoral epiphysis. J Pediatr Orthop 1993;13:154–158.

Loder RT, Richards BS, Shapiro PS, et al. Acute slipped capital femoral epiphysis: The importance of physeal stability. J Bone Joint Surg 1993;75:1134–1140.

Mann DC, Weddington J, Richton S. Hormonal studies in patients with slipped capital femoral epiphysis without evidence of endocrinopathy. J Pediatr Orthop 1988;8:543–545.

Wells D, King JD, Roe TF, et al. Review of slipped capital femoral epiphysis associated with endocrine disease. J Pediatr Orthop 1993;13:610–614.

Wilcox P, Weiner D, Leighly B. Maturation factors in slipped capital femoral epiphysis. J Pediatr Orthop 1988;8:196–200.

Sprains/Strains

Reider B. Sports Medicine: The School-Age Athlete. Philadelphia: WB Saunders, 1991.

Wojtys EM. Sports injuries in the immature athlete. Orthop Clin North Am 1987;18:689–708.

Occult Fractures

Aronson J, Garvin K, Seibert J, et al. Efficiency of the bone scan for occult limping toddlers. J Pediatr Orthop 1992;12:38–44.

Mellick LB, Reesor K. Spiral tibial fractures of children: A commonly accidental spiral long bone fracture. Am J Emerg Med 1990;8:234–237.

Oudjhane K, Newman B, Oh KS, et al. Occult fractures in preschool children. J Trauma 1988;28:858–860.

Tenenbien M, Reed MH, Black GB. The toddler's fracture revisited. Am J Emerg Med 1990;8:208–211.

Neoplasia

Campanacci M, Capanna R, Picci P. Unicameral and aneurysmal bone cyst. Clin Orthop 1986;204:25–36.

Dubousset J, Missenard G, Kalifa C. Management of osteogenic sarcoma in children and adolescents. Clin Orthop 1991;270:52–59.

Hall TR, Kangarloo H. Magnetic resonance imaging of the musculoskeletal system in children. Clin Orthop 1989;244:119–130.

Healy JH, Gheluran B. Osteoid osteoma and osteoblastoma: Current concepts and recent advances. Clin Orthop 1986;204:76–85.

Heinrich SD, Gallagher D, Warrior R, et al. The prognostic significance of the skeletal manifestations of acute lymphoblastic leukemia of childhood. J Pediatr Orthop 1994;14:105–111.

Jaffe N. Advances in the management of malignant bone tumors in children and adolescents. Pediatr Clin North Am 1985;32:801–810.

Makley JT, Carter JR. Eosinophilic granuloma of bone. Clin Orthop 1986;204:37–44.

Schubiner JM, Simon MA. Primary bone tumors in children. Orthop Clin North Am 1987;18:577–596.

Osteomyelitis/Septic Arthritis

Fletcher BD, Scoles PV, Nelson AD. Osteomyelitis in children: Detection by magnetic resonance. Radiology 1984;150:57–60.

Green NE, Edwards K. Bone and joint infection in children. Orthop Clin North Am 1987;18:555–576.

Scoles PV. Antimicrobial therapy of childhood skeletal infections. J Bone Joint Surg 1984;66:1487–1492.

Shaw BA, Kasser JR. Acute septic arthritis in infancy and childhood. Clin Orthop 1990;257:212–225.

Hip Monoarticular Synovitis

Hauseisen DC, Weiner DS, Weiner SD. The characterization of "transient synovitis of the hip" in children. J Pediatr Orthop 1986;6:11–17.

Landin LA, Danielsson LG, Wattsgard C. Transient synovitis of the hip: Its incidence, epidemiology and relation to Perthes disease. J Bone Joint Surg 1987;69:238–242.

Developmental Dysplasia of the Hip

Bernard AA, O'Hara JN, Bazin S, et al. An improved screening system for the early detection of congenital dislocation of the hip. J Pediatr Orthop 1987;7:277–282.

Forlin E, Choi IH, Guille JT, et al. Prognostic factors in congenital dislocation of the hip treated with closed reduction. J Bone Joint Surg 1992;74:1140–1152.

Gabuzda GM, Renshaw TS. Current concept review: Reduction of congenital dislocation of the hip. J Bone Joint Surg 1992;74:624–631.

Hensinger RD. Congenital dislocation of the hip: Treatment in infancy to walking age. Orthop Clin North Am 1987;18:597–616.

Kumar SJ, MacEwen GD. The incidence of hip dysplasia with metatarsus adductus. Clin Orthop 1982;164:234–235.

Mankey MG, Arntz CT, Staheli LT. Open reduction through a medial approach for congenital dislocation of the hip: A critical review of the Ludloff approach in sixty-one hips. J Bone Joint Surg 1993;75:1334–1345.

Weinstein S. Natural history of congenital hip dislocation and hip dysplasia. Clin Orthop 1987;225:62–65.

47 Back Pain in Children and Adolescents

Peter V. Scoles

Healthy children rarely have severe or persistent back pain. When children do report back pain, symptoms most often are of brief duration and subside spontaneously. Back pain is a more common complaint in adolescent patients and is frequently related to sports or work activities. Usually the duration of symptoms is brief and the precipitating cause is known. The pain is most often mild and does not interfere greatly with the daily activities of the patient. When no abnormalities are present on physical examination, there is no need for laboratory or imaging studies. Little treatment beyond rest, gradual resumption of activity, and a program of conditioning exercises is required. Back pain that persists, becomes more severe, or is associated with abnormalities on physical examination is a very serious finding in children and adolescents and requires thorough evaluation.

EVALUATION OF THE PEDIATRIC SPINE

Examination of the spine should be part of both the routine physical examination in the healthy child and adolescent and the overall examination performed for the work-up of patients with other organ system illness. Primary evaluation is not difficult; no specialized equipment is necessary, and the most important diagnostic skill required is careful observation. Even in patients who present with back pain as a chief complaint, the most important diagnostic steps are a detailed history and a thorough and systematic examination (Table 47–1).

When findings on screening examinations are abnormal or when a patient presents with complaints of back pain, a more detailed examination is required. The spinal column, spinal cord, and spinal nerves are intimately related, and disorders affecting any one of these elements produce symptoms and signs in the others. Detailed examination of strength in the muscles of the spine and lower extremities (Fig. 47–1), sensation (Fig. 47–2), abdominal and lower extremity reflexes, anal sphincter tone, and perianal sensation should be performed when the primary examination suggests involvement of the neural structures that pass through the spinal column. *Persistent or severe back pain is uncommon in children and adolescents and is often associated with serious underlying disease.*

Interpretation of the results of patient evaluation requires an understanding of the normal sequence of growth and development of the spine, a knowledge of normal spinal alignment, and an understanding of the age-related differential diagnosis of potential spinal disorders in children.

Normal Growth and Development of the Spine

Formation of the vertebral column begins during the third week of gestation and is complete by the end of the first trimester.

Although further growth and primary ossification of the spinal column occurs during the second and third trimesters, the cartilaginous model of the spine is complete by week 12 of embryonic development. Subsequent vertebral growth occurs in an orderly fashion throughout childhood and adolescence. As a general rule, 50% of vertebral column height is present by age 2 years. Growth of the trunk is linear throughout childhood. Acceleration of vertebral growth occurs during the adolescent growth spurt but contributes less to total height than does lower limb growth; the sitting height of early and late adolescent siblings is often remarkably similar. Spinal growth slows at menarche in females and at the time of voice change in males and is usually complete 2 to 3 years later. Developmental abnormalities of the column, such as idiopathic scoliosis, most commonly first appear just before the growth spurt. Alterations in spinal configuration caused by congenital deformities of vertebral segments change most rapidly during

Table 47–1. Guidelines for Primary Examination of the Back

History

Is there a history of back pain? If so, what is the:
 Frequency
 Duration
 Relationship to activity
 Antecedent trauma
Is there associated pain in legs?
Is there incontinence or enuresis?
Is walking painful?
Have there been systemic signs of chronic illness?
Is there a family history of deformity?
Is there a family history of disc disease?

Physical Examination

General Appearance

Are the right and left sides of the trunk symmetric?
Are there hairy patches, nevi, sinuses, or dimpling over the
 midline of the spine?
Are the pelvis and shoulders level?
Is there normal kyphosis and lordosis?
On forward bending, is a rib hump present?

Motion

Can the patient easily bend forward and touch his or her toes?
Is normal hamstring flexibility present?

Lower Extremities

Are leg lengths equal?
Is strength normal in the major motor groups of the lower limbs?
Is sensation normal in the lower limbs?
Are reflexes normal at the knees and ankles?
Are pathologic reflexes present?

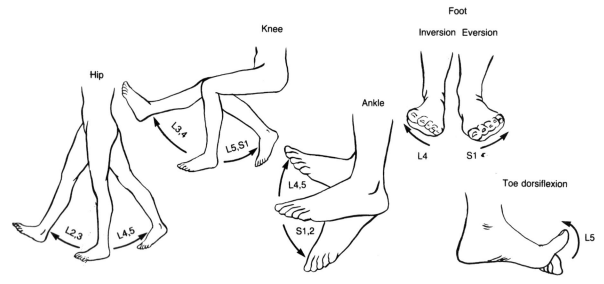

Figure 47–1. Motor control of the lower extremity. (From Reilly BM. Practical Strategies in Outpatient Medicine, 2nd ed. Philadelphia: WB Saunders, 1991:926.)

periods of rapid spinal growth: before age 2 years and at the time of the growth spurt.

Development of the spinal column is intimately connected to the development of other organ systems; there is a high association of genitourinary tract, cardiac, and neural abnormalities in patients with congenital abnormalities of the spine. Warning signs in patients with congenital spine deformities include leg-length inequality, foot-size asymmetry, high arches, hairy patches over the spine, sacral dimpling, enuresis, lower extremity reflex asymmetry, and lower extremity weakness.

Normal Spinal Alignment

The normal trunk is symmetric when viewed from the front or the back (Fig. 47–3). The shoulders and pelvis are parallel to each other and to the ground. The distance between the right and left elbows and the sides of the trunk is equal. When the trunk is viewed from the side, a series of curves is present (see Fig. 47–3). In the cervical region, a convex anterior lordotic curve is present. In the thoracic region, the spine is concave anteriorly in a kyphotic

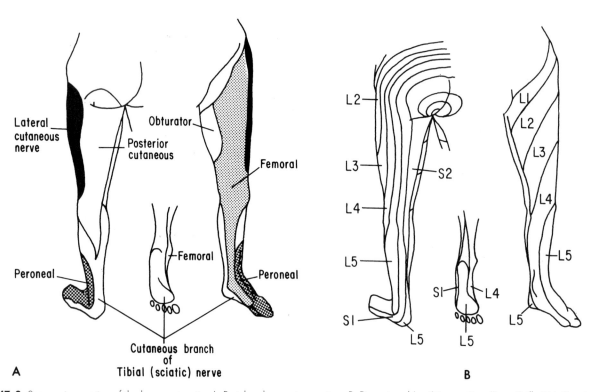

Figure 47–2. Sensory innervation of the lower extremity. *A,* Peripheral nerve innervation. *B,* Dermatomal (root) innervation. (From Reilly BM. Practical Strategies in Outpatient Medicine, 2nd ed. Philadelphia: WB Saunders, 1991:927.)

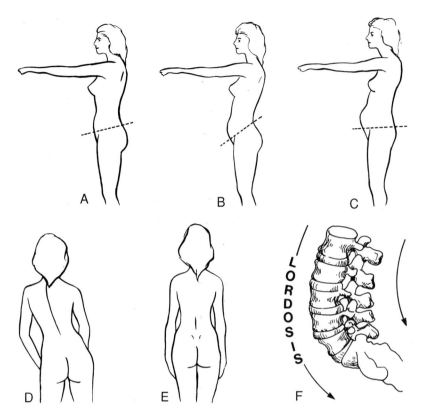

Figure 47–3. *A*, Normal posture with normal lumbar lordosis. *B*, Exaggerated lumbar lordosis due to pelvic tilting. *C*, "Paunchy" posture. *D*, Spastic scoliosis due to muscle spasm. *E*, Normal posture without scoliosis. *F*, The *normal orientation* of the lumbar spine is that of mild lordosis. Exaggerated lordosis may predispose the patient to mechanical back pain. (From Reilly BM. Practical Strategies in Outpatient Medicine, 2nd ed. Philadelphia: WB Saunders, 1991:908.)

pattern. The normal lumbar spine is lordotic, and the sacrum and coccygeal regions are kyphotic. Normal adult sagittal alignment develops gradually; children younger than 10 years of age typically have less cervical lordosis and more lumbar lordosis than adults.

Healthy children often are quite swaybacked. Injuries, infections, tumors, and developmental abnormalities of the spine often produce alterations in these expected contours. Range of motion is demonstrated in Figure 47–4.

Figure 47–4. Back range of motion. *A*, Flexion. Note the normal reversal of lumbar lordosis during flexion *(arrow)*. *B*, Extension. *C*, Persistent lordosis during back flexion due to muscle spasm *(arrow)*. *D*, Lateral flexion. *E*, Lateral torsion (rotation). (From Reilly BM. Practical Strategies in Outpatient Medicine, 2nd ed. Philadelphia: WB Saunders, 1991:909.)

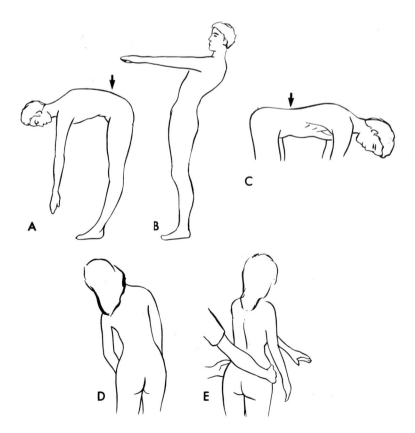

BACK PAIN OF BRIEF DURATION

Emergency department surveys and sports medicine studies indicate that very few children under age 10 years sustain significant injuries of the spinal column or associated musculature in routine play and organized sports activities. Extremity injuries are far more common in this age group. When the trunk is involved, contusions and abrasions are much more common than ligament sprains and muscle strains.

When a child presents with back pain of brief duration following a play or sports-related injury, a careful examination should be performed. If there are no other associated injuries and the screening examination shows no alterations in trunk configuration or lower extremity strength or sensation (see Figs. 47–1 and 47–2), no further work-up is necessary. A brief period of rest of 1 to 2 days, followed by gradual resumption of activities, is appropriate treatment. Routine radiographic evaluation is not necessary when the duration of symptoms is short and the physical examination normal.

Acute back injuries occur more frequently in adolescence, as the size of participants and potential forces generated in recreational activities increase. If there are no other associated injuries and the screening examination is normal, no further radiologic work-up is necessary. A period of rest followed by gradual resumption of activities is appropriate treatment. The importance of a comprehensive and balanced conditioning exercise program should be stressed to young athletes. Most sports-related injuries can be prevented by preparticipation conditioning, appropriate warm-up, careful supervision, and rest when fatigued.

Trauma sufficient to cause spine fractures may occur as a result of motor vehicle or bicycle accidents, falls, and diving and gymnastic injuries. The frequency and severity of spine trauma rises in later adolescence as exposure to potentially violent forces in sports and motor vehicles increases. In such cases, there is a clear relationship between the accident and the onset of symptoms. *Injury to the spinal column should be suspected in all individuals whose level of consciousness is impaired following an accident, regardless of the presence or absence of symptoms.*

Children with suspected acute spinal injury should be immobilized on back boards designed for children until definitive imaging studies can be performed and interpreted. Immobilization of the child's cervical spine on a solid back board should be avoided. The child's occiput projects farther posteriorly than that of the adult, and flexion of the neck will occur if the child's neck is immobilized on a standard back board. Spinal immobilization boards for children are readily available and have a cut-out section to accommodate the occiput. When such boards are not available, a blanket or firm mattress should be interposed between the trunk and the back board to prevent neck flexion.

PERSISTENT BACK PAIN

Persistent or severe back pain is uncommon in young children and only slightly more common in adolescents. The implications of severe or persistent back pain are more serious in younger patients than in older children and adolescents. Persistent back pain in young children is usually never the result of congenital spinal deformity or developmental disorders of the spine. As a child enters and passes through the adolescent growth spurt, back pain may arise from a small number of congenital and developmental disorders of the spinal column. Degenerative disorders of the spine such as intervertebral disc herniation are uncommon causes of back pain in childhood.

The differential diagnosis of persistent back pain in children less than 10 years of age includes intervertebral discitis and osteomyelitis, neoplasia of the spinal column, primary neoplasia of the spinal cord, and metastatic neoplasia (Table 47–2). In older children and adolescents, congenital variations in the formation of the lower lumbar spine are sometimes responsible for chronic back pain (see Table 47–1). Developmental round back is occasionally associated with midthoracic back pain in middle and late adolescence. Discitis, skeletal neoplasia, and tumors of the spinal cord and nerves also occur in adolescence. Special attention must be given in the history taking to the nature of the onset of symptoms, the presence of radiating pain in the legs, bowel and bladder function, associated abdominal pain, and the presence or absence of fever.

Table 47–2. Differential Diagnosis of Back Pain

Inflammatory Diseases

Discitis*
Vertebral osteomyelitis (pyogenic, tuberculosis)
Spinal epidural abscess
Pyelonephritis*
Perinephric abscess
Pancreatitis
Paraspinal muscle abscess—myositis
Psoas abscess
Endocarditis

Rheumatologic Diseases

Pauciarticular juvenile rheumatoid arthritis*
Reiter syndrome
Ankylosing spondylitis
Psoriatic arthritis
Ulcerative colitis—Crohn disease
Fibrositis—fibromyalgia

Developmental Diseases

Spondylolysis (in adolescence)*
Spondylolisthesis (in adolescence)*
Scheuermann syndrome (in adolescence)*
Scoliosis (unusual unless severe)

Mechanical Trauma and Abnormalities

Hip/pelvic anomalies
Herniated disc (rare)
Juvenile osteoporosis (rare)
Overuse syndromes (common with athletic training and in gymnasts and dancers)*
Vertebral stress fractures
Lumbosacral sprain*
Seat-belt injury
Trauma (direct injury—e.g., motor vehicle accident)*

Neoplastic Diseases

Primary vertebral tumors (osteogenic sarcoma, Ewing sarcoma)
Metastatic tumor (neuroblastoma)
Primary spinal tumor (neuroblastoma, lipoma, cysts)
Malignancy of bone marrow (ALL, lymphoma)
Benign tumors (eosinophilic granuloma, osteoid osteoma)

Other

Disc space calcification (idiopathic, ?S/P discitis)
Conversion reaction
Sickle cell anemia*
Hemolysis (acute)
Hematocolpos
S/P lumbar puncture

Modified from Behrman R, Kliegman R (eds). Nelson Essentials of Pediatrics, 2nd ed. Philadelphia, WB Saunders, 1994:711.
*Common.
Abbreviations: ALL = acute lymphocytic leukemia; S/P = status post.

SPECIFIC DIAGNOSIS

Intervertebral Discitis

Intervertebral discitis is the term applied to a number of processes that are characterized by back or leg pain and radiographically by narrowing of the intervertebral joint space between two adjacent vertebral segments (Figs. 47–5 and 47–6). The etiology of discitis is controversial. Bacterial infection of the intervertebral disc is undoubtedly responsible for many cases of discitis, but the benign nature of the process in other children suggests that, at times, less virulent infection or trauma may be responsible for the clinical signs and radiographic findings. Patients may respond to rest and immobilization alone, with little or no antibiotic therapy. Surgical drainage, a critical component of effective treatment of other closed-space infections of the musculoskeletal system, is rarely required in intervertebral discitis, even when an infectious etiology is established.

Discitis most often develops through hematogenous seeding across adjacent vertebral end plates. *Staphylococcus aureus* is the most commonly isolated organism (when one is isolated). Tuberculous infection of the spine is uncommon in the United States but must be considered in children exposed to tuberculosis and in immunocompromised children.

CLINICAL FINDINGS

Inflammatory lesions of the intervertebral disc in children produce a variety of clinical syndromes, depending on the age of the child involved. In children less than 3 years of age, irritability, decreased appetite, and refusal to walk are common findings. Examination often shows loss of lumbar lordosis, tenderness on palpa-

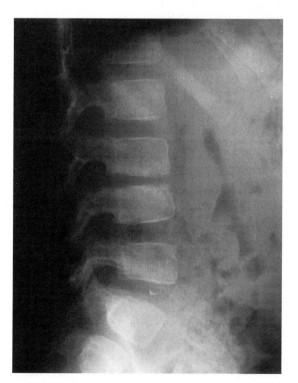

Figure 47–5. Intervertebral discitis. There is loss of intervertebral disc space height between lumbar vertebral segments 3 and 4, with early end-plate erosion on the anteroinferior surface of L-3 and anterosuperior surface of L-4.

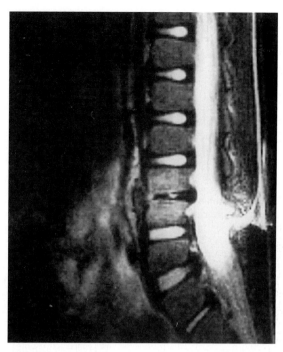

Figure 47–6. Intervertebral discitis, magnetic resonance image. Note the increased marrow signal from the vertebral bodies adjacent to the narrowed L-4 intervertebral disc. There is loss of the normal bright signal from the involved disc itself, and evidence of soft tissue abscess formation anterior to the involved disc space.

tion of the specific spine, and pain on flexion and extension of the hips. In older children, back pain is a more frequent complaint, but fussiness, loss of appetite, and refusal to walk are common findings. Loss of lordosis, muscle spasm, and pain on motion of the spine are more common in this older group of patients. In adolescents, back or leg pain is the most common associated complaint. Some patients are afebrile at the time of presentation.

LABORATORY AND IMAGING STUDIES

Elevation of the white blood cell count may or may not be present; the erythrocyte sedimentation rate is usually elevated. Radiographs of the spine are usually normal early in the process; later, intervertebral disc space narrowing and erosion of vertebral end plates develop (see Fig. 47–5). Radionucleotide bone scans usually show focal increase in radioisotope uptake at the involved site as a consequence of the increased bone turnover in the vertebrae adjacent to the involved disc. Magnetic resonance imaging (MRI) studies are useful in questionable cases and provide an estimate of the extent of abscess formation present (see Fig. 47–6).

TREATMENT

The diagnosis of intervertebral discitis should be suspected in older children with fever and unexplained back or leg pain and in previously healthy younger children who become irritable and refuse to walk. After appropriate laboratory studies have been performed, including blood, sputum, and urine cultures, treatment should be started. A bacterial etiology is likely if there is fever, leukocytosis, and elevation of the sedimentation rate. Antibiotic therapy (nafcillin, methicillin) should be started in such cases, as

S. aureus is the most commonly responsible organism. In very young children, or in immunocompromised hosts, broader-spectrum antibiotic coverage is essential. If an organism is recovered, antibiotic coverage can be adjusted appropriately. Initial therapy should be intravenous; oral antibiotics can be considered as pain decreases and laboratory studies return to normal ranges. A total of 4 to 6 weeks of therapy is recommended for patients with infectious intervertebral discitis.

Immobilization of the spine is a key factor in the treatment of discitis whether or not antibiotics are used. Patients without systemic signs of infection and in whom laboratory studies show no leukocytosis and only moderate elevation of the sedimentation rate may be managed by immobilization alone. Bed rest, spica casts, and thoracolumbar orthoses have all been employed. Four to 6 weeks is the minimum period of immobilization required.

Patients who remain ill or worsen after the initiation of rest and antibiotic treatment should undergo surgical biopsy and drainage. Biopsy should also be performed in patients suspected of tuberculous intervertebral disc space infection.

The evolution of radiographic findings lags behind clinical findings in intervertebral discitis. Although most patients with intervertebral discitis eventually experience disc space narrowing and endplate erosion during the course of treatment, normal radiographs and bone scans at the time of initial evaluation do not preclude the diagnosis. Radiographic changes continue long after the inflammatory process has resolved. Progressive disc space narrowing, intervertebral disc space calcification, and spontaneous intervertebral arthrodesis are common late findings.

Lack of focal increased isotope uptake on bone scans obtained 2 to 3 weeks after the onset of symptoms significantly lessens the likelihood of intervertebral discitis. In such patients, careful study for other potential diagnoses is essential. Tumors of the spinal cord may present in a similar fashion without causing the changes in the vertebral segments necessary to produce alterations on bone scanning. In such patients, MRI is invaluable.

Spondylolysis and Spondylolisthesis

Abnormalities of the lower lumbar and lumbosacral spine occur in about 6% of the North American population. The most common abnormalities, spina bifida occulta at L-5 or S-1 and spondylolysis at L-5, are often noted as incidental radiologic findings in entirely asymptomatic individuals. A few individuals with spondylolysis (defect in the pars interarticularis) experience back pain and progressive slippage deformity, known as spondylolisthesis.

As a consequence of the normal lordotic tilt of the lumbar spine, shear forces are generated between the L-5 and S-1 vertebral segments. Forward displacement of L-5 on S-1 is normally prevented by the stable articulation of the superior facets of S-1 and the inferior facets of L-5. Defective formation of the posterior elements of the lumbosacral joint or defects in the bony connection between the body and the arch of the fifth lumbar vertebra render the anterior junction of L-5 and S-1 unstable and may lead to relative displacement.

ETIOLOGY

Spondylolysis and spondylolisthesis in children and adolescents usually involves the fifth lumbar and first sacral units. Spondylolysis is not present at birth, but by age 6 years it is present in about 5% of children. Defects develop later in childhood and adolescence in another 1%. Spondylolysis appears to be less common in blacks and much more common in some North American Eskimo groups; the lowest incidence has been reported in black females, and the highest in white males. The disorder appears to be multifactorial; both hereditary and mechanical factors have been implicated. Relatives of patients with spondylolysis are much more likely to be affected than individuals in the general population, although the degree of slippage correlates less well.

Fatigue fracture of the posterior elements of L-5 may be responsible for acutely painful spondylolysis in some preadolescent and adolescent athletes. Activities that involve repeated trunk flexion and extension have been implicated; adolescent divers and gymnasts are reported to be susceptible to spondylolysis and spondylolisthesis.

Acute fracture-dislocation of vertebral units resulting from violent trauma in a strict sense is one form of spondylolisthesis, but because it differs so greatly from other types of spondylolisthesis in etiology, presentation, and treatment, it is usually considered as a separate entity.

PRESENTATION

Symptoms in patients with spondylolysis and spondylolisthesis are quite variable. Some patients with minimal slips have extreme pain, while others with moderate to severe slips have little or no discomfort. When present, pain is usually ill defined and poorly localized. Most patients complain of aching in the lumbar and lumbosacral regions. Buttock and posterior thigh pain may be present, but radicular symptoms of nerve root compression are usually absent. Discomfort is usually increased by exercise and relieved by rest.

Signs vary with the severity of spondylolisthesis. Asymptomatic patients with slips of mild severity may have no outward manifestations of vertebral abnormality. Patients with moderate to severe slips usually have tenderness on palpation of the lumbar spine and increased lumbar lordosis. Spasm of the hamstring muscles may extend the sacral spine, causing the buttocks to seem flattened or heart-shaped in appearance. In severe slips, a step-off of L-5 on S-1 can be palpated. A flexible scoliotic deformity caused by paraspinal muscle spasm may be present.

Neurologic examination is usually normal in children with spondylolysis. Symptoms and signs of nerve root compression and mechanical instability are much more common in the adult patient with progressive or severe untreated adolescent spondylolisthesis.

Hamstring muscle spasm is a common finding in patients with symptomatic spondylolisthesis and at times may be the chief presenting problem. Affected patients are unable to flex far enough forward to touch their toes without bending their knees. When severe, hamstring spasm causes a loss of normal lumbar lordosis and a flattened appearance of the low back. Hamstring muscle spasm also interferes with gait; stride length is shortened, and patients run with a peculiar stiff-legged posture. The cause of hamstring spasm in spondylolisthesis is unclear; it does not appear to be caused by compression of spinal nerves, and it is rarely accompanied by other signs of nerve root compromise. Most believe it is a result of abnormal strain on the hamstring muscles caused by mechanical instability of the lumbosacral junction.

RADIOGRAPHIC ASSESSMENT

When the history and physical examination suggest the possibility of spondylolysis and spondylolisthesis, radiographic assessment is justified. Initial studies should consist of standing anteroposterior and lateral views of the spine from T-1 to S-1. If these suggest that spondylolisthesis or spondylolysis is present, a spot lateral view of the lumbosacral junction and oblique views of the lumbosacral junction should be requested.

The degree of displacement in both dysplastic and spondylolytic spondylolisthesis can be estimated by noting the position of the

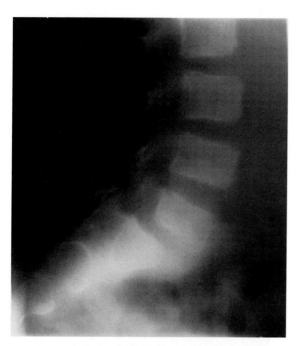

Figure 47–7. Spondylolisthesis. Slippage of L-5 on the underlying body of S-1 has occurred as a consequence of defective formation of the posterior elements of L-5. In this case, slippage is moderate, measuring slightly more than 25% of the width of the S-1 vertebral segment.

posterior border of the L-5 vertebral body with respect to the body of the first sacral vertebra (Fig. 47–7). Slips less than 25% of the width of the first sacral body are considered mild; slips between 25% and 50% are considered moderate; slips greater than 50% are considered severe. At times, slippage may be so severe that L-5 may be located in front of S-1. This is termed spondyloptosis.

When physical examination suggests that compromise of the lumbar or sacral nerve roots may be present, MRI scans of the lumbar spine should be obtained. Myelography, tomography, and computed tomography (CT) are not usually necessary for evaluation or for treatment planning. In cases in which the history and physical examination are suggestive of spondylolysis but radiographic studies are not clear, a radionucleotide bone scan may be helpful. Isolated increased uptake at the lower lumbar spine is consistent with spondylolysis.

TREATMENT

The management of patients with spondylolysis and spondylolisthesis depends on the age of the patient, symptoms, degree of slip, and associated neurologic findings. Asymptomatic children with minimal slips require no active treatment. Many of these children are discovered to have spondylolysis only as an incidental finding on roentgenogram made for other reasons. There is little reason to restrict activities when patients are asymptomatic. Since progression occurs in a small proportion of these patients, radiologic follow-up at 6- to 12-month intervals from the time of discovery through adolescence is indicated.

Asymptomatic children and adolescents with moderate degrees of spondylolisthesis should be carefully followed up. It is reasonable to restrict such patients from participation in contact sports and gymnastics. If progression occurs, stabilization is justified.

Symptomatic children with mild to moderate spondylolisthesis in most cases should be given a trial of nonoperative treatment. A period of bed rest, sometimes in a plaster body jacket, often relieves pain and associated muscle spasm. Gradual resumption of activities

can be permitted after 4 to 8 weeks. A lumbosacral spine brace may be useful in older children after the initial period of immobilization. Those sports that require trunk flexion and extension may have to be restricted.

In most cases, fusion of L-5 to S-1 stops progression and eliminates pain. Fusion from L-4 to the sacrum may be necessary in more severe slips. Reduction of the deformity is rarely necessary. Nerve root decompression, often needed in adults with spondylolisthesis, is rarely necessary in children.

Idiopathic Kyphosis

Abnormal increases in expected thoracic kyphosis in children and adolescents produce round back deformities (Fig. 47–8). These

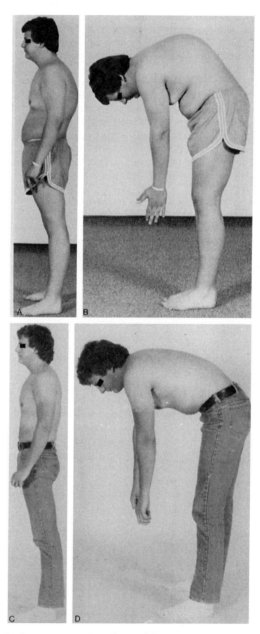

Figure 47–8. Preoperative *(A and B)* and postoperative *(C and D)* views of an adolescent boy with severe kyphosis secondary to Scheuermann's disease. He required both anterior and posterior spinal fusion. He now has a markedly improved appearance and no further progression of the kyphosis. (From Renshaw TS. Pediatric Orthopedics. Philadelphia: WB Saunders, 1986:53.)

may be congenital, neuromuscular, or idiopathic in origin. Mild to moderate increases in kyphosis cause little deformity and few symptoms. Severe kyphosis is disfiguring, often causes back pain, and may lead to spinal cord compromise.

Round back posture is often encountered in otherwise healthy adolescents at school screening examinations. Affected patients are usually asymptomatic, although their parents often report poor posture. A history should be obtained and physical examination performed. *Complaints of severe back pain or leg pain, enuresis, or findings of lower extremity weakness or increased reflex tone in patients with round back are ominous findings and warrant referral.*

If accentuated kyphosis is present, radiographic follow-up is indicated. Two radiologic patterns are common. The majority of individuals, especially younger adolescents, have thoracic kyphotic curves of 40 to 60 degrees, with no underlying structural vertebral changes. Usually such curves correct easily on passive or active hyperextension. For such children, no treatment except for a thoracic hyperextension exercise program and periodic follow-up examination is necessary.

More severe kyphosis with accompanying structural changes in vertebral bodies at the apex of the deformity is present in a small subset of adolescents with kyphosis. The association of developmental kyphosis, wedging of thoracic vertebrae, and back pain in adolescents and young adults was noted by Scheuermann in 1920. Affected individuals often have kyphotic curves greater than 60 degrees and show little correction with hyperextension. Roentgenograms show vertebral wedging, end-plate irregularity, and kyphosis (Fig. 47–9).

Scheuermann's kyphosis occurs in approximately 5% to 8% of the population, affecting males 5 to 10 times more often than females. The etiology remains unclear, but it may very well be the result of increased pressure on the anterior portion of the growing vertebral body and consequent growth retardation in individuals with extreme degrees of postural round back. It does not appear to be the result of any known metabolic, infectious, or traumatic disorder. Back pain is usually mild; many patients have no pain at all. The deformity in most is minimal and only rarely is cosmetically unacceptable. Late neurologic complications are extremely rare.

Treatment depends on the degree of deformity and the age of the patient. Skeletally immature individuals with significant deformity may improve with a program of exercise and Milwaukee brace use. Older patients with back pain usually respond to a back strengthening exercise program. Patients with unacceptable deformity who are too old for brace treatment require surgical correction. Often this requires a combination of anterior release and posterior spinal instrumentation and fusion.

Congenital vertebral malformations that produce kyphotic deformities develop during the first trimester of pregnancy and, like other congenital abnormalities of the spine, are often associated with abnormalities of the genitourinary tract or the spinal cord. Kyphosis that results from congenital vertebral deformities is often obvious early in life and may be rapidly progressive (Fig. 47–10). The spinal cord may become tented over the apex of the deformity, producing symptoms and signs of spasticity in the lower extremity and bladder. Progression of deformity is dangerous; congenital kyphosis is the spinal deformity most often associated with paraplegia. Patients should be promptly referred for orthopedic evaluation.

Intervertebral Disc Herniation

Intervertebral disc rupture is much less common in children than in adults. Since most such patients are treated nonoperatively, the absolute incidence of the disorder is not known. In the United States, fewer than 1% of patients undergoing discectomy are

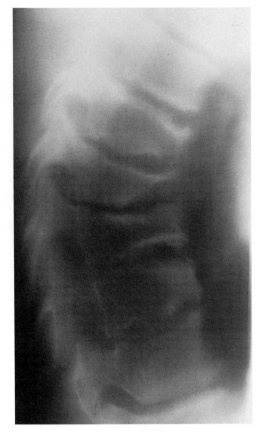

Figure 47–9. Scheuermann's kyphosis. Lateral radiographs of the midthoracic spine in an asymptomatic 16-year-old boy with moderately severe round back. There is severe wedging, loss of vertebral height, and end-plate irregularity present on these films. His radiographic findings appear far worse than his symptoms and signs. If further collapse develops and his kyphosis becomes more severe, surgical intervention will be necessary.

younger than 16 years of age. The frequency of symptomatic intervertebral disc herniation may be more common in Asian people than in Caucasians, perhaps because of the smaller size of the spinal canal.

Symptoms of intervertebral disc herniation in adolescents are similar to those in adults. The majority of affected patients report back pain; most have sciatica. About 30% complain of decreased sensation or paresthesia in the lower extremities. On physical examination, lumbar muscle spasm, scoliosis, and a decreased range of lumbar motion are common findings. A positive straight-leg-raising test is present in most patients. Abnormal reflex patterns and lower extremity weakness are much less likely to be present in young patients than in adults. A history of trauma is occasionally present; patients tend to be taller and slightly heavier than their peers. A positive family history for intervertebral disc disease is frequently present.

Radiographs often show loss of lumbar lordosis and lumbar scoliosis. Loss of intervertebral disc height is rarely noted on plain films. MRI is currently the study of choice for localization of the lesion.

Most patients respond to bed rest followed by gradual resumption of activities. When sciatica, loss of reflexes, or weakness persist, surgical excision of the intervertebral disc is indicated. Fusion is not necessary unless there is accompanying evidence of spinal instability. Good results can be expected about 75% of the time. The incidence of recurrent symptoms requiring repeated surgery is about 25%.

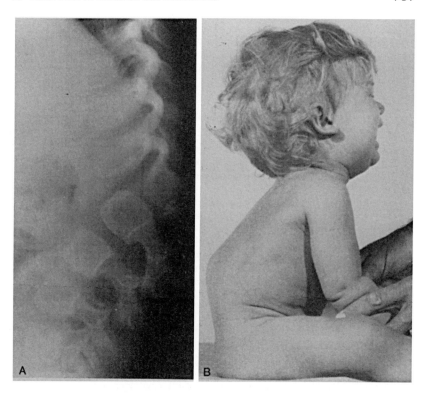

Figure 47–10. *A,* Congenital kyphosis secondary to failure of vertebral bodies to form at T-12 and L-1. *B,* The clinical appearance of the child. Thoracolumbar kyphosis is obvious. (From Renshaw TS. Pediatric Orthopedics. Philadelphia: WB Saunders, 1986:44.)

Scoliosis

Idiopathic scoliosis, a combination of lateral deviation and rotation of vertebral bodies, does not produce back pain. When painful scoliosis is present, a careful search for the cause of the symptoms must be undertaken. Infection, tumor, a spinal cord syringomyelia, and occult fractures may produce clinical findings that resemble idiopathic scoliosis but, unlike in idiopathic scoliosis, cause pain as well.

ETIOLOGY

Idiopathic scoliosis begins in the immature spine, although progression of preexisting curvatures may occur in adult life. The etiology of idiopathic scoliosis remains unknown. No consistent biochemical, neurologic, or traumatic abnormalities have been identified. Hormonal factors appear to play a role in curve progression, since severe curves occur much more often in girls. Some studies have demonstrated abnormalities of proprioception and vibratory sensation in affected patients, suggesting that abnormalities of posterior column function may contribute to the development of curvature. Other investigators have implicated cerebellar or muscular (myopathy) dysfunction as a possible cause of spinal imbalance.

No clear genetic pattern has been established. Curves occur more frequently in individuals with affected first-degree relatives, but transmission is not mendelian. Although curvature is more likely to develop in the daughters of affected mothers than in other children, the magnitude of curvature in an affected individual is not related to the magnitude of curvature in relatives. It appears likely that a combination of genetic predisposition and other undefined factors are responsible for development and progression of idiopathic scoliosis.

CLASSIFICATION

Idiopathic curves are grouped into infantile, juvenile, and adolescent categories on the basis of age of onset of curvature. The infantile form differs enough from the other varieties to be considered a distinct entity. The distinction between juvenile and adolescent scoliosis is not as sharp.

Infantile Idiopathic Scoliosis

Infantile idiopathic scoliosis is rare in the United States, probably accounting for less than 1% of new cases of idiopathic scoliosis. The majority of patients are male, and most curves are convex toward the left, rather than the right as in the other varieties of idiopathic scoliosis. Some infants suspected of having idiopathic deformity in reality have subtle congenital vertebral abnormalities. The diagnosis of idiopathic deformity is appropriate only when radiographic studies show no evidence of congenital vertebral anomalies (e.g., hemivertebra) and there are no signs of spinal dysraphism or neuropathic or myopathic disorders.

Although many infantile curves resolve spontaneously, others progress relentlessly and are very difficult to treat effectively. Observation is appropriate until age 6 months in infants with idiopathic scoliosis, but prompt referral should be made if curves persist or increase during the period of observation.

Juvenile Idiopathic Scoliosis

Juvenile idiopathic scoliosis begins prior to the adolescent growth spurt. Some curves are probably undetected cases of infantile scoliosis. Others, particularly those that occur in older children, may be early manifestations of adolescent idiopathic scoliosis. Some curves remain small and, in fact, may resolve spontaneously. Others remain stable until the onset of the growth spurt and then progress unless treated. Still others progress steadily throughout childhood and adolescence. There is no reliable method to predict behavior of juvenile curves at the time of diagnosis, but in general, high-magnitude curves in young patients are more likely to increase with growth than smaller curves in older children.

The majority of patients with juvenile curves greater than 30 degrees at the time of diagnosis require some form of active treatment. Treatment must begin at the time progression is first documented if severe deformity is to be prevented.

Adolescent Idiopathic Scoliosis

Most cases of idiopathic scoliosis in North America develop around the time of the adolescent growth spurt (Figs. 47–11 and 47–12). Often parents and children are unaware of the presence of curvature at outset. Nerve root impingement, intervertebral disc disease, and spinal cord compression are uncommon in young patients with idiopathic scoliosis. Pain is so rare that children and adolescents with painful curves must be carefully studied to exclude neoplastic and inflammatory processes of the spinal column or neural canal. *Idiopathic scoliosis is a painless disorder during childhood and adolescence. Even severe structural curves cause no pain until degenerative changes develop in adult life.*

SCHOOL SCREENING PROGRAMS

School screening for spinal deformity has been common in North America. Most programs concentrate on children in the late juvenile and early adolescent period. The most common screening method employed is the forward-bend test, based anatomically on the vertebral rotation that accompanies lateral spinal deviation

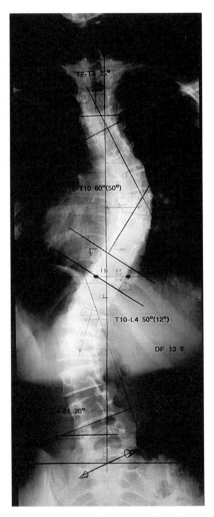

Figure 47–12. Adolescent idiopathic scoliosis. This 13-year-old girl has a severe double-curve pattern with significant accompanying deformity but no pain. Surgical treatment is warranted to halt progression and restore spinal alignment.

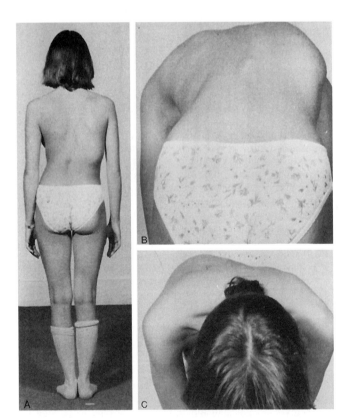

Figure 47–11. *A,* Adolescent idiopathic scoliosis viewed from the back. Note the right-sided thoracic prominence. When the patient bends forward *(B),* the rib prominence is even more apparent. This is secondary to rotation of the ribs and spine. When viewed from the front *(C),* the rib prominence is also quite evident. (From Renshaw TS. Pediatric Orthopedics. Philadelphia: WB Saunders, 1986:47.)

(see Fig. 47–11). Associated findings include shoulder asymmetry, unequal distances between the medial borders of the elbows and the flanks, and apparent leg-length inequality or pelvic tilt. Breast asymmetry, caused by forward rotation of the chest wall on the side of the curve concavity and backward displacement of the chest wall on the convex side of the curve, is often present.

The threshold for ''identification'' on screening examination is subjective, and not surprisingly the incidence of spine asymmetry detected by school screening programs varies with the method of screening and the experience of the examiner. A range of 3% to 18% has been reported. Follow-up radiographic studies of children thought to be abnormal on school screening examinations indicate an incidence of scoliosis in screened children of less than 15% (range, 0.4% to 14%). The incidence of curves greater than 20 degrees at the time of primary screening is probably less than 0.5%. Efforts to standardize the screening procedure with simple devices such as the ''scoliometer'' have not been proven to be effective, and the use of optical scanning systems such as Moire topography is expensive.

The first response to a positive school screening examination should be a repeated physical examination. If asymmetry is confirmed, a single standing posteroanterior spine film, including vertebral levels T1-S1, should be obtained. Lateral films, bending films, and oblique views are not necessary. Referral is appropriate for skeletally immature children or adolescents with curves greater than 20 degrees.

NATURAL HISTORY

The natural history of curvature in patients with spine asymmetry is highly variable. It is impossible to predict with certainty the behavior of a curve in specific patients, but factors that appear to be associated with risk of progression include the magnitude of curvature at the time of detection, the chronologic and skeletal age of the patient, the pattern of curvature, and the menarcheal status. Immature patients with large-magnitude curves are far more likely to experience progression than more mature patients with small curves. Progression of curves after skeletal growth is uncommon in idiopathic thoracic curves of less than 30 degrees at the end of growth but is likely to occur in patients with curves greater than 60 degrees at maturity.

Uncontrolled curve progression causes significant problems in adult life. Unacceptable deformity, back pain, chronic fatigue, and decreased work capacity are common. Premature degenerative arthritis and nerve root impingement caused by deformity and osteophytic spurring occur in patients with lumbar curves or double thoracic-lumbar curves. Asymptomatic decreased vital capacity is common in patients with thoracic curves; symptomatic cardiopulmonary (cor pulmonale) compromise may develop in patients with curves greater than 80 degrees.

TREATMENT

The goals of treatment in idiopathic scoliosis are to bring a patient to skeletal maturity with a cosmetically acceptable, balanced, and stable curve that is unlikely to progress in adult life. Mature adolescents with curves less than 30 degrees need no treatment beyond initial evaluation. Further progression of curvature is unlikely in these individuals. Patients with juvenile scoliosis and less mature adolescents with curves between 10 and 20 degrees should be followed at 6-month intervals with single standing posteroanterior spine radiographs. If progression occurs, they should be referred for orthopedic care.

Active treatment is indicated for growing patients with curves greater than 30 degrees. Brace treatment remains the standard method of nonoperative treatment of idiopathic curvature. Surgical treatment is appropriate for patients with curves too severe for brace treatment. Documented progression in spite of nonoperative treatment is another indication for surgical intervention.

Improved instrumentation and internal fixation devices, intraoperative monitoring of spinal cord function, and autologous transfusion have improved the safety and efficacy of surgical correction. In most cases, patients can be out of bed within 3 to 4 days of surgery and are walking within 5 days of surgery. Return to school is usually possible within 3 weeks; most activities of normal life, including sports, can be resumed within 6 months. In many instances, no postoperative immobilization is required; in other cases, a removable lightweight plastic orthosis can be employed. Prolonged periods of immobilization in a plaster cast are uncommon.

Tumors of the Spinal Column

Persistent back pain, muscle spasm, and abnormal trunk posture are ominous findings in children. Neoplastic disease must be considered in patients with no other obvious source of pain (see Table 47–2).

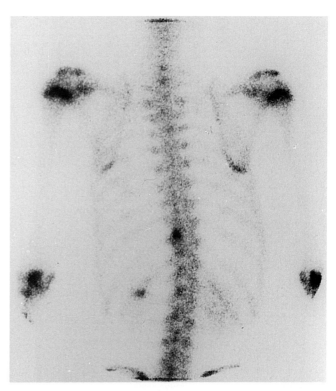

Figure 47-13. Osteoid osteoma of the spine. Technetium bone scanning shows increased uptake in the T-10 vertebral body in this 15-year-old boy. Note the scoliosis that accompanies this painful lesion. He did not respond to anti-inflammatory medications, and surgical excision was necessary.

PRIMARY LESIONS OF BONE

The most common primary bone tumors affecting the spinal column in children are osteoid osteoma (Fig. 47–13), osteoblastoma (Fig. 47–14), and aneurysmal bone cysts (see Chapter 46). Though benign, these lesions may cause considerable back pain and local bone destruction. Osteogenic sarcoma, a malignant lesion of bone, occurs less commonly in the spine than in the long bones of children. Unexplained pain is the hallmark of spinal neoplasia and is usually the presenting complaint. At times, pain may be severe and unresponsive to non-narcotic analgesics. In other instances, as in patients with osteoid osteoma, the relief of symptoms that occurs with nonsteroidal anti-inflammatory agents is so characteristic that it is considered a diagnostic test. Paraspinal muscle spasm, tenderness in the soft tissues on the side of the spinal column, and alterations in spinal configuration are common. Scoliosis, loss of lumbar lordosis, or accentuations of thoracic round back may be present.

Initial evaluation of patients with suspected spinal tumors should include standard anteroposterior and lateral radiographs of the spine (see Fig. 47–14). These may not show small lesions hidden in vertebral pedicles or posterior elements; other studies are often necessary. Technetium bone scanning is particularly useful (see Fig. 47–13). MRI and CT are usually necessary to localize lesions for surgical treatment. Prompt referral is essential when the diagnosis of spinal neoplasia is suspected. The success of treatment depends in large part on early discovery and intervention.

TUMORS OF NEURAL ELEMENTS

Back pain, lower extremity weakness, and sphincter disturbances are common manifestations of neoplasms of the spinal cord. Al-

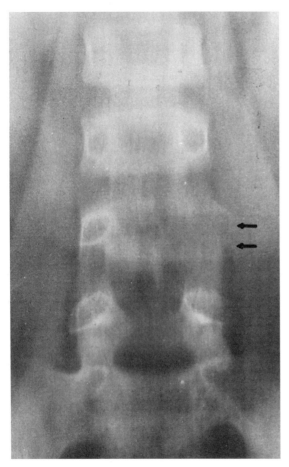

Figure 47–14. This patient presented with left-sided lumbar back pain. Note the destruction of the vertebral pedicle at L-4 *(arrows)*. This proved to be an osteoblastoma. Children with back pain should be suspected of having a tumor of the spine or spinal cord until proven otherwise. (From Renshaw TS. Pediatric Orthopedics. Philadelphia: WB Saunders, 1986:57.)

though such lesions are rare, they must be suspected in children with unexplained back or leg pain, weakness, sensory or reflex abnormalities, bowel or bladder incontinence, or unexplained gait abnormalities. Neuroblastoma is the most common lesion, but sarcomas (including Ewing sarcoma, rhabdomyosarcoma, and hemangiosarcoma) and astrocytomas also occur in the neural contents of the spinal canal.

In such patients, standard radiography often shows only loss of lordosis or scoliosis secondary to muscle spasm. MRI demonstrates the abnormality, but definitive diagnosis usually requires biopsy. The success of treatment is often related to prompt diagnosis. Early referral of patients with unexplained back pain is essential for appropriate treatment.

LEUKEMIA

Skeletal involvement is common in patients with leukemia; back pain or limb pain may be the presenting symptom in some children. Proliferation of abnormal hematopoietic tissue in the marrow of long bones or vertebral bodies causes pain and weakens their structure.

Clinical symptoms and signs in children with leukemic skeletal involvement may be confusing. Fever, localized pain and swelling, and elevations of the white blood cell count and erythrocyte sedi-

mentation rate may be mistaken for septic arthritis, osteomyelitis, or intervertebral disc space infection. The presence of abnormal white cells on the peripheral blood count or thrombocytopenia increases the likelihood of bone marrow tumor rather than infection.

Osteopenia, periosteal elevation, and metaphyseal lucencies are common radiographic findings in leukemic involvement of long bones. These may be difficult to detect in patients with spinal involvement. Vertebral compression and wedging are sometimes present and may mimic acute fracture or occasionally osteomyelitis (Fig. 47–15). The absence of a history of trauma should alert the examiner to search for other causes of the radiographic abnormality. Preservation of intervertebral disc space height with collapse of adjacent vertebral segments is an indication that the vertebral bodies rather than the intervertebral disc is the sight of the abnormality. Technetium bone scanning is useful to detect other areas of involvement, although it is not as reliable in leukemia as in other spinal lesions. MRI is useful to detect areas of spinal involvement not visible on plain radiographs and to assess the extent of intraspinal infiltrate or spinal cord compression present.

The diagnosis of leukemia can be established by bone marrow aspiration. Biopsy of involved vertebral segments is rarely necessary. Support of the spine in a custom-fabricated orthosis is useful to relieve pain and prevent further vertebral collapse during the initial phases of treatment. Prolonged brace treatment may be necessary to prevent vertebral compression fractures that may accompany the osteopenia resulting from steroid therapy. Surgical

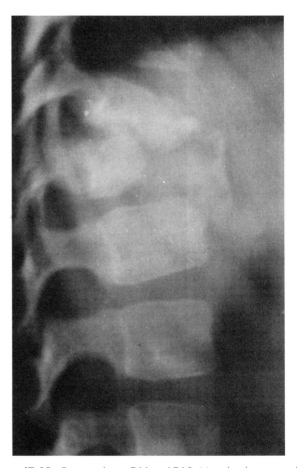

Figure 47–15. Osteomyelitis at T-11 and T-12. Note the destruction of the disc space and vertebral bodies with beginning of anterior ossification. This patient went on to spontaneous fusion and is now asymptomatic. (From Renshaw TS. Pediatric Orthopedics. Philadelphia: WB Saunders, 1986:59.)

decompression and fusion may be required in rare cases of acute vertebral compression and spinal cord compromise.

SUMMARY AND RED FLAGS

Back pain in children may be due to referred pain from intra-abdominal or retroperitoneal disease (see Table 47–2) and direct involvement of the spinal cord, vertebral bodies, or paraspinal musculature. In most children with a normal examination, back pain is benign, short-lived, and responsive to rest or nonsteroidal anti-inflammatory agents.

Chronic persistent back pain, pain associated with lower extremity or bowel and bladder neurologic deficits, systemic signs (as in inflammatory bowel disease, leukemia, osteomyelitis), acute pain, and tenderness with neurologic dysfunction after trauma are red flags. Signs of cord involvement are particularly ominous and emergent. Spinal cord involvement above T-10 produces symmetric weakness, increased deep tendon reflexes, up-going toes, and an appropriate sensory loss; conus medullaris involvement (T10-L2) produces symmetric weakness, increased knee and decreased ankle deep tendon reflexes, a saddle-type anesthesia, and up- or down-going toes on Babinski testing; while cauda equina (below L-2) produces asymmetric weakness, loss of deep tendon reflexes, and down-going toes. Such findings are an acute emergency requiring immediate imaging (MRI) and therapy, which may include high-dose corticosteroids, radiation therapy, or laminectomy to prevent permanent paralysis.

REFERENCES

Bell DF, Erlich MG, Zaleske DJ. Brace treatment for symptomatic spondylolisthesis. Clin Orthop 1988;236:192–198.

Conrad EU, Olszewski AD, Berger M, et al. Pediatric spinal cord tumors with spinal cord compromise. J Pediatr Orthop 1992;12:454–460.

Crawford AH, Kucharzyk DW, Ruda R, et al. Diskitis in children. Clin Orthop 1991;266:70–79.

Epstein JA, Epstein NE, Marc J, et al. Lumbar intervertebral disc herniation in teenage children: Recognition and management of associated anomalies. Spine 1984;9:427–432.

Fraser RD, Peterson DC, Simpson DA. Orthopedic aspects of spinal cord tumors in children. J Bone Joint Surg 1977;59-B:143–151.

Frennerd AK, Danielson BI, Nachemson AL. Natural history of symptomatic isthmic low-grade spondylolisthesis in children and adolescents: A seven year follow up study. J Pediatr Orthop 1991;11:209–213.

Hensinger RN. Back pain in children. J Bone Joint Surg 1989;71-A:1098–1107.

Jackson DW. Low back pain in young athletes. Evaluation of stress reaction and discogenic problems. Am J Sports Med 1979;7:364–366.

Letts MH, Haasbeek J. Hematocolpos as a cause of back pain in premenarchal adolescents. J Pediatr Orthop 1990;10:731–732.

Lonstein JE. Natural history and school screening for scoliosis. Orthop Clin North Am 1988;19:227–237.

Lowe TG. Scheuermann disease. J Bone Joint Surg 1990;72-A:940–945.

Pizzutillo PD, Hummer CD. Nonoperative treatment of painful adolescent spondylolysis or spondylolisthesis. J Pediatr Orthop 1989;9:538–540.

Rogalsky RJ, Black GB, Reed MH. Orthopedic manifestations of leukemia in children. J Bone Joint Surg 1986;68-A:494–501.

Sachs B, Bradford D, Winter RB, et al. Scheuermann kyphosis. Follow-up of Milwaukee brace treatment. J Bone Joint Surg 1987;69-A:50–57.

Seitsalo SK, Osterman H, Hyvarinen K, et al. Progression of spondylolisthesis in children and adolescents. A long term followup of 272 patients. Spine 1991;16:417–421.

Thompson GH. Back pain in children. J Bone Joint Surg 1993;75-A:928–938.

Tursz A, Crost M. Sports related injuries in children. Am J Sports Med 1986;14:294–299.

Varlotta GP, Brown MD, Kelsey JL, et al. Familial predisposition for herniation of a lumbar disc in patients who are less than twenty one years old. J Bone Joint Surg 1991;73-A:124–128.

Hematologic Disorders

48 Lymphadenopathy

27.7.97

John R. Schreiber   Brian W. Berman

Lymphadenopathy, defined as enlarged lymph nodal tissue measuring more than 1 cm in diameter, is a common presenting symptom in children. Enlarged nodes are a common feature of many childhood illnesses because of the role of the nodes in filtering pathogens, the anatomy of the lymph node chains, and the cellular proliferation that occurs in nodal tissue after exposure to infectious agents or by infiltration with malignant cells. Most of the illnesses manifesting with enlarged lymph nodes represent common pediatric bacterial or viral infections that improve either spontaneously or after appropriate antimicrobial therapy. By contrast, some serious childhood illnesses, particularly malignancy, can first manifest as lymphadenopathy. A careful history, physical examination, and knowledge of the anatomy of tissues drained by lymph nodes as well as the type of adenopathy caused by various illnesses usually lead to the appropriate diagnosis without the need for complex diagnostic procedures.

MECHANISM OF LYMPHADENOPATHY

The lymphatic system consists of lymphatic vessels (afferent and efferent) that connect lymphatic tissues, including lymph nodes, to the peripheral circulation via postcapillary venules. The lymph nodes contain both B and T cells, which lie in a supportive framework

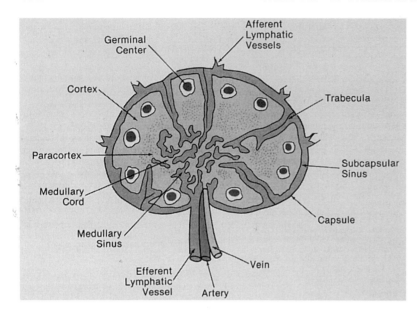

Figure 48–1. Diagrammatic representation of the structure of a lymph node. (From Faller DV. Diseases of the lymph nodes and spleen. *In* Wyngaarden JB, Smith LH, Bennett JC [eds]. Cecil Textbook of Medicine, 19th ed. Philadelphia: WB Saunders, 1992:979.)

within a connective tissue capsule (Fig. 48–1). The lymphatic fluid or "lymph"-containing antigens, bacteria, or other pathogens as well as various lymphocytes and macrophages enter through afferent lymphatic vessels; the cells within the node then interact with antigens. This interaction allows production of T-cell and/or humoral immune responses in the host's effort to clear the antigen or the pathogen. Efferent lymphatic vessels then carry lymph-containing antigen-sensitized lymphocytes from the nodes and eventually back to the peripheral circulation via the thoracic duct. Thus, enlargement of the nodes can be caused by several factors.

First, when nodes fulfill their normal function, hyperplasia occurs as a consequence of proliferation by nodal and newly arrived lymphoid cells. This proliferation is a response to antigenic stimulation. Such responses are particularly active in children, which explains the frequent observation of lymphadenopathy associated with some pediatric infections.

Second, bacteria or their products that have traveled to the nodes may stimulate the arrival of inflammatory cells, such as neutrophils, and cause enlargement as well as symptoms of lymphadenitis (erythema and tenderness).

Third, malignant cells either may arise in the node itself and proliferate, causing enlargement, or may arrive from distant cancerous sites and also infiltrate the nodal tissue.

Finally, in rare genetic storage diseases, macrophages laden with abnormally metabolized lipids may lodge in lymph nodes and cause clinically apparent lymphadenopathy.

The regional areas drained by each lymph node group are also important in determining the etiology of lymphadenopathy. The superficial cervical lymph nodes, for example, drain lymph from distinct areas of the head, neck, and throat (Fig. 48–2) and may enlarge if a local infection is present. These nodes, in turn, drain into the deep cervical nodes and eventually the thoracic duct.

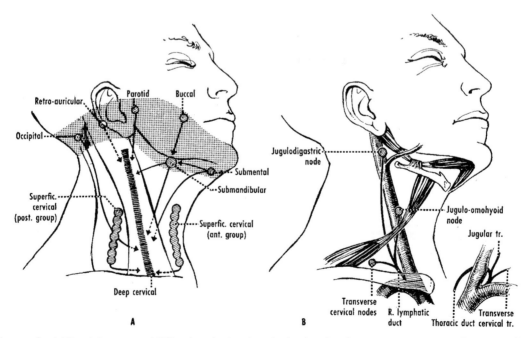

Figure 48–2. The superficial *(A)* and deep cervical *(B)* lymph nodes that drain the head and neck. post. = posterior; superfic. = superficial; ant. = anterior; R. = right; tr. = tributary. (From O'Rahilly RO. Gardner, Gray, O'Rahilly Anatomy—A Regional Study of Human Structure, 5th ed. Philadelphia: WB Saunders, 1986:719.)

Because viral and bacterial pharyngitis and otitis media are two of the most common infections in children, the cervical and occipital areas, respectively, are some of the more common sites for lymphadenopathy in small children. By contrast, the inguinal nodes drain the areas surrounding and including the urethra, the vagina, and the penis and may be enlarged, particularly in adolescents and adults with venereal diseases. The inguinal nodes also drain the distal extremities and may enlarge with soft tissue infections of the lower extremity in small children.

HISTORY

The history is important in the evaluation of lymphadenopathy and often yields distinct clues to the appropriate diagnosis. First, the character and temporal course of the adenopathy are important. Rapid onset of unilateral lymphadenopathy in the groin after trauma to the lower extremity, for example, suggests infection originating in the traumatized extremity. In contrast, nodes noticed with progressive enlargement in several areas of the body that are associated with weight loss, fevers, night sweats, or other systemic illness suggest diseases associated with involvement of multiple organ systems, such as lymphoma or tuberculosis. Second, the age of the child who has the enlarged lymph node or nodes is important in the consideration of the cause (Table 48–1).

Neonates with adenopathy usually have been exposed to an infectious agent *in utero* (e.g., cytomegalovirus [CMV], syphilis, toxoplasmosis). By contrast, toddlers with adenopathy (depending on whether it is regional or diffuse) tend to have either focal infections that drain into the affected nodal chain (cervical chain lymphadenopathy with pharyngitis) (see Fig. 48–2) or a systemic viral infection that results in enlarged nodes that are not regionalized. Similarly, malignancy manifested as adenopathy is rare in neonates but more common in toddlers and older children. The medical history should focus on presence of chronic illness, an immunodeficiency that would predispose to opportunistic infection or tumor, and the use of medications (procainamide, sulfasalazine, phenytoin, or tetracycline) that may be associated with lupus-like illnesses and adenopathy.

The family history may reveal the presence of infection, such as human immunodeficiency virus (HIV) or tuberculosis, in the parents or group A streptococcal infection or mononucleosis in a sibling. The family history should include place of birth and travel history to determine whether the child is from or has been exposed to geographic areas with high rates of infections (e.g., tuberculosis, histoplasmosis). Activities during travel are also important, particularly the consumption of unprocessed cheeses or unpasteurized milk products that may contain pathogens, such as *Brucella* or mycobacteria.

The social history may provide further clues to the cause of the lymphadenopathy. Is the child from a socioeconomic or immigrant ethnic group that epidemiologically has a more intense exposure to such infections as tuberculosis? Is there an adult in the household who is currently ill or taking medication? Does the family diet include raw meat that may predispose to acquisition of toxoplasmosis (a more common cause of toxoplasmosis than exposure to kitty litter in the United States)?

The presence of animals in the household or in households the child frequents may play a significant role in the lymphadenopathy. The presence of cats or, more often, kittens that scratch the child, for example, is often omitted from the parent's history of the patient unless such questions are specifically asked.

Adolescents should be questioned about sexual activity and other risk factors for HIV or other sexually transmitted diseases, such as syphilis or lymphogranuloma venereum, that may cause diffuse or inguinal lymphadenopathy.

PHYSICAL EXAMINATION

Careful visual inspection yields an overall impression of size and distribution of significant lymphadenopathy as well as the presence of an associated infection. Overall physical appearance may indicate whether systemic symptoms, such as weight loss and cachexia, have been present. Palpation of the nodes, however, is required to appreciate the actual size and regions of lymphadenopathy. All areas that commonly present with lymphadenopathy should be palpated, including the cervical, auricular, axillary, epitrochlear,

Table 48–1. Differential Diagnosis of Systemic Lymphadenopathy

Infant	Child	Adolescent
Common Causes		
Syphilis	Viral infection	Viral infection
Toxoplasmosis	EBV	EBV
CMV	CMV	CMV
HIV	HIV	HIV
	Toxoplasmosis	Toxoplasmosis
		Syphilis
Rare Causes		
Chagas disease (congenital)	Serum sickness	Serum sickness
Congenital leukemia	Lupus	Lupus
Congenital tuberculosis	Leukemia/lymphoma	Leukemia/lymphoma
Reticuloendotheliosis	Tuberculosis	Tuberculosis
Metabolic storage disease	Sarcoidosis	Sarcoidosis
	Fungal infection	Fungal infection
	Plague	Plague
	Langerhans cell histiocytosis	
	Chronic granulomatous disease	
	Sinus histiocytosis	

Abbreviations: CMV = cytomegalovirus; EBV = Epstein-Barr virus; HIV = human immunodeficiency virus.

Table 48–2. Common Sites of Local Lymphadenopathy and Associated Diseases

Cervical
  Oropharyngeal infection (viral or group A streptococcal,
    staphylococcal)
  Scalp infection
  Mycobacterial lymphadenitis
  Viral infection (EBV, CMV, HHV-6)
  Cat-scratch disease
  Kawasaki disease
  Thyroid disease
Anterior Auricular
  Conjunctivitis
  Eye infection
  Oculoglandular tularemia
Posterior Auricular
  Otitis media
  Viral infection (especially rubella, parvovirus)
Supraclavicular
  Malignancy or infection in the mediastinum (right)
  Metastatic malignancy from abdomen (left)
  Lymphoma
  Tuberculosis
Epitrochlear
  Hand infection, arm infection*
  Lymphoma†
  Sarcoid
  Syphilis
Inguinal
  Urinary tract infection
  Venereal disease (especially syphilis or lymphogranuloma
    venereum)
  Lower extremity suppurative infection
  Plague
Hilar (not palpable, found on chest x-ray study)
  Tuberculosis†
  Histoplasmosis†
  Blastomycosis†
  Coccidioidomycosis†
  Leukemia/lymphoma†
  Hodgkin disease†
  Metastatic malignancy*
  Sarcoidosis†
Axillary
  Cat-scratch disease
  Arm infection
  Malignancy of chest wall
  Leukemia/lymphoma
  Brucellosis

*Unilateral.
†Bilateral.
Abbreviations: CMV = cytomegalovirus; EBV = Epstein-Barr virus; HHV-6 = human herpesvirus 6.

inguinal, and supraclavicular areas, because lymphadenopathy in certain regions is linked to systemic or local illness (Table 48–2). The location of the lymphadenopathy is crucial to the determination of its cause.

Regional lymphadenopathy usually reflects pathology within the lymphatic drainage distribution of that particular nodal chain. Enlarged cervical nodes, for example, commonly indicate the presence of infection in the oropharyngeal cavity and lead the physician to a careful examination of the oropharynx. Similarly, posterior auricular nodes are commonly seen with scalp infections and otitis media but are also common in rubella and some other viral illnesses such as parvovirus (Fifth's disease). The diagnosis of rubella or

parvovirus infection is considered if there is a rash and fever. Supraclavicular nodes are usually pathologic and are red flags for serious illness. Supraclavicular nodes that are palpated on the right side often reflect a mediastinal tumor or invasive mediastinal infection, such as histoplasmosis. Palpable supraclavicular nodes on the left side are often the result of metastatic spread of an abdominal tumor. The presence of either type of node mandates an emergency work-up to determine the presence or absence of such pathology. Epitrochlear nodes, if unilateral, commonly point toward the hand or arm as a source of distal infection, which may be obvious at further examination. Palpable bilateral epitrochlear lymph nodes usually reflect systemic illness, such as syphilis, sarcoidosis, or lymphoma. Inguinal node enlargement is common and is probably due to the frequent occurrence of minor trauma and infections in the legs and feet. Significantly enlarged inguinal nodes, however, may be present with venereal diseases, such as syphilis, nonspecific chlamydial urethritis, lymphogranuloma venereum, or with urinary tract infection or lymphoma or abdominal tumors.

In addition to the location, the characteristic feel of the nodes often yields some clues as to the cause of the adenopathy:

1. Erythema, tenderness, and warmth: acute bacterial infection with adenitis.
2. Tenderness, non-erythematous, soft: viral infection or other systemic infection.
3. Firm, hard, rubbery, nontender: lymphoma or other infiltrating tumor.
4. Hard, matted, immobile, nontender: tumor, metastatic or local; fibrosis following acute infection.

LABORATORY AND IMAGING EVALUATION

Most children with acute lymphadenopathy require few, if any, laboratory or imaging studies. No laboratory testing may be required in well-appearing children whose acute, localized adenopathy can be attributed to an infection in the vicinity of the node. Otitis media and rubella are examples of illnesses that do not usually require laboratory studies. Patients with localized cutaneous infections causing adenopathy may not need supportive laboratory investigations before the initiation of antimicrobial therapy.

Acute cervical adenopathy accompanying pharyngitis in children over the age of 2 years may require a throat culture. The addition of hepatomegaly or splenomegaly should raise suspicions of Epstein-Barr viral (EBV) infections. The clinician could obtain a complete blood count with white cell differential (to identify lymphocytosis and atypical lymphocytes) and EBV titers (or a monospot test in children older than 8 years).

Supraclavicular adenopathy, acute cervical adenopathy accompanied by respiratory distress, or prolonged cervical adenopathy warrant a chest radiograph and complete blood count with white blood cell differential. Placement of a purified protein derivative (PPD) is routine in such individuals.

Children presenting with prolonged diffuse lymphadenopathy, hepatomegaly or splenomegaly, weight loss, night sweats, fevers, recurrent infections, or failure to thrive should be more thoroughly studied. Only after the complete blood count and differential and chest radiograph are analyzed should other diagnostic studies be considered. HIV, EBV, and cytomegalovirus studies (culture or serology) may be obtained on some children. Because the diagnosis of leukemia (bone marrow aspiration, biopsy), lymphoma (bone marrow aspiration, biopsy), systemic lupus erythematosus (antinuclear antibody, double-stranded DNA antibodies), and cat-scratch disease (biopsy) require more invasive and expensive tests, the physician should first consider all aspects of the history and physical examination before ordering laboratory studies.

DIFFERENTIAL DIAGNOSIS

Infections of the Oropharynx

Pharyngeal infection is the most common cause of local lymphadenopathy in children (see Chapter 6). Many of these pharyngeal infections are associated with cervical lymphadenopathy, are viral in origin, and include adenovirus, parainfluenza, influenza, rhinovirus, and enterovirus as possible causes. EBV and cytomegalovirus also can cause pharyngitis and cervical lymphadenopathy. The chief complaint usually includes pain with swallowing (particularly pain with swallowing of acidic juices) and talking as well as tender, enlarged lymph nodes in the neck. Systemic complaints, such as fever, muscle aches, and rhinorrhea, also may be present. An examination of the throat usually yields a symmetric erythematous posterior pharynx with enlarged tonsils, often with exudates. Exudates can be seen with both viral and bacterial causes of pharyngitis and adenopathy and thus does not discriminate between the two causes.

Herpes stomatitis (mucocutaneous involvement) or pharyngitis (oropharyngeal vesicles) is associated with bilaterally enlarged, tender, non-erythematous cervical nodes. Bacterial infection of the pharynx is also commonly associated with enlarged, tender cervical lymph nodes. Group A beta-hemolytic streptococcus is the most common pathogen to cause such infections and is difficult to differentiate clinically from viral causes of pharyngitis and lymphadenopathy, making throat culture or rapid antigen detection necessary. An associated sandpapery skin rash or beefy-red tonsils with palatal petechiae are not usually seen with viral pathogens and should make the examiner consider group A streptococci and toxin-mediated scarlet fever as a likely cause. Other bacteria also can cause pharyngitis and cervical adenopathy, including non–group A streptococci as well as anaerobic organisms, such as *Fusobacterium*. These organisms can lead to painful oral gingivitis or stomatitis and pharyngitis (Vincent's angina) that may progress to peritonsillar abscess. Asymmetry in the tonsils and the pharyngeal tissue surrounding the tonsils may be seen with peritonsillar abscesses, along with unilateral tender, enlarged cervical lymph nodes.

Acute cervical lympadenopathy or lymphadenitis (inflammation of the cervical lymph nodes with tender enlargement) is much more likely to occur, however, with group A streptococcal infection or with *Staphylococcus aureus* infection as well as with oral bacteria, including non–group A streptococci and anaerobes, presumably with the pharynx as the portal of entry. Other common sites for acute lymphadenitis include the submandibular nodes. Usually, these nodes quickly diminish in size after institution of oral or intravenous antibiotics with appropriate coverage for these pathogens (e.g., amoxicillin/clavulanic acid, ampicillin/sulbactam, nafcillin, clindamycin).

Suppuration of the nodes with drainage is less common than adenitis and generally rules out viral infection as the primary cause. Acute suppurative cervical adenitis can be seen in infections of the face and scalp and is usually due to group A streptococcal or *S. aureus* infection. Management of suppuration includes incision and drainage or excision of the suppurative node; Gram stain; bacterial, fungal and mycobacterial cultures of the drainage; and institution of appropriate antimicrobial therapy (Fig. 48–3). Total excision should be performed if mycobacterial infection is suspected.

Infections of the Extremities

Bacterial infections of the skin and soft tissues (erysipelas, abscess, cellulitis, fasciitis) of the extremities in children are common causes of lymphadenopathy and adenitis. These infections, primarily caused by group A beta-hemolytic streptococci or *S. aureus*, may drain into and inflame single or multiple regional lymph nodes.

Occasionally, injuries to the feet that occur in wet areas or through damp sneakers or shoes may yield infections with other bacteria, such as *Pseudomonas aeruginosa*. These infections usually present with cellulitis or osteomyelitis; lymphadenopathy is noted during the physical examination. The most common sites of infection include the foot or leg, leading to unilateral inguinal lymphadenitis, and the hand or arm, causing axillary lymphadenitis or, less commonly, unilateral inflammation of the epitrochlear nodes (see Fig. 48–3).

Epstein-Barr Virus Infection

Childhood infection with the EBV is a common cause of both regional and diffuse lymphadenopathy. This virus classically causes a "mononucleosis" syndrome in adolescents and young adults (Fig. 48–4), consisting of acute pharyngitis that may have a prolonged course, with tender firm cervical adenopathy (but sometimes with generalized adenopathy), malaise, fever, weight loss, and anorexia. Approximately 10% of patients become jaundiced; over 80% have mild hepatitis that is clinically silent but can be documented with liver function studies. Splenomegaly is present in more than 50% of patients and may rarely cause splenic rupture. A small number also have such parapharyngeal lymphoid hyperplasia, which causes difficulty swallowing or breathing that can produce significant problems, leading to dehydration or airway obstruction. Small children with EBV infection often present in a variable and atypical fashion or may be completely asymptomatic. Nonspecific rash (often after ampicillin therapy), fever, and mild cervical adenopathy may be the major symptoms on presentation, or the child may be significantly ill with high fever and pharyngitis. Young children with acute EBV infection are more likely to have hepatosplenomegaly, rash, and eyelid edema than are young adults.

The diagnosis of EBV infection in older children focuses on the aforementioned clinical syndrome and a relative lymphocytosis seen in the differential white blood cell count (40% to 50%), which shows a substantial percent of atypical lymphocytes (10% to 20%). Heterophile IgM antibodies, which are non-EBV–directed, and agglutinate sheep and horse red blood cells are found in more than 80% of young adults with EBV and are at maximal titer 3 to 4 weeks after infection. Heterophile antibodies are rarely found in young children (less than age 5 years) with EBV infections, and the monospot or other heterophile antibody test is not useful in this age group. In young children, antibody titers directed to specific EBV antigens are necessary to confirm the diagnosis (Fig. 48–5). IgM antibodies against viral capsid antigen (VCA) followed by IgG directed to VCA and early antigens (EAs) are the most common antibody profile. Antibodies to nuclear antigens (EBNA) develop weeks later, and if present with EA IgG are indicative of infection in the recent past. Approximately 20% of children present after the VCA IgM has already declined—these children will have VCA and EA IgG present.

Because group A streptococcal infection can present in a similar fashion to, or be present simultaneously with, EBV, and because other viruses can initially cause pharyngitis and tender, enlarged cervical lymph nodes, differentiating these various causes of pharyngitis and lymphadenopathy is important. Acute streptococcal pharyngitis improves after institution of penicillin therapy; EBV infections do not and also have a more prolonged clinical course. In addition, severe malaise and splenomegaly do not occur with most bacterial or viral causes of pharyngitis and cervical lymphadenopathy. These findings prompt the clinician to examine a peripheral white blood cell count and differential and to perform serologic confirmation of EBV infection. Similarly, most viral causes of cervical adenopathy and pharyngitis (except CMV) are not associated with the brisk atypical lymphocytosis commonly seen with EBV infections, and they are not usually associated with abnormal liver function results.

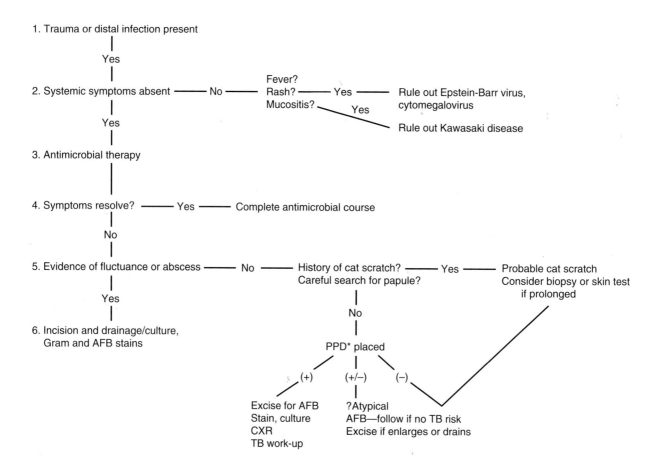

1. Trauma or distal infection present
   |
   Yes
   |
2. Systemic symptoms absent ——— No ——— Fever?
                                         Rash? ——— Yes ——— Rule out Epstein-Barr virus,
                                         Mucositis? ——— Yes   cytomegalovirus
   | Rule out Kawasaki disease
   Yes
   |
3. Antimicrobial therapy
   |
   |
4. Symptoms resolve? ——— Yes ——— Complete antimicrobial course
   |
   No
   |
5. Evidence of fluctuance or abscess ——— No ——— History of cat scratch? ——— Yes ——— Probable cat scratch
   | Careful search for papule?   Consider biopsy or skin test
   Yes | if prolonged
   | No
6. Incision and drainage/culture, |
   Gram and AFB stains   PPD* placed
                                                            |
                                            (+)   (+/−)   (−)
                                   Excise for AFB   ?Atypical
                                   Stain, culture   AFB—follow if no TB risk
                                   CXR   Excise if enlarges or drains
                                   TB work-up

*15 mm induration or more in a low-risk child with tuberculosis.

Figure 48–3. Paradigm for the management of typical acute regional lymphadenopathy (e.g., cervical, axillary, inguinal) in children. AFB = acid-fast bacillus—tuberculosis (TB); CXR = chest x-ray; PPD = purified protein derivative.

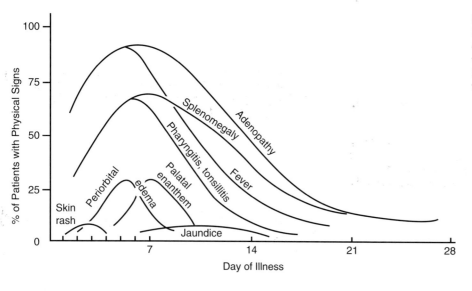

Figure 48–4. The clinical course of acute Epstein-Barr mononucleosis. Adenopathy occurs early in the infection and can persist for weeks. (Modified from Rapp CE, Hewston JF. Infectious mononucleosis and the Epstein-Barr virus. Am J Dis Child 1978; 132:78.)

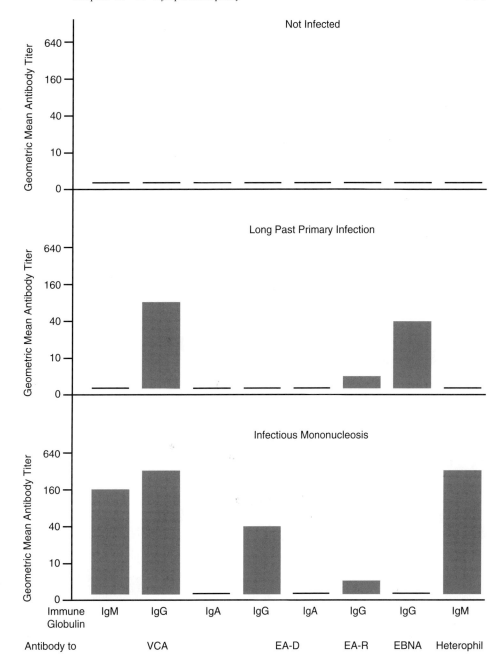

Figure 48–5. Serologic patterns in individuals not infected with the Epstein-Barr virus (EBV) *(top)*, infected with EBV in the past *(middle)*, and acutely infected with EBV *(bottom)*. EA = early antigen; EBNA = Epstein-Barr nuclear antigen; VCA = viral capsid antigen test. (From Res Staff Phys 1981:37.)

Cytomegalovirus Infection

Cytomegalovirus infection in children can be associated with a mononucleosis-like syndrome and lymphadenopathy. CMV mononucleosis is associated with fever and malaise similar to that seen in EBV; in contrast to EBV, however, CMV mononucleosis does not usually cause severe, exudative tonsillopharyngitis or the production of heterophil-specific or EBV-specific antibodies. CMV mononucleosis can be associated with an atypical lymphocytosis and diffuse lymphadenopathy in the normal host. Women of childbearing age who are pregnant when they have primary CMV (cervical or viremia) infections (usually through sexual contact) are at risk of delivering a child with congenital infection with CMV through transplacental infection or through contact with infected cervical secretions at the time of delivery. Infants with congenital CMV may have many complications and clinical findings. Lymphadenopathy is not a common finding in these congenitally infected infants.

The diagnosis in older children is usually made serologically, in tests measuring both IgM and IgG antibodies directed to CMV or by obtaining a throat or blood specimen for culture (leukocyte) that is positive for CMV. Congenital infection is confirmed by identifying CMV in the urine of the neonate in the first week of life.

Human Herpesvirus 6 Infection

Infection with the human herpesvirus 6 (HHV-6), in addition to causing roseola, has been associated with a mononucleosis-like syndrome with diffuse or cervical adenopathy in individuals who are seronegative for EBV and CMV. In addition, elevated or rising titers of antibodies to HHV-6 have been found in patients with documented acute EBV and CMV infections. It is unclear whether these seroconversions represent false-positive results caused by cross-reactive antigens between EBV, CMV, and HHV-6 or whether the HHV-6 rising antibody titers may represent a reactivation of old HHV-6 disease caused by another viral infection.

Cat-Scratch Disease

Cat-scratch disease (CSD) is an infection whose primary symptom is lymphadenopathy caused by a small gram-negative bacillus, *Bartonella henselae* (formerly *Rochalimaea henselae*). This organism has been isolated from patients with CSD, and serologic studies have shown that most patients with clinical CSD have antibodies to it. *B. henselae* also causes bacillary angiomatosis in patients with acquired immunodeficiency syndrome (AIDS). Cat-scratch disease occurs several days after exposure to a scratch or, less commonly, a bite of a cat or kitten (more than 90% of patients with clinical CSD report contact with cats). A papule at the site of the trauma usually develops, followed in 7 to 14 days by regional lymphadenopathy. Most patients with CSD have a single enlarged, often tender, lymph node. Axillary nodes are the most likely to be enlarged, probably because of the upper extremities being the most likely part of the body to be scratched or bitten. The next most common sites are in the neck and jaw, followed by the inguinal region. Although single nodes are most commonly affected, regional adenopathy involving several nodes may also occur. Generalized lymphadenopathy is extremely rare in CSD presenting in the normal host.

Approximately half the patients have low-grade fever and malaise; a small number have high fevers (>39.5°C) and more severe systemic symptoms. In most patients, the swollen, inflamed nodes regress spontaneously within several weeks; approximately 10% go on to have purulent fluid drainage that is culture-negative by standard techniques. Uncommon complications include encephalopathy that resolves spontaneously; erythema nodosum; oculoglandular syndrome of Parinaud, in which the CSD organism is inoculated into the eye and causes conjunctivitis and preauricular adenopathy; thrombocytopenia; hepatitis; or splenitis with granulomas; transverse myelitis; encephalitis; and rarely, osteolytic bone lesions.

The diagnosis is based on the history of contact with kittens or cats and the classic clinical presentation, including a careful search for an entrance site papule.

The gold standard for diagnosis is the pathology of tissue from a biopsy specimen of the involved node, which shows granulomas, central necrosis, and organisms seen on Warthin-Starry silver stain. The decision to perform a biopsy is usually reached when there is no clear history of cat scratch or when the presentation is atypical and cannot be differentiated from other, more serious illness, such as mycobacterial adenitis.

The treatment of CSD has not been adequately subjected to rigorous, randomized studies. Various antibiotics have been used in an uncontrolled fashion. There are anecdotal reports of clinical improvement after administration of several antibiotics, including rifampin, gentamicin, ciprofloxacin, and trimethoprim-sulfamethoxazole. Because CSD is a self-limited illness in most children, most clinicians do not routinely use antimicrobial therapy.

Chronic Granulomatous Disease

Chronic granulomatous disease (CGD) (see Chapter 52) comprises a group of rare inherited disorders of neutrophil function, characterized by recurrent pyogenic infections, which are often accompanied by lymphadenopathy and/or abscess formation. Most cases are inherited in an X-linked fashion; 30% are transmitted as an autosomal recessive trait. Chronic granulomatous disease should be considered in a young child (often male) who presents with recurrent fever and infection, pneumonia, adenopathy, and abdominal pain. Family history often reveals another relative with the disease or recalls a death from an infection in a young child.

The diagnosis is made by neutrophil nitroblue tetrazolium testing or by chemiluminescent studies, which demonstrate the defective neutrophil oxidation. Common pathogens contain catalase and include *S. aureus* and *Aspergillus*.

Human Immunodeficiency Virus

Human immunodeficiency virus (see Chapter 55) may present in children with diffuse lymphadenopathy. Many HIV-infected children also have failure to thrive, poor weight gain, and evidence of other infections, for example, oral thrush or opportunistic pneumonias such as that caused by *Pneumocystis carinii*. HIV-infected children are also more likely than normal hosts to have other infectious causes of lymphadenopathy, such as tuberculosis, or noninfectious causes, such as lymphoma. A history of transfusion or HIV risk factors is important to obtain. Regional lymphadenopathy is not a common presentation of HIV infections unless the adenitis represents another bacterial or mycobacterial infection.

Mycobacterial Infections

Tubercular cervical adenitis is not common in the United States, but in the past it was often associated with ingestion of raw, contaminated milk and infection with *Mycobacterium bovis*. With modern milk pasteurization and cattle inspection, *M. bovis* infection is very unusual. Regional or diffuse lymphadenopathy due to infection with *Mycobacterium tuberculosis* is also unusual in developed countries. Infection with *M. tuberculosis* is increasing in frequency in children in the United States as a result of an increase in the number of adults actively infected. This increase is associated with various problems, including underfunded tuberculosis control programs, the likelihood of some HIV-infected individuals to have a high mycobacterial burden, noncompliance by infected individuals with multidrug treatment regimens, and drug resistance by the organism. Most adenitis caused by mycobacteria in the United States is caused by atypical strains that are not serious pathogens in the normal host. With the increase in classic tuberculosis in the United States, however, differentiating tuberculosis infection that causes adenitis from that caused by atypical mycobacteria is becoming more and more important.

Several historical and clinical criteria can be used to differentiate tuberculosis adenitis from atypical mycobacterial infections. Most children with tuberculosis have a history of exposure to an adult with active tuberculosis, whereas those with atypical infections do not. Infection with atypical mycobacteria is more common in the southern parts of the United States. Children with tuberculosis adenitis often have hilar lymphadenopathy because the lungs are usually the source of primary infection, whereas those with cervical lymphadenitis due to atypical strains rarely have hilar adenopathy. Evidence of extra lymphatic disease also is common in children with tuberculosis and includes pneumonia, pleural effusions, bone marrow suppression, liver function abnormalities, and miliary disease. Disseminated tuberculosis may present with diffuse lymphadenopathy and should be considered if pulmonary infiltrates and systemic symptoms are present. Such extra lymphatic disease and diffuse lymphadenopathy is rare in normal children with adenitis caused by atypical mycobacteria but may occur in HIV-infected children infected with atypical mycobacteria.

The most common mycobacterial infection in children in the United States is infection of the lymph nodes with the atypical mycobacteria, primarily in the *Mycobacterium avium-intracellulare* complex as well as *Mycobacterium kansasii, Mycobacterium scrofulaceum,* and *Mycobacterium marinum.* The lymph nodes involved are unilateral and cervical in most infections, presumably because the organism enters via the oropharynx. Most frequently, a previously healthy child presents with unilateral lymphadenitis or adenopathy in the cervical, submandibular, or submaxillary region. Although fever may be present, significant systemic symptoms are usually not associated with local infection with atypical mycobacteria in the normal host. In a small number of patients, the affected node spontaneously ruptures and drains before presentation. The drainage is not usually grossly purulent and may be a clue that atypical mycobacteria are the cause of the infected node.

The gold standard for diagnosis of lymphadenitis due to atypical mycobacteria is acid-fast staining and culture of the excised node. Incision and drainage of these nodes may lead to chronically draining sinus tracts, which may scar; thus, this method is contraindicated. Fine needle aspiration may be beneficial if indicated. The usual clinical scenario involves a young, preschool-aged child with an enlarged cervical node that responds poorly to oral or intravenous antibiotics. The child has no history of cat scratch and is otherwise clinically well. A tuberculin skin test (which should be placed in children with lymphadenopathy) (see Fig. 48–3) often yields 5 to 9 mm of induration because atypical mycobacteria have cross-reactive antigens to those of tuberculosis. This amount of induration is considered indeterminate for tuberculosis in low-risk patients and suggests that the adenopathy is due to an atypical mycobacterium. Skin tests using antigens from the various atypical mycobacteria are very sensitive and specific for infection. These antigens are not consistently available in the United States. Rarely, infection with atypical mycobacteria yields skin test results in the positive range of more than 15-mm induration, which mandates a more extensive work-up that focuses on the possibility that the adenitis is due to *M. tuberculosis* infection. Gradual resolution of lymphadenitis may sometimes occur in children with atypical mycobacterial infections. Excisional biopsy is not necessary if the diagnosis is presumptively made from skin test results of less than 10 mm in induration, if other infections are ruled out, if resolution occurs, and if the child is at low risk for infection with *M. tuberculosis* (see Chapter 7). If the node does not improve, continues to enlarge, or spontaneously drains, fine needle aspiration (culture or acid-fast stain) or total excision is recommended and is usually curative.

Chemotherapy with antitubercular drugs is controversial for several reasons. First, most of the atypical mycobacteria tend to be resistant to the usual antitubercular drugs, and multiple, potentially toxic regimens are required. Second, because this is a self-limited infection that sometimes resolves or can be cured with excision, long courses of chemotherapy seem unwarranted. Finally, although there have been no controlled trials, use of antitubercular therapy in these children seems to have limited efficacy compared with that of excision. Antitubercular therapy should not be initiated without adequate cultures.

Toxoplasmosis

Toxoplasma gondii is a protozoan organism that is a parasite of cats. Many other animals, including humans, can be incidentally and chronically infected hosts in which the parasite cannot complete its life cycle. Human acquisition of toxoplasmosis in childhood can occur from contact with cat feces or soil containing oocysts, which infect the child when they are ingested. Alternatively, the ingestion of raw or undercooked meat, particularly lamb and pork that contain tissue cysts, may lead to infection. Adults in the United States are more likely to be infected from ingestion of raw meat than from contact with cat feces and soil oocysts. Finally, infection can be transmitted to the fetus, especially when a pregnant woman is acutely infected with toxoplasmosis. Although many of the fetal infections are asymptomatic, transplacental infection with toxoplasmosis can result in severe neurologic damage, retinochoroiditis, aseptic meningitis, and significant systemic illness presenting with the classic triad of hepatosplenomegaly, intracranial calcifications, and hydrocephalus. Although lymphadenopathy can occur in the newborn with congenital toxoplasmosis, lymphadenopathy is a more common presenting symptom of acute toxoplasmosis in older children and young adults.

The most common symptoms in children who acquire toxoplasmosis are lymphadenopathy, fever, malaise, myalgia, and pharyngitis. The nodes most commonly affected include anterior and posterior cervical and axillary, which may be tender; involvement is usually bilateral. The lymph node enlargement seen in toxoplasmosis is due to reticular hyperplasia and inflammation. Most laboratory results are normal, but the white blood cell count may show an absolute lymphocytosis with atypical lymphocytes, causing confusion with EBV or CMV mononucleosis.

The diagnosis is made primarily with serologic studies measuring IgG and IgM directed to antigens of the parasite. If tissue is available after biopsy, actual parasite forms can sometimes be demonstrated. Various diagnostic techniques can be used on the patient's serum, including indirect immunofluorescence, complement fixation, and enzyme-linked immunosorbent assay (ELISA). A fourfold rise in IgG titer or the presence of IgM antibodies is diagnostic. In neonatal infections, tests measuring IgM have become more sensitive and specific for the diagnosis of toxoplasmosis infection. Antigen tests and tests that grow the parasite are also available, but primarily on an investigational level.

Effective therapy for toxoplasmosis uses sulfonamides combined with pyrimethamine. Early treatment is especially important in the infant with congenital infection because treatment may yield improved neurologic outcome. Pregnant women known to be newly infected with toxoplasmosis can be treated with spiramycin, which concentrates in the placenta and interrupts transplacental infection of the fetus; sulfonamides and pyrimethamine also eradicate the parasite from the fetus. Preliminary data from France suggest that these therapies significantly improve the previously poor outcome of the congenitally infected infant.

Treatment of older children and adults with acute toxoplasmosis is more controversial. Many investigators do not treat immunologically normal individuals unless symptoms are persistent and severe. By contrast, individuals with T-cell deficiencies, such as those with AIDS, can develop severe disseminated toxoplasmosis, particularly involving the central nervous system and retina. Therefore, prolonged therapy is mandatory in these patients.

Syphilis

Syphilis, caused by the spirochete *Treponema pallidum,* is becoming more common in the United States. Numerous factors have caused this resurgent epidemic, including difficulty in eradicating the organism in patients with HIV, prostitution to obtain crack cocaine in the inner cities, and decreased public funding for syphilis control programs. Syphilis remains primarily a sexually transmitted disease. However, pregnant women with syphilis who are untreated readily transmit the disease to the fetus, causing congenital syphilis. Congenital syphilis leads to significant sequelae and represents a failure of the health care system to educate the population, detect disease, and treat young, sexually active people of child-bearing ages.

The natural course of syphilis in adults includes three major clinical manifestations:

- *Primary syphilis,* in which the individual develops a painless chancre at the site of inoculation

Table 48–3. Diagnostic Criteria for Kawasaki Disease*

A. Fever lasting for at least 5 days†
B. Presence of *four of the following five* conditions:
   1. Bilateral nonpurulent conjunctival injection
   2. Changes of the mucosa of the oropharynx, including infected pharynx, infected and/or dry fissured lips, strawberry tongue
   3. Changes of the peripheral extremities, such as edema and/or erythema of the hands or feet, desquamation, usually beginning periungually
   4. Rash, primarily truncal; polymorphous but nonvesicular
   5. Cervical lymphadenopathy
C. Illness not explained by other known disease process

*A consensus statement prepared by North Amerian participants of the Third International Kawasaki Disease Symposium, Tokyo, Japan, December, 1988. Pediatr Infect Dis J 8:663, 1989. © by Williams & Wilkins, 1989. Reprinted from Behrman RE. Nelson Textbook of Pediatrics, 14th ed. Philadelphia: WB Saunders, 1992:629.

†Many experts believe that, in the presence of classic features, the diagnosis of Kawasaki disease can be made (and treatment instituted) before the fifth day of fever by experienced individuals.

- *Secondary syphilis*, in which the organism hematogenously disseminates to many organs with protean manifestations
- *Tertiary syphilis*, in which end organs, such as the brain, heart, and bones, develop gummatous lesions

Lymphadenopathy can be seen as one of the manifestations of syphilis in several situations. In primary syphilis, in which the inoculation site is usually the genital area, regional lymphadenopathy with painless, firm nodes occurs at the time that a chancre is observed. Thus, inguinal adenopathy in an adolescent who is sexually active mandates further examination and work-up, to look for sexually transmitted diseases such as syphilis. In secondary syphilis, the organism has disseminated, causing multiple organs to be involved with the infection. The classic manifestations are protean and usually include nonvesicular rashes. Lymphadenopathy, regional or generalized, is common and often includes epitrochlear nodes (a hint that syphilis may be the diagnosis if no other explanation is found on the examination of the extremity). Systemic symptoms may be present with fever, malaise, anorexia, and weight loss. Syphilis, therefore, should be at the top of the differential diagnosis in sexually active adolescents with rash and lymphadenopathy. Finally, neonates with congenital syphilis may also have generalized lymphadenopathy, although this finding is less common than other systemic symptoms, such as hepatosplenomegaly, snuffles, and periosteal reactive disease.

The diagnosis of syphilis has been complicated by the inability to grow the organism *in vitro*. Dark-field examination of tissue from chancres or mucous lesions shows numerous spirochetes. Serology, however, continues to be the primary mode of diagnosis. Nontreponemal serologies rely on the production of antibodies to nonspecific lipoidal host-tissue antigens that probably arise as a result of infection with the spirochete. These tests include the Venereal Disease Research Laboratory (VDRL) test, the serologic test for syphilis, and the rapid plasma reagin (RPR) test. These antibodies decline after adequate treatment and are extremely useful in confirming eradication of the infection. False-positive reactions can occur, particularly in individuals with connective tissue disorders or mononucleosis. By contrast, the fluorescent treponemal antibody absorption (FTA-ABS) test measures antibodies directed specifically to *T. pallidum* and can be used as a confirmatory test in individuals with positive results on screening tests. These antibodies also remain present for the life of the infected individual, even if the patient receives adequate therapy. Thus, in contrast to the VDRL, the ''FTA-ABS'' has little use in following the efficacy of treatment.

The mainstay of treatment for syphilis remains penicillin. Neo-

nates may require relatively long courses of intravenous penicillin because of the difficulties in ruling out and treating presumed neurosyphilis. Persons with HIV infection also require prolonged high-dose penicillin therapies because syphilis appears to be particularly difficult to eradicate in immunodeficient individuals.

Kawasaki Disease
(Mucocutaneous Lymph Node Syndrome)

The diagnosis of Kawasaki disease is determined clinically in children who present with five consecutive days or more of high fever accompanied by cervical lymphadenopathy, mucosal erythema, conjunctivitis without exudates, skin rash, and desquamation of the skin on the fingers and toes (Table 48–3). Although not all features of the syndrome need be present, the history of prolonged fevers is universal, and adenopathy is common. Because the serious consequences from coronary artery vasculitis or aneurysms (myocardial infarction secondary to thrombosis) can be effectively prevented by treatment with high-dose aspirin (100 mg/kg/day) and intravenous gamma globulin (2 g/kg for one dose) therapy the diagnosis must not be overlooked. The differential diagnosis is listed in Table 48–4. The clinical course is divided into four stages, as noted in Table 48–5. Low-dose aspirin therapy (3 to 5 mg/kg/day) is offered in the convalescent phase.

Acute Leukemia, Lymphoma,
and Other Malignancies

In patients with leukemia or lymphoma, lymphadenopathy is frequently among their presenting findings. Enlarged lymph nodes may be noted in an isolated regional or generalized distribution with or without systemic symptoms, such as fever, malaise, night sweats, weight loss, and anorexia. Malignant nodes are usually firm and rubbery and nontender and may be matted. Unlike many of the acute lymphadenopathies caused by infectious agents, most lymph nodes that are malignant gradually increase in size over time. Approximately 50% of children with acute lymphoblastic leukemia have adenopathy at the time of diagnosis. Nodal disease may be either localized (often cervical) or generalized, nontender, rubbery, and frequently associated with other signs and symptoms, including fevers, malaise, weight loss, pallor, bone pain, petechiae, splenomegaly, or hepatomegaly. The complete blood count usually demonstrates anemia, thrombocytopenia, leukocytosis or leukopenia, circulating blasts, or some combination thereof. Some patients,

Table 48–4. Differential Diagnosis of Kawasaki Disease

Scarlet fever
Staphylococcal toxic shock syndrome
Stevens-Johnson syndrome (erythema multiforme)
Leptospirosis
Epstein-Barr virus
Juvenile rheumatoid arthritis
Measles
Acrodynia
Polyarteritis nodosa
Rocky Mountain spotted fever
Drug reaction
Scalded skin syndrome

From Kredicah DW. Rheumatic disease of childhood. *In* Behrman RE, Kliegman RM (eds). Nelson Essentials of Pediatrics, 2nd ed. Philadelphia: WB Saunders, 1994:293.

Table 48-5. Kawasaki Syndrome: Disease Phases, Complications, and Degree of Arteritis in Untreated Patients

	Acute	Subacute	Convalescent	Chronic
Clinical findings	Duration (1–11 days) Fever, conjunctivitis, oral changes, extremity changes, irritability, rash, cervical lymphadenopathy, high ESR	Duration (11–21 days) Irritability persists Prolongation of fever may occur Normalization of most clinical findings Palpable aneurysms may develop	Duration (21–60 days) Most clinical findings resolve Aneurysmal dilatation of peripheral vessels may persist Conjunctivitis may persist	Duration (? yr)
Complications	Early arthritis Myocarditis Pericarditis Mitral insufficiency Congestive heart failure Iridocyclitis Meningitis Sterile pyuria	Cononary aneurysms Late-onset arthritis Mitral insufficiency Gallbladder hydrops Fingertip and toe desquamation Thrombocytosis Coronary thrombosis with infarction	Arthritis may persist Coronary and peripheral aneurysms may persist Acute phase reactant normalization	Angina pectoris, coronary stenosis, or myocardial insufficiency may develop
Arterial correlates	Perivasculitis, vasculitis of capillaries, arterioles, venules Inflammation of intima of medium and large arteries	Aneurysms, thrombi, stenosis of medium-sized arteries, panvasculitis, edema of vessel wall Myocarditis less prominent	Vascular inflammation decreases	Scar formation Intimal thickening
Cause of death	Myocarditis	Myocardial infarction Rupture of aneurysm Myocarditis	Myocardial infarction Ischemic heart disease	Myocardial infarction

Modified from Hicks RV, Melish ME. Kawasaki syndrome. Pediatr Clin North Am 1986;33:1151. Reprinted from Behrman RE (ed). Nelson Textbook of Pediatrics, 14th ed. Philadelphia: WB Saunders, 1992:630.
Abbreviations: ESR = erythrocyte sedimentation rate.

however, may have initial normal peripheral blood laboratory results. Acute myelogenous leukemia is less common in children but may present in a similar fashion. Bone marrow biopsy and aspiration must be performed and are diagnostic.

Hodgkin disease often presents with painless cervical or supraclavicular lymphadenopathy in older school-aged children and adolescents. Nodes are firmer than those seen in patients whose nodes are enlarged in reaction to infections. In a small number of children with Hodgkin disease, the size of the nodes may wax and wane for several months before definitive diagnosis. Supraclavicular nodes usually indicate intrathoracic disease, which is present in 60% to 70% of patients at the time of diagnosis (confirmed by chest x-ray study and/or computed tomography [CT]). Axillary or inguinal nodes may also be the site of presenting lymphadenopathy. Approximately 30% of patients with Hodgkin disease have systemic symptoms at presentation, including fatigue, weight loss, fevers, night sweats, and poor appetite. Some patients with Hodgkin disease also have unusual symptoms, such as pruritus, hemolytic anemia, and chest pain after alcohol ingestion. Such systemic symptoms with lymphadenopathy are *red flags* for immediate work-up for malignancy. Diagnosis is confirmed by biopsy of involved nodes and/or bone marrow aspiration if the tumor has spread to the bone marrow.

Non-Hodgkin lymphoma is a relatively common childhood malignancy and often presents with mediastinal or pleural disease. Adenopathy in the supraclavicular, cervical, or axillary regions is usually present and may occur in the absence of chest involvement. Systemic symptoms are variable at the time of diagnosis. Lymph nodes, as with other malignancies, tend to be firm and rubbery. Their size may increase relatively rapidly over several weeks. Because lymphoblastic lymphoma may represent a variant of acute lymphoblastic leukemia, the signs and symptoms of leukemia and lymphoma may merge. Non-Hodgkin lymphoma of B-cell origin

(Burkitt and non-Burkitt lymphoma) in children in the United States usually originates in an intra-abdominal site, and regional adenopathy, if present, is then in the inguinal or iliac regions. The African variety of Burkitt lymphoma often presents as an expanding jaw mass.

Disseminated *neuroblastoma* may manifest as diffuse adenopathy in younger children. Such children often have primary adrenal or paraspinal masses with bony metastasis and have nonspecific systemic symptoms, abdominal mass, bone pain, and sometimes symptoms of spinal cord compression. Other tumors, such as rhabdomyosarcoma and thyroid cancer, may rarely present with lymphadenopathy due to local or disseminated metastasis.

Sinus Histiocytosis

Sinus histiocytosis is a rare disorder characterized by massive lymphadenopathy in the cervical region; it is associated with fever, elevated sedimentation rate, leukocytosis, and polyclonal hypergammaglobulinemia. The symptoms tend to resolve spontaneously after several months and are probably due to an immunoregulatory disorder. Diagnosis is made by biopsy of the involved nodes and pathologic examination.

MANAGEMENT STRATEGIES

Regional Lymphadenopathy

The typical child with acute regional lymphadenopathy (see Fig. 48-3) is previously healthy and presents with enlarged nodes, commonly in the cervical region. Careful history and physical examination should reveal whether nodes are definitively involved (compared with the parotid gland); whether other infected sites, such as the pharynx, are present; whether other causes (e.g., cat scratch) exist for the adenopathy; or whether the nodes have the characteristics of malignancy. In many cases, no other abnormalities are found on examination and systemic signs are minimal. Laboratory tests should include a complete blood count and differential as well as a sedimentation rate. In the child with fever and a tender cervical lymph node, oral antibiotics (with activity against mouth flora, streptococci, and staphylococci) should be started; if the lymphadenopathy persists or worsens, intravenous antibiotics are indicated. A PPD test should be placed, and if the results are negative and symptoms resolve, it is reasonable to complete the antimicrobial course orally.

By contrast, if the lymphadenopathy continues or becomes frank lymphadenitis with erythema and tenderness despite antimicrobial therapy, further work-up is indicated. Imaging the involved area is helpful but not always necessary. Although ultrasonography can reveal enlarged nodes or a fluid-filled abscess or cyst, CT of the area is the best method to define the extent of inflamed nodes and whether an abscess is present. If an abscess is found, incision and drainage followed by appropriate bacterial and mycobacterial cultures and stains are appropriate. If atypical mycobacteria are suspected based on a borderline positive PPD or clinical presentation, excisional biopsy is preferred because incision and drainage often leads to draining sinus tracts that are difficult to heal. Enlarged nodes that do not recede in several weeks with appropriate antimicrobial therapy also should raise the suspicion of malignancy.

Generalized Lymphadenopathy

In the child with generalized lymphadenopathy, the cause may be either infectious, immunologic, or malignant. Infectious causes, such as HIV, EBV, toxoplasmosis, secondary syphilis, and CMV infections, can generally be quickly determined via serologic testing. Noninfectious causes, such as systemic lupus erythematosus and serum sickness, can also generally be excluded by serologies and/or a careful history. If the generalized lymphadenopathy cannot be attributed to an infectious or other cause, and especially if there are systemic symptoms, malignancy should be considered. In addition, enlarging nodes that do not recede in several weeks, despite a diagnosis of a "viral" infection, should also raise concern for possible malignancy. An abnormal complete blood count demonstrating a depressed white cell, red cell, or platelet count or a chest x-ray study demonstrating mediastinal adenopathy or pleural disease is highly suggestive of malignancy. Because serious disseminated infections, such as tuberculosis and histoplasmosis, can present with a similar fashion, fine needle aspiration or biopsy of an involved node or bone marrow aspiration is crucial to obtaining a rapid diagnosis to differentiate malignancy from disseminated infection. Excision of a node is preferred in some cases to obtain adequate tissue for pathology, stains, or cultures.

SUMMARY AND RED FLAGS

Lymphadenopathy is one of the most common manifestations of childhood diseases. Most often, localized adenopathy is associated with a bacterial infection in the vicinity of the node or with a viral pharyngitis. Even generalized adenopathy in a child does not usually indicate a serious underlying disease. In children, adenopathy usually resolves either spontaneously or after appropriate antibiotic therapy. However, when adenopathy is accompanied by weight loss, recurrent fevers, night sweats, or other systemic signs or symptoms, a more serious cause must be vigorously sought. Obviously, adenopathy associated with hepatomegaly, splenomegaly, or an abdominal mass must be quickly investigated. Further, if the adenopathy does not diminish or resolve after antibiotic therapy or after 3 weeks, a more thorough evaluation is necessary. In children with known immunodeficiencies, the cause of the adenopathy is likely to be far more serious. These children are more prone to infections, and malignancies occur at a higher frequency in these children than in the general population.

REFERENCES

Cat-Scratch Disease

Carithers HA. Cat-scratch diseases: An overview based on a study of 1,200 patients. Am J Dis Child 1985;139:1124.
Schwartzman WA. Infections due to *Rochalimaea*: The expanding clinical spectrum. Clin Infect Dis 1992;15:893.

Cervical Adenopathy

Barton LL, Feigin RD. Childhood cervical lymphadenitis: A reappraisal. J Pediatr 1974;84:846.
Brook I. Aerobic and anaerobic bacteriology of cervical adenitis in children. Clin Pediatr 1980;19:693.

Epstein-Barr Viral Infections

Rapp CE, Heweston JF. Infectious mononucleosis and the Epstein-Barr virus. Am J Dis Child 1978;132:78.
Sumaya CV, Ench Y. Epstein-Barr virus infectious mononucleosis in children: I. Clinical and general laboratory findings. Pediatrics 1985;75:1003.

General References

Greenfield S, Jordan ML. The clinical investigation of lymphadenopathy in primary care practice. JAMA 1978;240:1388.
Grossman M, Shiramizu B. Evaluation of lymphadenopathy in children. Curr Opin Pediatr 1994;6:68–76.

Human Immunodeficiency Virus

Baroni CD, Uccini S. The lymphadenopathy of HIV infection. Am J Clin Pathol 1993;99:397–401.

Leukemia and Lymphoma

Graham M. Non-Hodgkin's lymphomas. Pediatr Ann 1988;17:192.

Mycobacterial Infections

Huebner RE, Schein MF, Cauthen GM, et al. Usefulness of skin testing with mycobacterial antigens in children with cervical adenopathy. Pediatr Infect Dis J 1992;11:450–456.
Schaad UB, Votteler TP, McCracken GH, Nelson JD. Management of atypical mycobacterial lymphadenitis in childhood: A review based on 380 cases. J Pediatr 1979;95:356.

Schuit KE, Powell DA. Mycobacterial lymphadenitis in childhood. Am J Dis Child 1978;132:675.

Sexually Transmitted Diseases

Morbid Mortal Wkly Rep Centers for Disease Control. 1993 Sexually transmitted diseases treatment guidelines: Syphilis. 1993;42:27–46.

Sinus Histiocytosis

Stones DK, Havenga C. Sinus histiocytosis with massive lymphadenopathy. Arch Dis Child 1992;67:521–523.

Toxoplasmosis

Frenkel JK. Toxoplasmosis. Pediatr Clin North Am 1985;32:917.

49 Pallor and Anemia

Brian W. Berman

PALLOR AND ANEMIA

Pallor, a perceptible deficit in the usual color and tone of the skin and/or mucosa, may result from alterations of cutaneous blood flow, anemia, or unknown mechanisms. Under normal circumstances, the pink appearance of the skin, lips, and mucosa is influenced by the nature and character of these tissues, the adequacy of vascular perfusion, and the concentration of hemoglobin. Pallor is a highly nonspecific finding that may be a manifestation of a wide diversity of disease, or it may be normal for a given individual. Parental perception of pallor frequently generates considerable anxiety. Although pallor is most often intuitively associated with anemia by families as well as by physicians, an open-minded, broad diagnostic perspective is appropriate (Table 49–1).

Anemia is a decrease in hemoglobin concentration (or hematocrit) of more than two standard deviations below the mean. Anemia is clinically relevant only when the low hemoglobin concentration results in a decreased oxygen-carrying capacity in the blood. By definition, 2.5% of the general population has a hemoglobin or a hematocrit level below the defined limits of normal. This fact must be kept in mind in the evaluation of children with mild anemia for which no explanation can be identified. Hemoglobin concentration varies considerably with age and sex (Table 49–2). Newborns have relatively high levels of circulating hemoglobin, which is an intrauterine adaptation to a relatively hypoxic environment. During the first 2 months of life, hemoglobin production markedly diminishes as a physiologic nadir is reached. The mean hemoglobin level rises gradually during childhood for both boys and girls until puberty is reached, when males achieve a level approximately 20% greater than that in females. The average hemoglobin level in black children is slightly lower (0.5 g/dl) than that in white or Asian children. *It is always appropriate to consider the hemoglobin concentration of a given patient in the context of age and sex.*

Anemia may result from intrinsic disorders of the bone marrow or red cell or from a wide range of superimposed factors. Anemia occurs as the result of one of three pathophysiologic mechanisms:

- Acute blood loss
- Impaired production of erythrocytes
- Increased destruction of red blood cells (hemolysis).

Under normal circumstances, the body's red blood cell (RBC) mass is maintained at a level appropriate to support tissue oxygen needs through the oxygen-sensing regulatory feedback stimulus of the hormone erythropoietin. Erythropoietin acts to stimulate the production of mature RBCs within the bone marrow. Over a 3- to 5-day period, RBC precursors mature into reticulocytes, the immediate precursor to the mature RBC, and are then released into the peripheral blood. In 24 to 48 hours, reticulocytes become mature RBCs, which then circulate in the peripheral blood for approximately 120 days. Senescent RBCs are removed from the circulation by reticuloendothelial cells within the spleen, liver, and bone marrow. A metabolic by-product of hemoglobin catabolism is bilirubin (see Chapter 24).

History

The child with pallor may not necessarily be anemic. An assessment of sun exposure and familial patterns of complexion is crucial because many patients are intrinsically pale by nature. A careful evaluation of the medical history is fundamental in the assessment of the pale patient (Table 49–3). In addition, one must determine the acuity of the anemia, its association with other symptoms, and the history of any chronic illness (weight loss, fever, malaise).

Dietary history is important as it relates to sources of iron. Infants, particularly those delivered prematurely and those consuming large amounts of cow's milk or formula unsupplemented with iron are at risk for iron deficiency anemia, as are children and adolescents who consume little meat. Patients or breast-fed infants of mothers who follow a strict vegan diet may become deficient in vitamin B_{12}. A history of pica suggests possible lead toxicity, iron deficiency, or both.

A neonatal history of hyperbilirubinemia supports a possible diagnosis of congenital hemolytic anemia, such as hereditary spherocytosis, which is further supported by a family history of anemia, splenectomy, and/or cholecystectomy (resulting from gallstones caused by chronic hyperbilirubinemia).

Medication history is pertinent because certain drugs induce oxidant-associated hemolysis in the patient deficient in glucose-6-

Table 49–1. Causes of Pallor in Children Based on Etiologic Mechanism

I. **Anemia**
II. **Decreased tendency of the skin to pigment**
    A. Physiologic (fair-skinned individuals)
    B. Limited sun exposure
III. **Alteration of the consistency of the subcutaneous tissue**
    A. Edematous states
        Increased intravascular hydrostatic pressure (e.g., congestive heart failure)
        Decreased intravascular oncotic pressure (hypoproteinemia)
        Increased vascular permeability (e.g., vasculitis)
    B. Hypothyroidism
IV. **Decreased perfusion of the cutaneous/mucosa vasculature**
    A. Hypotension
        Cardiogenic shock (pump failure or rhythm disturbance)
        Hypovolemia (blood loss, dehydration)
        Anaphylaxis
        Sepsis
        Acute adrenal insufficiency
        Vasovagal syncope
    B. Vasoconstriction
        Increased sympathetic activity (hypoglycemia, pheochromocytoma)
        Neurologic complications (head trauma, seizures, migraine)
V. **Chronic medical conditions**
    A. Malignant disease
    B. Atopy
    C. Chronic inflammatory disease
        Juvenile rheumatoid arthritis
        Inflammatory bowel disease
    D. Cardiopulmonary disease (including cystic fibrosis)
    E. Diabetes mellitus
    F. Congenital and acquired immunodeficiencies

From Reece RM. Manual of Emergency Pediatrics, 4th ed. Philadelphia: WB Saunders, 1992.

phosphate dehydrogenase (G6PD), whereas other medications may cause immune hemolysis (penicillin) or decreased RBC production (chloramphenicol). Travel history may suggest exposure to infections, such as malaria.

Physical Examination

The general appearance of the child gives a clue as to the acuity and chronicity of the problem. Severe anemia that develops slowly over weeks or months is often well tolerated. Vital signs (including orthostatic blood pressure), height, weight, and growth percentiles offer further insight into the severity of the problem. A thorough physical examination will define the degree of pallor (conjunctiva, palms, skin), detect the presence of underlying disease (all organ systems), and uncover signs of trauma. Isolated pallor in a well-appearing child who does not have evidence of systemic disease is usually much less ominous than that noted in a child with bruising, adenopathy, hepatosplenomegaly, or abdominal mass. Table 49–4 lists some clues that may assist in determining the underlying cause of the anemia.

Prominent cheekbones, dental malocclusion, and frontal bossing may occur in patients with chronic hemolytic anemias (sickle cell disease, thalassemia major) because of the expansion of bone marrow space. Tortuosity of conjunctival vessels occurs in the sickling

syndromes. Splenomegaly is often present in children with congenital hemolytic anemia (see Chapter 23). Lymphadenopathy and hepatosplenomegaly may indicate the presence of infiltrative disease of the bone marrow and visceral organs, such as leukemia. Purpura in the anemic child suggests associated thrombocytopenia, as may be seen in aplastic anemia or leukemia.

A wide array of congenital anomalies have been associated with hematologic syndromes. In Fanconi anemia (constitutional aplastic anemia), patients are often short and hyperpigmented with hypoplastic "finger-like" thumbs, radial bone anomalies, and structural renal abnormalities. Patients with Diamond-Blackfan anemia (congenital hypoplastic anemia) are often short and said to have a "curious, intellectual" facial expression.

When pallor is related to chronic inflammation or infection or systemic disease, a diligent general physical examination may yield substantive information (hypertension and short stature in the child with chronic renal disease, joint inflammation in the child with rheumatologic disorders, digital clubbing in the child with advanced cyanotic cardiopulmonary diseases, and poor nutritional status in the child with inflammatory bowel disease).

Recent onset of pallor suggests the possibility of anemia. The child who has always appeared somewhat pale but has been otherwise well, manifesting normal growth and development, may merely be expressing an intrinsic constitutional characteristic. In such instances, the child and other family members often have light hair and skin complexion. An unremarkable general medical history and physical examination support a physiologic explanation for pallor. Some children may appear pale as a result of limited sun exposure, as might occur during the winter in cooler climates.

Children may present with pallor, appear ill, and have other historical complaints or abnormalities on physical examination. Children with malignant disease or chronic illness (e.g., rheumatologic disorders, inflammatory bowel disease, chronic cardiopulmonary disorders, diabetes) may often have a pale appearance that is unrelated or out of proportion to the degree of associated anemia. Atopic children often have distinctly pale mucosa as a result of local edema. Children with generalized edema due to hypoproteinemia, congestive heart failure, or vasculitis often appear pale as a result of excess interstitial fluid within the mucosal or cutaneous

Table 49–2. Values (Normal Mean and Lower Limits of Normal) for Hemoglobin, Hematocrit, and MCV Determination

Age (yr)	Hemoglobin (g/dl)		Hematocrit (%)		MCV (fl)	
	Mean	*Lower Limit*	*Mean*	*Lower Limit*	*Mean*	*Lower Limit*
0.5–1.9	12.5	11.0	37	33	77	70
2–4	12.5	11.0	38	34	79	73
5–7	13.0	11.5	39	35	81	75
8–11	13.5	12.0	40	36	83	76
12–14:						
Female	13.5	12.0	41	36	85	78
Male	14.0	12.5	43	37	84	77
15–17:						
Female	14.0	12.0	41	36	87	79
Male	15.0	13.0	46	38	86	78
18–49:						
Female	14.0	12.0	42	37	90	80
Male	16.0	14.0	47	40	90	80

From Nathan DC, Oski F. Hematology of Infancy and Childhood, 4th ed. Philadelphia: WB Saunders, 1993.
Abbreviation: MCV = mean corpuscular volume.

Table 49–3. Historical Clues in Evaluation of Anemia

Variable	Comments
Age	Iron deficiency rare in the absence of blood loss prior to 6 mo in term or prior to doubling birth weight in preterm infants Neonatal anemia with reticulocytosis suggests hemolysis or blood loss; with reticulocytopenia, it suggests bone marrow failure Sickle cell anemia and beta-thalassemia appear as fetal hemoglobin disappears (4–8 mo of age)
Family history and genetic considerations	X-linked: G6PD deficiency Autosomal dominant: spherocytosis Autosomal recessive: sickle cell, Fanconi anemia Family member with early age of cholecystectomy (bilirubin stones) or splenectomy Ethnicity (thalassemia with Mediterranean origin), (G6PD deficiency in blacks, Greeks, and sephardic Jews) Race (beta-thalassemia in white, alpha-thalassemia in blacks and Orientals, and SC and SS in blacks)
Nutrition	Cow's milk diet and iron deficiency Strict vegetarian and vitamin B_{12} deficiency Goat's milk and folate deficiency Pica, plumbism, and iron deficiency Cholestasis, malabsorption, and vitamin E
Drugs	G6PD-susceptible agents Immune-mediated hemolysis (e.g., penicillin) Bone marrow suppression Phenytoin increasing folate requirements
Diarrhea	Malabsorption of vitamins B_{12} and E and iron Inflammatory bowel disease and anemia of chronic disease or blood loss Milk protein allergy–induced blood loss Intestinal resection and vitamin B_{12} deficiency
Infection	*Giardia* and iron malabsorption Intestinal bacterial overgrowth (blind loop) and vitamin B_{12} deficiency Fish tapeworm and vitamin B_{12} deficiency Epstein-Barr virus, cytomegalovirus, and bone marrow suppression *Mycoplasma* and hemolysis Parvovirus and bone marrow suppression Chronic infection Endocarditis Malaria and hemolysis Hepatitis and aplastic anemia

Adapted from Scott JP. Hematology. *In* Behrman RE, Kliegman RM (eds). Nelson Essentials of Pediatrics, 2nd ed. Philadelphia: WB Saunders, 1994:519.
Abbreviation: G6PD = glucose-6-phosphate dehydrogenase.

tissues. Patients with hypothyroidism are pale because of myxedematous changes in the skin, subcutaneous tissue, and mucosa. Rarely, children with pheochromocytoma can appear pale on the basis of catecholamine-induced vasoconstriction.

Laboratory Evaluation

The initial laboratory test in a child with pallor should be a complete blood count (CBC) with a white blood cell (WBC) differential and platelet count. Anemia as a cause of pallor does not occur until the hemoglobin level falls below 8 to 9 g/dl. "False anemia" (resulting from laboratory error, sampling error, or statistical value) should be considered whenever a child is said to be anemic, particularly when laboratory findings do not seem consistent with clinical impressions. Capillary blood sampling can be associated with substantial error, depending on the difficulty encountered in performing the procedure and the use of mechanical force necessary to promote blood flow. When laboratory or sampling errors are suspected, it is always appropriate to obtain a repeat venipuncture sample. Statistical anemia relates to the fact that by definition, 2.5% of a healthy population has hemoglobin

levels below the lower limit of normal. This phenomenon should be considered when mild, unexplained anemia is identified in a healthy child.

Nearly all laboratories perform complete blood counts with the use of automated technology systems. Hemoglobin concentration (g/dl), RBC count (cells/mm³), and mean corpuscular volume (MCV) expressed in femtoliters (fl), are directly measured. Hematocrit value, mean corpuscular hemoglobin, and mean corpuscular hemoglobin concentration are derived values and are less accurate. Other useful information reported includes red cell distribution width (RDW), WBC count (cell/mm³), and platelet count. Careful attention should be given to the hemoglobin value, the MCV, the RDW, the shape of the RBCs, and any abnormalities in the number of platelets or WBCs.

The reticulocyte count, reported as a percentage of total RBCs, is essential in categorizing anemia. An appropriately elevated reticulocyte count implies a response of the bone marrow to either hemolysis or acute or chronic blood loss. In cases of immediate blood loss, the reticulocyte count is not elevated for 3 to 4 days; a low value does not always imply underproduction. The reticulocyte count is most helpful for cases in which the anemia has been present for more than a few days.

The MCV may provide very helpful information but must always

Table 49–4. Physical Findings in the Evaluation of Anemia

System	Observation	Significance
Skin	Hyperpigmentation	Fanconi, dyskeratosis congenita
	Café-au-lait spots	Fanconi anemia
	Vitiligo	Vitamin B_{12} deficiency
	Partial oculocutaneous albinism	Chédiak-Higashi syndrome
	Jaundice	Hemolysis
	Petechiae, purpura	Bone marrow infiltration, autoimmune hemolysis with autoimmune thrombocytopenia, hemolytic uremic syndrome
	Erythematous rash	Parvovirus, Epstein-Barr virus
	Butterfly rash	SLE autoantibodies
Head	Frontal bossing	Thalassemia major, severe iron deficiency, chronic subdural hematoma
	Microcephaly	Fanconi anemia
Eyes	Microphthalmia	Fanconi anemia
	Retinopathy	SS, SC disease
	Optic atrophy, blindness	Osteopetrosis
	Blocked lacrimal gland	Dyskeratosis congenita
	Kayser-Fleisher ring	Wilson disease
	Blue sclera	Iron deficiency
Ears	Deafness	Osteopetrosis
Mouth	Glossitis	B_{12} deficiency, iron deficiency
	Angular stomatitis	Iron deficiency
	Cleft lip	Diamond-Blackfan syndrome
	Pigmentation	Peutz-Jeghers syndrome (intestinal blood loss)
	Telangiectasia	Osler-Weber-Rendu syndrome (blood loss)
	Leukoplakia	Dyskeratosis congenita
Chest	Shield chest or widespread nipples	Diamond-Blackfan syndrome
	Murmur	Endocarditis: prosthetic valve hemolysis
Abdomen	Hepatomegaly	Hemolysis, infiltrative tumor, chronic disease, hemangioma, cholecystitis
	Splenomegaly	Hemolysis, sickle cell disease (early), thalassemia, malaria, lymphoma, Epstein-Barr virus, portal hypertension
	Nephromegaly	Fanconi anemia
	Absent kidney	Fanconi anemia
Extremities	Absent thumbs	Fanconi anemia
	Triphalangeal thumb	Diamond-Blackfan syndrome
	Spoon nails	Iron deficiency
	Beau line (nails)	Heavy metal intoxication, severe illness
	Mees line (nails)	Heavy metals, severe illness, sickle cell anemia
	Dystrophic nails	Dyskeratosis congenita
	Edema	Milk-induced protein-losing enteropathy with iron deficiency
Rectal	Hemorrhoids	Portal hypertension
	Heme-positive stool	Intestinal hemorrhage
Nerves	Irritable, apathy	Iron deficiency
	Peripheral neuropathy	Deficiency of vitamins B_1, B_{12}, and E, lead poisoning
	Dementia	Deficiency of vitamins B_{12} and E
	Ataxia, posterior column signs	Vitamin B_{12} and E deficiency
	Stroke	Sickle cell anemia, paroxysmal nocturnal hemoglobinuria

Adapted from Scott JP. Hematology. *In* Behrman RE, Kliegman RM (eds). Nelson Essentials of Pediatrics, 2nd ed. Philadelphia: WB Saunders, 1994:520.
Abbreviation: SLE = systemic lupus erythematosus.

be viewed in conjunction with a review of the peripheral blood smear and reticulocyte count. A varied population of smaller and larger RBCs (e.g., reticulocytes) may yield a falsely normal MCV and be diagnostically misleading. *Microcytosis* may be associated with several commonly encountered anemias, including iron deficiency, thalassemia, lead toxicity, and anemia of chronic disease (Table 49–5). *Macrocytosis,* an unusual finding in children, is associated with vitamin B_{12} or folate deficiency, syndromes associated with elevated production of fetal-like RBCs (Fanconi, aplastic anemia), and some cases of hypothyroidism (see Table 49–5). Normal standards for MCV are age related—a simple rule of thumb

is that the lower normal limit of MCV is 70 fl plus the patient's age in years until the adult standards of 80 to 100 fl are reached (see Table 49–2).

An individual with small RBCs may have a normal or near-normal hemoglobin level if the RBC count is increased, as occurs in patients with thalassemia minor, who often have RBC counts of more than 5×10^6. The mean corpuscular hemoglobin concentration reflects the concentration of hemoglobin per cell and would be expected to be low in anemias in which RBCs are "underhemoglobinized," such as the hypochromic anemia of iron deficiency.

The RDW is derived from the histogram of RBC volumes. A

Table 49–5. **Causes of High or Low Mean Corpuscular Volume**

Low mean corpuscular volume
    Iron deficiency
    Thalassemias
    Lead toxicity
    Anemia of chronic disease
    Copper deficiency
    Sideroblastic anemia
    Hemoglobin E

High mean corpuscular volume
    Normal newborn
    Elevated reticulocyte count
    B_{12} or folate deficiency
    Diamond-Blackfan anemia (congenital hypoplastic anemia)
    Fanconi anemia
    Aplastic anemia
    Down syndrome
    Hypothyroidism (occasionally)
    Oroticaciduria
    Lesch-Nyhan syndrome
    Drugs (zidovudine, chemotherapy)
    Chronic liver disease

normal RDW (11.5% to 14.5%) implies that a uniform population of RBCs of similar size exists (β-thalassemia trait, in which a uniform population of small cells exists, hence a low MCV with a normal RDW). An elevated RDW implies a varying population of RBCs, as seen in iron deficiency (a variable population of small cells, hence a low MCV and an elevated RDW) or some hemolytic anemias (in which an elevated RDW is due to the presence of a population of large reticulocytes) (Table 49–6).

The basis for categorizing anemias relates to the adequacy of the reticulocyte response. The reticulocyte count, normally about 1%, is expressed as a percentage of the total number of RBCs; in some patients with moderate or severe anemia, the reticulocyte count may appear elevated, yet in absolute terms, it may be quite insufficient. Therefore, the reticulocyte count must be corrected:

$$\text{corrected reticulocyte count} =$$
$$\text{reticulocyte count} \times \text{hemoglobin/normal hemoglobin for age}$$

If the corrected reticulocyte count is greater than 2%, then the bone marrow is producing red cells at an accelerated pace (Fig. 49–1).

The WBC count, differential, and platelet count may provide extremely pertinent information. The presence of immature leukocytes on a smear, which may be associated with either a high or a low WBC count, suggests leukemia. Leukopenia and thrombocytopenia occurring in a patient with anemia of underproduction suggest aplastic anemia or infiltrative bone marrow disease, such as leukemia or neuroblastoma metastasis to the marrow.

When associated with a low hemoglobin level, *thrombocytosis* is seen in iron deficiency, blood loss, inflammatory disease, infection, malignancy, or asplenia.

The serum indirect bilirubin, lactate dehydrogenase (LDH), and urinary urobilinogen levels are elevated in patients with increased rates of RBC destruction. An elevated serum direct bilirubin level is seen only if hepatobiliary complications supervene (biliary tract stones, hepatitis). A low serum iron level, elevated total iron-binding capacity, and a low percentage of iron saturation and/or serum ferritin level are helpful in the diagnosis of iron deficiency. Determination of the level of free erythrocyte protoporphyrin (FEP), also known as zinc protoporphyrin (ZNP), is a very useful study in assessing patients with microcytosis because a normal value excludes iron deficiency and marked lead toxicity (>25 μg/

dl) and supports a diagnosis of thalassemia syndrome. The ZNP level may also be elevated in reticulocytosis, inflammatory or infectious states, and erythropoietic porphyria. Hemoglobin electrophoresis is necessary to define abnormal hemoglobins, such as sickle hemoglobin or hemoglobin C. Assessment of RBC enzyme levels (e.g., G6PD) may be necessary when one suspects infection-related or medication-related hemolytic anemia in a male of Mediterranean or African descent. True macrocytic anemia may require that serum vitamin B_{12} and folate levels be assessed. Bone marrow aspirate and biopsy are appropriate whenever leukemia or aplastic anemia is seriously suspected.

If autoimmune hemolytic anemia is suspected because jaundice, reticulocytosis (may be absent if antibody reacts with reticulocytes), splenomegaly (not universally), and RBC fragments are noted, a direct Coombs test should be performed to detect the presence of an autoantibody on the RBC surface.

Abnormalities of RBC morphology may be readily apparent on inspection of the peripheral blood smear (Table 49–7, Fig. 49–2).

From a practical clinical perspective, it is best to consider the differential diagnosis of pallor in the context of the acuteness and severity of the clinical findings (Fig. 49–3). The well-appearing child may need only a CBC, which might provide reassurance to the parents. The mild or moderately ill-appearing pale child requires a laboratory evaluation for anemia as well as studies to detect any suspected underlying disease. The seriously ill-appearing pale child requires urgent evaluation and appropriate therapeutic intervention. The only obligatory laboratory study is a CBC with other laboratory assessments, dictated on the basis of the suspected diagnosis (blood glucose, electrolyte, blood urea nitrogen (BUN), creatinine, blood culture). If hemorrhage or severe anemia is suspected, a type and cross-match must be sent to the blood bank; two large intravenous lines must be secured; and frequent serial evaluations of hemoglobin, blood pressure, pulse, perfusion, and end-organ function (central nervous system [mental status], renal function [urine output]) must be assessed.

Differential Diagnosis

CLASSIFICATION OF ANEMIA

The classification of anemia is presented in Figures 49–1 and 49–4.

Table 49–6. **Red Blood Cell Distribution Width (RDW) in Common Anemias of Childhood**

Anemia	MCV
Elevated RDW (Nonuniform Population of RBCs)	
Hemolytic anemia with elevated reticulocyte count	High
Iron deficiency anemia	Low
Anemias due to red cell fragmentation—DIC, HUS, TTP	Low
Megaloblastic anemias—vitamin B_{12} or folate deficiency	High
Normal RDW (Uniform Population of RBCs)	
Thalassemias	Low
Acute hemorrhage	Normal
Fanconi or aplastic anemia	High

Abbreviations: DIC = disseminated intravascular coagulation; HUS = hemolytic-uremic syndrome; TTP = thrombotic thrombocytopenic purpura; MCV = mean corpuscular volume; RBC = red blood cell.

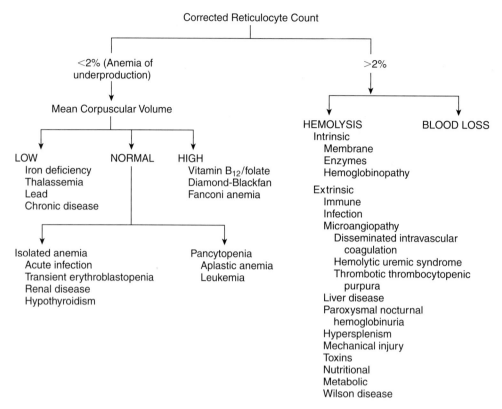

Figure 49–1. Diagnostic approach to anemia.

Table 49–7. **Peripheral Blood Morphologic Findings in Various Anemias**

Microcytes
Iron deficiency
Thalassemias
Lead toxicity
Anemia of chronic disease

Macrocytes
Newborns
Vitamin B_{12} or folate deficiency
Diamond-Blackfan anemia
Fanconi aplastic anemia
Liver disease
Down syndrome
Hypothyroidism

Spherocytes
Hereditary spherocytosis
Immune hemolytic anemia

Sickled Cells
Sickle cell anemias (SS disease, SC disease,
S–β-thalassemia)

Elliptocytes
Hereditary elliptocytosis

Target Cells
Hemoglobinopathies (especially hemoglobin C and thalassemia)
Liver disease

Basophil Stippling
Thalassemia
Lead intoxication

Red Blood Cell Fragments, Helmet Cells, Burr Cells
Disseminated intravascular coagulation
Hemolytic-uremic syndrome
Thrombotic thrombocytopenic purpura
Kasabach-Merritt syndrome
Waring blender syndrome
Uremia

Hypersegmented Neutrophils
Vitamin B_{12} or folate deficiency

Blasts
Leukemia (ALL or AML)
Severe infection (rarely)

Leukopenia/Thrombocytopenia
Aplastic or Fanconi anemia
Leukemia

Abbreviations: ALL = acute lymphocytic leukemia; AML = acute myeloid leukemia.

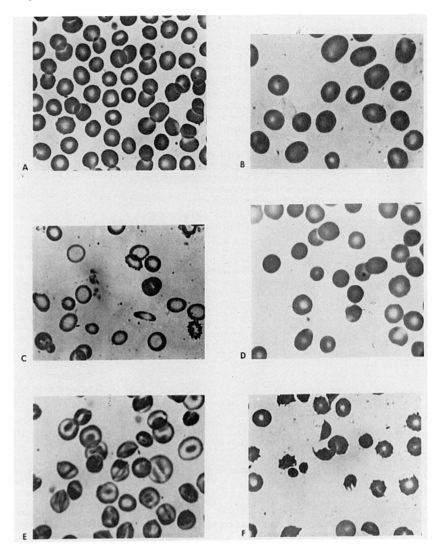

Figure 49-2. Morphologic abnormalities of the red blood cell. *A,* Normal. *B,* Macrocytes (folic acid deficiency). *C,* Hypochromic microcytes (iron deficiency). *D,* Spherocytes (hereditary spherocytosis). *E,* Target cells (hemoglobin CC disease). *F,* Schistocytes (hemolytic-uremic syndrome). (From Behrman RE, Kliegman RM [eds]. Nelson Essentials of Pediatrics, 2nd ed. Philadelphia: WB Saunders, 1994:521.)

ANEMIA

Anemia Due to Acute Blood Loss

Significant loss of blood on an acute or subacute basis leads to anemia. A period of 24 to 36 hours may be required for full intravascular equilibration after blood loss; the fall in hemoglobin level occurs gradually. In patients with severe acute blood loss, the primary concern is *intravascular volume,* which cannot be assessed by hemoglobin level. In this situation, the patient's condition is best assessed by measurement of blood pressure, heart rate, and adequacy of peripheral perfusion (capillary refill time). In most instances, an obvious history of blood loss is apparent (epistaxis, hematemesis, trauma), but severe occult blood loss may also occur. Large amounts of blood may accumulate in the gastrointestinal tract before the development of hematemesis, hematochezia, or melena. Intra-abdominal bleeding may occur after trauma or may result from an ulcer (see Chapters 18 and 21) and may be associated with progressive anemia in the absence of an obvious source of blood loss. The clinical history coupled with the physical examination (including rectal examination) and tests for occult blood in the stool generally define the source of blood loss.

In anemia associated with blood loss, the RBC size and morphology are normal, and after a period of 3 to 5 days, an appropriate elevation in the reticulocyte count is noted. Assuming that hemor-

rhage has ceased, one may expect the hemoglobin level to gradually rise unless supervening factors, such as iron deficiency, exist.

Severe hemorrhage associated with intravascular volume depletion requires immediate intervention; RBC transfusions are necessary until hemorrhage has ceased. Less severe hemorrhage may not be associated with intravascular volume depletion and may merely present with moderate to severe anemia. Transfusions are necessary when the oxygen-carrying capacity of the blood is diminished to the point of impending tissue hypoxia and is based on clinical parameters, including the presence of fatigue, lightheadedness, tachycardia, dyspnea, and heart failure. If hemorrhage has ceased, intravascular volume is replete, and the patient is not manifesting signs of cardiorespiratory compromise, transfusion therapy can often be avoided. In such instances, it is appropriate to supply therapeutic doses of iron to ensure adequacy of the reticulocyte response (see Table 49-10).

Anemia Due to Underproduction
(see Figs. 49-1 and 49-4)

The pathophysiologic feature of anemia due to underproduction is a suboptimal bone marrow response (reflected in a corrected reticulocyte count of <2%). The clinical context may predict anemia of underproduction, as in the patient with chronic renal disease,

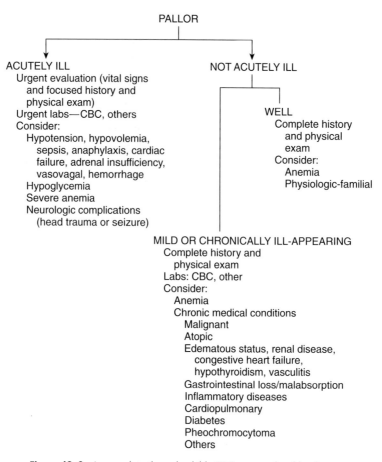

Figure 49–3. Approach to the pale child. CBC = complete blood count.

chronic inflammatory or infectious disease, or hypothyroidism. When anemia is not well explained based on initial clinical findings and the reticulocyte response is inadequate, one may consider subclassifying this group of anemias on the basis of RBC size—microcytic, normocytic, or macrocytic.

MICROCYTIC ANEMIAS

Hemoglobin, the chief intracellular component of the RBC, is composed of heme (iron and protoporphyrin IX) and globin chains (α and β). Any factors that diminish the availability or utilization of any of these components result in microcytic anemia. The automated MCV represents the mean RBC volume and does not address variations in cell size. The RDW, however, does describe the variation in cell size and, if normal, defines a relatively uniform population of cells. Review of the peripheral blood smear also provides additional evidence regarding variability in cell size and shape. It is important to recall that MCV is age related (see Table 49–2). When the diagnosis is not immediately apparent, it is helpful to carefully and judiciously select from a variety of available laboratory studies (Table 49–8).

IRON DEFICIENCY ANEMIA

Iron deficiency is the most common nutritional deficiency causing anemia. Iron deficiency results when nutritional intake is insufficient to meet demands associated with growth and in some in-

stances blood loss. Iron is a key component of the hemoglobin molecule; hence, its deficiency leads to anemia associated with underhemoglobinization (hypochromia) and small RBCs (microcytosis). At particular risk for the development of iron deficiency are infants, whose rapid growth and expanding blood volume impose considerable iron demands. Premature infants are particularly at high risk because most *in utero* iron is transferred to the fetus during the last trimester of pregnancy and postnatal growth rate is rapid. Adolescent females are at high risk because of menstrual blood loss and nutrition, which is often not optimal. *When iron deficiency occurs outside of the setting of infancy or female adolescence, a pathologic source of blood loss must be strongly considered (especially occult gastrointestinal bleeding).*

Nutritional sources of iron include iron-fortified infant formula (12 mg/L), iron-fortified infant cereal, breast milk (owing to its

Table 49–8. Laboratory Findings in Microcytic Anemia

	FEP	Fe	TIBC	Pb	Hgb A$_2$	Ferritin
Iron deficiency	↑	↓	↑	nl	nl	↓
α-Thalassemia	nl	nl	nl	nl	nl	nl
β-Thalassemia	nl	nl	nl	nl	↑	nl
Lead poisoning	↑	nl	nl	↑	nl	nl
Anemia of chronic disease	↑	↓	↓	nl	nl	nl or ↑

Adapted from Reece RM. Manual of Emergency Pediatrics, 4th ed. Philadelphia: WB Saunders, 1992.

Abbreviations: nl = normal; FEP = free erythrocyte protoporphyrin; Fe = iron; TIBC = total iron-binding capacity; Pb = lead; Hgb A$_2$ = hemoglobin A$_2$.

I. Acute blood loss with hemodilution

II. Anemia of RBC underproduction (i.e., inadequate reticulocyte count)
    A. Microcytic
        1. Iron deficiency
        2. Lead intoxication
        3. Thalassemia syndromes
        4. Anemia of chronic diseases
    B. Normocytic

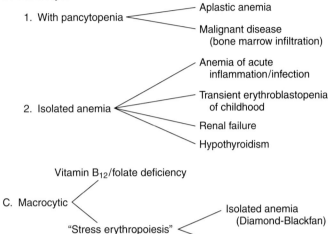

        1. With pancytopenia — Aplastic anemia / Malignant disease (bone marrow infiltration)

        2. Isolated anemia — Anemia of acute inflammation/infection / Transient erythroblastopenia of childhood / Renal failure / Hypothyroidism

    C. Macrocytic — Vitamin B_{12}/folate deficiency / "Stress erythropoiesis" — Isolated anemia (Diamond-Blackfan) / Pancytopenia-Fanconi or aplastic anemia

III. Anemia due to increased destruction = hemolysis (i.e., adequate reticulocyte count)
    A. Intrinsic RBC defect
        1. Hemoglobinopathies (sickle cell anemia, unstable hemoglobins)
        2. Membrane defects (hereditary spherocytosis or elliptocytosis)
        3. Enzymopathies (G6PD, pyruvate kinase deficiency)

    B. Extrinsic defects
        1. Immune hemolysis
        2. Infection (bacterial, viral, other)
        3. Microangiopathy (disseminated intravascular coagulation, hemolytic uremia syndrome, thrombotic thrombocytopenia purpura)
        4. Liver disease
        5. Paroxysmal nocturnal hemoglobinuria
        6. Hypersplenism
        7. Mechanical injury (e.g., burns)
        8. Toxins
        9. Nutritional (vitamin E deficiency)
      10. Metabolic (galactosemia)
      11. Wilson disease

Figure 49–4. Differential diagnosis of anemia. RBC = red blood cell; G6PD = glucose-6-phosphate dehydrogenase.

high bioavailability), beef, fish, and fowl. Ascorbic acid (vitamin C) markedly enhances the absorption of iron contained in vegetable products. Current nutritional guidelines proposed by the American Academy of Pediatrics recommend iron-fortified infant formula or breast milk until the age of 1 year and the introduction of foods rich in iron after 6 months of age. Low-iron formulas have an extremely small endowment of iron and are not recommended. Cow's milk is a very poor source of nutritional iron, and when ingested in large quantities, it is often a cause of occult gastrointestinal blood loss. Infants should receive no cow's milk until after 1 year of age and not more than 24 ounces per day. Iron supplementation is necessary in preterm infants, female adolescents, and pregnant women. Iron deficiency must be viewed as a systemic deficiency disorder, only one manifestation of which is anemia (Table 49–9).

Iron deficiency is usually detected by routine hemoglobin screen-ing performed between 9 and 18 months of age. Screening for iron deficiency anemia is complicated by the fact that infants with a current or recent viral illness often have mild transient anemia. The occurrence of anemia is two to three times higher in children who have experienced an infectious illness (including routine childhood illnesses) than in children who have been well in the preceding month.

Fewer than 2% of well-nourished 1-year-olds are anemic; hence, routine screening for iron deficiency is usually reserved for a high-risk population, including preterm infants, infants fed cow's milk or nonfortified formula before the age of 1 year or consuming more than 24 ounces of cow's milk per day, menstruating adolescent females, and children of lower socioeconomic status.

Symptomatic iron deficiency is infrequently seen, but when it occurs, it is generally noted in infants who consume large amounts of cow's milk who often have intestinal blood loss secondary

Table 49–9. Nonhematologic Consequences of Iron Deficiency

Impairment of cognitive development
Pica
Epithelial abnormalities (gastrointestinal mucosal lesion, glossitis; spoon-shaped nails)
Exercise intolerance
Behavioral manifestations
Abnormal immune response (?)
Growth retardation
Impaired collagen synthesis (blue sclera)

to milk protein–induced colitis. Such children may have pallor, irritability, fatigue, glossitis, blue sclera, and, in extreme cases, signs and symptoms of high-output cardiac failure (dyspnea, diaphoresis, pallor, tachycardia, gallop rhythm, and hepatomegaly).

Mild anemia in otherwise well infants between 6 and 24 months of age, particularly in association with ingestion of large amounts of cow's milk, is most likely due to iron deficiency. This is also true when mild anemia is detected in the well, menstruating adolescent. Empiric iron therapy is often prescribed in such circumstances (Table 49–10). If the hemoglobin level has normalized after 1 month of therapy, a presumptive diagnosis has been established, and the patient should receive an additional 3 to 4 months of therapeutic doses of iron to replete stores. An appropriate response to iron therapy is the diagnostic gold standard.

Laboratory confirmatory studies are necessary when iron deficiency anemia is suspected in patients who are not at high risk for nutritional deficiency or in those in whom anemia is moderately severe. A serum ferritin level of less than 12 ng/dl, an elevated ZNP in association with a normal lead level, or a iron saturation of less than 10% provides confirmation of diagnosis.

Parental iron therapy is rarely necessary, but in certain circumstances (iron malabsorption in patients with inflammatory bowel disease), it may be administered either intramuscularly or intravenously (recognizing that the intravenous use of iron has rarely been associated with anaphylactic reactions). The optimal approach to iron deficiency anemia in infants and children is prevention.

Thalassemia Syndromes

The thalassemia syndromes represent a heterogeneous group of inherited disorders of decreased globin production that lead to microcytic anemia, which is often mistaken for iron deficiency. The child with microcytic anemia who has no evidence of iron deficiency or lead toxicity likely has thalassemia.

β-THALASSEMIA MINOR (TRAIT)

Two genes code for the production of the β globin chains of hemoglobin one inherited from each parent. When one gene is affected by the β-thalassemia mutation, a moderate diminution in the production of the β globin chain occurs, resulting in mild microcytic anemia of underproduction. β-Thalassemia occurs most commonly in individuals of Mediterranean and African descent. Patients with β-thalassemia trait are asymptomatic and are frequently diagnosed when anemia and microcytosis are noted at the time of routine screening for iron deficiency or incidentally when a CBC is obtained for the assessment of acute or chronic symptoms. Typically, patients have mild anemia in association with a low MCV. For an equivalent degree of anemia, the MCV is usually lower than that seen in iron deficiency.

This phenomenon is reflected in the Mentzer index, calculated by dividing the MCV by the RBC count (in millions). An index of less than 13 is suggestive of thalassemia, whereas an index of more than 13 is often seen in iron deficiency anemia. *An MCV within the range of normal virtually excludes a diagnosis of β-thalassemia.* A normal RDW in thalassemia reflects the uniform population of microcytic red cells (as opposed to iron deficiency, wherein the RDW is elevated, reflecting the variation in cell size).

The peripheral blood smear demonstrates microcytosis, hypochromia, and target cells. Occasional fragments may be seen. The significance of β-thalassemia relates to (1) its confusion with iron deficiency (hence, patients may be treated unnecessarily with repeated courses of iron and undergo repeated unnecessary blood studies) and (2) its genetic implications. A mating between two individuals with β-thalassemia trait carries a 25% risk per pregnancy of an offspring with homozygous β-thalassemia (thalassemia major), an extremely serious disorder. Families with a child diagnosed with β-thalassemia minor should be appropriately screened and counseled. For purposes of screening, a normal age-adjusted MCV essentially excludes a diagnosis of β-thalassemia.

HOMOZYGOUS β-THALASSEMIA

Homozygous β-thalassemia, also known as β-thalassemia major, or Cooley anemia, results from the inheritance of the abnormal β-thalassemia mutation from each parent. This abnormality results in a severe deficiency of production of β globin chains. Excess α globin chains precipitate within developing erythroid elements in the marrow and lead to brisk intra-marrow destruction of developing erythroid elements (ineffective erythropoiesis). As a result, patients with homozygous β-thalassemia present during infancy (6 to 12 months of age) with severe anemia and an inadequate reticulocyte count. The child with β-thalassemia major typically presents with fatigue, irritability, pallor, jaundice, and marked hepatosplenomegaly (due to extramedullary hematopoiesis). Frontal bossing and prominent cheek bones (maxillary hyperplasia) may be noted and result from expansion of the marrow space in an attempt to compensate for severe anemia. Most patients are of Mediterranean (Italian or Greek) descent.

Laboratory findings include severe anemia and a decreased age-adjusted MCV. Peripheral blood smear is markedly abnormal, demonstrating severely underhemoglobinized red blood cells, target cells, and wide variability in cell shape and size. Long-term transfusion therapy sufficient to suppress ineffective erythropoiesis (main-

Table 49–10. Therapy for Iron Deficiency

Infants and children:
4 mg/kg of elemental iron/day, given as divided dose 2 or 3 times/day (mild nutritional anemia deficiency in infants may be treated with a single daily dose of 3 mg/kg/day before breakfast)

Adolescents:
3 mg/kg/day of elemental iron given as divided dose 2 or 3 times/day

Available iron preparations:
Ferrous sulfate drops: 15 mg of elemental iron/0.6 ml
Ferrous sulfate elixir: 44 mg of elemental iron/5 ml
Ferrous sulfate tablets: 65 mg of elemental iron/tablet

Duration of prescription:
Continue *therapeutic dose* of iron for 3 months after hemoglobin level has corrected (to replete stores), after which maintenance nutritional needs must be met

taining hemoglobin level greater than 10 g/dl) may be associated with relatively normal growth, development, and functional capabilities. Long-term desferoxamine iron chelation to prevent iron overload allows for prolonged survival and avoidance of transfusional hemosiderosis (hepatic, endocrine, and cardiac dysfunction), but it is a cumbersome treatment program that is associated with a substantial degree of poor compliance. Bone marrow transplantation, although associated with an approximate 10% risk of mortality, is curative and a potential treatment option for younger patients who have a human leukocyte antigen–identical, non-thalassemic sibling.

α-THALASSEMIA SYNDROMES

Four genes code for the α globin chains hemoglobin—two each on chromosome 16. Progressive deletions of one, two, three, or four of these genes account for the variable laboratory and clinical findings associated with the α-thalassemia syndromes. Decreased α globin chain production leads to an excess of β globin chains, which tend to precipitate within developing RBCs in the bone marrow, leading to destruction. Mature RBCs are mildly hypochromic and microcytic and may appear to be targeted.

Deletion of one gene occurs in about 30% of African-Americans as well as in some individuals of Asian descent. This is known as the ''silent carrier'' state because it is not associated with anemia or microcytosis.

Deletion of two genes represents α-thalassemia trait. Such patients manifest mild anemia and microcytosis, with MCVs generally in the mildly decreased range (less microcytosis than is generally seen in β-thalassemia trait).

A three-gene deletion leads to hemoglobin H disease, which is associated with moderate hemolytic anemia, microcytosis, reticulocytosis, and splenomegaly.

A four-gene deletion represents hemoglobin Bart disease, wherein the fetus is unable to produce any α chains; hence, nearly all *in utero* hemoglobin is Bart type (composed of four γ chains). Hemoglobin Bart has an extremely high oxygen affinity and leads to severe tissue hypoxemia and resultant fetal hydrops and death. Occasionally, babies with hemoglobin Bart disease have been saved by extraordinary measures (intrauterine transfusion and early delivery), but they are then committed to lifelong transfusion support.

Hemoglobin H disease and hemoglobin Bart disease occur almost exclusively in individuals of Asian descent. This inheritance relates to the distribution of the abnormal genes in Asian in contrast to individuals of African descent. When the α-thalassemia trait (two-gene deletion) occurs in the Asian population, deletions may occur in *cis* (both genes deleted from the same chromosome) or *trans* (each chromosome missing one gene). In individuals of African descent, the α-thalassemia trait (two-gene deletion) occurs only on the basis of a *trans* distribution; hence, a mating between two individuals with the African variety of α-thalassemia trait produces offspring with only two α genes deleted (α-thalassemia trait). A mating between two individuals of Asian descent who have the α-thalassemia trait may produce an offspring with all four genes deleted (Bart's hemoglobin disease). The implication of a diagnosis of α-thalassemia trait in individuals of African descent relates to its confusion with iron deficiency. There are no serious genetic implications. Asians must be appropriately guided regarding the potential for transmission of serious hematologic disease if a mating between two individuals with α-thalassemia occurs.

Lead Poisoning

The occurrence of elevated serum and total body burdens of lead is a public health problem, particularly in infants and young chil-

dren from lower socioeconomic families living in old housing with lead-based paint. Increasing serum levels of lead may decrease erythropoiesis because lead inhibits several enzymes along the path of protoporphyrin synthesis.

Anemia is usually seen in association with lead levels of greater than 70 μg/dl or higher. Anemia is mild, variably microcytic, and associated with prominent basophilic stippling of red cells. Coexistent iron deficiency is common because both conditions are more prevalent in lower socioeconomic populations, and iron deficiency promotes increased lead absorption. The ZNP (or FEP) level rises above the range of normal when lead levels increase to above 25 or 30 μg/dl; hence, a normal ZNP level is helpful in excluding only marked, but not less severe, lead intoxication. ZNP level determination is not recommended as the only screening for mildly to moderately elevated lead levels, given the concerns regarding the impact of modest increases in lead burden on permanent cognitive development in infants. A normal ZNP (FEP) level does, however, exclude lead toxicity as a cause of anemia because anemia occurs only in the child with a markedly increased lead burden. Lead chelation therapy is appropriate when lead levels are greater than 40 μg/dl. Additional features of significant lead toxicity include intestinal colic, lead lines in long bones, behavioral changes, renal tubular defects, and lead encephalopathy associated with marked increased intracranial pressures.

Anemia of Chronic Disease

Patients with a wide variety of chronic inflammatory or infectious disorders may have mild to moderate anemia. The MCV is often in the normal to mildly abnormal range. Chronic inflammation or infection impairs the transfer of iron from reticuloendothelial cells within the marrow to developing erythroid elements, resulting in some degree of iron deficient erythropoiesis even though stores of iron are quite adequate. Often the history and physical examination point to chronic illness, but occasionally patients have no obvious manifestations of systemic disease. The presence of unexplained mild microcytic anemia should alert the clinician to the possibility of occult systemic disease. An elevated erythrocyte sedimentation rate is usually noted in patients with chronic inflammatory or infectious states. Anemia of chronic disease is characterized by no specific abnormalities on peripheral smear other than mild hypochromia and microcytosis. Serum ferritin and ZNP levels are often elevated as a result of the inflammatory state and are thus a poor reflection of iron status. Serum iron level as well as total iron-binding capacity is generally decreased, but the percentage of iron saturation is often not outside of the normal range.

Rare Causes of Microcytic Anemia

Sideroblastic anemias are a group of very rare congenital (often X-linked) inherited diseases associated with impairment of protoporphyrin synthesis and variable microcytic anemia. The bone marrow examination demonstrates evidence of developing erythroid cells with excess iron deposited in mitochondria, which tend to form a circular appearance around the nucleus, hence the term ''ringed sideroblast.''

Copper deficiency is another rare cause of microcytic anemia. Associated features include neutropenia and scurvy-like bone changes (periosteal elevation). Only under unusual circumstances, when prominent microcytic anemia is otherwise unexplained, should these rare disorders be considered.

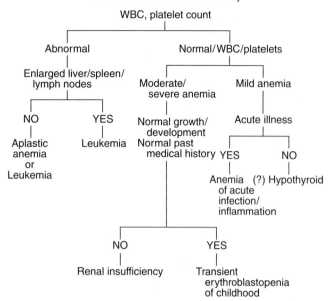

[ANEMIA, NORMAL MEAN CORPUSCULAR VOLUME, LOW RETICULOCYTE COUNT]

Figure 49–5. Diagnostic scheme of normochromocytic anemia of underproduction. WBC = white blood cell.

Normochromic Anemia of Underproduction

When patients with normochromic anemia of underproduction are identified, the key issue is whether anemia is occurring in isolation or is associated with other cytopenias (Figs. 49–4 and 49–5, Table 49–11). Normochromic anemia with an inadequate reticulocyte response and pancytopenia raises the possibility of serious primary or secondary bone marrow disease (see Table 49–11). The history and physical examination often predict the presence of associated thrombocytopenia (easy bruising, petechiae, ecchymosis). Adenopathy and hepatosplenomegaly raise a serious concern for the possibility of infiltrative malignancy disease invading the bone marrow.

Acquired aplastic anemia is a rare disorder of childhood characterized by pancytopenia (neutropenia, anemia, thrombocytopenia) and bone marrow that is markedly hypoplastic. Clinical presentation may include pallor, fatigue, purpura, bleeding (cutaneous petechiae and ecchymosis, epistaxis, gingival oozing), and/or recurrent infection. Physical examination may reveal purpura and pale mucosa and skin. Adenopathy and hepatosplenomegaly are distinctly *not* present. The cause is often obscure but may be related to prior infection (hepatitis, Epstein-Barr virus), toxin exposure (benzene, other volatile compounds), or medications (chloramphenicol, anticonvulsants). Postinfectious, drug-related, or idiopathic acquired aplastic anemia is most likely mediated by immunologic mechanisms. Peripheral blood smear demonstrates normal-appearing RBCs, an absence of polychromasia, and few leukocytes and platelets. A bone marrow biopsy demonstrates hypoplasia involving all cell lines. Severe acquired aplastic anemia is most appropriately treated by bone marrow transplantation when a human leukocyte antigen (HLA)–matched sibling marrow donor is available. Unrelated matched donors offer another possibility for bone marrow transplants. If marrow transplantation is not feasible, immunosuppressive therapy, including antilymphocyte globulin, corticosteroids, and cyclosporine, has been used with variable success. Aplastic anemia should always be considered when anemia occurs in association with thrombocytopenia and leukopenia.

Disorders associated with bone marrow infiltration, including *leukemia* and *metastatic malignancy,* often present with normochromic anemia of underproduction in association with thrombocytopenia and either leukopenia or leukocytosis. Teardrop erythrocytes may be present in the peripheral smear. Occasionally, the MCV is elevated. The child with leukemia frequently comes to medical attention because of pallor, fatigue, and purpura. Limping and skeletal pain are also commonly seen in childhood leukemia. Physical examination often discloses pallor, purpura, adenopathy, and hepatosplenomegaly. Peripheral blood smear may show leukemic blasts. Bone marrow examination is diagnostic. In children, 80% of childhood leukemia cases are of the lymphocytic variety (acute lymphocytic leukemia), the remaining being of myeloid origin. Modern chemotherapeutic treatment regimens have dramatically improved the long-term survival rates, such that two thirds of cases of acute lymphocytic leukemia are potentially curable. Some children with particularly favorable prognostic features have cure rates exceeding 85%. Acute myeloid leukemia represents an even greater therapeutic challenge. When available as an option, bone marrow transplantation may lead to a potential cure in about 65% of youngsters who have achieved a first remission. Chemotherapy treatment of myeloid leukemia, when transplantation is not an option, may improve survival.

When normochromic anemia of underproduction is isolated (unassociated with pancytopenia), several diagnostic entities must be considered. Mild anemia commonly accompanies *acute infections* (and inflammatory illness). Children are often incidentally found to be anemic several days to a few weeks after having childhood infectious illnesses, including viral upper respiratory tract infections, gastroenteritis, or undifferentiated febrile illnesses. Mild anemia has also been shown to occur 10 to 14 days after measles vaccination. Anemia reflects impaired erythrocyte production as a result of the suppressive effect of mediators of the immune/inflammatory response (including interferons, tumor necrosis factor). Cessation of RBC production leads to a fall in hemoglobin concentration of about 1 g/dl per week. Mild anemia discovered during or shortly after acute illness does not require an extensive evaluation, but rather a follow-up hemoglobin determination several weeks later. Persistent anemia requires further evaluation.

Transient erythroblastopenia of childhood represents a temporary arrest of erythropoiesis occurring predominantly in infants and toddlers on the possible basis of a undetermined post-viral humoral immunologic mechanism. Patients present with pallor and fatigue, which occurs gradually over several weeks to months. Because of the very gradual fall in hemoglobin level, most children are remarkably well compensated. Physical examination usually shows marked pallor and mild tachycardia. Adenopathy and hepatosplenomegaly are distinctly *not* present. Congestive heart failure occurs only if anemia is very severe. The CBC demonstrates a variable degree of normocytic anemia and profound reticulocytopenia. The WBC count and platelet count are normal in most patients; however, 25% of patients may have mild neutropenia at the time of presentation. The MCV and peripheral blood smear are unremarkable. Recovery is spontaneous. Blood transfusion is indicated only for patients with severe, symptomatic anemia. Transient erythroblastopenia of childhood may be difficult to differentiate from congenital hypoplastic anemia (Diamond-Blackfan anemia), particularly in children younger than 1 year of age (see Table 49–11). In the latter condition, which represents a constitutional RBC aplasia syndrome, MCV and fetal hemoglobin levels are usually elevated for the patient's age.

The patient with previously undiagnosed chronic hemolytic anemia (sickle cell anemia) may present with normocytic anemia and severe reticulocytopenia, if *transient RBC hypoplasia* occurs on the basis of viral infection (most commonly with parvovirus B19). Because of a shortened RBC life span in patients with chronic hemolysis, a transient arrest of production can manifest as progressively severe anemia evolving over several days. Patients may have

Table 49-11. Differentiation of Red Cell Aplasias and Aplastic Anemias

Disorder	Age of Onset	Characteristics	Treatment
Congenital			
Diamond-Blackfan syndrome (congenital hypoplastic anemia)	Newborn–1 mo; 90% <1 yr age	Pure red cell aplasia, autosomal recessive trait, elevated fetal hemoglobin, fetal i antigen present, macrocytic, thrombosis, short stature, web neck, cleft lip, triphalangeal thumb; late-onset leukemia	Prednisone, transfusion
Acquired			
Transient erythroblastopenia	6 mo–5 yr age; 85% >1 yr age	Pure red cell defect; no anomalies, fetal hemoglobin, or i antigen; spontaneous recovery, normal MCV	Expectant transfusion for symptomatic anemia
Idiopathic aplastic anemia (s/p hepatitis, drugs, unknown)	All ages	All cell lines involved; chloramphenicol, phenylbutazone, radiation	Bone marrow transplant, antithymocyte globulin, cyclosporine, androgens
Familial			
Fanconi syndrome	Before 10 yr age; mean is 8 yr	All cell lines; microcephaly, absent thumbs, *café-au-lait* spots, cutaneous hyperpigmentation, short stature; chromosomal breaks, high MCV and hemoglobin F; horseshoe or absent kidney; leukemic transformation; autosomal recessive trait	Androgens, corticosteroids, bone marrow transplant
Paroxysmal nocturnal hemoglobinuria	After 5 yr	Initial hemolysis followed by aplastic anemia; increased complement-mediated hemolysis; thrombosis; iron deficiency	Iron, bone marrow transplant, androgens, steroids
Dyskeratosis congenita	Mean 10 yr for skin; mean 17 yr for anemia	Pancytopenia; hyperpigmentation, dystrophic nails, leukoplakia; X-linked recessive; lacrimal duct stenosis; high MCV and fetal hemoglobin	Androgens, splenectomy, bone marrow transplant
Familial hemophagocytic lymphohistiocytosis	Before 2 yr	Pancytopenia; fever, hepatosplenomegaly, hypertriglyceridemia, CSF pleocytosis	Transfusion; often lethal VP-16 bone marrow transplantation
Infectious			
Parvovirus	Any age	Any chronic hemolytic anemia, typically sickle cell; new-onset reticulocytopenia	Transfusion
Epstein-Barr virus (EBV)	Any age; usually <5 yr	X-linked immunodeficiency syndrome, pancytopenia	Transfusion, bone marrow transplantation
Viral-associated hemophagocytic syndrome (CMV, HHV-6, EBV)	Any age	Pancytopenia; hemophagocytosis present in marrow	Transfusion, antiviral therapy, intravenous immunoglobulin

Adapted from Scott JP. Hematology. *In* Behrman RE, Kliegman RM (eds). Nelson Essentials of Pediatrics, 2nd ed. Philadelphia: WB Saunders, 1994:525.
Abbreviations: CMV = cytomegalovirus; CSF = cerebrospinal fluid; HHV-6 = human herpesvirus-6; MCV = mean corpuscular volume; s/p = status post.

a history of neonatal jaundice and intermittent icterus, and they often have splenomegaly and an abnormal peripheral smear related to their underlying hemolytic disease.

Isolated anemia of underproduction occurs in children with *chronic renal disease* due to a deficiency of erythropoietin. Clinical and laboratory findings often suggest a diagnosis of renal disease (poor growth, hypertension, edema, abnormal urinalysis, and elevated serum urea nitrogen level and creatinine). The anemia of chronic renal disease can be treated successfully by recombinant human erythropoietin administered by subcutaneous injection three times per week.

Macrocytic Anemia
(see Figs. 49–1 and 49–4)

Congenital hypoplastic anemia (Diamond-Blackfan anemia) is a constitutional pure RBC aplasia syndrome that presents during the first year of life with severe anemia and reticulocytopenia (see Table 49–11). The remainder of the CBC is otherwise unremarkable. Because synthesis of RBCs containing adult hemoglobin is markedly impaired, RBCs generally manifest fetal characteristics including elevated MCV, increased levels of fetal hemoglobin, and the ''i'' surface antigen. Bone marrow aspirate demonstrates pure RBC aplasia. Two thirds of patients with congenital hypoplastic anemia initially respond to corticosteroid treatment, and the remaining patients require long-term transfusion therapy. Patients who respond to steroid therapy may stop responding over time. Bone marrow transplantation has been curative in selected steroid-resistant patients.

Fanconi anemia usually presents with macrocytic anemia of underproduction in association with pancytopenia. It is a constitutional disorder frequently, but not invariably, associated with physical stigmata (see Table 49–11). Most patients do not present with overt hematologic manifestations until 4 or 5 years of age. Thumb and radial anomalies should alert the clinician to possible Fanconi anemia, even in the absence of cytopenias. Because of chronic bone marrow stress, RBCs tend to have fetal characteristics, including increased MCV and elevated fetal hemoglobin level. Patients usually respond initially to androgen therapy; however, mortality rates are high as a result of evolving resistance to treatment over time as well as a predisposition to myeloid leukemia and other malignancies. Bone marrow transplantation may be curative. Fanconi anemia is among the chromosomal breakage disorders wherein DNA is unusually fragile and susceptible to injury. The diagnostic laboratory abnormality is an increased chromosomal breakage when cells are cultured in the presence of a clastogenic agent, such as diepoxybutane.

Megaloblastic anemia (large RBCs with abnormalities of WBCs and platelets) due to vitamin B$_{12}$ or folate deficiency occurs rarely in children. In severe instances, pancytopenia may occur. In addition to large, ovoid RBCs, hypersegmented neutrophils (more than 5 lobes/cell) are often seen on peripheral smear (Fig. 49–6). It is appropriate to consider vitamin B$_{12}$ or folate deficiency in patients with otherwise unexplained macrocytic anemia. The presence of documented vitamin B$_{12}$ or folate deficiency requires an exhaustive etiologic search. Nutritional vitamin B$_{12}$ deficiency may occur in breast-feeding infants of mothers on strict vegetarian diets that exclude milk and egg products.

Congenital pernicious anemia is a rare syndrome associated with malabsorption that is caused by intrinsic factor deficiency. Children who have had resection of the terminal ileum, the site of absorption of vitamin B$_{12}$, may develop megaloblastic anemia. Vitamin B$_{12}$ malabsorption may occur with inflammatory disease involving the terminal ileum, such as Crohn disease or ulcerative colitis.

Unlike body stores of vitamin B$_{12}$, which may provide several years of reserve, folate stores are limited to several weeks' supply.

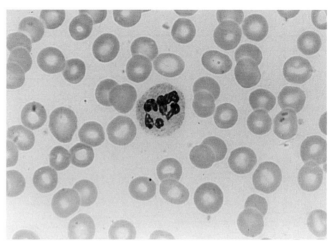

Figure 49–6. Hypersegmented polymorphonuclear leukocyte as seen in vitamin B$_{12}$ or folate deficiency.

Folate is ubiquitous in food sources; hence, nutritional deficiency is unusual. Although the deficiency is very rare today, infants fed unsupplemented goat's milk may develop profound folate deficiency. Malabsorption of folate can occur in children who have limited small-bowel absorptive capacity as a result of surgical resection or inflammatory disease. Patients with *chronic hemolytic anemia* (sickle cell disease) have an increased need for folate and occasionally manifest folate deficiency if they are receiving no supplementation and endure a period of poor nutrition of several weeks' duration.

Anemia Due to Increased Red Cell Destruction

The *hemolytic disorders* (see Figs. 49–1 and 49–4) are characterized by shortened RBC survival and reticulocytosis. Usually, RBCs survive approximately 120 days in the circulation. New RBCs are manufactured at a rate equivalent to the destruction of senescent RBCs, so that under normal circumstances an appropriate hemoglobin level is maintained. Various factors, some intrinsic to the RBC, others extrinsic, can lead to accelerated RBC destruction. Several clinical and laboratory hallmarks are associated with hemolysis (Table 49–12). It is imperative that a technically adequate peripheral blood smear be examined whenever hemolysis is suspected. Although normal RBC morphology does not exclude a diagnosis of hemolytic anemia, most hemolytic diseases are associated with morphologic abnormalities (Table 49–13). Depending on the cause of the hemolysis, RBCs may be removed from the circulation by reticuloendothelial cells (extravascular hemolysis) or may lyse within the circulation (intravascular hemolysis). In the latter circumstance, hemoglobin is released into the plasma and bound by the serum protein haptoglobin. In states of brisk intravascular hemolysis, the haptoglobin level may be depleted and free hemoglobin may be filtered by the kidney and appear in the urine. Under such circumstances, the urine appears pink. A urinary dipstick is positive for blood, but the microscopic examination of the urinary sediment does not demonstrate intact RBCs.

HEMOLYSIS DUE TO INTRINSIC RED BLOOD CELL DEFECTS

Three key components of the RBC exist: membrane, enzymes, and hemoglobin. Disturbances of any of these components may lead to ongoing or intermittent hemolysis.

Table 49–12. Clinical and Laboratory Features Suggesting Hemolytic Anemia

Pallor
Icterus
Splenomegaly
Gallstones
History of neonatal icterus
Positive family history of anemia, splenectomy, cholecystectomy
↑ Reticulocyte count
↑ RDW (due to reticulocyte count)
Abnormal RBC morphology
↑ Indirect bilirubin (normal direct bilirubin)
↓ Serum haptoglobin level
↑ Urinary urobilinogen level
Hemoglobinuria (+ dipstick test result for blood; no RBCs in urine)
↑ LDH level

Abbreviations: RDW = red cell distribution width; RBC = red blood cell; LDH = lactate dehydrogenase.

Hereditary Spherocytosis

The prototypic membrane defect is *hereditary spherocytosis,* which is an inherited disorder (autosomal dominant or less so recessive) occurring with a frequency of approximately 1 per 5000 live births. It is most typically seen in individuals of Northern European descent but may be identified in any population. The basic defect is an abnormality of the membrane protein spectrin that allows the RBC membrane to lose its redundancy and the usual biconcave disk shape, which is replaced by a small, dense cell of spheroid configuration. Hemolysis occurs because the spheroid RBCs are far less distensible and are unable to traverse the microcirculation of the spleen. Characteristic clinical findings include anemia, reticulocytosis, and the presence of abundant microspherocytes on peripheral smear. Associated findings of chronic hemolysis are often present, including pallor, icterus, and splenomegaly. The family history is often positive for anemia, splenectomy, or cholecystectomy.

Newborns with hereditary spherocytosis frequently develop jaundice within the first 24 hours of life, often necessitating phototherapy and occasionally exchange transfusion. Diagnosis may be confirmed by an osmotic fragility test, which reflects the limited capacity of the RBC to expand when incubated in a hypotonic environment. The clinic spectrum of disease is broad. Some patients have mild, well-compensated hemolysis, and their condition is detected during the adult years after the diagnosis in one of their children. Other patients may have brisk hemolysis during infancy, requiring intermittent transfusion support. Most patients have a disease characterized by mild to moderate anemia, reticulocytosis, and splenomegaly. Patients are susceptible to exacerbations of anemia as a result of the viral-related hyperhemolysis or transient RBC hypoplasia. Parvovirus B19 may cause superimposed transient RBC hypoplasia of about 1 week's duration.

Splenectomy has been used only for patients with moderate or severe disease. Patients who do not undergo splenectomy nearly always develop gallstones as time progresses. When splenectomy is performed, it should be deferred until the patient is 5 to 7 years of age except under extraordinary circumstances. The risk of postsplenectomy infection is markedly decreased if splenectomy is performed after the early years of life. Before splenectomy is performed it is critical that all patients be immunized with the pneumococcal, *Haemophilus influenzae* b, and meningococcal vaccines. Preventive penicillin or amoxicillin therapy (250 mg twice daily) is recommended in all patients who have undergone splenectomy and should be continued indefinitely. After splenectomy,

children who develop high fever should be evaluated for the possibility of bacteremia (usually caused by *Streptococcus pneumoniae,* less often by *H. influenzae,* meningococci, staphylococci, or gram-negative bacteria). Appropriate cultures and liberal use of empiric parenteral antibiotic therapy are indicated because a high fatality rate is associated with untreated bacteremia in patients who have undergone splenectomy.

Hereditary Elliptocytosis

Hereditary elliptocytosis represents a heterogeneous group of inherited disorders characterized by variable chronic hemolysis and abundant elliptoid cells on peripheral smear. The clinical and laboratory findings are similar to those seen in hereditary spherocytosis. Splenectomy is appropriate in patients with moderate to severe hemolytic disease.

Hereditary Pyropoikilocytosis

Hereditary pyropoikilocytosis is an autosomal recessive membrane disorder that presents in the newborn period and is characterized by marked jaundice and anemia, reticulocytosis, and striking aberrations of red cell morphology. Hemolysis lessens with advancing age.

Glucose-6-Phosphate Dehydrogenase Deficiency

The most common red blood cell enzyme defect is G6PD deficiency. An X-linked disorder, G6PD deficiency occurs most commonly in individuals of African and Mediterranean descent and should always be considered in the differential diagnosis of acute hemolytic anemia in males. Deficiency of G6PD activity renders hemoglobin susceptible to oxidant insult, leading to precipitation of hemoglobin, membrane damage, and, ultimately, RBC destruction. Oxidant injury may occur on the basis of intercurrent infection or ingestion of various substances, including medications, toxins, and foods (Table 49–14).

The African variety of G6PD mutant, G6PD A, is not associated with significant chronic hemolysis but manifests as acute hemolytic anemia related to specific precipitating factors. Rarely is hemolysis sufficiently severe to require transfusion therapy. Patients are often incidentally found to be anemic with evidence of an appropriate reticulocyte response. Peripheral blood smear often demonstrates bite cells as portions of the RBC (precipitates of hemoglobin) are removed by reticuloendothelial cells (Fig. 49–7). G6PD enzyme

Table 49–13. Hemolytic Anemia: Diagnostic Clues Based on Red Cell Morphology

Sickle cells: sickle cell disease
Target cells: hemoglobinopathies (hgb C, hgb S, thalassemia), liver disease
Burr cells/helmet cells/RBC fragments: microangiopathic hemolytic anemia-DIC, HUS, TTP
Spherocytes: hereditary spherocytosis, autoimmune hemolytic anemia
"Bite" cells: G6PD deficiency

Abbreviations: hgb = hemoglobin; RBC = red blood cell; DIC = disseminated intravascular coagulation; HUS = hemolytic-uremic syndrome; TTP = thrombotic thrombocytopenic purpura; G6PD = glucose-6-phosphate dehydrogenase.

Table 49–14. Factors Known to Promote Hemolysis in Patient with G6PD Deficiency

Viral or bacterial infection
Fava beans
Vitamin C (large doses)
Mothballs
Benzene and other volatiles
Medications
   Sulfonamides
   Antimalarial drugs
   Nitrofurantoin
   Nalidixic acid
   Chloramphenicol
   Vitamin K analogs
   Methylene blue

Abbreviation: G6PD = glucose-6-phosphate dehydrogenase.

assay is necessary for the establishment of a diagnosis, but the test must be performed on a sample that has been depleted of reticulocytes because newly released RBCs have large amounts of G6PD. The Mediterranean variety of G6PD deficiency tends to be more severe and may be associated with chronic hemolysis as well as superimposed acute events caused by infection or medication.

Pyruvate Kinase Deficiency

Pyruvate kinase deficiency is an uncommon autosomal recessive disorder characterized by chronic hemolytic anemia. Patients may have anemia, reticulocytosis, variable splenomegaly, and a peripheral blood smear that may demonstrate RBCs with spicules. Specific enzyme assay can be performed by specialized laboratories. Patients with moderate or severe hemolytic disease often improve after splenectomy. Some patients require intermittent transfusion support.

Hemoglobinopathies

Hemoglobinopathies usually occur as a result of a single amino acid substitution in the globin chain. Hemoglobinopathies are among the most common causes of chronic hemolytic disease. Sickle cell syndromes are the most frequently encountered disorders of hemoglobin.

Sickle Hemoglobinopathy Syndromes. The sickle hemoglobinopathy syndromes are a group of genetically determined disorders that are encountered most frequently in individuals of Central African descent and should be considered in the differential diagnosis of anemia in any African-American child. These disorders occur less frequently in individuals of Mediterranean or Arabic background.

Sickle cell anemia (SS disease) is an autosomal recessive disorder characterized by a single amino acid substitution of the β globin chain (valine for glutamic acid in the number 6 position). Sickle hemoglobin has a tendency to form insoluble fibers within the RBC on deoxygenation, which may ultimately lead to the formation of the characteristic crescent-shaped sickled erythrocyte (Fig. 49–8). Sickle hemoglobin may occur in the doubly heterozygous state in patients with hemoglobin C or β-thalassemia and may give rise to a disorder generally less severe than SS disease. Approximately 1 in 400 African-Americans are affected by sickle cell disease.

Sickle cell trait (the heterozygous state) occurs in about 8% of African-Americans and is rarely associated with clinical disease except under states of unusually severe arterial hypoxemia. Spontaneous hematuria occasionally occurs in sickle trait as a result of the induction of sickling in the extremely hypertonic environment of the renal medulla. Patients with sickle cell trait are distinctly *not* anemic and have a *normal* peripheral blood smear.

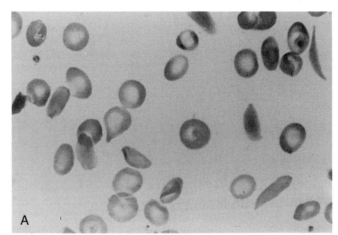
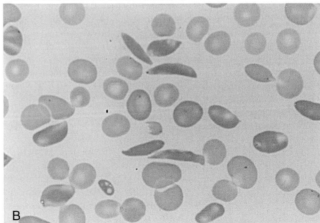

Figure 49–8. Sickle cell anemia. *A, B,* Sickled erythrocytes and target cells.

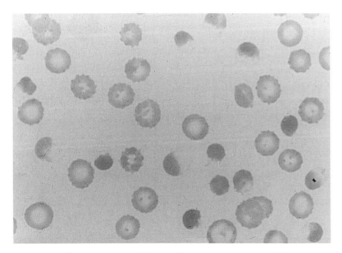

Figure 49–7. "Bite" cells and Burr cells as seen in G6PD deficiency hemolysis.

Table 49–15. Hemoglobin Electrophoresis Diagnosis of Sickle Hemoglobinopathy

Disease	Hemoglobin Type
Normal	A
SS disease	S (*no* hemoglobin A)
S trait	A + S (about equal proportions)
SC disease	S + C (about equal proportions)
S–β-thalassemia	S > A (S predominate hemoglobin)

The diagnosis of sickle cell anemia is usually straightforward. Children are variably anemic with reticulocytosis. The peripheral blood smear often demonstrates characteristic sickled erythrocytes (see Fig. 49–8). The hemoglobin solubility test (sickle preparation, Sickledex) result is positive in patients older than 6 months of age with sickle cell trait *and* disease. The definitive diagnosis must be established by hemoglobin electrophoresis (Table 49–15). Diagnosis in newborns is routinely and accurately performed in many locations within the United States.

The clinical manifestations of sickle hemoglobinopathy are (1) chronic hemolytic anemia, (2) vaso-occlusion resulting in ischemic injury to tissue, and (3) susceptibility to infection (Table 49–16). Infants younger than 4 to 6 months of age usually show no clinical manifestations, because of naturally high levels of fetal hemoglobin. By 1 to 2 years of age, most patients have had a specific sickling-related manifestation.

Patients may appear variably pale and icteric, depending on the degree of hemolysis. Enlargement of the spleen is routinely seen between 6 and 36 months of age in patients with SS disease and may persist into adolescence in some patients with milder variants (SC disease). Autoinfarction due to microvascular occlusion ultimately leads to fibrosis of splenic tissue. Maxillary hyperplasia and dental malocclusion occur commonly as a result of compensatory bone marrow expansion. Gallstones occur regularly and may lead to symptoms of cholelithiasis, acute cholecystitis, biliary tract obstruction, and/or pancreatitis. Many patients have delayed growth and pubertal development but ultimately achieve normal adult height. Exacerbation of anemia can occur as a result of infection-induced hyperhemolysis (in which case the patient may present with *increasing* jaundice, tachycardia, progressive anemia) or transient virus-induced RBC hypoplasia (manifesting as progressive pallor, fatigue, tachycardia, and *decreased* jaundice). Hyperhemolytic episodes may also occur in patients with concomitant G6PD deficiency. Red cell transfusions may be necessary when progressive anemia is accompanied by significant clinical symptoms.

The "painful crisis" is the most classic vaso-occlusive manifestation of the sickle hemoglobinopathy syndromes. Pain most often affects the extremities, axial skeleton, or abdomen. The hand-foot syndrome (dactylitis) is characterized by pain, swelling, and erythema involving the metacarpal and metatarsal bones in infants and young children. Painful events are variable with regard to frequency and severity. Most events are unprecipitated; others may be related to cold exposure, exercise, or trauma. Infarction of cortical bone may lead to localized extremity swelling, which may be difficult to differentiate from osteomyelitis. Abdominal pain may be confused with other intra-abdominal processes, including appendicitis, cholecystitis, or perforated viscus. Sickle-associated abdominal pain often occurs in the context of skeletal pain, and bowel sounds are usually preserved, helping to differentiate pain

Table 49–16. Clinical Manifestations of Sickle Cell Anemia*

Manifestation	Comments
Anemia	Chronic, onset 3–4 mo of age; may require folate therapy for chronic hemolysis. Hematocrit usually 18%–26%
Aplastic crisis	Parvovirus infection, reticulocytopenia; acute and reversible
Sequestration crisis	Massive splenomegaly, shock; treat with transfusion
Hemolytic crisis	May be associated with G6PD deficiency
Dactylitis	Hand-foot swelling in early infancy
Painful crisis	Microvascular painful vaso-occlusive infarcts of muscle, bone, bone marrow, lung, intestines
Cerebral vascular accidents	Large- and small-vessel sickling and thrombosis (stroke); requires chronic transfusion
Acute chest syndrome	Infection, infarction, hypoventilation, or bone marrow emboli, severe hypoxemia, infiltrate, dyspnea, rales
Chronic lung disease	Pulmonary fibrosis, restrictive lung disease, cor pulmonale
Priapism	Causes eventual impotence; treat with transfusion, oxygen, or corpora cavernosa to spongiosa shunt
Ocular	Retinopathy
Gallbladder disease	Bilirubin stones; cholecystitis
Renal	Hematuria, papillary necrosis, renal-concentrating deficit; nephropathy
Cardiomyopathy	Heart failure (fibrosis)
Leg ulceration	Seen in older patients
Infections	Functional asplenia, defects in properdin system; pneumococcal bacteremia, meningitis, and arthritis; deafness from meningitis in 35%; *Haemophilus influenzae* sepsis, *Salmonella,* and *Staphylococcus aureus* osteomyelitis; severe *Mycoplasma* pneumonia; *Escherichia coli* urinary tract infection; transfusion-acquired HIV, hepatitis A, B, C, D, and E, EBV, CMV
Growth failure, delayed puberty	May respond to nutritional supplements
Psychologic problems	Narcotic addiction, dependence unusual; chronic illness

Adapted from Scott JP. Hematology. *In* Behrman RE, Kliegman RM (eds). Nelson Essentials of Pediatrics, 2nd ed. Philadelphia: WB Saunders, 1994:530.

*Clinical manifestations with sickle cell trait are unusual but include renal papillary necrosis (hematuria), sudden death on exertion, intraocular hyphema extension, and sickling in unpressurized airplanes.

Abbreviations: CMV = cytomegalovirus; EBV = Epstein-Barr virus; HIV = human immunodeficiency virus; G6PD = glucose-6-phosphate dehydrogenase.

Table 49–17. Treatment of Severe Vaso-occlusive Painful Crisis in Sickle Cell Anemia

Correct dehydration

Maintenance rate plus correction for abnormal fluid losses and fever

5% dextrose in water plus ½ normal saline solution

No potassium chloride unless serum K^+ <3.5 mEq/L

Analgesics

Narcotics

Meperidine, 0.75–1.5 mg/kg IV, or morphine sulfate, 0.125–0.175 mg/kg IV, every 2 or 3 hours, depending on initial patient response (*not* p.r.n.)

plus

Nonsteroidal anti-inflammatory agent:

Ibuprofen or naproxyn sodium p.o.

or

Ketorolac parenteral therapy

Monitor

CNS—level of alertness

Respiratory status (respiratory rate and effort, pulse oximetry)

Vital signs (pulse, BP, temperature)

Abbreviations: IV = intravenously; p.o. = orally; p.r.n. = as necessary; CNS = central nervous system; BP = blood pressure.

from that due to an acute surgical complication. Chest pain may accompany pneumonia, pulmonary infarction, or fat embolus from infarcted bone marrow. Parenteral analgesic therapy is often requested when pain is severe (Table 49–17). Patients receiving parenteral narcotic therapy require careful monitoring of level of consciousness, respiratory status, and vital signs because narcotics may induce excessive sedation and/or decreased ventilatory effort, thus contributing to the development of the acute chest syndrome.

Acute Chest Syndrome. This syndrome represents an acute febrile pulmonary illness with radiographic infiltrates with or without pleural effusions. Signs of respiratory distress may appear rapidly (within 2 to 6 hours) and include increased respiratory rate and effort, flaring, and grunting in association with progressive hypoxemia. It is unclear in most cases whether the primary event represents pneumonia, intrapulmonary vaso-occlusive sickling, hypoventilation, or fat embolus, but local and systemic hypoxemia may promote further sickling with rapid expansion of infiltrates. The acute chest syndrome represents a major cause of mortality in children and adolescents and requires aggressive supportive respiratory care, broad-spectrum antibiotic (cefotaxime plus erythromycin) coverage, and, if symptoms are progressive, transfusion (simple or partial exchange) therapy. The incidence of acute chest syndrome may be reduced by incentive spirometry to reduce atelectasis.

Acute Splenic Sequestration. This disorder results from vascular occlusion of splenic sinusoids, leading to the trapping of blood within the substance of the spleen. Rapid enlargement of the spleen and progressive anemia occur. Patients may present with severe hypovolemic shock. Infants and young children are susceptible to this potentially lethal complication before autoinfarction of the spleen. Transfusion therapy is necessary in moderate to severe events.

Stroke. Stroke occurs in approximately 10% of patients with sickle hemoglobinopathy and may present with focal seizures, hemipare-

sis, gait disturbances, aphasia, or alterations in consciousness. Most events occur as a result of large cerebral vessel occlusion. Subarachnoid and intracerebral hemorrhage may occasionally occur in children. Patients with stroke require urgent evaluation and long-term transfusion to prevent recurrence. All children with sickle cell disease who have a seizure or focal neurologic symptoms or signs must be evaluated for possible stroke. Magnetic resonance imaging coupled with magnetic resonance angiography allows for rapid noninvasive assessment of brain and large cerebral vessel disease.

Priapism. Priapism, a persistent, painful penile erection caused by venous occlusion, occurs in teenagers and young adults and may lead to long-term impotence. In addition to analgesic and fluid therapy, exchange transfusion may be considered when detumescence does not occur in 24 to 48 hours.

Infection. Infection is the leading cause of death in young children with sickle cell disease. Dysfunction of the spleen, beginning at about 4 to 6 months of age, leads to a susceptibility to overwhelming infection (sepsis, meningitis), caused by encapsulated organisms, particularly *S. pneumoniae* and less commonly *H. influenzae* type b. Children older than 5 years of age are at less risk of infection, yet when infection does occur, gram-negative organisms account for about half of all episodes. *Escherichia coli* urinary tract infections and *Salmonella* infections (bacteremia, gastroenteritis, osteomyelitis) are also observed in children with sickle cell disease. Osteomyelitis may also occur as a result of *Staphylococcus aureus* infection and should be suspected in the patient who presents with focal skeletal pain and fever.

Preventive penicillin (or amoxicillin) therapy (in patients younger than the age of 3 years, 125 mg twice daily; in those older than 3 years, 250 mg twice daily) beginning at 3 months of age has dramatically decreased the incidence of serious infection and mortality. *All patients with sickle cell disease who present with fever of greater than 102°F should be considered bacteremic until proven otherwise, even if they do not appear ill.* Untreated bacteremia may rapidly lead to septic shock and death. Broad-spectrum antibiotic therapy (cefotaxime, ceftriaxone; vancomycin if penicillin-resistant pneumococcus is suspected) to eradicate susceptible organisms is instituted pending culture results.

Prognosis and Treatment. The course of sickle hemoglobinopathy is quite variable; a small percentage of patients account for a disproportionately large number of complications. Mortality during the first decade of life has dramatically declined as a result of comprehensive approaches to care, which include newborn diagnosis, extensive family education, preventive antibiotic therapy, and 24-hour access to medical care providers who are knowledgeable in the treatment of this disorder. Newer treatment modalities are being investigated, including bone marrow transplantation, which is curative but associated with a risk of morbidity and possible mortality. Attempts to elevate the fetal hemoglobin level in an effort to ameliorate the clinical course are actively being explored, including the use of hydroxyurea and butyrate therapies. The outlook for patients with sickle hemoglobinopathy has improved markedly during the past two decades. If the condition is diagnosed in the newborn period and comprehensive care is provided, the child may be expected to have a 10-year survival rate of greater than 98%. The doubly heterozygous states for sickle and hemoglobin C (SC disease) and sickle disease with β-thalassemia represent sickling syndromes of a generally lesser degree of severity than SS disease. Severe complications do, however, occur in patients with SC disease and S–β-thalassemia (including sepsis and acute chest syndrome); hence, comprehensive care and aggressive therapy for complications are justified.

Hemoglobin E. Hemoglobin E is seen with considerable frequency among individuals of Asian descent. Hemoglobin E trait is characterized by mild anemia and mild microcytosis. There are no significant clinical implications. The diagnosis is confirmed by hemoglobin electrophoresis. When hemoglobin E occurs in the double heterozygous state with β-thalassemia, patients often have a moderately severe thalassemic syndrome; hence, genetic counseling is advisable.

Autoimmune Hemolytic Anemia. This condition occurs infrequently in children and adolescents and may occur as a transient, post-viral process or in conjunction with underlying immunologic dysfunction (immunodeficiency, human immunodeficiency virus [HIV] infection, Hodgkin disease). Patients may present with pallor and, if hemolysis is brisk, with fatigue, tachycardia, and icterus. Splenomegaly is variably present. The degree of anemia is highly variable, and the reticulocyte count is elevated in most patients; however, a small percentage of patients present with a low reticulocyte count, caused by immune destruction of reticulocytes. The peripheral smear demonstrates microspherocytes; results of the direct Coombs test are positive. Patients with autoimmune hemolytic anemia should be studied for evidence of immunologic dysfunction, infection, and malignancy (immunoglobulin levels, T-cell and B-cell counts, HIV and Epstein-Barr virus studies, chest x-ray). Aggressive therapy is appropriate because life-threatening hemolysis is known to occur. If no underlying disease is uncovered, corticosteroids (prednisone, 2 mg/kg/day) should be administered, and the patient should be observed closely. Intravenous immunoglobulin (1 to 2 g/kg) and high-dose steroids (methylprednisone, 30 mg/kg intravenously to a 1-g maximum dose) should be considered in severe cases. Transfusion therapy is used only if absolutely necessary because cross-matching of blood may be difficult.

Anemia in the Neonate

It is appropriate to view neonatal anemia in the context of three possible pathophysiologic pathways (Table 49–18): (1) acute blood loss, (2) anemia of underproduction, and (3) anemia associated with increased destruction.

The term infant has a normal hemoglobin value (hemoglobin, 15 to 21 g/dl; hematocrit, 45% to 65%) that is substantially greater than that in older infants and young children. This finding represents a functional adaptation to the relatively hypoxic *in utero* environment. The reticulocyte count is elevated to about 7% to 8% during the first 3 days of life, after which there is an abrupt succession of erythropoiesis until a physiologic hemoglobin nadir of about 9.5 to 10 g/dl is reached at 2 months of age. This physiologic anemia of infancy is exaggerated in preterm infants, whose hemoglobin levels may fall to approximately 7 g/dl at about 1 to 1.5 months of age. This fall in hemoglobin value represents a physiologic response to the oxygen-rich extrauterine environment.

NEONATAL ANEMIA DUE TO BLOOD LOSS

Anemia due to blood loss is often obvious. It occurs in placenta previa, *abruptio placentae*, or large cephalohematoma. Other instances of hemorrhage may be occult and include intracranial and intrahepatic hematoma. Internal hemorrhage is much more likely to occur in difficult, traumatic deliveries. Twin-to-twin transfusion may occur, leading to anemia in one infant and polycythemia in the other. Fetal-maternal hemorrhage, although common, is sufficiently severe to cause anemia in only a small percentage of neonates. The Kleihauer-Betke test may detect the presence of fetal RBCs in

Table 49–18. Anemia in the Neonate

Blood loss (common)
  Placenta previs
  Abruptio placentae
  Twin-twin transfusion
  Fetal-maternal hemorrhage (acute versus chronic)
  Neonatal hemorrhage
Decreased RBC production (unusual)
  Diamond-Blackfan anemia
  Congenital leukemia
  Transient myeloproliferative syndrome in Down syndrome
  Osteopetrosis
Hemolysis
  Intrinsic RBC defect (uncommon)
    Membrane (hereditary spherocytosis or elliptocytosis)
    Enzyme (G6PD, PK)
    Hemoglobin (alpha or gamma chain abnormality)
  Extrinsic RBC defect
    Immune (ABO, Rh, minor group incompatibilities)
      (common)
    Infection (intrauterine infection, bacterial, viral protozoal)
    DIC
    Kasbach-Merritt syndrome
    Galactosemia

Abbreviations: RBC = red blood cell; G6PD = glucose-6-phosphate dehydrogenase; PK = pyruvate kinase; DIC = disseminated intravascular coagulation.

the maternal circulation but may yield falsely negative results, particularly in mothers with type O blood who have antibodies against infant A, B, or AB blood cells. Fetal-maternal hemorrhage must always be suspected when otherwise unexplained anemia occurs in a newborn.

The time course and extent of blood loss dictates the clinical presentation. If blood loss has been mild or chronic, infants may appear normal or may be somewhat pale and tachycardic. In the event of severe acute blood loss, the newborn infant may present with signs of acute illness including lethargy, tachycardia, hypotension, and respiratory distress. The hemoglobin value is a poor index of the severity of acute blood loss because equilibration of fluid compartments may take 24 to 36 hours. Blood loss as a cause of anemia should always be suspected in cases of obstetric complications, multiple births, or difficult and traumatic delivery. In cases of severe blood loss, emergent transfusion therapy is appropriate. In the neonate who is hemodynamically stable but has experienced significant blood loss, a more conservative approach is recommended.

NEONATAL ANEMIA DUE TO DECREASED RBC PRODUCTION

Anemia due to decreased RBC production in the newborn is distinctly unusual. Infants with congenital hypoplastic anemia (Diamond-Blackfan anemia) are, at most, mildly anemic during the newborn period. Congenital leukemia is a rare disorder characterized by infiltration of the bone marrow, leading to anemia, thrombocytopenia, and leukocytosis in association with hepatosplenomegaly and, occasionally, cutaneous leukemic infiltrates manifesting as blue papular lesions ("blueberry muffin" spots). Infants with Down syndrome may present with a clinical and hematologic picture identical to that of congenital leukemia, which is a transient myeloproliferative process that spontaneously remits over several months. Infantile osteopetrosis (marble bone disease),

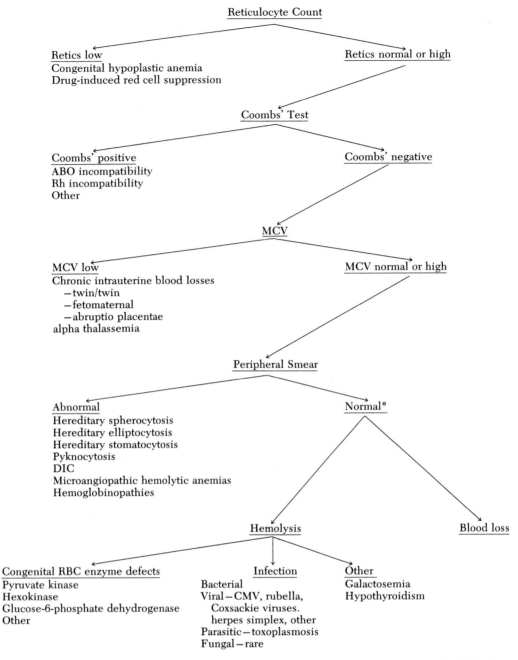

Figure 49–9. Diagnostic approach to anemia in the newborn based on reticulocyte count. The *asterisk* Indicates a peripheral blood smear with no specifically diagnostic abnormalities. MCV = mean corpuscular volume; DIC = disseminated intravascular coagulation; CMV = cytomegalovirus; RBC = red blood cell. (From Nathan DC, Oski F. Hematology of Infancy and Childhood, 4th ed. Vol 1. Philadelphia: WB Saunders, 1993.)

a disorder characterized by a limited ability to degrade bone, usually does not cause pancytopenia until a few months after birth.

NEONATAL ANEMIA DUE TO INCREASED RBC DESTRUCTION

Anemia due to increased RBC destruction (hemolytic anemia) places the neonate at risk for indirect hyperbilirubinemia as a result of the limited hepatic bilirubin-conjugating ability during the first weeks of life. Even relatively small increases in the rate of RBC destruction can lead to marked increases in serum bilirubin level.

All infants who have elevations of indirect bilirubin levels above the normal range during the first 3 days of life should be evaluated for possible hemolysis, with a hemoglobin level, reticulocyte count, peripheral blood smear, maternal and infant blood types, and direct Coombs test.

Intrinsic disorders of the erythrocyte may present in the neonate. Infants with *hereditary spherocytosis* or *elliptocytosis* may develop anemia and extreme hyperbilirubinemia that requires phototherapy and, in some cases, exchange transfusion. A peripheral blood smear and family history may be helpful in identifying an intrinsic RBC membrane defect.

G6PD deficiency can occur in male newborns of African or Mediterranean descent. Because of the increased susceptibility of neonatal RBCs to oxidant injury, anemia, reticulocytosis, and hyperbilirubinemia may occur without an obvious precipitating insult. *Hemoglobinopathies* rarely manifest during the neonatal period. β Globin chain defects, such as sickle cell syndromes and thalassemia, are not clinically apparent until about 4 months of life, as a result of the predominance of fetal hemoglobin in the perinatal period.

Severe α-thalassemia (hemoglobin Bart disease) can affect the fetus. Such infants develop severe *in utero* anemia, with resultant hydrops, because of the limited ability of hemoglobin Bart to release oxygen to tissues.

Isoimmune hemolytic anemia is the most common cause of anemia in the newborn. It is caused by incompatibility between maternal and fetal blood groups, including Rh, ABO, or minor blood group antigens. In Rh incompatibility, the mother is Rh negative, and the infant is Rh positive (inherited from the father). If the mother has been exposed to Rh-positive blood cells through prior pregnancy, miscarriage, therapeutic abortion, or mismatched blood transfusion, IgG antibodies may develop, which transverse the placenta and cause immune destruction of fetal Rh-positive cells. In such instances, hemolysis occurs *in utero* and in the newborn period. In severe circumstances, the fetus may be extremely anemic, resulting in hydrops and fetal death. In less serious instances, infants may be born quite anemic and brisk hyperbilirubinemia, which can lead to *kernicterus* (bilirubin encephalopathy), may develop. The severity of Rh immune hemolytic disease increases with repetitive pregnancies. This disorder is uncommon, because of the routine practice of administering Rh immune globulin to Rh-negative mothers at 28 to 30 weeks' gestation and within 72 hours of delivery (and after spontaneous or therapeutic abortion). Prenatal management of the affected fetus may include spectrophotometric assessment of amniotic fluid as an assessment of fetal bilirubin level, and, in high-risk situations, serial fetal hemoglobin levels obtained by ultrasound-guided aspiration of umbilical cord blood (cordocentesis). When the fetus demonstrates progressive *in utero* severe anemia, intrauterine intravascular blood transfusion therapy has been shown to decrease the risks of fetal death. Management of the neonate relates largely to the severity of the hemolysis. Hyperbilirubinemia must be aggressively treated with phototherapy, and if the condition is severe, exchange transfusion. Red blood cell transfusions are appropriate for symptomatic anemia.

Occasionally, anemia may be detected several weeks after Rh hemolysis, and may be associated with a profoundly depressed reticulocyte count. This late anemia is of uncertain etiology, but inappropriately low erythropoietin levels have been noted. Symptomatic infants may require transfusion therapy. Affected infants have been successfully treated with human recombinant erythropoietin.

Immune incompatibility due to the ABO system is common and usually occurs in mothers whose blood type is O and newborns whose blood type is A or B. The degree of hemolysis is usually much less severe than in Rh disease. Fetal hydrops is extremely rare. Most babies with ABO incompatibility manifest increased jaundice (indirect hyperbilirubinemia) during the first 1 to 2 days of life. Hemoglobin levels are often within the normal to mildly anemic range, but moderate anemia may occasionally occur. The reticulocyte count is usually mildly elevated, and the peripheral blood smear may show microspherocytes. The blood types of mother and infant demonstrate a "set up" (type O mother with infant who is either type A or B). Results of the Coombs test are usually weakly or moderately positive, but false-negative results do occur.

Treatment is generally directed toward hyperbilirubinemia and may require phototherapy. Exchange transfusion is rarely necessary. Anemia may require blood transfusion.

Immune incompatibility may also occur on the basis of minor blood groups, such as the Duffy or Kell antigen systems. Clinical and laboratory findings are similar to those in ABO hemolytic disease, except that the direct Coombs test result is strongly positive.

Other causes of hemolytic anemia in the newborn include bacterial sepsis, and, less often, intrauterine infection (cytomegalovirus, toxoplasmosis, herpes, rubella, and syphilis). Intrauterine infectious syndromes can cause mild to moderate hemolytic anemia of several months' duration. Such infants may demonstrate physical stigmata, including small size for gestational age, microcephaly, chorioretinitis, hepatosplenomegaly, intracranial calcifications, and "celery stalking" of the long bones on x-ray study.

Microangiopathic hemolytic anemia can occur in the newborn as a result of *disseminated intravascular coagulation* (DIC). In the neonate, DIC is usually caused by serious infection, hypoxemia due to respiratory distress syndrome in the preterm infant, or ischemic tissue injury related to birth asphyxia. Newborns with hemolysis due to infection or DIC are often extremely ill and require RBC transfusion support.

Microangiopathic hemolytic anemia and consumptive thrombocytopenia can occur in the *Kasabach-Merritt syndrome,* which is associated with *cavernous hemangiomas* and localized intravascular coagulation. Some infants have obvious expansive cutaneous and subcutaneous lesions, but occult visceral hemangiomas, particularly hepatic, can occur. The peripheral blood smear demonstrates evidence of RBC fragments and burr cells. Kasabach-Merritt syndrome may require treatment with plasma and platelet transfusions (if consumptive coagulopathy is severe). Corticosteroids and interferon therapy have been helpful in such infants.

The diagnostic approach to anemia in the neonate requires a careful assessment of maternal, prenatal, and perinatal history, as well as the clinical status of the neonate (Fig. 49–9). CBC, reticulocyte count, peripheral blood smear, maternal and infant blood types, and direct Coombs tests are virtually always necessary laboratory studies. Other studies must be dictated by the clinical and initial laboratory findings.

SUMMARY AND RED FLAGS

Anemia is a common finding in children. A complete and thorough evaluation of clinical findings (history and physical examination) is the single most important element in the establishment of a diagnosis and in defining appropriate therapy.

Anemia may be a primary event reflecting intrinsic hematologic disease, or it may be a manifestation of a wide variety of disorders involving virtually any organ system. Anemia always deserves to be fully evaluated, given the potential diagnostic and therapeutic implications. Patients who appear *acutely ill* should have a more thorough evaluation because *acute blood loss* needs to be treated

Table 49–19. Red Flags

Anemia accompanied by:
Neutropenia and/or thrombocytopenia
High MCV with normal RDW
Blasts on the peripheral smear
Firm adenopathy
Bruising or bleeding
Weight loss, failure to thrive
Shortness of breath, fatigue
Organomegaly
Edema
Abnormal vital signs

Abbreviations: MCV = mean corpuscular volume; RDW = red cell distribution width.

quickly. If acute blood loss is not suspected, *acute hemolysis* or *splenic sequestration* of RBCs must be considered.

Anemia is often a sign of *underlying* or *chronic disease.* In such cases, anemia is not usually an isolated finding. Therefore, symptoms such as shortness of breath, extreme pallor, weight loss, fevers, lethargy, and fatigue should prompt a thorough evaluation of the patient.

On physical examination, the findings of abnormal vital signs, failure to thrive, bleeding or bruising, adenopathy, or organomegaly should lead the examiner to suspect that a potentially serious underlying disorder is present (Table 49–19).

When a CBC is obtained, a low hemoglobin value accompanied by any abnormality of MCV, WBC, or platelet count should be taken seriously and should be more thoroughly investigated.

REFERENCES

Work-Up of Anemia

Bessman JD, Jilmer PR, Gardner FH. Classification of red cell disorders by MCV and RDW. Am J Clin Pathol 1983;80:322.

Hoffman R, Benz EJ, Shattil SJ, et al. Hematology, Basic Principles and Practice, 2nd ed. New York: Churchill Livingstone, 1995.

Miller DR, Baehner RL. Blood Diseases of Infancy and Childhood, 6th ed. St. Louis: CV Mosby, 1990.

Nathan DG, Oski FA. Hematology of Infancy and Childhood, 4th ed. Philadelphia: WB Saunders, 1993.

Novak RW. Red blood cell distribution within pediatric microcytic anemias. Pediatrics 1987;80:251.

Segall GB. Anemia. Pediatr Rev 1988;10:77.

Yip R, Binkin NJ, et al. Declining prevalence of anemia among low income children in the United States. JAMA 1987;258:1619.

Anemia with Acute and Chronic Disease

Abshire TC, Reeves JD. Anemia of acute inflammation in children. J Pediatr 1985;105:874.

Jansson LT, Kling S, Dallman PR. Anemia in children with acute infection seen in a primary pediatric outpatient clinic. Pediatr Infect Dis J 1968;5:424.

Lee RG. The anemia of chronic disease. Semin Hematol 1983;20:61.

Hemolytic Anemia

Addiego JE, Hurst D, Lubin BH. Congenital hemolytic anemia. Pediatr Rev 1985;6:201.

Beutler E. Glucose-6-phosphotase dehydrogenese deficiency. N Engl J Med 1991;324:169.

Forget BG. Hemolytic anemias: Congenital and acquired. Hosp Pract 1980;15:66–78.

Manno CS, Cohen AR. Splenectomy in mild hereditary spherocytosis: Is it worth the risk? Am J Pediatr Hematol Oncol 1989;11:300.

Hypoplastic Anemia

Glader BE. Diagnosis in management of red cell aplasia in children. Hematol Oncol Clin North Am 1987;1:431.

Glader BE. Red blood cell aplasias in children. Pediatr Ann 1990;19:3.

Halperin DS, Freedman MH. Diamond-Blackfan anemia: Etiology, pathophysiology, and treatment. Am J Pediatr Hematol Oncol 1989;11:380.

Hays T, Lane PA Jr, Shafer F. Transient erythroblastopenia of childhood. Am J Dis Child 1989;143:605.

Wine WC, Mentzer WC. Differentiation of transient erythroblastopenia of childhood from congenital hypoplastic anemia. J Pediatr 1967;88:784.

Iron Deficiency

Committee on Nutrition (American Academy of Pediatrics). Iron-fortified formulas. Pediatrics 1989;84:1114.

Lozoff B, Jimenez E, Wolf AW. Long-term small developmental outcome of infants with iron deficiency. N Engl J Med 1991;325:687.

Oski FA. Iron deficiency in infancy and childhood. N Engl J Med 1993;329:190.

Sickle Cell Disease

Charache S, Lubin B, Reid CD. Management and therapy of sickle cell disease. Washington D.C.: United States Department of Health and Human Services NIH Publ No. 84-2117, 1984.

Pearson HA. Sickle cell disease: Diagnosis and management in infancy and childhood. Pediatr Rev 1987;9:121.

Wethers D, Pearson H, Gaston M. Newborn screening for sickle cell disease and other hemoglobinopathies. Pediatrics 1989;83:813.

50 Neck Masses in Childhood

Robin E. M. Miller   Michael L. Nieder

Although the vast majority of neck masses represent benign inflammatory lesions, there are grave consequences associated with misdiagnosing the rare malignant neoplasm. While some lesions are most successfully managed with antibiotics or close observation, others require early referral and surgical intervention. A working knowledge of the regional anatomy combined with a thorough, directed history and physical examination forms the basis of the approach to neck masses.

Childhood neck masses should be considered in two broad diagnostic categories: congenital and acquired lesions. Of those masses that are acquired, the most common causes include infectious, inflammatory, and neoplastic conditions. Within these categories, each possibility must be considered with respect to its most likely anatomic location, age range at first presentation, and commonly associated historical features and physical findings. In this way the differential diagnosis can be narrowed and the appropriate diagnostic testing performed (Table 50–1; see Chapter 48).

CLINICAL HISTORY

The history should identify the most likely diagnostic category. A history of high fevers suggests an inflammatory or infectious etiology. Malignancy or a granulomatous process should be considered when fever is accompanied by constitutional symptoms such as night sweats and weight loss. In general, slowly enlarging lesions are more likely benign. Masses that are painless and that enlarge very rapidly suggest malignancy, while masses associated with infections are sometimes quite painful. Presence of the mass since birth, a prior lesion in a similar position, or a finding of chronic drainage from the region indicates congenital cysts or clefts.

Recent upper respiratory illnesses (otitis, pharyngitis) should be noted as well as any recent trauma or other infection in the head and neck region. A dental history can be particularly revealing because toothaches, bleeding gums, prior dental problems, and mouth trauma, with resultant odontogenic abscesses, are often associated with cervical lymphadenopathy. Information must be sought regarding all relevant exposures to illness, including tuberculosis contacts and travel history. The patient and family should be queried about pertinent risk factors for human immunodeficiency virus (HIV) such as intravenous drug abuse, high-risk sexual activity, and previous transfusions. Contact with cats, which serve as vectors for both cat-scratch disease and toxoplasmosis, should be identified. A history of pica could also be linked with toxoplasmosis.

A detailed review of systems can be extremely helpful. Symptoms such as palpitations, heat intolerance, or weight loss should be noted, since hyperthyroidism can result not only in midline goiter but in lymphadenopathy as well (Table 50–2). Similarly, manifestations of hypothyroidism should be noted (Table 50–3). The age-related causes of hypothyroidism are noted in Table 50–4.

Also important to consider is a history of symptoms associated with connective tissue disease (rashes, joint pain and stiffness). Symptoms indicating extrinsic compression of the trachea, esophagus, or recurrent laryngeal nerve (vocal cord paralysis) must be identified, as progression of the mass could result in life-threatening

---

Table 50–1. Differential Diagnosis of Childhood Neck Masses

Congenital Lesions	Systemic Disorders
Branchial cleft cyst	Kawasaki disease
Thyroglossal duct cyst	Sarcoidosis
Cystic hygroma	Immunodeficiency
Hemangioma	Juvenile rheumatoid arthritis
Congenital muscular torticollis	Systemic lupus erythematosus
Laryngocele	Hyperthyroidism
Dermoid or teratoma	*Medications*
Acquired Lesions	Phenytoin
Infections	Isoniazid
	Allopurinol
Viral and bacterial reactive adenitis	Hydralazine
Acute suppurative lymphadenitis	*Neoplasms*
Atypical mycobacterial infection	
Tuberculosis	Hodgkin and non-Hodgkin lymphoma
Cat-scratch disease	Leukemia
HIV	Rhabdomyosarcoma
Sialadenitis	Thyroid tumors
Toxoplasmosis	Neuroblastoma
Abscess secondary to mastoiditis	Nasopharyngeal carcinoma

Table 50–2. **Clinical Manifestations of Hyperthyroidism**

Increased catecholamine effects	Nervousness Palpitations Tachycardia Atrial arrhythmias Systolic hypertension (wide pulse pressure) Tremor Brisk reflexes Hyperdynamic precordium
Hypermetabolism	Increased sweating Shiny, warm, smooth skin Heat intolerance Fatigue Weight loss—increased appetite Increased bowel movement (hyperdefecation)
Myopathy	Weakness Periodic paralysis Cardiac failure—dyspnea
Miscellaneous	Proptosis, stare, exophthalmos, lid lag Hair loss Inability to concentrate Personality change (emotional lability) Goiter Thyroid bruit Onycholysis Acute thyroid storm (hyperpyrexia, tachycardia, coma, high-output heart failure, shock)

From Styne DM, Sperling MA, Chernausek SP. Endocrine disorders. *In* Behrman RE, Kliegman RM (eds). Nelson Essentials of Pediatrics, 2nd ed. Philadephia: WB Saunders, 1994:632.

Table 50–3. **Symptoms and Signs of Hypothyroidism***

Ectodermal	Poor growth Dull facies—thick pale lips, large tongue, depressed nasal bridge, periorbital edema Dry scaly skin Sparse brittle hair Diminished sweating Carotenemia Vitiligo
Circulatory	Sinus bradycardia/heart block Cold extremities Cold intolerance Pallor ECG changes—low-voltage QRS complex
Neuromuscular	Muscle weakness Hypotonia—constipation, potbelly Myxedema coma (CO_2 narcosis, hypothermia) Pseudohypertrophy of muscles Myalgia Physical and mental lethargy Delayed relaxation of reflexes Paresthesia (nerve entrapment: carpal tunnel syndrome) Umbilical hernia Hearing loss Cerebellar ataxia
Metabolic	Myxedema (tongue, face, extremities) Serous effusions (pleural, pericardial, ascites) Hoarse voice (cry) Weight gain (in adolescent) Menstrual irregularity Arthralgia Elevated CPK Macrocytosis (anemia)

From Styne DM, Sperling MA, Chernausek SP. Endocrine disorders. *In* Behrman RE, Kliegman RM (eds). Nelson Essentials of Pediatrics, 2nd ed. Philadephia: WB Saunders, 1994:631.

*Other features in infants and children: delayed bone maturation; long bone growth delay and epiphyseal dysgenesis; delayed dentition; elevated cholesterol; elevated prolactin; and, occasionally, ''precocious puberty.''

Abbreviations: CPK = creatine phosphokinase; ECG = electrocardiogram.

Table 50–4. Causes of Hypothyroidism in Infancy and Childhood

Age	Manifestation	Cause
Newborn	No goiter	Thyroid gland dysgenesis,* panhypopituitarism, TSH deficiency, TSH unresponsiveness
	Goiter	Inborn defect in hormone synthesis (iodine trapping defect, iodine organification defect [peroxidase deficiency—Pendred syndrome], iodotyrosine deiodination defect, thyroglobulin synthesis defect)
		Maternal goitrogens, including propylthiouracil, methimazole, iodides, amiodarone, radioiodine
		Severe iodide deficiency (endemic)
1–10 yr	No goiter	Thyroid gland dysgenesis, TSH deficiency, TSH unresponsiveness
		Cystinosis
		Hypothalamic-pituitary insufficiency
	Goiter	Inborn defect in hormone synthesis or effect
		Hashimoto thyroiditis: chronic lymphocytic thyroiditis*
		Goitrogenic drugs
		Endemic cretinism (iodine deficiency)
10–18 yr	No goiter	Hypothalamic-pituitary disorders (neoplasms, eosinophilic granuloma, other granulomatous processes, therapeutic CNS irradiation, idiopathic)
	Goiter	Hashimoto thyroiditis*
		Inborn defect in hormone synthesis or effect
		Goitrogenic drugs (lithium, amiodarone, foods)
		Surgical after thyrotoxicosis or thyroglossal duct cysts

*Most common for age group indicated.
Abbreviations: CNS = central nervous system; TSH = thyroid-stimulating hormone.

airway compromise. In addition to pain, such symptoms might include dyspnea, orthopnea, dysphagia, or stridor.

Other serious conditions associated with neck masses include the various types of immunodeficiency syndromes. It is important to obtain a history of recurrent infections (thrush, sinopulmonary infections, cellulitis, recurrent cutaneous abscesses). Although not found only in patients with immunodeficiencies or autoimmune disorders, a mass that becomes more painful with eating (and with associated dry mouth [xerostomia]) could represent infection of a salivary gland.

ANATOMIC CONSIDERATIONS

The precise location of the neck mass is crucial to making the correct diagnosis. The neck is commonly divided into two anatomic triangles, anterior and posterior (Fig. 50–1). The mandible forms the superior border of the anterior triangle, which extends along the sternocleidomastoid muscle to the anterior midline. The posterior border of the sternocleidomastoid, the distal two thirds of the

clavicle, and the midline posteriorly form the boundaries of the posterior triangle. Certain lesions are much more likely to occur in specific regions of the neck. Some normal structures of the neck can be confused with a pathologic mass. These include the angle of the mandible, the mastoid tip, the styloid process, the transverse processes of C-2 and C-6, and the greater cornu of the thyroid.

CONGENITAL MASSES

A congenital lesion should be suspected if a mass has been present since birth, if an area of chronic drainage is present, or in those in whom recurrent episodes of swelling occur in the same location. Initially, the presentation of congenital lesions is difficult to differentiate from infectious lymphadenitis. Congenital masses are often difficult to palpate and remain undetected until becoming acutely infected. Identifying these lesions is crucial, since surgical excision is usually required. Because most of these congenital lesions result from failure of embryologic structures to completely regress (and thus have very characteristic locations), anatomic con-

Figure 50–1. Triangles of the neck. (From Richardson MA. The neck: Embryology and anatomy. *In* Bluestone CD, Stool SE [eds]. Pediatric Otolaryngology, 2nd ed. Vol 2. Philadelphia: WB Saunders, 1990:1273.)

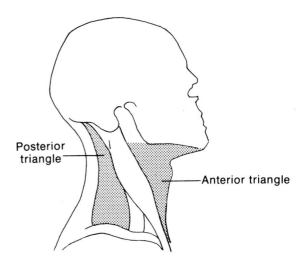

Table 50–5. Diagnosis of Congenital Neck Masses by Location and Physical Findings

Diagnosis	Location	Physical Findings
Thyroglossal duct cyst	Anterior midline	Retracts with tongue protrusion; may be inflamed
Branchial cleft cyst	1st—Mandibular angle or postauricular 2nd—Anterior border of sternocleidomastoid	± Fistula; may be inflamed
Hemangioma	Any location	Red or bluish hue; soft and spongy; increases with Valsalva maneuver; does not transilluminate
Cystic hygroma	Posterior neck; submental; submandibular	Soft and spongy; transilluminates; increases with Valsalva maneuver
Congenital torticollis	Belly of sternocleidomastoid	Firm, solid; head tilts toward mass; head rotated away from mass
Laryngocele	Area of thyrohyoid membrane; midline or just lateral	Compressible; transilluminates; hoarseness; increases with Valsalva maneuver; air-fluid level on radiograph
Dermoid	Midline	Doughy, smooth; nontender; does not transilluminate
Teratoma	Lateral	Doughy, irregular; calcifications on radiograph

siderations are of particular importance in securing the diagnosis (Table 50–5).

Thyroglossal Duct Cysts

The thyroglossal duct cyst is the most common neck mass of embryologic origin, arising from remnants of the thyroglossal tract. The fetal thyroid descends as a hollow tract originating from the foramen cecum at the base of the tongue and extending to the final position of the thyroid gland in the anterior neck (Fig. 50–2). Failure of the thyroglossal tract to atrophy can result in cyst formation anywhere along the course of descent. The majority of cysts are found near or below the level of the hyoid bone, either in the midline or slightly off center.

A thyroglossal duct cyst is usually a painless, asymptomatic mass and most typically exhibits a bimodal presentation from the ages of 2 to 3 years and mid adolescence. Because the tract originates at the tongue base, protrusion of the tongue may cause the cyst to move upward. Although this is a helpful physical finding if seen, its absence is not a reliable assurance against the diagnosis. The initial presentation of the thyroglossal duct cyst may be with acute inflammation, often associated with upper respiratory tract infection. Because these cysts often have associated lymphoid tissue, infection with a variety of bacterial pathogens, including oral anaerobes, is common. Although these lesions are not known to form congenital fistulas, recurrent inflammation can result in a draining sinus.

Diagnosis of the thyroglossal duct cyst is usually accomplished with reasonable certainty by its characteristic findings on physical examination (Fig. 50–3). Prior to surgical intervention, a thyroid scan should be considered to rule out ectopic thyroid gland, especially if a normal thyroid is not easily palpated in the usual position. Ultrasound has been used to differentiate cystic from solid lesions. If the cyst contains the only active thyroid tissue, surgical removal will leave the patient hypothyroid with the need for lifelong thyroid hormone replacement.

Management of the thyroglossal duct cyst requires complete surgical excision, including a core of tissue from the base of the tongue and the central portion of the hyoid bone as well as the cyst itself (Sistrunk procedure). Less extensive resection often results in recurrence. When infection is present, a course of systemic antibiotics should be given prior to resection.

Branchial Cleft Anomalies

The four major branchial arches first appear during the fourth to fifth weeks of fetal development (Fig. 50–4). The arches consist of mesoderm and are separated from one another externally by ectodermal clefts or grooves and internally by endodermal pouches. This system gives rise to most of the paired structures of the head and neck. Branchial anomalies are laterally located and may appear as cysts, sinuses, or fistulas. They result from failure of these fetal

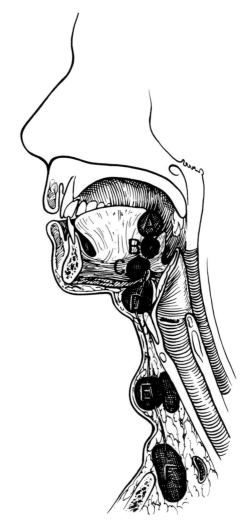

Figure 50–2. Thyroglossal duct cysts. These cysts can be located anywhere from the base of the tongue to behind the sternum. A and B: Lingual (rare). C and D: Adjacent to hyoid bone (common). E and F: Suprasternal fossa (rare). (From Welch K, et al. Pediatric Surgery. Chicago: Year Book Medical Publishers, 1986:549.)

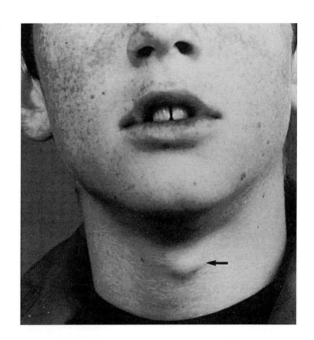

Figure 50–3. Thyroglosssal duct cyst *(arrow)* located in the midline of the neck. (From Lusk RP. Neck masses. *In* Bluestone CD, Stool SE [eds]. Pediatric Otolaryngology, 2nd ed. Vol 2. Philadelphia: WB Saunders, 1990:1298.)

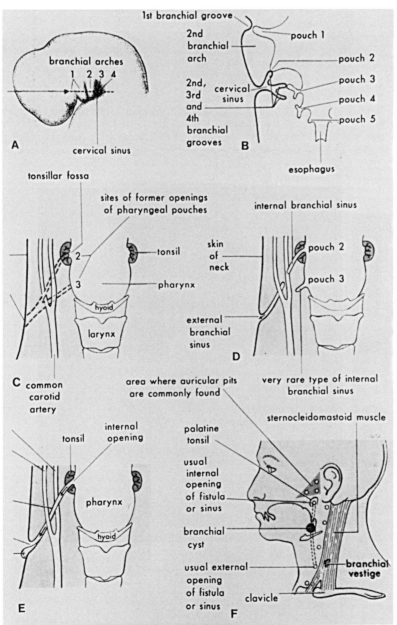

Figure 50–4. *A,* The head and neck region of a 5-week embryo. *B,* Horizontal section through the embryo illustrating the relationship of the cervical sinus to the branchial arches and pharyngeal pouches. *C,* The adult neck region indicating the former sites of openings of the cervical sinus and the pharyngeal pouches. The broken lines indicate possible courses of branchial fistulas. *D,* The embryologic basis of various types of branchial sinuses. *E,* A branchial fistula resulting from persistence of parts of the second branchial cleft and the second pharyngeal pouch. *F,* Possible sites of branchial cysts and openings of branchial sinuses and fistulas. A branchial vestige is also illustrated. (From Moore KL. The Developing Human: Clinically Oriented Embryology. Philadelphia: WB Saunders, 1977.)

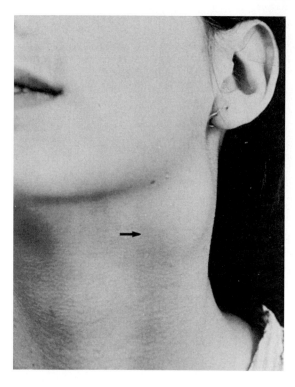

Figure 50–5. Branchial cleft cyst *(arrow)* along the anterior border of the sternomastoid muscle. (From Lusk RP. Neck masses. *In* Bluestone CD, Stool SE [eds]. Pediatric Otolaryngology, 2nd ed. Vol 2. Philadelphia: WB Saunders, 1990:1298.)

structures to regress as the mature organs are formed. Sinuses, which may drain either internally or externally, are thought to represent residual clefts or pouches, while a cyst represents a trapped residual of a cleft or pouch. Fistulas occur when residual clefts and pouches communicate, forming a tract with both internal and external openings.

Although developmental anomalies can arise from any of the first four branchial structures, more than 90% are associated with

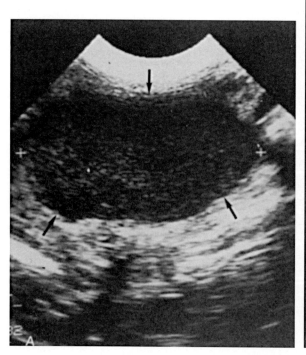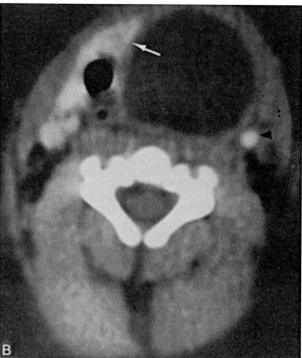

Figure 50–6. *A,* The longitudinal coronal sonogram of a 2-week-old boy with a nontender left neck mass *(arrows)* that is uniformly hypoechoic with good through transmission. *B,* The CT scan reveals low attenuation of the mass anteromedial to the carotid *(arrowhead)* sheath. The trachea and the esophagus are displaced to the right. The epicenter of this branchial cleft cyst is inferior to the left lobe of the thyroid gland *(arrow),* which is elevated and displaced to the right. (From Lima JA, Graviss ER. Methods of examination. *In* Bluestone CD, Stool SE [eds]. Pediatric Otolaryngology, 2nd ed. Vol 2. Philadelphia: WB Saunders, 1990:1290.)

the second branchial arch. Approximately 8% of branchial abnormalities affect the first arch, while anomalies of the third and fourth branchial structures are rare. Tracts or sinuses draining to the outside are usually quite apparent and therefore most frequently present during the first decade of life. Cysts often remain undiagnosed into the second decade unless a supervening acute infection within the cyst brings it to medical attention.

Cysts affecting the first branchial cleft (see Fig. 50–4) may occur either in close proximity to the external ear or in the anterior neck (always superior to the hyoid bone). If present, drainage from a sinus or fistula may be seen within the external ear canal or just behind the mandibular ramus.

The locations of cysts related to the second branchial clefts (Figs. 50–5 and 50–6) are typically noted along the anterior border of the sternocleidomastoid muscle below the level of the hyoid bone, with external sinuses draining in the same general region. A less common presentation is characterized by an internal sinus opening in the area of the tonsillar fossa.

In the absence of infection or visible external mucoid drainage, branchial cleft cysts typically show very slow enlargement and often are not discovered until early adulthood. Like thyroglossal duct cysts, occasionally branchial cleft cysts in children may show acute, painful enlargement and inflammation associated with upper respiratory tract infections. Sinuses and fistulas with external openings commonly become infected with bacterial organisms that colonize the skin, such as *Staphylococcus aureus* and group A streptococci. First branchial cleft anomalies, when infected, may present as chronic drainage from an ear without apparent middle ear disease. This situation might arise in either the presence or the absence of a mass in the neck. Rarely, recurrent abscess formation may occur from infection of an internally draining sinus. This type of infection would more likely be due to anaerobic organisms found in the oropharynx. Third and fourth branchial anomalies are more commonly associated with internal drainage and have also been associated with acute suppurative thyroiditis.

Complete excision of branchial cleft anomalies is required once adequate treatment of any acute infection or inflammation is completed. Unless absolutely necessary for control of infection, incision and drainage should be avoided, as this procedure may result in chronic fistula formation. A noninfected cyst or sinus in a very

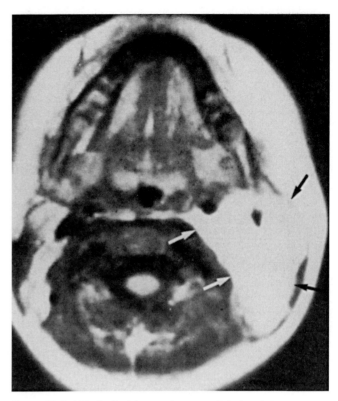

Figure 50–8. MRI clearly delineates the extent of the lymphangioma. Arrows mark the borders of the lymphangioma. (From Clary RA, Lusk RP. Neck masses. *In* Bluestone CD, Stool SE, Kenna MA [eds]. Pediatric Otolaryngology, 3rd ed. Vol 2. Philadelphia: WB Saunders, 1996:1494.)

young child may be followed conservatively for several years to permit growth, thus decreasing the risk of surgical damage to surrounding structures such as the facial nerve. In general, no radiologic procedures are required for diagnosis of these lesions, though the surgeon may request computed tomography (CT), magnetic resonance imaging (MRI), or fistulography to better delineate the anatomy.

Cystic Hygromas

Cystic hygromas (Figs. 50–7 and 50–8), otherwise known as lymphangiomas, are cystic masses consisting of dilated, anomalous lymphatic channels. Approximately 90% of these lesions are found in the posterior triangle of the neck. They have been found in many other areas, such as the submandibular or submental region, axilla, groin, or mediastinum. The majority are present at birth, rarely coming to attention later than the second year of life. These lesions are usually quite easy to identify on physical examination. They are soft, easily compressible, often diffuse, multiloculated cysts that are nontender and commonly transilluminate. They may increase in size with straining or crying.

Diagnosis assisted by ultrasound may be needed in the rare cases in which etiology of the mass remains unclear. Large lymphangiomas may cause serious airway compromise and feeding problems. The clinician should be alert for any stridor or other signs of respiratory difficulty. Mediastinal extension may occur with cervical lymphangiomas, especially those involving the lower neck. A chest radiograph should be considered to exclude this potentially life-threatening situation, even in the asymptomatic patient.

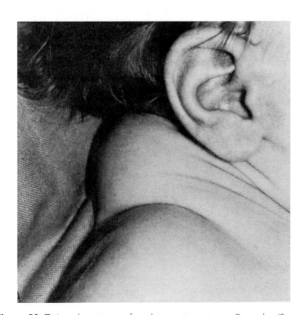

Figure 50–7. Lymphangioma of neck in patient at age 2 weeks. (From Clary RA, Lusk RP. Neck masses. *In* Bluestone CD, Stool SE, Kenna MA [eds]. Pediatric Otolaryngology, 3rd ed. Vol 2. Philadelphia: WB Saunders, 1996:1494.)

Cystic hygromas rarely undergo spontaneous regression. Most often, they show gradual increase in size with rapid enlargement associated with infection or hemorrhage into the cyst. Again, complete surgical excision is necessary to prevent recurrence, although this is sometimes quite difficult with very extensive lesions. Recurrence rates range from 5% to 15%, and multiple surgical resections are sometimes required. Early excision is advisable, before additional enlargement, infection, or hemorrhage complicates the situation.

Hemangiomas

Hemangiomas are congenital vascular anomalies that very commonly affect the head and neck region. They are usually present at birth, although they may initially be quite small. As the child grows in the first year of life, hemangiomas often enlarge, sometimes to massive proportions. Diagnosis is usually made on physical examination. Since hemangiomas are vascular lesions, they are similar in feel to cystic hygromas: soft, easily compressible, spongy masses. However, the hemangioma typically has a red or purplish hue and does not transilluminate. The hemangioma tends to enlarge with Valsalva maneuver (or crying in the infant) to an even greater degree than the cystic hygroma. A bruit may be heard, especially over very large lesions.

After the first year of life, the natural history of these lesions is spontaneous regression, usually by age 4 or 5 years. Thus, surgery is generally avoided except in cases in which enlarging lesions are impinging on vital structures or in those that fail to involute and cause severe cosmetic deformity. Large hemangiomas may result in the Kasabach-Merritt syndrome, characterized by thrombocytopenia, hemolytic anemia, and consumptive coagulopathy. This syndrome has a significant associated mortality, and urgent treatment is required. Hemangiomas have been treated successfully with steroids and interferon-α.

Congenital Muscular Torticollis

Progressive torticollis is generally noted within the first few weeks of life. On examination, a firm, fibrous, noninflamed area is palpable within the substance of the sternocleidomastoid muscle. Torticollis results in a head tilt in the direction of the mass with chin rotation in the opposite direction. It is thought to be caused by trauma or more likely abnormal positioning *in utero* with subsequent hematoma, fibrosis, or contracture formation within the muscle.

The parents can be taught to perform stretching exercises on the child at home, as this therapy is usually sufficient. In severe cases when exercise treatment fails, surgical correction is necessary. If prolonged, torticollis can result in significant deformity of the face and skull.

Dermoid Cysts and Teratomas

Dermoid cysts and teratomas are benign congenital neoplasms, most often found in the cervical region. Dermoids occur along lines of fusion of embryonic structures and are usually found in the midline. This location can make them difficult to differentiate from thyroglossal duct cysts. They tend to be nontender, smooth, and doughy or rubbery in texture. Differentiating between dermoids and thyroglossal duct cysts can be important, since the treatment of choice for dermoid cysts is simple excision of the cyst, while thyroglossal duct cysts require a much broader resection. Some authorities advocate interpretive aspiration of the cyst to differentiate, while others perform the more extensive operation when the diagnosis is in question.

Teratomas usually present early, either at birth or during the first year of life, and are commonly midline or paramedian masses. They tend to be firm and irregular, do not transilluminate, and may be quite large, resulting in airway compromise. Occasionally, they are associated with maternal polyhydramnios and can be detected on prenatal ultrasound. Radiologically, the teratoma may demonstrate calcifications. Imaging studies with CT or MRI are helpful in determining the extent of the lesion prior to surgical excision, which is the treatment of choice.

Laryngoceles

Laryngoceles are cystic dilatations of the laryngeal ventricle, the space located between the true and the false vocal cords. Externally, they present as soft, easily compressible masses just lateral to the midline in the region of the thyrohyoid membrane. Laryngoceles may enlarge with Valsalva maneuver, and they produce hoarseness and stridor if they extend internally. They are nontender unless infected (laryngopyocele), in which case the causative organism is usually one of the endogenous respiratory bacterial flora. An air-fluid level on radiograph may assist in the diagnosis. Laryngoceles, if symptomatic or infected, require surgical excision.

ACQUIRED NECK MASSES

Lymphadenopathy

Lymphadenopathy (see Chapter 48), with its wide range of etiologies, is by far the most common cause of cervical masses in children. When considering enlarged lymph nodes as a diagnostic possibility, one must have a thorough knowledge of the regional nodal anatomy (see Fig. 48–2) as well as an appreciation for the findings that fall outside the realm of normal variation. The majority of children over the age of 2 years have palpable cervical lymph nodes, and up to 30% of normal neonates may have a palpable node. These nodes are generally small (<1 cm in diameter) and nontender. Most lymph nodes are present without any associated signs or symptoms. In examining the neck, the examiner should carefully note the location of the involved nodes, their relation to surrounding nodes and structures, their consistency, size, shape, and mobility, as well as the presence or absence of overlying discoloration, warmth, or suppuration.

NONSUPPURATIVE LYMPHADENOPATHY

The most frequent, and also the most benign, cause of childhood cervical adenopathy is the viral upper respiratory tract infection. Associated nodes tend to be small and shotty, bilateral, minimally tender, soft, and nonsuppurative. Although their appearance tends to parallel that of the infection, these nodes may often persist for some time or recur in children with frequent upper respiratory tract illnesses. The clinician should become familiar enough with this type of lymphadenopathy to convincingly reassure the worried family.

Certain specific viral infections are well known to cause significant lymphadenopathy. Among these is the Epstein-Barr virus (EBV), which typically presents with culture-negative exudative pharyngitis, fatigue, fever, malaise, and often splenomegaly in addition to adenopathy. Lymph nodes are typically quite large, bilateral, and distributed throughout the anterior and posterior regions of the neck. The character of these nodes (matted or large size) may raise concern for lymphoma; however, the overall clinical picture, with lethargy, splenomegaly, and pharyngitis, usually leads to the correct diagnosis (see Chapter 48).

OTHER CAUSES OF LYMPHADENOPATHY

See Chapter 48.

ACUTE SUPPURATIVE LYMPHADENITIS

Recognizing an acute bacterial lymphadenitis is generally not difficult, as the presentation tends to be quite dramatic. A patient with fever and a swollen, tender, warm, and erythematous mass in the neck is most likely suffering a bacterial infection. These lesions are usually unilateral and involve only one or a few nodes. Submandibular and anterior cervical nodes are most commonly involved. An elevated white blood cell count and erythrocyte sedimentation rate are usually present. By far the predominant causative organisms are *S. aureus* and group A streptococci; initial antibiotic therapy should be selected accordingly. In neonates, group B streptococcus is another potential pathogen (see Chapter 48).

SALIVARY GLAND INFLAMMATION

Salivary gland inflammation, a clinical rarity in children, can easily be confused with lymphadenitis. Although there are many causes, most are uncommon in children. The parotid glands are most commonly involved (enlargement obscuring the angle of the jaw), although enlargement of the submandibular or minor glands also occurs. Mumps is a classic cause of parotid inflammation. Salivary gland enlargement may be seen in patients with HIV infection, collagen-vascular disease, lymphoma, anorexia nervosa (emesis induced), acute asthma, cystic fibrosis, recurrent parotitis, and acute infection of the gland.

Suppurative parotitis is usually due to *S. aureus* and may be heralded by the presence of purulent drainage from the Stensen duct. HIV infection should be suspected in a young patient with bilateral parotid enlargement, especially when it is associated with lymphadenopathy. Blockage of a duct by a stone (often associated with anticholinergic-antihistamine type drugs) or a congenital stenosis may also lead to enlargement. An entity known as recurrent idiopathic parotitis typically presents in episodic fashion, with each bout characteristically lasting 2 to 3 weeks. Usually, there is spontaneous resolution of the symptoms, but recurrences are common. An increase in pain with eating coupled with an elevated serum amylase is strongly suggestive of salivary gland inflammation.

SUBACUTE AND CHRONIC INFLAMMATION

Subacutely inflamed lymph nodes may enlarge slowly over days or weeks, are minimally tender, and are seldom associated with systemic symptoms. The most common causes of this so-called "cold" inflammation are atypical mycobacterial infection and cat-scratch disease. Tuberculosis must always be considered (see Chapter 48).

Lymphadenitis secondary to atypical mycobacteria is typically caused by *Mycobacterium avium-intracellulare, M. scrofulaceum,* and *M. kansasii.* These are acid-fast bacilli commonly found in soil, dust, water, and foods including eggs, milk, and vegetables. Transmission between humans is not known to occur. Children infected with these organisms usually experience a superficial lymphadenitis without any associated systemic illness. Typically, these infections involve nodes in a unilateral pattern in the upper neck: submandibular, preauricular, or anterior cervical nodes. The nodes are usually firm, rubbery, nontender, and without warmth. Characteristically with time, the overlying skin becomes thickened and discolored and may eventually break down, resulting in chronic drainage of the lesion to the surface. Spontaneous resolution may occur over several months or years.

Cat-Scratch Disease

To diagnose cat-scratch disease, a careful, specific history must be taken. The disease occurs most frequently in the fall and winter months. The majority of patients report having had close contact, usually a scratch, with a cat several days to a few weeks prior to illness. Often a single erythematous, painless, and nonpruritic papule is noted at the site of the scratch, which may form a pustule prior to healing. After this, the lymph node or nodes that drain the affected area typically become swollen and tender. Suppuration may occur together with associated fever and malaise, although the majority of patients are otherwise asymptomatic. The natural history of this illness is one of gradual resolution of the lymphadenitis over several weeks to months. Many unusual manifestations have been reported, including the oculoglandular syndrome of Parinaud (conjunctivitis associated with preauricular adenopathy), encephalopathy, and erythema nodosum.

Often because of the protracted nature of the nodal involvement, biopsies are performed to rule out more serious pathology. Needle aspiration may also prove to be diagnostic in cases in which suppuration is seen (see Chapter 48).

SYSTEMIC DISORDERS (See Chapter 48)

Neoplasms

For the child with a neck mass, the primary concern is the possibility of malignancy. Although most children presenting with neck masses do not have malignant neoplasms, it is critical that the clinician be alert to those signs and symptoms that should initiate a prompt and thorough evaluation (Table 50–6).

Approximately 25% of pediatric cancers involve the head and neck. Most malignant tumors found in the head and neck of

Table 50–6. "Red Flags": Signs and Symptoms Suspicious for Malignancy or Decompensation

Supraclavicular adenopathy
Adenopathy in posterior triangle without evidence of scalp inflammation
Nodes fixed to underlying tissue
Size > 3 cm
Matting of nodes into single indistinct mass
Slow, steadily progressive painless enlargement
Signs of airway obstruction
Constitutional symptoms in association with above:
    Fever
    Weight loss
    Night sweats

children are lymphomas, both Hodgkin and non-Hodgkin, and soft tissue sarcomas such as rhabdomyosarcoma. Rarer neoplasms in the head and neck region include thyroid carcinoma, neuroblastoma, and salivary gland tumors. Leukemias often present with generalized lymphadenopathy, which also involves the cervical region.

In general, any patient with supraclavicular adenopathy must be considered to have a malignancy until excisional biopsy proves otherwise. Symptoms such as persistent fevers, weight loss, and night sweats raise the suspicion of malignancy or another systemic disorder. Unless a specific cause can be identified based on signs, symptoms, and initial laboratory evaluation, excisional biopsy should be strongly considered. Entirely nontender, enlarged nodes are not inflammatory. Nodes that are firm, greater than 3 cm in size, matted together into an indistinct mass, or fixed to underlying tissue are particularly ominous, although this description can sometimes apply to cat-scratch disease and atypical mycobacterial infections.

Laboratory studies in patients, if there is suspicion of malignancy, should include a complete blood count with differential and examination of the peripheral blood smear. Signs of anemia, thrombocytopenia, white blood cell immaturity, or other abnormalities can be associated with both malignancy and inflammatory processes. Blood chemistries, with particular attention to the lactate dehydrogenase, alkaline phosphatase, and uric acid levels should be performed, as these values are often elevated in the presence of malignancy with a large tumor burden.

In children who present without a clear focus of inflammation, the underlying etiology of the adenopathy should be sought expeditiously. These patients should be evaluated with a chest radiograph to rule out mediastinal adenopathy, a finding very suspicious for lymphoma. Children with enlarged lymph nodes in the supraclavicular and lower neck regions are the most likely to also have abnormalities in the mediastinum.

Any node thought to be representative of an infectious or inflammatory condition that is not responsive to treatment or following the expected pattern of resolution should be considered for biopsy. All such nodes should be closely followed with serial measurements. Although there are no standard guidelines, a patient on antibiotic therapy whose node continues to increase in size over the first 2 weeks of follow-up or has not begun to shrink within 4 to 6 weeks deserves further investigation.

HODGKIN DISEASE

Hodgkin disease is rare in children younger than age 5; its incidence gradually rises through the teenage years, finally peaking in young adulthood. Patients usually present with painless enlargement of supraclavicular or cervical nodes, or both. These nodes are generally firm or rubbery. They can be slightly tender, which may make them more difficult to separate from inflammatory nodes. There is often associated mediastinal adenopathy, and a chest radiograph should be obtained whenever Hodgkin disease is suspected. The chest radiograph serves both to aid in diagnosis and to assess patency of the airway. Either anemia of chronic disease or a hemolytic anemia may occur. Patients are often anergic. Approximately 30% have associated systemic symptoms such as fevers, night sweats, and weight loss. These so-called ''B'' symptoms have prognostic significance.

Diagnosis is usually made through biopsy of an involved node, at which point a complete diagnostic work-up for staging purposes should begin. Survival for patients with Hodgkin disease has improved dramatically over the past two decades. Treatment depends on the age of patient and stage of the disease; radiotherapy and chemotherapy are the mainstays of current therapy.

NON-HODGKIN LYMPHOMA

Non-Hodgkin lymphoma (NHL), of which there are three main variants in children, occurs more commonly in younger children than does Hodgkin disease. NHL, particularly lymphoblastic lymphoma, may also present with cervical adenopathy. The nodes are usually firm and painless, sometimes noted in the supraclavicular region. However, children with NHL usually have other associated findings, the most common of which is the presence of a mediastinal mass. These tumors can grow extremely rapidly, making early diagnosis important. Patients with a mediastinal mass may quickly experience superior vena cava syndrome or life-threatening airway obstruction. Patients may also have bone marrow or meningeal involvement.

Diagnosis of NHL is usually made by biopsy of an involved node or mass, after which a staging work-up is done. Chemotherapy alone is the treatment of choice, as the role of radiation therapy in NHL has become relegated to emergencies occurring at the time of diagnosis.

These patients require close monitoring at initiation of therapy, as tumor lysis syndrome usually occurs. Tumor lysis syndrome may result in renal failure (uric acid nephropathy) and severe metabolic derangements (hypocalcemia, hyperphosphatemia, hyperkalemia).

LEUKEMIAS

Leukemias are the most common of all childhood malignancies. In children with leukemia, 80% of cases are acute lymphocytic leukemia. The majority of the remaining cases are acute nonlymphoblastic leukemia. Chronic leukemias are very rare in childhood.

Although children with leukemia often have diffuse lymphadenopathy at the time of diagnosis, there are almost always other ominous signs, symptoms, or laboratory values. Common relevant symptoms usually include weakness, bone pain, fever, and weight loss. Examination may reveal excess bruising or petechiae, pallor, and splenomegaly. The hemogram often demonstrates anemia and thrombocytopenia. The white blood cell count may be either high or low, frequently with circulating blast cells.

The diagnosis is made by bone marrow examination. A chest radiograph and spinal tap should be performed on all patients to diagnose the presence of mediastinal mass and central nervous system involvement, respectively. Although leukemia must be included in the differential diagnosis of cervical lymphadenopathy, there generally are other findings that, if sought, make the diagnosis more obvious.

RHABDOMYOSARCOMA

Rhabdomyosarcoma is the most common soft tissue sarcoma of childhood. Within the head and neck, these lesions originate in the nasopharynx (chronic sinusitis, nasal discharge), ear, or orbit (proptosis) and may present with serosanguinous drainage from the nose or ear refractory to medical therapy. Typically, it is associated with painless enlargement of cervical nodes. Therefore, a thorough examination of the nasopharynx is warranted in patients with cervical adenopathy. Median age at diagnosis is approximately 6 years.

Rhabdomyosarcoma is a very aggressive tumor, and treatment involves a combination of modalities, including surgery, chemotherapy, and radiation. Because total excision is an extremely important factor in determining prognosis, early diagnosis is very important.

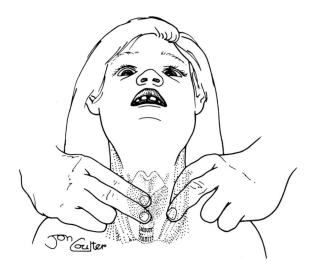

Figure 50–9. Palpation of the thyroid gland. The examiner stands behind the patient. A slight retraction of the sternocleidomastoid muscle away from the midline with one hand permits the other hand to outline the surface of the lobe. (From Lima JA, Graviss ER. Methods of examination. *In* Bluestone CD, Stool SE [eds]. Pediatric Otolaryngology, 2nd ed. Vol 2. Philadelphia: WB Saunders, 1990:1284.)

THYROID MASS

Masses discovered in the thyroid area in children should be considered malignant until proven otherwise, since a solitary thyroid nodule has approximately a 19% to 24% chance of being malignant. A history of therapeutic irradiation to the head or neck is an important risk factor for thyroid carcinoma. A rapidly growing, hard, solitary nodule that is nontender and associated with regional adenopathy is highly suggestive of malignant disease. Tenderness (diffuse) in the thyroid area is more suggestive of an inflammatory enlargement, such as that due to Hashimoto thyroiditis or hyperthyroidism (Graves disease). Examination of the thyroid gland is shown in Figure 50–9.

Thyroid function tests should be obtained in all patients with thyroid nodules or enlargement (Table 50–7). Thyroid radionuclotide scan should be performed in these patients, both to determine if the nodule is functional or nonfunctional ("hot" or "cold") and to look for any anomalies of the gland that could account for palpable enlargement. Although all nodules must be removed, patients with "hot" nodules (on nuclear medicine thyroid scans) may require treatment with antithyroid drugs prior to surgery to prevent thyroid storm. These nodules are also less likely to be malignant. High titers of circulating antithyroid antibodies suggest the presence of chronic lymphocytic thyroiditis.

Ultrasound may be used to differentiate cystic from solid nodules. However, thyroid malignancies can occasionally have a cystic component. Histologic examination must be done to make etiologic determination, which may be done using fine needle aspiration or open biopsy.

PAROTID GLAND ENLARGEMENT

Although parotid gland enlargement in children is usually due to inflammatory causes, neoplasms may occur. Most of these are benign, such as hemangiomas, hamartomas, or pleomorphic adenomas. However, malignancies do occur, of which mucoepidermoid carcinoma is the most common, with rhabdomyosarcoma only rarely reported. A solid, nontender, firm mass that continues to increase in size over several weeks to months should be sampled for biopsy by fine needle aspiration or excised.

OTHER MALIGNANCIES

Other malignancies that may involve the neck region include neuroblastoma and nasopharyngeal carcinoma. In the neck, neuroblastoma may be metastatic or primary and should be suspected in patients presenting with Horner syndrome, iris heterochromia (lesion on the side of the blue iris), and a cervical mass. Although neuroblastoma is a common childhood malignancy, its presentation is rarely isolated to the cervical area. Children presenting with neuroblastoma of the head and neck region often have the "raccoon eyes" resulting from orbital tumors.

DIAGNOSTIC APPROACH

The clinician should first try to establish the most likely broad diagnostic category by history and physical examination. Only when a diagnosis is suspected should the clinician attempt to narrow the differential by using the appropriate diagnostic testing. It is particularly important to decide which patients can be observed or managed medically by the primary care physician and which should be referred to a hematologist/oncologist, otolaryngologist, or pediatric surgeon. The physical examination is often the most valuable diagnostic tool.

A general approach to the patient with a neck mass is presented in the form of a decision tree in Figure 50–10. First, one must decide if the history and physical findings are suggestive of a congenital lesion. If so, after initiating treatment of any associated infection, the patient should be immediately referred to a surgical specialist for appropriate surgical management.

If the lesion is not congenital, the next step should be to deter-

Table 50–7. Laboratory Test Results in Various Types of Thyroid Function Abnormalities in Children

	Serum Total T$_4$	Free T$_4$	Serum TSH	Serum T$_3$ Resin Uptake	Serum TBG
Primary hypothyroidism	↓	↓	↑	↓	N
Hypothalamic (TRH) hypothyroidism	↓	↓	N	↓	N
Pituitary (TSH) hypothyroidism	↓	↓	N	↓	N
TBG deficiency	↓	N	N	↑	↓
TBG excess	↑	N	N	↓	↑

From Endocrine disorders. *In* Behrman RE, Kliegman RM (eds). Nelson Essentials of Pediatrics, 2nd ed. Philadelphia: WB Saunders, 1994:629.
Abbreviations: T$_3$ = triiodothyronine; T$_4$ = thyroxine; TBG = thyroxine-binding globulin; TRH = thyrotropin-releasing hormone; TSH = thyroid-stimulating hormone.
Key: ↓ = decreased; ↑ = increased; N = normal.

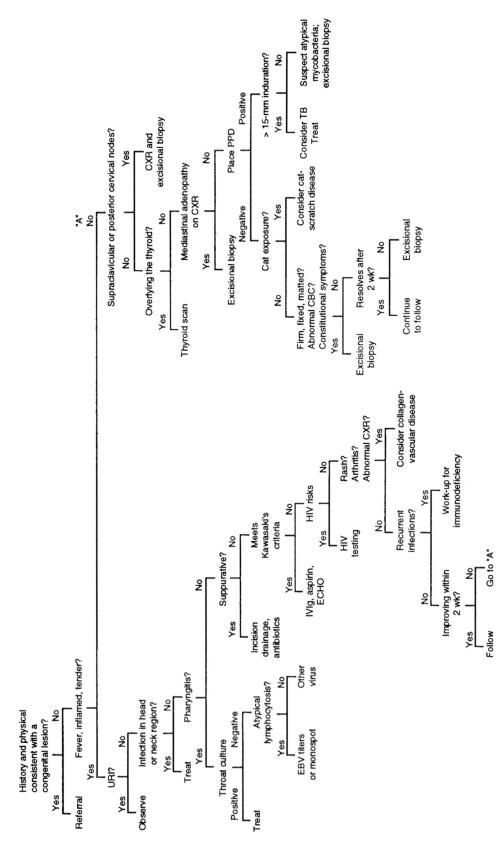

Figure 50-10. Diagnostic decision tree for childhood neck masses. CBC = complete blood count; CXR = chest x-ray; EBV = Epstein-Barr virus; ECHO = echocardiogram; HIV = human immunodeficiency virus; IVIg = intravenous immunoglobulin; PPD = purified protein derivative; TB = tuberculosis; URI = upper respiratory infection.

mine if the lesion appears inflamed or infected. If so, associated systemic infections (upper respiratory) or local infections (dental abscess, scalp lesion) should be sought. If pharyngitis is present, a throat culture should be considered to rule out group A streptococcal infection. If the culture result is negative and symptoms persist, the physician should consider a viral infection with EBV or cytomegalovirus (CMV), and appropriate serologic testing may be done. Toxoplasmosis or cat-scratch disease can be contemplated as well. A complete blood count with differential may be helpful at this point, since EBV is often associated with an atypical lymphocytosis.

If the inflamed lesion becomes fluctuant, referral should be made for incision and drainage both as a therapeutic maneuver and to provide material for culture and sensitivity testing. In any patient with a high fever or who appears toxic, a blood culture should be obtained.

The diagnosis of Kawasaki disease should be considered in any patient with an inflammatory node that does not suppurate and for which there is not an immediate explanation (see Chapter 48). If the patient fits the criteria for Kawasaki disease, intravenous immunoglobulin and salicylate therapy should be initiated promptly as well as consultation obtained with a pediatric cardiologist. In patients who do not fit these criteria, other systemic disorders should be considered. The patient and family should be questioned for HIV risk factors and tested if appropriate. Signs and symptoms of connective tissue disease should be sought and a chest radiograph obtained. If the patient is found to have a history remarkable for recurrent infections, further work-up for immunodeficiencies should be considered (see Chapter 52). If after all of these steps are taken the diagnosis remains unknown, the lesion may be followed expectantly for 2 to 3 weeks. If at follow-up regression of the mass has not occurred, further evaluation should be pursued as outlined below for the noninflamed mass.

If on examination the mass does not appear to be inflammatory and if it is located in the supraclavicular or posterior cervical region, a complete blood count should be performed and a chest radiograph obtained. Because of the high incidence of malignancy associated with these findings, an immediate referral should be made for incisional biopsy. If the lesion is overlying the thyroid and presentation is not consistent with thyroglossal duct cyst, thyroid function tests and thyroid scan should be performed and referral for fine needle aspiration or excisional biopsy should be made.

For lesions lying outside of these regions, a PPD should be part of the initial work-up. In patients who are skin test–positive with greater than 5 to 15 mm of induration (depending on risk group), tuberculosis is the most likely diagnosis (see Chapter 7). In patients with tuberculosis, associated lesions are frequently seen on chest radiograph. Treatment with INH and rifampin (or other appropriate agents, depending on the prevalence of drug resistance) should be initiated. If the patient is at low risk for tuberculosis and the skin test yields a ''positive'' reaction with less than 15 mm of induration, infection with atypical mycobacteria should be suspected. These cases should be referred for excisional biopsy and the material obtained for culture of acid-fast bacteria. If the patient is found to be anergic, immunodeficiencies and malignancies should be suspected.

If the PPD does not react, the diagnosis of cat-scratch disease may be entertained. Patients with a history of cat exposure and physical findings consistent with this diagnosis may be observed for a period of 2 to 3 weeks. If the nodes continue to enlarge, excisional biopsy with Warthin-Starry staining of the biopsy specimen is appropriate. In patients with noninflammatory nodes, especially with a history of cat exposure, toxoplasmosis should also be considered and titers may be sent.

In the patient whose clinical picture is not consistent with cat-scratch disease and whose diagnosis has not been established during the above evaluation, the possibility of malignancy must be

strongly considered. The clinician should consider several questions that indicate *red flags*:

Are the nodes firm, matted, or fixed to underlying tissue?
Are there associated constitutional symptoms?
Are there abnormalities on the complete blood count that would suggest malignancy or on the chest radiograph such as mediastinal adenopathy or mass?

If the answer is yes to any of these questions, immediate referral should be made for excisional biopsy. If not, the mass may again be followed with serial measurements for 2 to 3 more weeks. Masses that continue to increase in size should be sampled for biopsy. Those that do not regress over the next several weeks should also be sampled for biopsy.

By following the above approach, one can expeditiously arrive at the diagnosis for the majority of neck masses without using excessive invasive testing. Other masses will resolve within an acceptable period of observation, although the diagnosis may never be known. With increasing experience, the clinician will often be able to bypass many of these steps and suspect the correct diagnosis immediately by recognizing characteristic historical features and physical findings.

REFERENCES

General

Bamji M, Stone RK, Kaul A, et al. Palpable lymph nodes in healthy newborns and infants. Pediatrics 1986;78:573–652.

Barton LL, Feigin RD. Childhood cervical lymphadenitis: A reappraisal. J Pediatr 1974;84:842–852.

Burton DM, Pransky SM. Practical aspects of managing non-malignant lumps of the neck. J Otolaryngol 1992;21:398–403.

Carithers HA. Cat-scratch disease. Am J Dis Child 1985;139:1124–1133.

Cunningham MJ. The management of congenital neck masses. Am J Otolaryngol 1992;13:78–92.

Friedberg J. Pharyngeal cleft sinuses and cysts, and other benign neck lesions. Pediatr Clin North Am 1989;36:1451–1469.

Margileth AM. Management of nontuberculous (atypical) mycobacterial infections in children and adolescents. Pediatr Infect Dis J 1985;4:119–121.

Margileth AM. Antibiotic therapy for cat-scratch disease: Clinical study of therapeutic outcome in 268 patients and a review of the literature. Pediatr Infect Dis J 1992;11:474–478.

May M. Neck masses in children: Diagnosis and treatment. Ear Nose Throat J 1978;57:12–54.

Myers EN, Cunningham MJ. Inflammatory presentations of congenital head and neck masses. Pediatr Infect Dis J 1988;7:S162–168.

Pounds LA. Neck masses of congenital origin. Pediatr Clin North Am 1981;28:841–844.

Taha AM, Davidson PT, Bailey C. Surgical treatment of atypical mycobacterial lymphadenitis in children. Pediatr Infect Dis J 1985;4:664–667.

Telander RL, Filston HC. Review of head and neck lesions in infancy and childhood. Surg Clin North Am 1992;72:1429–1447.

Zitelli BJ. Evaluating the child with a neck mass. Contemp Pediatr 1990;7:90–112.

Nonthyroid Tumors

Bonilla JA, Healy GB. Management of malignant head and neck tumors in children. Pediatr Clin North Am 1989;36:1443–1450.

Ezekowitz RA, Mulliken JB, Folkman J. Interferon alfa-2a therapy for life-threatening hemangiomas of infancy. N Engl J Med 1992;326:1456–1463.

Knight PJ, Mulne AF, Vassy LE. When is lymph node biopsy indicated in children with enlarged peripheral nodes? Pediatrics 1982;69:391–396.

Raney RB Jr, Hays DM, Tefft M, et al. Rhabdomyosarcoma and the undifferentiated sarcomas. *In* Pizzo PA, Poplack DG (eds). Principles and Practice of Pediatric Oncology, 2nd ed. Philadelphia: JB Lippincott, 1993:769–794.

Silverman RA. Hemangiomas and vascular malformations. Pediatr Clin North Am 1991;38:811–834.

Ward RF, April M. Teratomas of the head and neck. Otolaryngol Clin North Am 1989;22:621–629.

Thyroid

Franklyn JA. The management of hyperthyroidism. N Engl J Med 1994; 330:1731–1738.

Garcia CJ, Daneman A, Thorner P, et al. Sonography of multinodular thyroid gland in children and adolescents. Am J Dis Child 1992;146:811–816.

Gharib H, Goellner JR. Fine-needle aspiration biopsy of the thyroid: An appraisal. Ann Intern Med 1993;118:282–289.

Hung W, Anderson KD, Chandra RS, et al. Solitary thyroid nodules in 71 children and adolescents. J Pediatr Surg 1992;27:1407–1409.

Jaksic J, Dumic M, Filipovic B, et al. Thyroid diseases in a school population with thyromegaly. Arch Dis Child 1994;70:103–106.

Mazzaferri EL. Management of a solitary thyroid nodule. N Engl J Med 1993;328:553–558.

Noyek AM, Friedberg J. Thyroglossal duct and ectopic thyroid disorders. Otolaryngol Clin North Am 1981;14:187–201.

Uderzo C, van Lint MT, Rovelli A, et al. Papillary thyroid carcinoma after total body irradiation. Arch Dis Child 1994;71:256–258.

Viswanathan K, Gierlowski TC, Schneider AB. Childhood thyroid cancer. Characteristics and long-term outcome in children irradiated for benign conditions of the head and neck. Arch Pediatr Adolesc Med 1994; 148:260–265.

51 Bleeding and Thrombosis

J. Paul Scott

Hemostasis is a process that maintains normal blood flow through healthy vessels but also permits rapid generation of a clot at sites of vascular injury. In addition to flow, the major components of the hemostatic mechanism are the platelets, the anticoagulant proteins, the procoagulant proteins, and various components of the vascular wall. Normal hemostasis is an interactive process in which each element cooperates closely and is capable of a rapid, cohesive, focused reaction. An abnormality of one element destabilizes the system, but significant clinical symptoms often manifest only when two components are affected. Typical examples include the hemophilia patient who sustains trauma and the antithrombin III–deficient patient who becomes pregnant with resultant compromise of vascular flow in the lower extremities. One has to be aware of situations that may exacerbate preexisting conditions. Conversely, pretreatment of known predisposing conditions can prevent complications, as exemplified by infusion of factor VIII concentrate prior to and after surgery to the patient with hemophilia A to achieve normal preoperative factor VIII levels and to prevent untoward bleeding.

Table 51–1 shows common bleeding symptoms: mucocutaneous bleeding, deep (internal)/surgical bleeding, and generalized bleeding and the most common disorders that trigger these symptoms.

THE COAGULATION CASCADE

Two opposing systems serve to generate local clots yet limit extension of thrombi only to areas of vascular damage. Figure 51–1 shows the sequence of activation of coagulation. The cascade is capable of rapid response, in that generation of a small number of activated factors at the "top" of the cascade leads to thousands of molecules of thrombin. Deficiencies of proteins at or below factors XI or VII result in clinical bleeding symptoms, whereas deficiencies of factor XII, prekallikrein, and high-molecular-weight kininogen do not. The coagulation mechanism is continuously generating a small amount of thrombin, probably via autocatalysis of factor VII to factor VIIa. If there is trauma, tissue factor and factor VII combine to activate factor X to Xa both directly and indirectly via factor IX. Factor Xa then forms a complex on a membrane surface (provided by the activated platelet) with factor V and calcium and results in more thrombin generation. The plate-

Table 51–1. Common Causes of Clinical Bleeding Symptoms

Mucocutaneous Bleeding
Acute
Immune thrombocytopenic purpura
Child abuse
Trauma
Chronic/insidious
von Willebrand disease
Platelet function defect
Marrow infiltration/aplasia
Deep/Surgical Bleeding
Hemophilia
Vitamin K deficiency
von Willebrand disease
Generalized Bleeding
Disseminated intravascular coagulation
Vitamin K deficiency
Liver disease
Uremia

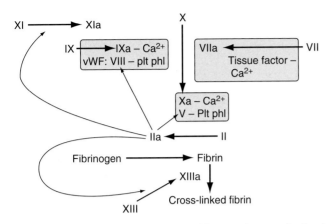

Figure 51–1. The coagulation cascade and the critical positive feedback role of factor IIa (thrombin) on multiple aspects of the coagulation cascade. In addition, thrombin aggregates platelets and thereby contributes to platelet plug formation. Enzymatic complexes that form on membranes are depicted in the shaded blocks. Plt phl = platelet phospholipid surface.

let surface accelerates thrombin generation and fibrin formation at sites of injury by localizing to areas of vascular damage.

Thrombin exerts a positive feedback on the system by:

1. Acting on factor XI to trigger the intrinsic system.
2. By cleaving factors V and VIII to activate them, thereby accelerating thrombin generation.
3. By aggregating platelets.

In this model, coagulation is always "turned on" and, therefore, is capable of a much more rapid response than if it were static and had to suddenly initiate a series of reactions to trigger clot formation. This dynamic concept underscores the impact of deficiencies of anticoagulant proteins, since the system is continuously generating thrombin. A deficiency of an inhibitory enzyme or a cofactor would accelerate ongoing thrombin generation.

COAGULATION INHIBITORS

Three key systems interact to inhibit the coagulation mechanism:

- Antithrombin III
- Protein C/S system
- Fibrinolytic system

Antithrombin III

Antithrombin III (ATIII) is a member of the serine protease inhibitor family (*Serpins*) that inhibits thrombin, factor Xa, and, less efficiently, factors IXa and XIa. Factors inhibited by ATIII are enclosed within a square in Figure 51–2. When ATIII is bound to heparin, this reaction is accelerated 1000-fold. ATIII is the active anticoagulant operative during heparin therapy, and if ATIII is deficient, heparin therapy often fails. Heparin-like molecules are synthesized by endothelial cells and interact with ATIII on the vessel wall to inhibit coagulation. Both congenital and acquired ATIII deficiencies are associated with a predisposition toward thrombosis.

Protein C/Protein S System

The protein C/protein S system is complex and limits clot extension by inactivating the rate-limiting coenzymes of the coagulation cascade, factors VIII and V. To prevent extension of the clot, the anticoagulant mechanism must limit thrombin formation to areas of vascular damage. This is accomplished by the protein C/protein S system.

As a first step, thrombin binds to the protein thrombomodulin on intact endothelial cells. Thrombomodulin-bound thrombin then converts protein C into its activated form, activated protein C (APC). APC then combines with protein S to inactivate factors VIII and V. In addition, APC may also promote fibrinolysis. In such a manner, thrombin itself is inactivated when bound to thrombomodulin and simultaneously augments the anticoagulant response by generating APC. APC limits the amount of thrombin that can be generated subsequently. The importance of deficiencies of ATIII, protein C, and protein S has been best defined by observations that congenital and acquired deficiencies of these proteins are associated with a predisposition toward thrombotic disease. The sites where protein C and protein S function within the coagulation cascade are circled in Figure 51–2. Resistance to APC because of a mutation in factor V (factor V Leiden) is a common cause of inherited tendency for spontaneous thrombosis.

The tissue factor pathway inhibitor (TFPI) is an inhibitor of factor VIIa. The role of TFPI as a physiologic inhibitor of coagulation is unclear at present (see Fig. 51–2).

Fibrinolytic System

The fibrinolytic system dissolves and removes clots from the vascular system so that normal flow through vessels can be restored. Endothelial cells synthesize two activators of plasminogen: tissue-type plasminogen activator (TPA) and urokinase (UK), both of which convert plasminogen to plasmin, the enzyme that degrades fibrin.

Normally, plasminogen activator and its inhibitor, plasminogen activator inhibitor (PAI), are synthesized in equimolar amounts and are released from endothelial cells in parallel, leading to minimal amounts of active fibrinolysis. Increased activation or damage to

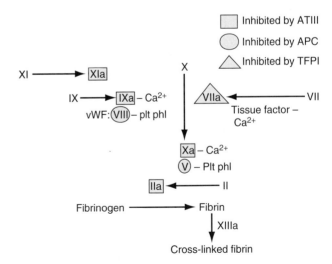

Figure 51–2. Physiologic anticoagulants. Sites of inhibition of coagulation by the anticoagulant proteins: antithrombin III (ATIII) *(squares)*, activated protein C (APC)/protein S *(circles)*, and the tissue factor pathway inhibitor (TFPI) *(triangles)*.

Blood Vessel

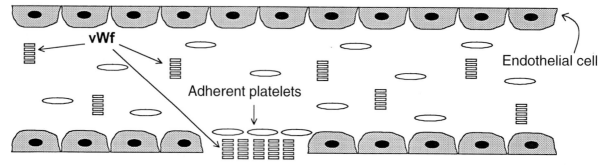

Adherence of platelets to damaged endothelium is vWf-dependent

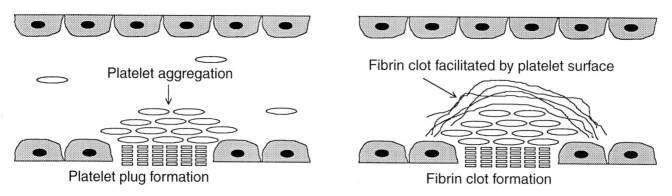

Figure 51–3. The endothelial cell/platelet/von Willebrand factor (vWf) interaction that results in initiation of the normal platelet plug by the adhesion of platelets to damaged endothelium mediated by vWf with subsequent formation of the platelet plug and fibrin clot. (Courtesy of R. R. Montgomery.)

the vascular system can alter this balance and result in increased TPA release, thus generating plasmin and lysing local clots.

When fibrin is degraded by plasmin, fibrin degradation products (FDPs) are formed. These can be measured in the clinical laboratory by immunologic assays that detect the presence of proteolysed fibrin(ogen) (FDPs) or that detect the breakdown products of plasmin action on cross-linked fibrin (D-dimer). Plasminogen activator has been synthesized in a recombinant form (rTPA) and is an effective pharmacologic fibrinolytic agent *in vivo*.

THE PLATELET-ENDOTHELIAL CELLS AXIS

Clotting is initiated when platelets adhere to damaged endothelium (Fig. 51–3). In areas of vascular damage, the adhesive protein, von Willebrand factor (vWf), binds to the exposed subendothelial collagen matrix and undergoes a conformational change. vWf then binds to its platelet receptor glycoprotein Ib (GPIb) and activates platelets. Activated platelets secrete adenosine diphosphate, which induces nearby circulating platelets to aggregate. Platelet-to-platelet cohesion is mediated by the binding of fibrinogen to its platelet receptor glycoprotein IIb/IIIa (GPIIb/IIIa). Therefore, both vWf and fibrinogen play essential roles in normal platelet function *in vivo*. Simultaneously with the platelet adhesion-aggregation response, coagulation is being activated. The platelet membrane brings the reactants of the cascade into close proximity, promoting rapid effective factor catalysis and accelerating the reactions 1000-fold faster than would occur in the absence of the appropriate surface.

Normally, endothelial cells provide an antithrombotic surface through which blood flows without interruption. Nevertheless, the endothelial cell is capable of a rapid change in function and character so that it can augment coagulation following stimulation with a variety of modulating agents, including lymphokines and cytokines as well as noxious agents such as endotoxin and infectious viruses (Fig. 51–4). Widespread alteration of endothelial cell function can shift and dysregulate the hemostatic response and promote activation of clotting. This is likely the mechanism by which sepsis induces the clinical syndrome of disseminated intravascular coagulation (DIC).

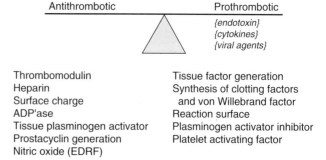

Figure 51–4. Endothelial balance. The pivotal role of the endothelium in maintaining a balance between antithrombotic and prothrombotic activities as influenced by endotoxins, viruses, and immunomodulatory cytokines. ADPase = adenosine diphosphatase; EDRF = endothelium-derived relaxing factor.

DEVELOPMENTAL HEMOSTASIS

Hemostatic disorders in newborns are common, more so than at any other age in pediatrics. The neonate is relatively deficient in most procoagulant and anticoagulant proteins. Platelet function may also be deficient. Blood flow characteristics in the newborn are unique because of the high hematocrit, small-caliber vessels, low blood pressure, and special areas of vascular fragility. Table 51–2 presents the normal values for coagulation screening tests and procoagulant proteins in preterm and term infants as well as in older children. Table 51–3 presents age-specific values for the anticoagulant and fibrinolytic proteins.

Factors V, VIII, fibrinogen, vWf, and platelets achieve normal levels by 28 weeks of gestation. Normal functional levels of protein S also appear to be attained, but levels of other anticoagulant proteins, especially protein C, ATIII, and plasminogen, are low in term infants and are even lower in the premature neonate. The levels of most procoagulant and anticoagulant proteins increase throughout gestation; therefore, the most immature infant has the lowest levels of these proteins and is at the highest risk of either bleeding or thrombotic complications (see Table 51–3). The hemostatic balance of the neonate, especially the premature neonate, is precarious and shifted toward bleeding, thrombosis, or both.

Vitamin K deficiency is a particular problem of the newborn. Vitamin K is a fat-soluble vitamin that induces the post-translational γ-carboxylation of the vitamin K–dependent factors (factors II, VII, IX, and X; protein C and protein S). This carboxylation step occurs after the protein is synthesized in the liver and must occur for that coagulation factor to bind calcium, the bridge to the membrane surface on which these proteins form complexes with other members of the clotting cascade and catalyze subsequent reactions. Vitamin K deficiency effectively renders these proteins unable to bind to a surface. Most of the vitamin K in adults originates from the diet and from bacterial production in the intestine. The neonate is at high risk for vitamin K deficiency because human milk is relatively deficient in vitamin K, the neonatal liver itself is immature, and the newborn's gut requires several days to develop normal bacterial flora.

Infants at highest risk for bleeding from vitamin K deficiency, known as *hemorrhagic disease of the newborn* (HDN), are breast-fed babies who do not receive intramuscular vitamin K prophylaxis at birth. Such infants may experience diffuse bleeding and even central nervous system hemorrhage at 3 to 5 days of life. Currently in the United States, HDN is an extraordinarily rare event because of nearly universal neonatal administration of vitamin K. One should confirm that vitamin K has been administered in any bleeding neonate. Patients with disorders of the gastrointestinal tract, those taking broad-spectrum antibiotics, those born of mothers who received phenobarbital or phenytoin during pregnancy, and those with cholestasis and malabsorption are at higher risk for vitamin K deficiency.

Clues from the History and Physical Examination

HISTORY

Table 51–4 provides an outline of historical questions that are important to the diagnosis of bleeding disorders. To obtain the history, it is critical to obtain quantifiable precise information: a documented need for transfusion after surgery due to unexplained bleeding, nosebleeds that require cautery, large (>2 inches in diameter), raised bruises in areas not usually associated with trauma. Although easy bruising and nosebleeds are common in children, the presence of large bruises at multiple sites, prolonged nosebleeds, and hematoma formation are rare in "nonbleeders" but are seen in 20% to 38.5% of "bleeders." The yield of evaluating children with an isolated history of easy bruising in a commonly traumatized area is quite low, whereas there is a much higher likelihood of pathology with a history of large bruises at multiple sites. Similar criteria likely apply to epistaxis in which frequent, *prolonged* (>15 to 30 minutes) epistaxis, especially without trauma or a history of allergy or infection, is much more likely caused by anatomic or hemostatic deficiencies. Epistaxis that requires cautery or packing, that results in iron deficiency is highly indicative. Some helpful questions include: "What was the biggest bruise you ever had, and what caused it?" "Which finger do you pick your nose with?" "Have you ever noted little red dots (petechiae) on your skin?"

A personal or family history of gynecologic bleeding is often valuable. Menorrhagia causing iron deficiency anemia, bleeding after childbirth, or requiring transfusion or early hysterectomy because of bleeding is often inappropriately assumed to be due to anatomic causes. One must ascertain the number of pads used per day in addition to the length and the frequency of each menstrual cycle (see Chapter 32). If the majority of women in a family have an underlying bleeding disorder, then that family's "normal menstrual periods" may be quite abnormal.

Historical information is equally important in deciding who requires evaluation for a congenital predisposition to thrombosis. Virtually all pediatric patients in whom a blood clot develops in the absence of major vascular instrumentation deserve careful laboratory screening for a prothrombotic state (a hereditary or acquired disorder that predisposes to clotting). The only group for whom there is insufficient evidence to judge whether studies need to performed are those neonates with catheters in place in whom venous or arterial thrombi develop related to the catheter. Even in these situations, a detailed family history should be taken for early-onset stroke, heart attack, and blood clots in the veins, arteries, or lungs.

PHYSICAL EXAMINATION

The most important determination is whether the patient appears acutely or chronically ill, including vital signs and growth parameters. The nose should be examined for ulcers or anatomic bleeding sites, and the heart should be examined for the presence of murmurs (endocarditis). Joints should be examined for chronic arthropathy (hemophilia) or joint laxity (Ehlers-Danlos syndrome), the extremities are examined for thumb or radial anomalies (thrombocytopenia–absent radius [TAR] syndrome, Fanconi anemia). The abdomen and lymph nodes should be examined for the presence of hepatosplenomegaly and adenopathy.

The examination of the skin should include a search for hematomas, petechiae, ecchymoses, telangiectasias, poor wound healing (scars), lax (loose) skin, and varicose veins (possible deep venous thrombosis). *Petechiae* are pinpoint, flat, dark-red lesions caused by capillary bleeding into the skin. *Ecchymoses* are larger lesions (bruises) that are nonraised and usually not palpable. *Hematomas* are an accumulation of blood in the skin or deeper tissues; in the skin, hematomas are raised and palpable. Bruises should be described in detail, including whether hematomas are associated with bruises and whether petechiae are present. Petechiae and ecchymoses are usually painless.

Purpura refers to any group of disorders characterized by the presence of dark-red, purplish, or brown lesions of the skin and mucous membranes. The discoloration is caused by the leakage of red blood cells from affected vessels. Purpuric lesions can be caused by abnormalities of the platelets, coagulation proteins, or vessel walls.

Table 51–2. Reference Values for Coagulation Tests in Healthy Children*

Tests	19–27 Weeks' Gestation†	28–31 Weeks' Gestation†	30–36 Weeks' Gestation	Full Term	1–5 Years	6–10 Years	11–18 Years	Adult
PT (sec)	—	15.4 (14.6–16.9)	13.0 (10.6–16.2)	13.0 (10.1–15.9)	11 (10.6–11.4)	11.1 (10.1–12.0)	11.2 (10.2–12.0)	12 (11.0–14.0)
INR	—	—	1.0 (0.61–1.7)	1.00 (0.53–1.62)‡	1.0 (0.96–1.04)	1.01 (0.91–1.11)	1.02 (0.93–1.10)	1.10 (1.0–1.3)
APTT (sec)	—	108 (80–168)	53.6 (27.5–79.4)‡ §§	42.9 (31.3–54.3)‡	30 (24–36)	31 (26–36)	32 (26–37)	33 (27–40)
Fibrinogen	1.00 (±0.43)	2.56 (1.60–5.50)	2.43 (1.50–3.73)‡ §	2.83 (1.67–3.99)	2.76 (1.70–4.05)	2.79 (1.57–4.0)	3.0 (1.54–4.48)	2.78 (1.56–4.0)
Bleeding time (min)	—	—	—	—	6 (2.5–10)‡	7 (2.5–13)‡	5 (3.8)‡	4 (1–7)
II	0.12 (±0.02)	0.31 (0.19–0.54)	0.45 (0.20–0.77)‡	0.48 (0.26–0.70)‡	0.94 (0.71–1.16)‡	0.88 (0.67–1.07)‡	0.83 (0.61–1.04)‡	1.08 (0.70–1.46)
V	0.41 (±0.10)	0.65 (0.43–0.80)	0.88 (0.41–1.44)§	0.72 (0.34–1.08)‡	1.03 (0.79–1.27)	0.90 (0.63–1.16)‡	0.77 (0.55–0.99)‡	1.06 (0.62–1.50)
VII	0.28 (±0.04)	0.37 (0.24–0.76)	0.67 (0.21–1.13)‡	0.66 (0.28–1.04)‡	0.82 (0.55–1.16)‡	0.86 (0.52–1.20)‡	0.83 (0.58–1.15)‡	1.05 (0.67–1.43)
VIII procoagulant	0.39 (±0.14)	0.79 (0.37–1.26)	1.11 (0.5–2.13)	1.00 (0.50–1.78)	0.90 (0.59–1.42)	0.95 (0.58–1.32)	0.92 (0.53–1.31)	0.99 (0.50–1.49)
vWf	0.64 (±0.13)	1.41 (0.83–2.23)	1.36 (0.78–2.10)	1.53 (0.50–2.87)	0.82 (0.60–1.20)	0.95 (0.44–1.44)	1.00 (0.46–1.53)	0.92 (0.50–1.58)
IX	0.10 (±0.01)	0.18 (0.17–0.20)	0.35 (0.19–0.65)‡ §	0.53 (0.15–0.91)† ‡	0.73 (0.47–1.04)‡	0.75 (0.63–0.89)‡	0.82 (0.59–1.22)‡	1.09 (0.55–1.63)
X	0.21 (±0.03)	0.36 (0.25–0.64)	0.41 (0.11–0.71)‡	0.40 (0.12–0.68)‡	0.88 (0.58–1.16)‡	0.75 (0.55–1.01)‡	0.79 (0.50–1.17)	1.06 (0.70–1.52)
XI	—	0.23 (0.11–0.33)	0.30 (0.08–5.2)‡ §	0.38 ±(0.40–0.66)‡	0.30 (0.08–0.52)‡ §	0.38 (0.10–0.66)	0.74 (0.50–0.97)‡	0.97 (0.56–1.50)
XII	0.22 (±0.03)	0.25 (0.05–0.35)	0.38 (0.10–0.66)‡ §§	0.53 (0.13–0.93)‡	0.93 (0.64–1.29)	0.92 (0.60–1.40)	0.81 (0.34–1.37)‡	1.08 (0.52–1.64)
PK	—	0.26 (0.15–0.32)	0.33 (0.09–0.89)‡	0.37 (0.18–0.69)‡	0.95 (0.65–1.30)	0.99 (0.66–1.31)	0.99 (0.53–1.45)	1.12 (0.62–1.62)
HMWK	—	0.32 (0.19–0.52)	0.49 (0.09–0.89)‡	0.54 (0.06–1.02)‡	0.98 (0.64–1.32)	0.93 (0.60–1.30)	0.91 (0.63–1.19)	0.92 (0.50–1.36)
XIIIa‖	—	—	0.70 (0.32–1.08)‡	0.79 (0.27–1.31)‡	1.08 (0.72–1.43)	1.09 (0.65–1.51)	0.99 (0.57–1.40)	1.05 (0.55–1.55)
XIIIb‖	—	—	0.81 (0.35–1.27)‡	0.76 (0.30–1.22)‡	1.13 (0.69–1.56)‡	1.16 (0.77–1.54)‡	1.02 (0.60–1.43)	0.98 (0.57–1.37)

Data from Andrew M, et al. Am J Pediatr Hematol Oncol 1990; 12:95–104; and Blood 1992; 80:1998–2005.

*All factors except fibrinogen are presented as units/ml (fibrinogen in mg/ml) where pooled normal plasma contains 1 unit/ml. All data are expressed as the mean followed by the upper and lower boundary encompassing 95% of the normal population.

†Levels for 19–27 weeks and 28–31 weeks are from multiple sources and cannot be analyzed statistically.

‡Values are significantly different from those of adults.

§Values are significantly different from those of full-term infants.

‖Value given as CTA units/ml.

Abbreviations: PT = prothrombin time; INR = international normalized ratio; APTT = activated partial thromboplastin time; VIII = factor VIII procoagulant activity; vWf = von Willebrand factor; PK = prekallikrein; HMWK = high-molecular-weight kininogen.

Table 51–3. Reference Values for the Inhibitors of Coagulation in Healthy Children Compared with Adults*

	19–27 Weeks' Gestation†	28–31 Weeks' Gestation†	30–36 Weeks' Gestation	Full Term	1–5 Years	6–10 Years	11–18 Years	Adult
ATIII	0.24 (±0.03)‡	0.28 (0.20–0.38)‡	0.38 (0.14–0.62)‡ §	0.63 (0.39–0.87)‡	1.11 (0.82–1.39)	1.11 (0.90–1.31)	1.06 (0.77–1.32)	1.0 (0.74–1.26)
Protein C	0.11 (±0.03)‡	—	0.28 (0.12–0.44)‡ §	0.35 (0.17–0.53)‡	0.66 (0.40–0.92)‡	0.69 (0.45–0.93)‡	0.83 (0.55–1.11)‡	0.96 (0.64–1.28)
Protein S								
Total (U/ml)	—	—	0.26 (0.14–0.38)‡ §	0.36 (0.12–0.60)‡	0.86 (0.54–1.18)	0.78 (0.41–1.14)	0.72 (0.52–0.92)	0.81 (0.61–1.13)
Free (U/ml)	—	—	—	—	0.45 (0.21–0.69)	0.42 (0.22–0.62)	0.38 (0.26–0.55)	0.45 (0.27–0.61)
Plasminogen (U/ml)	—	—	1.70 (1.12–2.48)‡ ‖	1.95 (1.25–2.65)‡ ‖	0.98 (0.78–1.18)	0.92 (0.75–1.08)	0.86 (0.68–1.03)‖	0.99 (0.77–1.22)
TPA (ng/ml)	—	—	8.48 (3.00–16.70)	9.6 (5.0–18.9)	2.15 (1.0–4.5)‡	2.42 (1.0–5.0)‡	2.16 (1.0–4.0)‡	1.02 (0.68–1.36)
a₂AP (U/ml)	—	—	0.78 (0.40–1.16)	0.85 (0.55–1.15)	1.05 (0.93–1.17)	0.99 (0.89–1.10)	0.98 (0.78–1.18)	1.02 (0.68–1.36)
PAI-1	—	—	5.4 (0.0–12.2)‡	6.4 (2.0–15.1)	5.42 (1.0–10.0)	6.79 (2.0–12.0)‡	6.07 (2.0–10.0)‡	3.60 (0–11.0)

Data from Andrew M, et al. Am J Pediatr Hematol Oncol 1990; 12:95–104; and Blood 1992; 80:1998–2005.

*All values are expressed in units/ml where pooled plasma contains 1 unit/ml, with the exception of free protein S, which contains a mean of 0.4 unit/ml. All values presented as the mean by the upper and lower boundary encompassing 95% of the population.

†Levels for 19–27 weeks and 28–31 weeks are from multiple sources and cannot be analyzed statistically.

‡Values are significantly different from those of adults.

§Values are significantly different from those of full-term infants.

‖Value given as CTA units/ml.

Abbreviations: ATIII = antithrombin-III; TPA = tissue plasminogen activator: α₂AP = α₂-antiplasmin; PAI-1 = plasminogen activator inhibitor type 1.

Table 51–4. History of a Bleeding Disorder

I. History of Disorder
  A. *Onset* of symptoms
    1. age
    2. acute versus lifelong
    3. triggering event
    4. timing of bleeding after injury: immediate vs. delayed
  B. *Sites* of bleeding
    1. **Mucocutaneous***
      a. Epistaxis
        (1) Duration, frequency, seasonal tendency
        (2) Associated trauma (nose picking, allergy, infection)
        (3) **Resultant anemia, emergency department evaluation, cautery**
      b. Oral (gingiva, tongue lacerations, bleeding after tooth brushing, after dental extractions requiring sutures/packing)
      c. Bruising (number, sites, size, **raised** [other than extremities] spontaneous versus trauma, knots within center, skin scarring)
      d. Gastrointestinal bleeding
    2. **Deep**
      a. Musculoskeletal
        (1) Hemarthroses, unexplained arthropathy
        (2) Intramuscular hematomas
      b. Central nervous system hemorrhage
      c. Genitourinary tract
    3. **Surgical**
      a. Minor (sutures, lacerations, poor or delayed wound healing)
      b. Major
        (1) Tonsillectomy and adenoidectomy
        (2) Abdominal surgery
  C. **Perinatal History**
      a. Superficial (bruising, petechiae)
      b. Deep
        (1) Circumcision
        (2) Central nervous system bleeding
        (3) Gastrointestinal bleeding
        (4) Cephalohematoma
        (5) Unexplained anemia or hyperbilirubinemia
        (6) Delayed cord separation, bleeding after cord separation
      c. Vitamin K administration
      d. Maternal drugs
  D. **Obstetric/gynecologic bleeding**
    1. Menorrhagia
      (1) Onset, duration, amount (number of pads), frequency, persistence after child birth
      (2) **Resultant anemia, iron deficiency**
    2. Bleeding at childbirth (onset, duration, **transfusion requirement,** history of traumatic delivery, recurrences with subsequent pregnancies, spontaneous abortions)
  E. **Medications**
      a. Aspirin and nonsteroidal anti-inflammatory drugs
      b. Anticoagulants
      c. Antibiotics
      d. Anticonvulsants
II. Family History
    Draw family tree. The above questions should be applied to immediate family members, especially a history of easy bruising, epistaxis, excessive bleeding after surgery, menorrhagia, excessive bleeding after childbirth, a family history of others with diagnosed or suspect bleeding disorders. Attempt to deduce inheritance pattern.

*Significant historical information is presented in bold type.

Coagulation Screening Tests

After obtaining a history and performing a physical, examination, one must decide the need for an evaluation. The presence of significant symptoms should trigger a work-up. The history is likely to be the most sensitive screening tool for a significant bleeding disorder, although the history is often nonspecific. Its use in a very young child, especially prior to the toddler age, is limited, and attention must shift to the perinatal history and the family history.

For patients who are to be evaluated because of clinical clues or planned surgery, the initial screening studies should evaluate the clotting factors and platelet and vessel wall interaction, including vWf function. No set of screening tests is complete and capable of detecting the panorama of hemorrhagic disorders, but the screen should include:

- A prothrombin time (PT, protime).
- A partial thromboplastin time (PTT).
- A functional fibrinogen level or thrombin time.
- A platelet count.
- A bleeding time.
- A measure of vWf function (ristocetin cofactor activity)

PT AND PTT

The PT (Fig. 51–5) and PTT (Fig. 51–6) measure all of the coagulation factors except factor XIII. Fibrinogen function should

be measured as fibrinogen activity or thrombin time. The bleeding time provides an indirect measure of platelet number, platelet function, and the platelet–vessel wall interaction. The PTT is the screening test that checks for deficiency of all clotting factors except factors VII and XIII. The PTT can be prolonged either by a deficiency of a clotting factor or by the presence of an agent in the plasma that delays the clotting time (an inhibitor). The PT is sensitive to deficiencies of factor VII.

To test for an inhibitor, one part of the patient plasma is mixed

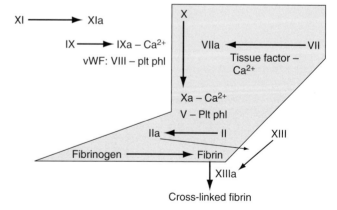

Figure 51–5. Elements of the coagulation cascade measured by the prothrombin time in the shaded area.

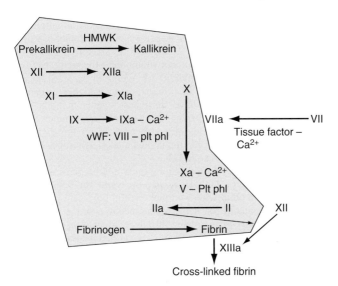

Figure 51–6. Elements of the coagulation cascade measured by the partial thromboplastin time (PTT) in the shaded area. HMWK = high-molecular-weight kininogen; vWf = von Willebrand factor. Note that PK, HMWK, and factor XII are shown in this figure and not in the depiction of the coagulation cascade in Figure 51–1, since a deficiency of PK, HMWK, or factor XII can cause a prolongation of the PTT but low levels of these proteins are not usually associated with a clinical bleeding disorder.

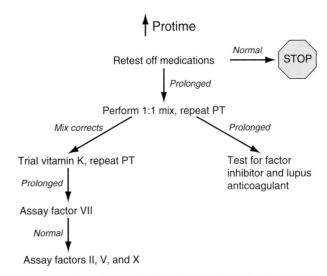

Figure 51–7. Flow diagram for the evaluation of an isolated prolongation of the prothrombin time (protime, PT).

with one part pooled normal plasma obtained from a pool of 20 to 50 healthy adults. Pooled normal plasma provides a 100% level of each clotting factor. If mixed 1:1 with plasma that is deficient in one or several factors, the mixture should possess at least a 50% level of each factor and the PTT should correct to the normal range. If an inhibitor is present, the PTT usually does not correct to normal. The most common types of inhibitors include anticoagulants, such as heparin, and autoantibodies directed against either specific clotting factors (factor VIII inhibitors) or the phospholipid substances used in the PTT (lupus-type anticoagulants).

The PTT is especially sensitive to deficiencies of factors VIII, IX, and XI (hemophilia A, B, and C, respectively). A prolonged PTT in an asymptomatic child is most commonly caused by factor XII deficiency or by an inhibitor. The PTT can yield a false result:

1. When poor venipuncture technique by adding tissue factor to the blood artifactually shortens the PTT.

2. When insensitive laboratory reagents fail to detect clinically significant deficiencies (commonly factor IX).

3. When the citrate concentration is not corrected for blood with a high hematocrit (neonates, cyanotic congenital heart disease).

BLEEDING TIME

The bleeding time is performed by placing a blood pressure cuff on the arm and inflating it to 40 mmHg; lower pressures have been used for infants. An incision of predetermined length and depth is made on the volar surface of the arm below the antecubital fossa using a standardized automated device. The wound is blotted with filter paper, and the time until the blood stops oozing is measured with a stopwatch.

The bleeding time may be an indirect measure of platelet number and a more direct measure of platelet function, vascular integrity, and platelet interaction with the vascular subendothelium. As such, the bleeding time should be abnormal in patients with thrombocytopenia, platelet function abnormalities, abnormal collagen (Ehlers-

Danlos syndrome), and von Willebrand disease. Unfortunately, because of its insensitivity and high level of variability, the bleeding time is a relatively poor tool to detect the milder forms of these hemostatic disorders and cannot be used to rule out von Willebrand disease or mild or moderate platelet function deficits. Figures 51–7 to 51–9 provide an approach to evaluate the patient with an isolated prolongation of the PT, PTT, or bleeding time, respectively.

THROMBIN TIME AND REPTILASE TIME

The thrombin time and reptilase time are two tests that measure the conversion of fibrinogen to fibrin. The thrombin time is sensitive to heparin effect, whereas the snake venom reptilase is not; the reptilase time remains normal in the presence of heparin. Both the thrombin time and the reptilase time are prolonged by uremia, by dysfibrinogenemia, and by FDPs formed by the action of plasmin on fibrin(ogen).

Both FDPs and D-dimer represent products formed when the fibrinolytic enzyme plasmin degrades fibrin. FDPs are a measure of plasmin action on fibrin and fibrinogen and should be less

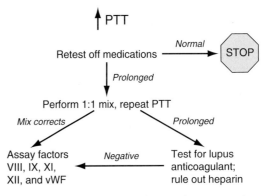

Figure 51–8. Flow diagram for the evaluation of a patient with a prolonged partial thromboplastin time (PTT). To rule out heparin effect, the thrombin time is compared with the reptilase time. If the thrombin time is significantly longer than the reptilase time, heparin is present in the sample. vWf = von Willebrand factor.

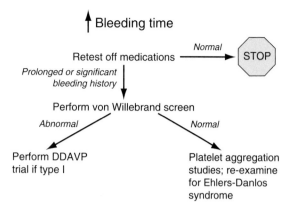

Figure 51–9. Evaluation for an isolated prolongation of bleeding time. DDAVP = desmopressin.

specific than the D-dimer assay, which measures the breakdown products of cross-linked fibrin.

MUCOCUTANEOUS BLEEDING

Mucocutaneous bleeding is bleeding within the skin or mucous membranes. Common complaints include prolonged, frequent nosebleeds, gum bleeding, bleeding after tooth extraction, menorrhagia, and easy bruising with or without petechiae formation. Mucocutaneous bleeding is usually associated with abnormalities of platelet number or function, platelet cofactors, or the vessel wall.

The well-appearing child who presents with the acute onset of petechiae and purpura often in association with nosebleeds or bleeding gums and an otherwise normal examination typically has *acute immune thrombocytopenic purpura* (ITP). Fifty percent to 65% of these children have an antecedent viral illness. Following exposure to the viral infection, an antibody develops in the child that binds to the platelet membrane, leading to the premature destruction of the antibody-coated platelets in the spleen.

The peak ages for the presentation of ITP are 1 to 4 years of age and adolescence. Females are more commonly affected in adolescence but not in childhood. The work-up of the child should include a careful history aimed to detect symptoms (weight loss, fever, bone pain, anorexia) of other preexisting illnesses (leukemia, systemic lupus erythematosus [SLE], endocarditis, human immunodeficiency virus [HIV]), exposures to drugs or toxins, and a personal or family history of thrombocytopenia. The physical examination must be detailed and include a search for signs of malignancy (lymphadenopathy, hepatosplenomegaly), chronic illness, and congenital malformations. When evaluating the complete blood count (CBC), one should ensure that the hemoglobin, white blood cell count, differential, indices, and smear are normal, thus making the diagnosis of a hematologic malignancy or other marrow failure syndrome unlikely. The presence of large platelets on the smear suggests accelerated thrombopoiesis and increased platelet destruction. The differential diagnosis of thrombocytopenia is noted in Table 51–5.

Following the presumptive diagnosis of ITP, requisite laboratory studies other than the CBC, smear, and platelet count can be debated. Some would obtain a Coombs test to rule out a simultaneous autoimmune hemolytic anemia, but the significance of this finding in a patient with a normal hemoglobin is undefined. The role of studies for platelet antibodies is unclear. There are no data indicating that these studies are either diagnostic or prognostic in children. If the child is male, young, and has a history of eczema or recurrent infection, immunoglobulins to rule out Wiskott-Aldrich syndrome are indicated (see Chapter 52). Similarly, in older chil-

dren, especially girls as they approach adolescence, an antinuclear antibody (ANA) to rule out SLE presenting as thrombocytopenia is warranted. Some clinicians would perform an ANA on all newly diagnosed patients, whereas others would defer the study, as fewer than 2% of adults and children are found to have SLE after presenting with acute ITP. In contrast, a much higher percentage of individuals with SLE have thrombocytopenia at some time during their illness (see Chapter 45). An ANA has a much higher likelihood of positivity if the test is performed for those children with chronic ITP. Acquired immunodeficiency syndrome (AIDS) may occasionally manifest as ITP.

In the past, a bone marrow aspiration would be performed prior to any treatment for ITP. However, the yield for bone marrow examination in a child with a normal, careful physical examination (no lymphadenopathy or hepatosplenomegaly) and a completely normal CBC, other than isolated thrombocytopenia, is negligible.

Once a diagnosis of ITP is made, several therapeutic options are available, including simple observation and education. The family should be advised that the child must avoid activities that increase the risk of head injury. Treatment should be reserved for those children at high risk for clinical bleeding (a platelet count < 20,000 to 25,000/mm³ and children with petechiae and mucosal hemorrhages). Some argue that those with mucous membrane purpura are at higher risk and definitively require treatment. The major mortality of ITP is related to intracranial hemorrhage, which has been observed in less than 0.5% to 1% of patients. Table 51–6 provides a perspective on treatment alternatives for ITP. Transfusion of platelets should be reserved for life-threatening bleeding because transfused platelets are rapidly destroyed. Initial therapy for those in need of treatment includes intravenous immune globulin (IVIG), prednisone, and IV anti-D (RhoGAM). IV anti-D appears to be equally effective as IVIG for the Rh-positive patient and is much less expensive. IV anti-D has fewer side effects than prednisone does.

Ten percent to 20% of children with acute ITP have persistence of thrombocytopenia for more than 6 months (chronic ITP). These patients are more likely to be older (adolescents) and female or to have had an insidious onset of symptoms. One must look carefully for predisposing causes, including SLE, HIV, or medications. The treatment of chronic ITP is evolving and includes IVIG or IV anti-D. Improved medical therapy has limited splenectomy to those patients with severe refractory chronic ITP.

Neonatal Thrombocytopenia

Thrombocytopenia is common, especially in sick newborns. The differential diagnosis of neonatal thrombocytopenia includes most of the causes seen in older children in addition to those peculiar to the newborn (see Table 51–5 and Fig. 51–10 in the shaded areas). When evaluating the thrombocytopenic newborn, the physician must know perinatal history. One should ask about the mother's health during this and previous pregnancies, including any current or previous history of low platelets or children dying of hemorrhage. A maternal history of viral infections (cytomegalovirus, rubella), sexually transmitted diseases (syphilis, AIDS), medications, toxemia, or collagen-vascular disease (SLE) is informative. The family history should be evaluated for bleeding disorders, recurrent infections, or malignancies, especially in children.

During examination of the newborn, the most important element to determine is the child's general well-being. The examiner should look especially for signs of systemic illness as well as lymphadenopathy, hepatosplenomegaly, mass lesions, hemangiomas, bruits, and congenital anomalies, especially of the radial bones.

One should carefully evaluate the hemoglobin, the white blood cell count, and the differential for the presence of abnormal cells (blasts). Red blood cell morphology should be examined for signs

Table 51-5. Differential Diagnosis of Thrombocytopenia in Children

I. Destructive Thrombocytopenias
Primary Platelet Consumption Syndromes

Immunologic
- Idiopathic thrombocytopenia purpura
- Drug-induced thrombocytopenia
- Infection-induced thrombocytopenia (human immunodeficiency virus)
- Post-transfusion purpura
- Autoimmune or lymphoproliferative disorders
- Neonatal immune thrombocytopenias
- Allergy and anaphylaxis
- Post-transplant thrombocytopenia

Nonimmunologic
- Chronic microangiopathic hemolytic anemia and thrombocytopenia
- Hemolytic-uremic syndrome
- Thrombotic thrombocytopenic purpura
- Catheters, prostheses, or cardiopulmonary bypass
- Congenital or acquired heart disease

Combined Platelet and Fibrinogen Consumption Syndromes
Disseminated intravascular coagulation
Kasabach-Merritt syndrome
Other causes of local consumption coagulopathy

Miscellaneous Causes

Specific to the neonate
- Phototherapy
- Perinatal aspiration syndromes
- Persistent pulmonary hypertension
- Rhesus alloimmunization
- Post–exchange transfusion
- Polycythemia
- Metabolic disorders
- Maternal HELLP syndrome

Glomerular disease
Preeclampsia
Fatty acid–induced thrombocytopenia

II. Impaired or Ineffective Production
Congenital and Hereditary Disorders

Primary hematologic processes
- TAR syndrome
- Other congenital thrombocytopenias with megakaryocytic hypoplasia
- Fanconi aplastic anemia
- Bernard-Soulier syndrome*
- May-Hegglin anomaly*
- Wiskott-Aldrich syndrome*
- Miscellaneous hereditary thrombocytopenias (X-linked or autosomal)*
- Mediterranean thrombocytopenia

Associated with trisomy 13 or 18

Metabolic disorders
- Methylmalonic acidemia
- Ketotic glycinemia
- Holocarboxylase synthetase deficiency
- Isovaleric acidemia

Acquired Disorders
Aplastic anemia
   Marrow infiltrative processes
   Drug- or radiation-induced
   Nutritional deficiency states (iron, folate, or vitamin B$_{12}$)

III. Sequestration
Hypersplenism
Hypothermia

Modified from Schultz Beardsley D. Platelet abnormalities in infancy and childhood. *In* Nathan DG, Oski FA (eds). Hematology of Infancy and Childhood, 4th ed. Vol 2. Philadelphia: WB Saunders, 1993:1566.
*These hereditary thrombocytopenias can be associated with normal or increased bone marrow megakaryocytes.
Abbreviations: HELLP = hypertension, elevated liver enzymes, low platelets; TAR = thrombocytopenia–absent radius.

Table 51–6. Common Treatment Alternatives for the Therapy of Childhood Immune Thrombocytopenic Purpura (ITP)

	Pro	Con	Cost Analysis for 15-kg 3-Year-Old
IVIG	Intravenous	Expensive	1 g/kg initial dose, 4-hr infusion as outpatient = $1500
	Rapid onset of action	Frequently needs multiple doses	
	Bone marrow not required	Does not alter long-term outcome	
	Noninfectious	IV in place for several hours	
	High frequency of response		
Prednisone	Inexpensive	Corticosteroid side effects	2-wk course, 2 mg/kg/day = $21
	Oral	May need multiple courses	
	Effective in 75%–80% of patients	No effect on long-term outcome	
	Relatively rapid onset of action	Requires bone marrow aspiration	$800–$1000 for procedure and histologic examination
IV anti-D	Relatively inexpensive	IV	1 dose, 50 μg/kg = $600
		Limited to Rh positive patients	
	Relatively rapid onset of action	Mild fall in hemoglobin	
	Highly effective	Ineffective after splenectomy	
Splenectomy	Curative in 80% of patients	Expensive, invasive	$10,000
		Impairs host defense versus encapsulated organisms	
		Reserved for *chronic, severe* ITP	
		Spontaneous remissions of ITP may occur late	

of microangiopathy. Small platelets suggest abnormal thrombopoiesis, whereas large platelets are found with accelerated platelet destruction. Mechanistically, thrombocytopenia can be caused by synthetic failure, sequestration, or destructive processes. The destructive processes are most common and are either immune or nonimmune in origin. Nonimmune causes of platelet consumption—for example, DIC, sepsis, congenital infections, or thrombotic events—are usually associated with obvious clinical findings. When evaluating the ill-appearing child or neonate for thrombocytopenia, one should perform coagulation studies to detect fibrinogen consumption (fibrinogen level, D-dimer, FDPs). Neonates with immune-mediated platelet destruction usually appear healthy.

After a careful history and physical examination are performed and the CBC is evaluated, the initial step in management of the child with thrombocytopenia depends on the etiology and severity of the thrombocytopenia. In the neonate with severe thrombocytopenia (platelet count < 30,000 to 40,000/mm³) delivered vaginally, an ultrasound study of the head should be done to rule out intracranial bleeding. When platelets are transfused for severe thrombocytopenia or clinical bleeding, or both, a platelet transfusion can serve as both a therapeutic and a diagnostic maneuver because those patients whose thrombocytopenia is due to a synthetic failure will have normal survival of transfused platelets, whereas those whose thrombocytopenia is due to consumption will have rapid destruction. For this reason, platelet transfusions are usually contraindicated in thrombocytopenic states due to accelerated platelet destruction, as in ITP and hemolytic-uremic syndrome. The yield and survival of the transfused platelets should be monitored with serial platelet counts after transfusion.

Antibody-mediated thrombocytopenia in the neonate is caused by transfer of maternal immunoglobulin G (IgG) antibodies that react with the neonate's platelets. A mother with active ITP or a previous history of ITP is at risk for delivering a thrombocytopenic baby. There is no definitive noninvasive method to determine the newborn's risk of thrombocytopenia, although the actual risk of severe bleeding during delivery appears small. In contrast, mothers who are sensitized to alloantigens present on the fetal platelets have a higher risk of perinatal hemorrhage and symptomatic

thrombocytopenia. *Neonatal alloimmune thrombocytopenic purpura* (NATP), the platelet equivalent of maternal Rh isoimmunization, differs from Rh disease, in that firstborn children are commonly affected. The importance of this diagnosis is that it is commonly associated with prenatal intracranial hemorrhage with a resultant high morbidity and mortality (15%). Therefore, recognition of the diagnosis in the first pregnancy can have a major impact on the management of subsequent pregnancies. In addition, therapy is available for the affected fetus and neonate to prevent untoward bleeding. Transfusion of washed maternal platelets that lack the paternal antigen toward which the maternal antibody is directed provides a rapid increase in platelet count and prevents further bleeding. Random donor platelets are rapidly destroyed.

Although the initial diagnosis of NATP is usually made by the studying the reaction of maternal sera against paternal platelets, prenatal diagnosis can now be performed using molecular biologic techniques to detect the allelic differences between the mother and the infant on amniotic cell DNA, thus allowing prenatal intervention with maternal treatment with IVIG to support the fetal platelet count. In addition, postnatal treatment of the neonate with IVIG and corticosteroids may be helpful after restoration of a normal platelet count by transfusion of washed maternal platelets. All blood products in a neonate with thrombocytopenia should be radiated to prevent graft-versus-host disease, as some patients may have a congenital immunodeficiency syndrome manifested by thrombocytopenia.

Child Abuse

The most common cause of remarkable bruising and bleeding with normal hemostatic screening studies is child abuse (see Chapter 37).

Chronic/Insidious Onset of Mucocutaneous Bleeding

When symptoms of skin and mucous membrane bleeding are lifelong, the most common cause is von Willebrand disease. Con-

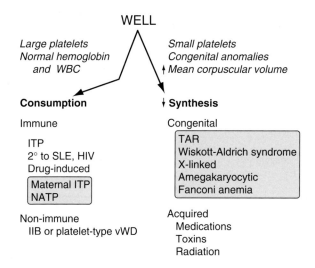

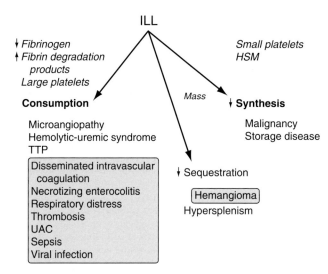

Figure 51–10. Differential diagnosis of childhood thrombocytopenic syndromes. The syndromes are initially separated by their clinical appearance. Clues leading to the diagnosis are presented in italics. The mechanisms and common disorders leading to these findings are shown in the lower part of the figure. Disorders that commonly affect neonates are listed in the shaded boxes. HIV = human immunodeficiency virus; ITP = idiopathic immune thrombocytopenic purpura; NATP = neonatal alloimmune thrombocytopenic purpura; SLE = systemic lupus erythematosus; TTP = thrombotic thrombocytopenic purpura; TAR = thrombocytopenia–absent radius (syndrome); WBC = white blood cell; UAC = umbilical artery catheter; HSM = hepatosplenomegaly.

genital platelet function defects, congenital thrombocytopenic syndromes, and abnormalities of the vessel wall are much less common. *Von Willebrand disease,* the deficiency of vWf, is the most common hereditary bleeding disorder, with a prevalence of approximately 1% of all children.

The inheritance of von Willebrand disease is usually autosomal dominant. vWf is a large multimeric protein that functions as the bridge between platelets and damaged vessel walls; therefore, deficient or dysfunctional vWf causes delayed formation of the platelet plug (see Fig. 51–3). In addition, vWf serves as a carrier protein for factor VIII. A profound deficiency of vWf is associated with low levels of factor VIII, as well as low vWf levels, so that the patient with severe von Willebrand disease has both a deficiency of vWf and simultaneously moderate to severe hemophilia A.

The presentation of von Willebrand disease is highly variable. Mucocutaneous bleeding or no symptoms are the most common findings. Since neonatal vWf levels are often elevated following vaginal delivery, the onset of clinical symptoms for mild and moderate von Willebrand disease is usually that of the toddler stage or older. The only presenting complaint may be abnormal preoperative coagulation studies. The laboratory diagnosis of the disease is particularly challenging because there is no single test that optimally measures vWf function.

The PTT and bleeding time were thought to be adequate screening tests to detect von Willebrand disease. The disease can be detected in 92% of affected individuals with a battery that includes the PTT, bleeding time, and vWf activity, but in only 58% of von Willebrand disease patients are both the PTT and bleeding time abnormal. Physician judgment is critical, and the need for additional work-up is defined by the clinical clues, including the patient's personal history of bleeding, the family history, and the potential for surgery.

The diagnosis of von Willebrand disease is further complicated by the fact that vWf is a labile protein and levels can be increased by stress, medication, trauma, pregnancy, and difficult venipuncture. In addition, vWf levels are blood type–dependent and must be interpreted on the basis of the patient's blood type. It remains unclear whether there is a physiologically different hemostatic level of vWf for different blood groups. Age has been shown to influence vWf levels in adults, and this has not been adequately investigated in children. Furthermore, there are multiple variants of von Willebrand disease. As a result, the clinician should repeat studies if there is a high index of suspicion or abnormal positive screening tests, or both.

Von Willebrand disease can be classified either as type 1 (classic disease with mild or moderate deficiency), type 2 (a dysproteinemia), or type 3 (severe disease—virtual absence of vWf and low levels of factor VIII). The treatment of the disease is dependent on the type and the response to DDAVP (desmopressin). DDAVP is a synthetic vasopressin analog that induces the release of vWf and factor VIII. Levels of these factors rise three-fold to fourfold after a dose of 0.3 μg/kg. *For most cases of von Willebrand disease, DDAVP is the treatment of choice.* A therapeutic trial with measurements of vWf before and both 1 hour and 4 hours after DDAVP should be performed to document the efficacy of DDAVP prior to surgery. Patients with rare variant forms of von Willebrand disease (type 2A, 2B, and platelet type) may have no response or an adverse response to DDAVP, so full studies to identify the subtype are needed prior to a trial of DDAVP. These studies correlate functional levels of vWf with the amount of protein measured antigenically (the vWf antigen), the multimeric size of the protein (vWf multimers), and the aggregation response of the patient's platelet-rich plasma to high and low concentrations of ristocetin.

Most patients with mild and moderate type 1 von Willebrand disease have a satisfactory response to DDAVP; hemostasis for most surgical procedures can be provided with daily doses of DDAVP on consecutive days. For severely affected patients or those with variant forms of the disease noted previously (2A, 2B, platelet type), treatment should be individualized. Some type 2A patients respond to DDAVP. Severely affected patients with von Willebrand disease and those with the 2B variant should receive a clotting factor concentrate containing a full complement of normal vWf multimers (Humate-P) in doses similar to those outlined for factor VIII in Table 51–7.

Platelet Function Defects

For patients with mucocutaneous bleeding but a normal platelet count and normal von Willebrand studies, platelet aggregation studies should be performed to evaluate for a primary or secondary platelet function defect. A large number of medications alter plate-

Table 51–7. Characteristics of Factors VIII and IX and Respective Modes of Treatment for Bleeding Caused by Hemophilia A or B

		Factor VIII	Factor IX
Yield		1.5%–2%/unit/kg infused	1%/unit/kg infused
Half-life		8–12 hr	24 hr
Therapeutic	Life- and limb-threatening	80%–100%	80%–100%
level	Routine: hemarthrosis	40%	30%
Dose computation		Dose = level desired × weight × 0.5	Dose = level desired × weight × 1.0
Therapeutic alternatives		DDAVP*	Monoclonal factor IX concentrate
		Recombinant factor VIII concentrate	Highly purified factor IX concentrate
		Highly purified factor VIII concentrate	Prothrombin complex concentrate (PCC)†

*After adequate levels have been demonstrated.
†Repeated doses associated with thromboembolic risk.

let function and may induce an acquired abnormality of platelet function. A careful history to elicit exposure to medications and to determine whether clinical symptoms correlate with exposure to specific drugs is critical. Common medications that alter platelet functions are aspirin, nonsteroidal anti-inflammatory drugs, alcohol, penicillin in high doses, valproic acid, and miscellaneous other agents.

Most primary platelet function defects cause relatively mild mucocutaneous bleeding symptoms. In these disorders, there is most commonly an abnormality of the storage granules or release mechanism within the platelet causing delayed or diminished response to agonists that induce platelet aggregation like collagen. Platelet function defects, like most other hemostatic defects, are accentuated by medications that impair platelet function. In rare instances, a patient demonstrates impressive petechiae and hematomas at birth because of an absence of one of the essential platelet membrane receptors for the adhesive proteins vWF or fibrinogen. These disorders, *Glanzmann thrombocytopenia* (deficiency of GPIIb/IIIa—the fibrinogen receptor) and *Bernard-Soulier syndrome* (deficiency of glycoprotein Ib—the von Willebrand receptor), provide the most severe types of platelet function defects. The platelet count is normal in Glanzmann thrombocytopenia, but patients with Bernard-Soulier syndrome usually have thrombocytopenia with remarkably large platelets. Patients with mild or moderate platelet function defects often respond to DDAVP, but more severe bleeding may require platelet transfusions.

Chronic Thrombocytopenic Syndromes

Patients with long-standing thrombocytopenia usually present with mucocutaneous bleeding. Mechanisms of the thrombocytopenia include impaired marrow synthesis, sequestration, and increased destruction (see Fig. 51–10). These can be acquired or congenital.

In general, the congenital thrombocytopenic syndromes usually present at the time of birth or early in infancy. These syndromes may be associated with congenital anomalies (TAR syndrome and Fanconi anemia) or as part of a complex hereditary syndrome (Wiskott-Aldrich syndrome with small platelets, and eczema and immunodeficiency) in addition to thrombocytopenia. Small platelets are a frequent finding in many of the syndromes associated with decreased platelet production. During the physical examination of patients with suspect congenital thrombocytopenia, one must search not only for the signs of bleeding but also for subtle congenital anomalies, including abnormal growth parameters, the presence of skin lesions, and anomalies of the limbs, axial skeleton, and urinary tract.

The acquired causes of thrombocytopenia due to decreased production usually have an insidious onset of symptoms and are often associated with other abnormalities in the blood count. The *aplastic syndromes* (congenital aplastic anemia and acquired aplastic anemia) are associated with the gradual onset of thrombocytopenia, usually in association with a falling granulocyte count and anemia (see Chapter 49). Platelets are small, and the mean corpuscular volume is usually elevated.

Infiltration of the marrow by malignant cells or storage cells interferes with normal thrombopoiesis and commonly results in thrombocytopenia. Common malignancies associated with thrombocytopenia include acute lymphoblastic leukemia, lymphomas, histiocytosis X, and metastatic solid tumors (neuroblastoma). Abnormalities of other blood elements as well as findings of adenopathy, hepatosplenomegaly, or masses are clues to the presence of an infiltrative disorder.

Disorders of the vessel walls may present either acutely or chronically. *Vasculitic disorders* often present with lesions of the skin and mucous membranes that appear hemorrhagic and are associated with clinical symptoms related to involvement of other organ systems (gastrointestinal, renal, central nervous system). Paradoxically, patients with these disorders usually have normal coagulation. Henoch-Schönlein purpura is an example and presents with a purpuric rash, including both petechiae and larger palpable purpuric lesions of the lower extremities and buttocks often found in association with arthritis, cramping abdominal pain, and focal glomerulonephritis (see Chapters 57 and 58).

Petechiae and ecchymosis are also common symptoms of disorders of the collagen matrix. Patients with Ehlers-Danlos syndrome have lax joints, hyperelastic skin, and abnormal wound healing. These patients frequently present with ecchymoses and rarely with petechiae. Hemostatic studies are often nondiagnostic, other than that the bleeding time is usually prolonged. The diagnosis is made on the basis of clinical findings, although platelet aggregation studies may be mildly abnormal.

DEEP BLEEDING

Bleeding into the tissues of the muscles or joints is characteristic of hemophilia. The presentation of the patient with hemophilia varies with severity, age, and exposure to trauma. Surprisingly, only one third of boys with hemophilia bleed at circumcision, and neonatal intracranial bleeding is rare despite the trauma of a vaginal delivery. After the neonatal period, children with hemophilia usually present as toddlers with either intramuscular hematomas or hemarthroses. In the toddler stage, the most commonly affected joints are the ankles and elbows, with the knees, hips, and shoulders affected later. The affected boys usually bruise easily, and hematomas frequently develop over common areas of trauma—the forehead, arms, and legs, especially over the pretibial area. Other common bleeding sites include the frenulum and sites of venipuncture. Sites of life-threatening bleeding include the central nervous system (the most common cause of death due to hemorrhage); the mouth and throat, resulting in airway obstruction; and the retroperitoneal area or gastrointestinal tract, leading to exsanguination.

The deficiency of factor VIII (hemophilia A) or factor IX (hemophilia B) causes bleeding because delayed thrombin formation results in a large friable clot. Often there is an initial hemostatic plug that breaks down hours later (secondary bleeding). Because factors VIII and IX are necessary for normal wound healing, patients with inadequate replacement or untreated hemophilia frequently have poorly healed wounds.

Hemophilia A occurs in 1 in 10,000 live births and hemophilia B in about 1 in 40,000. The PTT is prolonged and should correct on 1:1 mix with normal plasma. Specific assays for factors VIII and IX should be done to identify the deficient factor. Severity is determined by the level of the deficient clotting factor. Severe hemophilia is defined as less than 1% factor activity, moderate as 1% to 5% activity, and mild as greater than 5% activity. These factor levels correlate roughly with clinical symptoms, as patients with severe deficiency bleed spontaneously, patients with moderate deficiency bleed with minor trauma, and patients with mild deficiency bleed only after significant trauma and may go undiagnosed for many years.

Because hemophilia A and hemophilia B are transmitted as X-linked traits, the family history may be informative if there is a history of the maternal grandfather or other males on the maternal side with a history of a bleeding disorder. Approximately 33% have new mutations and therefore have a negative family history. Bleeding complications have rarely occurred in carrier females, especially at surgery, thus all carriers should have factor levels measured. The random inactivation of the X chromosome (the *Lyons hypothesis*) predicts that some carriers should be symptomatic because they represent the lower end of the predicted bell-shaped distribution of factor levels for carrier females.

Treatment of hemophilia requires prompt replacement or correction of the deficient factor with the safest available material. Table 51–7 provides dosing information and therapeutic alternatives for factor VIII and IX deficiency. Coverage of bleeding episodes should be maintained until the wound has healed. For factor VIII, the current optimal replacement product appears to be recombinant factor VIII or, as second choice, monoclonally purified factor VIII. For mild hemophilia A patients who respond to DDAVP with adequate levels, DDAVP is the treatment of choice. For factor IX deficiency, highly purified, virally inactivated factor IX concentrates are available. Even when recombinant material is available, all children with bleeding disorders should receive hepatitis B vaccine.

The common complications of hemophilia treatment can be divided into those of immunologic origin and those due to infectious organisms. In 15% to 25% of patients with hemophilia A and in a small percentage of patients with hemophilia B, inhibitors to clotting factor replacement material develop. These inhibitors, usually IgG antibodies, lead to rapid inactivation and clearance of infused replacement material. The presence of an inhibitor should be suspected and tested for in any patient with hemophilia who does not respond appropriately to infusion therapy. The treatment of inhibitors is problematic, includes immune modulation, and should be relegated to experts in hemophilia care.

Infectious complications of hemophilia therapy were once exceedingly common but have fortunately been curtailed by donor screening, sophisticated viral inactivation processes, and chemical purification techniques used in the preparation of replacement material. Recombinant factor VIII represents the culmination of these efforts. Older patients treated prior to 1983 with concentrates were exposed to HIV, hepatitis C (HCV), and sometimes to hepatitis B and the delta agent. Most patients exposed to HIV became infected and manifest the spectrum of signs and symptoms of HIV infection (see Chapter 55). Viral inactivation techniques in conjunction with intense donor screening for HCV antibody has greatly decreased the risk of HCV exposure. Nevertheless, chronic non-A, non-B hepatitis is a common finding in older patients treated with concentrates. Hepatitis B infection was a particular problem for young children treated in the 1970s with concentrates prior to careful donor screening, laboratory testing, and viral inactivation, as children demonstrated a propensity for development of the chronic carrier state for hepatitis B.

Surgical Bleeding

After technical causes, most surgical bleeding results from a failure to recognize a preexisting coagulopathy. Von Willebrand disease and primary or secondary platelet dysfunction are the most common causes of bleeding after ear, nose, and throat surgery. Significant hemorrhaging after general surgery is often a manifestation of previously undiagnosed mild or moderate hemophilia or vitamin K deficiency.

When elective surgery is planned, the decision to perform preoperative hemostatic screening is influenced by the patient's age (and therefore previous exposure to trauma), personal and family history of bleeding, and type of surgery. Certain surgical procedures (tonsillectomy, scoliosis repair, central nervous system surgery) provide major challenges to hemostasis, having a high frequency of bleeding complications. In contrast, most general surgical procedures (hernia repair) rarely involve clinical bleeding. The yield of preoperative studies prior to tonsillectomy and adenoidectomy has been studied and debated at length. In such studies, the frequency of detecting significant hemostatic abnormalities in children with no prior diagnosis of a hemostatic disorder has varied from 0.5% to 11.5%. Most of these studies have not included von Willebrand activity levels as part of the laboratory screening tests.

GENERALIZED BLEEDING

Generalized bleeding is a manifestation of a major disorder of hemostasis, usually due to a deficiency of multiple factors in association with deficient or dysfunctional platelets. Generalized bleeding occurs most commonly in the context of a consumption coagulopathy in seriously ill patients, with the most severe form termed disseminated intravascular coagulation (DIC). Rarely, rat poison (warfarin) intoxication produces such bleeding.

DISSEMINATED INTRAVASCULAR COAGULATION (DIC)

DIC is a generalized consumption of clotting factors, anticoagulant proteins, and platelets triggered by a critical illness and usually accompanied by ischemia, hypoxia, and shock (Table 51–8). DIC may be either a hemorrhagic or a thrombotic disorder, or both, as the clinical manifestations of this generalized coagulopathy are highly variable. Laboratory studies usually demonstrate a prolonged PT, decreased fibrinogen, and decreased platelets (these are the most reliable indicators of DIC) in addition to increased FDPs (and elevated D-dimer) and a prolonged PTT.

Several mechanisms can trigger acute DIC, including widespread endothelial damage induced directly or indirectly by infectious organisms and release of procoagulant material after trauma. Virtu-

Table 51–8. Causes of Disseminated Intravascular Coagulation

Infectious
  Meningococcemia (purpura fulminans)
  Other gram-negative bacteria *(Haemophilus, Salmonella, Escherichia coli)*
  Gram-positive bacteria (group B streptococci, staphylococci)
  Rickettsia (Rocky Mountain spotted fever)
  Virus (cytomegalovirus, herpes, hemorrhagic fevers)
  Malaria
  Fungus

Tissue Injury
  Central nervous system trauma (massive head injury)
  Multiple fractures with fat emboli
  Crush injury
  Profound shock or asphyxia
  Hypothemia or hyperthermia
  Massive burns

Malignancy
  Acute promyelocytic leukemia
  Acute monoblastic or myelocytic leukemia
  Widespread malignancies (neuroblastoma)

Venom or Toxin
  Snake bites
  Insect bites

Microangiopathic Disorders
  ''Severe'' thrombotic thrombocytopenic purpura or hemolytic-uremic syndrome
  Giant hemangioma (Kasabach-Merritt syndrome)

Gastrointestinal Disorders
  Fulminant hepatitis
  Severe inflammation bowel disease
  Reye syndrome

Hereditary Thrombotic Disorders
  Antithrombin III deficiency
  Homozygous protein C deficiency

Newborn
  Maternal toxemia
  Group B streptococcal infections
  Abruptio placentae
  Severe respiratory distress syndrome
  Necrotizing enterocolitis
  Congenital viral disease (cytomegalovirus, herpes)
  Erythroblastosis fetalis

Miscellaneous
  Severe acute graft rejection
  Acute hemolytic transfusion reaction
  Severe collagen-vascular disease
  Kawasaki disease
  Heparin-induced thrombosis
  Infusion of ''activated'' prothrombin complex concentrates
  Hyperpyrexia/encephalopathy, hemorrhagic shock syndrome

Modified from Montgomery RR, Scott JP. Hemostasis: Diseases of the fluid phase. *In* Nathan DG, Oski FA (eds). Hematology of Infancy and Childhood, 4th ed. Vol 2. Philadelphia: WB Saunders, 1993:1639.

ally any life-threatening illness can trigger DIC. In acute DIC, activation of the clotting mechanism leads to consumption of specific clotting factors, especially fibrinogen, prothrombin (II), factor V, factor VIII, platelets, and the anticoagulant proteins that serve to modulate hemostasis, especially protein C, ATIII, and plasminogen. Table 51–9 presents a comparison of laboratory findings in DIC

compared with other acquired coagulopathies that potentially could be confused with DIC. Because DIC is virtually always seen in a child with a life-threatening illness, the clinical diagnosis is usually made on the basis of the child's clinical appearance in association with laboratory abnormalities. Clotting factor and anticoagulant protein levels are confirmatory but seldom necessary to reach a diagnosis of DIC. The only diagnosis difficult to differentiate from DIC in the laboratory is that of severe hepatic disease with impending liver failure. The patient with severe liver disease is invariably markedly jaundiced; thrombocytopenia is relatively mild.

The treatment of DIC focuses on its pathophysiology and complications (the disorder that caused the DIC), the aberrations in homeostasis that sustain the coagulopathy, and the bleeding or thrombotic complications that ensue. Shock itself plays a critical role in DIC because shock reduces the reticuloendothelial clearance of activated clotting factors and complexes. Reduced hepatic blood flow causes decreased synthesis of depleted clotting and anticoagulant proteins.

To summarize the treatment of DIC:

1. Treat the trigger.
2. Optimize cardiorespiratory status by correcting acidosis and improving perfusion.
3. Replace deficient platelets, clotting factors, and anticoagulant proteins (Table 51–10). Specific indications for replacement are variable and depend on the patient's clinical condition and severity of bleeding.

The following are rough guidelines for treatment:

- Fresh frozen plasma, 10 to 15 cc/kg every 6 to 12 hours to provide clotting factors
- Platelets, one bag/5 kg for platelet count <50,000 mm³
- Cryoprecipitate, one bag/5 kg for fibrinogen <100 mg/dl

The role of anticoagulant therapy in DIC has not been proven in controlled prospective studies. Heparin has been used for the treatment of purpura fulminans, acute promyelocytic leukemia, and thromboses that develop in conjunction with DIC. Although most patients with DIC have a coagulopathy that consumes procoagulant proteins and causes clinical oozing or bleeding, in a small percentage of patients thrombosis develops. In these patients, anticoagulant therapy may decrease morbidity and should be utilized in a manner similar to that used for those patients who have major vascular thrombosis (Table 51–11). Deficient clotting factors and platelets should be transfused to prevent further development of thrombosis or bleeding during anticoagulation. In the syndrome known as *purpura fulminans,* microvascular thromboses develop in the skin, and heparin has been helpful in preventing the progression of the illness. In rare cases of partially compensated DIC, heparin therapy has been used to slow the coagulopathy, but there are no studies that document the benefits of heparin in such circumstances.

Finally, in some patients with DIC and poor peripheral perfusion, particularly those in whom the extremities are cool and cyanotic, low-dose heparin (5 to 10 units/kg/hour) has been tried to prevent small- and large-vessel thromboses. In the future, such patients may be treated with infusion of protein C or ATIII concentrates, or both, to restore normal levels of circulating anticoagulant proteins.

Neonatal Purpura Fulminans

The neonate who presents with multiple purpuric lesions over the buttocks, trunk, extremities, and face (nose, ears) that change from dark red to purple and black over a few minutes in association with abnormal neurologic findings or an abdominal mass presents a special case.

Although the differential diagnosis of these findings should include sepsis with DIC or a generalized viral infection, or both, the

Table 51–9. Differential Diagnosis of Coagulopathies That Can Be Confused with Disseminated Intravascular Coagulation (DIC)

	Prothrombin Time	Partial Thromboplastin Time	Fibrinogen	Platelets	Fibrinogen Degradation Products	Clinical Keys
DIC	↑	↑	↓	↓	↑	Shock (see Table 51–8)
Liver failure	↑	↑	↓	Normal or ↓	↑	Jaundice
Vitamin K deficiency	↑	↑	Normal	Normal	Normal	Malabsorption, liver disease
Sepsis without shock	↑	↑	Normal	Normal	↑ or normal	Fever

key finding in such a child is the presence of painful petechiae and purpura (purpura fulminans). The most likely diagnosis with this presentation is homozygous protein C deficiency. After viral and bacterial cultures, diagnostic studies should include CBC, platelet count, and coagulation screen for DIC as well as measurements of protein C, protein S, ATIII, and plasminogen.

To confirm this diagnosis, one must differentiate DIC from congenital protein C deficiency. DIC is characterized by the consumption of clotting factors, anticoagulant proteins, and platelets. Although protein C levels fall in DIC, patients with congenital protein C deficiency have strikingly low levels of protein C, in contrast to depressed but measurable levels of protein S, ATIII, and plasminogen. Anticoagulant proteins are routinely consumed in situations of widespread activation of the clotting mechanism. Therefore, the mildly depressed levels of protein S, ATIII, and plasminogen would be expected when there is generalized intravascular coagulation. In congenital protein C deficiency, the protein C level is strikingly lower than that of the other anticoagulant proteins, increasing the likelihood that the deficiency of protein C represents the primary cause of the coagulopathy. To clarify the situation, the next step is to obtain blood samples from the parents to define whether either or both demonstrate a deficiency of a specific anticoagulant protein, especially protein C. The usual adult case of protein C, or protein S or ATIII, deficiency presents as venous thromboembolic disease in early adulthood and is inherited as a codominant trait. Congenital severe, symptomatic protein C deficiency is usually inherited in an autosomal recessive manner from asymptomatic parents.

Therapy must be instituted promptly to replace the deficient anticoagulant protein with fresh frozen plasma. Fresh frozen plasma contains all of the clotting factors in an unconcentrated form. Protein C has a short half-life and may need to be infused every 6 to 12 hours to maintain measurable levels. This unfortunately leads to problems with fluid and protein overload if repeated doses of plasma are necessary. A new protein C concentrate is under development and, when available, the patient should be treated with protein C concentrate to correct the deficiency. The patient should also be heparinized to limit further thromboses. A striking improvement following administration of protein C, either as plasma or as concentrate, is strong evidence suggestive of the diagnosis. Warfarin therapy has been effective in managing these patients on a chronic basis.

Other Causes of Generalized Bleeding

A coagulopathy is a common complication of severe *liver disease* as a result of a deficiency of multiple clotting factors in association with increased FDPs formed due to hyperfibrinolysis. FDPs inhibit platelet function.

Uremia also results in a diffuse bleeding diathesis, with mucosal

Table 51–10. Commonly Used Hemostatic Agents

Component	Contents	Usual Dose	Comments/Disadvantages
FFP (unit)	1 unit/cc of each clotting factor	10–15 cc/kg	Large volume
Cryoprecepitate (bag)	100 units factor/bag 150 mg fibrinogen/bag Factor XIII, fibronectin	0.2 bag/kg 16 μg/5 kg	Infectious risk
Platelets (unit)	5.0–7.0 × 10¹⁰ platelets in 30–60 cc plasma	0.2 units/kg	Infectious risk
Factor concentrates	Units as labeled	Factor VIII 20–50 units/kg Factor IX 30–80 units/kg	Virally inactivated
DDAVP	10–50 μg vial	0.3 μg/kg/dose	Increase factor VIII, vWf 3- to 4-fold; useful for platelet function defects
ATIII concentrate	Units as labeled	$\dfrac{(\text{Desired—baseline ATIII}) \times \text{weight}}{1.4}$	Plasma-derived viral inactivated

Key Points to Transfusion

1. Determine deficiency state.
2. Use appropriate dose and material.
3. Measure response 1–2 hr and 24 hr after transfusion.

Abbreviations: FFP = fresh frozen plasma: DDAVP = desmopressin; vWf = von Willebrand factor; ATIII = antithrombin III.

Table 51–11. Comparison of Fibrinolytic and Anticoagulant Agents Used in the Treatment of Thromboembolic Disease

	Fibrinolytic Therapy	Heparin	Warfarin
Indication	Recent onset of life- or limb-threatening thrombus	Thrombus of indeterminate age	Long-term oral anticoagulation
Dose	TPA 0.1–0.2 mg/kg/hr IV UK 4400 units/kg/hr IV	50 units/kg/bolus, 20–25 units/kg/hr by continuous infusion	0.1–0.2 mg/kg/day p.o.
Adjustment	↑ Dose by 10% until "lytic" state is achieved	↑ Dose by 5–10% q6hr until adequate level of PTT achieved	Daily until stable INR
Course	12–72 hr	5–14 days	Weeks to months
Monitors	"Lytic state" ↑ FDP or D-dimer (TPA) ↓ Fibrinogen by 25% (UK) ↑ Thrombin time (UK)	PTT 2–2½ times control, thrombin time infinity Heparin level 0.3–0.7 unit/dl	INR 2.0–3.0
Mechanism	Activation of plasminogen to plasmin	Accelerates ATIII-dependent inactivation of factors IIa, Xa	Impairs vitamin K–dependent carboxylation of factors II, VII, IX, X
Risk of bleeding	Medium/high	Low	Low

Abbreviations: TPA = recombinant tissue type plasminogen activator; UK = urokinase; IIa = thrombin; INR = international normalized ratio; PTT = partial thromboplastin time; FDP = fibrin degradation product.

bleeding (epistaxis, gastrointestinal bleeding) as a major manifestation. These symptoms have been ascribed to the adverse effects of uremic toxins on platelet function, although there may be coexistent abnormalities of endothelial cells and perhaps clotting factors. Patients with bleeding due to uremia or liver disease frequently respond to DDAVP.

Vitamin K deficiency may be manifested as generalized bleeding into the skin, gastrointestinal tract, and central nervous system. Patients at highest risk are neonates, malnourished individuals, those receiving broad-spectrum antibiotics, and children with cholestatic liver disease and subsequent vitamin K malabsorption. The treatment of patients with vitamin K deficiency as the cause of generalized bleeding is parenteral vitamin K. The response is usually rapid, but in emergent situations fresh frozen plasma corrects the coagulopathy. Differentiation of some of these syndromes from DIC is presented in Table 51–9.

THROMBOSIS

Thromboembolic disease in pediatrics has a bimodal age distribution. Venous and arterial thrombi are common in the newborn and especially in the premature neonate because of the combination of low levels of anticoagulant proteins, decreased blood flow, elevated blood viscosity because of high hematocrit, and, especially, because of the placement of intravascular catheters for monitoring and nutrition. The second peak of thromboembolic disease, usually venous in character, is in adolescence, when patients with primary deficiencies of anticoagulant proteins typically present and when secondary disorders (e.g., vasculitis, pregnancy, surgery, major trauma, collagen-vascular disorders, and infection) induce a higher frequency of venous thrombosis.

Venous Thromboembolic Disease

DIAGNOSTIC APPROACH

Venous thromboembolic disease classically presents with a warm, swollen, tender extremity or affected organ. The differential

diagnosis in such cases includes trauma, infection, stasis without thrombosis, lymphedema, and neoplasm. In children and adolescents, thrombi may develop within major internal organs with distinctive clinical presentations, including sagittal sinus thrombosis with resultant increased intracranial pressure, hepatic vein thrombosis with the Budd-Chiari syndrome, portal vein thrombosis associated with splenomegaly and varices, and renal vein thrombosis with a resultant abdominal mass, hematuria, and proteinuria.

One should obtain a careful history for antecedent trauma, infection, or other predisposing causes of thromboembolic disease (Table 51–12). The abdomen and extremities should be carefully examined for mass lesions leading to venous stasis. The presence of a bruit or hemihypertrophy of the affected limb is a clue to an arteriovenous malformation. In addition, masses within the bone, abdominal tumors, and lymphatic obstruction should be considered. Initial laboratory studies should include a CBC, platelet count, and evaluation for DIC as well as cultures of the blood if the patient is febrile. During the process of a localized thrombosis, there may be consumption of clotting factors, but rarely is the consumption significant enough in older children and adults to induce abnormal routine coagulation screening tests (platelets, PT, PTT, fibrinogen). Tests for fibrin breakdown (FDPs, D-dimer) may be positive. Unfortunately, these tests are nonspecific and not necessarily diagnostic of vascular thrombosis. The diagnostic approach to a patient with suspected venous thrombosis is presented in Figure 51–11.

SPECIFIC DIAGNOSTIC STUDIES

Venography remains the gold standard for the diagnosis of venous thromboembolic disease. Doppler flow studies, compression ultrasonography, and various forms of plethysmography have been studied with variable results.

Doppler studies detect the flow of red blood cells through the artery or vein being examined. Plethysmography measures the change in blood volume within the extremity that occurs with respiration. If there is obstruction to flow, the normal physiologic variation is diminished.

Compression ultrasonography simply assesses the ability of the

Table 51–12. Hypercoagulable States

Primary Disorders (Congenital)
Antithrombin III deficiency
Protein C deficiency
Protein S deficiency
Dysfibrinogenemia
Plasminogen deficiencies
Resistance to activated protein C (factor V Leiden)

Secondary Disorders
Coagulopathies
   Nephrotic syndrome
   Oral contraceptives (estrogen)
   Malignancy
   Therapy with activated prothrombin complex
      concentrates
   Pregnancy
   Lupus anticoagulant (antiphospholipid antibody)
   Autoimmune disorders

Platelet Disorders
   Diabetes mellitus
   Myeloproliferative disorders
   Thrombocythemia
   Paroxysmal nocturnal hemoglobinuria

Flow and Vessel Disorders
   Polycythemia–hyperviscosity
   Homocystinuria
   Marfan syndrome
   Vasculitis
   Vessel grafts
   Vascular stasis
   Trauma
   Indwelling catheters
   Surgery
   Immobilization

Adapted from Schafer A. The hypercoagulable states. Ann Intern Med 1985; 102:814; and from Behrman RE, Kliegman RM (eds). Nelson Essentials of Pediatrics, 2nd ed. Philadelphia: WB Saunders, 1994:56.

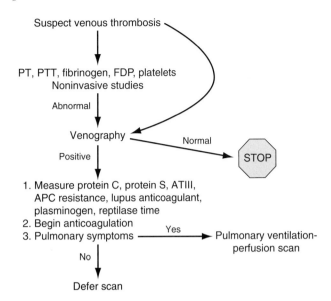

Figure 51–11. Flow diagram for the approach to a patient with venous thromboembolic disease. APC = activated protein C; ATIII = antithrombin III; PT = prothrombin time; PTT = partial thromboplastin time.

ultrasound probe to fully compress (completely lose the image of the lumen) when pressure is applied to the probe overlying the vessel in question. Fluid-filled vessels are readily compressible, whereas those in which a clot is present in the lumen are not. When these have been compared with venography, variable results have been obtained, suggesting significant differences in the techniques employed. Although repetitive Doppler studies and plethysmography appear to be relatively sensitive and specific, their sensitivity and specificity in children have not been documented. Prior to committing a child to long-term anticoagulant therapy, it is best to document the presence of thrombosis by the most accurate tool currently available, contrast venography.

Levels of the circulating anticoagulant proteins, protein C, protein S, ATIII, and plasminogen, should be measured to determine whether a congenital deficiency is present. Unfortunately, levels of protein C, ATIII, and plasminogen may be depleted after development of deep venous thrombosis or pulmonary emboli, or both. As such, low levels do not necessarily imply a congenital deficiency of protein C, plasminogen, or ATIII. If low levels are found, studies should be performed on the parents to establish the inheritance of the deficiency, as these are all inherited as autosomal codominant traits. Tests for resistance to activated protein C (factor V Leiden), as well as studies for the lupus anticoagulant, should also be performed. The lupus anticoagulant typically yields a prolonged PTT that fails to correct on mixing with normal plasma because of the presence of an antibody that reacts with the phospholipid

reagent in the PTT but does not bind *in vivo* to the platelet membrane. Paradoxically, the lupus anticoagulant has been clinically associated with venous and arterial thromboembolic disease and spontaneous abortions but is usually not a cause of clinical bleeding. If these studies are negative, a thrombin time or a comparison of functional and antigenic levels of fibrinogen should be done to detect a *dysfibrinogenemia*.

Abnormalities of protein C or protein S may be identified in 25% of the children with deep venous thrombosis. Furthermore, 40% to 60% of patients with familial or recurrent thrombotic disease have a congenital resistance to activated protein C as the cause of their prothrombotic condition. This resistance results from a structural abnormality of factor V, rendering it resistant to proteolysis by activated protein C.

After a diagnosis of deep venous thrombosis has been made, one must assess the risk of propagation and embolization of the thrombus. Calf vein thrombi rarely embolize and therefore are usually treated symptomatically. More proximal thrombi have a much higher likelihood of propagation and embolization and thus demand systemic anticoagulation. If the patient has respiratory symptoms of any sort, a ventilation-perfusion scan to evaluate for pulmonary emboli is warranted. Patients with symptoms suspicious of pulmonary disease require closer monitoring and more vigorous therapy (see Chapter 8).

Arterial Thrombosis

Arterial thrombi are remarkably rare in older children and adolescents and are frequently a manifestation of a systemic disorder resulting in vascular damage or embolic disease (sickle cell anemia, Kawasaki disease, bacterial endocarditis, periarteritis nodosa). The presence of an intra-arterial catheter is an obvious nidus for thrombosis.

Anticoagulant Therapy

HEPARIN

Heparin is the most commonly used agent for the initial treatment of venous or arterial thrombosis. Heparin functions as an anticoagulant by binding to ATIII and accelerating the ATIII-dependent inactivation of thrombin and factor Xa as well as factors IXa and XIa. Although most studies of heparin pharmacokinetics have been performed in adults, there are important differences in the pharmacology of heparin in children and especially neonates. Thirty-nine percent of children achieve a prolongation of the PTT within the target range following a bolus dose of 50 units/kg. Children under 1 year of age required an average of 28 units/kg/hour to maintain a therapeutic level of the PTT. In contrast, most children older than 1 year of age are satisfactorily maintained on 20 units/kg/hour of heparin. One protocol recommends an initial bolus of 50 units/kg of heparin, with 20 to 25 units/kg/hour for a minimum of 5 days to maintain a PTT of approximately 2 to 2½ times the control value. The heparin dose should be adjusted every 4 to 6 hours until a satisfactory level is attained. Reports in adults suggest that the heparin level is a better monitor for appropriate heparin therapy. Heparin levels can be especially useful in the premature and term newborn who may have a "normal" prolonged PTT. A therapeutic range of 0.3 to 0.6 units/dl appears to be effective.

The import of measuring heparin levels and the PTT to achieve prompt therapeutic levels has been underscored by studies in adults that have documented an increased risk of recurrent thrombi in patients who failed to achieve adequate anticoagulant levels promptly. Low-molecular-weight heparins may be equally effective with a lower risk of bleeding. Warfarin can be started soon after the institution of heparin therapy; 5 days of heparin therapy is as good as longer courses of treatment for routine venous thrombotic disease.

FIBROLYTIC THERAPY

Fibrinolytic therapy is indicated for serious and potentially life-threatening thrombosis. Fibrinolytic therapy provides for more rapid lysis of clots than standard anticoagulant treatment with heparin and is clinically effective in both arterial and venous clots. Because bleeding complications are many-fold higher than heparin in older individuals, the clinical severity of the clot must justify the use of lytic therapy. For smaller thrombi or those in nonvital locations, heparin is safe and effective. Lytic therapy is best used early in the evolution of the thrombus. If the clot has been long-standing, it is unlikely that fibrinolytic therapy will be efficacious.

The presence of any intracranial process, recent major surgery, or recent significant bleeding is an absolute contraindication to fibrinolytic therapy and a relative contraindication to heparin treatment. With a normal cranial sonogram (or CT) and complete occlusion of the aorta or evidence of compromise of major organ function, fibrinolytic therapy has been safely and successfully administered with very careful monitoring. Table 51–11 outlines dose and monitoring studies for two commonly used fibrinolytic agents, rTPA and urokinase (UK). Fibrinolytic therapy appears to result in a more rapid return of pulmonary artery flow following pulmonary emboli and may decrease the likelihood of postphlebitic syndrome after deep venous thrombosis.

WARFARIN

Warfarin (Coumadin) is the anticoagulant of choice for long-term oral therapy. Warfarin acts by blocking the vitamin K–dependent post-translational modification of factors II, VII, IX, and X as well as protein C and protein S. The usual dose is 0.05 to 0.2 mg/kg/day. Younger children appear to require higher doses to achieve a therapeutic level of the international normalized ratio

(INR).* If warfarin therapy is started early in the course of heparin therapy for thrombotic disease, effective oral anticoagulant effect will often have been achieved by day 5, at which time levels of all the vitamin K–dependent factors should be depressed by warfarin.

Early in the course of treatment with warfarin, the PT is affected first because factor VII has the shortest half-life of the vitamin K–dependent procoagulants and factor VII levels fall briskly following warfarin treatment. The aim of warfarin therapy for venous thromboembolic disease is to achieve a stable INR of 2.0 to 3.0.

For prevention of embolization from prosthetic valves, an INR of 3.0 to 4.0 is preferable. Patients with protein C or protein S deficiency are at risk for warfarin-induced skin necrosis when warfarin therapy is initiated, particularly if high doses are used. These individuals should be heparinized before warfarin is started, and they should not receive a loading (high) dose.

SUMMARY AND RED FLAGS

Bleeding and thrombotic problems are often familial but may be acquired. A family history and personal history that quantitate bleeding episodes are of utmost help in planning an evaluation. Red flags include signs of end-organ bleeding, particularly the central nervous system (coagulopathy, trauma, vascular malformation, thrombocytopenia), signs of a systemic disorder (pancytopenia, hypotension, rash, liver-renal-pulmonary system involvement), and signs of hemorrhagic shock.

REFERENCES

General

Andrew M, Paes B, Johnston M. Development of the hemostatic system in the neonate and young infant. Am J Pediatr Hematol Oncol 1990;12:95–104.

Andrew M, Vegh P, Johnston M, et al. Maturation of the hemostatic system during childhood. Blood 1992;80:1998–2005.

Burk CD, Miller L, Handler SD, et al. Preoperative history and coagulation screening in children undergoing tonsillectomy. Pediatrics 1992;89:691–695.

Hathaway WE, Goodnight S. Disorders of Hemostasis and Thrombosis: A Clinical Guide. New York: McGraw-Hill, 1993:50–57, 68–72, 219–229.

Kitchens CS. Approach to the bleeding patient. Hematol Oncol Clin North Am 1993;6:983–989.

Manno CS. Difficult pediatric diagnoses: Bleeding and bruising. Pediatr Clin North Am 1991;38:637–655.

Nosek-Cenkowska B, Cheang MS, Pizzi NJ, et al. Bleeding and bruising symptomatology in children with and without bleeding disorders. Thromb Haemost 1991;65:237–241.

Coagulopathy

Corrigan JJ Jr, Jordan CM, Bennett B. Disseminated intravascular coagulation in septic shock. Report of three cases not treated with heparin. Am J Dis Child 1974;126:629.

Desposito F, Arkel Y. Inhibitors of coagulation in children. Crit Rev Oncol Hematol 1987;7:53–69.

---

*The INR corrects the PT for institutional differences in reagents and instruments. When on a stable warfarin dose, the INR is calculated by a ratio of the patient's PT to the control PT raised to a correction factor (the ISI) that allows for comparison of different PT reagents and machines in different laboratories. All patients on chronic warfarin therapy should have their anticoagulant therapy measured as the INR. The INR level should be maintained between 2.0 and 3.0 for effective, safe anticoagulant therapy. An INR (>3.0) has been associated with increased risk of bleeding without improved therapeutic effects for patients with venous thromboembolic disease.

Furie BC. The molecular basis of blood coagulation. Cell 1988;53:505.

Kasper CK. Complications of hemophilia A treatment: Factor VIII inhibitors. Ann N Y Acad Sci 1991;614:97–105.

Mannucci PM. Desmopressin: A non-transfusional form of treatment for congenital and acquired bleeding disorders. Blood 1988;72:1449–1455.

Montgomery RR, Hilgartner MW. Understanding Von Willebrand Disease. New York: National Hemophilia Foundation, 1991:1–19.

Scott JP, Montgomery RR. The treatment of von Willebrand disease. Semin Thromb Hemost 1993;19:37–47.

Werner EJ, Abshire TC, Giroux DS, et al. Relative value of diagnostic studies for von Willebrand disease. J Pediatr 1992;121;34–38.

Yeowell HN, Pinnell SR. The Ehlers-Danlos syndromes. Semin Dermatol 1993;12:229–40.

Platelets

Beardsley DS. Immune thrombocytopenia in the perinatal period. Semin Perinatol 1990;14:368–373.

Bussel JB. Thrombocytopenia in newborns, infants, and children. Pediatr Ann 1990;19:181–193.

Bussel JB, Graziano JN, Kimberly RP, et al. IV anti-D treatment of ITP: Analysis of efficacy, toxicity, and mechanism of effect. Blood 1991;77:1884–1893.

Halperin D, Doyle JJ. Is bone marrow examination justified in idiopathic thrombocytopenic purpura. Am J Dis Child 1988;142:508–512.

Thrombosis

Andrew M, David M, Adams M, et al. Venous thromboembolic complications (VTE) in children: First analyses of the Canadian Registry of VTE. Blood 1994;83:1251–1257.

Bauer KA, Rosenberg RD. The pathophysiology of the prethrombotic state in humans: Insights gained from studies using markers of hemostatic system. Blood 1987;70:343.

Dahlback B, Hildebrand B. Inherited resistance to activated protein C is corrected by anticoagulant cofactor activity found to be a property of factor V. Proc Natl Acad Sci USA 1994;91:1396–1400.

David M, Andrew M. Venous thromboembolic complications in children. J Pediatr 1993;123:337–346.

Love PE, Santoro SA. Antiphospholipid antibodies: Anticardiolipin and the lupus anticoagulant in systemic lupus erythematosus (SLE) and in non-SLE disorders. Ann Intern Med 1990;112:682–688.

Schafer AI. The hypercoagulable states. Ann Intern Med 1985;102:814.

Therapy

Andrew M, Marzinotto V, Brooker LA, et al. Oral anticoagulation therapy in pediatric patients: A prospective study. Thromb Haemost 1994;71:265–269.

Andrew M, Marzinotto V, Massicotte P, et al. Heparin therapy in pediatric patients: A prospective cohort study. Pediatr Res 1994;35:78–83.

Hull RD, Raskob GE, Rosenbloom D, et al. Heparin for 5 days as compared with 10 days in the initial treatment of proximal venous thrombosis. N Engl J Med 1990;322:1260–1264.

Levy M, Benson LN, Burrows PE, et al. Tissue plasminogen activator for the treatment of thromboembolism in infants and children. J Pediatr 1991;118:467–472.

Limentani SA, Roth DA, Furie BC, et al. Recombinant blood clotting proteins for hemophilia therapy. Semin Thromb Hemost 1993;19:62–72.

Mannucci PM. Modern treatment of hemophilia: From the shadows towards the light. Thromb Haemost 1993;70:17–23.

Marder VJ, Sherry S. Thrombolytic therapy: Current status. N Engl J Med 1988;318:1512.

McDonald MM, Hathaway WE. Anticoagulant therapy by continuous heparinization in newborn and older infants. J Pediatr 1982;101:451.

Weinmann E, Salzman E: Deep-vein thrombosis. N Engl J Med 1994;331:1630.

Infectious Disorders

52 Recurrent Infection

Laurence A. Boxer   R. Alexander Blackwood

The function of the immune system is to prevent and retard the local establishment or systemic dissemination of bacteria, viruses, fungi, and protozoa. The immune system is composed of four primary components:

1. *Antibody-mediated immunity* (B-cell immunity) produces antibody in the secretions, plasma, and interstitial spaces after activation of bone marrow–derived lymphocytes (B cells).

2. *Cell-mediated immunity* (T-cell immunity) carries out its function by means of thymus-derived lymphocytes (T cells) in the blood and peripheral lymphoid tissue. The B cells are precursors of immunoglobulin-producing cells. Neither T cells nor mononuclear cells produce immunoglobulin, but they are necessary for B-cell function. T cells regulate the production of antibody, and macrophages are necessary for antigen presentation, which allows a normal immune response to occur.

3. The *phagocytic system* consists of macrophages, monocytes, and neutrophils within the blood and in the tissue engaged in phagocytosing and killing microorganisms.

4. The *complement system* acts synergistically with the remainder of the immune system to amplify resistance to microbial infection.

Defects in each of these systems are associated with immunodeficiency states and at times produce characteristic infections (Table 52–1).

Table 52–1.   **Risk Factors and Related Pathogens Affecting Immunocompromised Patients**

GRANULOCYTOPENIA (e.g., aplastic anemia, congenital, myelophthisis, myelosuppressive agents, bone marrow transplant)
Bacteria
  Gram-Negative Organisms
    Escherichia coli (sepsis, pneumonia, pyelonephritis)
    Klebsiella pneumoniae (sepsis, pneumonia)
    Pseudomonas aeruginosa (sepsis, pneumonia, cutaneous lesions)
    Mixed anaerobic and aerobic enteric bacteria (typhlitis, perianal abscess)
  Gram-Positive Organisms
    Staphylococcus aureus (sepsis, cellulitis, soft tissue infection)
    Staphylococcus epidermidis (sepsis, line infection)
    Corynebacterium JK (sepsis)
    α-Hemolytic streptococci (sepsis)
Fungi
  Candida (sepsis, pneumonia, ophthalmitis, liver and spleen abscesses)
  Aspergillus (sepsis, pneumonia, sinusitis, central nervous system [CNS] infection, cutaneous lesions)
  Mucormycosis (pneumonia, sinusitis, CNS infection)
  Fusarium (sepsis, cutaneous lesions, pneumonia)
  Pseudoallescheria (sepsis, cutaneous lesions, pneumonia)
  Alternaria (sepsis, cutaneous lesions)

PHAGOCYTIC DYSFUNCTION (e.g., chronic granulomatous disease, hyperimmunoglobulin E syndrome, leukocyte adhesion defects)
Bacteria
  S. aureus (soft tissue, skeletal, and solid organ abscesses; pneumonia, sepsis)
  Streptococci (soft tissue, skeletal, and solid organ abscesses; pneumonia, sepsis)
  Serratia marcescens (soft tissue and solid organ abscesses, pneumonia, sepsis)
  E. coli (soft tissue and solid organ abscesses, pneumonia, sepsis)
  Pseudomonas cepacia (soft tissue abscess, pneumonia, sepsis)
  Salmonella (enteritis)
  Nocardia (soft tissue and solid organ abscesses, pneumonia)
Fungi
  Candida (soft tissue, skeletal, and solid organ abscesses, pneumonia, sepsis)
  Aspergillus (soft tissue abscess, pneumonia, sepsis)

CELLULAR IMMUNE DEFICIENCY (e.g., congenital, acquired immunodeficiency syndrome, immunosuppression, corticosteroid use, transplantation, Hodgkin disease)
Bacteria
  Listeria monocytogenes (sepsis, meningitis)
  Salmonella (sepsis)
  Mycobacterium tuberculosis (pneumonia, disseminated disease)
  Atypical mycobacteria *(M. avium, M. intracellulare)* (sepsis, pneumonia, disseminated disease)
  Nocardia (pneumonia, CNS infection)
  Legionella (pneumonia)
Fungi
  Cryptococcus neoformans (sepsis, meningitis)
  Histoplasma capsulatum (pneumonia, disseminated disease)
  Coccidioides immitis (pneumonia, meningitis)
Viruses
  Varicella-zoster (cutaneous and CNS infection, pneumonia, hepatitis)
  Cytomegalovirus (bone marrow infection, hepatitis, pneumonia, retinitis, esophagitis, colitis, CNS infection)
  Herpes simplex (CNS infection, pneumonia, esophagitis, hepatitis, disseminated disease)
  Epstein-Barr virus (lymphoma)
  Measles (pneumonia, encephalitis)
  Polyomavirus BK (hemorrhagic cystitis, ureteric stenosis, renal insufficiency)
  Polyomavirus JC (progressive multifocal leukoencephalopathy)
Protozoa
  Pneumocystis carinii (pneumonia, rare extrapulmonary spread)
  Toxoplasma gondii (CNS infection, myocarditis)
  Cryptosporidium (enteritis)
Helminth
  Strongyloides stercoralis (enteritis, pneumonia, sepsis, meningitis)

Table 52–1. **Risk Factors and Related Pathogens Affecting Immunocompromised Patients** *Continued*

HUMORAL DEFECTS (e.g., congenital, immunoglobulin, complement, properdin deficiencies)
Bacteria
  Streptococcus pneumoniae (sepsis, meningitis, sinopulmonary infection)
  Haemophilus influenzae (sepsis, meningitis, arthritis, sinopulmonary infection)
  Neisseria meningitidis (sepsis, meningitis, arthritis)
  Neisseria gonorrhoeae (sepsis, meningitis, arthritis)
  Mycoplasma pneumoniae (arthritis)
  Campylobacter (enteritis)
Virus
  Enterovirus including polio vaccine (encephalitis, paralysis, myositis, arthritis)
  Rotavirus (enteritis)
Protozoa
  Giardia lamblia (enteritis)

SPLENIC DYSFUNCTION (e.g., asplenia, sickle cell anemia, splenectomy: a combined immunoglobulin and reticuloendothelial cell deficiency)
Bacteria
  S. pneumoniae (sepsis, meningitis)
  H. influenzae type b (sepsis, meningitis)
  N. meningitidis (sepsis, meningitis)
  Capnocytophaga canimorsus (sepsis, meningitis)
Protozoa
  Babesiosis
  Malaria

Adapted from Behrman RE (ed). Nelson Texbook of Pediatrics, 14th ed. Philadelphia: WB Saunders, 1992:671.

The differential diagnosis for a patient presenting with recurrent infections is formidable, given the complexity of the immune system (Table 52–2). Similarities in the clinical presentation of neutrophil, antibody, and complement disorders can further complicate attempts to establish their diagnosis. Infants and children who are brought to the physician for ''repeated infections'' must be carefully evaluated. Often these patients ultimately have no identifiable underlying disease, and they frequently have respiratory allergy or other risks for recurrent infections (Table 52–3). Most patients with recurrent infections do not have an identifiable phagocyte defect or immune deficiency. Given the low probability of identifying a discrete immune defect, the physician faces the difficult decision of which patients merit a complete evaluation.

In general, evaluation should be initiated for those who have at least one of the following clinical features: (1) more than two systemic bacterial infections (sepsis, meningitis, osteomyelitis); (2) three serious respiratory infections (pneumonia, sinusitis) or bacterial infections (cellulitis, draining otitis media, lymphadenitis) per year; (3) the presence of an infection at an unusual site (hepatic or brain abscess); (4) infections with unusual pathogens (*Aspergillus* pneumonia, disseminated candidiasis, or infection with *Serratia marcescens*, *Nocardia* sp, *Pseudomonas cepacia*); and (5) infections of unusual severity.

It is important to remember two caveats: (1) respiratory allergy, such as asthma or allergic rhinitis, can mimic respiratory infections, and (2) a single chronic infection may wax and wane with intermittent, inadequate treatment and may appear to parents as a series of infections.

Nevertheless, many nonimmune disorders are characterized by an increased susceptibility to infection, and these must be considered in the child who presents with a complaint of recurrent infections (see Table 52–3).

HISTORY AND PHYSICAL EXAMINATION

History

The clinical history should emphasize the frequency, location, severity, and complications of the infections; the accuracy of how infections were documented; the presence or absence of a symptom-free interval; the microbiology of any isolate; and the response to antibiotic therapy. Further historical data include the following categories.

Perinatal History. The response may reveal exposure to a maternal viral infection (human immunodeficiency virus [HIV], cytomegalovirus, herpes simplex virus, rubella) during pregnancy or a history of prematurity, or respiratory distress syndrome (with bronchopulmonary dysplasia), blood transfusions, or other neonatal illnesses. Infants previously placed on respirators may develop chronic obstructive lung disease (bronchopulmonary dysplasia), predisposing them to pulmonary infections, and blood transfusions may lead to the acquired immunodeficiency syndrome (AIDS) as well as to infections by other blood-borne pathogens (see Table 52–3). Although screening of blood for HIV antibody has reduced the number of infections with HIV, other opportunistic infections may be acquired after infusion of blood or blood products. Most perinatal HIV infection is seen in children of high-risk mothers who had multiple sex partners or who used cocaine or injected drugs (see Chapter 55). Neonatal cytomegalovirus acquisition occurs more frequently in babies with a birth weight of less than 1250 g. It also occurs more frequently in babies born to cytomegalovirus seronegative mothers, in infants who have been hospitalized for more than 4 weeks or who have received multiple blood transfusions or a single transfusion with a total volume exceeding 50 ml, and in neonates who received blood from a seropositive donor. Attention should be paid to the time of umbilical cord separation. Infants with a history of delayed umbilical cord separation and recurrent episodes of sepsis or pneumonia should be evaluated for the leukocyte adhesion deficiency. Additional clues to the diagnosis are noted in Table 52–4.

Recurrent Infections or Signs of Immunologic Disorders in Other Family Members. The response to this question could suggest either hereditary or familial disorders or a common pattern of exposure. For instance, a parental history of blood transfusion or a lifestyle that suggests promiscuity, bisexuality, or illicit drug use

Table 52–2. Etiology and Mechanism of Recurrent Infection in Immunodeficiency States

Disorder	Pathogen	Deficiency
Primary Immunodeficiencies		
Humoral immunodeficiency syndromes (predominantly B-cell defects)	Bacterial pathogens, sinopulmonary infections; enteroviruses	Reduced phagocytic efficiency, failure of lysis and agglutination of bacteria, inadequate neutralization of bacterial toxins
Cellular immunodeficiency syndromes (predominantly T-cell defects)	CMV, VZV, *Strongyloides stercoralis; Mycobacterium, Listeria, Nocardia, Cryptococcus,* and *Candida* sp, and *Pneumocystis carinii*	Absence or impaired delayed hypersensitivity response; absent T-cell cooperation for B-cell synthesis of antibodies to T cell-specific antigens
Severe combined immunodeficiency syndrome	Many bacteria, fungi, and viruses	Absence of T-cell and B-cell responses
Wiskott-Aldrich syndrome	Gram-negative enteric organisms: CMV, HSV, staphylococci; *Streptococcus pneumoniae, Haemophilus influenzae, P. carinii*	Decreased antibody production to carbohydrate antigens
Ataxia-telangiectasia	Sinopulmonary infections with saprophytes	T helper cell deficiency, immunoglobulin deficiency
Splenic insufficiency or absence	*Salmonella* sp, *S. pneumoniae,* gram-negative organisms	Defective opsonization, defective clearing of organisms
Neutropenia (ANC <500/mm³)	Pyogenic bacteria or fungi, *Pseudomonas* sp, *S. aureus*	Decreased neutrophil numbers
Chédiak-Higashi syndrome	*S. aureus, Candida albicans,* gram-negative organisms	Defective neutrophil bactericidal activity secondary to impaired chemotaxis and degranulation
Specific granule deficiency	*S. aureus, C. albicans,* gram-negative organisms	Defective neutrophil bactericidal activity secondary to impaired chemotaxis and deficiency of granule constituents
Leukocyte adhesion deficiency	Gram-negative organisms, *P. aeruginosa, S. aureus*	Impaired neutrophil bactericidal activity secondary to impaired neutrophil adhesion and chemostaxis
Hyperimmunoglobulin E syndrome	*S. aureus*	Defective neutrophil chemotaxis: impaired opsonization of *S. aureus*
Chronic granulomatous disease	Catalase-positive organisms, e.g., *S. aureus, Serratia* sp, *Pseudomonas cepacia, Nocardia, Candida, Aspergillus* sp	Impaired neutrophil bactericidal activity secondary to impaired production of hydrogen peroxide
Myeloperoxidase deficiency	*Candida* sp in diabetic patients	Failure to kill *Candida* by neutrophils
Complement deficiencies	*Streptococcus pyogenes, S. pneumoniae, S. aureus, H. influenzae, Neisseria meningitidis, Klebsiella* sp	Defective chemotaxis, impaired opsonization
C5–C8 properidin deficiencies	*N. meningitidis, Neisseria gonorrhoeae*	Defective membrane attack mechanism
Secondary Immunodeficiencies		
AIDS	CMV, VZV, adenovirus, HBV, *C. albicans, Giardia lamblia, Entamoeba histolytica, Mycobacterium avium-intracellulare, Toxoplasma gondii, Mycobacterium tuberculosis, Crypotococcus neoformans, P. carinii, Campylobacter, Candida, Isospora, Aspergillus, Nocardia, Strongyloides,* and *Cryptosporidium* sp	Retrovirus infections transmitted by bodily fluids that impair T-cell response, reduced T helper cell numbers
Cancer	VZV, HSV, *Escherichia coli, Pseudomonas, Klebsiella, Listeria, Cryptococcus, Pneumocystis,* and *Mycobacterium* sp	Neutropenia, lymphopenia, impaired cellular immunity
Immunosuppression	HSV, VZV, CMV, EBV, *Polyomavirus,* hepatitis virus; *Pseudomonas* sp, *E. coli, Klebsiella, Acinetobacter, Serratia, Candida, Aspergillus, Mucor,* and *Cryptococcus* sp	Dependent on agent used, leads often to impaired cellular immunity and neutropenia
Transplantation	CMV, HSV, VZV, hepatitis virus, *S. aureus, Pseudomonas, Klebsiella, Candida, Aspergillus, Nocardia,* and *Pneumocystis* sp, EBV	Probably related to use of immunosuppressive agents
Malnutrition	Measles, HSV, VZV, *Mycobacterium* sp	Impaired T-cell function, reduction in complement activity

Abbreviations: CMV = cytomegalovirus; VZV = varicella-zoster virus; HSV = herpes simplex virus; EBV = Epstein-Barr virus; ANC = absolute neutrophil count; AIDS = acquired immunodeficiency syndrome; HBV = hepatitis B virus.

Table 52–3. Infections in Patients Without Primary Immunodeficiency Syndromes

Alteration of Mucocutaneous Barrier	Organism and Type of Infection
Indwelling Catheter	
Central venous catheter (Broviac, Hickman)	*Staphylococcus aureus, Staphylococcus epidermidis, Corynebacterium* JK, *Candida:* bacteremia, fungemia
Urinary catheter	*Escherichia coli,* enterococcus, *Staphylococcus saprophyticus:* pyelonephritis
Tenckhoff catheter (continuous ambulatory peritoneal dialysis)	*S. epidermidis, S. aureus, E. coli, Pseudomonas aeruginosa, Candida:* peritonitis
Cerebrospinal fluid shunts	*S. epidermidis, S. aureus,* diphtheroid, *Bacillus* sp: meningitis
Aspirated pulmonary foreign body	*S. aureus,* anaerobes: pneumonia, pulmonary abscess, empyema
Burns	*P. aeruginosa, S. epidermidis, Candida:* cutaneous lesions, sepsis
Inhalation Therapy	
Contaminated solutions	*P. aeruginosa, Serratia marcescens, Legionella:* pneumonia
Surgical Wounds	
Abdominal	Gram-negative bacteria, *S. aureus, S. epidermidis, Candida*
Nongastrointestinal	*S. aureus, S. epidermidis,* streptococci, gram-negative bacteria: wound abscess, sepsis
Fistula-Sinus Communications	
Neurocutaneous fistula	*S. aureus, S. epidermidis, E. coli:* meningitis
Neuroenteric fistula	Gram-negative bacteria: meningitis
Otic, facial sinus-meningeal sinus tract	Pneumococcus: meningitis
Facial sinus fracture (CSF rhinorrhea)	Pneumococcus: meningitis
Intravenous Drug Abuse	*S. aureus, P. aeruginosa,* streptococci: endocarditis; osteomyelitis; hepatitis B, C, D virus; AIDS
Prosthetic Devices	
Cardiac valves	*S. epidermidis,* streptococci, *S. aureus,* diphtheroid, *Candida:* endocarditis
Pacemaker	*S. epidermidis, S. aureus, Candida:* subcutaneous pocket endocardial infection
Chronic Disease	
Malnutrition	Measles, tuberculosis, herpes simplex; bacterial, parasitic, and viral diarrhea, gram-negative bacterial pneumonia
Cystic fibrosis	*S. aureus, Haemophilus influenzae,* mucoid *P. aeruginosa, Pseudomonas cepacia:* pneumonia
Diabetes mellitus	Urinary tract infections, *Mucor* and other fungi, sinus-orbital infection
Nephrotic syndrome	Pneumococcus, *E. coli:* peritonitis
Uremia	*S. aureus,* gram-negative bacteria, fungi: sepsis, soft tissue infection
Cirrhosis, ascites	Pneumococcus, *E. coli:* peritonitis
Prolonged broad-spectrum antibiotic therapy	*Candida,* enterococcus, multidrug-resistant gram-negative or gram-positive bacteria: sepsis
Spinal cord injury	Gram-negative or gram-positive bacteria: pneumonia, pyelonephritis, pressure sores, abscesses, osteomyelitis
Sickle cell anemia	Pneumococcus: sepsis, meningitis, osteoarticular infection *Salmonella, S. aureus:* osteomyelitis
Congenital heart disease	*S. aureus, Streptococcus viridans* group: endocarditis
Urinary tract anomaly	*E. coli, S. saprophyticus,* enterococus: pyelonephritis
Kartagener syndrome (dysmotile cilia)	*H. influenzae, M. catarrhalis,* pneumococcus: pneumonia, sinusitis
Eczema	*S. aureus,* streptococcus, varicella, herpes simplex, molluscum, warts: cutaneous infection, cellulitis
Protein-losing enteropathy (lymphangiectasia)	Pneumococcus: sepsis, peritonitis *Giardia:* diarrhea
Periodontitis	*Fusobacterium:* cellulitis, facial space infection
Chronic blood product transfusion	CMV; EBV; parvovirus; HHV-6; hepatitis A (rare), B, C, D virus: hepatitis, syphilis, bacteremia *(P. aeruginosa),* HIV, Chagas disease, malaria; direct inoculation → primary disease

Modified from Behrman RE (ed). Nelson Textbook of Pediatrics, 14th ed. Philadelphia: WB Saunders, 1992:670.
Abbreviations: AIDS = acquired immunodeficiency syndrome; CSF = cerebrospinal fluid; HIV = human immunodeficiency virus; CMV = cytomegalovirus; EBV = Epstein-Barr virus; HHV-6 = human herpesvirus-6.

could possibly predispose the child to exposure to AIDS via one of the family members. A history of unexplained infant deaths may be due to inherited disorders of immunity. Additional clues are noted in Table 52–4.

Exposure to Tobacco or Marijuana. A positive response to this question may explain an increased incidence of respiratory disease in children exposed to cigarette smoke or other noxious fumes in the home.

Exposure to Animals, Chemicals, Farms, or Plants at Home, School, or Day Care. Often, respiratory and dermatologic findings

Table 52–4. Clinical Clues to the Diagnosis of Immunodeficiency

Suggestive of T cell deficit
Systemic illness following vaccination with any live virus or BCG; unusual life-threatening complication following infection with ordinarily benign viruses (e.g., giant cell pneumonia with measles; varicella pneumonia)
Chronic oral candidiasis after 6 mo of age
Chronic mucocutaneous candidiasis
Features of cartilage-hair hypoplasia (fine, thin hair; short-limbed dwarfism with characteristic roentgenographic features)
Intrauterine graft-versus-host disease—most characteristic feature is scaling erythroderma and total alopecia (absence of eyebrows quite striking)
Graft-versus-host disease after blood transfusion
Hypocalcemia in newborn (DiGeorge anomaly, especially with characteristic facies, ears, and cardiac lesion)
Small (less than 10 μm diameter) lymphocytes: counts persistently less than 1500/mm³, must rule out gastrointestinal loss or loss from lymphatics

Suggestive of B cell defect
Recurrent proved bacterial pneumonia, sinusitis, sepsis, or meningitis
Nodular lymphoid hyperplasia

Suggestive of B and T cell defect (combined immunodeficiency disease [CID])
Features of all above except chronic mucocutaneous candidiasis and nodular lymphoid hyperplasia
Features of Wiskott-Aldrich syndrome (draining ears, thrombocytopenia, and eczema)
Features of ataxia-telangiectasia

Suggestive of immunodeficiency without clearly implicating T or B cell defect
Pneumocystis carinii pneumonia
Intractable eczema
Ulcerative colitis in infants less than 1 yr of age
Intractable diarrhea
Unexplained hematologic deficiency (RBC, WBC, platelet)
Severe generalized seborrheic dermatitis (Leiner disease) suggests C5 deficiency; seborrhea common in combined immunodeficiency disease
Recurrent pyogenic infections seen in C3 deficiency

Suggestive of biochemical defect
Features of combined immunodeficiency with characteristic bony lesions (adenosine deaminase deficiency)
Features of Diamond-Blackfan aplastic anemia (nucleoside phosphorylase deficiency)

Suggestive of abnormality of polymorphonuclear leukocytes
Primarily skin infections (if associated with asthma, eczema, and coarse facies, think of Buckley syndrome*)
Chronic osteomyelitis with *Klebsiella* or *Serratia* sp, draining lymph nodes (chronic granulomatous disease)

Suggestive of secondary deficiency
Concomitant or preceding viral infection
Lymphoid malignancy (chronic lymphatic leukemia, Hodgkin disease, myeloma)

Modified from Hong R. Immunodeficiency. *In* Rose NR, Friedman H (eds). Manual of Clinical Immunology. Washington, DC: American Society for Microbiology, 1976. Reprinted from Behrman RE (ed). Nelson Textbook of Pediatrics, 14th ed. Philadelphia: WB Saunders, 1992:551.
Abbreviations: BCG = bacille Calmette-Guérin; RBC = red blood cell; WBC = white blood cell.
*Data from Buckley RH, et al: Extreme hyperimmunoglobulinemia E and undue susceptibility to infection. Pediatrics 1972; 49:59.

are seen as a result of exposure to environmental allergens and toxins.

Family History of Allergic Diseases. A family history that includes one allergic parent or two allergic parents predisposes the child to allergic reactions by 25% and 50%, respectively.

Travel to Foreign Countries, Camp, or Rural Areas. An affirmative answer may suggest exposure to unusual organisms, such as parasites, bites, or contaminated water.

Changes in the Daily Routine or Sleeping Arrangements. A move to a new house or to a new nursery school or exposure to a new baby sitter, pet, or housekeeper may suggest possible allergic and infectious exposures to new environmental agents.

Recurrent Episodes of High Fever with Purulent Secretions. The presence of fever and purulent secretions suggests bacterial infec-

tion, which could be caused by broad categories of immune deficiencies (see Table 52–1). The presence of serious bacterial infections without purulent formation suggests inability of neutrophils to migrate to sites of infection.

Health of the Patient Between Infections. If the patient is generally healthy between infections, including adequate appetite and growth, the patient is unlikely to have an underlying serious systemic illness.

Location and Severity. If the episodes are similar in location and severity, the patient may have an allergy or local mechanical problems, such as obstruction or foreign bodies.

History of Skull Fracture, Dermal Sinus Tracks, or Dermoids or Insertion of a Central Nervous System Shunt (see Table

52–3). Each of these problems may predispose patients to central nervous system infection from leakage of cerebrospinal fluid from a basilar skull fracture or from dermal sinus tracks that communicate with the subarachnoid space or neural tissue. Other conditions predisposing patients to opportunistic infection of the central nervous system include penetrating foreign body, cerebrospinal fluid shunts, myelomeningocele, encephalocele, treated or untreated local infections of the sinuses or of the middle ear that spread to contiguous structures to form cerebral abscesses or subdural-epidural empyema, intravenous drug abuse, bacterial endocarditis, heart disease with right-to-left shunt, lymphoma, leukemia, immunosuppression, AIDS, and transplantation.

Recurrent Pulmonary Infections After a Hospitalization. Endotracheal intubation during hospitalization with or without a history of organ transplantation, exposure to smoking, gastroesophageal reflux with aspiration, neurologic impairments, recent course of chemotherapy, or exposure to inhalation burns or smoke may predispose the patient to recurrent pulmonary infections with nosocomial organisms. Additional risks for recurrent pneumonia are noted in Table 52–5.

Physical Examination

The physical examination may provide clues to an underlying condition (see Table 52–4). Height and weight measurements are essential for the identification of failure to thrive or recent weight loss. Other important findings include scarred tympanic membranes, postnasal drip, and cervical adenopathy, which would suggest chronic respiratory infections. Transverse nasal creases, circles under the eyes, and posterior pharyngeal cobblestoning are consistent with respiratory allergy. Recurrent cough, wheezing, digital

Table 52–5. Differential Diagnosis of Recurrent Pneumonia

Hereditary Disorders
Cystic fibrosis
Sickle cell disease

Disorders of Immunity
Acquired immunodeficiency syndrome
Bruton agammaglobulinemia
Selective IgG subclass deficiencies
Common variable immunodeficiency syndrome
Severe combined immunodeficiency syndrome

Disorders of Leukocytes
Chronic granulomatous disease
Hyperimmunoglobulin E syndrome (Job syndrome)
Leukocyte adhesion defect

Disorders of Cilia
Immotile cilia syndrome
Kartagener syndrome

Anatomic Disorders
Sequestration
Bronchopulmonary dysplasia
Lobar emphysema
Esophageal reflux
Foreign body
Tracheoesophageal fistula (H type)
Gastroesophageal reflux
Bronchiectasis

Modified from Kercsmar CM. The respiratory system. *In* Behrman RE, Kliegman RM: Nelson Essentials of Pediatrics, 2nd ed. Philadelphia: WB Saunders, 1994:458.

clubbing, or chest deformity are suggestive of pulmonary disease. Auscultation of the apex of the heart in the right thorax (dextrocardia) may be accompanied by ciliary motility abnormalities. Lymphadenopathy, hepatosplenomegaly, pallor, wasting, or recent weight loss suggest systemic disease. Absent lymph tissue (tonsils, lymph nodes, or thymus on chest x-ray study) suggests T-cell, or B-cell, or combined cellular immunity deficiency states.

When a discrepancy exists between the severity of an illness as reported by the parent and the child's physical appearance, it is often prudent to delay a detailed evaluation until more objective evidence of recurrent fevers, severe respiratory disease, and unusual skin infections are documented by repeat examinations during acute episodes.

DIAGNOSTIC CATEGORIES

The information obtained from the history and physical examination is usually sufficient to make a tentative classification. Children with recurrent infections can be classified into four basic categories:

1. The probably well child.
2. The atopic or allergic child.
3. The chronically ill child with a nonimmunologic defect in host defense (see Table 52–3).
4. The immunodeficient child with a neutrophil defect, lymphocyte abnormality, antibody deficiency, or complement deficiency (see Tables 52–1 and 52–2).

The Probably Well Patient

A large number of patients have recurrent infection or recurrent fever. Although nearly all patients with well-characterized phagocytic or immune abnormalities have recurrent respiratory infections, the converse is seldom the case. Approximately 50% of children with a complaint of recurrent infections are probably well, and their problem is characterized by a relatively brief history of recurrent infections or a single prolonged illness from which recovery has been delayed. Most upper respiratory tract infections last less than 7 days; a duration of greater than 14 days is unusual. Most children under 1 year of age who have a large family or who attend day care develop respiratory or gastrointestinal infections about six times during the first year of life.

The well child has normal growth and development before the illness and usually a normal physical examination. The onset of the recurrent infection may coincide with entry into day care, preschool, or kindergarten. Such children usually have appropriate-sized tonsils and lymph nodes for their age. Minimal laboratory tests, which might include a complete blood cell count and erythrocyte sedimentation rate, are used to exclude rheumatic disorders, and culture and x-ray study of the affected area provide additional data. With parental reassurance, these children recover spontaneously. Simple measures, rather than a complex set of laboratory studies, are often the only treatment required.

The Allergic Patient

Approximately 30% of children with recurrent respiratory sinopulmonary symptoms can be categorized as atopic or allergic children and have normal growth and development. Episodes of recurrent illness are nonfebrile, respond poorly to antibiotics, and present with upper respiratory symptoms, such as coughing and wheezing. The family history includes atopy, or the patient's history includes food intolerance, colic, blotchy skin, or infantile eczema. The physical examination of allergic school-aged children may reveal the characteristic appearance of pallor, circles under the eyes, open mouth with dry lips, coated tongue, evidence of nasal obstruction, transverse nasal crease, boggy nasal mucosa, mucus in the pharynx, posterior pharyngeal cobblestoning, and postnasal drip. Other features may include cervical lymphadenopathy and an increase in the chest anteroposterior diameter, pectoral hypertrophy, chest asymmetry, chronic sinusitis, chronic respiratory obstruction, dry skin, eczema, and dermatographism.

The laboratory evaluation of the allergic child should include a complete blood count, erythrocyte sedimentation rate, nasal smear for eosinophils, spirometry before and after bronchodilators are given, sinus x-ray studies, with or without a chest x-ray, and quantitative immunoglobulins determination, including an IgE level. In particular, an IgE level of greater than 50 IU/ml in an infant younger than 1 year of age or an IgE level exceeding 100 IU/ml in a child older than 1 year suggests an allergic disorder.

The Chronically Ill Patient with an Anatomic or Obstructive Abnormality

Approximately 10% of children who present with a history of recurrent infections have an underlying chronic disease or a structural defect that predisposes them to recurrent infections (see Table 52–3). Many chronic illnesses may directly or indirectly alter immune function, resulting in recurrent infections. Malnutrition and specific vitamin deficiencies may alter immune cell function. Protein-losing enteropathies may lead to hypocomplementemia and hypogammaglobulinemia. Structural or anatomic defects often result in recurrent infections that are generally localized to the affected organ system. Eustachian tube abnormalities (as in cleft palate) result in recurrent or chronic otitis media, congenital heart disease results in an increased risk of endocarditis, and posterior urethral valves or ureteral pelvic junction obstruction results in recurrent urinary tract infections. Pneumonia may result from congenital malformations (tracheoesophageal fistulas or sequestration), from aspiration of a foreign body (peanut, small toys) or chronic aspiration (gastroesophageal reflux), and bronchopulmonary dysplasia (see Table 52–5). Chronic illnesses that result in recurrent pulmonary infections of nonimmunologic origin include cystic fibrosis, immotile cilia syndrome, or α_1-antitrypsin deficiency.

Children with anatomic or obstructive abnormalities are often ill-appearing with poor growth, although they may be normal. Patients with recurrent pneumonia usually have chronic cough with rales and digital clubbing; others may have failure to thrive, chronic diarrhea, abdominal distention, hepatosplenomegaly, muscle wasting, and pallor. Most children with a possible nonimmunologic cause for recurrent infection should undergo laboratory tests such as a complete blood count, chest x-ray, sweat test, and cultures of involved sites. Tests for quantitative immunoglobulin should also be performed to rule out an antibody deficiency. Possible nonimmunologic diagnoses for recurrent infections are listed in Table 52–3.

The Immunodeficient Patient

Approximately 10% of children with recurrent infection have an underlying immunodeficiency. Frequently, the onset of infections in these patients usually begins in the second half of the first year of life. The infections often vary in type, location, and severity, although pneumonias predominate (see Table 52–1). Unusual organisms and unexpected complications are often present. Such children usually respond to antibiotics but become ill when the

medications are discontinued. Affected patients also have failure to thrive (see Chapter 17).

DIAGNOSTIC APPROACH TO THE PATIENT WITH RECURRENT INFECTIONS

Patients with pyogenic infections involving multiple sites or organ systems should be investigated for an immune deficiency. Children who have had two or more severe infections by 9 months of age and older children who have had frequent infections with concomitant growth failure should be evaluated. Recurrent pulmonary infection, hepatic abscesses, and perirectal abscesses also alert the clinician to consider further diagnostic evaluation of possible neutrophil dysfunction and opsonic defects involving antibody or complement production.

A number of physical findings may be present in the child with immune deficiency, including absent or diminished tonsils or lymph nodes, which indicate cellular immune deficiency; skin abnormalities such as alopecia, eczema, pyoderma, and telangiectasia; evidence of hematologic disease, such as pallor, petechia, jaundice, and mouth ulceration; and generalized lymphadenopathy and splenomegaly, which may suggest HIV disease, a phagocyte disorder, or a possible associated hematologic disorder (Tables 52–6 and 52–7, see also Table 52–4).

The initial and advanced laboratory tests for children who may have a deficiency are outlined in Figure 52–1. Because 80% of patients with primary immune deficiency also have an antibody deficiency, tests for antibody function as well immunoglobulin level determinations are appropriate. Patients with an unusually convincing history of recurrent infections should undergo other tests for immunodeficiency, even if the initial screening tests are normal. Subsequent testing must be individualized, based on the results of the investigations for each patient. A very low neutrophil count might indicate severe congenital neutropenia, cyclic neutropenia, idiopathic neutropenia, marrow failure, or replacement of marrow by leukemia or a tumor if other hematopoietic cell lines are affected. Once initial immunoglobulin level screening is completed, other tests may include antibody responses to Pneumovax vaccine; IgG subclass levels for IgG1, IgG2, IgG3, and IgG4; and a delayed hypersensitivity skin test. Table 52–6 presents the characteristic clinical features of some of the primary immunodeficiencies according to patient age.

LYMPHOCYTE DISORDERS

Lymphocyte disorders are a heterogeneous group of primary disorders involving both the cell-mediated and humoral arms of the immune system. Disorders affecting T-cell function (cell-mediated immunity) tend to be more severe than primary B-cell disorders, and combined deficits carry the poorest prognosis.

The antibody immunodeficiency states can be divided into those that are due to genetic defects in B-lymphocyte maturation, occurring primarily at the pre–B cell or immature B-lymphocyte stage, and those that are due to defective interaction between T and B lymphocytes, occurring at the mature B-lymphocyte stage.

Children with altered lymphocyte function have recurrent infections (see Tables 52–1 and 52–7) or unusual responses to usually benign infectious agents, or they develop infections with unusual organisms. *Pneumocystis carinii*, cytomegalovirus, measles, and varicella often cause fatal pneumonia in these patients. Pneumonitis occurring with any of these agents should suggest a potential immunodeficiency. Affected children also have a higher incidence of malignancy and autoimmune disorders. A partial list of primary disorders of lymphocyte function is shown in Table 52–7; their

Table 52–6. Clinical Patterns in Some Primary Immunodeficiencies

Features	Diagnosis
Newborns and Infants to Age 6 Months	
Hypocalcemia, heart disease, unusual facies	DiGeorge syndrome
Cyanosis, heart disease, midline liver	Congenital asplenia
Delayed umbilical cord separation, leukocytosis, recurrent infections	Leukocyte adhesion deficiency syndrome
Diarrhea, pneumonia, thrush, failure to thrive	Severe combined immunodeficiency
Maculopapular rash, alopecia, lymphadenopathy, hepatosplenomegaly	Severe combined immundeficiency with graft-versus-host disease
Melena, draining ears, eczema	Wiskott-Aldrich syndrome
Oculocutaneous albinism, recurrent infections, neutropenia	Chédiak-Higashi syndrome
Recurrent pyogenic infections, sepsis	C3 deficiency
Chronic gingivitis, recurrent aphthous ulcers and skin infections, severe neutropenia	Severe congenital neutropenia
Infants and Children Age 6 Months to 5 Years	
Severe progressive infectious mononucleosis	X-linked lymphoproliferative syndrome
Paralytic disease following oral polio immunization	X-linked agammaglobulinemia
Recurrent cutaneous and systemic staphylococcal infections, coarse facial features	Hyperimmunoglobulin E syndrome
Persistent thrush, nail dystrophy, endocrinopathies	Chronic mucocutaneous candidiasis
Recurrent deep-seated skin abscesses	Specific granule deficiency
Children > Age 5 Years and Adults	
Progressive dermatomyositis with chronic ECHO virus encephalitis	X-linked agammaglobulinemia
Sinopulmonary infections, neurologic deterioration, telangiectasia	Ataxia-telangiectasia
Lymphadenopathy, dermatitis, pyloric-antral obstruction, pneumonias, small bone osteomyelitis	Chronic granulomatous disease
Recurrent *Neisseria* meningitis	C5, C6, C7, and C8 deficiency
Sinopulmonary infections, malabsorption, splenomegaly, autoimmunity	Common variable immunodeficiency

Abbreviations: ECHO = enteric cytopathogenic human orphan virus.

evaluation is described in Figure 52–1. Acquired immunodeficiency caused by HIV is described in Chapter 55.

Disorders of Antibody Production, X-linked Agammaglobulinemia

Bruton agammaglobulinemia is an X-linked recessive disorder characterized by an arrest in B-cell differentiation. This arrest in B-cell differentiation leaves these children severely deficient in serum immunoglobulins and at serious risk for developing recurrent life-threatening infections.

Although some children have remained asymptomatic until 2 years of age, most children with X-linked agammaglobulinemia show symptoms in infancy between 6 and 9 months of age, when transplacentally derived maternal antibodies disappear. They develop repeated infections (recurrent otitis media, sinusitis, pneumonia, meningitis) with highly pathogenic bacteria, such as pneumococci, staphylococci, streptococci, and *Haemophilus* sp. They handle most simple viral infections well, and immunizations do not tend to cause problems, with the following exceptions: the use of live polio vaccine has resulted in paralysis, and exposure to other enteroviruses has led to chronic diarrhea, hepatitis, pneumonitis, and meningoencephalitis.

Patients with X-linked agammaglobulinemia have marked hypoplasia of lymphoid tissue (adenoids, tonsils, lymph nodes) with absent germinal centers and rare, if present, plasma cells. The diagnosis can be suspected if serum IgG, IgM, and IgA levels are all less than 5% of age-adjusted control values in a patient with normal T-cell function. Occasionally, children with X-linked agam-

maglobulinemia present with elevated IgA or IgG level but do not respond to immunizations with specific antibody production. Treatment of X-linked agammaglobulinemia includes aggressive antibiotic management of infections and replacement of immunoglobulin, although chronic pulmonary and gastrointestinal diseases still occur in some patients (Table 52–8).

Common Variable Immunodeficiency

Common variable immunodeficiency (CVID) is a heterogeneous group of disorders characterized by the development of severe hypogammaglobulinemia, resulting in chronic respiratory infections, including sinusitis, bronchitis, and pneumonia, and severe gastrointestinal disease. Common variable immunodeficiency is associated with a sprue-like syndrome, which occurs in up to 60% of patients with these disorders. These patients experience heavy bacterial overgrowth of their small bowel, jejunal villous atrophy, and intestinal nodular lymphoid hyperplasia. The bacteria overgrowth in the gut often leads to diarrhea, steatorrhea, malabsorption, and protein-losing enteropathy. Patients can also develop noncaseating granulomas of the liver, spleen, lungs, and skin. *Giardia lamblia* infection is common and appears to play some role in the gastrointestinal problems because many patients improve with metronidazole therapy. As in X-linked agammaglobulinemia, the most common manifestations of CVID are chronic infections of the upper and lower respiratory tracts. Hematologic abnormalities include immune-mediated thrombocytopenia, anemia, leukopenia, and systemic lupus erythematosus. There appears to be an increased

Table 52–7. Disorders of Lymphocyte Function

Disorder	Genetics	Onset	Manifestations	Pathogenesis	Associated Features
Bruton agammaglobulinemia	X-linked (Xq21.3–q22)	Infancy (6–9 months)	Recurrent high-grade infections, sinusitis pneumonia, meningitis	Arrest in B-cell differentiation (pre-B-B level)	Lymphoid hypoplasia
Common variable immunodeficiency	AR; AD	Second to third decade	Sinusitis, bronchitis, pneumonia, chronic diarrhea	Arrest in B-cell to plasma cell differentiation	Autoimmune disease, RA, SLE, Graves disease, ITP, malignancy
Transient hypogamma-globulinemia of infancy		Infancy (4–9 months)	Recurrent viral and pyogenic infections	Delayed development of plasma cell maturation	Frequently in families with immunodeficiencies
IgA deficiency	X-linked, AR, ? 6p21.3	Variable	Sinopulmonary infections Gastrointestinal infections; may be normal	Failure of IgA expressing B-cell differentiation	IgG subclass deficiency, common variable immunodeficiency, autoimmune diseases
IgG subclass deficiency	AR 2p11; 14q32.3	Variable	Variable (normal to recurrent sinopulmonary infections and gastrointestinal infections)	Defect in isotype IgG production	IgA deficiency
IgM deficiency	AR	First year	Recurrent septicemia, pneumococcus, *Haemophilus influenzae*	Defective helper T-cell–B-cell interaction	Whipple disease, regional enteritis, lymphoid hyperplasia
Immunodeficiency with increased IgM	X-linked, AR, ? (Xq24–q26)	2–3 years	Recurrent pyogenic infections (otitis media, sinusitis, tonsillitis, pneumonia)	Defect in IgG and IgA synthesis	Hematologic autoimmune disease
DiGeorge anomaly	? (22)	Early infancy	Variable	Hypoplasia of third and fourth pharyngeal pouch	Hypoparathyroidism, aortic arch anomalies, micrognathia, hypertelorism
Wiskott-Aldrich syndrome	X-linked (Xp11–p11.3)	Early infancy	Recurrent otitis media, pneumonia, meningitis with encapsulated organisms	Unknown	Recurrent infections, atopic dermatitis, platelet dysfunction, thrombocytopenia
Ataxia-telangiectasia	AR (11q22.3)	2–5 years	Sinopulmonary infections	Unknown (defect in DNA repair)	Neurologic and endocrine dysfunction, malignancy, telangiectasias
Cartilage-hair hypoplasia (short-limbed dwarf)	AR	Birth	Variable	Unknown	Metaphyseal dysplasia, short extremities
Severe combined immunodeficiency	X-linked (Xq13.1–q21.1) AR	1–3 months	Candidiasis, all types of infections (bacterial, viral, fungal, protozoal)	IL-2R γ depletion (severe T-cell depletion)	Severe graft-versus-host disease from maternal fetal transfusions
Severe combined immunodeficiency (ADA deficiency)	AR (20q13-ter)	1–3 months	Candidiasis, all types of infections (bacterial, viral, fungal, protozoal)	Enzyme deficiency results in dATP-induced lymphocyte toxicity	Multiple skeletal abnormalities, chondro-osseous dysplasia
Severe combined immunodeficiency (PNP deficiency)	AR 14q13.1	1–3 months	Candidiasis, all types of infections (bacterial, viral, fungal, protozoal)	Enzyme deficiency results in dGTP-induced T-cell toxicity	Neurologic disorders, severe graft-versus-host disease from transfusions
Severe combined immunodeficiency (reticular dysgenesis)	AR	1–3 months	Candidiasis, all types of infections (bacterial, viral, fungal, protozoal)	Defective maturation of common stem cell affecting myeloid and lymphoid cells	Agamma-globulinemia, alymphocytosis, agranulocytosis

Abbreviations: ADA = adenosine deaminase; AR = autosomal recessive; RA = rheumatoid arthritis; SLE = systemic lupus erythematosus; ITP = idiopathic thrombocytopenic purpura; IL-2R γ = interleukin-2 receptor gamma chain; dATP = deoxy-adenosine triphosphate; dGTP = deoxy-guanosine triphosphate; PNP = purine nucleoside phosphorylase.

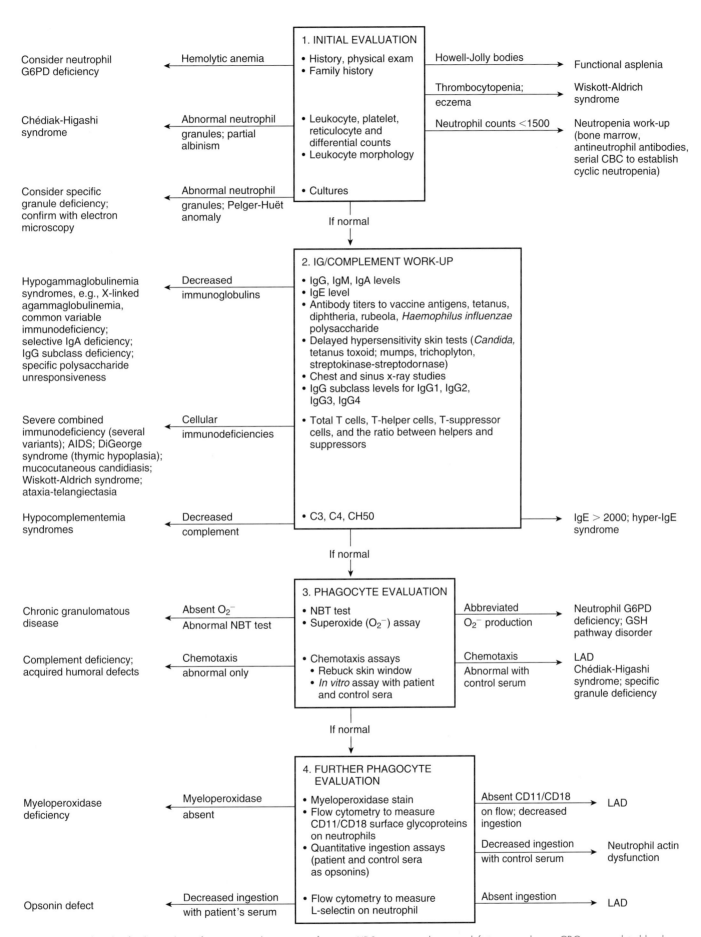

Figure 52–1. Algorithm for the work-up of a patient with recurrent infections. AIDS = acquired immunodeficiency syndrome; CBC = complete blood count; Ig = immunoglobulin; G6PD = glucose-6-phosphate dehydrogenase; GSH = reduced glutathione; NBT = nitroblue tetrazolium; LAD = leukocyte adhesion deficiency syndrome.

Table 52–8. Management of Infections in the Host Compromised by B and T Lymphocyte Defects

Immunodeficiency Syndrome	Treatment of Infection	Prevention of Infection
Humoral defects (predominant B cell deficiency)	Intravenous immunoglobulin 0.4 g/kg Bacterial and viral culture Incision and drainage of abscess Bactericidal antibiotics based on culture and sensitivity of microorganism Intraventricular immunoglobulin for echovirus encephalitis	Maintenance intravenous immunoglobulin 0.3–0.5 g/kg q 3–4 wk Avoid live virus vaccines in patient and relatives Respiratory care, postural drainage, monitor for cor pulmonale Chronic antibiotic prophylaxis is controversial

Cellular defects (predominant T cell deficiency)	Bacterial, viral, fungal, protozoal culture, microscopy, and stains
	Incision and drainage of abscess
	Biopsy, bronchoalveolar lavage if indicated
	Antibacterial, antiviral, antifungal, antiprotozoal therapy as appropriate for culture, sensitivity, stains, and symptoms
	Intravenous immunoglobulin if helper T lymphocyte–associated antibody deficiency, or if severe combined immunodeficiency syndrome
		Prophylactic trimethoprim-sulfamethoxazole for *Pneumocystis carinii*
		No live virus vaccines or bacillus Calmette-Guérin
		Careful screening for tuberculosis
		Irradiated blood products decrease risk of GVH
		CMV-negative blood products
		Varicella-zoster immune globulin used for those with varicella exposure
		Immunologic reconstitution performed with
		  1. Bone marrow transplant
		  2. Fetal thymus transplant
		  3. Polyethylene glycol ADA enzyme infusion
		  4. Potential ADA genetic reconstitution

From Behrman RE (ed). Nelson Textbook of Pediatrics, 14th ed. Philadlephia: WB Saunders, 1992.
Abbreviations: ADA = adenosine deaminase enzyme; CMV = cytomegalovirus; GVH = graft-versus-host disease, which increases risk of infection.

susceptibility to lymphoreticular malignancies and carcinoma of the stomach in adults.

Patients with CVID have low circulating levels of IgG, IgM, and IgA; however, they have normal to increased numbers of circulating B cells and greatly reduced numbers of plasma cells in the intestinal lamina propria. B cells fail to respond to normal maturational signals.

Transient Hypogammaglobulinemia of Infancy

Although the fetus is capable of producing IgM or IgG by the 20th week of gestation when adequately stimulated, under normal conditions, newborn levels of IgG are a reflection of prior maternal immunity; significant antibody production does not normally begin until the second or third month of life. Because maternal antibodies have a half-life of approximately 30 days, the infant may develop a variable physiologic hypogammaglobulinemia between the fourth to ninth month of life. If profound in extent or duration, this transient hypoglobulinemia may lead to recurrent viral and pyogenic infections. Infants with such infections are capable of making specific antibodies (tetanus, diphtheria toxoids), they respond to immunizations, and they have normal numbers of circulating B and T cells. Lymph nodes from these infants are small, and germinal centers are reduced in size and number. The abnormality in antibody production may be from decreased maturation of B cells to antibody-producing plasma cells. Most patients do not require gamma globulin therapy and achieve normal immunoglobulin levels between 12 and 36 months of life.

IgA Deficiency

IgA deficiency is the most common primary immunodeficiency. The mode of transmission appears to be variable, either autosomal

recessive or autosomal dominant with variable penetrance. The defect causes an arrest in B-cell maturation. Clinically, patients with IgA deficiency may be asymptomatic or may present with recurrent sinopulmonary and gastrointestinal infections. IgA deficiency is also often associated with IgG2 or IgG4 subclass deficiency, which worsens the prognosis. There is also a high incidence of autoimmune disorders and an association with CVID.

Most patients with IgA deficiency do not require treatment other than antibiotic management of their infections. Blood products that include immunoglobulins are often contraindicated because many patients develop antibodies against IgA, possibly precipitating anaphylactic reactions.

IgG Subclass Deficiency

Four different subclasses of IgG (IgG1 [65%], IgG2 [25%], IgG3 [5% to 10%], and IgG4 [5%]) have been identified. Different types of antigens are likely to elicit a particular subclass of IgG response (e.g., protein antigens tend to elicit an IgG1 response, whereas carbohydrates elicit an IgG2 response). Children younger than 2 years of age have difficulty eliciting an antibody response to carbohydrate antigens, which explains why IgG2 is the slowest subclass to reach adult levels.

The clinical spectrum of IgG subclass deficiency is variable. Some patients do well, whereas others have recurrent upper and lower respiratory infections, otitis media, sinusitis, and gastroenteritis, with both bacteria and viruses. In some children, immune function improves with age, often reaching normal levels by the age of 7 or 8 years. Quantitative immunoglobulin determinations do not reveal these disorders, because total IgG level is usually normal, and only on examination of IgG subclasses can the defect be detected. Determination of antibody titers to polysaccharide antigens (*Streptococcus pneumoniae, Haemophilus influenzae* type b) aids in the assessment of immunologic function and the specific need for medical intervention. Many children with subclass deficiency do well with no treatment, others respond to prophylactic antibiotics, and still others require intravenous immunoglobulin replacement.

IgM Deficiency

IgM deficiency is a rare autosomal recessively inherited disorder (see Table 52–7).

Immunodeficiency with Increased IgM Level

Immunodeficiency with increased IgM level is a heterogeneous group of disorders characterized by normal or increased concentrations of IgM and IgD, but absent or decreased levels of IgG, IgA, and IgE (see Table 52–7).

Combined Disorders of T and B Cells

T lymphocytes are the effectors for cell-mediated immunity. T lymphocytes also serve as regulators of the humoral and the cell-mediated immune system; they modulate the activities of nonlymphocyte cells, such as monocytes. Differentiation of T lymphocytes occur in the thymus.

DiGeorge Syndrome

DiGeorge anomaly is caused by a maldevelopment of structures that are derived from the first through the sixth branchial pouches during embryogenesis, resulting in variable hypoplasia of the thymus, parathyroid glands, face, ear, aortic arch, and heart. DiGeorge syndrome usually presents in early infancy with symptoms unrelated to immunodeficiency. Congenital heart defects, including truncus arteriosus, ventricular septal defect, interrupted aortic arch, and tetralogy of Fallot, are common features. Hypocalcemia tetany is often the initial problem in the first and second month of life. Facial abnormalities include microstomia, hypertelorism, and low-set ears. If patients survive the neonatal period, they manifest increased susceptibility to infections, including repeated pneumonias, chronic diarrhea, and oral candidiasis.

The degree of immunodeficiency is related to the extent of residual thymic function. Some patients have infections with opportunistic organisms (*P. carinii*, viruses, fungi), whereas others exhibit normal immune function. Serum immunoglobulin levels tend to be appropriate, but antibody response after antigenic challenge may be diminished. Intradermal delayed hypersensitivity may be absent, decreased, or normal, whereas lymph node paracortical areas and thymic dependent regions of the spleen show variable degrees of cell depletion, depending on the degree of thymic deficiency. The total lymphocyte count may vary from severely depressed to normal, but T-cell levels are usually more consistently depressed. Management of DiGeorge syndrome is noted in Table 52–8.

Wiskott-Aldrich Syndrome

Wiskott-Aldrich syndrome is an X-linked recessive disorder that is associated with abnormalities in lymphocyte, platelet, and phago-cyte function (see Table 52–7). It is characterized by a triad of symptoms: (1) recurrent infections involving encapsulated bacteria as well as opportunistic pathogens, (2) hemorrhage secondary to thrombocytopenia and platelet dysfunction, and (3) atopic dermatitis. Presenting in early infancy with pneumonia, otitis media, and meningitis, these children are particularly susceptible to encapsulated organisms. Later on, they develop fungal and *P. carinii* infections but are also at risk for disseminated herpes simplex and cytomegalovirus infections. Patients have selective defects in multiple arms of their immune system. Serum IgG levels are typically normal, with elevated IgA and IgE and decreased IgM levels. Patients respond normally to some antigens, such as tetanus, but are completely incapable of forming antibodies to polysaccharide antigens, particularly polysaccharides. Immunoglobulin serum half-life appears to be decreased. Features of Wiskott-Aldrich syndrome include abnormalities in cellular immunity manifested by anergy, despite having normal numbers of T cells and a normal T helper to T suppressor cell ratio.

Thrombocytopenia characterized by small platelets is a unique feature of this disease. Prolonged bleeding at circumcision or profuse bloody diarrhea is frequently observed. Many children with this disorder succumb to bleeding disorders or infection; 12% die of secondary lymphomas.

Ataxia-Telangiectasia

Ataxia-telangiectasia is an autosomal recessive disorder characterized by neurologic dysfunction, endocrine abnormalities, oculocutaneous telangiectasia, immunodeficiency, and a high rate of malignancy (see Table 52–7). Cerebellar ataxia is usually the first presenting sign, occurring when the child begins to walk. The patient's neurologic status often worsens, and choreoathetosis, involuntary myoclonic jerks, and oculomotor abnormalities develop. Telangiectasias first appear in the bulbar conjunctivae between 2 and 5 years of age and later spread to areas of trauma. Endocrine abnormalities, such as insulin-resistant diabetes mellitus, and hypogonadism are common. There is a 15% risk of malignancy; non-Hodgkin lymphoma is the most common.

Patients with ataxia-telangiectasia are extremely sensitive to ionizing radiation. They have an alteration in DNA repair, which accounts for the high incidence of chromosomal translocations involving chromosomes 7 and 14 at the site of T-cell receptor genes and immunoglobulin heavy-chain genes. The degree of immunodeficiency is quite variable; both B-cell and T-cell abnormalities occur. The most common B-cell abnormalities include IgA deficiency (75%), IgE deficiency (85%), and monomeric IgM (80%). IgG subclass deficiency occurs in about 50% of patients, with IgG2 and IgG4 deficiencies being the most common. T cells show abnormal, delayed-type hypersensitivity reaction; proliferative response to mitogens; and allograft rejection. The thymus is abnormally small, and although circulating T-lymphocyte numbers appear to be normal, peripheral lymphoid tissue reveals depletion in resident T cells. Patients with ataxia-telangiectasia have sinopulmonary infections. Administration of blood products that include immunoglobulin replacement can lead to anaphylactic reactions because IgA-deficient patients often produce autoantibodies to IgA.

Cartilage-Hair Hypoplasia (Short-Limbed Dwarfism)

Cartilage-hair hypoplasia is an autosomal recessive disease characterized by metaphyseal dysostosis; sparse, unpigmented hair; and variable immunodeficiency (see Table 52–7). Lymphocyte numbers may be normal or dramatically depressed. Proliferative responses to mitogens are generally depressed; immune function may deteriorate with time. The immunodeficiency can range from mild to severe; in most cases, it is relatively mild and benefits at most from replacement immunoglobulin.

Severe Combined Immunodeficiency Syndromes

Severe combined immunodeficiency (SCID) is a heterogeneous group of disorders characterized by profound abnormalities in B-cell and T-cell function. Patients generally present in the first few months of life with recurrent pneumonia, failure to thrive, and chronic diarrhea. They often have candidiasis of the mouth, esophagus, face, and diaper area, in addition to other infections (bacterial, viral, fungal, and protozoal). Adenovirus and cytomegalovirus frequently progress into chronic pneumonitis; disseminated, life-threatening varicella and measles infections occur; live vaccines can result in a fatal infection such as bacille Calmette-Guérin (BCG) or smallpox; and severe graft-versus-host disease frequently develops after blood transfusions that contain live donor lymphocytes.

Most patients exhibit severe deficits in immunoglobulin synthesis, which ranges from agammaglobulinemia to isolated subclass deficiencies; responses to specific antigens are usually impaired. B cells may be absent or increased, but T-cell abnormalities are always present. T-cell numbers are generally fewer than 10% of normal in over 80% of patients with SCID. Patients are anergic, and T cells show decreased proliferative responses to mitogens, decreased cytotoxicity, and decreased immunoregulatory activity. Residual host natural killer cell activity may account for graft failure in SCID treated with haploidentical bone marrow transplantation.

X-LINKED RECESSIVE

X-linked recessive SCID is the most common form of SCID and is characterized by T-cell depletion in the presence of normal numbers of B cells. This disorder arises from a lack of T-cell interleukin-2 receptor (IL-2R), which is necessary for thymic maturation of T cells. Female carriers can be identified because lymphocytes and natural killer cells exhibit nonrandom inactivation of their X chromosome. The management of X-linked recessive SCID is noted in Table 52–8.

RETICULAR DYSGENESIS

Severe combined immunodeficiency with reticular dysgenesis is the most severe form. There may be a defect in a common stem cell that affects myeloid as well as lymphoid cell lines. This disease is characterized by agammaglobulinemia, lymphopenia, and neutropenia, but erythroid and platelet precursors are normal. Patients die shortly after birth of overwhelming infection, unless they are treated successfully with bone marrow transplantation (see Table 52–8).

SWISS TYPE

Swiss-type SCID is a rare form of autosomal recessive SCID that is characterized by failure of lymphoid cell development and absence of both T and B cells. The genes for B-cell and T-cell antigen receptors, which are necessary for the development of immunocompetent lymphocytes, may be absent.

BARE LYMPHOCYTE SYNDROME

Failure of T cells to express specific surface histocompatibility molecules is also associated with SCID. Histocompatibility class II deficiency is an autosomal recessive disorder that accounts for 5% of SCID. Class II molecules are required for the positive selection of T-helper cells in the thymus, for T-cell recognition of antigen-presenting cells, and for T-helper cell interactions with B cells. Patients with this form of SCID have decreased T-helper cells, and their humoral deficiency arises from a T-cell antigen recognition.

ADENOSINE DEAMINASE DEFICIENCY

Adenosine deaminase (ADA) catalyzes the conversion of adenosine and deoxyadenosine to inosine and deoxyinosine, respectively. Its deficiency, which is autosomal recessive, results in the accumulation of deoxyadenosine, which is phosphorylated to deoxy-adenosine triphosphate (ATP) (see Table 52–7). Deoxy-ATP is toxic to lymphocytes, leading to their demise and subsequent SCID. Patients with this enzyme deficiency have different degrees of agammaglobulinemia and lymphopenia. Treatment is noted in Table 52–8.

PURINE NUCLEOSIDE PHOSPHORYLASE DEFICIENCY

Purine nucleoside phosphorylase (PNP) deficiency is caused by a lack of the enzyme that follows ADA in the purine salvage pathway, and catalyzes the conversion of inosine and guanosine to hypoxanthine and guanine, respectively, and leads to the intracellular buildup of deoxy-guanosine triphosphate (GTP), which is toxic to T cells; the number of B cells remain normal. Serum immunoglobulin and isohemagglutinin levels are normal. Specific antibody production is impaired because T helper function is abnormal. A low serum uric acid level is suggestive of PNP deficiency in patients with SCID.

INTERLEUKIN-2 DEFICIENCY

Several cases of SCID have been described with either a decreased production of, or response to, a variety of cytokines. Patients with IL-2 deficiency, have normal numbers of T cells; they exhibit an abnormal proliferative response to mitogen stimulation. In these cases, IL-2 replacement improves the immunodeficiency associated with the SCID.

NATURAL KILLER CELL DEFICIENCY

Natural killer cells are large, granular lymphocytes that lack cell receptors and are important mediators of cell lysis of virally infected and tumor cells. Patients deficient in natural killer cells have difficulty with recurrent herpes virus infections.

COMPLEMENT SYSTEM DEFICIENCIES

The complement system has an integral role in the regulation of the immune system and its response to infectious agents. As the complement cascade is activated and progresses, all arms of the immune system are affected; C4a and C2a regulate vascular permeability, C3b and C3bi regulate phagocytosis, C5a mediates the release of cytokines from monocytes and is chemotactic for neutrophils, and C9 complex formation mediates cell lysis.

Activation of the *classic pathway* begins with fixation of C1, by way of Clq to the Fc receptor of an antigen-antibody complex. A conformational shift results in the activation of C1s, which activates C4 then C2. The C142 complex acts as a C3 convertase, which activates C3 from C3b, whereas, in the *alternative pathway,* BbC3b activates C3. C3bi, an important opsonin, is formed by cleavage of C3b by C3b inactivator. C3b formation results in the sequential activation of C5 through C9. C9 activation results in the formation of the *membrane attack complex,* consisting of 12 to 18 C9 molecules that form a transmembrane channel, resulting in cell lysis. Teichoic acid from bacterial cell wall, endotoxic lipopolysaccharides, and aggregates of immunoglobulin, especially IgA, are potent activators of the alternative pathway. Although protein deficiencies or abnormalities have been identified for all 11 components in the classical complement pathway, the severity and the type of infection varies because of the considerable overlap between the two pathways (Table 52–9).

In addition, C1 inhibitor deficiency is an autosomal dominant disorder that results in dysregulation of the classic complement pathway. Activation of the classic pathway results in *angioneurotic edema* secondary to the uncontrolled formation of C4a and C2a, two vasoactive proteins. After minor trauma, patients develop swelling and edema without urticaria, pain, or erythema. The swelling usually lasts 24 to 48 hours before subsiding spontaneously. Angioedema involving the larynx or upper airways can be life-threatening, and involvement of the bowel leads to abdominal pain, vomiting, and diarrhea. Affected children often do not present until after puberty; androgens such as danazol or stanozolol are generally very effective at preventing attacks.

Secondary Complement Deficiencies

IgG binds to C1q, protecting it from rapid catabolism; therefore, children with hypogammaglobulinemia develop partial C1q deficiency. Patients with chronic membranoproliferative glomerulonephritis and partial lipodystrophy may develop nephritic factor, an antibody that protects the BbC3b complex from inactivation, resulting in the consumption of C3 and a relative C3-deficient state. These patients are at risk for developing pyogenic infections, including meningitis, if their serum C3 levels fall below 10% of normal levels. Patients with acute postinfectious glomerulonephritis and systemic lupus erythematosus may develop an antibody similar to nephritic factor, which protects the C3 convertase of the classic pathway.

Most newborn infants are relatively deficient in all components of the classic pathway as well as of factor B and properdin in the alternative pathway; thus, their ability to generate serum-derived chemotactic factors and opsonization is markedly diminished. Complement activity is even lower in premature infants. Malnutrition and anorexia nervosa may lead to decreased levels of all components of complement, whereas cirrhosis of the liver is associated with decreased synthesis of C3.

Immune complex disease (systemic lupus erythematosus, postinfectious nephritis) can result in increased complement consumption and relative deficiency. Increased consumption has also been demonstrated in lepromatous leprosy, subacute bacterial endocarditis, malaria, dengue fever, acute hepatitis B, and infectious mononucle-

Table 52–9. **Genetic Deficiencies of Complement Components**

		Associated Clinical Findings	
Component	**Genetics**	*Associated Diseases*	*Recurrent Infections*
C1q	Autosomal recessive	SLE, MPGN, vasculitis	Septicemia, meningitis, pyoderma, dermatitis
C1s	Autosomal recessive	SLE	Recurrent pneumonia, meningitis
C1r	Autosomal recessive	SLE, CGN, vasculitis	Recurrent pneumonia, meningitis
C1 inhibitor	Autosomal dominant	Hereditary angioedema, SLE	
C4	Autosomal recessive	SLE, HSP, Sjögren syndrome	Recurrent pneumonia, meningitis
C2	Autosomal recessive	SLE, HSP, ITP, CGN, dermatomyositis, vasculitis, MPGN	Recurrent septicemia, especially pneumococcal; meningitis; pneumonia
C3	Autosomal recessive	SLE, MPGN, vasculitis	Severe pyogenic infection due to meningococci and pneumococci
C5	Autosomal recessive	SLE	Disseminated gonococcal and meningococcal disease, pyoderma, meningitis
C6	Autosomal recessive	SLE, MPGN, Sjögren syndrome, Raynaud phenomenon	Disseminated gonococcal and meningococcal disease
C7	Autosomal recessive	SLE, scleroderma, ankylosing spondylitis, rheumatoid arthritis, Raynaud phenomenon	Disseminated gonococcal and meningococcal disease
C8	Autosomal recessive	SLE	Disseminated gonococcal and meningococcal disease
C9	Autosomal recessive		Meningococcal meningitis, extragenital gonococcal infections
C3bi	?		Recurrent pyogenic infections
Factor D	X-linked		Recurrent sinusitis, bronchitis
Factor I	Autosomal recessive		Pyogenic infections, septicemia
Factor H	Autosomal recessive	Hemolytic-uremic syndrome	Pyogenic infections, septicemia
Properdin	X-linked		Septicemia

Abbreviations: CGN = chronic glomerulonephritis; SLE = systemic lupus erythematosus; ITP = idiopathic thrombocytopenia purpura; MPGN = membranoproliferative glomerulonephritis; HSP = Henoch-Schönlein purpura.

Table 52–10. Disorders of Phagocyte Dysfunction

Disorder	Etiology	Impaired Function	Clinical Consequences
Degranulation Abnormalities			
Chédiak-Higashi syndrome	Autosomal recessive; disordered coalescence of lysosomal granules	Decreased neutrophil chemotaxis, degranulation, bactericidal activity; platelet storage pool defect; impaired NK function, failure to disperse melanosomes	Neutropenia; recurrent pyogenic infections; propensity to develop marked hepatosplenomegaly in the accelerated phase; pigment dilution in skin and fundus
Specific granule deficiency	Autosomal recessive; abnormal regulation of expression of various myeloid granule genes by a transacting factor	Impaired chemotaxis and bactericial activity; bilobed nuclei in neutrophils; reduced content of neutrophil defensins, gelatinase, collagenase, vitamin B_{12} binding protein, lactoferrin	Recurrent deep-seated skin abscesses
Adhesion Abnormalities			
Leukocyte adhesion deficiency	Absence of CD11/CD18 surface adhesive glycoprotein (β_2 integrins) on leukocyte membranes arising from failure to express CD18 mRNA	Decreased binding of complement to C3bi and endothelial ICAM 1 and ICAM 2	Neutrophilia, recurrent bacterial infections without pus
Leukocyte adhesion deficiency 2	Absence of sialyl-Lewis X	Decreased adhesion to inflamed endothelium	Neutrophila, recurrent bacterial infections without pus
Neutrophil actin dysfunction	Impaired polymerization of neutrophil cytoplasmic actin perhaps arising from the presence of an inhibitor to F-actin formation	Impaired neutrophil chemotaxis, adhesion, and bacterial killing	Neutrophilia, recurrent bacterial infections without pus
Disorders of Chemotaxis			
Defects in the generation of chemotactic signals	IgG deficiencies, C3 deficiency, and properdin deficiency can arise from genetic or acquired abnormalities	Deficiency of serum chemotaxis and opsonic activities	Recurrent pyogenic infections
Intrinsic defects of the neutrophil	Diminished ability to express neutrophil β_2 integrins and qualitative impairment in β_2 integrin function	Diminished chemotaxis	Mild propensity to develop pyogenic infections
Direct inhibition of neutrophil mobility by drugs	Ethanol, glucocorticoids, cyclic adenosine monophosphate	Impaired locomotion and ingestion, impaired adherence	Possible cause for frequent infections, neutrophilia seen with epinephrine is the result of cyclic AMP release from endothelium
Immune complexes	Bind to Fc receptors on neutrophils in patients with rheumatoid arthritis, systemic lupus erythematosus, other inflammatory states	Impaired chemotaxis	Recurrent pyogenic infections
Hyperimmunoglobulin E syndrome	(?) Autosomal dominant; variable expression of a soluble inhibitor from mononuclear cells affecting neutrophil chemotaxis; high levels of antistaphylococcal IgE	Impaired chemotaxis at times, impaired IgG opsonization of *Staphylococcus aureus*	Recurrent skin and sinopulmonary infections
Defects of Microbicidal Activity			
Chronic granulomatous disease	Failure to express functional gp91-phox in the membrane in X-linked CGD; failure to express functional protein in the membrane in p22-phox (AR), other AR CGD arises from failure to express protein p47phox or p67phox	Failure to activate neutrophil respiratory burst, leading to failure to kill catalase-positive microbes	Recurrent pyogenic infections with catalase-positive microorganisms

Table 52–10. Disorders of Phagocyte Dysfunction *Continued*

Disorder	Etiology	Impaired Function	Clinical Consequences
G6PD deficiency	Less than 5% of normal activity of G6PD	Failure to activate NADPH-dependent oxidase	Infections with catalase-positive microorganisms
Myeloperoxidase deficiency	Multiple causes, e.g., failure to process post-translationally modified precursor protein missense mutation; failure to express mRNA	H_2O_2-dependent antimicrobial activity not potentiated by myeloperoxidase	None
Deficiencies of glutathione reductase and glutathione synthetase	Failure to detoxify hydrogen peroxide	Excessive formation of hydrogen peroxide	Minimal problems with recurrent pyogenic infections
Impaired Spleen Function Splenic absence or splenic dysfunction	Congenital absence of spleen, removal of spleen, vascular occlusion of spleen	Removal or impaired function of splenic macrophage	Propensity to infection with encapsulated bacteria

From Boxer LA. Qualitative abnormalities of granulocytes. *In* Williams WJ, Beutler E, Erslev AJ, Lichtman MA (eds). *In* Hematology, 5th ed. New York: McGraw-Hill, 1995:828–843.

Abbreviations: X = X-linked; AR = autosomal recessive; G6PD = glucose-6-phosphate dehydrogenase; CGD = chronic granulomatous disease; ICAM = intracellular adhesion molecule; NK = natural killer; C = complement; m = messenger; H_2O_2 = hydrogen peroxide; NADPH = nicotinamide-adenine dinucleotide phosphate; AMP = adenosine monophosphate.

osis. Burn injuries can induce massive activation of complement, accounting at least partially for the increased risk of infection in burn patients. In patients with erythropoietic protoporphyria or porphyria cutanea tarda, hypocomplementemia develops because certain wavelengths of light activate complement, resulting in abnormal consumption.

Diagnosis and Management

The most useful screening test is the total hemolytic complement activity (CH_{50}). The CH_{50} measures the ability of all 11 components of the classic pathway to lyse antibody-coated red blood cells. This assay does not identify abnormalities in the alternative pathway, but in factor H and I deficiency, increased consumption of C3 is identified by a decrease in CH_{50}. The alternative pathway can be screened by use of a hemolytic assay that uses rabbit erythrocytes as both the activating surface and the target. Measurements of C3 and C4 can help distinguish complement deficiencies. In hereditary angioneurotic edema, C4 levels are generally low, but C3 levels are normal. Low C3 and C4 levels are seen when the classic pathway is activated, whereas activation of the alternative pathway characteristically results in low C3 levels and normal C4 levels.

No specific therapy exists for any of the genetic disorders of complement. Replacement factors are not available. Some patients with angioedema respond to androgen therapy, especially in short-term use. For patients at increased risk for infection as a result of other deficiencies in the complement system, appropriate immunizations and aggressive management of infections are the bulwark of therapy.

NEUTROPHIL DISORDERS

Neutrophils are particularly important in protecting the skin, mucous membrane, and lining of the respiratory and gastrointestinal tracts. As such, they form the first line of defense against microbial invasion. During the critical 2- to 4-hour period after

invasion by pathogenic organisms, phagocytic cells must arrive at the site of invasion if infection is to be contained. If not, the resulting infection leads to a larger local lesion or disseminates throughout the host.

To be effective and arrive at the site of inflammation, phagocytic cells must attach (adhere) to the vascular endothelium near the site of invasion or inflammation, engage in diapedesis through the vessel wall and move in a unidirectional fashion toward the site (chemotaxis), adhere and ingest (phagocytosis) the offending organisms, and activate biochemical pathways important in intracellular microbial killing (degranulation and oxidative metabolism). Microbial killing is accomplished by two mechanisms: (1) *de novo* synthesis of highly toxic and often unstable derivatives of molecular oxygen by an enzyme known as the respiratory burst oxidase, and (2) delivery into the phagocytic vacuoles containing the ingested microbes of preformed polypeptide antibiotics and proteases stored within several types of lysosomal granules.

Patients whose neutrophils have defects in adhesion or cell motility generally have cutaneous abscesses with common pathogens such as *Staphylococcus aureus* or have mucous membrane lesions caused by agents such as *Candida albicans* or oral anaerobic bacterial flora. If the defect in adhesion and chemotaxis is profound, lesions may contain few if any neutrophils. Disorders of phagocyte microbicidal activity (chronic granulomatous disease) are associated with cutaneous abscesses, lymphadenitis, pulmonary infections, and gastrointestinal problems, such as antral obstruction. These patients tend to have more deep-seated and chronic infections involving the liver and lung (Table 52–10).

Disorders of Neutrophil Motility

CONGENITAL LEUKOCYTE ADHERENCE DEFICIENCY

Leukocyte adherence deficiency is a rare autosomal recessive disorder of leukocyte function that is characterized by recurrent soft tissue infections, delayed wound healing, and severely impaired pus formation, despite striking blood neutrophilia ranging from 15 to 60 × 10⁹/L. Patients with this disorder have a decreased or absent expression of a family of leukocyte surface glycoproteins designated CD11/CD18 complex (also referred to as the B2 integrin family of leukocyte adhesive proteins) (see Table 52–10). These proteins include LFA-1 (CD11a/CD18), Mol-1 or Mac-1 (CD11b/CD18), and P150,95 (CD11c/CD18). Diminished or absent surface expression of these proteins accounts for a profound impairment of neutrophil and monocyte adhesion-dependent functions *in vitro*, including cell migration and complement-mediated phagocytosis.

Activated neutrophils of patients with the most severe clinical form of leukocyte adherence deficiency express fewer than 0.3% of the normal amount of the β_2 integrins, whereas those of the patients with the moderate phenotype may express 2% to 7% of normal numbers of β_2 integrin molecules. Patients with severe involvement have recurrent and gangrenous soft tissue infections of subcutaneous tissues or mucous membranes caused by *S. aureus*, *Pseudomonas* sp and other gram-negative enteric rods, or *Candida* species. Patients with moderate involvement have fewer and less severe infections. The diagnosis is made most readily by flow cytometric measurement of surface CD11b in stimulated and unstimulated neutrophils using monoclonal antibodies directed against CD11b.

CHÉDIAK-HIGASHI SYNDROME

The Chédiak-Higashi Syndrome (CHS) is a rare autosomal recessive disorder that is characterized by partial ocular cutaneous albinism, neutropenia, and morphologic disorder, in which all leukocytes contain giant cytoplasmic granules (see Table 52–10). CHS is recognized as a generalized cellular disease that affects all granule-bearing cells. Giant azurophil and specific granules are found in circulating neutrophils. Many of the abnormal myeloid precursors die in the marrow, resulting in a moderate neutropenia with white cell counts of about 2.5 × 10⁹/L. Despite normal ingestion of particles and active oxygen metabolism, these neutrophils kill microorganisms relatively slowly. This delay reflects a slow but inconsistent delivery of dilute amounts of hydrolytic enzymes from the giant granules into the phagosomes. Monocytes from patients with CHS have the same functional derangements as neutrophils. Recurrent infections that are usually encountered in CHS affect the skin, respiratory tract, and mucous membranes and are caused by both gram-positive and gram-negative bacteria as well as fungi; *S. aureus* is the most common organism. Natural killer function also is impaired. Despite normal platelet counts, patients with CHS have prolonged bleeding times, which is related to a platelet storage pool abnormality. Neuropathy may be present, which can be sensory or motor; ataxia may be a prominent feature.

A propensity for lymphohistiocytic proliferation, known as the *accelerated phase*, occurs in the reticuloendothelial systems of patients with CHS, which intensifies the already existing neutropenia and leads to pancytopenia. This proliferation is associated with recurrent bacterial and viral infections and fever and usually results in death. The onset of the accelerated phase may be related to the inability to contain and control the Epstein-Barr virus and leads to features that simulate viral-mediated hemophagocytic syndrome.

SPECIFIC GRANULE DEFICIENCY

Specific granule deficiency is a rare disorder that affects both sexes and is likely inherited as an autosomal recessive disease (see Table 52–10). Clinically, patients with this disorder have recurrent infections involving the skin and lungs. *S. aureus* is the most commonly observed pathogen, although *C. albicans* and a variety of gram-negative bacteria have also been isolated. Specific granulo-deficient neutrophils lack proteolytic activity in the tertiary granules, vitamin B₁₂ binding protein, lactoferrin and collagenase in the specific granules, and the bactericidal proteins known as defensins in the primary granules. Neutrophils from these patients have abnormal chemotaxis and a mild defect in bactericidal activity.

The diagnosis of specific granule deficiency is suggested by the presence of neutrophils that are devoid of specific granules but contain azurophil granules on the blood film. The diagnosis can be confirmed by demonstration of a severe deficiency in either lactoferrin or vitamin B₁₂ binding proteins by immunoperoxidase staining or by quantitation of the proteins themselves. The nuclei of the neutrophils are also bilobed. An acquired form of specific granule deficiency can be observed in thermally injured patients or in individuals with myelodysplasia.

OTHER DISORDERS OF NEUTROPHIL MOTILITY

Depressed neutrophil chemotaxis has been observed in a wide variety of clinical conditions (see Table 52–10). Patients with chemotactic disorders may be infected by various microorganisms, including fungi and gram-positive or gram-negative bacteria; *S. aureus* is the most common offender. Typically the skin, gingival mucosa, and regional lymph nodes are involved. Respiratory tract infections are common, but sepsis is rare. Delayed or inappropriate signs and symptoms of inflammation are common. With mild chemotactic disorders, the cells can be demonstrated to move slowly in chemotactic assays; they accumulate in sufficient numbers to produce pus. Detection of patients with neutrophils that have profound defects in chemotaxis is usually made through other phagocytic assays, such as monitoring of adhesion and phagocytosis.

Hyperimmunoglobulin E Syndrome

The hyperimmunoglobulin E syndrome is characterized by markedly elevated levels of serum IgE, chronic dermatitis, and serious recurrent bacterial infections (see Table 52–10). The skin infections are remarkable for their absence of surrounding erythema, leading to the formation of "cold abscesses." Neutrophils and monocytes from patients with this syndrome exhibit a variable but at times profound chemotactic defect that appears extrinsic to the neutrophil. Clinical manifestations of hyperimmunoglobulin E begin as early as 1 to 8 weeks of age. The syndrome is characterized by chronic eczematoid rashes, which are typically papular and pruritic. The rash generally involves the face and extensor surfaces of arms and legs; skin lesions are frequently sharply demarcated and usually lack surrounding erythema. By 5 years of age, all patients have had a history of recurrent skin abscesses and recurrent pneumonias, along with chronic otitis media and sinusitis. Patients may also develop septic arthritis, cellulitis, or osteomyelitis. The major offending pathogen is *S. aureus*. Other associated features include coarse facial features manifested by a broad nasal bridge, prominent nose, and irregular proportional checks and jaw. Growth retardation is found in a small number of patients and appears to be related to the presence of chronic illness.

All patients have serum IgE levels that exceed 2500 IU/ml. Unlike atopic patients, who occasionally have similar elevated IgE levels, patients with hyperimmunoglobulin E syndrome have their serum IgE antibody directed to *S. aureus*. Usually, patients have normal concentrations of IgG, IgA, and IgM and pronounced blood and sputum eosinophilia. At times, the neutrophils and monocytes of affected patients have a profound chemotactic defect. The molecular basis for this syndrome remains unknown. Some investigators believe that the immunologic basis of hyperimmunoglobulin E arises from suppressor T cells that are insufficient to inhibit IgE production. Alternatively, a predisposition to bacterial infections may arise from production of a chemotactic inhibitor, released by mononuclear cells, that inhibits normal neutrophil and monocyte chemotaxis.

Disorders of Neutrophil Oxidative Metabolism

CHRONIC GRANULOMATOUS DISEASE

Chronic granulomatous disease (CGD) is a rare disease with an incidence of approximately one in 1 million. It is characterized by the ability of neutrophils and monocytes to ingest but their inability to kill catalase-positive microorganisms because of a defect in the generation of antimicrobial oxygen metabolites (see Table 52–10). CGD is caused by mutations involving one of several genes that encode a component of nicotinamide-adenine dinucleotide phosphate (NADPH) oxidase.

Several laboratory tests are used to classify the forms of CGD. The initial diagnosis is usually made through the nitroblue tetrazolium dye test, in which the yellow water-soluble tetrazolium dye is not reduced to a blue and soluble formazan pigment because of the failure of the CGD neutrophil to generate superoxide anion.

The inability of phagocytes to generate superoxide anion is caused by the absence of one of the components of the NADPH oxidase system. Approximately 65% of affected children lack the membrane-bound component of the oxidase cytochrome b_{558}. The gene for this protein is located on the X chromosome. Not surprisingly, the family histories of children with the X-linked variety of CGD often include male maternal relatives who died of infections at a young age. Virtually all other patients with CGD lack one of the two identified cytosolic factors, either a 47-kD protein or 67-kD protein. These deficiencies are inherited in an autosomal recessive manner.

Although the clinical presentation is variable, several clinical features suggest the diagnosis of CGD (Table 52–11). Any patient

Table 52–11. Clinical Manifestations of Chronic Granulomatous Disease

Incidence	1:1,000,000
Male/female ratio	6:1
Clinical disorders*	
Pneumonitis	(77%)
Dermatitis	(68%)
Lymphadenitis	(60%)
Hepatic abscess	(39%)
Osteomyelitis	(32%)
Persistent diarrhea	(18%)
Septicemia/meningitis	(17%)
Persistent rhinitis	(15%)
Perianal abscess	(14%)
Stomatitis	(14%)
Gastric antral narrowing (rare)	
and pyelonephritis secondary to ureteral (rare) obstruction, pericarditis (rare)	

Data from Forrest CB, Forehand JR, Axtell RA, et al. Clinical features and current management of chronic granulomatous disease. Hematol Oncol Clin North Am 1988; 2:2.

*The number in parenthesis represents the percentage of patients affected.

with recurrent lymphadenitis should be considered to have CGD. Patients with bacterial hepatic abscesses, osteomyelitis at multiple sites or in the small bones of the hands and feet, a family history of recurrent infections, or unusual catalase-positive microbial infections all require clinical evaluation. The onset of clinical signs and symptoms may occur from early infancy to young adulthood, and the attack rate and severity of infections are variable. The most common pathogen is *S. aureus*. Infection with *Serratia marcescens Pseudomonas cepacia, Aspergillus* sp or *C. albicans* occurs frequently. Pneumonia, lymphadenitis, and skin infections are the most common infections encountered. Infections are characterized by microabscesses and granuloma formation. Patients may develop the sequelae of chronic infection, including the anemia of chronic disease, lymphadenopathy, hepatosplenomegaly, hypergammaglobulinemia, chronic purulent dermatitis, restrictive lung disease, gingivitis, hydronephrosis, and gastrointestinal narrowing.

Treatment includes antibiotics and drainage for infections or abscesses, prophylactic trimethoprim-sulfamethoxazole, and long-term continuous gamma interferon therapy. Steroids and antibiotics are used to treat granulomatous obstructing lesions of the gastrointestinal or urinary tract. Granulocyte transfusion may be needed to treat life-threatening, poorly responsive infection (*Aspergillus* pneumonia).

Leukocytes from patients with CGD have normal glucose-6-phosphate dehydrogenase (G6PD) activity. However, a few individuals with apparent CGD have been described to have neutrophils that lack or almost lack in G6PD activity. These patients also have a hemolytic anemia because their erythrocytes are affected by the lack of G6PD, which distinguishes these patients from those with classic CGD. In cases of severe neutrophil G6PD deficiency, an attenuated respiratory burst progressively decreases as a result of the depletion of intracellular NADPH, the primary substrate for the respiratory burst to oxidase.

MYELOPEROXIDASE DEFICIENCY

Myeloperoxidase deficiency is the most common hereditary disorder of neutrophil function; its incidence is one in 2000. The lack of myeloperoxidase, an enzyme that catalyses the production of hypochlorous acid in the phagosome, causes microbicidal deficiency of the neutrophils early after ingestion of microorganisms (see Table 52–10). Although killing of the bacteria is slower than normal, eventually effective killing of bacteria occurs. The most significant clinical manifestation in a few patients with diabetes mellitus and myeloperoxidase deficiency has been severe infection with *C. albicans*. Most patients with this genetic disorder have not been unusually susceptible to pyogenic infections and do not require therapy.

ASPLENIA

The spleen plays a particularly important role in attenuating infection, especially during the first year of life before specific immunity to certain bacteria has developed. Bacteria such as pneumococci and *H. influenzae* are filtered exclusively by the spleen when they are not opsonized with antibody. Clearance of the bacteria is rapidly followed by the development of some humoral immunity, which may be detectable within a day after exposure. In addition to its function of removing microbes, the spleen also produces antibodies. Individuals without a spleen (anatomic or functional) are subject to a severe form of sepsis that is rapid in onset and can lead to sudden death if it is not recognized and treated promptly (see Tables 52–1 and 52–10). Pneumococci are responsible for more than 50% of such infections; *H. influenzae* in about 25%; and *S. aureus,* group A streptococci, gram-negative enteric bacilli, and meningococci in the remaining patients (see Table 52–1).

The diagnosis of anatomic or functional asplenia is suggested by the presence of red cell inclusions, particularly Howell-Jolly bodies on peripheral blood smear. The diagnosis is confirmed when no spleen is noted on ultrasonography of the abdomen or by the failure of uptake of ^{99}Tc-sulfur colloid, which is normally taken up by the entire reticuloendothelial system. Pitted or pocked erythrocytes are also noted in asplenic patients.

Functionally asplenia occurs in children with sickle cell disease, initially as a result of vascular occlusion by the sickle cells in the splenic circulation. Congenital absence of the spleen may occur alone or as part of an *asplenia syndrome* with congenital heart disease (see Chapters 15 and 16). The usual presentation in the asplenia syndrome is that of a cyanotic newborn, often with respiratory distress and a midline liver. Clues to the presence of the asplenia syndrome are often found on the chest x-ray study. This condition should be considered when the cardiac position is distorted with that of the stomach and liver, especially if pulmonary vascular markings are very diminished as a result of pulmonary atresia or if pulmonary edema secondary to obstructive pulmonary veins is present.

The risk of fulminant infection in patients who have undergone splenectomy (from surgery or trauma) or in those with functional asplenia or congenital asplenia is greatest in the first few years. The risk is less in older children and in adults, probably because they have developed opsonizing antibodies through previous exposure. The management of functional or anatomic asplenia lies mainly in prevention. When splenectomy becomes necessary, partial protection against life-threatening infections can be obtained by immunizing patients with polyvalent pneumococcal vaccines and possibly with *H. influenzae* type b vaccines. Booster immunization may be needed because of waning immunity with time. Prophylactic antibiotics may be given continuously in a single daily dose for 1 to 3 years or up to the age of 16 years (some authorities suggest longer periods or even for life) after splenectomy in children who are not old enough to complain of mild symptoms; with older children, parents are advised to have the child seen by a physician or to administer the antibiotics at the first sign of a febrile respiratory illness.

SUMMARY AND RED FLAGS

Recurrent benign infections are common, especially in large families or in day care settings, where children may manifest six to 10 upper respiratory tract infections or gastroenteritis episodes a year. These infections should usually last less than 1 week. The child continues to grow and develop normally, and his or her activities are not restricted.

Red flags include absent lymphoid tissue, failure to thrive, chronic diarrhea, prolonged infections, infections with unusual organisms, repeated serious infections, eczematous dermatitis, a family history of early childhood deaths (presumably from infection), and other diseases associated with increased risks for infection (sickle cell anemia, malignancy, asplenia).

REFERENCES

Family History and Physical Examination

Stiehm ER. They're back: Recurrent infections in pediatric practice. Contemp Pediatr 1990;7:20.

Diagnostic Approach

Buckley RH. Immunodeficiency diseases. JAMA 1992;268:2797.

Castigli E, Geha RS, Chatila T. Severe combined immunodeficiency with selective T-cell cytokine genes. Pediatr Res 1993;33:S20–22.

Claman HN. The biology of the immune response. JAMA 1992;268:2790.

Hirschhorn R. Overview of biochemical abnormalities and molecular genetics of adenosine deaminase deficiency. Pediatr Res 1993;33:S35–41.

Noguchi M, Yi H, Rosenblatt HM, et al. Interleukin-2 receptor gamma chain mutation results in X-linked severe combined immunodeficiency in humans. Cell 1993;73:147.

Strober W, Eisenstein E, Jaffe JS, et al. Immunologic and genetic studies in common variable immunodeficiency. Ann Intern Med 1993;118:720.

Wengler GS, Allen RC, Parolini O, et al. Nonrandom X chromosome inactivation in natural killer cells from obligate carriers of X-linked severe combined immunodeficiency. J Immunol 1993;150:700.

Complement System Deficiency

Rother K, Rother V. Hereditary and acquired complement deficiencies in animals and man. Prog Allergy 1986;39:1.

Walport MJ. Inherited complement deficiency: Clues to the physiological activity of complement in vivo. Q J Med 1993;86:355.

Neutrophil Disorders

Boxer LA. Qualitative abnormalities of granulocytes. *In* Williams WJ, Beutler E, Erslev AJ, et al. (eds). Hematology, 5th ed. New York: McGraw-Hill, 1995:828–843.

Smolen JE, Boxer LA. Function of granulocytes. *In* Williams WJ, Beutler E, Erslev AJ, et al. (eds). Hematology, 5th ed. New York: McGraw-Hill, 1995:779–797.

Leukocyte Adhesion Deficiency

Arnaout MA. Dynamics and regulation of leukocyte-endothelial cell interactions. Curr Opin Hematol 1993;1:113.

Fischer A, Lisowska-Cirospierre B, Anderson DC, et al. Leukocyte adhesion deficiency: Molecular basis and functional consequences. Immunodefic Rev 1988;1:39.

Chédiak-Higashi Syndrome

Boxer LA, Smolen JE. Neutrophil granule constituents and their release in health and disease. Hematol Oncol Clin North Am 1988;2:101.

Ganz T, Metcalf JA, Gallin JI, et al. Microbicidal/cytotoxic proteins of neutrophils are deficient in two disorders: Chédiak-Higashi syndrome and ''specific'' granule deficiency. J Clin Invest 1988;82:552.

Specific-Granule Deficiency

Boxer LA, Coates TD, Haak RA, et al. Lactoferrin deficiency associated with altered granulocyte function. N Engl J Med 1982;307:404.

Johnston JJ, Boxer LA, Berliner N. Correlation of mRNA levels with protein defects in specific granule deficiency. Blood 1992;80:2088.

Disorders of Neutrophil Motility

Boxer LA, Allen JM, Baehner RL. Diminished polymorphonuclear leukocyte adherence: Function dependent on release of cyclic AMP by endothelial cells after stimulation of b-receptors by epinephrine. J Clin Invest 1980;66:268.

Weston BW, Axtell RA, Todd RF III, et al. Clinical and biologic effects of granulocyte-colony stimulating factor in the treatment of myelokathexis. J Pediatr 1991;188:229.

Hyperimmunoglobulin E Syndrome

Jeppson JD, Jaffe HS, Hill HR. Use of recombinant human interferon gamma to enhance neutrophil chemotactic responses in Job syndrome of hyperimmunoglobulin E and recurrent infections. J Pediatr 1991;3:383.
Leung DYM, Geha RS. Clinical and immunologic aspects of the hyperimmunoglobulin E syndrome. Hematol Oncol Clin North Am 1988;2:81.

Chronic Granulomatous Disease

Forrest CB, Forehand JR, Axtell RA, et al. Clinical features and current management of chronic granulomatous disease. Hematol Oncol Clin North Am 1988;2:253.
Moury R, Fischer A, Vilmer E, et al. Incidence, severity and prevention of infections in chronic granulomatous disease. J Pediatr 1989;114:555.

The International Chronic Granulomatous Disease Study Group. A controlled study of interferon gamma to prevent infections in chronic granulomatous disease. N Engl J Med 1991;324:509.

Myeloperoxidase Deficiency

Nauseef WM. Myeloperoxidase deficiency. Hematol Pathol 1990;4:165.

Asplenia

Gikonyo DK, Tandon R, Lucas RF Jr, et al. Scimitar syndrome in neonates: Report of four cases and review of the literature. Pediatr Cardiol 1986;6:193.
Reid M. Splenectomy, sepsis, immunisation and guidelines. Lancet 1994;344, 970.
Rose V, Izukawa T, Moes CAF. Syndromes of asplenia and polysplenia: A review of cardiac and noncardiac malformation in 60 cases with special reference to diagnosis and prognosis. Br Heart J 1975;37:840.

53 Meningismus and Meningitis

Jay H. Mayefsky

A stiff neck (nuchal rigidity) may be due to many causes (Table 53–1) but most often appropriately invokes the consideration of *meningitis*. Patients with meningitis usually do not complain solely of a stiff neck, as most have symptoms of fever, alterations of consciousness, or seizures. Alternately, most patients who have only a stiff neck do not have meningitis. In meningitis (bacterial, aseptic), the stiffness is caused by inflammation of the cervical dura and reflex spasm of the extensor muscles of the neck. Consequently, there is pain and limitation of motion on flexion of the neck. Lateral movement of the neck is often normal and pain-free. Although meningeal irritation may also be found in other conditions (tumor, subarachnoid hemorrhage), when this type of stiff neck is found, especially in the presence of fever, meningitis must be excluded and, if present, treated.

The child with a stiff neck may also present with the head drawn

to one side and rotated, with the chin pointing to the contralateral side. Spasm (torticollis) of the strap muscles of the neck may be found. Usually the neck can be flexed, but rotation or lateral movement is limited and causes pain. Torticollis is rarely a presentation of meningitis; investigations into the various causes of torticollis may be warranted (Table 53–2). A child may present with a painful neck that is not stiff. In this instance, the neck can be moved, albeit with pain, in all directions. This finding is seen in children with a variety of disorders, including lymphadenopathy, neuritis, and acute strains of the neck musculature.

Meningismus, also called meningism, is not synonymous with stiff neck and is a specific syndrome with a stiff neck and other meningeal signs (headache, Kernig and Brudzinski signs) (Fig. 53–1). Meningismus may be associated with an acute viral or bacterial infection outside the central nervous system (CNS). The stiff neck is often present at the onset but may not appear for up to a week after the onset of the infection. Examination of the cerebrospinal fluid (CSF) reveals no abnormalities except for an occasional increase in pressure. CSF cultures are negative.

The pathophysiology of this disorder is unclear. It may be due to a disturbed equilibrium in the osmotic relationship between the blood and CSF, the syndrome of inappropriate antidiuretic hormone secretion (SIADH), or increased formation of CSF. The symptoms are usually short-lived, and the spinal tap that is done to rule out meningitis is often curative, in that it results in the disappearance of the meningeal signs.

Before initiating an evaluation for nuchal rigidity, the physician must know that the disease process causing a stiff neck may originate in any of the structures of the neck—cervical dura, mus-

Table 53–1. Overview of the Differential Diagnosis of a Stiff Neck

Meningitis: bacterial, aseptic
Upper lobe pneumonia
Torticollis
Neck trauma (accidental, intentional, overuse)
Inflammatory-induced slipped cervical vertebra
Neck inflammation (lymphadenopathy, lymphadenitis, thyroiditis, deep neck cellulitis, jugular thrombophlebitis)
Retropharyngeal abscess

Table 53–2. Differential Diagnosis of Torticollis

Congenital
  Muscular torticollis
  Positional deformation
  Hemivertebra (cervicosuperior dorsal spine)
  Unilateral atlanto-occipital fusion
  Klippel-Feil syndrome
  Unilateral absence of sternocleidomastoid
  Pterygium colli

Trauma
  Muscular injury (cervical muscles)
  Atlanto-occipital subluxation
  Atlantoaxial subluxation
  C2-C3 subluxation
  Rotary subluxation
  Fractures

Inflammation
  Cervical lymphadenitis
  Retropharyngeal abscess
  Cervical vertebral osteomyelitis
  Rheumatoid arthritis
  Spontaneous (hyperemia, edema) subluxation with adjacent
    head and neck infection (rotary subluxation syndrome)
  Upper lobe pneumonia

Neurologic
  Visual disturbances (nystagmus, superior oblique paresis)
  Dystonic drug reactions (phenothiazines, haloperidol,
    metoclopramide)
  Cervicial cord tumor
  Posterior fossa brain tumor
  Syringomyelia
  Wilson disease
  Dystonia musculorum deformans
  Spasmus nutans

Other
  Acute cervical disc calcification
  Sandifer syndrome (gastroesophageal reflux, hiatal hernia)
  Benign paroxysmal torticollis
  Bone tumors (eosinophilic granuloma)
  Soft-tissue tumor
  Hysteria

From Behrman RE (ed). Nelson Textbook of Pediatrics, 14th ed. Philadelphia: WB Saunders, 1992:1718.

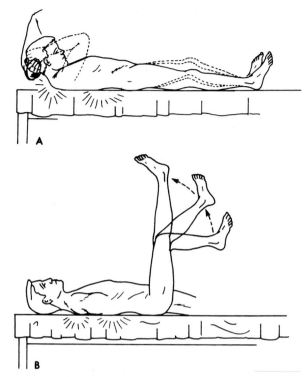

Figure 53–1. *A,* Brudzinski's sign. The patient lies supine, and the head is passively elevated from the table by the examiner. The patient complains of neck and low back discomfort and attempts to relieve the meningeal irritation by involuntary flexion of the knees and hips. *B,* Kernig's sign. The patient lies supine, with the hips and knees flexed. The knees are then gradually extended. Complaints of pain in the lower back, neck, and/or head are suggestive of meningeal irritation. (From Reilly BM. Practical Strategies in Outpatient Medicine, 2nd ed. Philadelphia: WB Saunders, 1991:95.)

cles, ligaments, bones, fascia, lymph nodes, glands, or viscera. With this knowledge, a complete history, physical examination, and laboratory investigation can be performed and an appropriate differential diagnosis formulated.

BACTERIAL MENINGITIS

Clinical Presentation

Bacterial meningitis is usually a disease of infants and young children. The highest attack rate occurs between 3 and 8 months of age; 66% of cases occur in children younger than 5 years of age. Bacterial meningitis is seen during all seasons; however, there may be a seasonal correlation between the presence of preceding respiratory pathogens (viral, mycoplasmal) in the upper respiratory tract and the subsequent development of bacterial meningitis. Bacterial meningitis usually occurs sporadically. Clusters of cases have

been noted in day care centers and other closed communities. Bacterial meningitis occurs more frequently in children with traumatic fractures of the cribriform plate or paranasal sinuses (pneumococcal); in children who have had neurosurgical procedures (*Staphylococcus aureus, Staphylococcus epidermidis, Corynebacterium*); in children with congenital or acquired immunodeficiencies (pneumococcus, *Listeria monocytogenes,* meningococcus); in children with anatomic or functional asplenia (pneumococcus, meningococcus); and in children with sickle cell disease (pneumococcus) and other hemoglobinopathies. There may be a genetic predisposition in some groups for the development of meningitis, as there is an increased incidence of *Haemophilus influenzae* type b meningitis in Navajo Indians, Eskimos, and children with HLA-B12.

Bacterial meningitis presents in two patterns. In the first, the symptoms may develop slowly over several days, with the initial symptoms being those of gastroenteritis or an upper respiratory infection. Subsequently, the signs and symptoms of meningitis develop. In the second pattern, the disease may develop suddenly and quickly, with the first indications of illness being the signs and symptoms of sepsis syndrome and meningitis.

The manifestations of meningitis depend on the child's age and the response to the pathogen. In infants, the findings are usually nonspecific and may be subtle. Infants may present with vomiting, diarrhea, irritability, lethargy, poor appetite, respiratory distress, seizures, hypothermia, or jaundice. Only 50% have fever; some present only with fever. It is uncommon for a young infant to have a stiff neck, and only 30% have a bulging fontanelle.

Older children present with more specific meningeal signs. They complain of a headache that is described as being severe, general-

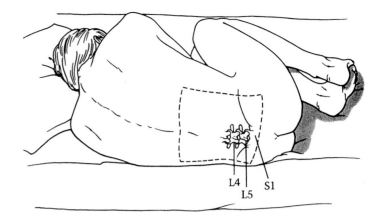

Figure 53–2. Lateral decubitus position for a lumbar puncture. L4-L5 position is determined by a vertical line drawn between the superior iliac crests. (From Davidson RI. Lumbar puncture. *In* Vander Salm TJ, Cutler BS, Wheeler HB [eds]. Atlas of Bedside Procedures, 2nd ed. Boston: Little, Brown, 1992:443.)

ized, deep-seated, and constant. They also complain of nausea, vomiting, anorexia, and photophobia. On examination, they demonstrate irritability, mental confusion or altered consciousness, nuchal rigidity, and occasionally hyperesthesia and ataxia.

Nuchal rigidity is demonstrated by feeling resistance and observing a painful response while flexing the child's neck. The stiffness may not be recognized until the end of flexion. The neck is stiff only to flexion and usually can be rotated without symptoms. In the child who is crying and tensing the muscles, nuchal rigidity may be demonstrated if the examiner places the hand under the occiput of the supine patient and lifts the child. If the neck does not flex, it is stiff. Alternatively, a sitting child may be observed following an object as it falls to the floor. The child who flexes the neck to look at the object does not have nuchal rigidity. In the presence of meningitis, flexion of the neck causes spontaneous flexion of the legs at the hips and knees. This is known as the *Brudzinski sign* (see Fig. 53–1). The *Kernig sign* is elicited when the patient lies supine and, with the knee flexed, the leg is flexed at the hip. The knee is then extended. A positive sign is present if this movement is limited by contraction of the hamstrings and causes pain. Absence of nuchal rigidity is found in 1.5% of cases of meningitis in older children; it may be absent in children who have overwhelming infections (meningococcemia), are deeply comatose, or who have focal or global neurologic impairment.

Fifteen percent of children with bacterial meningitis present initially in a comatose or semicomatose state (see Chapter 41). Focal neurologic signs are found in 15% of children at some point during their illness. These signs include hemiparesis, quadriparesis, cranial nerve palsies, endophthalmitis, visual field defects, cortical blindness, ataxia, deafness, and vestibular nerve dysfunction. Because of the short duration and inconsistent development of increased intracranial pressure, papilledema is usually not seen at presentation. When it is present, venous sinus thrombosis, subdural effusion, or an intracranial abscess must be considered. Seizures occur prior to admission in 20% of children.

The child with meningitis may also present with cutaneous findings. Although commonly associated with meningococcal disease, purpura, petechiae, or a diffuse nonspecific maculopapular rash may be present in meningitis caused by any of the common bacterial pathogens. Meningitis has also been reported in 8% of toddlers with coincident buccal (facial) cellulitis and in 1% of children with periorbital cellulitis (10% if there is bacteremia). This creates a problem for the physician who must decide whether to perform a spinal tap on a child with facial cellulitis. When the child is younger than 2 to 3 years of age, has meningeal signs, or appears toxic or if *H. influenzae* type b is suspected, the child should be evaluated for meningitis.

Bacterial meningitis has also been reported in 20% of children with septic arthritis. This has been assumed to be due to simultaneous infection following a bacteremia. Reactive arthritis due to immune complex deposition is also seen with bacterial meningitis.

This arthritis affects one large joint and appears 5 to 7 days after treatment for meningitis has started. In general, arthritis occurring acutely with meningitis should be assumed to be infectious (see Chapter 45).

Various eye disorders have also been described with acute bacterial meningitis, including transient cataracts, paralysis of the extraocular muscles, pupillary dysfunction, dendritic ulcers, and conjunctivitis.

Laboratory Studies

Although the clinical presentation suggests meningitis, the definitive diagnosis is based on the examination of the CSF. The CSF is usually obtained via a lumbar puncture (spinal tap). The indication for a lumbar puncture is clinical suspicion for the presence of meningitis.

The spinal tap is usually performed by introducing a small-bore, short-beveled, and styletted spinal needle into the subarachnoid space at the L3-4 or L4-5 levels (Figs. 53–2 to 53–4). A styletted needle is used in order to minimize the risk of introducing into the subarachnoid space a nest of epidermal cells that may later grow into a cord-compressing epidermoid tumor. Approximately 3 ml of fluid is removed for analysis.

There are a few contraindications for the performance of a spinal

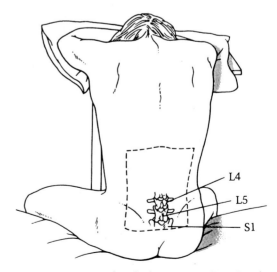

Figure 53–3. Sitting position for a lumbar puncture. (From Davidson RI. Lumbar puncture. *In* Vander Salm TJ, Cutler BS, Wheeler HB [eds]. Atlas of Bedside Procedures, 2nd ed. Boston: Little, Brown, 1992:443.)

Cauda equina

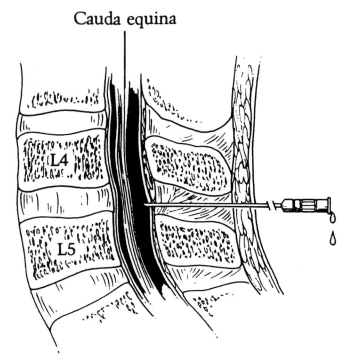

Figure 53–4. Advance the needle and stylet into the subarachnoid space. On penetration into the space, one often feels a give or pop after moving through the dura. After the needle enters into the subarachnoid space, remove the stylet and collect the cerebrospinal fluid. (From Davidson RI. Lumbar puncture. *In* Vander Salm TJ, Cutler BS, Wheeler HB [eds]. Atlas of Bedside Procedures, 2nd ed. Boston: Little, Brown, 1992:447.)

tap. The first is cardiorespiratory compromise. Performance of the spinal tap requires that the child be held in flexion to open the intervertebral spaces. In seriously ill children or children with significant underlying cardiac or pulmonary disease, this positioning may be enough to cause hypoxemia. The lumbar puncture may need to be postponed until the child stabilizes. Alternatively, the procedure may be done cautiously with continuous oxygen saturation monitoring by pulse oximetry or in the sitting position.

Second, children with increased intracranial pressure have a high risk of cerebral herniation following a spinal tap. Therefore, if signs or symptoms of increased intracranial pressure are present, the spinal tap should be postponed until the increased pressure is lowered with appropriate treatment (hyperventilation, mannitol). If a lumbar puncture is delayed (for suspected increased intracranial pressure or to obtain a computed tomography [CT] scan), appropriate antibiotic therapy should be initiated without further delay. Signs of increased intracranial pressure include ptosis, anisocoria, sixth cranial nerve palsy, Cushing triad (hypertension, bradycardia, irregularities of respiration), and papilledema.

Third, a spinal tap should not be done if the spinal needle must pass through an area of infection on its way to the subarachnoid space. To do so might introduce pathogens into the CNS that could cause meningitis.

Finally, epidural hematomas causing lower limb paralysis may be a complication of lumbar punctures in children with bleeding disorders. Therefore, in children with hemophilia or thrombocytopenia, extra care should be taken to avoid a traumatic spinal tap. Such children should be monitored after the procedure for the development of neurologic deficits in the legs. If time permits, the coagulopathy may be corrected prior to performing the spinal tap.

The CSF is examined for red blood cells (RBCs), white blood cells (WBCs) and differential, glucose, protein, and the presence

(by culture, by Gram stain or other stain, or by antigen or DNA testing for specific agents) of pathogenic organisms. Because children who are undergoing spinal taps are usually struggling or critically ill and because pressure measurement adds little to the evaluation of the patient, routine opening and closing pressures are not obtained. Children with bacterial meningitis usually have a mean opening pressure of 180 ± 70 mm H_2O. However, normal opening pressure in a recumbent child is up to 150 mm H_2O; it is higher in the sitting child.

Normal CSF is clear and colorless (Table 53–3). Blood in the CSF indicates a traumatic spinal tap or a CNS hemorrhage. Differentiation between the two can be achieved by centrifugation of the CSF sample. When blood has been present in the CSF for several hours, the CSF will be xanthochromic after centrifugation. However, if the blood was recently mixed with CSF as in the case of a traumatic tap, the supernatant will be clear. Xanthochromic CSF can also be due to icterus or an elevated CSF protein concentration. Obtaining a RBC count on tubes 1 and 3 may also differentiate the two conditions, as the count is unchanged in CNS hemorrhage but may decline in traumatic taps.

The normal values for WBCs in the CSF are shown in Table 53–3. Most children with bacterial meningitis have at least 1000/mm³ WBCs in their CSF, but generally more than 6/mm³ WBCs in children beyond the neonatal period is considered abnormal. An absolute neutrophil count ≥1/mm³ (neutrophils may be as high as 35%) is also considered abnormal and evidence of a bacterial infection. Although there are case reports of children with proven (usually rapidly fulminant meningococcal) bacterial meningitis who do not have CSF pleocytosis, the CSF of 98% of children with meningitis has pleocytosis and greater than 50% neutrophils. It takes at least 400/mm³ WBCs to turn CSF turbid. Therefore, even though the CSF obtained may be clear to the naked eye, the sample must be examined under the microscope. Neonates may have 0 to 30 (mean, 9) WBCs in the CSF; most of these cells are not neutrophils.

On occasion, the spinal needle is advanced too far and passes through the subarachnoid space and penetrates the richly vascularized ventral epidural space. Blood is thereby introduced into the subarachnoid space and the spinal fluid appears bloody. This is often called a *traumatic tap*. It is then difficult to know whether the WBCs seen on examination of the CSF are due to CSF pleocytosis or are peripheral blood WBCs contaminating the CSF. To aid in this determination, the ratio of WBCs to RBCs in the CSF is compared with the ratio of WBCs to RBCs in the patient's peripheral blood. A higher ratio in the CSF indicates the presence of CSF pleocytosis. When the CSF ratio is at least 10 times greater than the blood ratio, bacterial meningitis is indicated with a sensitivity of 88% and a specificity of 90%. Conversely, the negative predictive value for the presence of bacterial meningitis of a less than 10-fold difference between the ratios is 99%. Traumatic taps usually do not alter the CSF glucose, Gram stain, or culture, which are often abnormal with bacterial meningitis. When there is doubt about the validity of the cell count following a bloody tap, the lumbar puncture should be repeated after several hours by introducing the spinal needle one intervertebral space above the original tap.

In normal CSF, the glucose level is two-thirds that in serum. CSF glucose is low in most infected infants and younger children and in 45% of school-aged children with bacterial meningitis. In children older than 2 months of age, a CSF/serum glucose ratio of ≤0.4 is 80% sensitive and 98% specific for the presence of bacterial meningitis. The presence of RBCs in a CSF sample that is promptly analyzed does not affect the glucose level.

The normal CSF protein level is less than 45 mg/dl in children beyond the first 2 months of life. CSF protein is elevated in greater than 90% of younger children with bacterial meningitis but in only 60% of school-age and older children. Every thousand RBCs in

Table 53-3. Cerebrospinal Fluid Findings in Various Central Nervous System Disorders Associated with Fever

Condition	Pressure (mm H$_2$O)	Leukocytes/mm³	Protein (mg/dl)	Glucose	Comments
Normal	50–80	<5; 75% lymphocytes	20–45	>50 mg/dl or 75% blood glucose	
Acute bacterial meningitis	Usually elevated	100–60,000+; usually a few thousand; PMNs predominate	Usually 100–500	Depressed compared with blood glucose; usually <40 mg/dl	Organism may be seen on Gram stain and recovered by culture
Partially treated bacterial meningitis	Normal or elevated	1–10,000; PMNs usual but mononuclear cells may predominate if pretreated for extended period of time	100+	Depressed or normal	Organisms may or may not be seen; in disease due to *Haemophilus influenzae*, organism may grow despite pretreatment; pretreatment may render sterile CSF of patients with meningococcal disease
Tuberculous meningitis	Usually elevated; may be low due to block in advanced stages	10–500; PMNs early but lymphocytes predominate through most of course	100–500; may be higher in presence of block	<50 mg/dl usual in most cases; decreases with time if treatment is not provided	Acid-fast organisms may be seen on smear; organism can be recovered in culture
Fungal meningitis	Usually elevated	25–500; mononuclear cells predominate except PMNs early	25–500	<50 mg/dl, decreases with time if treatment is not provided	Budding yeast may be seen; organism may be recovered in culture; India ink preparation may be positive in cryptococcal disease
Syphilis (acute) and leptospirosis	Usually elevated	200–500, usually lymphocytes	50–200	Generally normal	Positive CSF serology; spirochetes not demonstrable by usual techniques of smear or culture; dark-field examination may be positive
Viral meningitis or meningo-encephalitis	Normal or slightly elevated	PMNs early; rarely more than 1,000 cells except in Eastern equine encephalomyelitis, in which counts of up to 20,000 have been recorded; mononuclear cells predominate during most of course	50–200	Generally normal; may be depressed to <40 mg/dl in various viral diseases, particularly mumps (15%–20% of cases)	Enteroviruses may be recovered from CSF by appropriate viral cultures
Chemical (drugs, dermoids, cysts, myelography dye)	Usually elevated	100–1,000+; PMNs predominate	50–100	20–40 mg/dl	Epithelial cells may be seen within CSF in some children with dermoids by use of polarized light
Subdural empyema	Usually elevated	100–5,000 PMNs predominate	100–500	Normal	No organisms on smear or culture of CSF unless meningitis also present; organism found on tap of subdural fluid
Brain abscess	Usually elevated	10–200; fluid rarely acellular; lymphocytes predominate; if abscess ruptures into ventricle, PMNs predominate and cell count may reach >100,000	75–500	Normal unless abscess ruptures into ventricular system	No organisms on smear or culture unless abscess ruptures into ventricular system
Cerebral epidural abscess	Normal to slightly elevated	0–500; lymphocytes predominate	50–200	Normal	No organisms on smear or culture
Spinal epidural abscess	Usually low, with spinal block	10–100; lymphocytes predominate	50–400	Normal	No organisms on smear or culture
Collagen-vascular disease	Slightly elevated	0–500; PMNs may predominate; lymphocytes may be present	100	Normal or slightly depressed	No organisms on smear or culture; LE preparation may be positive
Tumor, leukemia	Slightly elevated to very high	0–100+; mononuclear or blast cells	50–1,000	May be depressed to 20–40 mg/dl	Cytology may be positive

Adapted from Behrman RE (ed). Nelson Textbook of Pediatrics, 14th ed. Philadelphia: WB Saunders, 1992:656.
Abbreviations: PMNs = polymorphonuclear leukocytes; CSF = cerebrospinal fluid; LE = lupus erythematosus cell.

the CSF (from a traumatic tap) increases the protein level by 1 mg/dl.

The presence of bacterial pathogens in the CSF should be investigated in several ways. Microscopic examination of a Gram-stained sample of the fluid is performed first. The sensitivity of this test is directly related to the number of organisms in the CSF and is inversely related to the age of the patient. The Gram stain identification of certain organisms, such as *H. influenzae*, may be problematic. A decision whether to treat a child for bacterial meningitis should not be based on the Gram stain alone. The definitive diagnosis of bacterial meningitis is based on the CSF culture. Rapid diagnostic tests may also be helpful in the diagnosis of bacterial meningitis, especially in patients who had received antibiotics prior to lumbar puncture. The commonly used techniques are countercurrent immunoelectrophoresis and latex particle agglutination for the detection of bacterial antigens. These tests are available for the common pathogens of bacterial meningitis and may be performed on CSF, urine, and serum. The tests vary in sensitivity. In general, the most sensitive test is latex agglutination on CSF. False-positive and indeterminate results are common.

COMPUTED TOMOGRAPHY

Routine CT scans of the head are not indicated in children with suspected meningitis. Even though most children with bacterial meningitis have increased intracranial pressure, most CT scans are normal. In addition, most spinal taps do not result in cerebral herniation. Requiring a CT prior to lumbar puncture delays definitive diagnosis and possibly initiation of treatment. CT scans should be reserved for children who show *clinical signs* suggesting herniation or who may have an intracranial mass causing signs and symptoms similar to meningitis. In these children, a blood specimen should be obtained for culture, broad-spectrum parenteral antibiotics started, a CT scan performed when the patient is stable, and a spinal tap performed subsequently when appropriate. Even in the management of the child with proven meningitis, the CT scan is not routinely indicated because it seldom provides information that leads to a specific intervention and adds little to the clinical evaluation in the prediction of long-term outcome. CT aids in the evaluation of focal neurologic signs or in children suspected of a brain abscess or subdural empyema.

OTHER LABORATORY TESTS

Usually, the peripheral blood WBC and platelet counts are elevated with bacterial meningitis. A low WBC count and thrombocytopenia may also be seen and are associated with overwhelming infection and a poor outcome. The differential WBC count has been studied with the hope of predicting which infants do not have meningitis and therefore do not need a spinal tap based on the absence of a left shift. However, the sensitivity, specificity, and negative predictive value (70%, 54%, and 81%, respectively) are too low to render the differential WBC examination useful in making this decision.

Blood cultures may be useful in identifying the bacterial pathogen of meningitis. However, a negative blood culture may be found in up to 33% of children with meningococcal meningitis, 20% of pneumococcal cases, and 10% of patients with *H. influenzae* type b meningitis. This number increases with prior antibiotic therapy. In addition, there is a negative correlation between the length of illness prior to diagnosis and the rate of positive blood cultures.

Treatment

The mainstay of treatment for bacterial meningitis is antibiotic therapy. Antibiotics should be started as soon as possible after the spinal tap is performed. Therefore, in most instances antibiotic therapy is initiated before the etiologic agent is definitively identified. Consequently, therapy should be directed toward all the common pathogens for the age of the patient. Later, when the bacterium is identified and antibiotic sensitivities are determined, the single most appropriate drug or combination of drugs should be used. Table 53–4 lists the antibiotics commonly used for meningitis and their dosing schedules.

In newborn infants, the most cases of meningitis are caused by group B streptococci. Other common pathogens are *Escherichia coli*; enterococci, *Klebsiella, Enterobacter, Salmonella*, and *Serratia* species; and *L. monocytogenes*. In older infants and children, the usual pathogens are *H. influenzae* type b, *Streptococcus pneumoniae*, and *Neisseria meningitidis*. Since the introduction of *H. influenzae* vaccine, the incidence of meningitis due to this organism has declined considerably.

Other bacteria can cause meningitis. When uncommon bacteria

Table 53–4. Antibiotics Used for the Treatment of Bacterial Meningitis*

| Drug | Neonates | | Infants and Children |
	0–7 Days	*8–28 Days*	
Amikacin†‡	15–20 div q12h	20–30 div q8h	20–30 div q8h
Ampicillin	150–200 div q12h	150–200 div q8h or q6h	200–400 div q6h
Cefotaxime	100 div q12h	150–200 div q8h or q6h	200–250 div q8h or q6h
Ceftriaxone§	—	—	100–150 div q12h or q24h
Ceftazidime	150 div q12h	150 div q8h	150 div q8h
Chloramphenicol‡	25 once daily	50 div q12h	75–100 div q6h
Gentamicin†‡	5 div q12h	7.5 div q8h	7.5 div q8h
Methicillin or nafcillin	100–150 div q8h or q12h	150–200 div q8h or q6h	200–300 div q6h
Penicillin G	150,000–250,000 div q12h	250,000 div q8h or q6h	250,000–300,000 div q6h or q4h
Tobramycin†‡	5 div q12h	7.5 div q8h	7.5 div q8h
Vancomycin†‡	30 div q12h	30–45 div q8h	40–60 div q6h

Modified from Klein JO. Antimicrobial treatment and prevention of meningitis. Pediatr Ann 1994;23:76.
*Doses in mg/kg (units/kg for penicillin G) per day.
†Smaller doses and longer dosing intervals, especially for aminoglycosides and vancomycin for very-low-birth-weight neonates may be advisable.
‡Monitoring of serum levels is recommended to ensure safe and therapeutic values.
§Use in neonates is not recommended because of inadequate experience in neonatal meningitis.

cause meningitis, it is usually in a child with a predisposing factor such as prematurity, immunosuppression, other focus of infection, or a congenital anomaly of the CNS. Nonetheless, uncommon organisms have also been reported in normal children and should be considered when the child does not respond to the usual empiric antibiotic therapy.

In meningitis during the first month of life, initial treatment should consist of intravenous ampicillin in combination with cefotaxime or, less often, an aminoglycoside. Cefotaxime is preferred because it has high CSF levels and less toxicity than aminoglycosides; routine monitoring of drug levels is not required. Cefotaxime is the cephalosporin of choice in newborns because it is not excreted in the bile and therefore has less inhibitory effect on bowel flora.

Infants between 1 and 3 months of age may be infected by neonatal organisms or the common childhood pathogens. Therefore, empiric treatment should consist of ampicillin in combination with either ceftriaxone or cefotaxime. Chloramphenicol could also be paired with ampicillin; however, most pediatric infectious disease specialists prefer cephalosporins. Their benefits over chloramphenicol are that (1) there is no need to monitor levels, (2) they may be used in the presence of hepatic or renal insufficiency, (3) they do not interact with drugs metabolized by the liver, such as phenobarbital and phenytoin, (4) they have greater *in vitro* activity against the common pathogens, (5) they have greater bactericidal activity in CSF, and (6) they need to be given less frequently.

In older infants and children, treatment should be initiated with cefotaxime, ceftriaxone, or ampicillin and chloramphenicol. When the pathogen and its antibiotic sensitivities are identified, definitive treatment can be employed. For *H. influenzae* type b, the cephalosporin should be continued. If ampicillin and chloramphenicol were started, either one alone may be used, depending on sensitivities (about 30% of *H. influenzae* type b cases are ampicillin-resistant).

Increasing numbers of *S. pneumoniae* have been found to be resistant to penicillins. If intermediate resistance is detected, cephalosporins may be continued, as the organism is most likely susceptible to them. However, the minimal inhibitory concentration (MIC) to the cephalosporin should be determined to ensure efficacy. If high resistance is found or if the child has recently been treated with a beta lactam antibiotic, intravenous vancomycin or vancomycin and rifampin should be added.

Treatment of *N. meningitidis* meningitis may be with a penicillin, ceftriaxone, or cefotaxime. Since penicillin-resistant strains are being encountered in certain areas, antibiotic sensitivities must be checked.

The duration of antibiotic treatment for bacterial meningitis has not been studied thoroughly. In the past, guidelines were arbitrarily decided, based in part on anecdotal reports of patient outcome. In the past decade, three studies have shown that 7 days of antibiotic therapy is sufficient. Because of problems with these studies in their sample size and length of follow-up, the commonly accepted length of treatment for *H. influenzae* and pneumococcal meningitis is 7 to 10 days, based on clinical response. Because the meningococcus responds very quickly to antibiotic treatment, 7 days is considered adequate. Gram-negative meningitis is treated for 3 weeks, and longer if there is delayed sterilization of the CSF. In the newborn, group B streptococcal and *Listeria* meningitis are treated for 14 to 21 days.

In addition to these antibiotics, the child with *H. influenzae* type b meningitis must receive oral rifampin in a dose of 20 mg/kg/day in one dose for 4 days (maximum dose, 600 mg/day) to eradicate nasopharyngeal carriage of the organism. The rifampin should be administered before the child is discharged. If the child is being treated with chloramphenicol, the rifampin should not be given until the course of chloramphenicol is completed because rifampin may lower serum chloramphenicol levels. Additionally, if there are any household members younger than 48 months of age who are not fully immunized against *H. influenzae*, or are immunosup-

pressed, all members of the household should receive rifampin prophylaxis. If the child is in attendance more than 25 hours a week in a day care center where all children are older than 2 years of age and two cases of invasive *H. influenzae* type b disease have occurred within 60 days, all attendees and personnel should receive rifampin. If there are incompletely vaccinated children younger than 2 years of age in day care, they should receive rifampin, even when only one case of invasive *H. influenzae* disease has occurred. In addition they must receive any missing doses of the vaccine.

In regard to meningococcal meningitis, the patient, all household, day care, and nursery contacts, as well as persons who have contact with the patient's oral secretions and medical personnel who have had intimate contact with the patient prior to antibiotic therapy, should receive prophylaxis to eradicate nasopharyngeal carriage. Treatment may include oral rifampin (10 mg/kg [maximum dose, 600 mg] every 12 hours for four doses); intramuscular ceftriaxone (125 mg in children under age 12 years and 250 mg in older children and adults); or oral sulfisoxazole for 2 days when the infecting strain is susceptible (500 mg daily for infants under 1 year, 500 mg every 12 hours in children 1 to 12 years, and 1 g every 12 hours for older children and adults). In addition, meningococcal vaccine should be considered for contacts when the infection is caused by a vaccine serotype.

The high morbidity rate associated with bacterial meningitis is due to neuronal tissue damage. This damage is the result of interactions involving both the pathogen and the host immune system. Dexamethasone therapy in patients with meningitis reduces the local synthesis of tumor necrosis factor–α, interleukin-1, platelet activating factor, and prostaglandins and inhibits the activation of leukocyte and endothelial cells. These result in decreased blood-brain barrier permeability, meningeal inflammation, and tissue damage. Consequently, the therapeutic effect of dexamethasone in reducing the adverse sequelae of bacterial meningitis has been extensively studied.

Several studies have looked at both the efficacy and the safety of dexamethasone. These studies and two meta-analyses have yielded conflicting reports. In some, dexamethasone decreased the incidence of neurologic abnormalities, including hearing loss. However, two of these studies have been faulted for the unusually high incidence of permanent neurologic damage in the placebo group. Other studies did not find a therapeutic effect for dexamethasone. These studies suffer from small sample size, and a true difference between dexamethasone and placebo may have been missed. Several studies used different antibiotics and drug dosage regimens and may not be generalizable to other regimens.

The only adverse effect reported from the use of dexamethasone has been gastrointestinal bleeding. This usually manifests as melena, but bleeding requiring transfusion has been reported. Theoretically, dexamethasone, by reducing inflammation and thus blood-brain barrier permeability, may cause lower CSF antibiotic levels, which may produce delayed sterilization of the CSF, particularly in the presence of resistant or relatively resistant pneumococcus.

Most cases in the dexamethasone trials were *H. influenzae* type b meningitis. A retrospective review of 97 children with pneumococcal meningitis treated with dexamethasone showed a significant reduction in the incidence of neurologic sequelae, and in the experimental model the neuronal tissue damage due to pneumococcus is mediated by the same factors that mediate the damage associated with *H. influenzae* type b. No information is available about the safety and efficacy of dexamethasone in neonatal (first 6 weeks of life) meningitis.

With the concern of emerging pneumococcal and now meningococcal antibiotic-resistant strains, the use of dexamethasone remains controversial. The first dose of dexamethasone (if used at all) should be started before or at the time of the initial dose of antibiotics. The dose is 0.15 mg/kg per dose four times a day for 4 days. If resistant organisms are suspected, vancomycin should be added to the therapy.

Clinical Course

The child with bacterial meningitis must be observed very carefully during the first few days of the illness, for it is during this time that life-threatening complications may occur. The complications may be due to septicemia, such as septic shock or disseminated intravascular coagulation, or to meningitis itself. The most serious complication is cerebral edema leading to increased intracranial pressure and herniation (see Chapter 41). Consequently, vital signs and the child's mental status must be monitored frequently, and the child should be transferred to an intensive care unit for more intensive monitoring and therapy should these problems arise.

Fever normally persists for 3 to 5 days and for as long as 9 days in 13% of children. Dexamethasone therapy usually suppresses fever, which may recur after this steroid is discontinued. Prolonged or recurrent fever is often associated with a subdural effusion, infections at other sites such as joints or the lungs, thrombophlebitis secondary to intravenous lines, abscess formation from intramuscular injections, or drug fever. A secondary rise in fever is usually due to a nosocomial viral infection (respiratory syncytial virus, rotavirus) or a subdural effusion. If no source for an abnormally prolonged or secondary fever is found and based on the clinical status of the patient, a repeated spinal tap to assess the response to antibiotics should be considered. This is especially relevant if there is suspicion of antimicrobial resistance.

Baseline and serial neurologic evaluations should be performed, as alterations of mental status, seizures, and focal neurologic deficits may be found on admission or during the course of the illness. These are due to direct neuronal damage by inflammatory mediators and to disruption of normal cerebral blood flow by cerebral edema, vasculitis, thrombosis, and loss of cerebral autoregulation. The presence of focal neurologic abnormalities on admission is associated with long-term neurologic deficits.

Twenty percent to 30% of children have seizures prior to admission or during the first 2 days of hospitalization. These seizures should be treated aggressively with benzodiazepines, phenytoin, or phenobarbital because of the risk of cerebral injury from prolonged seizures. When these seizures are generalized and easily controlled, they are not associated with permanent neurologic deficits or subsequent seizures. Anticonvulsant medication may be discontinued at the time of discharge. However, seizures that are difficult to control or that persist or develop after the first 4 days of hospitalization, as well as focal seizures, are associated with permanent neurologic sequelae. In addition, when seizures start after the second day of hospitalization, investigations for possible causes such as hyponatremia (inappropriate ADH), venous sinus thrombosis, and intracranial abscess should be initiated.

Fever with seizure may represent a *benign febrile seizure* or a seizure with meningitis. Febrile seizures are common between 1 and 5 years of age, are short and nonfocal, and may be familial. There is no nuchal rigidity, alteration of consciousness, or signs of increased intracranial pressure. Any seizure with fever in a child less than 6 to 12 months old must be considered meningitis until proven otherwise, whereas seizures with fever and abnormal neurologic signs must also be considered meningitis.

About 30% of infants and children experience subdural effusions secondary to bacterial meningitis. The effusion may be detected by transillumination in infants. This procedure has been shown to be as sensitive for detecting subdural fluid as CT or radionuclide scans. Previously, effusions were considered to be a complication of meningitis that required detection and intervention. In most patients, however, the effusions cause no symptoms and the incidence of long-term sequelae following meningitis is not related to the presence of subdural effusions. The intense meningeal inflammation in severe cases of meningitis that leads to the development of neurologic signs (seizures, hemiplegia) also leads to the formation of subdural effusions. Tapping the effusion is warranted only when it appears that the effusion is causing problems such as increased intracranial pressure or a rapidly increasing head circumference.

Fluid management in children with bacterial meningitis is complex. Because of the evolving mental status of these children, their propensity to vomit, and the need to closely monitor fluid intake, they should not be fed orally for the first few days of their hospitalization. Historically, all patients with meningitis were kept on a fluid restriction of two-thirds maintenance to prevent the development and complications of SIADH. The complications are the worsening of cerebral edema due to fluid retention and the precipitation of seizures due to hyponatremia. SIADH is defined by the presence of hyponatremia with corresponding serum and extracellular fluid hypo-osmolality in the presence of continued renal sodium excretion, clinical absence of volume depletion, inappropriate elevation of urine osmolality, and normally functioning kidneys and adrenal glands. The incidence of SIADH has been reported to be 4% to 88% in bacterial meningitis and 9% to 64% in viral meningitis. However, a large subgroup of children with meningitis have elevated ADH without having SIADH. In these children, the elevated ADH is due to hypovolemia caused by increased fluid losses due to vomiting and fever, sepsis-induced hypotension, and decreased oral intake. Restriction of fluid in these children may reduce perfusion to the brain.

The presence of long-term neurologic abnormalities is correlated to both the degree and the duration of hyponatremia. Consequently, the initial evaluation of a child with meningitis must include a clinical assessment of hydration status as well the following laboratory tests: serum electrolytes and osmolality, urine electrolytes and osmolality, and urine specific gravity. If the child shows signs of dehydration and has elevated urine sodium and osmolality, he or she should receive replacement and full maintenance fluids calculated to restore euvolemia over 24 hours. The patient must also be frequently re-evaluated for the development of SIADH.

If the child is not dehydrated and the serum sodium concentration is less than 135 mEq/L, fluids should be restricted to two-thirds maintenance. The child should be observed closely, and as the sodium normalizes, the fluids may be liberalized. If severe hyponatremia and seizures occur, hypertonic saline (3% NaCl) should be administered.

The child in shock requires vigorous fluid resuscitation to maintain blood pressure, cerebral perfusion, and urine output. However, too much fluid (especially hypotonic crystalloid solutions) may increase cerebral edema and precipitate seizures. Therefore, the child must be monitored carefully. In addition, the use of intravenous colloid and vasopressors (dopamine, epinephrine) may decrease fluid requirements while maintaining perfusion.

Diabetes insipidus and cerebral salt wasting have also been rarely reported with meningitis. Therefore, fluid management should be tailored to each patient based on the initial and serial assessments of weight, fluid intake and output, neurologic status, and serum electrolyte levels.

Outcome

The sequelae of bacterial meningitis are listed in Table 53–5. The average mortality rate due to meningitis is about 10%. The percentage is higher (approaching 20%) in neonates and somewhat lower than 10% in infants and older children. The reported incidence of other sequelae varies from 14% to 50%. The difference in rates can be attributed to the age and socioeconomic status of the patients, the specific organism causing the meningitis, the therapy used, and, most important, the length of follow up. Studies have shown that even major neurologic deficits can resolve with time. One study found that 33% of children had neurologic abnormalities at discharge but only 11% of abnormalities persisted 5 years later.

One of the most common complications of bacterial meningitis is sensorineural hearing loss. The reported incidence of hearing loss is between 2% and 29%. When hearing loss is present, it is

Table 53–5. Sequelae of Bacterial Meningitis

Death
Cranial nerve dysfunction (usually transient)
Hemiparesis
Quadriparesis
Spinal cord infarction
Brain infarction
Hypertonia
Hypotonia
Ataxia (cerebellar or vestibular)
Permanent seizure disorder
Sensorineural hearing loss
Cortical blindness
Obstructive hydrocephalus
Diabetes insipidus
Transient cataracts
Transverse myelitis
Pericardial effusion (immune complex or septic)
Joint effusion (immune complex or septic)
Polyarteritis
Behavioral problems
Language delay
Mental retardation

permanent in about 10% of cases. Because the damage that causes hearing deficits occurs early in the course of the illness, early diagnosis and administration of antibiotics do not affect its incidence. It is thought that the administration of dexamethasone will.

Bacterial Meningitis in Children with Intraventricular Shunts

One subgroup of children with bacterial meningitis is children with ventriculoperitoneal shunts placed for the treatment of hydrocephalus. Between 20% and 30% of individuals with shunts experience a shunt infection at some time during their life. The majority (70%) of these infections occur within 2 months of the surgery to insert the shunt; 80% occur within 6 months.

Children with shunt infections differ from other children with bacterial meningitis in several ways. The most common pathogens of meningitis in children with shunts are *S. epidermidis* (coagulase-negative staphylococcus) and *S. aureus* (coagulase-positive staphylococcus). Gram-negative enteric bacteria and the common pathogens of childhood meningitis are less common. Only 30% present with meningeal signs. Instead, they present with erythema along the subcutaneous tract, fever, nausea, vomiting, malaise, headache, abdominal pain (from infected CSF irritating the peritoneum), and signs of increased intracranial pressure. Diagnosis is best made by percutaneous needle aspiration of the shunt, not by lumbar puncture. The degree of CSF pleocytosis is usually much less than in children without shunts. The number of WBCs in the CSF of patients with shunt infections may average less than 100. The CSF glucose concentration is only mildly depressed, and the protein is often normal.

Usual treatment for a shunt infection includes appropriate systemic antibiotics, supportive care, removal of the infected shunt, external ventricular drainage, and intraventricular antibiotics.

Partially Treated Bacterial Meningitis

On occasion during the early phase of the illness, before symptoms suggest meningitis, a child will receive oral or, rarely, paren-teral antibiotics. These have usually been prescribed for a presumed or identified focus of infection outside the CNS, such as otitis media. After the antibiotics have been started, the child exhibits meningeal signs or other symptoms suggestive of CNS infection. When the CSF from such a child is examined, organisms are often not seen on Gram stain or recovered on culture. The CSF cell count is elevated, and a predominance of usually neutrophils or less often mononuclear cells may be seen. The CSF protein remains elevated, and the glucose remains depressed.

In this instance, presumptive treatment for bacterial meningitis should be initiated. If an organism is identified by culture or antigen detection, definitive antibiotic treatment is administered. If no organism grows in culture and the CSF profile is compatible with bacterial meningitis, a full course of antibiotics should be administered.

Other disorders that may give the CSF picture of partially treated meningitis are tuberculous meningitis (Table 53–6) and parameningeal infections such as intracranial abscesses, sinusitis, mastoiditis, cranial osteomyelitis, and dermal sinus tract infections. Many of these are obvious or have a more chronic (>7 days) duration of CNS manifestations.

Repeated Bacterial Meningitis

Recurrent meningitis is defined as repetition of bacterial meningitis after convalescence. Fifty percent of patients who have recurrences have only one recurrence; others may have up to ten. The conditions associated with recurrent meningitis are listed in Table 53–7. Most patients with congenital fistulous communication between the CNS and the middle ear are also deaf.

The most common organisms causing recurrent meningitis are pneumococcus, *H. influenzae* type b, and meningococcus. In children with dermal sinus tracts, most cases of meningitis are caused by *S. aureus* and *E. coli*. Many of the patients with immunodeficiencies have had personal or family histories of recurrent infections at other sites (see Chapter 52). Therefore, a congenital or traumatically acquired CNS fistula should be suspected in a child with recurrent meningitis caused by the common pathogens; a dermal sinus tract should be suspected if the meningitis is caused by a staphylococcus or a gram-negative enteric organism; and immunodeficiency should be considered when the patient or a family member has a history of recurrent infections outside the CNS.

Definitive treatment involves antibiotic therapy for the acute infection followed by surgical repair of the fistula or prophylactic treatment for the immunodeficiency.

Recrudescence is the reappearance of meningitis during the ther-

Table 53–6. Differential Diagnosis of Tuberculous Meningitis

Fungal meningitis (cryptococcosis, histoplasmosis, blastomycosis, coccidioidomycosis)
Neurobrucellosis
Neurosyphilis
Neuroborreliosis
Focal parameningeal infection (sphenoid sinusitis, endocarditis)
Pyogenic brain abscess
Central nervous system (CNS) toxoplasmosis
Partially treated bacterial meningitis
Neoplastic meningitis (lymphoma, carcinoma)
Cerebrovascular accident
CNS sarcoidosis

Modified from Leonard JM, Des Prez RM. Tuberculous meningitis. Infect Dis Clin North Am 1990;4:769–787.

Table 53–7. Conditions Associated with Recurrent Bacterial Meningitis

Congenital Cerebrospinal Fluid (CSF) Fistula

Stapes footplate fistula
Oval window fistula
Cochlear aqueduct defect
Giant apical air cell syndrome
Basiethmoidal or cribriform plate defect
Cranial or spinal dermal sinus
Meningocele
Encephalocele
Neurenteric cyst
Klippel-Feil syndrome

Traumatic or Surgical CSF Fistulae

Skull fracture involving paranasal sinuses, cribriform plate, petrous bone
Postoperative (particularly following nasal surgery)

Immunodeficiency

Immunoglobulin deficiency
Complement component deficiency
Hemoglobinopathy
Congenital or acquired asplenia
Leukemia
Lymphoma

Parameningeal Infection

Mastoiditis
Sinusitis
Skull bone osteomyelitis

Idiopathic

Adapted from Kline MW. Review of recurrent bacterial meningitis. Pediatr Infect Dis J 1989; 8:630.

apy of the initial episode of CNS infection; antibiotic resistance (acquired, selected) should be suspected. *Relapse* occurs between 3 days and 3 weeks after successful therapy and usually represents persistent infection in sequestered sites (subdural empyema, ventriculitis, cerebral abscess, mastoiditis, cranial osteomyelitis, orbit). Relapse may be secondary to inadequate choice, duration, or dose of antibiotics.

ASEPTIC MENINGITIS

Aseptic meningitis must be included in the differential diagnosis of stiff neck. Aseptic meningitis is defined as an acute illness characterized by signs and symptoms of meningeal irritation; CSF pleocytosis, usually with a predominance of mononuclear cells; a normal or, less frequently, elevated CSF protein concentration; normal or, less often, low CSF glucose concentration; and no organisms demonstrable by Gram stain or routine bacterial cultures. There are many causes of aseptic meningitis (Table 53–8). By far the most common cause is viral infection of the meninges; up to 90% of cases are due to enteroviruses and arbovirus. The definitive diagnosis is made by viral isolation from the CSF. However, the virus is not always recovered, and the other etiologies must be ruled out by history, presence or absence of associated symptoms, and appropriate laboratory tests (Table 53–9).

Enteroviral meningitis occurs most often during the spring and summer months. Transmission is via the oral-fecal route, and young children exhibit increased transmission of the viruses and more severe disease. Initially, patients have gastrointestinal tract infec-

tion, which may manifest as a nonspecific febrile illness or be asymptomatic. Viral infection of the meninges occurs 7 to 10 days after initial exposure. Consequently, the clinical course is often biphasic. Virus from the oropharynx can be cultured only during the first 5 to 7 days of the illness but may be excreted in stool for 6 to 8 weeks.

Children with viral meningitis present with low-grade fever, nuchal rigidity, headache, and vomiting. Less commonly seen symptoms are anorexia, drowsiness, photophobia, myalgia, and malaise. As in bacterial meningitis, young infants often lack meningeal signs and present only with fever and irritability. In addition, children may have an altered sensorium, but focal neurologic signs are rare. Seizures are more common in infants.

The number of WBCs in the CSF varies from zero to several thousand (see Table 53–3). Up to 75% of initial (early in the illness) CSF specimens contain a predominance of polymorphonuclear cells. Mononuclear cells predominate by 2 days after the onset of symptoms. In children with enteroviral meningitis, 18% may have decreased CSF glucose concentrations while 12% may have elevated CSF protein. When the clinician is in doubt as to whether a patient has viral or bacterial meningitis and the patient is not ill appearing, it may be worthwhile to withhold antibiotics and repeat the spinal tap after several hours.

Treatment of viral meningitis is symptomatic and supportive. Admission may be required while bacterial meningitis is being ruled out and for intravenous hydration. Analgesics for headache and antipyretics may also be indicated. The initial spinal tap performed to diagnose viral meningitis is often helpful in ameliorating the acute symptoms of the illness. The mechanism for this is not clear.

Outcome is quite good for common viral pathogens causing aseptic meningitis. Sequelae in older children are rare. Adverse outcomes are more common (but unusual) in children who have viral meningitis during the first year of life. Speech and language development may be affected.

Treatment and outcome for the other types of aseptic meningitis depend on the underlying cause. If there is a depressed level of consciousness, treatable causes of aseptic meningitis-encephalitis must be considered (Table 53–10). In particular, *herpes simplex virus type 1* is a treatable and common cause of endemic (as contrasted to epidemic enterovirus or arbovirus) meningoencephalitis or encephalitis. Clues to the etiology of herpes simplex infection in non-neonates include depressed levels of consciousness, aseptic CSF profile with increased numbers of erythrocytes in the CSF, a temporal lobe focus on the CT scan or EEG and a positive CSF polymerase chain reaction to detect herpes simplex DNA. CSF culture is often negative; presumptive therapy for herpes simplex with intravenous acyclovir is indicated in any patient with aseptic meningitis and alterations in the level of consciousness in whom an obvious diagnosis is not evident. In neonates, herpes simplex (type 2 > > type 1) usually manifests as encephalitis, systemic infection, or local cutaneous, mouth, or eye (keratitis) disease. The onset is usually within the first 2 weeks of life, and 65% to 75% of patients have cutaneous vesicles (usually not present in older children with herpes simplex virus type 1 encephalitis). Treatment is with acyclovir.

Tuberculous meningitis is an important treatable cause of "aseptic" meningitis. During the primary pulmonary tuberculous infection and subsequent bacteremic spread to extrapulmonary sites, tubercle bacterium produces local microscopic granulomas in the CNS and meninges. If this primary CNS infection is not contained by host defense mechanisms (T lymphocytes, monocytes), or if host defense mechanisms fail at a later period, tuberculous meningitis may reactivate. Meningitis occurs weeks to months after the primary pulmonary process.

The symptoms of tuberculous meningitis are insidious and subacute (weeks to months; average, 2 weeks). Stage 1 is a prodrome with nonspecific manifestations (apathy, poor school function, irri-

Table 53–8. Clinical Conditions and Infectious Agents Associated with Aseptic Meningitis

Agents/Conditions	Example
Viruses	Enteroviruses (coxsackieviruses, echoviruses, polioviruses)
	Arboviruses (Eastern equine encephalitis, Western equine, encephalitis, Venezuelan equine encephalitis, St. Louis encephalitis, California encephalitis, Colorado tick fever)
	Mumps (native, vaccine)
	Herpes simplex (type 1, 2, 6)
	Others (human immunodeficiency virus, varicella, Epstein-Barr virus, lymphocytic choriomeningitis, measles, rubella, rabies, influenza, parainfluenza)
Bacterial meningitis	*Mycobacterium tuberculosis*
	Pyogenic or inadequately treated
	Leptospira sp. (leptospirosis)
	Treponema pallidum (syphilis)
	Borrelia sp. (relapsing fever)
	Borrelia burgdorferi (Lyme disease)
	Nocardia sp. (nocardiosis)
	Cat-scratch disease
Bacterial parameningeal focus	Sinusitis, mastoiditis, brain abscess, subdural-epidural empyema, cranial osteomyelitis
Rickettsia	*R. rickettsii* (Rocky Mountain spotted fever), *Ehrlichia*
Mycoplasma	*M. pneumoniae, M. hominis*
Chlamydia	*C. trachomatis*
Fungi	*Coccidioides immitis* (coccidioidomycosis)
	B. dermatitidis (blastomycosis)
	Cryptococcus neoformans (cryptococcosis)
	Histoplasma capsulatum (histoplasmosis)
	Candida albicans
Protozoa	*Toxoplasma gondii* (toxoplasmosis)
	Acanthamoeba; Naegleria
	Malaria
Other parasites	*Angiostrongylus cantonensis* (eosinophilic)
	Trichinella spiralis (trichinosis)
	Strongyloides stercoralis (hyperinfection)
	Schistosomiasis
Malignancy	Leukemia, lymphoma, central nervous system tumor (e.g., craniopharyngioma, dermoid-epidermoid cyst, glioma)
Postinfectious causes	Vaccines: rabies, influenza, measles; demyelinating or allergic encephalitis
Immune diseases	Kawasaki disease, sarcoidosis, Behçet syndrome, lupus erythematosus, vasculitis, Vogt-Koyanagi-Harada syndrome, Wegener granulomatosis, familial Mediterranean fever
Drugs	Intrathecal injections (contrast media, serum, antibiotics, antineoplastic agents)
	Nonsteroidal anti-inflammatory agents
	OKT3 monoclonal antibodies
	Carbamazepine
	Trimethoprim-sulfamethoxazole
	Azathioprine
	INH
	Intravenous immunoglobulins
Miscellaneous	Heavy metal poisoning (lead, arsenic)
	Foreign bodies (shunt, reservoir)
	Subarachnoid hemorrhage
	Postictal state
	Post migraine state
	Mollaret syndrome (recurrent)
	Intraventricular hemorrhage (neonate)
	Familial hemophagocytic syndrome
	Post neurosurgery state (posterior fossa syndrome)

Modified from Cherry JD. Aseptic meningitis and viral meningitis. *In* Feigin RD, Cherry JD (eds). Textbook of Pediatric Infectious Diseases, 2nd ed. Philadelphia: WB Saunders, 1987:479. Reprinted and modified from Behrman RE (ed). Nelson Textbook of Pediatrics, 14th ed. Philadelphia: WB Saunders, 1992:655.

Table 53–9. Characteristics of the Most Common Causes of the Aseptic Meningitis Syndrome

Organism	Peak Groups	Peak Season	Clues in Presentation	Epidemiologic Clues
Enteroviruses	Infants, younger children, uncommon after age 40	Summer, fall	Exanthem, myopericarditis, conjunctivitis, pleurodynia, hand-foot-mouth disease, herpangina	Known epidemic
Mumps	5–9 yr Male > female	Late winter–early spring	Parotitis, orchitis, oophoritis, pancreatitis, hyperamylasemia, hypoglycorrhachia in 25%	Known exposure to mumps, recent vaccination
Lymphocytic choriomeningitis virus	Older children, young adult	Fall, early winter	Late orchitis, alopecia, CSF leukocytes may be > 1000, hypoglycorrhachia in 25%	Exposure to rodents (mice, hamsters) or their excreta
Human immunodeficiency virus (HIV)	Adult (seen at all ages)	Year-round	Mononucleosis-like syndrome	HIV risk factors
Leptospira	Young adult	Late summer, early fall	Conjunctivitis, splenomegaly, jaundice, nephritis, rash, severe headache	Exposure to animals, water contaminated with animal urine
Borrelia burgdorferi (Lyme disease)		Primary: spring–late fall; secondary: follows exposure by weeks to months	Rash, radiculitis, cranial nerve or other focal findings, cardiac manifestations	Tick exposure (bite often unrecognized), endemic area
Herpes simplex virus type 2	Young adult	Year-round	Syndrome of primary genital herpes	Sexual history
Arthropod-borne viruses	California, children; St. Louis, adults; equine, children, elderly	Summer, early fall		Geographic area, contact with insect vector, encephalitis in community, disease in horses
Mycobacterium tuberculosis	Adults in U.S. (reactivation), children in endemic areas	Year-round	Cranial nerve findings, altered mentation, pulmonary disease in children, SIADH, low CSF glucose, chloride	History of TB or known exposure, HIV risk factors

Modified from Connolly KJ, Hammer SM. The acute aseptic meningitis syndrome. Infect Dis Clin North Am 1990; 4:599–622.
Abbreviations: SIADH = syndrome of inappropriated antidiuretic hormone secretion; CSF = cerebrospinal fluid; TB = tuberculosis.

tability, weight loss, fever, night sweats, nausea); stage 2 is heralded by the onset of neurologic signs (headache, cranial neuropathy, nuchal rigidity, signs of increased intracranial pressure); and stage 3 manifests with alterations of the level of consciousness (lethargy, stupor, coma). Meningismus is not present in all patients.

The diagnosis of tuberculous meningitis is suggested by a history of contacts with adults with active tuberculosis, a chronic cough, human immunodeficiency virus (HIV) disease, poverty, or homelessness, in addition to a chest radiograph in the patient compatible with active or, more often, quiescent tuberculosis (parenchymal-hilar node calcifications, infiltrates, hilar adenopathy, and, rarely, endobronchial or cavitary lesions) and a positive tuberculin skin test (see Chapter 7). The CSF results are noted in Table 53–3 and include profound hypoglycorrhachia, a high CSF protein, lymphocyte- or monocyte-predominant cells (usually 500 cells/mm³), increased opening pressure, and, on occasion, positive results on acid-fast staining to identify tubercle organisms. Polymerase chain reaction amplification of *Mycobacterium tuberculosis* DNA aids in making a rapid diagnosis culture of CSF, sputum (acid-fast stain also), or gastric aspirates, which traditionally (culture) may require

2 to 6 weeks to identify the *M. tuberculosis.* The differential diagnosis is noted in Table 53–6.

Treatment includes general supportive care for coma and increased intracranial pressure, including the use of intravenous corticosteroids. Antituberculous therapy includes the use of isoniazid (10 to 20 mg/kg/day), rifampin (10 to 20 mg/kg/day), pyrazinamide (20 to 40 mg/kg/day), and streptomycin (20 to 40 mg/kg/day) for 2 months on a daily basis, followed by 10 months of daily INH and rifampin (alternately INH and rifampin could be given twice weekly). If streptomycin resistance is suspected, capreomycin (15 to 30 mg/kg/day) or kanamycin (15 to 30 mg/kg/day) may be substituted. If INH or rifampin resistance is suspected, ethambutol (15 to 25 mg/kg/day) may be considered.

Recurrent Aseptic Meningitis

Several causes of recurrent aseptic meningitis have been reported (Table 53–11). Representative of these is *Mollaret meningitis,* the

Table 53-10. **Classification of Encephalitis by Etiology and Source**

I. **Infections—viral**
  A. Spread person to person only
    1. Mumps: frequent in an unimmunized population; often mild
    2. Measles: may have serious sequelae
    3. Enteroviruses frequent at all ages; more serious in newborns
    4. Rubella: uncommon; sequelae rare except in congenital rubella
    5. Herpesvirus group
      a. Herpes simplex (types 1 and 2, possibly 6): relatively common; sequelae frequent; devastating in newborns
      b. Varicella-zoster virus: uncommon; serious sequelae not rare
      c. Cytomegalovirus—congenital or acquired: may have delayed sequelae in congenital type
      d. Epstein-Barr virus (infectious mononucleosis): not common
    6. Pox group
      a. Vaccinia and variola: uncommon, but serious central nervous system (CNS) damage occurs
    7. Parvovirus (erythema infectiosum): not common
    8. Influenza A and B
    9. Adenovirus
    10. Other: reoviruses, respiratory syncytial, parainfluenza, hepatitis B
  B. Arthropod-borne agents
    Arboviruses: spread to man by mosquitoes or ticks; seasonal epidemics depend on ecology of the insect vector; the following occur in the United States:

Eastern equine	California
Western equine	Powassan
Venezuelan equine	Dengue
St. Louis	Colorado tick fever

  C. Spread by warm-blooded mammals
    1. Rabies: saliva of many domestic and wild mammalian species
    2. Herpesvirus simiae ("B" virus): monkeys' saliva
    3. Lymphocytic choriomeningitis: rodents' excreta

II. **Infections—nonviral**
  A. Rickettsial: in Rocky Mountain spotted fever and typhus; encephalitic component from cerebral vasculitis
  B. *Mycoplasma pneumoniae:* interval of some days between respiratory and CNS symptoms
  C. Bacterial: tuberculous and other bacterial meningitis; often has encephalitic component
  D. Spirochetal: syphilis, congenital or acquired; leptospirosis; Lyme disease
  E. Cat-scratch disease
  F. Fungal: immunologically compromised patients at special risk: cryptococcosis; histoplasmosis; aspergillosis; mucormycosis; candidosis; coccidioidomycosis
  G. Protozoal: *Plasmodium* sp.; *Trypanosoma* sp.; *Naegleria* sp.; *Acanthamoeba; Toxoplasma gondii*
  H. Metazoal: trichinosis; echinococcosis; cysticercosis; schistosomiasis

III. **Parainfectious—postinfectious, allergic**
  Patients in whom an infectious agent or one of its components plays a contributory role in etiology, but the intact infectious agent is not isolated *in vitro* from the nervous system. It is postulated that in this group the influence of cell-mediated antigen-antibody complexes plus complement is especially important in producing the observed tissue damage.
  A. Associated with specific diseases (these agents may also cause direct CNS damage—see I and II above)

Measles	Rickettsial infections
Rubella	Influenza A and B
Mumps	Varicella-zoster
Mycoplasma pneumoniae	

  B. Associated with vaccines

Rabies	Measles
Vaccinia	Yellow fever

IV. **Human slow-virus diseases**
  Accumulating evidence that viruses frequently acquired earlier in life, not necessarily with detectable acute illness, participate in later chronic neurologic disease (similar events also known to occur in animals)
  A. Subacute sclerosing panencephalitis; measles; rubella?
  B. Creutzfeldt-Jakob disease (spongiform encephalopathy)
  C. Progressive multifocal leukoencephalopathy
  D. Kuru (Fore tribe in New Guinea only)
  E. Human immunodeficiency virus

V. **Unknown—complex group**
  This group constitutes more than two thirds of the cases of encephalitis reported to the Centers for Disease Control and Prevention, Atlanta, Georgia. The yearly epidemic curve of these undiagnosed cases suggests that the majority are probably due to enteroviruses and/or arboviruses.

  There is also a miscellaneous group that is based on clinical criteria: Reye syndrome is one current example. Others include the extinct von Economo encephalitis (epidemic from 1918–1928); myoclonic encephalopathy of infancy; retinomeningoencephalitis with papilledema and retinal hemorrhage; recurrent encephalomyelitis (? allergic or autoimmune); pseudotumor cerebri; and epidemic neuromyasthenia—Iceland disease.

  An encephalitic clinical pattern may follow ingestion or absorption of a number of known and unknown toxic substances. These include ingestion of lead and mercury and percutaneous absorption of hexachlorophene as a skin disinfectant and gamma benzene hexachloride as a scabicide.

Modified from Behrman RE (ed). Nelson Textbook of Pediatrics, 14th ed. Philadelphia: WB Saunders, 1992:667.

Table 53–11. **Etiology of Recurrent Aseptic Meningitis**

Mollaret syndrome
Intracranial tumor
Vein of Galen aneurysm
Sarcoidosis
Behçet syndrome
Vogt-Koyanagi-Harada syndrome
Chronic benign lymphocytic meningitis
Systemic lupus erythematosus
Mixed connective tissue disease
Epstein-Barr virus infection
Lyme disease
Nonsteroidal anti-inflammatory drugs
Trimethoprim-sulfamethoxazole

etiology of which is unknown but may be due to recurrent leak of a CNS epidermal cyst into the CSF or due to chronic herpes simplex infection. The cellular debris released from the cyst may cause meningeal inflammation and the clinical picture of meningitis. In Mollaret syndrome, brief episodes of meningitis alternate with asymptomatic periods. Headache, nuchal rigidity, fever, nausea, and vomiting are presenting symptoms. After several years, the illness may suddenly disappear. CSF examination reveals pleocytosis that is initially predominately polynuclear but switches to mononuclear after the first day. The protein is elevated, and the glucose is depressed. The CSF returns to normal in a few days.

Evaluation of the child with recurrent aseptic meningitis includes a thorough history and physical, CT or magnetic resonance imaging of the head and spine, and other tests as indicated.

OTHER CAUSES OF NUCHAL RIGIDITY

The other conditions that present with neck stiffness are listed in Table 53–12. They may be differentiated from meningitis by the presence of specific neurologic signs or symptoms; the presence of signs and symptoms characteristic of another disease; the absence of signs and symptoms other than a stiff and painful neck; a history of predisposing factors; or a thorough head and neck examination.

Neurologic Signs and Symptoms

When a child presents with a stiff neck and a neurologic deficit, the nature of the deficit directs the physician to the proper evaluation. For example, in a child who presents with altered sensorium, encephalitis or a CNS hemorrhage is considered. Alternatively, if there is cranial nerve involvement, the differential diagnosis would include intracranial masses. Weakness or pain in the upper extremities directs the physician to investigate for causes of pressure on cervical nerve roots, such as an abscess, tumor, or trauma to the cervical spine. Ascending paralysis associated with a stiff neck is characteristic of Guillain-Barré syndrome. Muscular rigidity is expected in poliomyelitis, dystonia musculorum deformans, spasmodic torticollis, and Huntington chorea. Dystonic movements are also present in the last three.

Ocular torticollis is due to either superior oblique muscle weakness or congenital nystagmus. Torticollis and neck stiffness develop in the infant to compensate for abnormal eye movement. A good eye examination helps to make this diagnosis.

Other Diseases

Meningismus as the cause of neck stiffness is common in viral and bacterial illnesses. Neck stiffness is caused by spread of inflammation to the soft tissues of the neck, as in pharyngitis, deep neck infections, or upper lobe pneumonia. Spasm of the neck muscles due to the underlying disease is another etiology. Examples of this are black widow spider bites and reflux esophagitis. In juvenile rheumatoid arthritis, neck stiffness may be due to cervical spine involvement or encephalopathy.

Neck Pain

A child's unwillingness to move the neck because of pain may be confused with nuchal rigidity. An examination of the neck for muscle spasm and muscle or bone tenderness; a history of trauma, unusual positioning of the neck, or exposure to a draft; radiation of pain to shoulder and arm muscles; and the ability of the physician to flex and rotate the child's neck, plus the absence of other signs and symptoms, help to make the diagnosis. If a cervical subluxation, fracture, or dislocation is suspected, the neck should be immobilized and appropriate radiographs obtained.

Treatment is directed to the underlying cause. For the most common causes, minor trauma and myositis, analgesic and anti-inflammatory medication along with local heat and a soft cervical collar constitute the appropriate treatment.

History of Predisposing Factors

Two conditions that cause neck stiffness: postinfectious encephalomyelitis and post–upper respiratory infection subluxation of the first cervical vertebra on the second vertebra, in which the diagnosis depends on the history, a paucity of other physical findings, and the exclusion of other diseases.

There are three types of postinfectious encephalomyelitis:

1. *Acute toxic encephalopathy* (ATE) is most common in children under 2 years of age. ATE follows common viral illnesses. It presents with a sudden onset of fever, headache, stiff neck, vomiting, and mental status changes and may progress to coma. The CSF is normal except for elevated pressure. Treatment is symptomatic and supportive.

2. *Acute disseminated encephalomyelitis* (ADE) is most commonly found in children over the age of 2 years. It follows viral and bacterial infections as well as drug and plasma administration. Symptoms begin 4 to 21 days after the acute event and include fever, headache, neck stiffness, anorexia, vomiting, and mental status changes, including coma, seizures, and focal neurologic signs. CSF may be completely normal or show elevated pressure, WBCs, or protein. Again, treatment is symptomatic and supportive.

3. *Acute hemorrhagic leukoencephalitis* has similar antecedent conditions and presentation as the other forms. Onset is 1 to 20 days after the acute event. The CSF shows increased pressure, polymorphonuclear cell pleocytosis, and increased protein. Treatment is symptomatic and supportive.

Atlantoaxial subluxation may occur about 1 week after an upper respiratory tract infection. The cause is softening and stretching of spinal ligaments secondary to inflammation. It is most common in children between the ages of 6 and 12 years. Patients present with reduced range of motion in the neck and tenderness over the upper third of the cervical spine in the absence of cervical myalgia. The subluxation can be seen on radiographs of the cervical spine. In some children, manual traction may reduce the subluxation.

Table 53–12. Causes of Nuchal Rigidity Other Than Meningitis Categorized by Presentation

Neurologic Signs and Symptoms

Encephalitis
Guillain-Barré syndrome
Acute cerebellar ataxia
Brain abscess
Epidural abscess
Dystonia musculorum deformans
Spasmodic torticollis
Paroxysmal torticollis
Huntington chorea
Cervical cord syringomyelia
Multiple sclerosis
Poliomyelitis
Tic and Tourette syndrome
Vestibular dysfunction
Vascular Abnormalities
Subarachnoid hemorrhage
Cerebral aneurysms
Venous and venous sinus thrombosis
Neoplasms
Posterior fossa tumors
Brainstem tumors
Tumors of 3rd ventricle
Intraspinal tumor
Leaking craniopharyngioma
Superior oblique muscle weakness
Congenital nystagmus
Cervical Spine Trauma
Subluxation
Dislocation
Fractures
Sprain
Disc injury

Signs and Symptoms of a Specific Disease

Upper lobe pneumonia
Epiglottitis
Pharyngitis-tonsillitis
Otitis media-mastoiditis
Tuberculosis
Cat-scratch disease
Herpes zoster
Tetanus
Trichinosis
Chagas disease
Diphtheria
Rabies
Wilson disease
Fibrodysplasia ossificans progressiva
Spasmus nutans
Benign paroxysmal vertigo
Reflux esophagitis (Sandifer syndrome)
Black widow spider bite
Scorpion sting
Kawasaki syndrome
Systemic lupus erythematosus
Sarcoidosis
Vogt-Koyanagi-Harada syndrome
Juvenile rheumatoid arthritis
Deep Neck Infections
Lateral pharyngeal space
Retropharyngeal space
Masticator space
Visceral space
Ludwig angina
Dental infection
Carotid sheath and jugular vein thrombosis
Sialoadenitis
Parotitis
Bezold abscess (mastoiditis)
Congenital cysts and fistulas
Primary deep cervical adenitis

Neck Pain

Cervical spine or rib osteomyelitis
Discitis
Osteoid osteoma
Eosinophilic granuloma
Intraspinal tumor
Osseous tumor of cervical spine
Rhabdomyosarcoma
Lymphoma
Facet syndrome
Disc syndrome
Acute cervical myalgia
Myositis (due to draft or positioning)
Fibromyositis
Tension headache
Functional torticollis
Calcification of discs
Neuritis of spinal accessory nerve
Esophageal foreign body
Clavicular fracture
Cervical spine trauma

History

Postinfectious Encephalomyelitis
Acute toxic encephalopathy
Acute disseminated encephalomyelitis
Acute hemorrhagic leukoencephalitis

Other

Congenital
Ligamentous laxity of transverse ligament
Hemivertebrae
Klippel-Feil syndrome
Sprengel deformity
Arnold-Chiari malformation
Basilar impression
Congenital torticollis
Congenital absence of transverse ligament
Congenital absence or hypertrophy of cervical muscles
Intrauterine constraint
Hereditary stiff baby syndrome
Infantile Gaucher disease
Maple syrup urine disease
Glutaric aciduria
Cerebral palsy
Kernicterus
Intoxications
Phenothiazines
Strychnine
Lead
Methanol
Vitamin A

Subsequently, the children should wear a soft cervical collar for 1 week or until cervical range of motion is painless. Other children may require bed rest and traction.

Congenital Causes

There are several congenital causes of nuchal rigidity. They are caused by inborn errors of metabolism resulting in muscle stiffness or neurologic disorders, congenital anomalies of bone, perinatal problems, and primary neurologic disorders. They are diagnosed by age of onset and associated signs and symptoms.

One common cause is *congenital torticollis* (see Table 53–2). The infant presents in the weeks after birth with limited range of motion in the neck and a fibrous mass in the body of one sternocleidomastoid muscle. The head is tilted toward the affected side and the chin rotated to the opposite side. The mass initially increases in size and then resolves in 2 to 6 months, leaving a fibrotic and shortened sternocleidomastoid muscle. Treatment includes massage and stretching of the affected muscle and results in resolution of the disorder in 70% of cases.

REFERENCES

Bacterial Meningitis

Adams WG, Deaver KA, Cochi SL, et al. Decline of childhood *Haemophilus influenzae* type b (Hib) disease in the Hib vaccine era. JAMA 1993;269:221.

American Academy of Pediatrics Committee on Infectious Diseases. Treatment of bacterial meningitis. Pediatrics 1988;81:904.

American Academy of Pediatrics Committee on Infectious Diseases. Dexamethasone therapy for bacterial meningitis in infants and children. Pediatrics 1990;86:130.

Bonadio WA. The cerebrospinal fluid: Physiologic aspects and alterations associated with bacterial meningitis. Pediatr Infect Dis J 1992;11:423.

Bonadio WA, Mannenbach M, Krippendorf R. Bacterial meningitis in older children. Am J Dis Child 1990;144:463.

Bradley JS, Connor JD. Ceftriaxone failure in meningitis caused by *Streptococcus pneumoniae* with reduced susceptibility to beta-lactam antibiotics. Pediatr Infect Dis J 1991;10:871.

Brown LW, Feigin RD. Bacterial meningitis: Fluid balance and therapy. Pediatr Ann 1994;23:93.

Carraccio CL, Lomonico MP, Fisher MC. Limp as a presenting sign of meningitis. Pediatr Infect Dis J 1990;9:673.

Ciarallo LR, Rowe PC. Lumbar puncture in children with periorbital and orbital cellulitis. J Pediatr 1993;122:355.

Dodge PR. Neurological sequelae of acute bacterial meningitis. Pediatr Ann 1994;23:101.

Faillace WJ, Warrier I, Canady A. Paraplegia after lumbar puncture in an infant with previously undiagnosed hemophilia A. Clin Pediatr 1989;28:136.

Feigin RD, McCracken GH, Klein JO. Diagnosis and management of meningitis. Pediatr Infect Dis J 1992;11:785.

Friedland IR, Paris MM, Rinderknecht S, et al. Cranial computed tomographic scans have little impact on management of bacterial meningitis. Am J Dis Child 1992;146:1484.

Friedland IR, Shelton S, Paris M, et al. Dilemmas in diagnosis and management of cephalosporin-resistant *Streptococcus pneumoniae* meningitis. Pediatr Infect Dis J 1993;12:196.

Geiseler PJ, Nelson KE. Bacterial meningitis without clinical signs of meningeal irritation. South Med J 1982;75:448.

Givner LB, Kaplan SL. Meningitis due to *Staphylococcus aureus* in children. Clin Infect Dis 1993;16:766.

Gumerlock MK, Spollen LE, Nelson MJ. Cervical neurenteric fistula causing recurrent meningitis in Klippel-Feil sequence: Case report and literature review. Pediatr Infect Dis J 1991;10:532.

Havens PL, Wendelberger KJ, Hoffman GM, et al. Corticosteroids as adjunctive therapy in bacterial meningitis. A meta-analysis of clinical trials. Am J Dis Child 1989;143:1051.

Jafari HS, McCracken GH. Dexamethasone therapy in bacterial meningitis. Pediatr Ann 1994;23:82.

Kacica MA, Lepow ML. Meningitis: Clinical presentation and workup. Pediatr Ann 1994;23:69.

Kaplan SL, Catlin FI, Weaver T, et al. Onset of hearing loss in children with bacterial meningitis. Pediatrics 1984;73:575.

Kaplan SL, Patrick CC. Cefotaxime and aminoglycoside treatment of meningitis caused by gram-negative enteric organisms. Pediatr Infect Dis J 1990;9:810.

Kessler SL, Dajani AS. Listeria meningitis in infants and children. Pediatr Infect Dis J 1990;9:61.

Klein JO. Antimicrobial treatment and prevention of meningitis. Pediatr Ann 1994;23:76.

Kline MW. Review of recurrent bacterial meningitis. Pediatr Infect Dis J 1989;8:630.

Law DA, Aronoff SC. Anaerobic meningitis in children: Case report and review of the literature. Pediatr Infect Dis J 1992;11:968.

Mayefsky JH, Roghmann KJ. Determination of leukocytosis in traumatic spinal tap specimens. Am J Med 1987;82:1175.

Meirovitch J, Kitai-Cohen Y, Keren G, et al. Cerebrospinal fluid shunt infections in children. Pediatr Infect Dis J 1987;6:921.

Metrou M, Crain EF. The complete blood count differential ratio in the assessment of febrile infants with meningitis. Pediatr Infect Dis J 1991;10:334.

Moore PS, Hierholzer J, DeWitt W, et al. Respiratory viruses and mycoplasma as cofactors for epidemic group A meningococcal meningitis. JAMA 1990;264:1271.

Nagata M, Hara T, Aoki T, et al. Inherited deficiency of ninth component of complement: An increased risk of meningococcal meningitis. J Pediatr 1989;114:260.

Phillips CF. Epidemiology of bacterial meningitis. Pediatr Ann 1994;23:67.

Pike MG, Wong PK, Bencivenga R, et al. Electrophysiologic studies, computed tomography, and neurologic outcome in acute bacterial meningitis. J Pediatr 1990;116:702.

Polk DB, Steele RW. Bacterial meningitis presenting with normal cerebrospinal fluid. Pediatr Infect Dis J 1987;6:1040.

Pomeroy SL, Holmes SJ, Dodge PR, et al. Seizures and other neurologic sequelae of bacterial meningitis in children. N Engl J Med 1990;323:1651.

Powell KR, Sugarman LI, Eskenazi AE, et al. Normalization of plasma arginine vasopressin concentrations when children with meningitis are given maintenance plus replacement fluid therapy. J Pediatr 1990;117:515.

Radetsky M. Duration of treatment in bacterial meningitis: A historical inquiry. Pediatr Infect Dis J 1990;9:2.

Radetsky M. Duration of symptoms and outcome in bacterial meningitis: An analysis of causation and the implications of a delay in diagnosis. Pediatr Infect Dis J 1992;11:694.

Rodewald LE, Woodin KA, Szilagyi PG, et al. Relevance of common tests of cerebrospinal fluid in screening for bacterial meningitis. J Pediatr 1991;119:363.

Rowley AH, Chadwick EG, Kabat K, et al. Failure of a single dose of ceftriaxone to eradicate nasopharyngeal colonization of *Haemophilus influenzae* type b. J Pediatr 1987;110:792.

Rush PJ, Shore A, Inman R, et al. Arthritis associated with *Hemophilus influenzae* meningitis: Septic or reactive? J Pediatr 1986;109:412.

Snedeker JD, Kaplan SL, Dodge PR, et al. Subdural effusion and its relationship with neurologic sequelae of bacterial meningitis in infancy: A prospective study. Pediatrics 1990;86:163.

Taylor HG, Mills EL, Ciampi A, et al. The sequelae of *Haemophilus influenzae* meningitis in school-age children. N Engl J Med 1990;323:1657.

Tesoro LJ, Selbst SM. Factors affecting outcome in meningococcal infections. Am J Dis Child 1991;145:218.

Unhanand M, Mustafa MM, McCracken GH, et al. Gram-negative enteric bacillary meningitis: A twenty-one-year experience. J Pediatr 1993;122:15.

Ward E, Gushurst CA. Uses and technique of pediatric lumbar puncture. Am J Dis Child 1992;146:1160.

Aseptic Meningitis

Achard JM, Lallement PY, Veyssier P. Recurrent aseptic meningitis secondary to intracranial epidermoid cyst and Mollaret's meningitis: Two distinct entities or a single disease? A case report and nosologic discussion. Am J Med 1990;89:807.

Amir J, Harel L, Frydman M, et al. Shift of cerebrospinal polymorphonuclear cell percentage in the early stage of aseptic meningitis. J Pediatr 1991;119:938.

Aufricht C, Tenner W, Stanek G. Aseptic meningitis in the decennium of *Borrelia burgdorferi* infection (Lyme disease). Pediatrics 1991;87:268.

Auxier GG. Aseptic meningitis associated with administration of trimethoprim and sulfamethoxazole. Am J Dis Child 1990;144:144.

Baker RC, Lenane AM. The predictive value of cerebrospinal fluid differential cytology in meningitis. Pediatr Infect Dis J 1989;8:329.

Bia FJ, Barry M. Parasitic infections of the central nervous system. Neurol Clin 1986;4:171.

Dagan R, Jenista JA, Menegus MA. Association of clinical presentation, laboratory findings, and virus serotypes with the presence of meningitis in hospitalized infants with enterovirus infection. J Pediatr 1988;113:975.

Dorfman DH, Glaser JH. Congenital syphilis presenting in infants after the newborn period. N Engl J Med 1990;323:1299.

Feigin RD, Shackelford PG. Value of repeat lumbar puncture in the differential diagnosis of meningitis. N Engl J Med 1973;289:571.

Golden SE. Aseptic meningitis associated with *Ehrlichia canis* infection. Pediatr Infect Dis J 1989;8:335.

Gutierrez K, Abzug MJ. Vaccine-associated poliovirus meningitis in children with ventriculoperitoneal shunts. J Pediatr 1990;117:424.

Harrison SA, Risser WL. Repeat lumbar puncture in the differential diagnosis of meningitis. Pediatr Infect Dis J 1988;7:143.

Jaffe M, Srugo I, Tirosh E, et al. The ameliorating effect of lumbar puncture in viral meningitis. Am J Dis Child 1989;143:682.

Kitai I, Navas L, Rohlicek C, et al. Recurrent aseptic meningitis secondary to an intracranial cyst: A case report and review of clinical features and imaging modalities. Pediatr Infect Dis J 1992;11:671.

Newton RW. Tuberculous meningitis. Arch Dis Child 1994;70:364.

Rantala H, Uhari M, Tuokko H, et al. Poliovaccine virus in the cerebrospinal fluid after oral polio vaccination. J Infect 1989;19:173.

Rao SP, Teitelbaum J, Miller ST. Intravenous immune globulin and aseptic meningitis. Am J Dis Child 1992;146:539.

Ratzan KR. Viral meningitis. Med Clin North Am 1985;69:399.

Sabetta JR, Andriole VT. Cryptococcal infection of the central nervous system. Med Clin North Am 1985;69:33.

Sugiura A, Yamada A. Aseptic meningitis as a complication of mumps vaccination. Pediatr Infect Dis J 1991;10:209.

Waecker NJ, Connor JD. Central nervous system tuberculosis in children: A review of 30 cases. Pediatr Infect Dis J 1990;9:539.

Whitley RJ, Cobbs CG, Alford CA, et al. Diseases that mimic herpes simplex encephalitis. Diagnosis, presentation, and outcome. JAMA 1989;262:234.

Wilhelm C, Ellner JJ. Chronic meningitis. Neurol Clin 1986;4:115.

Other Causes of Nuchal Rigidity

Abbassioun K. Fever, meningeal reaction and increased intracranial pressure. Clin Pediatr 1971;10:332.

Beniz J, Forster DJ, Lean JS, et al. Variations in clinical features of the Vogt-Koyanagi-Harada syndrome. Retina 1991;11:275.

Bredenkamp JK, Maceri DR. Inflammatory torticollis in children. Arch Otolaryngol Head Neck Surg 1990;116:310.

Kiwak KJ. Establishing an etiology for torticollis. Postgrad Med 1984;75:126.

Krueger DW, Larson EB. Recurrent fever of unknown origin, coma, and meningismus due to a leaking craniopharyngioma. Am J Med 1988;84:543.

Lund L, Nielsen D, Andersen ES. Meningismus as main symptom in toxic shock syndrome. Acta Obstet Gynecol Scand 1988;67:395.

Reik L. Disorders that mimic CNS infections. Neurol Clin 1986;4:223.

Rizzo JD, Rowe SA. Meningism in a ten-month-old infant during OKT3 therapy. J Heart Transplant 1990;9:727.

Shumrick KA, Sheft SA. Deep neck infections. *In* Paparella MM, Shumrick DA, Gluckman JL, et al (eds). Otolaryngology, 3rd ed. Philadelphia: WB Saunders, 1991:2454.

Stein MT, Trauner D. The child with a stiff neck. Clin Pediatr 1982;21:559.

54 Bites

Martha Wright

Bites and stings by animals and insects are a common cause of human injury. The spectrum of disease following these injuries is broad; the recognizable clinical syndromes result from direct trauma, effects of toxins, immune phenomena, and transmitted infections.

MAMMALIAN BITES

Between 1 and 3.5 million mammalian bites occur each year in the United States and account for 1% of all emergency department visits. Children are at particular risk for significant injury, with 70% of dog bite–related fatalities occurring in victims under 10 years of age. Between 1% and 15% of all children are injured by animal bites each year.

Types of Bites

Dog. Dog bites account for 80% to 90% of animal bite wounds. Demographic studies reveal that German shepherds and pit bulls are implicated in a disproportionate number of attacks and that the typical pediatric victim is a boy between 5 and 9 years old who provoked a family or neighborhood dog. In young children, 60% to 80% of bites involve the head and neck; in older children and adults, the extremities are most commonly injured.

The animal's large teeth and strong jaw muscles are responsible for the observed patterns of injuries. Dogs tear and crush tissue, producing lacerations, abrasions, and avulsions. Wound infection occurs in 1.6% to 30% of bites, and other complications such as sepsis, septic arthritis, meningitis, osteomyelitis, tenosynovitis, endophthalmitis, rabies, and tetanus have been reported. In children, scarring and disfigurement may result because of the predilection for bites to the face.

Cat. Cats are responsible for about 10% of reported animal bites annually. Victims of cat bite are more frequently female and are older than dog bite victims (mean age, 19.5 years). In more than 50% of cases, the child is bitten by an unknown or stray animal. The cat's sharp teeth and claws and relatively weak jaw forces predispose the victim to scratches and puncture wounds. In adults, more than 80% of cat bites are inflicted on the upper extremities and hands; in children, a third of bites occur on the face and neck. Complications are similar to those seen following dog bites, although wound infections are more common and occur in 29% to 50% of cat bites. In addition, cats are the leading domestic carrier of rabies. Furthermore, cat bites and scratches may lead to cat-scratch disease (see Chapter 48).

Human. Human bites are much less common than dog and cat bites but can be associated with significant complications. In the pediatric population, more than 50% of human bites occur during fights in children older than 10 years of age. Other causes of ''tooth-skin'' contact include sports events, play activities, and child abuse. In contrast to injury patterns seen in adults, in whom deep hand lacerations and avulsions predominate, the types of injuries noted in children are usually abrasions involving the hands (knuckles), face, and neck. Wound infection, tenosynovitis, osteomyelitis, amputation, and transmission of various infectious pathogens, including hepatitis B and syphilis, are known complications of human bites.

Rodent. Rat bites are a problem primarily among laboratory workers and children living in poverty. Children younger than 10 years of age are at greatest risk, accounting for 69% of rat bites in one study. The characteristic rat bite is a puncture wound on the finger or hand that occurs during sleep or while attempting to handle the animal. Rat bites may result in wound infection in fewer than 10% of cases and transmission of a variety of diseases, including plague (bubonic, pneumonic, septicemic, and meningeal), rat bite fever, leptospirosis, melioidosis, and tetanus. Rabies transmission by rodents has not been reported in the United States.

Diagnostic Strategies

Information, including the type and immunization status of the animal responsible for the bite, report of unusual behavior in the animal, the time and circumstances of the injury, the immunization status of the victim, and any other victim characteristics that would predispose to infection (splenectomy, immunosuppression), focuses patient care.

The physical examination should include careful inspection and exploration of the bite wound, with special attention to altered neurovascular function and joint capsule integrity. Laboratory tests are rarely indicated in the evaluation of the acute noninfected wound. Pretreatment cultures in this setting have a low predictive value for causative organisms in wounds that subsequently become infected. Wounds with evidence of infection, however, should be cultured both aerobically and anaerobically. Radiologic studies may be indicated if concern exists for fracture or the presence of a foreign body in the wound (e.g., a tooth).

Treatment Strategies

The differential diagnosis of a mammalian bite wound is rarely in question. Instead, the dilemma is how to proceed with treatment. Current literature lacks large prospective studies to support many of the recommendations made for wound preparation, laceration repair, and use of prophylactic antibiotics. The aims of mammalian bite wound management include prevention of infection, maintenance and restoration of function of the injured area, and promotion of wound healing. These goals are effectively accomplished by meticulous wound care combining copious irrigation and debridement of devitalized tissue. Tetanus immunization status should be updated according to standard guidelines. With the exception of bites to the hand, surgical closure can be accomplished safely without apparent increase in infection risk. Delayed primary closure is recommended for hand bites.

Epidemiologic studies have identified several types of bites that appear to be at higher than average risk for infection. These include cat puncture wounds, closed-fist and other hand injuries from humans, dogs, or cats, and all bites in immunocompromised patients. Rodent bites, most dog bites, and abrasions or minor lacerations caused by any species in an immunocompetent victim are at no higher risk for infection than other non-bite wounds.

The use of prophylactic antibiotics in both high-risk and low-risk bite wounds has been studied, but consensus regarding efficacy is lacking because of study limitations. Of the randomized clinical trials published to date, the majority had a small sample size, high rate of patients lost to follow-up, lack of standardized wound

Table 54–1. Microorganisms Associated with Mammalian Bite Wound Infections

Common	Uncommon
Dogs	
Mixed infection	*Acinetobacter* sp.
Pasteurella multocida	*Aeromonas hydrophila*
Staphylococcus aureus	Alpha, beta, gamma streptococci
Staphylococcus epidermidis	Bacteroides sp.
	Brucella canis
	Capnocytophaga canimorsus (formerly DF-2)
	Enterobacter cloacae
	Enterococcus
	Escherichia coli
	Klebsiella sp.
	Moraxella sp.
	Peptococcus sp.
	Peptostreptococcus sp.
	Pseudomonas sp.
Cats	
Pasteurella multocida	*Acinetobacter* sp.
Staphylococcus aureus	*Bacteroides* sp.
	Corynebacterium sp.
	Enterobacter cloacae
	Fusobacterium sp.
	Streptococcus sp.
	Staphylococcus epidermidis
Humans	
Alpha, beta, gamma streptococci	*Enterococcus*
Bacteroides sp.	*Eubacterium* sp.
Corynebacterium sp.	*Klebsiella pneumoniae*
Eikenella corrodens	*Neisseria* sp.
Fusobacterium sp.	*Peptococcus* sp.
Mixed infection	*Pseudomonas* sp.
Peptostreptococcus sp.	*Veillonella* sp.
Staphylococcus aureus	

Table 54–2. Rabies Postexposure Prophylaxis Guide, United States 1991

Animal Type	Evaluation and Disposition of Animal	Postexposure Prophylaxis Recommendations
Dogs and cats	Healthy and available for 10-day observation Rabid or suspected rabid Unknown (escaped)	Should not begin prophylaxis unless animal develops symptoms of rabies* Immediate vaccination Consult public health officials
Skunks, raccoons, bats, foxes, and most other carnivores; woodchucks	Regarded as rabid unless geographic area is known to be free of rabies or until animal proven negative by laboratory tests†	Immediate vaccination
Livestock, rodents, and lagomorphs (rabbits and hares)	Consider individually	Consult public health officials. Bites of squirrels, hamsters, guinea pigs, gerbils, chipmunks, rats, mice, other rodents, rabbits, and hares almost never require antirabies treatment.

From Centers for Disease Control. Rabies prevention—United States, 1991. MMWR 1991;40 (RR-3):1–19.
*During the 10-day holding period, begin treatment with human rabies immune globulin (HRIG) and HDCV (human diploid cell rabies vaccine) or RVA (rabies vaccine absorbed) at first sign of rabies in a dog or cat that has bitten someone. The symptomatic animal should be killed immediately and tested.
†The animal should be killed and tested as soon as possible. Holding for observation is not recommended. Discontinue vaccine if immunofluorescence test results of the animal are negative.

preparation, and failure to document patient compliance. These studies suggest that prophylactic antibiotics in uninfected, low-risk, carefully prepared wounds do not decrease the likelihood of infection. No conclusions can be drawn regarding high-risk wounds because of small sample sizes and inconsistent findings.

All infected wounds require antibiotic therapy. Recommended antibiotics include those whose spectrum can address the expected organisms (Table 54–1). Penicillin is active against *Streptococcus* species, the gram-negative anaerobic rod *Eikenella corrodens,* and *Pasteurella multocida,* the infecting agent in 50% to 80% of cat bites and in 15% to 36% of dog bites. Semisynthetic penicillins and first- and second-generation cephalosporins treat *Staphylococcus* species. Dicloxacillin in combination with penicillin, amoxicillin/clavulanate, and erythromycin in the penicillin-allergic patient are each effective in this setting. Amoxicillin/clavulanate has the disadvantage of associated gastrointestinal side effects but eliminates the need for two drugs and is palatable in suspension. The broad-spectrum intravenous agents cefotaxime, ceftriaxone, imipenem/cilastin or ticarcillin/clavulanate are currently recommended for severe wound infections or septic complications.

Concern for rabies infection causes many people to seek medical attention following an animal bite. Risk for rabies is greatest after wild animal exposure, particularly to raccoons, skunks, and bats, although most postexposure rabies prophylaxis given in the United States follows dog or cat bites. Treatment guidelines are outlined in Tables 54–2 and 54–3.

RED FLAGS

Dog bite wounds to the head and face in young children have been associated with brain injury and meningitis. Compressive forces of 400 pounds per square inch (psi) generated by a dog's

Table 54–3. Rabies Postexposure Prophylaxis Schedule, United States 1991

Vaccination Status	Treatment	Regimen*
Not previously vaccinated	Local wound cleansing	All postexposure treatment should begin with immediate thorough cleansing of all wounds with soap and water
	HRIG	10 IU/kg body weight. If anatomically feasible, up to one-half the dose should be infiltrated around the wound(s) and the rest should be administered IM in the gluteal area. HRIG should not be administered in the same syringe or into the same anatomic site as vaccine. Because HRIG may partially suppress active production of antibody, no more than the recommended dose should be given.
	Vaccine	HDCV or RVA, 1.0 ml IM (deltoid area†), one each on days 0, 3, 7, 14, and 28
Previously vaccinated‡	Local wound cleansing	All postexposure treatment should begin with immediate thorough cleansing of all wounds with soap and water
	HRIG	HRIG should not be administered
	Vaccine	HDCV or RVA, 1.0 ml IM (deltoid area†), one each on days 0 and 3

From Centers for Disease Control. Rabies prevention—United States, 1991. MMWR 1991;40(RR-3):1–19.
*These regimens are applicable for all age groups, including children.
†The deltoid area is the only acceptable site of vaccination for adults and older children. For younger children, the outer aspect of the thigh may be used. Vaccine should never be administered in the gluteal area.
‡Any person with a history of pre-exposure vaccination with HDCV (human diploid cell rabies vaccine) or RVA (rabies vaccine absorbed); prior postexposure prophylaxis with HDCV or RVA; or previous vaccination with any other type of rabies vaccine and a documented history of antibody response to the prior vaccination.
Abbreviations: HRIG = human rabies immune globulin; IM = intramuscularly.

jaws can easily fracture an infant's skull. A computed tomography (CT) scan of the head is a useful adjunct in the assessment of the integrity of the skull and facial bones.

P. multocida typically produces a rapidly progressive, painful cellulitis that develops within 24 hours of the bite. Infections that develop after 24 hours are more frequently caused by *Staphylococcus* or *Streptococcus* species.

Closed-fist injuries contaminated with human oral flora can result in severe, disabling soft tissue infection and osteomyelitis. These wounds need scrupulous wound care and may benefit from evaluation by a hand surgeon.

SNAKEBITE

Of the 45,000 snakebites reported each year in the United States, approximately 8000 are caused by venomous snakes, with a disproportionate number seen in 5- to 19-year-old males. Only 10 to 15 deaths are recorded yearly, but no data are available on morbidity or resulting disability. Most of these attacks occur in the southeastern and southwestern United States, although the two families of indigenous poisonous snakes, Crotalidae and Elapidae, are distributed throughout the continental United States (Table 54–4).

Diagnostic Strategies

The challenge for clinicians treating snakebite victims is first to ascertain that the bite was inflicted by a poisonous snake and then to determine whether envenomation occurred. The differentiation of poisonous from nonpoisonous snakes can be done by directly inspecting the (preferably dead) snake or from a witness's description. Nonpoisonous snakes have round pupils, small teeth instead of fangs, a rounded snout, and no rattle on the tail (Fig. 54–1). Other information that influences the patient's management includes time elapsed since the bite, therapy rendered in the field, development of symptoms, and victim characteristics such as tetanus immunization status.

Inspection of the bite site usually confirms envenomation. Twenty percent of pit viper bites are "dry" and require nothing more than wound care. An envenomated pit viper wound, however, is immediately painful, with erythema and swelling developing at the site in minutes (Fig. 54–2). Over the next several hours, vesicles

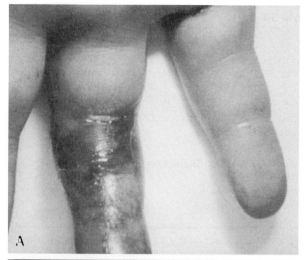
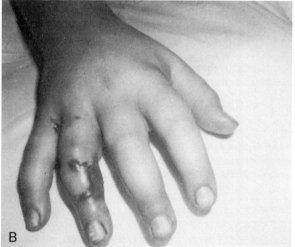

Figure 54–2. *A,* Crotalid envenomation, photograph taken 60 minutes after bite. Marked swelling and ecchymosis are apparent. Fang marks are barely visible. *B,* In the same patient, the back of the hand shows extensive swelling. (From Wolf MD. Envenomation. *In* Holbrook PR. Textbook of Pediatric Critical Care. Philadelphia: WB Saunders, 1993:1028.)

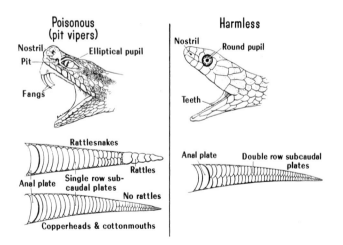

Figure 54–1. Characteristics that differentiate poisonous pit vipers from nonpoisonous snakes. (From Parrish HM. Public Health Rep 1966;81:269.)

and hemorrhagic bullae develop as the swelling increases, in some cases involving the entire limb and ipsilateral trunk. In addition to wound inspection, a complete physical assessment is necessary. Crotalidae venoms are snake-specific combinations of hemotoxic, neurotoxic, nephrotoxic, and cardiotoxic peptides and necrotizing proteinases that can result in multiple organ system dysfunction. Coral snake venom contains a potent neurotoxin that causes the gradual onset of weakness and flaccid paralysis. These symptoms occur in the absence of local tissue destruction or pain at the bite site.

Laboratory evaluation of the patient with an envenomated snakebite should include complete blood count (CBC), coagulation studies, type and cross-match, serum electrolytes, blood urea nitrogen (BUN)/creatinine, and urinalysis.

Differential Diagnosis

The symptoms exhibited after a snakebite may overlap other clinical entities and cause considerable confusion in the absence of

Table 54–4. **Characteristics of Snakes Indigenous to the United States**

	Crotalidae	Elapidae

Representative species	Rattlesnakes *(Crotalus, Sistrurus sp.)*
	 Copperhead *(Agkistrodon contortrix)*
	 Water moccasin *(Agkistrodon piscivorus)*
		Coral snakes
		  Eastern: *Micrurus fulvius*
		  Arizona: *Micruroides euryxanthus*

Geographic location	Rattlesnakes: throughout United States Copperhead: Southeast, northeast, west to Texas Water moccasin: Southeast to southern Illinois	Eastern coral snake: Midatlantic and southeastern states east of Mississippi Arizona coral snake: Arizona and New Mexico
Physical characteristics	Triangular-shaped head Elliptical pupils Two curved maxillary fangs Pits located on side of head between eye and nostril Some species with ''rattles''	Round head 2-ft length Typical color pattern: black snout with alternating red and black bands; bands bordered by narrow yellow rings Two maxillary fangs
Percentage of all snake bites in United States	99%	1%
Clinical characteristics of envenomation		
Local	Intense pain Fang marks (1–2 cm apart) Erythema Swelling Hemorrhagic vesicles Cutaneous necrosis	Minimal pain and swelling Small puncture marks (7–8 mm apart)
Systemic	Coagulopathy, hemolytic anemia Seizures, coma Weakness, paralysis Shock, hypotension Respiratory failure, pulmonary edema Oliguria, hematuria, hemoglobinuria	Malaise Bulbar palsies Generalized weakness Paralysis Respiratory failure
Antivenin	Antivenin (Crotalidae) polyvalent (Wyeth)	Antivenin for *Micrurus fulvius* (Wyeth)

history of snakebite. Pit viper envenomation can mimic septic shock, severe hemolytic anemia, hemolytic-uremic syndrome, and necrotic arachnidism. The weakness and flaccid paralysis of coral snake envenomation are similar to the neurologic manifestations seen in botulism, polio, Guillain-Barré syndrome, transverse myelitis, and spinal cord compression syndromes.

Treatment Strategies

The goals of snakebite therapy are treatment of systemic and local venom effects, venom inactivation, and prevention of long-term disability. An approach combining supportive care, conscientious wound management, and the appropriate use of antivenin (Fig. 54–3) is the most successful. Very little controlled scientific data on methods of treatment exist, and many of the current recommendations are based on anecdotal reports.

Following a snakebite, the patient should be transported rapidly to a medical facility. Validated first aid measures, such as continuous suction over the wound using appropriate equipment and use of constriction bands (2- to 4-cm bands placed loosely above the bite to restrict lymphatic flow while allowing arterial and venous blood flow), should be instituted. Suction, if begun within 5 to 10 minutes of a bite, removes 30% to 50% of radiolabeled venom in animal models. Fang mark incisions are no longer advocated, as these do not hasten venom removal and can cause additional tissue and tendon damage if improperly performed. Tourniquets are contraindicated.

In a medical facility, assessments of the wound and major organ function are the first priorities. Treatment of cardiovascular and respiratory dysfunction must be performed urgently. Following stabilization, wound care should proceed with irrigation, loose dressing, splinting for comfort, and tetanus immunization. Prophylactic use of broad-spectrum antibiotics has not been studied prospectively and remains controversial. Fasciotomies are rarely necessary despite the impressive nature of the swelling, and their use should be based on an objective direct measure of elevated compartment pressure. Previously recommended therapies, including early wide excision of the wound and use of steroids, do not improve outcome, and cryotherapy and electroshock therapy have proved harmful.

Treatment with antivenin depends on the type of snakebite and the clinical manifestations (Fig. 54–3). For pit viper envenomation, a single polyvalent antivenin is effective against all indigenous species (antivenin [Crotalidae] polyvalent, Wyeth). Dosage is based on wound appearance, presence of systemic symptoms, and laboratory test abnormalities. Because anaphylaxis can complicate antivenin use, all patients require skin testing prior to administration of therapeutic doses. Treatment with pit viper antivenin is not routinely advocated in all cases, as there are a number of reports describing both copperhead and rattlesnake bite victims who had excellent outcomes with supportive care alone. In addition, more than 50% of antivenin recipients experience serum sickness following treatment. To date, there are no human clinical trials evaluating the efficacy of this therapeutic modality.

Although antivenin treatment after crotalid envenomation is controversial, use after known or suspected Eastern coral snakebite is

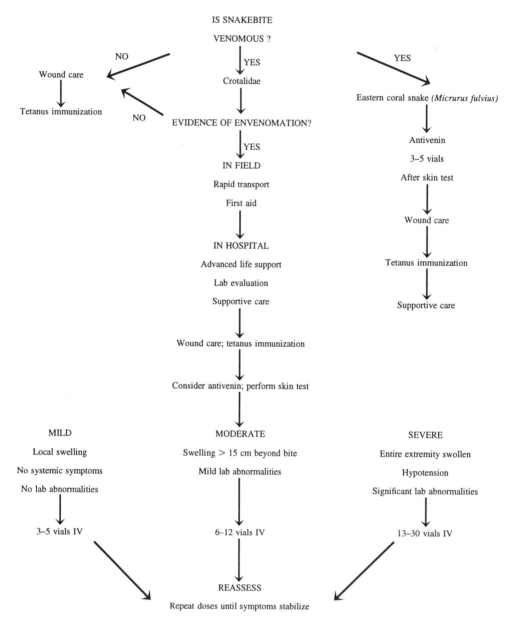

Figure 54–3. Treatment of snakebite. Symptoms of moderate envenomation include weakness, paresthesias, tachycardia, and hypotension; laboratory findings include hemoconcentration, low fibrinogen level, and thrombocytopenia. Symptoms of severe involvement include hypotension, shock, hemorrhage, and respiratory distress; laboratory findings include anemia, acidosis, and coagulopathy.

advocated regardless of the wound characteristics. Administration of three to five vials of *Micrurus fulvius* antivenin given intravenously after skin testing neutralizes the maximum amount of venom injected by this snake and should be given prior to the progression of neurologic signs. There is no antivenin available for the treatment of Arizona coral snake bites.

RED FLAGS

Coral snakes and some pit vipers, such as the Mojave rattler, cause unimpressive cutaneous reactions but life-threatening systemic effects. Snakebites in children are generally more severe than in adults because children receive a larger dose of venom per body weight. These patients should be monitored closely in intensive care settings. Knowledge of locally indigenous snakes is helpful when deciding to use antivenin following pit viper bites.

MARINE ANIMAL BITES

The exact incidence of injuries to children from marine animals is not known, but geographic proximity to the marine environment and family leisure activities along the coasts increase the chance of exposure to and injury by these creatures.

Types of Bites

Stingray. A deep puncture wound of the lower extremity in a person wading in a warm tidal pool is the typical injury inflicted by this marine vertebrate. The aptly named stingray is responsible for more human stings than any other marine vertebrate. Eleven species are found in United States coastal waters, accounting for as many as 2000 injuries yearly. When disturbed in its location on the sandy bottoms of secluded bays and lagoons, the ray reflexively whips its tail upward, jabbing a serrated, retropointed spine into the victim (Fig. 54–4). A heat-labile venom containing serotonin, phosphodiesterase, and 5′-nucleotidase is injected into the wound.

The spine creates a lacerated puncture wound on the lower extremity that is contaminated by debris, slime, and spinous fragments. Abdominal and chest wounds can occur and are associated with major organ damage. Pain at the site is intense, worsening over 30 to 90 minutes and lasting as long as 2 days. Systemic signs and symptoms such as nausea, seizures, hypotension, and muscle cramps frequently develop, whereas arrhythmias, paralysis, and death, though reported, are rare.

Jellyfish. Of the 100 species of coelenterates that are hazardous to humans, the majority are located in the Indo-Pacific oceans. In the United States, significant injuries are seen following contact with the Atlantic *(Physalia physalis)* and the Pacific *(P. utriculus)* Portuguese man-of-war and the lion's mane *(Cyanea capillata)*. Found in the warm coastal waters during the summer months, these large jellyfish inject venom into the victim from nematocysts that line their 75-foot-long tentacles.

The components of the venom are species-specific and affect the cardiovascular, autonomic, and central nervous systems by destabilizing cell membranes and altering calcium channel function. Tentacles and nematocysts leave evidence of a jellyfish attack on the skin in a characteristic ''whip mark'' pattern associated with urticaria, erythema, and vesiculation. Children are more likely to experience systemic effects, such as fever, chills, muscle spasms, hypotension, paralysis, and centrally mediated respiratory failure, because of the injection of a larger dose of venom relative to body weight.

Anemones, Corals. Hard and soft corals and anemones found along the United States coasts present minimal risk of serious envenomation to snorkelers and swimmers. Although these animals possess nematocysts that sting, the venom is rarely responsible for more than a burning sensation and a pruritic wheal at the site of injury. The greater risk for morbidity arises from abrasions and lacerations caused by contact with the rough exoskeletons of hard corals that become infected with organisms from the marine or cutaneous environment.

Echinoderms. Sea urchins and starfish species indigenous to United States coastal waters are not dangerously venomous like their tropical relatives, but they do present a risk for puncture wounds to the curious child who unwittingly steps on or handles these animals. Puncture wounds from the spines are intensely painful, erythematous, and edematous. Wound tattooing from the purple or black spines may result. Systemic effects are exceedingly rare and are similar to those seen following jellyfish envenomation. Late complications include granuloma formation, delayed inflammatory reactions, and infection.

Diagnostic Strategies

Information regarding the circumstances of the injury may help to identify the offending animal. The victim's tetanus status and immunocompetence should be ascertained. Inspection of the wound for the characteristics previously described guides therapy. Attention to cardiovascular and neurologic parameters is important, as systemic effects of venoms typically affect these organ systems.

Differential Diagnosis

The differential diagnosis of these injuries is frequently complicated by the victim's inability to identify the animal. However, the type of wound produced, the location of the wound, and the systemic symptoms following the bite or sting may narrow the diagnostic focus. Painful puncture wounds and lacerations are produced by stingrays, echinoderms, and a variety of poisonous fish, including scorpion fish and stonefish. Cutaneous urticaria and vesicle formation, especially in a linear pattern, are usually the result of contact with jellyfish, anemones, or soft coral.

Figure 54–4. Venomous apparatus of the stingray. Venom is stored in acini below the skin of the caudal appendage and is released after puncture by the spine. (Adapted from Kreuzinger R. In Halstead BW (ed). Poisonous and Venomous Marine Animals of the World. Princeton, NJ: The Darwin Press, 1978. Reprinted from Wolf MD. Envenomation. In Holbrook PR: Textbook of Pediatric Critical Care. Philadelphia: WB Saunders, 1993:1037.)

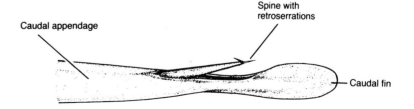

Treatment Strategies

Treatment of marine envenomations is directed at maintaining cardiovascular and neurologic stability, pain control, and venom inactivation. Wound care should be performed to prevent secondary infection, and tetanus immunization should be given if necessary. Treatment of stingray, echinoderm, and scorpion fish wounds begins with sea water irrigation to dilute the venom and wash away debris. Soaking the affected area in hot (40° to 45°C) water for 30 to 90 minutes provides pain relief and inactivates the heat-labile venom. Additional analgesia can be provided by narcotics. Wounds should be irrigated profusely with sterile saline, explored, and debrided. Radiographs may be necessary if foreign debris is suspected. Outcome following surgical repair of lacerations has not been studied prospectively, but several authors suggest leaving wounds open or using delayed primary closure.

Efficacy of prophylactic antibiotics in otherwise healthy patients is unproven. Antibiotics are indicated, however, for infected wounds and wounds in immunocompromised patients who are at high risk for overwhelming infection with *Vibrio* species. Broad-spectrum agents should cover the expected organisms (Table 54–5). Trimethoprim-sulfamethoxazole is a reasonable choice for children, and tetracycline or ciprofloxacin is used in older patients.

Following jellyfish wounds, irrigation with 5% acetic acid (vinegar) or 40% to 70% isopropyl alcohol for 30 minutes inactivates the venom and provides analgesia. Rinsing with fresh water and scrubbing the injured areas should be avoided, as these practices cause embedded nematocysts to release additional venom. Following irrigation, nematocysts can be removed by shaving the affected area. Topical steroids can provide local relief, and narcotics and diazepam may be necessary for relief from persistent pain and muscle spasms.

ARTHROPOD BITES

Of the one million species in the insect kingdom, the order Hymenoptera and the class Arachnida contain the few members that pose the greatest medical threat to humans.

Hymenoptera

Honeybees, wasps, yellow jackets, and fire ants are found throughout the United States and are responsible for the largest number of insect bites brought to medical attention. These insects envenomate their victim with immunoreactive substances that cause

Table 54–5. Microorganisms Associated with Infection in Marine-Acquired Wounds

Aeromonas hydrophila
Bacteroides fragilis
Chromobacterium violaceum
Clostridium perfringens
Erysipelothrix rhusiopathiae
Escherichia coli
Mycobacterium marinum
Pseudomonas aeruginosa
Salmonella enteritidis
Staphylococcus aureus
Streptococcus sp.
Vibrio vulnificus
Vibrio parahaemolyticus

Adapted with permission from Auerbach PS. Marine envenomations. New England Journal of Medicine 1991;325:486.

annoying local reactions and, in some cases, trigger synthesis of immunoglubulin E (IgE) antibodies that can mediate systemic anaphylaxis on subsequent re-exposure to the venom. Non-IgE immune-mediated reactions may also follow exposure to Hymenoptera venom and include a serum sickness–like syndrome, Guillain-Barré syndrome, acute glomerulonephritis, thrombocytopenic purpura, and transverse myelitis.

Bees. Bees attack their victims with barbed stingers that remain in the wounds and must be removed carefully to prevent further envenomation from the attached venom gland. A bee sting causes immediate pain and gradual development of local swelling, erythema, and pruritus. Systemic reactions, including nausea, vomiting, diarrhea, and fever, have been noted in adults following attacks by swarms.

Wasps, Hornets, Yellow Jackets. These insects have smooth stingers that can be used repeatedly to inject venom. Local and systemic reactions are similar to those seen following bee stings.

Fire Ants. Fire ants are found throughout the southern United States. These insects swarm from their hill when disturbed and attack the victim *en masse,* injecting venom that causes severe pain and burning. Each ant sting produces a small erythematous wheal surrounding a sterile pustule.

DIAGNOSTIC STRATEGIES

Knowledge of previous allergic reactions, insect type, time and circumstances of the sting, and development of symptoms guides patient treatment. Following Hymenoptera stings, patients should be assessed for cardiovascular and respiratory dysfunction and other signs of anaphylaxis.

DIFFERENTIAL DIAGNOSIS

Anaphylaxis is the syndrome resulting from antigen-triggered, IgE-mediated release of histamine and other vasoactive substances from mast cells. Sixty to 80 deaths from insect sting–induced anaphylaxis occur yearly, mostly in adults. Between 0.5% and 5% of the United States population has had a significant allergic reaction to bee stings, yet up to 80% of all deaths are reported in persons with no prior history of hypersensitivity.

The clinical syndrome of anaphylaxis develops within 30 minutes of a sting and is characterized by symptoms in two or more organ systems (Table 54–6). Death results either from hypoxemia secondary to airway obstruction or from cardiac failure secondary to shock. The differential diagnosis of anaphylaxis includes asthma, hereditary angioneurotic edema (HANE), vasovagal syncope, other types of distributive shock, upper airway infections, sepsis, and scombroid fish poisoning.

TREATMENT STRATEGIES

Anaphylaxis therapy is directed at relieving airway edema (epinephrine, intubation) or bronchospasm (epinephrine, beta-agonist aerosols [albuterol]) and improving perfusion (intravenous fluids, epinephrine). This therapeutic approach is then followed by relieving the other systemic effects of histamine (antihistamines H_1 and H_2 blockers) and other mediators (corticosteroids), suppressing

Table 54–6. Clinical Manifestations of Anaphylaxis

Skin	*Gastrointestinal*
Urticaria	Nausea
Flushing	Vomiting
Angioedema	Diarrhea
Pruritus	*Neurologic*
Pulmonary	Disorientation
Bronchospasm	Feeling of impending doom
Upper airway obstruction	
Cardiovascular	
Hypotension	
Dysrhythmias	
Shock	

further histamine release and mediator synthesis, and blocking histamine tissue receptors (H_1 and H_2 receptor antagonists) (Fig. 54–5). In mild cases, patient comfort and relief from pruritus are achieved using antihistamines. In severe cases, however, cardiovascular and respiratory support may be required. Patients experiencing bee sting anaphylaxis should be skin tested and offered desensitization therapy. Progressive desensitization is highly effective at preventing future anaphylactic reactions from Hymenoptera stings.

RED FLAGS

Anaphylaxis can have a biphasic clinical course in which the patient's initial histamine-related symptoms resolve, only to return several hours later. These late symptoms are due to synthesized mediators, such as prostaglandins, leukotrienes, and kinins. When one is planning disposition for a patient following an acute anaphylactic reaction, the potential for symptom recurrence should be considered.

Arachnidae

Spiders. In the United States, only two spiders have been responsible for fatal outcomes, the black widow (*Latrodectus mactans*) and the brown recluse (*Loxosceles reclusa*). All spiders are venomous, but only the black widow and a handful of others, of which the brown recluse is the best known, are capable of causing serious symptoms following envenomation.

Black Widow. The black widow spider is a nonaggressive insect that lives under rocks and in wood piles throughout the continental United States. Only the female, which injects a potent neurotoxin at the time of the bite, is poisonous to humans. This spider measures 15 to 18 mm, has a shiny black body, and has the characteristic red "hourglass" marking on her abdomen (Fig. 54–6).

Although the bite itself is usually painless, patients may describe a vague burning sensation at the site. Within an hour after envenomation, severe muscle spasms of the abdomen, back, and chest, hypertension, and descending paresthesia, especially in the soles of the feet, develop. Cholinergic symptoms may be present and include diaphoresis, increased salivation, lacrimation, vomiting, and diarrhea. These symptoms, due to venom-mediated synaptic acetylcholine and norepinephrine release, generally resolve in 24 to 48 hours.

As the spider is rarely recovered for identification and the bite may be undetected, the diagnosis is based on clinical features. The observed symptom complex must be differentiated from appendicitis, peritonitis, electrolyte disturbances, and cholinergic crisis from organophosphate poisoning or other toxins.

Treatment is directed at circulatory support and muscle spasm relief. Calcium gluconate and the muscle relaxants methocarbamol and diazepam are recommended in a number of anecdotal reports for pain relief; however, the effect is transient and little experience with pediatric envenomation has been described. Antivenin is available (Merck, Sharpe and Dohme), and a single dose of one vial is recommended following skin testing for patients under 12 years and over 65 years, as these age groups tend to be the most severely affected by the venom.

Brown Recluse. The brown recluse spider is the most familiar representative of a group of spiders responsible for the syndrome known as "necrotic arachnidism." These spiders inject an enzyme-rich venom that causes extensive local skin necrosis and a variety of systemic symptoms.

The brown recluse is found in the southeastern and midwestern United States, especially Missouri, Arkansas, Oklahoma, and Kansas, where it can be found in dark areas under rocks and in woodpiles. It is not aggressive, but it bites defensively when disturbed. This brown spider displays a characteristic violin-shaped marking on its dorsal cephalothorax (Fig. 54–7).

The bite of a necrotizing spider frequently goes unnoticed by the victim for several hours, when local itching, redness, and pain develop. Over the next several days, the center of the lesion turns

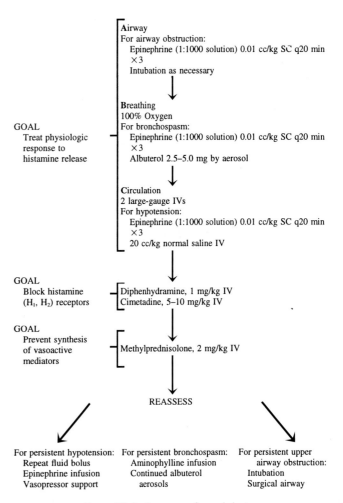

Figure 54–5. Treatment of anaphylaxis.

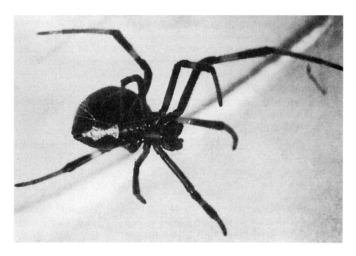

Figure 54–6. The female black widow spider has a shiny, black, globular body with a red hourglass mark on the abdomen. (From Paton BC. Surg Clin North Am 1963;43:537.)

black, and a slowly healing ulcer remains after the eschar sloughs. Nausea, vomiting, fever, headache, arthralgias, and myalgias are common features of this syndrome. Severe hemolytic anemia, seizures, renal failure, and shock are reported rarely. Children are bitten more frequently than adults and are more likely to have severe manifestations, especially hemolytic anemia.

Treatment of brown recluse spider bites requires conscientious wound care with skin grafting as necessary, tetanus prophylaxis, and management of systemic symptoms. Specific modalities, such

as local steroid injection, systemic corticosteroids, early wide excision of the lesion, local infiltration with phentolamine, and use of oral dapsone, which decreases the local infiltration of neutrophils into the envenomated area, have been advocated, but none have proven benefit in affecting the outcome of the lesion. Systemic steroids are useful in the management of hemolytic anemia resulting from envenomation.

Scorpions. Of the 650 species of scorpions in the world, only one species dangerous to humans is found in the United States. The scorpion *Centruroides exilicauda* makes its home in Arizona, Texas, Southern California, and Northern Mexico and is responsible for the majority of deaths reported from scorpion envenomation. The scorpion is an insect that contains a potent neurotoxin in specialized glands at the base of its tail. Humans are stung when they disturb the scorpions in their hiding places under rocks and logs or in clothing and shoes. Children (<45 kg) are especially vulnerable to the effects of the venom.

Scorpion venom causes acetylcholine and catecholamine release and calcium channel dysfunction. Following a sting, there is vague discomfort, tingling, and hyperesthesia at the site. Within 60 minutes, hyperactivity, restlessness, roving eye movements, tachycar-

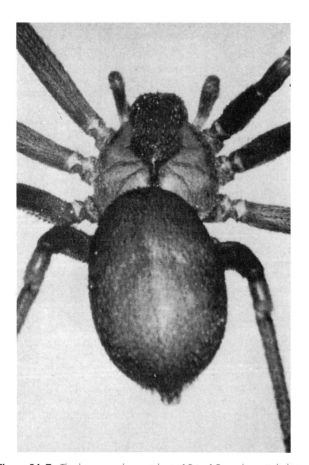

Figure 54–7. The brown recluse spider is 10 to 15 mm long, is light tan to dark brown in color, and has a species-specific dorsal, dark, violin-shaped band. (From Dillaha, CJ, Jansen GT, Honeycutt WM, Hayden CR. JAMA 1964;188:33.)

Table 54–7. **Scorpion Envenomation**

Grade 1:	Local discomfort and paresthesia
Grade 2:	Pain and paresthesia extend up the extremity
Grade 3:	Motor hyperkinesis Cranial nerve dysfunction Dysphagia Roving eyes Facial paresthesia Restlessness
Grade 4:	Cranial nerve dysfunction Drooling, uncontrollable eye movements Fasciculations, facial and distal muscles Neuromuscular hyperactivity Opisthotonos Convulsions Wheezing Hyperthermia Cyanosis

From Wolf MD. Envenomation. *In* Holbrook PR (ed). Textbook of Pediatric Critical Care. Philadelphia: WB Saunders, 1993:1024.

Table 54–8. Tick-Borne Diseases in the United States

Disease	Agent	Region
Lyme disease	*Borrelia burgdorferi*	Northeast, Wisconsin, Minnesota, California
Relapsing fever	*Borrelia* sp.	West
Tularemia	*Francisella tularensis*	Arkansas, Missouri, Oklahoma
Rocky Mountain spotted fever	*Rickettsia rickettsii*	Southeast, West, south central
Q fever	*Rickettsia burnetii*	Southwest, West
Ehrlichiosis	*Ehrlichia chaffeensis*	South central, South, Atlantic, upper midwest
Colorado tick fever	*Coltivirus* sp.	West
Babesiosis	*Babesia* sp.	Northeast

Adapted from Spach DH, Liles WC, Campbell GL, et al. Tick-borne diseases in the United States. New England Journal of Medicine 1993;329:936.

dia, and hypertension as well as cholinergic symptoms of salivation, lacrimation, vomiting, bronchorrhea, and wheezing develop and persist for as long as 36 hours (Table 54–7).

Marked agitation and restlessness are the most prominent clinical features and may suggest other causes, such as encephalitis, phenothiazine toxicity with dystonia, and movement disorders.

Treatment is directed at supporting cardiorespiratory function and pain control. Young children frequently require hospitalization, monitoring, and sedation as their symptoms resolve. Goat serum antivenin is available in Arizona but has not been approved by the Food and Drug Administration.

Ticks. Ticks threaten human health in their role as vectors for a variety of rickettsial, bacterial, and spirochetal diseases (Table 54–8) and through the toxin-mediated syndrome of tick paralysis. These arthropods inhabit grassy fields throughout the United States. The bite itself is rarely cause for alarm, although granuloma formation is known to occur at the site and certain spirochetal diseases may produce characteristic lesions (erythema chronicum migrans in Lyme disease; see Chapter 45). Generally, tick bites go unnoticed, and only about 50% of patients with proven tick-borne diseases relate a tick-bite history.

Tick paralysis is characterized by motor weakness or acute ataxia that progresses into an ascending flaccid paralysis. As the result of a neurotoxin elaborated at the bite site that blocks acetylcholine release at the neuromuscular junction, clinical symptoms disappear when the tick is removed. These neurologic symptoms must be distinguished from Guillain-Barré syndrome, poliomyelitis, spinal cord compression syndromes, and botulism (see Chapter 39).

REFERENCES

Mammalian Bites

Aghababian RV, Conte JE. Mammalian bite wounds. Ann Emerg Med 1980;9:79.
Avner JR, Baker MD. Dog bites in urban children. Pediatrics 1991;88:55.
Baker MD, Moore SE. Human bites in children: A six year experience. Am J Dis Child 1987;141:1285.
Boenning DA, Fleisher GR, Campos JM. Dog bites in children: Epidemiol-

ogy, microbiology, and penicillin prophylactic therapy. Am J Emerg Med 1983;1:17.
Brakenbury PH, Muwanga C. A comparative double blind study of amoxicillin/clavulanate vs placebo in the prevention of infection after animal bites. Arch Emerg Med 1989;6:251.
Brook I. Microbiology of human and animal bite wounds in children. Pediatr Infect Dis 1987;6:29.
Callaham ML. Prophylactic antibiotics in common dog bite wounds: A controlled study. Ann Emerg Med 1980;9:410.
Centers for Disease Control: Rabies prevention—United States, 1991. MMWR 1991;40(RR-3):1.
Dire DJ. Cat bite wounds: Risk factors for infection. Ann Emerg Med 1991;19:973.
Dire DJ, Hogan DE, Walker JS. Prophylactic oral antibiotics for low risk dog bite wounds. Pediatr Emerg Care 1992;8:194.
Elenbaas RM, McNabney WK, Robinson WA. Prophylactic oxacillin in dog bite wounds. Ann Emerg Med 1982;11:248.
Elenbaas RM, McNabney WK, Robinson WA. Evaluation of prophylactic oxacillin in cat bite wounds. Ann Emerg Med 1984;13:155.
Feder HM, Shanley JD, Barbasra JA. A review of 59 patients hospitalized with animal bites. Pediatr Infect Dis 1987;6:24.
Goldstein EJC, Citron DM, Wield B, et al. Bacteriology of human and animal bite wounds. J Clin Microbiol 1978;8:667.
Jones DA, Stanbridge TN. A clinical trial using cotrimoxazole in an attempt to reduce wound infection rates in dog bite wounds. Postgrad Med J 1985;61:593.
Kizer KW. Epidemiology and clinical aspects of animal bite injuries. J Am Col Emerg Physician 1979;8:134.
Marr JS, Beck AM, Lugo JA. An epidemiologic study of the human bite. Public Health Rep 1979;94:514.
Ordog GJ, Balasubramanium S, Wasserman J. Rat bites: 50 cases. Ann Emerg Med 1985;14:126.
Rosen RA. The use of antibiotics in the initial management of recent dog-bite wounds. Am J Emerg Med 1985;3:19.
Sacks JJ, Sattin RW, Bonzo SE. Dog bite related fatalities from 1979–1988. JAMA 1989;262:1489.
Schweich P, Fleisher G. Human bites in children. Pediatr Emerg Care 1985;1:51.
Skurka J, Willert C, Yogev R. Wound infection following dog bite despite prophylactic penicillin. Infection 1986;14:134.
Trott A. Care of mammalian bites. Pediatr Infect Dis 1987;6:8.

Snake Bites

Burch JM, Agarwal R, Mattox KL, et al. The treatment of crotalid envenomation without antivenin. J Trauma 1988;28:35.
Kunkel DB, Curry SC, Vance MV, et al. Reptile envenomations. J Toxicol Clin Toxicol 1984;21:503.
Wagner CW, Golladay ES. Crotalid envenomation in children: Selective conservative management. J Pediatr Surg 1989;24:128.

Marine Animal Bites

Auerbach PS. Marine envenomations. New Engl J Med 1991;325:486.
Brown CK, Shepherd SM. Marine trauma, envenomations, intoxications. Emerg Med Clin North Am 1992;10:385.

Arthropod Bites

Eitzen EM, Seward PN. Arthropod envenomations in children. Pediatr Emerg Care 1988;4:266.
Likes K, Banner W, Chavez M. Centruroides exilicauda envenomation in Arizona. West J Med 1987;141:634.
Rauber A. Black Widow spider bites. J Toxicol Clin Toxicol 1983;21:473.
Rimsza ME, Zimmerman DR, Bergeson PS. Scorpion envenomation. Pediatrics 1980;66:298.
Spach DH, Liles WC, Campbell GL, et al. Tick-borne disease in the United States. N Engl J Med 1993;329:936.
Valentine MD, Lichtenstein LM. Anaphylaxis and stinging insect hypersensitivity. JAMA 1987;258:2882.
Wasserman GS, Anderson PC. Loxoscelism and necrotic arachnidism. J Toxicol Clin Toxicol 1983–84;21:451.

55 Fever and AIDS

Philip Toltzis Robert N. Husson

The evaluation of the febrile, human immunodeficiency virus (HIV)–infected child is both difficult and frustrating because fever may arise from many sources and typically the evaluation needs to be performed many times throughout the life of the patient. The proper evaluation of the HIV-infected child with fever requires, first an accurate assessment of the patient's risk of acquiring a serious complication of HIV infection; second, the identification of the anatomic source of the infection through physical and laboratory examination; and third, the judicious use of tests and procedures to identify the infecting microorganism.

DEFINITIONS

Nearly all HIV infection in children is the result of vertical transmission from mother to child. Approximately 15% to 35% of infants born to HIV-infected mothers become infected; zidovudine therapy for pregnant mothers and their newborn infants (for 6 weeks after birth) may reduce the rate of vertical transmission to less than 10%. Diagnosis based on IgG antibody to HIV by Western blot analysis may produce false-positive results in infants younger than 18 months of age as a result of transplacental passage of maternally derived antibodies. Therefore, other tests are useful, including those allowing the detection of HIV viral antigens p24 or gp120, HIV virus by co-culture of the patient's lymphocytes, or more often HIV proviral DNA or RNA by polymerase chain reaction (PCR) amplification. In older children (>18 months) positive results on the Western blot antibody test proves infection. Acquisition of HIV infection may occur through transfusion of red blood cells and other blood-derived replacement products; this mode of transmission has become rare since the application in 1985 of routine blood bank screening for HIV. Disease in older children and adolescents may be acquired through sexual contact or through drug abuse–related needle contact. In a small number of instances, the mode of transmission is uncertain.

Vertically acquired HIV infection is characterized by many of the signs, symptoms, and complications seen in adult disease but with some peculiar characteristics of its own. Most infants experience a period of clinical latency after infection. HIV infection advances more rapidly in children; infants infected perinatally usually become symptomatic within the first 24 months of life. A small proportion of HIV-infected children have severe, rapidly progressive disease resulting in HIV-related manifestations in the first few months of life. Many infants infected with HIV demonstrate persistent mucocutaneous candidiasis, chronic or recurrent diarrhea, lymphadenopathy, and abdominal organomegaly (Table 55–1). Infants with HIV may fail to grow at the expected velocity. Direct HIV infection of tissue in the central nervous system results in an encephalopathy characterized by developmental delay, hypertonia, and spasticity. The Centers for Disease Control and Prevention (CDC) has developed a classification system that is specific for HIV disease in children (Tables 55–2 and 55–3).

HIV infects cells bearing the CD4 surface marker. The principal CD4-bearing cell that is the target for HIV infection is the helper T lymphocyte. In healthy persons, the CD4 molecule on helper T cells interacts with the major histocompatibility complex (MHC) class II/antigen complex presented by the macrophage or monocyte, a critical event in the pathogen-specific immune cascade. In HIV infection, the CD4 molecule binds to the HIV surface glycoprotein gp120 on free virus or on the surface of HIV-infected cells, facilitating viral entry into the cell. In addition, macrophages themselves and central nervous system (CNS) microglial cells express CD4 on their surface and may be similarly infected. Infection of the CD4-bearing helper T cell leads to its dysfunction and ultimate destruction. The consequences of this destruction are profound because the CD4$^+$ helper T cells, through cytokine production, orchestrate a host of additional immunologic mechanisms, including the induction of cytotoxic T cells, natural killer, and B lymphocytes. The dysfunction and ultimate depletion of the CD4 helper T cell population leave the patient defenseless against a broad range of opportunistic pathogens.

In addition to T-cell dysfunction, B-lymphocyte abnormalities are prominent in children infected with HIV, through both altered control by helper T cells and intrinsic dysfunction independent of diminished T-cell support. Many HIV-infected children demonstrate a *polyclonal hypergammaglobulinemia* beginning early in the course of their disease. Specific antibody responses to vaccinated or infecting antigens, both protein and polysaccharide, are poor. This defect is particularly detrimental in perinatally infected children who have had no chance to develop a repertoire of antibody-

Table 55–1. Principal Manifestations of Pediatric HIV Infection

Common
Hepatosplenomegaly
Diffuse lymphadenopathy
Persistent or recurrent oral candidiasis
Failure to thrive
Chronic or recurrent diarrhea
Lymphoid interstitial pneumonia
Recurrent bacterial infections
Developmental delay/encephalopathy
Opportunistic infection (*Pneumocystis carinii* penumonia, others)
Cardiomyopathy
Thrombocytopenia

Less Common
Nephropathy
Arteropathy
Parotitis
B-cell lymphoma and other HIV-related tumors

Modified from Rubinstein A. Pediatric AIDS. Curr Probl Pediatr 1986; 16:361–409.

Table 55–2. Immunologic Classification of Pediatric HIV Infection

	Age of Child					
	<12 mo		**1–5 yr**		**6–12 yr**	
Immunologic Category	*μL*	*(%)*	*μL*	*(%)*	*μL*	*(%)*
1: No evidence of suppression	≥1500	(≥25)	≥1000	(≥25)	≥500	(≥25)
2: Evidence of moderate suppression	750–1499	(15–24)	500–999	(15–24)	200–499	(15–24)
3: Severe suppression	<750	(<15)	<500	(<15)	<200	(<15)

From MMWR Morb Mortal Wkly Rep 1994;43:RR-12.

secreting cells against common pathogens. Consequently, they are particularly susceptible to repeated bacterial infections.

UNDERLYING CAUSES OF FEVER IN THE HIV-INFECTED CHILD

Recurrent bacterial and, in some instances, intercurrent viral infections are far more prominent in children than in adults. These infections occur in sites common to non–HIV-infected children: sinuses and middle ear, lungs, blood, gastrointestinal tract, CNS, urinary tract, and skin. Most of these infections are caused by bacteria or viruses that are typically found at the respective site: pneumococci in the respiratory tract, blood, and CNS; enteric gram-negative organisms in the urinary tract; and *Staphylococcus aureus* on the skin. Unusual pathogens are implicated only occasionally, particularly in children who acquire infection in the hospital and are critically ill. With the exception of *Pneumocystis carinii* pneumonia (PCP), it is unusual for children with HIV infection to present with

Table 55–3. Symptomatic Classification of Pediatric HIV Infection (1994)

Category N: Not Symptomatic

Children who have no signs or symptoms considered to be the result of HIV infection or who have only one of the conditions listed in category A.

Category A: Mildly Symptomatic

Children with two or more of the conditions listed below but none of the conditions listed in categories B and C.

- Lymphadenopathy (≥0.5 cm at more than two sites; bilateral = one site)
- Hepatomegaly
- Splenomegaly
- Dermatitis
- Parotitis
- Recurrent or persistent upper respiratory infection, sinusitis, or otitis media

Category B: Moderately Symptomatic

Children who have symptomatic conditions other than those listed for category A or C that are attributed to HIV infection. Examples of conditions in clinical category B include but are not limited to

- Anemia (<8 g/dl), neutropenia (<1000/mm³), or thrombocytopenia (<100,000/mm³) persisting ≥30 days
- Bacterial meningitis, pneumonia, or sepsis (single episode)
- Oropharyngeal candidiasis (thrush), persisting (>2 months) in children >6 months of age
- Cardiomyopathy
- Cytomegalovirus infection, with onset before 1 month of age
- Diarrhea, recurrent or chronic
- Hepatitis
- Herpes simplex virus stomatitis, recurrent (> two episodes within 1 year)
- Herpes simplex virus bronchitis, pneumonitis, or esophagitis with onset before 1 month of age
- Herpes zoster (shingles) involving at least two distinct episodes or more than one dermatome
- Leiomyosarcoma
- Lymphoid interstitial pneumonia or pulmonary lymphoid hyperplasia complex
- Nephropathy
- Nocardiosis
- Persistent fever (>1 month)
- Toxoplasmosis, onset before 1 month of age
- Varicella, disseminated (complicated chickenpox)

Category C: Severely Symptomatic

Children who have any condition listed in the case definition for acquired immunodeficiency syndrome as outlined in Table 55–4.

From MMWR Morb Mortal Wkly Rep 1994;43:RR-12.
Abbreviation: HIV = human immunodeficiency virus.

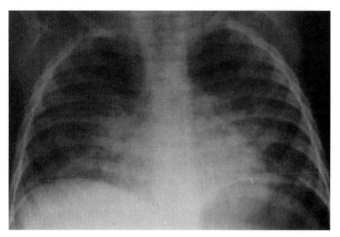

Figure 55–1. Typical diffuse interstitial infiltrates seen in a 20-month-old child with severe combined immune deficiency disease at the time of presentation with clinical *Pneumocystis carinii* pneumonitis. (From Hughes WT, Anderson DC. *Pneumocystis carinii* pneumonia. *In* Feigin RD, Cherry JD [eds]. Textbook of Pediatric Infectious Diseases, 3rd ed. Philadelphia: WB Saunders, 1992:293.)

opportunistic infections (Fig. 55–1). Although the incidence of opportunistic infections increases as the disease and immunodeficiency progress, some children die of inanition without ever experiencing an opportunistic infection. The range of opportunistic infection in children is more narrow than it is in adults, presumably because of lack of exposure at a young age. Cerebral toxoplasmosis and cryptococcal infection, for example, although quite common among adult AIDS patients, are infrequently seen in young children. Finally, HIV-associated cancers are unusual in children. Consequently, new-onset fever in the HIV-infected young child is most commonly associated with an intercurrent bacterial or viral infection, less so with an opportunistic infection, and rarely with an HIV-related malignancy. Adolescents with hemophilia who develop HIV infection may act more like adults with HIV infection.

DIAGNOSTIC STRATEGIES

History

The principal task in evaluating the febrile, HIV-infected child is to determine the likelihood that the fever represents an unusual or serious complication. All of the historical data that help to distinguish serious from insignificant febrile illness in the non–HIV-infected patient apply: contact with someone with a similar illness, duration and severity of fever, ability or willingness to eat and drink, and level of activity and presence of lethargy, as well as the appearance of symptoms suggesting a focus of infection (cough, dyspnea, diarrhea, vomiting, headache), are all assessed (see Chapter 59).

In addition, other data are frequently available regarding the HIV-infected child that define the child's risk for a serious complication. These factors are important in determining the extent of the initial work-up in the febrile HIV-infected child. These parameters are CD4 cell count, prophylaxis, history of previous infection, and age.

CD4 CELL COUNT

The number of circulating CD4 lymphocytes is the most frequently used laboratory marker for the staging of HIV disease (see

Table 55–2). In both children and adults, there is a relentless diminution of CD4 cells throughout the course of the infection. In adults, a CD4 count of less than 200 cells/mm^3 has been associated with a high risk of acquiring PCP and other opportunistic infections. The normal CD4 count of infants younger than 1 year of age is approximately 3000 cells/mm^3, two to three times higher than that in adults; consequently, infants whose counts are 1500 cells/mm^3 or even higher, well within the normal range for adults, may be at risk for PCP. In addition, the percent of CD4 cells in comparison to the total lymphocyte count is also prognostic: less than 20% places the child at increased risk for opportunistic infection regardless of the absolute number of cells.

PROPHYLAXIS

Prophylactic therapies against PCP significantly decrease the likelihood of its occurrence. The agent of choice is trimethoprim-sulfamethoxazole (TMP-SMX), with 75 mg/M^2 of the TMP component being administered twice a day three times a week. TMP-SMX has proved to be extremely effective in reducing the risk of PCP; breakthrough episodes are very uncommon (<5% per year). Alternative regimens, particularly oral dapsone (2 mg/kg/day in a single daily dose) or, in older children and adults, aerosolized pentamidine (300 mg/month), are available for patients who cannot tolerate TMP-SMX because of allergic reactions or bone marrow suppression. Although these therapies are also quite effective, breakthrough episodes of PCP are more common than with TMP-SMX. PCP must still be seriously considered in the CD4-depleted child with fever and hypoxia, even if the child is receiving PCP prophylaxis.

A second type of prophylactic therapy is monthly infusion of intravenous immune globulin (IVIG) to prevent bacterial and viral infections. A large multicenter placebo-controlled, blinded trial indicated that monthly IVIG decreases the incidence of serious bacterial infection in a subset of HIV-infected children with CD4 counts greater than 200 cells/mm^3. Bacterial infections clearly occur despite such therapy, however, and a history of IVIG infusions cannot be used to discount the possibility of serious bacterial disease. Rifabutin prophylaxis has been recommended for *Mycobacterium avium* complex disease in adults and children with very low CD4 counts. Breakthrough infection with *M. avium* complex is common, however, and this infection should always be considered in the child with very low CD4 counts (≤50 cells/mm^3) who presents with fever.

PREVIOUS INFECTIONS

A history of any AIDS-defining condition (Table 55–4) identifies the child as being at risk for opportunistic infections, regardless of his or her CD4 count. In addition, it has been suggested that a history of persistent oral candidiasis that has responded poorly to local antifungal agents is also a sign of poor T-cell immunity, indicating an increased risk of an AIDS-defining event. The pattern and natural history of bacterial infections in HIV-infected children are not sufficiently defined to determine whether a child with one or more such episodes will continue to have them throughout life. Based on anecdotal experience, however, it does appear that children prone to bacterial pneumonias and sinusitis have frequent recurrences.

AGE

The febrile HIV-infected infant younger than 2 to 3 months of age is difficult to evaluate clinically and must be approached with

Table 55–4. AIDS-Determining Conditions

Candidiasis of bronchi, trachea, or lungs
Candidiasis, esophageal
Cervical cancer, invasive
Coccidioidomycosis, disseminated or extrapulmonary
Cryptococcosis, extrapulmonary
Cryptosporidiosis, chronic intestinal (≥1 month's duration)
Cytomegalovirus disease (other than liver, spleen, or nodes)
Cytomegalovirus retinitis (with loss of vision)
Encephalopathy, HIV-related
Herpes simplex: chronic ulcer(s) (≥1 month's duration); or bronchitis, pneumonitis, or esophagitis
Histoplasmosis, disseminated or extrapulmonary
Isosporiasis, chronic intestinal (≥1 month's duration)
Kaposi's sarcoma
Lymphoma, Burkitt's (or equivalent term)
Lymphoma, immunoblastic (or equivalent term)
Lymphoma, primary, of brain
Mycobacterium avium complex or *M. kansasii*, disseminated or extrapulmonary
Mycobacterium tuberculosis, any site (pulmonary or extrapulmonary)
Mycobacterium, other species or unidentified species, disseminated or extrapulmonary
Pneumocystis carinii pneumonia
Pneumonia, recurrent
Progressive multifocal leukoencephalopathy
Salmonella septicemia, recurrent
Toxoplasmosis of brain
Wasting syndrome due to HIV

From MMWR Morbid Mortal Wkly Rep 41 (No. RR-17), December 18, 1992.
Abbreviation: HIV = human immunodeficiency virus.

greater caution than the older child. Opportunistic infections become more common in HIV-infected children as they grow older; this association is presumably the result of their worsening immune status and the greater likelihood of their exposure to an opportunistic pathogen. The most notable exception to this pattern is *P. carinii.* Exposure to pneumocystis occurs early in life, and the peak incidence of illness due to this pathogen is in the first year; PCP frequently occurs within the first 3 to 4 months. The incidence of PCP declines significantly after about 2 years of age, and then, similarly to other opportunistic infections, its incidence gradually increases again with increasing age, symptoms, and immunodeficiency.

Physical Examination

The physical examination of febrile, HIV-infected children is not significantly different from that of their non–HIV-infected counterparts. It is important to assess the child's overall appearance. Signs of chronic illness in the HIV-infected child, particularly poor weight gain and encephalopathy, may make the child appear "ill," suggesting sepsis, meningitis, or dehydration, even when the child is febrile with a minor intercurrent infection. Input from the child's regular caregiver may provide insight into the patient's baseline condition. Anxious appearance, an inability to focus on parent or examiner, a weak cry or poor response to noxious stimuli (such as a needle stick), or tachypnea or retractions with respirations are all alarming signs and suggest the presence of a serious infection.

The remainder of the physical examination is oriented toward identifying a focus of infection, thoroughly covering all major

systems. The anterior fontanelle, if open, is assessed for its softness and for evidence for meningeal signs. The tympanic membranes are carefully examined. Purulent rhinorrhea with fever and pain over the involved sinuses are typical findings of *acute bacterial sinusitis.* Pain and drainage may not be apparent, and patients may present only with fever or with cough or other atypical manifestations of sinusitis. Physical examination may reveal poor transillumination of the maxillary and ethmoid sinuses, or tenderness on firm palpation of the face over the ethmoid/maxillary region or, in older children, over the frontal sinuses. The pharynx should be examined to look for evidence of inflammation or tonsillitis as well as to assess the presence and degree of candidiasis or herpes simplex infection; if evidence of either problem is present, extension beyond the pharynx is suggested by hoarseness or dysphagia.

The *lung examination* is particularly important because many of the complicating infections affect the pulmonary tree. Pneumonia may present with signs of respiratory distress in the absence of abnormal auscultatory findings; respiratory rate, retractions and flaring frequently indicate significant pneumonic disease, even in the presence of clear chest sounds. Many acute illnesses in the HIV-infected child are associated with diffuse abdominal tenderness, including infection caused by many of the intraluminal pathogens (*Salmonella, Giardia*), disseminated infection with nontuberculous mycobacteria, pancreatitis (either primary or resulting from drug therapy with didanosine [ddI], zalcitabine [ddC], or pentamidine), urinary tract infection, or lower-lobe pneumonia. The skin should be examined in an orderly fashion to uncover evidence of cellulitis as well as manifestations from disseminated viral illness, such as varicella, disseminated zoster, or herpes simplex. Joints and long bones should be individually inspected to determine swelling or tenderness on active or passive range of motion, and gait or willingness to bear weight should be assessed.

Diagnostic Formulation

The initial diagnostic evaluation should complement the physical examination in locating the source of infection, and when appropriate, identifying the microbial agent.

FEVER WITHOUT AN APPARENT SOURCE OF INFECTION

The limits of evaluation of the febrile HIV-infected child without an apparent source of infection depend on the stage of the underlying HIV infection. In general, the following guidelines may be used.

In *low-risk* patients, namely, those who are asymptomatic from their HIV infection, appear well, are CD4 replete, and have had no major infections in the past, most fevers without source are due to intercurrent viral infections. Such patients may be followed up anticipatorily without need for diagnostic tests if follow-up is assured.

Mid-risk patients are those who have a CD4 count in the normal range and do not have a history of significant infectious complications but (1) are in the infant age group or (2) have mild HIV-related symptoms (lymph node or abdominal organ enlargement) or (3) appear ill. Such patients should be given a minimal initial work-up. The work-up usually includes a complete blood count, to screen for severe depletion of lymphocytes or neutrophils; a blood culture for routine bacterial pathogens; and urinalysis. A chest radiograph and pulse oximetry reading (or arterial blood gas) are usually added in small infants or in older children with evidence of cough, tachypnea, respiratory distress, or hypoxia.

In *high-risk* children, the limits of the evaluation are more difficult to define. This category includes children who suffer significant HIV-related symptoms (such as growth delay, encephalopathy, or persistent thrush), who have low CD4 counts, or who already have a history of serious infectious events. Even in these children, although many febrile events are due to minor intercurrent infections, the possibility of a disseminated opportunistic infection is significant. Table 55–5 lists the opportunistic pathogens most likely to be discovered in such children. These infections also may occur in the absence of fever and may be accompanied by nonspecific symptoms only, such as weight loss, anorexia, and decreased activity.

The opportunistic pathogens that cause disseminated infection are characteristically associated with prolonged fevers and are usually not rapidly progressive. Because their diagnosis often requires specialized testing and because in some instances the fever is due to infection with routine bacterial pathogens, it is reasonable to begin the evaluation of the high-risk child with the tests listed for the mid-risk child, namely, bacterial blood and urine cultures, pulse oximetry, and chest x-ray study. It is also reasonable to observe the stable, febrile high-risk patient for 2 to 3 days to allow time for resolution of self-limited intercurrent infections before embarking on a more extensive evaluation. Depending on the patient's appearance, the child may be given broad-spectrum oral or parenteral antibiotic therapy while the results of this evaluation are pending.

The diagnostic tests most commonly employed to identify disseminated opportunistic infections in the high-risk child are listed in Table 55–5. Blood and urine samples reveal most pathogens. Routine blood cultures are sufficient to identify bacteremic events and frequently detect blood-borne fungi. In addition, a blood specimen should be obtained to culture for *Mycobacterium* and serum should be tested for *Cryptococcus* by antigen detection. Circulating antigen tests are available in some centers for histoplasmosis as well. Blood-borne cytomegalovirus (CMV) is most expeditiously

identified through the shell-vial assay, in which blood or other normally sterile material (bronchoalveolar lavage fluid, biopsy material) is centrifuged onto a small cell-culture monolayer and tested soon after for the appearance of early CMV antigens by monoclonal fluorescent antibody. The presence of CMV may also be tested by the polymerase chain reaction or by direct antigen testing of blood. A urine culture positive for CMV suggests disseminated infection in the high-risk febrile child, but the definitive diagnosis of disseminated disease requires that the pathogen be detected in blood or tissue. In the absence of a positive shell-vial assay, disseminated CMV disease may be diagnosed noninvasively by detection of typical retinal disease on funduscopic examination.

If these tests are unrevealing, the microbiologic diagnosis may require more invasive procedures. Many of these pathogens disseminate to bone marrow, and aspiration and culture of this material may yield a diagnosis in the absence of positive blood cultures. Fungal, CMV, and mycobacterial disease as well as the HIV-related cancers all may affect the liver and gastrointestinal tract. Therefore, endoscopy, computed tomography (CT), magnetic resonance imaging (MRI), radionuclide scans, or biopsy may be appropriate, particularly in the presence of hepatomegaly, abnormal liver function tests, or prominent or nonspecific abdominal complaints.

FEVER WITH OTITIS MEDIA AND SINUSITIS

Otitis media and sinusitis are among the most common infections in HIV-infected children. Acute otitis media caused by typical bacterial pathogens occurs frequently in young children with HIV. Recurrent and chronic otitis media, however, is diagnosed in many HIV-infected children well beyond the age at which such infections occur in most immunocompetent children.

Although detailed microbiologic studies of otitis media in children with HIV infection have not been performed, the usual pathogens are thought to predominate: *Streptococcus pneumoniae, Moraxella catarrhalis,* and nontypable *Haemophilus influenzae.* Unusual pathogens rarely may be encountered as the cause of otitis media, including *Pseudomonas aeruginosa* and other gram-negative bacteria, fungi, and *Nocardia* species. *P. carinii* has been identified as a cause of otitis media in a number of case reports, typically presenting with pain and hearing loss in adult patients with AIDS. In the case of chronic otitis media or otitis media that is poorly responsive to therapy, aspiration of middle ear fluid or biopsy of mass lesions may provide a microbiologic or pathologic diagnosis. In children with recurrent or chronic otitis media, audiologic evaluation should be undertaken to evaluate hearing loss.

Paranasal sinusitis is common in children with HIV infection. Radiographic abnormalities of the sinuses can be seen on CT scan in most HIV-infected patients, even in the absence of symptoms. Although the patient with the triad of fever, pain, and purulent rhinorrhea may be treated for sinusitis on clinical grounds, radiographic evaluation is useful to confirm or exclude the diagnosis in less clear-cut cases. In addition, patients with systemic toxicity, neurologic signs, or evidence of soft tissue extension should undergo radiographic evaluation of the sinuses for evidence of bony erosion or extension of infection.

Acute sinusitis is likely to be the result of typical pathogens: *S. aureus* and other *Staphylococcus* species, *S. pneumoniae,* nontypable *H. influenzae,* and other respiratory flora. A number of uncommon organisms, including *Legionella,* fungi, and pneumocystis have been reported as rare causes of sinusitis in adults with AIDS. Aspiration of the involved sinus provides a microbiologic diagnosis in patients who present with systemic illness, have neurologic signs, or are poorly responsive to initial antibiotic therapy, or in those who have chronic or recurrent sinusitis.

Table 55–5. Conditions Associated with Fever Without Source

Condition	Diagnostic Tests*
Routine bacteremia	Blood culture
Mycobacterium tuberculosis	PPD, chest radiograph, blood culture,† gastric aspirate culture, BAL for stain and culture, bone marrow histology and culture
Mycobacterium avium complex	Blood culture,† stool culture, bone marrow histology and culture, liver/GI tract histology and culture
Disseminated fungus	Blood culture,† blood antigen,‡ bone marrow histology and culture
Cytomegalovirus	Blood culture,† retinitis by ophthalmologic examination, bone marrow or deep tissue histology, PCR and culture, (urine culture)§
Malignancy (B-cell lymphoma, Kaposi sarcoma)	Histology

*Tests are listed in order of preference.
†Special blood culture techniques are required.
‡Antigen tests are available for *Cryptococcus* and *Histoplasma.*
§Urine culture is supportive, but not diagnostic, of disseminated cytomegalovirus infection.

Abbreviations: BAL = bronchoalveolar lavage; PCR = polymerase chain reaction; GI = gastrointestinal; PPD = purified protein derivative.

FEVER WITH A PULMONARY SOURCE OF INFECTION

Pulmonary infections constitute the most common serious complications in pediatric HIV disease; lung disease develops in 80% at some time in these patients. Many organisms can cause these infections, and the diagnostic evaluation must proceed in an orderly, stepwise manner, beginning with the chest radiograph (Table 55–6, Fig. 55–2). Many of these entities present with various radiographic patterns, and, particularly in patients with diffuse disease, the radiograph may reflect pneumonia caused by two or more pathogens. Therefore, the radiographic distinctions of greatest practical utility are focal, hyperinflated, and multifocal or diffuse patterns. Focal pneumonia in a clinically stable child usually can be assumed to be bacterial and can be treated with a clinical trial of antibiotics without further diagnostic testing unless the patient worsens despite therapy over 24 to 48 hours. The patient with hyperinflation and perihilar infiltrates with upper respiratory tract symptoms typical of viral bronchiolitis can usually avoid invasive diagnostic testing, particularly if a viral diagnosis can be confirmed by culture or immunofluorescence.

Diffuse pneumonia, however, particularly in a child at high risk and especially in a patient who is hypoxic (arterial oxygen saturation ≤ 92% in room air), mandates a more aggressive approach. Some authorities have suggested empiric antipneumocystis (and antibacterial) therapy in patients with multilobular or diffuse interstitial pneumonia, saving invasive procedures only for those whose disease progresses or does not respond after a day or two. Others prefer aggressive diagnostic management consisting of bronchoalveolar lavage or biopsy shortly after the patient presents to the physician. Especially in infants, rapid disease progression and slow response to anti-PCP therapy warrant early invasive diagnostic procedures.

Special consideration should be taken for tuberculosis in the febrile HIV-infected child with pulmonary symptoms and diffuse

---

Table 55–6. Agents Associated with a Pulmonary Focus of Infection

Unilobar Infiltrates
Streptococcus pneumoniae
Haemophilus influenzae
Staphylococcus
Group A *Streptococcus*
Moraxella catarrhalis
Pseudomonas aeruginosa
Non-*Pseudomonas* gram-negative organisms

Hyperinflated on Perihilar Infiltrates
Respiratory syncytial virus
Other respiratory viruses
  Influenza
  Parainfluenza
  Adenovirus
Pneumocystis carinii

Multilobar or Diffuse Infiltrates
Pneumocystis carinii
Mycobacterium tuberculosis
Mycobacterium avium complex
Herpes simplex virus
Legionella
Fungi
  Aspergillus
  Histoplasmosis
  Coccidioidomycosis
  Cryptococcus

---

or multilobular disease, as seen on chest radiography (Figs. 55–3 and 55–4). The incidence of tuberculosis in all children has increased, and a substantial portion of the increase in adults has occurred in HIV-infected urban dwellers who are often the primary caretakers of HIV-infected children. A detailed history of possible contacts, particularly household contacts with active tuberculosis or with chronic cough, is essential. A Mantoux purified protein derivative (PPD) skin test (intradermal injection of 5 tuberculin units of PPD) should be placed, along with control skin tests (*Candida*, tetanus, or mumps), and the results of prior PPDs and anergy testing should be ascertained. Although the probability of a false-negative PPD result is higher in children with HIV infection, a substantial proportion of HIV-infected individuals, including those with acquired immunodeficiency syndrome (AIDS), react to a PPD. A negative PPD result should not be used to exclude the diagnosis of tuberculosis, but a positive result (>5 mm of induration 48 to 72 hours after placement in a child with HIV infection) is extremely useful information to support this diagnosis.

The patient with diffuse pattern on chest radiography and hypoxia and a negative or unknown PPD result, or the low-risk patient who does not respond to antibacterial or antipneumocystis therapy, should proceed in rapid succession first to sputum induction, then to bronchoscopy with bronchoalveolar lavage, and finally to lung biopsy. Induced sputum is quite accurate for diagnosing PCP and bacterial pathogens. It has been described in only a small number of children and requires considerable cooperation and effort from the child; the younger child who coughs deeply but who cannot expectorate the sputum may require oral and nasotracheal suctioning so that the material can be obtained for testing. In the very young or uncooperative child or the patient with rapidly progressive disease, the procedure has little chance of success and may only delay the diagnosis.

Bronchoalveolar lavage has become the method most frequently employed to evaluate the febrile HIV-infected child with diffuse pulmonary disease. The sensitivity of bronchoalveolar lavage alone for pneumocystis is approximately 90% or greater in both adults and children. The sensitivity of this procedure for other pathogens (bacteria, mycobacteria, CMV and respiratory viruses, and fungi) is less well defined but is probably lower (approximately 60% to 80%). In practice, bronchoalveolar lavage yields almost all the diagnostic information required for patient management: several recent series involving HIV-infected patients have indicated that patients with negative lavage results frequently improve with empirical antibiotic therapy and that few additional diagnoses are revealed by subsequent lung biopsy or autopsy. Transient worsening of hypoxia may occur and occasionally requires supplemental oxygen or intubation after the procedure; this condition usually resolves after about 24 hours.

Lung biopsy is required in the unusual patient whose bronchoalveolar lavage results are unrevealing and who has not improved with 24 to 48 hours of empirical antibacterial and antipneumocystis therapy. The specimens from some patients demonstrate only nonspecific lung injury, because of sampling error, resolution of the initial process by empirical therapy before the biopsy, or a noninfectious underlying pathology. Although open lung biopsy is often dismissed as the child's respiratory status deteriorates, the operative risk (consisting of pneumothorax and hemorrhage) from this procedure, even under these circumstances, is small. Biopsies may be performed through small thoracotomies in the intensive care unit with no significant morbidity.

Lung biopsy may be particularly helpful in the febrile patient with *lymphoid interstitial pneumonia* (Fig. 55–5). This common pediatric HIV-related process, characterized by a chronic, diffuse interstitial or nodular pattern on chest radiography and mild to moderate hypoxemia with few symptoms of respiratory distress, is not in itself associated with fever. Lymphoid interstitial pneumonia cannot be definitively diagnosed without a lung biopsy; nevertheless, in the absence of acute illness, many HIV caregivers assign

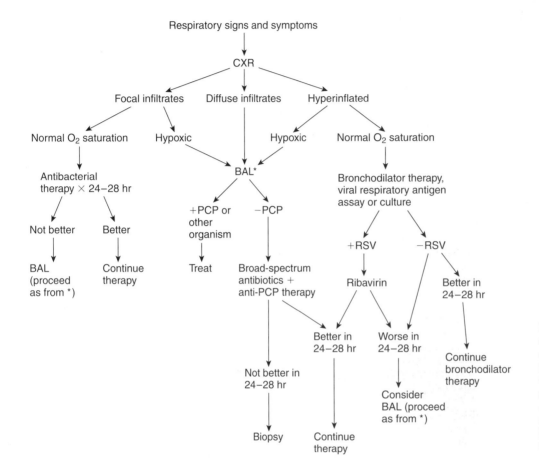

Respiratory signs and symptoms

CXR

Focal infiltrates   Diffuse infiltrates   Hyperinflated

Normal O₂ saturation   Hypoxic   Hypoxic   Normal O₂ saturation

Antibacterial
therapy × 24–28 hr   BAL*   Bronchodilator therapy,
                                        viral respiratory antigen
                                        assay or culture

Not better   Better   +PCP or   –PCP   +RSV   –RSV
                        other
                        organism

BAL   Continue   Treat   Broad-spectrum   Ribavirin   Better in
(proceed   therapy   antibiotics +   24–28 hr
as from *)   anti-PCP therapy

                            Better in   Worse in   Continue
                            24–28 hr   24–28 hr   bronchodilator
                                                    therapy

                    Not better in   Consider
                    24–28 hr   BAL (proceed
                                            as from *)

                    Biopsy   Continue
                            therapy

Figure 55–2. Algorithm for evaluating the febrile, HIV-infected child with respiratory symptoms. BAL = bronchoalveolar lavage; CXR = chest x-ray study; O₂ = oxygen; PCP = *Pneumocystis carinii* pneumonitis; RSV = respiratory syncytial virus. (Adapted from Cunningham. Pediatr Emerg Care 1991; 7:32–37.)

Figure 55–3. Radiographic abnormalities of tuberculosis in HIV-infected patients. *A,* Lower lobe infiltrate mimicking *Pneumocystis carinii* pneumonia. *B,* Mediastinal lymphadenopathy without parenchymal abnormalities. *C,* Pleural effusion in patient with disseminated tuberculosis. (From Cohn DL. Treatment and prevention of tuberculosis in HIV-infected persons. Infect Dis Clin North Am 1994;8:399–412.)

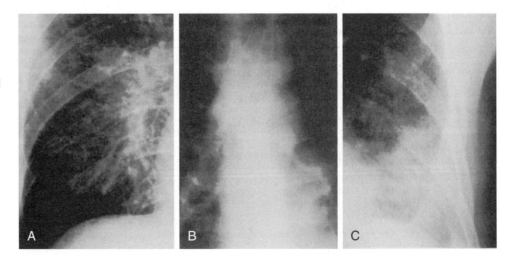

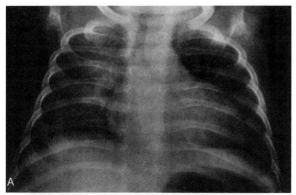

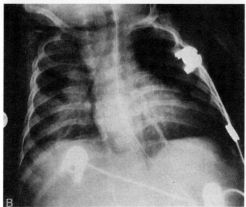

Figure 55–4. A 2-month-old HIV-positive infant of a drug-abusing mother who had multidrug-resistant tuberculosis. Extensive infiltrates in the right lung were caused by tuberculosis (A). The patient expired at 4 months of age. Note progression of the extensive infiltration in the right lung with hilar adenopathy (B). (From Marquis JR, Bardeguez AD. Imaging of HIV infection in the prenatal and postnatal period. Clin Perinatol 1994;21:125–147.)

this diagnosis by exclusion if the child is clinically stable and nonhypoxic and the bronchoalveolar lavage reveals no pathogens. The radiographic pattern of lymphoid interstitial pneumonia is frequently indistinguishable from that produced by pneumocystis or other opportunistic infections. In the febrile child with lymphoid pneumocystis pneumonia, therefore, it may be impossible to determine whether there is a superinfecting lung pathogen without examining tissue. Even under these circumstances, if a comparison of the current radiograph to previous radiographic examinations reveals a stable or improving pattern, lung biopsy may be avoided.

FEVER WITH GASTROINTESTINAL MANIFESTATIONS

Gastrointestinal complaints, particularly odynophagia, diarrhea, or abdominal pain, occur in 50% to 90% of patients with HIV infection some time during the course of their illness. Many patients have several loose stools a day for months; in some instances, this pattern persists throughout life. HIV infection itself results in diarrhea in the absence of a superinfecting pathogen in some patients. Biochemical evidence of HIV infection can be detected in the lymphoid elements in the gastrointestinal tract in association with chronic inflammatory changes and mucosal villous atrophy. The changes can be associated with disaccharidase deficiency (and lactose intolerance) and malabsorption; these in turn may result in malnutrition and may exacerbate deficiencies in growth and

development and in immune function. Abdominal complaints in HIV-infected children may emanate from commonly used therapy. In particular, zidovudine (AZT) is frequently associated with nausea and anorexia, particularly early in the course of therapy, and didanosine and, to a lesser extent, zalcitabine, may result in pancreatitis with associated abdominal pain and anorexia. Particularly in adult patients, abdominal complaints may result from gastrointestinal involvement with HIV-associated lymphoma or Kaposi sarcoma.

Gastrointestinal complaints in the HIV-infected child also may result from infection with one or more enteric pathogens (Table 55–7). The abdominal symptoms are often subacute or chronic and not associated with fever; occasionally, the episodes are intense and febrile. The evaluation of such a patient can be difficult for three reasons:

1. Many of the pathogens can affect more than one site in the gastrointestinal tract.
2. A given patient may be infected with multiple pathogens.
3. Some of the pathogens are difficult to identify even with invasive procedures.

In the patient with esophageal symptoms (odonophagia, dysphagia, or substernal chest pain), the definitive microbiologic diagnosis requires endoscopy and biopsy (Fig. 55–6). For the child who is not acutely ill and who suffers from a heavy growth of candidal organisms in the mouth, it is reasonable to begin an empirical course with an oral antifungal agent, such as ketoconazole or fluconazole, without an endoscopic examination, saving this invasive procedure for patients who do not respond. *Candida*, CMV, and herpes simplex virus frequently can be discriminated at endoscopy by the gross appearance of the lesions. Candidal infection produces large, white or yellow plaques throughout the esophagus. In contrast, both CMV and herpes simplex virus are associated with mucosal ulcerations; those produced by cytomegalovirus tend to be large, widespread, and superficial, whereas those produced by herpes simplex are characteristically fewer in number and deep. The microbiologic diagnosis of the organisms can be confirmed though histopathology, fungal stains, and culture.

The laboratory evaluation of the child with abdominal complaints

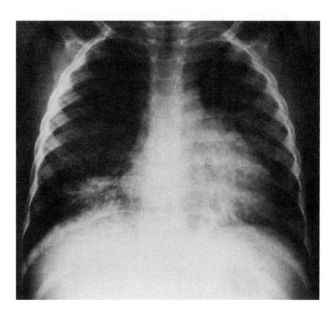

Figure 55–5. A 20-month-old HIV-positive male. Diffuse nodules throughout the lungs are typical of lymphoid interstitial pneumonia/pulmonary lymphoid hyperplasia (PLH) in the proper clinical setting. (From Marquis JR, Bardeguez AD. Imaging of HIV infection in the prenatal and postnatal period. Clin Perinatol 1994;21:125–147.)

Table 55–7. Infections of the Gastrointestinal Tract in Patients with AIDS

Site of Infection	Signs and Symptoms	Common Organisms	Uncommon Organisms
Esophagus	Dysphagia, odynophagia, retrosternal pain	*Candida albicans,* CMV, herpes simplex	*Histoplasma capsulatum* *Leishmania donovani* *Nocardia asteroides* *Toxoplasma gondii*
Stomach	Abdominal pain	CMV, MAC	*Leishmania donovani*
Liver/gallbladder	Abdominal pain, jaundice, biliary colic	CMV, *Cryptosporidium,* Hepatotropic viruses, MAC	*Toxoplasma gondii* *Rochalimaea quintana*–like organism *Pneumocystis carinii* *Encephalitozoon cuniculi* Adenovirus *Penicillium marneffei* *Leishmania donovani*
Small intestine	Diarrhea, abdominal pain, weight loss, nausea, vomiting	*Campylobacter* sp, *Cryptosporidium* sp CMV, *Enterocytozoon bieneusi,* *Giardia lamblia,* *Isospora belli,* MAC, *Salmonella* sp, *Strongyloides stercoralis*	*Aeromonas hydrophila* *Blastocystis hominis* *Chlorella*-like organisms (blue-green algae)
Large intestine	Diarrhea, abdominal pain, tenesmus	*Campylobacter jejuni,* *Clostridium difficile,* CMV, *Entamoeba histolytica,* herpes simplex, MAC, *Shigella* sp, *Salmonella* sp	Enteric adenovirus *Histoplasma capsulatum*

Adapted from Pickering LK, Cleary KR. Pediatric AIDS: The Challenge of HIV Infection in Infants, Children, and Adolescents, 2nd ed. Baltimore: Williams & Wilkins, 1994:378.
Abbreviations: CMV = cytomegalovirus; MAC = *Mycobacterium avium* complex.

should begin with a stool culture for bacterial pathogens and an examination for stool white and red blood cells and parasites. Culture of bacterial intestinal pathogens (*Salmonella, Campylobacter, Shigella*) is routine; additional culture and staining of the

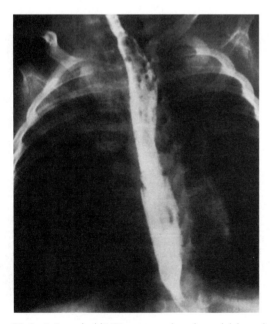

Figure 55–6. A 6-month-old HIV-positive male with candidal esophagitis on barium esophagram. Note bilateral upper lobe infiltrates. (From Marquis JR, Bardeguez AD. Imaging of HIV infection in the prenatal and postnatal period. Clin Perinatol 1994;21:125–147.)

stool for atypical mycobacteria may reveal gastrointestinal involvement with these organisms as well. Identification in the stool of the four most common parasites afflicting HIV-infected patients, namely, *Cryptosporidium, Microsporidium, Giardia,* and *Isospora,* is difficult and is best performed in a laboratory that routinely conducts such tests. The ability to identify these microorganisms is significantly enhanced by concentration techniques that separate the stool samples into parasite-rich fractions. Although patients with HIV infection may excrete larger numbers of parasites than do their immunocompetent counterparts, multiple stool specimens may be required before the pathogen can be successfully identified.

If the patient remains symptomatic and the stool culture and examination are unrevealing, endoscopy and biopsy of the small intestine or large intestine, or both, should be pursued. Histopathologic examination itself may reveal the diagnosis in parasitic and fungal disease (through direct staining of the organism), herpes simplex and CMV disease (through identification of inclusion bodies or through immunofluorescent stains using virus-specific monoclonal antibodies), and mycobacterial disease (through detection of the bacilli and granulomas, although formation of granulomas in HIV-infected patients may be poor). Culture material for fungus, virus, and routine bacteria and mycobacteria also is obtained from specimens taken directly from the bowel wall. *Cryptosporidium* and CMV can infect the biliary tree, where they produce symptoms typical of cholangitis (fever, right upper quadrant tenderness, abnormal liver function tests). Sampling of bile during endoscopy may reveal these diagnoses when other test results are negative.

Fever with Central Nervous System Manifestations

Neurologic manifestations are prominent in pediatric HIV disease. Primary HIV infection of the CNS is by far the most common

Table 55–8. Conditions Associated with Fever and Central Nervous System Source in Children

Meningoencephalitis	Focal Deficit
More Common	
Primary human immunodeficiency virus infection	
Streptococcus pneumoniae	
Haemophilus influenzae	
Meningococcus	
Mycobacterium tuberculosis	
Less Common	
Cryptococcus	Lymphoma
Cytomegalovirus	Toxoplasmosis
Rare	
Syphilis	Progressive multifocal
Histoplasmosis	leukoencephalopathy
Coccidioidomycosis	Brain abscess

cause of cognitive and motor abnormalities in children with HIV infection. New-onset neurologic findings associated with fever should prompt a search for complicating CNS infections.

Although all of the CNS opportunistic infections associated with HIV infection in adults can be seen in children, in general they are much less common. The initial approach to the HIV-infected child with fever and CNS findings is similar to that of the HIV-uninfected child. Rapid assessment and stabilization should be followed by blood culture and lumbar puncture to obtain cerebrospinal fluid (CSF) for a wide range of diagnostic tests. If the clinical presentation suggests focal brain involvement or if there are signs of increased intracranial pressure, CT or MRI of the brain should be performed before lumbar puncture to assess the possibility of mass effect from an intracranial lesion. If CNS imaging is deemed necessary and cannot be obtained emergently, empirical antibiotic therapy for routine CNS bacterial pathogens should not be delayed.

The underlying causes of fever and CNS symptoms in the HIV-infected child are listed in Table 55–8. It is useful to distinguish them by their propensity to cause meningoencephalitis or focal deficits.

MENINGOENCEPHALITIS

Although HIV infection does not appear to be a predisposing factor for meningitis in bacteremic children, the high incidence of bacteremia in HIV-infected children should prompt a strong consideration of bacterial meningitis in any HIV-infected child presenting with fever and meningismus, altered mental status, or seizures. A purulent CSF (elevated total white blood cell count with a marked polymorphonuclear neutrophil predominance, elevated protein level, and low glucose level) supports the diagnosis of bacterial meningitis. Diagnosis is confirmed by culture of CSF or blood (see Chapter 53).

Although disseminated infection with organisms of the *M. avium* complex is common in children with advanced AIDS, this organism rarely invades the CNS. In contrast, meningitis is common in primary or disseminated infection caused by *Mycobacterium tuberculosis*, particularly in younger children. Diagnosis of tuberculous meningitis is difficult but should be considered in any HIV-infected child with culture-negative meningitis in the absence of a documented alternative diagnosis. Because tubercular meningitis is a manifestation of disseminated tuberculosis and because the portal of entry for *M. tuberculosis* is the lung, a concomitant chest radiograph demonstrating segmental or diffuse infiltrates, particu-

larly in the presence of hilar adenopathy, may provide support for the diagnosis of tubercular meningitis (see Chapter 53). PPD skin testing provides strong supportive evidence for this diagnosis when the results are positive. The CSF profile in tubercular meningitis varies over time. Early, when symptoms are mild, there may be few cells, neutrophils may predominate, and the glucose level may be normal and the protein level only slightly elevated. With time, the CSF cellular response becomes primarily mononuclear (although the total number of cells rarely exceeds a few hundred), while the protein level rises to levels in excess of 200 mg/dl, and the glucose level falls to markedly low levels. Culture of the organism is the gold standard for the diagnosis of tuberculosis. A large volume of CSF should be inoculated by an experienced mycobacteriology laboratory. Culture of *M. tuberculosis* from other sources (blood, morning gastric aspirates, bronchoalveolar lavage) should also be pursued. PCR amplification of *M. tuberculosis* DNA can provide the diagnosis more rapidly than culture.

Cryptococcal meningitis, although uncommon, should be considered in the HIV-infected child with meningitis. Older HIV-infected children and adolescents in particular may present with this infection. Its onset may be insidious or acute; although typical signs of meningitis may occur in some patients, many adults present only with persistent headache and fever. The CSF profile in cryptococcal meningitis usually shows a mild inflammatory response, often with less than 20 cells/mm³, normal to mildly elevated protein level, and normal to mildly decreased glucose level. In some patients, all CSF parameters are normal.

Cryptococcal antigen testing on CSF is rapid and sensitive (>90%) and can provide semiquantitative information that can be used to follow treatment response. Serum also can be tested for cryptococcal antigen and strongly supports the diagnosis of cryptococcal meningitis in patients with consistent symptoms. The India ink test of the CSF is not as sensitive as the antigen test (Fig. 55–7). Fungal culture is usually positive when the antigen is positive, but requires 2 to 3 days. Other fungal diseases of the CNS are rare in HIV-infected adults and children.

Viral causes of fever and CNS manifestations other than HIV infection are difficult to document, and our knowledge of the manifestation of even the common viral agents is incomplete. CMV can infect the CNS; pathologic examination suggests that it plays a role in at least some HIV-infected children with encephalitis. Measles encephalitis has been demonstrated in HIV-infected children, including those with a history of prior measles vaccination. Herpes simplex and varicella zoster viruses rarely cause encephali-

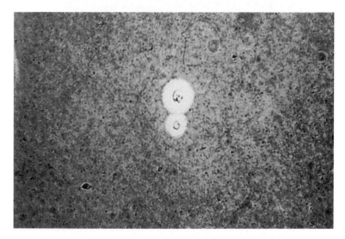

Figure 55–7. India ink stain of cerebrospinal fluid from a patient with cryptococcal meningitis. The dark stain outlines the capsule of *Cryptococcus neoformans* as it buds from a narrow base. (From White MH, Armstrong D. Cryptococcosis. Infect Dis Clin North Am 1994;8:383–398.)

tis, despite the frequency of reactivation of mucocutaneous disease in HIV-infected children. Progressive multifocal leukoencephalitis, caused by JC virus, has been reported in older HIV-infected children but is extremely rare.

FOCAL DEFICITS

Intracranial mass lesions may present in HIV-infected children, either through the new onset of focal neurologic abnormalities or through seizures. CNS lymphoma is the most common mass lesion seen in HIV-infected children (Fig. 55–8). Cerebral toxoplasmosis, although relatively common in adults with AIDS, is rare in children, although it may be seen in older children and adolescents. Focal lesions are not often associated with fever. Fever from an intercurrent infection may trigger the first episode of seizures associated with one of these lesions. The rare child with progressive multifocal leukoencephalitis may also present with focal neurologic signs or seizures.

The diagnostic approach to the HIV-infected child with a new onset of seizures or focal neurologic signs is straightforward, although obtaining a definitive diagnosis may be difficult. Neuroimaging studies should be obtained on an urgent basis. Although each type of lesion may have typical features on MRI or CT, diagnosis based on imaging alone is not definitive. A single lesion, location in the periventricular white matter, and diffuse enhancement favor the diagnosis of lymphoma, whereas multiple lesions, cortical or deep nuclear location, and ring-like enhancement are more typical of toxoplasmosis. Although empirical treatment for toxoplasmosis in an adult with multiple enhancing lesions is accepted practice, in young children strong consideration should be given to early biopsy of CNS lesions to document their cause because of both the rarity of toxoplasmosis and the toxicity of therapy for toxoplasmosis and lymphoma. Positive serologic results for toxoplasmosis provide support for this diagnosis in adults and may be useful in older children or adolescents. CSF evaluation may provide useful diagnostic information, particularly if abnormal

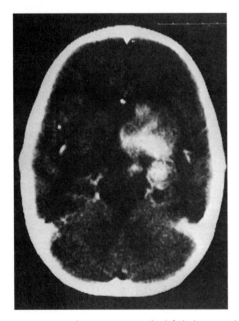

Figure 55–8. Contrast enhancing mass in the left thalamus and parietal lobe in a 6-year-old male with perinatally infected HIV. At surgery, a lymphoma was found. (From Marquis JR, Bardeguez AD. Imaging of HIV infection in the prenatal and postnatal period. Clin Perinatol 1994;21:125–147.)

cells consistent with lymphoma are found cytologically. The ability to perform a lumbar puncture, however, is often limited by mass effect of the brain lesions, and neuroimaging should be performed before lumbar puncture to assess the risk of this procedure.

THERAPEUTIC STRATEGIES (Table 55–9)

Fever without a Source of Infection

If the source of infection in the HIV-infected febrile child is not apparent by routine physical examination, the caregiver must confront the decision of whether or not to start empirical antibiotics until the culture results are known. In the approach to such a patient, it is again useful to distinguish low-, mid-, and high-risk patients:

- Low-risk patients who are asymptomatic and immunologically replete and have a benign past history can usually be safely observed without empirical therapy.
- In mid-risk patients who demonstrate some symptoms of HIV disease, the decision to offer empirical therapy pending culture results rests largely on the age of the patient (infants are treated more conservatively than are older children) and the patient's overall appearance.
- High-risk patients, namely those who are CD4-cell depleted, who have significant stigmata of infection, or who have a history of serious complicating infections, are frequently given empirical oral or intravenous antibiotics pending the results of the evaluation unless there is clear evidence of a benign intercurrent illness. This therapy usually includes cefotaxime, ceftazidime, ceftriaxone, or newer penicillins with β-lactamase inhibitors. Intravenous vancomycin is added if the patient has a central venous catheter.

Usually, the response of children with routine bacteremia to appropriate antibiotics is rapid, and the outcome is good. Patients may be safely converted from parental to oral therapy after 3 to 4 days to complete a 10-day course. Therapy of disseminated, drug-susceptible tuberculosis is curative, and the response of HIV-positive patients is similar to that of HIV-negative patients. Other infections respond less well (M. avium complex), and cure is often an unattainable goal. Consequently, lifelong suppressive therapy usually is required once the acute infection has been controlled. Therapy for these latter infections is very complex and includes many toxic agents.

Fever with Otitis Media and Sinusitis

Initial therapy for these infections is similar to therapy for the HIV-uninfected child. Because of the higher frequency of recurrence in children with HIV infection, prolonged therapy with second-line agents with a broad spectrum, such as second-generation cephalosporins or amoxicillin-clavulanate, are often required. Lack of response to these agents should lead to further diagnostic evaluation (sinus puncture aspiration, tympanocentesis) by an otolaryngologist to obtain a microbiologic diagnosis. Indications for placement of tympanostomy tubes in HIV-infected children with persistent or recurrent otitis media are not established; some patients poorly responsive to antimicrobial therapy may benefit from this procedure.

Fever with a Pulmonary Source of Infection

The HIV-infected child with pneumonia caused by routine bacteria usually responds rapidly to antibiotics. The initial choice of antimicrobial agents should cover *S. pneumoniae* and *H. influenzae*; as in the non-HIV infected child, antistaphylococcal therapy should be added in cases of severe pneumonia, and therapy for gram-negative organisms must be considered in severely ill, hospitalized children. The decision to give parenteral over oral therapy depends largely on the degree of the child's illness. However, brief hospitalization and an initial course of intravenous antibiotics allows one to observe the patient's response and to assess the need for further diagnostic tests or additional antibiotics.

The treatment of choice for *P. carinii* pneumonia is TMP-SMX. Intravenous pentamidine should be offered to patients who do not respond to TMP-SMX after approximately 4 to 5 days or who have a significant hypersensitivity response to the sulfa drug. Other regimens that have been applied to adults with PCP, including trimethoprim plus dapsone, clindamycin plus primaquine, atovaquone, and trimetrexate have not been extensively used in children. Adjunctive therapy with steroids has been shown to decrease the severity of PCP in adult patients with AIDS if steroids are initiated before the onset of respiratory failure. Reports of steroid use in small numbers of children indicate a similar benefit, but controlled trials are lacking. Pneumocystis in young children most likely represents primary rather than reactivated infection, and mortality is approximately 30% to 50%, even with expeditious treatment; survival in cases requiring mechanical ventilation may be 25% or lower.

Respiratory syncytial virus pneumonia can be particularly severe in the HIV-infected child, and aerosolized ribavirin therapy is currently recommended. Therapy for the other respiratory viral pathogens is supportive, including intravenous hydration and supplemental oxygen or mechanical ventilation, as necessary.

Fever with Gastrointestinal Manifestations

Frequently, the most critical aspect of therapy for gastrointestinal disease in the child with HIV infection is the provision of adequate nutritional support. Although the infection itself may pose no danger to the patient's well-being, anorexia, frequent and voluminous stools, and unremitting weight loss may be life-threatening. Enteral or, if necessary, parental calories must be given to the patient and may require the expert advise of a nutritionist or gastroenterologist. In some instances, profuse watery (secretory) diarrhea has responded to somatostatin analogs.

Therapies are available for most common gastrointestinal pathogens in the HIV-infected patient. Response to therapy for candida and herpes simplex esophagitis usually is quite good, whereas the response of gastrointestinal CMV to antiviral agents, whether in the esophagus or elsewhere in the gastrointestinal tract, is not as satisfactory. Treatment of bacterial pathogens of the small and large bowel is identical to that for non–HIV-infected children. Intraluminal *Salmonella* infection is unaffected by administration of antibiotics. Therapy should be withheld from the afebrile, well-appearing HIV-infected child who has a salmonella diarrheal disease. In the child who presents with bloody diarrhea and high fever, blood cultures should be obtained and consideration should be given to treating the patient with intravenous antibiotics until the blood culture results for salmonella are known. If the results are negative, antibiotic therapy should be discontinued.

Treatment of giardiasis and *Isospora belli* in HIV-infected children is similar to that given to non-HIV infected children, except that long-term suppressive therapy for *Isospora* usually is required. Numerous therapies, including the macrolide spiramycin and ingested immune globulin, have been attempted for cryptosporidiosis, with disappointing results. The nonabsorbable aminoglycoside paromomycin appears promising; this drug and azithromycin are under study. There is no effective therapy for microsporidiosis.

Fever with Central Nervous System Manifestations

Because of the variety of causes of CNS disease in HIV-infected children, therapy must be guided by the results of the diagnostic work-up. If other causes are not identified and if the findings are consistent with HIV infection as the cause of CNS complications, initiation or change in antiretroviral therapy may result in substantial symptomatic improvement.

BACTERIAL MENINGITIS

Pneumococcal infection is by far the most common cause of bacterial meningitis in the HIV-infected child; therefore, treatment should be active against this organism as well as against the wide variety of other pathogens that occasionally cause meningitis. Because of the rapidly increasing incidence of penicillin-resistant pneumococcal infection, some of which is resistant to cephalosporins, current empirical regimen for bacterial meningitis should include a third-generation cephalosporin, such as cefotaxime plus vancomycin, until culture and sensitivity results are known.

TUBERCULOUS MENINGITIS

Treatment should be initiated in the child with a history, clinical presentation, and CSF findings suggestive of this diagnosis because of the poor outcome associated with a delay in treatment. At present, initial therapy of tuberculous meningitis includes a minimum of four drugs: isoniazid, rifampin, pyrazinamide, and streptomycin (see Chapter 53). In drug-susceptible tuberculous meningitis, initial multidrug therapy for 2 months can be followed by isoniazid and rifampin therapy for an additional 10 months. If antibiotic resistance is suspected, additional agents should be included.

Treatment of drug-resistant tuberculous meningitis is difficult; specific regimens can be tailored to the susceptibility of the patient's or the source's isolate. Corticosteroids should be considered in children with tuberculous meningitis; daily administration for the first few weeks is followed by gradual tapering.

CRYPTOCOCCAL MENINGITIS

Intravenous amphotericin B is the standard treatment for acute disease; fluconazole is recommended by some experts for patients with mild symptoms and is associated with fewer side effects. Although most patients respond to appropriate antifungal therapy, eradication of the infection generally is not possible in individuals with AIDS, necessitating lifelong suppressive therapy with fluconazole or amphotericin B.

CEREBRAL TOXOPLASMOSIS

A regimen of pyrimethamine and sulfadiazine with folinic acid for 3 to 6 weeks is the treatment of choice for this disease. One of several alternative regimens may be employed in patients who cannot tolerate these agents. Because of the high frequency of relapse, secondary prophylaxis is recommended after treatment of acute infection.

Table 55–9. Therapy for the Common Causes of Fever in Children Infected with the Human Immunodeficiency Virus[a]

Organisms	Disease	Treatment Immediate	Response
Bacteria, routine	Otitis Sinusitis Bacteremia Pneumonia Meningitis	Identical to that for non–HIV-infected children	Good
Cryptosporidium	Diarrhea	? Paromomycin *or* ? Azithromycin	Variable[b, c]
Cytomegalovirus	Disseminated infection Pneumonia Gastroenteritis *or* Esophagitis Encephalitis	Ganciclovir 5 mg/kg IV b.i.d. × 14–21 d Foscarnet 60 mg/kg IV q 8 hr × 21 d[e]	Variable[b, d]
Enteric bacteria	Diarrhea	Identical to that for non–HIV-infected children	Good[b]
Fungus *Candida*	Esophagitis	Fluconazole 6–10 mg/kg IV/p.o. 1 ×/d × 7–14 d (until improvement) *or* Amphotericin B IV 0.3–0.5 mg/kg 1 ×/d × 7–14 d (until improvement)	Good[b, d]
Cryptococcus	Meningitis Pneumonia Disseminated infection	Amphotericin B 0.5–1.0 mg/kg 1 ×/d, followed by suppressive therapy with fluconazole 6–10 mg/kg p.o. 1 ×/d	Variable[b, d]
Aspergillus *Histoplasma* Coccidioidomycosis	Pneumonia Encephalitis Disseminated infection	Amphotericin B 0.5–1.0 mg/kg 1 ×/d	Poor–variable[b, d, f, g, h]
Giardia	Diarrhea	Identical to that for non–HIV-infected children	Good
Herpes simplex virus	Esophagitis Pneumonia	Acyclovir 5.0–10.0 mg/kg IV q 8 hr × 7–21 d *or* Foscarnet 40 mg/kg IV q 8 hr × 21 d[e]	Variable–good[b]

Organism	Clinical manifestation	Therapy	Response
Isospora	Diarrhea	TMP-SMX 2.5 mg TMP component/kg IV/p.o. q 6 hr × 10 d	Variable[b, d, i]
Microsporidium	Diarrhea	No therapy available	—
Mycobacterium avium complex	Pneumonia Gastroenteritis Disseminated infection	Clarithromycin 7.5–15 mg/kg p.o. b.i.d. *plus* Ethambutol 15 mg/kg p.o. 1 ×/d *plus* rifampin 10 mg/kg p.o. 1 ×/d *plus* clofazimine 1 mg/kg p.o. 1 ×/d	Poor–variable[b, j]
Mycobacterium tuberculosis	Pneumonia Meningitis Disseminated infection	Isoniazid 15 mg/kg p.o. 1 ×/d *plus* rifampin 10 mg/kg p.o. 1 ×/d *plus* pyrazinamide 30 mg/kg p.o. 1 ×/d *plus* either streptomycin 12–15 mg/kg IM/IV 1 ×/d *or* Ethambutol 15 mg/kg p.o. 1 ×/d	Good[k, l]
Pneumocystis carinii	Pneumonia Disseminated infection	TMP-SMX 5 mg/kg TMP component IV/p.o. q 6 h × 21 d *or* Pentamidine 4 mg/kg 1 ×/day × 21 d	Variable[m]
Respiratory syncytial virus	Pneumonia	Ribavirin 1 vial (6 g) aerosolized by SPAG-2 generator/d × 5 d	Variable
Toxoplasma	Encephalitis	Pyrimethamine 0.5 mg/kg p.o. q 12 hr *plus* sulfadiazine 30 mg/kg p.o. q 6 hr *plus* folinic acid × 6 wk	Variable–good

[a] Recommendations for therapy of HIV-related infections are changing rapidly. Consultation with an expert is strongly encouraged.

[b] Relapses are common.

[c] Dose and efficacy are still under evaluation.

[d] Prolonged suppressive therapy after acute treatment frequently is required.

[e] Foscarnet is reserved for patients whose disease progresses while they are receiving a first-line drug or for those who suffer dose-limiting toxicity to a first-line drug.

[f] Duration of therapy for deep tissue fungal disease depends on the pathogen and the patient response.

[g] Coccidioidomycosis meningitis requires adjunctive intraventricular amphotericin B.

[h] Acute treatment for histoplasmosis is followed by suppressive therapy with itraconazole.

[i] *Isospora* requires suppressive therapy 3 ×/wk with TMP/SMX (5 mg/kg of the TMP component) after acute treatment.

[j] Four-drug regimens, including amikacin (IV) or ciprofloxacin (p.o.), have also been used in adult patients.

[k] After an initial two months of four-drug therapy, drug-susceptible tuberculosis should be treated with an additional 10 months of isoniazid and rifampin.

[l] Evaluation for multi–drug resistant *M. tuberculosis* is *critical*. If multi–drug resistance is suspected or documented in the patient or his or her contact, a minimum of four initial drugs is required, and consultation with an expert is essential.

[m] Adjunctive corticosteroids are of probable, but undocumented, benefit in children with *P. carinii* pneumonia.

Abbreviations: b.i.d. = twice daily; d = day; IM = intramuscularly; IV = intravenously; HIV = human immunodeficiency virus; p.o. = orally; q = every; SPAG = small-particle aerosol generator; TMP-SMX = trimethoprim-sulfamethoxazole.

917

RED FLAGS

Children with HIV infection often become infected with the same bacterial and viral pathogens that commonly infect their age-adjusted non–HIV-infected peers. A major red flag is failure to respond in an expected time after the initiation of therapy. Such poor responses frequently suggest opportunistic infection with unusual organisms or antimicrobial resistance. A more aggressive approach, including bronchoalveolar lavage, biopsy, and special techniques, is then needed to identify the pathogen and to begin appropriate therapy.

REFERENCES

HIV Infection

Pizzo P, Wilfert C. Pediatric AIDS: The Challenge of HIV Infection in Infants, Children and Adolescents, 2nd ed. Baltimore: Williams & Wilkins, 1994.

Working Group on Antiretroviral Therapy: National Pediatric HIV Resource Center. Antiretroviral therapy and medical management of the human immunodeficiency virus-infected child. Pediatr Infect Dis J 1993;12:513–522.

Bacterial Infection

Barnett ED, Klein JO, Pelton SI, et al. Otitis media in children born to human immunodeficiency virus-infected mothers. Pediatr Infect Dis J 1992;11:360–364.

Benson CA, Ellner JJ. *Mycobacterium avium* complex infection and AIDS: Advances in theory and practice. Clin Infect Dis 1993;17:7–20.

Bernstein LJ, Krieger BZ, Novick B, et al. Bacterial infection in the acquired immunodeficiency syndrome of children. Pediatr Infect Dis J 1985;4:472–475.

Flores G, Stavola JJ, Noel GJ. Bacteremia due to *Pseudomonas aeruginosa* in children with AIDS. Clin Infect Dis 1993;16:706–708.

Hoyt L, Oleske J, Holland B, et al. Nontuberculous mycobacteria in children with acquired immunodeficiency syndrome. Pediatr Infect Dis J 1992;11:354–360.

Janoff EN, O'Brien J, Thompson P, et al. *Streptococcus pneumoniae* colonization, bacteremia, and immune response among persons with human immunodeficiency virus infection. J Infect Dis 1993;167:49–56.

Kemper CA, Meng T-C, Nussbaum J, et al. Treatment of *Mycobacterium avium* complex bacteremia in AIDS with a four-drug oral regimen. Ann Intern Med 1992;116:466–472.

Levine WC, Buehler JW, Bean NH, et al. Epidemiology of nontyphoidal *Salmonella* bacteremia during the human immunodeficiency virus epidemic. J Infect Dis 1991;164:81–87.

National Institute of Child Health and Human Development Intravenous Immunoglobulin Study Group. Intravenous immune globulin for the prevention of bacterial infections in children with symptomatic human immunodeficiency virus infection. N Engl J Med 1991;325:73–80.

Viral Infection

Drew WL. Cytomegalovirus infection in patients with AIDS. Clin Infect Dis 1992;14:608–615.

Chatis PA, Miller CH, Schrager LE, et al. Successful treatment with foscarnet of an acyclovir-resistant mucocutaneous infection with herpes simplex virus in a patient with acquired immunodeficiency syndrome. N Engl J Med 1989;320:297–300.

Jura E, Chadwick EG, Josephs SH, et al. Varicella-zoster virus infections in children infected with human immunodeficiency virus. Pediatr Infect Dis J 1989;8:586–590.

Pulmonary Infection

Bozzette SA. The use of corticosteroids in *Pneumocystis carinii* pneumonia. J Infect Dis 1990;162:1365–1369.

Bye MR, Bernstein L, Shah K, et al. Diagnostic bronchoalveolar lavage in children with AIDS. Pediatr Pulmonol 1987;3:425–428.

Centers for Disease Control. Guidelines for prophylaxis against *Pneumocystis carinii* pneumonia for children infected with human immunodeficiency virus. JAMA 1991;265:1637–1644.

Chandwani S, Borkowsky W, Krasinski K, et al. Respiratory syncytial virus infection in human immunodeficiency virus-infected children. J Pediatr 1990;117:251–254.

Committee on Infectious Diseases, American Academy of Pediatrics. Chemotherapy for tuberculosis in infants and children. Pediatrics 1992;89:161–165.

Graybill JR. Histoplasmosis and AIDS. J Infect Dis 1988;158:623–626.

Khouri YF, Mastrucci MT, Hutto C, et al. *Mycobacterium tuberculosis* in children with human immunodeficiency virus type 1 infection. Pediatr Infect Dis J 1992;11:950–955.

Mardola J, Pace B, Bonforte RJ, et al. Pulmonary manifestations of HIV infection in children. Pediatr Pulmonol 1991;10:231–235.

Murray JF, Mills J. Pulmonary infectious complications of human immunodeficiency virus infection. Am Rev Respir Dis 1990;141:1356–1372; 1582–1598.

Schneider MME, Hoepelman IM, Schattenkerk JK, et al. A controlled trial of aerosolized pentamidine or trimethoprim-sulfamethoxazole as primary prophylaxis against *Pneumocystis carinii* pneumonia in patients with human immunodeficiency virus infection. N Engl J Med 1992;327:1836–1841.

Gastrointestinal Infection

Galgiani JN, Ampel NM. Coccidioidomycosis in human immunodeficiency virus-infected patients. J Infect Dis 1990;162:1165–1169.

Johanson JF, Sonnenberg A. Efficient management of diarrhea in the acquired immunodeficiency syndrome (AIDS). Ann Intern Med 1990;112:942–948.

Laine L, Dretler RH, Conteas CN, et al. Fluconazole compared with ketoconazole for the treatment of candida esophagitis in AIDS. Ann Intern Med 1992;117:655–660.

Molina J-M, Sarfati C, Beauvais B, et al. Intestinal microsporidiosis in human immunodeficiency virus-infected patients with chronic unexplained diarrhea: Prevalence and clinical and biologic features. J Infect Dis 1993;167:217–221.

Peterson C. Cryptosporidiosis in patients infected with the human immunodeficiency virus. Clin Infect Dis 1992;15:903–990.

Smith PD, Quinn TC, Strober W, et al. Gastrointestinal infections in AIDS. Ann Intern Med 1992;116:63–77.

Wilcox CM, Diehl DL, Cello JP, et al. Cytomegalovirus esophagitis in patients with AIDS. Ann Intern Med 1990;113:589–593.

Central Nervous System Infection

Berenguer J, Moreno S, Laguna F, et al. Tuberculous meningitis in patients infected with the human immunodeficiency virus. N Engl J Med 1992;326:668–672.

Larsen RA, Leal MAE, Chan LS. Fluconazole compared with amphotericin B plus flucytosine for cryptococcal meningitis in AIDS—a randomized trial. Ann Intern Med 1990;113:183–187.

Luft BJ, Remington JS. Toxoplasmic encephalitis in AIDS. Clin Infect Dis 1992;15:211–222.

Powderly WG. Cryptococcal meningitis and AIDS. Clin Infect Dis 1993;17:837–842.

Other Infection

Grandon JD, Timpone JG, Schnittman SM. Emergence of unusual opportunistic pathogens in AIDS: A review. Clin Infect Dis 1992;15:134–157.

56 Fever of Unknown Origin

W. Thomas Corder   Stephen C. Aronoff

Fever in the pediatric population is usually grouped into four categories:

- Fever in the neonate
- Fever with localizing signs
- Fever without localizing signs
- Fever of unknown origin (FUO)

DEFINITIONS

The core temperature is a balance between the heat generated from the body's metabolic processes and the heat-dissipating mechanisms. Heat is generated by inefficient cellular metabolism. The body is cooled by a combination of heat loss by radiation, conduction, evaporation, and convection. Cooling takes place mainly by radiation and evaporation from the skin. The lungs also contribute to cooling but to a lesser degree.

An elevation in temperature is a result of fever or hyperthermia. *Fever* is the physiologic resetting of the normal regulating mechanism in the hypothalamic set point resulting in an elevated body temperature. *Hyperthermia* is failure of the body's cooling mechanisms to dissipate excessive heat production (malignant hyperthermia, heat stress, heat stroke). Fever often results from the direct action of systemically produced cytokines (interleukin-1β, tumor necrosis factor-α) acting on the hypothalamus. These proteins are synthesized as the response to inflammation, infection, or malignancy and elevate the hypothalamic set point.

In adults, FUO is defined as an illness of more than 3 weeks' duration, fever higher than 38.3°C (101°F) on several occasions, and diagnosis uncertain after 1-week study in hospital. In pediatrics, the definition is variable, as the duration of elevated temperature ranges from 8 days to 3 weeks. This may be dependent on the age of the patient, with shorter periods of fever in young infants and more traditional adult standards for adolescent patients. We will use the definition of FUO as an immunologically normal host with oral or rectal temperature greater than 38°C (100.4°F) at least twice a week for more than 3 weeks, a noncontributory history and physical examination, a normal chest roentgenogram, and normal findings on urinalysis. With this definition, the differential diagnosis remains large (Table 56–1).

In adults, infections account for 30% to 40% of cases of FUO, followed by neoplasms (20% to 30%), autoimmune disease (10% to 15%), and miscellaneous or undiagnosed diseases (10% to 20%). Four pediatric series of FUO are summarized in Table 56–2. An infectious etiology accounted for 33% to 52% of cases of pediatric FUO, followed by autoimmune diseases (6% to 20%), neoplasias (2% to 13%), and miscellaneous or undiagnosed causes (11% to 67%).

Infection is the most common cause of FUO in children of all ages. Respiratory infections account for 50% of infections. Most often these infections are atypical presentations of common childhood bacterial or viral pathogens rather than the more unusual or uncommon disorders noted in Table 56–1. Infections may occur twice as often in children under 6 years of age, while connective tissue disease occurs more often in children older than 6 years of age. Mortality in adult studies is higher than that in pediatric series (32% versus 9%). This mortality is usually due to untreatable primary diseases (cancer) rather than undiagnosed lethal diseases.

EVALUATION

Evaluation of the child with FUO requires a detailed history and physical examination. The history should be repeated, since parents often remember important details after the initial interview. The physical examination may also change during the course of the investigation and reveal important clues (Fig. 56–1).

History

The history should include the time of day of the fever, who measured the temperature, and the instrument that was used to measure the temperature. Unlike rectal measurements, axillary temperatures and aural and forehead liquid crystal thermometers do not always correlate with core temperature. Increased temperatures after exercise and in the afternoon may be due to normal variations. The appearance of the child while febrile is also important. Increased temperature without sweating might be seen in a child with ectodermal dysplasia or factitious temperature.

The pattern of fever should be noted. Sustained fever, intermittent fever, and relapsing fever have been associated with different disease states.

Sustained or *remittent fever* remains elevated with little variation during the day and has been associated with typhoid fever, tularemia, malarial infections, and rickettsial diseases such as typhus and Rocky Mountain spotted fever.

Intermittent fever normalizes at least once a day and is associated with tuberculosis, abscess, lymphoma, juvenile rheumatoid arthritis (JRA), and some forms of malaria.

Children with *relapsing fever* have afebrile days between febrile episodes. Relapsing fever has been associated with rat-bite fever, malaria, brucellosis, subacute bacterial endocarditis, African trypanosomiasis, lymphomas, and Lyme disease.

Saddle-back or *double-hump fever* lasts a few days followed by an afebrile day or two with subsequent return of fever and has been associated with some viruses and dengue fever.

Double quotidian fever (two fever spikes each day) occurs in kala-azar, malaria, and gonococcal endocarditis.

Unfortunately neither the fever pattern nor the duration is consistently helpful in identifying an etiology. FUO lasting for more than 1 year is usually not infectious and suggests factitious fever, collagen-vascular or granulomatous disorders, familial diseases, or malignancy.

A history of rash is important in Lyme disease, JRA, and acute

Table 56–1. Causes of Fever of Unknown Origin in Children

Infections

Bacterial Diseases

Specific organism causing systemic disease
  Bartonellosis
  Brucellosis
  Campylobacter
  Cat-scratch disease
  Gonococcemia (chronic)
  Meningococcemia (chronic)
  Salmonellosis
  Streptobacillus moniliformis
  Tuberculosis
  Tularemia
Localized infections
  Abscesses: abdominal, dental, hepatic, pelvic,
    perinephric, rectal, subphrenic, splenic,
    periappendiceal
  Cholangitis
  Endocarditis
  Mastoiditis
  Osteomyelitis
  Pneumonia
  Pyelonephritis
  Sinusitis

Spirochete

Borrelia (borreliosis: *B. recurrentis, B. burgdorfei*)
Leptospirosis
Lyme disease
Spirillium minor
Syphilis

Viral Diseases

Cytomegalovirus
Hepatitis
Human immunodeficiency virus (and its
  opportunistic-associated infections)
Infectious mononucleosis (Epstein-Barr virus)
Unidentified presumed virus

Chlamydial Diseases

Lymphogranuloma venereum
Psittacosis

Rickettsial Diseases

Ehrlichia canis
Q fever
Rocky Mountain spotted fever

Fungal Diseases

Blastomycosis (nonpulmonary)
Coccidioidomycosis (disseminated)
Histoplasmosis (disseminated)

Parasitic Diseases

Extraintestinal amebiasis
Babesiosis
Giardiasis
Malaria
Toxoplasmosis
Trypanosomiasis
Visceral larva migrans

Autoimmune Hypersensitivity Diseases

Drug fever
Hypersensitivity pneumonitis
Juvenile rheumatoid arthritis (systemic onset, Still
  disease)
Polyarteritis nodosa
Rheumatic fever
Serum sickness
Systemic lupus erythematosus
Undefined vasculitis

Neoplasms

Atrial myxoma
Ewing sarcoma
Hepatoma
Hodgkin disease
Leukemia
Lymphoma
Neuroblastoma

Granulomatous Diseases

Granulomatous hepatitis
Sarcoidosis
Crohn disease

Familial-Hereditary Diseases

Anhidrotic ectodermal dysplasia
Cyclic neutropenia
Deafness, urticaria, amyloidosis syndrome
Fabry disease
Familial dysautonomia
Familial Mediterranean fever
Hypertriglyceridemia
Ichthyosis

Miscellaneous

Behçet syndrome
Chronic active hepatitis
Diabetes insipidus (central and nephrogenic)
Factitious fever
Hemophagocytic syndromes
Histiocytosis syndromes
Hypothalamic-central fever
Infantile cortical hyperostosis
Inflammatory bowel disease
Kawasaki disease
Pancreatitis
Periodic fever
Postoperative (pericardiotomy, craniectomy)
Pulmonary embolism
Spinal cord injury-crisis
Thyrotoxicosis
Central fever

Undiagnosed Fever

Persistent
Recurrent
Resolved

Modified from Behrman RE (ed). Nelson Textbook of Pediatrics, 14th ed. Philadelphia: WB Saunders, 1992:653.

Table 56–2. **Comparison of Four Pediatric Fever of Unknown Origin Studies**

	McClung	Pizzo	Lohr	Steele
Year reported	1972	1975	1977	1991
Definition of fever	>38.9°C	>38.5°C	>38.3°C	≥38°C
Duration of fever on multiple occasions	3-wk outpatient or 1-wk inpatient	>2 wk	3-wk outpatient or 1-wk inpatient	3 wk
No. of patients	99	100	54	109
Diagnosis (%)				
Infection	29 (29)	52 (52)	18 (33)	23 (21)
Autoimmune disease	11 (11)	20 (20)	8 (15)	7 (6)
Inflammatory bowel disease	3 (3)		3 (6)	1 (1)
Neoplasm	8 (8)	6 (6)	7 (13)	2 (2)
Miscellaneous	16 (16)	10 (10)	8 (15)	2 (2)
No diagnosis made	11 (11)	12 (12)	10 (19)	73 (67)

rheumatic fever (see Chapter 57). A history of pica is associated with visceral larva migrans and toxoplasmosis. Exposure to domestic and wild animals should be identified to exclude zoonoses (see Chapter 54). The food history should be detailed and should include water source, use of game meats and cooking practices, and use of unpasteurized whole milk.

Domestic or foreign travel is critically important in the establishment of a differential diagnosis. Areas visited, accommodations, activities, prophylactic treatments, animal and insect exposure, and water and food supply should be reviewed. Coccidioidomycosis, histoplasmosis, malaria, Lyme disease, and Rocky Mountain spotted fever have regional distributions. Emigrant children are at increased risk for endemic diseases and *Mycobacterium tuberculosis*.

Previous medical records should be reviewed. Weight loss is important in many chronic diseases such as lymphoma, tuberculosis, and inflammatory bowel disease. Poor weight gain and growth, with or without gastrointestinal symptoms, may be the only historical clue to inflammatory bowel disease (see Chapter 19). Human immunodeficiency virus (HIV) risk factors should be reviewed in the parents and child (see Chapter 55). Many parents are unaware if their child has had a transfusion. Past and current medications should be reviewed. Family history may give clues to familial Mediterranean fever and other familial disorders (see Table 56–1). The review of systems may reveal heat intolerance, palpitations, tremors, and declining school work in a child with hyperthyroidism. A history of severe head trauma may be associated with hypothalamic dysfunction and central fevers.

Physical Examination

A complete physical examination may reveal clues to the illness. Whenever possible, the patient should be examined during a febrile episode. A high fever in the absence of an increased pulse may be present in a patient with factitious fever. To verify this diagnosis, the temperature of an immediate voided urine may be recorded. Tremor, high heart rate, palpitations, exophthalmos, lid lag, eyelid retraction, and smooth, flushed skin with diaphoresis suggest hyperthyroidism.

EYES

The ophthalmologic examination should include acuity, extraocular motion, visual field integrity, and gaze as well as inspection of external structures and funduscopic examination (see Chapter

44). *Conjunctivitis* or iritis-uveitis-scleritis, or both, may be seen in a variety of infectious diseases, including Epstein-Barr virus (EBV), leptospirosis, rickettsial infection, and cat-scratch disease. Conjunctivitis or uveitis, or both, is also seen in Kawasaki syndrome, systemic lupus erythematosus (SLE), polyarteritis nodosa, and rheumatoid arthritis. *Sarcoidosis* may be associated with conjunctival and uveal tract nodules. A thorough funduscopic evaluation (and, if needed, slit-lamp examination) should be performed. Sarcoidosis may show vascular occlusions, hemorrhages, vascular sheathing, and preretinal inflammatory exudates. Cytomegalovirus (CMV) produces chorioretinitis associated with white dots near vessels and confluent depigmented areas. Histoplasmosis causes small atrophic spots and, rarely, focal granulomas of the retina and choroid. *Toxoplasma gondii* is a common cause of recurrent retinochoroiditis. Retinal changes also occur with bacterial endocarditis. Tuberculosis can form choroidal tubercles and also ulcerative palpebral conjunctival lesions. Slit-lamp examination may also reveal iridocyclitis in JRA, Behçet syndrome, and inflammatory bowel disease.

SINUSES

The frontal and maxillary sinuses should be transilluminated and palpated for tenderness. The nares should be inspected for inflamed mucosa and purulent discharge. Tympanic membranes should be viewed and insufflated (see Chapter 9). The mouth should be checked for lesions, inflammation, and tooth tenderness. Behçet syndrome is rare in children but may present with oral aphthous lesions. Inspection of teeth and gums may reveal a dental abscess. Exudative and nonexudative pharyngitis is associated with EBV infection, tularemia, leptospirosis, and CMV. *Candida* in the mouth of children over 2 years of age may be due to immunodeficiency such as HIV or the use of inhaled steroids.

NECK

The neck should be examined for adenopathy or thyroid enlargement (see Chapter 50). The rest of the lymphatic system should be carefully examined (see Chapter 48). A single tender node may be seen with cat-scratch disease. Generalized adenopathy can be seen in CMV infection, EBV infection, and systemic JRA (see Chapter 48).

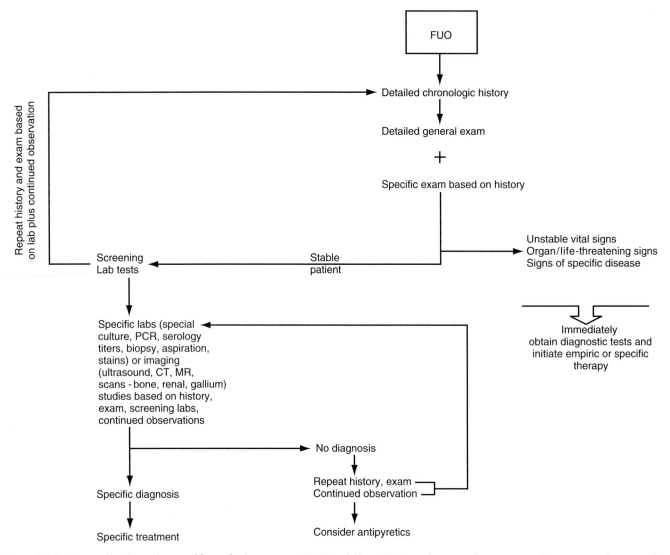

Figure 56–1. Approach to the evaluation of fever of unknown origin (FUO) in children. PCR = polymerase chain reaction; CT = computed tomography; MR = magnetic resonance.

HEART AND LUNGS

Careful auscultation of the heart and lungs is essential. A mitral or aortic regurgitant murmur may be the initial finding of endocarditis or of carditis in children with acute rheumatic fever. A pericardial friction rub may also suggest JRA, SLE, rheumatic fever, malignancy, or viral pericarditis. The abdomen must be carefully palpated for evidence of masses (see Chapter 26) or hepatosplenomegaly (see Chapters 22 and 23). A rectal examination should be performed, and stool should be tested for occult blood. Sexually active females should have a pelvic examination. Abdominal tenderness may be present in abdominal abscesses, hepatosplenomegaly, and inflammatory bowel disease. Pain on movement of the uterus during the pelvic examination may indicate pelvic inflammatory disease.

MUSCULOSKELETAL EVALUATION

The musculoskeletal examination should include strength, active and passive range of motion, and evaluation for warmth, tenderness, or swelling of joints. Irritability and pain to palpation over a

bone or disuse pseudoparalysis may be the first clues to osteomyelitis. Bone pain may also result from neoplastic infiltration of the bone marrow or sickle cell anemia. Unexplained fever, arthralgias, and arthritis may be present in acute rheumatic fever, Kawasaki syndrome, SLE, periarteritis nodosa, and Behçet syndrome (see Chapter 45). Myalgias may be present in rickettsial diseases, periarteritis nodosa, Takayasu arteritis, and dermatomyositis and occur quite commonly in viral diseases such as influenza.

SKIN

The skin must be inspected for evidence of rashes, lesions, and petechiae (see Chapter 57). JRA may present with an evanescent pink macular rash over the trunk and joints that may appear and disappear rapidly and be evident only during febrile periods. Dermatomyositis has a characteristic heliotropic rash of the upper eyelids and an erythematous eruption (vasculitis) over the extensor surfaces (Gottron sign). SLE may present with a butterfly rash over the nose and malar regions or signs of photosensitivity in sun-exposed areas or vasculitis. The rash of Kawasaki syndrome is erythematous and may present in many forms. In Rocky Mountain spotted fever there are macular erythematous spots on the palms and soles that develop into petechiae on wrists and ankles. Endocarditis may be associated with splinter hemorrhages or Janeway lesions.

Lyme disease usually presents with erythema chronicum migrans. This rash begins at the site of the tick bite and is erythematous with a pale center. The rash radiates out from the bite in a circular fashion and persists for weeks; satellite secondary lesions may also appear.

Tularemia, salmonellosis, listeriosis, and EBV infections may feature generalized maculopapular rashes.

Laboratory and Special Studies

Laboratory evaluation should proceed in a stepwise, focused manner with emphasis placed on identifying serious illness with defined interventions (see Fig. 56–1). Initial studies should include a complete blood count with differential, an erythrocyte sedimentation rate (ESR), blood cultures, urinalysis, urine culture, tuberculin skin tests with controls (anergy panel), and chest radiograph. Since EBV is common in childhood, viral-specific antibody titers may also be obtained at the initial evaluation (see Chapter 48). Further studies should be directed by information obtained from detailed histories and physical examinations. Specific serologies aid in the diagnosis of CMV, toxoplasmosis, brucellosis, tularemia, hepatitis A, B, and C, and leptospirosis. Biopsies of lymph node, skin, liver, or bone marrow may be indicated. Radiologic studies that may be of benefit if directed by the history, physical, and initial laboratory studies include sinus films, abdominal ultrasound, abdominal computed tomography (CT) or magnetic resonance imaging (MRI), gallium or indium scans, upper gastrointestinal series with small bowel follow-through, and technetium bone scanning. Aspiration of presumed abscess material or fluid collections (pleural, ascitic) is best performed under CT or ultrasound guidance.

The complete blood cell count with differential is not specific or diagnostic. There may be a predominance of neutrophils in patients with collagen-vascular disease or bacterial infections and in some viral infections. Approximately 30% of patients have abnormal white blood cell counts; 46% may have a "left shift," lymphocytosis, atypical lymphocytes, or blasts. Except for leukemic blasts, abnormalities are not specific for disease categories.

An elevated ESR indicates inflammation. The ESR is usually (70% to 90% of the time) high in children with FUO due to infectious etiologies, malignancies, and collagen-vascular diseases. Ninety percent of patients with an ESR less than 10 mm/hour usually have a self-limited or viral disease.

Urinalysis and urine culture identify occult infections, particularly in young females. The urinalysis may also be abnormal in patients with endocarditis and collagen-inflammatory disorders.

Unexpected consolidations, calcifications, interstitial changes, perihilar adenopathy, or cardiomegaly (heart failure, pericarditis) may be found on chest radiographs. Chest films are abnormal in 10% to 15% of patients.

Specialized radiologic studies performed without specific diagnostic clues from the history, physical, or initial laboratory evaluation have a surprisingly low yield. In one report, abnormal findings were discovered in 8 of 43 abdominal ultrasounds, 3 of 14 abdominal CT scans, 5 of 11 indium scans, 1 of 4 gallium scans, and 2 of 15 technetium bone scans.

ETIOLOGY

Infection

Infections identified in large series of children with FUO include subacute bacterial endocarditis, urinary tract infections, sinusitis,

abscesses, osteomyelitis, and rheumatic fever (postinfectious) (see Table 56–1).

SUBACUTE BACTERIAL ENDOCARDITIS

Subacute bacterial endocarditis is rare in children but increases with advancing age and history of preexisting heart disease (see Chapter 16). Murmurs or a change in the characteristic of the prior murmur may not be initially evident. Vegetations also may not be visible initially by transthoracic echocardiography; a transesophageal approach is much more sensitive and specific. Serial blood cultures using anaerobic and aerobic media are necessary for definitive diagnosis.

URINARY TRACT INFECTION

Both upper and lower urinary tract infections may be asymptomatic, and leukocytes may not always be present in urine (see Chapter 27). Sterile pyuria may be present in tuberculosis, Kawasaki syndrome, Reiter syndrome, and collagen-vascular syndromes. Renal ultrasonography may show areas of decreased echogenicity, enlarged echogenic kidneys, and renal or perinephric abscesses. Kidneys may be enlarged with acute pyelonephritis. With an enhanced CT scan, infected parenchyma may show nonenhancing lucency. Renal scans also identify active areas of infection and old scars.

SINUSITIS

Factors that decrease the size and patency of the ostium or impair the mucociliary transport system predispose a child to sinusitis. Ethmoid and maxillary sinuses are present at birth. The frontal sinuses usually appear near 5 or 6 years of age but may be asymmetric or absent. Sphenoid sinuses may be seen radiographically by 9 years of age (see Chapter 38). Prolonged nasal congestion, headache, purulent nasal discharge, sore throat, daytime cough, tender teeth, and halitosis may be present in children with sinusitis. Radiographic sinus series consisting of Waters, Caldwell, lateral, and submental vertex views may show opacification, air-fluid levels, or mucosal thickening. CT studies may be more helpful. Rhinoscopy may show purulent material at the ostium of an affected sinus. Infectious complications of sinusitis include dural space empyema or brain abscesses.

ABSCESSES

Hepatic, perinephric, pelvic, and subphrenic abscesses may present with FUO. Liver abscess may present with right upper quadrant tenderness and hepatomegaly. Blood cultures and liver function studies are often normal. The diagnosis may be made with MRI, CT, ultrasound, or gallium scan. Perinephric abscesses may have normal intravenous pyelograms, while CT or ultrasound is diagnostic. CT or ultrasound guidance may be used to direct percutaneous drainage of most abscesses. Pelvic abscesses should be suspected in children with abdominal, rectal, or pelvic tenderness.

OSTEOMYELITIS

Osteomyelitis usually follows bacteremia but may follow penetrating injury. Tenderness of bone to palpation over the infected site is common. Technetium scans show early changes (1 week) while abnormalities in plain films appear later (2 weeks). The blood or bone culture is often positive, and the ESR is often elevated and may be followed during therapy.

RHEUMATIC FEVER

Acute rheumatic fever may cause FUO; the diagnosis is made by fulfillment of the modified Jones criteria (see Chapter 16). Initially, a child may present with polyarthralgia and an increased ESR. Elbows, wrists, knees, and ankles are frequently involved. The later migratory nature of the true arthritis differentiates rheumatic fever from JRA.

BACTERIAL SYNDROMES

Bacterial syndromes that cause FUO in children include agents of:

- Lyme disease
- Cat-scratch disease
- Rat-bite fever
- Tularemia
- Brucellosis
- Leptospirosis
- Chronic bacteremias (meningococcus, gonococcus)

Lyme Disease

Lyme disease is caused by the spirochete *Borrelia burgdorferi* and is transmitted by the *Ixodes dammini* and *Ixodes pacificus* ticks. The usual presentation is with erythema chronicum migrans, an erythematous, annular, expanding rash with central clearing. The rash resolves 1 to 30 days (usually 2 weeks) after exposure. Patients may exhibit fever, chills, fatigue, headaches, malaise, myalgias, arthralgias, and lymphadenopathy. Two to 8 weeks after exposure, facial nerve palsy, peripheral neuropathy, cardiac conduction defects, myocarditis, and aseptic meningitis may occur. Months to years after exposure, arthritis and chronic neurologic symptoms can be seen (see Chapter 45). Diagnosis is usually made clinically; antibody titers, Western blot, and T-cell response are unreliable and often falsely positive. Polymerase chain reaction is in development.

Cat-Scratch Disease

Cat-scratch disease is a febrile illness associated with cats (usually kittens) and more rarely dogs. *Bartonella henselae*, which may be transmitted by the cat flea, is currently believed to be the etiologic agent. After a scratch or bite, a papule forms and may persist from days to months. Regional lymphadenopathy with one or more nodes occurs proximal to the skin site 1 to 9 weeks after inoculation. The node or nodes become enlarged and tender and may have overlying erythema. The lymphadenopathy usually resolves after 2 months but may last up to 3 years. Children may have adenopathy and also fever, headache, malaise, anorexia, sore throat, and conjunctivitis (see Chapter 48).

Rat-Bite Fever

Rat-bite fever is a relapsing fever caused by *Streptobacillus moniliformis* or *Spirillum minus*. *S. moniliformis* is a pleomorphic gram-negative bacillus transmitted by rat bite or contamination of food or water. In 1 to 10 days, patients may exhibit fever, chills, malaise, and muscle aches. A rash may form on the extremities; arthralgias and arthritis may occur. Endocarditis is a late manifestation. Diagnosis is made by blood culture. A fourfold increase in antibody titers may also be seen. Treatment is with penicillin.

Tularemia

Francisella tularensis is the causative agent of tularemia. The disease is spread by contact with wild animals, such as rabbits and squirrels, insects who bite these animals, such as mosquitoes, ticks, and deer flies, and contaminated water. A maculopapular nodule forms at the portal of entry and later becomes ulcerated. The child may present with fever, chills, and headache. Lymphadenopathy, pharyngitis, conjunctivitis, hepatosplenomegaly, and pneumonia may also occur. Diagnosis is made by serology. Treatment is with streptomycin or gentamicin.

Brucellosis

Brucellosis is caused by gram-negative coccobacilli: *Brucella abortus, B. melitensis, B. suis,* or *B. canis.* The microorganisms are found in sheep, goats, cattle, swine, and dogs. Infection may occur by airborne spread or by ingestion of meat or milk. The child may present with fever, chills, malaise, arthralgias, or myalgias. Pneumonia and cardiac and central nervous system (CNS) involvement occur rarely. Diagnosis is made by special culture techniques and serology.

Leptospirosis

Leptospirosis is caused by members of the spirochete *Leptospira* genus. Infection is spread by contact with urine of wild or domestic animals. After 1 to 2 weeks, patients experience the abrupt onset of fever, chills, malaise, myalgias, and headache. Conjunctival suffusion and rash are common findings. Liver, renal, and CNS involvement may also occur. Diagnosis is made by special culture techniques and microscopic agglutination.

FUNGAL INFECTIONS

Fungal causes of FUO include:

- Blastomycosis
- Histoplasmosis
- Coccidioidomycosis
- Cryptococcoses

Blastomyces dermatitidis is a fungus that has a yeast and mycelial form and is found in the soil in North America. Infections with this fungus may be disseminated or pulmonary. The diagnosis is made by visualization of single-budding yeast in clinical material, culture on Sabouraud agar, or serologic tests. Amphotericin B is used for treatment.

Histoplasma capsulatum is a yeast found in soil in the Ohio

River valley that causes pulmonary and disseminated disease. Diagnosis is made by the demonstration of the microorganism in biopsy specimens or by complement fixing antibody. Treatment is with amphotericin B.

Coccidioides immitis is found in soil in the southwestern United States. Human infections are associated with a febrile pulmonary disease characterized by cough, rash, and chest pain. Diagnosis is usually made serologically.

Cryptococcus neoformans is often found in pigeon droppings and can cause a variety of diseases. The diagnosis is made by culture or by identification of encapsulated yeast in collected specimens. Treatment is with amphotericin B.

CHLAMYDIAL INFECTION

Psittacosis and *lymphogranuloma venereum* are chlamydial causes of FUO. *Chlamydia psittaci* may be transmitted by infected birds and produces respiratory illness with fever. Cardiac, liver, CNS, and thyroid involvement are rare. Diagnosis is made serologically. *Chlamydia trachomatis* is a sexually transmitted organism that causes urogenital infections, perihepatitis, invasive lymphadenopathy (lymphogranuloma venereum), neonatal conjunctivitis, and neonatal pneumonia. Diagnosis is by cell culture and rapid antigen tests. Treatment is with erythromycin.

Q FEVER

Q fever is caused by *Coxiella burnetii* and presents with headache, fever, chills, malaise, and occasionally respiratory symptoms. Hepatic, cardiac, and CNS involvement may occur. Rash is usually not seen. Domestic farm animals, cats, rodents, and marsupials may be infected. Pasteurization destroys the organism in milk. Treatment is with tetracycline or chloramphenicol.

ROCKY MOUNTAIN SPOTTED FEVER

Rocky Mountain spotted fever presents with fever, headache, intense myalgias, and abdominal symptoms. A characteristic rash is usually present by the sixth day of illness. The rash covers the palms, wrists, soles, and ankles and progresses from macular to petechial. The disease can last up to 3 weeks. Many end organs can be involved, including heart, kidneys, and CNS. Transmission occurs by tick bite. Treatment is with chloramphenicol or tetracycline.

EHRLICHIOSIS

Human ehrlichiosis is presumed to be caused by *Ehrlichia chaffeensis*. The illness is usually seen in the southeastern and upper midwestern United States and has a presentation similar to Rocky Mountain spotted fever. The patient presents with headache, myalgias, fever, chills, nausea, vomiting, weight loss, thrombocytopenia, and leukopenia. Rash is inconsistent but may be seen after 1 week. Pulmonary and renal complications can occur. Mental status changes are less frequent. Tetracycline is used for treatment. Chloramphenicol may also be effective. Diagnosis is presumed by serology.

CYTOMEGALOVIRUS INFECTION

Cytomegalovirus may cause a mononucleosis-like syndrome in children. Generalized or cervical adenopathy may be seen along with fatigue, malaise, fever, hepatosplenomegaly, and abdominal pain (see Chapter 48). A morbilliform rash may also be present. Retinitis, hepatitis, colitis, and pneumonia may occur in children with impaired immune systems. The virus is transmitted by contact with secretions. Infection is diagnosed by culture (nasopharyngeal, blood, urine) or specific immunoglobulin G and immunoglobulin M antibodies.

INFECTIOUS MONONUCLEOSIS

Infectious mononucleosis is typically caused by Epstein-Barr virus and may present with fever, exudative pharyngitis, malaise, and fatigue (see Chapter 48). The appearance of rash is usually preceded by ampicillin therapy. Tender lymphadenopathy and hepatosplenomegaly may occur. The diagnosis may be made by nonspecific tests (heterophile antibody or monospot) in older patients, but these studies are unreliable for young children. Specific antibody tests against viral capsid antigen, early antigen, and nuclear antigen are recommended in younger children. Treatment is supportive.

HIV INFECTION

Infection with human immunodeficiency virus (HIV) is another cause of FUO in children (see Chapter 55).

PARASITES

FUO in children may be caused by parasitic infections, including (1) babesiosis, (2) toxoplasmosis, and (3) toxocariasis.

Babesiosis is caused by *Babesia microtia* and is a parasite of rodents transmitted to humans by tick bite. Infection may result in fever, chills, nausea, vomiting, night sweats, myalgias, and arthralgias. Identification of the organism in a thick smear of red blood cells is diagnostic.

Toxoplasma gondii is a protozoan parasite. Children become infected from eating contaminated, undercooked meat or from exposure to the feces of domestic cats. If acquired in adulthood, the disease is usually asymptomatic and self-limited. *Toxoplasma* infection resembles a mononucleosis-like illness (see Chapter 48).

Toxocariasis (visceral larva migrans) results from ingestion of larvae of *Toxocara canis* or *T. catis* shed in dog and cat feces. Infection results in fever, intense eosinophilia, hepatomegaly, and hypergammaglobulinemia. Lung, heart, and CNS involvement is rare. The eye may become infected. Diagnosis is presumed with increased eosinophils and hypergammaglobulinemia. Elevated titers of antibodies to A and B blood groups are often seen. Treatment is largely supportive.

In a child who has traveled outside the United States, consideration must be given to the areas traveled, water sources, and activities. Some causes of FUO following travel to a foreign country include malaria, hepatitis, typhoid fever, tuberculosis, amebic liver abscess, and filariasis.

MALARIA

Malaria is transmitted by the bite of an infected mosquito carrying *Plasmodium falciparum, P. vivax, P. ovale,* or *P. malariae.*

The patient experiences chills, rigors, fever, diaphoresis, and headaches. Incubation varies among species, from 1 week to 1 month. Demonstration of the parasite on thick peripheral blood smear is diagnostic. Treatment is given according to species involved and area where the patient was exposed.

HEPATITIS

Hepatitis A may be contracted by ingestion of contaminated food or water. Hepatitis B and C are transmitted through blood products and sexual contact. Diagnosis is by serologic testing. Symptoms can include fever, malaise, jaundice, nausea, and anorexia. Hepatitis B and C can become chronic. Treatment is supportive, although interferon-α has been used for chronic illness.

TYPHOID FEVER

Typhoid fever is caused by infection with *Salmonella typhi*. After ingestion of contaminated water or food, incubation is from 1 to 6 weeks. Persistent fever, rose spots, and glomerulonephritis are clinical hallmarks of typhoid fever. Diagnosis is by blood or, rarely, bone marrow culture. Treatment is with ceftriaxone or cefotaxime.

TUBERCULOSIS

Tuberculosis may present as FUO in children (see Chapters 7, 48, and 55). The child may have pulmonary or extrapulmonary disease. The signs and symptoms of pulmonary disease may vary greatly, from weight loss, skin test conversion, and low-grade fever to mass effect from mediastinal lymphadenopathy and fulminant disseminated pulmonary involvement with miliary infiltrates or, rarely, cavitation. Nonpulmonary tuberculosis more commonly presents as FUO, since positive chest radiograph findings and pulmonary signs may initiate an early work-up for tuberculosis. Hematogenous spread may cause liver, heart, or renal involvement. Ingested bacilli may result in gastrointestinal tuberculosis. The diagnosis requires demonstration of acid-fast bacilli from sputum, gastric aspirate, or the affected organ. Skin testing may be negative even with positive controls.

AMEBIC INFECTION

Intestinal infection with *Entamoeba histolytica* may produce invasion of the mucosal lining and spread to other organs such as the liver. Amebic liver abscess may present with fever, weight loss, right upper quadrant pain, and anorexia. The patient may have painful hepatomegaly without splenomegaly. The abscess may be localized with abdominal ultrasonography. Diagnosis is by serology. Treatment is with metronidazole.

FILARIASIS

Filariasis may result from the bite of a mosquito infected with *Wuchereria bancrofti*, *Brugia malayi*, or *B. timori*. Disease results from inflammation and obstruction of lymph channels by the developing nematode. Patients may present with fever, myalgias, lymph-adenitis, and lymphangitis. Diagnosis is by observing microfilariae in blood or adult worms in tissue biopsy material.

Rheumatologic Causes of Fever of Unknown Origin

Collagen-vascular diseases as a cause of FUO are more common in children over 6 years of age. The diagnosis is often difficult and may take months to establish. JRA, polyarteritis, SLE, and Behçet syndrome may all present as FUO (see Chapter 45).

ARTHRITIS

Juvenile rheumatoid arthritis is a diagnosis that requires time to identify all of its manifestations and the exclusion of other entities. JRA is defined by arthritis (swelling or both pain and limitation of motion) of unknown origin that begins in a child under 16 years of age and persists for a minimum of 6 weeks. JRA is divided into three subtypes: systemic, polyarticular, and pauciarticular. The systemic form (Still disease) often presents with prolonged high fever. Affected children often have a daily fever and may have a fine macular rash, arthralgias, arthritis, hepatosplenomegaly, or pericardial involvement. Polyarticular JRA may present with arthritis, low-grade fever, morning stiffness, anorexia, and weight loss.

POLYARTERITIS

Polyarteritis is a necrotizing vasculitis that may present with myalgia, arthralgia, fever, vasculitic skin lesions, and abdominal pain. Cardiac, CNS, and renal involvement may also occur. The ESR is usually markedly elevated. Biopsy and antibodies to proteinase 3 and myeloperoxidase (antineutrophil cytoplasmic antibodies) are helpful. Treatment is with prednisone or cyclophosphamide.

SYSTEMIC LUPUS ERYTHEMATOSUS

Systemic lupus erythematosus may present with fever, photosensitivity, mouth sores, weight loss, rash, myalgias, malaise, and hepatosplenomegaly. Patients may also have serositis and renal involvement. Laboratory tests that are helpful include LE cell preparation, antinuclear antibody, anti-Sm, anti-RNP, Ro (SS-A), and La (SS-B).

BEHÇET DISEASE

Behçet disease is very rare in children but may present with FUO. Patients may have aphthous stomatitis, arthritis, genital ulcers, uveitis, and erythema nodosum.

NEOPLASMS

Hodgkin disease, lymphoma, neuroblastoma, and leukemia may all present as FUO. In young children, leukemia, neuroblastoma, and lymphoma should be suspected, while Hodgkin disease and Ewing sarcoma are more common as causes of FUO in adolescents.

Hodgkin Disease

Hodgkin disease may present with firm, nontender adenopathy, fever, night sweats, and weight loss. Diagnosis is by biopsy. Treatment is with radiation and chemotherapy.

Lymphoma

Non-Hodgkin lymphoma may present as painless adenopathy, cough from mediastinal mass, abdominal mass, nerve compression, bone pain, fever, and weight loss. Diagnosis is by biopsy. Treatment depends on site and extent of tumor. Surgery, radiation, and chemotherapy may be used.

Neuroblastoma

Neuroblastoma may present as abdominal, thoracic, or pelvic masses, spinal cord compression, bone pain, hypertension, hepatomegaly, diarrhea, and fever (see Chapter 26). Diagnosis is aided by radiologic studies and urinary catecholamines and confirmed by biopsy. Surgery, radiation, and chemotherapy are used for treatment.

Leukemia

Acute lymphocytic leukemia and acute nonlymphocytic leukemia may both present with lethargy, pallor, bleeding, fever, bone pain, lymphadenopathy and arthralgias. Diagnosis is made by blood smear and bone marrow aspirate with biopsy. Treatment is with chemotherapy.

Miscellaneous Causes of Fever of Unknown Origin

There are many other causes of FUO.

FAMILIAL MEDITERRANEAN FEVER

Familial Mediterranean fever is an autosomal recessive trait seen in Sephardic Jews and people of Middle Eastern origin. The fever may be accompanied by joint, abdominal, and chest pains.

ANHIDROTIC ECTODERMAL DYSPLASIA

Anhidrotic ectodermal dysplasia is an X-linked recessive disorder associated with decreased ability to sweat, dental abnormalities, and sparse hair. Eyebrows and eyelashes may be absent. Fever may result from inability of the body to cool itself. Diagnosis is made by skin biopsy showing absence of eccrine glands.

DRUG FEVER

Drug fever is a diagnosis of exclusion. Some drugs are more likely than others to cause drug fever (alpha-methyldopa, quinidine,

penicillins). There is no characteristic fever pattern. There is a highly variable lag time between initiation of drug and onset of fever, and there is an infrequent association with rash or eosinophilia. Some drugs may cause fever by virtue of physiologic side effects. Anticholinergic drugs may decrease sweating and diminish the body's ability to cool itself. Chronic salicylate intoxication can cause increased heat production by uncoupling oxidative phosphorylation.

KAWASAKI SYNDROME

Kawasaki syndrome may present with a variety of signs, including rash, lymphadenopathy, conjunctival hyperemia, strawberry tongue, erythematous lips, swelling of hands and feet, arthralgia, arthritis, myocarditis, late desquamation of hands, feet, and perineal area, and sterile pyuria (see Chapters 48 and 57). Fever may be high and spiking. Diagnosis is by fulfillment of clinical criteria. ESR may be greatly elevated. While blood cells may be increased with left shift. Platelets are also elevated. Treatment is with intravenous gamma globulin and aspirin.

INFLAMMATORY BOWEL DISEASE

Inflammatory bowel disease (ulcerative colitis, Crohn disease) may present with FUO. Ulcerative colitis may present with bloody diarrhea, fever, fecal urgency, and straining (see Chapter 19). Pyoderma gangrenosum, arthritis, and erythema nodosum can also be seen. Diagnosis is made by radiographic studies and colonoscopy. Treatment is supportive and includes topical or systemic steroids or enteric anti-inflammatory agents. Crohn disease (regional enteritis) may present with abdominal pain, fever, anorexia, and growth failure. Diarrhea may develop later. Arthritis, erythema nodosum, and finger clubbing may also occur. Diagnosis is by radiographic studies. ESR is usually elevated. Treatment is with prednisone.

PHEOCHROMOCYTOMA

Pheochromocytomas are rare catecholamine-secreting tumors; 10% occur in children. These tumors manifest with paroxysmal or sustained hypertension, headache, excessive sweating, fever, hyperglycemia, and palpitations. The tumors are usually in the adrenal medulla, but 35% of those occurring in children are multiple or extra-adrenal. Diagnosis is by 24-hour urinary metanephrine collection. Localization of tumor is by CT, MRI, or ^{131}I-metaiodobenzylguanidine scanning. Treatment is surgical removal. Preoperative volume loading with alpha- and beta-adrenergic blockade is indicated.

THYROTOXICOSIS

Hyperthyroid states may present with FUO. Children usually have multiple symptoms, such as irritability, tremor, eyelid lag, and exophthalmos. Diagnosis is made by thyroid function studies.

FACTITIOUS FEVER

Factitious fever may be a form of Munchausen syndrome or Munchausen syndrome by proxy (see Chapter 37). A variety of techniques have been used to falsely elevate a recorded temperature. A mercury thermometer may be rubbed between hands or placed near a light bulb when the patient is unobserved. Hot liquids may be placed in the mouth before an oral temperature is taken. Hot rectal douches have also been reported to raise a rectally taken temperature. Even with pathologic fevers there is some circadian rhythm to the temperature curve; with factitious fever there is no rhythm. In addition, there is usually no vasoconstriction, sweating, tachypnea, or tachycardia. If factitious fever is suspected, temperature should be obtained while observing the patient. Temperature of freshly voided urine can also be recorded.

Other patients may produce actual diseases that cause true fevers, such as by injecting infected pyogenic material subcutaneously or intravenously or by taking toxic levels of thyroid hormone. Once the diagnosis is documented, psychiatric care is indicated.

PATIENTS IN WHOM NO DIAGNOSIS IS MADE

If no diagnosis is made, most patients are clinically well and asymptomatic on follow-up. Some may be determined to be healthy from the start, most are in good health at follow-up, while few have symptoms at the end of evaluation. Some may have relapses of fever for a few months.

SUMMARY AND RED FLAGS

Work-up of patients with FUO should proceed in a stepwise manner. It should be kept in mind that many patients with FUO have unusual, atypical, or complicated manifestations of common childhood illness (mainly infectious). Initial evaluation should include blood and urine cultures, chest radiograph, complete blood count with differential, ESR, purified protein derivative with controls, and EBV titers (see Fig. 56–1). Further testing should be done only if directed by repeated histories and physical examinations. The outcome of undiagnosed patients appears to be favorable in general, and these should be followed clinically.

Red flags include weight loss, night sweats, exposure to infected patients, locations, animals, medications, focal findings on examination, signs of organ system dysfunction or failure (bone marrow, liver, renal), a positive family history, and unstable vital signs suggestive of sepsis. Only in this latter category should a rapid diagnostic approach be performed and empirical antibiotic therapy initiated. In most situations, immediate or empirical antimicrobial therapy is not indicated. However, once the diagnosis of FUO is suspected and the fever pattern documented, the febrile response may be attenuated with nonaspirin nonsteroidal anti-inflammatory agents or acetaminophen in antipyretic doses.

REFERENCES

Brevis EG. Undiagnosed fever. Br Med J 1965;9:107–109.

Brusch JL, Weinstein L. Fever of unknown origin. Med Clin North Am 1988;72:1247–1261.

Doyle M, Pickering LK. Is this child's fever a worry? Postgrad Med 1989;85:207–222.

Feigin RD, Shearer WT. Fever of unknown origin in children. Curr Probl Pediatr 1976;10:2–65, quoting Hoeprich PD. Manifestations of infectious diseases. *In* Hoeprich PD (ed). Infectious Diseases. New York: Harper & Row, 1972:57.

Fisher MC. Conjunctivitis in children. Pediatr Clin North Am 1987; 34:1447–1456.

Gartner JC Jr. Fever of unknown origin. Adv Pediatr Infect Dis 1992;7:1–24.

Jacobs JC. Pediatric Rheumatology for the Practitioner. New York: Springer-Verlag, 1993;76, 245, 435, 530, 562, 566.

Lange WR, Warnock-Eckhart E, Bean ME. Mycobacterium tuberculosis infection in foreign born adoptees. Pediatr Infect Dis J 1989;8:625–629.

Lohr JA, Hendley JO. Prolonged fever of unknown origin. Clin Pediatr 1977;16:768–773.

Mackowiak PA, LeMaistre CF. Drug fever: A critical appraisal of conventional concepts. Ann Intern Med 1987;106:728–733.

Manger WM, Gifford RW. Pheochromocytoma: Current diagnosis and management. Cleve Clin J Med 1993;60:365–378.

McClung MC. Prolonged fever of unknown origin in children. Am J Dis Child 1972;124:544–550.

McCrea W, Findley LJ, Melia WM. A case of factitious fever and 'epilepsy.' J R Army Med Corps 1992;138:135–137.

Petersdorf RG, Beeson PB. Fever of unexplained origin: Report on 100 cases. Medicine 1961;40:1–30.

Pizzo PA, Lovejoy FH, Smith DH. Prolonged fever in children: Review of 100 cases. Pediatrics 1975;55:468–473.

Rakover Y, Adar H, Tal I, et al. Behçet disease: Long-term follow-up of three children and review of the literature. Pediatrics 1989;83:986–992.

Reid BS, Bender TM. Radiographic evaluation of children with urinary tract infection. Radiol Clin North Am 1988;26:393–407.

Saxe SE, Gardner P. The returning traveler with fever. Infect Dis Clin North Am 1992;6:427–439.

Steele RW, Jones SM, Lowe BA, et al. Usefulness of scanning procedures for diagnosis of fever of unknown origin in children. J Pediatr 1991;119:526–530.

57 Fever and Rash

Robert M. Lembo

Fever and rash are each protean manifestations of multiple diseases. Their coexistence suggests a more narrow spectrum of pathologic entities for diagnostic consideration. This spectrum includes both local and disseminated infection with a wide range of microbial pathogens; toxin-mediated disorders, including those associated with bacterial superantigen production; and the vasculitides (see Chapter 58), including hypersensitivity disorders. The essential elements for accurate diagnosis in the infant, child, or adolescent presenting with fever and rash include a detailed history, a careful systematic observation of the patient for evidence of toxicity, and a thorough physical examination. Because this approach lacks perfect sensitivity, however, the laboratory plays an important role.

A morphologic nomenclature of cutaneous manifestations helps in documentation, classification, and communication regarding this group of disorders (Figs. 57–1 to 57–8). For more detail, see Chapter 58.

ASSESSMENT

History

The history generates hypotheses regarding etiology based on the specific features and temporal aspects of the present illness combined with a thorough understanding of the pathobiology, epidemiology, and clinical course of specific diseases that might have caused it. The history also includes an analysis of host immunocompetence through a careful elicitation of the patient's medical history and the family history, a review of systems, and an analysis of risk through a careful epidemiologic and social history.

Key elements of the history are summarized in Table 57–1. Information about the features of the rash includes when it occurred in relation to the fever, its evolution or progression, and its location

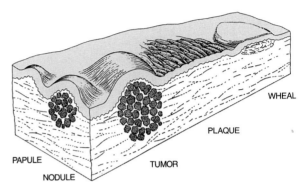

Figure 57–2. Primary lesions. Palpable, elevated, solid masses. (From Swartz MH. Textbook of Physical Diagnosis: History and Examination. Philadelphia: WB Saunders, 1989:92.)

and distribution. Information from the epidemiologic and social history should include exposure to known ill contacts at home, day care, school, or, for some adolescents, work; recent travel or exposure to individuals from different geographic areas; exposure to pets, wildlife, or insects; recent immunizations; a detailed list of medications both prescribed specifically for the patient and medications available to the patient in the home; blood transfusion; and, for the adolescent patient, intravenous drug use and sexual activity.

The past medical and family history should assess the overall health of the patient over time as well as that of family members to determine the possibility of underlying disorders associated with primary or acquired immunodeficiency or diseases associated with autoimmunity or chronic inflammation. A history of increased susceptibility to infection, as manifested by chronic or recurrent infectious illnesses after infancy, such as pneumonia, sinusitis, bronchitis, otitis media, diarrhea, and bacteremia, is an important indicator of underlying immunodeficiency disease (see Chapter 52).

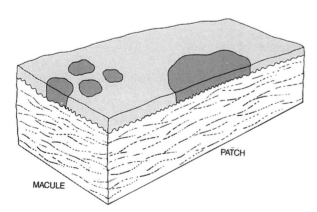

Figure 57–1. Primary lesions. Flat, nonpalpable. (From Swartz MH. Textbook of Physical Diagnosis. History and Examination. Philadelphia: WB Saunders, 1989:92.)

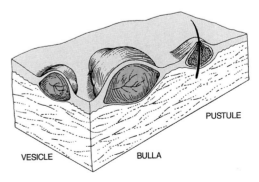

Figure 57–3. Primary lesions. Palpable, elevated, fluid-filled masses. (From Swartz MH. Textbook of Physical Diagnosis: History and Examination. Philadelphia: WB Saunders, 1989:93.)

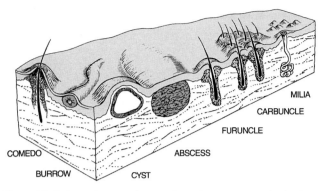

Figure 57–4. Special primary lesions. (From Swartz MH. Textbook of Physical Diagnosis: History and Examination. Philadelphia: WB Saunders, 1989:93.)

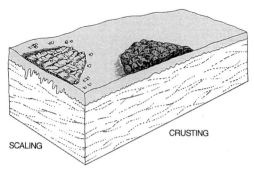

Figure 57–6. Secondary lesions above the skin plane. (From Swartz MH. Textbook of Physical Diagnosis: History and Examination. Philadelphia: WB Saunders, 1989:94.)

Additionally, the occurrence of an unusually severe infection or an infection with a pathogen of low virulence (e.g., *Pneumocystis carinii*) should raise suspicion of an immunodeficiency state. A history of hemolytic anemia, leukopenia, thrombocytopenia, or arthritis suggests an autoimmune disorder or malignancy, which may also be associated with an impairment in immune function (see Chapter 45).

A thorough systems review should assess the probability of a subacute or chronic underlying infectious, inflammatory, or malignant disease by inquiring about such symptoms as anorexia, nausea, vomiting, weight loss, night sweats, fatigue, cough, and exercise intolerance. Symptoms suggesting multisystem disease, such as myalgias, arthralgia, headache, precordial pain or pain with inspiration, abdominal pain, jaundice, skin photosensitivity, peripheral edema, alopecia, Raynaud phenomenon, and hematuria, should also be sought. In patients with symptoms that suggest the presence of multisystem disease, a thorough survey of the functional status of the central, peripheral, and autonomic nervous systems is clinically relevant. Specific inquiries into visual disturbances, photophobia, disordered mentation, neck stiffness, paraesthesia, weakness, or seizure activity are essential and may reveal potentially life-threatening infection within the central nervous system or the vasculature of the brain, or a systemic vasculitis involving the nervous system, such as systemic lupus erythematosus (SLE) or polyarteritis nodosa.

Examination

The physical examination of the patient with fever and rash is used to refine the probability of underlying serious illness, as estimated by the history and the Acute Illness Observation Score, which is especially useful in infants younger than 24 months of age with fever. The examination should narrow the range of etiologic considerations by gathering information specific to a particular diagnosis. Key elements of the physical examination are summarized in Table 57–2 (see also Chapters 58 and 59).

A critical first step is an assessment of the patient's vital signs. The highest point of the fever is an important indicator of underlying serious illness. Approximately 7.3% of children younger than 24 months of age with a fever of 40°C (104°F) or greater (with or without a rash) at the time of initial presentation are bacteremic, and the sensitivity and specificity of this finding for bacteremia in this age group are approximately 57% and 75%, respectively. Therefore, for purposes of clinical decision making, all children with hyperpyrexia should be considered to be at high risk for bacteremia or other serious illnesses.

Table 57–1. Essential Elements of the History in the Clinical Assessment of Fever and Rash

Demographic Data
  Age
  Gender
  Race
  Season
  Geographic area

Exposures
  Ill contacts (home, day care, school, work place)
  Sexual contacts
  Travel
  Pets, wildlife, insects (especially ticks)
  Medications and drugs
  Transfusions
  Immunizations

Features of Rash
  Temporal associations (onset relative to fever)
  Progression and evolution
  Location and distribution
  Pain or pruritis

Associated Symptoms
  Focal (suggesting organ-specific illness)
  Systemic (suggesting generalized or multisystem illness)

Prior Health Status
  Past medical and surgical history
  Growth and development
  Recurrent infectious illnesses

Family History

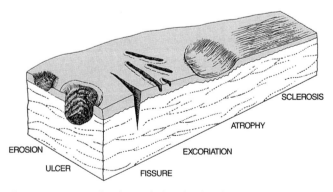

Figure 57–5. Secondary lesions below the skin plane. (From Swartz MH. Textbook of Physical Diagnosis: History and Examination. Philadelphia: WB Saunders, 1989:94.)

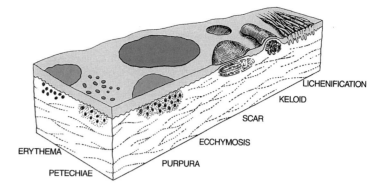

Figure 57–7. Other important dermatologic terms. (From Swartz MH. Textbook of Physical Diagnosis: History and Examination. Philadelphia: WB Saunders, 1989:95.)

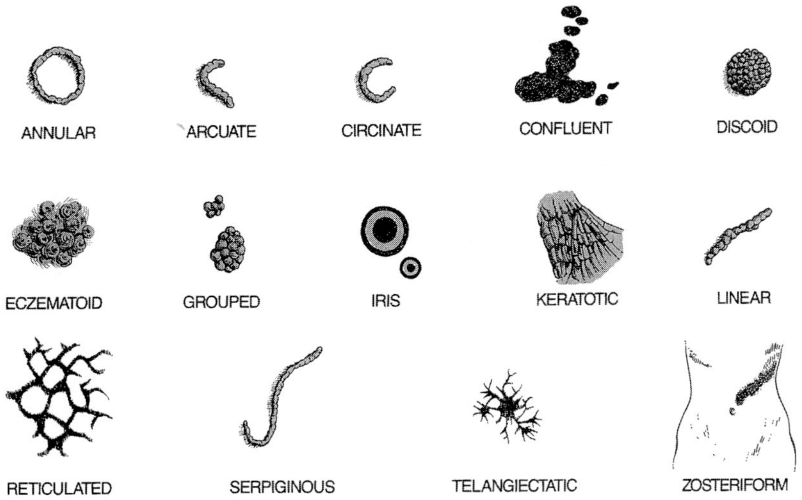

ANNULAR   ARCUATE   CIRCINATE   CONFLUENT   DISCOID

ECZEMATOID   GROUPED   IRIS   KERATOTIC   LINEAR

RETICULATED   SERPIGINOUS   TELANGIECTATIC   ZOSTERIFORM

Lesion	Description	Example
Annular	Ring shaped	Ringworm
Arcuate	Partial rings	Syphilis
Bizarre	Irregular or geographic pattern not related to any underlying anatomic structure	Factitial dermatitis
Circinate	Circular	
Confluent	Lesions run together	Childhood exanthems
Discoid	Disc shaped without central clearing	Lupus erythematosus
Discrete	Lesions remain separate	
Eczematoid	An inflammation with a tendency to vesiculate and crust	Eczema
Generalized	Widespread	
Grouped	Lesions clustered together	Herpes simplex
Iris	Circle within a circle; a bull's-eye lesion	Erythema multiforme (iris)
Keratotic	Horny thickening	Psoriasis
Linear	In lines	Poison ivy dermatitis
Multiform	More than one type of shape or lesion	Erythema multiforme
Papulosquamous	Papules or plaques associated with scaling	Psoriasis
Reticulated	Lace-like network	Oral lichen planus
Serpiginous	Snake-like, creeping	Cutaneous larva migrans
Telangiectatic	Relatively permanent dilatation of the superficial blood vessels	Osler-Weber-Rendu disease
Universal	Entire body involved	Alopecia universalis
Zosteriform*	Linear arrangement along a nerve distribution	Herpes zoster

*Also known as dermatomal.

Figure 57–8. Descriptive dermatologic terms. (From Swartz MH. Textbook of Physical Diagnosis: History and Examination. Philadelphia: WB Saunders, 1989:96.)

Table 57–2. Essential Elements of the Physical Examination in the Clinical Assessment of Fever and Rash

Degree of Toxicity (Acute Illness Observation Score)
  ≤10: Low risk of underlying serious illness
    (approximately 3%)
  11–15: Moderate risk of underlying serious illness
    (approximately 25%)
  >16: High risk of underlying serious illness
    (approximately 92%)

Vital Signs
  Height of fever
  Tachycardia or bradycardia
  Tachypnea
  Hypotension or hypertension

Characteristics of Rash
  Macular
  Papular
  Maculopapular
  Petechiae or purpura
  Diffuse erythroderma
    Accentuation in flexural creases
    Desquamation with stroking (Nikolsky sign)
  Localized erythroderma
    Expansile
    Painful
  Urticaria
  Vesicles, pustules, bullae
  Nodules
  Ulcers

Distribution and Localization of Rash
  Generalized or localized
  Symmetric or asymmetric
  Centripedal or centrifugal

Associated Enanthem
  Buccal mucosa
  Palate
  Pharynx and tonsils

Associated Findings (Isolated or in Clusters)
  Ocular
  Cardiac
  Pulmonary
  Gastrointestinal
  Musculoskeletal
  Reticuloendothelial
  Neurologic

The presence of tachycardia and tachypnea with a stable blood pressure in any patient with fever and rash suggests the presence of sepsis. Evidence of alteration in mental status suggests either the sepsis syndrome, which is associated with major alterations in organ system perfusion, or primary meningoencephalitis. The presence or development of hypotension usually indicates septic shock, which may lead rapidly and irreversibly to multiorgan dysfunction syndrome, although other disorders, such as toxic shock syndrome, dengue hemorrhagic shock syndrome, hemorrhagic fever with renal syndrome due to Hantavirus, and the hemorrhagic shock–encephalopathy syndrome, must also be considered in this context. Hypertension may be noted in association with vasculitic disorders involving small to medium-sized arteries, such as polyarteritis and SLE.

The clinical characteristics of the rash may be useful in establishing an etiologic diagnosis. An *exanthem* is defined as a skin eruption occurring as a sign of a generalized disease. An *enanthem* is an eruption on the mucous membranes that occurs in the context

of generalized disease, usually in association with an exanthem. Exanthems and enanthems may be macular, maculopapular, vesicular, urticarial, petechial, or diffusely erythematous. Because a wide variety of infectious agents, including viruses, bacteria, and the rickettsiae, can cause exanthems and enanthems, very few are pathognomonic (Table 57–3). Tables 57–4 and 57–5 summarize the clinical features of several common, recognizable exanthems and enanthems.

Certain skin lesions may be clues to potentially life-threatening infections. All clinicians must be particularly concerned about a patient with fever and a petechial rash, especially an infant or child younger than 24 months of age. Between 8% and 20% of these patients have an underlying bacterial infection; 7% to 10% have sepsis due to *Neisseria meningitidis* infection, whereas others may have infection with enteroviruses, particularly ECHO (enteric cytopathogenic human orphan virus) 9, *Streptococcus pneumoniae*, *Haemophilus influenzae* type b, *Rickettsia rickettsii*, and, occasionally in the western United States, *Yersinia pestis*, or they may have another disorder, such as bacterial endocarditis or a noninfectious vasculitis. Although patients with concurrent cough or emesis and petechiae confined to areas above the nipple line may be at lesser risk for bacteremic or invasive infectious disorders, this manifestation does not preclude life-threatening illness.

PURPURA

Larger areas of bleeding into the skin produce purpura. This may accompany disorders associated with disseminated intravascular coagulation (DIC), profound thrombocytopenia, or both, but can occur in their absence, as in the noninfectious vasculitides (see Chapter 58) or idiopathic thrombocytopenic purpura (ITP) associated with an intercurrent infection (see Chapter 51). Purpura followed by subsequent necrosis of skin is referred to as *purpura fulminans*, which has been reported after relatively benign infections, such as varicella or more serious disorders (meningococcemia).

DIFFUSE PURPURIC LESIONS

Diffuse purpuric lesions may be noted in a wide variety of disorders. These include, but are not limited to, infectious diseases associated with organisms with a predilection for vascular endothelium, such as *N. meningitidis* and *R. rickettsii*; virus-associated diseases, such as dengue hemorrhagic fever and the hemorrhagic fever with renal syndrome caused by the Hantavirus; infrequently encountered bacterial diseases, such as Brazilian purpuric fever due to *Haemophilus aegyptius*; and the hemorrhagic shock–encephalopathy syndrome. Discrete, raised purpuric lesions (palpable purpura) distributed predominantly over the buttocks and lower extremities also may be noted in the noninfectious vasculitis syndrome of Henoch-Schönlein. Pragmatically, however, all febrile patients presenting with diffuse or discrete purpuric lesions must be considered to be at risk for a potentially life-threatening bacteremia (Fig. 57–9).

URTICARIAL RASHES

See Chapter 58.

VESICULAR RASHES

Vesicular rashes (sharply demarcated, raised lesions containing clear fluid), bullae (vesicles exceeding 1 cm in diameter), or pus-

Text continued on page 938

Table 57–3. Differential Diagnosis of Fever and Rash

Lesion	Pathogen or Associated Factor
Maculopapular or macular rash	*Viruses* Measles (confluent)*, rubella (discrete)*, roseola (human herpesvirus-6)*, fifth disease (parvovirus)*, Epstein-Barr virus*, enteroviruses*, hepatitis B virus (papular acrodermatitis or Gianotti-Crosti syndrome), human immunodeficiency virus, dengue virus, adenovirus *Bacteria* Rheumatic fever (group A streptococcus), scarlet fever, erysipelas, *Arcanobacterium haemolyticus*, secondary syphilis, leptospirosis, *Pseudomonas,* meningococcal infection (early), *Salmonella,* Lyme disease, *Mycoplasma pneumoniae*, Listeria monocytogenes* *Rickettsia* Early Rocky Mountain spotted fever, typhus (scrub, endemic), ehrlichiosis *Other* Kawasaki disease*, *Coccidioides immitis*
Diffuse erythroderma	*Bacteria* Scarlet fever (group A streptococcus)*, other streptococci, toxic shock syndrome *(Staphylococcus aureus)*, staphylococcal scarlet fever *Fungi* *Candida albicans*
Urticarial rash	*Viruses* Epstein-Barr virus, hepatitis B, human immunodeficiency virus, enteroviruses *Bacteria* *Mycoplasma pneumoniae,* group A streptococci, *Shigella,* meningococcus, *Yersinia* *Other* Various parasites, insect bites, food-drug allergens (usually afebrile)
Vesicular, bullous, pustular	*Viruses* Herpes simplex*, varicella-zoster*, coxsackieviruses A and B*, ECHO virus *Bacteria* Staphylococcal scalded skin syndrome, staphylococcal bullous impetigo, group A streptococcal crusted impetigo *Other* Toxic epidermal necrolysis, erythema multiforme (Stevens-Johnson syndrome)*, rickettsialpox
Petechial-purpuric	*Viruses* Atypical measles, congenital rubella, cytomegalovirus, enterovirus, human immunodeficiency virus, hemorrhagic fever viruses, hemorrhagic varicella *Bacteria* Sepsis (meningococcal*, gonococcal, pneumococcal*, *Haemophilus influenzae*)*, endocarditis, *Pseudomonas aeruginosa* *Rickettsiae* Rocky Mountain spotted fever*, epidemic typhus, ehrlichiosis *Other* Vasculitis, thrombocytopenia, Henoch-Schönlein purpura*, malaria
Erythema nodosum	*Viruses* Epstein-Barr, hepatitis B *Bacteria* Group A streptococcus, tuberculosis, *Yersinia,* cat-scratch disease *Fungi* Coccidioidomycosis, histoplasmosis *Other* Sarcoidosis, inflammatory bowel disease, estrogen-containing oral contraceptives, systemic lupus erythematosus, Behçet disease
Distinctive rashes Ecthyma gangrenosum	*Pseudomonas aeruginosa*
Erythema chronicum migrans	Lyme disease
Necrotic eschar	Aspergillosis, mucormycosis
Erysipelas	Group A streptococcus
Koplik spots	Measles

Modified from Prince A. Infectious diesases. *In* Behrman RE, Kliegman RM (eds). Nelson Essentials of Pediatrics, 2nd ed. Philadelphia: WB Saunders, 1994:299.
*Common.
Abbreviation: ECHO = enteric cytopathogenic human orphan virus.

Table 57-4. Common Bacterial Exanthems

Disease	Etiology	Age	Season	Transmission	Incubation (Days)	Prodrome	Features and Rash Morphology	Enanthem	Complications	Prevention	Comments
Scarlet fever	Group A streptococcus	School age	Fall, winter, spring	Direct contact, droplets	1–4	Sore throat, headache, abdominal pain, cervical lymphadenopathy; fever, 0–2 days, acute onset	Diffuse erythema with "sandpaper" feel and "goose flesh" appearance; accentuation of erythema in flexural creases (Pastia lines); circumoral pallor; lasts 2–7 days; may exfoliate	Palatal petechia, strawberry tongue	Peritonsillar abscess, rheumatic fever, glomerulonephritis	Prevent rheumatic fever with penicillin within 10 days of onset of pharyngitis; treat with penicillin	Similar rash may be noted with *Arcanobacterium haemolyticum* in adolescents; group A streptococci may also produce toxic shock or true bacteremic shock syndromes in addition to cellulitis, lymphangitis, and erysipelas; *S. aureus* may produce a scarlatiniform rash
Scalded skin syndrome (see Fig. 57–11)	*Staphylococcus aureus* producing exfoliative toxin	Neonates and infants	Any	Colonization, contact	Unknown	None	Sudden onset, tender erythroderma progressing to diffuse flaccid bullae; significant perioral, perinasal peeling; eventual diffuse exfoliation (positive Nikolsky sign); possibly fever, conjunctivitis, rhinorrhea	Unusual	Shock	Treat with intravenous nafcillin or vancomycin if methicillin-resistant *S. aureus*	
Toxic shock syndrome	*S. aureus* producing toxic shock syndrome toxins	Usually adolescent females if menstrual; others variable	Any	Colonization, contact	Variable, often 1–5	Myalgias or preceding viral croup or pneumonia if biphasic. May be secondary to wound infection	Diffuse sunburn-like erythroderma; hypotension (may be orthostatic), diarrhea, emesis, mental confusion; late desquamation	Conjunctivitis	Shock, multisystem organ dysfunction. Systemic inflammatory response syndrome	Treat with intravenous nafcillin (vancomycin if resistant), plus intravenous fluids, dopamine; possible IVIG or steroids; prevent by frequent changes of tampon	

934

Disease	Organism	Age	Season	Transmission	Incubation (days)	Symptoms	Rash	Petechiae	Complications	Treatment/Prevention	Differential Diagnosis
Meningococcemia (see Fig. 57–9)	*Neisseria meningitidis*	Any (<5 yr)	Winter/spring, follows influenza epidemics	Close, prolonged contact	5–15	Fever, malaise, myalgia, 1–10 days	Erythematous, nonconfluent, discrete papules (early); petechiae, purpura, ecchymosis present on trunk, extremities, palms, soles	Petechiae	Shock, meningitis, pericarditis, arthritis, endophthalmitis, gangrene. DIC	Contacts—rifampin; general—vaccine; treat with ceftriaxone, cefotaxime, penicillin (if sensitive)	*Neisseria gonorrhoeae*, pneumococcus, *H. influenzae* type b, group A streptococci may produce similar clinical manifestations
Rocky Mountain spotted fever	*Rickettsia rickettsii*	Any (>5 yr) Males > female	Summer	Carrier ticks	3–12	Fever, myalgia, headache, malaise, ill appearance, 2–4 days	Early maculopapular, then petechial or rarely purpuric; present on extremities, palms and soles, trunk	Petechiae variable	Shock, myocarditis, encephalitis, pneumonia	Remove ticks as soon as possible; use tick repellants; treat with doxycycline	*Ehrlichia canis* and other rickettsiae may produce similar illnesses with or without a rash
Rickettsialpox	*Rickettsia akari*	Any	Any	Blood-sucking mite	7–14	Fever, chills, headache, malaise, 4–7 days	At primary bite site, eschar; secondary papulovesicles in same stage throughout illness; fewer vesicles than in chickenpox (5–30); present on trunk and proximal extremities	Unknown	Usually none	Treat with doxycycline	Often confused with chickenpox—may be more common than expected, especially in crowded urban settings with poor housing

Abbreviations: DIC = disseminated intravascular coagulation; IVIG = intravenous immune globulin.

935

Table 57-5. Common Viral Exanthems

Disease	Etiology	Age	Season	Transmission	Incubation (Days)	Prodrome	Features and Rash Morphology	Enanthem	Complications	Prevention	Comments
Measles (rubeola)	Measles virus	Infants, adolescents	Winter/spring	Respiratory droplet	10–12	High fever, cough, coryza, conjunctivitis, 2–4 days	Maculopapular (confluent), begins on face, spreads to trunk; lasts 3–6 days Brown color develops; fine desquamation; toxic, uncomfortable appearance, photophobia; rash may be absent in HIV infection	Koplik spots on buccal mucosa before rash	Febrile seizures, otitis, pneumonia, encephalitis, laryngo-tracheitis, thrombocytopenia; delayed subacute sclerosing panencephalitis	General: measles vaccine at 12–15 months, and again by 12 yr Exposure: measles vaccine if within 72 hr; immune serum globulin if within 6 days (must then wait 5–6 mo to vaccinate)	Reportable to public health department; epidemics reported, contagious 3 days before symptoms and to 4 days after rash
Rubella (German measles (minor measles) (see Fig. 57-14)	Rubella virus	Infants, young adults	Winter/spring	Respiratory droplet	14–21	Malaise, low-grade fever (<101°F), posterior auricular-cervical, occipital adenopathy, 0–4 days	Discrete, nonconfluent, rose-colored macules and papules, begins on face and spreads downward; lasts 1–3 days	Variable erythematous macules on soft palate	Arthritis, thrombocytopenia, encephalopathy; fetal embryopathy	General: rubella vaccine at 12–15 months and again by 12 yr; exposure: possibly immune serum globulin	Reportable to public health department; epidemics reported, contagious 2 days before symptoms and 5–7 days after rash
Roseola (exanthem subitum)	Human herpesvirus-6	Infants- (6 mo–2 yr)	Any	Unknown; saliva of asymptomatic carrier?	5–15 (?)	Irritability, high fever 3–4 days, cervical, occipital adenopathy	Discrete macules on trunk, neck; sudden onset rash with defervescence; lasts 0.5–2 days; some have no rash	Variable erythematous macules on soft palate	Single or recurrent febrile seizures; hemophagocytic syndrome; encephalopathy; dissemination (e.g., liver, CNS, lung) in immunosuppressed patients	None	No epidemics
Fifth disease (erythema infectiosum) (see Fig. 57-12)	Parvovirus B19	Prepubertal children, school teachers	Winter/spring	Respiratory droplets; blood transfusion, placenta	5–15	Headache, malaise, myalgia, often afebrile	Local erythema of cheeks (slapped cheeks); lacy pink-red erythema of trunk and extremities, ± pruritus; rash may lag prodrome by 3–7 days; lasts 2–4 days, may recur 2–3 wks later	None	Arthritis, aplastic crisis in patients with chronic hemolytic anemia (e.g., sickle cell), fetal anemic hydrops, vasculitis, Wegener granulomatosus	Isolation of patients with aplastic crisis but not normal host with fifth disease	Epidemics reported; once rash is present, the normal host is not contagious; patients with aplastic crisis often have no rash

Disease	Agent	Age	Season	Transmission	Incubation (days)	Prodrome	Rash	Enanthem	Complications	Prevention	Comments
Chickenpox (varicella) (see Fig. 57–10)	Varicella-zoster virus	1–14 yr	Late fall, winter, early spring	Respiratory droplet	12–21	Fever	Pruritic papules, vesicles in various stages; 2–4 crops then crusts; distributed on trunk, then face, extremities; lasts 7–10 days; recurs years later in dermatomal distribution (zoster, shingles)	Oral mucosa, tongue	Staphylococcal or streptococcal skin infection, arthritis, cerebellar ataxia, thrombocytopenia, Reye syndrome (with aspirin), myocarditis, nephritis, hepatitis, pneumonia; dissemination in immuno-compromised patients; fetal embryopathy	VZIG for exposed immunosuppressed patients, susceptible pregnant women, preterm neonates, and infants at birth whose mother developed varicella 5 days before and 2 days after birth; active immunization possible with live attenuated vaccine	Acyclovir for therapy for immuno-suppressed and possibly normal patients (controversial); contagious 1–2 days before rash and 5 days after rash (usually no longer contagious when all lesions are crusted and no new lesions appear)
Enteroviruses	Coxsackievirus, ECHO and others	Infants, young children	Summer/fall	Fecal-oral	4–6	Variable—irritable, fever, sore throat, myalgias, headache	Hand-foot-mouth—vesicles in those locations; others: nonspecific, usually fine, nonconfluent, macular or maculopapular rash, rarely petechial, urticarial, or vesicular; lasts 3–7 days	Yes	Aseptic meningitis, hepatitis, myocarditis, pleurodynia, paralysis: usually in younger patients	None	Rash may appear with fever or after defervescence; rash may be present in <50% of entero-viral illnesses; epidemics possible, contagious up to 2 wk
Mononucleosis	Epstein-Barr virus	Children, adolescents	Any	Close contact, saliva, blood transfusion	28–49	Fever, adenopathy, eyelid edema, sore throat, hepatosplenomegaly, malaise. Lymphocytosis	Maculopapular, or morbilliform on trunk, extremities. May be confluent. Often elicited by simultaneous administration of ampicillin or allopurinol. Rash in 15%, and in 50% with drug-induced form; lasts 2–7 days	Variable	Anemia, thrombocytopenia, aplastic anemia, hepatitis; rarely hemophagocytic syndrome, lymphoproliferative syndrome	None	Cytomegalovirus and toxoplasmosis also produce mononucleosis-like illnesses; monospot or heterophile tests will be negative
Gianotti-Crosti syndrome (papular acrodermatitis of childhood)	Hepatitis B, Epstein-Barr, other	1–6 yr	Any	Variable. Fecal, sexual, blood products for hepatitis B.	Unknown. 50–180 days for hepatitis B.	Usually none except for specific viral disease; arthritis-arthralgia for hepatitis B	Papules, papulovesicles, discrete or confluent. Face, arms, extremities, often spares trunk; lasts 4–10 days	Variable	As per specific disease	Hepatitis B = HBIG plus vaccine	

Abbreviations: VZIG = varicella-zoster immune globulin; HBIG = hepatitis B virus immune globulin; CNS = central nervous system; HIV = human immunodeficiency virus.

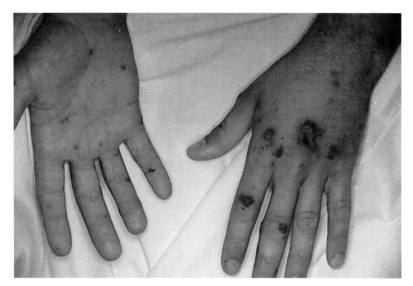

Figure 57-9. Purpuric lesions with sharply marginated borders on the hands of a patient with meningococcemia. (Courtesy of Department of Dermatology, Yale University School of Medicine.)

tules (raised lesions containing cloudy fluid composed of serum and inflammatory cells) may suggest focal or disseminated infection with various pathogens. Localized vesicles may signify infection with herpes simplex virus type 1 or 2 (especially if the vesicles are grouped on an erythematous base) or varicella-zoster virus (especially if grouped vesicles are distributed in a dermatomal pattern) (Fig. 57–10), or infection with nonviral pathogens, such as *Rickettsia akari* (the cause of rickettsialpox) and *Rickettsia tsutsugamushi* (the cause of scrub typhus). Localized pustules and bullae usually suggest pyodermas caused by *Staphylococcus aureus,* but pustular lesions distributed on the palms and soles in the context of fever may represent infective emboli with microabscess formation (Janeway lesions), which is often due to *S. aureus* bacteremia, or represent disseminated infection with *Neisseria gonorrhoeae* in a sexually active menstruating female.

Vesicles distributed in a more generalized pattern, especially with a concentration of lesions over the head and trunk, suggest primary varicella-zoster virus infection (chickenpox), whereas a more generalized pattern with a concentration over the extremities suggests enteroviral infection, especially with coxsackievirus A16 (hand-foot-mouth disease). The clinician evaluating the sexually active patient presenting with asymmetric generalized vesicles or pustules should also consider the diagnosis of disseminated infection with *N. gonorrhoeae.* Diffuse vesiculobullae also may be noted in Stevens-Johnson syndrome, a hypersensitivity syndrome with significant constitutional symptoms.

NODULES

Nodules (discrete, raised, firm, well-demarcated lesions without fixation to the overlying skin) may be associated with a number of

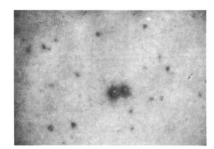

Figure 57-10. Skin lesions of chickenpox. Note the varying stages of development (macules, papules, and vesicles) present at the same time. (Courtesy of P. F. Lucchesi, M.D.)

underlying infectious or inflammatory disorders, such as polyarteritis and, rarely in children, Sweet syndrome (febrile neutrophilic dermatosis). Importantly, red, pink, or plum-colored nodules distributed in a seemingly random fashion over the skin surface may represent leukemic infiltrates.

Erythema nodosum (erythematous and painful nodules usually distributed over the extremities) may be associated with bacterial infectious agents, such as *S. pneumoniae* and *Yersinia* species, mycobacterial infections, fungal infections with *Candida* species, *Histoplasma capsulatum, Cryptococcus neoformans,* or *Coccidioides immitis,* or drug reactions, especially in response to sulfonamides. Non-erythematous and nontender subcutaneous nodules may also be noted in acute rheumatic fever, polyarticular JRA, and dermatomyositis.

ULCERS

Ulcers are depressed lesions in which the epidermis and some or all of the dermis has been destroyed. In immunocompromised hosts, infection with herpes simplex virus may present with shallow erosive or ulcerative, as opposed to vesicular, lesions. In immunocompetent hosts, cutaneous ulcerations may be noted in noninfectious disorders associated with vasculitis, such as SLE, polyarteritis nodosa, and Henoch-Schönlein purpura.

Pyoderma gangrenosum and *ecthyma gangrenosum* are painful cutaneous ulcerative lesions with an erythematous, raised edge. The lesion usually begins as a papule and breaks down rapidly with central necrosis. It may be seen in immunocompromised patients with systemic infections due to bacterial pathogens, such as *Pseudomonas aeruginosa* and *Xanthomonas maltophila* (ecthyma). In immunocompetent patients, the lesion may present in the context of inflammatory bowel disease (pyoderma gangrenosum) or rheumatoid arthritis. Digital ulcerations may be noted in patients with small-vessel vasculitis, such as SLE. Oral ulcerations may be noted in those with common infections with herpes simplex or coxsackievirus (hand-foot-mouth disease) or as a manifestation of inflammatory bowel disease.

ERYTHEMA

Diffuse erythema is most likely associated with toxin-mediated disorders characterized by superantigen production (see Tables

57–3 and 57–4). Nonspecific T-cell stimulation caused by superantigen production results in several acute rash-fever disorders, such as the staphylococcal scalded skin syndrome (Fig. 57–11), streptococcal scarlet fever, staphylococcal and streptococcal toxic shock syndromes, and possibly, Kawasaki syndrome.

Localized erythema in the context of acute fever is strongly suggestive of cellulitis or abscess. The presence of warmth and tenderness on palpation and, on occasion, associated lymphangitis is highly indicative. Organisms causing cellulitis or abscess formation are usually inoculated directly into the skin as a result of trauma. However, bacteremic localization is well described among young children with preseptal or facial cellulitis associated with *H. influenzae* type b or *S. pneumoniae*.

Patients with SLE may present with an isolated erythematous malar rash (butterfly rash), which is exacerbated by exposure to sunlight. However, the acute onset of intense "slapped cheek" erythema of the face suggests erythema infectiosum, a recognizable exanthem caused by parvovirus B19, and should be differentiated easily from the malar rash of SLE, which usually manifests other characteristics, such as hyperkeratosis and follicular plugging. Additionally, patients with erythema infectiosum tend to have a maculopapular lace-like rash over the arms, which may spread to the buttocks and thighs (Fig. 57–12; see also Table 57–5).

Patients with dermatomyositis may have localized lilac-colored lesions over the eyelids (heliotrope rash), which may be associated with periorbital edema. Such patients characteristically, but not invariably, have an erythematous, scaly eruption on the face, neck, knees, elbows, and phalanges. When the rash is localized over the knuckles, it resembles dripped wax and has been referred to as "Gottron papules."

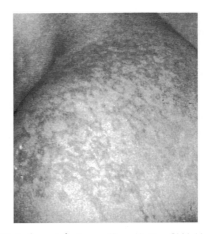

Figure 57–12. Erythema infectiosum. (From Korting GW. Hautkrankheiten bei Kindern und Jugendlichen, 3rd ed. Stuttgart, Germany: FK Schattauer Verlag, 1982.)

ERYTHEMA MULTIFORME

Erythema multiforme refers to a hypersensitivity syndrome that manifests skin lesions, with or without mucosal involvement (see Chapter 58). The lesions are erythematous and demonstrate polymorphous characteristics. The basic lesions are macular (flat and discrete), urticarial, and vesiculobullous and are symmetrically distributed, especially over the palms, soles, and extensor surfaces of

the extremities. The primary lesion is an erythematous macule or urticarial lesion in which a central papule, vesicle, or fine petechiae develops. Subsequently, the central portion clears and a target ("iris") lesion, with concentric rings of alternating erythema and cyanosis, is apparent (Fig. 57–13). The presence of these characteristic lesions on the skin and, at most, one mucosal surface (usually the oral mucosa) in the acutely febrile child is characteristic of erythema multiforme minor. The presence of predominantly vesicobullous skin lesions involving two or more mucosal surfaces is characteristic of erythema multiforme major, a more severe form

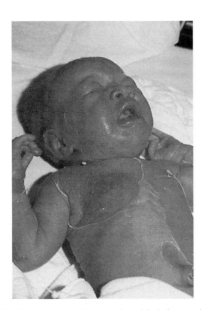

Figure 57–11. Infant with staphylococcal scalded skin syndrome. (From Behrman RE (ed). Nelson Textbook of Pediatrics, 14th ed. Philadelphia: WB Saunders, 1992.)

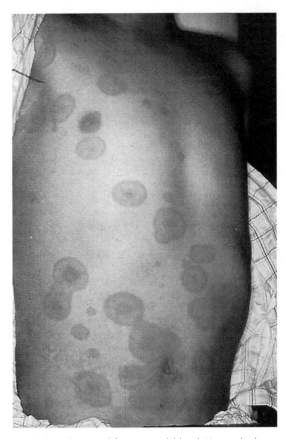

Figure 57–13. Erythema multiforme in a child with Kawasaki disease. (Courtesy of Tomisaku Kawasaki, M.D.)

of this hypersensitivity syndrome (Stevens-Johnson syndrome). Recurrent erythema multiforme minor has been associated with herpes simplex virus infection, whereas the development of erythema multiforme major has been associated with *M. pneumoniae* infection and exposure to drugs, including penicillins, sulfonamides, and anticonvulsants.

TOXIC EPIDERMAL NECROLYSIS

Toxic epidermal necrolysis, an exfoliative dermatosis characterized by diffuse cutaneous erythema and full-thickness necrosis of the epidermis resembling a scald injury may be an extremely severe form of erythema multiforme major. It is usually associated with exposure to drugs and differs histopathologically from staphylococcal scalded skin syndrome, which also presents clinically with diffuse erythema and blistering, in its cleavage plane (see Table 57–4). In scalded skin syndrome, blistering is produced more superficially by disruption of the epidermal granular cell layer in response to one of two staphylococcal epidermolytic toxins (ET-A or ET-B). This results in easy disruption of skin with firm rubbing (Nikolsky sign).

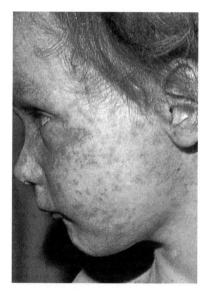

Figure 57–14. Rash of rubella (German measles). (From Korting GW. *Hautkrankheiten bei Kindern und Jugendlichen*, 3rd ed. Stuttgart, Germany: FK Schattauer Verlag, 1982.)

NONSPECIFIC MACULOPAPULAR ERUPTIONS

Unfortunately, most fever-rash syndromes are characterized by nonspecific maculopapular eruptions, which rarely assist the clinician in establishing a specific diagnosis or in decision making. Although some experienced clinicians believe that characterizing the maculopapular eruption as *rubelliform* (generalized discrete maculopapular rash) or *morbilliform* (generalized confluent maculopapular rash) is of help diagnostically, prospective use of this classification suggests that the clinical features of the rash at presentation are unhelpful in defining the causative agent.

STAR COMPLEX

A valuable cluster of associated findings is the STAR complex—*s*ore throat (pharyngitis), elevated *t*emperature, moderate to severe *a*rthritis, and *r*ash, which may be pruritic or urticarial, in the absence of signs of carditis, serositis, meningitis, adenopathy, or reticuloendothelial hyperplasia on physical examination. Short-duration (<3 weeks) STAR complex is associated usually with an infection caused by known viral agents, such as rubella (Fig. 57–14), parvovirus B19, hepatitis B virus, adenovirus, Epstein-Barr virus, and the enteroviruses; Lyme disease; or serum sickness associated with exposure to cefaclor, penicillin, or the combination of trimethoprim and sulfamethoxazole. STAR complex of intermediate duration (3 to 6 weeks) suggests acute rheumatic fever, and that of long duration (>6 weeks) suggests systemic JRA.

OTHER CLUSTERS OF FINDINGS

Other clusters of findings that are of diagnostic importance include:

1. The mucocutaneous-lymph node cluster (bilateral conjunctival injection, palmar-plantar erythema/indurative edema of the hands and feet, erythema of the oropharyngeal mucosa/ "strawberry" tongue, cervical lymphadenopathy), which suggests

Kawasaki syndrome, toxic shock syndrome, Stevens-Johnson syndrome, streptococcal scarlet fever, Rocky Mountain spotted fever, dengue, and leptospirosis.

2. The reticuloendothelial cell hyperplasia cluster (hepatosplenomegaly with or without generalized adenopathy), which suggests disseminated infectious disease of a bacterial (*Salmonella typhi* or other enteric fever pathogens), viral (cytomegalovirus, human immunodeficiency virus-1 [HIV-1], Epstein-Barr virus), rickettsial (*R. tsutsugamushi* in "scrub typhus"), protozoal (malaria), or fungal (*H. capsulatum, C. immitis*) cause; disseminated malignancy; sarcoidosis; or collagen-vascular disease.

3. The mononucleosis-like syndrome cluster (exudative pharyngitis and regional adenopathy with or without splenomegaly), which suggests infection due to group A streptococcus, *Francisella tularensis,* Epstein-Barr virus, toxoplasmosis, cytomegalovirus, or coxsackievirus, or hypersensitivity reactions due to drugs such as phenytoin.

The presence of isolated lower respiratory tract findings (decreased breath sounds, rales, expiratory wheezing) on examination should suggest underlying pulmonary infection with an organism such as measles, respiratory syncytial virus, adenovirus, *M. pneumoniae,* or *Legionella pneumophila.* Although sarcoidosis, collagen vascular disease, and systemic vasculitis (Wegener granulomatosus, Henoch-Schönlein purpura) may involve the lower respiratory tract, isolated pulmonary findings are infrequently indicative of these disorders in the context of acute fever and rash.

JOINT MANIFESTATIONS

Joint manifestations, such as pain, swelling, tenderness, and limited range of motion involving one joint, multiple joints, or migrating from joint to joint, or discrete pain at the insertion of tendons, ligaments, or fascia (enthesopathy), should suggest either a primary infectious illness, a "reactive" (immunologically mediated) disorder, or a systemic inflammatory condition (see Chapter 45). Primary infectious illnesses associated with this finding include *N. gonorrhoeae, B. burgdorferi,* parvovirus, and rubella, including vaccine-associated strains. Reactive disorders, such as Reiter syndrome (arthritis/enthesitis, conjunctivitis, urethritis) may be associated with infection caused by enteric pathogens, such as *Salmonella* and *Shigella* or genital pathogens, such as *N. gonorrhoeae* or *Chlamydia*, but may also include diseases of unknown etiology, such as inflammatory bowel disease, in which the rash is usually erythema nodosum. Systemic inflammatory conditions include Kawasaki syndrome, polyarteritis, SLE, systemic-onset JRA, acute rheumatic fever, and familial Mediterranean fever.

CARDIAC MANIFESTATIONS

Isolated cardiac manifestations may accompany acute rheumatic fever, bacterial endocarditis, or systemic-onset JRA (see Chapter 16). The presence of tachycardia out of proportion to the severity of the fever may be indicative of the carditis accompanying acute rheumatic fever, although this is not an invariable finding. A precordial friction rub is suggestive of pericarditis, which is noted frequently in patients with JRA. The presence of a new murmur or a changing murmur on auscultation is suggestive of bacterial endocarditis, whereas the detection of the apical systolic murmur of mitral regurgitation or the diastolic murmur of aortic insufficiency is suggestive of acute rheumatic fever. A gallop rhythm on auscultation should suggest underlying myocarditis, which may accompany coxsackievirus infection, rheumatic disease, or Kawasaki syndrome.

OCULAR MANIFESTATIONS

Isolated ocular manifestations, such as conjunctival injection and frank conjunctivitis, may suggest infection with measles or adenovirus, leptospirosis, Kawasaki syndrome, erythema multiforme, or Reiter syndrome. Anterior uveitis (redness with accompanying photophobia or pain or change in vision) may indicate Kawasaki syndrome, systemic JRA, sarcoidosis, ulcerative colitis, or, uncommonly, an infection such as leptospirosis (see Chapter 44). Retinal hemorrhages seen on funduscopy may indicate bacterial endocarditis.

NEUROLOGIC MANIFESTATIONS

Neurologic findings accompanying fever and rash may be indicative of specific infectious or immunologically mediated disorders. Mental status findings that indicate recent-onset psychosis may indicate cerebritis, which can accompany SLE. Significant alteration in mental status accompanied by seizure or focal motor impairment or cerebellar dysfunction may suggest primary infectious encephalitis associated with arborvirus, herpes simplex, measles, varicella-zoster virus, rickettsiosis, or *M. pneumoniae* infection. Nuchal rigidity, Kernig sign, or Brudzinski sign suggests meningeal irritation, which may accompany infection caused by the enteroviruses, encapsulated bacteria such as *H. influenzae* type b, *S. pneumoniae*, and *Neisseria meningitidis*, fungi such as *H. capsulatum*, *Borrelia burgdorferi*, or inflammation due to underlying SLE, sarcoidosis, or Kawasaki syndrome (see Chapter 53). Cranial nerve palsies, ataxia, or peripheral neuropathy may accompany infection with *B. burgdorferi* early in the course of Lyme disease (especially Bell palsy), or it may indicate an underlying vasculitis, such as SLE. Movement abnormalities, particularly chorea, may suggest either SLE or acute rheumatic fever.

Laboratory Tests

Laboratory tests should be ordered as adjuncts to the history and physical examination, which together set the prior probability of a specific disease. In the context of a very high or very low prior probability of a specific disease, testing adds very little clinically useful information and neither an unexpectedly positive nor an unexpectedly negative test result significantly modifies the posterior probability such that the initial clinical impression is invalidated (see Chapter 3). Thus, testing is most useful clinically when the prior probability of disease is equivocal.

The clinician should perform a Gram stain of any ulcerative, pustular, petechial, or purpuric lesion. The identification of bacteria suggests pyogenic infection, which may be localized or disseminated. The presence of only polymorphonuclear white blood cells in fluid of pustular lesions does not exclude bacterial infection from consideration, especially disseminated infection with *N. gonorrhoeae*. Specimens of these lesions or any fluid from a pustule for specific bacterial pathogens should also be obtained for culture.

Vesicular and bullous lesions in the febrile child with an uncertain diagnosis should be unroofed, scraped at the base, and submitted for microscopic examination after Tzanck preparation by an experienced observer (see Chapter 58). If the patient has an obvious case of chickenpox, herpes simplex, or bullous impetigo, most would not perform a microscopic examination but would observe or treat the condition empirically. The presence of multinucleated giant cells indicates infection with herpes virus or varicella-zoster virus. The sensitivity of the Tzanck preparation for cutaneous herpes simplex infection, compared with recovery of the virus directly from the lesion by culture, is 64%, and the specificity is 86%. Because the sensitivity of the procedure is relatively low, a negative result does not exclude the diagnosis of herpes simplex infection. Thus, to isolate the virus, a specimen of the lesion should also be obtained for culture. The diagnostic yields of both the viral culture and the Tzanck preparation are also a function of the type of lesion sampled. The rates of viral recovery from culture and positive microscopy are highest when vesicular lesions are sampled (100% and 67%, respectively) and lowest when crusted ulcers are sampled (33% and 17%, respectively).

Punch biopsy for light and electron microscopy and immunohistologic studies should be considered for diagnostic purposes for patients presenting with fever and bullous lesions that are clearly not typical pyodermas, fever and nodular lesions, or lesions suggestive of vasculitis (palpable purpura, livido reticularis). A punch biopsy with indirect immunofluorescent antibody staining may also be useful for patients with petechial lesions, especially in an acral distribution, for the early (days 4 to 8 of illness) diagnosis of infection due to *R. rickettsii*. This procedure has a sensitivity of 53% and a specificity of 100%. The low sensitivity of the test probably is related to the rickettsiostatic effect of antimicrobial treatment before presentation, but it indicates clearly that decision making in the acute care setting is limited by the high rate of false-negative classifications expected with this procedure.

Arriving at a diagnosis of systemic infectious illnesses may necessitate the use of specific bacterial, viral, or fungal culture techniques; paired acute and convalescent phase serology using complement fixation, indirect hemagglutination, hemagglutination inhibition, or neutralization techniques; or antigen detection systems, such as direct or indirect immunofluorescence, enzyme-linked immunosorbent assay (ELISA), latex particle agglutination, or immunoblot techniques. Culture techniques are most specific when normally sterile tissue or body fluids are sampled and inoculated directly into liquid or solid media. Interpretation of bacterial cultures obtained from nonsterile sites, such as the tonsils and nasopharynx, are subject to increased rates of false-positive results because of recovery of organisms that colonize these areas.

Serologic techniques are used to establish a diagnosis of a specific infection by demonstrating a fourfold rise in titer between samples obtained during the acute and convalescent phases of illness. Detection of a recent infection with group A streptococci may be accomplished by demonstrating a fourfold rise in antibodies to streptolysin-O (ASO titer) or by demonstrating the presence of other extracellular antigens produced by the streptococci (deoxyribonuclease B, hyaluronidase, streptokinase, nicotinamide adenine dinucleotidase) with the Streptozyme agglutination test. Occasionally during the acute phase of illness, a single titer that exceeds a certain threshold value (ASO titer > 1:333 or complement fixation titer > 1:256 for *M. pneumoniae*) may strongly suggest a specific diagnosis at presentation.

Antigen detection systems are employed for the purpose of rapid diagnosis. A solid phase detection system, such as ELISA, has the advantage of being independent of the need for intact cellular material but is affected by antigen or antibody cross-reactivity in the sample (which limits specificity) and by poor antigen-antibody affinity (which limits sensitivity). Nonetheless, ELISA is the preferred technique for the serologic diagnosis of a wide spectrum of infectious agents, including *B. burgdorferi,* the causative agent of Lyme disease, and hepatitis B virus.

Latex particle agglutination is an alternative solid phase antigen detection system that does not require intact cellular material and offers the advantages of rapidity of use and ease of interpretation. Latex particle agglutination is used for the rapid identification of patients with group A streptococcal pharyngitis or with invasive disease caused by encapsulated bacteria, such as *S. pneumoniae, H. influenzae* type b, *N. meningitidis,* group B streptococci, and *Escherichia coli*–K1. Latex particle agglutination is limited by factors similar to those affecting ELISA. Latex agglutination tests for group A streptococci have specificities of more than 90%, which facilitates their use for clinical confirmation of infection, but their sensitivities are only 60% to 90%, which limits their efficacy for case finding.

Confirmation of infection with the rickettsiae is best accomplished through serologic techniques demonstrating a fourfold increase in titer because culture systems (guinea pig or monocyte culture) are not widely available. Confirmation of infection with specific viral pathogens by culture is clinically appropriate.

The identification of patients with noninfectious systemic illness due to underlying collagen vascular disease, immune complex disease, or vasculitis is best accomplished through serologic techniques combined with other indirect laboratory evidence of active inflammation or tissue injury (see Chapter 45).

DIAGNOSIS AND DECISION MAKING

Accurate diagnosis depends on careful synthesis of selected data obtained from the clinical assessment. Because most children with acute episodes of fever and rash generally have a common, self-limited infectious disease, a specific diagnosis can often be established simply by pattern recognition after the history and physical examination in the absence of any laboratory assessment (visual recognition of the common exanthema of childhood or the specific lesion of erythema chronicum migrans), or with minimal use of adjunctive testing (a rash consistent with scarlet fever supported by a positive latex agglutination test for group A streptococcal antigen). Because the spectrum of infectious pathogens is broad, however, presenting complaints or features of the rash may be atypical and, occasionally, the diagnosis may not yield easily to simple pattern recognition. In these situations, empiric use of the laboratory for purposes of case finding may prove useful to the clinician.

In a prospective series of 100 febrile children presenting or referred for evaluation of generalized erythematous rashes of various patterns (macules, papules, maculopapules, urticaria, microvesicles, or petechiae) that were not indicative of a specific disorder by history or examination, Goodyear and colleagues were able to establish an infectious cause in 65% after performing a set of laboratory tests consisting of a throat swab and culture for streptococci (including non–group A streptococci) and serologic studies to detect rubella, measles, hepatitis A and B virus, Epstein-Barr

virus, parvovirus B19, and *M. pneumoniae.* This strategy of case finding, employing a limited repertoire of laboratory tests, was based on physician knowledge of the age-specific and/or seasonal incidence of infectious pathogens in the population studied. Case finding may be preferable to "watchful waiting" and serial clinical follow-up as a diagnostic approach when the patient is judged on the basis of epidemiologic considerations to be at risk for a treatable illness that is associated with significant subsequent morbidity (streptococcal infection, leading to acute rheumatic fever), or when specific information is required to advise parents of the risk of contagion to other children, especially immunocompromised contacts, or to pregnant women.

Although not every patient presenting with fever and rash who cannot have a diagnosis established through simple pattern recognition requires a laboratory assessment for the aforementioned reasons, the subset of patients who appear toxic, have unstable vital signs or altered mental status, or manifest a petechial or purpuric component to their rash must have a comprehensive evaluation and a diagnosis confirmed as quickly as possible to detect potentially life-threatening underlying infection and to plan appropriate therapy. The diagnostic approach to the child with a petechial or purpuric rash includes a complete blood count with a differential white blood cell count, a coagulation profile, and cultures of throat, blood, and cerebrospinal fluid (CSF). If the patient has a normal mental status, no nuchal rigidity, and no toxicity, a lumbar puncture may not be needed. Patients older than 36 months with primary complaints of sore throat and fever and clinical evidence of pharyngitis may be evaluated more conservatively, with a complete blood count and differential and a throat swab for rapid streptococcal antigen detection and culture.

Patients with a normal platelet count and coagulation profile but with a total peripheral white cell count of greater than 15,000/mm^3, an absolute band count of greater than 500 cells/mm^3, or a CSF examination demonstrating greater than 7 cells/mm^3 in the context of fever and petechiae or purpura have a 48% likelihood of invasive bacterial or rickettsial infection and should be admitted to a hospital for appropriate antimicrobial therapy. Patients with thrombocytopenia and an abnormal coagulation profile should be admitted for further evaluation and treatment of DIC, which may have an underlying infectious or inflammatory etiology. Patients with thrombocytopenia and a normal coagulation profile may have infection with Epstein-Barr virus, an autoimmune disease such as SLE, or a primary hematologic-oncologic disorder, such as idiopathic thrombocytopenic purpura or leukemia associated with an intercurrent infection, and should be evaluated for these disorders. However, irrespective of the suspected underlying cause, all such patients with platelet counts below 50,000/mm^3 should be admitted to the hospital for observation and consultation with a hematologist. Furthermore, many authorities recommend treating all patients with parenteral antibiotics if they manifest fever without a focus and petechiae that cannot be explained by significant and repeated coughing or emesis.

In certain instances, the diagnostic approach to disorders manifesting with fever and rash is wholly dependent on an aggregation of nonspecific signs, symptoms, and laboratory results. These disorders either have many underlying causes presenting with overlapping features that represent a final common pathway of clinical expression or have unknown causes for which no confirmatory tests have yet been devised. Diagnosis by formalized aggregation is termed *syndromic diagnosis* and must be considered an essential part of the comprehensive approach to the patient with fever and rash. Although syndromic diagnosis is based on explicit clinical criteria, some of the clusters of signs, symptoms, and laboratory findings were established originally for epidemiologic purposes (case definition) to facilitate exploration of an underlying cause. As such, although they are usually quite specific, these criteria may be less sensitive when they are applied in the acute care setting for the purposes of clinical diagnosis and misclassifications may occur.

Syndromic diagnosis is applicable to the following disorders: toxic shock syndrome, acute rheumatic fever (see Chapter 16), SLE (see Chapter 45), Kawasaki syndrome (mucocutaneous lymph node syndrome) (see Chapter 48), Stevens-Johnson syndrome (erythema multiforme major), hypersensitivity reactions (serum sickness), and dermatomyositis.

TOXIC SHOCK SYNDROME

The diagnosis of toxic shock syndrome is confirmed from criteria established by the Centers for Disease Control and Prevention (CDC) in 1980. The criteria include:

1. Fever greater than 39.2°C.
2. Diffuse macular erythroderma.
3. Desquamation predominantly localized on palms and soles during convalescence.
4. Hypotension, defined as systolic blood pressure less than the fifth percentile for age among children or adolescents, or orthostatic hypotension.
5. Evidence of multisystem involvement as manifested by dysfunction in more than three organ systems (gastrointestinal—diarrhea, vomiting; musculoskeletal—myalgia, elevated CPK; hyperemic—vagina, pharynx, conjunctiva; renal—sterile pyuria, BUN or creatinine > twice normal; liver—bilirubin, AST or ALT > twice normal; hematologic—thrombocytopenia; CNS—altered mental status).
6. Negative evidence of underlying bacterial infection, as indicated by sterile cultures of blood, urine, and cerebrospinal fluid, and a negative throat culture for significant growth of group A streptococci.
7. Negative serologic studies for measles virus, the rickettsiae, and the leptospirae.

Because toxic shock syndrome is most likely the result of superantigen production by either staphylococci or streptococci, both menstrual and nonmenstrual cases have been described, and a history of tampon use is of limited assistance to the pediatric clinician. Younger children present with symptoms of acute-onset hyperpyrexia and complaints of myalgia, headache or dizziness, sore throat, or gastrointestinal upset manifested by vomiting, ab-

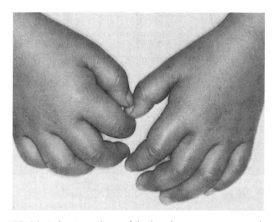

Figure 57–16. Indurative edema of the hands in mucocutaneous lymph node syndrome (Kawasaki disease). (Courtesy of Tomisaku Kawasaki, M.D.)

dominal pain, or diarrhea. A co-focus of infection (tracheitis, pneumonia, wound, nasal packing) may be identified on examination, which may be the only clue that the patient has nonmenstrual toxic shock syndrome.

KAWASAKI SYNDROME

The Kawasaki syndrome, also known as the *mucocutaneous lymph node syndrome,* is an acute, febrile illness of unknown etiology that has a worldwide distribution and tends to affect young children, irrespective of race, most frequently under the age of 5 years (see Chapter 48).

Six criteria have been established for the diagnosis of Kawasaki syndrome:

1. Fever of more than 38°C persisting for more than 5 days.
2. Bilateral bulbar nonexudative conjunctival injection.
3. Polymorphous rash, which may be accentuated in the perineal or perianal region.
4. Changes in the extremities, including indurative edema of the hands or feet, or palmar or plantar erythema, or desquamation, especially in the periungual region.
5. Changes in the oral mucosa, including cracking or fissuring of the lips, strawberry tongue, or diffuse oropharyngeal erythema.
6. Enlargement of a single or of multiple cervical lymph nodes to greater than 1.5 cm in diameter (Figs. 57–13 and 57–15 to 57–19).

The presence of fever and more than four of the remaining five

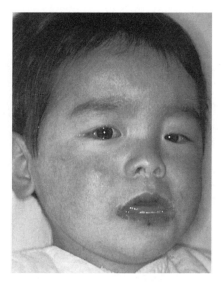

Figure 57–15. Kawasaki disease (mucoculaneous lymph node syndrome) Note characteristic facies with congestion of the bulbar conjunctivae and hemorrhagic crusts and erosions of the lips. (Courtesy of Tomisaku Kawasaki, M.D.)

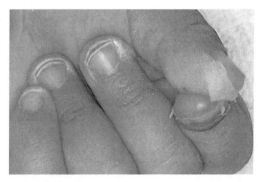

Figure 57–17. Desquamation of the fingers in a patient with mucocutaneous lymph node syndrome (Kawasaki disease). (Courtesy of Tomisaku Kawasaki, M.D.)

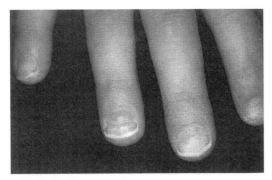

Figure 57–18. Beau's lines, a horizontal groove on the nails of a patient with Kawasaki disease. (From Hurwitz S. Clinical Pediatric Dermatology: A Textbook of Skin Disorders of Childhood and Adolescence, 2nd ed. Philadelphia: WB Saunders, 1993:549.)

criteria are sufficient for clinical confirmation in a patient who has no clinical or laboratory evidence of another disease, such as a common infectious exanthema, Epstein-Barr virus infection, scarlet fever, toxic shock syndrome, leptospirosis, rickettsiosis, or the Stevens-Johnson syndrome.

Associated features in Kawasaki syndrome include aseptic meningitis, urethritis, jaundice, hepatitis, and hydrops of the gallbladder. Supportive but nondiagnostic laboratory data include peripheral blood leukocytosis, mild nonhemolytic anemia, thrombocytosis (platelet count > 650,000/mm³ in second or third week of disease), elevated sedimentation rate, elevated bilirubin or hepatic transaminase levels, hypoalbuminemia, hyponatremia, and sterile pyuria. Cardiologic studies, such as electrocardiography, may demonstrate prolonged PR or QT intervals or nonspecific changes in the ST-T waves, whereas echocardiography may reveal pericardial effusion, decreased myocardial contractility, or valvar insufficiency early and aneurysms later in the course of illness. Because cardiovascular sequelae similar to those in classic Kawasaki syndrome have been found in young patients, especially those younger than 6 months of age, who present with incomplete or atypical features of this disorder, patients with prolonged febrile illnesses (>5 days) should be considered at high risk and should be monitored by serial clinical examination, electrocardiography, and echocardiography for any evidence of cardiovascular dysfunction or early coronary artery abnormalities.

STEVENS-JOHNSON SYNDROME

Stevens-Johnson syndrome is a hypersensitivity reaction diagnosed when blistering of two or more mucosal surfaces is accompa-

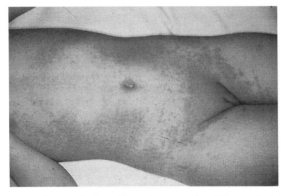

Figure 57–19. A scarlet fever–like rash in a child with Kawasaki disease. (Courtesy of Tomisaku Kawasaki, M.D.)

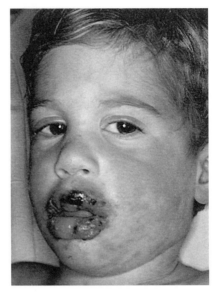

Figure 57–20. Stevens-Johnson syndrome. Mucous membrane involvement with severe swelling and hemorrhagic crusting of the lips. The hypersensitivity syndromes. (From Hurwitz S. Clinical Pediatric Dermatology: A Textbook of Skin Disorders of Childhood and Adolescence. Philadelphia: WB Saunders, 1993:527.)

nied by the typical cutaneous lesions of erythema multiforme (see Fig. 57–13). The rash is symmetric and involves the soles, palms, backs of the hands and feet, and extensor surfaces of the arms and legs. Extensive disease involves the trunk and face. The key feature that distinguishes this syndrome from the others is the presence of blistering lesions, which may involve the lips, eyes, nasal mucosa, genitalia, or rectum (Figs. 57–20 and 57–21). Extensive ocular involvement, including corneal ulceration, uveitis, and panophthalmitis, may develop. Pulmonary and renal involvement have also been reported.

SERUM SICKNESS

Serum sickness is a systemic hypersensitivity reaction resulting from immune complex deposition in or around blood vessels that

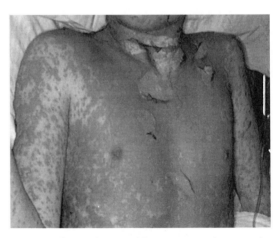

Figure 57–21. Bullous erythema multiforme (Stevens-Johnson syndrome). Confluent erythema, target lesions, blisters, and exfoliation of the epidermis are present. The hypersensitivity syndromes. (From Hurwitz S. Clinical Pediatric Dermatology: A Textbook of Skin Disorders of Childhood and Adolescence. Philadelphia: WB Saunders, 1993:528.)

causes tissue damage through complement activation and may follow the administration of foreign proteins or drugs. Because other disorders, such as SLE, are characterized by immune complex type hypersensitivity, serum sickness manifests clinical features that are nonspecific and include complaints of abdominal pain, nausea, vomiting, malaise and arthralgia, polyarticular arthritis and tender lymphadenopathy associated with fever, and an urticarial or erythematous palmar or plantar serpiginous rash. Uncommon findings include peripheral neuropathy, angioedema, and clinical evidence of myopericarditis. Critical to the diagnosis of the syndrome of serum sickness is a history of exposure to drugs or heterologous protein antitoxins; agents include antimicrobial agents, such as the penicillins, sulfonamides, and cephalosporins; anticonvulsants, such as phenytoin; antihypertensive agents, such as hydralazine and propranolol; and antivenins, given from 1 day to 2 weeks before the onset of illness. Characteristically, illness associated with a primary exposure evolves less rapidly than illness associated with a secondary exposure, reflecting the time required for immune complexes generated in response to the exposure to reach a critical level for clinical manifestations to develop.

Laboratory testing plays a minor direct role in the diagnosis of serum sickness but may be helpful when eosinophilia is noted on the peripheral blood smear or when the level of total hemolytic complement in serum is found to be depressed. Although glomerulonephritis may occur, it is usually clinically silent or mild, and urinalysis demonstrates cylindruria or minimal, but not heavy, proteinuria. This latter finding, if present on urinalysis, should suggest an alternative diagnosis. Serologic laboratory testing may be of assistance in excluding other, more specific disorders that mimic serum sickness, such as SLE, rubella, hepatitis B, and Epstein-Barr virus. A watchful waiting approach may support the diagnosis, inasmuch as the syndrome should resolve within approximately 4 weeks if exposure to the purported offending agent has been curtailed. Persistence of findings beyond this period should suggest another disorder associated with immune complex–mediated vasculitis (see Chapters 45 and 58).

OTHER DISORDERS

In addition to these syndromic diagnoses, certain disorders presenting with fever and rash can be approached as diagnoses of exclusion or as diagnoses requiring tissue confirmation. These disorders are generally encountered with varying frequency in clinical practice but all are well described and have finite morbidity, making accurate and timely diagnosis imperative. Diagnoses of exclusion include systemic-onset (chronic) JRA (see Chapter 45), and Henoch-Schönlein purpura (Fig. 57–22). Representative diagnoses requiring tissue confirmation are sarcoidosis, and other vasculitides, such as polyarteritis nodosa (antineutrophil cytoplasm antibodies are often present).

Henoch-Schönlein purpura is a vasculitic syndrome of unknown etiology that affects vessels in the skin, joints, gastrointestinal tract, and kidneys. The clinical manifestations include a rash, which initially is urticarial and then frequently evolves into a maculopapular eruption; this eruption subsequently develops petechiae and then purpuric plaques distributed predominantly on the buttocks and over the lower extremities (see Fig. 57–22). These plaques usually are raised from the skin surface giving the rash its characteristic feature of ''palpable purpura.'' Associated findings that are not invariably present include arthralgias and arthritis; edema of the feet, hands, face, scrotum, and scalp; melena, which may accompany intussusception; and an abnormal urinalysis that demonstrates hematuria and proteinuria.

Laboratory testing is of use to the clinician in excluding the infectious or hematologic causes of purpura. Specifically, the results of both the platelet count and the coagulation profile are

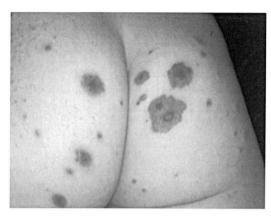

Figure 57–22. Henoch-Schönlein purpura (anaphylactoid purpura). Hemorrhagic macules, papules, and urticarial lesions appear in a symmetric distribution over the buttocks of a young child. (From Hurwitz S. Clinical Pediatric Dermatology: A Textbook of Skin Disorders of Childhood and Adolescence. Philadelphia: WB Saunders, 1993:540.)

normal, excluding DIC or a hemorrhagic diathesis, and blood cultures are sterile. A Gram stain of the lesion is not usually needed, but the results are negative, and skin biopsy demonstrates the characteristic leukocytoclastic vasculitis involving the vessels in the dermis. However, this finding is not specific for Henoch-Schönlein purpura, nor is it required for clinical confirmation.

MANAGEMENT

Treatment of patients with fever and rash follows logically after accurate diagnosis and includes both anticipatory guidance and therapeutic considerations. Anticipatory guidance alone usually suffices in the treatment of patients who have an identifiable acute, self-limited, and noninvasive infectious disorder. Parents should be informed of the probable duration of illness, the expected evolution of clinical manifestations, potential complications and how to recognize them, and when and how to recontact the physician (passive surveillance) (see Tables 57–4 and 57–5). Active surveillance by the physician to detect complications through follow-up telephone contact or a return visit to the office or clinic may be appropriate when there is concern that the caretakers may not be reliable observers, or when the patient manifests a higher level of clinical toxicity (higher Acute Illness Observation Score) than anticipated at presentation. Among patients in whom the diagnosis is equivocal, the strategy of active surveillance is clinically prudent.

Therapeutic interventions may be supportive, empiric, or definitive.

Supportive interventions are appropriate for all patients but especially for those with recognizable derangements in physiologic homeostasis at presentation. These interventions are aimed at preventing or replacing fluid losses, which may be related to fever, hyperpnea, vomiting or diarrhea; maintaining adequate systemic oxygenation, ventilation, and perfusion; and supporting metabolism through maintenance of adequate levels of blood glucose. For most patients, fluid maintenance or replacement may be achieved via the enteral route, but for patients with altered mental status or cardiovascular instability, the parenteral approach is more appropriate.

The use of antipyretics for supportive therapy in patients with fever remains controversial. Arguments in favor of such therapy include decreasing symptomatic discomfort associated with the febrile state and reducing the undesirable metabolic and cardiopulmonary effects. A concern exists, however, regarding the choice of antipyretic agents for treating fever and rash. Reye syndrome has been reported in association with aspirin consumption in patients with varicella or other viral illnesses. Given the high likelihood that patients with an acute fever-rash illness have an underlying viral illness, aspirin should probably be avoided for antipyresis; acetaminophen, 10 to 15 mg/kg/dose, should be used instead. However, in patients with fever and rash caused by systemic inflammatory disorders (JRA, SLE), aspirin and the nonsteroidal anti-inflammatory agents do play an important role in both control of fever and modulation of disease activity.

Empirical therapy is employed when the diagnosis of a treatable disorder associated with unacceptable rates of morbidity or mortality is suspected on the basis of epidemiologic, clinical, or nonspecific laboratory data but when confirmation is lacking, either because more specific test results are pending at the time of presentation or no specific tests exist to guide management further. Empiric therapy is thus an appropriate management strategy for patients with fever and signs of focal cutaneous infection, such as cellulitis and erythema chronicum migrans, for patients with petechial or purpuric rash who are thought to have invasive infectious disorders, or for patients with fever and nonspecific rash who appear toxic or manifest signs of cardiovascular instability on examination.

Cellulitis is associated with a broad spectrum of bacterial organisms in immunocompetent hosts. The most common organisms related to direct inoculation after local trauma (even microscopic, less obvious trauma) are coagulase-positive *S. aureus* and group A streptococci. The most common organisms related to bacteremic localization unassociated with trauma in children younger than 4 years of age (preseptal or buccal cellulitis) are *H. influenzae* type b and *S. pneumoniae*. In immunocompromised hosts, *P. aeruginosa* and the gram-negative enteric rods are also frequently recovered. Empiric treatment of the immunocompetent host with cellulitis after local trauma should include either an antistaphylococcal penicillin or a first-generation cephalosporin. A third-generation cephalosporin, such as ceftriaxone or cefotaxime, should be given for secondary cellulitis believed to be related to a primary bacteremia. The immunocompromised host should be treated empirically with a combination of an aminoglycoside and a third-generation cephalosporin, such as ceftazidime. For both categories of patients, initial therapy should be parenteral, with consideration given to use of enteral agents for immunocompetent hosts once a significant clinical response, indicated by resolution of erythema or heat, is noted. Bacteremic patients may require a complete 7- to 10-day course of parenteral therapy.

Empirical treatment of the patient with fever and petechiae or purpura should be directed at correcting underlying DIC (see Chapter 51), if present, and at providing broad-spectrum antimicrobial therapy against both gram-positive and gram-negative bacteria. Should epidemiologic evidence or clinical features of the rash suggest infection with any of the *Rickettsia* species, the antimicrobial regimen must include a rickettsiostatic drug appropriate for the age of the patient (in patients ≥ 8 years, use doxycycline; in those younger than 8 years, use chloramphenicol). Ongoing monitoring of coagulation status, platelet counts, and renal function is essential for appropriate management.

The choice of antimicrobial agents is guided by the age of the patient and the presence of any underlying focus of infection, such as meningitis. Young infants (<2 months) are frequently infected by group B streptococcus; gram-negative enteric rods; and, to a lesser extent, by *Listeria monocytogenes* or the encapsulated pathogens, such as *S. pneumoniae*, *H. influenzae* type b, *N. meningitidis*, and *N. gonorrhoeae*. Rickettsial infections are unusual in this age group, but disseminated herpes simplex infection or herpes meningoencephalitis should be considered especially in the patient presenting with a vesicular rash and laboratory evidence of DIC, or with a sterile CSF pleocytosis. Older infants, children, and adolescents are frequently infected by the encapsulated pathogens and by *Salmonella* species.

For young infants (<30 days), the combination of intravenous ampicillin (100 to 200 mg/kg/day divided every 6 hours) and an aminoglycoside or, more often, a third-generation cephalosporin, such as cefotaxime (150 to 200 mg/kg/day divided every 6 to 8 hours) are appropriate empiric therapy (see Chapters 53 and 59). Consideration should be given to the parenteral administration of acyclovir in a daily dosage of 30 mg/kg divided every 8 hours if herpes simplex is a possibility. For older patients, parenteral monotherapy with a third-generation cephalosporin, such as ceftriaxone (100 mg/kg/day given every 12 hours) or cefotaxime (150 to 200 mg/kg/day divided every 6 to 8 hours), will suffice (see Chapters 53 and 59). For empiric therapy of the rickettsiae, parenteral chloramphenicol in a daily dosage of 100 mg/kg (maximum of 3 g) divided every 6 hours, or, for children equal to or older than the age of 8 years, parenteral tetracycline or doxycycline in a daily dosage of 20 mg/kg divided every 6 to 12 hours, is appropriate.

Patients for whom a diagnosis is established by pattern recognition, case finding, syndromic aggregation, biopsy, or exclusion may receive *definitive interventions*, as available, if the treatment benefits outweigh the risks. Because definitive interventions may not always be curative, they include prescription of antimicrobial agents, anti-inflammatory drugs, or immunosuppressants.

Streptococcal infections or associated disorders, such as acute rheumatic fever and toxic shock syndrome, should be treated with penicillin. Standard therapy for pharyngitis associated with scarlet fever or acute rheumatic fever is penicillin given orally or as an intramuscular injection of benzathine penicillin (see Chapters 6 and 16).

Infections due to herpes simplex virus or varicella-zoster virus may be treated with oral or intravenous acyclovir. Intravenous therapy is particularly appropriate for immunocompromised or immunosuppressed patients (see Chapter 31). The benefits of acyclovir therapy for herpes simplex virus or varicella in immunocompetent hosts are less clear.

Pharmacologic interventions in the systemic inflammatory disorders of unknown etiology include anti-inflammatory agents, such as the nonsteroidal drugs and corticosteroids (Table 57–6). Anti-inflammatory therapy has been reported to be beneficial in reducing mortality in acute rheumatic fever manifesting severe carditis (congestive heart failure), systemic-onset JRA, SLE, dermatomyositis, and the vasculitides. Patients with acute rheumatic fever without carditis, Henoch-Schönlein purpura, Stevens-Johnson syndrome, or serum sickness may also benefit symptomatically from anti-inflammatory therapy, but the efficacy of such therapy in the reduction or prevention of morbidity remains controversial.

Immunosuppressant or modulating agents include intravenous immunoglobulin (IVIG), cyclosporine, azathioprine, and cyclophosphamide. Although the latter drugs may be used adjunctively with corticosteroids as interventions for SLE or the necrotizing vasculitides, IVIG administration is considered a definitive intervention in all patients with Kawasaki syndrome to reduce morbidity by preventing coronary aneurysm formation. The most cost-effective approach to IVIG in these patients is the one-dose regimen of 2 g/kg given intravenously over 10 hours. Concurrent therapy with aspirin at a total daily dosage of 80 to 100 mg/kg for the initial 14 days of illness, followed by a reduction in daily dosage to 3 to 5 mg/kg for 6 to 8 weeks in the absence of coronary artery aneurysms, is appropriate to control inflammation and to prevent thrombotic complications (see Chapter 48).

SUMMARY AND RED FLAGS

Most childhood episodes of fever and rash represent benign viral illnesses with little sequelae. *Red flags* include fever without a

Table 57-6. Drugs Used to Control Inflammation in Children

Name	Total Daily Dosage (mg/kg)	Dosing Interval (hours)	Therapeutic Range	Preparations
NSAID*				
Aspirin	80–100	4–6	20–30 mg/dl	Tablets (81, 325 mg)
Ibuprofen	20–50 (max, 3200/day)	6–8	Not known	Suspension (100 mg/5 ml), tablets (200, 300, 400 mg)
Naproxen	10–15 (max, 1500/day)	12	30–90 μg/ml	Suspension (125 mg/5 ml), tablets (250, 375, 500 mg)
Tolmetin sodium	15–30 (max, 1800 day)	6–8	Not known	Tablets (200, 400, 600 mg)

Name	Relative Potency	Relative Mineralocorticoid Effect	Route of Administration
Corticosteroids†			
Hydrocortisone	1	1	Oral, intravenous
Prednisone‡	4	0.8	Oral
Prednisolone	4	0	Oral, intravenous
Methylprednisolone	5	0	Oral, intravenous
Dexamethasone	25	0	Oral, intravenous

*All drugs have been reported to have the following adverse effects: gastric irritation, platelet inhibition, gastrointestinal bleeding, hepatitis, and nephropathy.

†Chronic administration has been associated with cushingoid changes, growth failure, osteopenia, cataracts, gastrointestinal bleeding, glucose intolerance, myopthy, and increased risk of generalized infection.

‡Recommended dosage for initiation of therapy to achieve rapid control of inflammation is 1–2 mg/kg, not to exceed 60 mg/day.

Abbreviation: NSAIDs = nonsteroidal anti-inflammatory drugs.

focus in infants younger than 2 years of age, and petechiae (suggesting bacteremia), manifestations of treatable diseases with significant sequelae (rheumatic fever, Kawasaki syndrome, Rocky Mountain spotted fever, SLE, JRA), and contagious illnesses that are of concern for either immunocompetent or immunosuppressed patients. Unstable vital signs (tachycardia, hypotension) and meningismus are additional red flags.

REFERENCES

American Academy of Pediatrics. Lyme disease. *In* Report of the Committee on Infectious Diseases, 23rd ed. Elk Grove Village, Ill: American Academy of Pediatrics; 1994:297–300.

American Heart Association Committee on Rheumatic Fever, Endocarditis, and Kawasaki Disease. Diagnostic guidelines for Kawasaki disease. Am J Dis Child 1990;144:1220–1222.

Baker RC, Seguin JH, Leslie N, et al. Fever and petechiae in children. Pediatrics 1989;84:1051–1055.

Balfour HH, Rotbart HA, Feldman S, et al. Acyclovir treatment of varicella in otherwise healthy adolescents. J Pediatr 1992;120:627–633.

Baraff LJ, Bass JW, Fleisher GR, et al. Practice guidelines for the management of infants and children 0–36 months of age with fever without source. Pediatrics 1993;92:1–12.

Bialecki C, Feder HM, Grant-Kels JM. The six classic childhood exanthems: A review and update. J Am Acad Dermatol 1989;21:891–903.

Boh DD, Millikan LE. Vesiculobullous diseases with prominent immunologic features. JAMA 1992;268:2893–2898.

Brazilian Purpuric Fever Study Group. *Haemophilus aegyptius* bacteremia in Brazilian purpuric fever. Lancet 1987;2:761–763.

Burns J, Wiggins J, Toews W, et al. Clinical spectrum of Kawasaki disease in infants younger than 6 months of age. J Pediatr 1986;109:759–763.

Cone LA, Woodard DR, Schlievert PM, et al. Clinical and bacteriologic observations of a toxic-like syndrome due to *Streptococcal pyogenes*. N Engl J Med 1987;317:146–149.

Eichenfield LF, Honig PJ. Blistering disorders in childhood. Pediatr Clin North Am 1991;38:959–976.

Frieden IJ, Resnick SD. Childhood exanthems: Old and new. Pediatr Clin North Am 1991;38:859–887.

Goodyear HM, Laidler PW, Price EH, et al. Acute infectious erythemas in children: A clinico-microbiological study. Br J Dermatol 1991;124:433–438.

Hurwitz S. Erythema multiforme: A review of its characteristics, diagnostic criteria, and management. Pediatr Rev 1990;11:217–222.

Jones EM, Callen JP. Collagen vascular disease of childhood. Pediatr Clin North Am 1991;38:1019–1039.

Jundt JW, Creager AH. STAR complexes: Febrile illnesses associated with sore throat, arthritis, and rash. South Med J 1993;86:521–528.

Kingston ME, Mackey D. Skin clues in the diagnosis of life-threatening infections. Rev Infect Dis 1986;8:1–11.

Levy M, Koren G. Atypical Kawasaki disease: Analysis of clinical presentation and diagnostic clues. Pediatr Infect Dis J 1990;9:122–126.

Malane MS, Grant-Kels JM, Feder HM, et al. Diagnosis of Lyme disease based on dermatologic manifestations. Ann Intern Med 1991;114:490–498.

McCarthy PL, Sharpe MR, Spiesel SZ, et al. Observation scales to identify serious illness in febrile children. Pediatrics 1982;70:802–809.

Newburger JW, Takahashi M, Beiser AS, et al. A single intravenous infusion of gamma globulin as compared with four infusions in the treatment of acute Kawasaki syndrome. N Engl J Med 1991;324:1633–1639.

Pattishall EN, Strope GL, Spinola SM, et al. Childhood sarcoidosis. J Pediatr 1986;108:169–177.

Solomon AR, Rasmussen JE, Varani J. The Tzanck smear in the diagnosis of cutaneous herpes simplex. JAMA 1984;251:633–635.

Walker DH, Cain BB, Olmstead PM. Laboratory diagnosis of Rocky Mountain spotted fever by immunofluorescent demonstration of *Rickettsia rickettsii* in cutaneous lesions. Am J Clin Pathol 1978;69:619–623.

Weiner LB. Management of young children with fever and rash. Pediatr Infect Dis J 1991;10:416–417.

Amy Jo Nopper   Linda G. Rabinowitz

Approximately 20% to 30% of pediatric office visits involve a primary or secondary dermatologic complaint. In addition to the myriad of primary skin disorders encountered during infancy and childhood, the skin is frequently a marker of underlying systemic disease. Cutaneous findings often aid in the diagnosis of many hereditary disorders that require evaluation for associated systemic abnormalities and genetic counseling.

HISTORY

Obtaining a careful and focused history is often necessary to establish diagnoses of pediatric skin disorders. It may be helpful to examine the patient first and then proceed with a relevant line of questioning. Important questions to ask include the following:

1. When did the eruption begin?
2. How did the eruption evolve (distribution, spread, change in morphology of individual lesions)?
3. Are the lesions pruritic or painful?
4. Have there been previous similar episodes?
5. Are there associated systemic symptoms?
6. Are there exacerbating or alleviating factors?
7. Has treatment been rendered? If so, what effect has it had?
8. Are there affected family members or close contacts?
9. Is there a family history of skin disease?

PHYSICAL EXAMINATION

It is necessary to identify the primary skin lesion, secondary skin lesions or changes, size, color, distribution, and configuration of the eruption. In addition, several specific signs are pathognomonic for certain diseases. Examination of the hair, nails, and mucosal surfaces should be included. Palpation of cutaneous lesions provides additional information, such as firmness, tenderness, mobility, temperature, and ability to blanch with pressure. Precise morphologic descriptions are critical for establishing a differential diagnosis (see also Chapter 57).

Primary Lesions

Macules and Patches. Macules are flat, circumscribed lesions that are detected because of a change in color. Pink or red macules may be caused by inflammation or vasodilatation. Brown, black, or white lesions may be due to alterations in melanin synthesis. Purple hues may represent extravasation of blood into the skin. Macules larger than 1 cm in diameter are usually described as patches.

Papules, Nodules, Plaques, Tumors. *Papules* are circumscribed, palpable, elevated solid lesions. Typically less than 0.5 to 1 cm in diameter, these lesions may be epidermal or dermal in origin and may be flat-topped or dome-shaped. Papules that are 0.5 to 2 cm are described as nodules. *Nodules* are epidermal, dermal, or subcutaneous lesions that may, in some cases, evolve from preexisting papules. *Plaques* are elevated flat-topped lesions, larger than 1 cm, and often formed by coalescence of papules. *Tumors* are larger nodules that are usually solid and well circumscribed.

Vesicles and Bullae. Vesicles are elevated fluid-filled lesions. Bullae are large vesicles, usually greater than 1 cm. The tenseness or flaccidity of the blister indicates whether the level of separation is intra- or subepidermal (Fig. 58–1 and Table 58–1).

Pustules. Pustules are white or yellow well-circumscribed lesions

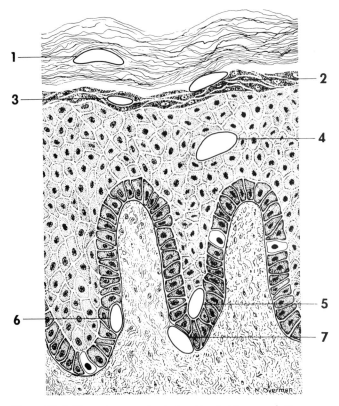

Figure 58–1. Blister cleavage sites in the skin. *1,* Intracorneal. *2,* Subcorneal. *3,* Granular layer. *4,* Intraepidermal. *5,* Suprabasal. *6,* Junctional (between the basal cell membrane and basement membrane). *7,* Subepidermal. (From Esterly NB. The skin. *In* Behrman RE [ed]. Nelson Textbook of Pediatrics, 14th ed. Philadelphia: WB Saunders, 1992:1640.)

Table 58-1. Sites of Blister Formation and Diagnostic Studies for the Vesicobullous Disorders

Disorder	Blister Cleavage Site	Cutaneous Diagnostic Studies
Acrodermatitis enteropathica	IE	—
Bullous impetigo	GL	Smear, culture
Bullous pemphigoid	SE (junctional)	Direct and indirect immunofluorescence studies
Candidosis	SC	KOH preparation, culture
Chronic bullous dermatosis of childhood	SE	Direct immunofluorescence studies
Dermatitis herpetiformis	SE	Direct immunofluorescence studies
Dermatophytosis	IE	KOH preparation, culture
Dyshidrotic eczema	IE	—
Epidermolysis bullosa (EB) simplex	IE	Electron microscopy; immunofluorescence mapping
Hands and feet	IE	Electron microscopy; immunofluorescence mapping
Junctional EB (Letalis)	SE (junctional)	Electron microscopy; immunofluorescence mapping
Recessive dystrophic EB	SE	Electron microscopy; immunofluorescence mapping
Dominant dystrophic EB	SE	Electron microscopy; immunofluorescence mapping
Epidermolytic hyperkeratosis	IE	—
Erythema multiforme	SE	—
Erythema toxicum	SC, IE	Smear for eosinophils
Incontinentia pigmenti	IE	Smear for eosinophils
Insect bites	IE	—
Mastocytosis	SE	Smear for mast cells
Miliaria crystallina	IC	—
Pachyonychia congenita	IC	—
Pemphigus foliaceus	GL	Direct and indirect immunofluorescence studies Tzanck smear
Pemphigus vulgaris	SB	Direct and indirect immunofluorescence studies Tzanck smear
Pseudomonas infection	IE, SE	Smear, culture
Scabies	IE	Scraping
Staphylococcal scalded skin syndrome	GL	Frozen section biopsy
Syphilis	SE	Dark-field preparation
Toxic epidermal necrolysis (Lyell)	SE	Frozen section biopsy
Transient neonatal pustular melanosis	SC, IE	Smear for cells
Viral blisters	IE	Tzanck smear for herpesvirus infections

From Esterly NB. The skin. *In* Behrman RE, Kliegman RM (eds). Nelson Textbook of Pediatrics, 14th ed. Philadelphia: WB Saunders, 1992:1641.
Abbreviations: GL = granular layer; IC = intracorneal; IE = intraepidermal; SB = suprabasal; SC = subcorneal; SE = subepidermal.

that contain purulent material. Pustules do not always signify an infectious etiology.

Wheals. Wheals are edematous, elevated lesions that are transient in nature and variable in shape and size. They may be white or erythematous and often have central pallor.

Telangiectases. These are ectatic superficial blood vessels of the skin that typically blanch when pressure is applied.

Secondary Lesions

Secondary lesions may represent the natural evolution of primary lesions or changes that result from external manipulation, such as scratching.

Crusts. Crusts represent serum, pus, blood, or exudate that has dried on the skin surface.

Scales. Scales appear as yellow, white, or brownish flakes on the skin surface that represent desquamation of stratum corneum.

Erosions. Erosions are moist, erythematous, circumscribed lesions that result from partial or complete loss of the epidermis. They are often due to rupture of a blister. Unlike ulcers, erosions do not involve the dermis or subcutaneous tissue and, therefore, heal without scarring.

Ulcers. Ulcers are deep erosions into the dermis or fat that usually heal with scarring.

Lichenification. Lichenification, or thickening of the skin, usually results from chronic scratching or rubbing. Accentuation of skin markings is observed.

Fissures. A fissure is a linear crack in the epidermis extending to the dermis.

Atrophy. Atrophy represents loss of substance of the skin. Epidermal atrophy is characterized by loss of skin markings, increased wrinkling, and transparency with visibility of underlying vasculature. Dermal or subcutaneous atrophy results in depression of the skin with minimal, if any, epidermal changes.

Excoriations. Excoriations are linear erosions on the skin due to scratching.

DIAGNOSTIC TECHNIQUES

Potassium Hydroxide Test

A common diagnostic procedure performed in the office setting is the potassium hydroxide (KOH) preparation. This simple and rapid test can confirm the diagnosis of dermatophyte or candidal infections. Scale is scraped with a curved blade onto a microscope slide. Hair or nail fragments can also be examined microscopically. A glass coverslip is then placed on the slide after adding one to two drops of 10% to 20% KOH. The slide is heated gently, avoiding boiling, which can result in KOH crystallization and subsequent difficulty in interpretation. Dermatophyte infections are confirmed by identifying fungal hyphae, which appear as long, branching septate filaments. Pseudohyphae or budding spores are characteristic of candidiasis. Short, broad hyphae and clusters of budding cells, resembling "spaghetti and meatballs," are diagnostic of tinea versicolor.

Tzanck Smear

A Tzanck smear is useful for diagnosis of viral blistering diseases, such as varicella-zoster virus and herpes simplex virus infections. The smear is prepared by unroofing a blister with a curved blade and gently scraping the blister base and underside of the roof. The material is spread in a thin layer onto a glass slide. The slide is air-dried and stained with a Giemsa or Wright stain. Identification of multinucleated giant cells, a syncytium of epidermal cells with multiple overlapping nuclei, establishes the diagnosis of a viral infection. These cells may have 2 to 15 nuclei and are much larger than other inflammatory cells. Although a positive Tzanck preparation is confirmatory, a negative test does not rule out viral infection. Viral specimens should be obtained for culture to differentiate herpes simplex from varicella-zoster virus infections.

Scabies Test

A scabies preparation exhibiting the mite, egg, or feces (scybala) confirms the diagnosis of scabies infestation. The mite is most often found within burrows (serpiginous or elongated papules), which may have a vesicle or pustule at one end. A drop of mineral oil should be applied to the lesion so that the scraped material adheres to the blade. The site is then scraped firmly with a curved blade, which occasionally induces minimal bleeding. The material is applied to a microscope slide, another drop of mineral oil is added, and a glass coverslip is placed. Mites are eight-legged arachnids that are easily identified under low magnification. Eggs are frequently observed as smooth ovals approximately one-half the size of the mite. Feces are smaller than ova and appear as red-brown pellets, often in clusters.

Gram Stain

A Gram stain can be useful in the diagnosis and treatment of suspected bacterial infections. After the site is disinfected, the pustule or blister roof is carefully removed with a needle or straight blade. The contents of the pustule are removed in a sterile fashion and thinly spread onto a glass slide. The specimen is air-dried or heat-fixed and stained with crystal violet and iodine. The slide is decolorized and counterstained with safranin, dried, and examined microscopically. Results help determine which antibiotic, if any, is indicated. Bacterial cultures are typically obtained simultaneously.

Wood's Lamp Examination

A Wood's lamp emits low-intensity ultraviolet light at 365 nm and is useful for accentuating pigmentary alterations and detecting several fungal or bacterial infections. The examination is performed in a darkened room, and the lamp is held 4 to 6 inches from the patient's skin. Characteristic color changes are outlined in Table 58–2.

Skin Biopsy

A skin biopsy can be performed by a dermatologist when a clinical diagnosis is unclear. Histologic evaluation of a small skin specimen may reveal changes in the epidermis, dermis, or subcutaneous tissue that confirm or rule out specific disorders. Direct immunofluorescence testing can be extremely helpful in the diagnosis of collagen-vascular and inflammatory bullous diseases (Table 58–3).

NEONATAL DERMATOLOGY

Neonatal dermatology comprises conditions unique to the newborn infant. Many entities are due to physiologic phenomena in response to the transition to the new environment. Most are benign and self-limited. There are also specific skin disorders, such as subcutaneous fat necrosis, that are primarily seen in this age group. Other conditions, such as congenital infections, require prompt recognition and intervention.

Table 58–2. Wood's Lamp Findings

Fluorescence	Clinical Appearance	Organisms/Disease
Coral, red, pink	Brown or red thin plaques in groin, axillae, or toe webs	Erythrasma (*Corynebacterium minutissimum*)
Pale green	Hypopigmented or hyperpigmented macules and plaques on trunk	Tinea versicolor (*Pityrosporum orbiculare*, *Malassezia furfur*)
Bright yellow-green	Infection of the toe web space, often in burn patients	*Pseudomonas aeruginosa*
Yellow-green	Scaling of scalp with patchy hair loss	Tinea capitis (*Microsporum canis*, *M. audouinii*)

Table 58-3. Immunofluorescent Findings in Immune-Mediated Cutaneous Diseases

Disease	Involved Skin	Uninvolved Skin	Direct IF	Indirect IF	Other Antibodies
Dermatitis herpetiformis	Negative	Positive	Granular IgA ± C in papillary dermis	None	IgA antireticulum in 20–70%. Antigliadin antibodies with celiac disease
Bullous pemphigoid	Positive	Positive	Linear IgG and C band in BMZ, occasionally IgM, IgA, IgE	IgG to BMZ in 70%	None
Pemphigus (all variants)	Positive	Positive	IgG in intercellular spaces of epidermis between keratinocytes	IgG to intercellular space	None
Pemphigus foliaceus	Positive	Positive	IgG to desmosomal glycoprotein, desmoglein	Same as direct IF	None
Herpes gestations	Positive	Positive	C3 at BMZ, occasionally IgG	IgG anti-BMZ	None
Linear IgA bullous dermatosis (chronic bullous dermatosis of childhood)	Positive	Positive	Linear IgA at BMZ, occasionally C	Low titer, rare IgA, anti-BMZ	None
Discoid lupus erythematosus	Positive	Negative	Linear IgG, IgM, IgA, and C3 at BMZ (lupus band)	None	Antinuclear antibody (ANA) negative
Systemic lupus erythematosus	Positive	Variable: exposed to sun, 30–50%; nonexposed, 10–30%	Linear IgG, IgM, C3 at BMZ (lupus band)	None	ANA Anti-Ro (SSA) Anti-RNP Anti-DNA Anti-Sm
Henoch-Schönlein purpura	Positive	Negative	IgA around vessel walls	None	IgA rheumatoid factor, occasionally

From Esterly NB. The skin. *In* Behrman RE (ed). Nelson Textbook of Pediatrics, 14th ed. Philadelphia: WB Saunders, 1992:1623.
Abbreviations: BMZ = basement membrane zone at the dermoepidermal junction; C = complement; IF = immunofluorescence; Ig = immunoglobulin.

Physiologic Changes of the Skin

ACROCYANOSIS

The normal newborn infant usually displays a bluish-purple discoloration of the hands, feet, and lips. Referred to as acrocyanosis, this typically occurs in association with crying or cold stress. It results from increased peripheral arteriolar tone, which leads to vasospasm and subsequent venous pooling. Acrocyanosis should be differentiated from cyanosis associated with pulmonary or cardiac disease, which is noted on mucosal surfaces (see Chapter 15).

Physiologic acrocyanosis gradually resolves spontaneously during the neonatal period.

CUTIS MARMORATA

Cutis marmorata is also associated with neonatal cold stress. Characterized by symmetric reticulated cyanosis involving the trunk and extremities, this marbled appearance usually resolves on rewarming. When this vascular pattern is seen in older infants or children, it may be associated with Down syndrome, Cornelia de Lange syndrome, or hypothyroidism.

Cutis marmorata should be differentiated from *cutis marmorata telangiectatica congenita* (CMTC), a condition also referred to as *congenital phlebectasia*. The persistent cutis marmorata of CMTC is characteristically asymmetric, often dermatomal, and more localized than physiologic cutis marmorata. In addition, the reticulated mottling of CMTC is darker in color and does not resolve with rewarming. Although CMTC improves with age, the abnormal vascular pattern is more persistent than that seen in physiologic cutis marmorata. It may be an isolated entity or associated with mesodermal or neuroectodermal anomalies.

HARLEQUIN COLOR CHANGE

The harlequin color change is a distinctive condition observed in infants lying on their sides. It is characterized by marked erythema on the dependent side of the infant's body with simultaneous blanching of the nondependent side. This phenomenon occurs more often in premature infants but may be observed in full-term newborns. The change may be due to hypothalamic immaturity, which results in altered peripheral vascular tone.

Although it typically occurs within the first 3 weeks of life, harlequin color change is most often noted at 2 to 5 days of age. The changes develop abruptly and usually resolve within 20 minutes.

Common Neonatal Dermatoses

ERYTHEMA TOXICUM NEONATORUM

Erythema toxicum neonatorum is a benign condition that occurs in 30% to 70% of white full-term infants. Erythema toxicum occurs less frequently in premature infants for reasons that are unclear. The eruption is characterized by blotchy, erythematous macules with central papules, pustules, or vesicles, which give the infant a "flea-bitten" appearance (Fig. 58–2). The lesions develop most commonly between the second and fourth days of life; however, they may appear during the first 2 to 3 weeks of life. They are self-limited and usually resolve within several days. Typical sites of involvement include the face, trunk, and proximal extremities. There may be very few to hundreds of lesions.

A Giemsa or Wright stain of the intralesional contents reveals sheets of eosinophils with a relative absence of neutrophils. Peripheral eosinophilia may be present in up to 20% of affected infants. Erythema toxicum may occasionally be confused with transient neonatal pustular melanosis, congenital cutaneous candidiasis, impetigo neonatorum, milia, herpes simplex, or miliaria rubra (prickly heat).

TRANSIENT NEONATAL PUSTULAR MELANOSIS

Transient neonatal pustular melanosis (TNPM), seen in up to 4% of neonates, occurs more often in African-American infants. Typically present at birth, the initial lesions are 2- to 5-mm pustules distributed over the face, neck, and upper chest and less often on the sacrum, trunk, thighs, palms, and soles. Unlike the lesions of

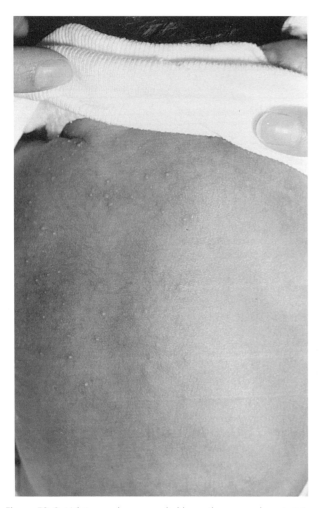

Figure 58–2. White papules surrounded by erythema are characteristic of erythema toxicum.

erythema toxicum, there is no erythema surrounding each pustule, and Wright stain of pustular contents reveals many neutrophils and few, if any, eosinophils. In both disorders, the pustules are sterile and should be distinguished from those seen in potentially serious infections caused by herpes simplex virus, *Staphylococcus aureus,* or candidal species.

The superficial pustules of TNPM rupture spontaneously within the first few days of life, leaving hyperpigmented macules that have collarettes of fine scale. It is common to see only hyperpigmented macules at birth. These brown spots slowly fade over several weeks to months.

MILIARIA

Miliaria results from sweat retention and is exacerbated by heat and humidity. Affected newborn infants are frequently in incubators or receiving phototherapy. Keratinous plugging of the eccrine ducts and subsequent release of eccrine sweat into the surrounding skin produce two distinct clinical presentations with different sites of eccrine duct obstruction. In *miliaria crystallina,* obstruction occurs just below the stratum corneum, resulting in superficial, noninflammatory 1- to 2-mm vesicles. In *miliaria rubra,* or "prickly heat," obstruction occurs in the mid epidermis. This is associated with an inflammatory response exhibited by vesicles, papules, or papulovesicles surrounded by a rim of erythema. The lesions occur in clusters on the trunk, face, scalp, and intertriginous regions.

Neither type of miliaria warrants therapy, but improvement occurs with cooling of the skin and avoidance of excessive warmth and moisture.

MILIA

Milia are pinpoint white or yellow papules that are present in 40% to 50% of neonates. Located predominantly on the face, they may also be seen in the oral cavity, where they are referred to as *Epstein's pearls* (palate) or *Bohn's nodules* (gingiva). The lesions represent keratin-filled epidermal inclusion cysts, which usually resolve spontaneously during the first few weeks of life. Unusually widespread or persistent lesions may be associated with defects such as hereditary trichodysplasia, oral-facial-digital syndrome, or particular subtypes of epidermolysis bullosa.

NEONATAL ACNE

Neonatal acne may develop in approximately 20% of newborn infants. Typically, it is not present at birth but usually appears during the first month of life. Characterized by papules, pustules, and closed or open comedones located on the face, chest, back, or groin, lesions usually resolve within the first several months of life. Therapeutic intervention is rarely required. It is believed that both maternal and endogenous androgens play a role in the development of neonatal acne. It remains unclear whether or not these infants are at greater risk for severe adolescent acne.

SEBACEOUS GLAND HYPERPLASIA

Sebaceous gland hyperplasia is characterized by the presence of multiple flesh- to yellow-colored tiny papules primarily on the nose and cheeks of full-term infants. The increased sebaceous cell size and number as well as sebaceous gland volume may result from maternal androgen stimulation. Spontaneous resolution occurs within the first 4 to 6 months of life.

SEBORRHEIC DERMATITIS

Seborrheic dermatitis, common during infancy, typically has its onset within the first several weeks of life. Characterized by erythema and a yellow, greasy scale, it usually resolves spontaneously within several months. The eruption occurs at sites where sebaceous glands are concentrated, such as the face, chest, and posterior auricular and intertriginous areas. "Cradle cap" is seborrhea that is confined to the scalp of infants. Involvement of the diaper area is characterized by salmon-colored patches that arise in skin folds and spread to the genitalia, suprapubic area, and upper medial thighs. Unlike atopic dermatitis, this eruption is not very pruritic. Secondary candidal or bacterial infection is common.

Diagnosis

The diagnosis of seborrheic dermatitis is established clinically. Presence of greasy yellow scale and salmon-colored patches, involvement of the scalp and intertriginous areas, early onset, and lack of pruritus or atopic history help distinguish seborrheic from atopic dermatitis. Seborrheic dermatitis should also be differentiated from *Letterer-Siwe disease* (histiocytosis), in which the lesions, often in a seborrheic distribution, are typically purpuric, erosive, or crusted. Skin biopsy findings as well as hepatosplenomegaly, purpura, lymphadenopathy, anemia, thrombocytopenia, interstitial pneumonia, and osseous lesions further distinguish this serious condition from seborrheic dermatitis.

Treatment

Treatment of the scalp consists of mild keratolytic shampoos, such as those containing selenium sulfide, zinc pyrithione, or tar. Mineral oil may be helpful in removing thick, adherent scale. The scalp and diaper dermatitis may be treated with low-potency topical corticosteroids. Topical antifungal or antibacterial agents should be used for coexisting candidiasis or impetigo.

DIAPER DERMATITIS

Diaper dermatitis (Table 58–4) is one of the most common dermatologic disorders of infants and toddlers. It comprises a group of inflammatory conditions that characteristically involve the lower abdomen, genitalia, upper thighs, and buttocks. Clinical manifestations include erythema, edema, erosions, vesicles, or pustules. Secondary changes of postinflammatory hyperpigmentation or hypopigmentation are common.

Although urinary ammonia was originally thought to be the primary factor in the development of diaper dermatitis, feces now appear to play a more important role in its pathogenesis. Fecal ureases, by converting urea to ammonia, cause elevation of skin pH, which, in turn, increases fecal protease and lipase activity. These proteases and lipases cause disruption of the epidermal barrier. Skin wetness, friction, maceration, and contact with feces, urine, and microbes further compromise epidermal integrity. This results in increased permeability of the skin to irritants such as soaps, powders, and detergents. Diaper dermatitis usually develops

between 1 and 2 months of age and may become a chronic or recurrent problem.

Developmental Defects

APLASIA CUTIS CONGENITA

Aplasia cutis congenita is a heterogeneous group of disorders in which there is a congenital absence of skin. It is characterized by localized absence of epidermis, dermis, or subcutaneous tissues (Fig. 58–3). The most common lesion is a 1- to 2-cm circular or oval defect on the vertex of the scalp. These ulcerative lesions are easily identifiable by their classic punched-out appearance. The defect is usually solitary; however, in a minority of patients, multiple sites may be affected. Aplasia cutis can also occur on the trunk and limbs, where the defects are often bilateral and symmetric.

Gradual epithelialization usually occurs spontaneously; however, large, deep, or widespread lesions may require surgical intervention.

NEVUS SEBACEUS

Nevus sebaceus of Jadassohn is an asymptomatic, well-circumscribed, hairless plaque of sebaceous gland derivation. Typically present at birth, these lesions are variable in size, usually solitary, and located on the scalp, face, and neck. During infancy, they are yellowish-orange smooth, velvety, or waxy plaques. These nevi tend to thicken and become verrucous during puberty.

Because 10% to 15% of these lesions develop secondary neoplasms during adolescence or adulthood (most commonly basal cell carcinomas or sweat gland tumors), prophylactic surgical excision is recommended.

Miscellaneous Neonatal Lesions

Subcutaneous fat necrosis is an uncommon condition of otherwise healthy infants that is sometimes associated with preceding

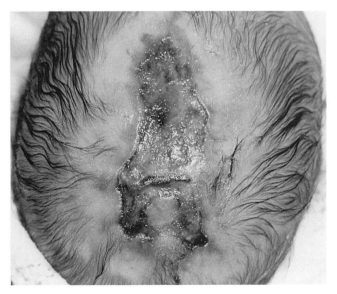

Figure 58–3. Congenital absence of skin (aplasia cutis congenita) on the scalp of a neonate.

Table 58–4. Diaper Dermatitis

Disease	Clinical Presentation	Other Features	Treatment
Friction	Inner surface of thighs, genitalia, buttocks, abdomen Mild erythema with a shiny glazed surface, occasional papules	Course waxes and wanes, aggravated by talc	Responds well to frequent diaper changes, avoidance of diapers, simple drying measures
Irritant	Confined to convex surfaces of buttocks, perineal area, lower abdomen, proximal thighs Sparing of intertriginous creases	Exacerbated by excessive heat, moisture, sweat retention	Gentle cleansing Lubricants (petrolatum) Barrier pastes (zinc oxide) Low-potency corticosteroids
Allergic contact	Often confined to the convex surfaces in direct contact with the offending agent, with sparing of the intertriginous skin Mild cases—diffuse erythema, papules, vesicles, edema, scaling Severe cases—papules, vesicles, psoriasiform lesions, annular plaques, secondary erosions, ulcerations, infiltrated nodules	May complicate an irritant dermatitis or arise *de novo* Often attributable to topical antibiotics or to preservatives, plus emulsifiers in topical baby products	Removal of offending agent Judicious use of low-potency topical corticosteroids
Seborrheic	Salmon-colored patches with greasy, yellow scale Involves intertriginous areas Fissures, maceration, weeping occasionally seen	May involve axillae, scalp "Cradle cap" Infants remain healthy and asymptomatic Significant hypopigmentation may be prominent in black infants	Low-potency topical corticosteroids Anticandidal agents for coexistent infection
Candidiasis	Typically involves skin creases Bright-red eruption, well demarcated; may have white scale at borders Characteristic satellite papules and pustules	Occasionally associated with oral thrush Occurs commonly after treatment with antibiotics	Aluminum acetate dressings Topical anticandidal medications, including Nystatin and clotrimizole (Lotrimin)
Intertrigo	Well-demarcated areas of maceration and oozing Intergluteal region and fleshy folds of the thigh	Often associated with miliaria	Avoidance of excessive heat Cool clothing
Psoriasis	Bright red, scaly, well demarcated May persist for months or recur frequently Less responsive to topical therapy	May have red scaly lesions on trunk or extremities Nail changes	Topical corticosteroids Emollients
Staphylococcal infection	Characterized by many thin-walled pustules on erythematous bases that leave a collarette of scale after rupturing		Antistaphylococcal therapy
Acrodermatitis enteropathica	Early lesions are vesicular and pustular More often see well-demarcated, dry, scaly, crusty lesions in periorificial distribution Often mimics candidiasis	Irritability or listlessness Failure to thrive, alopecia, diarrhea	Secondary to zinc deficiency Treat with zinc replacement
Histiocytosis (Letterer-Siwe)	Persistent seborrhea-like eruption; clusters of infiltrated papules, which are often hemorrhagic or purpuric Ulceration may be seen	Involvement of axillae and retroauricular skin Reddish-yellow papules and patches on the head and neck Anemia, thrombocytopenia, hepatosplenomegaly, osseous lesions	Chemotherapy

trauma or hypoxia. Single or multiple violaceous indurated nodules or plaques arise on the buttocks, thighs, back, cheeks, and arms. Occasionally, the lesions liquefy, ulcerate, and drain an oily substance. Intact lesions heal spontaneously within several months, while ulcerated lesions require a longer healing time and result in scarring.

Hypercalcemia may accompany this disorder, and treatment may include restriction of vitamin D intake, low-calcium diet, hydration, and administration of furosemide. Systemic corticosteroids can lower serum calcium levels, but prolonged therapy is not necessary.

DERMATOLOGIC DISORDERS IN OLDER INFANTS AND CHILDREN

Scaling Disorders

The term *papulosquamous* refers to conditions in which the primary lesions are papules or plaques associated with scale. These disorders are typically benign but can be chronic and therapeutically challenging.

PITYRIASIS ROSEA

Pityriasis rosea is an acute, common, self-limited eruption that has no sex predilection. Although the precise cause is unknown, a viral etiology is suspected because there have been reports of epidemics, clusters of cases among closely related individuals, and low recurrence rates. Furthermore, a prodrome of malaise, headache, and respiratory symptoms is occasionally observed.

The eruption usually begins with a solitary oval, pink scaly plaque, approximately 3 to 5 cm in diameter, that is typically located on the trunk or proximal extremities. Referred to as the *herald patch,* this finding is observed in 50% to 70% of cases. When the herald patch has an elevated red border and central clearing, it resembles tinea corporis. These two conditions can be differentiated by performing a KOH preparation, which is negative in pityriasis rosea. Within 1 to 2 weeks after appearance of the herald patch, numerous small, pink scaly papules or plaques arise over the trunk and proximal extremities, sparing the face and distal extremities. The lesions classically have a fine cigarette-paper–like peripheral collarette of scale. These oval 0.5- to 2-cm lesions have their long axis oriented along skin lines and, when present on the trunk, result in a ''Christmas-tree'' pattern. Young children, particularly African-Americans, may have an ''inverse'' type of pityriasis rosea, with most lesions distributed on the distal extremities, face, neck, and intertriginous regions. Other variants seen in children demonstrate lesions that are papular, vesicular, pustular, purpuric, or lichenoid.

Pityriasis rosea is most severe during the first month and gradually abates over the ensuing 12 to 14 weeks. Some cases resolve within a few weeks. Therapy is unnecessary; however, topical corticosteroids or oral antihistamines help relieve pruritus, when present. In addition, pityriasis rosea improves significantly with exposure to ultraviolet light. Postinflammatory hypopigmentation or hyperpigmentation may persist for several months, especially in dark-skinned individuals. Other dermatoses that resemble pityriasis rosea include secondary syphilis, guttate psoriasis, drug eruptions, dermatophyte infections, seborrheic dermatitis, nummular eczema, Mucha-Habermann disease, and cutaneous T-cell lymphoma. In sexually active adolescents, a rapid plasma reagin (RPR) test (VDRL test) should be obtained to rule out the possibility of secondary syphilis, which may have an identical clinical appearance. Persistence of the eruption beyond 3 to 4 months requires a search for another diagnosis.

PSORIASIS

Psoriasis, another common papulosquamous disease of children and adolescents, is characterized by well-demarcated erythematous scaly papules and plaques located most often on the scalp, elbows, knees, genitalia, and lumbosacral regions. The course is more chronic and unpredictable than that of pityriasis rosea. Psoriasis occurs in approximately 1% to 3% of the population and is estimated to present before the age of 20 years in about 25% of patients. It affects males and females equally in adulthood, but childhood psoriasis is more prevalent in girls. It is uncommon in Native Americans and African-Americans. The etiology is multifactorial, but there is a genetic predisposition in many affected individuals. There is a family history of psoriasis in approximately 30% of cases.

Psoriasis encompasses a broad spectrum of clinical manifestations, ranging from mild, asymptomatic, virtually undetectable disease to extensive, chronic, debilitating disease. The course is usually marked by recurrent flares and remissions and is often exacerbated by stress, trauma, infection, climate, hormonal factors, and particular medications. The lesions of psoriasis are due to a marked increase in epidermal cell proliferation and turnover. The rate of epidermal cell turnover is increased fourfold to sevenfold compared with normal skin.

Clinical Presentations

Although morphologic variations exist, the classic lesions of psoriasis are well-demarcated erythematous papules or plaques with a silvery-white scale (Fig. 58–4). The lesions usually begin as small erythematous papules that gradually enlarge and coalesce to form plaques up to several centimeters in diameter. The micaceous (mica-like) scale of the psoriatic plaque is more adherent centrally than peripherally. Removal of this scale results in multiple small bleeding points. This is referred to as the *Auspitz sign* and is secondary to disruption of the dilated blood vessels that are located high in the papillary dermis. Although this finding is seen in psoriasis, it is not pathognomonic.

The *Koebner phenomenon,* another characteristic feature of psoriasis, is an isomorphic response (development of new or larger lesions) occurring at sites of injury or trauma such as scratching, sunburn, or surgery. Koebnerization is also observed in lichen planus, lichen nitidus, vitiligo, and verrucae. Psoriatic lesions tend to be distributed symmetrically. Although extensor surfaces are typically involved, a variant of psoriasis, known as *inverse psoriasis,* affects flexural surfaces, such as the axillae and groin.

Scalp lesions are present in the majority of children with psoriasis. Diffuse, thick white scale may be accompanied by erythema. In contrast to seborrhea, psoriasis often extends beyond the hairline, affecting the forehead, ears, and neck. The lesions are variably pruritic and are generally not associated with hair loss. Scalp psoriasis tends to be more resistant to therapy than seborrheic dermatitis.

Nail abnormalities are seen in 25% to 50% of patients. Nail pits are the most common finding, identified by multiple pinpoint depressions that are irregularly distributed over the nail plate. Although nail pitting is characteristic of psoriasis, it is not a pathognomonic sign. It is also associated with atopic dermatitis, alopecia areata, and trauma. Other nail changes include separation of the nail plate from the nail bed (onycholysis), subungual hyperkeratosis, discoloration, crumbling, and ''oil spots'' on the nail plate. This latter finding is seen more often in older patients and are yellowish-brown spots on the nail thought to be due to glycoprotein accumulation.

Guttate psoriasis, characterized by numerous drop-like lesions,

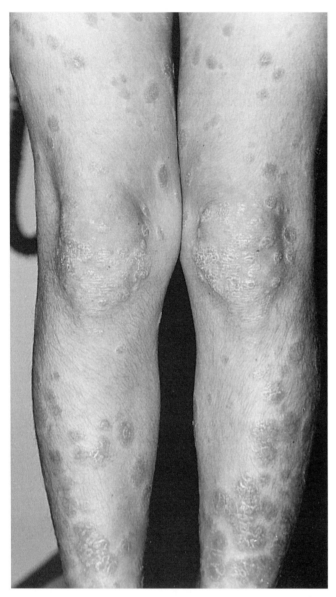

Figure 58–4. Well-demarcated erythematous, scaly plaques of psoriasis.

is a variant commonly seen in children and young adults. The round to oval, pinkish-red, somewhat scaly papules arise in crops and are widely distributed, particularly on the trunk. Two thirds of patients have a history of an upper respiratory tract infection, usually streptococcal in origin, that was present 1 to 3 weeks prior to the onset of lesions. Clinical improvement is seen following appropriate antibiotic therapy. Guttate psoriasis, in contrast to large-plaque psoriasis, is unlikely to become a chronic condition.

Diagnosis

Psoriasis is usually diagnosed by the clinical appearance of skin lesions. However, when the diagnosis is unclear, a skin biopsy may be helpful because specific histologic findings are usually observed. Differential diagnosis of psoriasis includes seborrheic dermatitis, dermatophytosis, pityriasis rosea, lichen planus, atopic dermatitis, and subacute cutaneous lupus erythematosus.

Treatment

The course of psoriasis is marked by recurrent flares and remissions. Although unpredictable, there appears to be a subset of individuals whose disease gradually improves over time. Various therapeutic modalities are available and may range from simple topical regimens to aggressive systemic management.

For mild cases, topical corticosteroids, tar, anthralin, and emollients may be sufficient. Moderate- to high-potency topical corticosteroids are usually effective within 2 to 3 weeks of therapy. However, remissions may be temporary because tachyphylaxis often develops. Care should be taken with the chronic, generalized application of topical corticosteroids in children, as systemic absorption may occur. Tar solutions and shampoos may be helpful for removal of scale from the scalp, especially when used in conjunction with topical corticosteroid preparations.

Other useful topical medications include salicylic acid, anthralin, and calcipotriene. Salicylic acid can be combined with topical corticosteroids, emollients, or oils to enhance scale removal. Anthralin is a tricyclic hydrocarbon that, when applied daily for 15 to 30 minutes and then washed thoroughly, can be highly effective. A topical synthetic vitamin D_3 derivative, calcipotriene (Dovonex), is a promising therapeutic alternative in some patients.

Ultraviolet light therapy is generally effective in the management of psoriasis. This can be in the form of natural sunlight or ultraviolet B light (UVB) therapy via a light box. Care must be taken, however, to avoid sunburn, which can result in exacerbation of the disease. For moderate to severe cases, daily use of crude coal tar in combination with UVB therapy, referred to as *Goeckerman therapy,* can result in complete clearing and long-term remissions after 2 to 4 weeks of treatment. In recalcitrant or severe debilitating psoriasis, photochemotherapy (psoralen plus ultraviolet A [PUVA]), oral retinoids, methotrexate, and cyclosporine can be used with caution, but side effects limit their usefulness in children. The use of oral corticosteroids should be avoided in psoriasis, as withdrawal may result in severe erythroderma or flares of their disease.

LICHEN PLANUS

Lichen planus occurs in patients of all ages but is less commonly seen in children than adults. It is characterized by *p*urple, *p*olygonal, *p*lanar, *p*ruritic *p*apules (the five Ps). The primary lesion is a shiny, violaceous flat-topped papule, often with angulated borders, measuring from 2 mm to greater than 1 cm in diameter. The lesions are very pruritic and demonstrate the Koebner phenomenon, resulting in development of new lesions (often in a linear configuration) at sites of scratching. Distribution may be localized or generalized, and lesions may number from few to numerous. Sites of predilection include the volar wrists, forearms, legs, genitalia, and mucous membranes. A reticulated pattern of delicate white lines or streaks *(Wickham striae),* seen on the buccal mucosa or skin, aids in confirming the diagnosis of lichen planus.

Nail changes are seen in approximately 10% of patients with lichen planus. These include longitudinal ridging, generalized nail destruction, red or brown discoloration, subungual hyperkeratosis, and thinning of the nail plate. Pterygium formation results from the overgrowth of fibrous tissue, which extends from the proximal nail fold to the tip of the nail, obliterating the nail plate. Medications that can produce a lichenoid eruption that is indistinguishable from lichen planus include beta blockers, antituberculous agents, tetracycline, furosemide, dapsone, phenothiazines, and carbamazepine.

Diagnosis

It is often possible for the experienced clinician to diagnose lichen planus strictly on clinical grounds. However, a skin biopsy specimen can reveal specific findings seen in lichen planus. The clinical differential diagnosis includes psoriasis and drug eruptions. If oral lesions are present, one needs to consider aphthous stomatitis, erythema multiforme, herpes simplex, and leukoplakia as diagnostic possibilities.

Treatment

Topical corticosteroids are the treatment of choice in most cases. Lichen planus usually resolves spontaneously over 1 to 2 years, but some cases may persist for many years. Generalized eruptions may respond to a short course of systemic corticosteroids. Oral antihistamines provide symptomatic relief.

ICHTHYOSIS

The ichthyoses are a group of inherited disorders characterized by scaling of the skin. The term *ichthyosis*, derived from the Greek word *ichthus*, meaning fish, was initially chosen to describe the fish scale–like appearance of the skin. This reference is offensive to some patients; thus, the ichthyoses are also referred to as *disorders of cornification*. The pathogenesis of these conditions appears to be multifactorial.

The ichthyoses can be divided into four main subtypes based on mode of inheritance, clinical features, histology, and biochemical markers. The most common of these subtypes, *ichthyosis vulgaris,* has a prevalence of 1 in 300 persons. It is transmitted in an autosomal dominant fashion and is the mildest form of ichthyosis. The scaling of ichthyosis vulgaris is usually not apparent at birth but appears after 3 months of age. Approximately 50% of affected patients have concomitant atopic dermatitis. The scales are fine and white and appear to be "pasted on." Sites of involvement include the extensor surfaces of the limbs and the trunk, whereas flexural surfaces are characteristically spared. Ichthyosis vulgaris usually worsens during winter months but tends to improve with age.

Emollients and keratolytics are the mainstay of therapy. Ichthyosis vulgaris can usually be managed with lubricants such as petroleum jelly and alpha-hydroxy acids (lactic and glycolic acid) or urea-containing preparations that improve binding of water to the epidermis. In addition, salicylic acid is a useful keratolytic agent but may result in irritation or burning. These side effects may also be noted with use of urea, lactic acid, and glycolic acid. Systemic retinoids are reserved for treatment of severe forms of ichthyosis because of the potential for serious side effects.

The presence of a collodion membrane at birth is sometimes seen in normal infants but may be the first sign of underlying ichthyosis, particularly *lamellar ichthyosis.* This type of ichthyosis is inherited in an autosomal recessive fashion and is clinically manifested by large plate-like scales and ectropion (Fig. 58–5).

Other forms of ichthyosis have different clinical features and inheritance patterns.

SEBORRHEIC DERMATITIS

Seborrheic dermatitis is characterized by an erythematous, scaly, symmetric eruption that occurs most often in hair-bearing and intertriginous regions. Seborrhea of infancy is discussed in the text

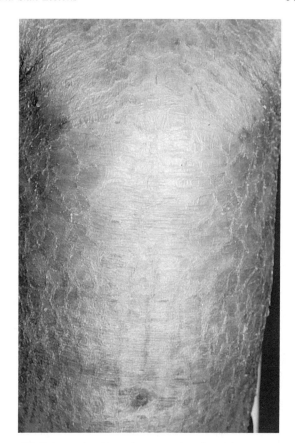

Figure 58–5. Large plate-like scales seen in lamellar ichthyosis, an autosomal recessive disorder.

on neonatal dermatology. In adolescents, yellowish, greasy scale of the scalp, eyebrows, nasolabial folds, nasal bridge, postauricular regions, and mid chest may be accompanied by mild erythema. Immunodeficiency disorders and neurologic dysfunction may be associated with severe, recalcitrant seborrheic dermatitis.

Therapy consists of low-potency topical corticosteroids. Antiseborrheic shampoos containing selenium sulfide, salicylic acid, zinc pyrithione, and tar are helpful for controlling scaling. Ketoconazole cream or shampoo can be used in patients who are not responding to topical corticosteroid preparations. Although individuals usually respond well to therapy, recurrences are common.

ATOPIC DERMATITIS

Atopic dermatitis (atopic eczema) is a chronic condition characterized by pruritus, a personal or family history of atopy, and an age-dependent distribution. It is common during infancy and childhood (3% to 5% of young children); approximately 80% of children outgrow the condition by puberty. Ninety percent of affected individuals have signs of atopic dermatitis prior to 5 years of age.

Typical lesions of acute atopic dermatitis are red crusted or scaly plaques consisting of tiny vesicles or papules. Some individuals have follicular accentuation, particularly on the trunk, manifested by a goose bump-like texture. Lichenification (thickened skin with exaggerated skin markings) is a feature of chronic atopic dermatitis and results from repeated rubbing and scratching. Excoriations are secondary lesions caused by scratching. Postinflammatory pigmentary changes are frequently noted, especially in darker-skinned individuals. Associated findings are noted in Table 58–5.

Table 58-5. Atopic Dermatitis: Associated Findings

Ichthyosis vulgaris	Affects 20% of patients with atopic dermatitis Primarily involves legs and trunk
Keratosis pilaris	Asymptomatic hyperkeratotic follicular papules found mainly on extensor surface of upper arms and anterior thighs, also facial in children
Pityriasis alba	Hypopigmented patches on the cheeks and occasionally upper body
Hyperlinear palms/soles	Common physical finding in atopic individuals
Dennie-Morgan folds	A double line found under the lower eyelids, commonly seen in atopic individuals Not pathognomonic
Lichen spinulosus	More commonly seen in black skin Pruritic grouped hyperkeratotic follicular spires
Eye findings	Keratoconjunctivitis, cataracts, keratoconus (abnormally shaped cornea), retinal detachment (rare)
Dyshidrotic eczema	Firm vesicles found on the palms and soles, lateral aspects of digits Frequently associated with hyperhidrosis
Nummular eczema	Well-demarcated, scaly, coin-shaped lesions usually on the lower extremities Associated with xerosis
Juvenile plantar dermatosis	Occasionally exudative lesions Painful erythema, scaling, cracking, and fissuring of feet Often associated with hyperhidrosis Improvement after puberty

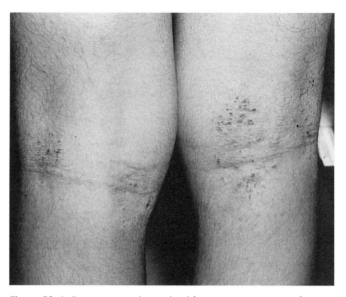

Figure 58-6. Excoriations in the popliteal fossae, a common site of involvement of childhood atopic dermatitis.

need occasional treatment with antistaphylococcal antibiotics to eradicate secondary infection. Presence of pustules, extensive excoriations, or weeping and crusted lesions suggest the need for antibiotic therapy. Topical therapy with mupirocin may be sufficient for limited areas; however, widespread involvement may necessitate the use of oral antimicrobials.

Secondary infection with herpes simplex virus is referred to as *eczema herpeticum,* or *Kaposi varicelliform eruption.* This occurs following inoculation of the eczematous skin with the herpes simplex virus. For example, transmission may occur during routine child care from a caretaker with a herpetic fever blister. The hallmark of this condition is the rapid development of numerous umbilicated vesicles and pustules. The infection may be associated with fever and other constitutional symptoms, and expedient treatment with acyclovir is required. Hospitalization may be necessary in young infants or severely affected individuals.

The distribution of the lesions tends to be age-dependent. The *infantile* form typically begins between 2 and 6 months of age. The cheeks, face, scalp, trunk, and extensor surfaces of the arms and legs are characteristically involved. The diaper region is usually spared because the skin is well hydrated from occlusive diapers.

Childhood atopic dermatitis occurs between 2 and 10 years of age. The neck, wrists, ankles, and flexural surfaces of the extremities are predominant sites of involvement (Fig. 58–6). After puberty, atopic dermatitis has a predilection for the face, neck, hands, and feet. The morphology of the skin lesions is not specific to this condition, as other eczematous eruptions (contact dermatitis, seborrheic dermatitis) have a similar appearance. Laboratory tests are of limited value, and histologic findings reveal a nonspecific spongiotic dermatitis. The distribution of lesions, age of onset, and history are most important for establishing the diagnosis of atopic dermatitis. Obtaining a complete personal and family history of atopic diatheses such as asthma, allergies, hay fever, allergic rhinitis, and eczema is necessary.

Diagnosis

The differential diagnosis is presented in Table 58–6.

Treatment

Management of atopic dermatitis is noted in Table 58–7.

Adverse Effects from Prolonged or High-Potency Topical Corticosteroid Use

1. Cutaneous atrophy
2. Telangiectases
3. Easy bruisability
4. Development of contact dermatitis rare, usually secondary to vehicle
5. Systemic absorption
   a. Growth retardation
   b. Electrolyte abnormalities
   c. Hyperglycemia
   d. Hypertension
   e. Increased susceptibility to infection

Complications

Secondary infections are the most common complication of atopic dermatitis. Individuals with atopic dermatitis have increased colonization with *Staphylococcus aureus.* Most affected children

Table 58–6. Differential Diagnosis of Atopic Dermatitis

Condition	Similarities	Differences
Seborrheic dermatitis	Scaly plaques May see erythroderma when severe	Earlier onset Pruritus minimal or absent Well-demarcated lesions Characteristic yellowish-salmon greasy lesions with intertriginous distribution
Contact dermatitis		
Primary irritant	Common in infants, young children May have similar distribution depending on the irritant, i.e., cheeks, chin, neck	Usually less pruritic and less eczematoid Diaper area distribution uncommon in atopic dermatitis
Allergic	Pruritic Erythematous, papulovesicular eruption	Well circumscribed Uncommon in first few months of life Involutes spontaneously on removal of offending agent
Psoriasis	Scaly, red lesions	Deeper red-violaceous hue Thick micaceous scale Characteristic nail changes Sharply demarcated lesions Distinct distribution Pruritus may be less intense
Scabies	Frequent eczematous changes secondary to scratching, rubbing, or irritating therapy Can be very difficult to distinguish in infancy	Presence of hyperpigmented nodules Presence of burrows Isolation of mite from skin scrapings Acute onset Affected household members
Letterer-Siwe disease (histiocytosis)	Scaly, erythematous eruption Usually begins during first year of life	Primarily children <3 yr of age Presence of purpuric papules Associated hematologic abnormalities, hepatosplenomegaly
Acrodermatitis enteropathica	Vesiculobullous eczematoid lesions Onset during infancy	Acral, periorificial distribution Associated features: failure to thrive, diarrhea, alopecia, nail dystrophy Low serum zinc levels
Wiskott-Aldrich syndrome	Severe eczematous dermatitis	X-linked recessive disorder Associated features of thrombocytopenia, defects in cellular and humoral immunity, bloody diarrhea
Phenylketonuria	Eczematous eruption	Hereditary Mental retardation, seizures, diffuse hypopigmentation, blond hair, photosensitivity Elevated blood phenylalanine levels
Hyper-IgE syndrome	Symptoms begin in first 3 mo of life Eczematous dermatitis involving the face and extensor surfaces Personal or family history of atopy	Coarse facial features, irregularly proportioned jaw and cheeks, broad nasal bridge, prominent nose, severe oral mucositis Lifelong history of severe streptococcal or staphylococcal infections of the skin, limbs, joints Exceptionally high serum IgE levels Diminished neutrophil chemotaxis

Corticosteroid "No-No's"

1. Use of high-potency topical corticosteroids on the face, diaper area, and intertriginous skin.
2. Extended use of high-potency preparations.
3. Use of high-potency preparations with occlusion.
4. Administration of large quantities of corticosteroids with unlimited refills (should prescribe only sufficient quantity to last between appointments).
5. Indiscriminate use of topical corticosteroids on all cutaneous eruptions. May exacerbate some conditions such as tinea corporis or acne.

LUMPS AND BUMPS

The presence of cutaneous or subcutaneous nodules and tumors can present a diagnostic challenge for the clinician. They are also a source of great concern to parents, who fear the possibility of malignancy. Fortunately, most nodules and tumors in children are benign and cutaneous malignancies are rare. The clinical features and appropriate management of dermal lumps and bumps as well as tumors of the epidermal appendages are noted in Table 58–8.

Granuloma Annulare

Granuloma annulare is characterized by skin-colored to mildly erythematous dermal papules and nodules that may expand and coalesce into rings. These asymptomatic annular plaques measure from 1 to 4 cm in diameter and are most commonly located on the dorsal hands and feet or extensor surfaces of the extremities (Fig. 58–7). The centers of these lesions usually appear normal but occasionally can be hyperpigmented or violaceous in color. The

Table 58–7. Management of Atopic Dermatitis

Therapeutic Modality	Indications and Recommendations
Bathing	Recommended daily for 10–15 min using warm, not hot, water. May use fragrance-free bath oils. Hydrates the skin.
Soaps	Mild, fragrance-free cleansers are essential, such as Dove, Basis, Aveenobar, Olay, Cetaphil, or Aquanil.
Emollients	Best applied immediately after bathing/showering. Should be used as often as possible. Petroleum jelly is ideal emollient—contains no water, additives, or preservatives and prevents evaporative water loss from skin. Thick creams such Eucerin, Nivea, and Cetaphil are some alternatives.
Compresses	Indicated for acute weeping lesions of atopic dermatitis. Helps cool and dry the skin, reduces inflammation. Use cool tap water or aluminum acetate solutions for 20 min, 2–4 times daily. Follow with topical corticosteroid application when appropriate.
Topical corticosteroids	Indicated to reduce pruritus and inflammation. Potency of topical corticosteroid determined by age of patient, site of involvement, severity of dermatitis, and duration of therapy. Facial and intertriginous skin should be treated with low-potency preparations. Apply prior to emollient. Use lowest potency that is effecive. Monitor closely for potential side effects, such as striae and cushingoid features.
Antihistamines	Controversial whether or not effective in this condition. If helpful, recommend oral, not topical, administration. May help some patients sleep. Hydroxyzine (2 mg/kg/day) often more effective than diphenhydramine (5 mg/kg/day). May induce drowsiness. Nonsedating antihistamines such as terfenadine or astemizole helpful in older children and adolescents, but avoid dangerous drug interactions.
Antibiotics	Patients have increased colonization with *Staphylococcus aureus*. Use if multiple excoriations, crusts, or pustules suggest secondary infection or if severe or resistant eczema is present. Treat with antistaphylococcal antibiotics. *Caution:* 1. Increased erythromycin resistance in many regions of United States. 2. Do not use erythromycin with the nonsedating antihistamines—increased risk of cardiac arrhythmia.
Ultraviolet light	Useful for severe, uncontrollable atopic dermatitis. May administer ultraviolet B light (UVB), or ultraviolet A light in conjunction with oral 8-methoxpsoralen (PUVA). Tanning beds not effective.
Tars	Useful for chronic, dry, lichenified lesions, not for acute dermatitis.
Environmental conditions	Environmental factors may influence the severity of the dermatitis. Some helpful measures: Avoid fragrances in all topicals and laundry products Avoid wool, feathers, dust exposure Reduce house dust mites Eliminate animal dander Use plastic mattress covers Reduce stress/anxiety Increase environmental humidity to reduce skin evaporative losses

overlying epidermis is unaffected. Multiple lesions are common, particularly in children. Granuloma annulare may be seen in all age groups, but at least 40% of cases occur before 15 years of age.

Etiology and Diagnosis

The etiology is unclear. Some cases have been associated with preceding trauma, such as insect bites. Histologically, there is dermal infiltration of lymphocytes and histiocytes surrounding degenerated collagen. Some postulate that the condition may result from a cell-mediated immune response.

The differential diagnosis includes tinea corporis, sarcoidosis, rheumatoid nodules, necrobiosis lipoidica diabeticorum, annular lichen planus, secondary syphilis, and leprosy. The eruption is most commonly confused with tinea corporis, but tinea has epidermal changes such as scaling, vesiculation, or pustules.

There are several variants of granuloma annulare. Generalized granuloma annulare is characterized by hundreds of asymptomatic papules symmetrically distributed. The ring-like lesions may coalesce into reticulated or circinate forms. The features of subcutaneous granuloma annulare are multiple deep nodules on the extremities, buttocks, and scalp. This entity is most frequently mistaken for rheumatoid nodules; however, the latter are usually larger.

Treatment and Prognosis

Granuloma annulare resolves spontaneously over several months to years. Although more than 50% of cases clear within 2 years, recurrences are common. Treatment is generally unnecessary, but the use of topical or intralesional corticosteroids may hasten resolution.

DISORDERS OF PIGMENTATION

These conditions are often cosmetically disfiguring and persistent. They can be markers of serious systemic diseases. Pigmentary disorders may be localized or generalized, congenital or acquired, and transient, stable, or progressive.

Congenital Disorders of Hypopigmentation and Depigmentation

PIEBALDISM

Piebaldism, or partial albinism, is characterized by circumscribed areas of depigmentation in the newborn. The leukoderma is usually

Table 58–8. Lumps and Bumps: Distinguishing Features

Diagnosed Lesion	Usual Onset	Color	Size	Site	Comments	Therapy
Epidermal cyst	Birth, childhood, adolescence	Skin-colored	1–3 cm	Face, scalp, neck, trunk	Potential for inflammation and infection	Elective excision
Dermoid cyst	Birth	Skin-colored	1–4 cm	Face, scalp, lateral eyebrow	When midline, may have sinus tract	Elective excision
Pilomatricoma	Any age 50% before adolescence	Skin-colored Reddish-blue Bluish-gray	0.5–3 cm	Head, neck	Malignant transformation possible but rare	Elective excision
Dermatofibroma	Adulthood 20% before age 20 yr	Skin-colored Tan, brown, black	0.3–1 cm	Extremities	May follow trauma	Elective excision
Neurofibroma	Occasionally at birth Usually childhood or adolescence	Usually skin-colored Also pink, blue	2 mm to several centimeters	Any body site	May be associated with neurofibromatosis May see *café au lait* spots	Elective excision
Juvenile xanthogranuloma	Birth Childhood	Yellow to reddish-brown	0.5–4 cm	Head, neck, trunk, proximal extremities	Extracutaneous lesions involving eye	Ophthalmology consult needed if numerous lesions
Keloids	Peak between puberty and age 30	Pink to violaceous	Variable	Any site of injury Commonly earlobes following piercing	Often tender or pruritic Familial tendency	Difficult Intralesional steroids Excision
Granuloma annulare	Childhood Adolescence	Skin-colored to red	1–4 cm	Distal extremities	May be generalized in approximately 15% of cases	Observe Topical steroids
Lipoma	Puberty Adulthood	Skin-colored	Variable May be >10 cm	Any, but usually neck, shoulders, back, abdomen	Malignant change very rare	Observe Excision
Solitary mastocytoma	Birth Early infancy	Skin-colored to light brown or tan Occasionally pink or yellowish hue	1–5 cm	Any site, but most often on arms, neck, trunk	+ Darier sign	Usually resolves spontaneously; antihistamines may be helpful
Erythema nodosum	Usually >10 yr of age Peak in third decade	Begin bright to deep red than develop a brownish-red to violaceous bruise-like appearance	1–5 cm	Symmetric distribution over pretibial region, legs Occasionally arms	Tender Association with many infectious agents (group A streptococci, tuberculosis, mycoplasma), inflammatory diseases (sarcoidosis, inflammatory bowel disease), medications (birth control pills)	Thorough evaluation and treatment of underlying cause Anti-inflammatory agents Bed rest/elevation of legs

located on the frontal scalp and is associated with a white forelock; however, the depigmented patches may involve any area of the body. This rare condition is transmitted in an autosomal dominant pattern. The disorder is usually present at birth but may not be recognized in early infancy because of the light color of neonatal skin. A Wood's lamp may enhance the contrast between depigmented and normal skin.

Piebaldism is a stable condition throughout life, and most affected individuals are otherwise normal. There are, however, several rare syndromes associated with partial albinism. Sun protection and cosmetic camouflage of the depigmented skin are the mainstays of therapy.

WAARDENBURG SYNDROME

Waardenburg syndrome, a rare autosomal dominant disorder, is considered a variant of piebaldism. It is characterized by a white forelock, areas of leukoderma, congenital sensorineural deafness, heterochromia of the irides, and lateral displacement of the medial canthi. Other features may include a flattened nasal bridge, confluent eyebrows, hypoplasia of the nasal alae, speech impairment that may or may not be related to presence of a cleft lip or palate, and various skeletal abnormalities.

ALBINISM

Albinism is manifested by diffuse congenital hypopigmentation or depigmentation of the skin, hair, and eyes. This heterogeneous group of disorders is composed of approximately ten types of oculocutaneous albinism and five forms of ocular albinism. Most types of oculocutaneous albinism are inherited in an autosomal recessive pattern. The variants of ocular albinism are transmitted in an X-linked or autosomal recessive mode of inheritance.

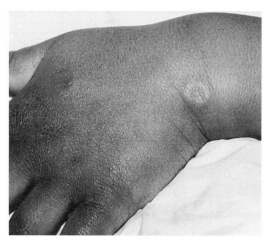

Figure 58–7. Ring of confluent dermal papules, typical of granuloma annulare.

Diagnosis

The various forms of albinism can usually be diagnosed by findings on physical examination. These features include absent or reduced skin and hair pigmentation and ophthalmologic findings such as foveal hypoplasia, nystagmus, photophobia, transillumination of the irides, fundal depigmentation, and decreased visual acuity. In whites, the skin is usually milk white and the hair is white, blond, or light brown. The pupils are usually pink and the irides are blue or gray. In African-Americans, the skin may appear tan or white and is frequently freckled. The hair is usually blond or red, and the eyes are blue or hazel.

Treatment

Treatment of albinism includes photoprotection and sun avoidance. Individuals are predisposed to severe actinic damage and should be monitored closely for the development of actinic keratoses, basal cell carcinomas, squamous cell carcinomas, and melanomas.

TUBEROUS SCLEROSIS

Ash leaf spots are hypopigmented macules, present at birth, that allow early identification of individuals with tuberous sclerosis. Although infrequently observed in normal infants, the characteristic lesions are present in up to 90% of patients with tuberous sclerosis. They are usually 2 to 3 cm in size and are located on the trunk and extremities. The macules may be lancet-shaped or may have a confetti-like or irregularly shaped appearance (Fig. 58–8). Wood light examination may facilitate identification of these lesions. Although tuberous sclerosis is an autosomal dominant disorder, spontaneous mutations are responsible for up to 50% of new cases. Other cutaneous findings include facial angiofibromas (adenoma sebaceum), periungual or subungual fibromas, gingival fibromas, shagreen patches (connective tissue hamartomas), and fibrous plaques (typically on the forehead). Systemic manifestations include seizures, mental retardation, cardiac rhabdomyomas, renal angiomyolipomas and cysts, optic gliomas, and pulmonary cysts. Imaging studies of the brain may demonstrate cortical tubers or subependymal nodules, which are pathognomonic for tuberous sclerosis. Other neurocutaneous disorders are noted in Table 58–9.

Acquired Disorders of Hypopigmentation or Depigmentation

POSTINFLAMMATORY HYPOPIGMENTATION

Postinflammatory hypopigmentation is a common cause of acquired hypopigmentation and may follow any inflammatory skin condition, including bullous disorders, infections, eczema, psoriasis, pityriasis rosea, secondary syphilis, and burns. More frequently detected in dark-skinned individuals, the clinical findings consist of irregularly shaped hypopigmented patches of variable size, often with a mottled appearance, located at sites of preceding inflammation.

Postinflammatory hypopigmentation usually resolves gradually over several months, and no treatment is necessary.

PITYRIASIS ALBA

Pityriasis alba is characterized by poorly demarcated, slightly scaly, oval hypopigmented macules located on the face, upper trunk, or extensor surfaces of the arms. The lesions generally vary from 0.5 to 2 cm, are often multiple, and are usually asymptomatic. Pityriasis alba may resemble tinea versicolor but can be differentiated by its negative KOH examination. The hypopigmentation typically persists for several months to years.

Although no therapeutic intervention is required, the use of emollients and low-potency topical corticosteroids may be effective.

VITILIGO

Vitiligo is an acquired disorder characterized by complete loss of pigment of the involved skin. The condition often presents during childhood and is believed to occur in genetically predisposed individuals.

Etiology

The precise etiologic agent of vitiligo remains unclear. Many believe that it is an autoimmune process with circulating antibodies that destroy melanocytes. There is an increased incidence of autoimmune diseases in affected individuals and their families, includ-

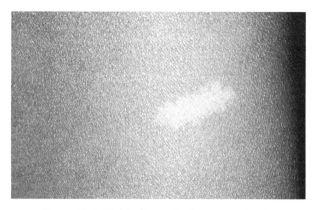

Figure 58–8. "Ash-leaf" macule of tuberous sclerosis.

Table 58–9. Neurocutaneous Syndromes

Syndrome	Mode of Inheritance	Cutaneous Findings	Systemic Findings
Tuberous sclerosis	Autosomal dominant	Ash leaf macules Angiofibromas (adenoma sebaceum) Shagreen patches Periungual/subungual fibromas Gingival fibromas	CNS involvement (seizures, mental retardation, cortical tubers) Cardiac rhabdomyomas Retinal gliomas Renal carcinoma or hamartoma Renal or pulmonary cysts Skeletal abnormalities
Neurofibromatosis (NF1 >85% cases)	Autosomal dominant	*Café au lait* macules (>6 measuring ≥1.5 cm) Axillary freckling (Crowe sign) Neurofibromas Blue-red macules and pseudoatrophic macules (involuted neurofibromas) Lisch nodules (melanocytic hamartomas of the iris)	Acoustic neuroma in NF2 Optic glioma, may result in exophthalmos, decreased visual acuity Mental retardation Seizure disorders Tumors (astrocytomas) Hyperactivity Learning disabilities Osseous defects (up to 50%) Intestinal neurofibromas Endocrine disorders
Incontinentia pigmenti	X-linked dominant	Phase 1—inflammatory vesicles/bullae in crops over trunk and extremities, may persist weeks to months Phase 2—irregular linear verrucous lesions on ≥1 extremity, resolves spontaneously within several months Phase 3—brown to blue-gray hyperpigmentation, swirl-like formations on extremities and trunk; increases in intensity through second year of life, then remains stable for many years Phase 4—streaked hypopigmented lesions	Eosinophilia CNS involvement (seizures, spasticity, ↓ IQ) Spastic abnormality Ophthalmic changes (strabismus, cataracts, optic atrophy, retinal damage) Alopecia Skeletal abnormalities Dental abnormalities

Abbreviations: CNS = central nervous system; IQ = intelligence quotient.

ing Hashimoto thyroiditis, alopecia areata, pernicious anemia, myasthenia gravis, parathyroid abnormalities, and other polyendocrine deficiencies. The incidence of vitiligo in persons with diabetes mellitus is also higher than that of the general population. The onset of vitiligo may be precipitated by sunburn or other trauma.

Diagnosis

Physical findings are usually sufficient for establishing the diagnosis of vitiligo. Well-demarcated depigmented macules that are often bilateral and symmetric are distributed on the extremities, on the periorificial areas, and within skin folds. In some cases, depigmentation may have a segmental or generalized distribution.

Prognosis

The clinical course is unpredictable. Spontaneous complete repigmentation is unusual; however, partial repigmentation may be seen during the summer months, especially within lesions of less than 2 years duration. Repigmentation proceeds gradually and is more likely to occur in children than in adults.

Treatment

Treatment options include daily application of topical corticosteroids, which may be effective in more limited diseases after several

months of therapy. For more cosmetically disfiguring vitiligo in motivated, compliant patients, photochemotherapy may provide the best chance of repigmentation. Psoralen can be administered either topically or systemically, and UVA light can be provided by natural sunlight or via an ultraviolet light box. This form of therapy is often effective in children or young adults, especially in lesions of recent onset. Care must be taken to avoid burning, as this can further exacerbate disease activity. Photochemotherapy usually requires several months until appreciable improvement is noted. Other intervention may consist of camouflage with cosmetics and careful photoprotection at sites of depigmentation in order to prevent development of cutaneous malignancy. Bleaching agents are another option in individuals with depigmentation of greater than 50% of their cutaneous surface.

Disorders of Hyperpigmentation

EPIDERMAL MELANOCYTIC LESIONS

Lentigines

Lentigines are 1- to 5-mm macules that are darker than freckles and may occur on any cutaneous site, including the mucous membranes. They do not have a predilection for sun-exposed skin. Lentigines have no seasonal variance, and those that present during early childhood often disappear during adulthood. A lentigo may be clinically indistinguishable from a junctional nevus (mole); however, these lesions are histologically distinct.

Several syndromes are associated with multiple lentigines. *Lentiginosis profusa* is an entity characterized by multiple deeply pigmented macules that are usually present at birth or early infancy. These individuals have no associated systemic or developmental abnormalities, unlike children with the *LEOPARD syndrome,* which also presents during infancy. As the acronym suggests, these children may have multiple lentigines (L), electrocardiograph abnormalities (E), ocular hypertelorism (O), pulmonic stenosis (P), abnormal genitalia (A), growth retardation (R), and neural deafness (D). Multiple lentigines located on the mucous membranes, especially the vermilion border of the lips and buccal mucosa, should alert the clinician to the possibility of *Peutz-Jeghers syndrome,* which is characteristically associated with intestinal polyposis and subsequent risk of malignant transformation and intussusception.

Café au Lait Macules

Café au lait macules are well-circumscribed tan macules that usually measure greater than 0.5 cm but may be as large as 15 to 20 cm in diameter. The lesions are found on any cutaneous site and may present at birth or appear during early childhood. Although *café au lait* spots are seen in 10% to 20% of normal individuals, the presence of many macules should raise the clinical suspicion of neurofibromatosis (Table 58–9). The presence of 6 or more *café au lait* spots (>0.5 cm in prepubertal children; >1.5 cm in postpubertal children) fulfills one of the diagnostic criteria for type 1 neurofibromatosis. Although the lesions are not pathognomonic, they are present in 90% of patients with neurofibromatosis and tend to be larger and greater in number. *Café au lait* spots have also been associated with tuberous sclerosis, McCune-Albright syndrome, Turner syndrome, Bloom syndrome, ataxia-telangiectasia, Russell-Silver syndrome, Fanconi anemia, epidermal nevus syndrome, Gaucher disease, and Chédiak-Higashi syndrome.

DERMAL MELANOCYTIC LESIONS

Mongolian Spots

Mongolian spots are large, poorly demarcated, slate-gray to blue-black macules usually located over the buttocks or lumbosacral region of normal infants. The condition occurs in approximately 80% to 90% of black infants, 75% of Asian infants, and 10% of white neonates. Mongolian spots may be single or multiple and frequently measure up to 10 to 20 cm in diameter. This benign disorder is present at birth, usually fades during early childhood, and requires no therapeutic intervention. Rarely, the lesions may persist into adulthood and may benefit from therapy with lasers that treat dermal pigmentation. These lesions should not be confused with bruising or child abuse.

The *nevus of Ota* and *nevus of Ito* are special variants of mongolian spots seen most commonly in Japanese and black individuals. In contrast to mongolian spots, these conditions tend to persist throughout adulthood. The nevus of Ota is a slate-gray to blue-black macular lesion located in the distribution of the trigeminal nerve. The condition is usually unilateral and involves the forehead, temple, periorbital region, nose, and cheek. Pigmentation of the eye occurs in about 50% of affected individuals. The disorder may be cosmetically disfiguring, and laser treatment may be promising in some cases. The nevus of Ito is a similar process occurring in the distribution of the lateral supraclavicular and brachial nerves. The condition is usually unilateral and involves the shoulder, neck,

upper arm, scapular, and/or deltoid regions. It may be seen alone or in conjunction with the nevus of Ota.

Postinflammatory Hyperpigmentation

Postinflammatory hyperpigmentation is the most common cause of hyperpigmentation in children. This pigmentary alteration can follow any inflammatory insult and is seen commonly after insect bites, diaper dermatitis, acne, drug reactions, or other skin trauma. The clinical features are usually more striking in darkly pigmented individuals and often may be more pronounced than the original inflammatory lesions. No treatment is required, as the increased pigmentation usually resolves gradually over several months to years.

MELANOCYTIC NEVI AND MELANOMA

Congenital Nevi

Congenital melanocytic nevi are pigmented macules or plaques that are present at birth or early infancy in approximately 1% of children. The lesions are often tan at birth and become darker and hairier during infancy (Fig. 58–9). Congenital nevi can be divided into small (<2 cm), medium (2 to 10 cm), and giant (>10 cm) lesions. Most nevi are small to medium in size, with giant congenital nevi occurring in only 1 in 20,000 newborns.

The malignant potential of congenital nevi remains an area of great controversy. A recent study concluded that the risk of malignant transformation is significantly lower in blacks. Risk of malignant transformation before 15 years of age is 1 in 10,000, and maximum risk increases to 1 in 3700 between the ages of 15 and 35 years in black patients. The risk of malignant transformation in the general population for small and medium congenital nevi is unknown, and there are no universal guidelines for their management. Some experts advocate prophylactic excision of these lesions, whereas others advocate close observation of the nevi. Most dermatologists agree that removal of these nevi can wait until later childhood, when local anesthesia and outpatient surgery are feasible.

The risk of malignant transformation of giant congenital nevi is

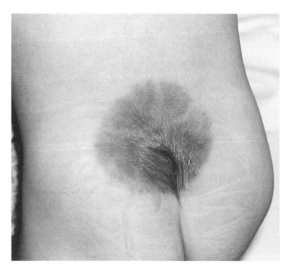

Figure 58–9. This hairy congenital melanocytic nevus was associated with a normal MRI of the lumbosacral spine.

another controversial issue and is reported to be between 2% and 15%, as compared to the general population's lifetime risk of melanoma of 1%. These large lesions warrant close observation and serial photography. Careful annual or semiannual examinations with palpation of the nevi is essential, as melanoma can arise from deep portions of the nevi with little or no apparent surface alterations. Most authors suggest that giant congenital nevi be completely removed whenever possible. This may require extensive grafting as well as soft tissue expansion procedures.

Pediatricians caring for infants or children with giant congenital nevi should also be aware of the potential for *neurocutaneous melanosis,* that is, the coexistence of large or multiple congenital melanocytic nevi and benign or malignant pigment cell tumors. The prevalence of this condition is unknown but appears to occur more commonly with congenital melanocytic nevi located on the scalp, face, or neck. Signs and symptoms of neurocutaneous melanosis usually present during the first 2 years of life; however, they may become apparent during the second or third decades of life. Affected individuals may present with neurologic manifestations of increased intracranial pressure, spinal cord compression, or mass lesions. The development of leptomeningeal melanoma has a very poor prognosis and is usually fatal. Diagnostic procedures such as cerebrospinal fluid cytology and magnetic resonance imaging with gadolinium contrast should be considered in children with giant congenital nevi.

Acquired Nevi

Acquired melanocytic nevi arise during early childhood as 1- to 2-mm hyperpigmented macules occurring most often on sun-exposed skin. These flat moles usually represent junctional nevi, in which nests of nevus cells are located along the dermoepidermal junction. Over time, some nevus cells may spread into the dermis, forming compound melanocytic nevi, which clinically appear somewhat larger and more papular than junctional nevi. In some nevi, the nevus cells may become restricted to the dermis. These intradermal nevi are usually fleshy or even pedunculated in appearance. Located usually on the head, neck, or upper trunk, these nevi may clinically resemble skin tags.

There is a gradual increase in the number of nevi during childhood and adolescence. The average individual acquires approximately 20 to 40 melanocytic nevi. This number peaks at 25 years of age. In general, fair-skinned persons have a greater number of nevi than darkly pigmented individuals. Later in adulthood, many of these pigmented lesions gradually fade away. Often, the moles develop peripheral circumferential hypopigmentation/halo effect during regression.

Melanoma

Although melanomas are very rare in childhood, their incidence in adults is increasing. The overall lifetime risk of melanoma development is approximately 1%, with about 2% of cases presenting before the age of 20 years. Melanoma can arise *de novo* or from preexisting congenital or acquired nevi. It appears that congenital nevi possess a greater risk of malignant transformation. Nevi should therefore be observed for specific changes that may be indicative of malignancy. These alterations include:

1. Rapid growth.
2. Changes in texture, including nodularity, crusting, ulceration, bleeding, or loss of normal skin lines.
3. Changes in pigmentation, especially the development of red, white, or blue hues.

4. Border irregularity, especially notched or scalloped edges.
5. Symptoms of itching, tenderness, or pain.

In general, melanomas occur more frequently in lightly pigmented individuals and in those with a family history of melanoma. Melanomas usually appear as darkly pigmented nodular masses greater than 6 mm in diameter. They are often asymmetric and tend to have irregular borders and surface characteristics. Malignant melanomas must be differentiated from other benign pigmented lesions, including congenital and acquired melanocytic nevi, blue nevi, Spitz nevi, vascular lesions such as hemangiomas and pyogenic granulomas, and pigmented lesions due to trauma. Suspicious lesions should be referred to a dermatologist for further evaluation and potential excisional biopsy.

The mortality rate of melanoma is estimated to be between 10% and 20%. The prognosis depends on the thickness of the lesion. For lesions less than 0.75 mm in depth, the prognosis is excellent. Surgical excision is the treatment of choice.

BULLOUS LESIONS (Table 58–10)

Erythema Multiforme Major (Stevens-Johnson Syndrome)

Stevens-Johnson syndrome is characterized by blisters, erosions, erythema, and hemorrhagic crusting of mucous membranes of the mouth, nose, eyes, and/or genitalia (Fig. 58–10). At least two of these sites must be involved to establish this diagnosis. Cutaneous target lesions, typical of erythema multiforme minor, may be present as well. Fever and prostration accompany this condition, which is seen more often in children than in adults (see Chapter 57).

Etiology

Although many factors have been implicated in the etiology of Stevens-Johnson syndrome, infections and medications are the most common causes in children (Table 58–11). In particular, penicillins, sulfonamides, anticonvulsants, and *Mycoplasma* infections are frequent triggers of this hypersensitivity reaction.

Treatment

Supportive therapy is the mainstay of treatment; few physicians believe that systemic corticosteroids are helpful in cases that are drug-induced. Careful ophthalmologic monitoring is necessary, since corneal scarring may lead to blindness. Maintenance of hydration and prevention of secondary bacterial infection are goals of treatment. Removal of the triggering factor is important.

Toxic Epidermal Necrolysis

Toxic epidermal necrolysis is a more severe hypersensitivity reaction than Stevens-Johnson syndrome but is often considered to be within the same disease spectrum. As with Stevens-Johnson syndrome, it is also triggered by underlying infection or medications, particularly sulfonamides, penicillins, phenobarbital, phenytoin, and allopurinol. Clinically, patients experience tender erythema of the skin that progresses to blistering and subsequent denudation. Malaise and fever accompany these skin changes. Mu-

Table 58–10. Vesiculobullous Eruptions

Entity	Clinical Clues
I. *Hereditary*	
A. Epidermolysis bullosa (AR, AD)	Bullae at birth in more severe forms
	Localized or widespread
	Dystrophic nails in some forms
	Bullae induced by trauma, friction; may occur spontaneously
	Mucosal involvement in severe forms
B. Incontinentia pigmenti (X-linked recessive)	Crops of blisters at birth or early infancy
	Often linear
	May have coexistent streaky hyperpigmentation
	Eosinophilia
	Associated CNS, dental, ocular, cardiac, skeletal abnormalities
	Females affected; males may have Klinefelter syndrome
C. Porphyria cutanea tarda (AD or acquired)	On dorsal hands, other sun-exposed skin
	Heal with milia formation
	Increased fragility of skin
	Hypertrichosis
D. Epidermolytic hyperkeratosis (bullous congenital ichthyosiform erythroderma) (AR)	Verruciform scales in flexural surfaces
	Bullae within first week of life
	Hyperkeratosis after third month
	Collodion membrane at birth in some cases
II. *Autoimmune*	
A. Linear IgA disease (chronic bullous disease of childhood)	Onset usually before age 6 yr
	Sites of predilection: perioral, periocular, lower abdomen, buttocks, anogenital region
	Annular or rosette configuration of tense blisters—''cluster of jewels''
	Mucous membranes commonly involved
	Spontaneous remission
	DIF shows linear deposits of IgA at DEJ
B. Bullous pemphigoid	Large, tense subepidermal bullae
	Lower abdomen, thighs, face, flexural areas
	Oral lesions common
	DIF shows linear deposits of C3 and IgG at DEJ
C. Pemphigus vulgaris	Flaccid bullae, persistent erosions
	Seborrheic distribution
	Mucosal involvement very common, usually the initial manifestation
	Positive Nikolsky sign
	DIF with intercellular (desmosomal) deposits of IgG, C3
D. Pemphigus foliaceus	Small flaccid bullae or shallow erosions with scaling, crusting
	Back, scalp, face, upper chest, abdomen
	Oral lesions uncommon
	May resemble a generalized exfoliative dermatitis
	DIF shows intercellular deposition of IgG, C3 in superficial epidermis
E. Dermatitis herpetiformis	Intensely pruritic
	Associated with gluten-sensitive enteropathy
	Extensor surfaces elbows, knees, buttocks, shoulders, neck
	Hemorrhagic lesions palms and soles
	DIF shows granular deposition of IgA in dermal papillae
III. *Infectious*	
A. Bacterial	
1. Staphylococcal scalded skin syndrome (SSSS)	Generalized, tender erythema
	Positive Nikolsky sign
	Occasionally associated with underlying infection such as osteomyelitis, septic arthritis, pneumonia
	Desquamation, moist erosions observed
	More common in children <5 yr of age
2. Bullous impetigo	Localized SSSS
B. Viral	
1. Herpes simplex virus	Grouped vesicles on erythematous base
	May be recurrent in same site—lips, eyes, cheeks, hands
	Reactivated by fever, sunlight, trauma, stress
	Positive Tzanck smear, herpes culture

Table 58–10. Vesiculobullous Eruptions *Continued*

Entity	Clinical Clues
2. Varicella	Crops of vesicles on erythematous base—"dewdrops on rose petal" Highly contagious May see multiple stages of lesions simultaneously Associated with fever Positive Tzanck smear, varicella-zoster culture
3. Herpes Zoster	Grouped vesicles on erythematous base limited to one or several adjacent dermatomes Usually unilateral Burning, pruritus Positive Tzanck smear; varicella-zoster culture Thoracic dermatomes most commonly involved in children
4. Hand-foot-mouth syndrome (coxsackievirus)	Prodrome of fever, anorexia, sore throat Oval blisters in acral distribution, usually few in number Shallow oval oral lesions on erythematous base Highly infectious Peak incidence late summer, fall
C. Fungal	
1. Tinea corporis	Annular scaly plaques, usually with central clearing Pustule formation common Positive KOH, fungal culture
2. Tinea pedis	Vesicles and erosions on instep Interdigital fissuring Positive KOH, fungal culture
D. Scabies	Burrow formation Interdigital web spaces, genitalia, ankles, lower abdomen, wrist Intensely puritic Very contagious Positive scabies preparation
IV. *Hypersensitivity*	
A. Erythema multiforme major (Stevens-Johnson syndrome)	Prodrome of fever, headache, malaise, sore throat, cough, vomiting, diarrhea Involvement of two mucosal surfaces, usually see hemorrhagic crusts on lips Target lesions progress from central vesiculation to extensive epidermal necrosis; may have sheets of denuded skin Associated with infection, drugs
B. Toxic epidermal necrolysis	Possible extension of erythema multiforme major involving >30% of body surface Severe exfoliative dermatitis Older children, adults Frequently related to drugs (e.g., sulfonamides, anticonvulsants) Positive Nikolsky sign
V. *Extrinsic*	
A. Contact dermatitis	Irritant or allergic Distribution dependent on the irritant/allergen Distribution helpful in establishing diagnosis
B. Insect bites	Occur occasionally following flea or mosquito bites May be hemorrhagic bullae Often in linear or irregular clusters Very pruritic
C. Burns	Irregular shapes and configurations May be suggestive of abuse Vary from first to third degree, bullae with second and third degree
D. Friction	Usually on acral surfaces May be related to footwear Often activity related
VI. *Miscellaneous*	
A. Urticaria pigmentosa	Positive Darier sign Coexistent pigmented lesions Usually presents during infancy Dermatographism commonly seen
B. Miliaria crystallina	Clear, 1–2-mm superficial vesicles occurring in crops, rupture spontaneously Intertriginous areas, especially neck and axillae

Abbreviations: AR = autosomal recessive; AD = autosomal dominant; CNS = central nervous system; Ig = immunoglobulin; DIF = direct immunoflouresence; DEJ = dermoepidermal junction; KOH = potassium hydroxide.

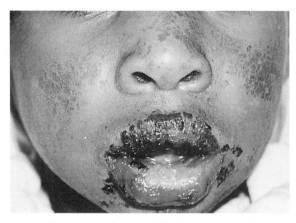

Figure 58-10. Erosions and crusting of the lips in Stevens-Johnson syndrome.

cous membranes are typically involved, and lesions are similar to those seen in Stevens-Johnson syndrome.

Patients are cared for as if they sustained a severe burn; fluid and electrolyte balance, temperature control, protein loss, and prevention of infection are serious concerns. With meticulous supportive care, most children do well; however, there is a high mortality rate associated with this condition.

Staphylococcal Scalded Skin Syndrome

Staphylococcal scalded skin syndrome (SSSS) comprises a spectrum of exfoliative dermatitis produced by staphylococcal epidermolytic toxins. The condition is most common in children younger than 5 years of age but is also seen in adults, especially in individuals with underlying immunosuppression or renal insufficiency. The condition may be localized or generalized, and approximately 80% to 85% of childhood SSSS is secondary to *S. aureus* phage group

Table 58-11. Potential Etiologies of Erythema Multiforme

Infectious Agents	*Antibiotics*
Herpes simplex 1, 2*	Penicillin
Mycoplasma pneumoniae†	Sulfonamides†
Tuberculosis	INH
Group A streptococcus	Tetracyclines
Hepatitis B vaccine	
BCG vaccine	*Anticonvulsants*
Yersinia	Phenytoin†
Enteroviruses	Phenobarbital†
Histoplasmosis	Carbamazepine†
Coccidioidomycosis	
	Other drugs
Chemicals	Phenylbutazone
Terpenes	Captopril
Perfumes	Etoposide
Nitrobenzene	Aspirin
Specific Diseases	*Other*
Leukemia	Radiation therapy
Lymphoma	

Modified from Esterly NB. The skin. *In* Behrman RE (ed). Nelson Textbook of Pediatrics, 14th ed. Philadelphia: WB Saunders, 1992:1641.
*Recurrent erythema multiforme.
†Erythema multiforme major (Stevens-Johnson syndrome: toxic epidermal necrolysis).
Abbreviations: BCG = bacille Calmette-Guérin; INH = isoniazid.

II. In children, most cases have been associated with exfoliative toxin A, with a minority of SSSS cases secondary to exfoliative toxin B.

Bullous impetigo is considered to be a localized form of SSSS. On the other end of the spectrum, SSSS can be a generalized, rapidly progressive disorder.

Diagnosis

The diagnosis should be considered in children with generalized tender erythema. A positive *Nikolsky sign* is seen in most cases and signifies the ability to laterally spread a blister or slough the skin with the application of light tangential pressure. The initial sites of involvement are the face, neck, groin, and axillae. One may see flaccid bullae, sheets of desquamating skin, or moist red erosions that heal within several days. Healing, without residual scarring, occurs within 1 to 2 weeks, as the level of cleavage is high within the epidermis. Unlike in Stevens-Johnson syndrome or toxic epidermal necrolysis, the mucosal surfaces are usually unaffected.

The diagnosis is usually established by the clinical presentation. *S. aureus* may be isolated from a minority of blood cultures. The organism is more likely to be isolated from distant sites, such as the nares, throat, and conjunctivae, than from the bullae themselves. In some children, the toxin may be produced by an underlying infection, such as pneumonia, osteomyelitis, or septic arthritis.

Treatment and Prognosis

The condition is usually self-limited in otherwise healthy children. Oral antistaphylococcal antibiotics may be indicated in localized SSSS. Children with widespread involvement usually require hospitalization, treatment with intravenous antistaphylococcal antibiotics, and supportive management. The skin should be handled very carefully, and adhesives should be avoided. Pain control is frequently necessary. Underlying infection should be suspected and investigated on an individual basis.

The prognosis is good in immunocompetent children, and the mortality rate is much lower than in affected adults.

Allergic Contact Dermatitis

Allergic contact dermatitis is a classic example of a type IV delayed hypersensitivity reaction. This T-cell–mediated immune response occurs after contact of the responsible antigen with the skin. Initially, the reaction becomes apparent 7 to 14 days after antigenic exposure. Future contact with the same antigen provokes an inflammatory response within hours to 1 to 3 days.

Acute contact dermatitis is usually characterized by the sudden onset of erythema, vesiculation, edema, and intense pruritus. Chronic contact dermatitis results in the development of lichenification, scaling, and hyperpigmentation and possible bacterial infection. *Poison ivy,* or *Rhus* dermatitis, is the most common cause of allergic contact dermatitis in the United States. Direct contact of the skin with the sap of poison ivy, oak, or sumac may result in dermatitis. Contact with clothing or pets that have been exposed to the plant resin or smoke from the fire of plants being burned are other forms of exposure. The eruption of poison ivy is usually seen as linear vesicles and papules or plaques. The spread to body sites is due to exposure to the plant resin, not the blister fluid. Therefore, scratching affected skin or contact with affected individuals should not result in spreading of the eruption.

Other common forms of allergic contact dermatitis result from exposure to cosmetics, fragrances, hair dyes, and nickel. Nickel dermatitis often results from prolonged contact with the nickel in jewelry or belt buckles. The eczematous changes are usually localized to the sites of contact, including the earlobes, neckline, wrists, or waistline.

Diagnosis

The diagnosis of contact dermatitis can usually be determined by history and clinical examination. When allergic contact dermatitis is suspected but the responsible agent is unclear, patch testing with a selected group of antigens may provide useful information. Prevention of future exposure to inciting antigens is necessary.

Treatment

Usually, treatment with topical corticosteroids is sufficient to control the eruption. However, widespread dermatitis or severe involvement of the face may require administration of systemic corticosteroids. A 3-week course of prednisone usually results in complete resolution of the eruption. Wet compresses aid in the drying of weeping, vesicular lesions and provide symptomatic relief. Antihistamines and other antipruritic agents are also useful. Secondary bacterial infection should be treated, if present.

Epidermolysis Bullosa

Epidermolysis bullosa (EB) is a heterogeneous group of inherited blistering disorders characterized by spontaneous and post-traumatic bulla formation. It is estimated to occur in approximately 1 in 50,000 births; however, the severe variants are seen less frequently. There are presently 23 distinct variants that are distinguished by the inheritance pattern, cutaneous manifestations, histologic findings, and ultrastructural abnormalities.

In *epidermolysis bullosa simplex,* the level of blister cleavage is intraepidermal. This form results from a defect in the basal cell keratins 5 and 14, which have been localized to chromosomes 12 and 17, respectively, and are necessary for epidermal integrity. Most of the simplex forms are mild and are autosomal dominant conditions. Bullae formation may be localized or generalized.

In the localized *Weber-Cockayne variant,* blisters are usually confined to the hands and feet, which develop after significant friction or trauma. This form may not become apparent until adolescence or adulthood and may present after strenuous activities such as hiking, military training, or golf. There are also generalized forms of epidermolysis bullosa simplex in which the bullae are much more extensive and usually apparent at birth and during early infancy. In general, the various subtypes are characterized by bullae that heal without scarring, mild or absent nail changes, and minimal mucosal involvement. There are usually no associated extracutaneous manifestations.

In *junctional epidermolysis bullosa,* the cleavage plane occurs at the level of the lamina lucida of the dermoepidermal junction. This variant results from defects in the protein laminin 5, which is localized to the anchoring filaments, which are fibrillar structures within the lamina lucida. The junctional form is transmitted in an autosomal recessive mode of inheritance. There is a wide spectrum of subtypes, ranging from mild involvement to a more severe, potentially fatal variant. Most forms are clinically apparent at birth. In general, there are widespread bullae that heal with atrophy, not scarring. Dysplastic nails, severe oral lesions, and enamel

dysplasia are usually seen. The most severe variant has been referred to as *epidermolysis bullosa letalis of Herlitz.* Often fatal by 2 years of age, this variant is characterized by exuberant granulation tissue on the face and around the mouth. Its extracutaneous manifestations include pyloric atresia, chronic anemia, and laryngeal involvement often necessitating tracheostomy.

In *dystrophic epidermolysis bullosa,* tissue separation occurs below the dermoepidermal junction at the level of the lamina densa. The lamina densa is made up of anchoring fibrils composed of type VII collagen. Individuals with the dystrophic form have qualitative or quantitative abnormalities due to mutations in the gene for type VII collagen. Dystrophic epidermolysis bullosa is further separated into variants that may be inherited in either an autosomal dominant or recessive pattern. Usually apparent at birth, there is a wide array of clinical presentations, but in general the condition is characterized by nail dystrophy and generalized blisters that heal with scarring and milia formation. In the more severe recessive dystrophic form, affected individuals usually have severe interdigital scarring, which results in syndactyly between fingers and eventual encasement of fingers and thumbs known as the *mitten deformity.* Severe mucosal involvement is a constant feature of recessive dystrophic epidermolysis bullosa, and esophageal stenosis and obstruction is a significant cause of morbidity and mortality. These patients have multiple extracutaneous manifestations as well as very high frequency of aggressive and recurrent squamous cell carcinomas. The dominant dystrophic forms are usually more localized and have a better prognosis.

Diagnosis

It is usually impossible to distinguish the variants on the basis of clinical manifestations alone. Skin biopsies are mandatory for determining the correct subtype. Transmission electron microscopy remains the gold standard for diagnosis by demonstrating the ultrastructural level of cleavage. Immunofluorescent antigenic mapping is helpful in determining the precise level of blister formation; EB-specific monoclonal antibodies may provide further data.

Treatment

Treatment modalities are dependent on the severity of the particular variant. In general, the emphasis is on wound care, prevention of infection, and prevention of mechanical factors likely to induce blister formation. Topical antibiotics and nonadhesive semipermeable dressings may be necessary for recalcitrant wounds. All adhesives should be avoided. In patients with the severe variants of epidermolysis bullosa, a multidisciplinary approach is imperative and should focus on preventive care. All patients should undergo genetic counseling.

PURPURA AND PETECHIAE (Table 58–12)

Purpura results from leakage of blood from vessels into the skin or mucous membranes (see Chapter 51). Purpuric lesions do not blanch when pressure is applied. Small lesions that are pinpoint or a few millimeters in diameter are called *petechiae.* Large lesions may be referred to as *ecchymoses.* Raised or palpable purpura is diagnostic of vasculitis and can be seen in conditions such as Henoch-Schönlein purpura, lupus erythematosus, and Rocky Mountain spotted fever (Table 58–13). Inflammation and destruction of blood vessel walls are responsible for the raised quality of these lesions. Nonpalpable purpura can be seen with platelet abnormali-

Table 58–12. Causes of Purpura

Infections	Drugs
Rocky Mountain spotted fever	Aspirin
Sepsis	Corticosteroids
Subacute bacterial	Penicillins
endocarditis	Sulfonamides
Streptococcal infection	Thiazides
Gonococcemia	**Other**
Meningococcemia	Scurvy
Hepatitis	Trauma
Echovirus 9	Cryoglobulinemia
Atypical measles	Henoch-Schönlein purpura
Collagen-Vascular Diseases*	PLEVA
Lupus erythematosus	Polyarteritis nodosa
Dermatomyositis	Malignancy
Rheumatoid arthritis	
Hematologic Disorders	
Idiopathic thrombocytopenic	
purpura	
Acute lymphocytic leukemia	
Aplastic anemia	
DIC	
Clotting factor deficiencies	
Coumadin or heparin use	

*Usually livedo pattern.
Abbreviations: DIC = disseminated intravascular coagulation; PLEVA = pityriasis lichenoides et varioliformis acuta.

ties, leukemia and other thrombocytopenic conditions (see Chapter 51), capillaritis (pigmented purpuras), scurvy, viral exanthems, and physical exertion. Petechiae on the upper body (above the nipple line) can result from crying, vomiting, or coughing. Careful clinical examination is important for detecting these lesions and establishing a proper diagnosis.

Henoch-Schönlein Purpura

Henoch-Schönlein (anaphylactoid) purpura is a small-vessel vasculitis that usually occurs in children and young adults. The skin, joints, kidneys, and gastrointestinal tract can be involved. It is an immune complex–mediated disorder that typically demonstrates immunoglobulin A (IgA) deposition in affected tissues. The antigens responsible for this hypersensitivity reaction may be bacteria or viruses, but drugs and foods have been implicated as well. The precise nature of the immunologic reaction is unclear.

The dermatologic features include purpuric macules, papules, or urticarial lesions that have a predilection for the buttocks and extensor aspects of the extremities. Hemorrhagic bullae and ulcerations can also be present. In infants, edema of the hands, feet, genitalia, and face may be seen. Systemic involvement is present in approximately 66% of patients. Gastrointestinal features include vomiting, colicky abdominal pain, nausea, diarrhea, bleeding, and, rarely, intussusception (see Chapter 18). Arthritis or arthralgias are most often noted in the elbows and knees. There may be purpura overlying the affected joints. Joint effusions are rare. Renal involvement is the most serious complication and can be manifested by hematuria (see Chapter 29).

The clinical course is characterized by acute onset of cutaneous lesions, often associated with fever and malaise. Attacks usually last for several weeks. Recurrences are common, but spontaneous resolution almost always occurs.

Diagnosis

The diagnosis of HSP is made on clinical grounds, but a biopsy of the skin confirms the presence of leukocytoclastic vasculitis. Direct immunofluorescence staining of the skin biopsy specimen reveals IgA and C3 deposition.

Treatment

Treatment includes supportive care and analgesics for joint pains as needed. Systemic corticosteroids may be indicated when there is significant gastrointestinal pain. The prognosis is excellent. Mortality is rare and is usually due to severe renal involvement.

Table 58–13. Types of Vasculitis and Associated Skin Lesions

Type of Vasculitis	Blood Vessels Involved	Type of Skin Lesion
Leukocytoclastic or hypersensitivity angiitis: Henoch-Schönlein purpura, cryoglobulinemia, hypocomplementemic vasculitis	Dermal capillaries, venules, and occasional small muscular arteries in internal organs	Purpuric papules, hemorrhagic bullae, cutaneous infarcts
Rheumatic vasculitis: systemic lupus erythematosus, rheumatoid vasculitis	Dermal capillaries, venules, and small muscular arteries in internal organs	Purpuric papules: ulcerative nodules; splinter hemorrhages; periungual telangiectasia and infarcts
Granulomatous vasculitis		
Churg and Strauss allergic granulomatous angiitis	Dermal small and larger muscular arteries and medium muscular arteries in subcutaneous tissue and other organs	Erythematous, purpuric, and ulcerated nodules, plaques, and purpura
Wegener granulomatosis	Small venules, arterioles of dermis, and small muscular arteries	Ulcerative nodules, peripheral gangrene
Periarteritis: classic type limited to skin and muscle	Small and medium muscular arteries in deep dermis, subcutaneous tissue, and muscle	Deep subcutaneous nodules with ulceration; livedo reticularis; ecchymoses
Giant cell arteritis: temporal arteritis, polymyalgia rheumatica, Takayasu disease	Medium muscular arteries and larger arteries	Skin necrosis over scalp

From Wyngaarden JB, Smith LH (eds). Cecil Textbook of Medicine, 18th ed. Philadelphia: WB Saunders, 1988.

VASCULAR LESIONS

Hemangiomas

Vascular birthmarks are classified as hemangiomas (Table 58–14) or vascular malformations. Hemangiomas, primarily composed of capillaries, are characterized by endothelial cell proliferation, whereas malformations have normal endothelial cell turnover. Hemangiomas are the most common benign tumors occurring in children. These lesions develop in 10% to 12% of white infants by 1 year of age. Girls are affected three times as often as boys. The incidence is higher in premature infants. The natural course of hemangiomas includes proliferative and involutional phases that result in complete, spontaneous regression in most cases.

Classification

There are three types of hemangiomas:

- *Superficial* hemangiomas, once referred to as strawberry marks, are the most common type and are bright red with well-demarcated borders (Fig. 58–11).
- *Deep* hemangiomas (called *cavernous* in the past) are the least common of the three types and are blue-violet or covered by normal-appearing skin.
- *Mixed* hemangiomas possess both superficial and deep components.

Pathogenesis

Most hemangiomas occur on the head and neck, but any area of the body may be involved. Although the etiology of hemangiomas is not clear, their natural course has been well documented. They are present at birth in only 30% of cases but typically develop by 3 to 4 weeks of life. The initial lesion may be a white macule with central thread-like telangiectases or a red macule resembling a port-wine stain. A peripheral zone of pallor representing vasoconstriction may be noted at this stage. Within the first few months of life, the macule becomes raised and enlarges. During the first 6 months of life, hemangiomas proliferate at a rapid rate. After 6 months, the lesion grows at a slower rate and peaks at 10 to 12 months. Involution begins around this time and is heralded by a color change from bright cherry red to dull red-violet. Deep hemangiomas start to lose their blue-violet hue. In time, the central portion of the superficial hemangioma develops a grayish-white color that eventually extends to the periphery of the lesion. It is not possible to predict precisely how long a hemangioma will take to involute. Statistically, 50% of lesions are gone by 5 years of age, 70% by 7 years, and 90% by 9 years. By 10 to 12 years of age, 95% to 97% of hemangiomas have disappeared. Once resolved, residual skin changes such as hypopigmentation and scarring may be present.

Treatment

For most hemangiomas, no treatment is needed. If there are extensive, disfiguring lesions or ones that compromise vital functions, systemic corticosteroids may be used. The pulsed dye laser can be effective for treating superficial hemangiomas, particularly when they are macular and treated early in their natural course. Interferon is effective in blocking endothelial cell motility and proliferation *in vitro* and inhibiting the process of angiogenesis.

Vascular Malformations

SALMON PATCHES

Salmon patches are the most common vascular lesion in infancy. These lesions consist of ectatic capillaries and are present at birth

Table 58–14. Syndromes Associated with Hemangiomas

Syndrome	Clinical Features	Age of Onset	Evaluation	Treatment	Prognosis
Kasabach-Merritt	Rapidly enlarging hemangioma Thrombocytopenia Microangiopathic hemolytic anemia DIC	First few months of life Rarely in older children	CBC Peripheral blood smear PT/PTT Platelets Fibrinogen level Fibrin split products	Prednisone (2–4 mg/kg/day) Heparin Cryoprecipitate, FFP Epsilon-amino-caproic acid Interferon-α2a Surgery	20–40% mortality
Benign neonatal hemangiomatosis	Widespread cutaneous hemangiomas No visceral involvement	Birth or first few weeks of life	Careful physical examinations and follow-up	None	Excellent
Diffuse neonatal hemangiomatosis	Widespread cutaneous hemangiomas May have visceral hemangiomas, multisystem involvement, hepatomegaly, anemia, high-output cardiac failure	Birth or first few weeks of life	If indicated by clinical examination: CBC, platelets PT/PTT Stool guaiac, urinalysis Chest radiography, ECG Liver function tests, abdominal ultrasound MRI (brain)	Prednisone (2–4 mg/kg/day) If indicated, diuretics, digoxin	High mortality rate

Abbreviations: DIC = disseminated intravascular coagulation; CBC = complete blood count; PT = prothrombin time; PTT = partial thromboplastin time; FFP = fresh frozen plasma; ECG = electrocardiogram; MRI = magnetic resonance imaging.

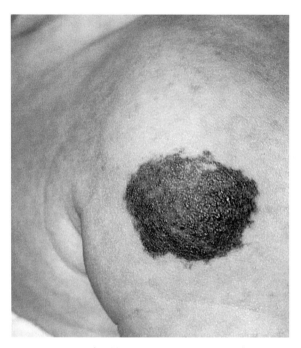

Figure 58–11. A superficial hemangioma early in its proliferative phase.

in about 40% of infants. These pink to red macules can be located on the nape of the neck, glabella, forehead, upper eyelids, and nasolabial regions.

No treatment is necessary, as most of these fade by 1 to 2 years of age. Persistent lesions can be treated successfully with the pulsed dye laser.

PORT-WINE STAINS

Port-wine stains *(nevus flammeus)* occur in 0.3% of all newborns. They are present at birth and represent progressive ectasia of the superficial vascular plexus. These lesions, in contrast to salmon patches, do not undergo spontaneous resolution. They are usually unilateral and segmental but can be bilateral. The face and neck are the most commonly affected sites (Fig. 58–12). Port-wine stains are typically pink during infancy and darken to reddish-purple hues

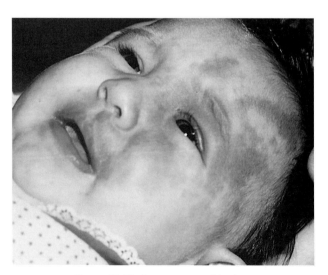

Figure 58–12. Port-wine stain of the face.

with advancing age. Adults frequently have thickened, nodular port-wine stains that may be associated with soft tissue hypertrophy. Port-wine stains occur as isolated cutaneous lesions or in conjunction with other abnormalities. Sturge-Weber, Klippel-Trenaunay, Parkes-Weber, and Cobb syndromes all feature port-wine stains as one of the clinical manifestations.

Treatment is best accomplished with the pulsed dye laser. This laser operates at 585 nm and specifically destroys blood vessels without damaging surrounding tissue.

Pyogenic Granuloma

Pyogenic granulomas are acquired vascular lesions that arise from the connective tissue of the skin or mucous membranes. These vascular nodules may be associated with antecedent trauma and represent a reactive, proliferative process. They are usually solitary, but multiple lesions rarely occur. Arising as small red papules, pyogenic granulomas grow rapidly and can ulcerate, leading to profuse bleeding.

Treatment involves destruction by laser therapy, electrodesiccation, surgical removal or cryotherapy. These lesions, in contrast to hemangiomas, do not regress spontaneously.

Spider Angioma (Nevus Araneus)

Telangiectases are dilated capillaries that appear as red linear stellate or punctate lesions. There are many causes of primary telangiectasias (spider angiomas, Osler-Weber-Rendu syndrome, cutis marmorata telangiectatica congenita) and secondary telangiectasias, such as collagen-vascular diseases. Spider angiomas are the most common of the telangiectasias. In the pediatric age group, these lesions are typically not associated with systemic disease.

Spider angiomas are seen most often on the face, trunk, and upper extremities. They are acquired lesions that develop after 2 years of age. Small vessels radiate from a central punctum (arteriole), giving the appearance of a "spider." When pressure is applied to the central punctum, the lesion blanches. Treatment, if desired, consists of gentle electrodesiccation or pulsed dye laser therapy. In some cases, spider angiomas clear without treatment.

ALOPECIA

Alopecia (hair loss) is the most common hair abnormality seen in children.

History and Physical Examination

An accurate history alone can lead to a presumptive diagnosis. Information regarding duration of loss, rate of shedding, drug intake, trauma, family history of hair disorders, symptoms such as pruritus or burning, breakage, and hair care is particularly important. The scalp should be examined for the pattern and distribution of hair loss, erythema, scaling, scarring, pustules, and crusts. Abnormal or broken hairs as well as texture, length, and color should be noted. Associated abnormalities of the teeth, nails, and sweat glands may occur. Hair pulls (gentle pulling on small tufts of hair) and microscopic examination of removed hairs should be performed. Appropriate tests (KOH, culture, scalp biopsy) are done to confirm clinical suspicions.

Classification

Classification of alopecia is somewhat arbitrary, but it is helpful to determine whether hair loss is acquired or congenital and localized or diffuse. The four disorders responsible for most cases of childhood alopecia are (1) alopecia areata, (2) tinea capitis, (3) trauma/trichotillomania, and (4) telogen effluvium. All are acquired conditions and, in most cases, associated with localized hair loss.

ALOPECIA AREATA

Alopecia areata is a common disorder that affects all ages, particularly children. Although the exact pathogenesis is unclear, it is generally thought that it is an autoimmune condition associated with lymphocytic inflammation around hair follicles. A family history of alopecia areata is present in approximately 20% of affected individuals.

Clinically, there is acute onset of hair loss that is occasionally preceded by burning or itching of the scalp. Localized areas of alopecia result, and the scalp is normal or slightly inflamed. The exclamation point hairs are pathognomonic and are due to breakage of abnormally growing hairs. When the disease is active, dystrophic anagen hairs can be easily pulled from the periphery of lesions. Nail pitting is seen in some cases.

Prognosis

Although the course is unpredictable, about one half of patients have a recurrence. Factors that portend a poor prognosis for regrowth include extensive loss (alopecia totalis, alopecia universalis), early onset, nail involvement, atopic background, and an ophiasis pattern (involvement of the hairline). Girls tend to have a better prognosis, as do those individuals whose alopecia has not been longstanding.

Treatment

Treatment consists of topical, intralesional, or systemic corticosteroids, topical minoxidil, anthralin, sensitization to contact allergens, PUVA (psoralen plus ultraviolet A light), camouflage, hairpieces, and support groups. In some cases, hair regrows without medical intervention.

TINEA CAPITIS

Tinea capitis (ringworm) is another common cause of alopecia in children, although it may not always be associated with hair loss or breakage. The "seborrheic" type is manifested by diffuse scaling without scalp inflammation. Alopecia is often not noted, but broken hairs may be present occasionally. This type of alopecia is frequently misdiagnosed as dandruff. Tinea capitis can also present as localized scaly patches, kerions, and "black-dot" patches. This latter type features hairs that have broken at the surface of the scalp, resulting in a black-dot appearance.

Kerions are boggy, inflammatory plaques on the scalp that are due to hypersensitivity to the offending dermatophyte (Fig. 58–13). Pustules and drainage are common, but the purulent material is typically sterile. Cervical lymphadenopathy, fever, and elevated white blood cell counts may accompany kerions.

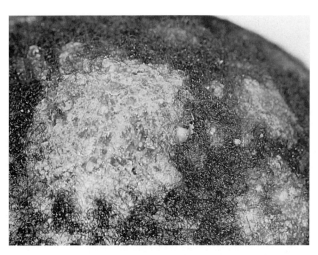

Figure 58–13. Boggy, purulent, crusted plaques typical of kerions.

Etiology

The most common etiologic agent of tinea capitis is *Trichophyton tonsurans,* a dermatophyte that produces endothrix infections. Because spores are not present on the surface of the hair shafts, Wood's lamp examination is not useful. If, however, the infection is caused by *Microsporum canis* or another dermatophyte that produces an ectothrix infection, Wood's lamp examination results in positive fluorescence. Fungal cultures should be performed in all suspected cases of tinea capitis. KOH preparations can be useful if positive, but false-negative results are possible.

Treatment

Treatment consists of oral griseofulvin for 6 to 8 weeks. The standard dose is 15 to 20 mg/kg/day of microsized preparations, and this can be given in single or divided doses. Griseofulvin should be administered with fat-containing foods, since fat is required for optimal absorption. Selenium sulfide 2.5% shampoo should be used to decrease surface spores and reduce spread to other individuals.

Occasionally, there is a secondary bacterial infection that requires antibiotic therapy. Kerions respond to griseofulvin; in severe cases, systemic corticosteroids may be added to decrease inflammation and drainage. Incision and drainage are not indicated.

TRAUMATIC ALOPECIA

Etiology

Various types of trauma can lead to alopecia in children and adolescents. *Traction alopecia* is seen in individuals whose hair is tightly braided or pulled into ponytails. Chronic tension on the hair shafts leads to breakage and gradual hair loss. Avulsion (forcible removal) is another type of trauma that is commonly associated with childhood alopecia. This condition, termed *trichotillomania,* or manipulative alopecia, affects approximately 8 million Americans of all ages. Individuals pull, break, or twist hair from one or several hair-bearing areas. Eyebrows, eyelashes, pubic hair, and scalp hair may be involved. In young children, this condition is a harmless habit that is outgrown. Older children and adolescents have a less favorable prognosis. The disorder is often refractory to treatment in teenagers and adults.

Diagnosis

On physical examination, there are hairs of varying lengths in bizarre, often geometric, patterns. The occiput is often spared. Hairs have blunt tips because of the mechanical breakage. If the diagnosis is unclear or denied, scalp biopsy findings can be confirmatory.

Treatment

Treatment is directed toward identifying underlying psychosocial stressors. Evaluation of the home and school environments should be considered. Although therapy is often supportive, behavior modification, self-hypnosis, or medications such as clomipramine can be beneficial.

TELOGEN EFFLUVIUM

Telogen effluvium is characterized by excessive shedding of telogen (resting) hairs. This may be due to medications, febrile illness, crash diets, parturition, surgical procedures or anesthesia, endocrine disorders, or severe emotional stress. A large number of growing hairs enter the resting phase, resulting in a threefold to fivefold increase in the number of resting hairs. Gradually, these numerous telogen hairs are shed over 6 to 24 weeks. Affected individuals notice sparser scalp hair 2 to 4 months after they have been exposed to the inciting factor.

The prognosis for this type of diffuse alopecia is excellent. Patient education is important, as is reassurance that regrowth can be expected within approximately 6 months. Women who have telogen effluvium after parturition may experience partial regrowth of hair.

No treatment is indicated.

INFECTIONS AND INFESTATIONS

Impetigo

Impetigo is the most frequently diagnosed bacterial skin infection. It is a contagious superficial skin infection, occurring most often in infancy and early childhood. The two major pathogens, *S. aureus* and group A beta-hemolytic streptococcus (*Streptococcus pyogenes*), can cause lesions at any body site.

CLASSIFICATION

Nonbullous Impetigo

Nonbullous impetigo accounts for the majority of cases and is secondary to infection with either of the aforementioned pathogens. The predominance of each organism has varied over the past several decades, with streptococcus representing the primary pathogen in the 1960s and 1970s. However, in the 1980s, staphylococcal infections became more prevalent. Clinically, the lesions of nonbul-

lous impetigo caused by either organism are indistinguishable. The lesions typically arise on the face or extremities, following trauma such as insect bites, cuts, abrasions, or varicella. The primary lesion is usually a vesicle or a pustule that develops secondary changes of honey-colored crusting, the clinical hallmark of this condition. In general, the lesions are smaller than 2 cm and may be single or multiple (Fig. 58–14). Surrounding erythema is often absent. Although patients are generally asymptomatic, regional lymphadenopathy is sometimes present.

The differential diagnosis of nonbullous impetigo includes herpes simplex infections, nummular eczema, varicella, kerions, and scabies. Nonbullous impetigo usually resolves spontaneously within 2 weeks. It is highly contagious, however, and should therefore be treated with appropriate antimicrobial agents to decrease outbreaks in day care centers and schools.

Bullous Impetigo

Bullous impetigo is always caused by *S. aureus,* usually phage group II. It develops on intact skin and is a localized form of staphylococcal scalded skin syndrome. The initially transparent flaccid bullae are more likely to occur on covered body sites such as the trunk and perineum than are the lesions of nonbullous impetigo. They do, however, occur on the face and extremities as well. Intact vesicles or bullae may be observed, or moist erythematous shallow erosions may be the sole clinical finding following disruption of the bullae. Bullous impetigo should be differentiated from allergic contact dermatitis, burns, erythema multiforme, and inflammatory bullous diseases.

TREATMENT

Impetigo may be treated with topical or oral antibiotics. Topical antibiotics are inferior to oral agents in the treatment of cutaneous infections with the exception of mupirocin (Bactroban). Mupirocin is bactericidal at concentrations that result from topical administration and has been found to be comparable or even superior to oral erythromycin in several studies. Furthermore, this topical antibiotic has fewer side effects than oral erythromycin. The major adverse effect is an allergic contact sensitivity to the propylene glycol in its vehicle. Treatment guidelines recommend application three times daily for 7 to 10 days.

There are many oral antibiotics with good antistreptococcal and antistaphylococcal activity. Some of the more cost-effective choices

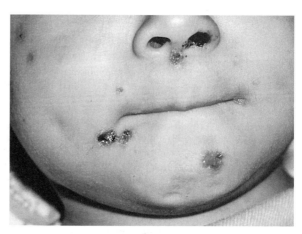

Figure 58–14. Multiple honey-colored crusted lesions of impetigo.

include cephalexin and dicloxacillin. The incidence of erythromycin-resistant strains of *S. aureus* has increased dramatically in many regions of North America, and this agent should be reserved for regions where resistance is not yet a problem. Oral antibiotics should be used when there is widespread involvement or evidence of soft tissue involvement. A 7-day course is usually satisfactory. Recurrent impetigo is often secondary to carriage of *S. aureus*. Although intranasal carriage is common, colonization can also involve the axillae and perineum. Intranasal application of mupirocin four times daily for 5 days may eradicate the organism; however, recolonization occurs over time.

COMPLICATIONS

Potential complications of impetigo include pneumonia, cellulitis, osteomyelitis, septic arthritis, and septicemia. More specifically, streptococcal infections can result in scarlet fever, guttate psoriasis, lymphadenitis, and lymphangitis. Furthermore, nephritogenic strains can result in poststreptococcal glomerulonephritis, which is generally seen in children aged 3 to 7 years (see Chapter 29). The latency period following impetigo is approximately 3 weeks. Treatment does not prevent poststreptococcal glomerulonephritis but does prevent the spread of the organism to others.

Molluscum Contagiosum

Molluscum contagiosum, caused by a large DNA poxvirus, is most often seen in children and adolescents. The characteristic well-circumscribed, skin-colored to pearly papules usually arise in crops on the face, trunk, and extremities but have a predilection for the axillary, antecubital, and crural regions. Generally ranging in size from 1 to 5 mm, these asymptomatic papules have a central umbilication. In some individuals, eczematous changes develop at sites of the molluscum lesions, probably representative of a delayed hypersensitivity response. This dermatitis may be localized or more extensive.

Diagnosis

The diagnosis is made by the clinical appearance of the lesions. However, skin biopsies or microscopic examination of the core of the lesions can confirm the diagnosis by revealing molluscum bodies, which are masses of virus-infected epidermal cells. The condition should be differentiated from warts, closed comedones, and milia.

Incubation

Molluscum contagiosum is both contagious and autoinoculable. The incubation period ranges from 2 weeks to 6 months, and multiple family members are often affected. Immunosuppressed individuals are at risk for more aggressive disease, especially patients infected with human immunodeficiency virus (HIV) infection. Patients with preexisting atopic dermatitis are also at greater risk for widespread molluscum lesions because of altered cutaneous T-cell immunity.

Treatment

Treatment options include curettage, liquid nitrogen, and topical application of trichloroacetic acid. Topical cantharidin is effective

and relatively painless, making it a good choice for treating children. It is applied to individual lesions and washed off when blistering occurs. As with other poxvirus infections, these lesions occasionally result in scarring.

Warts

Warts are intraepidermal tumors caused by human papillomavirus (HPV), a small DNA virus. They may be present in up to 10% of the general population. There are more than 60 types of HPV. The virus produces four major types of warts: common, flat, plantar, and genital (condyloma acuminatum).

The incubation period generally varies from 1 to 6 months, depending on the size of the inoculum, the site of infection, and the host's immune status. The duration of the wart is variable as well, with approximately 65% of the lesions resolving spontaneously within 2 years. Warts can be spread between persons and between body sites by direct or indirect contact. Most warts are located on the fingers, hands, and elbows because trauma to these sites promotes inoculation of the virus. Warts also display the Koebner phenomenon, resulting in linear configurations of lesions at sites of shaving or scratching.

CLASSIFICATION

Common Warts

Verruca vulgaris, or the common wart, is found most commonly on the dorsal surface of the hands or fingers, although it may be located at any body site. The lesions may be solitary or multiple and measure from several millimeters to greater than 1 cm. Varying in color from yellowish tan to grayish black, the common wart has a distinct rough, papillated surface (Fig. 58–15). Punctate thrombosed capillaries, clinically manifested by black dots, may be seen on the surface.

Flat Warts

Verrucae plana, or flat warts, are 2 to 5-mm flat-topped papules that are typically skin-colored, tan, or brown. They are distributed on the face, neck, and extremities. They often appear grouped, especially when koebnerized secondary to shaving or other trauma. These lesions are most often confused with lichen planus or lichen nitidus, since these disorders also feature flat-topped papules.

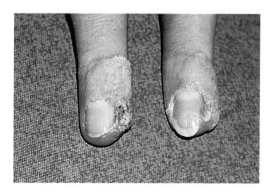

Figure 58–15. Periungual warts are common in children and are often difficult to treat.

Plantar Warts

Verrucae plantaris, or plantar warts, develop on the weight-bearing areas of the toes, heels, and mid-metatarsal region. The lesions are pushed into the skin in such a manner that the verrucous surface is even with the surrounding skin. These warts are often very tender and produce significant discomfort with ambulation. Plantar warts may be difficult to distinguish from corns and callouses.

Genital Warts

Condylomata acuminata, or genital warts, are fleshy papillomatous growths found on the genitalia. Their growth can be exuberant in some patients, resulting in cauliflower-like masses. In early or mild cases, the only physical finding may be subtle skin-colored, flat-topped papules. These genital warts should be differentiated from moist papular or nodular lesions of secondary syphilis (condylomata lata). Although nonvenereal transmission may occur, the presence of genital warts in young children may be associated with sexual abuse (see Chapter 31).

TREATMENT

Treatment is designed to be cytodestructive and varies, depending on type of wart, site of the lesion, age of the patient, immune status, and extent of involvement. Topical treatment includes keratolytic preparations, such as salicylic and lactic acid. Salicylic acid is available in a variety of paints and plasters that can be applied daily for several weeks and leads to maceration of the infected skin, which can then be easily removed. Cantharidin can be applied in the office setting and washed off several hours later after blisters have formed. It results in effective and relatively painless eradication of the wart virus. Liquid nitrogen, or cryotherapy, is another effective modality, but its burning sensation may limit its usefulness in small children. Podophyllin is reserved for the treatment of genital warts because it is most effective on mucosal surfaces.

Extremely recalcitrant warts may necessitate surgical or laser treatment or intralesional bleomycin. Multiple or serial treatments may be necessary, and recurrences are common.

Herpes Simplex Virus

Herpes simplex virus (HSV) is a large DNA virus that is divided into two major antigenic subtypes. Type 1 (HSV-1) has been traditionally associated with oral and nongenital herpes infections; type 2 (HSV-2) is generally responsible for genital infection. The clinical lesions are indistinguishable but can be differentiated by serologic tests. HSV infections are categorized as either primary or recurrent. Primary infections usually follow an incubation period of approximately 1 week. They range from subclinical infections to localized or generalized vesicular eruptions to life-threatening systemic infections. Primary herpetic infections can involve any cutaneous or mucosal surface.

The classic clinical presentation consists of grouped umbilicated vesicles on an erythematous base. The lesions usually begin as papules, which evolve into vesicles, or sometimes pustules, within approximately 48 hours. The vesicles rupture and form a crust over the next 5 to 7 days and generally heal within 2 weeks. The cutaneous eruption is often accompanied by fever, regional lymphadenopathy, or flu-like symptoms.

Following the primary infection, the virus remains dormant until reactivated. Recurrent infections occur in previously infected individuals and are characterized by localized vesicular eruptions and symptoms such as itching or burning at the same site. Recurrent HSV infections are usually less severe than primary herpes. Reactivation of the virus may be triggered by sunburn, cutaneous trauma, febrile illnesses, menstruation, or emotional stress. If administered during the prodromal period before the onset of lesions, oral acyclovir may abort or shorten recurrent episodes.

Herpetic gingivostomatitis is typically seen in infants and toddlers. Multiple vesicles and subsequent erosions develop on the lips, gingivae, anterior tongue, or hard palate. The condition is very painful and is often accompanied by inability to eat and drink. Fever, irritability, and cervical lymphadenopathy are frequently observed in affected children. The fever typically resolves within 3 to 5 days, whereas the oral lesions may persist for up to 2 weeks. The eruption may resemble aphthous ulcers, which are usually more localized and are not accompanied by systemic symptoms as with herpetic gingivostomatitis. Enteroviruses may produce similar oral manifestations; however, they tend to spare the gingivae and often affect the posterior pharynx.

The diagnosis of HSV infection can be established by a positive Tzanck smear, a viral culture, or immunofluorescent staining.

Treatment is supportive, with an emphasis on pain control and fluid replacement. Oral acyclovir may hasten resolution of the lesions and shorten the course of the illness.

Neonatal herpes is a potentially fatal infection (HSV-2), often with severe central nervous system (CNS) involvement. Intravenous acyclovir as well as vigilant supportive care is required. Immunocompromised children in whom a herpetic infection develops should also receive intravenous acyclovir and be monitored carefully for evidence of pulmonary, hepatic, and CNS involvement. Another high-risk group consists of children with underlying atopic dermatitis who, if exposed to HSV, are susceptible to rapid spread of herpetic blisters. Referred to as eczema herpeticum or Kaposi varicelliform eruption, the condition may be accompanied by fever and malaise. Oral or intravenous acyclovir as well as supportive care is indicated.

Varicella

Varicella (chickenpox) is a common, very contagious, but usually self-limited infection caused by the varicella-zoster virus. When this infection occurs in adults, it is usually much more serious and has the potential to involve the lungs, liver, and CNS.

INCUBATION

Transmitted by close contact and respiratory droplets, varicella has an incubation period of 10 to 21 days. The cutaneous presentation in healthy children is characterized by crops of lesions (usually two or three crops of 50 to 100 lesions each) that initially appear as 2- to 3-mm red macules and then evolve through a papular, vesicular, and finally a pustular stage within approximately 24 hours. Although the vesicular stage has traditionally been described as resembling "dewdrops on a rose petal," it is common to see lesions in various stages at the same anatomic site. All vesicles become crusted and resolve over several days. Chickenpox usually heals without scarring, except for lesions that have been excoriated or secondarily infected. The eruption is usually accompanied by fever, intense pruritus, and malaise.

Diagnosis

When the diagnosis is unclear, confirmatory tests include immunofluorescent staining and viral culture. A positive Tzanck smear supports the diagnosis but is not specific for varicella.

Treatment

Symptomatic treatment consists of oral antihistamines, oatmeal baths, calamine lotion, and cool compresses. Lesions should be observed for signs of secondary bacterial infection. Immunocompromised individuals or those receiving systemic corticosteroids usually require intravenous acyclovir. Some pediatricians advocate the use of oral acyclovir for healthy children in whom varicella develops or who have sibling contacts. If given, oral acyclovir should be administered within 24 hours of onset of the eruption.

High-risk individuals (immunosuppressed, immunocompromised, those with malignancies) who have been exposed to varicella should receive gamma globulin prophylaxis (VZIG) as soon as possible. If varicella develops in the mother within 5 days before delivery or 48 hours after delivery, the infant should also be treated with VZIG. The generalized use of the varicella vaccine has been advocated by the American Academy of Pediatrics and is to be given to children between 12 and 18 months of age.

Herpes Zoster

Similar to herpes simplex virus, the varicella-zoster virus remains dormant in the dorsal root ganglia following initial infection. Reactivation of the virus results in the clinical manifestations of herpes zoster, or shingles. The infection usually presents as a linear or band-like papulovesicular eruption affecting one or several dermatomes (Fig. 58–16). Commonly, there is a prodrome of burning, pruritus, or pain of the affected skin that may last several days prior to the appearance of cutaneous lesions. Vesicles become crusted, and all lesions resolve within a few weeks. The most common dermatomes involved are within the thoracic regions. Up to six to ten satellite lesions may be encountered outside the primary dermatomes in uncomplicated zoster. An increased number of satellite lesions is observed in generalized zoster, which carries a greater risk of systemic involvement. Widespread vesicles should raise the suspicion of an underlying immunodeficiency disorder.

Immunocompromised patients, especially children with lymphoreticular malignancies, are at increased risk for zoster and should be treated with either oral or intravenous acyclovir. As in herpes simplex infections, lesions of the nasal tip are suggestive of ocular involvement. Ocular complications occur in approximately 50% of the patients with ophthalmic zoster. The potential for deep keratitis, uveitis, secondary glaucoma, and loss of vision warrants prompt ophthalmologic evaluation. Patients with zoster should avoid contact with high-risk individuals who are susceptible to development of varicella.

Scabies

Scabies is extremely common, occurs in persons of all ages, and results from infestation of the superficial layers of skin by the human mite *Sarcoptes scabiei*. The infestation is highly contagious and is therefore seen frequently among individuals living in crowded conditions. Humans are the only source of the mite, which can be passed from one person to another. Fomites can also play an important role in transmission. In previously unexposed individuals, the incubation period varies from 2 to 6 weeks. This period is significantly shortened in individuals who have been exposed to the mite.

Although the morphologic appearance of scabies can vary dramatically, the hallmark lesion is the burrow. A burrow is a serpiginous or linear papule caused by movement of the mite through the epidermis. Although considered to be characteristic of scabies, the burrow is apparent in only a minority of patients. Other typical lesions include papules, vesicles, and pustules, the distribution of which is age-dependent. In infants, the distribution is generalized and involves the scalp, face, neck, axillae, palms, and soles (Fig. 58–17). Because the eruption is extremely pruritic, secondary infection and eczematization are common, leading to misdiagnoses of impetigo and atopic dermatitis. In older children, adolescents, and adults, the lesions characteristically involve the volar aspects of the wrists, ankles, interdigital web spaces, buttocks, genitalia, groin, abdomen, and axillae. Unlike infantile scabies, the lesions always spare the head.

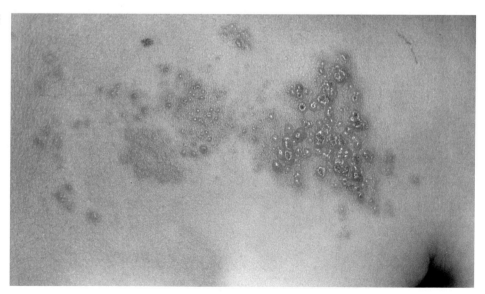

Figure 58–16. A dermatomal distribution of umbilicated vesicles is characteristic of herpes zoster.

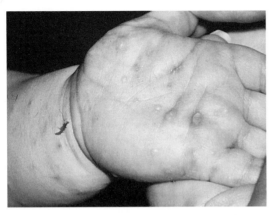

Figure 58–17. Lesions of the palms and soles are typical of scabies in infants.

Diagnosis

The diagnosis of scabies can be confirmed by scraping the newer lesions, ideally a burrow, with a blade after the application of mineral oil. The scraping may be viewed microscopically and is considered diagnostic if mites, ova, or feces are present. Although the yield may be low, particularly in children, suspicious lesions should be scraped and an attempt to identify the mite should be made.

Treatment

Topical 5% permethrin cream (Elimite) is the treatment of choice. It has been established to be highly effective in eradicating the mite and is safer than topical lindane (Kwell). Lindane is still an effective treatment; however, the potential for neurotoxicity, although minimal, makes it second-line therapy for infants and young children. Permethrin cream is applied to the body and thoroughly washed off after 8 to 12 hours. This treatment may be repeated 1 to 2 weeks later.

It is critical that all household members as well as close contacts, such as babysitters, be treated simultaneously to prevent reinfestation. All linens and clothes should be washed and dried in an electric drier, as heat kills the mite (>50°C). Bulkier linens, such as bedspreads, and stuffed toys can be placed in plastic bags for several days. Mites do not survive without a human host for more than 2 to 3 days. The topical antiscabietics can cause an irritant dermatitis that may last for several weeks and may improve with emollients and judicious use of topical corticosteroids.

Pediculosis

Lice are six-legged ectoparasitic insects. *Pediculus humanus capitis,* the head louse, causes the most common form of louse infestation. This occurs more often in whites; girls are more susceptible than boys. Because the head louse can survive for more than 2 days off the host's scalp, the condition can be transmitted via shared hats, combs, brushes, and even clothing or bedding.

Diagnosis

On physical examination, the nits (ova) can be found close to the scalp on the proximal hair shafts. They appear as small, oval, whitish bodies approximately 0.5 mm in length. They are tightly adherent to the hair shaft and are not easily removed. The nits can be more readily identified by their fluorescence under a Wood's lamp. Microscopic examination of the proximal hair shaft may further aid in recognition of the nits. The infestation is characterized by intense pruritus, especially at night.

Treatment

Treatment of pediculosis capitis consists of topical application of permethrin (Nix) or lindane (Kwell) shampoos applied to the scalp for 5 to 10 minutes, rinsed, and repeated 1 week later. It is extremely important to wash and dry (on a hot cycle) all exposed bedding and clothing. All combs and brushes should be soaked with the pediculicide for 15 minutes, and all items that cannot be machine-washed with hot water or dry-cleaned should be placed in plastic bags for 2 weeks. Family members and other close contacts should be examined and subsequently treated if there is any evidence of pediculosis.

Candidiasis

Candidal species, in particular *Candida albicans,* may be considered part of the normal cutaneous flora in most individuals. However, predisposing factors such as endocrinologic disorders, genetic disorders, immunosuppressive conditions, and the administration of systemic corticosteroids or antibiotics may allow for overgrowth of this organism and subsequent infection. *Candidiasis* refers to an acute or chronic infection of the skin, mucous membranes, or internal organs caused by this pathogenic yeast. Other conditions, such as warmth, moisture, and disruption of the epidermal barrier, further promote invasion and overgrowth of this resident flora.

Cutaneous candidiasis can have a variety of clinical manifestations, depending on the site of infection. Some of the most common presentations include (1) oral candidiasis (thrush), (2) candidal diaper dermatitis, (3) vulvovaginitis, and (4) paronychia.

Oral candidiasis is a common condition of infancy and immunosuppressed individuals. It is characterized by painful inflammation of the oral cavity with multiple, often confluent, white plaques on an intensely erythematous base. The condition is often acquired during vaginal delivery and passage through an infected vaginal canal; however, it is often not apparent until the second week of life. The disorder usually responds to treatment with oral nystatin suspension, which is applied to the oral mucosa four times daily until 2 days after the lesions have completely resolved. Extensive involvement or failure to respond to treatment should suggest an underlying immunodeficiency disease.

Cutaneous lesions in the intertriginous and diaper areas are frequently coexistent with thrush.

Candidal paronychia presents with erythema and edema of the proximal and lateral nail folds, which is usually not associated with tenderness, unlike acute bacterial paronychia. The condition is seen commonly in thumb suckers. Treatment with topical nystatin applied nightly under occlusion for several weeks usually results in clinical resolution.

Dermatophytoses

CLASSIFICATION

The dermatophytes are a group of fungi that infect the hair, skin, and nails and result in a collection of clinical syndromes referred to as dermatophytoses. The clinical conditions are referred to as *tinea* (or ringworm), and the affected body site determines the name of the entity. For example, tinea faciei involves the face, tinea pedis affects the feet, tinea manuum refers to infection of the hands, and tinea corporis involves the body. Tinea cruris ("jock itch"), tinea unguium (nails), and tinea capitis (scalp) are additional clinical entities. This group of infections is caused by species of *Trichophyton, Microsporum,* and *Epidermophyton.* Dermatophyte infections are usually confined to the epidermis. Serum has fungistatic properties, making disseminated infection rare except in immunocompromised individuals.

Tinea Capitis

Tinea capitis is discussed in the section on alopecia.

Tinea Corporis

Tinea corporis is characterized by one or multiple annular erythematous patches that can occur anywhere on the body (Fig. 58–18). The lesions typically have a papular scaly border and demonstrate central clearing. Vesiculation and pustulation, especially peripherally, are commonly observed. The borders are usually sharply demarcated. Identification of fungal hyphae by KOH examination of scrapings of the lesion's scaly border confirms the diagnosis. Psoriasis, secondary syphilis, the herald patch of pityriasis rosea, and the annular plaques of granuloma annulare may resemble tinea corporis. Nummular eczema often mimics tinea corporis (Fig. 58–19).

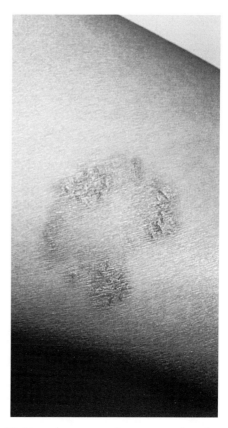

Figure 58–19. Nummular eczema, also seen as scaly, red, annular patches or plaques, can mimic tinea corporis.

Tinea Pedis

Tinea pedis is diagnosed most often in postpubertal adolescents. The clinical presentation is variable, but multiple vesicles or erosions on the insteps are characteristic. Other variants include fissures and maceration of the web spaces and "moccasin foot" tinea pedis, in which there is generalized scaling of one or both soles with extension onto the lateral aspect of the foot. The differential diagnosis includes atopic or contact dermatitis, juvenile plantar dermatosis, psoriasis, and scabies. A positive KOH scraping or fungal culture rules out these other entities.

Tinea Faciei

Tinea faciei, a dermatophyte infection of the face, is commonly seen in children. Erythematous, scaly, and often in a malar distribution, the condition may resemble lupus erythematosus. Atopic, contact, and seborrheic dermatitis may have similar cutaneous manifestations. Again, the diagnosis can be confirmed by a positive KOH scraping or fungal culture.

Tinea Cruris

Tinea cruris, uncommon before adolescence, is an erythematous, scaly eruption involving the inguinal creases and medial thighs. The eruption is usually symmetric, and sometimes the margins are papular. This infection may resemble candidiasis, in which there is also scrotal erythema. *Erythrasma,* an uncommon superficial bacte-

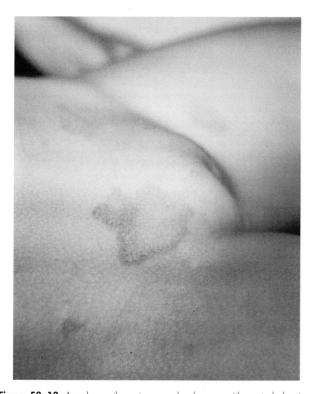

Figure 58–18. Annular erythematous, scaly plaques with central clearing are seen in tinea corporis.

rial infection caused by *Corynebacterium minutissimum,* may also mimic tinea cruris. The coral red fluorescence seen on Wood's light examination is diagnostic of erythrasma, which can be further differentiated by a negative KOH preparation and fungal culture.

TREATMENT

Tinea infections of the skin can usually be successfully managed with topical antifungal agents such as clotrimazole, econazole, ciclopirox, tolnaftate, or terbinafine creams or lotions. These medications are applied twice daily for approximately 4 weeks. They should be continued for several days after clinical resolution is apparent. Widespread eruptions or treatment failures may necessitate systemic antifungal therapy, such as griseofulvin, ketoconazole, fluconazole, or itraconazole.

Tinea Versicolor

Occurring more frequently in adolescents and adults, tinea versicolor is a superficial fungal infection characterized by multiple, slightly scaly macules and patches located on the upper trunk, neck, proximal extremities, and occasionally the face. The macular lesions vary in hue (pink, tan, brown, white), hence the name "versicolor." In darkly pigmented or tanned individuals, the macules appear hypopigmented; in fair-skinned persons or during winter months, the lesions usually appear tan brown.

Etiology

Tinea versicolor is caused by *Pityrosporum orbiculare,* also called *Malassezia furfur,* a dimorphic fungus that is a skin saprophyte. It is generally present in its yeast form, which does not produce a rash. When proliferation of the filamentous form occurs, the organism produces the characteristic lesions of tinea versicolor. Because the responsible agent is a saprophyte, the condition is not transmissible. Usually asymptomatic or only slightly pruritic, tinea versicolor is primarily a cosmetic disturbance that occurs most commonly in warm and humid environments.

Diagnosis

Although the diagnosis is established by the distinctive clinical presentation, a KOH scraping of the fine scale reveals multiple round spores and short, curved hyphae, giving the characteristic "spaghetti and meatballs" appearance typical of this disorder. Wood's light examination may demonstrate a yellow, orange, or blue-white fluorescence, further supporting the diagnosis. The differential diagnosis includes postinflammatory pigment alteration, pityriasis alba, vitiligo, contact dermatitis, seborrheic dermatitis, and pityriasis rosea.

Treatment

Tinea versicolor is a chronic condition. Although usually responsive to therapy, recurrences are common. Application of 2.5% selenium sulfide shampoo to the affected skin 15 to 20 minutes daily for 1 to 2 weeks, or overnight application on a weekly basis for 1 to 2 months, can be very effective. Other topical treatments include broad-spectrum antifungal creams or lotions; however, the expense of widespread application may be prohibitive. In extremely widespread or recalcitrant cases, or in immunosuppressed individuals, treatment with oral ketoconazole or itraconazole may be indicated. After successful treatment, the lesions remain temporarily hypo- or hyperpigmented.

MISCELLANEOUS DISORDERS

Acne Vulgaris

Acne is a very common condition seen in adolescents, but all age groups can be affected. Open and closed comedones, inflammatory papules, pustules, and nodules are characteristic primary lesions (Fig. 58–20). Scarring and sinus tracts are present in moderate to severe forms. Androgens stimulate the sebaceous follicles, leading to hyperkeratosis of the follicular epithelium. The microscopically plugged follicle is clinically apparent as a comedo. Sebaceous gland contents (sebum) accumulate, and if the follicle walls rupture, releasing sebaceous material into the surrounding dermis, inflammatory papules and pustules result. *Propionibacterium acnes,* an

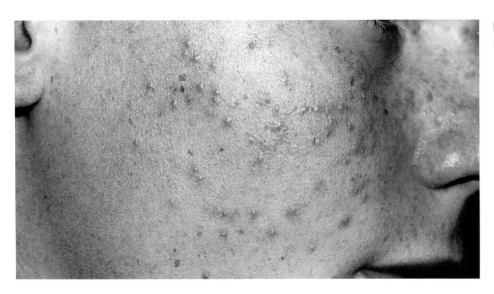

Figure 58–20. Inflammatory papules and pustules of acne vulgaris.

anaerobic follicular diphtheroid, contributes to the inflammatory process.

Diagnosis

The diagnosis of acne is a clinical one; skin biopsies and other diagnostic studies are not necessary. In some cases, endocrinologic evaluation may be needed to further elucidate the hormonal factors contributing to formation of acne lesions. Drug-induced acne can be seen in all age groups and may be due to glucocorticoids, androgens, hydantoin, and isoniazid.

Treatment

Treatment of acne varies, depending on the types of lesions present and individual tolerance to acne medication (Table 58–15). In general, soaps are not helpful. Antibacterial soaps and cleansers may help reduce surface bacteria. Benzoyl peroxide products can be used as an adjunct to tretinoin therapy, but tretinoin is more effective in reducing and preventing abnormal keratinization of the follicular canal. Benzoyl peroxide has antibacterial and mild comedolytic effects. Inflammatory acne requires use of antibiotics, either topically or systemically. Minocycline, tetracycline, erythromycin, and sulfonamides are some of the more frequently used oral antibiotics for treating acne. Numerous topical antibiotic preparations are available; most contain either erythromycin or clindamycin.

Nodular acne is best treated with isotretinoin, a synthetic vitamin A derivative, which is prescribed by a physician experienced with this medication. Side effects such as cheilitis, dry skin and mucous membranes, vertebral hyperostoses, reversible alopecia, and elevated triglyceride levels may be seen. Visual complaints and headaches may also occur. Teratogenicity has been well documented; there is a 25-fold increased risk of fetal malformations from isotretinoin. Pregnancy testing is mandatory for all women with childbearing potential, and effective contraception must be used for all sexually active patients taking this drug. The risks, benefits, and possible side effects must be discussed with each patient (and parent), and treatment must be individualized.

Urticaria

Urticaria (hives) is characterized by transient pruritic wheals that are pink, red, or white "swellings" of the skin (Table 58–16). These lesions may be small or large (giant) and can produce geographic patterns. The raised portions of wheals are due to edema caused by extravasation of fluid from small blood vessels. Urticaria, by definition, produces lesions that last for less than 24 to 36 hours. The lesions often give the appearance of moving over a short period of time; they are not fixed. If urticarial lesions persist, other diagnoses, such as urticarial vasculitis, should be

Table 58–16. Types of Urticaria

Due to ingestants (IgE mechanism in some cases)
  Foods, particularly fish, shellfish, nuts, eggs, and peanuts; food additives (tartrazine, azo dyes, benzoates)
  Drugs (penicillin, aspirin, sulfonamides, codeine)
Due to contactants (IgE mechanism in some cases)
  Plant substances (e.g., stinging nettle)
  Animal—insect (tarantula hairs, Portuguese man-of-war, cat scratch, moth scales)
  Drugs applied to the skin
  Animal saliva
Due to injectants (IgE mechanism in some cases)
  Drugs (particularly penicillin), transfused blood, therapeutic antisera, insect stings and bites (papular urticaria), allergenic extracts
Due to inhalants (IgE mechanism)
  Pollens, danders, and ? molds
Due to infectious agents (mechanism unknown)
  Parasites
  Viruses (e.g., hepatitis, infectious mononucleosis)
  Bacteria (streptococcus, mycoplasma)
  ? Fungi
Due to physical factors (mechanism mostly unknown)
  Cold urticaria
  Pressure urticaria
  Solar urticaria
  Aquagenic urticaria
  Local heat urticaria
  Dermographism
  Exercise-induced
  Vibratory angioedema
Episodic angioedema with eosinophilia (? a distinct entity)
Cholinergic urticaria (a distinct entity)
Associated with systemic diseases (mechanism mostly unknown)
  Collagen-vascular (systemic lupus erythematosus, cryoglobulinuria, Sjögren syndrome)
    Cutaneous vasculitis
    Serum sickness–like disease
  Malignancy (leukemia-lymphoma)
  Hyperthyroidism
  Urticaria pigmentosa (systemic mastocytosis)
Associated with genetic disorders (various mechanisms)
  Familial cold urticaria
  Hereditary angioedema
  Amyloidosis with deafness and urticaria
  C3b inactivator deficiency
Chronic urticaria and angioedema (mechanism unknown)
Psychogenic urticaria (existence as an entity uncertain)

Adapted from Behrman RE (ed). Nelson Textbook of Pediatrics, 14th ed. Philadelphia: WB Saunders, 1992:600.

considered. When hives resolve, there is no residual hyperpigmentation, scale, or scarring. Pruritus is due to histamine release from mast cells, which is caused by antibody reactions to an antigen. Urticaria is usually an allergic reaction to a specific immunoglobulin E (IgE) antibody. Immune complexes of IgG plus antigen can also produce urticaria as part of a serum sickness reaction.

Angioedema is a form of urticaria affecting deeper tissue planes and frequently involves the lips, dorsum of the hand or feet, scalp, scrotum, or periorbital tissue. Treatment consists of antigen avoidance and medical blockade of histamine receptors.

Urticaria is either acute or chronic. *Acute* urticaria has a duration of less than 6 weeks. When hives continue to develop for more than 6 weeks, urticaria is considered to be chronic. The etiology is often unknown. Acute urticaria is often due to drugs (many, partic-

Table 58–15. A Simple Approach to Treatment of Acne

Open comedones	Tretinoin
Closed comedones	Tretinoin
Inflammatory papules (few)	Tretinoin + topical antibiotics
Inflammatory papules (many)	Tretinoin + oral antibiotic
Pustules (many)	Tretinoin + oral antibiotic
Nodules	Oral isotretinoin

ularly antibiotics), foods (milk, nuts, eggs, fish), infections (*Streptococcus, Mycoplasma,* Epstein-Barr virus), or physical stimuli (cold, exercise, vibration).

The cause of *chronic* urticaria is typically difficult to determine. In some cases, chronic urticaria can be a sign of underlying systemic disease such as malignancy, connective tissue disorders, or hepatitis.

Although hives are usually self-limited, treatment of pruritus consists of elimination of identifiable causes and administration of antihistamines. Hydroxyzine and diphenhydramine are used often but do produce drowsiness. Nonsedating antihistamines are popular, but prescribers must be aware of potential interactions with concurrent medications.

REFERENCES

Atton A, Tunnessen W. Alopecia in children: The most common causes. Pediatr Rev 1990;12:25–30.

Baker R, Sequin J, Leslie N, et al. Fever and petechiae in children. Pediatrics 1989;84:1051–1055.

Dajan R. Impetigo in childhood: Changing epidemiology and new treatments. Pediatr Ann 1993;22:235–240.

Darmstadt GL, Lane AT. Impetigo: An overview. Pediatr Dermatol 1994;11:293–303.

Feldman SR. Bullous dermatoses associated with systemic disease. Dermatol Clin 1993;11:597–608.

Fine JD, Bauer EA, Briggaman RA, et al. Revised clinical and laboratory criteria for subtypes of inherited epidermolysis bullosa. J Am Acad Dermatol 1991;24:119–135.

Frieden IJ. Aplasia cutis congenita: A clinical review and proposal for classification. J Am Acad Dermatol 1986;14:646–660.

Hebert AA, Esterly NB. Bacterial and candidal cutaneous infections in the neonate. Dermatol Clin 1986;4:3–20.

Hurwitz S. Clinical Pediatric Dermatology. Philadelphia: WB Saunders, 1993.

Kadonaga JN, Frieden IJ. Neurocutaneous melanosis: Definition and review of the literature. J Am Acad Dermatol 1991;24:747–755.

Kahn RM, Goldstein EJ. Common bacterial skin infections. Postgrad Med 1993;93:175–182.

Mulliken J, Young A. Vascular Birthmarks: Hemangiomas and Malformations. Philadelphia: WB Saunders, 1988.

Rabinowitz LG, Esterly NB. Inflammatory bullous diseases in children. Dermatol Clin 1993;11:565–581.

Rabinowitz LG, Esterly NB. Atopic dermatitis and ichthyosis vulgaris. Pediatr Rev 1994;15:220–226.

Rice TD, Duggan AK, DeAngelis C. Cost-effectiveness of erythromycin versus mupirocin for the treatment of impetigo in children. Pediatrics 1992;89:210–214.

Shpall S, Frieden I, Chesney M, Newman T. Risk of malignant transformation of congenital melanocytic nevi in blacks. Pediatr Dermatol 1994;11:204–208.

Uitto J, Christiano AM. Inherited epidermolysis bullosa. Dermatol Clin 1993;11:549–563.

Williams ML. The ichthyoses—pathogenesis and prenatal diagnosis: A review of recent advances. Pediatr Dermatol 1983;1:1–24.

59 Fever Without Focus

Kenneth Graff*   David M. Jaffe

Fever is one of the most commonly encountered signs in pediatric practice, accounting for 20% of pediatric emergency department visits and for 35% of unscheduled ambulatory visits. Fever without focus (FWF) occurs when an elevated body temperature is the only sign of disease. It occurs in 5% to 10% of children presenting with fever. Most children with FWF have a self-limited viral process. A bacterial pathogen is causative in 3% to 5%. The diagnostic challenge in managing the febrile child with no focus of infection is to identify this small but important group and to avoid the morbidity of serious bacterial disease. This goal can be met through careful assessment, epidemiologic considerations, selected laboratory evaluation, and individualization of treatment options.

DEFINITIONS

The hypothalamus is the thermoregulatory center for the body. *Fever* results when a shift in the hypothalamic set point causes a controlled elevation of body temperature above the normal range. This normal set point for most humans has a daily circadian rhythm, ranging between 36°C and 37.8°C, with the peak occurring in the afternoon. The diurnal variation becomes more pronounced with age; the variation is small in infants, increasing to 0.9°C in children 2 to 6 years of age and rising to 1.1°C in children above 6 years old. Most well individuals do not have a rectal temperature ≥ 38.0°C (100.4°F); this is the usual value defining fever.

Fever production begins when an infectious agent, toxin, immune complex, or other inflammatory agent stimulates macrophages or endothelial cells to produce endogenous pyrogens, such as interleukin-1 and tumor necrosis factor. These circulating endogenous pyrogens induce the endothelium in the anterior hypothalamus to produce prostaglandin E_2 and other arachidonic acid metabolites, which in turn act on the hypothalamic thermoregulatory neurons to raise the thermostat set point. Various efferent nerves are signaled by this change in set point and cause peripheral vasoconstriction, an increase in metabolic rate, and shivering. Behavioral changes are also initiated, such as seeking warmer temperatures, adding warmer clothing, and assuming a posture to minimize heat loss. These physiologic and behavioral efforts persist until the body temperature matches the new set point.

Fever is distinct from *hyperthermia*. Hyperthermia is an elevation of body temperature above the hypothalamic set point. Hyperthermia occurs when heat loss mechanisms are overwhelmed by conditions such as high ambient temperatures (*heat stroke*) or

---

*Deceased.

excessive metabolic heat production (*malignant hyperthermia*) or when heat dissipation mechanisms (vasodilation and sweating) are impaired by drugs (atropine) or disease (ectodermal dysplasia) (Table 59–1). Hyperthermia is usually marked (≥40.5°C), does not respond to antipyretic agents, and is usually not associated with diaphoresis.

Fever without focus is defined as the acute onset of fever (rectal temperature ≥ 38.0°C) in a child in whom no probable cause for the fever is evident after a careful history and physical examination. Synonyms for FWF include *fever without source* and *fever without localizing signs*.

Occult bacteremia (OB) occurs when pathogenic bacteria are present in the blood culture from a febrile child with no apparent focus of infection and no signs of sepsis. Occult bacteremia is distinct from the more obvious sepsis in which there are clear and demonstrable signs of serious illness, such as shock, hypotension, or purpura (Table 59–2). The sequelae of occult bacteremia are referred to as *serious bacterial illnesses* (SBIs) and include meningitis, sepsis, bone and joint infections, urinary tract infections, pneumonia, and enteritis.

FWF is also distinct from *fever of unknown origin* (FUO) (see Chapter 56). FUO invokes a different set of diagnostic possibilities. Fever with rash is discussed in Chapter 57.

DATA COLLECTION
History

In a child with fever without focus, the parent reports the presence of fever with no associated symptoms, except at times mild,

---

Table 59–1. Etiology of Hyperthermia

Excessive Heat Production

Exertion
Heat stroke (exertion)
Malignant hyperthermia (anesthesia induced)
Neuroleptic malignant syndrome
Catatonia
Tetanus
Status epilepticus
Delirium
Endocrine disorders (hyperthyroidism, pheochromocytoma)
Drugs (cocaine, amphetamines, ephedrine, phencyclidine, tricyclic antidepressants, LSD, lithium, thyroid hormone, salicylates)

Diminished Heat Dissipation

Heat stroke
Occlusive dressings
Dehydration
Extensive burns (including severe sunburn)
Anhidrotic ectodermal dysplasias
Anticholinergic-like drugs (atropine, antihistamines, phenothiazines, tricyclic antidepressants)
Autonomic neuropathy
Spinal cord level paralysis (spinal crisis)
Possible overbundling (especially in a warm environment)
Therapeutic hyperthermia

*Hypothalamic Dysfunction**

Stroke
Encephalitis
Granulomatous processes (sarcoid, tuberculosis, eosinophilic)
Trauma
Central—idiopathic
Phenothiazines
Hemorrhage

*Usually associated with hypothermia.

---

nonpurulent rhinorrhea. A detailed history may reveal a focus for infection. Important historical variables to be assessed include (1) onset and duration of fever, (2) degree of temperature (if taken, and by what method and in what anatomic site), (3) medications given, including antipyretics and home remedies, (4) environmental exposures, either ambient or toxin-related, (5) associated symptoms, (6) the presence of similar symptoms in siblings or playmates, and (7) the date of last immunizations.

The child's medical history may have important implications for management, including recurrent febrile illnesses or conditions predisposing the patient to severe infection, such as sickle cell disease, asplenia, malignancy, or primary immunodeficiency, and medications that alter host defenses such as chemotherapeutic agents.

Physical Examination

TEMPERATURE ASSESSMENT

Core temperature is best assessed by rectal thermometry. Oral and axillary temperatures correlate with rectal temperature but are less accurate measures of core temperature. Oral thermometry requires that the child hold the thermometer between the tongue and the floor of the mouth with the mouth closed. This method may be unreliable in children under 2 years old or in those with nasal congestion. Oral temperature can be influenced by hot or cold substances ingested immediately prior to measurement. Axillary measurement also may be inaccurate, especially in an environment of low ambient temperature or in a patient with peripheral vasoconstriction. Rectal temperature assessment is the standard but should be avoided in neutropenic immunocompromised patients, in whom rectal manipulation may seed the blood stream with bacteria.

Temperature assessment using electronic thermometers has achieved popularity because a steady-state reading can be obtained in less than 30 seconds rather than the 3 to 4 minutes required by traditional mercury thermometers. Most models lack a means of calibration, making accuracy uncertain; liquid crystal methods to measure skin temperature can often underestimate core temperature. Tympanic thermometry is another method that allows rapid temperature measurement. The tympanic membrane shares vascular supply with the hypothalamus, and it has been shown in adult intensive care unit patients that tympanic membrane readings correlate well with core temperature. The presence of otitis media or cerumen does not appear to affect reliability. Several early studies in children support the accuracy of tympanic thermometry in comparison to rectal temperatures. Others have found that tympanic temperature correlates poorly with oral and rectal glass thermometry in children under 3 months of age. Tympanic thermometry is useful for older children; however, rectal temperatures are preferable in all children and particularly in infants younger than 3 months of age.

Bundled Infants

A common belief is that core temperature may become elevated in a heavily wrapped infant. Guidelines suggest that a bundled infant with an elevated temperature be unclothed and rechecked for fever. One study demonstrated that bundled children had significant elevation of skin temperature but not of rectal temperature compared with controls. Another study found that rectal temperature increased 0.56°C after 150 minutes of bundling. These investigators conclude that wrapping and ambient heat should be accounted for when estimating core temperature. However, only 2 of 12 infants

Table 59–2. Definitions of Related Infectious and Shock States

Infection: Microbial phenomenon characterized by an inflammatory response to the presence of microorganisms or the invasion of normally sterile host tissue by those organisms.

Bacteremia: The presence of viable bacteria in the blood.

Systemic Inflammatory Response Syndrome: The systemic inflammatory response to a variety of severe clinical insults. The response is manifested by two or more of the following conditions:

    Temperature > 38°C or < 36°C
    Heart rate > 90 beats/min*
    Respiratory rate > 20 breaths/min* or $PaCO_2$ < 32 torr
    WBC > 12,000 cells/min³, <4000 cells/mm³, or >10% immature (band) forms

Sepsis: The sytemic response to infection. This systemic response is manifested by two or more of the following conditions as a result of infection:

    Temperature > 38°C or < 36°C
    Heart rate > 90 beats/min*
    Respiratory rate > 20 breaths/min* or $PaCO_2$ < 32 torr
    WBC >12,000 cells/mm³, <4000 cells/mm³, or >10% immature (band) forms

Severe Sepsis: Sepsis associated with organ dysfunction, hypoperfusion, or hypotension. Hypoperfusion and perfusion abnormalities may include, but are not limited to, lactic acidosis, oliguria, or an acute alteration in mental status.

Septic Shock: Sepsis with hypotension, despite adequate fluid resuscitation, along with the presence of perfusion abnormalities that may include, but are not limited to, lactic acidosis, oliguria, or an acute alteration in mental status. Patients, who are on inotropic or vasopressor agents may not be hypotensive at the time that perfusion abnormalities are measured.

Hypotension: A systolic blood pressure of <90 mm Hg* or a reduction of >40 mmHg from baseline in the absence of other causes for hypotension.

Multiple Organ Dysfunction Syndrome: Presence of altered organ function in an acutely ill patient such that homeostasis cannot be maintained without intervention.

From American College of Chest Physicians/Society of Critical Care Medicine Consensus Conference. Definitions for sepsis and organ failure and guidelines for the use of innovative therapies in sepsis. Crit Care Med 1992;20:864.
*Adult standards for vital signs; adjust accordingly for children norms.

reached a temperature of 38.0°C, and none exceeded this temperature. Although additional study is needed to evaluate the extent that wrapping can elevate core temperature, the available evidence suggests that a rectal temperature above 38°C may not be attributable to bundling. There are few data but much anecdotal evidence that overbundling and high ambient temperatures may elevate the temperature of neonates during the first week of life.

Fever by History

Another issue concerns the child with a history of fever at home who is afebrile on presentation. Among infants admitted to the hospital with history of fever, more than 50% are afebrile on presentation. In one study, none of 26 patients with a history of tactile fever had subsequent documented fever while 8 of 40 (20%) with a history of elevated rectal temperature had subsequent fever. Five of the infants who were afebrile on presentation had SBI (27% of all SBIs), including one with a history of tactile fever. Patients with a history of measured elevated temperature may be managed just as those with fever documented in the acute care setting. Infants with a history of tactile fever who have repeated normal temperature and a normal clinical evaluation may not require further evaluation. However, all need close follow-up.

GENERAL APPEARANCE

The physical examination of a child with FWF is, by definition, nonlocalizing. The appearance of that child is a vital component of the evaluation and has important prognostic implications. In one model, patients can be divided into two categories: toxic and nontoxic. A toxic child is one who is lethargic, irritable, or has evidence of shock (weak peripheral pulses, poor perfusion, respiratory distress, cyanosis, mottling). Infants younger than 12 weeks of age who appear toxic have an incidence of SBI of 17.3%, including 10.7% bacteremia and 3.9% meningitis. Nontoxic infants in this age group have an incidence of 8.6% for SBI, 2.0% for bacteremia, and 1.0% for meningitis.

Often a child cannot easily be classified as toxic or nontoxic but appears to be in the gray area between the two. Experienced physicians develop observational skills to gain a sense of the degree of a child's illness. The ability to identify serious illness by observation is variable. One study found that experienced pediatricians diagnosed trivial illness in 52% of infants with culture-proven bacteremia. Another study examined physician assessment for bacteremia and found a sensitivity of only 47%, a specificity of 83%, and a positive predictive value (PPV) of 14%. Private pediatricians are able to identify serious illness with a sensitivity of 74% and a specificity of 75%.

To aid in the assessment of serious illness, McCarthy and coworkers defined observation variables contributing to the judgment of severity of illness. These variables were examined for utility as predictors of serious illness in febrile children. The Acute Illness Observation Scale (AIOS) (Table 59–3) identified six items as key predictors. Each item is graded on a scale of 1, 3, or 5, signifying normal, moderate impairment, or severe impairment, respectively. A score above 10 had a sensitivity of 88% and a specificity of 77% for serious illness. Serious illness occurred 13 times more frequently in those with a score above 10. In another study, the AIOS in combination with a careful history and physical examination had higher sensitivity and correlation for serious illness than did the traditional history and physical. Three of 36 patients with SBI were identified only by the AIOS. In this study, the history and physical examination identified 78% of serious illness, while history, physical examination, and observation identified 86% of serious illness.

In young infants (4 to 8 weeks of age), the AIOS may be less accurate. Twenty-two percent of such infants with a score at or below 10 (well appearing) may have serious illness but only 45% with scores at or above 16 (ill appearing) have serious illness. The sensitivity for the score in this setting was 46%, the specificity was 80%, the PPV was 49%, and the negative predictive value (NPV) was 78%. Young infants may not have developed the social gestures and may lack the typical clinical findings of serious illness that are more reliable in older children. Alternatively, viral illnesses may produce more severe behavioral symptoms in younger infants.

RESPONSE TO ANTIPYRETICS

The temperature response of children given antipyretic therapy does not help distinguish trivial from serious illness. Neither the

Table 59–3. Acute Illness Observation Scale

Observation Item	1 Normal	3 Moderate Impairment	5 Severe Impairment
Quality of cry	Strong with normal tone *or* Content and not crying	Whimpering *or* Sobbing	Weak *or* Moaning *or* High-pitched
Reaction to parent stimulation	Cries briefly then stops *or* Content and not crying	Cries off and on	Continual cry *or* Hardly responds
State variation	If awake → stays awake *or* If asleep and stimulated → wakes up quickly	Eyes close briefly → awake *or* Awakes with prolonged stimulation	Falls to sleep *or* Will not rouse
Color	Pink	Pale extremities *or* Acrocyanosis	Pale *or* Cyanotic *or* Mottled *or* Ashen
Hydration	Skin normal, eyes normal *and* Mucous membranes moist	Skin, eyes normal *and* Mouth slightly dry	Skin doughy *or* Tented *and* Dry mucous membranes *and/or* Sunken eyes
Response (talk, smile) to social overtures	Smiles *or* Alerts (≤2 mo)	Brief smile *or* Alerts briefly (≤2 mo)	No smile, Face anxious, dull, expressionless *or* No alerting (≤2 mo)

From McCarthy PL, Sharpe MR, Spiesel SZ, et al. Observation scales to identify serious illness in febrile children. Pediatrics 1982; 70:802.

magnitude of temperature decrease nor physician assessment after acetaminophen is predictive for the presence or absence of bacteremia. As many as 88% of children with bacteremia and 83% without bacteremia respond to acetaminophen.

The use of antipyretics may hinder the ability to assess a child. Clinical appearance prior to administration of antipyretics may be a better indicator of SBI; routine administration of antipyretics may mask serious illness.

LABORATORY DATA AND INTERPRETATION

At the initial visit, clinical appearance does not always adequately separate serious from benign illness in febrile young children with no focus of infection. This problem has led to efforts to examine the utility of different laboratory tests to identify children at high risk for serious illness.

White Blood Cell Count

There is a direct relationship between the height of the white blood cell count (WBC) and the prevalence of bacteremia. Among children 3 to 36 months of age who had a temperature at or above 39.5°C, the prevalence of bacteremia for a WBC ≥ 30,000/mm³ was 42.9%, for a WBC between 15,000/mm³ and 30,000/mm³ was 16.6%, and for a WBC between 10,000/mm³ and 15,000/mm³ was 2.8%. For a WBC below 10,000/mm³, no patients had bacteremia. Other studies confirm this relationship. A WBC ≥ 15,000/mm³ may identify a group of children having at least a three times greater risk for bacteremia than those with a lower WBC: for a WBC ≥ 15,000/mm³, the risk of bacteremia is 13.0%, while for a WBC below 15,000/mm³, the risk is 2.6%. With a WBC ≥ 15,000/mm³ as a positive test for disease, this test has a sensitivity of 84.5% and a specificity of 60.3%. The test has an NPV of 98.3%

and a PPV of 13.0%. The high NPV and low PPV are seen in most screening tests for bacteremia because the prevalence of bacteremia is low (3% to 5%) in children with FWF. Because of the low overall prevalence of bacteremia, even though 85% of children with bacteremia will have a WBC ≥ 15,000/mm³, 85% to 90% of children with a WBC ≥ 15,000/mm³ will not have bacteremia.

To develop user-specific selection of cutoff values for sensitivity and specificity, receiver operating characteristic (ROC) curves for temperature and WBC have been developed (Fig. 59–1). The sensitivity and specificity of WBC at 10,000/mm³ are 92% and 43%, respectively. For a WBC of 15,000/mm³, sensitivity was 65% and specificity 77%. For a WBC of 20,000/mm³, sensitivity was 38% and specificity 92%. The temperature curve was not found to be useful, and the combination of temperature and WBC curves offered no advantage over the WBC curve alone. The ROC curve can help individual practitioners to choose cutoff points for diagnostic testing tailored to their particular needs. One would choose a lower WBC (high sensitivity) to avoid missing children with bacteremia and choose a higher WBC (high specificity) if avoiding unnecessary treatment was an important objective.

Despite its direct relationship with bacteremia, using a WBC to assess risk of bacteremia has limitations. Up to 50% of children with *Haemophilus influenza* type b (Hib) bacteremia will have a WBC of 5000/mm³ to 15,000/mm³. Children with *Neisseria meningitidis* may be leukopenic. A WBC ≥ 15,000/mm³ and absolute band count ≥ 500/mm³ are not predictive of bacteremia in infants under 8 weeks of age. Because of these shortcomings, other screening tests have been examined for their utility in categorizing children with FWF.

Neutrophils, Bands, and Other Acute-Phase Reactants

The ability of polymorphonuclear neutrophils (PMNs) and absolute band counts to identify bacterial disease in febrile children

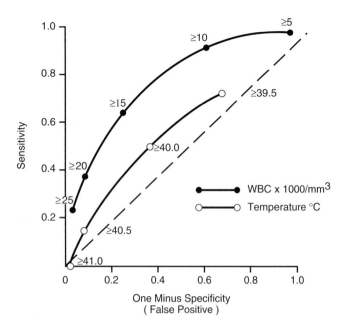

Figure 59–1. Receiver operating characteristic curves of white blood cell count (WBC) and temperature. (Data from Jaffe and Fleisher.)

reveals PMNs $\geq$ 10,000/mm³ or bands $\geq$ 500/mm³ to be 75% sensitive and 80% specific. Others have found the combination of PMNs $\geq$ 10,000/mm³, bands $\geq$ 500/mm³, or PMNs + bands $\geq$ 10,500/mm³ to have a sensitivity of 87.5% and a specificity of 92.8%. However, other studies have not supported these parameters as useful predictors of bacteremia above that of total WBC.

Vacuolization in neutrophils was thought to be a marker of SBI. However, vacuoles in neutrophils may be present in only 40% of children with bacteremia and in only 15% with sepsis. Vacuolization is present with similar frequency in bacterial and nonbacterial illnesses and is not specific or predictive. Vacuolization in ill neonates had a sensitivity of 81%, a specificity of 93%, and a PPV of 59% in detecting bacterial illness.

Erythrocyte sedimentation rate (ESR), C-reactive protein (CRP), and zeta sedimentation rate (ZSR) have also been used to assess risk. ESR $\geq$ 30 mm/hour is 75% sensitive and 66% specific in detecting serious illness, while CRP at 1:50 dilution is 77% specific but only 60% sensitive. The tests in combination may be 82% sensitive but only 54% specific for bacterial illness. In another investigation, children with temperature $\geq$ 40°C and a WBC $\geq$ 15,000/mm³ or an ESR $\geq$ 30 mm/hour were at five times the risk for serious bacterial illness than those with a temperature $\geq$ 40°C with laboratory results below these values (prevalence of SBI was 15% versus 3%, respectively). ESR $\geq$ 30 mm/hour may be 80% sensitive and 94% specific for predicting SBI in infants under 8 weeks of age.

PMNs, absolute band count, ESR, ZSR, and CRP have value in identifying children at risk for serious illness. The higher the value of these parameters, the greater the risk of bacteremia. However, with the exception of absolute band count, availability of these tests is limited. Additionally, there is no clearly demonstrated advantage over the WBC.

Antigen Testing

Latex agglutination and enzyme immunoassay antigen testing are rapid and exist for many of the organisms causing SBI in children, including *Streptococcus pneumoniae* and *H. influenzae*

type b. Unfortunately, these tests do not have sufficient sensitivity for routine clinical practice. Polymerase chain reaction methods may ultimately be used to detect bacterial-specific or viral-specific DNA or RNA. This technique is promising because it can detect low levels of DNA that are present in bacteremia.

Blood Cultures

Blood cultures are the gold standard for determination of bacteremia. They are relatively expensive, not always readily available in the private office, and do not provide immediate results. They provide essential information in the course of patient follow-up because they positively identify patients with bacteremia who are at risk for SBI. Because more rapid diagnostic tests do not permit positive identification, blood cultures remain an important part of the diagnostic and management strategy for many children with FWF.

False-negative blood culture results are due to prior treatment with antibiotics, missing an episode of bacteremia (if intermittent), and inoculation of too little (<1 ml) blood into the media. Occasionally, too much blood inoculated into a blood culture bottle may yield a false-negative result because of ongoing killing of bacteria by neutrophils. False-positive results are due to improperly cleaning the skin, resulting in contamination with skin flora.

Lumbar Puncture

Lumbar puncture is indicated if the diagnosis of sepsis (not occult bacteremia) or meningitis is considered. Normal cerebrospinal fluid (CSF) findings, including normal CSF chemistries, cell count, and Gram stain, help exclude the diagnosis of meningitis (see Chapter 53). Fewer than 1% of children with normal CSF results will have a positive culture (usually *N. meningitidis*). Thus, even in the presence of a normal CSF examination, close follow-up is important.

Urinalysis and Urine Culture

Another screening test is the urinalysis (UA) (see Chapter 27). UA aids in early identification of children with an occult urinary tract infection (UTI). However, 20% of young children with UTI have a normal urinalysis based on a negative reagent strip for leukocyte esterase or nitrites and a normal microscopic examination. A Gram-stained smear of urine may be a better screen, with reports of sensitivity from 89% to 99% and specificity from 80% to 90%. The combination of dipstick test (leukocyte esterase, nitrite tests) and microscopic analysis for bacteria (unstained or Gram stained) may have a sensitivity of 100% and an NPV of 100%. These data are based on symptomatic children over 1 year of age; the data may not be referable to children with occult UTI or young infants (see Chapter 27). Among infants under 8 weeks of age, 50% with a UTI may have a normal urinalysis (WBC < 5/high-power field of centrifuged urine and no bacteria on an unspun sample).

Although a screening urinalysis using dipstick and microscopy is of some value, a urine culture should routinely be obtained to confirm the diagnosis of UTI and to establish the diagnosis if the screening tests are negative. For children who are not toilet-trained, the best means to obtain urine for analysis and culture is to perform a catheterization of the bladder or a suprapubic aspiration. Urine collected through bag specimens can be contaminated with fecal or skin flora, which makes interpretation of results difficult.

Chest Radiographs

Chest radiographs (CXRs) are most often normal in children who have a fever without a focus. In studies of children who had a fever with no source, the percentage of children 2 years of age or younger with a positive CXR ranged from 0% to 2.7%. When children up to the age of 18 years are considered, the range is 0% to 15.0%. Respiratory signs or symptoms are good predictors of clinically significant positive CXR findings in the group under 2 months of age. Only 1% of infants without respiratory symptoms have a positive CXR, while 31% of those with symptoms have a positive CXR. The positive CXRs from asymptomatic children may show nonspecific mild peribronchial thickening and usually result in no management change.

The sensitivity of respiratory signs in predicting a positive CXR may be 93%, the specificity 73%, and the NPV 99%. In a bayesian meta-analysis, the mean probability of a positive CXR in a child with FWF is 3.3% (95% confidence interval [CI], 0.8% to 7.5%). Most of the infiltrates in the asymptomatic children were thought to be of viral etiology and did not change management.

Stool Analysis and Culture

Analysis and culture of stool are important if diarrhea is present. In this instance, it can be considered as a focus of infection. If the parent or guardian is uncertain about recent bowel habits, the clinician should consider gross examination of the stool for blood or mucus and microscopic examination for white blood cells. Bacterial enteritis is indicated by the presence of blood, mucus, or more than five white blood cells per high-power field. If these screening tests are positive, a confirmatory stool culture should be obtained.

DIFFERENTIAL DIAGNOSIS

The nature of fever without focus is such that a definitive diagnosis is not possible at the initial visit. Most of the children who present with FWF are eventually found to have acute, self-limited infectious diseases that are of viral origin. These children may be in the prodromal phase of a variety of infections, such as enterovirus, influenza, roseola, measles, Rocky Mountain spotted fever, or Kawasaki disease (see Chapter 57). Alternatively, in 3% to 5%, the fever may represent an occult bacterial infection in the blood, urine, or other site. Only continued care allows the clinician to make a final diagnosis (Table 59–4).

Other conditions presenting with FWF are extremely rare. Diseases such as malignancy and connective tissue disorders are usually accompanied by historical clues and systemic signs. Most series of acutely febrile children (3 months to 3 years old) with no focus have not reported patients with these processes. Unless specific clinical clues exist, these diagnoses should not be pursued. Fever caused by immunization may have no associated signs or symptoms but should be suspected on the basis of the history. Fever from a diphtheria-pertussis-tetanus (DPT) injection usually has an onset within 12 to 24 hours and may last 24 to 48 hours. Measles-mumps-rubella (MMR) immunization may cause fever for 7 to 10 days after injection and may be accompanied by a faint rash. Historical clues may lead the clinician to a diagnosis of heat illness or to drug poisoning (see Table 59–1).

In one prospective analysis to identify pathogens causing FWF in children under 3 months of age, a cause may be determined in 50% of patients using multiple cultures and antibody titers for bacteria and viruses. Viral agents are identified in 40% of patients and represent 73% of identifiable pathogens. The majority of the viruses will be nonpolio enteroviruses, with the remainder being parainfluenza, respiratory syncytial virus, adenovirus, and cytomegalovirus. A detailed viral investigation is not necessary unless FWF evolves into an FUO or fever with end-organ involvement (hepatitis, meningitis).

Bacterial etiology is identified in 15% and includes 11% with UTI (primarily *Escherichia coli*), 3% with salmonellosis, and rare cases of group B streptococcal meningitis. As stated earlier, bacteremia may be present in 3% to 5% of infants with FWF.

Urinary Tract Infection

The overall prevalence of occult UTI in children is 1.5% to 6.6%. The prevalence rate may be 11% in febrile children under 3

Table 59–4. Differential Diagnosis of Fever Without Focus

	Example	3 to 36 Months	0 to 3 Months
Common			
Viral infections		Enterovirus, parainfluenza adenovirus, RSV, CMV, roseola, fifth disease, influenza, other viruses	Same plus HSV
Bacterial infections	Occult bacteremia	*Streptococcus pneumoniae, Haemophilus influenzae, Neisseria meningitidis, Salmonella* sp.	Same plus group B streptococci, gram-negative organisms, *Listeria monocytogenes*
	Urinary tract infection	*Escherichia coli, Klebsiella,* other gram-negative organisms	Same
	Other site	Unlikely without signs	Meningitis (same organisms), salmonellosis
Rare			
Connective tissue diseases		Rheumatic fever, SLE, sarcoidosis, JRA	
Malignancies		Leukemia, lymphoma, neuroblastoma, Ewing sarcoma	
Poisoning		Atropine, salicylates, cocaine, anticholinergics	

Abbreviations: RSV = respiratory syncytial virus; CMV = cytomegalovirus; HSV = herpes simplex virus; SLE = systemic lupus erythematosus; JRA = juvenile rheumatoid arthritis.

months of age. A positive urine culture may be present in 15.8% of boys under 3 months of age who present with FWF. This incidence drops to 3.9% and 0.0% in 4- to 6-month-old and 7- to 35-month-old boys, respectively. For girls who have FWF, the rate of UTI may be 20.0%, 3.7%, 1.6%, and 0.0% in the age groups 0 to 3, 4 to 6, 7 to 12, and 13 to 36 months, respectively. However, other studies have reported an incidence of only 4.2% in girls younger than 8 weeks of age.

A UTI may be associated with a risk of bacteremia, especially in younger age groups. Six percent of infants under 2 months of age with UTI may have bacteremia. Other studies have found the prevalence rate to range from 21% to 36%. A referral bias of sicker patients may have increased the prevalence of bacteremia. The incidence of bacteremia with UTI may be based on age. For patients ≤1 month of age, the rate may be 21%. In the 1- to 2-month age group, it may be 13%; in 2- to 3-month-old children, 4%; and in 3- to 6-month-old children, 8%. Laboratory values did not distinguish those with bacteremia.

Occult Bacteremia

Occult bacteremia (OB) is the presence of a positive blood culture for pathogenic bacteria in a nontoxic-appearing but febrile patient without a focus for infection. Although OB may resolve spontaneously (particularly with pneumococcus), it also may precede the development of the serious bacterial infections. It is this group of patients whom the practitioner most wants to identify and treat.

PREVALENCE

Overall. The overall prevalence of bacteremia in children up to 3 years of age is approximately 5% (reported range, 2.8% to 11.1%). In the private practice setting, a prevalence of 10% has been reported in those children with a temperature ≥ 38.3°C and FWF. A prevalence rate of 3.2% to 4.4% in children with temperature ≥ 38.3°C has been reported from a walk-in clinic. Prevalence rates in different areas of Chicago reveal a prevalence of 3.5% in an inner-city hospital outpatient clinic, 1.9% in a suburban emergency department, and 5.9% in a private office.

By Age. Occult bacteremia has been reported in children of all age groups. One study found the highest prevalence of bacteremia to be in children between 7 and 12 months of age (11.1%). In patients 13 to 24 months old, the prevalence was 4.6%; in 2 to 4 year olds, it was 2.2%; and in those over 4 years of age, it was 3.0%. In this sample, the frequency of bacteremia in infants 6 months or younger was 1%. This study looked at all children with a temperature ≥ 38.3°C without regard to the presence or absence of a focus. In another study of children 3 to 36 months of age having a temperature ≥ 39.5°C and a WBC ≥ 15,000/mm³, the overall frequency was 11.6%. Frequency by age was 10.2% in those 3 to 12 months old, 11.8% in those 13 to 24 months, and 15.6% in those 25 to 36 months old.

By Organism. Occult bacteremia may be caused by a number of different organisms. The most common etiologic agents are *S. pneumoniae* (85% of cases), *H. influenzae* type b (10%), and *N. meningitidis* (3%). Invasive disease caused by Hib has decreased markedly since the introduction of routine immunization with the Hib vaccine, and the proportion of OB due to this organism will likely decrease. In a multicenter study completed in 1991, children

with a temperature above 39°C and no focus of infection had an overall risk of OB of 2.8%. *S. pneumoniae* accounted for 87%, Hib 5%, *N. meningitidis* 1%, and *Salmonella* 2%; 5% of cases were caused by other organisms.

Pathogens observed in neonates are different. During the first 2 months of life, group B streptococci and *E. coli* are the most common isolates in *sepsis*. In a 10-year review of isolates from neonates *with* sepsis, the incidence of group B streptococci was 24%, while *E. coli* was 17%, *Klebsiella pneumoniae* 7%, and Hib 3%. *Listeria monocytogenes* is another potential pathogen in this age group, as are the community-acquired pathogens, such as *S. pneumoniae, N. meningitidis,* and *Salmonella* species.

The incidence of organisms causing bacteremia varies in different regions of the world. The overall frequency of bacteremia in outpatient children in East Africa is 7.7%. Of the etiologic agents, salmonellae, streptococci, and staphylococci accounted for 57%, 16%, and 14%, respectively.

By Height of Fever. Height of fever has been related to the risk of occult bacteremia. Bacteremia is uncommon when temperature is below 39°C. In children 3 to 24 months old with temperature below 39°C, the prevalence is less than 1%, while in those with temperature ≥ 39°C, the prevalence is 3% to 5%. A prospective study of 600 febrile children seen consecutively at a walk-in clinic found that 0% of children with temperature under 38.9°C had a positive blood culture, while 3.9% of those with temperatures ≥ 38.9°C had bacteremia.

In another study, children with temperature above 40°C had an 8.2% rate of bacteremia and those with temperature above 40.5°C had a 10.5% rate. Among hyperpyrexic children seen in a pediatric emergency department, and with temperatures from 40.5°C to 41.0°C, 13% had positive blood cultures. Of those with temperature above 41.0°C, the rate was 26%. The rate of SBI (bacteremia plus other serious infections) in infants increases in direct proportion to fever height, or 3.2% when temperature is below 39°C, 5.2% when temperature is between 39°C and 39.9°C, and 26% when temperature is ≥40°C. In identifying SBI, the presence of hyperpyrexia (temperature ≥ 40°C) may be 21% sensitive and 97% specific and have a 25% PPV and a 96% NPV. A meta-analysis found that the probability of OB when temperature is ≥39°C is 4.3%; however, when only temperatures of ≥40.0°C are considered, the probability is 13%. Nonetheless, other investigations have not confirmed this association of height of fever and bacteremia. In one study, no patient with a temperature ≥ 41.0°C had bacteremia and the prevalence of bacteremia among children in all temperature groups between 39.0°C and 41.0°C did not exceed 5%.

The apparent discrepancy regarding height of fever and prevalence of bacteremia among these different reports may be due to selection bias. In the studies showing high bacteremia rates in hyperpyrexic children, blood specimens were not routinely obtained for all children but only for those children selected by the physician. In the studies showing no difference in prevalence rates, blood specimens were either obtained on all patients or control groups were included. In the reports using selected patients, high temperature may have been related to other factors (clinical appearance) that prompted a more thorough search for bacteremia (ascertainment bias). Although hyperpyrexia may be associated with a modestly increased risk of bacteremia, this risk has not been consistently substantiated.

By Presence of Other Foci of Infection. The finding of a focus of infection on examination does not make bacteremia less likely. One study found a prevalence of 9.9% if a focus such as otitis media or viral syndrome was diagnosed compared to 3.3% if no focus was identified. The rate of bacteremia in the presence of fever and otitis media may be 3%. This was comparable to the rate in the group with no focus on examination. Other studies have found febrile children with otitis media to have a bacteremia rate of 1.5% to 5.8%. These data suggest that children with otitis media are at risk for bacteremia at a rate similar to those children who have FWF.

By White Blood Cell Count. See laboratory data and interpretation.

NATURAL HISTORY

Occult bacteremia can result in four outcomes: spontaneous resolution, persistent bacteremia, sepsis (see Table 59–2), or focal infection, such as meningitis, arthritis, osteomyelitis, pneumonia, cellulitis, or other soft tissue infection. The rates of complications vary for the different etiologic agents.

Streptococcus pneumoniae. Approximately 40% of *S. pneumoniae* bacteremia resolves spontaneously, 7% to 22% of patients have continued fever with persistent bacteremia, and 6% to 10% go on to have meningitis. In a meta-analysis, the estimated risk of meningitis in occult pneumococcal bacteremia is 5.8% (95% CI, 3.4% to 8.8%).

***Haemophilus influenzae* Type b.** Hib bacteremia is much more likely to progress to focal disease than is *S. pneumoniae*. SBI develops in approximately 32% to 77% and meningitis in 23%. In a study on Hib bacteremia, of 20 children who did not receive initial antibiotic treatment, 50% had persistent bacteremia. Additionally, focal infections developed in 60%, including 20% with pneumonia, 10% with meningitis, epiglottitis, and cellulitis, and 5% with septic arthritis and otitis media. In another study, despite the observation that 48 patients (80%) had received antibiotics, 25 patients (42%) progressed to focal disease (meningitis, pneumonia, arthritis, pericarditis). Most of the children in whom invasive infection developed were ill or febrile at follow-up.

Children with Hib bacteremia are 12 times more likely to develop meningitis than those with *S. pneumoniae* bacteremia. The risk of Hib meningitis is not altered by treatment with oral antibiotics. In a meta-analysis, the risk of meningitis in Hib bacteremia is 26.6% (95% CI, 18.3% to 36.3%). Even if afebrile and well appearing, these children may still be at risk for serious sequelae. They deserve evaluation for focal infection and treatment with appropriate antimicrobial therapy.

Neisseria meningitidis. *N. meningitidis* bacteremia is frequently associated with serious sequelae. Children with *N. meningitidis* bacteremia are 85.6 times more likely to progress to meningitis than those with *S. pneumoniae* bacteremia. In a review of 12 children with unsuspected *N. meningitidis* bacteremia, among the four children who did not receive initial antibiotics, three had persistent bacteremia, including two who died and one in whom meningitis developed. Of the eight who received antibiotics, only four improved while meningitis developed in two. As with Hib bacteremia, children found to have *N. meningitidis* bacteremia warrant careful evaluation and therapy.

Salmonella. *Salmonella* bacteremia is often accompanied or preceded by an enteritis. In some instances, especially in young infants, the diarrhea is mild or even absent. The prevalence of *Salmonella* bacteremia among patients with *Salmonella* enteritis has been reported to be between 2% and 45%. In a prospective series, the prevalence is 6.5% in children up to 1 year of age. Fever is not uniformly present in *Salmonella* bacteremia. Furthermore, 50% who had persistent bacteremia may be afebrile at the return visit. In addition, approximately 55% on appropriate oral antibiotics had persistent bacteremia.

Among 47 cases of *Salmonella* bacteremia and 135 cases of *Salmonella* gastroenteritis, there were no serious sequelae in children with normal host defenses. Additionally, the nine patients with bacteremia who were not given antibiotics recovered spontaneously. The data indicate that *Salmonella* bacteremia frequently accompanies *Salmonella* enteritis. Though oral antibiotics may not adequately treat the bacteremia, serious complications in children with normal host defenses are uncommon. Infants under 3 months of age may be an exception; it is currently recommended that these young infants be treated.

TREATMENT STRATEGIES

Defining strategies for the management of febrile children without a focus of infection has been a perplexing issue in pediatrics. Because the prevalence of bacterial infections is low but the potential morbidity of those infections is high, the aim of management strategies is to identify and treat only those individuals at high risk for SBI and to avoid unnecessary treatment of low-risk children. The approach to these patients should vary with age because the ability to identify high-risk individuals changes between the neonatal period and childhood. Using clinical observation and selected laboratory screening tests, various authors have investigated different treatment plans.

Children Under 3 Months of Age (0 to 90 Days)

In children younger than age 3 months, particularly in those younger than 1 month, observational variables alone have serious shortcomings in assessment of risk for bacterial infection. The Acute Illness Observation Scale may fail to detect serious illness in febrile 4- to 8-week-old children. Nontoxic febrile infants still have a probability of SBI of 8.6%, including a 2.0% risk of bacteremia and a 1.0% risk of meningitis. In this group of infants, because observation is not sufficient to ensure low risk, laboratory evaluation is warranted. Yet screening tests do not identify all infants with a bacterial infection.

In an attempt to help direct management strategies, a group of prospective studies evaluated criteria developed in Rochester, New York, to identify infants younger than 2 months of age unlikely to have SBI. The criteria applied to previously healthy children who appeared well on presentation. Low-risk criteria included no history of prematurity, perinatal complications, prior antibiotics, or underlying conditions; no physical findings consistent with soft tissue, skeletal, or ear infection; a peripheral WBC between 5000 and 15,000/mm³; an absolute band count less than 1500/mm³; and a urinalysis with less than 10 white blood cells per high-power field in centrifuged sediment. Lumbar puncture results were not specifically used to classify infants, although any infants with abnormal CSF values were not considered low risk.

The original study missed one SBI, an infant with *Salmonella* gastroenteritis. In subsequent studies, infants with diarrhea received a stool examination for white blood cells. In a second study, low-risk criteria included all of the above and stool WBC < 5 per high power field. No cases of SBI were missed in the 148 infants classified as low risk. (The prevalence of SBI in the high-risk group was 24%.) Another study missed one SBI (*N. meningitidis* bacteremia) in 86 patients determined to be at low risk. Combining the data from these studies, of 430 febrile infants who met all low-risk criteria, two had SBI, one with *Salmonella* gastroenteritis and one with meningococcal bacteremia. With these data, the NPV of the Rochester criteria for SBI is 99.53% (95% CI, 98.14% to 99.92%).

In a review of studies evaluating diagnostic tests to identify infants younger than 3 months at low risk for SBI, it was determined that results pooled from the studies using the Rochester criteria had high methodologic validity, insignificant heterogeneity, and the best estimate of the negative likelihood ratio for SBI (i.e., how many times it is less likely for a patient with a negative result to have an SBI than it is for one with a positive result to have an SBI). That negative likelihood ratio was 0.03 (95% CI, 0.0% to 0.23%). It was calculated that if the probability for an infant with a fever to have an SBI is 7% prior to testing, if the Rochester criteria for low risk are satisfied, the probability for SBI decreases to 0.2% (95% CI, 0.0% to 1.7%). In other studies, however, the Rochester criteria correctly categorized only 26 of 80 patients (67%), while 3 of 70 low-risk infants had SBI. To date, the Rochester criteria have been the most carefully studied and provide the best means to assign infants under 3 months of age to a low-risk category. In a meta-analysis of studies of febrile children younger than 3 months of age using low-risk criteria similar to the Rochester criteria, it was found that if low-risk criteria are met (previously healthy, no focus on physical examination, WBC 5000 to 15,000/m³, band count less than 1500/m³, normal UA, and, if diarrhea is present, less than 5 white blood cells per high-power field), the probability of SBI is 1.4%, of OB is 1.1%, and of meningitis is 0.5%.

In another study, infants meeting low-risk criteria plus requirements for outpatient management (caregiver with adequate observational skills, telephone in home, and personal automobile) were managed as outpatients and given intramuscular (IM) ceftriaxone in a dose of 50 mg/kg. One of the 86 (1.2%) low-risk patients had an SBI (*N. meningitidis* bacteremia). This patient was subsequently hospitalized and recovered without complications.

In a different study, more liberal low-risk criteria were used in 1- to 3-month-old children to evaluate outpatient management. Low-risk patients were required to appear well, have a WBC <20,000/mm³, a urine screen negative for leukocyte esterase, and CSF WBC less than 10 × 10⁶/L. Low-risk patients received 50 mg/kg IM ceftriaxone at discharge and 24 hours later. SBI was found during follow-up in 27 of 503 (5.4% patients). Nine (1.8%) patients were bacteremic, 8 (1.6%) had UTI, and ten (2.0%) had bacterial gastroenteritis. Although these less stringent criteria classified more patients as low risk than the Rochester criteria, the authors stated that all were well at follow-up and recovered fully. However, one infant had *Staphylococcus aureus* osteomyelitis diagnosed 1 week after entry into the study. This infant reportedly recovered without complications.

The Milwaukee protocol was used in another prospective study for distinguishing the risk for SBI in 4- to 8-week-old infants. Criteria for low risk included well appearance, no focus of infection on examination, and a normal sepsis evaluation (urine, CSF, blood). A total of 143 of 534 patients were determined to be at low risk, given IM ceftriaxone (50 mg/kg), and seen for follow-up in 24 hours. SBI was seen in 1 patient (0.7%) in the low-risk group and in 23 patients (5.9%) in the high-risk group. The low-risk patient had a blood culture result positive for *Moraxella catarrhalis*. This child was afebrile and well at 24-hour follow-up, had a repeated blood culture, which was negative, and had no complications. The sensitivity of the Milwaukee protocol was determined to be 96% for SBI and to have an NPV of 99%.

In an effort to continue outpatient management of low-risk infants and to avoid unnecessary antibiotic administration, a 60-month prospective study was used to determine whether febrile infants 1 to 2 months of age identified at low risk for SBI could be effectively managed as outpatients without antibiotics. The study

evaluated 747 infants with temperature ≥ 38.2°C; SBI developed in 65 (8.7%). The criteria identified 64 of 65 patients—a sensitivity of 99% (95% CI, 98% to 100%). The misidentified infant had bacteremia, and the diagnosis was subsequently ectodermal dysplasia. Mean medical charges were $784 for the outpatient group compared with $5532 for hospital controls. Using strict selection criteria, one can safely manage these infants as outpatients without antibiotics; the result is a significant cost reduction without increasing risk. In a review of the literature, there were 11 infants between 1 and 3 months of age who had an SBI and yet were low risk according to the Rochester criteria and were initially managed without antibiotics (six with UTI, 3 with occult bacteremia, two with bacterial gastroenteritis). All of these patients did well despite the lag in starting antimicrobial agents.

The literature supports an outpatient management strategy in selected patients under 3 months of age. *At present, this strategy may not be applicable to infants younger than 1 month of age.* Most of the reports studied infants older than 27 days of age. Because there are insufficient data supporting outpatient treatment in this age group, conservative, in-hospital management is warranted. Guidelines published in 1993 by Baraff and colleagues suggested that all infants younger than 28 days of age should receive a complete evaluation for bacterial infection and be managed in the hospital on intravenous antimicrobial therapy until culture results are negative. The Baraff panel also suggested that infants meeting low-risk criteria may be hospitalized without starting antimicrobial therapy, provided that close observation for changes in examination are possible.

Outpatient management may be considered in the 1- to 3-month-old age group (28 to 90 days) if low-risk criteria are met and close follow-up is ensured. Low-risk patients should be defined as in the Rochester criteria. Although not explicitly stated in the Rochester criteria, infants with abnormal CSF values are not considered low risk. Infants who do not meet low-risk criteria should be hospitalized and given parenteral antibiotic therapy pending results of blood, urine, and CSF cultures.

If the child meets low-risk criteria, making outpatient management an option, several social factors need be considered to ensure careful follow-up and a return visit if there is a change in the child's condition. The guidelines suggested that the parents should have the following: (1) a thermometer, (2) a telephone in the home, (3) a car that is readily available, and (4) a travel time to the hospital of less than 30 minutes. Parental maturity also deserves assessment. Parents need to understand the practitioner's concerns for the child, to be able to observe the child, to keep return appointments, and to return for evaluation immediately if the child's condition deteriorates.

If outpatient management is chosen, the child should receive 50 mg/kg of IM ceftriaxone and have follow-up within 24 hours to examine the child for any signs of deterioration and to check for any growth in the blood culture, urine culture, and CSF culture. A proposed alternative strategy for low-risk infants is outpatient observation without antibiotics. The literature has not demonstrated a higher complication rate when treatment is delayed for this group. Another option suggested by Baraff's panel called for only a urine culture and careful outpatient observation for low-risk infants. The panel cautioned against the use of ceftriaxone if other specimens for culture are not obtained because of the difficulty in differentiating partially treated bacterial from viral infections if the clinical condition worsens.

In most paradigms, if the clinical condition deteriorates or the CSF culture or blood culture is positive, the infant should be admitted for parenteral antibiotic therapy. If the child is well appearing, all culture results are negative, and ceftriaxone was given initially, the IM injection should be repeated, close follow-up continued, and a return visit made in 18 to 24 hours.

Baraff's panel report also suggested a plan for management of specific conditions found at re-evaluation. Infants who on follow-up have a positive blood culture result for *S. pneumoniae* yet are afebrile and well by parental history and by physical examination may continue to be managed closely as outpatients. Because of concern regarding resistance to penicillin, these patients should receive a second injection of ceftriaxone until penicillin sensitivity is documented. At that time, patients may complete a 10-day course on oral penicillin (50 mg/kg/day) or an aminopenicillin (amoxicillin at 50 mg/kg/day) while continuing close follow-up.

Infants with only a positive urine culture who are afebrile and appear well at follow-up can continue closely monitored outpatient treatment with an oral antibiotic. Sensitivity testing should guide the choice of antimicrobial.

Children 3 to 36 Months of Age

The risk of occult bacteremia in children 3 to 36 months of age with temperature ≥ 39°C is between 3% and 11%, with a mean probability of 4.3% (95% CI, 2.6% to 6.5%). If temperature is below 39°C, the risk of bacteremia is less than 1%. For well-appearing children with no focus of infection and a rectal temperature under 39°C, screening studies are not necessary.

For the remainder of children, the challenge is to identify those patients at high risk for occult infection to avoid the complications of SBI. The WBC is currently the most useful screening test. The desired sensitivity and specificity for detection of OB can be individualized by physicians using the ROC curve (see Figure 59–1). The 1993 practice guidelines proposed by Baraff and co-workers use a WBC ≥ 15,000/mm³ to establish high risk. The relative risk of bacteremia around this WBC value is five (13.0% versus 2.6%). Risk assignment should also be based on urinalysis. Boys younger than 6 months of age and girls under 1 year of age are at increased risk of UTI (4% and 2%, respectively). Children younger than these ages should receive a urinalysis, and the urine specimen should be obtained via bladder catheterization or suprapubic aspiration to avoid contamination and indeterminate results from a bagged specimen. Urine culture is routinely recommended because of the imperfect sensitivity of urinalysis in detecting UTI. Stool analysis, specimens for culture, and CXR are recommended only if history and physical examination warrant them. After review of the appropriate tests, the patient can be assigned to a high-risk or low-risk category for further treatment.

A number of studies suggested that oral antibiotics (e.g., amoxicillin), when given presumptively for OB, reduced the incidence of focal complications. Pneumococcal bacteremia may persist in 29% of untreated patients but in only 6% of patients treated with oral antibiotics. In a review of 20 studies that compared outcome of bacteremia, children with bacteremia treated without antibiotics had a 55.8% risk of persistent fever, a 20.9% risk of persistent bacteremia, and 9.2% risk of meningitis. If oral antibiotics were administered, persistent fever, persistent bacteremia, and meningitis decreased to 15.6%, 3.8%, and 4.5%, respectively. This analysis used data from several trials that were uncontrolled, had inconsistent treatment regimens, or had poorly comparable groups.

In a randomized clinical trial comparing oral amoxicillin with placebo in children 3 to 36 months of age with temperature ≥ 39.0°C and no focus of infection, 27 of 955 (2.8%) patients had bacteremia. There was no difference in incidence of complications between the placebo and antibiotic group, 12.5% (1 of 8) versus 10.5% (2 of 19), respectively. Though the power for this comparison is low, these data do not support routine use of oral amoxicillin in febrile children without a focus of infection. In a retrospective review, 57% (16 of 28) of patients who received oral antimicrobial therapy for Hib infection had subsequent evidence of Hib infection at follow-up. Additionally, eight children who were afebrile and appeared well at follow-up had persistence of Hib disease.

Given the equivocal efficacy of oral therapy, other investigations

have examined the use of IM ceftriaxone in bacteremia. One prospective, randomized multicenter clinical trial compared oral amoxicillin/potassium clavulanate (AC), 40 mg/kg/day of amoxicillin) to IM ceftriaxone (75 mg/kg) for the treatment of children 3 to 36 months of age with temperature ≥ 39.5°C and WBC ≥ 15,000/mm³. In the AC group, 22% (4 of 22) of patients with pneumococcal bacteremia were still febrile at 24 hours. However, repeated cultures in all were negative and no additional morbidity was observed. All ceftriaxone (0 of 33) patients with pneumococcal bacteremia were afebrile at 24 hours and remained well. In one of the two patients with Hib bacteremia in the AC group, pneumonia developed. One of four with Hib bacteremia given IM ceftriaxone was irritable and lethargic on initial presentation. Although CSF values were normal the CSF culture grew Hib. Repeated CSF culture at 24 hours was sterile, and the patient recovered without sequelae. This patient was hospitalized at the time of the initial visit. One patient in each group had *N. meningitidis* bacteremia, both patients were afebrile and well at 24 hours, and repeated cultures were sterile. Diarrhea developed in significantly more AC patients (5.6% versus 0.5%). Both treatments are rational, but ceftriaxone has advantages in terms of reducing duration of fever, decreasing complications from Hib bacteremia, and minimizing side effects.

A multicenter trial comparing IM ceftriaxone (50 mg/kg) and oral amoxicillin (60 mg/kg/day) evaluated 6794 febrile patients (temperature > 39°C), of which 192 (2.8%) had OB. The ceftriaxone-treated group had complete elimination of bacteremia and no definite focal infections (0 of 102). In the amoxicillin treatment group, 5.6% (5 of 90) had definite focal infection (one persistent bacteremia, three meningitis, one pneumonia), and three of 90 patients (2 Hib, 1 *Salmonella*) had bacteria isolated from the blood after 24 hours. Ceftriaxone, in contrast to amoxicillin, reduces the incidence of subsequent focal bacterial infections and eradicates bacteria from the blood stream. These two prospective studies demonstrated that parenteral antimicrobial therapy with ceftriaxone reduced the duration of fever and led to fewer complications of occult bacteremia than oral therapy. The evidence from the aforementioned studies supports the use of parenteral ceftriaxone to prevent serious sequelae in the outpatient management of selected febrile children with no source of infection.

From these data, a rational management strategy can be derived for febrile children 3 to 36 months of age with no focus of infection. If the child appears well and has a temperature below 39.0°C, no diagnostic tests need to be initiated. The parent should be instructed to return if the fever persists for more than 48 hours or if the child's condition deteriorates. If the temperature is ≥39.0°C, a urine culture is suggested for boys under 6 months of age and for girls under 2 years of age. Additionally, consider a WBC, followed by IM ceftriaxone if the WBC ≥ 15,000/mm³. In the guidelines proposed by Baraff's panel, this algorithm was one suggested, although a second option consisted of blood culture and empiric antibiotics for all patients with a temperature ≥ 39°C. Children should be re-evaluated in 24 and 48 hours. If the child is afebrile and well on follow-up and the cultures show no growth, no further therapy is necessary. Children appearing toxic on initial evaluation or on follow-up should be admitted to the hospital and given parenteral antibiotics after completing a sepsis evaluation.

At the time of follow-up, children who have a positive blood culture for *S. pneumoniae*, yet are afebrile and well by history and physical examination, may continue to be managed closely as outpatients. Because of concern regarding resistance to penicillin, these patients should receive a second injection of ceftriaxone until penicillin sensitivity is documented. At that time, patients may complete a 10-day course of oral penicillin (50 mg/kg/day) or an aminopenicillin (amoxicillin at 50 mg/kg/day) while continuing close follow-up. Children whose blood cultures grow a pathogen other than *S. pneumoniae* should be hospitalized for sepsis evaluation and parenteral antibiotic therapy. Any children with positive

CSF cultures need hospital admission and parenteral antimicrobial therapy.

Children with only a positive urine culture and who are afebrile and appear well at follow-up can continue closely monitored outpatient treatment with an oral antibiotic. Sensitivity testing should guide the choice of antimicrobial agent.

PHARMACOLOGIC THERAPY

Ceftriaxone

Ceftriaxone is a parenteral third-generation cephalosporin that is useful for outpatient bacteremia therapy because adequate tissue levels are achieved for 24 hours with a single IM dose and because it is active against the typical pathogens causing SBI. The usual dose is 50 mg/kg/day when given intramuscularly. The risk of anaphylaxis is not known. In the patient with penicillin allergy, the risk is estimated to be between 10% and 15%. Signs or symptoms related to ceftriaxone therapy include tenderness, swelling, or bruising at the injection site. Dermatologic reactions are uncommon (1.5%), but gastrointestinal reactions (abdominal pain, diarrhea) occur in about 5% of children who receive ceftriaxone.

Cases of cephalosporin treatment failure in penicillin-resistant and cephalosporin-resistant *S. pneumoniae* meningitis have been reported. The efficacy of ceftriaxone therapy for outpatient management of occult bacteremia may change if the prevalence of these resistant strains increases.

Antipyretics

Despite considerable debate on the theoretical benefits of fever for host defense, there are few proven benefits in humans. There are known benefits in fever reduction. Children are symptomatically improved with fever reduction. Decreasing body temperature also reduces metabolic demands and the need for increased fluid intake. An increase in fluid of 100 ml/m²/day is needed for every 1°C rise in temperature above 37.8°C.

When fever is caused by an alteration in the hypothalamic set point, as in infection, therapy to inhibit prostaglandin production and reset the thermostat is appropriate. Acetaminophen is the standard agent for antipyresis in this setting. The recommended dose is 10 to 15 mg/kg given up to every 4 hours, with a maximum single dose of 650 mg. Aspirin is used infrequently because of its association with Reye syndrome and its ability to cause gastrointestinal upset and bleeding. Ibuprofen is a nonsteroidal anti-inflammatory agent that is effective in reducing fever, although it has not been shown to offer any clear advantage over acetaminophen. The suggested dose for ibuprofen is 10 mg/kg. This medication is safe for the vast majority of patients, yet it may have adverse effects on patients with renal disease or dehydration. Gastrointestinal upset has been reported in 0% to 16%.

Febrile children may not benefit from external cooling by tepid-water sponge bath. The mechanism of cooling by this method is heat loss through the energy of evaporation as water evaporates from the skin. Although this technique may transiently decrease body temperature, it does not alter the hypothalamic axis and the efferent neurons continue to produce an increase in body temperature. Methods of physical cooling are appropriate when hyperthermia (as in heat stroke) results in temperature elevation.

Another important aspect in the treatment of fever is parental education. Many parents are fearful of fever and worry about low-grade temperatures (<38.9°C). Most parents believe that a temperature below 40°C may lead to neurologic injury. Antipyretics

are given by 85% of parents when the temperature is ≤38.4°C. Parents may need education and reassurance on the reasons for and risks of fever in their children.

ADDITIONAL ISSUES

Costs and Complications of Hospitalization

One of the primary strategies in managing children with FWF is to avoid the costs and complications of unnecessary hospitalization. For low-risk infants 1 to 2 months of age observed as outpatients, the mean medical charges are $784; for hospitalized controls, the mean charges are $5532. A complication rate of 20% to 25% has been noted in febrile infants younger than 60 days of age admitted to the hospital. Complications included intravenous catheter infiltration, skin sloughing due to intravenous therapy, fluid overload, antibiotic overdose, diarrhea, candidiasis, fever due to high incubator temperature, distraught mothers secondary to multiple procedures, nosocomial infections (respiratory syncytial virus, rotavirus), and even stolen infants. Additionally, diagnostic misadventures (repeating diagnostic tests unnecessarily, following up on contaminated cultures, not following up on abnormal tests, and continuing hospitalization unnecessarily while awaiting consultation) are possible. Reducing costs and complications are potential benefits of outpatient treatment.

HOST CONSIDERATIONS

Special consideration applies to immunocompromised children presenting with FWF. Such patients include those with malignancies, those with primary and acquired immunodeficiency syndromes, and those receiving cytotoxic therapies. Immunocompromised hosts are at increased risk of life-threatening infection (see Chapters 49, 52, 55, and 60).

Neutropenia

Children with neutropenia make up one group at high risk for serious infections (see Chapter 60). Granulocytopenia can occur in response to cytotoxic therapy for malignancy or from bone marrow failure. The relation between neutropenia and serious infection has been clearly demonstrated. The rate of infection starts to rise when absolute neutrophil count drops below 1000/mm³, it increases significantly below 500/mm³, and it is most marked when it falls below 100/mm³. In a study of 1000 consecutive pediatric oncology patients, 80% of febrile episodes occurred with the absolute neutrophil count ≤ 500/mm³ (see Chapter 60).

Sickle Cell Hemoglobinopathy

Mortality in children with sickle cell hemoglobinopathy (SCH) (see Chapter 49) is most commonly due to infection. The risk of sepsis or meningitis in children under 5 years of age is 15%, and the resultant mortality is 30%. The risk of pneumococcal sepsis is 400 times that of unaffected children, and for Hib sepsis the risk is two to four times as great. The types of organisms responsible for infection are not atypical and usually involve the polysaccharide-encapsulated organisms *S. pneumoniae*, Hib, *Neisseria* species, and *Salmonella* species; *E. coli* is associated with UTIs, while *S. aureus* and *Salmonella* are noted in patients with osteomyelitis. With SCH, the ability of the host to contain the infecting agent is altered. The immunologic functions of the spleen—antibody synthesis and clearing organisms ineffectively opsonized by complement—are impaired. Repeated episodes of sickling and infarction lead to functional asplenia in the first year of life. Most patients are permanently asplenic by the age of 7 years.

Children between 6 months and 5 years old with SCH and fever have an overall bacteremia rate of 5.4%. When temperature is above 39.5°C, 11% may have bacteremia; and when the temperature is above 40.6°C, 62% have bacteremia. The WBC, band count, and degree of splenomegaly are not useful indicators of bacterial infection. Patients with SCH are at high risk when they present with fever, as this may be the initial sign of an overwhelming infection. For these patients, a blood specimen and a complete blood count should be obtained and a urinalysis and urine culture should be strongly considered. A lumbar puncture and a CXR should be done if clinically indicated. Because of their high-risk status, admission of these patients is recommended along with administration of parenteral antibiotics active against the polysaccharide-encapsulated organisms.

Outpatient management of children with SCH has not been well studied. In one report of outpatient management of 211 febrile children under 5 years of age with SCH, in which all patients received intravenous ceftriaxone before disposition, 3% of patients had bacteremia; none of these were initially managed as outpatients. This study was uncontrolled and nonrandomized, and while it provides preliminary data, further study is indicated to determine the safety of outpatient management.

SUMMARY AND RED FLAGS

The majority of febrile infants and children with no focus of infection have a self-limited disease process. Only 4% have an invasive bacterial infection. Although there is no single, rapid test that correctly categorizes all patients, clinical and laboratory screening criteria have been developed to help identify a level of risk in children of different ages. These criteria have been presented along with current suggested guidelines to help the practitioner institute a safe and effective management strategy.

Red flags include the criteria in Table 59–2, neutropenia (overwhelming infection), leukocytosis, ill appearance, petechiae (see Chapter 57), normal CSF chemistries and cell count with positive CSF Gram stain, and signs of focal end-organ involvement.

REFERENCES

General

Dinarello CA, Cannon JG, Wolff SM. New concepts on the pathogenesis of fever. Rev Infect Dis 1988;10:108.

Bundled Infants

Berera G, Berkowitz CE, Seidel J, et al. The effects of bundling on infant temperature (abstr). Am J Dis Child 1993;147:457.
Cheng TL, Partridge JC. Effect of bundling and high environmental temperature on neonatal body temperature. Pediatrics 1993;92:238.

General Appearance

Baker MD, Avner JR, Bell LM. Failure of infant observation scales in detecting serious illness in febrile 4- to 8-week-old infants. Pediatrics 1990;85:1040.
Bonadio WA, Henner H, Smith D, et al. Reliability of observation variables in distinguishing infectious outcome of febrile young infants. Pediatr Infect Dis J 1993;12:111.
McCarthy PL, Sharpe MR, Spiesel SZ, et al. Observation scales to identify serious illness in febrile children. Pediatrics 1982;70:802.
McCarthy PL, Lembo RM, Fink HD, et al. Observation, history, and physical examination in diagnosis of serious illnesses in febrile children ≤ 24 months. J Pediatr 1987;110:26.

Response to Antipyretics

Baker RC, Tiller T, Bausher JC, et al. Severity of disease correlated with fever reduction in febrile infants. Pediatrics 1989;83:1016.
Torrey SB, Henretig F, Fleisher, et al. Temperature response to antipyretic therapy in children: Relationship to occult bacteremia. Am J Emerg Med 1985;3:190.
Yamamoto LT, Wigder HN, Fligner DJ, et al. Relationship of bacteremia to antipyretic therapy in febrile children. Pediatr Emerg Care 1987;3:223.

Laboratory Data and Interpretation

Baraff LJ, Bass JW, Fleisher GR, et al. Practice guideline for the management of infants and children 0 to 36 months of age with fever without source. Pediatrics 1993;92:1.
Bass JW, Steele RW, Wittler RR, et al. Antimicrobial treatment of occult bacteremia: A multicenter cooperative study. Pediatr Infect Dis J 1993;12:466.
Jaffe DM, Fleisher GR. Temperature and total white blood cell count as indicators of bacteremia. Pediatrics 1991;87:670.

Neutrophils, Bands, and Other Acute-Phase Reactants

Bennish M, Beem MO, Ormiste V. C-reactive protein and zeta sedimentation ratio as indicators of bacteremia in pediatric patients. J Pediatr 1984;104:729.
Crocker PJ. Occult bacteremia in the emergency department. Ann Emerg Med 1984;13:45.
Liu CH, Lehan C, Speer ME, et al. Degenerative changes in neutrophils: An indicator of bacterial infection. Pediatrics 1984;74:823.
McCarthy PL. Comparison of acute phase reactants in pediatric patients with fever. Pediatrics 1978;62:716.
McCarthy PL, Jekel JF, Dolan TF. Temperature greater or equal to 40°C in children less than 24 months of age: A prospective study. Pediatrics 1977;59:663.

Chest Radiographs

Crain EF, Bulas D, Bijur PE, et al. Is a chest radiograph necessary in the evaluation of every febrile infant less than 8 weeks of age? Pediatrics 1991;88:821.
Leventhal JM. Clinical predictors of pneumonia as a guide to ordering chest roentgenograms. Clin Pediatr 1982;21:730.
Patterson RJ, Bisset GS, Kirks DR, et al. Chest radiographs in the evaluation of the febrile infant. Am J Roentgenol 1990;155:833.

Differential Diagnosis

General

Krober MS, Bass JW, Powell JM, et al. Bacterial and viral pathogens causing fever in infants less than 3 months old. Am J Dis Child 1985;139:889.

Urinary Tract Infection

Bachur R, Caputo GL. Bacteremia with urinary tract infections (abstr). Am J Dis Child 1993;147:463.

Bauchner H, Philipp B, Dashefsky B, et al. Prevalence of bacteriuria in febrile children. Pediatr Infect Dis J 1987;6:239.

Crain EF, Gershel JC. Urinary tract infections in febrile infants less than 8 weeks of age. Pediatrics 1990;86:363.

Krober MS, Bass JW, Powell JM, et al. Bacterial and viral pathogens causing fever in infants less than 3 months old. Am J Dis Child 1985;139:889.

Lohr JA, Portilla MG, Geuder TG, et al. Making a presumptive diagnosis of urinary tract infection by using a urinalysis performed in an on-site laboratory. J Pediatr 1993;122:22.

Occult Bacteremia

Alpert G, Hibbert E, Fleisher GR. Case-control study of hyperpyrexia in children. Pediatr Infect Dis J 1990;9:161.

Baraff LJ, Oslund S, Prather M. Effect of antibiotic therapy and etiologic microorganism on the risk of bacterial meningitis in children with occult bacteremia. Pediatrics 1993;92:140.

Baron MA, Fink HD. Bacteremia in private pediatric practice. Pediatrics 1980;66:171.

Bass JW, Steele RW, Wittler RR. Antimicrobial treatment of occult bacteremia: A multicenter cooperative study. Pediatr Infect Dis J 1993;12:466.

Ghiorghis B, Geyid A, Haile M. Bacteremia in febrile out-patient children. East Afr Med J 1992;69:74.

McCarthy PL, Dolan TF, Jr. Hyperpyrexia in children: Eight-year emergency room experience. Am J Dis Child 1976;130:849.

McCarthy PL, Grundy GW, Spiesel SZ, et al. Bacteremia in children: An outpatient review. Pediatrics 1976;57:861.

McGowan JE, Bratton L, Klein JO, et al. Bacteremia in febrile children seen in a "walk-in" pediatric clinic. N Engl J Med 1973;288:1309.

Schutzman SA, Petrycki S, Fleisher GR. Bacteremia with otitis media. Pediatrics 1991;87:48.

Teele DW, Pelton SI, Grant MJ, et al. Bacteremia in febrile children under 2 years of age: Results of cultures of blood of 600 consecutive febrile children in a "walk-in" clinic. J Pediatr 1975;87:227.

Streptococcus pneumoniae

Carroll WL, Farrell MK, Singer JI, et al. Treatment of occult bacteremia: A prospective randomized clinical trial. Pediatrics 1983;72:608.

Feder HM. Occult pneumococcal bacteremia and the febrile infant and young children. Clin Pediatr 1980;19:457.

Rosenberg N, Cohen SN. Pneumococcal bacteremia in pediatric patients. Ann Emerg Med 1982;11:11.

Haemophilus influenzae Type B

Anderson AB, Ambrosino DM, Siber GR. *Haemophilus influenzae* type b unsuspected bacteremia. Pediatr Emerg Care 1987;3:82.

Forman PM, Murphy TV. Reevaluation of the ambulatory pediatric patient whose blood culture is positive for *Haemophilus influenzae* type b. J Pediatr 1991;118:503.

Korones DN, Marshall GS, Shapiro ED. Outcome of children with occult bacteremia caused by *Haemophilus influenzae* type b. Pediatr Infect Dis J 1992;11:516.

Marshall R, Teele DW, Klein JO. Unsuspected bacteremia due to *Haemophilus influenzae*: Outcome in children not initially admitted to hospital. J Pediatr 1979;95:690.

Shapiro ED, Aaron NH, Wald ER, et al. Risk factors for development of bacterial meningitis among children with occult bacteremia. J Pediatr 1986;109:15.

Teele DW, Marshall R, Klein JO. Unsuspected bacteremia in young children. Pediatr Clin North Am 1979;26:773.

Neisseria meningitidis

Dashefsky B, Teele DW, Klein JO. Unsuspected meningococcemia. J Pediatr 1983;102:69.

Salmonella

Katz BZ, Shapiro ED. Predictors of persistently positive blood cultures in children with "occult" *Salmonella* bacteremia. Pediatr Infect Dis 1986;5:713.

Meadow WL, Schneider H, Beem MO. *Salmonella* enteritidis bacteremia in childhood. J Infect Dis 1985;152:185.

Torrey S, Fleisher G, Jaffe D. Incidence of *Salmonella* bacteremia in infants with *Salmonella* gastroenteritis. J Pediatr 1986;5:718.

Treatment Strategies

Avner JR, Crain EF, Baker MD. Failure to validate the Rochester Criteria for evaluation of febrile infants (abstr). Am J Dis Child 1993;147:441.

Baraff LJ, Oslund SA, Schriger DL, et al. Probability of bacterial infections in febrile infants less than three months of age: A meta-analysis. Pediatr Infect Dis J 1992;11:257.

Baraff LJ, Bass JW, Fleisher GR, et al. Practice guideline for the management of infants and children 0 to 36 months of age with fever without source. Pediatrics 1993; 92:1.

Baskin MN, O'Rourke EJ, Fleisher GR. Outpatient treatment of febrile infants 28 to 89 days of age with intramuscular administration of ceftriaxone. J Pediatr 1992;120:22.

Bonadio WA, Shallow K, Smith D. Efficacy of the Milwaukee Protocol in distinguishing risk for serious bacterial infections in febrile young infants (abstr). Am J Dis Child 1993;147:441.

Dagan R, Sofer S, Phillip M, et al. Ambulatory care of febrile infants younger than 2 months of age classified as being at low risk for having serious bacterial infections. J Pediatr 1988;112:355.

Klassen TP, Rowe PC. Selecting diagnostic tests to identify febrile infants less than 3 months of age as being at low risk for serious bacterial infection: A scientific overview. J Pediatr 1992;121:671.

McCarthy CA, Powell KR, Jaskiewicz JA, et al. Outpatient management of selected infants younger than two months of age evaluated for possible sepsis. Pediatr Infect Dis J 1990;9:385.

Wasserman GM, White CB. Evaluation of the necessity for hospitalization of the febrile infant less than three months of age. Pediatr Infect Dis J 1990;9:163.

Children 3 to 36 Months of Age

Baraff LJ, Lee SI. Fever without source: Management of children 3 to 36 months of age. Pediatr Infect Dis J 1992;11:146.

Bass JW, Steele RW, Wittler RR. Antimicrobial treatment of occult bacteremia: A multicenter cooperative study. Pediatr Infect Dis J 1993;12:466.

Bratton L, Teele DW, Klein JO. Outcome of unsuspected pneumococcemia in children not initially admitted to the hospital. J Pediatr 1977;90:703.

Fleisher GR, Platt R, Occult Bacteremia Study Group. Intramuscular antibiotic therapy for prevention of bacterial sequelae in children with occult bacteremia (abstr). Pediatr Res 1992;31:161A.

Jaffe DM, Tanz RR, David AT. Antibiotic administration to treat possible occult bacteremia in febrile children. N Engl J Med 1987; 317:1175.

Korones DN, Marshall GS, Shapiro ED. Outcome of children with occult bacteremia caused by *Haemophilus influenzae* type b. Pediatr Infect Dis J 1992;11:516.

Pharmacologic Therapy

Fleisher GR, Platt R, Occult Bacteremia Study Group. Intramuscular antibiotic therapy for prevention of bacterial sequelae in children with occult bacteremia (abstr). Pediatr Res 1992;31:161A.

McCarthy CA, Powell KR, Jaskiewicz JA, et al. Outpatient management of selected infants younger than two months of age evaluated for possible sepsis. Pediatr Infect Dis J 1990;9:385.

Schmitt BD. Fever phobia: Misconceptions of parents about fevers. Am J Dis Child 1980;134:176.

60 Fever and Neutropenia*

Brigitta U. Mueller   Philip A. Pizzo

Neutropenia is a decreased number of circulating neutrophils. The absolute neutrophil count (ANC) is calculated by multiplying the white blood cell (WBC) count by the percentage of polymorphonuclear leukocytes and band forms. An ANC of less than 1000 cells/mm³ in white children between the ages of 2 weeks and 1 year or an ANC of less than 1500 cells/mm³ in older infants is considered to be neutropenia. African-American children tend to normally have ANCs that are 200 to 600 cells/mm³ lower than those of white children. A neutrophil count below 500 cells/mm³ is associated with an increased risk for infection; this risk is highest with profound neutropenia (ANC < 100 cells/mm³) or prolonged neutropenia (>1 week). Patients who present with an ANC between 500 and 1000 cells/mm³ but whose ANC is expected to fall below 500 cells/mm³ within the following 24 to 48 hours are also at risk for an infection and should be promptly evaluated and treated. *Fever* is usually defined as a single oral temperature of at least 38.5°C or three successive readings of at least 38°C in a 24-hour period.

This chapter concentrates on patients who have repeated or prolonged episodes of neutropenia that are most often due to cancer therapy–induced myelosuppression. Numerous congenital and other acquired disorders cause neutropenic states (Table 60–1, Fig. 60–1). Patients with these disorders often have recurrent mucocutaneous infections due to *Staphylococcus aureus* or group A streptococci; those with severe and prolonged neutropenia tend to develop bacterial sepsis (see Chapter 52). Patients with chemotherapy-induced neutropenia have other disorders of host defense, such as mucosal breakdown from mucositis, monocytopenia, lymphopenia, and qualitative B-lymphocyte and T-lymphocyte defects. The use of high-dose cytotoxic chemotherapy for neoplastic diseases as well as the use of zidovudine (AZT) in patients infected with the human immunodeficiency virus (HIV) has led to an increase in the prevalence of febrile, neutropenic episodes. Much of our understanding and approach to febrile neutropenic children has been developed in patients with malignancies and chemotherapy-induced neutropenia.

DIAGNOSIS

Patient history, physical examination, and laboratory investigations are the mainstays of the diagnosis and monitoring of chemotherapy-induced neutropenic patients in whom fever develops. These assessments should be performed at least once daily during the period of fever and neutropenia (Table 60–2). In addition to the degree and duration of neutropenia, other aspects of the patient's cellular and humoral immune defense as well as the reason for the neutropenia (iatrogenic versus congenital versus infectious) also greatly influence the risk for infection. The onset of fever in the neutropenic patient should be considered an emergency and should be evaluated immediately. Rapid therapy is mandatory to prevent the development of, or to treat the presence of, high-grade bacteremia caused by an invasive organism that may

quickly produce sepsis, shock, and death. Antibiotic treatment may initially be empirical and then modified by findings obtained through repeated patient assessments. Negative laboratory or radiographic findings do not exclude an infectious focus for the fever, because the diminished inflammatory response resulting from the neutropenia may alter the classic signs and symptoms of infection. Pain, tenderness, and induration may nevertheless be present in soft tissue infections.

History

The history follows traditional guidelines but may be weighted individually (Table 60–3). For accurate detection of fever in a

---

Table 60–1. Etiologic Factors in Neutropenia

Congenital Neutropenias
 Kostmann syndrome (severe congenital autosomal recessive
  neutropenia)
 Chronic benign (idiopathic) neutropenia (occasionally familial
  and autosomal dominant)
 Fanconi anemia
 Schwachman syndrome (chronic moderate neutropenia,
  pancreatic insufficiency)
 Cartilage-hair hypoplasia (moderate neutropenia, short-limb
  dwarfism, abnormal cellular immunity, fine hair)
 Dyskeratosis congenita (neutropenia in ⅓ of patients, nail
  dystrophy, leukoplakia, skin hyperpigmentation)
 Neutropenia associated with metabolic disturbances (organic
  acidemias)
 Reticular dysgenesis
 Cyclic neutropenia
 Neutropenia with agammaglobulinemia and
  dysgammaglobulinemia

Acquired Neutropenias
 Aplastic anemia
 Reticuloendothelial sequestration (hypersplenism)
 Infections (sepsis, HIV infection, tuberculosis, acute viral or
  rickettsial infections)
 Autoimmune or neonatal isoimmune neutropenia, systemic
  lupus erythematosus
 Bone marrow infiltration and replacement with malignant cells
  (leukemia, neuroblastoma)
 Drug induced (chemotherapy for cancer treatment,
  immunosuppression for other diseases, antibiotics—especially
  sulfa drugs, anticonvulsants, antipsychotics, antithyroid
  agents, cardiovascular agents, antihistamines, NSAID, AZT,
  antivirals)
 Radiation therapy
 Osteopetrosis

Abbreviations: AZT = zidovudine; NSAID = nonsteroidal anti-inflammatory drug;
HIV = human immunodeficiency virus.

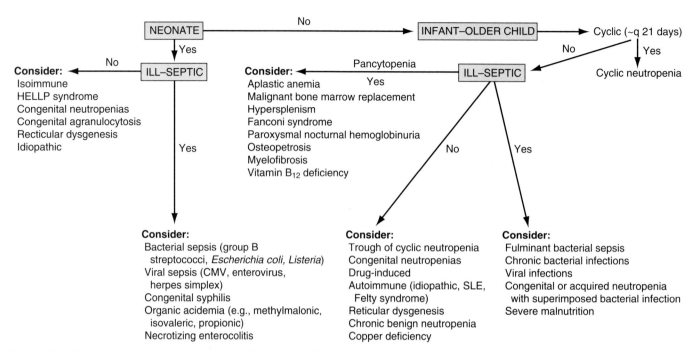

Figure 60–1. Diagnostic approach to neutropenia. CMV = cytomegalovirus; HELLP = preeclampsia induced neutropenia with hemolysis elevated liver enzymes and low platelets; SLE = systemic lupus erythematosus.

neutropenic patient, oral temperatures should be checked at least three times daily. Patients at risk for neutropenia should understand the importance of fever and should be seen by a physician within 2 hours of its onset. More than a third of the patients may present with other infectious or noninfectious conditions (e.g., dehydration, systemic hypotension, inadequate pain control, bleeding), which complicate the presentation.

The *duration of neutropenia* is crucial in the evaluation of the risk for infections. It is also important to note whether this is the first episode of fever during the current episode of neutropenia or whether the patient has a recurrent or persistent fever (described later). Determining the nature and timing of the antecedent chemotherapy is important. For example, certain cytotoxic agents are only mildly myelosuppressive and recovery from neutropenia is relatively rapid in these cases. Other drug combinations (or even use of fewer myelosuppressive agents in patients who have received high-dose chemotherapy) cause a profound and prolonged dose-dependent neutropenia. Furthermore, particular infectious syndromes can be associated with certain chemotherapeutic agents. Cytosine arabinoside typically causes oral mucositis, which is associated with an increased frequency of *Streptococcus mitis* infections. It is also important to recognize that the concurrent use of other medications can be a cofactor in the development of neutropenia (e.g., the use of antibiotics like trimethoprim-sulfamethoxazole for prophylaxis against *Pneumocystis carinii* pneumonia or the use of therapeutic antiviral agents for treatment of HIV infection). The use of a bone marrow–stimulating cytokine, such as granulocyte-macrophage colony-stimulating factor (GM-CSF) or granulocyte colony-stimulating factor (G-CSF) can reduce the expected duration and depth of neutropenia. Chronic steroid therapy not only increases the risk for infection but may blunt the ability of the patient to develop a fever in response to an infection.

Questions regarding the patient's past medical history should include information about previous episodes of fever and neutropenia; their course, duration, and complications; and whether a specific organism was isolated. The underlying illness also influences the choice and dosage of empirical antibiotic therapy (e.g., avoiding imipenem-cilastatin in a patient with a brain tumor because of the risk of seizures).

Patients with HIV disease are often severely immunocompromised in addition to being neutropenic. They appear to be at a higher risk for certain opportunistic infections. They may suffer chronic or recurrent bacterial or viral infections, even after an adequate course of antibiotic therapy has been completed (see Chapter 55). Patients with cancer or aplastic anemia are at much higher risk for developing invasive fungal infections with *Aspergillus* sp. or *Candida* sp.

An exposure history is important in determining the pathogens most likely to be involved. A hospitalized patient usually becomes colonized with multi–drug-resistant organisms common to that environment. The balance of the patient's own endogenous flora is often shifted toward more resistant and virulent bacteria. Infections with gram-positive bacteria, especially with coagulase-negative staphylococci resistant to β-lactam antibiotics, are common. The number of infections with *Pseudomonas aeruginosa* has decreased. If a fever occurs while the patient is an outpatient, it is important to know whether other close contacts have been sick. However, most infections in the immunocompromised host arise from the patient's endogenous flora and cannot be avoided.

An in-depth review of systems can reveal minor complaints that may help to determine the cause of the fever. Such complaints may be minimal but can indicate a possible focus of infection. Information about perianal tenderness or pain associated with defecation is not usually volunteered by patients but can be indicative of perianal cellulitis or abscess. The presence of any foreign bodies (e.g., central venous catheters, intraventricular reservoirs or shunts, prosthetic devices, patches after cardiac surgery) must be noted and considered when antimicrobial therapy is chosen.

Physical Examination

A meticulous physical examination must be repeated daily as long as the patient is febrile and neutropenic. Particular attention must be directed to common but often occult sites of infection, such as the oral cavity, the periungual area, and the perianal area. However, the examination of the perirectal area should usually be limited to careful inspection and external palpation. A careful rectal

Table 60–2. Evaluation of the Febrile Neutropenic Patient with Chemotherapy-Induced Neutropenia

	Time Point of Evaluation	Comment
History and physical examination	Daily	See Table 60–3 for history
Laboratory Studies		
Complete blood count with differential	At pretreatment evaluation and then daily	Less frequently in patients with known protracted neutropenia (after bone marrow transplant, aplastic anemia)
Chemistry profile, electrolyte levels	At pretreatment evaluation and then at least weekly	To monitor kidney and liver function
Drug levels	Within 36 hours of initiation of certain antibiotics	In patients receiving aminoglycosides, vancomycin, or flucytosine
Blood cultures	Daily, until negative Daily, until afebrile Daily if there is a new fever	Blood cultures should be drawn from each port if a multilumen central venous line is used Peripheral cultures at least initially and once daily if there is a new fever
Urine culture	At pretreatment evaluation With any urinary tract symptoms	
Throat culture	At pretreatment evaluation	
Cultures of sites of infection	At pretreatment evaluation	Exit site of central venous catheters, skin lesions, drainage fluid
Radiographic Studies		
Chest radiograph	At pretreatment evaluation Weekly with persistent fever With new fevers or symptoms	At initial evaluation in all patients, regardless of symptoms (complaints can be minimal)
Only in Selected Patients		
Lumbar puncture	Not routinely necessary except in special patient populations	Indicated in febrile (neutropenic) newborns and infants Indicated in patients with intraventricular foreign bodies (shunt, reservoir) if no evidence of increased intracranial pressure present In symptomatic patients (headache, meningismus)
Virus cultures	At pretreatment evaluation in symptomatic patients In patients with protracted fever of unknown origin	URI symptoms: respiratory viruses Prolonged fever: cytomegalovirus, herpes simplex, HHV-6 Skin lesions: herpes simplex, varicella-zoster Hematuria: adenovirus
Sputum examination	Daily in intubated patients Limited yield in most non-intubated patients	Induced sputum or bronchoalveolar lavage may be helpful in patient with chronic lung infections or HIV infection and respiratory symptoms
Endoscopy	Avoid if possible during neutropenia	Empiric treatment often preferable
Other radiographic evaluations (MRI, CT, ultrasonography)	Indicated in selected patients or clinical settings	CT of lung is more sensitive than plain chest films to detect fungal lesions CT or MRI of liver and or spleen helpful to diagnose hepatosplenic candidiasis (see Chapter 23) Sinus films or CT in patients with symptoms or fever for >7 days Esophagogram in patients with symptoms (mucositis, odynophagia, retrosternal pain)
Nuclear medicine evaluations	Indium white cell scan Gallium scan Bone scan	Only with specific localizing symptoms Often unreliable because of the lack of an inflammatory response

Abbreviations: CT = computed tomography; MRI = magnetic resonance imaging; URI = upper respiratory infection; HIV = human immunodeficiency virus; HHV-6 = human herpes virus 6.

Table 60–3. Important Aspects of the History in the Febrile Neutropenic Patient

Chief complaint	Complaints are often minimal and frequently focused on the rapid onset of general malaise
History of present illness	Duration of fever, duration of neutropenia Current drugs (especially prophylactic antibiotics and cytokines) Date and type of last chemotherapy
Past medical history	Previous episodes of fever and neutropenia (were any complications defined?) Underlying illness; its duration, stage, and treatment
Family history	Exposure history (other members of family sick?)
Review of systems	Headaches? Sinus pain? Earache? Rhinorrhea? Sore throat? Mouth ulcers? Pain with swallowing? Cough? Chest pain? Abdominal pain (constant, colicky, localized?) Tenderness in perirectal area? Diarrhea (mucoid, bloody, watery?) Dysuria? Frequency? Vaginal discharge? Tenderness around exit site of central venous catheter? Other skin lesions? Joint pain? Fingernail-toenail pain? Foreign bodies present?

examination should be performed only when symptoms strongly suggest a localized infection (e.g., tenderness or fluctuance). The area around the exit site of a central venous catheter should be inspected and palpated daily; attention must be given to skin lesions and tenderness around the fingernails and toenails.

Laboratory Evaluation

Cultures of blood, urine, and any site of presumed infection are essential for the treatment of the patient with fever and neutropenia. Despite cultures, the cause of the fever may not be identified initially in nearly 70% of patients.

Therapy in chemotherapy-induced neutropenia with fever must never be delayed because of the lack of a proven infectious organism. Often, therapy is initiated empirically in such cases. Some centers recommend routine surveillance cultures in patients with prolonged neutropenia, with the rationale that most organisms causing infections in the immunocompromised host arise from the endogenous flora or are acquired in the hospital. However, the predictive yield of these cultures is low. Possible exceptions include cultures from the anterior nares to diagnose colonization with methicillin-resistant *S. aureus* or *Aspergillus* sp.

At least two sets of blood specimens should be obtained for culture from all patients. If a central venous catheter is present, a culture from each lumen is warranted before antibiotic therapy is initiated. Although only about 5% of documented bacteremic episodes are caused by anaerobic bacteria, aerobic and anaerobic cultures are important. Cultures for bacteria and fungi as well as a Gram stain should be obtained from any infectious site, including the exit site of a central venous catheter. If a lesion is chronically infected, special stains and cultures for *Mycobacterium* should be performed as well. Diarrheal stool should be assessed for *Clostridium difficile* toxin, bacteria, viruses, and parasites. Urine culture and analysis are part of the routine evaluation. Pyuria may be absent in the neutropenic patient with a urinary tract infection.

The value of virus cultures in the initial evaluation of the febrile neutropenic patient is less defined. For patients with respiratory symptoms, specimens should be obtained to look for respiratory viruses, and for patients with mucositis, even if they are presumed to have chemotherapy-induced stomatitis, specimens should be obtained to look for herpes simplex infection. Specimens of vesicular skin lesions should be obtained to detect herpes viruses, and a Tzanck preparation should be performed. The initiation of empirical antibacterial therapy should not, however, be postponed because of the possibility of a viral etiology of the fever.

Deep-seated tissue infections can be diagnostically and therapeutically challenging. Infections of the liver and spleen (e.g., hepatosplenic candidiasis) are sometimes difficult to visualize with radiographic methods when a patient is neutropenic. When such infections are highly suspected, a computed tomography (CT)–directed or an open or laparoscopic biopsy can be considered. Pulmonary lesions can have an infectious (bacterial or fungal) origin or an embolic etiology, or they can represent a complication of the underlying disease (metastases). Unfortunately, endoscopy can be associated with a high risk of bacteremia in the neutropenic patient who may also have friable mucosa. The presence of mucositis and thrombocytopenia often makes surgical interventions and biopsies less feasible. A definitive diagnosis of deep tissue infections may need to be postponed until the neutropenia has resolved.

Imaging

A chest x-ray study is usually obtained at presentation and thereafter as clinically indicated or at least weekly in the patient with persistent neutropenia. Radiologic findings may be subtle in the neutropenic patient but become more prominent once the neutrophil count recovers. This phenomenon occurs even when the patient is clinically improving. Chest x-ray studies are usually normal in patients without respiratory symptoms but can be useful in the diagnosis of pulmonary aspergillosis. However, chest CT can be helpful in patients with normal chest x-ray studies, especially in the setting of prolonged fever of unknown origin. Ultrasonography, CT, and magnetic resonance imaging (MRI) are used to identify the presence of hepatosplenic candidiasis, but the results can remain inconclusive until the granulocyte count recovers.

Bone scans with ^{99}Tc may be helpful in a symptomatic patient, but their interpretation can be difficult in patients with bony metastases. Because of the diminished inflammatory response, a gallium scan is usually not helpful in the neutropenic patient.

DIFFERENTIAL DIAGNOSIS

Two important factors must be considered in the differential diagnosis of fever and neutropenia: age and underlying immune status of the patient (see Fig. 60–1, Table 60–1, and Table 60–4).

Neutropenia in the Child Without Immunodeficiency

NEONATES

Neonatal neutropenia occurs most frequently during the first week of life; 43% of such episodes are reported on day one. Fewer than 40% of these neonates have an identifiable infectious cause (Table 60–4). An elevated temperature is not always present in the infected neonate, and empirical antibiotic therapy is often initiated for 2 to 3 days and stopped if cultures remain negative. If the neutropenia is prolonged, there is an increased risk of infections with nosocomial, endogenous, or fungal organisms, as seen in children with neonatal isoimmune neutropenia. The latter is due to the presence of maternal IgG antineutrophil antibodies after the mother becomes sensitized to the paternal antigens on the fetal neutrophil. This autoimmune neutropenia is analogous to hemolytic disease of the newborn. The organisms recovered in neonates vary according to several factors: onset of fever and neutropenia (first day of life versus later), degree of general supportive care necessary (regular well baby nursery versus intensive care unit), and duration of neutropenia.

Primary acquired autoimmune neutropenia in infancy is associated with a higher incidence of infections, particularly otitis media, upper respiratory tract infections, and benign skin infections, but routine antibiotic therapy is usually sufficient for treatment.

Table 60–4. Fever and Neutropenia in the Child Without Underlying Immunodeficiency

Neonate

Infectious Etiology (in 40%)

In 35%, bacterial infections, onset of neutropenia on first day of life, duration 2–4 days

Symptoms: Sepsis, shock, respiratory distress, meningitis

Organisms: Group B streptococci, *Escherichia coli, Klebsiella, Listeria monocytogenes,* enterococci, *Haemophilus influenzae, Streptococcus pneumoniae*

In 20%, postnatal viral infections, onset of neutropenia at day 3 of life, prolonged duration, more common in neonates who have undergone multiple transfusions

Symptoms: Hepatitis, thrombocytopenia, respiratory distress

Organisms: Most commonly cytomegalovirus

In 35%, associated with necrotizing enterocolitis in premature neonates, onset of neutropenia day 20 of life, duration 1–2 weeks

Organisms: Often none recovered; possible association with *Clostridium perfringens, E. coli, Staphylococcus epidermidis,* rotavirus

Idiopathic (in 40%)

Isoimmune Etiology (neutrophil count normalized by 7 weeks of age)

Symptoms: Mostly cutaneous infections

Organisms: *Staphylococcus aureus, E. coli,* α-hemolytic streptococci

Other Causes (associated with maternal preeclampsia, post-operatively, post-exchange transfusion)

Infant and Child

Transient Neutropenia, Autoimmune Neutropenia

Symptoms: Severe infectious complications are rare; otitis media, skin infections, upper respiratory tract infections are most common

Organisms: *H. influenzae, S. pneumoniae, Staphylococcus aureus,* group A streptococci

---

OLDER CHILDREN

The risk for infectious complications in well-appearing children with transient neutropenia and without an underlying immune defect is low but increases with the duration of neutropenia. In a study of 119 otherwise immunocompetent patients with a median duration of neutropenia of 13 days (range, 1 to 491 days), only four patients (whose neutropenia lasted more than 30 days) developed an infectious complication (stomatitis in two, cellulitis in one, pneumonia in one). In another study, of 68 immunocompetent children with transient neutropenia, five of the 17 children who appeared ''ill'' at presentation had a serious bacterial infection (bacteremia or meningitis), but none of the 51 ''well''-appearing children had an infectious focus.

Neutropenia in the Child with an Immunodeficiency

Fever in the immunocompromised neutropenic patient is often of undetermined origin; evaluation and therapy must follow an empirical approach. The spectrum of likely infections varies according to underlying disease, especially in the patient with prolonged neutropenia. In the patient with an unknown source for fever (Table 60–5), diagnostic studies may be quite helpful.

S. aureus and the coagulase-negative staphylococci have become the most commonly recovered isolates (Table 60–6). The most common gram-negative organisms in neutropenic cancer patients are *Escherichia coli* and *Klebsiella pneumoniae*; the incidence of infections caused by *Enterobacter* sp. appears to be rising in some centers. This is particularly worrisome because these organisms can induce bacterial β-lactamase production and rapidly develop resistance to cephalosporins and penicillins. It is unclear why the frequency of infections with *P. aeruginosa* has decreased in cancer patients. Children with HIV infection, especially if they have an indwelling central venous catheter, have a relatively high incidence of infections with this organism. Anaerobes are usually found only in patients with polymicrobial infections, especially if extensive mucosal damage is present (necrotizing gingivitis, perianal cellulitis).

Cancer patients with prolonged neutropenia and especially children with aplastic anemia are at risk for fungal infections (Table 60–6). An aggressive search for possible foci should be initiated in the patient with prolonged (more than 5 to 7 days) neutropenia and persistent or recurrent fevers. The patient is also at risk for fungal infections if prolonged and repeated periods of neutropenia occurred in the past.

Candida sp. can cause a local infection (thrush, esophagitis), fungemia, or deep tissue infection (hepatosplenic candidiasis). Risk factors for the development of candidemia are previous bacteremia, prolonged neutropenia, fever, and/or administration of antimicrobial agents. *Candida* sp. recovered from blood should never be considered a contaminant, because it can be the only manifestation of an invasive tissue infection. Hepatosplenic candidiasis can be very difficult to document until the neutrophil count recovers. This infection should be suspected in the patient with low-grade, recurrent fevers and a rise in serum alkaline phosphatase levels. Infection with *Aspergillus* sp. is a major concern in patients with aplastic anemia or relapsed leukemia or in patients recovering from bone marrow transplants. Invasive pulmonary aspergillosis is associated with a mortality as high as 95%. A common extrapulmonary site of aspergillosis is the paranasal sinuses, and an infection here can progress to the central nervous system (CNS) and be fatal.

Table 60–5. Fever of Unknown Origin in the Immunocompromised Neutropenic Patient

	Organism	Evaluation
Cancer or Aplastic Anemia		
Early during neutropenia	Bacteria	Cultures, CXR
Prolonged neutropenia (≥7 days)	Bacteria, fungi *(Candida, Aspergillus);* less commonly viruses and/or parasites	Cultures; CXR; sinus films; CT of chest; CT, MRI, or ultrasound study of abdomen
Bone Marrow Transplant		
	Bacteria (gram-positive and gram-negative) during the period of neutropenia	Cultures (including surveillance cultures); CXR; sinus films; CT of chest; CT, MRI, or ultrasound study of abdomen
	Streptococcus pneumoniae infection in the chronic period (>100 days after allogeneic transplant)	
	Herpes simplex early after transplant; cytomegalovirus approximately 50 days after transplant and varicella-zoster virus approximately 100 days after transplant	
	Fungi *(Candida, Aspergillus)* during the immediate post-transplantation period	
HIV Infection		
	Bacterial (gram positive, gram negative)	Cultures of blood and bone marrow, CXR, sinus films, CT of chest and abdomen
	Viral (CMV, HIV)	
	Mycobacterial, including *Mycobacterium avium-intracellulare* and *Mycobacterium tuberculosis*	
	Fungal *(Cryptococcus, Candida, Aspergillus)*	

Abbreviations: CXR = chest x-ray; HIV = human immunodeficiency virus; CMV = cytomegalovirus; CT = computed tomography; MRI = magnetic resonance imaging.

Specific Symptoms

In the neutropenic patient with or without fever, even subtle complaints or seemingly trivial findings on physical examination may indicate the presence of an infectious focus. Important findings not to be missed and *red flags* are listed in Table 60–7.

HEADACHES

Infections of the CNS are relatively uncommon in children with cancer, and a routine lumbar puncture to evaluate such patients with fever and neutropenia is therefore not warranted except in the neonate or young infant. However, if symptoms are suggestive of a CNS process, the evaluation of the cerebrospinal fluid should include a Gram stain, routine bacterial and fungal cultures, and cryptococcal antigen determination in addition to cell count with cytology and protein and glucose level determinations. Patients with intraventricular devices (shunts or Ommaya reservoirs) are at an increased risk for infections with bacteria that commonly colonize the skin (coagulase-positive and coagulase-negative staphylococci, *Corynebacterium* sp. and enterococci). In one study, *Propionibacterium acnes* was the most common pathogen, sometimes producing no clinical symptoms. *Listeria monocytogenes* can cause meningitis in patients with impaired T-lymphocyte function; patients often present with low-grade fevers and personality changes. In the severely immunosuppressed patient, regardless of neutrophil count, the presence of infections with fungal *(Cryptococcus)*, viral (herpes simplex, varicella-zoster, cytomegalovirus, Epstein-Barr), or parasitic *(Toxoplasma gondii)* pathogens should be considered. A brain abscess can occur rarely in such patients.

EARS AND NOSE

The most likely pathogens to cause ear infections in children with fever and neutropenia are the same as in the immunocompe-

tent host *(Streptococcus pneumoniae, Haemophilus influenzae, Moraxella* sp.). In addition, the gram-positive and gram-negative organisms that colonize the oropharynx and nasopharynx must also be considered.

Sinusitis in the granulocytopenic patient is often accompanied by only mild localized tenderness or minimal (often non-purulent) nasal discharge. Bacterial infections are usually caused by the same organisms as in the immunocompetent host. Fungal infections are an additional concern in the patient with prolonged neutropenia *(Aspergillus* sp., *Mucor, Fusarium* sp.). In addition to the radiologic documentation (sinus x-ray studies, CT, and/or MRI), the diagnosis must often be established through a sinus aspirate or biopsy. Because such infections may progress by intracranial extension, an aggressive diagnostic approach is mandatory. Surgical debridement and early institution of antifungal therapy are essential for patient survival.

MOUTH OR THROAT PAIN, PAIN WITH SWALLOWING

Although mucositis in cancer patients can be caused by chemotherapy, it is necessary to exclude herpes simplex and *Candida albicans* infections. Gingivitis or periodontitis is usually caused by a mixed infection with aerobic and anaerobic pathogens. Esophagitis can present as retrosternal pain, dysphagia, odynophagia, emesis, or refusal to eat and drink.

COUGH, CHEST PAIN, ABNORMAL CHEST RADIOGRAPH

Infections of the respiratory tract are common in the immunocompromised patient. Symptoms and findings on physical examination can be minimal. Symptoms often worsen transiently, even with appropriate antibiotic treatment, when the neutrophil count is

Table 60–6. Predominant Organisms in the Cancer Patient with Fever and Neutropenia

Organism	Comment
Gram-Positive Bacteria	
Staphylococcus aureus	Emergence of methicillin-resistant organisms
Coagulase-negative staphylococci	Predominant pathogen in many centers, often associated with an infected intravascular catheter
α-Hemolytic streptococci	Oral mucositis; bacteremia can be associated with adult respiratory distress syndrome
Enterococci	Increased incidence, perhaps from the use of third-generation cephalosporins, which do not cover enterococci
	Emergence of vancomycin-resistant enterococci
Corynebacterium JK	Arises often from cutaneous defects (intravascular catheter, cellulitis)
	More common after prolonged neutropenia and hospitalization
Clostridium difficile	Common infection after antibiotic therapy, may be nosocomial
Gram-Negative Bacteria	
Enterobacteriaceae (*Escherichia coli, Klebsiella pneumoniae*)	Predominant gram-negative organisms
Pseudomonas aeruginosa	Decreased incidence in cancer patients, but possibly increasing in HIV-infected patients
Enterobacter sp., *Citrobacter, Serratia*	Less common, but potentially serious because of the risk of developing resistance to β-lactam antibiotics
Anaerobes	Often as part of polymicrobial infection, especially in the oral cavity, gastrointestinal tract, and perianal area
Fungi	
Candida sp.	Most common; thrush, esophagitis, candidemia, hepatosplenic candidiasis, endophthalmitis
Aspergillus sp.	Incidence varies with center; sinusitis and pulmonary infections in patients with prolonged profound neutropenia
Cryptococcus	Solitary pulmonary lesions can be misdiagnosed as metastasis; patients with prolonged immunosuppression (human immundeficiency virus infection, aplastic anemia) are at risk for meningitis
Mucor	Can cause invasive, necrotic sinusitis; orbital infections; erosive palate lesions; with central nervous system involvement in the patient with prolonged neutropenia (aplastic anemia)
Histoplasma capsulatum, Blastomyces dermatidis, Coccidioides immitis	Pulmonary or disseminated disease in immunocompromised hosts (in endemic areas)
Trichosporon beigelii, Fusarium sp.	Less common; can cause disseminated disease
Viruses	
Herpes simplex virus	Oral gingivostomatitis, esophagitis
Varicella-zoster virus	Not specifically associated with neutropenia, rather with underlying immune status
Cytomegalovirus	In bone marrow transplantation patients and patients with aplastic anemia; can be associated with serious infection (especially pneumonitis, hepatitis, colitis)
Parasites	
Pneumocystis carinii, Strongyloides stercoralis, Cryptosporidium sp.	Not specifically associated with neutropenia, rather with underlying immune status.

recovering. Although bacterial and viral infections are the most common pathogens, fungal organisms or parasites are occasionally recovered. Most symptoms can be caused by any of these microorganisms, but some should prompt immediate attention:

1. *Chest pain.* Although a noninfectious process (pulmonary embolus) can be responsible, an infection with *Aspergillus* sp. should be suspected and an aggressive diagnostic approach is warranted.

2. *Nonproductive cough, chest pain, effusion on chest radiograph.* These symptoms may be caused by *Legionella* or *Mycoplasma* infection (direct fluorescent antibody test or culture on special media is necessary for the diagnosis). In addition, infection with *S. pneumoniae* or gram-negative bacteria (e.g., *P. aeruginosa*) must also be considered.

3. *Hypoxemia and diffuse interstitial infiltrate on chest radiograph.* *P. carinii* should be seriously considered in the hypoxic patient with minimal or diffuse findings on chest radiographs. However, the patient with HIV infection rarely presents with the "typical" radiographic picture.

Bacterial pathogens predominate in patients with pneumonia whose neutropenia lasts less than 14 days, whereas fungal and other opportunistic infections are more commonly seen with prolonged neutropenia and lymphopenia. A chest radiograph may not initially show an infiltrate, even if the patient has clinical evidence of pneumonia. However, if an infiltrate is present, the distinction between patchy or diffuse infiltrates may help guide the differential diagnosis (Table 60–8). Bronchoalveolar lavage or even an open lung biopsy should be considered if the patient fails to respond to empirical antimicrobial therapy.

ABDOMINAL PAIN, DIARRHEA, PERIRECTAL TENDERNESS

Acute or subacute right lower quadrant pain and fever in the neutropenic patient who is being treated for malignancy (especially acute leukemia) may indicate the presence of *typhlitis,* a necrotizing

Table 60–7. Symptoms Not to Be Missed and "Red Flags"

Symptom	Consider
With Short Neutropenia (<7 Days)	
Sinus tenderness	Bacterial sinusitis
Oral and esophageal mucositis	Infection with herpes simplex or *Candida*
Pulmonary infiltrate	Bacterial or viral pneumonia
Abdominal pain	Typhlitis
Tenderness around exit site of catheter	Exit site or tunnel infection
Crepitus	Gas gangrene
Diarrhea	*Clostridium difficile* colitis
Perirectal tenderness	Anaerobic mixed cellulitis
With Prolonged Neutropenia (>7 Days)	
Sinus tenderness, stuffy nose	Fungal sinusitis
Oral and esophageal mucositis	Infection with herpes simplex or *Candida*
Chest pain with patchy infiltrate	Pulmonary aspergillosis
Abdominal pain with rising alkaline phosphatase level and leukocytosis at time of neutrophil recovery	Hepatosplenic candidiasis
Small, erythematous skin lesions	Disseminated candidiasis
Crepitus	Gas gangrene
Diarrhea	*C. difficile* colitis
Perirectal tenderness	Mixed cellulitis

cellulitis involving the cecum. The etiologic organisms include anaerobes and gram-negative bacilli, most notably clostridia and *P. aeruginosa.* These organisms may also cause pneumatosis intestinalis, noted on abdominal x-ray studies as cystic, gas-filled submucosal or subserosal bleb-like lesions. In patients whose symptoms are progressing despite optimal antibiotic therapy, surgical intervention may be necessary (even if the patients are profoundly neutropenic).

Diarrhea with or without colicky abdominal pain is often caused by infection with *C. difficile,* a pathogen that produces toxins in association with prior or concurrent antibiotic therapy. *C. difficile* can be diagnosed with culture and toxin assay.

Mild abdominal pain, low-grade persistent fever, and a rising alkaline phosphatase level in a patient who has had prolonged periods of neutropenia (>7 days) should alert the physician that hepatosplenic candidiasis may be the cause. Radiographic studies may be unrevealing while the patient remains neutropenic.

Even minor lacerations, erosions, or ulcerations in the perianal area can result in a cellulitis, most commonly with gram-negative organisms, *S. aureus,* and anaerobes. During episodes of neutropenia, symptoms and findings may be minimal (tenderness, mild erythema, rarely fluctuance). These symptoms can become more prominent when the neutrophil count rises. The progression of the symptoms and signs does not necessarily indicate that the current treatment is inadequate. In addition to receiving systemic antibiotics, the patient should be treated with sitz baths, stool softeners, and a high degree of personal hygiene.

URINARY TRACT COMPLAINTS

Urinary tract infections are relatively uncommon in children with fever and neutropenia, although the risk is increased in children

Table 60–8. Common Pathogens Causing Pulmonary Infiltrates in the Febrile Neutropenic Patient*

Localized Infiltrate	Diffuse Infiltrate
Bacteria	**Bacteria**
Common: *Streptococcus pneumoniae, Haemophilus influenzae*	Common: *S. pneumoniae, H. influenzae*
Rare: *Klebsiella, Pseudomonas* sp., *Staphylococcus aureus, Mycobacterium, Nocardia*	Rare: *Legionella, Chlamydia, Nocardia* sp., *Mycobacterium*
Fungi	**Mycoplasma**
Common: *Aspergillus, Cryptococcus, Histoplasma*	
Rare: Zygomycetes, *Candida* sp.	**Fungi**
	Common: *Aspergillus* sp., *Pneumocystis carinii, Cryptococcus* sp., *Histoplasma* sp.
	Rare: Zygomycetes, *Candida* sp.
	Parasites
	Toxoplasma gondii, Strongyloides
Viruses	**Viruses**
Herpes simplex, varicella-zoster virus	Herpes simplex, varicella-zoster virus, cytomegalovirus, measles, influenza, parainfluenza, respiratory syncytial virus, adenovirus

*Pathogens presented in order of frequency.

with an obstructive urologic process, a neurogenic bladder dysfunction, or an indwelling bladder catheter. The diagnosis is complicated by the fact that the neutropenic patient does not usually have pyuria, even in the presence of an active infection. In addition to bacterial infections, the urinary tract can also become infected with *C. albicans,* either as a superficial mucositis in the bladder or as part of a disseminated infection. The presence of pseudohyphae in the urine is not diagnostic.

MISCELLANEOUS SYMPTOMS AND COMPLAINTS

Musculoskeletal infections are unusual in patients with cancer and can be difficult to diagnose because of the lack of an inflammatory response and the possibility of a complication associated with the underlying disease. Pain from leukemic infiltrate or metastases must be distinguished from signs of infection. Immediate surgical intervention and antibiotic therapy are necessary if crepitus and soft tissue tenderness are present because these symptoms suggest an infection with *Clostridium* or toxin-producing *Bacillus cereus.*

Localized cutaneous infections can occur, primarily because the integrity of the epidermis is often iatrogenically disrupted by needle punctures, surgery, and radiation. Although uncommon, tropical myositis has been observed in immunocompromised children with cancer or HIV infection. Special attention should be paid to the exit site of central venous catheters because even extensive central catheter tunnel infections sometimes present with only minimal erythema and swelling. Such infections are usually characterized by tenderness along the subcutaneous tract of the catheter. Pathogens most commonly include staphylococci, streptococci, and *Candida* sp. In addition, the skin can become infected as part of a systemic infection with bacteria (*P. aeruginosa*), fungi (*Candida*), or viruses (herpes simplex, varicella-zoster virus).

TREATMENT STRATEGIES

An important aspect of the treatment of the febrile neutropenic patient is prompt initiation of empirical broad-spectrum antibiotics immediately after a careful evaluation of the patient. Decisions about which antibiotics to use initially or to add to the regimen depend on the duration of the neutropenia and changes in the patient's clinical and laboratory manifestations (Fig. 60–2, Table 60–9). An empirical regimen should include coverage for both gram-positive and gram-negative bacteria, including *P. aeruginosa.* The specific regimen used depends on the dominant isolates and the sensitivity pattern at the patient's treatment center. Common regimens include the use of either a third-generation cephalosporin (ceftazidime or cefoperazone) or a carbapenem (imipenem-cilastin) alone or in combination with an aminoglycoside or another β-lactam antibiotic. Whether vancomycin should be added to the initial empirical therapy for gram-positive coverage or reserved until a specific isolate has been identified has been widely debated. In a randomized study of 550 episodes of fever and neutropenia, no treatment failures were observed when vancomycin was added only after a gram-positive infection had been documented. In centers where there is a high frequency of methicillin-resistant *S. aureus,* enterococci, or severe viridans streptococci (e.g., *S. mitis*), it is appropriate to include vancomycin in the initial antibiotic regimen. The most commonly used antimicrobial agents are listed in Table 60–10.

Modifications or additions to the initial empirical treatment are often required in patients with continued fever and neutropenia (Table 60–9). Reasons to modify the initial regimen include the lack of a clinical response (e.g., persistent or new fever after a week of empirical therapy or evidence that the patient's condition is deteriorating), the isolation of a pathogen that is not optimally covered by the current regimen, the development of specific findings on physical examination, or the emergence of a fungal, viral, or parasitic infection. Those antimicrobial drugs most often added include:

• Vancomycin for *Staphylococcus epidermidis,* methicillin-resis-

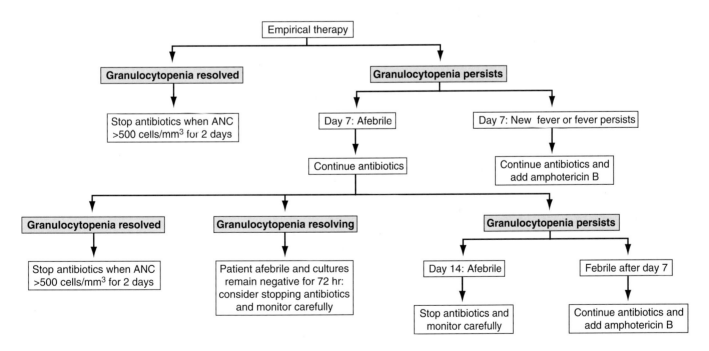

Figure 60–2. Treatment schema for fever of unknown origin and neutropenia in immunosuppressed patients (cancer, bone marrow transplantation). If a microbial agent is isolated, the duration and type of antibiotic coverage need to be adjusted appropriately. ANC = absolute neutrophil count.

Table 60–9. When to Add Antibiotics or Change Initial Empirical Treatment

Indication	Modification
Fever:	
Persistent for >7 days, or new in patient with persistent neutropenia	Add empirical antifungal therapy (amphotericin B) (see also Fig. 60–2)
Positive blood cultures	
Gram-positive organism	Add vancomycin, pending sensitivities
Gram-negative organism	Isolated before antibiotic therapy, isolate sensitive to empiric antibiotics and patient stable: maintain regimen
	If *Pseudomonas aeruginosa, Enterobacter,* or *Citrobacter:* add aminoglycoside or an additional β-lactam antibiotic
	Isolated during antibiotic therapy: change to new combination therapy (imipenem plus gentamicin and vancomycin, or vancomycin, piperacillin, and gentamicin)
From central venous catheter	Attempt to treat, rotate administration of antibiotics in each lumen in patients with multiple-lumen catheters. Exception: in patients with positive cultures for bacillus species or *Candida,* the catheter should be removed and the patient treated appropriately
Necrotizing gingivitis	Add antianaerobic antibiotic (clindamycin or metronidazole)
Mucositis with vesicular or ulcerative lesions	Culture for herpes simplex and treat with acyclovir
Sinus tenderness, nasal ulcerative lesions	Suspect fungal infection, try to establish diagnosis, treat with amphotericin B
Painful swallowing	Suspect herpes simplex or *Candida* infection. Add antifungal therapy, and if patient not improving, consider adding acyclovir
Abdominal pain, perianal tenderness	Optimize anaerobic coverage
Diarrhea	If positive for *Clostridium difficile* toxin, treat with metronidazole
Pulmonary infiltrates	See Table 60–8
Exit site infection	Add vancomycin if gram-positive organism isolated
	Remove catheter and treat appropriately if rapidly growing mycobacteria *(Mycobacterium chelonei, Mycobacterium fortuitum)* or *Aspergillus* is isolated
Tunnel infection	Remove catheter and treat appropriately

tant *S. aureus, Corynebacterium* sp., or α-hemolytic streptococci
- Aminoglycosides for *P. aeruginosa, Enterobacter, Serratia,* or *Citrobacter* sp. because these organisms are more likely to break through single agent coverage as a result of inducible β-lactamases or mutations
- Clindamycin or metronidazole, when the initial regimen does not have adequate anti-anaerobic coverage and a site of presumably mixed infection is defined (e.g., necrotizing gingivitis, perianal abscess)
- Amphotericin B for suspected or proven fungal infection in patients remaining febrile and neutropenic for 7 or more days
- Acyclovir for suspected or proven herpes infection

Many patients with cancer or HIV infection have indwelling central venous catheters, which can be associated with local infections (exit site infection, tunnel infection), bacteremia, or fungemia. The incidence of infectious complications appears to be similar in patients with externalized catheters (Hickman, Broviac) or subcutaneously implanted devices (port-A-Cath, MediPort), and such infections can occur whether or not the patient is neutropenic. An exit site infection can usually be managed without removal of the catheter, except for infections with *Mycobacterium* or *Aspergillus* sp. However, tunnel infections usually persist unless the foreign body is removed. Most bacteremias can be treated without removal of the catheter, if three important rules are followed:

- The catheter has to be removed if *Candida* sp. or *Bacillus* sp. is isolated, if there is evidence of a tunnel infection, or if cultures remain persistently positive, despite adequate therapy.
- Antibiotics must be given through *all* lumens of the catheter in a rotating fashion, and specimens should be drawn for culture from all lumens as well.
- If the placement of a new catheter is necessary, this should be performed only after at least 24 to 48 hours of antibiotic

therapy have been completed and preferably when the patient is no longer neutropenic.

The duration of empirical therapy without positive cultures or findings on physical examination depends on the recovery of the neutrophil count (see Fig. 60–2). For most proven infections, an adequate duration of treatment is a total of 10 to 14 days after the first negative culture. Therapy should be monitored with blood levels where indicated (vancomycin, aminoglycosides); kidney and liver function should be evaluated regularly so that antibiotic dosages can be adjusted.

PREVENTIVE STRATEGIES

Three approaches have been explored to prevent infections in patients with neutropenia:

1. *Preventing exogenous infections.* The most important preventive strategy remains careful hand washing by all those caring for neutropenic patients. Various isolation methods have been studied, but the results are controversial. The use of high-efficiency particulate air-filtered or laminar air-flow rooms is expensive, and their use is probably limited to the patient who is anticipated to have a very prolonged neutropenia (e.g., a patient who has undergone bone marrow transplantation or other profound immunosuppression).

2. *Preventing endogenous infections.* Most infections in the febrile neutropenic host are derived from endogenous flora. Several studies have evaluated the use of regimens attempting "gut decontamination" with oral nonabsorbable antibiotics, but most trials have failed to demonstrate a clear benefit. However, specific indications for prophylaxis exist, including the use of trimethoprim-sulfamethoxazole for the prevention of *P. carinii* pneumonia in

Table 60–10. Commonly Used Antimicrobial Agents and Their Dosages in the Febrile Neutropenic Patient

Antibiotic	Daily Dose (mg/kg)	Schedule	Maximal Daily Dose	Major Indications	Comments
Third-Generation Cephalosporins					
Ceftazidime	90	q 8 hr	6–8 g	Gram-positive (not enterococci, methicillin-resistant staphylococci, *Corynebacterium jekeium, Listeria monocytogenes*) Gram-negative: *Escherichia coli, Proteus, Klebsiella, Haemophilus influenzae,* Enterobacteriaceae, *Pseudomonas aeruginosa* Anaerobes (not *Bacteroides fragilis*)	Broad spectrum, can be used as initial monotherapy Reaches high bactericidal levels with adequate CSF levels Emergence of resistance (variable from center to center)
Cefoperazone	25–100	q 6–8 hr	4–6 g	Gram-positive (not methicillin-resistant staphylococci, *C. jekeium, L. monocytogenes*) Gram-negative: similar to ceftazidime (not *Acinetobacter* sp.) Anaerobes (not *B. fragilis*)	Broad spectrum, has anti-*Pseudomonas* activity Reaches high bactericidal levels Poor penetration into CSF
Carbapenems					
Imipenem-cilastin	40–60	q 6 hr	3–4 g	*Staphylococcus aureus,* group D streptococci, some coagulase-negative staphylococci (not methicillin-resistant staphylococci) Enterobacteriaceae, *P. aeruginosa* (but not other pseudomonads) Anaerobes	Very broad spectrum, including *P. aeruginosa,* can be used as initial monotherapy If *P. aeruginosa* is isolated, aminoglycoside must be added, because of rapid emergence of resistance *Clostridium difficile* colitis common Should not be used in patients with brain tumors or seizure disorder (reduces seizure threshold, dose-dependent)
Extended-Spectrum Penicillins					
Piperacillin	300	q 4–6 hr	18–24 g	Streptococci, enterococci, not staphylococci Gram-negative: *Pseudomonas, Proteus, H. influenzae, E. coli, Klebsiella* (not *Acinetobacter, Serratia*) Anaerobes, including *B. fragilis*	Should be combined with aminoglycoside or third-generation cephalosporin (high risk for development of resistance)
Azlocillin	300	q 4–6 hr	18–24 g	Same as piperacillin	Same as piperacillin
Mezlocillin	300	q 4–6 hr	18–24 g	Same as piperacillin	Same as piperacillin
Monobactams					
Aztreonam	100–150	q 6 hr	6–8 g	Gram-positive: none Gram-negative: broad, not *Acinetobacter* Anaerobes: none	Alternative for patients with allergy to β-lactam antibiotics Should be combined with vancomycin (± aminoglycoside) for empiric coverage
Quinolones					
Ciprofloxacin	20–30	q 12 hr	1–2 g	Gram-positive: not streptococci, enterococci, methicillin-resistant staphylococci Gram-negative: broad, including *P. aeruginosa* Anaerobes: none	Not approved for children Possibly of use for low-risk patients Do not use for prophylaxis (to avoid resistance)

Table continued on following page

Table 60–10. Commonly Used Antimicrobial Agents and Their Dosages in the Febrile Neutropenic Patient *Continued*

Antibiotic	Daily Dose (mg/kg)	Schedule	Maximal Daily Dose	Major Indications	Comments
Vancomycin	40	q 6 hr	2 g	Gram-positive: emergence of resistant enterococci Gram-negative: none Anaerobes: none	Monitor levels with IV therapy 125 mg q.i.d. p.o. for treatment of *C. difficile* colitis Pathogen-directed therapy As part of empiric therapy only in centers with a high incidence of methicillin-resistant staphylococci
Aminoglycosides					
Gentamicin	5–7.5	8 hr	Levels	Enterobacteriaceae, *P. aeruginosa,* enterococci (with ampicillin)	Monitor levels
Tobramycin	3–6	8 hr	Levels	Similar to gentamicin, but more effective against *P. aeruginosa*	Monitor levels
Amikacin	15–20	q 8 hr	Levels	Similar to gentamicin, plus *Serratia, Proteus, Providencia*	Monitor levels
Macrolides					
Clindamycin	40	q 8 hr	2–4 g	Gram-positive (not enterococci, methicillin-resistant staphylococci) Anaerobes	Can cause *C. difficile* colitis
Metronidazole	30	q 6 hr	4 g	Anaerobes	Can be added to initial therapy if anaerobic infection is suspected
Antifungals					
Amphotericin B	0.5–1.5	q 24 hr		*Candida, Aspergillus, Torulopsis,* zygomycetes, *Cryptococcus, Histoplasma*	Best treatment 0.6 mg/kg/day for *Candida albicans,* and *Cryptococcus;* 1 mg/kg/day for *Candida tropicalis;* 1.5 mg/kg/day for *Aspergillus*
Fluconazole	100–150 (mg/m²)	q 24 hr		*Candida, Cryptococcus*	Very effective for thrush or esophagitis, under investigation for systemic mycoses
5-Flucytosine	40–80	q 6 hr	Levels	*Cryptococcus, Candida, Torulopsis,* chromomycosis	Monitor levels Commonly used in combination with amphotericin B
Antivirals					
Acyclovir	750 or 1500 (mg/m²)	q 8 hr		Herpes simplex Varicella-zoster virus	Low dose for herpes simplex High dose for varicella-zoster infection, give intravenously Monitor kidney function, good hydration
Ganciclovir	5–10	q 12 hr		Cytomegalovirus	Monitor kidney function
Foscarnet	60–90	q 12–24 hr		Cytomegalovirus, varicella-zoster virus, resistant herpes simplex virus	Second-line drug
Antiparasitic					
Trimethoprim-sulfamethoxazole (as TMP)	20	q 6 hr		*S. aureus, S. pneumoniae, Pneumocystis carinii, Nocardia* Gram-negative (not *P. aeruginosa*)	Best drug for *P. carinii* prophylaxis (75 mg/m² b.i.d. for 3 days/week)
Intravenous pentamidine	4	q 24 hr		*P. carinii*	Alternative treatment for *P. carinii* Aerosolized form (300 mg q 2–4 weeks) is an alternative but is less effective prophylaxis

Abbreviations: CSF = cerebrospinal fluid; p.o. = orally; b.i.d. = twice daily; q = every; IV = intravenous; q.i.d. = four times daily.

patients with leukemia or acquired immunodeficiency syndrome (AIDS), and the use of acyclovir and gancyclovir for the prevention of herpes infections (herpes simplex virus and cytomegalovirus, respectively) in the patient undergoing a bone marrow transplant.

3. *Improving the host defense.* Immunizations against bacterial and viral pathogens play an important role in the prevention of infections in the immunocompetent host, but active immunization is usually unsuccessful or unreliable in the immunocompromised patient. Passive immunization with intravenous immunoglobulins has no proven benefit in preventing fever or infection in patients with neutropenia but may be of benefit in preventing infections in children with HIV. Hematopoietic growth factors (cytokines) shorten the duration of neutropenia. In addition, cytokines and certain cytotoxic agents (cyclophosphamide) are currently also being investigated for their ability to increase the number of circulating progenitor cells that can be harvested and infused during times of neutropenia.

SUMMARY AND RED FLAGS

The early initiation of empirical broad-spectrum antibiotic therapy combined with the careful monitoring of physical findings and an aggressive diagnostic approach have significantly decreased morbidity and mortality from fever and neutropenia. Modifications of the current approach may be necessary as the spectrum of pathogens changes or strategies that improve host defense mechanisms become more effective. Nonetheless, simple measures, such as hand washing and educating the patient and caregivers about the importance to contact the physician in the event of fever and neutropenia, continue to be some of the most important interventions in the care of the patient at risk for fever and neutropenia.

All episodes of fever and neutropenia are medical emergencies and require immediate evaluation, treatment, and hospitalization of the patient. *Red flags* include hypotension, poor capillary perfusion, reduced level of consciousness, and development of petechiae; these suggest fulminant bacterial infection. Other red flags are noted in Table 60–7.

REFERENCES

Neonatal Neutropenia

Baley ME, Stork EK, Warketin PI, et al. Neonatal neutropenia: Clinical manifestations, cause, and outcome. Am J Dis Child 1988;142:1161.

Cadnapaphornchai M, Faix RG. Increased nosocomial infection in neutropenic low birth weight (2000 grams or less) infants of hypertensive mothers. J Pediatr 1992;121:956–961.

Mouzinho A, Rosenfeld CR, Sanchez PJ, et al. Effect of maternal hypertension on neonatal neutropenia and risk of nosocomial infection. Pediatrics 1992;90:430–435.

Neutropenia in Older Children

Alario AJ, O'Shea JS. Risk of infectious complications in well-appearing children with transient neutropenia. Am J Dis Child 1989;143:973.

Dunkel IJ, Bussel JB. New developments in the treatment of neutropenia. Am J Dis Child 1993;147:994–1000.

Glasser L, Duncan BR, Corrigan JJ. Measurement of serum granulocyte colony-stimulating factor in a patient with congenital agranulocytosis (Kostmann's Syndrome). Am J Dis Child 1991;145:925–928.

Hammond WP, Price TH, Souza LM, et al. Treatment of cyclic neutropenia with granulocyte colony-stimulating factor. N Engl J Med 1989;320:1306–1311.

Jonsson OG, Buchanan GR. Chronic neutropenia during childhood: A 13-year experience in a single institution. Am J Dis Child 1991;145:232–235.

Logue GL, Shastri KA, Laughlin M, et al. Idiopathic neutropenia: Antineutrophil antibodies and clinical correlations. Am J Med 1991;90:211–216.

Roilides E, Butler KM, Husson RN, et al. *Pseudomonas* infections in children with human immunodeficiency virus infection. Pediatr Infect Dis J 1992;11:547.

Roilides E, Marshall D, Venzon D, et al. Bacterial infections in human immunodeficiency virus type 1-infected children: The impact of central venous catheters and antiretroviral agents. Pediatr Infect Dis J 1991;10:813.

Shastri KA, Logue GL. Autoimmune neutropenia. Blood 1993;81:1984–1995.

Weinberger M, Elattar I, Marshall D, et al. Patterns of infections in patients with aplastic anemia and the emergence of *Aspergillus* as a major cause of death. Medicine 1992;71:24.

Yang KD, Hill HR. Neutrophil function disorders: Pathophysiology, prevention, and therapy. J Pediatr 1991;119:343–354.

Young NS. Agranulocytosis. JAMA 1994;271:935–938.

Fever and Neutropenia in Cancer Patients

Browne MJ, Dinndorf PA, Perek D, et al. Infectious complications of intraventricular reservoirs in cancer patients. Pediatr Infect Dis J 1987;6:182.

Chanock S. Evolving risk factors for infectious complications of cancer therapy. Hematol Oncol Clin North Am 1993;4:771.

Dichter JR, Levine SJ, Shelhamer JH. Approach to the immunocompromised host with pulmonary symptoms. Hematol Oncol Clin North Am 1993;4:887.

Fergie JE, Patrick CC, Lott L. *Pseudomonas aeruginosa* cellulitis and ecthyma gangrenosum in immunocompromised children. Pediatr Infect Dis J 1991;10:496–500.

Gorelick MH, Owen WC, Seibel NL, et al. Lack of association between neutropenia and the incidence of bacteremia associated with indwelling central venous catheters in febrile pediatric cancer patients. Pediatr Infect Dis J 1991;10:506–510.

Pizzo PA, Rubin M, Freifeld A, et al. The child with cancer and infection: II. Nonbacterial infections. J Pediatr 1991;119:845.

Shelhamer JH, Toews GB, Masur H, et al. Respiratory disease in the immunosuppressed patient. Ann Intern Med 1992;117:415–431.

Thaler M, Pastakia B, Shawker TH, et al. Hepatic candidiasis in cancer patients: The evolving picture of a syndrome. Ann Intern Med 1988;108:88.

Wingard JR, Santos GW, Saral R. Differences between first and subsequent fevers during prolonged neutropenia. Cancer 1987;59:844.

Treatment of Fever and Neutropenia in Cancer Patients

Bow EJ, Ronald AR. Antibacterial chemoprophylaxis in neutropenic patients: Where do we go from here? Clin Infect Dis 1993;17:333–337.

Browne MJ, Potter D, Gress J, et al. A randomized trial of open lung biopsy versus empiric antimicrobial therapy in cancer patients with diffuse pulmonary infiltrates. J Clin Oncol 1990;8:222.

Buchanan GR. Approach to the treatment of the febrile cancer patient with low-risk neutropenia. Hematol Oncol Clin North Am 1993;5:919.

EORTC International Antimicrobial Therapy Cooperative Group. Empiric antifungal therapy in febrile granulocytopenic patients. Am J Med 1989;86:668–672.

Freifeld AG. The antimicrobial armamentarium. Hematol Oncol Clin North Am 1993;4:813.

The GIMEMA Infection Program. Prevention of bacterial infection in neutropenic patients with hematologic malignancies: A randomized, multicenter trial comparing norfloxacin with ciprofloxacin. Ann Intern Med 1991;115:7–12.

Hughes WT, Armstrong D, Bodey GP, et al. Guidelines for the use of antimicrobial agents in neutropenic patients with unexplained fever. J Infect Dis 1990;161:381–396.

The International Antimicrobial Therapy Cooperative Group of the European Organization for Research and Treatment of Cancer. Efficacy and toxicity of single daily doses of amikacin and ceftriaxone versus multiple daily doses of amikacin and ceftazidime for infection in patients with cancer and granulocytopenia. Ann Intern Med 1993; 119:584–593.

Katz JA, Mustafa MM. Management of fever in granulocytopenic children with cancer. Pediatr Infect Dis J 1993;12:330–339.

Malik IA, Abbas Z, Karim M. Randomised comparison of oral ofloxacin alone with combination of parenteral antibiotics in neutropenic febrile patients. Lancet 1992;339:1092–1096.

Pizzo PA. Management of fever in patients with cancer and treatment-induced neutropenia. N Engl J Med 1993;328:1323.

Pizzo PA, Rubin M, Freifeld A, et al. The child with cancer and infection: I. Empiric therapy for fever and neutropenia, and preventive strategies. J Pediatr 1991;119:679–694.

Riikonen P. Imipenem compared with ceftazidime plus vancomycin as

initial therapy for fever in neutropenic children with cancer. Pediatr Infect Dis J 1991;10:918–923.

Riikonen P, Saarinen UM, Makipernaa A, et al. Recombinant human granulocyte-macrophage colony-stimulating factor in the treatment of febrile neutropenia: A double blind placebo-controlled study in children. Pediatr Infect Dis J 1994;13:197–202.

Rubin M, Hathorn JW, Marshall D, et al. Gram-positive infections and the use of vancomycin in 550 episodes of fever and neutropenia. Ann Intern Med 1988;108:30.

Viscoli C, Moroni C, Boni L, et al. Ceftazidime plus amikacin versus ceftazidime plus vancomycin as empiric therapy in febrile neutropenic children with cancer. Rev Infect Dis 1991;13:397–404.

Walsh TJ, Lee J, Lecciones J, et al. Empiric therapy with amphotericin B in febrile granulocytopenic patients. Rev Infect Dis 1991;13:496–503.

Winston DJ, Ho WG, Bruckner DA, et al. Beta-lactam antibiotic therapy in febrile granulocytopenic patients. Ann Intern Med 1991;115:849–859.

Endocrine/Metabolic Disorders

61 Disorders of Puberty

Ruth P. Owens

Puberty is a process as well as the phase of life through which one attains adult sexual development, function, and fertility. This process is controlled in part by maturation of the hypothalamic-pituitary-gonadal axis. Hypothalamic gonadotropin-releasing hormone (GnRH) is produced in such a way as to stimulate pituitary production of luteinizing hormone (LH) and follicle-stimulating hormone (FSH), which in turn stimulate the gonads to develop and produce sex steroids. Sex steroids cause development of internal and external reproductive organs and secondary sexual characteristics by binding to receptor proteins in the cells of target tissues.

NEUROENDOCRINE EVOLUTION

Perinatal Development

Maternal estrogens stimulate breast development in both male and female fetuses. Maternal estrogens also stimulate uterine developmental and endometrial growth; at birth, withdrawal of the high levels of maternal estrogen and placental progesterone causes the infant endometrium to regress or even slough and manifests as vaginal bleeding. At birth, levels of LH and FSH in both sexes rise markedly and remain elevated for months. In the female, FSH stimulates ovarian granulosa cells to produce 17β-estradiol sufficient to maintain prenatal breast development for up to 8 months of life. Estrogen-induced vaginal cornification is generally evident as abundant vaginal discharge at birth and is maintained as long as infant estrogens are produced, as demonstrated by the vaginal smear maturation index determined microscopically by increased

parabasal round, large nuclei, and pyknotic nuclei of superficial squamous cells.

Male breast development regresses rather quickly after birth. Cornification of urethral cells is apparent while the estrogens persist (maturation index of cells of first 5 ml of urine). Elevated LH levels after birth stimulate Leydig cell production of testosterone for 6 to 12 months, leading to further genital development. Penis length increases from a length of 3 to 5 cm in the full-term newborn to 4.5 to 6 cm by 2 to 3 years.

Infantile Development

The average gonadal volume for both sexes in infancy is 1 to 2.0 cm³. Ovarian size from birth to 3 months ranges from 0.7 up to 3.6 cm³, decreasing to up to 2.7 cm³ by 12 months and to 1.7 cm³ by 24 months; this size persists until the onset of puberty. Ultrasound studies of the ovaries in normal infants show many microcysts.

In males, penis length increases from 3–5 cm in full-term neonates to 4.5–6 cm by 2–3 years of age.

Prepubertal Development

Over the next 8 to 10 years, the hypothalamic and pituitary sensitivity to sex steroid feedback appears to decrease so that progressively higher levels of LH and FSH are produced, which leads to progressively higher levels of sex steroids. Yet sex steroid levels are still not enough to produce sexual development. Because sexual development is not seen, the system appears to be "quiescent." During this quiescent time, the pituitary gonadotrophs are relatively less responsive to stimuli and usually do not respond to administration of exogenous GnRH.

PUBERTY (GONADARCHE)

As the hypothalamus matures further, the pulses of GnRH generated are of greater amplitude and frequency and the pituitary is up-regulated to respond with increasing baseline levels and pulses of LH and FSH. At this point, gonadotropins are released during deep sleep and in response to exogenous GnRH. In the presence of adequate growth hormone (GH), gonadotropins stimulate the gonads to enlarge and produce sex steroids. Maturation of the hypothalamus has occurred within a balance of potentiating and inhibiting factors, with the maturational process apparently proceeding in correlation with maturation of the body in general. On average, the onset of increased GnRH pulses and increased LH and FSH appears to correlate with maturation of the skeleton to a bone age of about 11 years. This maturation coincides less tightly with maturation of dentition, but eruption of the 12-year molars in boys frequently correlates with enlargement of the testes. Gonadal growth and sex hormone production constitute gonadarche.

SEX STEROID EFFECTS

In response to FSH, both testes and ovaries enlarge, starting gonadarche. Ovarian granulosa cells produce 17β-estradiol, which causes estrogen effects that generally occur in a fixed order (Table 61–1). Growth increase is one of the early effects of estrogen. Growth is stimulated by estrogen-stimulated increased production of GH and insulin-like growth factor–1 (IGF-1). In girls, the growth of puberty is fastest in the first 2 years, but slower growth usually continues for 2 to 3 more years. Estrogen along with GH and thyroid hormones increases bone mineralization and growth.

In response to LH, testicular Leydig cells produce testosterone, which is converted to dihydrotestosterone (DHT), leading to androgen signs that generally occur in the same order (Table 61–2).

Note that growth is not stimulated early by rising testosterone; in fact, during the phase when testosterone levels are beginning to rise, growth is usually slowed perceptibly from prepubertal height velocity of perhaps 5 cm/year to a velocity as slow as 3 cm/year for 12 to 18 months. As levels of testosterone increase closer to 400 ng/dl and testis volume increases to between 9 and 10 cm³, boys finally make the transition to rapid growth. Rapid growth for boys thus occurs for about 2 years in mid puberty and slower growth continues for 2 to 3 more years.

Gynecomastia (breast development) often occurs at the middle phase of puberty, when the testes have reached perhaps 9 to 10 cm³ in volume; enough estrogen relative to the amount of testosterone is produced so that breast development occurs. Gynecomastia is very common, usually starts on one side, and is usually self-limited in duration to less than 8 months.

Table 61–1. Estrogen Effects

1. Vaginal and urethral cornification
2. Breast development, often asymmetric
3. Growth
4. Fat development
5. Uterine development
6. Menarche: 2 to 2½ yr after breast buds

Table 61–2. Androgen Effects

1. Psychologic changes
2. Skin and hair oils, sweat odors
3. Areolar growth and pigment
4. Sexual skin pigment and folding
5. Phallic growth
6. Voice change
7. Sexual hair growth
8. Hairline recession
9. More psychologic changes
10. Statural growth
11. Muscle mass/strength

ADRENARCHE

The pituitary is thought to produce an adrenal androgen-stimulating hormone (AASH) that has not yet been isolated. AASH is thought to induce adrenal androgen production, with dehydroepiandrosterone sulfate (DHEAS) being a major androgen. These adrenal androgens produce androgen effects occurring in the same order as listed in Table 61–2. Growth velocity is not affected in either sex by these adrenal androgens of adrenarche, and in males penis size and muscle size are not affected by the normal levels of adrenal androgens. Adrenarche, the effects of adrenal androgens, is thus a separate endocrine process; it may become active either before or after the hypothalamic-pituitary-gonadal system of puberty (gonadarche). Adrenarche usually starts when the bone age is 8 to 10 years.

TIMING OF PUBERTY

The range of ages for onset of normal puberty in the general population is large. The first event of puberty is always enlargement of the gonads.

Girls

In females, correlation of estrogen levels and physical signs with ovarian size, as determined by ultrasound, shows that estrogen is produced as soon as the ovaries enlarge. In estrogen-deficient girls, estrogen treatment produces vaginal cornification and discharge within 1 week, increased arm, leg, and buttock fat within 1 month, and breast budding and increased growth velocity very soon thereafter. The uterus also begins to develop early, but menses come much later.

In spontaneous puberty, events follow the same general timetable. The interval between breast budding and menses is generally 2 to 2½ years. The average age of onset of menses in the general population is between 12 and 12½ years. Therefore, on average, breast development would be expected to be starting by 9½ to 10 years of age. The normal range of age for onset of menses is from 9 to 16 years; this should imply that the range of age for onset of breast development would be from 7 to 14 years. The range frequently described for breast budding (8 to 13 years) is more limited.

Boys

In males, the size of the testes can be determined. The average age for starting testicular enlargement to greater than infant size is

11 to 11½ years, or at about the time when 12-year molars begin to erupt. The normal range of age for beginning testicular enlargement is said to be 9 to 14 years. Testosterone levels rise with testicular enlargement and androgen physical signs appear. Although androgen signs can be from either adrenal (adrenarche) or testicular (gonadarche) androgen, the growth of penis, muscle mass, or increased height velocity requires greater amounts of testosterone, normally from a testicular source. Whereas height velocity generally slows at the beginning of testicular enlargement, the growth spurt of males begins when testicular volume reaches 9 to 10 cm³ and serum testosterone nears 400 ng/dl (6.6 mmol/L).

Family Patterns

There are generally at least two family patterns for growth and development for each parent's family and thus several possibilities for the child. If the mother's menses began at 9 years, 4 months of age (probable onset of breast development by 7 to 7½ years) and she completed her growth by 11 years of age, and if the father was shaving daily in the seventh grade and completed his growth by the ninth grade (at age 15), "early" onset of puberty in their child would actually be "normal" for their family. On the other hand, if the mother's menses began at 16 years of age, and the father grew 8 inches after getting his driver's license and 2 inches after completing high school *(constitutional delay)*, the onset of puberty in the couple's children would be expected to be late.

PSYCHOLOGIC FACTORS

No matter when puberty is occurring, the individual adolescent generally does not feel "normal." The adolescent has no idea of "what is supposed to be happening," and whatever *is* happening is worrisome. Adolescents question the adequacy of their parts, the normality of their development and feelings, and their identity, yet they are increasingly resistant to accepting opinions, advice, and answers from others. Adolescents are agonizingly aware of having no control over what is happening. They may attempt to gain some degree of "control," for instance, with diet and weight lifting. Estrogens have no direct psychologic effects, but girls recognize that they are maturing and usually take more responsibility and plan for the future. The androgens may produce tearfulness, frustration, and anger. Adolescents may be defiant or best friends; they may eat excessively or diet and exercise; they often join groups to get a sense of belonging somewhere outside the family; and they may want to earn money so that they can gain more independence. Medical evaluation, in itself, of pubertal changes may be stressful to the adolescent because of the focus on sexual changes and genitalia.

DELAYED PUBERTY

A "delay" in puberty is signified by:

- No estrogen signs by 13 years of age in girls
- No androgen signs by 14 years of age in boys
- Onset of puberty markedly later than in other members of the family

Differential Diagnosis (Tables 61–3 and 61–4)

One may approach the analysis of the hypothalamic-pituitary-gonadal axis in reverse, keeping androgen and estrogen signs separate.

Table 61–3. Classification of Delayed Puberty and Sexual Infantilism

Constitutional Delay in Growth and Puberty (Delayed Activation of Hypothalamic GnRH Pulse Generator)

Hypogonadotropic Hypogonadism
  Central nervous system disorders
    Tumors (craniopharyngioma, germinoma, glioma)
    Congenital malformations
    Radiation therapy
    Other causes
  Isolated gonadotropin deficiency
    Kallmann syndrome (anosmia-hyposmia)
    Other disorders
  Idiopathic and genetic forms of mulitple pituitary hormone deficiencies
  Miscellaneous disorders
    Prader-Willi syndrome
    Laurence-Moon-Biedl syndrome
    Functional gonadotropin deficiency
      Chronic systemic disease and malnutrition
      Hypothyroidism
      Cushing disease
      Diabetes mellitus
      Hyperprolactinemia
      Anorexia nervosa
      Psychogenic amenorrhea
      Impaired puberty and delayed menarche in female athletes and ballet dancers (exercise amenorrhea)

Hypergonadotropic Hypogonadism
  Klinefelter syndrome (syndrome of seminiferous tubular dysgenesis) and its variants
  Other forms of primary testicular failure
  Anorchia and cryptorchidism
  Syndrome of gonadal dysgenesis and its variants (Turner syndrome)
  Other forms of primary ovarian failure
  XX and XY gonadal dysgenesis
    Familial and sporadic XX gonadal dysgenesis and its variants
    Familial and sporadic XY gonadal dysgenesis and its variants
  Pseudo-Turner syndrome
  Galactosemia

From Styne DM, Grumbach MM. Disorders of puberty in the male and female. *In* Yen SSC, Jaffe RB (eds). Reproductive Endocrinology, 3rd ed. Philadelphia: WB Saunders, 1991:513.

ABSENCE OF ANDROGEN SIGNS

The physician should first determine whether androgens are deficient or whether there is a deficiency of androgen receptors.

If a female has advanced breast development but no androgen signs, she may have a deficiency of androgen receptors. If she has any signs of androgen, she has some androgen receptors, although their levels may be deficient. In females, the androgens predominantly come from the adrenals (adrenarche). If the bone age has not passed 8 years when DHEAS generally increases, adrenarche may simply be delayed in that person *(delayed adrenarche)*. If bone age is advanced, however, there is a deficiency in androgen production. There may be an inherited problem in androgen synthesis from an enzyme deficiency, or the adrenal may be damaged secondary to autoimmune, infectious, or hypoxic injury. In these latter conditions, other signs of adrenal insufficiency would be evident (see Chapter 33).

If adrenal steroid production pathways appear to be intact, there could be a deficiency of AASH. Currently, such a pituitary defi-

Table 61-4. Differential Diagnostic Features of Delayed Puberty and Sexual Infantilism

	Stature	Plasma Gonadotropins	GnRH Test: LH Response	Plasma Gonadal Steroids	Plasma DHEAS	Karyotype	Olfaction
Constitutional Delay in Growth and Adolescence	Short for chronologic age, usually appropriate for bone age	Prepubertal, later pubertal	Prepubertal, later pubertal	Low, later normal	Low for chronologic age, appropriate for bone age	Normal	Normal
Hypogonadotropic Hypogonadism							
Isolated gonadotropin deficiency	Normal, absent pubertal growth spurt	Low	Prepubertal or no response	Low	Appropriate for chronologic age	Normal	Normal
Kallmann syndrome	Normal, absent pubertal growth spurt	Low	Prepubertal or no response	Low	Appropriate for chronologic age	Normal	Anosmia or hyposmia
Idiopathic multiple pituitary hormone deficiencies	Short stature and poor growth since early childhood	Low	Prepubertal or no response	Low	Usually low	Normal	Normal
Hypothalamo-pituitary tumors	Decrease in growth velocity of late onset	Low	Prepubertal or no response	Low	Normal or low for chronologic age	Normal	Normal
Primary Gonadal Failure							
Syndrome of gonadal dysgenesis and variants	Short stature since early childhood	High	Hyper-response for age	Low	Normal for chronologic age	XO or variant	Normal
Klinefelter syndrome and variants	Normal to tall	High	Hyper-response at puberty	Low or normal	Normal for chronologic age	XXY or variant	Normal
Familial XX or XY gonadal dysgenesis	Normal	High	Hyper-response for age	Low	Normal for chronologic age	XX or XY	Normal

From Styne DM, Grumbach MM. Disorders of puberty in the male and female. *In* Yen SSC, Jaffee RB (eds). Reproductive Endocrinology, 3rd ed. Philadelphia: WB Saunders, 1991:513.

Abbreviations: DHEAS = dehydroepiandrosterone sulfate; GnRH = gonadotropin-releasing hormone; LH = luteinizing hormone.

ciency of AASH cannot be detected; however, other pituitary hormones should be evaluated for possible pituitary deficiency.

If a male is lacking androgen signs of puberty, a lack of receptors is not possible because he has already developed as a boy; therefore, this may be delayed adrenarche. The bone age may not have passed 8 years. Enzymatic deficiency for androgen production is not a question in this phenotypically developed boy. Adrenal insufficiency may have been acquired, limiting adrenal androgen (as well as cortisol) production. If the testes are larger than at prepubertal age but there are no signs of androgens, the cause may be either fragile X syndrome or intact FSH (which stimulates testicular volume) with deficient LH (which stimulates Leydig cell testosterone production).

If the testes are small, they may have been damaged by torsion, sickle cell disease, infection, autoimmune disease, chemotherapy, or radiation and may not be able to respond to LH stimulation. If the bone age is greater than 12 years and the hypothalamus has probably matured, the serum LH may then be high. However, the hypothalamic-pituitary-testis system may take longer to mature and, in some cases, gonadotropins do not "turn on" until older bone ages. This type of delayed puberty is a normal variant.

When the testis size is prepubertal, if LH is present but testosterone is not increasing, there may be a problem with the LH receptor or there may be a deficiency of GH necessary for LH effectiveness.

In this latter case, deficient growth velocity should be apparent from growth records. Growth slowing in patients with GH deficiency with decreased androgen production from prepubertal testes should not be confused with the decreased growth velocity of early puberty in which there would be testicular enlargement and early androgen signs.

LH deficiency may be due to deficient pituitary synthesis, or isolated LH deficiency or multiple pituitary hormone deficiencies. The latter may be due to pituitary damage from trauma, radiation, infection, sickle cell disease, compression by infiltrate or tumor, or autoimmune processes, or there can be a lack of pituitary stimulation by GnRH. In differentiating primary pituitary deficiency from that secondary to hypothalamic deficiency, one should remember that all pituitary hormones are stimulated by hypothalamic-releasing hormones *except* prolactin, which is inhibited by hypothalamic prolactin inhibitory factor (PIF). Therefore, if all pituitary hormones, *including* prolactin, are deficient, the problem is in the pituitary. If prolactin levels are present or even elevated while the other pituitary hormones are deficient, the problem is above the pituitary in the stalk or hypothalamus.

Lack of proper pulses of GnRH from the hypothalamus to the pituitary may result from interruption of the portal blood supply from hypothalamus to pituitary. The GnRH pulse generator may be disrupted by an interfering substance, such as excess prolactin (with or without hypothyroidism), and an interfering factor associated with stress, chronic illness, malnutrition, excessive physical activity, or endogenous opioids. Some interfering drugs include neuroleptics, antidepressants, opiates, verapamil, and cimetidine. The hypothalamic arcuate nucleus may have been damaged by trauma, radiation, infection, infiltration (histiocytosis X), pressure, or surgery. The most common tumors are craniopharyngiomas, gliomas, germinomas, and cysts. Congenital conditions or malformations may have allowed enough GnRH for infantile development but not enough for pubertal needs.

One malformation associated with deficient sense of smell and sometimes ichthyosis constitutes *Kallmann syndrome,* which is linked to Xp 22.3 deletion. *Lawrence-Moon-Biedl syndrome* is a recessively transmitted condition with deficient GnRH for stimulation of LH and FSH, mild mental retardation, retinitis pigmentosa, polydactyly, syndactyly, obesity, and other anomalies. The hypogonadism of *Prader-Willi syndrome* also appears to be hypothalamic in origin; patients have neonatal hypotonia, later-onset hyperphagia, obesity, and mental retardation as well.

ABSENCE OF ESTROGEN SIGNS

If a female is lacking estrogen signs, the first step is to consider whether or not there is a lack of estrogen receptors in the target tissue. Because estrogen is not involved in differentiation and development of the prepubertal female, there would be no clue to estrogen receptor deficiency. Estrogen receptor problems appear to be extremely rare. Therefore, if estrogen is deficient, one would assume a problem in production. The ovary may be unable to synthesize estrogen (an inherited metabolic defect, possibly associated with excess adrenal mineralocorticoid and hypertension); the ovary may not be formed well (dysgenesis), associated with XO, XX/XO, XY/XO, XO/XXY karyotypes; or the ovary may have been damaged by any of the factors listed for testicular damage but also including galactosemia.

The ovary may be intact but may not be stimulated by gonadotropins. The bone age may need to reach 13 to 14 years for the hypothalamus to have matured enough for gonadotropin production (delayed puberty, normal variant). If gonadotropins are present but not effective, there is either an FSH receptor problem or a growth hormone deficiency (GH facilitating FSH effect). In the latter case, growth deficiency should also be present. If gonadotropin levels are deficient, this deficiency may be secondary to any of the factors contributing to pituitary deficiency or to deficient GnRH stimulation, as outlined earlier.

TREATMENT OF SEX STEROID DEFICIENCY

The benefits of sex steroids for male skeletal mineralization are lost in pubertal delay, not only for the adolescent years but also for long-term skeletal mineral mass. Both estrogen and testosterone benefit bone mineral.

Boys

Testosterone leads to increased bone cortical mass. In addition, testosterone gives growth and sexual development if GH levels are adequate, and maturation of the hypothalamus in the case of delayed puberty, helping to speed the onset of natural puberty. Relatively low testosterone doses give good growth and development and allow adult height consistent with genetic endowment. With physiologic doses of testosterone, the risks appear to be no more than those of endogenous pubertal testosterone: increased low-density-lipoprotein (LDL) cholesterol and decreased high-density-lipoprotein (HDL) cholesterol.

Males with no androgen signs by age 14 benefit from treatment. Doses of testosterone enanthate of 25 mg IM every 2 weeks, or 50 mg every 4 weeks for 6 months, are generally well tolerated and effective. The male should be made aware of the expected androgen effects on complexion, psychologic upset, distraction by females, and increased erections. Two months after completing the course of treatment, the male can be reevaluated to see if spontaneous puberty will occur. Even when more prolonged testosterone treatment is needed, these doses preserve full adult stature potential while allowing good growth and sexual development.

Girls

Estrogen plays a role in all stages of female skeletal development and leads to increased trabecular bone mineral, contributing to mineralization of the lumbar spine. Bone mass for females is usually maximized by age 16. Small doses of estrogen can stimulate growth via increased GH and IGF-1 and incorporation of more calcium into the skeleton. There are lipid benefits as HDL cholesterol is increased and LDL cholesterol is decreased. Girls with no estrogen signs by age 13 usually benefit from estrogen treatment. Doses of conjugated estrogens of 0.15 to 0.3 mg/day for 6 months, are generally well tolerated and effective. There is no need for cycling or the use of progestin for this short time period. The risks of small estrogen doses to those with a family history of breast cancer are minimal compared with the benefits to bone and blood vessel.

Evaluation of Delayed Puberty

See Tables 61–4 and 61–5.
1. Medical history (trauma, illness, injury, medications, radiation, growth problems, stresses, sickle status, autoimmune problems, galactosemia, general health problem, infection, malnutrition)
2. Review of systems
   a. Psychologic factors, stress, school performance
   b. Growth records, head size since birth
   c. Vision problems, headache, vomiting
   d. Ability to detect odors
   e. Age of androgen signs, age of estrogen signs
   f. Small genitalia at birth
   g. Skin (ichthyosis; tanning of adrenal insufficiency)
   h. Need for deodorant, hair washing frequency
3. Family history
   a. Maternal childhood growth
      (1) Onset of menses
      (2) Final height
   b. Paternal childhood growth
      (1) Growth after driver's license
      (2) Growth after high school, final height
      (3) Age at initial shaving
   c. Siblings and cousins with delayed development
4. Physical examination
   a. Vital signs, especially temperature and blood pressure
   b. Height, arm span, skinfold thickness, weight, head circumference, tooth age
   c. Skin
      (1) Pigment (*café-au-lai spots*), tanning, ichthyosis, skinfold thickness
      (2) Androgen signs (oil, odor, complexion, sexual hair) (see Table 61–5)

Table 61-5. Staging of Puberty

Breasts

1. No areolar widening or pigment	No breast tissue palpable
2. Areola widening red or tan pigment	Breast bud beneath areola
3. Areola wider blends with breast contour	Breast tissue conical; contour blends with areola
4. Areola and papilla mounded on top of breast	Breast tissue rounded; areola mounded on top
5. Papilla projects above areola; areola blends with breast contour	Rounded breast tissue; areola blends with contour

Genitals

1. Appearance of 3- to 5-year old	1.5–3 cm³*	Pubic hair—none
2. Penis width increasing; scrotum more saccular	3–8 cm³*	Pubic hair—none
3. Penis wider, longer	8–14 cm³*	Crescent hair over penis and scrotal junction
4. Penis nearly adult; scrotum adult	14–22 cm³*	Triangular hair not up to symphysis
5. Penis adult	15–25 cm³*	Triangular hair to symphysis

Pubic Hair

1. No coarse hairs
2. One or more coarse or pigmented, longer hairs
3. A crescent of hairs around pubic junction
4. Triangular formation; not up to symphysis
5. Triangular formation filling area to symphysis
6. Extension above symphysis to linea alba or to medial thighs

*Approximate testis volume.

---

d. HEENT (head, eyes, ears, nose, and throat)
  (1) Visual fields
  (2) Ability to detect odors
  (3) *Fundi* discs
  (4) Retinitis pigmentosa
e. Breast development (note stage) (see Table 61–5)
f. Cardiac system
g. Pulmonary system (signs of underlying disease)
h. Abdomen (signs of underlying disease)
i. Genitalia
  (1) Vaginal cornification/discharge
  (2) Penis size, scrotal development
    (a) Testicular volume
    (b) Pubic hair stage (see Table 61–5)
j. Neurologic status, deep tendon reflexes
k. Psychosocial (affect or mood, intellectual ability)
l. Dysmorphic features
5. Studies
  a. Bone age always needed; puberty not to be expected until bone age above 11 years, sometimes age 13 to 14
  b. General (complete blood count, differential, sedimentation rate, sickle cell preparation)
  c. Urinalysis; chemistry profile after fasting
  d. Thyroid function (free thyroxine and thyroid-stimulating hormone)
  e. Prolactin
  f. If slow growth, IGF-1: possible need for pituitary GH testing
  g. If delayed androgens: DHEAS (and cortisol), testosterone
  h. If delayed estrogens: estradiol
  i. In either case, LH and FSH
    (1) If *high,* karyotype needed
    (2) If *low,* with anosmia, mental retardation, polydactyly, or hypotonia, genetic consultation needed
  j. If LH and FSH levels are low: GnRH test with LH level at 30 to 45 minutes
  k. If any neurologic symptoms or examination abnormality or if any pituitary deficiency, magnetic resonance imaging (MRI) of the head indicated

Treatment of Delayed Puberty

Care of adolescents with delayed sexual development involves attending to their feelings, fears, angers, and needs. Any underlying medical problem must be identified and treated. The evaluation may be complex, even uncomfortable. A diagnosis of constitutional delay can be made only when all other problems have been ruled out. If the problem turns out to be simply constitutional delay, that may be a relief, but treatment may still be needed.

Sex hormone treatments are to be recommended, but treatment can be offered only to the adolescent who chooses to take it. Some patients may refuse treatment, but most welcome the beneficial effects. If girls are lacking androgen signs and have no pubic hair, a limited course of mild androgen may also be helpful. Although exercise increases the benefits of sex steroids on bone as well as general health, excessive exercise may delay pubertal progress; therefore, moderation is to be encouraged. Advice about diet and calcium is particularly important for the rapid growth phase that the adolescent is entering during treatment (see Treatment of Sex Steroid Deficiency).

PRECOCIOUS PUBERTY

The term *precocious* in regard to puberty includes the following:

- Breast development before age 8 in girls
- Testis enlargement before age 9 in boys
- Markedly earlier development than in other members of the family

Isosexual development refers to compatibility with the predominant sex steroid of a child's own gonads.

Heterosexual development refers to compatibility with sex steroids of the opposite sex.

Thelarche refers to isolated breast development.

Early (precocious) adrenarche refers to the onset of adrenal androgen effects at or before age 7 years.

Differential Diagnosis (Tables 61–6 and 61–7)

ISOSEXUAL DEVELOPMENT IN FEMALES

Central Precocious Puberty

The first event of true central puberty (Fig. 61–1) (pituitary gonadotropin-dependent) is enlargement of the gonads. In females, the first visible sign is breast development. Breast tissue that is stimulated by estrogen is firm and tender and often initially occurs only on one side. Ovarian enlargement correlates with estrogen production and can sometimes be observed on ultrasonography.

As puberty begins, the ovaries' production of estrogen may seem "hesitant"—starting then stopping, then starting again. When estrogen production turns on, breast development starts along with vaginal cornification, uterine development, and statural growth. When estrogen turns off, the changes regress. The most prompt response to estrogen is in vaginal cornification, responding within 5 to 6 days to the presence or absence of estrogen. Thus, the vaginal smear is an excellent screening procedure for the presence or absence of estrogen.

When breast development clearly persists before 8 years of age, it may be precocious and its cause must be considered. However, breast development before 8 years of age may be part of a family pattern; for example, perhaps the mother had onset of menses at 9 years, 3 months, supposedly with onset of breast development at age 7, and the father had started to shave daily in the sixth grade. In the same context, breast development at age 10 might actually

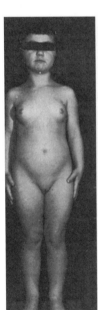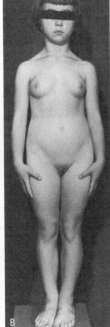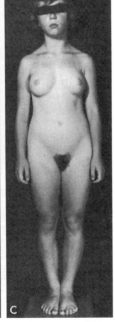

Figure 61–1. Idiopathic precocious puberty. Patient at 3 years, 11 months (A), 5 years, 8 months (B), and 8 years, 6 months (C). Breast development and vaginal bleeding began at 2½ years of age. Osseous age was 7½ years at 3 years, 11 months and 14 years at 8 years of age. Repeated estrogen assays varied between normal prepubertal and adult female levels. Urinary gonadotropins were not demonstrable until the child was 5 years old. Intelligence and dental age were normal for chronologic age. Growth was completed at 10 years; ultimate height was 142 cm (56 inches). (From DiGeorge AM. The endocrine system. *In* Behrman RE [ed]. Nelson Textbook of Pediatrics, 14th ed. Philadelphia: WB Saunders, 1992:1409.)

Table 61–6. Conditions Causing Precocious Puberty

True Precocious Puberty (Gonadotropin-Dependent)
  Idiopathic (constitutional, functional)
  Central nervous system lesion
    Hypothalamic hamartoma, brain tumors, hydrocephalus,
      postencephalitic scars, etc.
  Prolonged untreated primary hypothyroidism
  Therapy of congenital adrenal hyperplasia
  McCune-Albright syndrome—late
  Administration of gonadotropins

Precocious Pseudopuberty (Gonadotropin-Independent)
  Females
    Isosexual (feminization)
      Ovarian tumors
        Granulosa—theca cell tumor
          Associated with Ollier disease
        Teratoma, chorionepithelioma
        Sex-cord tumor with annular tubules (associated with
          Peutz-Jeghers syndrome)
      Autonomous functional cyst of ovary
      McCune-Albright syndrome
      Adrenocortical tumor
      Exogenous estrogen
    Heterosexual (virilization)
      Congenital adrenal hyperplasia
      Adrenocortical tumor
        Testosterone-secreting tumor
      Androblastoma (arrhenoblastoma)
      Androgen-producing teratoma
      Exogenous androgen
  Males
    Isosexual (masculinization)
      Male-limited autosomal dominant
      Congenital adrenal hyperplasia
      Adrenocortical tumor
      Leydig cell tumor
      Teratoma (containing adrenocortical tissue)
      hCG-secreting tumor
        CNS tumor
        Hepatoblastoma
        Mediastinal tumor
          Associated with Klinefelter syndrome
      Exogenous androgen
    Heterosexual (feminization)
      Adrenocortical tumor
      Exogenous estrogen
      Sertoli cell tumor
        Sex-cord tumor with annular tubules (associated with
          Peutz-Jeghers syndrome)

Partial Precocious Puberty
  Premature adrenarche
  Premature thelarche
  Premature menarche

Modified from DiGeorge AM. The endocrine system. *In* Behrman RE (ed). Nelson Textbook of Pediatrics, 14th ed. Philadelphia: WB Saunders, 1992:1408.

be premature in a family in which the mother had onset of menses at 16 and the father grew 8 inches after getting his driver's license.

Endogenous estrogen must be from either ovaries or adrenals. Ovarian size, as seen on a sonogram, is generally a reflection of ovarian estrogen production. In true central puberty, pituitary gonadotropins cause both ovaries to increase in size—stroma and follicles. The granulosa cells of the follicles respond to FSH to produce 17β-estradiol. Gonadotropins have been stimulated by

Table 61-7. Differential Diagnosis of Sexual Precocity

	Serum Gonadotropin Concentration	LH Response to GnRH	Serum Sex Steroid Concentrations	Gonadal Size	Miscellaneous
True Precocious Puberty (Premature Reactivation of Hypothalamic GnRH Pulse Generator)	Prominent LH pulses, initially during sleep	Pubertal	Pubertal values of testosterone or estradiol	Normal pubertal testicular enlargement or ovarian and uterine enlargement (by sonography)	MRI scan of brain to rule out CNS tumor or other abnormality
McCune-Albright syndrome	Prepubertal	Prepubertal	Pubertal	Enlarged	Skeletal survey
Incomplete Sexual Precocity (Pituitary Gonadotropin Independent)					
Males					
Chorionic gonadotropin–secreting tumor in males	High hCG	Prepubertal	Pubertal values of testosterone	Slight to moderate uniform enlargement of testes	Hepatomegaly suggests hepatoblastoma; CT scan of brain if chorionic gonadotropin–secreting CNS tumor suspected
Leydig cell tumor in males	Prepubertal	Prepubertal	Very high testosterone	Irregular asymmetric enlargement of testes	
Familial testotoxicosis	Prepubertal	Prepubertal	Pubertal values of testosterone	Testes symmetric and larger than 2.5 cm but smaller than expected for pubertal development; spermatogenesis occurs	Familial; probably sex-limited, autosomal dominant trait
Premature adrenarche	Prepubertal	Prepubertal	Prepubertal testosterone; DHEAS or urinary 17-ketosteroid values appropriate for pubic hair stage 2	Testes prepubertal	Onset usually after 6 yr of age; more frequent in brain-injured children
Females					
Granulosa cell tumor (follicular cysts may present similarly)	Low	Prepubertal	Very high estradiol	Ovarian enlargement on physical examination, MRI, CT, or sonography	Tumor often palpable on abdominal examination
Follicular cyst	Low	Prepubertal	Prepubertal to very high estradiol values	Ovarian enlargement on physical examination, MRI, CT, or sonography	Single or repetitive episodes; exclude McCune-Albright syndrome (skeletal survey)
Feminizing adrenal tumor	Low	Prepubertal	High estradiol and DHEAS values	Ovaries prepubertal	Unilateral adrenal mass
Premature thelarche*	Prepubertal	Prepubertal	Prepubertal or early pubertal estradiol	Ovaries prepubertal	Onset usually before 3 yr of age
Premature adrenarche	Prepubertal	Prepubertal	Prepubertal estradiol; DHEAS or urinary 17-ketosteroid values appropriate for pubic hair stage 2	Ovaries prepubertal	Onset usually after 6 yr of age; more frequent in brain-injured children

Modified from Wilson JD, Foster DW (eds.) Williams Textbook of Endocrinology, 8th ed. Philadelphia: WB Saunders, 1990:1205.
*Same pattern evident with exogenous estrogen administration.
Abbreviations: CT = computed tomography; DHEAS = dehydroepiandrosterone; LH = luteinizing hormone; GnRH = gonadotropin-releasing factor; hCG = human chorionic gonadotropin; MRI = magnetic resonance imaging.

greater amplitude and frequency pulses of GnRH. A bolus of exogenous GnRH causes an increase of serum LH in 30 to 45 minutes, confirming central puberty. When onset is before 8 years, this is central precocious puberty.

Evaluation. Central precocious puberty can be genetic, but a precipitating organic cause must be sought (see Tables 61–6 and 61–7). There may have been central nervous system trauma, radiation, or infection. Brain tumors (glioma, astrocytoma, neurofibroma, hamartoma) as well as hydrocephalus can lead to precocious puberty. Other causes include craniopharyngioma, pinealoma, and pineal cyst. Careful neurologic and vision examinations are imperative. An MRI study of the head (i.e., the hypothalamic, pituitary, and pineal areas) is essential.

Treatment. Because it is the pulses of GnRH that stimulate the pituitary gonadotrophs, a sustained increased level of GnRH can obscure the pulses and turn off gonadotroph stimulation. GnRH analogs have been produced that can turn off central precocious puberty (Table 61–8). During analog treatment, the size of the ovaries and uterus decreases. The GnRH analog is the treatment choice for central precocious puberty. The psychosocial benefits of analog treatment are great, as treatment turns off the early sexual development that brings with it psychologic stress and behavioral problems in the child and psychosocial problems, even abuse from those around them.

Peripheral Precocious Puberty (Gonadotropin-Independent)

Progressive breast development with *bilateral ovarian enlargement* and increased estradiol but *without* increased gonadotropins or any LH response to exogenous GnRH suggests *McCune-Albright syndrome*. The ovaries are autonomous and are not stimulated by FSH, but they act as if they were FSH-stimulated. In McCune-Albright syndrome, the FSH receptor G_s protein is constantly turned on and is not regulated. Production of estradiol is continuously stimulated and estradiol levels are high, whereas LH and FSH levels are very low. On ultrasonography, the ovaries show multiple large ovarian cysts. Since these ovaries are not dependent on pituitary gonadotropins, GnRH stimulation does not cause an increase of LH; GnRH analog treatment would be of no benefit.

Patients with McCune-Albright syndrome usually have *café-au-lait* areas of skin pigment with an irregular outline resembling the ''coast of Maine'' as well as multiple areas of bone dysplasia (polyostotic fibrous dysplasia). In these patients, autonomous function of other endocrine organs as well is also likely. One approach to the treatment of McCune-Albright syndrome is turning off this estrogen production by blocking estrogen synthesis with the aromatase inhibitor testolactone (see Table 61–8). This allows stopping estrogen effects, including breast development; prevents menses; stops excess growth and skeletal maturation; and allows greater adult stature. Pediatric endocrine evaluation and guidance are essential in this complex situation.

Progressive premature breast development with increased estrogen levels as well as androgen signs may result from an ovarian tumor. A sonogram would then show one enlarged ovary. Actually, such ovarian tumors are usually large enough to be palpable. These tumors can be completely resected.

The most common cause of premature progressive breast development is *simple premature thelarche*. In this case, a pelvic ultrasound study may show prepubertal ovaries varying from 1 to 3 cm^3 in volume with many small follicular cysts. Some cysts may be larger (persistent follicular cysts). Estradiol is produced by the granulosa cells lining the follicles and causes vaginal discharge and breast development. Estradiol may cause uterine development as well but generally does *not* cause increased growth velocity. LH and FSH levels are low. The follicular cysts regress spontaneously (90% of the time) within a few weeks to months, and the vaginal cornification is lost within 1 week of cyst regression. The breast tissue then softens but can remain for months. Thus, this premature thelarche of persistent follicular cysts is usually benign and self-limited; 10% of the cysts may persist and enlarge. Some follicular cysts may become large enough to threaten ovarian torsion and to necessitate surgical treatment (see Chapter 26).

Very rarely estrogens can be produced by *adrenal adenomas*. *Exogenous estrogens* can also cause breast development with

Table 61–8. Pharmacologic Therapy of Sexual Precocity

Disorder	Treatment	Action and Rationale
GnRH dependent true or central precocious puberty	GnRH agonists	Desensitization of gonadotropes; blocks action of endogenous GnRH
GnRH independent incomplete sexual precocity		
Girls		
Autonomous ovarian cysts	Medroxyprogesterone acetate	Inhibition of ovarian steroidogenesis; regression of cyst (inhibition of FSH release)
McCune-Albright syndrome	Medroxyprogesterone acetate*	Inhibition of ovarian steroidogenesis; regression of cyst (inhibition of FSH release)
	Testolactone* or fadrozole	Inhibition of P-450 aromatase; blocks estrogen synthesis
Boys		
Familial testotoxicosis	Ketoconazole*	Inhibition of P-450$_{c17}$ (mainly 17,20-lyase activity)
	Spironolactone* or flutamide *and* testolactone or fadrozole	Antiandrogen Inhibition of aromatase; blocks estrogen synthesis
	Medroxyprogesterone acetate*	Inhibition of testicular steroidogenesis

Modified from Grumbach MM, Kaplan SL. Recent advances in the diagnosis and management of sexual precocity. Acta Paediatr Jpn 1988; 30(Suppl):155.
*If true precocious puberty develops, a GnRH agonist can be added.
Abbreviations: FSH = follicle-stimulating hormone; GnRH = gonadotropin-releasing hormone.

low LH and FSH levels. Cosmetics and medications may contain estrogen, and there have been reports of effects from estrogen-treated poultry.

Vaginal Bleeding

The usual progression of puberty in girls dictates that breast and uterine development will begin about 2 years before the vaginal bleeding of menses. When the rate of pubertal progression is accelerated, menses may start as early as 1 to 1½ years after thelarche; if the rate is slow, menses may start perhaps 3 to 4 years after thelarche. In any case, vaginal bleeding is always a much later sign than breast development, and whenever vaginal bleeding occurs too early—especially if it ever occurs before breast development starts—it must be investigated thoroughly.

PRECOCIOUS ISOSEXUAL DEVELOPMENT IN MALES

Central Precocious Puberty

In true puberty (pituitary gonadotropin dependent) testes enlarge and androgen production increases (Fig. 61–2). The size of testes enlargement sufficient to determine puberty is debatable. Generally, prepubertal testes are less than 2 cm^3 in volume and 2 cm in length. A testis 3 cm^3 in volume and 2.5 cm in length is enlarging. If on examination *both* testes are enlarged and androgen signs are present, testosterone levels are increasing. If pituitary gonadotropins are increasing or if LH levels increase markedly after GnRH stimulation, the diagnosis is central precocious puberty.

Evaluation. Possible etiologic factors include trauma, radiation, infection, brain tumors (glioma, astrocytoma, germinoma, neurofibroma, hamartoma) and increased intracranial pressure (Fig. 61–2) (Tables 61–6 and 61–7). These factors lead to activation of the GnRH pulse generator. Since central precocious puberty is dependent on GnRH pulses, a bolus of GnRH will stimulate LH in 30 to 45 minutes. Careful neurologic, visual, and magnetic resonance imaging (MRI) examinations are indicated.

Treatment. The advantages of GnRH analog treatment for central precocious puberty are many, in that the analogs turn off psychologic as well as physical signs of androgens. In addition, adult stature is presumably preserved. The co-occurrence of central precocious puberty and GH deficiency must be watched for, in which case both GnRH analog and GH treatments are needed. The physician should remember family patterns of pubertal development in considering relative precocity of sexual development.

Peripheral Precocious Puberty

If *both testes are slightly increased* in volume and testosterone levels are increased but LH and FSH levels are low, there are two possibilities. Either the testes are being stimulated by human chorionic gonadotropin (hCG), which acts like LH and does not increase volume, as with FSH, or the testes are functioning autonomously. Beta-hCG levels must be determined and, if they are increased, tumors producing hCG must be found and removed;

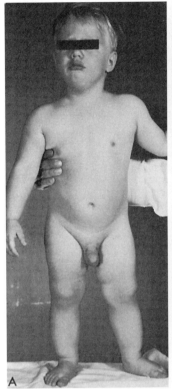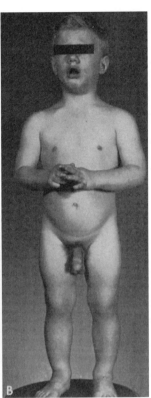

Figure 61–2. Precocious puberty with a central nervous system lesion. Photographs at 1½ years (A) and 2½ years (B). Accelerated growth, muscular development, osseous maturation, and testicular development were consistent with the degree of secondary sexual maturation. Urinary gonadotropins were repeatedly negative, 17-ketosteroids usually 2 to 3 mg/24 hours. In early infancy, the patient began having frequent spells of rapid, purposeless motion; later in life, he had episodes of uncontrollable laughing with ocular movements. At 7 years, he exhibited emotional lability, aggressive behavior, and destructive tendencies. Although a hypothalamic hamartoma had been suspected, it was not established until CT scanning became available, when the patient was 23 years old. Epiphyses fused at 9 years of age; final height was 142 cm (56 inches). (From DiGeorge AM. The endocrine system. *In* Behrman RE [ed]. Nelson Textbook of Pediatrics, 14th ed. Philadelphia: WB Saunders, 1992:1410.)

such tumors may include hepatoma, hepatoblastoma, teratoma, and choriocpithelioma.

If *both testes are producing testosterone autonomously without gonadotropin stimulus*, the condition of *testotoxicosis* is probable. This is perhaps similar to McCune-Albright syndrome (testosterone levels are high; FSH and LH levels are low); it can be familial and can be treated by blocking testosterone synthesis (see Table 61–8). Because these testes are not stimulated by pituitary gonadotropins and GnRH plays no role, GnRH does not stimulate LH and GnRH treatment would not be effective.

If *one testis* is *enlarged*, a Leydig cell adenoma in that testicle is probably producing excess testosterone; the tumor must be removed. The high levels of testosterone have suppressed LH and FSH, and the other testicle remains small. Depending on age, a testicular prosthesis may be inserted to replace the removed testicle.

If androgen signs are developing steadily but *neither testis has enlarged*, the androgen is presumed to be either from the adrenals or from an exogenous source. An adrenal source is either a tumor (that cannot be suppressed by dexamethasone) or a steroid synthesis enzymatic deficiency leading to excessive adrenal androgen production (that *can* be turned off by dexamethasone). An adrenal tumor would have affected growth whenever it started to function, but not necessarily beginning at birth. A defect in steroid synthesis due to an enzymatic deficiency would be congenital, as in congenital adrenal hyperplasia (CAH) (see Chapter 33), and the excess androgen production resulting from the enzymatic deficiency would have been produced from the time of birth, leading to increased growth velocity from early life. Children with congenital adrenal hyperplasia may have severe adrenal crises during an illness or surgery. A tumor can be identified by computed tomography (CT) or ultrasonography and must be removed.

Another source of androgen is the use of exogenous anabolic steroids. The use of anabolic steroids may start at any age when a male feels an excessive need for growth and muscle development. If anabolic steroids are taken at the age of puberty, secondary sexual development will progress but the testes will remain small. Psychologic problems in such boys can be major.

Scrotal hair has been a cause of some concern; it is sometimes thought of as an early sign of adrenarche. However, scrotal hair may grow without increased androgen levels and without any other androgen signs in sweat glands or face and hair glands and years before there is any true pubic hair growth. Thus, scrotal hair is usually benign and not related to adrenarche and does not affect growth or development.

HETEROSEXUAL DEVELOPMENT

Boys

Breast tissue frequently develops in males (gynecomastia) during mid puberty, when the production of estrogen from testosterone in the testes temporarily overbalances the testosterone effects. Only rarely does breast tissue develop in younger males, since the young male does not respond to transient gonadotropin stimulation with estrogen production. Therefore, in younger males, breast size, testis size, and testis growth must be watched to look for either a testis or adrenal source of estrogen and for any excess of gonadotropin or prolactin. Any excess of gonadotropins requires a karyotype. In *Klinefelter syndrome*, gynecomastia may occur before testes reach 8 cm³ in volume. Any excess of prolactin requires pituitary evaluation and MRI scanning. Use of marijuana may also stimulate breast development.

Girls

Androgen signs of adrenarche normally develop in females beginning by age 8 but sometimes as early as age 7, especially in taller girls. If there are earlier androgen signs, they may be due to early or premature adrenarche. Growth must be carefully monitored, because adrenarche does not increase growth velocity, whereas pathologic causes of excess androgen can speed growth. Androgen levels (DHEAS and testosterone) must be measured to ensure that they do not exceed the normal range. Normal androgen levels of normal premature adrenarche do not affect clitoral diameter (which should always be less than 5 mm) or height growth velocity. Excess androgen from ovary or adrenal pathology can cause clitoral widening and can speed growth.

Ovarian tumors producing androgens *(thecoma)* and sometimes also estrogen may be palpable on physical examination and are usually easily seen on a pelvic sonogram.

Adrenal tumors can be detected with ultrasonography or CT. Androgens produced by adrenal tumors are not suppressed by dexamethasone. Excessive adrenal androgens produced because of an *inherited enzymatic deficiency* (CAH) can be suppressed by dexamethasone (see Chapter 33). Such an enzymatic deficiency would have to be mild, since it did not cause ambiguity of genitalia; however, it might cause a very slowly increasing growth rate.

Exogenous androgens have been taken by female athletes in an attempt to improve muscle development, stamina, and performance. Such androgens can also produce clitoral enlargement (particularly in diameter), complexion problems, and hirsutism as well as emotional upsets. Serious psychologic problems may exist.

Labial hair has been a cause of concern, usually thought of as an early sign of adrenarche. However, labial hair may grow without any other androgen signs occurring in the sweat glands, face, or hair glands, and years before any true pubic hair growth. Thus, labial hair is usually benign, not related to adrenarche and not affecting growth or development.

Evaluation of Precocious Puberty

1. Medical history
   a. Growth patterns
   b. Excessive responses to illnesses (adrenal crisis)
   c. Hydrocephalus (myelodysplasia, neurofibromatosis)
   d. Exposure to exogenous sex steroids
2. Review of systems
   a. Growth records, head size since birth, clothing size
   b. Vision problems, headache
   c. Age of onset of androgen signs (e.g., behavior changes, need for hair washing, deodorant)
   d. Age at onset of estrogen signs (vaginal discharge, breast budding, underpants size)
   e. Skin
      (1) *Café-au-lait* areas
      (2) "Coast of Maine" (McCune Albright syndrome)
      (3) "Coast of California" (neurofibromatosis)
3. Family history
   a. Maternal growth
      (1) Onset of menses
      (2) Final height
   b. Paternal growth (how early growth completed)
   c. Initial age of shaving
   d. Siblings and cousins with early development
   e. Neurofibromatosis
4. Physical examination (special care, parent present)
   a. Vital signs
   b. Height, weight, head circumference, tooth age
   c. Skin
      (1) Pigment (*café-au-lait* spots, coast of Maine, coast of California)
      (2) Androgen signs (complexion, hair oil, pigment, odor)
      (3) Neurofibromata
   d. HEENT
      (1) Visual fields
      (2) Fundi
   e. Breast development (note stage) (see Table 61–5)
   f. Abdomen (masses, hepatomegaly)
   g. Genitalia
      (1) Vaginal cornification/discharge
      (2) Penis/clitoris size diameter
      (3) Testicular volume
      (4) Scrotal/labial development and pigmentation (see Table 61–5)
      (5) Pubic hair (see Table 61–5)
   h. Neurologic status (deep tendon reflexes)
   i. Extremities (bone abnormalities such as McCune-Albright syndrome, asymmetry of length)
   j. Psychosocial (affect or mood, intellectual ability)
5. Studies

Table 61–9. "Red Flags" That Must Be Evaluated

Vaginal bleeding before breast development
Girls with advancing breast development but no androgen signs
Headaches
Vision changes
Galactorrhea
Abnormal neurologic examination
Pelvic mass
Testicular asymmetry
Testicular underdevelopment
Polyuria or bed wetting

   a. Bone age (advancement dependent on amount of sex steroid and duration)
   b. If excess androgens, serum levels of:
      (1) DHEAS, 17-OH progesterone, androstenedione
      (2) 17-OH pregnenolone/17-OH progesterone after ACTH
      (3) Testosterone, free testosterone
      (4) β-hCG
   c. If excess estrogens, estradiol; if levels not increased, check total estrogens
   d. Prolactin
   e. LH/FSH
      (1) If levels increased, karyotype (gynecomastia in Klinefelter syndrome)
      (2) If low levels: GnRH test with LH level at 30 to 45 minutes
      (3) If a pubertal LH response to GnRH or if neurologic symptoms, MRI of the head indicated
   f. Ultrasound or CT of the pelvis for uterus and ovarian size, and of abdomen for liver or adrenal tumors
   g. Bone survey if possibly McCune-Albright syndrome

Treatment of Precocious Puberty

The stresses felt by children with precocious development require great support and a lot of time. All historical questions need to be asked in such a way as to not imply a "defect," an "abnormality," or something "wrong." These children are chronologically younger than their appearance suggests, and they need gentle help in spite of perhaps looking older. The tests and treatments may suggest to the child that something is wrong and unfair, since other children do not have to endure such indignities. The rapidly growing child needs all the help of those entering sexual development at a more usual time.

SUMMARY AND RED FLAGS

Disorders of sexual development may involve hypothalamus, pituitary, adrenal, gonadal or sex steroid receptor dysfunction. *Red*

Table 61–10. Things Not to Miss

Estrogen signs occurring in order
All growth records
Penis or clitoris diameter
Testicular volume
   Both enlarged
   One enlarged
   Neither enlarged
Size of testes in patients with gynecomastia

flags are listed in Table 61–9, and issues to note are presented in Table 61–10.

A detailed history and physical examination remain central features to the evaluation of such children. Imaging studies and various static or provocative hormone studies supplement the history and physical examination.

REFERENCES

Pubertal Development

Auchus RJ, Lynch SC. Treatment of post-orchiectomy gynecomastia with testolactone. The Endocrinologist 1994;4:429.

Bonjour JP, Theintz G, Buchs B, et al. Critical years and states of puberty for spinal and femoral bone mass accumulation during adolescence. J Clin Endocrinol Metab 1991;73:555.

Cohen HL, Shapiro MA, Mandel FS, Shapiro ML. Normal ovaries in neonates and infants: A sonographic study of 77 patients 1 day to 24 months old. AJR Am J Roentgenol 1993;160:583.

Kletter GB, Padmanabhan V, Brown MB, et al. Serum bioactive gonadotropins during male puberty: A longitudinal study. J Clin Endocrinol Metab 1993;76:432.

Metzger DL, Kerrigan JR, Rogol AD. Gonadal steroid hormone regulation of the somatotropic axis during puberty in humans: Mechanism for androgen and estrogen action. Trends Endocrinol Metab 1994;5:290.

Orsini LF, Salardi S, Pilu G, et al. Pelvic organs in premenarchal girls: Real time ultrasonography. Radiology 1984;153:113.

Delayed Puberty

Adan L, Souberbielle JC, Brauner R. Management of short stature due to pubertal delay in boys. J Clin Endocrinol Metab 1994;78:478.

Bonjour JP, Theintz G, Buchs B, et al. Critical years and states of puberty for spinal and femoral bone mass accumulation during adolescence. J Clin Endocrinol Metab 1991;73:555.

Hardelin JP, Levilliers J, Young J, et al. p22.3 deletions in isolated familial Kallmann syndrome. J Clin Endocrinol Metab 1993;76:827.

Ho KK, Weissberger AJ. Impact of short-term estrogen administration on growth hormone secretion and action: Distinct route-dependent effects on connective and bone tissue metabolism. J Bone Miner Res 1992;7:821.

Kulin HE. The assessment of gonadotropins during childhood and adolescence: An ongoing struggle. The Endocrinologist 1994;4:279.

Patton ML, Woolf PD. Hyperprolactinemia and delayed puberty: A report of three cases and their response to therapy. Pediatrics 1983;71:572.

Slemenda CW, Reister TK, Hui SL, et al. Influences on skeletal mineralization in children and adolescents: Evidence for varying effects of sexual maturation and physical activity. J Pediatr 1994;125:201.

Uruena M, Pantsiotou S, Preece MA, Stanhope R. Is testosterone therapy for boys with constitutional delay of growth and puberty associated with impaired final height and suppression of the hypothalamo-pituitary-gonadal axis? Eur J Pediatr 1992;151:15.

Precocious Puberty

Ambrosino MM, Hernanz-Schulman M, Genieser NB, et al. Monitoring of girls undergoing medical therapy for isosexual precocious puberty. J Ultrasound Med 1994;13:501.

Cara JF, Kreiter ML, Rosenfield RL. Height prognosis of children with true precocious puberty and growth hormone deficiency: Effect of combination therapy with gonadotropin releasing hormone agonist and growth hormone. J Pediatr 1992;120:709.

Foster CM. Endocrine manifestations of McCune-Albright syndrome. The Endocrinologist 1993;3:359.

Garibaldi LR, Aceto T Jr, Weber C. The pattern of gonadotropin and estradiol secretion in exaggerated thelarche. Acta Endocrinol 1993;128:345.

Herman-Giddens ME, Sandler AD, Friedman NE. Sexual precocity in girls: An association with sexual abuse? Am J Dis Child 1988;142:431.

Lee PA. Laboratory monitoring of children with precocious puberty. Arch Pediatr Adolesc Med 1994;148:369.

Nakamura M, Okabe I, Shimorzumi H, et al. Ultrasonography of ovary, uterus, and breast in premature thelarche. Acta Pediatr Jpn 1991;33:645.

Pasquino AM, Pucarelli I, Passeri F, et al. Progression of premature thelarche to central precocious puberty. J Pediatr 1995;126:11.

Rosenfield RL. Selection of children with precocious puberty for treatment with gonadotropin releasing hormone analogs. J Pediatr 1994;124:989.

Salardi S, Orsini LE, Cacciari E, et al. Pelvic ultrasonography in girls with precocious puberty, congenital adrenal hyperplasia, obesity, or hirsutism. J Pediatr 1988;112:880.

Silverman SH, Migeon CJ, Rosenberg E, Wilkins L. Precocious growth of sexual hair without other secondary sexual development. Pediatrics 1952;10:426.

Sonis WA, Comite F, Blue J, et al. Behavior problems and social competence in girls with true precocious puberty. J Pediatr 1985;106:156.

Van Winter JT, Noller KL, Zimmerman D, Melton LJ III. Natural history of premature thelarche in Olmsted County, Minnesota, 1940 to 1984. J Pediatr 1990;116:278.

Zachmann M, Sobradillo B, Frank M, et al. Bayley-Pinneau, Roche-Wainer-Thissen, and Tanner height predictions in normal children and in patients with various pathologic conditions. J Pediatr 1978;93:749.

62 Short Stature

Leona Cuttler

Short stature is a symptom, not a disease. It may represent a normal variant or may be a signal of serious physical or emotional illness. Since linear growth is a crucial component of childhood, in many ways it is an index of childhood well-being. Illnesses, even those not involving aberrations of growth-regulating hormones, often interfere with growth. Therefore, the measurement and charting of heights sequentially on standardized growth charts constitute a central part of a child's medical evaluation.

DEFINITION OF SHORT STATURE

The definition of short stature depends on both statistical and cultural variables. Heights below the first, third, or fifth percentile for age and sex are often utilized to distinguish short children from others. Similarly, the child who is more than 2 or 2.5 standard deviations below the mean for age may be considered to have short stature. Implicit in all such definitions is the understanding that height is a normally distributed characteristic; therefore, a proportion of normal individuals will have heights below each of these arbitrary cutoff points. The greater the deviation from the mean, the more likely the short stature reflects underlying pathology. In addition to actual height, poor linear growth can also be defined as a subnormal rate of growth or as stature that is inappropriately low for the child's genetic endowment (Figs. 62–1 and 62–2).

Whichever definition is utilized in the evaluation of short stature, the physician's diagnostic task is generally to distinguish normal children with short stature from those who have short stature due to an underlying medical condition; the more the child's height or growth rate deviates from age-related norms and family growth patterns, the greater the likelihood of an underlying medical condition (Table 62–1).

Cultural variables may also influence the degree to which a height is perceived as a medical problem. For example, historically, boys at the third or fifth percentile have been more likely to be evaluated for short stature than girls of equivalent height relative to peers.

Short stature should be distinguished from "failure to thrive." The latter term refers primarily to poor *weight* gain in infants and young children (although linear growth may be secondarily affected), whereas short stature refers primarily to subnormal linear growth throughout childhood and adolescence (see Chapter 17).

NORMAL PATTERNS OF GROWTH

Fetal Growth and Birth Size

Fetal growth and birth size normally reflect mainly maternal factors, including maternal or uterine size, parity and multiparity, nutrition, and uteroplacental blood flow. Many congenital disorders that markedly stunt postnatal growth (gonadal dysgenesis, congenital growth hormone [GH] deficiency) have a small effect on prenatal growth and birth size. Heredity, which plays a major role in postnatal growth, generally does not influence birth size. Birth size usually does not predict the eventual growth pattern in most children. An exception is the baby who is small for gestational age (SGA; intrauterine growth retardation [IUGR]), which is due to reduced prenatal and postnatal growth potential. Such disorders affect fetal cell number by reduced innate growth (chromosomal disorders [trisomy D, E] or syndromes [Russell-Silver]), infection (congenital rubella, cytomegalovirus), or toxins (alcohol) (Table 62–2). Infants with intrauterine growth retardation due to poor maternal nutrition, small maternal size, or reduced uteroplacental perfusion usually demonstrate postnatal catch-up growth and eventually achieve their true growth potential determined by parental genetic influences.

Postnatal Growth Patterns

The rate of linear growth is greatest in infancy (see Fig. 62–2). During infancy, genetic or familial influences begin to exert a profound effect on height. These influences cause approximately 66% of normal infants to shift linear growth percentiles during the

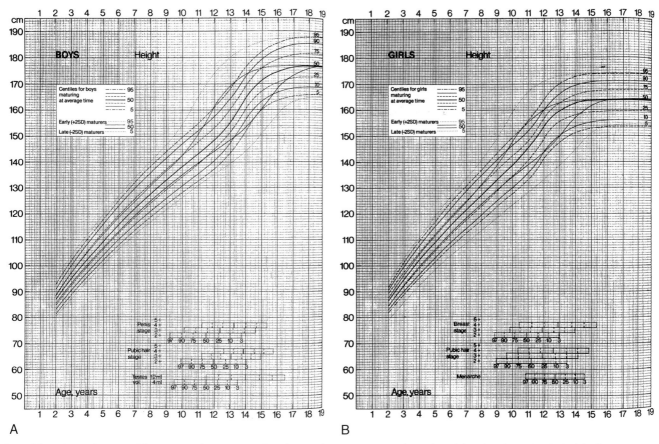

Figure 62–1. *A,* Height attained for American boys. Lines with early growth increment = 50th centile *(solid)* and 95th centile *(dashed)* for boys 2 standard deviations (SDs) of tempo early; lines with gradual and delayed increment = 50th centile *(solid)* and 5th centile *(dashed)* for boys 2 SD of tempo late. *B,* Height attained for American girls. Lines with early growth increment = 50th centile *(solid)* and 95th centile *(dashed)* for girls 2 SD of tempo early; lines with gradual and delayed increment = 50th centile *(solid)* and 5th centile *(dashed)* for girls 2 SD of tempo late. (Redrawn from Tanner J, Davies P. Clinical longitudinal standards for height and height velocity in North American children. J Pediatr 1985;107:317–329.)

period from birth to 18 to 24 months. By 24 months, these shifts are complete and most infants have "found their growth channel" or linear growth percentile relative to peers. After infancy, there is a strong tendency for normal children to maintain their growth channel; significant deviation from this channel is often an indication of illness.

Linear growth rate slows somewhat in childhood, between infancy and adolescence. The average rate of growth is approximately 6 cm/year during midchildhood; sustained rates below 4.5 cm/year are considered abnormal. Figure 62–2 illustrates norms for growth velocity at each age. Just before puberty, growth rates tend to slow to a nadir. In children with average tempo of puberty, the nadir may reach as low as 3.8 cm/year in males (third percentile). Just before puberty, the growth rate of girls may slow to 4.2 cm/year (third percentile).

Growth accelerates again at puberty. The timing of the pubertal growth spurt differs between girls and boys. Girls begin pubertal development at a mean age of 11 years (range, 9 to 13.3 years), with breast enlargement generally the first sign of puberty. In girls, the pubertal growth spurt starts coincident with breast development and peaks before menarche. For girls with an average tempo of puberty, a mean peak growth velocity (8 to 9 cm/year) is reached at 11 to 12 years of age. After menarche, the growth rate declines. In boys, testicular enlargement is generally the first sign of puberty and occurs at a mean age of 11.6 years (range, 9 to 14.3 years). In boys with an average tempo of pubertal development, peak growth velocity occurs at approximately 14 years, with an average rate of 10.3 cm/year. The ultimate taller stature of boys relative to girls is

due, in part, to their longer period of prepubertal growth and to their higher peak growth velocity before puberty.

There are large variations in the timing of puberty—and therefore in growth rates—among individuals of the same age. Therefore, assessments of growth rates during adolescence should be made using longitudinally derived norms rather than cross-sectional data (see Fig. 62–2). In late puberty, growth decelerates and eventually ceases when the epiphyses have fused. After menarche, girls generally grow approximately 7 cm before reaching adult height. On average, growth is complete by age 15 and 16 years in girls and boys, respectively, but there are significant individual variations.

There are also racial variations in growth patterns and puberty. African-American children from ages 5 to 12 years are approximately 2 cm taller than white American children matched for family income, but after age 14 years, the groups do not differ significantly in height. The median height of Asian-American males is about 5 cm below that of white males before puberty, although there is a tendency to catch up after 14 years. By contrast, Asian-American females tend to be shorter than their white counterparts throughout childhood and adolescence.

Because of these characteristic patterns of growth during childhood and adolescence, the rate of growth (cm/year or inches/year) is a key variable in evaluating a short child. Growth rates may vary somewhat with season and can be affected by transient illness, but they should enable a child to maintain the growth channel on the linear growth percentile charts. A child whose rate of growth is consistently at the third percentile will not be able to sustain a height parallel to the normal curve (i.e., will fall below the growth

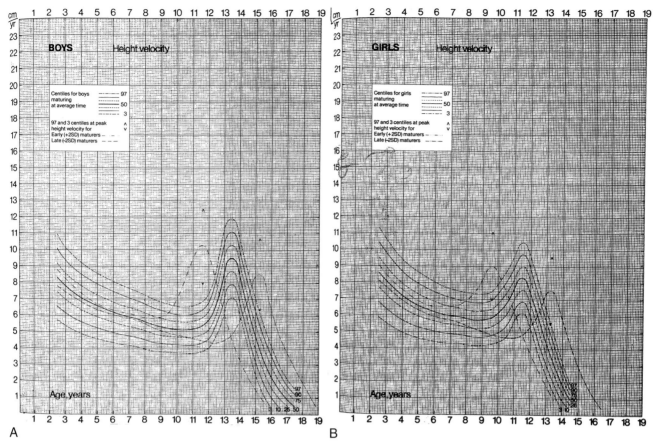

Figure 62–2. *A,* Height velocity for American boys. Lines with early velocity = 50th centile for boys 2 standard deviations (SD) of tempo early; lines with late or gradual velocity = 50th centile for boys 2 SD of tempo late. ∧ and ∨ = 97th and 3rd centiles for peak velocities of early and late maturers, respectively. *B,* Height velocity for American girls. Lines with early velocity = 50th centile for girls 2 SD of tempo early; lines with late or gradual velocity = 50th centile for girls 2 SD of tempo late. ∧ and ∨ = 97th and 3rd centiles for peak velocities of early and late maturers, respectively. (Redrawn from Tanner J, Davies P. Clinical longitudinal standards for height and height velocity for North American children. J Pediatr 1985;107:317–329.)

channel). A persistently slow rate of growth in relation to age-appropriate norms is alarming and is likely to reflect an underlying medical disorder. An exception is the adolescent boy with delayed puberty who may have an extended slow rate of growth.

MEASURING A CHILD

Stature is evaluated as supine length until 2 years of age and as standing height thereafter (Fig. 62–3). For measurement of supine length, the infant lies on an inflexible ruled horizontal surface, at one end of which the head is held in contact with a fixed board; a second person extends the infant's leg as much as possible and brings a movable plate in contact with the infant's heels. Recumbent measurements average 1 cm more than standing height. After 2 years of age, children are measured standing and barefoot with a device such as a Harpenden stadiometer; a vertical metal bar is affixed to an upright board or wall, with height being measured at the top of the head by a sliding perpendicular plate or block. In contrast to these techniques, measurements of length using pen marks at the head and foot of infants are often *grossly inaccurate,* as are height measurements using a flexible metal rod atop a standard weight scale.

With the use of optimal techniques, the variation in measurement among observers is less than 0.3 cm. It is then possible to determine changes in height over 3- to 4-month intervals to estimate the annualized growth rate. However, because of normal seasonal vari-

ations in growth rates, a longer interval between measurements (6 to 12 months) is more reliable.

Measurements are interpreted in terms of age-related norms for North American children. Heights (or length for infants) are plotted on standard growth charts for North American children (see Fig. 62–1). Calculated growth rates (cm/year or inches/year) should be evaluated in relation to age-related norms using growth velocity charts for North American children (see Fig. 62–2). These respective measurements enable assessment of the child's height in relation to age-specific norms and the child's growth rate in relation to age-matched peers. In addition, height may be plotted on charts relating the child's stature to mid-parental height to assess the child's height in relation to his or her genetic potential.

Other useful measurements in the assessment of the child's growth include the upper-to-lower segment ratio (U/L) (Fig. 62–4), the arm span, and the head circumference. The U/L is determined by measuring the lower segment (vertical distance between the symphysis pubis and the floor, with the child standing) and the upper segment (difference between the lower segment and height). The normal U/L is age-dependent (see Fig. 62–4) and differs among races. Disorders associated with short stature and abnormal body proportions include hypothyroidism (high U/L), certain skeletal dysplasias (high U/L), and irradiation-induced spinal damage (low U/L). *Arm span* refers to the distance between the outstretched middle fingertips with the child standing against a flat board or wall; disorders associated with short stature and abnormal arm span include certain skeletal dysplasias.

Weight should be considered in relation to a child's stature.

Table 62-1. Causes of Short Stature

Variations of Normal

Constitutional
Genetic

Endocrine Disorders

GH deficiency
  Congenital
    Isolated GH deficiency
    With other pituitary hormone deficiencies
    With midline defects
    Pituitary agenesis
    With IgG deficiency
  Acquired
    Hypothalamic/pituitary tumors
    Histiocytosis X
    CNS infections and granulomas
    Head trauma (birth and later)
    Hypothalamic/pituitary radiation
    CNS vascular accidents
    Hydrocephalus
    Autoimmune
    Psychosocial dwarfism (functional GH deficiency)
    Amphetamine treatment for hyperactivity (?)
Laron dwarfism (increased GH and decreased IGF-I)
Mutations in growth hormone receptor
Pygmies
Hypothyroidism
Glucocorticoid excess
  Endogenous
  Exogenous
Diabetes mellitus under poor control
Diabetes insipidus (untreated)
Hypophosphatemic vitamin D-resistant rickets
Virilizing congenital adrenal hyperplasia (tall child, short adult)

Skeletal Dysplasias

Osteogenesis imperfecta
Osteochondroplasias

Lysosomal Storage Diseases

Mucopolysaccharidoses
Mucolipidoses

Syndromes of Short Stature

Turner syndrome (gonadal dysgenesis)
Noonan syndrome (pseudo–Turner syndrome)
Autosomal trisomy 13, 18, 21
Prader-Willi syndrome
Laurence-Moon-Biedl syndrome
Autosomal abnormalities
Dysmorphic syndromes (Russell-Silver, Cornelia de Lange)
Pseudohypoparathyroidism

Chronic Disease

Cardiac disorders
  Left-to-right shunt
  Congestive heart failure
Pulmonary disorders
  Cystic fibrosis
  Asthma
Gastrointestinal disorders
  Malabsorption (e.g., celiac disease)
  Disorders of swallowing
  Inflammatory bowel disease
Hepatic disorders
Hematologic disorders
  Sickle cell anemia
  Thalassemia
Renal disorders
  Renal tubular acidosis
  Chronic uremia
Immunologic disorders
  Connective tissue disease
  Juvenile rheumatoid arthritis
  Chronic infection
  AIDS
Hereditary fructose intolerance

Malnutrition

Kwashiorkor, marasmus
Iron deficiency
Zinc deficiency
Anorexia due to chemotherapy of neoplasms

Modified from Styne DM. Growth disorder. *In* Fitzgerald PA (ed). Handbook of Clinical Endocrinology. Norwalk, Conn: Appleton & Lange, 1992:73–99.

Abbreviations: GH = growth hormone; IgG = immunoglobulin G; CNS = central nervous system; IgF = insulin-like growth factor; AIDS = acquired immunodeficiency syndrome.

Undernutrition is generally due to nonendocrine factors; less commonly, it is due to endocrinopathies such as poorly controlled diabetes mellitus or hyperthyroidism. Obesity in childhood is usually exogenous, reflecting in part overeating and sedentary habits rather than endocrine disturbances. Exogenous obesity is generally associated with an accelerated growth rate. By contrast, those endocrine disorders that do cause obesity (Cushing syndrome, hypothyroidism, and in some instances GH deficiency) as well as certain syndromes that cause obesity (Prader-Willi and Laurence-Moon-Biedl syndromes) are usually associated with slow growth. Therefore, the obese child who has a slow growth velocity is likely to have a serious underlying condition.

FACTORS THAT INFLUENCE LINEAR GROWTH IN CHILDHOOD

Familial and Genetic Factors

Both parental height and parental pattern of growth are key influences on a child's growth pattern. This strong familial influ-

ence on height is not detectable at birth but is manifested by 2 to 3 years of age. The correlation between child height and mid-parental height is 0.5 by 2 years of age. This trend becomes more pronounced with age, with the correlation coefficient of adult height with mid-parental height being 0.7.

In addition to the influence of actual height, parental patterns of growth are often repeated in their children. In particular, males who were "late bloomers" with delayed onset of puberty and delayed but normal growth spurts often have sons with a similar growth pattern. In addition to these normal familial or genetic influences on growth, other genetic disorders may interfere with growth (see Table 62–1).

Birth Size

See Fetal Growth and Birth Size earlier.

Nutrition

Adequate intake and metabolic utilization of nutrients are essential for normal growth. Poor nutritional intake or utilization first

Table 62-2. Potential Causes of Intrauterine Growth Retardation (IUGR)

Nutrition

Adolescents, especially those who are not married
Women with low prepregnancy weights
Women with inadequate weight gain during pregnancy
Women who have low income or problems purchasing food
Women with a history of frequent conceptions
Women with a history of infants having low birth weight
Women with diseases that influence nutritional status: diabetes, tuberculosis, anemia, drug addiction, alcoholism, or mental depression
Women known to be dietary faddists or with frank pica
Low maternal weight at mother's birth

Chronic Disease

Chronic maternal hypertension
Nephritis
Essential hypertension
Pregnancy-induced hypertension
Advanced maternal diabetes mellitus
Lupus anticoagulant
Severe cyanotic congenital heart disease
Eisenmenger's complex
Sickle cell anemia
Diminished environmental oxygen saturations at high altitudes

Drugs

Amphetamines
Antimetabolites (e.g., aminopterin, busulfan, methotrexate)
Bromides
Cigarettes (carbon monoxide, thiocyanate, nicotine)
Cocaine
Ethanol (acetaldehyde)
Heroin
Hydantoin
Isotretinoin
Methadone
Methylmercury
Phencyclidine
Polychlorinated biphenyls (PCBs)
Propranolol
Steroids (prednisone)
Toluene
Trimethadione (Tridione)
Warfarin

Placental Disorders

Twins (implantation site)
Twins (vascular anastomoses)
Chorioangioma
Villitis (TORCH)
Villitis (unknown etiology)
Avascular villi
Ischemic villous necrosis
Vasculitis (decidual arteritis)
Multiple infarcts
Syncytial knots
Chronic separation (abruptio placentae)
Diffuse fibrinosis
Hydatidiform change
Abnormal insertion
Single umbilical artery
Fetal vessel thrombosis
Circumvallate placenta

Fetal Disorders
Chromosomal Disorders Associated with IUGR

Trisomies 8, 13, 18, 21
Short-arm deletion 4
Long-arm deletion 13
Long-arm deletion 21
Triploidy
XO
XXY, XXXY, XXXXY
XXXXX

Metabolic Disorders Associated with IUGR

Agenesis of pancreas
Congenital absence of islets of Langerhans
Congenital lipodystrophy
Galactosemia (?)
Generalized gangliosidosis type I
Hypophosphatasia
I-cell disease
Leprechaunism
Maternal phenylketonuria
Maternal renal insufficiency
Maternal Gaucher disease
Menkes syndrome
Transient neonatal diabetes mellitus

Syndromes Associated with IUGR

Aarskog-Scott syndrome
Anencephaly
Bloom syndrome
Cornelia de Lange syndrome
Dubowitz syndrome
Dwarfism (e.g., achondrogenesis, achondroplasia)
Ellis–van Creveld syndrome
Familial dysautonomia
Fanconi pancytopenia
Meckel-Gruber syndrome
Microcephaly
Möbius syndrome
Mulitple congenital anomalads
Osteogenesis imperfecta
Potter disease
Prader-Willi syndrome
Progeria
Prune-belly syndrome
Radial aplasia; thrombocytopenia
Robert syndrome
Russell-Silver syndrome
Seckle syndrome
Smith-Lemli-Opitz syndrome
VATER and VACTERL syndromes
Williams syndrome

Congenital Infections Associated with IUGR

Rubella
Cytomegalovirus
Toxoplasmosis
Malaria
Syphilis
Varicella
Chagas disease

Abbreviations: TORCH = congenital intrauterine infections, toxoplasmosis, other (syphilis), rubella, cytomegalovirus, herpes; VATER = syndrome of vertebral, anal tracheoesophageal, renal anomalies; VACTERL = syndrome of vertebral, anal, cardiac, tracheoesophageal, renal and limb anomalies.

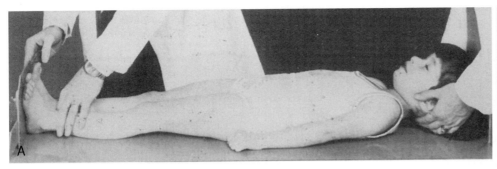
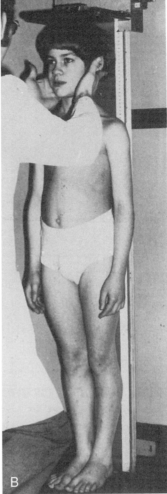

Figure 62–3. *A,* Technique for measuring length. *B,* Technique for measuring erect height. (From Wilson JD, Foster DW [eds]. Williams Textbook of Endocrinology, 8th ed. Philadelphia: WB Saunders, 1992:1106–1107.)

affects weight, and only when severe and prolonged does it affect height.

General Nonstatural Well-Being

As growth is a barometer of a child's health, general well-being and freedom from serious illness are necessary for a child to achieve the genetic growth potential. Chronic illnesses that are not primarily problems of stature often interfere with growth secondarily, and short stature may be the presenting feature of such conditions as inflammatory bowel disease, celiac disease, and rheumatoid arthritis.

Psychologic Factors

Under normal circumstances, emotional and psychologic factors do not have a great effect on growth. However, emotional distress under certain circumstances can interfere with growth (e.g., deprivation dwarfism).

Endocrine Influences

Growth hormone (GH) is essential for normal growth in childhood and adolescence. Its secretion from the pituitary gland is determined by a finely balanced interplay of stimulatory and inhibitory influences. The hypothalamic peptides, GH-releasing factor (GHRF) and somatostatin (somatotropin release inhibiting factor: SRIF) stimulate and inhibit GH secretion, respectively. GH is secreted episodically, with peak secretion occurring during sleep. It exerts its growth-promoting effect through stimulating the production of insulin-like growth factor I (IGF-I; also known as somatomedin C) as well as through a direct effect on bone. IGF-I, in turn, has a negative feedback effect to dampen pituitary GH release. Other factors (activin, Pit-1) also influence the production and secretion of GH. Deficiency of GH in a child markedly impairs height and growth rate.

Thyroid hormone is also essential for normal postnatal linear growth.

Glucocorticoids, in excess, stunt growth. Deficiency of glucocorticoids generally does not adversely affect growth if the child is otherwise healthy.

Sex steroids (estradiol and testosterone) mediate pubertal growth spurt in females and males, respectively. This probably involves direct effects of sex steroids on bone growth as well as indirect steroid-induced amplification of GH secretion. Sexual precocity (true precocious puberty, or congenital adrenal hyperplasia) tends to accelerate linear growth transiently due to premature or excessive production of sex steroids, or both. If not successfully treated, these conditions advance osseous maturation, leading to premature epiphyseal fusion and short adult height. Absence of sex steroids (hypogonadism) in the absence of other abnormalities does not tend to limit growth.

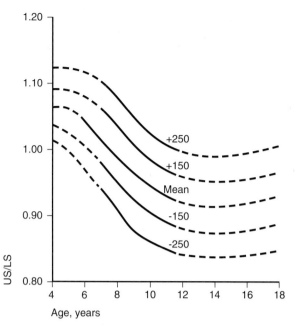

Figure 62–4. Normal upper to lower segment ratios (US/LS) for white children. (From McKusick V. Hereditable Disorders of Connective Tissue, 4th ed. St. Louis: CV Mosby, 1972.)

CAUSES OF SHORT STATURE

Understanding the factors that influence childhood growth leads directly to an understanding of the causes of short stature and to the differential diagnosis of short stature for an individual child (Tables 62–1 and 62–3). It is helpful to assess derangements of growth, in part, by the relationships among the child's chronologic age, growth rate, height age, weight age, and bone age (Table 62–4).

Familial or Genetic Causes

The two most frequent causes of short stature in children are familial and have been viewed as variants of normal. These are familial short stature and constitutional delay in growth and development.

FAMILIAL SHORT STATURE

The child with familial short stature comes from a short but otherwise normal family. The child's height is in keeping with the genetic endowment, and the child is otherwise healthy. Typically, one or both parents (and often other family members) are about 1.5 to 2 standard deviations below the mean in height. The child is usually noted to be small relative to peers by early childhood. Although the growth channel is low, it should parallel the normal growth curve. Continued deviation away from the normal growth curve (indicating a subnormal growth velocity) is not typical and should raise concerns about a disorder other than familial short stature (Fig. 62–5). Stature that is out of keeping with the family or that is extremely low (2.5 to 3 or more standard deviations below the mean) raises similar concerns. The review of systems is generally negative, as is the physical examination (aside from short stature). The height-to-weight ratio, body proportions, muscularity,

and pubertal development are normal for age. Abnormalities on review of systems or physical examination, or both, are unusual and prompt consideration of other diagnoses.

Laboratory studies are normal, including bone age. The normal bone age suggests that the short index child's "room for growth" is not greater than that of other children of the same age, indicating that the adult height is likely to be shorter than average. Actual predictions of adult height can be made, although the accuracy is variable; the predicted height is in keeping with family heights.

Familial short stature is generally believed to represent one end of the normal spectrum of height. It has been suggested that some of these children may have subtle disorders of GH or its receptor, but this has not been conclusively proven. In addition, inherited pathologic conditions, such as hypochondroplasia, may present in a manner similar to familial short stature and should be considered in the evaluation, particularly if the short stature is marked.

CONSTITUTIONAL DELAY

Constitutional delay in growth and development is a growth pattern that is traditionally also considered a variant of normal (see Fig. 62–5). It is recognized predominantly in boys and accounts for a high proportion of referrals for growth evaluation. The children often begin to show moderate short stature during early to

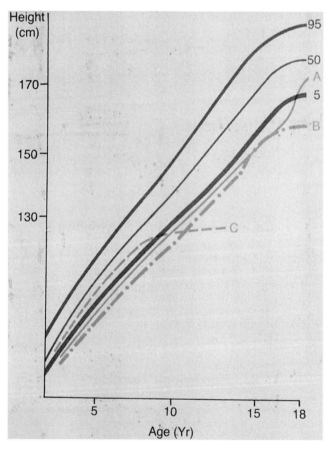

Figure 62–5. Patterns of linear growth. Normal growth percentiles (5th, 50th, 95th) are shown along with typical growth curves for constitutional delay of growth and adolescence (A), familial short stature (B), and acquired pathologic growth failure (C) (e.g., acquired primary hypothyroidism). (From Styne DM. Endocrine disorders. *In* Behrman RE, Kliegman RM [eds]. Nelson Essentials of Pediatrics, 2nd ed. Philadelphia: WB Saunders, 1994:616.)

Table 62–3. Differential Diagnosis and Therapy of Common Causes of Short Stature

	Hypopituitarism Including Gonadotropin Deficiency (Possibly with ACTH or TRH Deficiency)	Constitutional Delay	Familial Short Stature	Deprivational Dwarfism	Turner Syndrome	Hypothyroidism	Chronic Disease
Family history	Rare	Frequent	Always	No	No	Variable	Variable
Phenotypic sex	Both	Males > females	Both	Both	Female	Both	Both
Facies	Immature or with midline defect (e.g., cleft palate or optic hypoplasia)	Normal	Normal	Normal	Turner facies or normal	Coarse (cretin), or normal	Normal
Sexual development	Delayed	Delayed	Normal	Delayed	Prepubertal	Usually delayed, may be precocious if severe	Delayed
Bone age	Delayed	Delayed	Normal	Usually delayed; growth arrest lines	Delayed	Delayed	Delayed
Dentition	Delayed	Slight delay	Normal	Variable	Normal	Delayed	Normal
Hypoglycemia	Variable	No	No	No	No	No	No
Karyotype	Normal	Normal	Normal	Normal	45,X or partial deletion of X chromosome or mosaic	Normal	Normal
Free T_4	Low or normal	Normal	Normal	Normal or low	Normal: hypothyroidism may be acquired	Low	Normal
Stimulated growth hormone	Low	Normal	Normal	Possibly high	Usually normal	Low or normal	Variable
Insulin-like growth factor I	Low	Normal for bone age	Normal	Low or normal	Normal	Low or normal	Low or normal (depending on nutritional status)
Therapy	Replace deficiencies	Reassurance; sex steroids to initiate secondary sexual development in selected patients	None; GH therapy controversial	Change or improve environment	Sex hormone replacement, GH; oxandrolone appears useful	T_4	Treat malnutrition, organ failure (e.g., dialysis, transplant, cardiotonic drugs, insulin)

Modified from Styne DM. Endocrine disorders. *In* Behrman RE, Kliegman RM (eds). Nelson Essentials of Pediatrics, 2nd ed. Philadelphia: WB Saunders, 1994:618–619.
Abbreviations: ACTH = adrenocorticotropic hormone; TRH = thyrotropin-releasing hormone; T_4 = thyroxine; GH = growth hormone.

middle childhood but are otherwise healthy. They have delayed onset of puberty and therefore a delayed growth spurt. One or both parents (or other family members) usually have a history of delayed puberty, a late adolescent growth spurt, and cessation of growth at a late age. The affected parent usually is of normal adult stature. Otherwise, the history and review of systems are generally negative. The physical examination is generally normal except for delayed onset of puberty in children of an appropriate age.

Laboratory tests are normal, with the important exception of a delayed bone age (bone age < chronologic age). It suggests that

Table 62–4. Terms Used in the Evaluation of Short Children

Height age = the age for which the child's height would be average

Weight age = the age for which the child's weight would be average

Bone age = the age for which the child's osseous development, as assessed by radiographs of the wrist and sometimes the knee, would be average

Growth rate or growth velocity = the number of centimeters (or inches) the child grows in 1 yr

the child has more "room to grow" than the average age-matched child and that the child is likely to reach an adult height closer to the mean than the current height percentile. Some children have mixed familial short stature and constitutional delay in growth and development and tend to have both delayed puberty and a short predicted adult height.

Although constitutional delay is generally believed to represent a normal variant, it has been suggested that some children with this condition may have subtle dysregulation of GH secretion. Chronic illness may also mimic constitutional delay in growth and development and should be considered in the differential diagnosis. It is sometimes difficult to distinguish children with constitutional delay in growth and development from the more unusual condition of central (hypothalamic/pituitary) hypogonadism; a positive family history of delayed but normal puberty and growth, a normal sense of smell (to exclude Kallmann syndrome), and normal neurologic findings favor constitutional delay. Sometimes a gonadotropin-releasing hormone (GnRH) test, GnRH analog test, or sensitive assay of luteinizing hormone (LH) may help to distinguish the conditions.

The management of constitutional delay in growth development involves reassurance and sometimes a short course of low-dose sex steroids. The use of GH therapy in this condition is a subject of investigation.

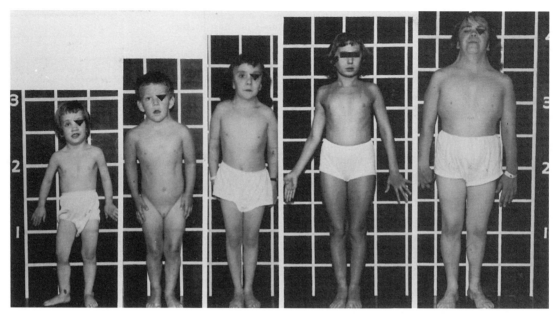

Figure 62–6. Five girls with 45,X syndrome illustrating the variability of features such as webbed neck and broad chest. (From Lemli L, Smith D. J Pediatr 1963;63:577.)

Chromosomal Abnormalities

A variety of genetic disorders and syndromes of unknown etiology are associated with short stature. Many chromosomal aberrations, bone dysplasias, and syndromes of unknown etiology are characterized by short stature. Important examples are described next and in Tables 62–1, 62–5, and 62–6.

TURNER SYNDROME

Turner syndrome and its variants (*gonadal dysgenesis*) are common causes of short stature in females, with an incidence of 1 in 2000 to 5000 liveborn female newborns. It is due to the absence or abnormality of an X chromosome, the classic form being 45,X. The major clinical features of Turner syndrome include short stat-

Table 62–5. Examples of Syndromes Associated with Short Stature*

Syndrome	Genetics	Major Features
Noonan (Turner-like)	Sporadic, occasionally AD	Short stature, mental retardation, webbed neck, cryptorchidism, pulmonic stenosis
Russell-Silver (Silver)	Sporadic, occasionally AD	Small stature of prenatal onset, asymmetry, occasionally chromosomal abnormalities, small triangular face, *café au lait* spots, occasionally fasting hypoglycemia in infancy, usually normal intelligence
Bloom	AR	Short stature of prenatal onset, malar hypoplasia, facial telangiectatic eczema, chromosomal fragility, malignancies
Williams	Sporadic	Moderate short stature of prenatal onset, cardiac anomalies (especially supravalvular aortic stenosis), hypercalcemia infrequent, unusual facies
Fetal alcohol	Environmental	Prenatal growth failure, microcephaly, short palpebral fissures, intellectual or behavioral impairment, joint and cardiac anomalies
Fanconi	AR	Short stature, radial hypoplasia, pigmentation, strabismus, small phallus/cryptorchidism, mental retardation, pancytopenia with time, chromosome fragility, leukemia
Laurence-Moon-Biedl	AR	Obesity, mental deficiency, poly/syndactyly, retinitis pigmentosa, hypogonadism
Prader-Willi	Deletion chromosome 15	Obesity, hypotonia, mental retardation, hypogonadism, small hands and feet

*Excluding those with chromosomal abnormalities and excluding bone dysplasias.
Abbreviations: AD = autosomal dominant; AR = autosomal recessive.

Table 62–6. **Examples of Bone Dysplasias (Osteochondrodystrophies)**

Disorder	Genetics	Characteristics
Achondroplasia	AD	Most common osteochondrodystrophy (1:26,000), short limbs, macrocephaly, low nasal bridge, caudal narrowing of spinal canal, occasionally hydrocephalus
Hypochondroplasia	AD	Short stature, short limbs, relative lack of craniofacial in comparison to achondroplasia
Acromesomelic dysplasia	AR	Short distal limbs, kyphosis, frontal prominence
Kniest syndrome	Sporadic	Flat facies, enlarged joints, platyspondyly
Kozowski spondylometaphyseal dysplasia	AD	Short spine, pectus carinatum, irregular metaphyses
Schmid metaphyseal chondrodysplasia syndrome	AD	Metaphyseal dysostosis, tibial bowing, flared lower ribs

Abbreviations: AD = autosomal dominant; AR = autosomal recessive.

ure and ovarian failure (Fig. 62–6). The birth size may be slightly small, a webbed neck may be evident, and there may be lymphedema beginning in the neonatal period (manifesting mainly as puffy hands and feet). By early childhood, marked short stature is usually noted and there is progressive deviation of height away from the normal growth curve. Linear growth is further attenuated during the teenage years. The natural history includes a mean adult height of 142 cm. Even in females with Turner syndrome, adult height is influenced by the height of the parents. Breast enlargement and menses generally fail to occur as a result of ovarian failure; rarely, females with mosaicism develop some of these secondary sex characteristics because of functioning ovarian tissue, and in a few cases fertility has been reported. In addition to short stature and ovarian failure, there are frequent dysmorphic features, including

webbed neck, low posterior hairline, increased carrying angle of the arm, pigmented nevi, short fourth metacarpals, nail abnormalities, and renal and cardiac anomalies (coarctation of the aorta).

A karyotype analysis is necessary to rule in or out the diagnosis of Turner syndrome in any girl with short stature of unknown etiology. Additional laboratory features may include abnormally high levels of the gonadotropins LH and follicle-stimulating hormone (FSH), indicative of ovarian failure; however, levels may be normal in midchildhood because of normal central nervous system suppression of gonadotropin secretion at that time.

Ovarian failure in Turner syndrome is managed by sex steroid replacement therapy, beginning near adolescence. GH therapy (alone or with low-dose oxandrolone) may increase the height of girls with Turner syndrome.

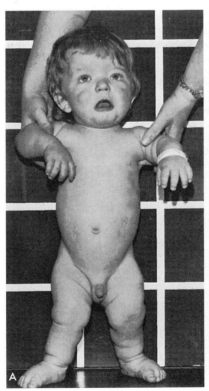 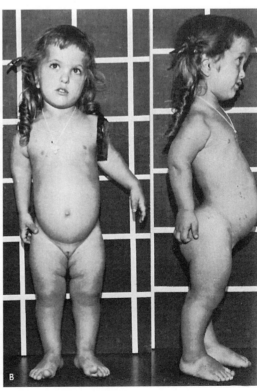

Figure 62–7. Achondroplasia. *A,* One-year-old boy with height age of 4 months. (From Smith DW. J Pediatr 1967;70: 504.) *B,* Four-year-old girl with height age of 20 months. (From Jones KL [ed]. Smith's Recognizable Patterns of Human Malformation, 4th ed. Philadelphia: WB Saunders, 1988.)

PRADER-WILLI SYNDROME

Prader-Willi syndrome is marked by infantile hypotonia, hypogonadism, mental retardation, acromicria, obesity with a voracious appetite, and short stature (average adult height, 147 cm and 155 cm in females and males, respectively). Abnormalities of chromosome 15 have been described.

DOWN SYNDROME

A prominent feature in Down syndrome is short stature. The cause of impaired growth is not known. It is independent of the hypothyroidism that may also occur in this condition. The short stature has traditionally not been amenable to treatment. GH therapy may increase linear growth in Down syndrome. However, this is very controversial—both because of a need for controlled studies and because of concern for possible untoward effects of GH in these children.

BONE DYSPLASIAS

Bone dysplasias (*osteochondrodystrophies*) constitute a group of disorders wherein there is innate failure of bone or cartilage to grow normally. Abnormal body proportions are characteristic of these conditions (disproportionate short stature), although there are some exceptions. Many bone dysplasias are inherited, often in an autosomal dominant pattern. Bone ages are not reliable indicators of osseous maturity in these conditions. Examples of bone dysplasias are described next and in Table 62–6.

Achondroplasia

Achondroplasia is the classic example of an osteochondrodystrophy (Fig. 62–7). The incidence is 1 in 26,000. Short stature, body disproportion with short limbs, and a relatively large head are often noted at birth. Progressive deceleration of growth rate begins in infancy, and the humerus and femur are particularly shortened. In addition, there may be hydrocephalus due to narrowing of the foramen magnum, kyphosis, stenosis of the spinal canal, and vertebral disc lesions. The diagnosis is clinical and is supported by characteristic radiologic features that include small cuboid vertebral bodies and anterior beaking of the first or second lumbar vertebra. There is currently no effective therapy for short stature in this condition.

Hypochondroplasia

Hypochondroplasia manifests with short stature and dysmorphic features that are often more mild than in achondroplasia. In particular, there are few craniofacial abnormalities and body disproportion may be subtle. Newborns may be slightly small, but short stature generally becomes apparent by age 3 years. The short stature is minimally disproportionate with relatively short limbs. The hands and feet are usually stubby. Genu varum may occur. Radiologic hallmarks include metaphyseal indentation and flaring as well as hypoplasia of the ilia with small greater sciatic notches. Some reports suggest a beneficial effect of GH.

Malnutrition

Worldwide, poverty and associated malnutrition are the commonest causes of short stature. In North America, malnutrition may arise from inadequate intake secondary to poverty or deprivation, poor intake secondary to overt or occult chronic illness (inflammatory bowel disease, renal failure), or inability to utilize food intake (malabsorption, see Chapter 19). Weight tends to be depressed to a greater degree than height (weight age < height age). The history should include review of the child's food intake (often best obtained by a 3-day diet record), appetite, and detailed review of systems. Specific nutritional disorders, such as rickets, may also lead to short stature.

Chronic Illness

Chronic illnesses, such as inflammatory bowel disease, celiac disease, renal dysfunction, and chronic inflammation, lead to short stature. The mechanisms of impaired growth include poor appetite or poor intake (inflammatory bowel disease, renal dysfunction), malabsorption (celiac disease), medications (chronic glucocorticoids for severe asthma), chronic acidosis (renal tubular acidosis), chronic inflammation (poor or excessive nutrient utilization), and secondary endocrine dysfunction (low levels of insulin-like growth factor [IGF] binding protein in renal failure). Although the primary disorder is evident in many cases, sometimes short stature is the presenting feature of the chronic disease. This occurs notably in inflammatory bowel disease, celiac disease, and renal dysfunction.

The history typically reveals that the child had been growing normally until some point. Then growth rate slowed, suggesting that an illness had been acquired. The history may reveal a clear earlier diagnosis of chronic illness or may instead include symptoms suggestive of the underlying disorder (for inflammatory bowel disease, loss of appetite, diarrhea, mouth sores, fevers). The physical examination typically shows that the weight is depressed more than the height. There may also be features indicative of the underlying disorder (pallor, buttock adipose tissue wasting, edema in celiac disease).

Laboratory studies that screen for chronic illness (complete blood count, erythrocyte sedimentation rate, chemistry profile, urinalysis) may at times provide clues to the diagnosis. If indicated by the clinical features and screening laboratory studies, definitive diagnosis requires directed tests (endoscopy and biopsy for inflammatory bowel disease or celiac disease, sweat chloride test for cystic fibrosis).

The management of these conditions rests on specific therapy directed at the underlying condition (gluten-free diet for celiac disease). When adequately treated, the growth rate often improves. GH therapy is approved for the treatment of short stature in children with renal failure before renal transplantation. GH is also under investigation for the treatment of short stature in association with some other chronic conditions.

Emotional Deprivation

Deprivation can stunt growth in two ways. First, a child may be deprived of food (an example of malnutrition); in this case the child's weight is generally depressed more than the height. Second, a child who is emotionally deprived may have profound short stature without apparent malnutrition. In this case, the height is depressed more than the weight (Fig. 62–8). The child may have the clinical features of GH deficiency and may in fact show laboratory evidence of hypopituitarism. When placed in a more nurturing

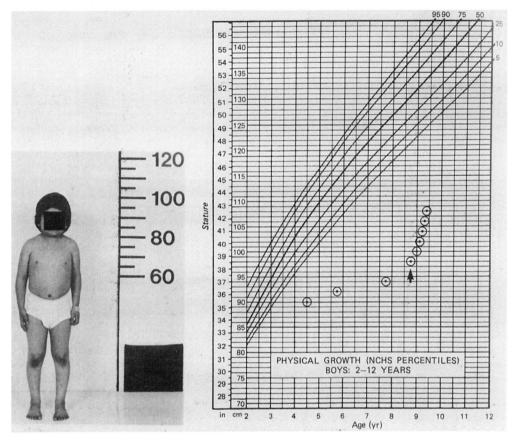

Figure 62–8. Photograph and growth chart of a boy with deprivation dwarfism (psychosocial dwarfism). Between ages 6 and 8⁷⁄₁₂ years, he had chemical evidence of growth hormone (GH) deficiency. After placement in a chronic care facility *(arrow)*, his growth rate improved markedly and his GH tests reverted to normal. (From Styne DM. Growth. *In* Greenspan FS, and Forsham PH [eds]. Basic and Clinical Endocrinology, 3rd ed. Los Altos, Calif: Appleton & Lange, 1991.)

environment, the child grows markedly and the GH tests revert to normal. This disorder may be difficult to diagnose, and the social history is critical. The diagnosis ultimately rests on significant improvement of growth once the environment improves.

Endocrine Disorders

GROWTH HORMONE DEFICIENCY

GH deficiency is a cause for short stature in some children. GH is essential for postnatal growth, and children who lack it will be extremely stunted. GH deficiency may be congenital or acquired. The congenital form may be idiopathic, associated with midline defects (absence of the septum pellucidum and optic nerve hypoplasia [septo-optic dysplasia], cleft palate, holoprosencephaly, single central incisor), or inherited (in association with defects of the GH gene or of the transcription factor Pit-1 that regulates the GH gene). Rarely, functional GH deficiency may occur due to an abnormal GH molecule. GH deficiency may be acquired secondary to birth injury, head injury, or other trauma, cranial irradiation, and midline tumors or masses (craniopharyngioma). Both congenital and acquired forms may be associated with isolated GH deficiency or with multiple pituitary hormone deficiencies (panhypopituitarism).

The presenting features may differ according to whether the condition is congenital or acquired and according to the etiology of GH deficiency. Infants are often normal in birth size, although statistical analysis suggests that, as a group, they are somewhat small. Some newborns with congenital GH deficiency show hypoglycemia in the newborn period; they may also have jaundice with a hepatitis-type picture; males may have micropenis (particularly if there is also gonadotropin deficiency). Other infants with congenital GH deficiency show no signs in the newborn period but later in infancy show slow growth. Poor linear growth usually becomes clear by age 3 years.

In acquired forms of GH deficiency, there may be a history of a precipitating event (cranial irradiation, head trauma) or a history suggesting an intracranial lesion (headaches, vomiting, visual disturbances). Such children often had normal growth until the point at which the disorder began; thereafter, their growth is attenuated.

On physical examination, children with GH deficiency are typically short and look younger than their actual age. The children are often chubby or cherubic, and their height is depressed more than their weight (height age < weight age). They often have high-pitched voices, delayed dentition, and poor musculature. In congenital GH deficiency, there may be midline defects and, in males, microphallus. In acquired GH deficiency, there may be evidence of the underlying disturbance (bitemporal hemianopsia, optic atrophy, or papilledema in midline tumors such as craniopharyngioma; dermatitis, scalp lesions, hepatosplenomegaly in histiocytosis X). Those with panhypopituitarism may show failure to enter or progress normally through puberty.

Classically, the diagnosis of GH deficiency is based on short stature, with a slow growth rate for age, delayed bone age (bone age = height age < chronologic age), and subnormal GH levels (<7 or 10 ng/ml) in response to two pharmacologic stimuli (clonidine, arginine, L-dopa with or without propranolol, insulin-induced hypoglycemia). Random GH levels are of no value in the diagnosis of GH deficiency. The GH tests must be done in a euthyroid individual. Levels of IGF-I tend to be low in GH deficiency but may be affected by age, puberty, and nutrition and therefore, are not diagnostic. IGF binding protein 3 levels may also provide clues to GH deficiency. Once the diagnosis of GH deficiency is made, magnetic resonance imaging scans are performed to assess the possibility of an intracranial tumor or structural abnormality causing the GH deficiency. Evaluation of other pituitary hormones is also needed. Children with classic GH deficiency respond well to

GH therapy and often more than double their rates of growth once treatment is begun. Treatment is needed until epiphyses have fused in order to maximize linear growth. Some studies suggest that GH-deficient individuals who have completed growth may benefit from GH therapy.

There is controversy about whether the classic definition of GH deficiency is too rigid and whether there may be children with mild or subtle forms of GH deficiency who are missed by the classic criteria. Some physicians advocate therapeutic trials of GH for selected individuals, but the criteria for undertaking and evaluating such trials are controversial.

In addition to GH deficiency, another defect of the GH axis is end-organ resistance to GH (*Laron syndrome*). This has been considered a rare condition that is associated with high circulating levels of GH and low levels of IGF-I. Laron syndrome may be more common than previously thought; studies to assess the effect of IGF-I therapy in this condition are underway.

HYPOTHYROIDISM

Hypothyroidism, or a deficiency of thyroid hormone, has been shown to impair linear growth (see Fig. 62–5). Thyroid deficiency may be congenital or acquired (Fig. 62–9). Given the usefulness of newborn thyroid screening programs, it is very uncommon for congenital hypothyroidism to cause short stature.

Acquired hypothyroidism in children is usually due to autoimmune thyroiditis (see Chapter 50). Children with Turner syndrome, Down syndrome, Klinefelter syndrome, or diabetes mellitus are at increased risk for autoimmune hypothyroidism, as are children with a family history of autoimmune disease. Acquired hypothyroidism tends to present most commonly in older children and teenagers. Often there are few complaints except for slow growth (after previously normal growth), weight gain, or a goiter, or a combination of these. Other symptoms (dry hair or skin, constipation, cold intolerance) are less common. Postmenarchal girls may have amenorrhea or, rarely, galactorrhea. School performance is generally not impaired. On physical examination, the major features are a height suggesting deceleration from the previous growth curve, a goiter, and relative obesity (weight age > height age). The physical examination may also reveal bradycardia, dry hair or skin, and delayed reflexes.

In acquired hypothyroidism, the laboratory tests often include a high level of thyroid-stimulating hormone (TSH) and a low or low-normal free thyroxine (T_4) or free thyroxine index (FTI). Positive thyroid antibodies (antithyroglobulin, antimicrosomal antibodies) are consistent with autoimmune thyroiditis. A low or normal TSH level in the presence of low free T_4 or FTI would suggest that the child does not have a primary thyroid problem but instead may have a hypothalamic/pituitary abnormality leading to deficiency of TSH (alternatively, the child could have euthyroid sick syndrome, a concomitant of serious illness). The bone age is often significantly delayed in hypothyroidism.

The treatment of hypothyroidism is thyroid replacement therapy (L-thyroxine). Monitoring of free T_4 (or FTI) and TSH is essential to optimize the dose of medication. Unduly large doses may advance osseous maturation or lead to symptoms of thyroid excess.

CUSHING SYNDROME

Cushing syndrome results from excessive levels of glucocorticoids. Whether endogenous or exogenous, glucocorticoids markedly stunt growth. Generally, because such conditions are acquired, the history reveals a child previously growing well whose growth velocity slows. The child typically continues to gain weight at a rapid rate, even though linear growth is attenuated. This contrasts with exogenous obesity in which children tend to grow at normal or rapid rate. The history may indicate that the child was treated with oral, topical (especially with occlusive dressings), or intradermal glucocorticoids in high doses or for long durations. Alternate-day oral steroids are much less likely to attenuate growth than daily steroids. In endogenous Cushing syndrome, the history may include acne, evidence of virilization, large appetite or hyperpig-

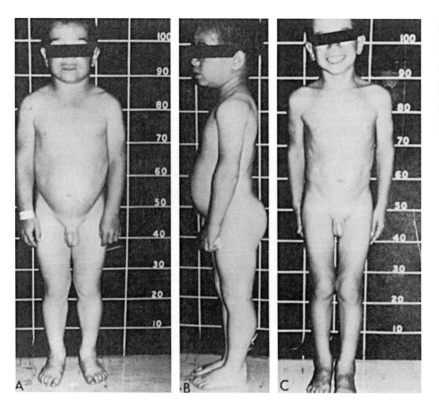

Figure 62–9. *A and B*, A 10-year-old boy with acquired hypothyroidism before treatment. Note short stature, immature body proportions, sleepy expression, generalized myxedema, and protuberant abdomen. *C*, After 4 months of thyroid hormone therapy, the child has grown, has lost myxedema, and has a bright facial expression. (From Kaplan SA [ed]. Clinical Pediatric and Adolescent Endocrinology. Philadelphia: WB Saunders, 1982.)

mentation (due to excess adrenocorticotropic hormone [ACTH] in Cushing syndrome due to pituitary tumors or ectopic ACTH production).

The physical examination usually reveals short stature with relative obesity. The child often has the moon face and plethora characteristic of Cushing syndrome. A buffalo hump, striae, acne, and hypertension may also be present. Marked virilization is worrisome, as it may suggest an adrenal tumor.

The diagnosis of endogenous Cushing syndrome is based on demonstrating abnormally high glucocorticoid production (on 24-hour urine sample for free cortisol, normalized to creatinine) and failure to suppress cortisol production adequately in response to exogenous glucocorticoid. A screening test for capacity to suppress cortisol secretion in response to exogenous glucocorticoid is the overnight dexamethasone suppression test. This involves the child taking 0.3 mg/m² of dexamethasone at 11 P.M. (the standard dose of dexamethasone in adults is 1 mg), followed by a measurement of circulating cortisol the following morning; a normal cortisol level after dexamethasone is less than 5 μg/ml. False-positive results may occur in obesity, chronic illness, or stress. If cortisol production is excessive or is not suppressed in an overnight dexamethasone test, formal high- and low-dose dexamethasone tests are needed to define the presence and nature of hypercortisolism. If the child shows biochemical evidence of Cushing syndrome, further investigations, including computed tomography and magnetic resonance imaging scans and ACTH levels are needed to determine whether it is due to a pituitary tumor (commonest cause), an adrenal tumor, or ectopic ACTH production. Exogenous Cushing syndrome is usually evident from the history and physical examination; when necessary, the diagnosis can be confirmed by failure of the child to secrete cortisol normally after administration of ACTH (ACTH stimulation test) together with clinical evidence of Cushing syndrome.

Treatment involves the removal of excess glucocorticoids either by reducing or discontinuing exogenous steroids if medically feasible or, in the case of endogenous hypercortisolism due to a pituitary or adrenal tumor, by surgery.

DIABETES

Diabetes mellitus, when poorly controlled, can lead to slow linear growth. This is probably due to lack of biologically available nutrients. The diagnosis should be apparent by history. However, given the risk of autoimmune thyroiditis, slow-growing children with diabetes should also be checked for hypothyroidism.

Diabetes insipidus, when poorly controlled or untreated, may lead to slow growth. This is presumed to reflect poor caloric intake associated with intense thirst and should be alleviated with adequate replacement of vasopressin.

Iatrogenic Causes

Treatments for medical conditions may secondarily impair growth. The classic example is glucocorticoids. Spinal irradiation for treatment of malignancies may stunt growth by limiting further spinal growth; this is associated with a high U/L. It has also been suggested that certain treatments for hyperactivity (sympathomimetic agents suppress appetite) may interfere with growth.

EVALUATING THE CHILD WITH SHORT STATURE (Tables 62–7 and 62–8)

History

PREGNANCY AND BIRTH HISTORY

Did the mother have illnesses or take medication during the pregnancy? Maternal illness or use of certain drugs can cause poor fetal growth.

What was the birth weight and length? IUGR tends to lead to continuing small stature.

Table 62–7. Growth Failure: Screening Test

Test	Rationale
CBC	*Anemia:* nutritional, chronic disease, malignancy, Fanconi's *Leukocytosis:* inflammation, infection *Leukopenia:* bone marrow failure syndromes *Thrombocytopenia:* malignancy, infection, Fanconi's
ESR and CRP	Inflammation of infection, inflammatory diseases, malignancy
SMA 20 (electrolytes, liver enzymes, BUN)	Signs of acute or chronic hepatic, renal, adrenal dysfunction; hydration and acid-base status
Carotene and prothrombin time	Assess malabsorption of vitamin A and K
Urinalysis	Signs of renal dysfunction, hydration, water and salt homeostasis; renal tubular acidosis
Karyotype	Determines Turner or other chromosomal syndromes
Cranial imaging (MRI, CT)	Assesses hypothalamic-pituitary tumors (craniopharyngioma, glioma, germinoma) or congenital midline defects
Bone age	Compare with height age, and eventual height potential
IGF-I, IGF BP3	Reflects GH status
Free thyroxine	Detects panhypopituitarism or isolated hypothyroidism
Prolactin	Elevated in hypothalamic dysfunction or destruction

From Styne DM. Endocrine disorders. *In* Behrman RE, Kliegman RM (eds). Nelson Essentials of Pediatrics, 2nd ed. Philadelphia: WB Saunders, 1994:618–620.
Abbreviations: CBC = complete blood count; ESR = erythrocyte sedimentation rate; CRP = C-reactive protein; MRI = magnetic resonance imaging; CT = computed tomography; IGF = insulin-like growth factor; BP3 = binding protein 3; GH = growth hormone.

Table 62–8. An Approach to Laboratory Tests in the Evaluation of Short Stature

If a child has significant short stature, a slow growth rate, and/or is short for midparental height:

a. If there is strong clinical evidence as to the etiology, may do specific directed studies (e.g., in a child with short stature, goiter, and clinical evidence of hypothyroidism, check free T_4 and TSH.)

b. If the cause of short stature is not evident clinically, do screening tests:
CBC with differential and platelet count, ESR, chemistry profile, urinalysis, free T_4 or free thyroxine index, TSH, bone age (IGF-I and IGF binding protein 3 are also checked by some physicians).

If the screening tests are normal, either:

a. Recheck growth rate in 3 to 6 mo. If growth rate is low, do further studies (karyotype in girls, GH stimulation tests).

   or

b. If the child is markedly short or there is other reason for immediate concern, may do above tests (e.g., karyotype, GH stimulation tests) as part of the initial evaluation (note: the child should be proven euthyroid before undertaking GH stimulation tests).

Abbreviations: T_4 = thyroxine; TSH = thyroid-stimulating hormone; CBC = complete blood count; ESR = erythrocyte sedimentation rate; IGF = insulin-like growth factor; GH = growth hormone.

Did the baby have perinatal problems such as unexplained hypoglycemia, prolonged jaundice, or, in boys, a small phallus? These suggest congenital GH deficiency.

Did the baby have other perinatal problems (hypoxia, puffy extremities)? These may provide clues to the underlying etiology of short stature (hypoxia might lead to hypopituitarism; puffy extremities in a female suggests Turner syndrome).

INFANCY AND CHILDHOOD

What was the child's growth pattern? Establishing a child's growth pattern is aided by obtaining previous height measurements and plotting them on standard growth charts. The child who has been short but growing at a normal rate and paralleling the fifth percentile is more likely to have familial or constitutional short stature. The child whose height deviates progressively away from the normal curve (especially after 24 months) is much more likely to have an underlying medical disorder. When this progressive deviation occurs from early childhood and continues, it often represents a congenital disorder (Turner syndrome, congenital GH deficiency). However, if growth attenuation occurs after a sustained period of normal growth, it suggests that a disorder has been acquired (acquired GH deficiency, inflammatory bowel disease).

Two periods of life may be associated with crossing of percentiles in normal children. During the first 24 months of life, normal children may shift height percentiles while "finding their own growth channels" and thereafter tend to maintain that channel throughout childhood. It may be difficult to distinguish this normal "finding of one's own growth channel" from a true abnormality, and assessing the child's growth in relation to genetic endowment and general well-being may be helpful. Children with constitutional delay of growth and pubertal development may have a prolonged slowdown of growth before entering puberty.

What were the child's developmental milestones? How is the school performance? Slow development or poor school performance may suggest a central disorder or may represent part of a syndrome (Prader-Willi syndrome). Hypothyroidism acquired after age 3 years usually does not interfere with school performance, although inadequately treated congenital hypothyroidism often leads to intellectual impairment. This question may also elicit a history of emotional problems.

Has the child had any serious illnesses or been on medication? Chronic illness often impedes growth, as do certain medications (glucocorticoids). A history of nonendocrine medical problems may also provide clues to the underlying disorder (a history of aortic coarctation may suggest Turner syndrome).

What has been the impact of short stature on the child? This will help to assess the emotional ramifications of short stature on the child and may help to clarify the particular concerns or questions of the parents.

Review of Systems

How is the child's appetite? What does the child eat in a typical 3-day period (often best described by a formal diet record)? Adequate caloric intake is needed for growth. Inadequate intake may be a symptom of underlying chronic disease.

Does the child have abdominal pain, diarrhea, unexplained fevers, mouth or anal sores, or joint pain? These are among the symptoms that suggest occult inflammatory bowel disease.

Does the child have neck swelling, lethargy, constipation, cold intolerance, or weight gain without much increase in height? These are among the symptoms of acquired hypothyroidism.

Does the child have headaches, vomiting, or visual disturbances? Symptoms of central nervous system dysfunction or raised intracranial pressure, or both, suggest the possibility of acquired hypopituitarism in association with a central lesion such as a tumor or hydrocephalus.

Has the child begun pubertal development (appropriate for a child of pubertal age)? Puberty influences growth. Children with constitutional delay in growth and development have delayed puberty and often have an exaggerated nadir of growth velocity before puberty begins. However, the more puberty is delayed, the greater the likelihood of a medical disorder such as hypogonadism.

Delayed puberty may be a manifestation of hypogonadism (Turner syndrome) or be secondary to a growth-impeding disorder (hypothyroidism or hypopituitarism).

Family History

What were the heights of parents and other family members at the child's age, and when did they undergo puberty? What are the current heights of parents and family members? The most frequent causes of short stature are familial short stature and constitutional delay in growth and development. In the former, a family history of short stature is elicited. In the latter, a family history of delayed puberty is elicited. The child's height may be assessed more formally in relation to that of the parents using midparental height charts. Some familial disorders are associated with short stature (hypochondroplasia).

Who lives at home? Who are the primary caregivers? As deprivation can lead to stunted growth, it is important to have a sense of the family situation, although it is often extremely difficult to define this fully.

Physical Examination

Height and weight should each be plotted carefully on growth charts. The degree of short stature relative to peers is ascertained.

If previous height measurements are available, they provide an index of the child's pattern of growth. The height-to-weight ratio should be noted. If the weight is depressed more than height in a short child, it suggests chronic illness or malnutrition. By contrast, a child who is short but chubby is more likely to have an endocrine disorder or syndrome (GH deficiency, hypothyroidism, Cushing syndrome, Prader-Willi syndrome).

Exogenous obesity is usually associated with relatively tall stature. Disproportionate short stature (especially short legs and arms, leading to a high U/L or short arm span, or both) is characteristic of many osteochondrodystrophies. Short lower limbs may also occur in hypothyroidism.

The presence of *dysmorphic features* often suggests a syndrome or genetic disorder (e.g., Turner syndrome, Noonan syndrome). Midline defects suggest hypopituitarism.

Goiter, delayed dentition, bradycardia, dry hair or skin, or delayed reflexes may suggest hypothyroidism.

Cherubic or doll-like appearance, high-pitched voice, delayed dentition, poor musculature, and relative adiposity may suggest GH deficiency.

Bitemporal hemianopsia, papilledema or optic atrophy, or accelerating head circumference in a young child suggests a central nervous system abnormality (craniopharyngioma) causing hypopituitarism.

The *stage of puberty* is noted. Delayed puberty is compatible with constitutional delay in growth and development, hypogonadism, panhypopituitarism, severe hypothyroidism, or chronic illness. The degree of pubertal development also often correlates with the bone age, thus indicating the growth potential.

CLINICAL SYNTHESIS AND LABORATORY EVALUATION (see Tables 62–7 and 62–8)

If the child is moderately short (1.5 to 2 standard deviations below normal for age), is paralleling the normal height curve, has a family history of short stature or delayed puberty, and is otherwise healthy, it is reasonable to do no further investigations initially and simply to follow the growth carefully. A bone age may be helpful to indicate growth potential and to distinguish, to some degree, familial short stature from constitutional delay in growth and development.

The bone age is the age at which the observed degree of bone maturation would be typical. Bone growth is normally accompanied by a predictable sequence, rate, and morphology of bone maturation. Bone age correlates more closely with overall body maturation than height or chronologic age. The degree of bone maturation is inversely proportional to the amount of epiphyseal cartilage growth remaining and therefore can be used cautiously to predict adult height; the more delayed the bone age, the greater the growth potential as long as no medical disorder is present. Despite their usefulness, predictions of adult height have intrinsic variability.

If on follow-up it appears that the child's growth is decelerating, further studies may be needed.

If a child is more markedly short (>2 to 2.5 standard deviations below the mean), has a decelerating growth pattern (crossing percentiles), is short for the genetic endowment, or is unwell, further investigations are needed. The specific investigations depend on the clinical findings. If there is clear evidence of a specific disorder (disproportionate short stature suggesting osteochondrodystrophies, a goiter suggesting hypothyroidism, dysmorphic features suggesting Turner syndrome), the appropriate investigations are needed (skeletal survey, thyroid function tests, karyotype). If the specific disorder is not clear, screening tests are needed to assess growth potential (bone age), hypothyroidism (free T_4 [or FTI] and TSH), and the possibility of chronic illness as a cause of short stature (complete blood count, differential and platelet count, erythrocyte sedimenta-

tion rate, chemistry profile, urinalysis). Girls with unexplained short stature should be assessed for Turner syndrome by karyotype analysis. Levels of IGF-I and IGF binding protein 3 may provide clues to presence or absence of GH deficiency.

If these tests are normal, the child's height may be followed carefully at 3- to 4-month intervals to establish the growth velocity; a slow growth velocity for age warrants evaluation for possible GH deficiency (formal GH stimulation tests) or other disorders. Alternatively, if the child's stature or well-being is excessively impaired, GH stimulation tests may be undertaken as part of the initial evaluation once the child is established to be euthyroid.

THERAPEUTIC OPTIONS

Specific Treatment of the Primary Disorder

If the child is found to have a clear medical condition causing short stature and for which treatment is available (hypothyroidism, GH deficiency), the appropriate treatment (thyroid replacement therapy or GH therapy, respectively) improves growth markedly as long as the epiphyses remain open. Often, the child experiences accelerated growth (catch-up growth) for a period of time after appropriate treatment is instituted. The term "catch-up growth" refers to a period of rapid growth that occurs spontaneously after relief from an illness that had suppressed the rate of growth. Complete compensation for growth failure is unlikely if the disorder was many years in duration or occurred very close to the onset of normal puberty.

SEX STEROIDS

Sex steroid treatments may be utilized for adolescents with constitutional delay of growth and development. Boys with delayed puberty may be treated with testosterone enanthate (50 to 100 mg IM/month for approximately 3 to 6 months) to gradually bring about secondary sexual characteristics and some linear growth. This is often gratifying for boys and is followed by gradual spontaneous pubertal development. The low dose of testosterone is designed to avoid undue advancement of bone age and loss of growth potential. Bone age should be followed.

COUNSELING

Reassurance and counseling should be available for all patients. For many children with familial short stature or constitutional delay in growth and development, it is reassuring to be told that they are normal and are likely to reach a normal adult height or one in keeping with the family heights. This is particularly true for children with delayed puberty in whom the discrepancy in height compared to peers (who have gone through their pubertal growth spurts) is disconcerting. It is helpful if parents do not dwell on the child's height but focus on other areas of strength for the child. Gymnastics, wrestling, soccer, and swimming are often activities at which short children are not at a disadvantage and in which they may excel.

GROWTH HORMONE THERAPY

GH therapy for short children who do not have GH deficiency is controversial. The issues include whether there may be subtle

Table 62–9. "Red Flags" in the Evaluation of Short Stature

Height > 2–2.5 standard deviations below the mean for age
Subnormal growth velocity
Abnormal body proportions
Abnormal height:weight ratio
Dysmorphic features
Goiter
Abnormal central nervous system examination

forms of GH deficiency not detected by current methods and whether GH treatment may increase the height of short children who clearly do not have GH deficiency. The controversy centers on issues of efficacy, safety, and ethics.

GH therapy at this time has been approved for the treatment of growth failure due to lack of adequate endogenous GH and for growth failure associated with chronic renal insufficiency. GH has also been used in the treatment of Turner syndrome (alone or together with oxandrolone); it appears to increase growth rate and predicted adult height, and controlled studies of its effect on adult height are forthcoming. GH has also been tried with varying success for many other disorders, including IUGR, Prader-Willi syndrome, hypochondroplasia, and spina bifida. Controlled studies to adult height are generally not yet available for these conditions.

Potential side effects of GH have included fluid retention and pseudotumor cerebri, slipped capital femoral epiphyses (it is not clear whether this occurs secondary to rapid growth or GH treatment itself), GH-neutralizing antibodies (rarely of clinical impact), and glucose intolerance. Acute leukemia has been reported following GH therapy, but this may represent children with underlying predispositions to malignancy. As GH has been used for non–GH-deficient children for a relatively short time, currently unforeseen long-term side effects are possible.

Initial studies suggest that children with familial or constitutional short stature or idiopathic short stature will have an initial augmentation of growth velocity on GH treatment. The long-term effect on adult height is not known. Aside from a need to establish efficacy, there are also ethical issues; for example, is GH treatment

a way to maximize a child's potential, or does it represent a cosmetic tampering with an otherwise normal child? GH is very costly, leading to questions about optimal use of resources and distribution of therapy.

SUMMARY AND RED FLAGS

Short stature may be a variant of normal development or may indicate a serious underlying problem. When short stature is associated with obesity, vomiting, or a goiter, a search for systemic disease should be undertaken (Tables 62–9 and 62–10). Understanding how to measure a child accurately, performing simple proportional measurements, and calculating growth velocity are skills that all pediatricians must know in order to diagnose short stature and identify associated disease states and syndromes.

REFERENCES

Diagnosing Growth Disorders

American Academy of Pediatrics Section on Endocrinology and Committee on Genetics and the American Thyroid Association Committee on Public Health. Newborn screening for congenital hypothyroidism: Recommended guidelines. Pediatrics 1993;91:1203.

LaFranchi S. Diagnosis and treatment of hypothyroidism in children. Compr Ther 1987;13:20–30.

Rose SR, Ross JL, Uriarte M, et al. The advantage of measuring stimulated as compared with spontaneous growth hormone levels in the diagnosis of growth hormone deficiency. N Engl J Med 1988;319:201–207.

Savage MO, Blum WF, Ranke MB, et al. Clinical features and endocrine status in patients with growth hormone insensitivity (Laron Syndrome). J Clin Endocrinol Metab 1993;77:1465–1471.

Tanner J, Goldstein H, Whitehouse R. Standards for children's height at ages 2 to 9 yr, allowing for height of parents. Arch Dis Child 1970;45:755–762.

Tanner J, Davies P. Clinical longitudinal standards for height and height velocity for North American children. J Pediatr 1985;107:317–329.

Growth

Cuttler L, Van Vliet G, Conte F, et al. Somatomedin-C levels in children and adolescents with gonadal dysgenesis: Differences from age-matched normal females and effect of chronic estrogen replacement therapy. J Clin Endocrinol Metab 1985;60:1087–1092.

Jones KL. Smith's Recognizable Patterns of Human Malformation, 4th ed. Philadelphia: WB Saunders, 1988.

Kliegman R. Intrauterine growth retardation: Determinants of aberrant fetal growth. In Fanaroff AA, Martin RG (eds): Neonatal-Perinatal Medicine, 5th ed. St. Louis: Mosby–Year Book, 1992.

Thorner MO, Vance ML, Horvath E, et al. The anterior pituitary. In Wilson JD, Foster DW (eds): William's Textbook of Endocrinology, 8th ed. Philadelphia: WB Saunders, 1992.

Growth Hormone

Fradkin JE, Mills JL, Schonberger LB, et al. Risk of leukemia after treatment with pituitary growth hormone. JAMA 1993;270:2829–2832.

Goddard A, Covello R, Luoh S, et al. Mutations of the growth hormone receptor in children with idiopathic short stature. N Engl J Med 1995;333:1093–1098.

Hintz RL. Untoward events in patients treated with growth hormone in the USA. Horm Res 1992;38:44–49.

Table 62–10. Things Not to Miss

Hypoglycemia in a full-term newborn who is appropriate for gestational age and whose mother does not have diabetes mellitus	Rule out hypopituitarism
Hypoglycemia and microphallus in a newborn male	Rule out hypopituitarism
Obese child who is short	Rule out hypothyroidism, growth hormone deficiency, Cushing syndrome, Prader-Willi syndrome, Laurence-Moon-Biedl syndrome
Short child with a goiter	Rule out hypothyroidism
Short child with headache, vomiting, or visual disturbance	Rule out hypopituitarism secondary to central nervous system lesion, including craniopharyngioma or hydrocephalus

Lantos J, Siegler M, Cuttler L. Ethical dilemmas in growth hormone therapy. JAMA 1989;261:1148–1154.

Lippe BM, Nakamoto JM. Conventional and nonconventional uses of growth hormone. Recent Prog Horm Res 1994;48:179–225.

Rosenfeld RG, Frane J, Attie KM, et al. Six-yr results of a randomized, prospective trial of human growth hormone and oxandrolone in Turner Syndrome. J Pediatr 1992;121:49–55.

Spiliotis B, August G, Hung W, et al. Growth hormone neurosecretory dysfunction: A treatable cause of short stature. JAMA 1984;251:2223–2230.

63 Hypoglycemia

✓ 21/7/97

Satish C. Kalhan   Thomas F. Riley

Glucose is the primary metabolic fuel for the central nervous system (CNS), including the brain and peripheral nerve in addition to the red blood cells and possibly the renal medulla. Because circulating glucose is the primary source of glucose for the brain, and because the uptake of glucose by the brain depends on its concentration in the blood, a significant decrease in blood glucose concentration results in decreased cerebral glucose utilization and thus curtails CNS function. A lack or decreased supply of essential fuel to the brain results in rapid appearance of symptoms and signs attributed to hypoglycemia (neuroglucopenia) or the counterregulatory hormone—epinephrine—which attempts to increase blood glucose (Table 63–1).

DEFINITION

A uniform definition (one applicable to all age groups) of low blood glucose (hypoglycemia) is difficult. This is in part related to a large number of otherwise well patients, in particular newborn infants, who may have a low blood glucose level without any obvious signs and symptoms—the so-called *asymptomatic hypoglycemia.*

Table 63–1. Symptoms and Signs of Hypoglycemia

Features Associated with Epinephrine Release*	Features Associated with Cerebral Glucopenia
Perspiration	Headache
Palpitation (tachycardia)	Mental confusion
Pallor	Somnolence
Paresthesia	Dysarthria
Trembling	Personality changes
Anxiety	Inability to concentrate
Weakness	Staring
Nausea	Hunger
Vomiting	Convulsions
	Ataxia
	Coma
	Diplopia
	Stroke

From Styne DM. Endocrine disorders. *In* Behrman RE, Kliegman RM (eds). Nelson Essentials of Pediatrics, 2nd ed. Philadelphia: WB Saunders, 1994:651.

*These features may be blunted if the patient is receiving beta-blocking agents.

Attempts have been made to define hypoglycemia by taking either a statistical or a clinical approach. The former approach relates to defining hypoglycemia when the blood glucose concentration falls outside a described limit (2 standard deviations of the mean glucose concentration measured in that population); the latter approach defines the blood glucose concentration threshold at which clinical signs and symptoms appear. The wide range of blood glucose concentration at which clinically overt signs may appear has led to uncertainty in definition. Aggressive, clinical, and nutritional (oral or parenteral alimentation) care has resulted in changes in "normal" blood glucose concentrations, so that the glucose concentrations observed in the past are no longer seen with current clinical practice.

When comparing reported glucose values, one must recognize some technical factors. Unless a free-flow blood sample is obtained with minimal pain to the infant, the glucose values are likely to vary greatly. Second, whole blood glucose values are slightly less than those of plasma because of the dilution by the fluid in the red blood cells. In contrast to the previously reported nonspecific reducing substance assay methods, glucose-specific enzymatic methods are used by most laboratories. Finally, hematocrit also influences the blood glucose concentration. This is particularly important in neonates, whose hematocrit values can vary in a wide range. A high hematocrit level results in lower blood glucose concentration; the opposite is true for low hematocrit values.

NORMAL GLUCOSE LEVELS

Neonate

During the newborn period, plasma glucose concentrations vary not only with the gestational age of the infant but also with the chronologic age. In particular after birth, during the transitional period encompassing the immediate adaptation (0 to 6 hours of age) of the newborn to the extrauterine environment, as the infant initiates glucose production from hepatic glycogen stores from a state of no glucose production *in utero*, the plasma glucose concentration undergoes a sequential change in relation to the time after birth. At birth, the plasma glucose concentration reflects maternal blood glucose concentration and is 70% to 80% of maternal levels. This is followed by a decrease in plasma glucose concentration, which reaches the lowest level at 45 to 60 minutes after birth, then rises to a stable level by about 2 hours. In normal full-term infants born to normal mothers following an uncomplicated pregnancy and delivery, the "normal" plasma glucose concentration can be considered as follows: cord vein, 60 to 70 mg/dl; at 1 hour, 30 to 40 mg/dl; and at 2 hours, 40 to 50 mg/dl. In preterm infants, these levels are somewhat lower (~10 mg/dl lower). Currently, the average plasma glucose levels in the full-term infant on the first day after birth are between 45 and 65 mg/dl.

Controversy remains as to the definition of hypoglycemia in the newborn, particularly because (1) many infants remain asymptomatic even with very low glucose levels and (2) the follow-up data do not provide a convincing relationship between *transient* hypoglycemia in the infant and long-term sequelae. "Transient" implies a single plasma glucose value recorded in the low range. In the absence of a defined functional value for hypoglycemia in the neonate, investigators have relied on what is called a "statistical" definition of hypoglycemia: a plasma glucose value that falls outside 2 standard deviations of the observed mean. According to such a definition, a plasma glucose concentration below 30 to 40 mg/dl should be considered low in a full-term neonate 2 to 3 hours after birth. Such a definition also implies corrective action on the part of the physician taking care of the infant and therefore mandates monitoring the infant until the glucose level reaches the perceived normal range.

In contrast to the transient hypoglycemia, a consensus exists in regard to "persistent" hypoglycemia; persistent refers to a low glucose level for a *prolonged* time period. However, what is prolonged remains unknown: minutes, hours, or days. A low blood glucose level recorded on several consecutive observations has been shown to be associated with neurologic sequelae. Thus, *persistent hypoglycemia* can be defined as a low glucose concentration that persists for more than 30 to 60 minutes. Obviously, in a symptomatic infant the plasma glucose level, irrespective of the statistical definition, is significant and appropriate therapeutic intervention is warranted.

The definition of hypoglycemia in preterm and small-for-gestational-age infants should not be different from that of full-term healthy newborns. All neonates should be considered hypoglycemic if their plasma glucose concentration falls below 40 mg/dl. This is particularly underscored in view of studies showing the hazardous consequences of a low glucose level in premature infants.

Older Infants, Children, and Adolescents

Because there is a paucity of normative data in older infants and children, most of the information is derived from glucose values in adolescents and adults or from children being investigated for other problems not related to glucose. In addition, asymptomatic hypoglycemia, as described in the neonate, is not usually observed in older children. The mean plasma glucose concentration following an overnight fast in adolescents and adults is reported to be 90 mg/dl, with a range of 75 to 100 mg/dl. Hypoglycemic symptoms may appear if the level is less than 50 mg/dl.

REGULATION OF BLOOD GLUCOSE CONCENTRATION

The plasma blood glucose concentration is maintained at a steady level by the interaction of primarily two major components: (1) hepatic production and (2) peripheral tissue utilization.

Glucose Production

The liver is the primary organ responsible for the release of glucose into blood. The kidney has a small contribution, if any, to the production of glucose. Glucose either is released from stored glycogen via glycogenolysis or is newly formed from pyruvate by a process called *gluconeogenesis*. The major steps involved in these two processes are displayed in Figure 63–1. Pyruvate is the common entry point for a number of gluconeogenic substrates (e.g., lactate, amino acids). In addition, glycerol released from triglycerides during lipolysis contributes to glucose production via triose phosphate. The production of glucose (glycogenolysis, gluconeogenesis) is regulated by: (1) hormones, (2) key regulatory enzymes, and (3) availability of gluconeogenic substrates.

HORMONES

Insulin causes a rapid decrease, whereas glucagon and catecholamine cause a rapid increase in the production of glucose *in vivo*. These effects are mediated by their effects on glycogenolysis as well as gluconeogenesis. Thus, insulin causes a decrease in glycogen breakdown as well as a decrease in gluconeogenesis. Because insulin also suppresses fatty acid oxidation, hyperinsulinism produces hypoglycemia *and* an absence of ketonuria. Cortisol is a permissive hormone, as its presence is required for the normal activity of the various gluconeogenic enzymes. The exact effect of growth hormone (HGH) on hepatic glucose production remains unclear.

ENZYMES

Glycogenolysis and gluconeogenesis require the presence of the various enzymes to facilitate these processes. A decrease in the activity of any of the rate-limiting enzymes (gluconeogenic, glycogenolytic) as a result of genetic defects may result in decreased glucose production (described later). In addition, because most peripheral tissues (muscle, heart) also metabolize fat, enzyme defects in fatty acid oxidation may result in excessive glucose utilization and hypoglycemia without ketonuria.

SUBSTRATES

For glucose to be produced continuously via gluconeogenesis, a continuous supply of precursor substrates, such as lactate, glycerol,

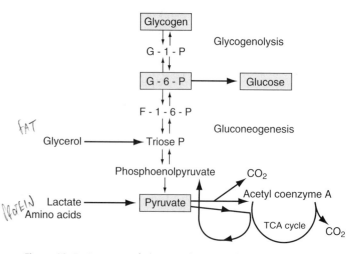

Figure 63–1. Processes of glycogenolysis and gluconeogenesis. TCA = tricarboxylic acid.

and amino acids, is required. Under certain circumstances, when supply of these precursors (alanine) is reduced, a decrease in glucose production has been observed (*ketotic hypoglycemia*).

Plasma glucose itself appears to normally influence glucose production—a high glucose level resulting in decreased production and a low glucose level having the opposite effect.

Glucose Utilization

The utilization of glucose is primarily regulated by certain hormones via their influence on glucose transporters. Insulin, secreted by the endocrine pancreas, results in increased glucose uptake primarily by the muscle; catecholamines cause a decrease in glucose uptake. Cortisol and growth hormone appear to have their effects by influencing the action of insulin. Glucose is taken up by the cell by a carrier-mediated process that involves specific glucose transport proteins called *glucose transporters*. At least six glucose transport proteins (Glut 1–6) have been identified. These proteins are differentially expressed in different tissues. A defect in the synthesis of such proteins could impair the uptake of glucose by that particular tissue, resulting in *intracellular hypoglycemia* in the presence of normal blood glucose concentrations.

CAUSES OF HYPOGLYCEMIA

Low plasma glucose levels may be the consequence of either decreased production of glucose by the liver or increased utilization by the peripheral tissues.

Characteristics of decreased hepatic glucose production are noted in defects in glycogenolysis and *hyperinsulinemic states*. An increase in plasma insulin concentration due to any cause results in a decreased production of glucose by the liver by suppressing both glycogen breakdown and gluconeogenesis (as well as suppressing lipolysis and fat oxidation, or hypoketonemia); hyperinsulinemia also increases peripheral glucose utilization. Clinical and pathologic situations in which increased insulin levels as a cause of hypoglycemia are observed are noted in Table 63–2.

Intrapartum Maternal Glucose Administration

Administration of excessive glucose quantities to the mother during labor results in maternal as well as fetal hyperglycemia.

Table 63–2. Hyperinsulinemic States

Intrapartum maternal glucose administration
Maternal drug therapy
   Hypoglycemic agents
   Beta sympathomimetic agents
Infants of diabetic mothers
Erythroblastosis fetalis
Beckwith-Wiedemann syndrome
Idiopathic hyperinsulinism (hypoxia)
Organic hyperinsulinism
   Pancreatic adenoma
   Pancreatic nesidioblastosis (often familial)*
Factitious (insulin or oral hypoglycemic agents)
Accidental ingestion (oral hypoglycemic agents)

*May previously have been classified as "leucine"-sensitive hypoglycemia.

Increased fetal glucose concentrations causes increased fetal insulin secretion and fetal hyperinsulinism. If the glucose has been administered to the mother immediately before the infant's birth, the infant will be born with high insulin levels. In addition, high fetal blood glucose and insulin levels may also cause an increase in fetal blood lactate concentration and metabolic acidosis. These effects are more pronounced if the mother has been infused with glucose for a prolonged time. An acute administration of large amounts of glucose-containing fluids (e.g., to prevent hypotension in women receiving conduction anesthesia) leads to fetal hyperglycemia, hyperinsulinism, and metabolic acidosis. The hyperinsulinism of the fetus continues transiently in the neonate and leads to hypoglycemia.

Maternal Drug Therapy

The various pharmacologic agents administered to the mother for the treatment of medical problems that can influence blood glucose levels in the newborn can be divided into two broad categories:

1. Drugs that can *directly* affect blood glucose, including oral hypoglycemic agents. Oral hypoglycemic agents, such as chlorpropamide and sulfonylureas, are used by some for the treatment of gestational diabetes. Because these drugs are easily transported across the placenta, the neonate is born with a certain amount of drug present in the circulation. These drugs, particularly those with prolonged effects, may result in profound hypoglycemia that tends to persist until the drug is removed, either by its own clearance or by exchange transfusion.

2. Drugs administered to the mother with *indirect* effects (the more common contributor to neonatal hypoglycemia). Beta sympathomimetic agents commonly used for the prevention and treatment of premature labor can result in maternal hyperglycemia by increasing hepatic glucose production and decreasing glucose utilization. Maternal hyperglycemia, in turn, can initiate fetal hyperglycemia and the hyperinsulinism syndrome and, consequently, can cause hypoglycemia in the neonate.

Infants of Diabetic Mothers

Newborn infants born to mothers with diabetes mellitus during pregnancy often develop transient hypoglycemia immediately after birth. In most instances, the hypoglycemia lasts a short period, 3 to 4 hours, with spontaneous improvement and recovery. Rigorous control of maternal metabolism during pregnancy and during the intrapartum period has significantly reduced the frequency of hypoglycemia. These infants have characteristic physical features, especially macrosomia (birth weight > 90th percentile) because of increased growth of insulin-responsive tissues (adipose tissue, visceromegaly). These infants may be plethoric because of a high hematocrit value, may have an enlarged heart from a specific cardiomyopathy (subaortic septal hypertrophy), and on occasion may have a congenital anomaly, such as sacral agenesis. Additional problems are noted in Table 63–3.

Hypoglycemia in these infants is related to fetal and neonatal hyperinsulinemia as a consequence of increased transfer of glucose and other nutrients from the diabetic mother to the fetus. Hyperinsulinism in the infants of diabetic mothers has been confirmed by demonstrating increased C peptide and insulin levels in the umbilical cord blood. After birth, these infants remain hyperinsulinemic and cannot mount an appropriate glucagon response, so that hypoglycemia appears to be a combined effect of increased insulin and lower glucagon concentration. The combined effect of these hormones results in decreased production of glucose by the liver.

Table 63–3. Pathophysiology of Morbidity and Mortality of the Infant of a Diabetic Mother

Problem	Pathophysiology
Fetal demise	Acute placental failure?
	Hyperglycemia—lactic acidosis—hypoxia?
Macrosomia	Hyperinsulinism
Respiratory distress syndrome	Insulin antagonism of cortisol
	Variant surfactant biochemical pathways
Wet lung syndrome	Cesarean delivery
Hypoglycemia	↓ Glucose and fat mobilization–hyperinsulinemia
Polycythemia	Erythropoietic "macrosomia"?
	Mild fetal hypoxia?
	↓ O_2 delivery to fetus–HbA_{1c}?
Hypocalcemia	↓ Neonatal parathyroid hormone
	↑ Calcitonin?
	↓ Magnesium
Hyperbilirubinemia	↑ Erythropoietic mass
	↑ Bilirubin production
	Immature hepatic conjugation?
	Oxytocin induction
Congenital malformations (central nervous system, heart, skeletal)	Hyperglycemia?
	Genetic linkage?
	Insulin as teratogen?
	Vascular accident?
Renal vein thrombosis	Polycythemia?
	Dehydration?
Neonatal small left colon syndrome	Immature gastrointestinal motility?
Cardiomyopathy	Reversible septal hypertrophy
	↑ Glycogen?
	↑ Muscle?
Family psychologic stress	High-risk pregnancy
	Fear of diabetes in infant
Subsequent development of insulin-dependent diabetes	Genetic HLA markers; risk is greater for infant of diabetic father

Adapted from Kliegman RM, Fanaroff AA. Developmental metabolism and nutrition. *In* Gregory GA (ed). Pediatric Anesthesiology. New York: Churchill Livingstone, 1983.
Abbreviations: Hb = hemoglobin; HLA = human leukocyte antigen.

Erythroblastosis Fetalis

An association between hypoglycemia and erythroblastosis fetalis due to rhesus incompatibility occurs in infants who are anemic at birth (cord hemoglobin < 10 g/dl). The low blood glucose levels in these infants have been attributed to high plasma insulin concentration. The cause of these high insulin levels remains undefined. The current prevention and management of rhesus sensitization have markedly reduced the incidence of erythroblastosis and fetal and neonatal anemia. Nonetheless, such infants require careful monitoring of plasma glucose concentration soon after birth.

Beckwith-Wiedemann Syndrome

The clinical features of infants born with Beckwith-Wiedemann syndrome consist of macroglossia, abdominal wall defects (omphalocele, umbilical hernia), diastasis recti, somatic gigantism, visceromegaly (liver, kidney, spleen), and hypoglycemia. Other features include ear anomalies, such as creases on the lobe; cardiac defects; hemihypertrophy; and neonatal polycythemia.

Early recognition of hypoglycemia is extremely important for appropriate clinical management. Any infant born with an omphalocele should be monitored for potential hypoglycemia. The mechanism of hypoglycemia has been related to hyperinsulinism. At autopsy, hypertrophy and hyperplasia of the islet of Langerhans have been observed. Other pathologic findings include adrenal cortical cysts, nephromegaly with prominent lobulation, persistent

nephrogenesis and medullary dysplasia, and medullary sponge kidney. These infants are prone to have intra-abdominal malignancies, in particular nephroblastomas, adrenal carcinoma, and neural crest tumors. Most cases of Beckwith-Wiedemann syndrome are sporadic, although familial cases have been reported. Chromosomal analysis has suggested partial duplication of chromosome 11p; however, this is not a consistent finding in all infants with this syndrome.

Hypoxia-Idiopathic Hyperinsulinism

Newborn infants recovering from birth asphyxia often develop hypoglycemia or require high rates of infusion of glucose to maintain normal blood glucose concentrations. The exact mechanism of this altered glucose homeostasis remains unclear, although some data suggest that hyperinsulinemia is a contributing factor. Hyperinsulinism has also been suggested as a contributor to hypoglycemia in some small-for-gestational-age neonates.

Primary Pancreatic Lesions (Nesidioblastosis, Pancreatic Tumors, Hyperplasia)

Infants born with primary pancreatic lesions have been exposed to high insulin levels for a prolonged period *in utero* and, depending on the severity, may present with features of chronic hyperinsulinism (large-for-gestational-age, as in infants of diabetic mothers; visceromegaly), and may develop persistent hypoglycemia. They require high rates of glucose infusion for prolonged periods (days) to maintain a normal blood glucose concentration.

The diagnosis is suspected when hypoglycemia develops immediately after birth and the newborn requires high rates of glucose infusion and cannot be weaned from the glucose infusion. In the presence of hyperinsulinemia, low blood glucose concentrations are accompanied by low plasma levels of free fatty acids, ketones, and branched chain amino acids. However, these changes may also be the consequence of glucose infusions. The diagnosis is confirmed only by the measurement of plasma insulin levels that are noted to be inappropriately high for the prevailing glucose concentration. Plasma levels of counterregulatory hormones (glucagon, catecholamine, cortisol, growth hormone) are usually within normal limits.

Other diagnostic techniques, such as ultrasound imaging of the pancreas, computed tomography (CT), and selective celiac angiography, are not very helpful in cases of nesidioblastosis.

Pancreatic lesions should be suspected in any infant or child with persistent intractable hypoglycemia that requires high rates of glucose infusion to maintain normoglycemia. Pathologic findings of nesidioblastosis include diffuse proliferation of disordered islet cells throughout the pancreas. In addition, there is an increase in cell numbers as well as in the size of the islet cells, even in the normally formed islets. Islet cell adenomas, although rare, have also been reported in infants and children. However, the histologic findings of the tumors in infants show discrete clusters of all the endocrine cells rather than the usual single cell type tumors.

HORMONE DEFICIENCIES

The glucose counterregulatory hormones (those having actions opposite to those of insulin when administered *in vivo*) increase plasma glucose concentration by increasing hepatic glucose production or by decreasing peripheral uptake. Deficiency of these hormones has been described either in isolation or as a result of congenital defects of the CNS (pituitary defects) and have been associated with hypoglycemia (Table 63–4).

Glucagon Deficiency

Isolated glucagon deficiency has been described in a few newborn infants and is associated with severe, persistent hypoglycemia. Infants appear normal at birth but hypoglycemia develops during the first 24 to 48 hours of life. Plasma glucagon levels in the basal

Table 63–4. Hormonal Deficiencies Causing Hypoglycemia

Glucagon (isolated)
Catecholamine (adrenal hemorrhage)
Growth hormone
  Isolated
  Panhypopituitarism
    Primary or "aplasia"
    Septo-optic dysplasia
    Midline central nervous system
      malformation
Cortisol
  Adrenal hemorrhage
  Adrenogenital syndrome

state or in response to a secretagogue, such as alanine, remain low. In response to exogenous glucagon, these infants respond normally by increasing their plasma glucose concentration.

Catecholamine (Epinephrine) Deficiency

Catecholamine deficiency is extremely rare and has been described in small-for-gestational-age infants secondary to adrenal hemorrhage. These infants may present for the first time during childhood with hypoglycemia during fasting. The diagnosis is confirmed by measurement of plasma or urinary catecholamine levels. Some children may show evidence, on abdominal films, of previous adrenal hemorrhage in the form of adrenal calcification.

Growth Hormone Deficiency

Deficiency of HGH, isolated or in association with multiple hormone deficiencies (as in panhypopituitarism) may present with hypoglycemia in the immediate newborn period or even in later childhood. A number of syndromes, such as midline craniofacial defects, septo-optic dysplasia, and Russel-Silver dwarfism, may be associated with hypopituitarism. In the newborn period, infants with hypopituitarism may present with hypoglycemia, hypotonia, and hyperbilirubinemia. Male infants characteristically have microphallus, which is a useful diagnostic sign.

INBORN ERRORS OF METABOLISM

Inborn errors of metabolism are classified into two groups (Table 63–5). The first consists of disorders primarily involving glucose

Table 63–5. Inborn Errors of Metabolism (Enzyme Defects)

I. Primary Defects of Glucose Metabolism

  A. Glycogen metabolism
    1. Type I glycogen storage disease: glucose-6-phosphatase deficiency
    2. Type III glycogen storage disease: debrancher enzyme deficiency
    3. Type VI or hepatic phosphorylase deficiency
    4. Others: glycogen synthase deficiency
  B. Galactosemia
    Galactose-1-phosphate uridyl transferase deficiency
  C. Defects in gluconeogenesis
    1. Fructose 1,6-diphosphatase deficiency
    2. Defects in pyruvate metabolism

II. Defects of Amino Acid and Fat Metabolism That Secondarily Cause Hypoglycemia

  A. Fatty acid metabolism
    1. Carnitine metabolism
    2. Acyl coenzyme A dehydrogenase deficiency (medium- and long-chain)
  B. Amino acid metabolism
    1. Maple syrup urine disease
    2. Branched chain keto-dehydrogenase deficiency
    3. Propionic acidemia
    4. Methylmalonic acidemia
    5. Tyrosinosis
    6. 3-Hydroxy, 3-methyl glutaryl coenzyme A deficiency

metabolism. In the second group, glucose metabolism is affected secondarily to a primary defect in amino acid or fatty acid metabolism; in addition, glucose release or production by the liver is affected either by accumulation of some metabolites or, in the case of fatty acid defects, by the lack of available energy to synthesize glucose from gluconeogenic precursors or to spare glucose utilization by peripheral tissues.

Glycogen Storage Diseases

Glucose is stored in the liver during feeding in the form of glycogen through a series of enzymatic reactions. The hepatic glycogen is then released as glucose, during fasting, involving a series of enzyme reactions (debrancher enzyme or amylo-1,6-glucosidase, hepatic phosphorylase, and, finally, glucose-6-phosphatase). Glucose-6-phosphatase is the final step where glucose-6-phosphate is converted to glucose, which is released into circulation. Hereditary defects that result in decreased activity or absence of these enzymes involved in glycogen breakdown result in accumulation of glycogen in the liver and decreased production of glucose. These are described in order of their frequency.

GLYCOGEN STORAGE DISEASE TYPE I (GLUCOSE-6-PHOSPHATASE DEFICIENCY)

Because glucose-6-phosphatase is the key enzyme involved in release of glucose from the liver, either from glycogen breakdown or from gluconeogenesis, absence of this enzyme results in severe and profound hypoglycemia characteristically immediately after feeding, when the enterally absorbed glucose disappears from the circulation. In addition, and as a consequence of hypoglycemia and counterregulatory hormone (catecholamine, glucagon) secretion, lipolysis and glycogenolysis are increased. However, since glucose-6-phosphate produced in the liver cannot be hydrolyzed to glucose, it is shunted toward pyruvate, resulting in profound lactic acidosis. Increased lipolysis from adipose tissue sites results in increased circulating fatty acids, ketones, and triglycerides. In addition, accumulation of triglycerides in the liver results in a large, firm, fatty liver. Increased uric acid production, coupled with decreased renal clearance of uric acid, results in hyperuricemia.

Newborns with glycogen storage disease type I present with severe hypoglycemia and lactic acidosis; thus, the diagnosis should be suspected in an infant who becomes hypoglycemic soon after feeding and is hyperventilating as a consequence of metabolic acidosis. Laboratory studies show elevated lactic acid levels, uricemia, high circulating triglyceride levels, uricemia, high circulating triglyceride levels, and high fatty acid levels. In the neonatal period, the infant may not show any physical findings (hepatomegaly, xanthomas). During infancy, however, an enlarged, firm liver, a typical doll-like face, and a failure to thrive with vomiting become evident.

Clinical diagnostic tests are aimed at demonstrating a lack of glucose response to orally administered galactose or to a glycogenolytic hormone, such as glucagon. The definitive diagnosis is confirmed by liver biopsy and measurement of enzyme activity.

GLYCOGEN STORAGE DISEASE TYPE III (DEBRANCHER ENZYME OR AMYLO-1,6-GLUCOSIDASE DEFICIENCY)

Because absence of this enzyme limits the breakdown or glycogen molecule up to the branch points by the action of phosphoryl-

ase, these infants and children can tolerate short periods of fasting without becoming hypoglycemic. A prolonged fast (beyond 4 to 6 hours in the neonate and beyond 8 to 10 hours in the older child), however, may result in hypoglycemia.

Children present with marked hepatomegaly and frequently with growth failure. In more severe forms, hypoglycemia may be the prominent feature, with elevated blood levels of triglycerides, ketones, and fatty acids. Increased glycogen content is demonstrated in liver and muscle, and the diagnosis is confirmed by measuring the enzyme activity in the liver.

Clinical diagnostic tests are suggestive when the response is compared during fasting and fed states. A glucagon challenge results in normal glycemic response soon after a feeding, but little or no increase in blood glucose is observed when glucagon is given after a short (4- to 6-hour) fast. Unlike the case with type I disease, administration of galactose and fructose results in a normal increase in blood glucose.

GLYCOGEN STORAGE DISEASE TYPE VI (HEPATIC PHOSPHORYLASE DEFICIENCY)

Phosphorylase is the key enzyme involved in breakdown of hepatic glycogen. It hydrolyses successive glucose residues from the glycogen molecule until it reaches the branch point at which the debrancher enzyme systems cause further cleavage. Defects of the hepatic phosphorylase system have been termed type VI glycogen storage disease, and resemble those in infants with type III disease. Typically, patients present with mild symptomatic hypoglycemia and failure to thrive.

Glycogen Synthase Deficiency

Glycogen synthase deficiency is extremely uncommon and is characterized by fasting hypoglycemia and lack of any demonstrable glycogen in the muscle, liver, kidney, and adrenal glands. Liver biopsy shows fatty infiltration and a lack of glycogen synthase activity.

Galactosemia (Galactose-1-Phosphate Uridyl Transferase Deficiency)

Galactosemia is a serious inborn error of metabolism wherein many of the long-term consequences of the metabolic defect can potentially be prevented by early intervention. For this reason, all infants born in the United States are screened for galactosemia in the newborn period. Absence of galactose-1-phosphate uridyl transferase prevents the conversion of galactose to glucose and results in accumulation of galactose-1-phosphate in the liver and other tissues. It has been suggested that accumulation of this metabolite inhibits the enzyme involved in the conversion of glucose-1-phosphate to glucose-6-phosphate and thus decreases the production of glucose from glycogen, hence producing hypoglycemia. Depending on the magnitude of the defect, these infants may present in the immediate newborn period or later in infancy. The patients do not tolerate galactose or lactose. Intolerance to milk, the major nutrient containing galactose, is evident soon after birth when feedings are initiated. The infant may present with vomiting, failure to thrive, hepatomegaly, and indirect or direct hyperbilirubinemia. In severe or untreated cases, lenticular opacities, amino aciduria, and mental retardation may occur. In untreated patients, progressive hepatomegaly, cirrhosis, and hepatic failure may develop. Infants are at increased risk for *Escherichia coli* sepsis.

Any infant with persistent jaundice, hepatomegaly, and failure to thrive should be tested for galactosemia. A presumptive diagnosis can be made by the presence of reducing sugar (Clinitest positive) that is not glucose (i.e., the glucose enzyme test is negative) in the urine. This test should be done while the infant is being fed a galactose-containing formula. The diagnosis should be confirmed by measuring the enzyme activity in the red blood cells.

Treatment consists of elimination of galactose from the diet. In spite of treatment, which results in prevention of hepatic disease and mental retardation, adult females with galactosemia develop ovarian failure whereas many older children demonstrate learning and behavior problems.

Defects in Gluconeogenesis

As hepatic glycogen stores are depleted during fasting, gluconeogenesis becomes the prominent source of glucose production. Pyruvate—or, more specifically, phosphoenolpyruvate—is the key entry point for gluconeogenic precursors in the formation of glucose. The only gluconeogenic substrate that does not enter the gluconeogenic pathway at phosphoenolpyruvate is glycerol. Primary defects of enzymes involved in gluconeogenesis are uncommon. Such children present with hypoglycemia during fasting and accumulation of pyruvate or lactate and metabolic acidosis.

Hepatic Fructose-1,6-Diphosphatase Deficiency

Patients may present with symptoms and signs similar to those of type I glycogen storage disease. Hypoglycemia, lactic acidosis, hyperlipidemia, and hyperuricemia are typically observed. The enlarged liver is a result of accumulation of lipids. Diagnosis is confirmed by liver biopsy. Because the defect involves gluconeogenesis and not the glycogen system (which is intact), affected children show a normal response to oral galactose. In addition, glucagon challenge yields a normal glycemic response soon after feeding but not after a fast. Administration of compounds that enter the gluconeogenic pathway below the level of fructose-1,6-diphosphatase (glycerol, fructose, amino acids) results in hypoglycemia and lactic acidosis.

Defects of Pyruvate Metabolism (Pyruvate Carboxylase Deficiency)

These defects are uncommon inborn errors of metabolism that present as unexplained metabolic acidosis and, in some instances, with mental retardation or acute encephalomyelopathy (Leigh encephalopathy). Hypoglycemia, at least in a severe form, is rare, perhaps because of the contribution of other gluconeogenic precursors that do not enter via pyruvate. The diagnosis should be suspected in any infant with persistent lactic acidosis. These disorders are difficult to treat and are usually suspected after the history has revealed that a patient's sibling has died early in infancy.

Defects of Amino Acids and Fat Metabolism

Defects that secondarily cause hypoglycemia by influencing gluconeogenesis are listed in Table 63–5. Most of these defects are associated with metabolic acidosis and are suspected by screening for the particular metabolic defect. Medium-chain acyl dehydrogenase deficiency is probably the most common and is characterized by hypoglycemia, relative hypoketonemia, emesis, coma, hypotonia, sudden death, and at times metabolic acidosis. Onset is at any age and may be precipitated by viral illnesses or fasting or may occur spontaneously.

SUBSTRATE DEFICIENCY

Substrate deficiencies are poorly characterized disorders that may present with hypoglycemia during fasting. The most common of disorders, *ketotic hypoglycemia,* is characterized by low blood glucose levels following a prolonged fast (15 to 24 hours) in children between the ages of 18 months and 5 years and is generally thought to remit by puberty. Hypoglycemia is associated with high levels of ketones in blood and urine. The symptoms can be precipitated by placing the child on a high-fat ketogenic diet or by prolonged fasting.

Ketotic syndrome has been attributed to gluconeogenic substrate (alanine) deficiency. It should be recognized that a ketotic response to fasting and a low blood glucose level is also observed in normal children and the observations in ketotic hypoglycemia are probably an exaggeration of normal fasting (''accelerated starvation''). The mechanism of alanine ''deficiency'' in this syndrome remains undefined and may be related to partial defects of amino acid metabolism in the muscle.

Other situations of substrate deficiency are seen in patients with severe malnutrition who, as a result of chronic depletion, cannot sustain gluconeogenesis during fasting.

OTHER HYPOGLYCEMIA SYNDROMES

Reactive Hypoglycemia

Reactive hypoglycemia is not a well-characterized syndrome; it is diagnosed by the development of low blood glucose at the end of an oral glucose tolerance test or a meal. In response to a glucose challenge, patients have a normal increase in blood glucose that is followed by a greater than normal decline, resulting in hypoglycemia. This phenomenon has been attributed to exaggerated insulin response, perhaps mediated by gastrointestinal insulinotropic hormones.

Defects of Glucose Transport in the Blood-Brain Barrier

One patient has been identified with symptoms of hypoglycemia who had normal blood glucose concentrations but consistently lower cerebrospinal glucose concentrations. A defect in the glucose transport protein in the blood-brain barrier was noted. In this context, this syndrome should be called *normoglycemic hypoglycemia.*

MANAGEMENT OF HYPOGLYCEMIA

As listed in Table 63–1, manifestations of hypoglycemia are relatively nonspecific. Particularly in the newborn, hypoglycemia should be included in the differential diagnosis of a number of clinical conditions (transient tachypnea, respiratory distress, sepsis, cyanosis, lethargy, jitteriness, seizures, hypotonia, feeding difficulties, apnea). In the older child, hypoglycemia should be suspected when these symptoms appear, particularly after a fast or in the presence of other mild intercurrent illness.

A diagnostic and therapeutic approach is noted in Figure 63–2 and is based on the presence or absence of Whipple's triad—a low blood glucose level, consistent signs or symptoms, and improvement after administration of glucose.

Diagnostic Studies

BLOOD GLUCOSE MEASUREMENT

Irrespective of the age group, blood glucose levels should be measured in the laboratory by a glucose specific enzymatic method. Bedside enzymatic sticks should be used only for screening and must be confirmed by laboratory measurement. Blood glucose levels should be measured in relation to symptoms in order to document the presence of hypoglycemia. Because hypoglycemia is common in newborns, blood glucose levels should be routinely monitored in at-risk infants (Table 63–6).

OTHER SUBSTRATES

Measurement of plasma ketones, free fatty acids, and branched chain amino acids are useful for documenting appropriate counter-regulatory responses. Levels of these metabolites are decreased in the presence of high insulin levels and are increased in normal subjects with low glucose and low insulin levels.

If metabolic acidosis exists and is characterized by an increased anion gap, measurement of blood lactate, pyruvate, and organic acids is useful as an indicator of inborn errors of metabolism.

HORMONES

Plasma insulin levels should be measured with prolonged hypoglycemia and related to prevailing glucose concentration; the blood sample should be obtained when glucose levels are low. An inappropriately high insulin level in the presence of a low glucose concentration is diagnostic of hyperinsulinemia. If hypopituitarism or hypoadrenalism is suspected, appropriate hormones (growth hormone, cortisol, catecholamines) should be measured. Because hypoglucagonemia is rare and because laboratory measurements are not easily available, glucagon levels are measured only when glucagon deficiency is strongly suspected.

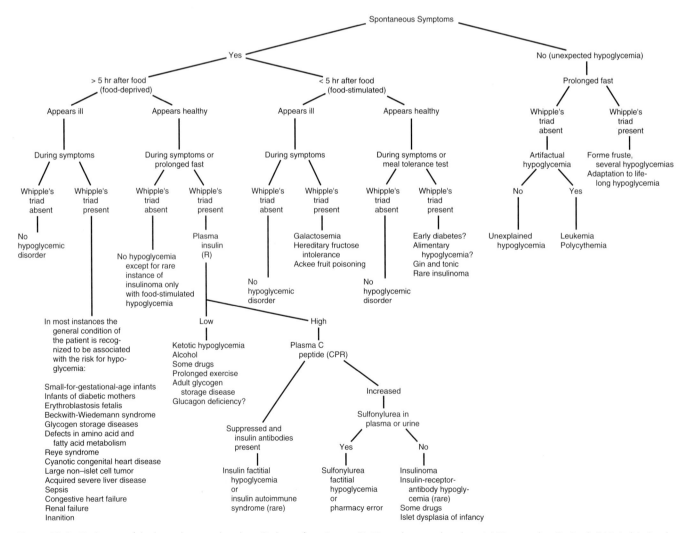

Figure 63–2. Evaluation of the hypoglycemic disorders. (Redrawn from Service FJ. Hypoglycemic disorders. *In* Wyngaarden JB, Smith LH Jr [eds]. Cecil Textbook of Medicine, 17th ed. Philadelphia: WB Saunders, 1995:1343.)

Table 63–6. Risk Factors for Neonatal Hypoglycemia

Factors	Mechanism
Common	
Prematurity	Limited glycogen stores
Infant of a diabetic mother	Hyperinsulinism
Intrauterine growth retardation	Limited glycogen stores, hyperinsulinism
Asphyxia-perinatal stress	Depleted glycogen stores
Hypothermia	Increased glucose utilization
Starvation	Depleted glycogen stores
Large for gestational age	Possible hyperinsulinism
Infant of obese mother	Possible hyperinsulinism
Maternal medications (tocolytics, propranolol, chlorpropamide, high-glucose infusion in labor)	Possible hyperinsulinism
Uncommon	
Erythroblastosis fetalis	Hyperinsulinism
Beckwith-Wiedemann syndrome	Hyperinsulinism
Islet cell adenoma	Hyperinsulinism
Nesidioblastosis	Hyperinsulinism
Familial hyperinsulinism	Hyperinsulinism
Polycythemia	Increased glucose utilization/ decreased production
Sepsis	Increased glucose utilization
Inborn errors of metabolism	Decreased glycogenolysis, gluconeogenesis or utilization of alternate fuels
Growth hormone deficiency	Increased glucose utilization, decreased gluconeogenesis
Adrenal insufficiency	Decreased glucose production (gluconeogenesis)

From Kliegman RM. Fetal and neonatal medicine. *In* Behrman RE, Kliegman RM (eds). Nelson Essentials of Pediatrics, 2nd ed. Philadelphia: WB Saunders, 1994:202.

FUNCTIONAL STUDIES

A number of functional tests have been proposed and used for clinical diagnostic purposes:

Glucagon Challenge Test

Because glucagon is a potent glycogenolytic hormone, its parenteral administration results in rapid breakdown of glycogen and increase in blood glucose concentration. A normal response is characterized by a 50% increase in blood glucose concentration and suggests normal glycogenolysis. Lack of an increase in the fed state strongly suggests a defect in any of the steps involved in glycogen breakdown. As a result of resistance to the effect of glucagon, newborn infants require a higher dose of glucagon (as much as 300 μg/kg) compared with adults to show a maximal increase in blood glucose. Infants with hepatic glycogen storage disease do not show increased blood glucose levels in response to glucagon, and lactic acidosis may develop.

Galactose, Fructose, and Glycerol Tolerance Tests

Tolerance tests have been used in the past in an attempt to make clinical diagnosis of defects of hepatic glucose metabolism.

Galactose, fructose, and glycerol tolerance tests are based on the principle that administration of these substrates at a point before the enzyme defect will result in lack of appropriate glucose response. Therefore, a galactose tolerance test in a patient with type I glycogen storage disease will not show a rise in blood glucose and a fructose or glycerol tolerance test administered in a patient with fructose-1,6-diphosphatase deficiency will show no increase in blood glucose. However, these tests are only screening procedures and may be dangerous; greater reliance is placed on tissue biopsy and direct measurement of the enzyme activity.

Glucose Tolerance Test

The glucose tolerance test is employed only when hypoglycemia occurs in the fed state in order to document a high insulin response to the glucose challenge.

Response to Fasting

In older infants and children, a response to a prolonged and observed fast provides the most useful information in understanding the altered physiologic state. The patient should be fasted in the hospital for an extended period and blood samples for the measurement of circulating hormones and metabolites obtained to document the metabolic profile. Blood samples should be obtained from indwelling cannulae, because the patient should not be subjected to pain as a result of repeated venipuncture. At the end of the fast (after 36 to 48 hours) or if a low glucose level or symptoms develop, other physiologic studies outlined earlier may be performed to delineate specific metabolic defects.

OTHER DIAGNOSTIC STUDIES

Tissue biopsies and fibroblast cultures are warranted for the measurement of enzyme activities. These tests are done according to the specific enzyme defect suspected on the basis of the clinical presentation and family history.

Clinical Management

The clinical management of the patient with hypoglycemia should be directed at correcting the low glucose level and treating the underlying cause. The newborn infant is rather unique because of the high frequency of transient hypoglycemia related to intrauterine or maternal factors. The transient hypoglycemia of the newborn disappears within the first 2 to 3 days, and thus only symptomatic therapy is required. However, this condition needs to be distinguished from the recurrent or persistent neonatal hypoglycemia. One algorithm for the management of transient hypoglycemia of the neonate is presented in Figure 63–3.

In every infant with hypoglycemia, the glucose level should be confirmed by a second quantitative laboratory measurement. In most asymptomatic healthy infants, the problem is resolved by administering early oral feedings. Blood glucose levels should be monitored to document persistent hypoglycemia or normoglycemia. If hypoglycemia recurs, further investigations would be necessary to determine the cause.

In the symptomatic infant, hypoglycemia should be treated immediately with intravenous glucose therapy. Glucose should be infused at 4 to 6 mg/kg/minute via a constant infusion pump to

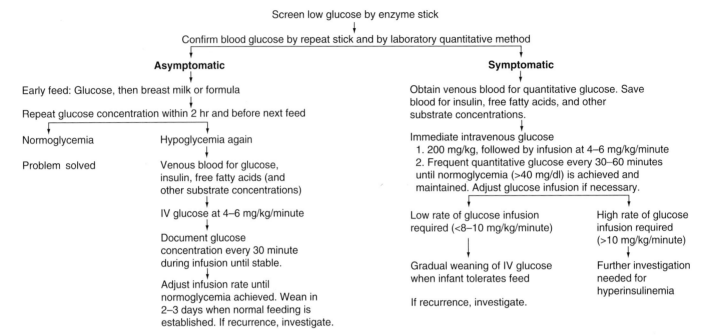

Figure 63–3. Approach to the clinical management of neonatal hypoglycemia.

avoid erratic infusion rates. At this rate, plasma glucose levels will reach the normal range within 15 to 20 minutes in most infants. With the constant infusion of glucose, a glucose bolus (200 mg/kg, or 2 ml/kg of 10% dextrose in water) should also be given in symptomatic patients. Large bolus administration of glucose is avoided to prevent rebound hypoglycemia. Following the initial correction of blood glucose, the rate of glucose infusion should be adjusted to maintain normal glucose concentration. Such a regimen can also be used in older infants and children.

Attempts should be made to wean the infant from the glucose infusion as soon as possible, (within 1 to 2 days). If the infant continues to require high rates of glucose infusion, a diagnosis of hyperinsulinism should be considered.

Pharmacologic agents have been used for the treatment of persistent hypoglycemia of the newborn. These include glucocorticoids, which may act by inducing gluconeogenesis, and diazoxide, which acts via inhibiting insulin secretion. A trial of oral diazoxide, 10–15 mg/kg/day, is effective as a temporizing measure in some patients with hyperinsulinism caused by nesidioblastosis. If diazoxide is ineffective, a long-acting somatostatin analog (octreotide) may be used to temporarily suppress insulin secretion prior to surgery in older patients. Eventually, most of these patients require subtotal pancreatectomy.

Other symptomatic measures to correct hypoglycemia include administration of glucose polymers (cornstarch) in patients with glycogen storage disease, frequent feedings, and constant infusion of glucose by nasogastric tube during periods of fasting, such as during sleep at night. The aim of all these measures is to maintain normoglycemia and suppress the counter regulatory responses.

SUMMARY AND RED FLAGS

Hypoglycemia has many manifestations and must be thought of as a cause of nonspecific signs in neonates or disordered consciousness, seizures, and signs of catecholamine excess. Untreated symptomatic hypoglycemia is life-threatening and can produce significant CNS injury.

Red flags include metabolic acidosis (inborn errors of metabolism, sepsis), a positive family history (inborn errors of metabolism, nesidioblastosis, hypoglycemic agents), hypoketonuria–high glucose infusion rates (hyperinsulinemia), adolescent onset (e.g., drugs or alcohol), hepatomegaly (glycogen storage disease, other inborn errors of metabolism), feeding intolerance (galactosemia), or repeated or a family history of emesis, lethargy, coma, or sudden infant death syndrome (medium-chain acyl dehydrogenase deficiency).

REFERENCES

Aynsley-Green A. Hypoglycaemia in infants and children. Clin Endocrinol Metab 1982;11:159–194.

Cornblath M, Schwartz R. Disorders of Carbohydrate Metabolism in Infancy, 3rd ed. Cambridge, Mass: Blackwell Scientific Publications, 1991.

Definition

Koh THHG, Eyre JA, Aynsley-Green A. Neonatal hypoglycaemia: The controversy regarding definition. Arch Dis Child 1988;63:1386–1388.

Hawdon JM, Ward Platt MP. Metabolic adaptation in small for gestational age infants. Arch Dis Child 1993;68:262–268.

Lucas A, Morley R, Cole TJ. Adverse neurodevelopmental outcome of moderate neonatal hypoglycaemia. Br Med J 1988;297:1304–1308.

Lubchenco LO, Bard H. Incidence of hypoglycemia in newborn infants classified by birth weight and gestational age. Pediatrics 1981;47:831–838.

Glucose Production

Cryer PE. Glucose conterregulation: Prevention and correction of hypoglycemia in humans. Am J Physiol 1993;264:E149–E155.

Hyperinsulinism

Epstein MF, Nicholls E, Stubblefield PG. Neonatal hypoglycemia after beta-sympathomimetic tocolytic therapy. J Pediatr 1979;94:449–453.

Philipson EH, Kalhan SC, Riha MM, et al. Effects of maternal glucose infusion on fetal acid-base status in human pregnancy. Am J Obstet Gynecol 1987;157:866–873.

Soltesz G, Aynsley-Green A. Hyperinsulinism in infancy and childhood. *In* Frick HP, von Harnack G-A, Kochsiek K, et al (eds). Advances in Internal Medicine and Pediatrics. Berlin: Springer-Verlag, 1984:152–202.

Zucker P, Simon G. Prolonged symptomatic neonatal hypoglycemia associated with maternal chlorpropamide therapy. Pediatrics 1968;42:824–825.

Infant of a Diabetic Mother

Cowett RM, Schwartz R. The infant of the diabetic mother. Pediatr Clin North Am 1982;29:1213–1231.

Schwartz R, Cornblath M. Infant of the diabetic mother. J Pediatr Endocrinol 1992;5:197–216.

Beckwith-Wiedemann Syndrome

Martinez RM, Martinez-Carboney R, Ocampo-Campos R, et al. Wiedemann-Beckwith syndrome: Clinical, cytogenetical and radiological observations in 39 new cases. Genet Couns 1992;3:67–76.

Ping AJ, Reeve AE, Law DJ, et al. Genetic linkage of Beckwith-Wiedemann Syndrome to 11p15. Am J Hum Genet 1989;44:720–723.

Hypoxia

Collins JE, Leonard JV, Teale D, et al. Hyperinsulinaemic hypoglycaemia in small for dates babies. Arch Dis Child 1990;65:1118–1120.

Nesidioblastosis

Bordi C, Ravazzola M, Pollak A, et al. Neonatal islet cell adenoma: A distinct type of islet cell tumor? Diabetes Care 1982;5:122–125.

Dahms BB, Landing BH, Blaskovics M, et al. Nesidioblastosis and other islet cell abnormalities in hyperinsulinemic hypoglycemia of childhood. Hum Pathol 1980;11:641–649.

Hirsch HJ, Loo S, Evans N, et al. Hypoglycemia of infancy and nesidioblastosis: Studies with somatostatin. N Engl J Med 1977;296:1323–1326.

Hormone Deficiency

Kollee LA, Monnens LA, Cejka V, et al. Persistent neonatal hypoglycaemia due to glucagon deficiency. Arch Dis Child 1978;53:422–424.

Zachmann M, Aynsley-Green A, Illig R, et al. Simultaneous occurrence of hypopituitarism and adrenal medullar insufficiency in a boy with hypoglycemia. Helv Paediatr Acta 1977;32:419–424.

Substrate Deficiency

Haymond MW, Ben-Galim E, Strobel KE. Glucose and alanine metabolism in children with maple syrup urine disease. J Clin Invest 1978;398–405.

Pagliara AS, Karl IE, DeVivo DC, et al. Hypoalaninemia: A concomitant of ketotic hypoglycemia. J Clin Invest 1977;51:1440–1426.

Management

Abu-Osba YK, Manasra KB, Mathew PM. Complications of diazoxide treatment in persistent neonatal hyperinsulinism. Arch Dis Child 1989;64:1496–1500.

Lilien LD, Grajwer LA, Pildes RS. Treatment of neonatal hypoglycemia with continuous intravenous glucose infusion. J Pediatr 1977;91:779–782.

Lilien LD, Pildes RS, Srinivasan G, et al. Treatment of neonatal hypoglycemia with minibolus and intravenous glucose infusion. J Pediatr 1980;97:295–298.

INDEX

Note: Page numbers in *italics* refer to illustrations; page numbers followed by t refer to tables.

A

ABCs, in coma management, 646, 648
Abdomen, examination of, 265, 387
    in abdominal pain, 265
    in cough, 69
    in gastrointestinal bleeding, 334
    in splenomegaly, 356
    in vomiting, 303, 305t
  injury to, in child abuse, 566, 567t
  tumors of, *388*
Abdominal epilepsy, vomiting in, 321
Abdominal mass, 387–398
  age-related etiology of, 390t
  clinical history in, 387, 390t
  imaging studies in, 390, *392, 393*
  laboratory tests in, 390
  location of, *388, 389*, 391t
  physical examination in, 387, 390
  red flags with, 391t, 397
Abdominal migraine, vomiting in, 319
Abdominal muscles, in cough, 68
Abdominal pain, 258–277
  acute, 260–261, 263–276
    abdominal examination in, 265
    activity level with, 261, 263
    age-related etiology of, 260t, 261t
    anorexia with, 263
    character of, 261
    computed tomography in, 268
    constipation with, 263
    contrast studies in, 268
    diarrhea with, 263
    etiology of, 259t, 260t, 261t
    family history in, 263
    gastrointestinal symptoms in, 263
    history in, 260–261, 260t
    in appendicitis, 269–270, *270*, 270t, *271, 272*
    in cholelithiasis, 274–275, *276*
    in ectopic pregnancy, *272*
    in pancreatitis, 270–271, 273t, 274, *275*
    in peptic ulcer disease, 275–276
    laboratory evaluation in, 265–267
    location of, 261, 263t
    management of, 268–269, *269*
    medical history in, 263, 264t
    nausea with, 263
    obturator sign in, 265, *266*
    pathophysiology of, 258, 260, *261, 262*
    physical examination in, 263–265

Abdominal pain *(Continued)*
    plain radiography in, 267, *267*
    psoas sign in, 265
    rebound pain in, 265
    rectal examination in, 265
    red flags in, 266t
    systemic symptoms with, 263, 264t
    time of onset of, 260–261
    ultrasonography in, 267–268, *268*
    urinalysis in, 267
    vomiting with, 263
  chronic, 261t, 276–277
  functional, 277
  in constipation, 382
  in neutropenia, 1001–1002
  parietal, 258, 260, *262*
  rebound, 265
  visceral, 258, *261*
Abetalipoproteinemia, ataxia in, 696t
ABO incompatibility, 368–369, 823
Abscess, 923, *930*
  appendiceal, *388*
  brain, cerebrospinal fluid findings in, 881t
  Brodie, in antalgic gait, 772t
  epidural, hypotonia with, 604
    spinal, cerebrospinal fluid findings in, 881t
  hepatic, 348, 350, *388*
  peritonsillar, 53t, 59, *59*, 127t
  retropharyngeal, 53t, 59, *60*, 127t
    in airway obstruction, 130–131
  splenic, 359, *359*
  tubo-ovarian, *388*, 455–456, 456t
Abuse. See *Child abuse; Sexual abuse; Substance abuse;* and under specific substances.
Accident, vs. child abuse, 562–564, 563t, 571t
Accommodation, disorders of, 706–707
  loss of, 707
  spasm of, 707
Accommodative esotropia, 724–725
Accuracy, of diagnostic test, 7–9, 8t, *18*
Acetaminophen poisoning, 327t, 328t, 658
Acetazolamide, for seizures, 635t, 637t
Achalasia, chest pain in, 193
  vomiting in, 316
Achilles tendon contracture, in toe-walking, 766
Achondroplasia, *1029*, 1029t
  hypotonia in, 603
  short stature in, 1030
Achromatopsia, 702, 708t
Acidemia, lactic, hepatomegaly and, 343
  organic, altered consciousness in, 660t

C

H

I

M

O

ISBN 0-7216-5161-5

90038